# ABRAMS'
# CLINICAL
# DRUG THERAPY
## Rationales for Nursing Practice

**Geralyn Frandsen, EdD, RN**
Assistant Director of Nursing
Professor of Nursing
Catherine McAuley School of Nursing
Maryville University
St. Louis, Missouri

**Sandra Smith Pennington, PhD, RN**
Chief of Staff, Office of the President
Rocky Mountain University of Health Professions
Provo, Utah
Professor Emeritus
Department of Nursing
Berea College
Berea, Kentucky

Wolters Kluwer

Philadelphia • Baltimore • New York • London
Buenos Aires • Hong Kong • Sydney • Tokyo

*Vice President, Nursing Segment*: Julie K. Stegman
*Manager, Nursing Education and Practice Content*: Jamie Blum
*Senior Acquisitions Editor*: Jonathan Joyce
*Senior Development Editor*: Meredith L. Brittain
*Editorial Coordinator*: Tim Rinehart
*Marketing Manager*: Brittany Clements
*Editorial Assistant*: Molly Kennedy
*Production Project Manager*: Sadie Buckallew
*Design Coordinator*: Steve Druding
*Art Director*: Jennifer Clements
*Manufacturing Coordinator*: Karin Duffield
*Prepress Vendor*: SPi Global

Twelfth Edition

**Cataloging-in-Publication Data available on request from the Publisher**

ISBN: 978-1-9751-3613-0

# Contributors

## CONTRIBUTORS TO THE 12TH EDITION

**Lisa Albers, MSN, RN**
Clinical Assistant Professor of Nursing
Catherine McAuley School of Nursing
Maryville University
Staff Nurse
SSM Health Cardinal Glennon Children's Hospital
St. Louis, Missouri
> Chapter 4: Pharmacology and the Care of Infants and Pediatric Patients

**Vicki C. Coopmans, PhD, CRNA, CHSE**
Associate Professor
Director of Clinical Education
Department of Nurse Anesthesia
Webster University
St. Louis, Missouri
> Chapter 50: Drug Therapy With Local Anesthetics
> Chapter 51: Drug Therapy With General Anesthetics

**Ryan D. Dunn, PharmD**
Division Infection Disease Pharmacist
HCA–West Florida Division
Largo, Florida
> Chapter 18: Drug Therapy With Beta-Lactam Antibacterial Agents
> Chapter 24: Drug Therapy for Fungal Infections

**Gary M. Frandsen, JD, MSN, RN**
Associate Teaching Professor
College of Nursing
University of Missouri–St. Louis
St. Louis, Missouri
> Chapter 22: Drug Therapy for Tuberculosis and *Mycobacterium Avium* Complex Disease
> Chapter 35: Nutritional Support Products, Vitamins, and Mineral Supplements
> Chapter 44: Drug Therapy to Regulate Calcium and Bone Metabolism

**Jennifer B. Miles, PharmD, MBA**
Vice President of Pharmacy Services
HCA West Florida Division
HealthTrust
Largo, Florida
> Chapter 19: Drug Therapy With Aminoglycosides and Fluoroquinolones
> Chapter 20: Drug Therapy With Tetracyclines, Sulfonamides, and Urinary Antiseptics
> Chapter 21: Drug Therapy With Macrolides and Miscellaneous Anti-infective Agents
> Chapter 31: Drug Therapy for Nasal Congestion and Cough
> Chapter 32: Drug Therapy to Decrease Histamine Effects and Allergic Response
> Chapter 33: Drug Therapy for Asthma, Airway Inflammation, and Bronchoconstriction

**Vicki Moran, PhD, RN, MPH, CNE, CDE, PHNA-BC, TNS**
Assistant Professor
Trudy Busch Valentine School of Nursing
Saint Louis University
St. Louis, Missouri
> Chapter 41: Drug Therapy for Diabetes Mellitus
> Chapter 42: Drug Therapy for Hyperthyroidism and Hypothyroidism

**Sharon Souter, RN, PhD, CNE**
Professor and Adjunct Faculty Member
University of Mary Hardin–Baylor
Belton, Texas
> Chapter 37: Drug Therapy for Peptic Ulcer Disease and Hyperacidity
> Chapter 52: Drug Therapy for Migraine and Other Headaches
> Chapter 54: Drug Therapy for Anxiety and Insomnia
> Chapter 57: Drug Therapy for Attention Deficit Hyperactivity Disorder and Narcolepsy

**Elizabeth Stuesse, MSN, RNC-OB, RNC-MNN, C-EFM, CLC, CCE, CHBE**
Clinical Assistant Professor
Catherine McAuley School of Nursing
Maryville University
Women & Children Educator RN
Women's Education
Mercy Hospital
St. Louis, Missouri
> Chapter 6: Pharmacology and the Care of Pregnant or Lactating Women

**Jennifer L. Taylor, PhD, RN, CNE**
Assistant Professor of Nursing, BSN Coordinator
Catherine McAuley School of Nursing
Maryville University
St. Lois, Missouri
> Chapter 26: Drug Therapy for Hypertension
> Chapter 27: Drug Therapy for Dysrhythmias
> Chapter 30: Drug Therapy for Heart Failure

**Dana Todd, PhD, APRN**
Professor
School of Nursing and Health Professions
Murray State University
Murray, Kentucky
> Chapter 7: Pharmacology and Women's Health

**Gladdi Tomlinson, RN, MSN**
Professor of Nursing
Harrisburg Area Community College
Harrisburg, Pennsylvania
> Chapter 47: Drug Therapy for Myasthenia Gravis, Alzheimer's Disease, and Other Conditions Treated with Cholinergic Agents
> Chapter 48: Drug Therapy for Parkinson's Disease, Urinary Spasticity, and Disorders Requiring Anticholinergic Drug Therapy

*I dedicate this edition to my husband and nursing colleague, Gary. I also dedicate this edition to the Maryville University nursing faculty, alumni, and students. Each one of you inspires me!*

Geralyn Frandsen

*To my family, my constant source of strength, inspiration, and gratitude.*

Sandy Pennington

# CONTRIBUTORS TO THE 11TH EDITION

**Lisa Albers, MSN, RN**
Clinical Assistant Professor of Nursing
BSN Coordinator
Catherine McAuley School of Nursing
Maryville University
RN Staff Nurse
Cardinal Glennon Children's Hospital
St. Louis, Missouri
> **Chapter 4: Pharmacology and the Care of Infants and Pediatric Patients**

**Jennifer Brunworth, MSN, RN**
Clinical Assistant Professor of Nursing
Catherine McAuley School of Nursing
Maryville University
St. Louis, Missouri
> **Chapter 26: Drug Therapy for Hypertension**

**Gary Frandsen, JD, MSN, RN**
Assistant Professor of Nursing
University of Missouri
St. Louis, Missouri
> **Chapter 22: Drug Therapy for Tuberculosis and Mycobacterium avium Complex Disease**
> **Chapter 35: Nutritional Support Products, Vitamins, and Mineral Supplements**
> **Chapter 44: Drug Therapy to Regulate Calcium and Bone Metabolism**

**Susan Golden, MSN, RN**
Nursing Program Director
Nursing Faculty
Eastern New Mexico University–Roswell
Roswell, New Mexico
> **Chapter 49: Drug Therapy With Opioids**

**Jennifer Binggeli Miles, PharmD, MBA, BCPS**
Director of Remote Order Entry Operations
Largo, Florida
> **Chapter 19: Drug Therapy With Aminoglycosides and Fluoroquinolones**
> **Chapter 20: Drug Therapy With Tetracyclines, Sulfonamides, and Urinary Antiseptics**
> **Chapter 31: Drug Therapy for Nasal Congestion and Cough**
> **Chapter 50: Drug Therapy With Local Anesthetics**
> **Chapter 51: Drug Therapy With General Anesthetics**
> **Chapter 58: Drug Therapy for Substance Abuse Disorders**

**Vicki Moran, PhD, RN, CNE**
Assistant Professor
School of Nursing
Saint Louis University
St. Louis, Missouri
> **Chapter 41: Drug Therapy for Diabetes Mellitus**
> **Chapter 42: Drug Therapy for Hyperthyroidism and Hypothyroidism**

**Jacqueline R. Saleeby, PhD, RN, PMHCS**
Associate Professor
Catherine McAuley School of Nursing
Maryville University
St. Louis, Missouri
> **Chapter 56: Drug Therapy for Psychotic Disorders**

**Sharon Souter, PhD**
Professor
College of Nursing
University of Mary Hardin Baylor
Belton, Texas
> **Chapter 37: Drug Therapy for Peptic Ulcer Disease and Hyperacidity**
> **Chapter 52: Drug Therapy for Migraines and Other Headaches**
> **Chapter 54: Drug Therapy for Anxiety and Insomnia**
> **Chapter 57: Drug Therapy for Attention Deficit Hyperactivity Disorder and Narcolepsy**

**Elizabeth Stuesse, MSN, RNC-OB, RNC-MNN, C-EFM, CLC**
Clinical Assistant Professor
Catherine McAuley School of Nursing
Maryville University
St. Louis, Missouri
> **Chapter 6: Pharmacology and the Care of Pregnant or Lactating Woman**

**Dana Todd, PhD, APRN**
Professor
Department of Nursing
Murray State University
Murray, Kentucky
> **Chapter 7: Pharmacology and Women's Health**

**Gladdi Tomlinson, MSN, RN**
Professor of Nursing
Harrisburg Area Community College
Harrisburg, Pennsylvania
> **Chapter 47: Drug Therapy for Myasthenia Gravis, Alzheimer's Disease, and Urinary Retention**
> **Chapter 48: Drug Therapy for Parkinson's Disease, Urinary Spasticity, and Disorders Requiring Anticholinergic Drug Therapy**

**Jeannette Zelhart-Smith, RN**
Maternity Course Coordinator
University of Saint Francis
Crown Point, Indiana
> **Chapter 36: Drug Therapy for Weight Management**
> **Chapter 43: Drug Therapy for Pituitary and Hypothalamic Dysfunction**

**Nina Zimmermann, MSN, APRN, ANP-BC, AE-C**
Assistant Director of Nursing
Director of the MSN Nurse Practitioner Program
Assistant Professor of Nursing
Catherine McAuley School of Nursing
College of Health Professions
Maryville University
St. Louis, Missouri
> **Chapter 33: Drug Therapy for Asthma and Bronchoconstriction**

# Reviewers

# Foreword

The 12th edition of *Abrams' Clinical Drug Therapy: Rationales for Nursing Practice* comes at a critical juncture in health care worldwide. Even as health care was in transition due to changes in delivery, access, and economics, the global pandemic related to COVID-19 shook traditional processes for everyone. News headlines around the world hailed nurses for their steadfastness and diligence in providing frontline care, frequently in dire circumstances. This unprecedented showcase of the work nurses do every day, pandemic or not, demonstrates the deep knowledge and skills that characterize professional nursing practice and the professional values and attitudes that drive nurses. Every day nurses are the primary administrators for medications. Quality safe medication administration, though, became a centerpiece of managing the COVID-19 outbreaks and highlighted the imperative of evidence-based nursing practice. The principles and practices in this book are a roadmap to guide nurses across health care settings to ensure a patient-centered approach to quality safe care for all populations and settings.

Now as never before, the challenges for quality safe medication administration hinge on nurses' knowledge, skills, and attitudes. Daily, nurses call on the basic pharmacologic knowledge honed in academic programs and refined in practice to address challenges in medication management across all environments, and particularly when following strict infection control guidelines.

To guide quality safe care practices, nurses have turned to the Quality and Safety Education for Nurses (QSEN) project, launched in 2006 as an evidence-based framework of six competencies: patient-centered care, teamwork and collaboration, evidence-based practice, safety, quality improvement, and informatics (Cronenwett et al., 2007, 2009). These six competencies are integrated into national curriculum standards for nursing so that all nurses are accountable for integrating safety and quality responsibilities into their daily work. Many schools of nursing apply the QSEN framework to guide their curriculum and course objectives. Each has a role in safe clinical drug therapy.

In the midst of COVID-19, nurses' stories from the frontlines of care revealed the role of these six competencies as nurses valiantly applied the knowledge, skills, and attitudes to keep their patients safe. But was this really any different from the holistic care nurses provide every day, except for the fact that it was now illuminated because of the exponential explosion of demand for intense care brought on by the influx of critically ill patients in nearly every country?

As noted in this evidence-based 12th edition, nurses are the primary administrators of medications in most settings. Every day, nurses administer pharmacologic interventions. Every day, they apply the six QSEN competencies by considering patient-centered preferences and situations, collaborating across interprofessional teams, applying evidence-based standards for each medication and within the patient's context, participating in continuous quality improvement, applying safety science concepts, and using informatics to plan and manage the pharmacology needs of their patients.

Medication administration is multifaceted, complex, team-based, patient-centered, and carries the possibility of multiple failures. One in nine emergency department admissions is related to an adverse drug event, 3.2 billion medication orders are prescribed each year, and 160 medication errors occur each year in primary care (AHRQ, 2018). These shocking statistics remind us that nurses may in fact be a last line of defense in safe medication administration.

Nurses are accountable for current knowledge of a particular patient's medication regimen. To achieve reliability, nurses must follow practices that ensure the right medication is administered in the right dose, by the right route, at the right time, and to the right patient, every time. Safety culture, a subset of the overall organizational culture, demands awareness of the potential for error, willingness to report errors and near misses, and action to correct system failures. Safety culture includes "just culture." In just culture, all personnel are responsible for reporting near misses and breakdowns in care but share accountability across the system to trace broken processes, analyze the action pathway for administering a medication, and implement improvement processes to prevent the same type of event from happening again.

This text serves as a reliable reference for safe medication administration. A key feature of *Abrams' Clinical Drug Therapy: Rationales for Nursing Practice* is the incorporation of disease characteristics with clinical drug knowledge in demonstrating a comprehensive approach to safe medication administration. Nurses are provided a step-by-step guide for medication safety through pharmacologic knowledge, evidence-based standards for administration, awareness of organizational challenge, instructions for careful medication administration, and knowledge of how to complete documentation. Learners at all levels are able to apply the learning actions included in this text to ensure reliability and safety by following the QSEN competencies.

- Patient-centered care means treating all patients and families with respect and honor. By including patients and families as partners in care, they become safety allies. Engaging patients and their family members in making decisions about the treatment plan encourages active engagement as team members so they help with choices about their care that are more likely to have the desired therapeutic effects.
- Teamwork and collaboration may include nurses, physicians, a nurse practitioner, a physician assistant, pharmacist, social worker, dietitian, physical therapist, occupational therapist, and speech–language pathologist. To help coordinate the complexities of safe medication administration, teamwork behaviors include flexible leadership, standardized communication, mutual support, and constant environmental scans.
- Evidence-based practice requires an enquiring mind to constantly seek the best available information in pharmacotherapeutics, which appears in the QSEN Alerts throughout the text. Safe medication administration uses evidence-based practice standards to ensure that appropriate precautions are taken to assess for adverse effects.
- Quality improvement processes measure care outcomes to compare with benchmark data to determine areas to improve. Teams apply quality improvement tools to raise performance.
- Safety is the constant awareness of the inherent risks in medication administration and how that risk can be miti-

gated through collaboration among physicians, pharmacists, nurses, and the patient and family.

- Informatics is the thread in all the competencies for managing care, documentation, and decision support tools.

Reflection before action (planning), reflection in action (pausing to problem solve), and reflection on action (debriefing) are processes for nurses to ask questions to examine their actions for constant improvement and growth. With a spirit of enquiry, nurses develop a habit of the mind for constant questioning as they follow clinical drug therapy in their practice. In using this text, central questions guide practice development.

- What are the roles and responsibilities for each team member in the complex steps in medication administration? How do I maintain awareness of the scope of responsibility for each discipline involved, particularly when patients have multiple providers?
- How do I ensure medication safety during transitions in care when I hand over my patient to another provider?
- Where do I find the information I need about this medication for safe administration?
- What communication skills will help me understand my patient's preferences and values related to medications?

Reflecting on questions like these develop a quality and safety mindset so that by following the guidance in this book, nurses will ensure that the next national medication safety measures will reflect improvement. The year 2020 will be remembered for the global COVID-19 pandemic but also the designation by WHO as the Year of the Nurse and Midwife. It is also the year the first *State of the World's Nursing* was released (WHO, 2020). It has and continues to be the year of the nurse; stories of the impact of nurses stand out in all media outlets. As the largest health care profession, nurses have a profound impact in universal access and in safety. Medication safety is a key area where nurses can truly make a difference for every patient, every time, every day.

*Gwen Sherwood, PhD, RN, FAAN, ANEF*
*Professor Emeritus*
*University of North Carolina at Chapel Hill School of Nursing*

## References

AHRQ. (2018). *Guide to improving patient safety in primary care settings by engaging patients and families.* Rockville, MD: Agency for Healthcare Research and Quality. Retrieved July 2018, from https://www.ahrq.gov/patient-safety/reports/engage.html

Cronenwett, L. Sherwood, G. Barnsteiner, J. Disch, J. Johnson, J. Mitchell, P., et al. (2007). Quality and safety education for nurses. *Nursing Outlook, 55*(3), 122–131.

Cronenwett, L. Sherwood, G. Pohl, J. Barnsteiner, J. Moore, S. Taylor Sullivan, D., et al. (2009). Quality and safety education for advanced practice nursing practice. *Nursing Outlook, 57*(6), 338–348.

World Health Organization. (2020). *State of the World's Nursing Report—2020: Investing in education, jobs, and leadership.* Geneva. Retrieved from https://www.who.int/publications-detail/nursing-report-2020

# Preface

*Abrams' Clinical Drug Therapy: Rationales for Nursing Practice* has a long tradition of guiding students and instructors through the practice of safe and effective medication administration. The 12th edition includes Quality and Safety Education for Nurses (QSEN) content in each chapter. Each chapter also includes information about the pathophysiology of disease and associated drug therapy for prevention and treatment of disease.

## GOALS AND RESPONSIBILITIES OF NURSING CARE RELATED TO DRUG THERAPY

Varied goals and responsibilities inherent in safe medication administration are identified in each chapter. The following information will guide you in developing your own goals and responsibilities inherent to safe and effective nursing practice.

- Preventing the need for drug therapy, when possible, by promoting health and preventing conditions that require drug therapy.
- Using nonpharmacologic interventions alone or in conjunction with drug therapy. When used with drugs, such interventions may promote lower drug dosage, less frequent administration, and fewer adverse effects.
- Administering drugs accurately and taking into consideration patient characteristics such as age, weight, and hepatic and renal function, which can influence drug response.
- Preventing or minimizing adverse effects by knowing the major adverse effects associated with particular drugs. It is important to assess patients with impaired hepatic and renal function closely for adverse effects. The early recognition of adverse effects allows for the implementation of interventions to minimize their severity. All drugs cause adverse effects, and nurses must maintain a high index of suspicion that the development of new signs and symptoms may be drug induced.
- The effect produced if medications are combined with other medications, herbs, or foods.
- Teaching patients and families about the effects of medications. The nurse must instruct patients and families about the role and importance of their medications in treating particular illnesses, accurate administration of medications, nonpharmacologic treatments to use with or instead of pharmacologic treatments, and when to contact their health care provider.

## ORGANIZATIONAL FRAMEWORK

The 10 sections of the textbook provide the reader with basic information about drug therapy as well as the administration of medications for the prevention and treatment of disease. The first section introduces the safeguards in place to promote drug safety, the Institute of Medicine Core Competencies, and medication administration. It also describes the nursing process and explains the application of the nursing process in the care of patients receiving drug therapy. The use of concept maps addresses priority considerations and nursing actions related to drug therapy. The second section addresses the effect medications have throughout the life span. The text introduces the effects of drugs on infants, children, older adults, pregnant and lactating women, and drugs affecting male and female health. The remaining sections provide information on drug therapy related to systems, infections, and disease processes.

Each chapter opens with a case study, and its use throughout the chapter helps the reader integrate information about a particular disease and its drug therapy so he or she can apply it. The chapters also have NCLEX-style questions distributed throughout to test knowledge of the content and its application to patient care. This approach will help the reader prepare for class examinations as well as the NCLEX itself.

The chapters that focus on drug treatment for specific diseases use the prototype approach, allowing the reader to see the similarity in medications within each broad drug classification. Introduction and Overview sections provide the basis for understanding the drug therapy that prevents or treats the disease. The presentation of disease pathophysiology helps the reader understand the effect of a particular medication on the prevention and treatment of disease. Drug therapy sections summarize the medications, identifying the pharmacokinetics, action, use, adverse effects, contraindications, and nursing implications—including administration, assessment, and patient teaching. Many chapters discuss the effect of herbal supplements on prescribed medications. This information has become crucial for the maintenance of patient safety. Boxes containing patient teaching guidelines for a drug or class of drugs highlight crucial information the nurse should teach the patient and family. Each chapter also includes a clinical reasoning case study to assist in the application of drug therapy in the care of patient.

## RECURRING FEATURES

This updated edition includes new and revised features to enhance learning.

### Chapter-Opening Features

- **Learning Objectives** summarize what the student should learn while reading the chapter and answering both the Clinical Application Case Study Questions and NCLEX Success questions, described below.
- A **Clinical Application Case Study** opens each chapter with a patient-focused clinical scenario. Throughout the chapter, the reader is asked **critical thinking questions** to apply chapter content, emphasizing a patient-centered and interdisciplinary approach to pharmacology.
- **Key Terms** with definitions help the reader understand the chapter's content.

### Special Features

- Each chapter introduces the disease process and the pertinent **pathophysiology**. This allows students to make connections between the pathophysiology and pharmacologic management of a disease.

- **QSEN Alerts**, presented in the context of the chapter discussion, alert the reader to important QSEN considerations and emphasize safety as a primary objective in patient care.
- **Black Box Warnings** highlight serious or life-threatening adverse effects identified by the FDA as being associated with a drug.
- **Drugs at a Glance Tables**—which include **Canadian drug names**—summarize the routes and dosage ranges (for adults and for children), as well as the pregnancy category, for each drug in the class. The prototype drug is indicated with an icon. Medications developed after 2015 reflect the new FDA Pregnancy Category guidelines.
- **Drug Interactions** and **Herb and Dietary Interactions** boxes highlight the risk of interactions as well as increased or decreased drug effects when drugs are combined with other medications, food, or herbal supplements.
- **Patient Teaching Guidelines** list specific information for the education of the patient and family.
- **NCLEX Success** sections interspersed throughout the chapter ask the student to answer NCLEX-style questions that pertain to the learning objectives and the information just presented. This feature helps students check and apply their knowledge as they read and assists them to prepare for patient care and for the NCLEX. The questions align to the terminology used on the NCLEX. The NCLEX Success questions exclusively use generic names for medications, which is consistent with the RN licensure examination.
- **Nursing Process Concept Maps** provide a succinct overview of drug therapy in terms of assessment, planning/goals, nursing interventions, and evaluation. Located at the end of each chapter, the nursing process concept maps provide the guidelines for drug therapy specifically related to nursing care. (Nursing diagnoses do not appear in these concept maps because nursing diagnoses are not tested on the NCLEX.)
- **Clinical Reasoning Case Studies** focus on the action of the medication prescribed and the associated assessment of medication outcomes.
- **Unfolding Patient Stories**, written by the National League for Nursing, are an engaging way to begin meaningful conversations in the classroom. These vignettes, which appear in relevant chapters, feature patients from Wolters Kluwer's *vSim for Nursing | Pharmacology* (co-developed with Laerdal Medical) and DocuCare products; however, each Unfolding Patient Story in the book stands alone, not requiring purchase of these products.
- **Concept Mastery Alerts** clarify common misconceptions as identified by Lippincott's Adaptive Learning Powered by prepU

## Chapter-Ending Features

- **Key Concepts** summarize the most salient content that appears in each chapter.
- **References and Resources** provide sources on which content is based and direction for further reading.

# A COMPREHENSIVE PACKAGE FOR TEACHING AND LEARNING

To further facilitate teaching and learning, a carefully designed ancillary package has been developed to assist faculty and students.

## Resources for Instructors

Tools to assist with teaching this text are available upon its adoption on thePoint® at http://thePoint.lww.com/Abrams12e.

- An **e-Book** gives you access to the book's full text and images online.
- The **Test Generator** lets you put together exclusive new tests from a bank containing more than 1,000 questions to help assess students' understanding of the material. Test questions are mapped to chapter learning objectives and page numbers.
- An extensive collection of materials is provided for each book chapter:
  - **Pre-Lecture Quizzes** (and answers) are quick, knowledge-based assessments that allow you to check students' reading comprehension.
  - **PowerPoint Presentations** provide an easy way for you to integrate the textbook with your students' classroom experience, either via slide shows or handouts. Multiple-choice and true/false questions are integrated into the presentations to promote class participation and allow you to use i-clicker technology.
  - **Guided Lecture Notes** walk you through the chapters, objective by objective, and provide you with corresponding PowerPoint slide numbers.
  - **Discussion Topics** (and suggested answers) can be used as conversation starters or in online discussion boards.
  - **Assignments** (and suggested answers) include group, written, clinical, and Web assignments.
  - **Case Studies** with related questions (and suggested answers) give students an opportunity to apply their knowledge to a client case similar to one they might encounter in practice.
- An **Image Bank** lets you use the photographs and illustrations from this textbook in your PowerPoint slides or as you see fit in your course.
- Sample **Syllabi** provide guidance for structuring your nursing pharmacology course.
- A **QSEN Competency Map** identifies content and special features in the book related to competencies identified by the QSEN Institute.
- A **BSN Essentials Competency Map** identifies book content related to the BSN Essentials.
- **Learning Management System Cartridges**.
- **Strategies for Effective Teaching** offer creative approaches.

Contact your sales representative or check out LWW.com/Nursing for more details and ordering information.

## Resources for Students

An exciting set of free resources is available to help students review material and become even more familiar with vital concepts. Students can access all these resources on thePoint® at http://thePoint.lww.com/Abrams12e, using the codes printed in the front of their textbooks.

- **NCLEX-Style Review Questions** for each chapter help students review important concepts and practice for NCLEX.
- **Concepts in Action Animations** bring physiologic and pathophysiologic concepts to life and enhance student comprehension.
- **Watch & Learn Video Clips** demonstrate nursing skills and appeal to visual and auditory learners.
- The following **online appendices**:
  - Appendix A: Answers for NCLEX Success
  - Appendix B: Answers for the Clinical Application Case Studies
  - Appendix C: Critical Thinking Questions and Answers
  - Appendix D: The International System of Units
  - Appendix E: Serum Drug Concentrations
  - Appendix F: Tables of Normal Values
- **Journal Articles** for each book chapter offer access to current research available in Wolters Kluwer journals.
- **Dosage Calculation Quizzes** provide opportunities for students to practice math skills and calculate drug dosages.
- A **Spanish–English Audio Glossary** provides helpful terms and phrases for communicating with patients who speak Spanish.
- Plus **Heart and Breath Sounds** and **Learning Objectives** from the textbook.

## ADAPTIVE LEARNING POWERED BY PREPU

Lippincott's Adaptive Learning Powered by PrepU helps every student learn more, while giving instructors the data they need to monitor each student's progress, strengths, and weaknesses. The adaptive learning system allows instructors to assign quizzes or students to take quizzes on their own that adapt to each student's individual mastery level. Visit http://thePoint.lww.com/prepU to learn more.

## VSIM FOR NURSING

vSim for Nursing, jointly developed by Laerdal Medical and Wolters Kluwer Health, offers innovative scenario-based learning modules consisting of Web-based virtual simulations, course learning materials, and curriculum tools designed to develop critical thinking skills and promote clinical confidence and competence. vSim for Nursing | Pharmacology includes 10 cases from the Simulation in Nursing Education—Pharmacology Scenarios. Students can progress through suggested readings, pre- and postsimulation assessments, documentation assignments, and guided reflection questions, and will receive an individualized feedback log immediately upon completion of the simulation. Throughout the student learning experience, the product offers remediation back to trusted Lippincott resources, including Lippincott Nursing Advisor and Lippincott Nursing Procedures—two online, evidence-based, clinical information solutions used in health care facilities throughout the United States. This innovative product provides a comprehensive patient-focused solution for learning and integrating simulation into the classroom.

Contact your Wolters Kluwer sales representative or visit http://thepoint.lww.com/vsim for options to enhance your pharmacology nursing course with vSim for Nursing.

## LIPPINCOTT DOCUCARE

Lippincott DocuCare combines Web-based academic electronic health record (EHR) simulation software with clinical case scenarios, allowing students to learn how to use an EHR in a safe, true-to-life setting, while enabling instructors to measure their progress. Lippincott DocuCare's nonlinear solution works well in the classroom, simulation lab, and clinical practice.

Contact your Wolters Kluwer sales representative or visit http://thepoint.lww.com/DocuCare for options to enhance your pharmacology nursing course with DocuCare.

## A COMPREHENSIVE, DIGITAL, INTEGRATED COURSE SOLUTION: *LIPPINCOTT® COURSEPOINT+*

The same trusted solution, innovation, and unmatched support that you have come to expect from *Lippincott CoursePoint+* is now enhanced with more engaging learning tools and deeper analytics to help prepare students for practice. This powerfully integrated digital learning solution combines learning tools, case studies, virtual simulation, real-time data, and the most trusted nursing education content on the market to make curriculum-wide learning more efficient and to meet students where they're at in their learning. And now, it's easier than ever for instructors and students to use, giving them everything they need for course and curriculum success!

*Lippincott CoursePoint+* includes the following:

- Engaging course content provides a variety of learning tools to engage students of all learning styles.
- A more personalized learning approach, including adaptive learning powered by PrepU, gives students the content and tools they need at the moment they need it, giving them data for more focused remediation and helping to boost their confidence.
- Varying levels of case studies, virtual simulation, and access to Lippincott Advisor help students learn the critical thinking and clinical judgment skills to help them become practice-ready nurses.
- Unparalleled reporting provides in-depth dashboards with several data points to track student progress and help identify strengths and weaknesses.
- Unmatched support includes training coaches, product trainers, and nursing education consultants to help educators and students implement CoursePoint+ with ease.

# Acknowledgments

The expertise of our contributors and reviewers is a great example of how the power of collaboration improves outcomes, and we thank them. We also wish to thank the team at Wolters Kluwer who provided their expertise to this edition.

# Contents

# SECTION 10
# DRUGS AFFECTING THE EYE, EAR, AND SKIN  1167

# AVAILABLE ON thePoint®

# Case Studies in This Book

*Note that each chapter has a Clinical Application Case Study that unfolds within that chapter. The page number for the introduction to the Clinical Application Case Study in each chapter is given here.

# SECTION 1

# The Conceptual Framework of Pharmacology

# The Foundation of Pharmacology: Quality and Safety

## LEARNING OBJECTIVES

*After studying this chapter, you should be able to:*

1. Define a prototype drug.
2. Distinguish between generic and trade names of drugs.
3. Describe the main categories of controlled substances in relation to therapeutic use, potential for abuse, and regulatory requirements.
4. Identify the multiple safeguards that are in place to promote drug safety in packaging, drug laws, and approval processes.
5. Recognize initiatives designated to enhance safe drug administration.
6. Develop personal techniques for learning about drugs and using drug knowledge in patient care.
7. Identify authoritative sources of drug information.

## CLINICAL APPLICATION CASE STUDY

Joan Clark, a senior nursing student, is preparing for the NCLEX-RN examination. As she reviews material, she examines safeguards in place to protect the public from injury due to medication administration.

## KEY TERMS

**Biotechnology:** process that may involve manipulating deoxyribonucleic acid [DNA] and ribonucleic acid [RNA] and recombining genes into hybrid molecules that can be inserted into living organisms [often *Escherichia coli* bacteria] and repeatedly reproduced

**Brand [trade] name:** manufacturer's chosen name for a drug, which is protected by a patent

**Controlled substances:** drugs that are categorized by federal law according to therapeutic usefulness and potential for abuse; also known as scheduled drugs

**Drug classifications:** groups of medications that are classified according to their effects on particular body systems, their therapeutic uses, and their chemical characteristics

**Generic name:** chemical or official name of the drug that is independent of the manufacturer and often indicates the drug group

**Over-the-counter [OTC] drugs:** medications available for purchase without a prescription

**Pharmacoeconomics:** costs of drug therapy, including costs of purchasing, dispensing, storage, administration, and laboratory and other tests used to monitor patient responses; also considers losses due to expiration

**Pharmacogenomics (also known as pharmacogenetics):** study of how a person's genetic heritage leads to variable responses to drugs; more generally refers to genetic polymorphisms that occur in a patient population, such as an ethnic group, as opposed to an individual person

**Pharmacotherapy:** use of drugs to prevent, diagnose, or treat signs, symptoms, and disease processes

**Placebo:** inert substance containing no medication and given to reinforce a person's expectation to improve

**Prescription drugs:** medications that are ordered in writing by a licensed health care provider

**Prototype:** often the first drug of a particular drug class to be developed; usually the standard against which newer, similar drugs are compared

## INTRODUCTION

Pharmacology is the study of drugs (chemicals) that alter the functions of living organisms. **Pharmacotherapy**, also known as drug therapy, is the use of drugs to prevent, diagnose, or treat signs, symptoms, and diseases. When prevention or cure is not a reasonable goal, relief of symptoms can greatly improve a patient's quality of life and ability to perform activities of daily living. Contemporary nursing guidelines require that nurses keep safety issues in mind when involved in the practice of pharmacotherapy.

Drugs given for therapeutic purposes are also called medications. These substances may be given for their local or systemic effects. Drugs with local effects, such as sunscreen lotions and local anesthetics, act mainly at the site of application. Those with systemic effects are taken into the body, circulated through the bloodstream to their sites of action in various body tissues, and eventually eliminated from the body. Most drugs are given for their systemic effects. Drugs may also be given for acute disorders, such as pain or infection, or to relieve signs and symptoms of long-term disease processes, such as hypertension or diabetes.

## DRUG SOURCES

Historically, drugs came from plants, animals, and minerals. Now, most drugs are synthetic compounds manufactured in laboratories. Chemists, for example, often create useful new drugs by altering the chemical structure of existing drugs. Such techniques and other technologic advances have enabled the production of new drugs as well as synthetic versions of many drugs originally derived from plants and animals. Synthetic drugs are more standardized in their chemical characteristics, more consistent in their effects, and less likely to produce allergic reactions. Semisynthetic drugs (e.g., many antibiotics) are naturally occurring substances that have been chemically modified.

**Biotechnology** is also an important source of drugs. This process may involve manipulating deoxyribonucleic acid (DNA) and ribonucleic acid (RNA) and recombining genes into hybrid molecules that can be inserted into living organisms (*Escherichia coli* bacteria are often used), which can be repeatedly reproduced. Each hybrid molecule produces a genetically identical molecule, called a clone. Cloning makes it possible to identify the DNA sequence in a gene and to produce the protein product encoded by a gene, such as insulin. Cloning also allows production of adequate amounts of the drug for therapeutic or research purposes. Biotechnology drugs constitute an increasing percentage of drugs now undergoing development, and this trend is expected to continue into the foreseeable future.

## DRUG CLASSIFICATIONS AND PROTOTYPES

Drugs are classified according to their effects on particular body systems, their therapeutic uses, and their chemical characteristics. For example, morphine can be classified as a central nervous system depressant and a narcotic or opioid analgesic. The names of therapeutic classifications usually reflect the conditions for which the drugs are used (e.g., antidepressants, antihypertensives). However, the names of many drug groups reflect their chemical characteristics rather than their therapeutic uses (e.g., adrenergics, benzodiazepines). Many drugs fit into multiple groups because they have wide-ranging effects on the human body.

An individual drug that represents groups of drugs is called a **prototype**. The prototype, often the first drug of a particular drug class to be developed, is usually the standard with which newer drugs in the class are compared. For example, morphine is the prototype of the opioid analgesics, and penicillin is the prototype of the beta-lactam antibacterial drugs.

**Drug classifications** and prototypes are quite well established, and most new drugs can be assigned to a group and compared with a recognized prototype. However, some groups lack a universally accepted prototype, and some prototypes are replaced over time by newer, more commonly used drugs. In this text, information about the prototype is provided for each drug class.

## DRUG NAMES

Individual drugs may have several different names, but the two that are most commonly used are the generic (official) name and the brand (trade) name. The **generic name** (e.g., amoxicillin) is related to the chemical or official name and is independent of the manufacturer. The generic name often indicates the drug group (e.g., drugs with generic names ending in "cillin" are penicillins). In the United States, the United States Adopted Names Council assigns the generic name. The **brand (trade) name** is designated and patented by the manufacturer. For example, amoxicillin is manufactured by several pharmaceutical companies, some of which assign a specific trade name (e.g., Amoxil, Larotid) and several of which use only the generic name.

In drug literature, trade names are capitalized, and generic names are presented in lowercase unless in a list or at the beginning of a sentence. Drugs may be prescribed and dispensed by generic or trade name. Generic equivalents are available for the majority of drugs and can be substituted for trade-named drugs unless the prescriber requests the trade-named medication by writing "do not substitute" on the prescription. Generic drugs are required to be therapeutically equivalent and are less expensive than trade-named drugs.

 **QSEN Alert: Safety**

Using different drug names (i.e., generic or trade names) increases confusion and the risk of misuse. If the drug name on the package does not match the one on the **prescription drug** label, an individual may take too much medication or not take it at all.

**NCLEX Success**

1. The nurse is caring for a woman who has strong beliefs about not putting anything unnatural into her body. It is most accurate to say that most modern medications are
   A. natural products derived from plants
   B. natural products derived from minerals
   C. synthetic products manufactured in laboratories
   D. synthetic modifications of natural products

2. The nurse is taking care of a man who is confused about the different medications he is prescribed. He notes that some of the drug names have changed over the course of time he has been taking them. When counseling him, it is most important to keep the following statement in mind:
   A. A drug can belong to only one group or classification.
   B. A prototype drug is the standard by which similar drugs are compared.
   C. Drug groups and prototypes change frequently, and knowledge about a prototype cannot guide knowledge about other drugs in the same class.
   D. The generic name of a drug changes among manufacturers.

## DRUG MARKETING

A patent protects a new drug for several years, during which time only the pharmaceutical manufacturer that developed it can market it. The company views this protection as a return on its investment in developing the drug, which might have required years of work and millions of dollars, and as an incentive to develop other drugs. Other pharmaceutical companies cannot manufacture and market the drug until the patent expires. However, for new drugs that are popular and widely used, other companies often produce similar drugs, with different generic and trade names.

## PHARMACOECONOMICS

**Pharmacoeconomics** involves the costs of drug therapy, including costs of purchasing, dispensing (i.e., salaries of pharmacists, pharmacy technicians), storage, administration (i.e., salaries of nurses, costs of supplies), and laboratory and other tests used to monitor patient responses, as well as losses due to expiration. Length of illness or hospitalization is also a consideration. The goal of most pharmacoeconomic research is to identify drug therapy regimens that provide the desired benefits at the lowest cost.

## PHARMACOGENOMICS

**Pharmacogenomics** is the study of how one's genetic inheritance affects the body's response to drugs. The term comes from the words *pharmacology* and *genomics* and is a combination of drugs and genetics. Because essentially all diseases and conditions have a genetic or genomic component, the use of this information in prevention, screening, diagnosis, and treatment and effectiveness enhances the likelihood of best practice in drug therapy.

## ACCESS TO DRUGS

### Prescription and Nonprescription Drugs

Legally, American consumers have two ways to access therapeutic drugs. They can obtain them as **prescription drugs**, which require a written order. A licensed health care provider such as a physician, dentist, or nurse practitioner writes the prescription. Alternatively, they can purchase **over-the-counter (OTC) drugs**, which do not require a prescription. Various laws regulate these routes. Acquiring and using prescription drugs for nontherapeutic purposes by people who are not authorized to have the drugs or for whom they are not prescribed is illegal.

### American Drug Laws and Standards

Current drug laws and standards have evolved over many years. Their main goal is to protect the public by ensuring that drugs marketed for therapeutic purposes are safe and effective. Table 1.1 further describes and summarizes the main provisions.

The Food, Drug, and Cosmetic Act of 1938 and its amendments regulate the manufacture, distribution, advertising, and labeling of drugs. The law also requires that official drugs (i.e., those listed in the United States Pharmacopeia and designated USP) must meet standards of purity and strength as determined by chemical analysis or by animal response to specified doses (bioassay). The Durham-Humphrey Amendment designates drugs that must be prescribed by a licensed physician or nurse practitioner and dispensed by a pharmacist. The U.S. Food and Drug Administration (FDA) is charged with enforcing the law. In addition, the Public Health Service regulates vaccines and other biologic products, and the Federal Trade Commission can suppress misleading advertisements of nonprescription drugs.

The Comprehensive Drug Abuse Prevention and Control Act was passed in 1970. Title II of this law, called the Controlled Substances Act, regulates the manufacture and distribution of narcotics, stimulants, depressants, hallucinogens, and anabolic

**TABLE 1.1**

## American Drug Laws and Amendments

| Year | Name | Main Provision(s) |
|------|------|-------------------|
| 1906 | Pure Food and Drug Act | Established official standards and requirements for accurate labeling of drug products<br>Established the forerunner of FDA |
| 1912 | Shirley Amendment | Prohibited fraudulent claims of drug effectiveness |
| 1914 | Harrison Narcotic Act | Restricted the importation, manufacture, sale, and use of opium, cocaine, marijuana, and other drugs that the act defined as narcotics |
| 1938 | Food, Drug, and Cosmetic Act | Revised and broadened FDA powers and responsibilities; gave the FDA control over drug safety<br>Required proof of safety from the manufacturer before a new drug could be marketed<br>Authorized factory inspections<br>Established penalties for fraudulent claims and misleading labels |
| 1945 | Amendment | Required governmental certification of biologic products, such as insulin and antibiotics |
| 1951 | Durham-Humphrey Amendment | Designated drugs that must be prescribed by a physician and dispensed by a pharmacist (e.g., controlled substances, drugs considered unsafe for use except under supervision by a health care provider, and drugs limited to prescription use under a manufacturer's new drug application) |
| 1962 | Kefauver-Harris Amendment | Required a manufacturer to provide evidence (from well-controlled research studies) that a drug was effective for claims and conditions identified in the product's labeling<br>Gave the federal government the authority to standardize drug names |
| 1970 | Comprehensive Drug Abuse Prevention and Control Act; Controlled Substance Act | Regulated distribution of narcotics and other drugs of abuse<br>Categorized these drugs according to therapeutic usefulness and potential for abuse<br>Title II, Controlled Substances Act<br>Updated or replaced all previous laws regarding narcotics and other dangerous drugs |
| 1978 | Drug Regulation Reform Act | Established guidelines for research studies and data to be submitted to the FDA by manufacturers<br>Shortened the time required to develop and market new drugs |
| 1983 | Orphan Drug Act | Decreased taxes and competition for manufacturers who would produce drugs to treat selected serious rare diseases |
| 1987 | | Established new regulations designed to speed up the approval process for high-priority medications |
| 1992 | Prescription Drug User Fee Act | Allowed the FDA to collect user fees from pharmaceutical companies, with each new drug application, to shorten the review time (e.g., by hiring more staff)<br>Specified a review time of 12 mo for standard drugs and 6 mo for priority drugs |
| 1993 | NIH Revitalization Act | Requires inclusion of women and minorities in NIH-funded research studies, including Phase III clinical drug trials |
| 1997 | FDA Modernization Act | Updated regulation of biologic products<br>Increased patient access to experimental drugs and medical devices<br>Accelerated review of important new drugs<br>Allowed drug companies to disseminate information about off-label (non–FDA-approved) uses and costs of drugs<br>Extended user fees |
| 2002 | Best Pharmaceuticals for Children Act | Encouraged pharmaceutical companies to conduct studies and label drugs for use in children<br>Provided funds for 5 y for pediatric drug studies |
| 2003 | Medicare Prescription Drug Improvement and Modernization Act | Afforded the largest overhaul of Medicare in the 38-y history of the program<br>Provided entitlement benefit for prescription drugs and other benefits for seniors and those with medical disabilities |
| 2005 | Combat Methamphetamine Epidemic Act | Established federal law that regulates retail over-the-counter sales of ephedrine, pseudoephedrine, and phenylpropanolamine products due to their use in the manufacturing of illegal drugs. Specifically, these drugs are:<br>• Kept behind the counter or in a locked case<br>• Limited in purchase to no more than 3.6 g a day and 9 g a month<br>• Dispensed after purchasers produce identification and sign a sales log<br>• Handled by employees who are properly trained<br>Geared at curtailing clandestine production of methamphetamine |

*(Continued)*

**TABLE 1.1**

## American Drug Laws and Amendments (Continued)

| Year | Name | Main Provision(s) |
|------|------|-------------------|
| 2008 | Ryan Haight Online Pharmacy Consumer Protection Act | Applies to all controlled substances in all schedules<br>Established federal law that it is illegal to deliver, distribute, or dispense a controlled substance by means of the Internet unless the online pharmacy holds a modification of DEA registration authorizing it to operate as an online pharmacy |
| 2018 | Substance Use-Disorder Prevention that Promotes Opioid Recovery and Treatment (SUPPORT) for Patients and Communities Act | Dedicates more federal resources to combat the opioid crisis through alternate strategies for pain management, including increased focus on nonopioid pain relief, expanded treatment options for people with substance abuse disorders, greater access to APRN-delivered care and telehealth services<br>Amends the Controlled Substances Act to permanently authorize Nurse Practitioners and provide a 5-y authorization for clinical nurse specialists, certified registered nurse anesthetists, and certified nurse-midwives to prescribe Medication-Assisted Treatments (MAT for opioid use disorders; expands Medicaid coverage for MAT) |

APRN, Advanced Practice Registered Nurses; DEA, Drug Enforcement Administration; FDA, U.S. Food and Drug Administration; MAT, medication-assisted treatment; NIH, National Institutes of Health.

steroids and requires the pharmaceutical industry to maintain physical security and strict record keeping for these drugs and substances. These drugs are categorized according to therapeutic usefulness and potential for abuse (Box 1.1) and are labeled as **controlled substances** (e.g., morphine is a C-II or Schedule II drug).

The Drug Enforcement Administration (DEA) enforces the Controlled Substances Act. Individual people and companies legally empowered to handle controlled substances must register with the DEA, keep accurate records of all transactions, and provide for secure storage. The DEA assigns prescribers a number, which they must include on all prescriptions they write for a controlled substance. Prescriptions for Schedule II drugs cannot be refilled; a new prescription is required. Nurses are responsible for storing controlled substances in locked containers, administering them only to people for whom they are prescribed, recording each dose given on agency narcotic sheets and on the patient's medication administration record, maintaining an accurate inventory, and reporting discrepancies to the proper authorities.

An approach known as medication-assisted treatment (MAT) may be used in the management of substance abuse disorders. MAT involves the use of FDA-approved medications in combination with counseling and behavioral therapies. The Substance Abuse and Mental Health Services Administration program provides a "whole-patient" approach to the treatment of substance use disorders that is consistent with the latest regulations that address the opioid crisis. The Substance Use-Disorder Prevention that Promotes Opioid Recovery and Treatment (SUPPORT) for Patients and Communities Act assists states in implementing updates to their plans of safe care and improving data sharing between states. It can help some people to sustain recovery.

**BOX 1.1** *Categories of Controlled Substances*

**Schedule I**

Drugs that have no accepted medical use, have lack of accepted safety, and have high abuse potentials: heroin, lysergic acid diethylamide (LSD), 3,4-methylenedioxy-methamphetamine (MDMA or ecstasy), mescaline, and peyote.

**Schedule II**

Drugs that are used medically and have high abuse potentials: opioid analgesics (e.g., codeine, hydromorphone, methadone, meperidine, morphine, oxycodone), central nervous system (CNS) stimulants (e.g., cocaine, methamphetamine), and barbiturate sedative–hypnotics (e.g., pentobarbital).

**Schedule III**

Drugs with less potential for abuse than those in Schedules I and II, but abuse of which may lead to psychological or physical dependence: androgens and anabolic steroids, some depressants (e.g., ketamine, pentobarbital), some CNS stimulants (e.g., methylphenidate), and mixtures containing small amounts of controlled substances (e.g., codeine, barbiturates not listed in other schedules). These drugs and substances have an accepted medical use in the United States.

**Schedule IV**

Drugs with an accepted medical use in the United States but with some potential for abuse: benzodiazepines (e.g., diazepam, lorazepam), other sedative–hypnotics (e.g., phenobarbital, chloral hydrate), and some prescription appetite suppressants (e.g., phentermine).

**Schedule V**

Products containing moderate amounts of controlled substances. They may be dispensed by the pharmacist without a physician's prescription but with some restrictions regarding amount, record keeping, and other safeguards. Included are cough suppressants containing small amounts of codeine and antidiarrheal drugs, such as diphenoxylate and atropine (Lomotil).

In addition to federal laws, state laws also regulate the sale and distribution of controlled drugs. These laws may be more stringent than federal laws; if so, the stricter laws usually apply.

# DRUG APPROVAL PROCESSES: FOOD AND DRUG ADMINISTRATION

The FDA is responsible for ensuring that new drugs are safe and effective before approving the drugs and allowing them to be marketed. The FDA reviews research studies (usually conducted or sponsored by pharmaceutical companies) about proposed new drugs; the organization does not test the drugs.

## Testing Procedure

Since 1962, newly developed drugs undergo extensive testing before being marketed for general use. A clinical trial proceeds through five phases if there is continuing evidence of drug safety and effectiveness. Initially, drug testing occurs in animals and small groups of humans (Phase 0), and the FDA's Center for Drug Evaluation and Research (CDER) reviews the test results. Next, researchers perform clinical trials in more humans (Phases 1–4), usually with a randomized, controlled experimental design that involves selection of subjects according to established criteria, random assignment of subjects to experimental groups, and administration of the test drug to one group and a control substance to another group.

In Phase 1, a few doses are given to a certain number of healthy volunteers to determine safe dosages, routes of administration, absorption, metabolism, excretion, and toxicity. In Phase 2, a few doses are given to a certain number of subjects with the disease or symptom for which the drug is being studied, and responses are compared with those of healthy subjects. In Phase 3, the drug is given to different populations and different dosages and by using the drug in combination with other drugs. In double-blind, placebo-controlled designs, half of the subjects receive the new drug and half receive a **placebo** (an inactive substance similar in appearance to the actual drug), with neither subjects nor researchers knowing who receives which formulation. In crossover studies, subjects serve as their own control; each subject receives the experimental drug during half of the study and a placebo during the other half. Other research methods include control studies in which some patients receive a known drug rather than a placebo; in subject matching, patients are paired with other individuals of similar characteristics. Phase 3 studies help determine whether the potential benefits of the drug outweigh the risks. Testing may be stopped during any of the early phases if inadequate effectiveness or excessive toxicity becomes evident. In Phase 4, the FDA allows the drug to be marketed and requires manufacturers to continue postmarketing monitoring and electronic report submission of the drug's safety and effectiveness.

Historically, drug research involved mainly young, white males. In 1993, Congress passed the National Institutes of Health (NIH) Revitalization Act, which formalized a policy of the NIH that women and minorities be included in human subject research studies funded by the NIH and that women and minorities be included in clinical drug trials. Now, major drug trials must recruit female subjects and include outcome data on women. In addition, all newly developed drugs must include gender-related effectiveness and safety information in the initial FDA application. Knowledge about the drug effects in women has increased but is still relatively limited because many commonly used drugs were developed before enactment of these regulations.

Subsequent withdrawal of approved and marketed drugs has occurred, usually because of serious adverse effects that become evident only when the drugs are used in a large, diverse population. In addition, over the past 25 years, the FDA has issued BLACK BOX WARNING (BBWs) ◆ about drugs that can cause serious adverse effects. The warning appears on the label, package insert, and any marketing literature; these BBWs are identified in this text (see Chap. 2 for additional information).

In response to growing public concern regarding health risks posed by approved drugs, the FDA requested that the Institute of Medicine (IOM) conduct an independent assessment of the FDA's drug safety system in the United States. Their 2006 report released in 2006 recounted major deficiencies and made recommendations to improve risk assessment, surveillance, and the safe use of drugs. Ongoing assessment of deficiencies and identification of additional error reduction strategies persists.

## Approval of Prescription and Nonprescription Drugs

The FDA's CDER approves many new prescription drugs annually, and it also approves drugs for OTC availability. With prescription drugs, a health care professional diagnoses the condition, often with the help of laboratory and other diagnostic tests, and determines a need for the drug. With OTC drugs, the consumer must make these decisions, with or without consultation with a health care provider. The CDER handles the transfer of drugs from prescription to OTC status and may require additional clinical trials to determine the safety and effectiveness of OTC use. For prescription drugs taken orally, the switch to OTC status may mean different indications for use and lower doses. FDA approval of a drug for OTC availability involves evaluation of evidence that the consumer can use the drug safely, using information on the product label, and shifts primary responsibility for safe and effective drug therapy from health care professionals to consumers.

Having drugs available OTC has potential advantages and disadvantages for consumers. Advantages include greater autonomy, faster and more convenient access to effective treatment, possibly earlier resumption of usual activities of daily living, fewer visits to health care providers, and possibly increased efforts by consumers to learn about their symptoms/conditions and recommended treatments. Disadvantages include inaccurate self-diagnoses and potential risks of choosing a wrong or contraindicated drug, delayed treatment by health care professionals, and development of adverse drug reactions and interactions. When a drug is switched from prescription to OTC status, sales and profits of pharmaceutical companies increase and costs of insurance companies decrease. Costs to consumers increase because health insurance companies do not cover most OTC drugs.

## Clinical Application 1.1

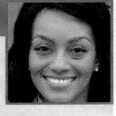

Ms. Clark analyzes drug safety, including the national organizations charged with ensuring it.

● What is the role of the U.S. Food and Drug Administration (FDA) in the drug approval process?
● What is the role of the Drug Enforcement Administration (DEA) and the nurse with regard to controlled substances?

## NCLEX Success

3. In understanding the use of controlled substances for patients, it is important that the nurse knows that controlled drugs are

   A. categorized according to prescription or nonprescription status
   B. regulated by state and local laws more than federal laws
   C. those that must demonstrate high standards of safety
   D. scheduled according to medical use and potential for abuse

4. A patient is asking what the difference is between a prescription for 800 mg of a medication that can be purchased on an OTC basis as a 200-mg tablet. To address this issue, it is important that the nurse knows that OTC drugs

   A. are considered safe for any consumer to use
   B. are not available for treatment of most commonly occurring symptoms
   C. often differ in indications for use and recommended dosages from their prescription versions
   D. are paid for by most insurance policies

## SAFETY IN DRUG ADMINISTRATION

At least 7 million preventable adverse drug events costing more than 21 billion dollars occur in the health care system each year (New England Health Institute). As described previously, multiple safeguards to promote drug safety in packaging, drug laws, and approval processes are in place. Just as critical are safeguards to promote the safe administration of drugs at the point of care.

## Rights of Medication Administration

Patient safety with medication administration begins by adhering to the rights of medication administration. The 10 rights of medication administration include the right drug, right dose, right patient, right route, right time, right reason, right documentation, right patient education, right evaluation, and right to refuse the medication. These rights are goals of the medication administration process, and discussion of the effort to reduce medication errors and harm has expanded over the years. However, the focus on rights has been on the nurse and not the system in which medication administration takes place. Chapter 3 discusses the medication rights and their application to the nursing process.

### ! QSEN Alert: Quality Improvement

Smetzer, Baker, Byrne, and Cohen (2010) reported on a nurse who mistakenly administered epidural pain medication intravenously to a pregnant woman in a birthing suite. Complications developed, and although cesarean section resulted in the delivery of a healthy infant, the teenage mother died from cardiovascular collapse. Media publicity called attention to the error when a nurse was charged with a criminal offense.

As part of the investigation of this issue, the hospital's medication and safety procedures were analyzed using a root cause analysis. In addition, an external review team evaluated the organization's medication system and processes, patterns of staffing, leadership, and institutional culture; identified problems; and suggested improvements. Enhanced safety initiatives included team training for staff working in the birthing suites, implementing consistent procedures for scanning-adherence tracking, and streamlining the bar code scanning tracking of medications. This incident identified system gaps and process failures within an organization that led to the death of a patient. Prudent nursing actions support an organization's culture of safety by complying with processes (safety nets and fail-safe mechanisms) that are aimed at preventing and/or reducing environmental effects to prevent medication errors.

New technology in medication administration has expanded required competencies for safe medication administration. Electronic charting, automated drug-dispensing systems, and bar code medication administration have required enhanced nursing skills to manage these complex systems. The entire process of medication administration in a hospital is distracting, causing the nurse to lose focus on the task at hand; multiple interruptions and the extended hours that nurses work inevitably lead to the possibility of unintended consequences.

### ! QSEN Alert: Safety

Error-reduction strategies during medication administration include the following:

● Having a "quiet zone" to prepare medications
● Placing "quiet zone" signs at the entrance to the medication room or above the automated medication-dispensing system
● Following protocols and checklist outlining medication administration
● Wearing a sash or vest to signal others to avoid interrupting the nurse during medication administration
● Educating staff to reduce interruptions of nurses administering medications
● Having a drug guide available during drug administration

Multiple national strategies have been implemented to reduce medication errors since the seminal work of the IOM (2000), which highlighted the breadth of preventable medical errors in the United States. Examining human factors and the response of nurses to workflow changes and technology have led to more successful system design, operation, and usability.

# Quality and Safety Education for Nurses Project

The Quality and Safety Education for Nurses (QSEN) project, sponsored by the Robert Wood Johnson Foundation, is committed to the continuous improvement in the quality and safety of health care systems by focusing on the needed knowledge, skills, and attitudes (KSA) required in the preparation of future nurses in six areas: patient-centered care, teamwork and collaboration, evidence-based practice, quality improvement, safety, and informatics. Using the IOM competencies for nursing, QSEN faculty outlined prelicensure and graduate quality and safety competencies for nursing. Additionally, recommended targets for the KSA that need to be developed in prelicensure nursing students for each competency have been established. The QSEN competencies in the six areas are highlighted throughout the text as they relate to medication administration. Box 1.2 outlines these competencies and their definitions.

# National Patient Safety Goals

The Joint Commission is also concerned with implementing strategies to enhance safety and annually updates targeted patient safety goals related to medication safety. Outlined below are two areas of particular interest to medication administration safety.

## *"Do Not Use" List of Abbreviations*

 **QSEN Alert: Quality Improvement**

The Joint Commission published a Sentinel Event Alert in 2001 regarding medical abbreviations. Since then, this organization has developed a standardized list of abbreviations, acronyms, dose designations, and symbols that are not to be used in a health care organization.

Table 1.2 lists these terms. This list was developed as part of the requirements for meeting one of the National Patient Safety Goals.

## *Targeted High-Risk Activities*

The Joint Commission also requires performance measures related to safety in drug administration. Specifically, a health care facility must demonstrate safe medication management using risk-reduction activities with medication labeling and use of anticoagulant medications.

In the perioperative area and other procedural settings, all medications must be labeled in syringes and basins if transferred from the original packaging. This practice focuses on an identified risk point in medication administration.

Health care institutions that provide anticoagulant therapy must establish a defined process that has a positive impact on patient safety with this class of medications (see Chap. 9) and leads to better outcomes. It is necessary to develop a process for anticoagulant use related to education, standardized ordering, dispensing, administration, and monitoring. Routine short-term use of anticoagulants for prevention of venous thromboembolism is not included as an element of performance when it is expected that the patient's laboratory values will remain within or close to normal limits with the therapy.

---

| BOX 1.2 | *Quality and Safety Education for Nurses (QSEN) Competencies and Definitions* |
|---|---|

### Patient-Centered Care

Recognize the patient or designee as the source of control and full partner in providing compassionate and coordinated care based on respect for patient's preferences, values, and needs

### Teamwork and Collaboration

Function effectively within nursing and interprofessional teams, fostering open communication, mutual respect, and shared decision-making to achieve quality patient care

### Evidence-Based Practice (Known as EBP)

Integrate best current evidence with clinical expertise and patient/family preferences and values for delivery of optimal health care

### Quality Improvement

Use data to monitor the outcomes of care processes, and use improvement methods to design and test changes to continuously improve the quality and safety of health care systems

### Safety

Minimizes risk of harm to patients and providers through both system effectiveness and individual performance

### Informatics

Use information and technology to communicate, manage knowledge, mitigate error, and support decision-making

Reprinted from Cronenwett, L., Sherwood, G., Barnsteiner, J., Disch, J., Johnson, J., Mitchell, P., et al. (Copyright 2007). Quality and safety education for nurses. *Nursing Outlook, 55*(3), 122–131, with permission from Elsevier.

---

# High-Alert Medications

The Institute for Safe Medication Practices (ISMP) identifies drugs that when used in error have a heightened risk of causing significant patient harm.

 **QSEN Alert: Technology**

To reduce the chance of errors, strategies such as automatic alerts, automated dispensing devices, bar codes, computerized physician order entry, point-of-care drug resources, and standardizations of processes are important.

Box 1.3 lists drug classes and specific drugs that appear on the ISMP high-alert list.

## TABLE 1.2

### Official "Do Not Use" List*

| Do Not Use | Potential Problem | Use Instead |
|---|---|---|
| U (unit) | Mistaken for "0" (zero), the number "4" (four), or "cc" | Write "unit" |
| IU (International Unit) | Mistaken for IV (intravenous) or the number 10 (ten) | Write "International Unit" |
| Q.D., QD, q.d., qd (daily) | Mistaken for each other | Write "daily" |
| Q.O.D., QOD, q.o.d., qod (every other day) | Period after the Q mistaken for "I" and the "O" mistaken for "I" | Write "every other day" |
| Trailing zero (X.0 mg)† Lack of leading zero (.X mg) | Decimal point is missed | Write X mg Write 0.X mg |
| MS | Can mean morphine sulfate or magnesium sulfate | Write "morphine sulfate" |
| MSO₄ and MgSO₄ | Confused with one another | Write "magnesium sulfate" |

*This list applies to all orders and all medication-related documentation that is handwritten (including free-text computer entry) or on preprinted forms.

†**Exception:** A "trailing zero" may be used only where required to demonstrate the level of precision of the value being reported, such as for laboratory results, imaging studies that report size of lesions, or catheter/tube sizes. It may not be used in medication orders or other medication-related documentation.

© The Joint Commission, 2018. Reprinted with permission.

## BOX 1.3    *High-Alert Medications*

### Classes/Categories of Medications

Adrenergic agonists, IV (e.g., epinephrine, phenylephrine, norepinephrine)

Adrenergic antagonists, IV (e.g., propranolol, metoprolol, labetalol)

Anesthetic agents, general, inhaled, and IV (e.g., propofol, ketamine)

Antidysrhythmics, IV (e.g., lidocaine, amiodarone)

Antithrombotic agents (anticoagulants), including warfarin, low molecular weight heparin, IV unfractionated heparin, factor Xa inhibitors (fondaparinux), direct thrombin inhibitors (e.g., argatroban, lepirudin, bivalirudin), thrombolytics (e.g., alteplase, reteplase, tenecteplase), and glycoprotein IIb/IIIa inhibitors (e.g., eptifibatide)

Cardioplegic solutions

Chemotherapeutic agents, parenteral and oral

Dextrose, hypertonic, 20% or greater

Dialysis solutions, peritoneal and hemodialysis

Epidural or intrathecal medications

Hypoglycemics, oral

Inotropic medications, IV (e.g., digoxin, milrinone)

Insulin, subcutaneous and IV

Liposomal forms of drugs (e.g., liposomal amphotericin B)

Moderate sedation agents, IV (e.g., midazolam)

Moderate sedation agents, oral, for children (e.g., chloral hydrate)

Narcotics/opiates, IV, transdermal, and oral (including liquid concentrates, immediate- and sustained-release formulations)

Neuromuscular blocking agents (e.g., succinylcholine, rocuronium, vecuronium)

Radiocontrast agents, IV

Sodium chloride for injection, hypertonic (greater than 0.9% concentration)

Sterile water for injection, inhalation, and irrigation (excluding pour bottles) in containers of 100 mL or more

Total parenteral nutrition solutions

### Specific Medications

Epoprostenol (Flolan), IV

Magnesium sulfate injection

Methotrexate, oral, nononcologic use

Opium tincture

Oxytocin, IV

Nitroprusside sodium for injection

Potassium chloride for injection concentrate

Potassium phosphate injection

Promethazine, IV

Vasopressin, IV or intraosseous

Reprinted with permission from the Institute for Safe Medication Practices (ISMP). (Copyright 2014). *ISMP's list of high-alert medications*. Retrieved August 7, 2017, from http://www.ismp.org/Tools/highalertmedications.pdf

### Unfolding Patient Stories: Junetta Cooper • Part 1

Junetta Cooper, a 75-year-old woman with atherosclerotic heart disease and hypertension, is hospitalized. Her morning medications include four oral medications, a transdermal patch, and an IV push medication. What measures can the nurse implement to prevent medication errors and ensure patient safety when preparing and administering these six medications? (Junetta Cooper's story continues in Chapter 26.)

Care for Junetta and other patients in a realistic virtual environment: *vSim for Nursing* (thepoint.lww.com/vSimPharm). Practice documenting these patients' care in DocuCare (thepoint.lww.com/DocuCareEHR).

## Pregnancy Categories for Safety

As discussed in detail in Chapter 2, the Pregnancy and Lactation Labeling Rule in 2015 provided a new system that documents exposed known or potential maternal or fetal adverse reactions with individual drugs. This classification scheme has replaced the pregnancy categories. The system is anticipated to improve communication on the best available evidence on risks associated with drug exposure in pregnancy for better-informed prescribing decisions. Because it will take years to transition to the new system, this text continues to contain the associated pregnancy category in the Drugs at a Glance tables for all drugs approved before 2015.

## Beers Criteria for Potentially Inappropriate Medications Used in Older Adults

The American Geriatrics Society Beers Criteria, a list of medications that are generally considered best avoided generally in older adults and specifically in those with certain diseases, confirm that toxic medication effects and drug-related problems affect the safety of older adults. For a wide variety of reasons, the medications listed tend to cause adverse effects in this population and have been linked to poor health outcomes, including confusion, falls, and death. Further discussion of the Beers Criteria, including the medications on the 2015 list and strategies used to identify age-related changes associated with drug administration, is found in Chapter 5.

### NCLEX Success

5. A man is very upset with a drug recall of a medication he has been taking for a long time. He states that he feels like he can no longer trust anyone to protect him. In response to his questions about the process of drug development, it is important to know that with a new drug, the U.S. Food and Drug Administration (FDA) is responsible for
   A. testing the drug with animals
   B. testing the drug with healthy people
   C. marketing the drug to health care providers
   D. evaluating the drug for safety and effectiveness

6. Error-reduction strategies during medication administration include which of the following? (Select all that apply.)
   A. quiet zone signs at entrance to the medication room
   B. protocols and checklist outlining medication administration
   C. wearing of a sash or vest to signal others to avoid interruptions of the nurse during medication administration
   D. carrying several patients' prescanned medications on a tray

## SOURCES OF DRUG INFORMATION

Sources of drug information include pharmacology and other textbooks, drug reference books, journal articles, point-of-care references, and Internet sites. Textbooks provide information regarding groups of drugs in relation to therapeutic uses. Drug reference books and point-of-care referencing tools are most helpful concerning individual drugs. Two authoritative sources are (1) the *American Hospital Formulary Service*, published by the American Society of Health-System Pharmacists and updated periodically, and (2) *Drug Facts and Comparisons*, published by the Facts and Comparisons division of Wolters Kluwer/Lippincott Williams & Wilkins and updated monthly (loose-leaf edition) or annually (hardbound edition). A less authoritative source is the *Physicians' Desk Reference*, published yearly, which compiles manufacturers' package inserts for selected drugs.

Numerous drug handbooks (e.g., *Lippincott Nursing Drug Guide*, published annually) and pharmacologic, medical, and nursing journals also contain information about drugs. Textbook chapters and journal articles often present information about drug therapy for patients with specific disease processes and may thereby facilitate application of drug knowledge in clinical practice.

Internet sites also contain drug information, but it is essential to assess their quality. A wide variety of information, ranging in accuracy, reliability, and value, is easily accessible. The Web site for *Lippincott Nursing Drug Guide* is a reliable clinical resource for drug information (see References and Resources). Additionally, point-of-care references, such as UpToDate, provide quick access to drug information that supports decision-making regarding drug therapy.

### Clinical Application 1.2

Ms. Clark also reviews additional strategies to promote the system safety in the administration of drugs at the point of care.
- What systemic issues in a hospital or nursing home have an impact on safe medication administration?
- What can the nurse do to avoid medication errors while dispensing medications?

# STRATEGIES FOR STUDYING PHARMACOLOGY

- Concentrate on therapeutic classifications and their prototypes. For example, morphine is the prototype of opioid analgesics (see Chap. 49). Understanding morphine makes learning about other opioid analgesics easier because they are compared with morphine.
- Compare a newly encountered drug with a prototype or similar drug when possible. Relating the unknown to the known aids learning and retention of knowledge.
- Try to understand how the drug acts in the body. This understanding allows prediction of therapeutic effects and prediction, prevention, or minimization of adverse effects by early detection and treatment.
- Concentrate study efforts on major characteristics. Such characteristics include the main indications for use, common and potentially serious adverse effects, conditions in which the drug is contraindicated or must be used cautiously, and related nursing care needs.
- Keep an authoritative, up-to-date drug reference readily available. A drug reference is a more reliable source of drug information than memory, especially for dosage ranges. Use the reference freely when learning about an unfamiliar drug or when answering a question about a familiar one. Also, nurses have access to computerized databases of drug information through multiple electronic sources, and these can provide a ready source of up-to-date information.
- Use your own words when taking notes or writing drug information cards. Also, write notes, answers to review questions, definitions of new terms, and trade names of drugs encountered in clinical practice settings directly into your pharmacology textbook. The mental processing required for these activities helps in both initial learning and later retention and application of knowledge.
- Rehearse applying drug knowledge in nursing care by asking (yourself), "What if I have a patient who is receiving this drug? What must I do to safely administer the drug? For what must I assess the patient before giving the drug, and for what must I observe in the patient after drug administration? What if my patient is an elderly person or a child?"

## KEY CONCEPTS

- Drug therapy or pharmacotherapy is the use of drugs to prevent, diagnose, or treat signs, symptoms, and disease processes.
- Drugs given for therapeutic purposes are called medications.
- Drugs may be given for local or systemic effects; most are given for systemic effects.
- A prototype is an example of a group of drugs, often the first one of the group to be developed.
- Trade names of drugs are determined by manufacturers; generic names are independent of manufacturers.
- Controlled drugs are categorized according to therapeutic usefulness and potential for abuse.
- Electronic charting, automated drug-dispensing systems, and bar code medication administration require enhanced nursing skills to manage administration of drugs in the clinical setting.
- Observe for the 10 rights of medication administration (right drug, right dose, right patient, right route, right time, right reason, right documentation, right patient education, right evaluation, and right to refuse medication).
- Error-reduction strategies that prevent and/or reduce environmental effects can assist in preventing medication errors.

## CLINICAL REASONING CASE STUDY

**The Scenario**

It is the first day of Pharmacology class at Maryville University. Dr. Frandsen splits her class into four groups. Each group is given one of the following questions to answer.
- Group One: Why is it important to learn pharmacology based on therapeutic broad classifications and their prototypes?
- Group Two: Why is it important to learn the generic and trade names of the medications?
- Group Three: What is Quality and Safety Education for Nurses (QSEN)? Why is it important?
- Group Four: What are the strategies for studying pharmacology?

**Assessing Drug Information**

- Group One should review their pharmacology textbook for information on the therapeutic broad classifications and prototypes.
- Group Two should review and distinguish the difference between generic and trade names.
- Group Three should review information regarding QSEN in the Forward by Dr. Gwen Sherwood and in Chapter 1, and visit the Web site www.qsen.org.
- Group Four should review the strategies for studying pharmacology.

**Nursing Actions**

Group One reports:
- The names of the therapeutic classifications reflect the condition the drugs are used to treat.
- This classification provides information on the effects of the body system.
- Drugs can fit in multiple groups due to their wide range of effects.
- The prototype is often the first drug developed in the class and is the standard for the development of other drugs in the class.

Group Two reports:
- The generic name is related to the chemical or official name and independent of the manufacturer.
- The brand or trade name is designated and patented by the manufacturer.

Dr. Frandsen reports:
- The generic name only will be used on the NCLEX-RN examination.

Group Three reports:
- QSEN is a project committed to continuous improvement in the quality and safety of health care systems by focusing on knowledge, skills, and attitudes.
- The QSEN competencies in medication administration are:
  - Patient-Centered Care: Include all patients and families in the care of the patient.
  - Teamwork and Collaboration: Work effectively within nursing and interprofessional teams to coordinate the complexities of safe medication administration.
  - Evidence-Based Practice: Use current evidence-based practice standards to ensure that appropriate precautions are taken to assess for adverse effects.
  - Quality Improvement: Monitor outcomes and incorporate improvement methods as an integral part of safe medication administration.
  - Safety: Maintain safe medication administration and determine strategies to prevent medication errors.
  - Informatics: Use information technology to manage medication administration and documentation.

Group Four reports:
- To effectively study pharmacology:
  - Learn the therapeutic classifications and their prototypes.
  - Recognize the drug action, uses, adverse effects, and nursing implications.

*Visit* thePoint® *at* **http://thePoint.lww.com/Frandsen12e** *for answers to NCLEX Success questions (in Appendix A), answers to Clinical Application Case Studies (in Appendix B), and more!*

## REFERENCES AND RESOURCES

Ahmad, F.B., Rossen, L.M., Spencer, M.R., Warner, M., & Sutton, P. (2018). *Provisional drug overdose death counts*. National Center for Health Statistics.

American Geriatrics Society 2015 Beers Criteria Update Expert Panel. (2015). American Geriatrics Society 2015 updated Beers Criteria for potentially inappropriate medication use in older adults. *Journal of the American Geriatrics Society, 2015*, 1–20.

Cronenwett, L., Sherwood, G., Barnsteiner, J., Disch, J., Johnson, J., Mitchell, P., et al. (2007). Quality and safety education for nurses. *Nursing Outlook, 55*(3), 122–131.

DiPiro, J., Talbert, R., Yee, G., Matzke, G., Wells, B., & Posey, L. M. (Eds.). (2017). *Pharmacotherapy: A pathophysiologic approach* (10th ed.). New York, NY: McGraw-Hill.

Institute for Safe Medication Practices. http://www.ismp.org

Institute of Medicine Committee on Quality of Health Care in America; Kohn, L. T., Corrigan J. M., & Donaldson, M. S. (Eds.). (2000). *To err is human: Building a safer health system*. Washington, DC: National Academies Press. doi: 10.17226/9728

Institute of Medicine. (2003). *Health professions education: A bridge to quality*. Washington, DC: National Academies Press.

Institute of Medicine. (2006). *Future of drug safety: Promoting and protecting the health of the public*. Washington, DC: National Academies Press.

Institute of Medicine. (2007). *Preventing medication errors*. Washington, DC: National Academies Press.

Karch, A. M. (2019). *Lippincott pocket drug guide for nurses*. Philadelphia, PA: Lippincott Williams & Wilkins.

Keers, R. N., Williams, S. D., Cooke, J., & Ashcroft, D. M. (2015). Understanding the causes of intravenous medication administration errors in hospitals: A qualitative critical incident study. *BMJ Open, 5*(3), e005948.

Larmené-Beld, K. H. M., Alting, E. K., & Taxis, K. (2018). A systematic literature review on strategies to avoid look-alike errors of labels. *European Journal of Clinical Pharmacology, 74*(8), 985–993. http://doi.org/10.1007/s00228-018-2471-z

New England Health Institute. *Preventing medication errors: A $21 billion opportunity*. Retrieved October 1, 2018, from http://www.nehi.net/bendthecurve/sup/documents/Medication_Errors_%20Brief.pdf

Quality and Safety Education for Nurses (QSEN). Retrieved from http://www.qsen.org

QSEN Institute. (2013). *Competencies*. Retrieved September 30, 2018, from http://qsen.org/competencies/

Scott, I. A., Pillans, P. I., Barras, M., & Morris, C. (2018). Using EMR-enabled computerized decision support systems to reduce prescribing of potentially inappropriate medications: A narrative review. *Therapeutic Advances in Drug Safety, 9*(9), 559–573. http://doi.org/10.1177/2042098618784809

Smetzer, J., Baker, C., Byrne, F. D., & Cohen, M. R. (2010). Shaping systems for better behavioral choices: Lessons learned from a fatal medication error. *Joint Commission Journal on Quality and Patient Safety/Joint Commission Resources, 36*(4), 152–163.

The Joint Commission. (2018). *National patient safety goals*. Retrieved September 28, 2018, from http://www.jointcommission.org/standards_information/npsgs.aspx

U.S. Food and Drug Administration. *Frequently asked questions*. Retrieved September 28, 2018, from http://www.fda.gov/ForIndustry/FDABasicsforIndustry/ucm234634.htm

Weant, K. A., Bailey, A. M., & Baker, S. N. (2014). Strategies for reducing medication errors in the emergency department. *Open Access Emergency Medicine: OAEM, 6*, 45–55. http://doi.org/10.2147/OAEM.S64174

# Basic Concepts and Processes

## LEARNING OBJECTIVES

*After studying this chapter, you should be able to:*

1. Discuss cellular physiology in relation to drug therapy.
2. Describe the main pathways and mechanisms by which drugs cross biologic membranes and move through the body.
3. Explain each process of pharmacokinetics.
4. Recognize individual differences in patient drug responses related to genomic variations.
5. Discuss the clinical usefulness of measuring serum drug levels.
6. Describe major characteristics of the receptor theory of drug action.
7. Differentiate between agonist drugs and antagonist drugs.
8. List drug-related and patient-related variables that affect drug actions.
9. Discuss mechanisms and potential effects of drug–drug interactions.
10. Identify signs and symptoms that may occur with adverse drug effects on major body systems.
11. Discuss initial management considerations related to drug overdose and toxicity.
12. Discuss selected drug antidotes.

## CLINICAL APPLICATION CASE STUDY

Doris Green, an 89-year-old widow with cardiovascular and renal disease, takes a number of medications, including three medications to control her hypertension. She has recently switched to a new antihypertensive medication. She prides herself on being independent and able to manage on her own, despite failing memory and failing health.

You, as a home health nurse, visit Mrs. Green to assess the therapeutic and adverse effects of her antihypertensive medications and her adherence to the prescribed medical regimen. You plan to measure her blood pressure to check that it is within normal limits (for Mrs. Green), as well as assess her understanding of her antihypertensive medications and dosing regimen.

## KEY TERMS

- **Absorption:** process that occurs from the time a drug enters the body to the time it enters the bloodstream to be circulated

- **Agonist:** drug that produces effects similar to those produced by naturally occurring hormones, neurotransmitters, and other substances

- **Antagonist:** drug that inhibits cell function by occupying receptor sites

- **Antidote:** substance that relieves, prevents, or counteracts the effect of a poison

**Bioavailability:** portion of a drug dose that reaches the systemic circulation and is available to act on body cells

**Biotransformation:** when drugs are altered from their original form into a new form by the body; also referred to as metabolism

**Distribution:** transport of drug molecules within the body; after a drug is injected or absorbed into the bloodstream, it is carried by the blood and tissue fluids to its sites of action, metabolism, and excretion

**Enterohepatic recirculation:** drugs or metabolites that are excreted in bile, reabsorbed from the small intestine, returned to the liver, metabolized, and eventually excreted in urine

**Enzyme induction:** production of larger amounts of drug-metabolizing enzymes by liver cells; process accelerates drug metabolism because larger amounts of the enzymes (and more binding sites) allow larger amounts of a drug to be metabolized during a given time

**Enzyme inhibition:** process in which a molecule binds to enzymes and inhibits their activity

**Excretion:** elimination of a drug from the body; effective excretion requires adequate functioning of the circulatory system and of the organs of excretion (kidneys, bowel, lungs, and skin)

**First-pass effect:** initial metabolism of some oral drugs as they are carried from the intestine to the liver by the portal circulatory system prior to reaching the systemic circulation for distribution to site of action

**Hypersensitivity:** immune-mediated reaction to a drug

**Loading dose:** dose larger than the regular prescribed daily dosage of a medication; used to attain a therapeutic blood level

**Maintenance dose:** quantity of drug that is needed to keep blood levels and/or tissue levels at a steady state or constant level

**Nephrotoxicity:** toxic or damaging effect of a substance on the kidney; potentially serious because renal damage interferes with drug excretion, causing drug accumulation and increased adverse effects

**Pharmacodynamics:** reactions between living systems and drugs; drug actions on target cells and the resulting alterations in cellular biochemical reactions and functions

**Pharmacogenomics (also known as pharmacogenetics):** the study of how a person's genetic heritage leads to variable responses to drugs; more generally refers to genetic polymorphisms that occur in a patient population, such as an ethnic group, as opposed to an individual person

**Pharmacokinetics:** drug movement through the body to reach sites of action, metabolism, and excretion

**Polymorphism:** the occurrence of two or more clearly different forms (or phenotypes) in a species important in drug therapy because it explains the functionally different response to drugs in a general patient population or a specific individual

**Prodrugs:** initially inactive drugs that exert no pharmacologic effects until they are metabolized

**Serum drug level:** laboratory measurement of the amount of a drug in the blood at a particular time

**Serum half-life:** time required for the serum concentration of a drug to decrease by 50%; also called elimination half-life

## INTRODUCTION

All body functions, all disease processes, and most drug actions occur at the cellular level. Drugs are chemicals that alter basic processes in body cells. They can stimulate or inhibit normal cellular functions; however, they cannot change the type of function that occurs normally. To act on body cells, drugs given for systemic effects must reach adequate concentrations in the blood and other tissue fluids surrounding the cells. Thus, they must enter the body and be circulated to their sites of action (target cells). After they act on cells, they must be eliminated from the body.

How do systemic drugs reach, interact with, and leave body cells? How do people respond to drugs? The answers to these questions are derived from cellular physiology, pathways, and mechanisms of drug transport, pharmacokinetics, pharmacodynamics, pharmacogenomics, and other basic concepts and processes that form the foundation of rational drug therapy and the content of this chapter.

Protoplasm, which constitutes the internal environment of body cells, is composed of water, electrolytes (potassium, magnesium, phosphate, sulfate, bicarbonate), proteins, lipids, and carbohydrates. Water makes up 70% to 85% of most cells; cellular enzymes, electrolytes, and other chemicals are dissolved or suspended in the water. Electrolytes provide chemicals for cellular reactions and are required for some processes (e.g., transmission of electrochemical impulses in nerve and muscle cells). Proteins consist of "physical" proteins that form the structure of cells and "chemical" proteins that function mainly as enzymes within the cell. Lipids, mainly phospholipids and cholesterol, form the membranes that separate structures inside the cell and the cell itself from surrounding cells and body fluids. Carbohydrates play a major role in cell nutrition. Glucose is present in extracellular fluid and is readily available to supply the cell's need for energy. In addition, a small amount of carbohydrate is stored within the cell as glycogen, which can be rapidly converted back to glucose when needed.

The nucleus regulates the types and amounts of proteins, enzymes, and other substances to be produced. The cytoplasm surrounds the nucleus and contains the working units of the cell. The cytosol, the clear fluid portion of the cytoplasm, contains dissolved proteins, electrolytes, and glucose. The endoplasmic reticulum (ER) contains ribosomes, which synthesize proteins, including enzymes that synthesize glycogen, triglycerides, and steroids and those that metabolize drugs and other chemicals. The ER is also important in the production of hormones by glandular cells and the production of plasma proteins by liver cells. Most proteins produced by the ribosomes are released into the cytosol where they act as enzymes or structural proteins of the cell. The Golgi complex stores the substances produced by the ER. It also packages these substances into secretory granules, which then move out of the Golgi complex into the cytoplasm and, after a stimulus, are released from the cell. Mitochondria generate energy for cellular activities and require oxygen. Lysosomes are membrane-enclosed vesicles that contain enzymes capable of digesting nutrients (proteins, carbohydrates, fats), damaged cellular structures, foreign substances (e.g., bacteria), and the cell itself. When a cell becomes worn out or damaged, the membrane around the lysosome breaks and the enzymes (hydrolases) are released. However, lysosomal contents also are released into extracellular spaces and may destroy surrounding cells. Normally, the enzymes are inactivated by enzyme inhibitors, and excessive tissue destruction is prevented.

The cell membrane, a complex structure of phospholipids, proteins, cholesterol, and carbohydrates, separates intracellular contents from the extracellular environment; provides receptors for hormones and other biologically active substances; participates in electrical events that occur in nerve and muscle cells; and helps regulate growth and proliferation.

The cell membrane, which covers the entire surface of the cell, consists of a thin, double layer of lipids interspersed with proteins. The lipid layer is composed of phospholipid (fatty acid and phosphate) molecules. The proteins are usually combined with a carbohydrate and called glycoproteins. Some proteins provide structural pores through which water and water-soluble substances (e.g., sodium, potassium, and calcium ions) can diffuse between extracellular and intracellular fluids. Other proteins act as carriers to transport substances through the cell membrane. Still others act to regulate intracellular function or as enzymes to catalyze chemical reactions within the cell.

Carbohydrates in the cell membrane occur mainly in combination with proteins (glycoproteins) or lipids (glycolipids). Glycoproteins (composed of carbohydrate around a small, inner core of protein and called proteoglycans) often are attached to and cover the entire outside surface of the cell. As a result, the carbohydrate molecules are free to interact with extracellular substances and perform several important functions. First, many have a negative electrical charge that repels other negatively charged substances. Second, the "carbohydrate coat" of some cells attaches to the carbohydrate coat of other cells and thereby connects cells to each other. Third, many of the carbohydrates act as receptor molecules for binding hormones (e.g., insulin). The receptor–hormone combination then activates the attached inner core of protein to perform its enzymatic or other functions in the cell.

## CELLULAR PHYSIOLOGY

Cells are dynamic, busy "factories" (Box 2.1; Fig. 2.1) that take in raw materials, manufacture products required to maintain bodily functions, and deliver those products to their appropriate destinations in the body. Although cells differ from one tissue to another, their common characteristics include the ability to

- Exchange materials with their immediate environment
- Obtain energy from nutrients
- Synthesize hormones, neurotransmitters, enzymes, structural proteins, and other complex molecules
- Reproduce
- Communicate with one another via various biologic chemicals, such as neurotransmitters and hormones

## DRUG TRANSPORT THROUGH CELL MEMBRANES

Drugs must reach and interact with or cross the cell membrane to stimulate or inhibit cellular function. Most drugs are given to affect body cells that are distant from the sites of administration (i.e., systemic effects). To move through the body and reach their sites of action, metabolism, and excretion (Fig. 2.2), drug molecules must cross numerous cell membranes. For example, molecules of most oral drugs must cross the membranes of cells in the gastrointestinal (GI) tract, liver, and capillaries to reach the bloodstream, circulate to their target cells, leave the bloodstream and attach to receptors on cells, perform their action, return to the bloodstream, circulate to the liver, reach

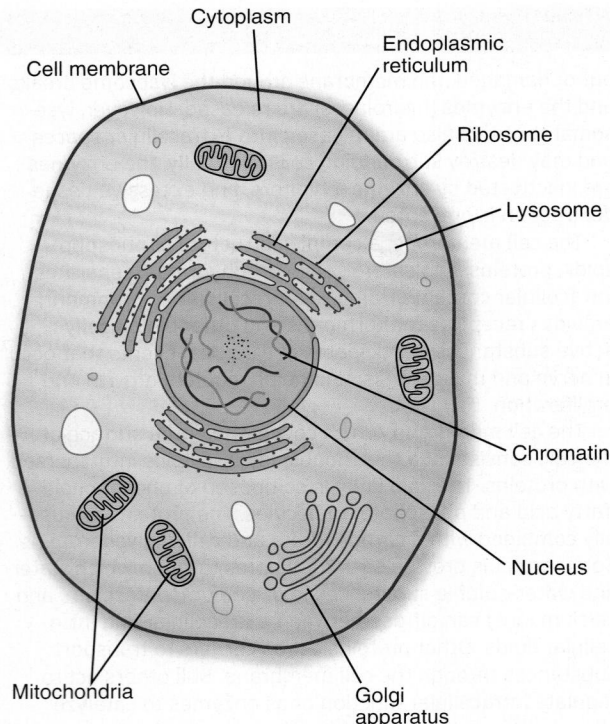

**Figure 2.1.** Cytoplasmic organelles of the cell.

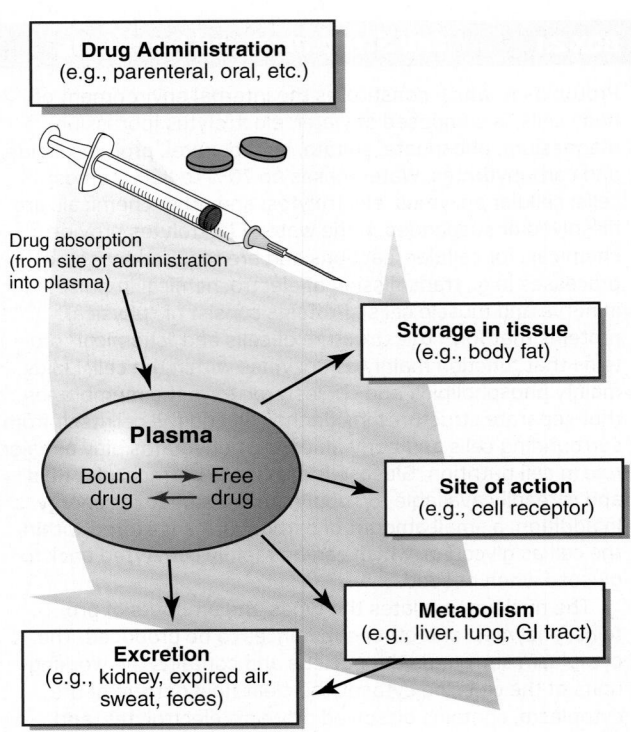

**Figure 2.2.** Entry and movement of drug molecules through the body to sites of action, metabolism, and excretion.

drug-metabolizing enzymes in liver cells, reenter the blood-stream (usually as metabolites), circulate to the kidneys, and be excreted in urine. Box 2.2 and Figure 2.3 describe the transport pathways and mechanisms used to move drug molecules through the body.

# PHARMACOKINETICS

**Pharmacokinetics** involves drug movement through the body (i.e., "what the body does to the drug") to reach sites of action, metabolism, and excretion. Specific processes are absorption,

---

**BOX 2.2**    *Drug Transport Pathways and Mechanisms*

### Pathways

There are three main pathways of drug movement across cell membranes. The most common pathway is direct penetration of the membrane by lipid-soluble drugs, which are able to dissolve in the lipid layer of the cell membrane. Most systemic drugs are formulated to be lipid soluble, so they can move through cell membranes, even oral tablets and capsules that must be sufficiently water soluble to dissolve in the aqueous fluids of the stomach and small intestine.

A second pathway involves passage through protein channels that go all the way through the cell membrane. Only a few drugs are able to use this pathway because most drug molecules are too large to pass through the small channels. Small ions (e.g., sodium and potassium) use this pathway, but their movement is regulated by specific channels with a gating mechanism (a flap of protein that opens briefly to allow ion movement and then closes).

The third pathway involves carrier proteins that transport molecules from one side of the cell membrane to the other. All of the carrier proteins are selective in the substances they transport; a drug's chemical structure determines which carrier will transport it.

### Mechanisms

Once absorbed into the body, drugs are transported to and from target cells by passive diffusion, facilitated diffusion, and active transport.

Passive diffusion, the most common mechanism, involves movement of a drug from an area of higher concentration to one of lower concentration. For example, after oral administration, the initial concentration of a drug is higher in the GI tract than in the blood. This promotes movement of the drug into the bloodstream. When the drug is circulated, the concentration is higher in the blood than in body cells, so that the drug moves (from capillaries) into the fluids surrounding the cells or into the cells themselves. Passive diffusion continues until a state of equilibrium is reached between the amount of drug in the tissues and the amount in the blood.

Facilitated diffusion is a similar process, except that drug molecules combine with a carrier substance, such as an enzyme or other protein.

In active transport, drug molecules are moved from an area of lower concentration to one of higher concentration. This process requires a carrier substance and the release of cellular energy.

Lipid-soluble drugs dissolve in the lipid layer of the cell membrane and diffuse into or out of the cell.

Cell membrane

Na²⁺

Gated channels regulate movement of ions.

Nucleus

K⁺

Cytoplasm

Carrier proteins attach to drug molecules and move them across cell membranes.

**Figure 2.3.** Drug transport pathways. Drug molecules cross cell membranes to move into and out of body cells by directly penetrating the lipid layer, diffusing through open or gated channels, or attaching to carrier proteins.

distribution, metabolism, and excretion. Metabolism and excretion are often grouped together as drug elimination or clearance mechanisms. Overall, these processes largely determine serum drug levels; onset, peak, and duration of drug actions; therapeutic and adverse effects; and other important aspects of drug therapy.

## Absorption    Body → Bloodstream

**Absorption** is the process that occurs from the time a drug enters the body to the time it enters the bloodstream to be circulated. Onset of drug action is largely determined by the rate of absorption; intensity is determined by the extent of absorption. Numerous factors affect the rate and extent of drug absorption, including dosage form, route of administration, blood flow to the site of administration, GI function, the presence of food or other drugs, and other variables. Dosage form is a major determinant of a drug's **bioavailability** (the portion of a dose that reaches the systemic circulation and is available to act on body cells). An intravenous (IV) drug is virtually 100% bioavailable. In contrast, an oral drug is virtually always less than 100% bioavailable because some of it is not absorbed from the GI tract and some goes to the liver and is partially metabolized before reaching the systemic circulation.

Most oral drugs must be swallowed, dissolved in gastric fluid, and delivered to the small intestine (which has a large surface area for absorption of nutrients and drugs) before they are absorbed. Liquid medications are absorbed faster than are tablets or capsules because they need not be dissolved. Rapid movement through the stomach and small intestine may increase drug absorption by promoting contact with absorptive mucous membrane; it also may decrease absorption because some drugs may move through the small intestine too rapidly to be absorbed. For many drugs, the presence of food in the stomach slows the rate of absorption and may decrease the amount of drug absorbed.

Drugs injected into subcutaneous or intramuscular (IM) tissues are usually absorbed more rapidly than are oral drugs because they move directly from the injection site to the blood-

stream. Absorption is rapid from IM sites because muscle tissue has an abundant blood supply. Drugs injected intravenously do not need to be absorbed because they are placed directly into the bloodstream.

Other absorptive sites include the skin, mucous membranes, and lungs. Most drugs applied to the skin are given for local effects (e.g., sunscreens). Systemic absorption is minimal from intact skin but may be considerable when the skin is inflamed or damaged. Also, some drugs are formulated in adhesive skin patches for absorption through the skin (e.g., clonidine, fentanyl, nitroglycerin). Some drugs applied to mucous membranes also are given for local effects. However, systemic absorption occurs from the mucosa of the oral cavity, nose, eye, vagina, and rectum. Drugs absorbed through mucous membranes pass directly into the bloodstream. The lungs have a large surface area for absorption of anesthetic gases and a few other drugs.

## Distribution    Transport w/ in body

**Distribution** involves the transport of drug molecules within the body. After a drug is injected or absorbed into the bloodstream, it is carried by the blood and tissue fluids to its sites of action, metabolism, and excretion. Most drug molecules enter and leave the bloodstream at the capillary level, through gaps between the cells that form capillary walls. Distribution depends largely on the adequacy of blood circulation. Drugs are distributed rapidly to organs receiving a large blood supply, such as the heart, liver, and kidneys. Distribution to other internal organs, muscle, fat, and skin is usually slower.

Protein binding is an important factor in drug distribution (Fig. 2.4). Most drugs form a compound with plasma proteins, mainly albumin, which act as carriers. Drug molecules bound to plasma proteins are pharmacologically inactive because the large size of the complex prevents their leaving the bloodstream through the small openings in capillary walls and reaching their sites of action, metabolism, and excretion. Only the free or unbound portion of a drug acts on body cells. As the free drug acts on cells, the decrease in plasma drug levels causes some of the bound drug to be released.

Protein binding allows part of a drug dose to be stored and released as needed. Some drugs also are stored in muscle, fat,

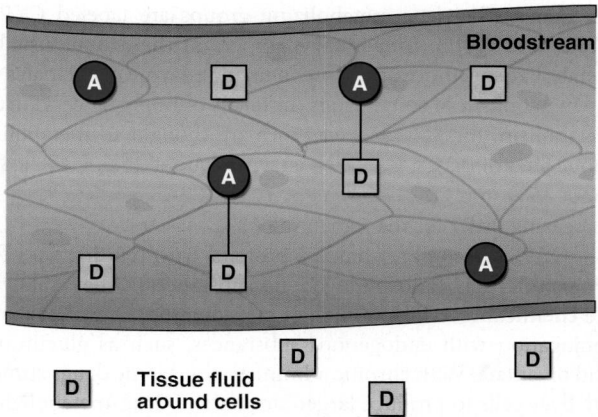

Bloodstream

A    D    A    D

A    D

D    D    A

D    D

Tissue fluid around cells

D    D

**Figure 2.4.** Plasma proteins, mainly albumin [A], act as carriers for drug molecules [D]. Bound drug [A–D] stays in the bloodstream and is pharmacologically inactive. Free drug [D] can leave the bloodstream and act on body cells.

or other body tissues and released gradually when plasma drug levels fall. These storage mechanisms maintain lower, more consistent blood levels and reduce the risk of toxicity. Drugs that are highly bound to plasma proteins or stored extensively in other tissues have a long duration of action.

Drug distribution into the central nervous system (CNS) is limited because the blood–brain barrier, which is composed of capillaries with tight walls, limits movement of drug molecules into brain tissue. This barrier usually acts as a selectively permeable membrane to protect the CNS. However, it also can make drug therapy for CNS disorders more difficult because drugs must pass through cells of the capillary wall rather than between cells. As a result, only drugs that are lipid soluble or have a transport system can cross the blood–brain barrier and reach therapeutic concentrations in brain tissue.

Drug distribution during pregnancy and lactation is also an important consideration (see Chap. 6). During pregnancy, most drugs cross the placenta and may affect the fetus. During lactation, many drugs enter breast milk and may affect the nursing infant.

## Metabolism → inactivated

Metabolism, or **biotransformation**, is the method by which drugs are inactivated or biotransformed by the body. Most often, an active drug is changed into inactive metabolites, which are then excreted. Some active drugs yield metabolites that are also active and that continue to exert their effects on body cells until they are metabolized further or excreted. Other drugs (called **prodrugs**) are initially inactive and exert no pharmacologic effects until they are metabolized. Most drugs are lipid soluble, a characteristic that aids their movement across cell membranes. However, the kidneys can excrete only water-soluble substances. Therefore, one function of metabolism is to convert fat-soluble drugs into water-soluble metabolites. Hepatic drug metabolism or clearance is a major mechanism for terminating drug action and eliminating drug molecules from the body. Genetic **polymorphisms** influence metabolism by producing functionally different responses to drugs in ethnic groups or specific individuals.

Cytochrome P-450 (CYP) enzymes in the liver metabolize most drugs. Red blood cells, plasma, kidneys, lungs, and GI mucosa also contain drug-metabolizing enzymes. The CYP system consists of several groups of enzymes, some of which metabolize endogenous substances and some of which metabolize drugs. The drug-metabolizing groups are labeled CYP1, CYP2, and CYP3. Individual members of the groups usually metabolize specific drugs; more than one enzyme participates in the metabolism of some drugs. In terms of importance in drug metabolism, the CYP3A4 enzymes are thought to metabolize about 50% of drugs; CYP2D6 enzymes about 25%; CYP2C8/9 about 15%; and CYP1A2, CYP2C19, CYP2A6, and CYP2E1 in decreasing order for the remaining 10%.

CYP enzymes are complex proteins with binding sites for drug molecules (and endogenous substances). They catalyze the chemical reactions of oxidation, reduction, hydrolysis, and conjugation with endogenous substances, such as glucuronic acid or sulfate. With chronic administration, some drugs stimulate liver cells to produce larger amounts of drug-metabolizing enzymes. This **enzyme induction** accelerates drug metabolism because larger amounts of the enzymes (and more binding sites) allow larger amounts of a drug to be metabolized during a given period. As a result, larger doses of the rapidly metabolized drug may be required to produce or maintain therapeutic effects.

Rapid metabolism may also increase the production of toxic metabolites with some drugs (e.g., acetaminophen). Drugs that induce enzyme production also may increase the rate of metabolism for endogenous steroidal hormones (e.g., cortisol, estrogens, testosterone, vitamin D). However, enzyme induction does not occur for 1 to 3 weeks after an inducing agent is started, because new enzyme proteins must be synthesized.

Metabolism also can be decreased or delayed in a process called **enzyme inhibition**, which most often occurs with concurrent administration of two or more drugs that compete for the same metabolizing enzymes. In this case, smaller doses of the slowly metabolized drug may be needed to avoid adverse effects and toxicity from drug accumulation. Enzyme inhibition occurs within hours or days of starting an inhibiting agent. Cimetidine, a gastric acid suppressor, inhibits several CYP enzymes (e.g., 1A, 2C, 2D, 3A) and can greatly decrease drug metabolism. The rate of drug metabolism also is reduced in infants (their hepatic enzyme system is immature), in people with impaired blood flow to the liver or severe hepatic or cardiovascular disease, and in people who are malnourished or on low-protein diets.

When drugs are given orally, they are absorbed from the GI tract and carried to the liver through the portal circulation. Some drugs are extensively metabolized in the liver, with only part of a drug dose reaching the systemic circulation for distribution to sites of action. This is called the **first-pass effect** or presystemic metabolism.

## Excretion

**Excretion** refers to elimination of a drug from the body. Effective excretion requires adequate functioning of the circulatory system and of the organs of excretion (kidneys, bowel, lungs, and skin). Most drugs are excreted by the kidneys and eliminated (unchanged or as metabolites) in the urine. Some drugs or metabolites are excreted in bile and then eliminated in feces; others are excreted in bile, reabsorbed from the small intestine, returned to the liver (called **enterohepatic recirculation**), metabolized, and eventually excreted in urine. Some oral drugs are not absorbed and are excreted in the feces. The lungs mainly remove volatile substances, such as anesthetic gases. The skin has minimal excretory function. Factors impairing excretion, especially severe renal disease, lead to accumulation of numerous drugs and may cause severe adverse effects if dosage is not reduced.

**NCLEX Success**

1. A nurse practitioner (NP) has just changed a patient's medication from an oral form to a patch formulation to avoid the first-pass effect. The NP has explained it to the patient, but the patient still has questions and asks the nurse to explain again what is meant by the first-pass effect. The nurse would be most correct in explaining that this has to do with how
   A. drugs initially bind to plasma proteins
   B. initial renal function is involved in drug excretion
   C. the way drugs first reach their target cells
   D. initial metabolism of an oral drug occurs before it reaches the systemic circulation

2. A nurse is reading a research report about use of a medication that describes the pharmacokinetics of a particular medication that a patient is taking. Pharmacokinetics involves

   A. drug effects on human cells
   B. drug binding with receptors
   C. drug absorption, distribution, metabolism, and elimination
   D. drug stimulation of normal cell functions

3. A nurse is caring for a man who has worsening liver disease. In monitoring his medication, it is important to know that a patient with liver disease may have impaired drug

   A. absorption
   B. distribution
   C. metabolism
   D. excretion

## Serum Drug Levels

A **serum drug level** is a laboratory measurement of the amount of a drug in the blood at a particular time (Fig. 2.5). It reflects dosage, absorption, bioavailability, half-life, and the rates of metabolism and excretion. A minimum effective concentration (MEC) must be present before a drug exerts its pharmacologic action on body cells; this is largely determined by the drug dose and how well it is absorbed into the bloodstream. A toxic concentration is a level at which toxicity occurs; what is toxic for some patients is not toxic for others (see subsequent discussion). Toxic concentrations may stem from a single large dose, repeated small doses, or slow metabolism that allows the drug to accumulate in the body. Between these low and high concentrations is the therapeutic range, which is the goal of drug therapy—that is, enough drug to be beneficial but not enough to be toxic.

For most drugs, serum levels indicate the onset, peak, and duration of drug action. When a single dose of a drug is given, onset of action occurs when the drug level reaches the MEC. The drug level continues to climb as more of the drug is absorbed, until it reaches its highest concentration and peak drug action occurs. Then, drug levels decline as the drug is eliminated (i.e., metabolized and excreted) from the body. Although there may still be numerous drug molecules in the body, drug action stops when drug levels fall below the MEC. The duration of action is the time during which serum drug levels are at or above the MEC. When multiple doses of a drug are given (e.g., for chronic conditions), the goal is usually to give sufficient doses often enough to maintain serum drug levels in the therapeutic range and avoid the toxic range.

In clinical practice, measuring serum drug levels is useful in several circumstances:

- When drugs with a narrow margin of safety are given, because their therapeutic doses are close to their toxic doses (e.g., digoxin, aminoglycoside antibiotics, lithium)
- To document the serum drug levels associated with particular drug dosages, therapeutic effects, or possible adverse effects
- To monitor unexpected responses to a drug dose such as decreased therapeutic effects or increased adverse effects
- When a drug overdose is suspected

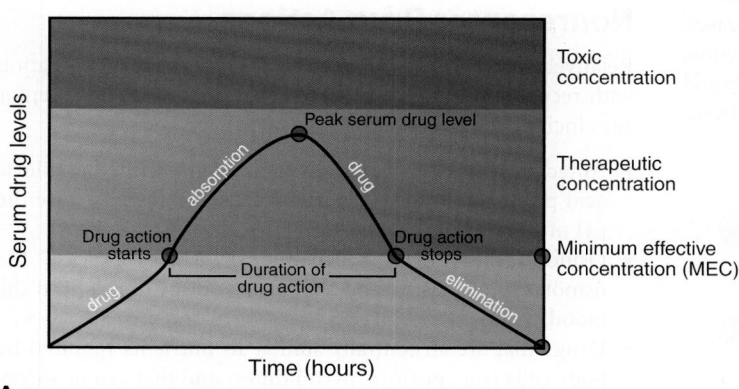

**A** Drug action in relation to serum drug levels and time after a single dose.

**Figure 2.5.** Serum drug levels with single **(A)** and multiple **(B)** oral drug doses. Drug action starts when enough drug is absorbed to reach the minimum effective concentration (MEC), continues as long as the serum level is above the MEC, wanes as drug molecules are metabolized and excreted (if no more doses are given), and stops when the serum level drops below the MEC. The goal of drug therapy is to maintain serum drug levels in the therapeutic range.

**B** Drug action in relation to serum drug levels with repeated doses.

## Serum Half-Life

**Serum half-life**, also called elimination half-life, is the time required for the serum concentration of a drug to decrease by 50%. It is determined primarily by the drug's rates of metabolism and excretion. A drug with a short half-life requires more frequent administration than one with a long half-life.

When a drug is given at a stable dose, four or five half-lives are required to achieve steady-state concentrations and to develop equilibrium between tissue and serum concentrations. Because maximal therapeutic effects do not occur until equilibrium is established, some drugs are not fully effective for days or weeks. To maintain steady-state conditions, the amount of drug given must equal the amount eliminated from the body. When a drug dose is changed, an additional four to five half-lives are required to reestablish equilibrium; when a drug is discontinued, it is eliminated gradually over several half-lives.

## PHARMACODYNAMICS

**Pharmacodynamics** involves drug actions on target cells and the resulting alterations in cellular biochemical reactions and functions (i.e., "what the drug does to the body").

## Receptor Theory of Drug Action

Like the physiologic substances (e.g., hormones, neurotransmitters) that normally regulate cell functions, most drugs exert their effects by chemically binding with receptors at the cellular level (Fig. 2.6). Most receptors are proteins located on the surfaces of cell membranes or within cells. Specific receptors include enzymes involved in essential metabolic or regulatory processes (e.g., dihydrofolate reductase, acetylcholinesterase); proteins involved in transport (e.g., sodium–potassium adenosine triphosphatase) or structural processes (e.g., tubulin); and nucleic acids (e.g., DNA) involved in cellular protein synthesis, reproduction, and other metabolic activities.

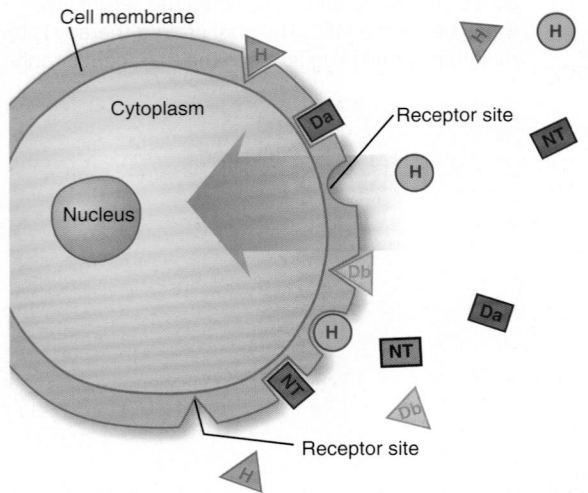

**Figure 2.6.** Cell membrane contains receptors for physiologic substances such as hormones [*H*] and neurotransmitters [*NT*]. These substances stimulate or inhibit cellular function. Drug molecules [*Da* and *Db*] also interact with receptors to stimulate or inhibit cellular function.

When drug molecules bind with receptor molecules, the resulting drug–receptor complex initiates physiochemical reactions that stimulate or inhibit normal cellular functions. One type of reaction involves activation, inactivation, or other alterations of intracellular enzymes. Because enzymes catalyze almost all cellular functions, drug-induced changes can markedly increase or decrease the rate of cellular metabolism. For example, an epinephrine–receptor complex increases the activity of the intracellular enzyme adenylyl cyclase, which then causes the formation of cyclic adenosine monophosphate (cAMP). In turn, cAMP can initiate any one of many different intracellular actions, the exact effect depending on the type of cell.

A second type of reaction involves changes in the permeability of cell membranes to one or more ions. The receptor protein is a structural component of the cell membrane, and its binding to a drug molecule may open or close ion channels. In nerve cells, for example, sodium or calcium ion channels may open and allow movement of ions into the cell. This movement usually causes the cell membrane to depolarize and excite the cell. At other times, potassium channels may open and allow movement of potassium ions out of the cell. This action inhibits neuronal excitability and function. In muscle cells, movement of the ions into the cells may alter intracellular functions, such as the direct effect of calcium ions in stimulating muscle contraction.

A third reaction may modify the synthesis, release, or inactivation of the neurohormones (e.g., acetylcholine, norepinephrine, serotonin) that regulate many physiologic processes. Box 2.3 describes additional elements and characteristics of the receptor theory.

## Nonreceptor Drug Actions

Relatively few drugs act by mechanisms other than combination with receptor sites on cells. Drugs that do not act on receptor sites include the following:

- Antacids, which act chemically to neutralize the hydrochloric acid produced by gastric parietal cells and thereby raise the pH of gastric fluid
- Osmotic diuretics (e.g., mannitol), which increase the osmolarity of plasma and pull water out of tissues into the bloodstream
- Drugs that are structurally similar to nutrients required by body cells (e.g., purines, pyrimidines) and that can be incorporated into cellular constituents, such as nucleic acids, which interfere with normal cell functioning. Several anticancer drugs act by this mechanism.
- Metal chelating agents, which combine with toxic metals to form a complex that can be more readily excreted

## VARIABLES THAT AFFECT DRUG ACTIONS

Historically, expected responses to drugs were based on those occurring when a particular drug was given to healthy adult men (18–65 years of age) of average weight (150 lb [70 kg]). However, other groups (e.g., women, children, older adults, different ethnic or racial groups, patients with diseases or symptoms that the drugs are designed to treat) receive drugs and

| BOX 2.3 | *Additional Elements of the Receptor Theory of Drug Action* |
| --- | --- |

- The site and extent of drug action on body cells are determined primarily by specific characteristics of receptors and drugs. Receptors vary in type, location, number, and functional capacity. For example, many different types of receptors have been identified. Most types occur in most body tissues, such as receptors for epinephrine (whether received from stimulation of the sympathetic nervous system or administration of drug formulations) and receptors for growth hormone, thyroid hormone, and insulin. Some occur in fewer body tissues, such as receptors for opioids in the brain and subgroups of receptors for epinephrine in the heart (beta$_1$-adrenergic receptors) and lungs (beta$_2$-adrenergic receptors). Receptor type and location influence drug action. The receptor is often described as a lock into which the drug molecule fits as a key, and only those drugs able to bond chemically to the receptors in a particular body tissue can exert pharmacologic effects on that tissue. Thus, all body cells do not respond to all drugs, even though virtually all cell receptors are exposed to any drug molecules circulating in the bloodstream.

  The number of receptor sites available to interact with drug molecules also affects the extent of drug action. Drug molecules must occupy a minimal number of receptors to produce pharmacologic effects. Thus, if many receptors are available but only a few are occupied by drug molecules, few drug effects occur. In this instance, increasing the drug dosage increases the pharmacologic effects. Conversely, if only a few receptors are available for many drug molecules, receptors may be saturated. In this instance, if most receptor sites are occupied, increasing the drug dosage produces no additional pharmacologic effect.

  Drugs vary even more widely than receptors. Because all drugs are chemical substances, chemical characteristics determine drug actions and pharmacologic effects. For example, a drug's chemical structure affects its ability to reach tissue fluids around a cell and bind with its cell receptors. Minor changes in drug structure may produce major changes in pharmacologic effects. Another major factor is the concentration of drug molecules that reach receptor sites in body tissues. Drug-related and patient-related variables that affect drug actions are further described later in this chapter.

- When drug molecules chemically bind with cell receptors, pharmacologic effects result from agonism or antagonism. **Agonists** are drugs that produce effects similar to those produced by naturally occurring hormones, neurotransmitters, and other substances. Agonists may accelerate or slow normal cellular processes, depending on the type of receptor activated. For example, epinephrine-like drugs act on the heart to increase the heart rate, and acetylcholine-like drugs act on the heart to slow the heart rate; both are agonists. **Antagonists** are drugs that inhibit cell function by occupying receptor sites. This strategy prevents natural body substances or other drugs from occupying the receptor sites and activating cell functions. After drug action occurs, drug molecules may detach from receptor molecules (i.e., the chemical binding is reversible), return to the bloodstream, and circulate to the liver for metabolism and the kidneys for excretion.

- Receptors are dynamic cellular components that can be synthesized by body cells and altered by endogenous substances and exogenous drugs. For example, prolonged stimulation of body cells with an excitatory agonist usually reduces the number or sensitivity of receptors. As a result, the cell becomes less responsive to the **agonist** (a process called receptor desensitization or down-regulation). Prolonged inhibition of normal cellular functions with an antagonist may increase receptor number or sensitivity. If the antagonist is suddenly reduced or stopped, the cell becomes excessively responsive to an agonist (a process called receptor up-regulation). These changes in receptors may explain why some drugs must be tapered in dosage and discontinued gradually if withdrawal symptoms are to be avoided.

respond differently from healthy adult men. As a result, newer clinical trials include more representatives of these groups. In any patient, however, responses may be altered by both drug-related and patient-related variables.

## Drug-Related Variables

### Dosage

Dosage refers to the frequency, size, and number of doses; it is a major determinant of drug actions and responses, both therapeutic and adverse. If the amount is too small or administered infrequently, no pharmacologic action occurs because the drug does not reach an adequate concentration at target cells. If the amount is too large or administered too often, toxicity (poisoning) may occur. Overdosage may occur with a single large dose or with chronic ingestion of smaller doses.

Dosages recommended in drug literature are usually those that produce particular responses in 50% of the people tested. These dosages usually produce a mixture of therapeutic and adverse effects. The dosage of a particular drug depends on many characteristics of the drug (reason for use, potency, pharmacokinetics, route of administration, dosage form, and so on) and of the recipient (age; weight; state of health; and function of cardiovascular, renal, and hepatic systems). Thus, recommended dosages are intended only as guidelines for individualizing dosages.

Even if the recommended dose controls a patient's symptoms, he or she may need a special **loading dose** at the beginning of drug therapy. This dose, which is larger than the regular prescribed daily dosage of a medication, is used to attain a more rapid therapeutic blood level of the drug. After the patient has been taking the drug for a few days, a **maintenance dose**, or quantity of drug that is needed to keep blood levels and/or tissue levels at a steady state, or constant level, is usually sufficient.

### Route of Administration

Routes of administration affect drug actions and patient responses largely by influencing absorption and distribution. For rapid drug action and response, the IV route is most effective because the drug is injected directly into the bloodstream. For some drugs, the IM route also produces drug action within a few minutes because muscles have a large blood supply. The oral route usually produces slower drug action than parenteral routes. Absorption and action of topical drugs vary according to the drug formulation, whether the drug is applied to the skin or mucous membranes, and other factors.

## Drug–Diet Interactions

A few drugs are used therapeutically to decrease food absorption in the intestinal tract. For example, orlistat (Xenical) decreases absorption of fats from food and is given to promote weight loss, and ezetimibe (Zetia) decreases absorption of cholesterol from food and is given to lower serum cholesterol levels. However, most drug–diet interactions are undesirable because food often slows absorption of oral drugs by slowing gastric emptying time and altering GI secretions and motility.

### QSEN Alert: Safety

Giving medications 1 hour before or 2 hours after a meal can minimize drug-diet interactions that decrease drug absorption.

In addition, some foods contain certain substances that react with certain drugs. One such interaction occurs between tyramine-containing foods and monoamine oxidase (MAO) inhibitor drugs. Tyramine causes the release of norepinephrine, a strong vasoconstrictive agent, from the adrenal medulla and sympathetic neurons. Normally, norepinephrine is quickly inactivated by MAO. However, because MAO inhibitor drugs prevent inactivation of norepinephrine, ingesting tyramine-containing foods with an MAO inhibitor may produce severe hypertension or intracranial hemorrhage. MAO inhibitors include the antidepressants isocarboxazid and phenelzine and the anti-Parkinson drugs rasagiline and selegiline.

### QSEN Alert: Safety

Tyramine-rich foods to be avoided by patients taking MAO inhibitors include aged cheeses, sauerkraut, soy sauce, tap or draft beers, and red wines.

Another type of interaction may occur between warfarin (Coumadin), an oral anticoagulant, and foods containing vitamin K. Because vitamin K antagonizes the action of warfarin, large amounts of spinach and other green leafy vegetables may offset the anticoagulant effects and predispose the person to thromboembolic disorders.

Another type of interaction occurs between the antibiotic tetracycline and dairy products, such as milk and cheese. The drug combines with the calcium in milk products to form a nonabsorbable compound that is excreted in the feces.

Still, another interaction involves grapefruit. Grapefruit contains a substance that strongly inhibits the metabolism of drugs normally metabolized by the CYP3A4 enzyme. This effect greatly increases the blood levels of some drugs (e.g., the widely used "statin" group of cholesterol-lowering drugs), and the effect lasts for several days. Patients who take medications metabolized by the CYP3A4 enzyme should be advised against eating grapefruit or drinking grapefruit juice.

## Drug–Drug Interactions

The action of a drug may be increased or decreased by its interaction with another drug in the body. Most interactions occur whenever the interacting drugs are present in the body; some, especially those affecting the absorption of oral drugs, occur when the interacting drugs are taken at or near the same time. The basic cause of many drug–drug interactions is altered drug metabolism. For example, drugs metabolized by the same enzymes compete for enzyme binding sites, and there may not be enough binding sites for two or more drugs. Also, some drugs induce or inhibit the metabolism of other drugs. Protein binding is also the basis for some important drug–drug interactions.

Interactions that can increase the therapeutic or adverse effects of drugs include the following:

- Additive effects, which occur when two drugs with similar pharmacologic actions are taken (e.g., ethanol + sedative drug increases sedative effects).
- Synergism, which occurs when two drugs with different sites or mechanisms of action produce greater effects when taken together (e.g., acetaminophen [nonopioid analgesic] + codeine [opioid analgesic] increases analgesic effects).
- Interference by one drug with the metabolism of a second drug, which may result in intensified effects of the second drug. For example, cimetidine inhibits CYP1A, CYP2C, and CYP3A drug-metabolizing enzymes in the liver and therefore interferes with the metabolism of many drugs (e.g., benzodiazepine antianxiety and hypnotic drugs, several cardiovascular drugs). When these drugs are given concurrently with cimetidine, they are likely to cause adverse and toxic effects because blood levels of the drugs are higher. The overall effect is the same as taking a larger dose of the drug whose metabolism is inhibited or slowed.
- Displacement (i.e., a drug with a strong attraction to protein-binding sites may displace a less tightly bound drug) of one drug from plasma protein-binding sites by a second drug, which increases the effects of the displaced drug. This increase occurs because the displaced drug, freed from its bound form, becomes pharmacologically active. The overall effect is the same as taking a larger dose of the displaced drug. For example, aspirin displaces warfarin and increases the drug's anticoagulant effects.

Interactions in which drug effects are decreased include the following:

- An **antidote** drug, which can be given to antagonize the toxic effects of another drug. For example, naloxone is commonly used to relieve respiratory depression caused by morphine and related drugs. Naloxone molecules displace morphine molecules from their receptor sites on nerve cells in the brain so that the morphine molecules cannot continue to exert their depressant effects.
- Decreased intestinal absorption of oral drugs, which occurs when drugs combine to produce nonabsorbable compounds. For example, drugs containing aluminum, calcium, or magnesium bind with oral tetracycline (if taken at the same time) to decrease its absorption and therefore its antibiotic effect.
- Activation of drug-metabolizing enzymes in the liver, which increases the metabolism rate of any drug metabolized mainly by that group of enzymes and therefore decreases the drug's effects. Several drugs (e.g., phenytoin, rifampin) and cigarette smoking are known enzyme inducers.

## Patient-Related Variables

### Age

The effects of age on drug action are especially important in neonates, infants, and older adults. In children, drug action depends largely on age and developmental stage.

During pregnancy, drugs cross the placenta and may harm the fetus. Fetuses have no effective mechanisms for eliminating drugs because their liver and kidney functions are immature. Newborn infants (birth to 1 month) also handle drugs inefficiently. Drug distribution, metabolism, and excretion differ markedly in neonates, especially premature infants, because their organ systems are not fully developed. Older infants (1 month to 1 year) reach approximately adult levels of protein binding and kidney function, but liver function and the blood–brain barrier are still immature.

Children (1–12 years) have a period of increased activity of drug-metabolizing enzymes so that some drugs are rapidly metabolized and eliminated. Although the onset and duration of this period are unclear, a few studies have been done with particular drugs. Theophylline, for example, is eliminated much faster in a 7-year-old child than in a neonate or adult (18–65 years). After about 12 years of age, healthy children handle drugs similarly to healthy adults.

In older adults (65 years and older), physiologic changes may alter all pharmacokinetic processes. Changes in the GI tract include decreased gastric acidity, decreased blood flow, and decreased motility. Despite these changes, however, there is little difference in drug absorption. Changes in the cardiovascular system include decreased cardiac output and therefore slower distribution of drug molecules to their sites of action, metabolism, and excretion. In the liver, blood flow and metabolizing enzymes are decreased. Thus, many drugs are metabolized more slowly, have a longer action, and are more likely to accumulate with chronic administration. In the kidneys, there is decreased blood flow, decreased glomerular filtration rate, and decreased tubular secretion of drugs. All these changes tend to slow excretion and promote accumulation of drugs in the body. Impaired kidney and liver function greatly increase the risks of adverse drug effects. In addition, older adults are more likely to have acute and chronic illnesses that require the use of multiple drugs or long-term drug therapy. Thus, possibilities for interactions among drugs and between drugs and diseased organs are greatly multiplied.

### Body Weight

Body weight affects drug action mainly in relation to dose. The ratio between the amount of drug given and body weight influences drug distribution and concentration at sites of action. In general, people who are heavier than average may need larger doses, provided that their renal, hepatic, and cardiovascular functions are adequate. Recommended doses for many drugs are listed in terms of grams or milligrams per kilogram of body weight.

### Pharmacogenomic Variations

Prescribers order drugs to cause particular effects in recipients. However, when some people receive the same drug in the same dose, by the same route, and in the same time interval, they may experience inadequate therapeutic effects or unusual or exaggerated effects, including increased toxicity. These interindividual variations in drug response are often attributed to genetic heritage, which produces differences in drug metabolism. The study of genetic variations in drug response is called **pharmacogenomics** (or pharmacogenetics).

Until recently, the emphasis of pharmacogenomics has been on forecasting adverse drug events in specific populations based on age, sex, or ethnicity. The focus has been on identifying inherited variability in metabolism among individuals that alters the uptake, effectiveness, and toxicity of drugs and makes some people react differently than anticipated.

Pharmacogenomic influences on drug response alter the pharmacologic effects of a drug. Specifically, the impact of genetic variability affects drug pharmacokinetics; pharmacodynamics; idiosyncratic reactions, such as hypersensitivity reactions; and/or the drug's effects on disease development, severity, or response to therapy.

Research has increased with awareness that genetic and ethnic characteristics are important factors and that diverse groups must be included in clinical trials. There is also increased awareness that each person is genetically unique and must be treated as an individual rather than as a member of a particular ethnic group.

### Genetics

When most drugs enter the body, they interact with proteins (e.g., in plasma, tissues, cell membranes, drug receptor sites) to reach their sites of action, and they interact with other proteins (e.g., drug-metabolizing enzymes in the liver and other organs) to be biotransformed and eliminated from the body. Genetic characteristics that alter any of these proteins can alter drug responses. For example, metabolism of isoniazid, an antitubercular drug, requires the enzyme acetyltransferase. People may metabolize isoniazid rapidly or slowly, depending largely on genetic differences in acetyltransferase activity. Clinically, rapid metabolizers may need larger-than-usual doses to achieve therapeutic effects, and slow metabolizers may need smaller-than-usual doses to avoid toxic effects.

In addition, several genetic variations (called polymorphisms) of the CYP drug-metabolizing enzymes have been identified. Specific variations may influence any of the chemical processes by which drugs are metabolized. For example, CYP2D6 metabolizes several antidepressant, antipsychotic, and beta-adrenergic blocker drugs. Some Caucasians (about 7%) metabolize these drugs poorly and are at increased risk for drug accumulation and adverse effects. Conversely, codeine is also metabolized by CYP2D6 and, as a prodrug, is not active until it is converted into morphine in the liver. For ultrarapid metabolizers, the conversion of codeine to morphine occurs quickly and poses a risk for serious adverse effects, such as respiratory depression. CYP2C19 metabolizes diazepam, omeprazole, and some antidepressants. As many as 15% to 30% of Asians may metabolize these drugs poorly and develop adverse effects if dosage is not reduced.

Still another example of genetic variation in drug metabolism is that some people are deficient in glucose-6-phosphate dehydrogenase, an enzyme normally found in red blood cells and other body tissues. These people may have hemolytic anemia when given antimalarial drugs, sulfonamides, analgesics, antipyretics, and other drugs.

An increasing number of published pharmacogenomic studies and integration of next-generation sequencing technology for pharmacogenomic testing into patient care has shaped drug therapy regimens that maximize the therapeutic effects and minimize the adverse effects. The U.S. Food and Drug Administration (FDA) has updated drug labels with information that highlights the pharmacogenomic implications of specific drugs and has released a table of genomic biomarkers that have established roles in determining drug response. Many of the recommended tests for individual drugs are not routinely used for clinical decisions in part due to lack of education on potential benefit, limited guidelines for implementation of findings, and the potential delay of therapy when waiting for results.

> **⚠ QSEN Alert: Safety**
>
> The FDA has included the effect of genomic variations in boxed warnings on drug labels highlighting known contraindications or precautions for individuals who require genotype-specific dosing. The nurse should recognize the role of pharmacogenomics in avoiding adverse drug reactions with an optimized drug dosage.

## Ethnicity

Most drug information had been derived from clinical drug trials using Caucasian men. Interethnic variations became evident when drugs and dosages developed for Caucasians produced unexpected responses, including toxicity, when given to people from other ethnic groups. One common variation is that African Americans respond differently to some cardiovascular drugs. For example, for African Americans with hypertension, angiotensin-converting enzyme (ACE) inhibitors and beta-adrenergic blocking drugs are less effective, and diuretics and calcium channel blockers are more effective. Also, African Americans with heart failure seem to respond better to a combination of hydralazine and isosorbide than do Caucasian patients with heart failure.

Another variation is that those of Asian descent usually require much smaller doses of some commonly used drugs, including beta-adrenergic blockers and several psychotropic drugs (e.g., alprazolam, an antianxiety agent, and haloperidol, an antipsychotic). Some other documented interethnic variations are included in later chapters.

## Sex

Most drug-related research has involved men, and the results have been extrapolated to women, sometimes with adjustment of dosage based on the usually smaller size and weight of women. Historically, sex was considered a minor influence on drug action except during pregnancy and lactation. Now, differences between men and women in responses to drug therapy are being increasingly identified, and since 1993, regulations require that major clinical drug trials include women. However, data on drug therapy in women are still limited. Some identified differences include the following:

- Women who are depressed are more likely to respond to the selective serotonin reuptake inhibitors (SSRIs), such as fluoxetine (Prozac), than to the tricyclic antidepressants (TCAs), such as amitriptyline (Elavil).
- Women with anxiety disorders may respond less well than men to some antianxiety medications.
- Women with schizophrenia seem to need smaller doses of antipsychotic medications than men. If given the higher doses required by men, women are likely to have adverse drug reactions.
- Women may obtain more pain relief from opioid analgesics (e.g., morphine) and less relief from nonopioid analgesics (e.g., acetaminophen, ibuprofen), compared with men.

Different responses in women are usually attributed to anatomic and physiologic differences. In addition to smaller size and weight, for example, women usually have a higher percentage of body fat, less muscle tissue, smaller blood volume, and other characteristics that may influence responses to drugs. In addition, women have hormonal fluctuations during the menstrual cycle. Altered responses have been demonstrated in some women taking clonidine, an antihypertensive; lithium, a mood-stabilizing agent; phenytoin, an anticonvulsant; propranolol, a beta-adrenergic blocking drug used in the management of hypertension, angina pectoris, and migraine; and antidepressants. In addition, a significant percentage of women with arthritis, asthma, depression, diabetes mellitus, epilepsy, and migraines experience increased symptoms premenstrually. The increased symptoms may indicate a need for adjustments in their drug therapy regimens. Women with clinical depression, for example, may need higher doses of antidepressant medications premenstrually, if symptoms exacerbate, and lower doses during the rest of the menstrual cycle.

There may also be differences in pharmacokinetic processes, although few studies have been done. With absorption, it has been noted that women absorb a larger percentage of an oral dose of two cardiovascular medications than men (25% more verapamil and 40% more aspirin). With distribution, women may have higher blood levels of medications that distribute into body fluids (because of the smaller amount of water in which the medication can disperse) and lower blood levels of medications that are deposited in fatty tissues (because of the generally higher percentage of body fat), compared with men. With metabolism, the CYP3A4 enzyme metabolizes more medications than other enzymes, and women are thought to metabolize the drugs processed by this enzyme 20% to 40% faster than men (and therefore may have lower blood levels than men of similar weight given the same doses). The CYP1A2 enzyme is less active in women so that women who take the cardiovascular drugs clopidogrel or propranolol may have higher blood levels than men (and possibly greater risks of adverse effects if given the same doses as men). With excretion, renally excreted medications may reach higher blood levels because a major mechanism of drug elimination, glomerular filtration, is approximately 20% lower in women.

In general, women given equal dosages or equal weight-based dosages are thought to be exposed to higher concentrations of medications compared to men. Although available data are limited, the main reasons postulated for the sex differences are that women have a lower volume of distribution, lower glomerular filtration, and lower hepatic enzyme activity (except for the medications metabolized by the CYP3A4 enzyme system, which is more active in women). As a result, all women should be monitored closely during drug therapy because they are more likely to experience adverse drug effects than are men.

### *Other Considerations*
#### Preexisting Conditions

Various pathologic conditions may alter some or all pharmacokinetic processes and lead to decreased therapeutic effects or increased risks of adverse effects. Examples include the following:

- Cardiovascular disorders (e.g., myocardial infarction, heart failure, hypotension), which may interfere with all pharmacokinetic processes, mainly by decreasing blood flow to sites of drug administration, action, metabolism (liver), and excretion (kidneys).
- GI disorders (e.g., vomiting, diarrhea, inflammatory bowel disease, trauma or surgery of the GI tract), which may interfere with absorption of oral drugs.
- Hepatic disorders (e.g., hepatitis, cirrhosis, decreased liver function), which mainly interfere with metabolism. Severe liver disease or cirrhosis may interfere with all pharmacokinetic processes.
- Renal disorders (e.g., acute or chronic renal failure), which mainly interfere with excretion. Severe kidney disease may interfere with all pharmacokinetic processes.
- Thyroid disorders, which mainly affect metabolism. Hypothyroidism slows metabolism, prolonging drug action and slowing elimination. Hyperthyroidism accelerates metabolism, shortening drug action and hastening elimination.

#### Psychological Factors

Psychological considerations influence individual responses to drug administration, although specific mechanisms are unknown. An example is the placebo response. A placebo is a pharmacologically inactive substance. Placebos are used in clinical drug trials to compare the medication being tested with a "dummy" medication. Recipients often report both therapeutic and adverse effects from placebos.

Attitudes and expectations related to drugs in general, a particular drug, or a placebo influence patient response. They also influence compliance or the willingness to carry out the prescribed drug regimen, especially with long-term drug therapy.

## Tolerance and Cross-Tolerance

Drug tolerance occurs when the body becomes accustomed to a particular drug over time so that larger doses must be given to produce the same effects. Tolerance may be acquired to the pharmacologic action of many drugs, especially opioid analgesics, alcohol, and other CNS depressants. Tolerance to pharmacologically related drugs is cross-tolerance. For example, a person who regularly drinks large amounts of alcohol becomes able to ingest even larger amounts before becoming intoxicated—this is tolerance to alcohol. If the person is then given sedative-type drugs or a general anesthetic, larger-than-usual doses are required to produce a pharmacologic effect—this is cross-tolerance.

Tolerance and cross-tolerance are usually attributed to activation of drug-metabolizing enzymes in the liver, which accelerates drug metabolism and excretion. They also are attributed to decreased sensitivity or numbers of receptor sites.

## ADVERSE EFFECTS OF DRUGS

As used in this book, the term "adverse effects" refers to any undesired responses to drug administration, as opposed to therapeutic effects, which are desired responses. Most drugs produce a mixture of therapeutic and adverse effects; all drugs can produce adverse effects. Adverse effects may produce essentially any symptom or disease process and may involve any body system or tissue. They may be common or rare, mild or severe, and localized or widespread—depending on the drug and the recipient. Some adverse effects occur with usual therapeutic doses of drugs (often called side effects); most are more likely to occur and to be more severe with high doses. Box 2.4 describes common or serious adverse effects. Although adverse effects may occur in anyone who takes medications, they are especially likely to occur with some drugs (e.g., insulin, warfarin) and in older adults, who often take multiple drugs.

> ### **!  QSEN Alert: Evidence-Based Practice**
>
> Although a list of drugs that should be avoided in older adults is available (Beers Criteria; see Chap. 5), older patients continue to experience significant use of potentially inappropriate medications (PIMs). Mattison, Afonso, Ngo, and Mukamal (2010) implemented a medication-specific warning system within a hospital's computerized provider order entry (CPOE) system that alerted providers regarding PIMs ordered for elders. The alert reduced the number of medications ordered in patients ages 65 years and older by offering recommendations regarding lowering the dose or suggesting an alternative medication. Older adults are at significant risk for adverse drug events, especially when hospitalized. Prompts, such as an alert in the CPOE system, allow for increased awareness of the risk associated with PIM and lead to safer drug therapy in elderly patients.

### Central Nervous System Effects

CNS effects may result from CNS stimulation (e.g., agitation, confusion, disorientation, hallucinations, psychosis, seizures) or CNS depression (e.g., impaired level of consciousness, sedation, coma, impaired respiration and circulation). CNS effects may occur with many drugs, including most therapeutic groups, substances of abuse, and over-the-counter preparations.

### Gastrointestinal Effects

GI effects (e.g., nausea, vomiting, constipation, diarrhea) commonly occur. Nausea and vomiting occur with many drugs as a result of local irritation of the GI tract or stimulation of the vomiting center in the brain. Diarrhea occurs with drugs that cause local irritation or increase peristalsis. More serious effects include bleeding or ulceration (most often with nonsteroidal anti-inflammatory agents such as ibuprofen) and severe diarrhea/colitis (most often with antibiotics).

### Hematologic Effects

Hematologic effects (excessive bleeding, clot formation [thrombosis], bone marrow depression, anemias, leukopenia, agranulocytosis, thrombocytopenia) are relatively common and potentially life threatening. Excessive bleeding is often associated with anticoagulants and thrombolytics; bone marrow depression is associated with anticancer drugs.

### Hepatic Effects

Hepatic effects (hepatitis, liver dysfunction or failure, biliary tract disorders) are potentially life threatening. The liver is especially susceptible to drug-induced injury because most drugs are circulated to the liver for metabolism and some drugs are toxic to liver cells. Hepatotoxic drugs include acetaminophen (Tylenol), isoniazid (INH), methotrexate (Trexall), phenytoin (Dilantin), and aspirin and other salicylates. In the presence of drug- or disease-induced liver damage, the metabolism of many drugs is impaired. Besides hepatotoxicity, many drugs produce abnormal values in liver function tests without producing clinical signs of liver dysfunction.

### Nephrotoxicity

**Nephrotoxicity** (nephritis, renal insufficiency or failure) occurs with several antimicrobial agents (e.g., gentamicin and other aminoglycosides), nonsteroidal anti-inflammatory agents (e.g., ibuprofen and related drugs), and others. It is potentially serious because it may interfere with drug excretion, thereby causing drug accumulation and increased adverse effects.

### Hypersensitivity

**Hypersensitivity** or allergy may occur with almost any drug in susceptible patients. It is largely unpredictable and unrelated to dose. It occurs in those who have previously been exposed to the drug or a similar substance (antigen) and who have developed antibodies. When readministered, the

drug reacts with the antibodies to cause cell damage and the release of histamine and other substances. These substances produce reactions ranging from mild skin rashes to anaphylactic shock. Anaphylactic shock is a life-threatening hypersensitivity reaction characterized by respiratory distress and cardiovascular collapse. It occurs within a few minutes after drug administration and requires emergency treatment with epinephrine. Some allergic reactions (e.g., serum sickness) occur 1 to 2 weeks after the drug is given.

### Drug Fever

Drugs can cause fever by several mechanisms, including allergic reactions, damaging body tissues, interfering with dissipation of body heat, or acting on the temperature-regulating center in the brain. The most common mechanism is an allergic reaction. Fever may occur alone or with other allergic manifestations (e.g., skin rash, hives, joint and muscle pain, enlarged lymph glands, eosinophilia). It may begin within hours after the first dose if the patient has taken the drug before or within about 10 days of continued administration if the drug is new to the patient. If the causative drug is discontinued, fever usually subsides within 48 to 72 hours unless drug excretion is delayed or significant tissue damage has occurred (e.g., hepatitis). Many drugs have been implicated as causes of drug fever, including most antimicrobials.

### Idiosyncrasy

Idiosyncrasy refers to an unexpected reaction to a drug that occurs the first time it is given. These reactions are usually attributed to genetic characteristics that alter the person's drug-metabolizing enzymes.

### Drug Dependence

Drug dependence may occur with mind-altering drugs, such as opioid analgesics, sedative–hypnotic agents, antianxiety agents, and CNS stimulants. Dependence may be physiologic or psychological. Physiologic dependence produces unpleasant physical symptoms when the dose is reduced or the drug is withdrawn. Psychological dependence leads to excessive preoccupation with drugs and drug-seeking behavior.

### Carcinogenicity

Carcinogenicity is the ability of a substance to cause cancer. Several drugs are carcinogens, including some hormones and anticancer drugs. Carcinogenicity apparently results from drug-induced alterations in cellular DNA.

### Teratogenicity

Teratogenicity is the ability of a substance to cause abnormal fetal development when taken by pregnant women. Drug groups considered teratogenic include antiepileptic drugs, "statin" cholesterol-lowering drugs, antidepressant drugs, nonopioid analgesics, and the antiflu drug oseltamivir (Tamiflu).

## Black Box Warnings

For some prescription drug groups and individual drugs that may cause serious or life-threatening adverse effects, the FDA requires drug manufacturers to place a warning formatted with a box or border around the text on the label of a prescription drug or in the literature describing it. The colloquial term,

**BLACK BOX WARNING (BBW)** ◆, often describes these FDA-required warnings, and this term is used in this text. A BBW is the strongest warning that the FDA can give consumers and often includes prescribing or monitoring information intended to improve the safety of using the particular drug or drug group. In recent years, BBWs have been added to antidepressant drugs, nonopioid analgesics, and immediate-release opioid analgesics.

*Concept Mastery Alert*

When administering a drug with a black box warning, the nurse should monitor the patient closely for adverse effects.

## Pregnancy Categories

Since 1979, the FDA has categorized drug risk in a range from A (safest) to X (known danger). In 2015, the FDA implemented the Pregnancy and Lactation Labeling Rule and launched the phaseout of these pregnancy categories from prescription drug labeling that stratified risk of fetal injury from drugs used as directed by the mother during pregnancy. Although simplistic, the categories were found to lead to false conclusions on which drug decisions were made. The new system includes pregnancy exposure registries that document exposed known or potential maternal or fetal adverse reactions pregnancy outcomes with individual drugs. This registry will provide the best available evidence on risks associated with drug exposure in pregnancy that should lead to better-informed prescribing decisions. Labeling for over-the-counter medications will not change.

The five categories that will be phased out over time are:

- Category A. Risk to the fetus in the first trimester (and in later trimesters) has not been demonstrated in well-controlled studies in pregnant women.
- Category B. Animal reproduction studies have not demonstrated risk to the fetus, and there are no well-controlled studies in pregnant women.
- Category C. Animal reproduction studies have not demonstrated risk to the fetus, and there are no well-controlled studies in pregnant women; however, potential benefits may outweigh potential risk in use of drug in pregnant women.
- Category D. Evidence of risk to the fetus has been demonstrated. However, the benefits may outweigh risk in pregnant women if the drug is needed in a life-threatening situation and other safer drugs cannot be used or are ineffective.
- Category X. Studies in humans or animals have demonstrated fetal abnormalities or evidence of fetal risk, and the risk clearly outweighs the benefit. The drug is contraindicated in women who are pregnant or in those who may become pregnant.

### Clinical Application 2.1

- During your most recent visit (3 days ago), you instructed Mrs. Green to take her medication with a large glass of water and set up a daily pill calendar. You also checked her vital signs; her blood pressure was 148/70 mm Hg. Today, you recheck her vital signs, and her blood pressure is 96/60 mm Hg. You ask her about her medication, and she tells you she has been taking each medication according to the calendar three times a day. What future actions should the home health nurse take?

In the new system, there is a new category—Pregnancy (including Labor and Delivery) and Lactation. In addition, a new labeling grouping, Females and Males of Reproductive Potential, outlines the need for pregnancy testing, contraception recommendations, and information about infertility with use of an individual drug.

Labeling changes for prescription drugs will be phased in gradually. Therefore, the Drugs at a Glance tables in this edition provide the pregnancy category for each listed drug FDA before June 30, 2015. Drugs approved after that date will have "unknown" and the year of drug approval in the Pregnancy Category column in the Drugs at a Glance tables.

## TOXICOLOGY: DRUG OVERDOSE

Drug toxicity (also called poisoning or overdose) results from excessive amounts of a drug and may damage body tissues. It is a common problem in both adult and pediatric populations. It may result from a single large dose or prolonged ingestion of smaller doses. Toxicity may involve alcohol or prescription, over-the-counter, or illicit drugs. Clinical manifestations are often nonspecific and may indicate other disease processes. Because of the variable presentation of drug intoxication, health care providers must have a high index of suspicion so that toxicity can be rapidly recognized and treated.

When toxicity occurs in a home or outpatient setting and the victim is collapsed or not breathing, emergency aid can be obtained by dialing 911. If the victim is responsive, a poison specialist is available 24 hours a day, 7 days through the National Poison Control Center by phone at 1-800-222-1222. The caller is connected to a local Poison Control Center and, if possible, needs to tell the responding pharmacist or physician the name of the drug or substance that was taken as well as the amount and time of ingestion. The poison control consultant may recommend treatment measures over the phone or taking the victim to a hospital emergency department.

It is possible that the patient or someone else may know the toxic agent (e.g., accidental overdose of a therapeutic drug, use of an illicit drug, a suicide attempt). Often, however, multiple drugs have been ingested, the causative drugs are unknown, and the circumstances may involve traumatic injury or impaired mental status that make the patient unable to provide useful information. The main goals of treatment are starting treatment as soon as possible after drug ingestion, supporting and stabilizing vital functions, preventing further damage from the toxic agent by reducing absorption or increasing elimination, and administering antidotes when available and indicated. Box 2.5 describes general aspects of care, Table 2.1 lists selected antidotes, and relevant chapters noted discuss specific aspects of care.

### QSEN Alert: Safety

Unconscious patients should not receive activated charcoal until the airway is secure to reduce the risk of pulmonary aspiration. To decrease the risk of bowel obstruction, many patients are given a laxative (e.g., sorbitol) to aid removal of the charcoal–drug complex.

| BOX 2.5 | *Enteral Management of Toxicity* |
|---|---|

- The first priority is support of vital functions, as indicated by rapid assessment of vital signs and level of consciousness. In serious poisonings, an electrocardiogram is indicated, and findings of severe toxicity (e.g., dysrhythmias, ischemia) justify aggressive treatment. Standard cardiopulmonary resuscitation (CPR) measures may be needed to maintain breathing and circulation. An intravenous (IV) line is usually needed to administer fluids and drugs, and invasive treatment or monitoring devices may be inserted.

  Endotracheal intubation and mechanical ventilation are often required to maintain breathing (in unconscious patients), correct hypoxemia, and protect the airway. Hypoxemia must be corrected quickly to avoid brain injury, myocardial ischemia, and cardiac dysrhythmias.

  Serious cardiovascular manifestations often require drug therapy. Hypotension and hypoperfusion may be treated with inotropic and vasopressor drugs to increase cardiac output and raise blood pressure. Dysrhythmias are treated according to advanced cardiac life support (ACLS) protocols.

  Recurring seizures or status epilepticus requires treatment with anticonvulsant drugs.
- For unconscious patients, as soon as an IV line is established, some authorities recommend a dose of naloxone (2 mg IV) for possible narcotic overdose and thiamine (100 mg IV) for possible brain dysfunction due to thiamine deficiency. In addition, a fingerstick blood glucose test should be done, and if hypoglycemia is indicated, a 50% dextrose solution (50 mL IV) should be given.
- After the patient is out of immediate danger, a thorough physical examination and efforts to determine the drug(s), the amounts, and the time lapse since exposure are needed. If the patient is unable to supply needed information, anyone else who may be able to do so should be interviewed. It is necessary to ask about the use of prescription and over-the-counter drugs, alcohol, and illicit substances.
- There are no standard laboratory tests for poisoned patients, but baseline tests of liver and kidney function are usually indicated. Screening tests for toxic substances are not very helpful because test results may be delayed, many substances are not detected, and the results rarely affect initial treatment. Specimens of blood, urine, or gastric fluids may be obtained for laboratory analysis. Serum drug levels are needed when acetaminophen, alcohol, aspirin, digoxin, lithium, or theophylline is known to be an ingested drug, to assist with treatment.
- For most orally ingested drugs, the initial and major treatment is a single dose of activated charcoal. Sometimes called the "universal antidote," it is useful in many poisonings because it adsorbs many toxins and rarely causes complications. When given within 30 minutes of drug ingestion, it decreases absorption of the toxic drug by about 90%; when given an hour after ingestion, it decreases absorption by about 37%. Activated charcoal (1 g/kg of body weight or 50–100 g) is usually mixed with 240 mL of water (25–50 g in 120 mL of water for children) to make a slurry, which is gritty and unpleasant to swallow. It is often given by nasogastric tube. The charcoal blackens subsequent bowel movements. If used with whole-bowel irrigation (WBI; see below), activated charcoal should be given before the WBI solution is started. If given during WBI, the binding capacity of the charcoal is decreased. Activated charcoal does not significantly decrease absorption of some drugs (e.g., ethanol, iron, lithium, metals).

  Multiple doses of activated charcoal may be given in some instances (e.g., ingestion of sustained-release drugs). One regimen is an initial dose of 50 to 100 g and then 12.5 g every 1, 2, or 4 to 6 hours for a few doses.

  Adverse effects of activated charcoal include pulmonary aspiration and bowel obstruction from impaction of the charcoal–drug complex.

  Ipecac-induced vomiting and gastric lavage are no longer routinely used because of minimal effectiveness and potential complications. Ipecac is no longer recommended to treat poisonings in children in home settings; parents should call a poison control center or a health care provider. Gastric lavage may be beneficial in serious overdoses if performed within an hour of drug ingestion. If the ingested agent delays gastric emptying (e.g., drugs with anticholinergic effects), the 1-hour time limit for gastric lavage may be extended. When used after ingestion of pills or capsules, the tube lumen should be large enough to allow removal of pill fragments.
- WBI with a polyethylene glycol solution (e.g., Colyte) may be used to remove toxic ingestions of long-acting, sustained-release drugs (e.g., many beta-adrenergic blockers, calcium channel blockers, and theophylline preparations); enteric-coated drugs; and toxins that do not bind well with activated charcoal (e.g., iron, lithium). It may also be helpful in removing packets of illicit drugs, such as cocaine or heroin. When used, 500 to 2000 mL/h are given orally or by nasogastric tube until bowel contents are clear. Vomiting is the most common adverse effect. WBI is contraindicated in patients with serious bowel disorders (e.g., obstruction, perforation, ileus), hemodynamic instability, or respiratory impairment (unless intubated).
- Urinary elimination of some drugs and toxic metabolites can be accelerated by changing the pH of urine (e.g., alkalinizing with IV sodium bicarbonate for salicylate overdose), diuresis, or hemodialysis. Hemodialysis is the treatment of choice in severe lithium and aspirin (salicylate) poisoning.
- Specific antidotes can be administered when available and as indicated by the patient's clinical condition. Available antidotes vary widely in effectiveness. Some are very effective and rapidly reverse toxic manifestations (e.g., naloxone for opioids, specific Fab fragments for digoxin).

  When an antidote is used, its half-life relative to the toxin's half-life must be considered. For example, the half-life of naloxone, a narcotic antagonist, is relatively short compared with the half-life of the longer-acting opioids such as methadone, and repeated doses may be needed to prevent recurrence of the toxic state.

*not going to ask about antidotes*

## TABLE 2.1

## Antidotes for Overdoses of Selected Therapeutic Drugs

| Overdosed Drug (Poison) | Antidote | Route and Dosage Ranges | Comments |
|---|---|---|---|
| Acetaminophen (see Chap. 16) | Acetylcysteine (10% or 20% inhalation/ oral solution, Acetadote 20% [200 mg/mL] injection solution) | PO 140 mg/kg initially, then 70 mg/kg every 4 h for 17 doses (72-h oral regimen) IV (Acetadote only): loading dose 150 mg/kg, diluted in 200 mL 5% dextrose, infused over 15 min. Maintenance dose one: 50 mg/kg, diluted in 500 mL 5% dextrose, infused over 4 h. Maintenance dose two: 100 mg/kg, diluted in 1000 mL 5% dextrose, infused over 16 h (21-h IV regimen) | Dilute oral solution to a 5% solution with a cola or other soft drink for oral administration. Follow instructions carefully and note that doses, amounts of diluent, and infusion times are different for the three total IV infusions. Only the 72-hour oral and 21-hour IV regimens are FDA approved for acetaminophen overdose |
| Anticholinergics (atropine; see Chap. 48) | Physostigmine | IV, IM 2 mg; give IV slowly, over at least 2 min | Infrequently used because of its toxicity; consulting a regional poison center recommended. Should not be given to patients with a seizure disorder, overdose of unknown drugs, or overdose of drugs known to cause seizures in overdose (e.g., cocaine, lithium). In such circumstances, the risks of seizures outweigh drug benefits |
| Benzodiazepines (see Chap. 54) | Flumazenil | IV 0.2 mg over 30 s; if no response, may give additional 0.3 mg over 30 s. Additional doses of 0.5 mg may be given at 1-min intervals up to a total amount of 3 mg | Should not be given to patients with overdose of unknown drugs or drugs known to cause seizures in overdose (e.g., cocaine, lithium) |
| Beta-adrenergic blockers (see Chap. 27) | Glucagon | IV 50–150 mcg/kg (5–10 mg for adults) over 1 min initially, then 2–5 mg/h by continuous infusion as needed | Glucagon increases myocardial contractility and raises blood pressure. It does not act on beta-adrenergic receptors and is therefore not affected by beta-adrenergic blocking drugs |
| Calcium channel blockers (see Chap. 26) | Calcium gluconate 10% | IV 1 g over 5 min; may be repeated | Increases myocardial contractility |
| Cholinergics (see Chap. 47) | Atropine | Adults: IV 2 mg, repeated as needed. Children: IV 0.05 mg/kg, up to 2 mg | If poisoning is due to organophosphates (e.g., insecticides), pralidoxime may be given with the atropine |
| Digoxin (see Chap. 30) | Digoxin immune Fab | IV 40 mg (one vial) for each 0.6 mg of digoxin ingested. Reconstitute each vial with 4 mL water for injection, then dilute with sterile isotonic saline to convenient volume and give over 30 min, through 0.22-μm filter. If cardiac arrest seems imminent, may give the dose as bolus injection | Recommended for severe toxicity; reverses cardiac and extracardiac symptoms in a few minutes. Note: Serum digoxin levels increase after antidote administration, but the drug is bound and therefore inactive |
| Heparin (see Chap. 9) | Protamine sulfate | IV 1 mg/100 units of heparin, slowly, over at least 10 min; a single dose should not exceed 50 mg | |
| Iron (see Chap. 35) | Deferoxamine | IM 1 g every 8 h PRN. IV 15 mg/kg/h if hypotensive | Indicated for serum iron levels >500 mg/dL or serum levels >350 mg/dL with GI or cardiovascular symptoms. Can bind and remove a portion of an ingested dose; urine becomes red as iron is excreted |

## TABLE 2.1

### Antidotes for Overdoses of Selected Therapeutic Drugs (Continued)

| Overdosed Drug (Poison) | Antidote | Route and Dosage Ranges | Comments |
|---|---|---|---|
| Isoniazid (INH) (see Chap. 22) | Pyridoxine (vitamin B6) | IV 1 g per gram of INH ingested, at rate of 1 g every 2–3 min. If amount of INH unknown, give 5 g; may be repeated | Indicated for management of seizures and correction of acidosis |
| Lead | Dimercaptosuccinic acid (succimer; Chemet) | Children: PO 10 mg/kg every 8 h for 5 d followed by 10 mg/kg/dose every 12 h for 14 d; maximum: 500 mg/dose Adults: at same dosing parameters as children (off-label use) | Dimercaptosuccinic acid is dialyzable although the lead chelates are not |
| Opioid analgesics (see Chap. 49) | Naloxone (Narcan) | Adults: IM or intranasal (preferred) 0.4–2 mg PRN Children: IV (preferred) 0.1 mg/kg per dose; maximum dose 2 mg | Can be given by alternate routes as indicated |
| Phenothiazine antipsychotic agents (see Chap. 56) | Diphenhydramine | Adults: IV 50 mg Children: IV 1–2 mg/kg, up to a total of 50 mg | Given to relieve extrapyramidal symptoms (movement disorders) |
| Thrombolytics (see Chap. 9) | Aminocaproic acid (Amicar) | PO, IV infusion, 5 g initially, then 1–1.25 g/h for 8 h or until bleeding is controlled; maximum dose, 30 g/24 h | |
| Tricyclic antidepressants (see Chap. 55) | Sodium bicarbonate | IV 1–2 mEq/kg initially, then continuous IV drip to maintain serum pH of 7.5 | To treat cardiac dysrhythmias, conduction disturbances, and hypotension |
| Warfarin (see Chap. 9) | Vitamin K1 | PO 5–10 mg daily IV (severe overdose) continuous infusion at rate no faster than 1 mg/min | |

Most overdosed patients are treated in emergency departments and discharged to their homes. A few are admitted to intensive care units (ICUs), often because of unconsciousness and the need for endotracheal intubation and mechanical ventilation. Unconsciousness is a major toxic effect of several commonly ingested substances such as benzodiazepine antianxiety and sedative agents, TCAs, ethanol, and opioid analgesics. Serious cardiovascular effects (e.g., cardiac arrest, dysrhythmias, circulatory impairment) are also common and warrant admission to an ICU.

### Clinical Application 2.2

- You see Mrs. Green again in a few days. She is taking three antihypertensive medications, and her blood pressure is 128/72 mm Hg. She tells you that she has been feeling better and that she is moving in with her daughter. What suggestions could you provide Mrs. Green's daughter regarding her mother's medication management?

## NCLEX Success

4. A nurse is looking up information about the effects of a drug on different receptors. Characteristics of receptors include which of the following?

   A. They are carbohydrates located in cell membranes or inside cells.
   B. They are constantly synthesized and degraded in the body.
   C. They bind with molecules of any drug circulating in the bloodstream.
   D. They regulate the actions of all drugs.

5. A patient with an overdose of an oral drug usually receives which of the following?

   A. specific antidote
   B. activated charcoal
   C. syrup of ipecac
   D. strong laxative

6. The mother of a 14-month-old girl calls a nurse working in a pediatric clinic and reports that her daughter ingested an unknown number of sleeping pills about 4 hours ago and is now drowsy. The mother asks what she should do. The best response to give the mother is
   A. "Administer a dose of syrup of ipecac to ensure vomiting"
   B. "Call the Poison Control Center immediately"
   C. "Administer a strong laxative and observe for a response"
   D. "Call 911 to transport your daughter to the nearest emergency department"

7. Differences in CYP-450 drug-metabolizing enzymes are known to cause genetic variation in the drug metabolism of certain drugs that increase the risk of adverse effects. These include which of the following? [Select all that apply.]
   A. CYP2D6 metabolism of several antidepressant, antipsychotic, and beta-adrenergic blocker drugs that increases the risk of drug accumulation and adverse effects.
   B. CYP2D6 metabolism of codeine in individuals who are ultrarapid metabolizers. The conversion of codeine to morphine occurs quickly and poses a risk of serious adverse effects, such as respiratory depression.
   C. CYP2C19 metabolism in some individuals of Asian descent. This may cause decreased drug metabolism of diazepam, omeprazole, and some antidepressants leading to adverse effects.
   D. Individuals with a deficiency of glucose-6-phosphate dehydrogenase, who may have hemolytic anemia when given antimalarial drugs, sulfonamides, analgesics, antipyretics, and other drugs.

## KEY CONCEPTS

- Drugs can stimulate or inhibit normal cellular activities; however, they cannot change the type of function that occurs normally.
- Most drugs exert their effects by chemically combining with receptors at the cellular level.
- Receptor proteins can be altered by endogenous substances and exogenous drugs.
- Pharmacokinetic processes involve absorption, distribution, metabolism, and excretion.
- Serum drug levels reflect dosage, absorption, bioavailability, elimination half-life, and the rate of elimination.
- Drug-related variables that affect drug action include dosage, route, and drug–diet and drug–drug interactions.
- Pharmacogenomic influences affect drug pharmacokinetics and pharmacodynamics; idiosyncratic reactions, such as hypersensitivity reactions; and a drug's effects on disease development, severity, or response to therapy.
- Patient-related variables that affect drug action include age, body weight, genetic and ethnic characteristics, sex, pathologic conditions, and psychological status.
- All drugs can produce adverse effects; adverse effects may produce essentially any symptom or disease process and may involve any body system.
- Drug toxicity results from excessive amounts of a drug, whether received in a single large dose or multiple smaller doses.
- Activated charcoal is considered the "universal" antidote; most drugs do not have specific antidotes for overdoses.
- Ipecac-induced vomiting and gastric lavage are no longer routinely used because of minimal effectiveness and potential complications.
- The current pregnancy categories, which identify risk of fetal injury due to drug therapy when used as directed by the mother during pregnancy, are being phased out. More evidence-based information on which to make better-informed prescribing decisions are replacing them.

## CLINICAL REASONING CASE STUDY

**The Scenario**

There are three groups of students in Dr. Frandsen's pharmacology class. Each group is given the same assignment. They are required to answer the following questions and post their answers to the discussion board.

- What are some factors that decrease absorption of an oral drug?
- Does protein binding speed or slow drug distribution to sites of action? Why?
- What are the implications of hepatic enzyme induction and inhibition in terms of drug metabolism and elimination from the body?

**Assessing Drug Information**

Dr. Frandsen reviews each group's posting and summarizes their results as follows:

- Changes in the cardiovascular system include decreased cardiac output and therefore slower distribution of drug molecules to their sites of action, metabolism, and excretion. In the liver, there is decreased blood flow and metabolizing enzymes. In the kidneys, there is decreased blood flow, decreased glomerular filtration rate, and decreased tubular secretion of drugs. Thus, many drugs are metabolized more slowly, have a longer action, and are more likely to accumulate with chronic administration. All these changes tend to slow excretion and promote accumulation of drugs in the body. Impaired kidney and liver function greatly increase the risks of adverse drug effects.
- Tissue penetration and half-life in drugs that are highly protein bound may differ significantly from those that are minimally bound. Protein binding can limit drug distribution because blood proteins are unable to leave the bloodstream and are confined to the blood vessels. A protein-bound drug is prevented from reaching the cells of the body tissue. Drugs that are highly bound to plasma proteins or stored extensively in other tissues have a long duration of action. If the drug's site of action is in the brain or other areas outside of the blood vessels, being bound to proteins decreases the drug's effectiveness. If the drug's site of action is directly on blood cells, such binding might enhance the drug's action.
- The increase in the rate of a specific enzyme synthesis from basal to maximum level caused by the presence of a substrate or substrate analog that acts as an inducer increases the activity of the hepatic enzymes. The inducer may be a substance that inactivates a repressor chemical in the cell. Enzyme induction is the effect some compounds have in increasing the activity of microsomal hepatic enzymes. This may cause alterations in the metabolism of concurrently administered drugs.

**Nursing Actions**

Dr. Frandsen reiterates the following information to her students:

- Knowledge of the factors that decrease oral absorption of a drug or binding of the drug influences the drug action potentially leading to changes in therapeutic and adverse drug effects. Additionally, understanding alterations in metabolism and elimination of drugs from the body also affect therapeutic and adverse drug effects.

*Visit* thePoint* *at* **http://thePoint.lww.com/Frandsen12e** *for answers to NCLEX Success questions (in Appendix A), answers to Clinical Application Case Studies (in Appendix B), and more!*

## REFERENCES AND RESOURCES

Christensen, K. D., Vassy, L. J., Jamal, L., Lehmann, L. S., Slashinski, M. J., Perry, D. L., et al. (2016). Are physicians prepared for whole genome sequencing? A qualitative analysis. *Clinical Genetics, 89*(2), 228–234.

Hinkle, J. L., & Cheever, K. H. (2017). *Brunner & Suddarth's textbook of medical-surgical nursing* (14th ed.). Philadelphia, PA: Lippincott Williams & Wilkins.

Karch, A. M. (2019). *2019 Lippincott pocket drug guide for nurses.* Philadelphia, PA: Lippincott Williams & Wilkins.

Mattison, M. L., Afonso, K. A., Ngo, L. H., & Mukamal, K. J. (2010). Preventing potentially inappropriate medication use in hospitalized older patients with a computerized provider order entry warning system. *Archives of Internal Medicine, 170*(15), 1331–1336.

National Human Genome Research Institute. (2016). *An overview of the Human Genome Project.* Retrieved from http://www.genome.gov/12011238

Olson, K. R. (2018). Poisoning. In M. Papadakis, S. J. McPhee, & M. W. Rabow (Eds.), *Current medical diagnosis & treatment 2019* (58th ed., pp. 1580–1610). New York: McGraw-Hill.

Roden, D. M., Van Driest, S. L., Wells, Q. S., Mosley, J. D., Denny, J. C., & Peterson, J. F. (2018). Opportunities and challenges in cardiovascular pharmacogenomics: From discovery to implementation. *Circulation Research, 122*(9), 1176–1190. doi: 10.1161/CIRCRESAHA.117.310965

Rodziewicz, T. L., & Hipskind, J. E. (Updated 2018 Mar 30). Medical error prevention. In *StatPearls* [Internet]. Treasure Island, FL: StatPearls Publishing; 2018. Retrieved from https://www.ncbi.nlm.nih.gov/books/NBK499956/

Rogers, M. A., Lizer, S., Doughty, A., Hayden, B., & Klein, C. J. (2017). Expanding RN scope of knowledge-Genetics/genomics: The new frontier. *Journal for Nurses in Professional Development, 33*, 56–63. https://doi.org/10.1097/NND.0000000000000340

Yee, G. C., Talbert, R. L., Matzke, G. R., DiPiro, J. T., & Wells, B. G.(Eds.). (2016). *Pharmacotherapy: A pathophysiologic approach* (10th ed.). New York: McGraw-Hill.

# Medication Administration and the Nursing Process of Drug Therapy

## LEARNING OBJECTIVES

*After studying this chapter, you should be able to:*

1. Apply the rights of medication administration in the care of a patient.
2. Illustrate knowledge needed to administer medications to a patient.
3. Identify and interpret drug orders for medication administration.
4. Demonstrate the ability to calculate drug dosages accurately.
5. Apply the steps of the nursing process in the administration of medications.
6. Demonstrate safe and accurate administration of medications.
7. Apply evidence-based practice research in the administration of medications.
8. Identify alternative or complementary therapy that may potentiate, negate, or cause toxicity with prescribed medications.

## CLINICAL APPLICATION CASE STUDY

Jacqueline Baranski has been admitted to the hospital for a total abdominal hysterectomy. This is the first postoperative day. She is currently taking lisinopril 10 mg PO daily and estradiol 1 mg PO. She is also receiving morphine sulfate by patient-controlled analgesia and heparin 5000 units subcutaneously every 12 hours for 7 days.

## KEY TERMS

**Assessment:** collection of patient data that affects drug therapy

**Controlled-release:** oral tablet or capsule formulations that maintain consistent serum drug levels

**Dosage form:** form in which drugs are manufactured; includes elixirs, tablets, capsules, suppositories, parenteral drugs, and transdermal systems

**Enteric-coated:** coating of a tablet or capsule that makes it insoluble in stomach acid

**Evaluation:** determining a patient's status in relation to stated goals and expected outcomes

**Evidence-based practice:** scientific evidence that yields the best practice in patient care

**Interventions:** planned nursing activities performed on a patient's behalf, including assessment, promotion of adherence to drug therapy, and solving problems related to drug therapy

**Medication history:** list of prescription medications, over-the-counter medications, herbal supplements, or illegal substances taken by the patient (both current and past)

**Nursing diagnosis:** description of patient problems based on assessment data

**Nursing process:** systematic way of gathering and using information to plan and provide individualized patient care

**Parenteral:** injected administration; subcutaneous, intramuscular, or intravenous route

**Planning/goals:** expected outcomes of prescribed drug therapy

**Rights of medication administration:** assist to ensure accuracy in drug therapy; rights include right drug, right dose, right patient, right assessment, right route, right time, right reason, right documentation, right patient education, right evaluation, and right to refuse the medication

**Topical:** application of drugs (e.g., solutions, ointments, creams, or suppositories) to skin or mucous membranes

**Transdermal:** adsorption of drugs (e.g., skin patches) through the skin

# INTRODUCTION

This chapter discusses the administration of medications and the implementation of the **nursing process** with medication administration. The purpose of administering medications is to evoke a therapeutic response. Giving medications to a patient is an important nursing responsibility in many health care settings, including ambulatory clinics, hospitals, long-term care facilities, schools, and homes. The basic requirements for accurate drug administration are the **rights of medication administration**, which are as follows:

- Right drug
- Right dose
- Right patient
- Right assessment
- Right route
- Right time
- Right reason
- Right to refuse the medication
- Right documentation
- Right patient education
- Right evaluation

These "rights" require knowledge of the drugs to be given and the patients who are to receive them as well as specific nursing skills and interventions. The implementation of the nursing process in the administration of medications provides a systematic way of gathering and using information to plan and provide individualized patient care as well as to evaluate the outcomes of that care. It involves both cognitive and psychomotor skills. Knowledge of, and skill in, the nursing process are required for drug therapy as in other aspects of patient care. The five steps of the nursing process are assessment, nursing diagnosis, planning and establishing goals for care, interventions, and evaluation as it is applied to medication administration. The nursing process is a way to assess a patient's needs, response to medications, and identification of adverse effects. In this edition of the textbook, the authors have chosen to eliminate the nursing diagnosis because it is not tested by the National Council of State Boards of Nursing. A concept map outlining the nursing process appears at the end of every chapter that discusses a specific group of drugs.

# GENERAL PRINCIPLES OF ACCURATE DRUG ADMINISTRATION

The nurse adheres to the following principles:

- Follow the "rights" associated with medication administration consistently.
- Learn essential information about each drug to be given (e.g., indications for use, contraindications, therapeutic effects, adverse effects, any specific instructions about administration).
- Interpret the prescriber's order accurately (i.e., drug name, dose, frequency of administration). Question the prescriber if any information is unclear or if the drug seems inappropriate for the patient's condition.
- In the event a verbal or telephone order is given by a prescriber, write down the order or enter it in the computer, and then read the order back to the prescriber.
- Read labels of drug containers for the drug name and concentration (usually in milligrams per tablet, capsule, or milliliter of solution). Many medications are available in different dosage forms and concentrations, and it is extremely important to use the correct ones.
- Use only approved abbreviations for drug names, doses, routes of administration, and times of administration. For example, do not use U to refer to units. Instead, write out *units*. This promotes safer administration and reduces errors. Consult the "Do Not Use List," the safety guidelines published by The Joint Commission (see Table 1.2). Check the organization's Web site for details.
- Calculate doses accurately. Current nursing practice requires few dosage calculations. The advent of high-technology infusion pumps has decreased the need for these calculations. In addition, a pharmacist calculates the dosage prior to filling the prescriber's order and the medication's delivery to the health care facility for administration. Nevertheless, it is important to assess the dosage for accuracy. For medications with a narrow safety margin or potentially serious adverse effects, ask another pharmacist or a colleague to do the calculation also, and compare the results. This is especially important when calculating children's dosages.
- Measure doses accurately. Ask a colleague to double-check measurements of insulin and heparin, unusual doses (i.e., large or small), and any drugs to be given intravenously.
- Use the correct procedures and techniques for all routes of administration. For example, use appropriate anatomic landmarks to identify sites for intramuscular (IM) injections, follow the manufacturers' instructions for preparation and

administration of intravenous (IV) medications, and use sterile materials and techniques for injectable and eye medications.

- Seek information about the patient's medical diagnoses and condition in relation to drug administration (e.g., ability to swallow oral medications; allergies or contraindications to ordered drugs; new signs or symptoms that may indicate adverse effects of administered drugs; heart, liver, or kidney disorders that may interfere with the patient's ability to distribute, metabolize, or eliminate drugs).
- Verify the identity of all patients before administering medications; check identification bands on patients who have them (e.g., in hospitals or long-term care facilities).
- Omit or delay doses as indicated by the patient's condition, and report or record omissions appropriately.
- Be especially vigilant when giving medications to children, because there is a high risk of medication errors. One reason is children's great diversity in age, from birth to 18 years, and in weight, from 2 to 3 kg to 100 kg or more. A second reason is that most drugs have not been tested in children. A third reason is that many drugs are marketed in dosage forms and concentrations suitable for adults. This often requires dilution, calculation, preparation, and administration of very small doses. A fourth reason is that children have limited sites for administration of IV drugs, and several may be given through the same site. In many cases, the need for small volumes of fluid limits flushing between drugs (which may produce undesirable interactions with other drugs and IV solutions).
- According to The Joint Commission and the World Health Organization, patient safety is the prevention of errors and adverse effects. Each nurse and health care institution is responsible for internal and external reporting requirements for adverse drug events (ADEs), adverse drug reactions, and medication errors.
- Maintain up-to-date skills for medication administration and knowledge of theoretical drug information.

### Clinical Application 3.1

- Prior to administering the medications to Ms. Baranski, how does the nurse incorporate the rights of medication administration into the patient's care?
- Why is The Joint Commission's "Do Not Use" list so important in the prevention of medication administration errors?

### NCLEX Success

1. A physician writes an order using the abbreviation MS. The order states "MS 10 mg IV push every 6 hours as needed for pain." According to The Joint Commission's "Do Not Use" list, what is the potential problem in this order?

   A. The order does not include a dosage.
   B. The drug could be magnesium sulfate or morphine sulfate.
   C. The potential problem is minimal, and the order is clear.
   D. The order does not include the route.

2. A prescriber has written an order for an oral antihypertensive medication for a patient who is in rehabilitation following a stroke. Prior to administering the medication, which of the following nursing interventions is most important? [Select all that apply.]

   A. allowing the patient to take the medication with thickened liquids
   B. placing the patient in the sitting position
   C. assessing the patient's blood pressure
   D. assessing the patient's ability to swallow

## LEGAL RESPONSIBILITIES

Registered and licensed practical nurses are legally empowered, under state nurse practice acts, to give medications ordered by licensed physicians, nurse practitioners, physician assistants, and dentists.

When giving medications, the nurse is legally responsible for safe and accurate administration. This means that the nurse may be held liable for not giving a drug or for giving a wrong drug or a wrong dose. In addition, the nurse is expected to have sufficient drug knowledge to recognize and question erroneous orders. If, after questioning the prescriber and seeking information from other authoritative sources, the nurse considers that giving a drug is unsafe, the nurse must refuse to give the drug. The fact that a physician wrote an erroneous order does not excuse the nurse from legal liability if he or she carries out that order.

The nurse also is legally responsible for actions delegated to people who are inadequately prepared for or legally barred from administering medications (e.g., nursing assistants). However, certified medical assistants (CMAs) may administer medications in physicians' offices, and certified medication aides (nursing assistants with a short course of training, also called CMAs) often administer medications in long-term care facilities.

The nurse who consistently follows safe practices in giving medications does not need to be excessively concerned about legal liability. The basic techniques and guidelines described in this chapter are aimed at safe and accurate preparation and administration. Most errors result when these practices are not followed.

Legal responsibilities in other aspects of drug therapy are less clear-cut. However, in general, nurses are expected to monitor patients' responses to drug therapy (e.g., therapeutic and adverse effects) and to teach patients safe and effective self-administration of drugs when indicated. The medical director of the Institute for Safe Medication Practices (ISMP) has recently referred to the process of preventing medication errors as *pharmacovigilance* (Hilton, 2018). The four guidelines that reportedly prevent errors in medication administration include using the following:

- Prefilled syringes, in which the syringes are prefilled when manufactured
- Bar codes, which contain information to maintain patient safety, such as the patient's allergies and contraindications related to the use of the medication (see Changes to Prevent Medication Errors)
- Tubing connectors for different routes of medications, which prevents the administration of a noncompatible medication
- Proper labeling, which is essential to prevent medication errors

The nurse recommends docusate, a stool softener, for Mary Richards, an 82-year-old with heart failure. The provider informs the nurse that the order will be placed in the computer. When the nurse reviews the provider orders, the only medication written is losartan 50 mg PO daily, which the nurse recognizes as an angiotensin receptor blocker used in the treatment of heart failure. Because losartan was not requested or discussed during patient rounds but sounds similar to docusate, how should the nurse proceed with this order? (Mary Richards' story continues in Chap. 26.)

Care for Mary and other patients in a realistic virtual environment: *vSim for Nursing* (thepoint.lww.com/vSim-Pharm). Practice documenting these patients' care in DocuCare (thepoint.lww.com/DocuCareEHR).

# MEDICATION ERRORS AND THEIR PREVENTION

Medication errors continue to receive increasing attention from numerous health care organizations and agencies. Much of this interest stems from a 1999 report of the Institute of Medicine (IOM), which estimated that 44,000 to 98,000 deaths occur each year in the United States because of medical errors, including medication errors. The 2004 report of the IOM, *Keeping Patients Safe: Transforming the Work Environment of Nurses*, reported that the extended hours nurses work contribute to medication errors. Potential adverse patient outcomes of medication and other errors include serious illness, conditions that prolong hospitalization or require additional treatment, and death. Medication errors commonly reported include giving an incorrect dose, not giving an ordered drug, and giving an unordered drug. Specific drugs often associated with errors and ADEs include insulin, heparin, and warfarin. The risk of ADEs increases with the number of drugs a patient uses.

ADEs are injuries that result from the use of medications (Zhu & Weingart, 2017). Medication errors may or may not lead to injury, but the process an outcome of an error may provide the risk management team with strategies to improve patient care. Many years ago, the labels of heparin were very similar. This similarity resulted in an overdosage of heparin, leading to patient death. These drug errors led to changes in medication labeling. Potential adverse drug reactions pose a risk to the patient. A potential adverse drug reaction can also be termed as near misses. The nonpreventable adverse drug reaction is related to the chemical and pharmacologic properties that can result in an allergic reaction or hypersensitivity reaction.

Medication errors may occur at any step in the drug distribution process, from the manufacturer to the patient, including prescribing, transcribing, dispensing, and administering. Many steps and numerous people are involved in giving the correct dose of a medication to the intended patient; each step or person has a potential for contributing to a medication error or preventing a medication error. All health care providers involved in drug therapy need to recognize risky situations, intervene to prevent errors when possible, and be extremely vigilant in all phases of drug administration. Recommendations for prevention of medication errors have been developed by several organizations, including the IOM, the Agency for Healthcare Research and Quality (AHRQ), The Joint Commission, the ISMP, and the National Coordinating Council for Medication Error Reporting and Prevention (NCCMERP). Some sources of medication errors and recommendations to prevent them are summarized in Table 3.1.

The NCCMERP (2018), an independent council of 27 organizations, works to maximize the safe use of medications. It increases awareness of medication errors and promotes strategies to prevent further errors. It has developed

**TABLE 3.1**

## Medication Errors: Sources and Prevention Strategies

| Sources of Errors | Recommendation to Prevent Errors |
|---|---|
| **Drug Manufacturers**<br>• Drugs may have similar names that can lead to erroneous prescribing, dispensing, or administration.<br>• For example, the antiseizure drug lamotrigine (Lamictal) has been confused with Lamisil, an antifungal drug; lamivudine, an antiviral drug; and others.<br>• The FDA estimates that 10% of all reported medication errors result from drug name confusion.<br>• In addition to similar names, many drugs, especially those produced by the same manufacturer, have similar packaging. This can lead to errors if container labels are not read carefully, especially if the products are shelved or stored next to each other.<br>• Long-acting oral dosage forms with various, sometimes unclear indicators (e.g., LA, XL, XR), may be crushed, chewed, or otherwise broken so that the long-acting feature is destroyed. This can cause an overdose. | • FDA evaluation of proposed trade names in manufacturers' new drug applications in seeking FDA approval for marketing.<br>• When choosing a trade name for a new drug, avoid names that are similar to drugs already on the market.<br>• Design packaging so that all drugs from an individual manufacturer do not look alike in terms of color, appearance, etc.<br>• Clearly designate long-acting drug formulations.<br>• Use "Tall Man" lettering on drug labels to distinguish between generic drug with similar names (e.g., NICARdipine, NIFEdipine; vinBLAstine, VinCristine). |

**TABLE 3.1**

## Medication Errors: Sources and Prevention Strategies (Continued)

| Sources of Errors | Recommendation to Prevent Errors |
|---|---|
| **Health Care Agencies**<br><br>• Prescribers, pharmacists, and nurses have a heavy workload, with resultant rushing of prescribing, dispensing, and administering medications.<br>• They may also experience distractions by interruptions, noise, and other events in the work environment that make it difficult to pay needed attention to the medication-related task. | • Provide prescribers with CPOE technology and standardized drug order sheets; discourage handwritten drug orders; minimize verbal orders and state procedures to follow when verbal orders are necessary.<br>• Provide computerized technology (e.g., bar coding for patients; handheld scanning devices for nursing staff) to verify the drug, the dose, and the patient identity before administration of a dose and to record administration after a dose.<br>• Provide sufficient pharmacy staff to dispense medications.<br>• Provide sufficient nursing staff to administer medications.<br>• Try to provide a quiet and orderly work environment, with limited traffic, telephones, and other distractions.<br>• Provide adequate equipment for the required medication-related tasks. For pharmacies, this includes an adequate computer system for accessing databases of drug information and for detecting risks of adverse drug effects and drug–drug interactions.<br>• Standardize drug administration materials and equipment (e.g., infusion pumps) throughout the agency.<br>• Be sure that all professional staff members know and follow safety standards and medication reconciliation processes mandated by The Joint Commission. |
| **Prescribers**<br><br>• May write orders illegibly<br>• Order a drug that is not indicated by the patient's condition<br>• Fail to order a drug that is indicated<br>• Fail to consider the patient's age, size, kidney function, liver function, and disease process when selecting a drug or dosage<br>• Fail to consider other medications the patient is taking, including prescription, over-the-counter, and herbal drugs<br>• Lack sufficient knowledge about the drug<br>• Fail to monitor for, or instruct others to monitor for, effects of administered drugs<br>• Fail to discontinue drugs appropriately | • Use CPOE when available.<br>• Be sure that any handwritten drug order is legible (e.g., printed in block letters if necessary), clear, and unambiguous.<br>• Avoid or minimize the use of abbreviations. Consult The Joint Commission's "Do Not Use" List.<br>• Use generic names of medications rather than brand names, and include the purpose of the drug.<br>• Avoid verbal orders when possible. If a verbal order is necessary, have the person taking the order write the order and read it back, spelling drug names, dosages, routes, and so forth when indicated.<br>• Review the patient's health status and other drugs being taken before ordering any new drug. Also, discontinue drugs appropriately when no longer needed.<br>• Maintain a current knowledge base about new drugs and changes in uses of drugs for the relevant area of clinical practice. |
| **Nurses**<br><br>• May have inadequate knowledge about a drug or about the patient receiving the drug<br>• Not follow the rights to medication administration<br>• Fail to question the medication order when indicated | • Be aware of agency policies and procedures about medication use, storage, administration, and recording.<br>• Maintain an up-to-date knowledge base about drugs and their administration.<br>• Make a diligent effort to learn about patients' health status and the drugs they are receiving.<br>• Question or clarify any unclear drug orders.<br>• Verify medication calculations with another nurse or a pharmacist, especially for children.<br>• Recheck a single dose any time the amount seems unusually large or small.<br>• Verify settings on drug infusion pumps with another nurse, when indicated.<br>• Follow the rights of medication administration consistently.<br>• Recheck the original drug order when a patient questions whether a particular drug dose should be taken. |

*(Continued on page 40)*

| TABLE 3.1 | |
|---|---|
| **Medication Errors: Sources and Prevention Strategies** (Continued) | |
| **Sources of Errors** | **Recommendation to Prevent Errors** |
| **Nurses (*Continued*)** | |
| | • Report errors, so that preventive efforts can be designed.<br>• Discuss patients' medications during change-of-shift reports, including new and discontinued drugs, patients' responses to their medications, patient teaching about medications, and medications given 1–2 hours before or after shift report. |
| **Patients and Consumers** | |
| • Outpatients may take drugs from several prescribers<br>• Fail to inform one prescriber about drugs prescribed by another health care provider<br>• Get prescriptions filled at more than one pharmacy<br>• Fail to get prescriptions filled or refilled<br>• Underuse or overuse an appropriately prescribed drug<br>• Take drugs left over from a previous illness or prescribed for someone else<br>• Fail to follow instructions for drug administration or storage<br>• Fail to keep appointments for follow-up care<br>• Fail to ask for information when needed | • Inform all health care providers about health status, any drug allergies, and all medications being taken (e.g., prescription, over-the-counter, herbal, and dietary supplements).<br>• Ask prescribers to include the purpose of a drug on the label of all prescription medications.<br>• If able, know names, strengths, doses, and the reason for use of all medications.<br>• Follow instructions about when and how to take medications; do not increase amount or frequency of any medication without checking with a health care provider. Ask questions or request written instructions if needed.<br>• If unable to take medications or if problems occur, discuss with a health care provider. Do not stop taking prescribed medications.<br>• Maintain a current list of all medications being taken. Take the list or the medications to each visit to a health care provider.<br>• Keep all medications in their original containers.<br>• Read labels of medication containers every time a dose is taken.<br>• Do not chew, crush, or break any tablets or capsules unless a health care provider says it is okay to do so. |

CPOE, computerized provider order entry; FDA, Food and Drug Administration.

an index for categorizing medication errors (Fig. 3.1) and an algorithm (Fig. 3.2). This categorization of medication errors can be adopted by health care institutions. Using A through I, this system ranks medication errors according to the severity of their outcomes. Category A identifies circumstances that have the capacity to cause an error, and Category I identifies an error that contributed to a patient's death. This system gives health care institutions the ability to track the rate of medication errors.

## Medication Systems

Each health care facility has a system for distributing drugs. The unit-dose system, in which most drugs are dispensed in single-dose containers for individual patients, is widely used. The pharmacist or pharmacy technician checks drug orders and stocks the medication in the patient's medication drawer. When a dose is due to be taken, the nurse removes the medication and gives it to the patient. Unit-dose wrappings of oral drugs should be left in place until the nurse is in the presence of the patient and ready to give the medication. It is essential that each dose of a drug be recorded on the patient's medication administration record (MAR) as soon as possible after administration.

Increasingly, institutions are using automated, computerized, locked cabinets for which each nurse on a unit has a pass-word or code for accessing the cabinet and obtaining a drug dose. The pharmacy maintains the medications and replaces the drug when needed.

Controlled drugs, such as opioid analgesics, are usually kept as a stock supply in a locked drawer or automated cabinet and replaced as needed. The nurse must sign for each dose and record it on the patient's MAR. He or she must comply with legal regulations and institutional policies for dispensing and recording controlled drugs.

## Changes to Prevent Medication Errors

Changes in medication systems are being increasingly implemented, largely in efforts to decrease medication errors and improve patient safety. These include the following:

• Computerized provider order entry (CPOE). In this system, a prescriber types a medication order directly into a computer. This decreases errors associated with illegible handwriting and erroneous transcription or dispensing. CPOE, which is already used in many health care facilities, is widely recommended as the preferred alternative to error-prone handwritten orders.
• Bar coding. In 2004, the Food and Drug Administration (FDA) passed a regulation requiring drug manufacturers to put bar codes on current prescription medications

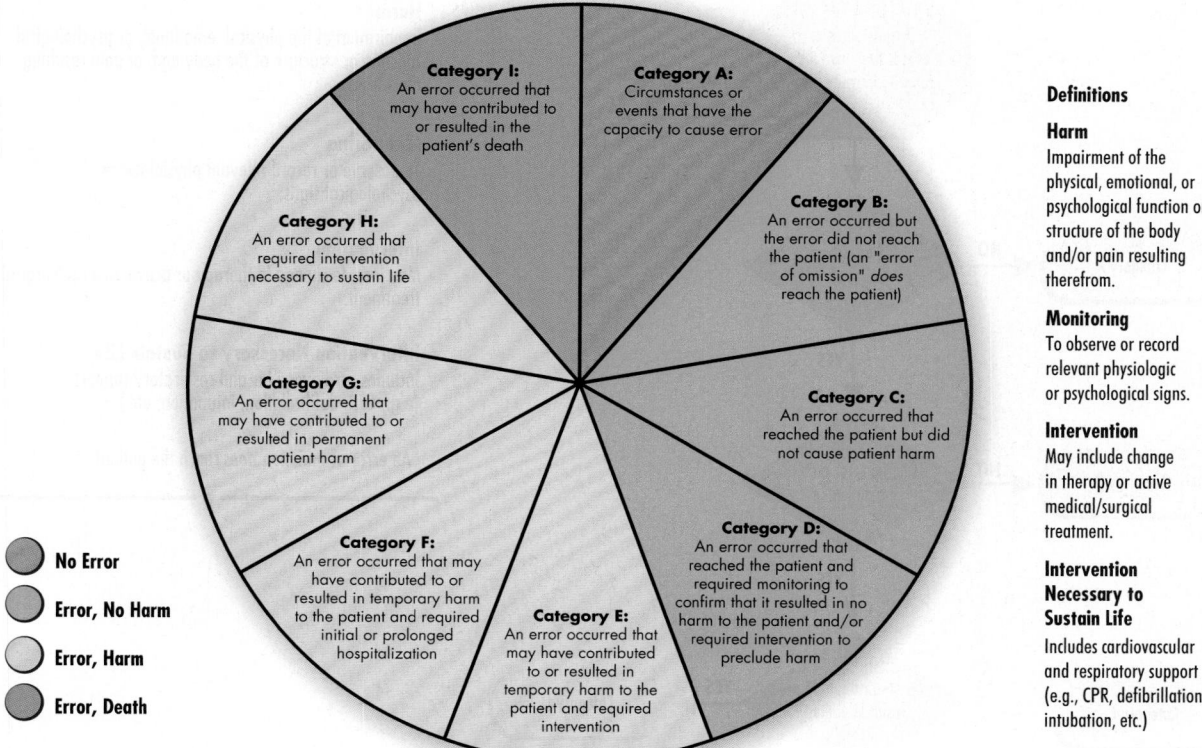

**Figure 3.1.** Index for categorizing medication errors, National Coordinating Council for Medication Error Reporting and Prevention. (NCC MERP Index for Categorizing Medication Errors. © 2017 National Coordinating Council for Medication Error Reporting and Prevention. All Rights Reserved. Retrieved from: https://www.nccmerp.org/sites/default/files/indexColor2001-06-12.pdf.)

and nonprescription medications that are commonly used in hospitals. New drugs must have bar codes within 60 days of their approval. In hospitals, bar codes operate with other agency computer systems and databases that contain a patient's medication orders and MAR. The bar code on the drug label contains the identification number, strength, and dosage form of the drug, and the bar code on the patient's identification band contains the MAR, which can be displayed when a nurse uses a handheld scanning device. When administering medications, the nurse scans the bar code on the drug label, on the patient's identification band, and on the nurse's personal identification badge. A wireless computer network processes the scanned information; gives an error message on the scanner or sounds an alarm if the nurse is about to give the wrong drug or the right drug at the wrong time; and automatically records the time, drug, and dose given on the MAR. The FDA estimates that it will take about 20 years for all US hospitals to implement this system of bar codes for medication administration.

For nurses, implementing the bar coding technology increases the time requirements and interferes with their ability to individualize patient care in relation to medications. Such a system works well with routine medications, but nonroutine situations (e.g., variable doses or times of adminis-

tration) may pose problems. In addition, in long-term care facilities, it may be difficult to maintain legible bar codes on patient identification bands. Despite some drawbacks, bar coding increases patient safety, and therefore nurses should support its development.

• Point of care. The Department of Veterans Affairs developed the point-of-care bar code–assisted software in August 1999 for the department's medical centers. Point of care is the time in which the nurse scans the bar-coded medication administered to the patient. This system uses bar code scanning that verifies the right drug, dose, patient, route, and time. The reason for the medication and subsequent documentation is the responsibility of the nurse administering the medication. This technology increases patient safety and accuracy of reporting. Using a handheld electronic device, the nurse scans the bar code and compares the medication being administered with what was ordered for the patient. Following receipt of the written order, the pharmacist enters, verifies, and profiles the order. Prior to administering the medication, the nurse confirms a match between the written and electronically profiled order. Before administering the medication, the nurse scans the patient's wrist band and medication. The device then verifies that it is the correct dose, correct time, and correct patient.

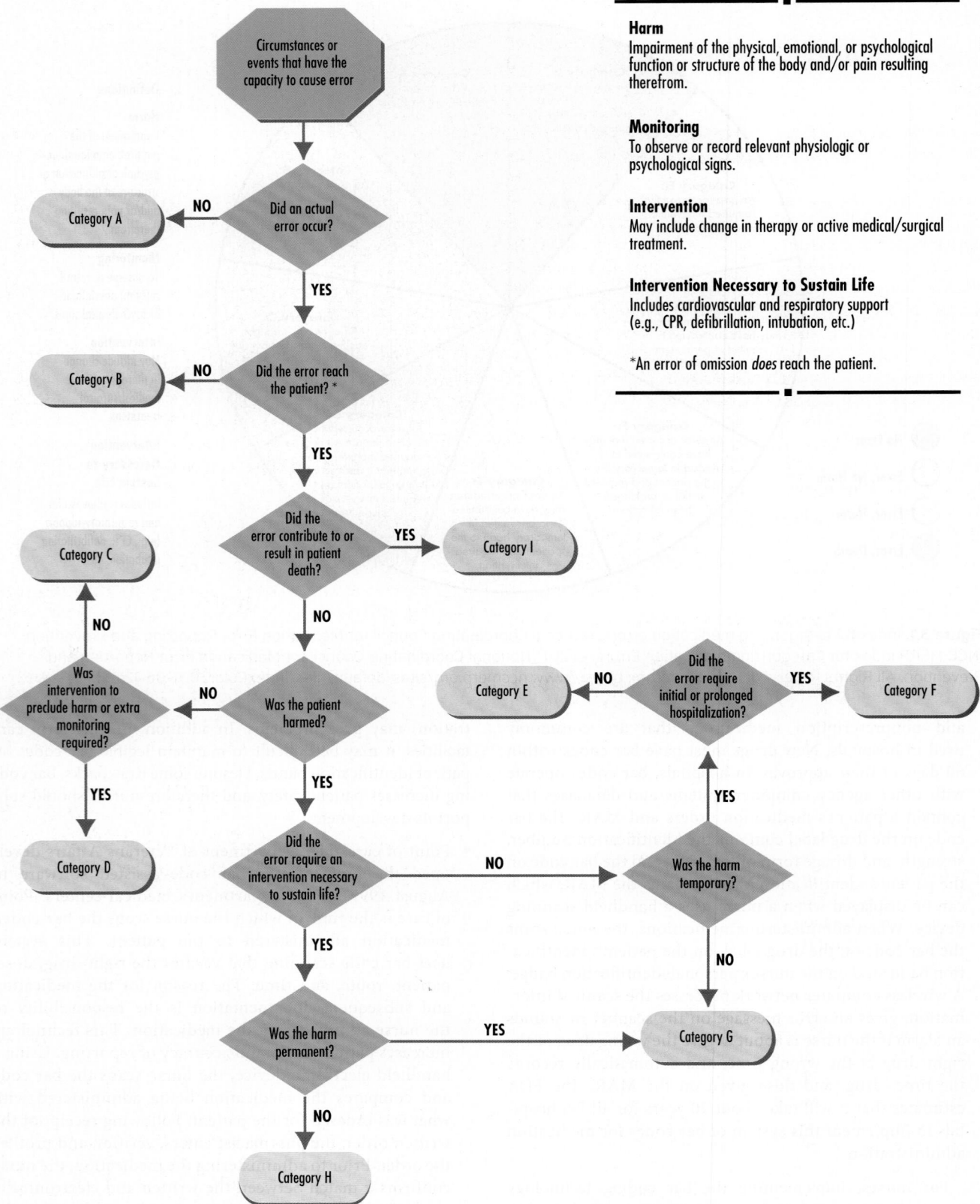

**Harm**
Impairment of the physical, emotional, or psychological function or structure of the body and/or pain resulting therefrom.

**Monitoring**
To observe or record relevant physiologic or psychological signs.

**Intervention**
May include change in therapy or active medical/surgical treatment.

**Intervention Necessary to Sustain Life**
Includes cardiovascular and respiratory support (e.g., CPR, defibrillation, intubation, etc.)

*An error of omission *does* reach the patient.

**Figure 3.2.** Algorithm for categorizing medication errors. [National Coordinating Council for Medication Error Reporting and Prevention. NCC MERP Index for Categorizing Medication Errors Algorithm. © 2017 National Coordinating Council for Medication Error Reporting and Prevention. All Rights Reserved. Retrieved from:https://www.nccmerp.org/sites/default/files/algorColor2001-06-12.pdf.]

According to the FDA, hospitals have reduced medication administration errors since 2006 with the use of the bar coding technology. Drawbacks to bar code technology have been identified. For example, bar codes on suppositories and IV solution bags can become unreadable. Also, as tubes of ointments are rolled from the bottom, the bar code may become difficult to decipher. Drug companies apply linear bar codes on pharmaceuticals. In 2011, President Barack Obama signed the executive order "Improving Regulation and Regulatory Review," requiring federal regulatory agencies to strengthen, complement, and modernize rules. The FDA chose to address the bar code rules.

Many countries use Bar Code Medication Administration (BCMA) to give medications. Strudwick et al. (2018) conducted an integrative review of the literature. The reviews revealed that in 11 studies conducted in the United States, United Kingdom, and Japan, a significant decrease in medical errors was reported 6 months after the installation of BCMA. The authors found "wrong time" errors in studies, which may be related to the increased time required to administer medications with the BCMA technology. New workstations on wheels allow the nurse to bring the technology closer to the patient. The administration of medications with the BCMA technology has ensured that the medications available were only ordered for that patient.

- Limiting use of abbreviations. The ISMP has long maintained a list of abbreviations that are often associated with medication errors, and The Joint Commission requires accredited organizations to maintain a "Do Not Use" list (e.g., u or U for units, IU for international units, qd for daily, qod for every other day) that applies to all prescribers and transcribers of medication orders. Other abbreviations are not recommended as well. In general, it is safer to write out drug names, routes of administration, and so forth and to minimize the use of abbreviations, symbols, and numbers that are often misinterpreted, especially when handwritten.
- Medication reconciliation. This is a process designed to avoid medication errors such as omissions, duplications, dosing errors, or drug interactions that occur when a patient is admitted to a health care facility, transferred from one department or unit to another within the facility, or discharged home from the facility. It involves obtaining an accurate medication history about all drugs (both prescription and over-the-counter [OTC]), vitamins, and herbal medications taken at home, including dose and frequency of administration, on entry into the health care facility (see later discussion). The list of medications developed from the medication history is compared to newly ordered medications, and identified discrepancies are resolved. The list is placed in the medical record so that it is accessible to all health care providers, including the prescriber who writes the patient's admission drug orders. When the patient is transferred, the updated list must be communicated to the next health care provider. When a patient is discharged, an updated list should be given to the next provider and to the patient. The patient should be encouraged to keep the list up-to-date when changes are made in the medication regimen and to share the list with future health care providers.

---

**! QSEN Alert: Evidence-Based Practice**

Oscanoa, Lizaraso, and Carvajal (2017) conducted a systematic review and meta-analysis of studies addressing adverse drug reactions in hospitalized patients over 60 years of age. The review of literature spanned from 1988 to 2015. Forty-two articles were selected with average hospital admission at rate at 8.7%. Reaction to nonsteroidal anti-inflammatory drugs (NSAIDs) was the most frequently noted adverse drug reactions leading to hospitalization. Other adverse drug reactions that led to hospitalization were beta blockers, antibiotics, oral anticoagulants, digoxin, angiotensin-converting enzyme inhibitors, anticancer drugs, calcium channel blockers, opioids, and oral antidiabetic agents. The authors noted that renal failure was a significant adverse drug reaction in 4 out of 8 studies. Also, female patients were at higher risk in 6 out of 21 studies.

---

**Clinical Application 3.2**

- The nurse is checking Ms. Baranski's patient-controlled analgesia of morphine sulfate. The medication cartridge is empty and needs to be changed. What are the nurse's legal responsibilities when changing an opioid medication?
- What nursing interventions prevent medication errors?

---

**NCLEX Success**

3. A prescriber has written an order for levothyroxine sodium 50 mg/day by mouth. The nurse knows that the standard dose is 50 mcg. What action should the nurse take?

   A. Call the prescriber and question the order.
   B. Administer 50 mcg instead.
   C. Consult the pharmacist about the order.
   D. Ask the patient what he or she usually takes.

4. The nurse is administering the first dose of an anti-infective agent. Which of the following assessments should the nurse make prior to administering the anti-infective agent?

   A. Assess the patient's temperature.
   B. Assess the patient's level of consciousness.
   C. Assess whether the patient is allergic to any anti-infective agent.
   D. Assess whether the patient has taken the medication previously.

5. Which of the following nursing actions will prevent adverse drug events?

   A. Use only the trade name when documenting medications.
   B. Crush long-acting medications if the patient has dysphagia.
   C. After receiving a verbal order, administer the medication and then write down the order.
   D. Use bar code technology according to institutional policy.

# MEDICATION ORDERS

Medication orders should include the full name of the patient; the name of the drug (preferably the generic name); the dose, route, and frequency of administration; and the date, time, and signature of the prescriber.

Orders in a health care facility may be typed into a computer (the preferred method) or handwritten on an order sheet in the patient's medical record. Occasionally, verbal or telephone orders are acceptable. When taken, they should be written on the patient's order sheet, signed by the person taking the order, and later countersigned by the prescriber. After the order is written, a copy is sent to the pharmacy, where the order is recorded and the drug is dispensed to the appropriate patient care unit. In many facilities, pharmacy staff prepares a computer-generated MAR for each 24-hour period.

For patients in ambulatory care settings, the procedure is essentially the same for drugs to be given immediately. For drugs to be taken at home, written prescriptions are given. In addition to the previous information, a prescription should include instructions for taking the drug (e.g., dose, frequency) and whether the prescription can be refilled. Prescriptions for Schedule II controlled drugs cannot be refilled.

To interpret medication orders accurately, the nurse must know commonly used abbreviations for routes, dosages, and times of drug administration (Table 3.2). As a result of medication errors that occurred because of incorrect or misinterpreted abbreviations, many abbreviations that were formerly commonly used are now banned or are no longer recommended by The Joint Commission, the ISMP, and other organizations concerned with increasing patient safety. Thus, it is safer to write out such words as "daily" or "three times daily"; "at bedtime," "ounce," "teaspoon," or "tablespoon"; or "right," "left," or "both eyes" rather than using abbreviations, in both medication orders and in transcribing orders to the patient's MAR. If the nurse cannot read the physician's order or if the order seems erroneous, he or she must question the order before giving the drug.

## TABLE 3.2

### Common Abbreviations

**Routes of Drug Administration**

| | |
|---|---|
| IM | intramuscular |
| IV | intravenous |
| PO | by mouth, oral |
| SL | sublingual |
| Sub-Q | subcutaneous |

**Drug Dosages**

| | |
|---|---|
| cc | cubic centimeter |
| g | gram |
| mg | milligram |
| mcg | microgram |
| mL | milliliter |
| oz | ounce |
| tbsp | tablespoon |
| tsp | teaspoon |

**Times of Drug Administration**

| | |
|---|---|
| ad lib | as desired |
| PRN | as needed |
| q4h | every 4 h |
| stat | immediately |

## NCLEX Success

6. **A nurse is administering an elixir. Which of the following measures is appropriate?**
   - A. microgram
   - B. milligram
   - C. milliliter
   - D. kilogram

7. **The nurse has administered lacosamide to the wrong patient. What is the first action the nurse should take?**
   - A. Assess the patient's vital signs and level of consciousness.
   - B. Notify the physician.
   - C. Fill out an incident report.
   - D. Call the respiratory therapist for administration of oxygen.

# DRUG PREPARATIONS AND DOSAGE FORMS

Drug preparations and dosage forms vary according to the drug's chemical characteristics, reason for use, and route of administration. Some drugs are available in only one dosage form, and others are available in several forms. Table 3.3 and the following section describe characteristics of various dosage forms.

**Dosage forms** of systemic drugs include liquids, tablets, capsules, suppositories, and transdermal and pump delivery systems. Systemic liquids are given orally, or PO (Latin *per os*, "by mouth"), or by injection. Those given by injection must be sterile.

Administration of tablets and capsules is PO. Tablets contain active drug plus binders, colorants, preservatives, and other substances. Capsules contain active drug enclosed in a gelatin capsule. Most tablets and capsules dissolve in the acidic fluids of the stomach and are absorbed in the alkaline fluids of the upper small intestine. **Enteric-coated** tablets and capsules are coated with a substance that is insoluble in stomach acid. This delays dissolution until the medication reaches the intestine, usually to avoid gastric irritation or to keep the drug from being destroyed by gastric acid. Tablets for sublingual (under the tongue) or buccal (held in cheek) administration must be specifically formulated for such use.

Several **controlled-release** dosage forms and drug delivery systems are available, and more continue to be developed. These formulations maintain more consistent serum drug levels and allow less frequent administration, which is more convenient for patients. Controlled-release oral tablets and capsules are called

**TABLE 3.3**

## Drug Dosage Forms

| Dosage Forms and Their Routes of Administration | Characteristics | Considerations/Precautions |
|---|---|---|
| **Tablets** | | |
| *Regular:* PO, gastrointestinal (GI) tube (crushed and mixed with water) | • Contain active drug plus binders, dyes, preservatives<br>• Dissolve in gastric fluids | 8 oz of water recommended, to promote dissolution and absorption |
| *Chewable:* PO | Colored and flavored, mainly for young children | Children may think tablets are candy; keep out of reach to avoid accidental overdose |
| *Enteric coated:* PO | Dissolve in the small intestine; mainly used for medications that cause gastric irritation | Do not crush; instruct patients not to chew or crush |
| *Extended release* (XL) (also called sustained release [SR], long acting [LA], and other names): PO | Slowly absorbed; effects prolonged, usually 12–24 hours<br>Contain relatively large amounts of active drug | **Warning:** Crushing to give orally or through a GI tube administers an overdose, with potentially serious adverse effects or death! *Never crush*; instruct patients not to chew or crush |
| *Sublingual:* Under the tongue | Dissolve quickly | |
| *Buccal:* Held in cheek | Medication absorbed directly into the bloodstream and exerts rapid systemic effects | Few medications formulated for administration by SL or buccal routes |
| **Capsules** | | |
| *Regular:* PO | Contain active drug, fillers, and preservatives | 8 oz of fluid recommended to promote dissolution and absorption |
| | Gelatin capsules dissolve in gastric fluid and release medication | |
| *Extended release* (XL); sustained release (SR); long-acting (LA): PO | Slowly absorbed; effects prolonged, usually 12–24 hours<br>Contain relatively large amounts of active drug | **Warning:** Emptying a capsule to give the medication orally or through a GI tube administers an overdose, with potentially serious adverse effects or death! Instruct patients not to bite, chew, or empty these capsules |
| **Solutions** | | |
| *Oral:* PO, GI tube | Absorbed rapidly because they do not need to be dissolved | Use of appropriate measuring devices and accurate measurement is extremely important |
| *Parenteral:* IV, IM, Sub-Q, intradermal | Medications and all administration devices must be sterile<br>IV produces rapid effects; Sub-Q is used mainly for insulin and heparin; IM is used for only a few drugs; intradermal is used mainly to inject skin-test material | Use of appropriate equipment and accurate measurement is extremely important. Insulin syringes should always be used for insulin, and tuberculin syringes are recommended for measuring small amounts of other drugs |
| **Suspensions** | | |
| PO, Sub-Q (e.g., NPH, Lente insulins) | Particles of active drug are suspended in a liquid; the liquid must be rotated or shaken before measuring a dose | Drug particles settle to the bottom on standing. If not remixed, the liquid vehicle is given rather than the drug dose |
| **Dermatologic Creams, Lotions, Ointments**<br>Topically to skin | Most are minimally absorbed through skin and exert local effects at the site of application; some (e.g., skin patches) are absorbed and exert systemic effects | *Formulations vary with intended uses and are not interchangeable.*<br>When removed from the patient, skin patches must be disposed of properly to prevent someone else from being exposed to the active drug remaining in the patch |

*(Continued on page 46)*

**TABLE 3.3**

**Drug Dosage Forms** (Continued)

| Dosage Forms and Their Routes of Administration | Characteristics | Considerations/Precautions |
|---|---|---|
| Solutions and Powders for Oral or Nasal Inhalation, Including Metered Dose Inhalers (MDIs) | Oral inhalations are used mainly for asthma; nasal sprays for nasal allergies (allergic rhinitis). Effective with less systemic effect than oral drugs Deliver a specified dose per inhalation | Several research studies indicate that patients often do not use MDIs correctly; correct use is essential to obtaining therapeutic effects and avoiding adverse effects. |
| Eye Solutions and Ointments | *Should be sterile* Packaged in small amounts for individual use | Can be systemically absorbed and cause systemic adverse effects |
| Throat Lozenges | Used for cough and sore throat | |
| Ear Solutions | Used mainly for ear infections | |
| Vaginal Creams and Suppositories | Used to treat vaginal infections | |
| Rectal Suppositories and Enemas | • Suppositories may be used to administer sedatives, analgesics, and laxatives <br> • Medicated enemas may be used for constipation or inflammatory bowel diseases | Effects somewhat unpredictable because absorption is erratic |

by a variety of names (e.g., timed release, sustained release, extended release), and their names usually include CR, SR, XL, or other indications that they are long-acting formulations. Most of these formulations are given once or twice daily. Some drugs (e.g., alendronate for osteoporosis, fluoxetine for major depression) are available in formulations that deliver a full week's dosage in one oral tablet. Because controlled-release tablets and capsules contain high amounts of drug intended to be absorbed slowly and act over a prolonged period of time, they should never be broken, opened, crushed, or chewed. Such an action allows the full dose to be absorbed immediately and constitutes an overdose, with potential organ damage or death. **Transdermal** (skin patch) formulations include systemically absorbed clonidine, estrogen, fentanyl, and nitroglycerin. These medications are slowly absorbed from the skin patches over varying periods of time (e.g., 1 week for clonidine and estrogen). Pump delivery systems may be external or implanted under the skin and refillable or long acting without refills. Pumps are used to administer insulin, opioid analgesics, antineoplastics, and other drugs.

Solutions, ointments, creams, and suppositories are applied topically to the skin or mucous membranes. They are formulated for the intended route of administration. For example, several drugs are available in solutions for nasal or oral inhalation; they are usually self-administered as a spray into the nose or mouth.

Many combination products containing fixed doses of two or more drugs are also available. Commonly used combinations include analgesics, antihypertensive drugs, and cold remedies. Most are oral tablets, capsules, or solutions.

## CALCULATING DRUG DOSAGES

When calculating drug dosages, the importance of accuracy cannot be overemphasized. Accuracy requires basic skills in mathematics, knowledge of common units of measurement, and methods of using data in performing calculations.

## Systems of Measurement

The most commonly used system of measurement is the metric system, in which the meter is used for linear measure, the gram for weight, and the liter for volume. One milliliter (mL) equals 1 cubic centimeter (cc), and both equal 1 gram (g) of water. The household system, with units of drops, teaspoons, tablespoons, and cups, is infrequently used in health care agencies but may be used at home. Table 3.4 lists some commonly used equivalent measurements.

**TABLE 3.4**

**Selected Equivalent Measurements**

| Metric | Household |
|---|---|
| **Weights** | |
| 1000 mcg = 1 mg | |
| 1000 mg = 1 g | |
| 30 g | 1 oz |
| 454 g | 1 lb |
| 1000 g = 1 kg | 2.2 lb |
| **Liquids** | |
| 1 mL = 1 cc | |
| 5 mL | 1 tsp |
| 30 mL | 2 tbsp or 1 oz |
| 250 mL | 1 cup or 8 oz |
| 500 mL | 1 pint |
| 1000 mL = 1 L | 1 quart |

A few drugs are ordered and measured in terms of units or milliequivalents (mEq). Units express biologic activity in animal tests (i.e., the amount of drug required to produce a particular response). Units are unique for each drug. For example, concentrations of insulin and heparin are both expressed in units, but there is no relation between a unit of insulin and a unit of heparin. These drugs are usually ordered in the number of units per dose (e.g., NPH insulin 30 units subcutaneously every morning or heparin 5000 units subcutaneously every 12 hours) and labeled in number of units per milliliter (U 100 insulin contains 100 units/mL; heparin may have 1000, 5000, or 10,000 units/mL). Milliequivalents express the ionic activity of a drug. Drugs such as potassium chloride are ordered and labeled in the number of milliequivalents per dose, tablet, or milliliter.

## Mathematical Calculations

Most drug orders and labels are expressed in metric units of measurement. If the amount specified in the order is the same as that on the drug label, no calculations are required, and preparing the right dose is a simple matter. For example, if the order reads "ibuprofen 600 mg PO" and the drug label reads "ibuprofen 600 mg per tablet," it is clear that one tablet is to be given.

What happens if the order calls for a 600-mg dose and 200-mg tablets are available? The question is, "How many 200-mg tablets are needed to give a dose of 600 mg?" In this case, the answer can be readily calculated mentally to indicate three tablets. This is a simple example that also can be used to illustrate mathematical calculations. This problem can be solved by several acceptable methods; the following formula is presented because of its relative simplicity for students lacking a more familiar method.

$$\frac{D}{H} = \frac{X}{V}$$

$D$ = desired dose (dose ordered, often in milligrams)
$H$ = on-hand or available dose (dose on the drug label; often in mg per tablet, capsule, or milliliter)
$X$ = unknown (number of tablets, in this example)
$V$ = volume or unit (one tablet, in this example)

$$\frac{600 \text{ mg}}{200 \text{ mg}} = \frac{X \text{ tablet}}{1 \text{ tablet}}$$

Cross multiply:

$$200 \, X = 600$$

$$X = \frac{600}{200} = 3 \text{ tablets}$$

What happens if the order and the label are written in different units? For example, the order may read "amoxicillin 0.5 g" and the label may read "amoxicillin 500 mg/capsule." To calculate the number of capsules needed for the dose, the first step is to convert 0.5 g to the equivalent number of milligrams or convert 500 mg to the equivalent number of grams. *The desired or ordered dose and the available or label dose must be in the same units of measurement.* Using the equivalents

(i.e., 1 g = 1000 mg) listed in Table 3.4, an equation can be set up as follows:

$$\frac{1 \text{ g}}{1000 \text{ mg}} = \frac{0.5 \text{ g}}{X \text{ mg}}$$

$$X = 0.5 \times 1000 = 500 \text{ mg}$$

The next step is to use the new information in the formula, which then becomes

$$\frac{D}{H} = \frac{X}{V}$$

$$\frac{500 \text{ mg}}{500 \text{ mg}} = \frac{X \text{ capsules}}{1 \text{ capsule}}$$

$$500 \, X = 500$$

$$X = \frac{500}{500} = 1 \text{ capsule}$$

The same procedure and formula can be used to calculate portions of tablets or doses of liquids. These are illustrated in the following problems:

1. Order: 25 mg PO
   Label: 50-mg tablet

$$\frac{25 \text{ mg}}{50 \text{ mg}} = \frac{X \text{ tablet}}{1 \text{ tablet}}$$

$$50X = 25$$

$$X = \frac{25}{50} = 0.5 \text{ tablet}$$

2. Order: 25 mg IM
   Label: 50 mg in 1 cc

$$\frac{25 \text{ mg}}{50 \text{ mg}} = \frac{X \text{ cc}}{1 \text{ cc}}$$

$$50X = 25$$

$$X = \frac{25}{50} = 0.5 \text{ cc}$$

3. Order: 4 mg IV
   Label: 10 mg/mL

$$\frac{4 \text{ mg}}{10 \text{ mg}} = \frac{X \text{ mL}}{1 \text{ mL}}$$

$$10X = 4$$

$$X = \frac{4}{10} = 0.4 \text{ mL}$$

## Other Useful Formulas

Two other methods can be used to calculate the proper amount of medication to be administered to the patient. One is referred to as the two-ratio method. The other is referred to as the formula method.

### Two-Ratio Method

The first ratio in this method is the known equivalent. The second ratio is the ordered dose.

Suppose a patient is having increasing pain at the end-of-life. The home care nurse notifies the physician of the patient's increased pain, and he or she orders morphine sulfate to be increased from 5 to 10 mg. The home care nurse has a prescription for morphine sulfate, 5 mg per tablet. How many tablets of morphine sulfate should the home care nurse administer to the patient? The ratio is as follows (using the same mathematical symbols given earlier):

$$\frac{V}{H} = \frac{D}{X}$$

$$\frac{5 \text{ mg}}{1 \text{ tablet}} = \frac{10 \text{ mg}}{X \text{ mg}}$$

$$5X = 10$$

$$X = \frac{10}{5} = 2 \text{ tablets}$$

### Formula Method

The easiest method to understand and use is the formula method. Supposing a nurse has acetaminophen 325 mg in 5 mL and needs to administer 650 mg orally. How many milliliters are administered? The drug formula is as follows (using the same mathematical symbols given earlier):

$$\frac{D}{H} \times V = X$$

$$\frac{650 \text{ mg}}{325 \text{ mg}} \times 5 \text{ mL} = X = 10 \text{ mL}$$

## ROUTES OF ADMINISTRATION

Routes of administration depend on drug characteristics, patient characteristics, and desired responses. The major routes are oral (by mouth), **parenteral** (injected), and **topical** (applied to skin or mucous membrane). Each has advantages, disadvantages, indications for use, and specific techniques of administration (Table 3.5). Common parenteral routes are subcutaneous (Sub-Q), IM, and IV injections. Injections require special drug preparations, equipment, and techniques. The following section discusses general characteristics of the IV route, and Box 3.1 presents specific considerations.

| TABLE 3.5 | | | |
|---|---|---|---|
| **Routes of Drug Administration** | | | |
| **Route and Description** | **Advantages** | **Disadvantages** | **Comments** |
| Oral | Simple and can be used by most people<br>Convenient; does not require complex equipment<br>Relatively inexpensive | Dosage is unknown because some drug is not absorbed and some is metabolized in the liver before reaching the bloodstream.<br>Slow drug action<br>Irritation of gastrointestinal (GI) mucosa by some drugs | The oral route should generally be used when possible, considering the patient's condition and ability to take or tolerate oral drugs. |
| GI tubes (e.g., nasogastric, gastrostomy) | Allows use of GI tract in patients who cannot take oral drugs<br>Can be used over long periods of time, if necessary<br>May avoid or decrease injections | With nasogastric tubes, medications may be aspirated into the lungs.<br>Small-bore tubes often become clogged.<br>Requires special precautions to give correctly and avoid complications | Liquid preparations are preferred over crushed tablets and emptied capsules, when available.<br>Tube should be rinsed before and after instilling medication. |
| Subcutaneous (Sub-Q) injection—injection of drugs under the skin, into the underlying fatty tissue | Relatively painless<br>Very small needles can be used.<br>Insulin and heparin, commonly used medications, can be given Sub-Q. | Only a small amount of drug (up to 1 mL) can be given.<br>Drug absorption is relatively slow.<br>Only a few drugs can be given Sub-Q. | Sub-Q route is commonly used for only a few drugs because many drugs are irritating to Sub-Q tissues. Such drugs may cause pain, necrosis, and abscess formation if injected Sub-Q. |
| Intramuscular (IM) injection—injection of drugs into selected muscles | May be used for several drugs<br>Drug absorption is rapid because muscle tissue has an abundant blood supply. | A relatively small amount of drug (up to 3 mL) can be given.<br>Risks of damage to blood vessels or nerves if needle is not positioned correctly. | It is very important to use anatomic landmarks when selecting IM injection sites. |

**TABLE 3.5**

## Routes of Drug Administration (Continued)

| Route and Description | Advantages | Disadvantages | Comments |
|---|---|---|---|
| Intravenous (IV) injection—injection of a drug into the bloodstream | Allows medications to be given to a patient who cannot take fluids or drugs by GI tract<br>Bypasses barriers to drug absorption that occur with other routes<br>Rapid drug action<br>Larger amounts can be given than by Sub-Q and IM routes<br>Allows slow administration when indicated | Time and skill required for venipuncture and maintaining an IV line<br>After it is injected, drug cannot be retrieved if adverse effects or overdoses occur.<br>High potential for adverse reactions due to rapid drug action and possible complications of IV therapy (i.e., bleeding, infection, fluid overload, extravasation)<br>Phlebitis and thrombosis may occur and cause discomfort or pain, take days or weeks to subside, and limit the veins available for future therapy. | The nurse should wear latex gloves to start IV infusions, for protection against exposure to blood-borne pathogens.<br>Phlebitis and thrombosis result from injury to the endothelial cells that form the inner lining (intima) of veins and may be caused by repeated venipunctures, the IV catheter, hypertonic IV fluid, or irritating drugs. |
| Topical administration—application to skin or mucous membranes. Application to mucous membranes includes drugs given by nasal or oral inhalation; by instillation into the lungs, eyes, or nose; and by insertion under the tongue (sublingual), into the cheek (buccal), and into the vagina or rectum. | With application to intact skin, most medications act at the site of application, with little systemic absorption or systemic adverse effects.<br>Some drugs are given topically for systemic effects (e.g., medicated skin patches). Effects may last several days, and the patches are usually convenient for patients.<br>With application to mucous membranes, most drugs are well and rapidly absorbed. | Some drugs irritate the skin or mucous membranes and cause itching, rash, or discomfort.<br>With inflamed, abraded, or damaged skin, drug absorption is increased, and systemic adverse effects may occur.<br>Application to mucous membranes may cause systemic adverse effects (e.g., beta-blocker eye drops, used to treat glaucoma, can cause bradycardia just as oral beta-adrenergic blockers can).<br>Specific drug preparations must be used for application to skin, eyes, and sublingual, buccal, vaginal, and rectal sites. | When available and effective, topical drugs are often preferred over oral or injected drugs, because of fewer and/or less severe systemic adverse effects. |

**BOX 3.1**    *Principles and Techniques With Intravenous Drug Therapy*

**Methods**

Intravenous (IV) injection or **IV** push is the direct injection of a medication into the vein. The drug may be injected through an injection site on IV tubing or an intermittent infusion device. Most IV push medications should be injected slowly. The time depends on the particular drug but is often 2 minutes or longer for a dose. Rapid injection should generally be avoided because the drug produces high blood levels and is quickly circulated to the heart and brain, where it may cause adverse or toxic effects. Although IV push may be useful with a few drugs or in emergency situations, slower infusion of more dilute drugs is usually preferred.

**Intermittent infusion** is administration of intermittent doses, often diluted in 50 to 100 mL of fluid and infused over 30 to 60 minutes. The drug dose is usually prepared in a pharmacy and connected to an IV administration set that controls the amount and flow rate. Intermittent infusions are often connected to an injection port on a primary IV line, through which IV fluids are infusing continuously. The purpose of the primary IV line may be to provide fluids to the patient or to keep the vein open for periodic administration of medications. The IV fluids are usually stopped for the medication infusion and then restarted. Drug doses may also be infused through an intermittent infusion device (e.g., a heparin lock) to conserve veins and allow freedom of motion between drug doses. The devices decrease the amount of IV fluids given to patients who do not need them [i.e., those who are able to ingest adequate amounts of oral fluids] and those who are at risk of fluid overload, especially children and older adults.

An intermittent infusion device may be part of an initial IV line or used to adapt a continuous IV for intermittent use. The devices include a heparin lock or a resealable adapter added to a peripheral or central IV catheter. These devices must be flushed routinely to maintain patency. If the IV catheter has more than one lumen, all must be flushed, whether being used or not. Saline is probably the most commonly used flushing solution; heparin may also be used if recommended by the device's manufacturer or required by institutional policy.

**Continuous infusion** indicates medications mixed in a large volume of IV fluid and infused continuously, over several hours. For example, vitamins and minerals [e.g., potassium chloride] are usually added to liters of IV fluids. Greater dilution of the drug and administration over a longer time decrease risks of accumulation and toxicity, as well as venous irritation and thrombophlebitis.

### Equipment

Equipment varies considerably from one health care agency to another. Nurses must become familiar with the equipment available in their work setting, including IV catheters, types of IV tubing, needles and needleless systems, types of volume-control devices, and electronic infusion devices [IV pumps].

**Catheters** vary in size [both gauge and length], design, and composition [e.g., polyvinyl chloride, polyurethane, silicone]. The most common design type is over the needle; the needle is used to start the IV, and then it is removed. When choosing a catheter to start an IV, one that is much smaller than the lumen of the vein is recommended. This allows good blood flow and rapidly dilutes drug solutions as they enter the vein. This, in turn, prevents high drug concentrations and risks of toxicity. Also, after a catheter is inserted, it is very important to tape it securely so that it does not move around. Movement of the catheter increases venous irritation and risks of thrombophlebitis and infection. If signs of venous irritation and inflammation develop, the catheter should be removed and a new one inserted at another site. Additional recommendations include application of a topical antibiotic or antiseptic ointment at the IV site after catheter insertion, a sterile occlusive dressing over the site, and limiting the duration of placement to a few days.

Many medications are administered through peripherally inserted central catheters [PICC lines] or central venous catheters, in which the catheter tips are inserted into the superior vena cava, next to the right atrium of the heart. Central venous catheters may have single, double, or triple lumens. Other products, which are especially useful for long-term IV drug therapy, include a variety of implanted ports, pumps, and reservoirs.

*If a catheter becomes clogged, do not irrigate it. Doing so may push a clot into the circulation and result in a pulmonary embolus, myocardial infarction, or stroke. It may also cause septicemia, if the clot is infected.*

**Needleless systems** are products with a blunt-tipped plastic insertion device and an injection port that opens. These systems greatly decrease needlestick injuries and exposure to blood-borne pathogens.

**Electronic infusion devices** allow amounts and flow rates of IV drug solutions to be set and controlled by a computer. Although the devices save nursing time because the nurse does not need to continually adjust flow rates, the biggest advantage is the steady rate of drug administration. The devices are used in most settings where IV drugs and IV fluids are administered, but they are especially valuable in pediatrics, where very small amounts of medication and IV fluid are needed, and in intensive care units, where strong drugs and varying amounts of IV fluid are usually required. Several types of pumps are available, even within the same health care agency. It is extremely important that nurses become familiar with the devices used in their work setting, so that they can program them accurately and determine whether or not they are functioning properly [i.e., delivering medications as ordered].

### Site Selection

IV needles are usually inserted into a vein on the hand or forearm; IV catheters may be inserted in a peripheral site or centrally. In general, recommendations are as follows:

- Start at the most distal location. This conserves more proximal veins for later use, if needed. Veins on the back of the hand and on the forearm are often used to provide more comfort and freedom of movement for patients.
- Use veins with a large blood volume flowing through them when possible. Many drugs cause irritation and phlebitis in small veins.
- When possible, avoid the antecubital vein on the inner surface of the elbow, veins over or close to joints, and veins on the inner aspect of the wrists. Reasons include the difficulty of stabilizing and maintaining an IV line at these sites and the fact that inner wrist venipunctures are very painful. *Do not perform venipuncture in foot or leg veins.* The risks of serious or fatal complications are too high.
- Rotate sites when long-term use [more than a few days] of IV fluid or drug therapy is required. Venous irritation occurs with longer duration of site use and with the administration of irritating drugs or fluids. When it is necessary to change an IV site, use the opposite arm if possible.
- Most IV drugs are prepared for administration in pharmacies, and this is the safest practice. When a nurse must prepare a medication, considerations include the following points.
- Only drug formulations manufactured for IV use should be given IV. Other formulations contain various substances that are not sterile, pure enough, or soluble enough to be injected into the bloodstream. *In recent years, there have been numerous reports of medication errors resulting from IV administration of drug preparations intended for oral use!* Such errors can and should be prevented. For example, when liquid medications intended for oral use are measured or dispensed in a syringe [as they often are for children, for adults

| BOX 3.1 | *Principles and Techniques With Intravenous Drug Therapy* [Continued] |
| --- | --- |

with difficulty in swallowing tablets and capsules, or for administration through a gastrointestinal [GI] tube], the syringe should have a blunt tip that will not connect to or penetrate IV tubing injection sites.

- Use sterile technique during all phases of IV drug preparation.
- Follow the manufacturer's instructions for mixing and diluting IV medications. Some liquid IV medications need to be diluted prior to IV administration, and powdered medications must be reconstituted with the recommended diluent. The diluent recommended by the drug's manufacturer should be used because different drugs require different diluents. In addition, be sure any reconstituted drug is completely dissolved to avoid particles that may be injected into the systemic circulation and lead to thrombus formation or embolism. A filtered aspiration needle should be used when withdrawing medication from a vial or ampule, to remove any particles in the solution. The filter needle should then be discarded, to prevent filtered particles from being injected when the medication is added to the IV fluid. Filters added to IV tubing also help to remove particles.
- Check the expiration date on all IV medications. Many drugs have a limited period of stability after they are reconstituted or diluted for IV administration.
- IV medications should be compatible with the infusing IV fluids. Most are compatible with 5% dextrose in water or saline solutions.
- If adding a medication to a container of IV fluid, invert the container to be sure the additive is well mixed with the solution.
- For any IV medication that is prepared or added to an IV bag, label the medication vial or IV bag with the name of the patient, drug, dosage, date, time of mixing, expiration date, and the preparer's signature.

- Most IV medications are injected into a self-sealing site in any of several IV setups, including a scalp–vein needle and tubing; a plastic catheter connected to a heparin lock or other intermittent infusion device; or IV tubing and a plastic bag containing IV fluid.
- Before injecting any IV medication, be sure the IV line is open and functioning properly [e.g., catheter not clotted, IV fluid not leaking into surrounding tissues, phlebitis not present]. If leakage occurs, some drugs are very irritating to subcutaneous tissues and may cause tissue necrosis.
- Maintain sterility of all IV fluids, tubings, injection sites, drug solutions, and equipment coming into contact with the IV system. Because medications and fluids are injected directly into the bloodstream, breaks in sterile technique can lead to serious systemic infection [septicemia] and death.
- When two or more medications are to be given one after the other, flush the IV tubing and catheter [with the infusing IV fluid or with sterile 0.9% sodium chloride injection] so that the drugs do not come into contact with each other.
- In general, administer slowly to allow greater dilution of the drug in the bloodstream. Most drugs given by IV push [direct injection] can be given over 2 to 5 minutes, and most drugs diluted in 50 to 100 mL of IV fluid can be infused in 30 to 60 minutes.
- When injecting or infusing medications into IV solutions that contain other additives [e.g., vitamins, insulin, minerals such as potassium or magnesium], be sure the medications are compatible with the other substances. Consult compatibility charts [usually available on nursing units] or pharmacists when indicated.
- IV flow rates are usually calculated in mL/hour and drops per minute.

## Drugs for Injection

Injectable drugs must be prepared, packaged, and administered in ways to maintain sterility. Vials are closed containers with rubber stoppers through which a sterile needle can be inserted for withdrawing medication. Single-dose vials usually do not contain a preservative and must be discarded after a dose is withdrawn. Multiple-dose vials contain a preservative and may be reused if aseptic technique is maintained.

Ampules are sealed glass containers, the tops of which must be broken off to allow insertion of a needle and withdrawal of the medication. Broken ampules and any remaining medication are discarded. When vials or ampules contain a powder form of the drug, a sterile solution of water or 0.9% sodium chloride must be added and the drug dissolved before withdrawal. When available, a filter needle is used to withdraw the medication from an ampule or vial because broken glass or rubber fragments may need to be removed from the drug solution. The filter needle is replaced with a regular needle before injecting the patient.

Many injectable drugs (e.g., morphine, heparin) are available in prefilled syringes with attached needles. These units are

inserted into specially designed holders and used like other needle–syringe units.

 **QSEN Alert: Safety**

It is important to note that many such units, especially those from the same manufacturer, are similar, and their use may lead to medication errors if the label is not read carefully.

## Equipment for Injections

Sterile needles and syringes are used to measure and administer parenteral medications; they may be packaged together or separately. Needles are available in various gauges and lengths. The term *gauge* refers to lumen size, with larger numbers indicating smaller lumen sizes. For example, a 25-gauge needle is smaller than an 18-gauge needle. Choice of needle gauge and length depends on the route of administration, the viscosity (thickness) of the solution to be given, and the size of the patient. Usually, a 25-gauge, 5/8-inch needle is used for Sub-Q injections, and a 22- or 20-gauge, 1½-inch needle is used for IM injections. Other needle sizes are available for special uses, such as for insulin or intradermal injections. When needles are used, avoid recapping them, and dispose of them in appropriate containers. Such containers are designed to prevent accidental needlestick injuries to health care and housekeeping personnel.

In many settings, needleless systems are used. These systems involve a plastic tip on the syringe that can be used to enter vials and injection sites on IV tubing. Openings created by the tip reseal themselves. Needleless systems were developed because of the risk of injury and spread of blood-borne pathogens, such as the viruses that cause acquired immunodeficiency syndrome and hepatitis B or C.

Syringes also are available in various sizes. The 3-mL size is often used. It is usually plastic and is available with or without an attached needle. Syringes are calibrated so that drug doses can be measured accurately. However, the calibrations vary according to the size and type of syringe.

Insulin and tuberculin syringes are used for specific purposes. Insulin syringes are calibrated to measure up to 100 units of insulin. Safe practice requires that *only* insulin syringes be used to measure insulin and that they be used for no other drugs. Tuberculin syringes have a capacity of 1 mL. They should be used for small doses of any drug because measurements are more accurate than with larger syringes.

## Sites for Injections

Common sites for subcutaneous injections are the upper arms, abdomen, back, and thighs (Fig. 3.3). Sites for IM injections are the deltoid, ventrogluteal, and vastus lateralis muscles. It should be noted that most health care agencies no longer allow the administration of IM injections in the dorsogluteal site. It is important to review the policies and procedures of the institution before administering medications utilizing that site. To select the proper injection sites, the anatomical landmarks are identified (Fig. 3.4). Common sites for IV injections are the veins on the back of the hands and on the forearms (Fig. 3.5). Less common sites include intradermal (into layers of the skin), intra-arterial (into arteries), intra-articular (into joints), and intrathecal (into spinal fluid). Nurses may perform intradermal and intra-arterial injections (if an established arterial line is present); physicians perform intra-articular and intrathecal injections.

**QSEN Alert: Safety**

In the past 10 years, it has been recommended that the dorsogluteal site for intramuscular (IM) injections not be utilized for the administration of IM medications. It has been determined that the dorsogluteal site poses an increased risk of injury due to the close proximity to the sciatic nerve. The ventrogluteal site is preferred because it is away from the sciatic nerve and large blood vessels. The ventrogluteal site is also less painful due to the lack of large blood vessels and nerve fibers.

### *Clinical Application 3.3*

- Ms. Baranski's IV line has infiltrated and will not be restarted. Her physician has ordered hydrocodone/acetaminophen (Vicodin) 500 mg by mouth every 6 hours as needed (PRN) for pain, as well as ketorolac. In the event the pain is severe, the nurse can administer ketorolac 15 mg IM every 6 hours PRN. Five hours after receiving the Vicodin, the patient rates her pain as 9 on a scale of 1 to 10. The nurse decides to administer the ketorolac. The only ketorolac available is 30 mg/1 mL. How much ketorolac should be administered?

### NCLEX Success

8. A patient is to receive lamotrigine 300 mg by mouth two times per day. The pharmacy has delivered 50-mg tablets. How many tablets should the nurse administer each time?

   A. 2 tablets
   B. 4 tablets
   C. 6 tablets
   D. 8 tablets

**Figure 3.3.** Subcutaneous injection sites.

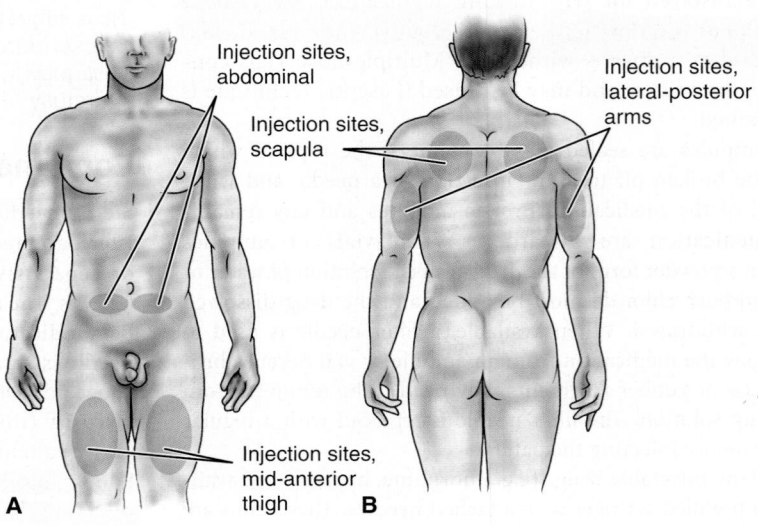

Injection sites, abdominal

Injection sites, scapula

Injection sites, lateral-posterior arms

Injection sites, mid-anterior thigh

A          B

**Figure 3.4.** Anatomic landmarks and intramuscular (IM) injection sites. **A.** Ventrogluteal muscle. **B.** Deltoid muscle. **C.** Vastus lateralis and rectus femoris muscle.

9. A nurse is preparing to administer a subcutaneous injection. What size needle should the nurse use to administer the injection?

   A. 18 gauge
   B. 20 gauge
   C. 23 gauge
   D. 25 gauge

10. A patient is to receive an intramuscular injection of ketorolac. Which of the following muscles should be avoided?

    A. deltoid
    B. dorsogluteal
    C. ventrogluteal
    D. vastus lateralis

# NURSING PROCESS IN DRUG THERAPY

As previously stated, the nursing process involves assessment, nursing diagnosis, planning and establishing goals for nursing care, interventions, and evaluation. Assessment and intervention are "action" phases, whereas analyzing assessment data, establishing nursing diagnoses and goals, and performing evaluations are "thinking" phases. However, knowledge and informed, rational thinking should underlie all data collection, decision making, and interventions.

## Assessment

**Assessment** involves collecting data about patient characteristics known to affect drug therapy. This includes

**Figure 3.5.** Veins of the hand and forearm that may be used to administer intravenous fluids and medications.

observing and interviewing the patient, interviewing family members or others involved in patient care, completing a physical assessment, reviewing medical records for pertinent laboratory and diagnostic test reports, and other methods. Initially (before drug therapy is started or on first contact), the nurse assesses age, weight, vital signs, health status, pathologic conditions, and ability to function in usual activities of daily living. In addition, the nurse assesses for previous and current use of prescription, nonprescription, and nontherapeutic (e.g., alcohol, caffeine, nicotine, cocaine, marijuana) drugs. A **medication history** (Box 3.2) is useful; it is possible to incorporate the information into any data collection tool. Specific questions and areas of assessment include the following:

- What are current drug orders?
- What does the patient know about current drugs? Is teaching needed?
- What drugs has the patient taken before? Include any drugs taken regularly, such as those for hypertension, diabetes mellitus, or other chronic conditions. Ask the patient about OTC drugs for colds, headaches, or indigestion, because some people do not think of these preparations as drugs.

- Has the patient ever had an allergic reaction to a drug? If so, what signs and symptoms occurred and how were they managed?
- Is the patient able to communicate verbally; can he or she swallow oral medications?
- Does the patient have pathologic conditions that influence drug therapy? For example, all seriously ill patients should be assessed for impaired function of vital organs.
- Assess for current use of herbal or dietary supplements (e.g., echinacea, glucosamine/chondroitin, vitamins). If so, ask for names, how much is taken and how often, for how long, their reason for use, and perceived benefits or adverse effects.

In addition to assessment data, the nurse uses progress notes (of any other health care providers), laboratory reports, and other sources to obtain baseline data for monitoring therapeutic or adverse drug effects. Laboratory tests of liver, kidney, and bone marrow function are often helpful because some drugs may damage these organs. Also, if liver or kidney damage exists, drug metabolism or excretion may be altered. The nurse consults authoritative sources for information about the patient's disease processes and ordered drugs, if needed.

After assessment data are obtained, they need to be analyzed to determine the patient's nursing care needs. Although listed as the first step in the nursing process for discussion purposes, assessment is a component of all steps and occurs with every contact with the patient. Ongoing assessment of a patient's health status and response to treatment is needed to determine whether nursing care requirements have changed. In general, nurses must provide care based on available information while knowing that assessment data are always relatively incomplete.

## Nursing Diagnosis

A **nursing diagnosis**, as developed by the North American Nursing Diagnosis Association, describes patient problems or needs. It is based on assessment data and individualized according to the patient's condition and the drugs prescribed. Thus, the number of nursing diagnoses needed to adequately reflect the patient's condition varies considerably. Because the NCLEX does not test nursing diagnoses, this textbook will focus on all aspects of the nursing process except nursing diagnoses.

## Planning/Goals

The **planning/goals** phase describes the expected outcomes of prescribed drug therapy. As a general rule, goals are stated in terms of patient behavior, not nurse behavior. For example, the patient will

- Receive or take drugs as prescribed
- Experience relief of signs and symptoms
- Avoid preventable adverse drug effects
- Self-administer drugs safely and accurately

| BOX 3.2 | *Medication History* |
|---------|---------------------|

Name _____ Age _____
Health problems, acute and chronic
Are you allergic to any medications?
If yes, describe specific effects or symptoms.

### Part 1: Prescription Medications

1. Do you take any prescription medications on a regular basis?
2. If yes, ask the following about each medication.

| | |
|---|---|
| Name | Dose |
| Frequency | Specific times |
| How long taken | Reason for use |

3. Do you have any difficulty in taking your medicines? If yes, ask to specify problem areas.
4. Have you had any symptoms or problems that you think are caused by your medicines? If yes, ask to specify.
5. Do you need help from another person to take your medicines?
6. Do you take any prescription medications on an irregular basis? If yes, ask the following about each medication.

| | |
|---|---|
| Name | Dose |
| Frequency | Reason |
| How long taken | |

### Part 2: Nonprescription Medications

Do you take over-the-counter medications?

| | | Medication | | |
|---------|--------|------|--------|-----------|
| Problem | Yes/No | Name | Amount | Frequency |
| Pain | | | | |
| Headache | | | | |
| Sleep | | | | |
| Cold | | | | |
| Indigestion | | | | |
| Heartburn | | | | |
| Diarrhea | | | | |
| Constipation | | | | |
| Other | | | | |

### Part 3: Social Drugs

| | Yes/No | Amount/day |
|---|--------|-----------|
| Coffee | | |
| Tea | | |
| Cola drinks | | |
| Alcohol | | |
| Tobacco | | |

### Part 4: Herbal or Dietary Supplements

Do you take any herbal or dietary supplements (e.g., ginkgo, glucosamine/chondroitin)? If so, ask for names, how much and how often taken, reason for use, perceived effectiveness, and any adverse effects.

- Verbalize essential drug information
- Keep appointments for monitoring and follow-up
- Use any herbal and dietary supplements with caution and report such use to health care providers

## Interventions

**Interventions** involve implementing planned activities and include any task performed directly with a patient or indirectly on a patient's behalf. Areas of intervention are broad and may include assessment, promoting adherence to prescribed drug therapy, and solving problems related to drug therapy, among others.

General interventions related to drug therapy include promoting health, preventing or decreasing the need for drug therapy, using nondrug measures to enhance therapeutic effects or decrease adverse effects, teaching, individualizing care, administering drugs, and observing patient responses. Some examples include

- Promoting healthful lifestyles in terms of nutrition, fluids, exercise, rest, and sleep
- Performing hand hygiene and other measures to prevent infection
- Ambulating, positioning, and exercising
- Assisting to cough and deep breathe
- Applying heat or cold
- Increasing or decreasing sensory stimulation
- Scheduling activities to promote rest or sleep
- Recording vital signs, fluid intake, urine output, and other assessment data

The intervention of teaching patients and caregivers about drug therapy is essential because most medications are self-administered and patients need information and assistance to use therapeutic drugs safely and effectively. Adequate knowledge, skill, and preparation are required to fulfill teaching responsibilities. Teaching aids to assist the nurse in this endeavor include Boxes 3.3, 3.4, and 3.5. Future chapters will address the patient teaching guidelines for medications discussed in each chapter.

Certain interventions exist with the administration of medications based on the route. No matter which route of medication administration is being implemented, it is important for the nurse to be uninterrupted during the time. The greatest number of failures within the medication administration system leading to medication errors occurs when the nurse is interrupted during administration of medications. Thomas, Donohe-Porter, and Fishbein (2017) conducted a study of the impact of interruptions, distractions, and cognitive load on procedure failures and medication errors. A minimum of one procedural error was noted in 81.3% of the medication administration episodes. In nurses who were interrupted while preparing or administering medications, errors occurred 67.1% of the time. The most common distractions reported by nurses were fatigue, unresolved patient issues, noise, and hunger. Nurses also reported greater frustration if they experienced distractions.

---

| **BOX 3.3** | ***Preparing to Teach a Patient or Caregiver*** |

- Assess learning needs, especially when new drugs are added or new conditions are being treated. This includes finding out what the person already knows about a particular drug. Do not assume that teaching is unneeded, even if the patient has been taking a drug for a while.
- Assess ability to manage a drug therapy regimen (i.e., read printed instructions and drug labels, remember dosage schedules, self-administer medications by ordered routes). A medication history (see Box 3.2) helps assess the patient's knowledge about drug therapy.
- From assessment data, develop an individualized teaching plan. This saves time for both nurse and patient by avoiding repetition of known material. It also promotes adherence to prescribed drug therapy.
- Try to decrease anxiety. Patients and caregivers may feel overwhelmed by complicated medication regimens. Provide positive reinforcement for effort.
- Choose an appropriate time (e.g., when the patient is mentally alert and not in acute distress from pain or other symptoms) and a place with minimal noise and distractions, when possible.
- Proceed slowly, in small steps; emphasize essential information; and provide opportunities to express concerns or ask questions.
- Provide a combination of verbal and written instructions, which is more effective than either alone. Minimize medical jargon, and be aware that patients may have difficulty understanding and retaining the material being taught because of the stress of the illness.
- When explaining a drug to a hospitalized patient, describe the name (preferably both the generic and a trade name), purpose, expected effects, and so on. The purpose can usually be stated in terms of symptoms to be relieved or other expected benefits. In many instances, the drug is familiar and can be described from personal knowledge. If the drug is unfamiliar, use available resources (e.g., drug reference books, computer drug databases, pharmacists) to learn about the drug and provide accurate information to the patient.
- When teaching a patient about medications to be taken at home, provide specific information and instructions about each drug, including how to take them and how to observe for beneficial and adverse effects. If adverse effects occur, teach them how to manage minor ones and which ones to report to a health care provider. In addition, discuss ways to develop a convenient routine for taking medications, so that usual activities of daily living are minimally disrupted. Allow time for questions, and try to ensure that the patient understands how, when, and why to take the medications.
- When teaching a patient about potential adverse drug effects, the goal is to provide needed information without causing unnecessary anxiety. Most drugs produce undesirable effects; some are minor, some are potentially serious. Many people stop taking a drug rather than report adverse reactions. If reactions are reported, it may be possible to continue the drug by reducing dosage, changing the time of administration, or other measures. If severe reactions occur, the drug should be stopped and the prescriber should be notified.
- Emphasize the importance of taking medications as prescribed throughout the teaching session and perhaps at times of other contacts. Common patient errors include taking incorrect doses, taking doses at the wrong times, omitting doses, and stopping a medication too soon. Treatment failure can often be directly traced to these errors.
- Reassess learning needs when medication orders are changed (e.g., when medications are added because of a new illness or stopped).

**BOX 3.4** *Patient Teaching Guidelines for Safe and Effective Use of Prescription Medications*

**General Considerations**

- Use drugs cautiously and only when necessary because all drugs affect body functions and may cause adverse effects.
- Use nondrug measures, when possible, to prevent the need for drug therapy or to enhance beneficial effects and decrease adverse effects of drugs.
- Do not take drugs left over from a previous illness or prescribed for someone else, and do not share prescription drugs with anyone else. The likelihood of having the right drug in the right dose is remote, and the risk of adverse effects is high in such circumstances.
- Keep all health care providers informed about all the drugs being taken, including over-the-counter (OTC) products and herbal or dietary supplements.
- Take drugs as prescribed and for the length of time prescribed; notify a health care provider if unable to take a medication. Therapeutic effects greatly depend on taking medications correctly. Altering the dose or time may cause underdosage or overdosage. Stopping a medication may cause a recurrence of the problem for which it was given or withdrawal symptoms. Some medications need to be tapered in dosage and gradually discontinued. If problems occur with taking a drug, report them to a health care provider. An adjustment in dosage or other aspect of administration may solve the problem.
- Follow instructions for follow-up care (e.g., office visits, laboratory or other diagnostic tests that monitor therapeutic or adverse effects of drugs). Some drugs require more frequent monitoring than do others. However, safety requires periodic checks with essentially all medications. With long-term use of a medication, responses may change over time with aging, changes in kidney function, and so on.
- Take drugs in current use (or an up-to-date list) to appointments with a health care provider.
- Get all prescriptions filled at the same pharmacy, when possible. This is an important safety factor in helping to avoid multiple prescriptions of the same or similar drugs and to minimize undesirable interactions of newly prescribed drugs with those already in use.
- Report any drug allergies to all health care providers, and wear a medical identification emblem that lists allergens.
- Ask questions (and write down the answers) about newly prescribed medications, such as the following:
  - What is the medicine's name?
  - What is it supposed to do (i.e., what symptoms or problems will it relieve)?
  - How and when do I take it, and for how long?
  - Should it be taken with food or on an empty stomach?
- While taking this medicine, should I avoid certain foods, beverages, other medications, or certain activities? (e.g., alcoholic beverages and driving a car should be avoided with medications that cause drowsiness or decrease alertness.)
  - What side effects are likely and what do I do if they occur?
  - Will the medication affect my ability to sleep or work?
  - What should I do if I miss a dose?
  - Is there a drug information sheet I can have?
- Store medications out of reach of children, and, to prevent accidental ingestion, never refer to medications as "candy."
- When taking prescription medications, talk to a doctor, pharmacist, or nurse before starting an OTC medication or herbal or dietary supplement. This is a safety factor to avoid undesirable drug interactions.
- Inform health care providers if you have diabetes or kidney or liver disease. These conditions require special precautions with drug therapy.
- If pregnant, consult your obstetrician before taking any medications prescribed by another physician.
- If breast-feeding, consult your obstetrician or pediatrician before taking any medications prescribed by another health care provider.

**Self-Administration**

- Develop a routine for taking medications (e.g., at the same time and place each day). A schedule that minimally disrupts usual activities is more convenient and more likely to be followed accurately.
- Take medications in a well-lighted area, and read labels of containers to ensure taking the intended drug. Do not take medications if you are not alert or cannot see clearly.
- Most tablets and capsules should be taken whole. If unable to take them whole, ask a health care provider before splitting, chewing, or crushing tablets or taking the medication out of capsules. Some long-acting preparations are dangerous if altered so that the entire dose is absorbed at the same time.
- As a general rule, take oral medications with 6 to 8 oz of water, in a sitting or standing position. The water helps tablets and capsules dissolve in the stomach, "dilutes" the drug so that it is less likely to upset the stomach, and promotes absorption of the drug into the bloodstream.
- Take most oral drugs at evenly spaced intervals around the clock. For example, if ordered once daily, take about the same time every day. If ordered twice daily or morning and evening, take about 12 hours apart.
- Follow instructions about taking a medication with food, on an empty stomach, or with other medications.
- If a dose is missed, most authorities recommend taking the dose if remembered soon after the scheduled time and omitting the dose if it is not remembered for several hours. If a dose is omitted, the next dose should be taken at the next scheduled time. Do not double the dose.

*(Continued on page 58)*

**BOX 3.4** *Patient Teaching Guidelines for Safe and Effective Use of Prescription Medications* (Continued)

- If taking a liquid medication (or giving one to a child), measure with a calibrated medication cup or measuring spoon. A dose cannot be measured accurately with household teaspoons or tablespoons because they are different sizes and deliver varying amounts of medication. If the liquid medication is packaged with a measuring cup that shows teaspoons or tablespoons, that should be used to measure doses, for adults or children.
- Use oral or nasal inhalers, eye drops, and skin medications according to instructions. If you are not clear how a medication is to be used, be sure to ask a health care provider. Correct use is essential for therapeutic effects.

- Report problems or new symptoms to a health care provider.
- Store medications safely, in a cool, dry place. Do not store them in a bathroom; heat, light, and moisture may cause them to decompose. Do not store them near a dangerous substance, which could be taken by mistake. Keep medications in the container in which they were dispensed by the pharmacy, where the label identifies it and gives directions. Do not mix different medications in a single container.
- Discard outdated medications; do not keep drugs for long periods. Drugs are chemicals that may deteriorate over time, especially if exposed to heat and moisture.

**BOX 3.5** *Patient Teaching Guidelines for Safe and Effective Use of Over-the-Counter Medications*

- Read product labels carefully. The labels contain essential information about the name, ingredients, indications for use, usual dosage, when to stop using the medication or when to see a health care provider, possible adverse effects, and expiration dates.
- Use a magnifying glass, if necessary, to read the fine print. If you do not understand the information on labels, ask a physician, pharmacist, or nurse.
- Do not take over-the-counter (OTC) medications longer or in higher doses than recommended.
- Note that all OTC medications are not safe for everyone. Many OTC medications warn against use with certain illnesses (e.g., hypertension). Consult a health care provider before taking the product if you have a contraindicated condition. If taking any prescription medications, consult a health care provider before taking any OTC drugs to avoid undesirable drug interactions and adverse effects. Some specific precautions include the following:
  - Avoid alcohol if taking sedating antihistamines, cough or cold remedies containing dextromethorphan, or sleeping pills. Because all these drugs cause drowsiness alone, combining any of them with alcohol may result in excessive and potentially dangerous sedation.
  - Avoid OTC sleeping aids if you are taking a prescription sedative-type drug (e.g., for anxiety or nervousness).
  - Ask a health care provider before taking products containing aspirin if you are taking an anticoagulant (e.g., warfarin).
  - Ask a health care provider before taking other products containing aspirin if you are already taking a regular dose of aspirin to prevent blood clots, heart attack, or stroke. Aspirin is commonly used for this

purpose, often in doses of 81 mg (a child's dose) or 325 mg.
- Do not take a laxative if you have stomach pain, nausea, or vomiting, to avoid worsening the problem.
- Do not take a nasal decongestant (e.g., pseudoephedrine [Sudafed], a multisymptom cold remedy containing phenylephrine products, that is, formulated to remove pseudoephedrine [e.g., Actifed], or an antihistamine–decongestant combination [e.g., Claritin D]) if you are taking a prescription medication for hypertension. Such products can raise blood pressure and decrease or cancel the blood pressure–lowering effect of the prescription drug. This could lead to severe hypertension and stroke. Loratadine (Claritin) is safe to take if you have hypertension.
- Store OTC drugs in a cool, dry place, in their original containers; check expiration dates periodically, and discard those that have expired.
- If pregnant, consult your obstetrician before taking any OTC medications.
- If breast-feeding, consult your pediatrician or family doctor before taking any OTC medications.
- For children, follow any age limits on the label.
- Measure liquid OTC medications with the measuring device that comes with the product (some have a dropper or plastic cup calibrated in milliliters, teaspoons, or tablespoons). If such a device is not available, use a measuring spoon. It is not safe to use household teaspoons or tablespoons because they are different sizes and deliver varying amounts of medication.
- Do not assume continued safety of an OTC medication you have taken for years. Older people are more likely to have adverse drug reactions and interactions because of changes in the heart, kidneys, and other organs that occur with aging and various disease processes.

The following sections present a list of guidelines for each route of medication administration. The process begins by checking the medication against the MAR (Fig. 3.6) and ends with the nurse documenting the medication administration (Fig. 3.7).

### Oral Medication Administration

- Position the patient to prevent aspiration (Fig. 3.8).
- Open the unit-dose package at the patient's bedside, and place the capsule or tablet in a medicine cup.
- For liquid medications, place the cup at eye level and pour the desired amount of solution (Fig. 3.9). (Shake the elixir before measuring, if recommended by the manufacturer.)
- Administer medications with or without food as indicated to enhance absorption.
- For infants and children, administer liquid medications with a syringe or dropper.
- Hold liquid medications if the patient cannot take anything orally (Latin *nil per os*, or nothing by mouth [NPO]) or is vomiting, sedated, or unconscious.

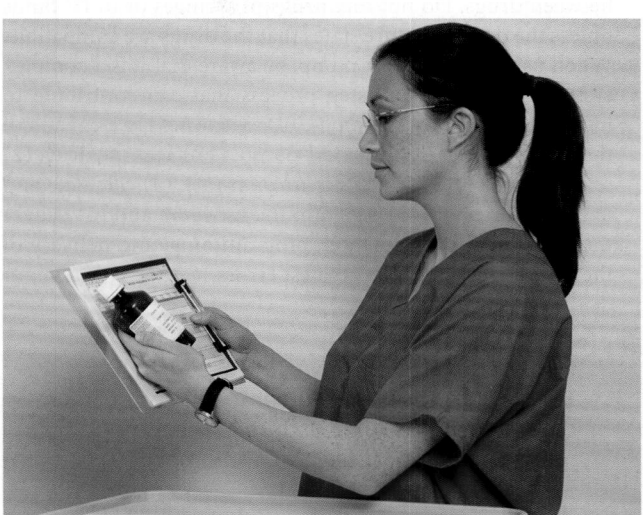

**Figure 3.6.** The nurse assesses the medication using the medication administration record.

**Figure 3.7.** The nurse documents the administration of the medication in the electronic medical record.

### Nasogastric or Gastrostomy Tube Medication Administration

- Administer liquid medications when available.
- Crush pills and dissolve in 30 mL of water. (Do not crush enteric-coated or extended-release medications, and do not empty the powdered medication in extended-release capsules.)
- Using a large catheter-tipped syringe, aspirate gastric fluid and assess pH.
- Rinse the tube and instill medication by gravity flow, and rinse the tube again with 50 mL of water. Do not allow the syringe to empty completely between additions of medication or water.
- Clamp off the tube from suction or drainage for at least 30 minutes.

### Subcutaneous Medication Administration

- Use only sterile drug preparations labeled or commonly used for subcutaneous injections.
- Use a 25-gauge, 5/8-inch needle for most subcutaneous injections.
- Select an appropriate injection site, based on patient preferences, drug characteristics, and visual inspection of possible

**Figure 3.8.** The nurse positions the patient to prevent aspiration.

**Figure 3.9.** The nurse pours the liquid medication at eye level.

sites. In long-term therapy, such as insulin, rotate injection sites. Avoid areas with lumps, bruises, or other lesions.
- Cleanse the site with an alcohol sponge.
- Tighten the skin or pinch a fold of skin and tissue between the thumb and fingers.
- Hold the syringe like a pencil, and insert the needle quickly at a 45- or 90-degree angle. Use enough force to penetrate the skin and subcutaneous tissue in one smooth motion.
- Release the skin so that both hands are free to manipulate the syringe. *Never aspirate when giving heparin subcutaneously.* The Centers for Disease Control and Prevention no longer recommends pulling back on the plunger to aspirate when administering a vaccine. However, in a 2016 study, Thomas, Mraz, and Rajcan (2016) surveyed 164 registered nurses and found that 74% still aspirate. "If parenteral medication has different administration rates, dose, viscosity, or other concerns when given intramuscularly versus intravenously, aspiration during IM administration should be implemented."
- Remove the needle quickly and apply pressure for a few seconds.

### Intramuscular Medication Administration
- Use only drug preparations labeled or commonly used for IM injections. Check label instructions for mixing drugs in powder form.
- Use a 1½-inch needle for most adults and 5/8- to 1½-inch needle for children, depending on the size of the patient.
- Use the smallest gauge needle that accommodates the medication. A 22-gauge is satisfactory for most drugs; a 20-gauge may be used for viscous medications.
- Select an appropriate injection site, based on the patient preferences, drug characteristics, anatomic landmarks, and visual inspection of possible sites. Rotate sites if frequent injections are being given, and avoid areas with lumps, bruises, or other lesions. *If the patient has had a mastectomy, do not administer any injection in the arm on the affected side.*
- Cleanse the site with an alcohol sponge.
- Tighten the skin, hold the syringe like a pencil, and insert the needle quickly at a 90-degree angle. Use enough force to penetrate the skin and subcutaneous tissue into the muscle in one smooth motion.
- Remove the needle quickly and apply pressure for several seconds.

### Clinical Application 3.4
- Ms. Baranski's pain is not controlled with the Vicodin, and administration of ketorolac is necessary. What is the proper procedure for giving an IM injection?

### Intravenous Medication Administration
- Use only drug preparations that are labeled for IV use.
- Check label instructions for the type and amount of fluid to use for dissolving or diluting the drug.
- Prepare drugs just before use, as a general rule. Also add drugs to IV fluids just before use.
- For venipuncture and direct injection into a vein, apply a tourniquet, select a site in the arm, cleanse the skin with an antiseptic (e.g., povidone–iodine or alcohol), insert the needle, and aspirate a small amount of blood into the syringe to be sure that the needle is in the vein. (*If the patient has had a mastectomy, do not administer any injection in the arm on the affected side.*) Remove the tourniquet, and inject the drug slowly. Remove the needle and apply pressure until there is no evidence of bleeding.
- For administration by an established IV line:
  1. Check the infusion for patency and flow rate. Check the venipuncture site for signs of infiltration and phlebitis before each drug dose.
  2. For direct injection, cleanse an injection site on the IV tubing, insert the needle, and inject the drug slowly.
  3. To use a volume-control set, fill it with 50 to 100 mL of IV fluid, and clamp it so that no further fluid enters the chamber and dilutes the drug. Inject the drug into the injection site after cleansing the site with an alcohol sponge and infuse, usually in 1 hour or less. After the drug is infused, add solution to maintain the infusion.
  4. To use a "piggyback" method, add the drug to 50 to 100 mL of IV solution in a separate container. Attach the IV tubing and needle. Insert the needle in an injection site on the main IV tubing after cleansing the site. Infuse the drug over 15 to 60 minutes, depending on the drug.
- When more than one drug is to be given, flush the line between drugs. Do not mix drugs in syringes or in IV fluids unless the drug literature states that the drugs are compatible.
- When using an IV smart pump, be aware that it is a complex system that has a multistep process that can contribute to medication errors. Giuliano (2018) identifies six elements of the process to set up the smart pump; (1) select the drug, (2) select the dose, (3) select the infusion rate, (4) calculate and order the infusion, (5) program the infusion, and (6) deliver the infusion. The calculation, programming, and delivery of the infusion result in the greatest errors.

### NCLEX Success

11. The patient receives regular insulin 5 units subcutaneously. To what degree is the syringe held for the injection? (Select all that apply.)
    A. 30 degrees
    B. 45 degrees
    C. 60 degrees
    D. 90 degrees

12. **How is a medication delivered by piggyback administered?**
    A. It is pushed into the IV line.
    B. It is retrograded into the IV line.
    C. It is injected intramuscularly after another medication.
    D. It is mixed with 50 to 100 mL of IV fluid in a separate container.

## Medication Administration to the Skin

- Use only drug preparations labeled for dermatologic use.
- Cleanse the skin, remove any previously applied medication, and apply the drug in a thin layer. For broken skin or open lesions, use sterile gloves, a tongue blade, or a cotton-tipped applicator to apply the drug.

## Medication Administration to the Eye

- Use drug preparations labeled for ophthalmic use. Wash hands, open the eye to expose the conjunctival sac, and drop the medication into the sac, without touching the dropper tip to anything. Provide tissue for blotting any excess drug. If two or more eye drops are scheduled at the same time, wait 1 to 5 minutes before instillations.
- With children, prepare the medication, place the child in a head-lowered position, steady the hand holding the medication against the child's head, gently retract the lower lid, and instill the medication in the conjunctival sac.

## Medication Administration to the Nose

- Have the patient hold his or her head back and drop the medication into the nostrils. Give the amount ordered.
- With children, place in a supine position with the head lowered, instill the medication, and maintain the position for 2 to 3 minutes. Then place the child in the prone position.

## Medication Administration to the Ear

- Open the ear canal in adults by pulling the ear up and back for adults.
- Open the ear canal in children by pulling the ear down and back for children.
- Drop the medication on the side of the ear canal.

## Medication Administration to the Rectum

- Lubricate the end with a water-soluble lubricant, wear a glove or finger cot, and insert into the rectum the length of the finger. Place the suppository next to the mucosal wall.
- If the patient prefers and is able, provide supplies for self-administration.

## Medication Administration to the Vagina

- Use gloves or an applicator for insertion. If an applicator is used, wash thoroughly with soap and water after each use.
- If the patient prefers and is able, provide supplies for self-administration.

## Evaluation

**Evaluation** involves determining the patient's response in relation to stated goals and expected outcomes. Some outcomes can be evaluated within a few minutes of drug administration (e.g., relief of acute pain after administration of an analgesic), but most require longer periods of time. Over time, the patient is likely to experience brief contacts with many health care providers, which increases the difficulty of evaluating outcomes of drug therapy. However, it is possible to manage difficulties by using appropriate techniques and criteria of evaluation.

General techniques include directly observing the patient's status; interviewing the patient or others about the patient's response to drug therapy; and checking appropriate medical records, including medication records and diagnostic test reports.

General criteria include progress toward stated outcomes, such as relief of symptoms, accurate administration, avoidance of preventable adverse effects, and compliance with instructions for follow-up monitoring by a health care provider. Specific criteria indicate the parameters that must be measured to evaluate responses to particular drugs (e.g., blood sugar with antidiabetic drugs, blood pressure with antihypertensive drugs).

## INTEGRATING EVIDENCE-BASED PRACTICE WITH THE NURSING PROCESS

Evidence-based nursing practice requires a conscientious and continuing effort to provide high-quality care to patients by obtaining and analyzing the best available scientific evidence from research. Then, the scientific evidence is integrated with the nurse's clinical expertise and the patient's preferences and values to yield "best practices" for a patient with a particular disease process or health problem.

**Evidence-based practice** (EBP) may include any step of the nursing process, and it does not accept tradition or "that's the way we've always done it" as sufficient rationale for any aspect of nursing care. Requirements for implementing EBP include

- Using research. Although professional nurses have always been encouraged to use research, EBP structures and formalizes the process. The nurse must use computer skills to search for the best evidence in making decisions about patient care. The search needs to be systematic; obtained data need to be critically analyzed for quality and relevance to the clinical situation.
- Keeping up-to-date in regard to research studies related to one's area of clinical practice. This includes reading research reports and analyzing them to determine their applicability.
- Considering levels of evidence to support clinical decision making. Level A is the strongest level.
- Interpreting research evidence in relation to one's clinical expertise and patient choices to provide a scientific rationale for one's clinical decisions.
- Applying the available information to improve nursing care of an individual or group of patients.
- Evaluating the effectiveness of application—did the intervention improve the patient's condition?

## HERBAL AND DIETARY SUPPLEMENTS

Complementary and alternative therapies, including herbal and dietary supplements, can be helpful in patient care. However, they can potentiate or negate the effects of prescribed medications, and it is important that the nurse evaluate the effects in a particular patient. Herbal and dietary supplements are commonly used, and patients who take them are likely to be encountered in any clinical practice setting. Herbal medicines, also called botanicals, phytochemicals, and nutraceuticals, are derived from plants. Other dietary supplements may be derived from a variety of sources. The 1994 Dietary Supplement Health and Education Act (DSHEA) defined a dietary supplement as "a vitamin, a mineral, an herb or other botanical used to supplement the diet." Under this law, herbs can be labeled according to their possible effects on the human body, but the products cannot claim to diagnose, prevent, relieve, or cure specific human diseases unless approved by the FDA.

It has become evident that nurses need to know about their patient's use of herbal and dietary supplements to provide safe care. An additional impetus came from the IOM, which released a report on complementary and alternative medicine (CAM) in 2005 in which it recommended that "health profession schools incorporate sufficient information about…CAM into the standard curriculum at all levels to enable licensed professionals to competently advise their patients about CAM." The National Center for Complementary and Integrative Health, an agency of the U.S. Department of Health and Human Services and National Institutes of Health, funds and conducts research on CAM therapies. It seeks to answer questions on complementary health approaches. As Saper (2018) states, the increased usage of herbs and supplements is related to the belief that these substances will enhance health, diminish memory loss, and decrease arthritic pain and fatigue. The FDA (2018) has also warned of the increased risk of drug interactions with the use of herbal supplements or complementary and alternative therapies. The dietary supplements can affect the absorption, metabolism, and distribution of prescribed or OTC medications. For example, combining St. John's Wort with a selective serotonin reuptake inhibitor will put the patient at risk for the development of serotonin syndrome.

More specifically, there are five major concerns associated with the nursing role in relation to herbal products and drug therapy, as follows:

1. Many of the products may not be safe because active ingredients and effects on humans are often unknown. Some contain heavy metals (e.g., lead) and other contaminants (e.g., pesticides); some contain prescription or nonprescription drugs. In addition, ingredients are not standardized and often differ from those listed on the product label.

2. Use of supplements may keep the patient from seeking treatment from a health care provider when indicated. This may allow disease processes to worsen and be more difficult to treat.

3. The products may interact with prescription drugs to decrease therapeutic effects or increase adverse effects. Dangerous interactions have been identified with St. John's wort and some herbs that affect blood clotting mechanisms.

4. Most products have not been studied sufficiently to evaluate their safety or effectiveness. In many studies, the products have not been standardized in terms of types or amounts of active ingredients. In addition, most reported studies have been short-term and with few subjects.

5. Many patients who use supplements do not tell their health care providers. This omission can lead to dangerous interactions when the supplements are combined with prescription or OTC drugs.

In general, nurses need to have an adequate knowledge base to assess and assist patients who use herbal products to do so safely. To develop and maintain a knowledge base, nurses (and patients) need to seek information from authoritative, objective sources rather than product labels, advertisements, or personal testimonials from family members, friends, or celebrities. Some resources are listed below:

- Commonly used supplements, some of which are described in Table 3.6. Later chapters describe selected supplements with some scientific support for their use in more detail. For example, Chapter 16 discusses some products reported to be useful in relieving pain, fever, inflammation, or migraines.

## TABLE 3.6

## Herbal and Dietary Supplements

| Name/Uses | Characteristics | Remarks |
|---|---|---|
| **Black Cohosh** | | |
| Most often used to relieve symptoms of menopause (e.g., flushes, vaginal dryness, irritability) | Well tolerated; in overdose may cause nausea, vomiting, dizziness, visual disturbances, and reduced pulse rate | The World Health Organization identified the treatment of profuse sweating, irritability, and sleep disorders (Boyle, 2018). |
| May also relieve premenstrual syndrome (PMS) and dysmenorrhea | Most clinical trials done with Remifemin, in small numbers of women; other trade names include Estroven and Femtrol | Not recommended for use longer than 6 months |
| **Capsaicin** | | |
| Used to treat pain associated with neuralgia, neuropathy, and osteoarthritis | A topical analgesic that may inhibit the synthesis, transport, and release of substance P, a pain transmitter | Applied topically |
| Self-defense as the active ingredient in "pepper spray" | Derived from cayenne pepper | |
| | Adverse effects include skin irritation, itching, redness, and stinging | |

## TABLE 3.6

## Herbal and Dietary Supplements (Continued)

| Name/Uses | Characteristics | Remarks |
|---|---|---|
| **Chamomile** | | |
| Used mainly for antispasmodic effects in the GI tract; may relieve abdominal cramping<br>Decreases serum LDL cholesterol and triglycerides while raising HDL cholesterol (Heidary et al., 2018) | Usually ingested as a tea; may delay absorption of oral medications<br>May cause contact dermatitis and severe hypersensitivity reactions, including anaphylaxis, in people allergic to ragweed, asters, and chrysanthemums<br>May increase risks of bleeding | Few studies and few data to support use and effectiveness in GI disorders |
| **Chondroitin** | | |
| Arthritis | Derived from the trachea cartilage of slaughtered cattle<br>Usually taken with glucosamine<br>Adverse effects may include GI upset, nausea, and headache | Several studies support use |
| **Creatine** | | |
| Athletes take creatine supplements to gain extra energy, to train longer and harder, and to improve performance | An amino acid produced in the liver and kidneys and stored in muscles<br>Causes weight gain, usually within 2 weeks of starting use<br>Legal and available in health food stores as a powder to be mixed with water or juice, as a liquid, and as tablets and capsules | Not recommended for use by children because studies have not been done and effects are unknown<br>Nurses and parents need to actively discourage children and adolescents from using creatine supplements |
| **Echinacea** | | |
| Most often used for the common cold but also advertised for many other uses (immune system stimulant, anti-infective) | Many species, but *E. purpurea* most often used medicinally<br>Effects on immune system include stimulation of phagocytes and monocytes<br>Contraindicated in persons with immune system disorders<br>Hepatotoxic with long-term use | Hard to interpret validity of claims because various species and preparations used in reported studies<br>Some evidence (level B) to support use in patients with the common cold, with possibly shorter durations and less severe symptoms |
| **Feverfew** | | |
| Migraines, menstrual irregularities, arthritis | May increase risk of bleeding<br>May cause hypersensitivity reactions in people allergic to ragweed, asters, daisies, or chrysanthemums<br>May cause a withdrawal syndrome if use is stopped abruptly | Some studies support use in patients with migraine |
| **Garli** | | |
| Used to lower serum cholesterol and for other uses | Active ingredient thought to be allicin<br>Has antiplatelet activity and may increase risk of bleeding<br>Adverse effects include allergic reactions (asthma, dermatitis), dizziness, nausea, and vomiting | Some evidence that garlic has a small cholesterol-lowering effect; no reliable evidence to support other uses |
| **Ginger** | | |
| Used mainly to treat nausea, including motion sickness and postoperative nausea | Inhibits platelet aggregation; may increase clotting time<br>Gastroprotective effects in animal studies | Should not be used for morning sickness associated with pregnancy—may increase risk of miscarriage |

*(Continued on page 64)*

## TABLE 3.6

## Herbal and Dietary Supplements [Continued]

| Name/Uses | Characteristics | Remarks |
|---|---|---|
| **Ginkgo Biloba**<br>Used mainly to improve memory and cognitive function in people with Alzheimer's disease; may be useful in treating peripheral arterial disease | May increase blood flow to the brain and legs, improve memory, and decrease intermittent claudication (leg pain with walking)<br>Inhibits platelet aggregation; may increase risks of bleeding with any drug that has antiplatelet effects (e.g., aspirin)<br>Adverse effects include GI upset, headache, bleeding, and allergic skin reaction | Good evidence (level A) for small effects in treating dementia and claudication<br>NIH is conducting a clinical trial with more than 3000 volunteers to see if ginkgo prevents the onset of dementia (specifically Alzheimer's disease), slows cognitive decline and functional disability, and reduces the incidence of cardiovascular disease |
| **Ginseng**<br>Used to increase stamina, strength, endurance, and mental acuity | Has various pharmacologic effects that vary with dose and duration of use<br>Adverse effects include hypertension, nervousness, depression, insomnia, skin rashes, epistaxis, palpitations, and vomiting<br>May increase risks of bleeding with any drug that has antiplatelet effects (e.g., aspirin)<br>Increases risk of hypoglycemic reactions if taken with antidiabetic drugs<br>Should not be taken with other herbs or drugs that inhibit monoamine oxidase (e.g., St. John's wort, selegiline); headache, mania, and tremors may occur | Insufficient evidence to support use for any indication<br>A ginseng abuse syndrome, with insomnia, hypotonia, and edema, has been reported<br>Caution patients to avoid ingesting excessive amounts<br>Instruct patients with cardiovascular disease, diabetes mellitus, or hypertension to check with their health care provider before taking ginseng.<br>Instruct any patient taking ginseng to avoid long-term use. Siberian ginseng should not be used longer than 3 weeks |
| **Glucosamine**<br>Osteoarthritis | Usually used with chondroitin<br>Has beneficial effects on cartilage<br>Adverse effects mild, may include GI upset, drowsiness | Several studies support use |
| **Melatonin**<br>Used mainly for treatment of insomnia and prevention and treatment of jet lag | Several studies of effects on sleep, energy level, fatigue, mental alertness, and mood indicate some improvement, compared with placebo<br>Contraindicated in persons with hepatic insufficiency or a history of cerebrovascular disease, depression, or neurologic disorders<br>Adverse effects include altered sleep patterns, confusion, headache, sedation, and tachycardia | Patients with renal impairment should use cautiously. |
| **St. John's Wort**<br>Used for treatment of depression, advertised as an "herbal Prozac" | Active component may be hypericin or hyperforin<br>Adverse effects include confusion, dizziness, GI upset, and photosensitivity<br>Interacts with many drugs; can decrease effectiveness of birth control pills, anticancer drugs, antivirals used to treat acquired immunodeficiency syndrome (AIDS), and organ transplant drugs (e.g., cyclosporine) | Good evidence (level A) for improvement in mild to moderate depression; not effective in major or serious depression<br><br>Should not be combined with monoamine oxidase inhibitors or selective serotonin reuptake inhibitor antidepressants<br>Use has declined since serious herb–drug interactions reported |

### TABLE 3.6

## Herbal and Dietary Supplements (Continued)

| Name/Uses | Characteristics | Remarks |
|---|---|---|
| **Saw Palmetto** | | |
| Used to prevent and treat urinary symptoms in men with benign prostatic hyperplasia | May have antiandrogenic effects<br>Adverse effects may include GI upset and headache; diarrhea may occur with high doses | Some evidence (Level B) of small beneficial effects with doses of 320 mg/d |
| **Valerian** | | |
| Used mainly to promote sleep and allay anxiety and nervousness; also has muscle relaxant effects | Adverse effects with acute overdose or chronic use include blurred vision, drowsiness, dizziness, excitability, hypersensitivity reactions, and insomnia; also, risk of liver damage from combination products containing valerian and from overdoses averaging 2.5 g<br>Additive sedation if taken with other CNS depressants | Should not be combined with sedative drugs and should not be used regularly<br>Many extract products contain 40%–60% alcohol<br>Insufficient evidence to support use for treatment of insomnia |

CNS, central nervous system; GI, gastrointestinal; HDL, high-density lipoprotein; LDL, low-density lipoprotein; NIH, National Institutes of Health.

- Basic teaching guidelines about herbal and dietary supplements, which are presented in Box 3.6. This chapter provides general information. Later chapters have guidelines that may emphasize avoidance or caution in using supplements thought to interact adversely with prescribed drugs or particular patient conditions.

- Assessment guidelines. This chapter presents general information about the use or nonuse of supplements. Later chapters discuss specific supplements that may interact with particular drug group(s). For example, some supplements are known to increase blood pressure or risk of excessive bleeding.

---

**BOX 3.6**  *Patient Teaching Guidelines for General Information About Herbal and Dietary Supplements*

- Herbal and dietary products are chemicals that have druglike effects in people. Unfortunately, their effects are largely unknown and may be dangerous for some people because there is little reliable information about them. For most products, little research has been done to determine either their benefits or their adverse effects.

- The safety and effectiveness of these products are not regulated by laws designed to protect consumers, as are pharmaceutical drugs. As a result, the types and amounts of ingredients may not be identified on the product label. In fact, most products contain several active ingredients, and it is often not known which ingredient, if any, has the desired pharmacologic effect. In addition, components of plants can vary considerably, depending on the soil, water, and climate where the plants are grown. Quality is also a concern, as heavy metals (e.g., lead), pesticides, and other contaminants have been found in some products.

- These products can be used more safely if they are manufactured by a reputable company that states the ingredients are standardized (meaning that the dose of medicine in each tablet or capsule is the same).

- The product label should also state specific percentages, amounts, and strengths of active ingredients. With herbal medicines especially, different brands of the same herb vary in the amounts of active ingredients per recommended dose. Dosing is also difficult because a particular herb may be available in several different dosage forms (e.g., tablet, capsule, tea, extract) with different amounts of active ingredients.

- These products are often advertised as "natural." Many people interpret this to mean the products are safe and better than synthetic products. This is not true; "natural" does not mean safe, especially when taken concurrently with other herbals, dietary supplements, or drugs.

- When taking herbal or dietary supplements, follow the instructions on the product label. Inappropriate use or taking excessive amounts may cause dangerous side effects.

- Inform health care providers when taking any kind of herbal or dietary supplement to reduce risks of severe adverse effects or drug–supplement interactions.

- Most herbal and dietary supplements should be avoided during pregnancy or lactation and in young children.

- The American Society of Anesthesiologists recommends that all herbal products be discontinued 2 to 3 weeks before any surgical procedure. Some products (e.g., echinacea, feverfew, garlic, ginkgo, ginseng, valerian, and St. John's wort) can interfere with or increase the effects of some drugs, affect blood pressure or heart rhythm, or increase risks of bleeding; some have unknown effects when combined with anesthetics, other perioperative medications, and surgical procedures.

- Store herbal and dietary supplements out of the reach of children.

## Clinical Application 3.5

- Ms. Baranski says that a friend suggested that she take black cohosh for the hot flashes she is experiencing with menopause instead of the estrogen preparation her prescriber ordered. What information should the nurse teach Ms. Baranski regarding black cohosh in menopause?

## NCLEX Success

13. **During an initial nursing assessment, the patient reports that he is allergic to a particular medicine. What should the nurse ask the patient?**

    A. What symptoms occurred when you had the allergic reaction?
    B. Did you need to take epinephrine (Adrenalin)?
    C. Did your physician think this information needed to be communicated?
    D. Have you ever overdosed on this medication?

14. **How do nursing interventions increase safety and effectiveness of drug therapy?**

    A. by avoiding the use of nondrug measures during drug therapy
    B. by using multiple drugs to relieve most symptoms or problems
    C. by teaching patients about their drug therapy
    D. by avoiding excessive instructions

15. **What should the nurse keep in mind when evaluating a patient's response to drug therapy?**

    A. Few drugs cause adverse effects.
    B. Drugs may cause virtually any symptom or problem.
    C. Patients always report adverse effects.
    D. Therapeutic effects are more important than adverse effects.

## KEY CONCEPTS

- The rights of safe and accurate medication administration are the right drug, right dose, right patient, right route, right time, right reason, right documentation, right patient education, right evaluation, and right to refuse the medication.
- Basic knowledge and techniques for accurate medication administration include knowledge of the medication, knowledge of the patient, interpretation of the prescriber orders and labels of medication container, calculations and measurements of doses, and correct techniques for all dosage forms and routes of administration.
- Each health care facility has a system for distributing drugs.
- Each nurse must follow the legal aspects of medication administration and the policies of the health care institution for the administration of medications.
- The nurse must accurately calculate dosages to be administered to prevent medication errors that are harmful to the patient.

- The nurse must identify potential sources of medication errors and intervene to prevent errors when possible.
- The nurse needs to apply the nursing process in drug therapy and all aspects of nursing care.
- The nurse is responsible for safe and effective administration of medications and the observation of the medication's response.
- Instructing patients and caregivers about medications is imperative for safe and effective patient care.
- Evidence-based nursing practice requires continued searching for and using best practice interventions, as based on research and other authoritative evidence.
- It is important for the nurse to understand the effect herbal remedies and dietary supplements have and the related interactions with medications.

## CLINICAL REASONING CASE STUDY

**The Scenario**

Marquita Jones is a nursing student at Maryville University. She is beginning her pediatric clinicals, on a neurological division, and is concerned about her ability to calculate pediatric drug dosages. Dr. Frandsen has developed the following case study and questions for Marquita to complete. The case study states, Isaiah Thomas is a 3-year-old child admitted to the pediatric neurological division following his first seizure. The prescriber has ordered a loading dose of phenytoin (Dilantin) orally. Isaiah is to receive a loading dose of 15 mg/kg. Isaiah weighs 36 lb. The medication is an elixir in a 125 mg/5 mL suspension.

- What is the rationale for administering a loading dose to Isaiah?
- How much phenytoin does the nurse administer to this patient in a loading dose?
- How does the nurse administer the medication to this 3-year-old patient?
- The patient eventually takes 5 mg/kg orally in two divided doses. How much phenytoin is the nurse then administering?

**Assessing Drug Information**

- A loading dose of phenytoin is administered to Isaiah following his first seizure to provide him with a larger than regular dosage of phenytoin. This will provide Isaiah with a more rapid therapeutic blood level of phenytoin. The loading dose of phenytoin will assist in preventing another seizure.
- To determine the proper loading dose, Marquita must complete the following steps to accurately calculate Isaiah's dosage of phenytoin.
  - Determine Isaiah's weight in kilograms.
  - Determine the number of milliliters to administer.
    - Divide the number of pounds by 2.2 kg to determine Isaiah's weight in kilograms.
  - Determine the number of milligrams to be administered.

  - $\dfrac{kg}{mg} = \dfrac{mg}{X}$

  - Determine the number of milliliters to administer.

    - D = Desired dose (dose in milligrams)
      H = On hand or available dose
      X = Unknown
      V = volume or unit
      $\dfrac{D}{H} = \dfrac{X}{V}$

**Nursing Actions**

- Marquita completed the following calculations:

  $\dfrac{36\ lb}{2.2\ kg} = 16.36\ (16.4)\ kg$, the patient's weight

  $\dfrac{1\ kg}{15\ mg} = \dfrac{16.4\ kg}{X\ mL}$   X = 246 mg, the amount of phenytoin

  $\dfrac{125\ mg}{5\ mL} = \dfrac{246\ mg}{X\ mL}$

  $X = \dfrac{1230}{125} = 9.84\ mL$ loading dose

- Marquita identifies the steps to administer phenytoin elixir to Isaiah.
  - She will obtain a 10 mL syringe and a tuberculin syringe.
  - She will draw up 9 mL of phenytoin in the 10 mL syringe.
  - She will draw up 0.84 mL in the tuberculin syringe.
  - She will place the 10 mL syringe in Isaiah's cheek and slowly push the plunger to administer the phenytoin in the side of his mouth, allowing him to swallow the phenytoin.
  - She will then do the same with the tuberculin syringe.

- Determine the total number of milligrams of phenytoin to be administered daily.

  $\dfrac{1\ kg}{5\ mg} = \dfrac{15\ kg}{X\ mg}$

  X = 82 mg

  $\dfrac{125\ mg}{5\ mL} = \dfrac{41\ mg}{X\ mL}$

  $X = \dfrac{205\ mg}{mL} \div 125\ mg$

  X = 1.64 mL per dose of phenytoin

Visit the Point® at **http://thePoint.lww.com/Frandsen12e** for answers to NCLEX Success questions (in Appendix A), answers to Clinical Application Case Studies (in Appendix B), and more!

## REFERENCES AND RESOURCES

Boyle, M. (2018). An evidence-based review of the botanicals: Bilberry fruit, black cohosh, and St. John's wort in clinical practice. *Journal of the Australian Traditional-Medicine Society, 24*(2), 89–93.

Centers for Disease Control and Prevention. (2018). *Epidemiology and prevention of vaccine-preventable diseases*. Retrieved from https://www.cdc.gov/vaccines/pubs/pinkbook/vac-admin.html

Giuliano, K. K. (2018). Intravenous smart pumps usability issues, intravenous medication administration error, and patient safety. *Critical Care Nurse Clinics of North America, 20*, 215–244.

Heidary, M., Yazdanpanahi, Z, Dabbaghmanesh, M. H., Parsanezhad, M., Emamghoreishi, M., & Akbarzadeh, M. (2018). Effect of chamomile on lipid and hormonal related parameters among women of reproductive age with polycystic ovary syndrome. *Journal of Research in Medical Sciences, 23*, 33. Retrieved from http://www.jmsjournal.net

Hilton, L. (2018). 4 tips to prevent errors: Applying certain technologies can help you avoid human error. *Dermatology Times*.

Hinkle, J. H., & Cheever, K. H. (2018). *Brunner & Suddarth's textbook of medical-surgical nursing* (14th ed.). Philadelphia, PA: Lippincott Williams & Wilkins.

Institutes of Medicine Committee on the Use of Complementary and Alternative Medicine in the United States. (2005). *Complementary and alternative medicine in the United States*. Washington, DC: National Academies Press. Retrieved April 25, 2016, from http://www.nap.edu/catalog/11182.html

Institutes of Medicine of the National Academies. (2004). *Keeping patients safe: Transforming the work environment of nurses*. Washington, DC: National Academies Press.

Institute of Medicine of the National Academies. (2007). *Preventing medications errors*. Washington, DC: National Academies Press.

National Center for Complementary and Integrative Health. (2015). About NCCIH.

Oscanoa, T. J., Lizaraso, F., & Carvagal, A. (2017). Hospital admissions due to adverse drug reactions in the elderly. *European Journal of Clinical Pharmacology, 73*, 759–770.

Saper, R. B. (2018). *Overview of herbal medicine and dietary supplements*. Up-To-Date, Wolters Kluwer.

Strudwick, G., Reisdorfer, E., Warnock, C., Kalia, K., Sulkers, H., Clark, C., et al. (2018). Factors associated with barcode medication administration technology that contribute to patient safety: An integrative review. *Journal of Nursing Care Quality, 33*(1), 79–85.

Taylor, C., Lynn, P., & Bartlett, J. L. (2019). *Fundamentals of nursing: The art and science of person-centered care* (9th ed.). Philadelphia, PA: Lippincott Williams & Wilkins.

The Joint Commission National Patient Safety Guidelines Do Not Use List. (2018). Retrieved November 4, 2018, from https://www.joint-commission.org/facts_about_do_not_use_list/

The Joint Commission Patient Safety Systems. (2016). Comprehensive Accreditation Manual for Hospitals Update 2. Retrieved from http://www.jointcommission.org/patient_safety_systems_chapter_for_the_hospital_program/

Thomas, L., Donohue-Porter, P., & Fishbein, J. S. (2017). Impact of interruptions, distractions, and cognitive load on procedural failures and medication administration errors. *Journal of Nursing Care Quality, 32*(4), 309–317.

Thomas, C. M., Mraz, M., & Rajcan, L. (2016). Blood aspiration during IM injection. *Clinical Nursing Research, 25*(4), 549–559.

U. S. Food & Drug Administration. (2018). *Mixing medications and dietary supplements can endanger your health*. Retrieved from https://www.fda.gov/ForConsumers/ConsumerUpdates/ucm420349.htm

Zhu, J., & Weingart, S. N. (2017). *Prevention of adverse drug events in hospitals*. Up-to-Date, Wolters Kluwer.

# Drug Therapy Throughout the Lifespan

# Pharmacology and the Care of Infants and Pediatric Patients

## LEARNING OBJECTIVES

*After studying this chapter, you should be able to:*

1. Identify key characteristics of pediatric pharmacotherapy in children from birth to 18 years of age.
2. Describe the evolution of pediatric pharmacotherapy and the purpose of federal legislation in the development of current practice standards.
3. Describe methods for determining accurate pediatric dosing.
4. Explain differences in pharmacodynamic variables between children and adults.
5. Explain pharmacokinetic differences between children and adults.
6. Describe nursing interventions, based on child growth and development standards, to help ensure safe and effective medication administration to children.

## CLINICAL APPLICATION CASE STUDY

Billy Lee, a 6-year-old boy, complains of shortness of breath. He is restless with expiratory wheezes. His mother reports that her son has a 2-day history of coldlike symptoms, with a productive cough and fever.

## KEY TERMS

**Blood–brain barrier:** barrier in the central nervous system composed of capillaries with tight bonds, which acts to prevent the passage of most ions and large-molecular-weight compounds, including some drugs, from the blood to the brain

**Body surface area:** surface of a human body expressed in square meters

**Child(ren):** person(s) between birth and 18 years of age

**Total body water:** amount of water within the body (both intracellular and extracellular)

## INTRODUCTION

**Children** naturally differ from adults. However, therapeutic indications and effects of drug therapy are similar in many ways. It is essential that nurses and other health care professionals understand the many ways children differ from adults because this presents a challenge in medication dosing, administration, and management. For example, physiologic changes throughout development influence both the pharmacodynamic and pharmacokinetic actions of medications. A child's immature organ systems mean that molecular binding, receptor reactions, and intended actions of medications may not mimic those known for adults. Variables in absorption, distribution, metabolism, and excretion further complicate the medication process, and taken together, these differences indicate a need for vigilance in nursing management of pediatric pharmacotherapy.

Pediatrics includes the evaluation and management of all children—patients from birth to age 18. This group is further divided into five subgroups (Table 4.1), and each developmental group is characterized by a select set of physiologic changes that affect pharmacotherapy. The younger the patient, the greater the variation in medication action. Of course, many pediatric patients cannot verbalize adverse effects, and good assessment skills are crucial in evaluating all pediatric patients. It is also important to remember that as patients go through puberty, they begin to respond more like adults physiologically, but they are still immature psychologically and may lack the ability to dose, administer, or evaluate the effectiveness of their medications.

## DRUG SAFETY IN PEDIATRICS

### Legislation and Drug Testing

Many challenges in pediatric medication management involve both the known physical differences in pediatric patients and the unknown action of drugs; these problems are often related to the lack of adequate information. Historically, researchers used only adults to test medications, and prescribers simply assumed that smaller doses would elicit the same results in smaller patients. However, since 1994, the pediatric pharmacotherapy began to change. In 1994, the U.S. Food and Drug Administration (FDA) enacted the Pediatric Rule, which compelled the pharmaceutical industry to submit all known data about the pharmacokinetics, safety, and efficacy of medications used for children (Boslaugh, 2016). The FDA continued the trend toward safer medication management for children when it passed the *U.S. Food and Drug Administration Modernization Act of 1997* (FDAMA) followed by the *2002 Best Pharmaceuticals for Children Act* (BPCA). These acts provide incentives to companies

who perform research to determine the safety, efficacy, dosage, and unique risks associated with medications for children (Avant, Wharton, & Murphy, 2018; USFDA, 2015).

The FDA continued to press for more research and better practice standards by issuing the *Pediatric Research Equity Act of 2003* and renewing the BPCA in 2007. Since these measures were put in place, the research has now uncovered other gaps in pediatric studies, including a need for pediatric formulations, preclinical studies, and pediatric outcome measures. The *Food and Drug Administration Safety and Innovation Act (FDASIA)*, enacted in 2012, gives an overview of laws and regulations and an assessment of the pediatric program and suggestions for improving pediatric research.

With the current emphasis on increased patient safety and decreased medication-related adverse events, it is especially important for pediatric practitioners to be at the forefront of current research and practice standards in pediatric pharmacotherapy. Prescribers must still treat pediatric patients with drugs for which they lack information; therefore, they must practice good assessment, dosing, and evaluation during the administration of any medication to a pediatric patient.

### Clinical Application 4.1

- Are Billy's medications chosen based on empiric evidence obtained from solid research performed on other 6-year-old boys?

### Calculating Drug Dosages

The basis of pediatric drug dosing is weight, and determining drug dosages is highly dependent on the growth and development changes that occur across the lifespan. The prescriber uses weight alone to calculate pediatric dosages in an expression such as gentamicin 5 mg/kg/24 h or determines the **body surface area** (BSA), the surface of a human body expressed in square meters, using the child's weight (Table 4.2). Then the prescriber calculates the dose based on a known adult dose by using the following equation: pediatric dose = BSA/1.73 × adult dose.

### TABLE 4.1
#### Pediatric Age Groups

| Group | Age |
|---|---|
| Premature infant | <38 wk gestational age |
| Neonate | From full-term newborn 0 to 4 wk of age |
| Infant | From >4 wk to 1 y of age |
| Child | From >1 to 12 y of age |
| Adolescent | 13–18 y of age |

### TABLE 4.2
#### Body Surface Area*

| Age | Average BSA (m²) |
|---|---|
| Neonate (newborn) | 0.25 |
| Child, 2 y | 0.50 |
| Child, 9 y | 1.07 |
| Child, 10 y | 1.14 |
| Child, 12–13 y | 1.33 |
| Man (older than 18 y) | 1.90 |
| Woman (older than 18 y) | 1.60 |

*The following formula is used to calculate BSA:

$$BSA \ (m^2) = \sqrt{\frac{body \ weight \ (kg) - body \ height \ (cm)}{3600}}$$

# PHARMACOTHERAPY IN PEDIATRICS

## Pharmacodynamics

Pharmacodynamics involves drug actions on target cells and the resulting alterations in cellular reactions and functions. These actions occur because of chemicals that bind with receptors at the cellular level. Most of these receptors are proteins on the surface or within cells. Therefore, pharmacodynamic variables in pediatric patients are related to differences in target cell sites and changing numbers of protein receptors. Immature systems and changing body compositions mean that drugs affect children differently. Causes of pharmacodynamic variability across the lifespan include differences in body composition, immature organ systems, and genetics. **Total body water**, fat stores, and protein levels change throughout childhood and greatly influence the effectiveness of drugs in the pediatric population (Kear, 2017).

One example of a drug that has different pharmacodynamic actions in adults and children is the fetal disaster caused by the drug thalidomide in the 1960s. Thalidomide worked wonders for decreasing morning sickness in pregnant women. However, it was soon apparent that it had severe teratogenic (adverse) effects on the fetus. This antiemetic drug, which was used to prevent vomiting in pregnant women, resulted in tragic limb abnormalities and often death for the fetus. Pharmacodynamic differences of positive drug action in adult females and negative toxic effects to their unborn fetuses illustrate one of the many challenges in medication management of children versus adults.

Another example of pharmacodynamic issues in younger patients involves antidepressants. Initially, prescribers assumed that these drugs, widely used successfully in treating adults, could be safely used therapeutically in adolescents and children. However, by 2004, the FDA had found that these medications needed a **BLACK BOX WARNING ◆** stating that antidepressants may play a causal role in inducing suicidality in pediatric patients. Ten years later, practitioners are still debating the use and risk of these drugs in children and adolescents because many feel the warning should be eliminated or amended based on recent research (Gupta, Gersing, Erkanli, & Burt, 2016).

---

### *Clinical Application 4.2*

- What nursing interventions would take priority in Billy's care?

---

### NCLEX Success

1. Billy's medications should be individualized to ensure the best outcome. Individualizing drug therapy for a child involves which one of the following?

   A. assessing the child's age and development level
   B. administering an adult drug selection and dosage and observing for adverse reactions
   C. deferring treatment until a better pediatric drug is developed
   D. determining the child's diet and exercise needs

2. Billy is unable to tolerate montelukast (Singulair) for his asthma and had a rash and abdominal pain. However, this drug works well for his father, who experiences no adverse effects. Billy's physician is aware that the boy's reaction to the medication is most likely a reflection of his

   A. inability to understand the purpose of the drug
   B. hope that he will not have to take the drug
   C. inability to swallow pills
   D. genetic variability

## Pharmacokinetics

Pharmacokinetics refers to the processes of drug absorption, distribution, metabolism, and elimination. The organ systems in pediatric patients vary widely in their growth and maturation compared with adult patients. This, in turn, greatly affects a prescriber's ability to dose pediatric drugs effectively. Newborn infants are a prime example because they process drugs very inefficiently. However, by age 12, children have grown and matured sufficiently to develop pharmacokinetic responses that resemble those of adults. To account for immature or impaired body systems in neonates and younger children, it is often necessary to dramatically change drug therapies. Drug effects are more varied in children and must be anticipated and carefully evaluated for after administration.

### *Absorption*

Drug absorption in pediatrics is affected by the age of the child, gastric emptying, intestinal motility, routes of administration, and skin permeability. Careful thought to proper route, good monitoring, and anticipation of potential adverse effects can help ensure intended outcomes are seen with administered drugs.

Age is one important factor in absorption of medications. During pregnancy, many drugs cross the placenta, and they may harm the fetus. The possible teratogenic risk is coded for each medication as a pregnancy risk category from A to X, with A being the safest and X known to be dangerous ("do not use"). During infancy, neonates have delayed, irregular gastric emptying and reduced gastric acidity. This delay potentially leads to greatly increased drug levels. The decreased acidity results in greater absorption of acid-labile medications or reduced absorption of weakly acidic medications.

In addition, the route of administration greatly affects absorption. Prescribers avoid the use of intramuscular (IM) injections in pediatric patients because of the associated pain and unpredictable absorption. Low blood flow to skeletal muscles and weak muscle contractions also contribute to the erratic absorption of IM injections. Thin and highly permeable skin increases the rate of absorption of topical drugs, and careful administration is important to avoid toxicity.

### *Distribution*

Distribution of drugs in pediatric patients is dependent on percentage of body water, liver function, degree of protein binding, and the development of the **blood–brain barrier**. Children differ from adults in the percentages of total body water. This includes the amount of water within the body, including in the intracellular and extracellular compartments, plus the water in the gastrointestinal and urinary tracts (Kear, 2017) (Fig. 4.1). In adults,

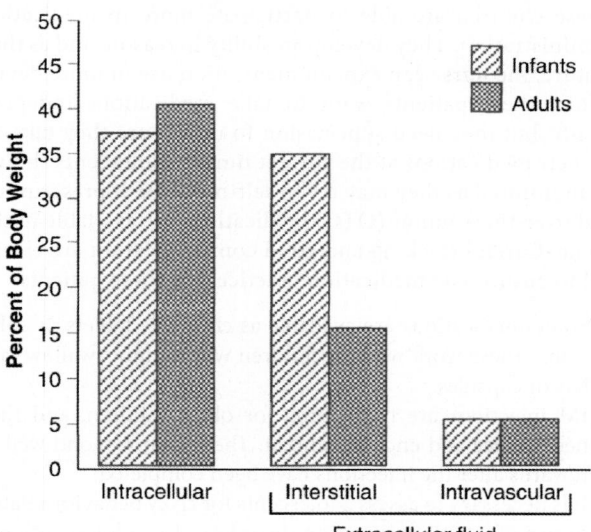

**Fluid Distribution in Body**

**Figure 4.1.** Graph indicating distribution on fluid in body compartments. Comparison between the infant and adult fluid distribution in body compartments shows that the adult total is about 60% of body weight, whereas the infant total is more than 70% of body weight. [Reprinted with permission from Hatfield, N. (2008). *Broadribb's introductory pediatric nursing* (7th ed., Fig. 6-5). Philadelphia, PA: Wolters Kluwer Health.]

total body water is approximately 60%, whereas in newborns, it is approximately 80%. This difference means that water-soluble drugs such as atenolol (Tenormin) and penicillin (Penicillin-G) are diluted easily and readily moved into intercellular tissue. As a result, serum drug concentrations are lower, and increased dosages of water-soluble drugs may be necessary to maintain therapeutic drug levels in neonates and premature infants.

In infants, immature liver function leads to very low plasma protein levels, which limits the amount of protein binding by drugs. Consequently, the serum concentrations of highly protein-bound drugs, including phenytoin (Dilantin), warfarin (Coumadin), ampicillin, and morphine (Duramorph), may be higher than expected, and toxicity may occur. By the end of the first year, protein-binding ability is at the adult level, and its effect on drug distribution is no longer a concern.

The blood–brain barrier, which is composed of capillaries with tight bonds in the central nervous system (CNS), prevents the passage of most ions and large-molecular-weight compounds—including certain drugs—from the blood to the brain. Although this barrier protects the CNS, it can make drug delivery to the neurons more difficult. In neonates, the blood–brain barrier is poorly developed; thus, drugs and other chemicals easily affect the CNS in young infants. The nurse must assess for increased drug effects or toxic results from drug administration and must be alert for other chemicals or drugs that may cause unwanted CNS effects such as vital sign irregularities, sedation, excitability, and seizures.

### Metabolism

The enzyme cytochrome P450 (CYP450) in the liver metabolizes most drugs. In neonates, the ability to metabolize drugs is very low because of the immaturity of the liver and the resultant inability to break down drugs. To avoid toxicity, the prescriber

needs to calculate drug doses carefully, and the nurse must monitor infants and young children closely until the liver is more mature—by the end of the second year.

### Elimination

Excretion of most drugs occurs via the kidneys, and elimination in the urine follows. Young children have immature kidneys, a reduced glomerular filtration rate, and slower renal clearance. Neonates are especially prone to increased levels of drugs that are eliminated primarily by the kidneys; the prescriber should dose appropriately and the nurse monitor carefully until renal function reaches maturity—between 1 and 2 years of age.

---

### Clinical Application 4.3

- How does the nurse know whether interventions designed to help Billy have been successful? What assessment data are warranted?

---

## NCLEX Success

3. For Billy's asthma, a prescriber has ordered albuterol (Proventil). Which one of the following important factors related to growth and development is most likely to affect absorption of this beta$_2$-adrenergic agonist?
   A. the ability of Billy to cough up his secretions
   B. the need to decrease the dose as Billy's age increases
   C. the need to monitor Billy for hypotension
   D. the ability of Billy and his caregivers to understand how to use the inhaler and spacer to administer the albuterol

4. A 3-month-old infant who receives fosphenytoin (Cerebyx) for a seizure disorder does not process this drug in the same way as an adult. Alterations in infant pharmacokinetics that influence drug action include which of the following concepts?
   A. Drug response in infants is slower and less rapid than that in adults.
   B. Neonates have a decreased response to drugs that affect the CNS.
   C. Infants have a decreased response to water-soluble drugs and an increased response to protein-bound drugs.
   D. By 3 months of age, drug response in infants is similar to that of adults.

## MEDICATION ADMINISTRATION IN PEDIATRICS

Administering medications to infants and children presents its own set of challenges because of difficulties in communication, cooperation, and adherence. Trends in growth and development serve as the basis for care across different age groups, and the nurse must continue to focus on safety in all activities involving drug administration.

## Infants

The focus in this age group is aimed at calculation of correct dosages, safety in administration, and teaching parents how to deliver medications correctly. This includes a few key points related to infant growth and development.

- Oral medications are administered with a dropper or oral syringe into the inner aspect of the cheek, giving children time to swallow the medication as it is instilled.
- Some practitioners prefer giving oral medications through a nipple with a small amount of formula or breast milk, but this is controversial. Some authorities believe that infants may then refuse feedings if they associate food with the taste of the medication.
- Infants lack well-developed muscles. Thus, care is practiced when medications or vaccinations can only be given by IM injections. Good practice involves using the smallest needle, preferably in the largest available muscle, the vastus lateralis.
- Many common medications come in suppository form, which makes administration easier in this age group.
- Comfort care is important with infants. They need holding and cuddling and are offered a pacifier with, or shortly after, medication administration.
- Intravenous (IV) sites for medication administration are often found in the scalp, hands, or feet and a 22- to 24-gauge needle is frequently used.

## Toddlers and Preschoolers

Toddlers are mobile and curious. Preschoolers are inquisitive and controlling. They love investigating but have short attention spans and want to exert their independence. The nurse involves toddlers and preschoolers in medication administration by having them hold items or choose the self-adhesive bandage or cup that will be used, but explanations should be short and simple, and adults need to control administration.

- To make oral medications more palatable, the nurse often mixes them with flavored syrups or fruit purees. Children may receive their favorite drink afterward.
- As the toddlers develop bigger muscle mass, IM injections can move from the vastus lateralis to the ventrogluteal area.
- Reaction to suppositories is strong. Therefore, explanations should be short, and for successful administration, an assistant may be necessary. For toddlers, IV sites in the scalp are still occasionally appropriate, but for older toddlers and preschoolers, the feet, the hands, or antecubital are preferable.

> **!** **QSEN Alert:** Safety for Infants and Toddlers
>
> The goal of the Pediatric Cough and Cold Safety Surveillance System, launched in 2008, was to understand the safety profile of cough and cold medications (CCMs). This led to voluntary relabeling of the dosing instructions of these products that specified "do not use in children less than 4 years old," a withdrawal of the concentrated infant formulations from manufacture, and reminders from the U.S. Food and Drug Administration to never use CCMs in children younger than 2 years of age.

## School-Aged Children and Adolescents

These children are able to participate more in medication administration. They develop an ability to reason, and as they mature, the nurse can explain medication use in more detail. Often, these patients want to take medications independently, but they need supervision to make sure they take all of their medications at the correct times. Adolescents should be monitored as they may try to self-medicate if prescription and over-the-counter (OTC) medications are available in the home. Careful tracking and good communication are essential to ensure safe medication practices for these patients.

- Some medications are available as chewable tablets or solutions. These work well for children who cannot swallow tablets or capsules.
- IM injections are frightening for older children, and they need praise and encouragement. They often respond well to rewards after the injections have been completed.
- It is necessary to assess adolescents for risky behavior related to use of laxatives in eating disorders. The adolescent's use of prescription and OTC medication abuse should also be assessed. It is important to assess the adolescent's use of alcohol or illegal drug use. Education on all of the effects of prescription, nonprescription, alcohol, and illegal drugs is imperative to promote patient safety.
- Important information about self-care related to medication administration are good teaching points for this age group. Adolescents need explanations about the use of acne medications and antibiotics, including adverse effects. The nurse should tell teenage girls who are taking birth control medications about possible decreased effectiveness with certain drugs and should also discuss the importance of preventive measures such as sun protection with many groups of medications.

> *Clinical Application 4.4*
>
> - What is the best way to teach Billy about his discharge plan, teach him how to use his inhaler, and review how to take his medications?

> **!** **QSEN Alert:** Safety for Pediatric Patients
>
> - Ensure that medications are dosed based on weight and calculated individually for each child.
> - Ensure that electronic medical records are standardized to allow only kilograms and centimeters for pediatric weight and height entries.
> - Use adequate measuring devices, graduated to tenths, for pediatric patients, and help make sure that these devices are available to caregivers.
> - Administer oral medications only in oral syringes.
> - Administer IV medications only in Luer lock syringes.
> - Order, dispense, and administer medications based on individual dosages in milligrams, micrograms, units, and so on, not on variables such as tablets or milliliters, for which the concentration may vary.
> - Administer IV medications using smart pump technology with safety systems enabled.

- Administer IV fluids and medications with syringe pump technology for smaller amounts over set times or at set rates, with safety systems enabled.
- Ensure a double-check system in prescribing, dispensing, and administering high-risk pediatric medications.
- Have access to current, pediatric-focused medication references.
- Collaborate with interdisciplinary team members on best practice solutions to pediatric medication management problems.
- Keep medications, including topicals and solutions, out of the reach of pediatric patients. Never store these in a crib or on a bedside table.
- Administer medications using a caring approach, involving knowledge of pediatric growth and development.
- Involve family or caregivers in the management of a child's medications, including teaching and demonstrating storage, safety, and proper administration of medications.

## NCLEX Success

1. **A nurse is teaching a parent how to administer analgesic eardrops at home to a toddler with acute otitis media. Which statements by the parent indicate that teaching has been successful?**
   A. "I will let my child squirt in the eardrops so he won't fight me and he can feel independent."
   B. "I will use the holding technique you showed me to administer the medication even if my child is fighting and screaming."
   C. "I will give my child cold medication so he won't keep getting stuffy ears."
   D. "I will give the eardrops in my child's mouth if he won't let me put it in his ear because that will work for the pain, too."
   E. "If my child is running a fever and in pain, I will give him an over-the-counter medication like acetaminophen (Tylenol) or ibuprofen (Motrin) according to the directions on the label."

## THE NURSING PROCESS

A concept map outlines the nursing process related to drug therapy considerations in this chapter. Additional nursing implications related to the disease process should also be considered in care decisions.

**Assessment**
- Record the age, weight, and height of the child. Drug dosages are based on these values.
- Assess allergies and determine family allergy history.
- Assess growth and development related to age, cognitive, psychosocial, physiologic, and nutritional status.
- Assess medication history.
- Assess family understanding and cognitive level.
- Assess ability of patient and family to adhere to medication regimen.

**Outcomes of Therapy**
The patient will
- Receive the correct drug dose based on weight (recorded in kilograms).
- Receive a drug by the best route based on growth and development and therapeutic expectations.
- With the parents or caregiver, understand medication administration, action, use, and adverse effects. The child should be involved in all aspects of medication management as warranted by cognitive and growth and development levels.
- Maintain medication adherence.

**Nursing Interventions**
- Use appropriate pediatric drug references.
- Monitor closely for side effects related to immature liver and kidney function.
- Teach patients, especially nonverbal, young, or developmentally delayed children, and parents and/or caregivers about medication dosage, administration, therapeutic effects, adverse effects, and precautions.
- Communicate with patients, based on cognitive and growth and development levels, as well as parents and/or caregivers about all aspects of medication management and planning for care.
- Communicate with interdisciplinary team to advocate for the pediatric patient and ensure therapeutic medication management.
- Instruct parents and/or caregivers about the risk of using over-the-counter and alternative therapies without first consulting a health care practitioner.
- Advise parents and/or caregivers about safety practices related to medication storage, access, and administration.

**Evaluation**
- Evaluate the patient's response to the medication regimen.
- Evaluate the patient's and caregiver's understanding of the medication regimen.
- Evaluate the ability of the patient and caregiver to adhere to the medication regimen.

## KEY CONCEPTS

- Federal legislation has resulted in increased testing, improved surveillance, and attention to medication effectiveness in the various pediatric age groups.
- Dosages of pediatric medications are calculated based on weight.
- Medications are dosed and administered, and their effectiveness is evaluated differently in pediatric patients because of physiologic differences across developmental levels.
- Pharmacodynamic variability is related to total body water, fat stores, and protein-carrying ability.
- Effects of drugs are longer and stronger in infants than in adults because of delayed gastric emptying and reduced gastric acidity.

- The risk of CNS effects related to drugs is higher in infants than in adults because of the immature blood–brain barrier.
- Water-soluble drugs lead to lower drug levels in infants than in adults. In contrast, protein-bound drugs lead to increased drug levels.
- Drug metabolism and excretion are decreased in infants compared with adults because of immature hepatic and renal function.
- The FDA has issued a **BLACK BOX WARNING** ◆ stating that antidepressants may play a causal role in inducing suicidality in pediatric patients.

## CLINICAL REASONING CASE STUDY

| | |
|---|---|
| **Meet the Patient** | Megan, a 7-month-old infant, has a 2-day history of vomiting and fever. She has only had one wet diaper today and just 8 oz of formula. Her mother is concerned that this illness may have started with an ear infection and is concerned about giving her daughter any medications. Megan lies on the examination table without crying but does smile and interact with her mother. Vital signs are temperature 102.4°F, heart rate 160 beats/minute, and respiratory rate 34/minute. In addition, she is pulling at her ears.<br>• What nursing interventions take priority?<br>• What medications does the nurse anticipate having to administer to Megan?<br>• What challenges are there in administering medications to Megan?<br>• What are key teaching points to address with Megan's mother? What outcomes will be expected from these nursing interventions?<br>• What outcomes will be expected from these nursing interventions? |
| **Assessing Drug Information** | • Obtain accurate height and weight.<br>• Monitor for changes in breathing or circulation.<br>• Assess level of pain using age-appropriate pain rating scale.<br>• Assess level of consciousness as a sign of worsening infection or dehydration.<br>• Assess supporting data: fussiness, restlessness, crying, parental input, vital signs, ability to take nutrition, and ability to sleep.<br>• Assess the response to the administration of analgesic ear drops, antipyretic agents, and antibiotic agents.<br>• Assess the patient's ability to breastfeed or tolerate formula.<br>• Assess skin turgor and urinary output. |
| **Nursing Actions** | • Administer analgesics such as acetaminophen to Megan.<br>  • Administer in liquid form if she is no longer vomiting.<br>  • Use rectal form if emesis continues. Cut or divide suppositories to deliver the proper dose, using adequate lubrication to an appropriate depth. Use proper technique to instill medication in the rectum.<br>• Demonstrate and teach the mother the proper holding and administration technique and allow verbalization of questions.<br>• Raise Megan's head or position her to lie on the unaffected ear.<br>• Demonstrate or explain proper use of heating pad, or compress to Megan's mother. Explain risk of burns or scalds if too hot or applied too long. Apply warm compress to affected ear.<br>• Administer analgesic eardrops. Use appropriate concentrations of liquid medications. Use a proper-sized administration device (such as the provided dropper) to administer correct dose. Use proper technique to instill liquid medication in the ear canal for age and developmental level.<br>• Explain to the mother that sucking with bottle or breastfeeding may cause pressure in the affected ear and increased pain. Pain assessment and treatment should emphasize maximizing feeding with peak of pain control medication effects.<br>• Administer antibiotics as directed.<br>• Educate the mother on all aspects of medication administration. |

Visit thePoint° at http://thePoint.lww.com/Frandsen12e for answers to NCLEX Success questions (in Appendix A), answers to Clinical Application Case Studies (in Appendix B), and more!

## REFERENCES AND RESOURCES

Alomari, A., Wilson, V., Davidson, P., & Lewis, J. (2015). Families, nurses and organisations contributing factors to medication administration error in paediatrics: A literature review. *International Practice Development Journal, 5*(1), 1–14.

Avant, D., Wharton, G., & Murphy, D. (2018). Characteristics and changes of pediatric therapeutic trials under the Best Pharmaceuticals for Children Act [BPCA]. *The Journal of Pediatrics, 192*, 8–12. doi:10.1016/j.jpeds.2017.08.048

Boslaugh, S. (2016). *The SAGE encyclopedia of pharmacology and society.* Los Angeles, CA: SAGE Publications, Inc.

Gillette, C., Rochich-Winston, N., Kuhn, J., Flesher, S., & Shepherd, M. (2016). Inhaler technique in children with asthma: A systematic review. *Academic Pediatrics, 16*(7), 605–615. doi:10.1016/j.acap.2016.04.006

Green, J., Wang, G., Reynolds, K., Banner, W., Bond, R., Kauffman, R., et al. (2017). Safety profile of cough and cold medication use in pediatrics. *Pediatrics, 139*(6), 1–8. doi:10.1542/peds.2016-3070

Gupta, S., Gersing, K. R., Erkanli, A., & Burt, T. (2016). Antidepressant regulatory warnings, prescription patterns, suicidality and other aggressive behaviors in major depressive disorder and anxiety disorders. *The Psychiatric Quarterly, 87*(2), 329–342. doi:10.1007/s11126-015-9389-8

Hockenberry, M., & Wilson, D. (2015). *Wong's nursing care of infants and children.* St. Louis, MO: Mosby Elsevier.

Institute for Safe Medication Practices (ISMP). (2015a). *2016–2017 Targeted medication safety best practices for hospitals.* Horsham, PA: ISMP.

Institute for Safe Medication Practices (ISMP). (2015b). *ISMP Part 1: Results of survey on pediatric medication safety, more is needed to protect hospitalized children from medication errors.* Retrieved from https://www.ismp.org/newsletters/acutecare/showarticle.aspx?id=110

Kear, T. M. (2017). Fluid and electrolyte management across the age continuum. *Nephrology Nursing Journal, 44*(6), 491–496.

Matalova, P., Urbanek, K., & Anzenbacher, P. (2016). Specific features of pharmacokinetics in children. *Drug Metabolism Reviews, 48*(1), 70–79. doi:10.3109/03602532.2015.1135941

Mosteller, R. D. (1987). Simplified calculation of body surface area. *The New England Journal of Medicine, 317*(17), 1098.

Paine, M. F. (2017). Therapeutic disasters that hastened safety testing of new drugs. *Clinical Pharmacology & Therapeutics, 101*(4), 430–434.

U.S. Department of Health and Human Services (USDHHS) & Agency for Healthcare Research and Quality Patient Safety (AHRQ). (2015). *Patient safety network (PSNet) Primer: Medication errors.* Retrieved from https://psnet.ahrq.gov/primers/primer/23

U.S. Food and Drug Administration (USFDA). (2015). *The Food and Drug Administration Safety and Innovation Act (FDASIA) Best Pharmaceuticals for Children Act and Pediatric Research Equity Act.* Retrieved from http://www.fda.gov/scienceresearch/specialtopics/pediatrictherapeuticsresearch/ucm509707.htm

# Pharmacology and the Care of Adults and Geriatric Patients

## CLINICAL APPLICATION CASE STUDY

Charles Franklin is a 75-year-old man with a diagnosis of an enlarged prostate. He has been experiencing insomnia for the past month and has begun taking acetaminophen in the form of Tylenol PM.

## KEY TERMS

**Adult:** person who ranges in age from 19 to 64 years

**Age-related changes:** physiologic events due to increasing age, which affect drug responses

**Older adult:** person who is 65 years of age or older

**Polypharmacy:** use of several drugs during the same period

**Risk-to-benefit ratio:** poor outcome (adverse effects of medications) in relation to good outcome (desired medication effects); increases with increasing age

# INTRODUCTION

Aging is a natural process that begins at birth. The most significant **age-related changes** begin in the **adult** years (19–64 years of age). These physiologic events, which can affect drug responses, are due to increasing age. Most commonly, they occur in middle age and are related to heart disease, pulmonary insufficiency, cancer, arthritis, diabetes mellitus, obesity, substance abuse, and depression.

**Older adults**, people who are 65 years of age or older, are the largest consumers of health care. Chronic conditions have roots in the aging process. The most common health problems in older adults include arthritis, heart disease, decreased sensory perception, bone disorders, and diabetes mellitus. Older adults are also more prone to antibiotic-resistant infections. The treatment of chronic illnesses and associated comorbidities results in **polypharmacy**, the use of multiple medications. The interactions of medications can lead to greater complications and diminished mental status. In addition, the **risk-to-benefit ratio**, the relationship between the negative effects and the positive effects of a medication, increases as the patient ages. The nurse and the prescriber must consider the risk of associated adverse effects of those medications as well as possible benefits these medications might have in changing physiologic processes related to disease. As Rochon (2018, p. 1) states, "Optimizing drug therapy is an essential part of caring for an older person." It is important for the nurse to evaluate an older adult's reaction to any medication or reaction to a combination of medications.

# PHARMACODYNAMICS IN OLDER ADULTS

Pharmacodynamics involves drug actions on target cells and the resulting alterations in cellular biochemical reactions and functions. In older adults, physiologic changes such as a reduced number of receptor sites for medications or affinity to receptors alter the medication's ability to produce the desired effect. Older adults are prone to adverse drug reactions because of a decrease in the number of receptors needed for drug distribution. Beta-adrenergic agonists are less effective as a result of the decreased function of the beta-receptor system.

Nurses must be aware of other physiologic changes associated with increased age. The volume of distribution of drugs may be increased based on the older adult's increase in body fat relative to the percentage of the skeletal muscle. The decline in renal function inhibits the adequate clearance of a drug. In addition, drug storage reservoirs increase with age. This physiologic change prolongs a drug's half-life, increasing the plasma drug concentrations (Rochon, 2018).

Cardiovascular disease is the number one cause of death in adults, including older adults. In patients with hypertension, the control of blood pressure is key to the prevention of cardiovascular disease and stroke. Hypertension affects 70% to 80% of older adults. Although a salt-reduction diet is often effective in the treatment of hypertension in younger adults, in older adults, lifestyle modifications alone may not be effective. Older adults who require antihypertensive medication should initially be prescribed a low-dose thiazide-type diuretic, angiotensin-converting enzyme inhibitor, angiotensin II receptor blocker, or long-acting calcium channel blocker. Beta-blockers should not be used as a primary treatment for systolic hypertension in the older adult population. Studies have shown that the use of beta-blockers may be worse than other agents in preventing stroke and may hasten death. This is particularly evident in older adults who have a history of smoking (Egan, 2019).

The use of digoxin (Lanoxin) in heart disease should not exceed 0.125 mg/day except when treating atrial fibrillation or supraventricular tachydysrhythmia. In atrial fibrillation, the maximum dose is 1.5 mg over 24 hours. In supraventricular tachydysrhythmia, the digitalizing dose is 0.75 to 1.5 mg, with a daily maintenance dose of 0.125 to 0.5 mg once daily. Digoxin has a low therapeutic index, placing patients at risk for adverse effects. Thus, administration of the medication with a reduced dose assists in maintaining safety.

## Beers Criteria

Dr. Mark Beers initially developed the Beers Criteria list of potentially inappropriate medications used by the older adult population in 1997, and the American Geriatrics Society updated this list in 2019. The Beers Criteria for Potentially Inappropriate Medication Use in Older Adults is updated every 3 years. It provides clinicians with the names of medications that are potentially inappropriate for use in older adults, listing drugs to be avoided and giving adjustments in dosages related to chronic kidney disease and diminished kidney function. An interdisciplinary panel of experts determines new criteria and updates existing criteria based on scientific evidence.

The 2019 update includes the two parts established in the 2015 review: (1) drugs for which dose adjustment is required based on kidney function and (2) drug–drug interactions (American Geriatrics Society 2019 Beers Criteria Updated AGS Beers Criteria for Potentially Inappropriate Medication Use in Older Adults, 2019). The list does not include medications administered in the hospice and palliative care delivery systems. It is important to consider patients' needs for opioids in the treatment of chronic pain. The use of opioids in older adults requires patient assessment of response to treatment.

In nursing practice, it is vital to implement strategies to identify age-related changes associated with medication administration. According to Rochon (2018), 2.4% to 6.5% of all medical admissions are related to adverse drug events. Adverse drug events leading to overdose occur in two thirds of the events. Table 5.1 lists the potentially inappropriate medication use in older adults as identified by the 2019 Beers Criteria.

---

> **! QSEN Alert: Patient-Centered Care**
>
> Drugs that contribute to or produce adverse effects in older adults include the following:
>
> - Amiodarone [Nexterone, Pacerone]: altered QT interval
> - Amitriptyline hydrochloride: anticholinergic effects and sedation
> - Cyclobenzaprine [Amrix]: anticholinergic effects and weakness
> - Dextromethorphan/quinidine: limited efficacy and increased risk of falls

*BAD older Pts* (handwritten)

- Digoxin (Lanoxin): digoxin toxicity
- Diphenhydramine hydrochloride: urinary retention
- Flurazepam hydrochloride: sedation
- Hydroxyzine hydrochloride: confusion and sedation
- Ketorolac: gastrointestinal bleeding
- Meperidine hydrochloride (Demerol): confusion
- Methocarbamol (Robaxin): anticholinergic effects and weakness
- Methyldopa: bradycardia and depression
- Nitrofurantoin (Macrodantin): renal toxicity

- Opioids with benzodiazepines and gabapentinoids: central nervous system (CNS) adverse effects and potential death
- Rivaroxaban: caution required in patients older than age 75, increased risk of bleeding
- Serotonin–norepinephrine reuptake inhibitors: avoid in patients who have experienced fractures or prone to falls
- Trimethoprim–sulfamethoxazole used with angiotensin-converting enzyme inhibitors or angiotensin receptor blockers: increased risk of hyperkalemia

## TABLE 5.1

### 2015 American Geriatrics Society Beers Criteria: Potentially Inappropriate Medication Use in Older Adults

| Drug* | Rationale | Recommendation | Quality of Evidence |
|---|---|---|---|
| **Anticholinergics** | | | |
| ***First-generation antihistamines*** Brompheniramine Carbinoxamine Chlorpheniramine Clemastine Cyproheptadine Dexbrompheniramine Dexchlorpheniramine Dimenhydrinate Diphenhydramine (oral) Doxylamine Hydroxyzine Meclizine Pyrilamine Triprolidine | Highly anticholinergic; clearance reduced with advanced age, and tolerance develops when used as hypnotic; risk of confusion, dry mouth, constipation, and other anticholinergic effects or toxicity Use of diphenhydramine in situations such as acute treatment of severe allergic reaction may be appropriate | Avoid | Moderate |
| **Antiparkinsonism agents** Benztropine (oral) Trihexyphenidyl | Not recommended for prevention of extrapyramidal symptoms with antipsychotics; more effective agents available for treatment of Parkinson's disease | Avoid | Moderate |
| **Antispasmodics** Atropine (excludes ophthalmic) Belladonna alkaloids Clidinium–chlordiazepoxide Dicyclomine Homatropine (excludes ophthalmic) Hyoscyamine Methscopolamine Propantheline Scopolamine | Highly anticholinergic, uncertain effectiveness | Avoid | Moderate |
| **Antithrombotics** Dipyridamole, oral short acting (does not apply to extended-release combination with aspirin) | May cause orthostatic hypotension; more effective alternatives available; intravenous form acceptable for use in cardiac stress testing | Avoid | Moderate |
| **Anti-infective** Nitrofurantoin | Potential pulmonary toxicity, hepatotoxicity, and peripheral neuropathy, especially with long-term use; safer alternatives available | Avoid in individuals with creatinine clearance <30 mL/min or for long-term suppression of bacteria | Low |

**TABLE 5.1**

## 2015 American Geriatrics Society Beers Criteria: Potentially Inappropriate Medication Use in Older Adults (Continued)

| Drug* | Rationale | Recommendation | Quality of Evidence |
|---|---|---|---|
| **Cardiovascular** | | | |
| ***Peripheral alpha-1 blockers*** <br> Doxazosin <br> Prazosin <br> Terazosin | High risk of orthostatic hypotension; not recommended as routine treatment for hypertension; alternative agents have superior risk–benefit profile | Avoid use as an antihypertensive | Moderate |
| ***Central alpha-blockers*** <br> Clonidine <br> Guanabenz <br> Guanfacine <br> Methyldopa <br> Reserpine (>0.1 mg/d) | High risk of adverse CNS effects; may cause bradycardia and orthostatic hypotension; not recommended as routine treatment for hypertension | Avoid as first-line antihypertensive <br> Avoid other CNS alpha-agonists as listed | Low |
| Disopyramide | May induce heart failure in older adults because of potent negative inotropic action; strongly anticholinergic; other antiarrhythmic drugs preferred | Avoid | Low |
| Dronedarone | Worse outcomes have been reported in patients taking dronedarone who have permanent atrial fibrillation or severe or recently decompensated heart failure | Avoid in individuals with permanent atrial fibrillation or severe or recently decompensated heart failure | High |
| Digoxin for treatment of atrial fibrillation or heart failure | In atrial fibrillation: should not be used as a first-line agent, because there are safer and more effective alternatives for rate control supported by high-quality evidence <br> In heart failure: evidence for benefits and harms of digoxin is conflicting and of lower quality, but most though not all of the evidence concerns use in HFrEF. There is strong evidence for other agents as first-line therapy to reduce hospitalizations and mortality in adults with HFrEF. Higher doses are not associated with additional benefit and may increase the risk of toxicity. Decreased renal clearance of digoxin may lead to increased risk of toxic effects; further dose reduction may be necessary in patients with stage 4 or 5 chronic kidney disease | Avoid as first-line therapy for atrial fibrillation <br> For atrial fibrillation or heart failure, avoid dosages >0.125 mg/d | Moderate with dosages >0.125 mg/d |
| Nifedipine, immediate release | Potential for hypotension; risk of precipitating myocardial ischemia | Avoid | High |
| Amiodarone | Effective for maintaining sinus rhythm but greater toxicities than other antiarrhythmics used in atrial fibrillation; may be reasonable first-line therapy in patients with concomitant heart failure or substantial left ventricular hypertrophy if rhythm control is preferred over rate control | Avoid as first-line therapy for atrial fibrillation unless patient has heart failure or substantial left ventricular hypertrophy | High |

*(Continued on page 82)*

**TABLE 5.1**

## 2015 American Geriatrics Society Beers Criteria: Potentially Inappropriate Medication Use in Older Adults (Continued)

| Drug* | Rationale | Recommendation | Quality of Evidence |
|---|---|---|---|
| **Central Nervous System** | | | |
| ***Antidepressants, alone or in combination*** <br> Amitriptyline <br> Amoxapine <br> Clomipramine <br> Desipramine <br> Doxepin (>6 mg/d) <br> Imipramine <br> Nortriptyline <br> Paroxetine <br> Protriptyline <br> Trimipramine | Highly anticholinergic, sedating, and cause orthostatic hypotension; safety profile of low-dose doxepin (≤6 mg/d) comparable with that of placebo | Avoid | High |
| ***Antipsychotics*** <br> (First-generation [conventional] and second-generation [atypical]) | Increased risk of cerebrovascular accident (stroke) and greater rate of cognitive decline and mortality in persons with dementia <br> Avoid antipsychotics for behavioral problems of dementia or delirium unless nonpharmacologic options (e.g., behavioral interventions) have failed or are not possible and the older adult is threatening substantial harm to self or others | Avoid, except for schizophrenia, bipolar disorder, or short-term use as antiemetic during chemotherapy | Moderate |
| **Barbiturates** <br> Amobarbital <br> Butabarbital <br> Butalbital <br> Mephobarbital <br> Pentobarbital <br> Phenobarbital <br> Secobarbital | High rate of physical dependence and tolerance to sleep benefits and greater risk of overdose at low dosages | Avoid | High |
| **Benzodiazepines** <br> *Short and immediate acting*: <br> Alprazolam <br> Estazolam <br> Lorazepam <br> Oxazepam <br> Temazepam <br> Triazolam <br> *Long acting*: <br> Clorazepate <br> Chlordiazepoxide (alone or in combination with amitriptyline or clidinium) <br> Clonazepam <br> Diazepam <br> Flurazepam <br> Quazepam | Older adults have increased sensitivity to benzodiazepines and decreased metabolism of long-acting agents; in general, all benzodiazepines increase risk of cognitive impairment, delirium, falls, fractures, and motor vehicle crashes in older adults <br> May be appropriate for seizure disorders, rapid eye movement sleep disorders, benzodiazepine withdrawal, ethanol withdrawal, severe generalized anxiety disorder, and periprocedural anesthesia | Avoid | Moderate |
| Meprobamate | High rate of physical dependence; very sedating | Avoid | Moderate |

**TABLE 5.1**

**2015 American Geriatrics Society Beers Criteria: Potentially Inappropriate Medication Use in Older Adults** [Continued]

| Drug* | Rationale | Recommendation | Quality of Evidence |
|---|---|---|---|
| **Nonbenzodiazepine, benzodiazepine receptor agonist hypnotics** (i.e., Z drugs) Eszopiclone Zolpidem Zaleplon | Have adverse events similar to those of benzodiazepines in older adults (e.g., delirium, falls, fractures); increased emergency department visits/hospitalizations; motor vehicle crashes; minimal improvement in sleep latency and duration | Avoid | Moderate |
| **Ergoloid mesylates** (dehydrogenated ergot alkaloids) Isoxsuprine | Lack of efficacy | Avoid | High |
| **Endocrine-related agents** Androgens Methyltestosterone Testosterone | Potential for cardiac problems; contraindicated in men with prostate cancer | Avoid unless indicated for confirmed hypogonadism with clinical symptoms | Moderate Weak |
| Desiccated thyroid | Potential for cardiac problems; safer alternatives | Avoid | Low |
| Estrogens with or without progestins | Evidence of carcinogenic potential (breast and endometrium); lack of cardioprotective effect and cognitive protection in older women; evidence that vaginal estrogens for the treatment of vaginal dryness are safe and effective; women with history of breast cancer who do not respond to nonhormonal therapies are advised to discuss risks and benefits of low-dose vaginal estrogen (doses of estradiol <25 μm twice weekly) with health care provider | Avoid oral and topical patch Acceptable to use low-dose intravaginal estrogen for management of dyspareunia, lower urinary tract infections, and other vaginal symptoms | Oral and patch: high Vaginal cream or tablets: moderate Oral and patch: strong Topical vaginal cream or tablets: weak |
| Growth hormone | Impact on body composition is small and associated with edema, arthralgia, carpal tunnel syndrome, gynecomastia, and impaired fasting glucose | Avoid except as hormone replacement after pituitary gland removal | High |
| Insulin, sliding scale | Higher risk of hypoglycemia without improvement in hyperglycemia management regardless of care setting; refers to sole use of short- or rapid-acting insulins to manage or avoid hyperglycemia in absence of basal or long-acting insulin; does not apply to titration of basal insulin or use of additional short- or rapid-acting insulin in conjunction with scheduled insulin (i.e., correction insulin) | Avoid | Moderate |
| Megestrol | Minimal effect on weight; increases risk of thrombotic events and possibly death in older adults | Avoid | Moderate |
| **Sulfonylureas, long duration** Chlorpropamide Glyburide (also known as glibenclamide) | Chlorpropamide: prolonged half-life in older adults; can cause prolonged hypoglycemia; causes syndrome of inappropriate antidiuretic hormone secretion Glyburide: higher risk of severe prolonged hypoglycemia in older adults | Avoid | High |
| **Gastrointestinal agents** Metoclopramide | Can cause extrapyramidal effects, including tardive dyskinesia; risk may be greater in frail older adults | Avoid, unless gastroparesis with duration of use not to exceed 12 wk except in rare cases | Moderate |

*(Continued on page 84)*

**TABLE 5.1**

### 2015 American Geriatrics Society Beers Criteria: Potentially Inappropriate Medication Use in Older Adults (Continued)

| Drug* | Rationale | Recommendation | Quality of Evidence |
|---|---|---|---|
| Mineral oil, given orally | Potential for aspiration and adverse effects; safer alternatives available | Avoid | Moderate |
| Proton pump inhibitors | Risk of *Clostridium difficile* infection and bone loss and fractures | Avoid scheduled use for >8 wk unless for high-risk patients (e.g., oral corticosteroids or chronic NSAID use), erosive esophagitis, Barrett's esophagitis, pathologic hypersecretory condition, or demonstrated need for maintenance treatment (e.g., due to failure of drug discontinuation trial or H₂ receptor antagonists) | High |
| **Pain medications**<br>Meperidine | Not effective oral analgesic in dosages commonly used; may have higher risk of neurotoxicity, including delirium, than other opioids; safer alternatives available | Avoid, especially in individuals with chronic kidney disease | Moderate |
| **Noncyclooxygenase-selective NSAIDs (oral)**<br>Aspirin (>325 mg/d)<br>Diclofenac<br>Diflunisal<br>Etodolac<br>Fenoprofen<br>Ibuprofen<br>Ketoprofen<br>Meclofenamate<br>Mefenamic acid<br>Meloxicam<br>Nabumetone<br>Naproxen<br>Oxaprozin<br>Piroxicam<br>Sulindac<br>Tolmetin | Increased risk of gastrointestinal bleeding or peptic ulcer disease in high-risk groups, including those aged older than 75 y or who are taking oral or parenteral corticosteroids, anticoagulants, or antiplatelet agents; use of proton pump inhibitors or misoprostol reduces but does not eliminate risk. Upper gastrointestinal ulcers, gross bleeding, or perforation caused by NSAIDs occurs in ~1% of patients treated for 3–6 mo and in 2%–4% of patients treated for 1 y; these trends continue with longer duration of use | Avoid chronic use unless other alternatives are not effective and patient can take gastroprotective agent (proton pump inhibitor or misoprostol) | Moderate |
| Indomethacin | More likely than other NSAIDs to have adverse effects (CNS problems and others); has the most adverse effects of all the NSAIDs | Avoid | Moderate |
| Ketorolac, includes parenteral | Increased risk of gastrointestinal bleeding, peptic ulcer disease, and acute kidney injury in older adults | | Moderate |
| **Skeletal muscle relaxants**<br>Carisoprodol<br>Chlorzoxazone<br>Cyclobenzaprine<br>Metaxalone<br>Methocarbamol<br>Orphenadrine | Most muscle relaxants poorly tolerated by older adults because some have anticholinergic adverse effects, sedation, and increased risk of fractures; effectiveness of dosages tolerated by older adults questionable | Avoid | Moderate |
| **Genitourinary agents**<br>Desmopressin | High risk of hyponatremia; safer alternative treatments | Avoid for treatment of nocturia or nocturnal polyuria | Moderate |

*Organized by organ system/therapeutic category.

CNS, central nervous system; HFrEF, heart failure with reduced ejection fraction; NSAID, nonsteroidal anti-inflammatory drug.

From American Geriatrics Society. (2019). American Geriatrics Society 2019 updated AGS Beers criteria for potentially inappropriate medication use in older adults. *Journal of the American Geriatrics Society, 67*(4), 674–694. doi:10.1111/jgs.15767. All rights reserved, used with permission.

## Prevention of Adverse Effects

Strategies to prevent adverse drug reactions include the following:

- Assess a patient's health history and list of medications taken by the patient, including prescription medications, over-the-counter (OTC) medications, and herbal supplements.
- Assess blood urea nitrogen and creatinine clearance (CrCl) levels to determine the patient's ability to excrete the medications.
- Assess the ratio of alanine aminotransferase to aspartate aminotransferase to determine the patient's liver function and ability to metabolize drugs.
- Assess therapeutic drug levels as ordered by the prescriber to determine the medication effectiveness and prevention of toxicity.
- Educate the patient and family about all medications and possible drug–drug, drug–herb, and drug–diet interactions.
- Educate the patient and family about the generic and trade names of medications to prevent overmedication.
- Educate the patient and family to use one primary care provider who prescribes medications in consultation with other health care specialists.
- Educate the patient and family to have all prescriptions filled at one pharmacy.
- Assess the patient's adherence to the prescribed medications.
- Provide the patient with medication administration aids to increase adherence.

### Clinical Application 5.1

- What urinary effect is Mr. Franklin prone to developing since he began taking Tylenol PM?

↓ *mental awareness*

### NCLEX Success

1. When administering a beta-adrenergic agonist to a patient older than 65 years of age, what response do you anticipate?
   A. The drug will work very rapidly to decrease blood pressure.
   B. The dosage will need to be increased to provide an effective response.
   C. The drug should be combined with atropine to enhance effectiveness.
   D. The dosage will need to be titrated over 20 minutes to increase blood pressure.

2. A 75-year-old woman is having difficulty remembering to take all of her medications. Which of the following nursing interventions will assist her to improve adherence to the medication schedule?
   A. Have her daughter administer the medications.
   B. Decrease the number of medications administered.
   C. Evaluate her ability to care for herself.
   D. Provide a medication administration aid.

## PHARMACOKINETICS IN OLDER ADULTS

Aging results in physiologic changes that affect the absorption, distribution, metabolism, and excretion of medications. The most relevant physiologic change is the decreased function of vital organs needed for the pharmacokinetic processes. Frail, elderly adults are at greatest risk for altered drug responses. The more physically active older adults are, the less likely they will experience altered drug responses.

Health care providers prescribe anticholinergic agents for many older adults. These agents are useful in the treatment of Parkinson's disease, irritable bowel syndrome, and allergic reactions. The anticholinergic drug scale (ADS), which was developed and revised in 2006 (Carnahan, Lund, Perry, Pollack, & Culp, 2006), measures anticholinergic effects on an ordinal scale of 0 to 3. Patients with ADS scores of three or above have a higher risk of cognitive impairment. The study by Nissan, Brill, and Hershkovitz (2019) reveals that anticholinergic drug prescription changes and rehabilitation outcomes were decreased with patients having lowered functional abilities.

Many studies have reported that anticholinergic agents produce negative health outcomes in older adults. These outcomes increase the risk of falls, confusion, and diminished mental alertness. In a longitudinal study of cognitively normal adults, Risacher et al. (2016) have shown that the use of anticholinergic drugs increases the risk of decline in cognitive ability and poses a risk to increase brain dysfunction. The greater the anticholinergic effects of the medication, the more severe the brain dysfunction. The study subjects scored lower mean scores on the Wechsler Memory Scale-Revised Logical Memory immediate test. The results of positron emission tomography (PET) and magnetic resonance imaging (MRI) scans revealed a reduction in glucose metabolism in the hippocampus and a reduction in the total cortical volume. Nurses should use this information when consulting with practitioners regarding reducing the prescribing and use of anticholinergic agents. This should include educating patients to avoid the use of medications containing anticholinergic drugs. OTC drugs that pose a concern are first-generation histamine $H_1$ antagonists. The most common OTC medication is the prototype of this class, diphenhydramine, which was once available as Benadryl. Many preparations, such as Advil PM, Aleve PM, and Tylenol PM, contain this medication.

## Absorption

In older adults, changes in the gastrointestinal (GI) tract include decreased gastric acidity, with an increase in the gastric pH, and delayed absorption or lack of absorption of medications that require this decreased pH. Other changes in the GI tract responsible for affecting drug absorption in older adults are decreased blood flow and decreased surface area to support absorption. Diminished gastric emptying also plays a role by causing the medication to be in the stomach for a longer period. This factor increases the risk of developing nausea and vomiting, thus causing elimination of the medication in emesis and promoting fluid volume deficit.

In older patients, decreased circulation means that parenteral medications are also slowly absorbed. Decreased muscle mass and altered circulation can result in abnormal blood concentrations of medications administered intramuscularly.

In all cases, a slow rate of absorption can result in changes in peak serum drug levels. This factor may require greater dosages to be administered to produce therapeutic results.

## Distribution

In older adults, physiologic factors that contribute to alterations in distribution of medications include diminished cardiac output, increased body fat, decreased body mass and body fluid, and decreased serum albumin. Aging results in body mass changes; the proportion of body fat increases while lean body mass decreases. These changes may have the following consequences:

- Lipid-soluble drugs such as the anesthetic agents stay in the fat tissue for a longer period of time. This places older adults at risk for respiratory depression following surgery.
- The amount of body fluid decreases in proportion to total body weight. Water-soluble drugs such as antibiotics are distributed in smaller volumes due to the decrease in total body fluid volume. This increases the risk of toxicity because drug concentrations are greater.
- Many medications require serum albumin to bind, transport, and distribute the medication to the target organ. In the event that the amount of serum albumin is insufficient, the amount of free drug rises, and the effect of the drug is more intense.
- Medications are not distributed adequately due to the decreased circulation and diminished cardiac output.

## Metabolism

Age-related physiologic changes of the liver affect the metabolism of medications. At approximately 60 years of age, the liver begins to decrease in size and mass. There is also a decrease in the hepatic circulation, lowering the rate of metabolism. The hepatic enzymes of the liver are decreased, altering the ability to remove metabolic by-products. It is important to understand that because older adults have a reduced metabolism, medications with a long half-life will remain in the body for a greater amount of time.

Some responses to drug therapy are genetically determined and may differ in various ethnic and racial populations. Caucasian Americans and African Americans are poor metabolizers of medication compared with Asian Americans; Asian Americans have the ability to metabolize and excrete medications more quickly than those of Caucasian and African descent. Circulating levels of medications in Caucasian Americans and African Americans are higher. For example, beta-adrenergic blockers are less effective in African Americans, whereas Asian Americans require a smaller dose due to the ethnic variation in medication response.

## Excretion

The elimination of medications is vital in the prevention of adverse drug reactions. In older adults, physiologic changes associated with alterations in medication excretion include diminished renal blood flow, number of functioning nephrons, glomerular filtration rate, and tubular secretion. The assessment of the patient's CrCl is an important indicator of the ability of the renal system to eliminate the medication and prevent adverse drug effects. Dosages of medications should be lower in medications with an increased half-life. In most older adults, the serum creatinine remains within the normal range due to decreasing creatinine levels in association with a decrease in muscle mass. The glomerular filtration rate is the most reliable measure for evaluation of renal function. However, this value is very costly to obtain and is often unavailable. An alternative to the 24-hour CrCl and the glomerular filtration rate is the Cockroft-Gault method. This method estimates the CrCl (Norris, 2019) (http://www.mdcalc.com/creatinine-clearance-cockcroft-gault-equation/).

$$\text{Estimated CrCl(mL / min)} = \frac{(140 - \text{age}) \times (\text{body weight in kg})}{(72 \times \text{serum creatinine in mg / dL})}$$

The result should be multiplied by 0.85 for women.

Prior to the administration of a medication excreted by the renal system, the nurse assesses the patient's glomerular filtration rate and hydration status by using the serum creatinine value to calculate the estimated CrCl. With a decreased CrCl, it is necessary to reduce the dosage of the medication. The average estimated glomerular filtration rate is 120 to 130 mL/min/1.73 m$^2$ for normal young healthy adults. The average estimated glomerular filtration rate declines with every decade of life; by 70 years of age, the average estimated glomerular filtration rate is 75 mL/min/1.73 m$^2$. The glomerular filtration rate is an overestimation of the CrCl, because creatinine is secreted by the proximal tubule and filtered by the kidneys. The glomerular filtration rate is lower in females as a result of their decreased muscle mass, and it is higher in African Americans, both males and females, because of their increased muscle mass (National Institute of Diabetes and Digestive and Kidney Diseases, http://www.niddk.nih.gov/health-information/health-communication-programs/nkdep/identify-manage/identify-evaluate/estimate-gfr/Pages/estimate-gfr.aspx). The National Kidney Disease Education Program (National Institute of Diabetes and Digestive and Kidney Diseases, 2019) strongly recommends using the modification of diet in renal disease study equation or the chronic kidney disease epidemiology collaboration equation to estimate the glomerular filtration rate. These equations identify impaired kidney function in both Caucasian and African American populations.

### Clinical Application 5.2

- What is the suspected effect of Mr. Franklin's race on his creatinine clearance and excretion of medications?

## NCLEX Success

3. A 68-year-old woman has been prescribed digoxin 0.125 mg. Based on her age, what condition is she at risk for developing?
   A. diarrhea
   B. digoxin toxicity
   C. edema
   D. pulmonary embolism

4. An 85-year-old woman is administered a general anesthetic for repair of a hip fracture. Which of the following properties of the anesthetic place her at risk for respiratory depression?
   A. solubility in lipids
   B. solubility in water
   C. binding to cytochrome P450
   D. binding to muscle tissue

### Clinical Application 5.3

Mr. Franklin has developed herpes zoster (shingles) and is complaining of severe neuropathic pain. His physician has ordered gabapentin (Neurontin) 300 mg twice daily by mouth. The recommended dosage with renal impairment is 200 to 700 mg twice daily if the creatinine clearance (CrCl) is greater than 30 to 59 mL/min. Mr. Franklin's serum creatinine is 2.2 mg/dL.
- What is the patient's estimated CrCl?
- Is this dosage of gabapentin appropriate?

## MEDICATION ADHERENCE AND AGING

As patients increase in age, they use a greater number of medications, both prescription and over the counter, along with alternative therapies such as vitamins or herbal supplements. (As previously mentioned, the use of increased medications is known as polypharmacy.) It is often difficult to remember medications or maintain appropriate administration schedules. Altered mental status and diminished visual acuity also contribute to improper medication use. Patients who have decreased vision may not be able to discriminate the dosing instructions or may not be able to see the amount of insulin drawn up in an insulin syringe.

Economic factors also contribute to nonadherence. Some older adults may have to choose between the cost of their medications and the ability to purchase food or pay for utilities. A multidisciplinary team approach is used to assist patients in obtaining medications. It is important for the prescriber to use generic medications and to order small quantities of medications initially so that an individual patient's reaction to the medication can be determined. In the event the medication needs to be changed, the great financial burden on the patient will not be too great.

Starting slow and with low doses improves adherence to the medication regimen. Patients may describe not feeling well after using the prescribed medications. Starting with smaller doses minimizes these adverse effects. The administration of several medications concurrently can result in adverse effects. When adverse effects are experienced by older patients, they may not adhere to the recommended administration guidelines.

Being asymptomatic may contribute to nonadherence to a medication regimen. Many patients begin to feel better with the initiation of therapy and then discontinue medications altogether or miss individual doses. Patients and their families should be educated about adherence to medication regimens. This is particularly evident in patients being treated for hypertension. Patients who do not take antihypertensives as prescribed have an increased risk of a cardiovascular event. It is important that health care providers educate patients and families about medications and their use. To improve adherence, nurses and other health care providers should keep the care inexpensive, using generic preparations, and easy to follow, using the fewest number of doses required. UpToDate recommends two types of patient education. "The Basics" recommends that patient education should be written in plain language at a fifth- to sixth-grade reading level. "Beyond the Basics" provides higher-level educational information that is at the 10th to 12th grade level (Egan, 2019).

### ⚠ QSEN Alert: Evidence-Based Practice

The elderly population is at a great risk for negative health outcomes related to polypharmacy and inappropriate drug use. Barzargan et al. (2017) conducted a study of 400 underserved African American adults living in South Los Angeles, California. In face-to-face interviews, the researchers collected data on medication administration, frequency, dosage, and indications for treatment of health conditions. Thirty-eight percent of participants had received five or more medications from three prescribers. Inappropriate drug use that was strongly correlated to polypharmacy affected 75% of the study participants. Polypharmacy led to poor coordination and management of medications among providers and pharmacists. This study recommended strategies to reduce inappropriate polypharmacy and potentially inappropriate medication use in underserved populations. More multidisciplinary assessment of medication outcomes should be implemented to identify adverse effects and inappropriate outcomes of medication response.

### Clinical Application 5.4

Mr. Franklin's primary health care provider has prescribed three medications for him. These include gabapentin (Neurontin), 300 mg twice daily by mouth; famciclovir (Famvir), 500 mg every 12 hours by mouth; and meperidine (Demerol), 50 mg every 6 hours PRN by mouth.
- Which of the following medications is inappropriate for this patient?
- How will you assist this patient to maintain medication adherence?

## NCLEX Success

5. A 68-year-old woman is receiving chemotherapy. What is the rationale for teaching her to drink eight glasses of water throughout the day following the administration of chemotherapy?
   A. Chemotherapy is toxic to the liver, and the water will reduce the adverse effects.
   B. The water will prevent the body from rejecting the medication.
   C. Chemotherapy is excreted in the kidneys and urine. The water will help eliminate it from the body.
   D. The water will prevent dehydration, an adverse effect of the medication.

6. A 78-year-old man is receiving treatment for hypertension. He has been having persistent headaches and difficulty with the medications he has been prescribed. This is the third prescription he has received. He states, "I can't afford to get this filled and then stop it in a few days." Which statement is most appropriate for the nurse to communicate to the patient?
   A. Have the pharmacist give you a few pills to start.
   B. Take your other medication and then switch.
   C. Take the other medications back to the pharmacy for a refund.
   D. Save all your pills; you may need them again.

## THE NURSING PROCESS

A concept map outlines the nursing process related to drug therapy considerations in this chapter. Additional nursing implications related to the disease process should also be considered in care decisions.

**Assessment**
- Assess the patient's knowledge of his or her medication regimen, including knowledge of the action and use of each medication administered.
- Assess the patient's ability to administer the medication correctly.
- Assess the patient for adverse effects of medications as well as drug–drug, drug–diet, and drug–herb interactions.
- Assess the patient's physiologic status with regard to the medication's pharmacokinetics (e.g., renal function, liver function, cardiovascular function).
- Assess physiologic changes, such as the patient's ability to swallow.
- Assess body mass and its effect on medication absorption and distribution.
- Assess the patient's ability to maintain medication adherence based on memory, self-care, and caregiver's ability to assist in care.

**Outcomes of Therapy**
The patient will
- Take medications as prescribed.
- Tolerate medications based on renal and liver function.
- Report adverse effects to primary care provider.
- Understand all aspects of medication administration, including action, use, and adverse effects.
- Maintain medication adherence.

**Nursing Interventions**
- Assess the patient's liver and renal function as well as his or her circulation and changes in body mass affecting pharmacokinetics.
- Assess the patient's response to medication regimen.
- Assess the patient's ability to maintain medication administration.
- Assess for adverse effects of medications.
- Assess for the patient's adherence to medications.
- Instruct the patient and family about the use of medication administration aids.
- Instruct the patient and family about the administration of medications.
- Instruct the patient and family about the action, use, and adverse effects of medications.

**Evaluation**
- Evaluate the patient's response to the medication regimen.
- Evaluate the patient's and family's understanding of the medication regimen.
- Evaluate the patient's adherence to the medication regimen.

## KEY CONCEPTS

- Pharmacodynamics involves drug actions on target cells and the resulting alterations in cellular biochemical reactions and functions.
- In older adults, physiologic changes alter the ability for the medication to provide the desired effect for which it is intended.
- In nursing practice, it is vital to implement strategies to identify age-related changes associated with medication administration.
- Aging results in physiologic changes affecting the absorption, distribution, metabolism, and excretion of medications.
- The most relevant physiologic change is the decreased function of vital organs needed for the pharmacokinetic processes.
- The GI tract changes affecting drug absorption include an increase in the gastric pH.

- A decrease in blood flow to the GI tract, a decrease in surface area to support absorption, and diminished gastric emptying also limit absorption.
- Alterations in distribution of medications include diminished cardiac output, increased body fat, and decreased body mass, body fluid, and serum albumin.
- Physiologic changes associated with alterations in medication excretion include diminished renal blood flow, number of functioning nephrons, glomerular filtration rate, and tubular secretion.
- The nurse implements strategies to increase medication adherence such as educating the patient about medication administration and adverse effects, providing medication administration aids, and assessing for adverse effects.

## CLINICAL REASONING CASE STUDY

### Meet the Patient

Maria Collins is a 70-year-old woman who is being treated with chemotherapy for breast cancer. She recently has developed neuropathic pain related to the chemotherapy agents. To decrease the neuropathic pain, her health care provider has ordered amitriptyline hydrochloride. This drug has anticholinergic effects.

- Since Ms. Collins is age 70, what age-related changes will affect the absorption of amitriptyline?
- Ms. Collins is 5 foot 3 inches and 238 lb. How does her obesity affect distribution?
- How does age-related physiologic changes affect metabolism?
- Why is the elimination of amitriptyline vital to the prevention of adverse effects?
- What anticholinergic effects does amitriptyline have?
- How should the nurse instruct Ms. Collins to reduce the adverse effects of amitriptyline?

### Assessing Drug Information

- Gastrointestinal changes related to increasing age will cause a decrease in gastric acid and increase in gastric pH.
- A decrease in blood flow to the gastrointestinal tract will diminish drug absorption.
- Diminished gastric emptying causes the medication to be in the stomach for a longer period, increasing the risk of nausea and vomiting that could result in elimination of medication in emesis and resulting in fluid volume deficit.
- In the event that fluid volume deficit results, Ms. Collins will have a decreased serum albumin due to dehydration. The inability to distribute any of the medications Ms. Collins is taking can result in increased adverse effects and diminished therapeutic effects.
- In addition, Ms. Collins' body weight may result in her medications being stored in fat tissue for a longer period of time. This places her at risk for adverse effects, such as sedation, with amitriptyline.
- At approximately 60 years of age, the liver begins to decrease in size and mass. There is a decrease in hepatic circulation, lowering the rate of metabolism. The result of hepatic changes in the older adult will lengthen the half-life of medications and cause them to remain in the body for a greater period of time.
- The elimination of medications is vital in preventing adverse drug reactions in the older adult. The alteration of renal function is related to diminished blood flow, the number of functioning nephrons, diminished glomerular filtration, and tubular secretion. Dosages of medications should be lowered with an increased half-life.
- The normal half-life of amitriptyline is 13 to 36 hours. With the associated age-related changes in elimination, Ms. Collins is at risk for the following adverse effects: falls, urinary retention, constipation, dry mouth, blurred vision, and increased intraocular pressure.

### Nursing Actions

- Assess Ms. Collins for adverse effects of all medications related to the physiologic changes that affect absorption, distribution, metabolism, and elimination of her medications.
- Instruct Ms. Collins that amitriptyline leads to increased thirst and sedation.
- Instruct Ms. Collins to do the following:
  - Stay well hydrated by drinking frequent sips of water or other fluid. Sucking on hard candy also helps reduce dry mouth.
  - Take frequent rests to help manage the sedative properties of the drug.
  - Consider taking a dose at bedtime in the event that she becomes too sedated during the day. Instruct Ms. Collins to consult her prescriber in the event she would like to take the amitriptyline at bedtime.
  - Protect against falls. When Ms. Collins rises from a supine position, dizziness and orthostatic hypotension may occur. Tell Ms. Collins to rise slowly when sitting or lying down.
  - Increase dietary fiber and fluid intake related to constipation.

*Visit* thePoint *at* **http://thePoint.lww.com/Frandsen12e** *for answers to NCLEX Success questions (in Appendix A), answers to Clinical Application Case Studies (in Appendix B), and more!*

## REFERENCES AND RESOURCES

American Geriatrics Society. (2019). American Geriatrics Society 2019 updated AGS Beers criteria for potentially inappropriate medication use in older adults. *Journal of the American Geriatrics Society, 67*(4), 674–694. doi:10.1111/jgs.15767

Barzargan, M., Smith J., Movassaghi, M., Martin, D., Yazdanshenas, H., Mortazavi, S. S., et al. (2017). Polypharmacy among underserved older African American adults. *Journal of Aging Research,* 1–8. Retrieved May 23, 2017, from https://doi.org/10.1155/2017/6026358

Carnahan, R. M., Lund, B. C., Perry, P. J., Pollack, B. G., & Culp, K. R. (2006). The Anticholinergic Drug Scale as a measurement of drug-related anticholinergic burden: Associations with serum anticholinergic activity. *Journal of Clinical Pharmacology, 46,* 1481–1486. doi:10.1177/0091270006292126

Egan, B. M. (2019). Treatment of hypertension in the elderly patient, particularly isolated systolic hypertension. *UpToDate.* Philadelphia, PA: Wolters Kluwer.

National Institute of Diabetes and Digestive and Kidney Diseases. (2019). Estimate glomerular filtration rate. Retrieved May 7, 2019, from http://www.niddk.nih.gov/health-information/health-communication-programs/nkdep/identify-manage/identify-evaluate/estimate-gfr/Pages/estimate-gfr.aspx

Nissan, R., Brill, S., & Hershkovitz, A. (2019). Association between anticholinergic drug prescription changes and rehabilitation outcome in post-acute hip fractured patients. *Disability and Rehabilitation.* 1–6. April 12, 2019. doi:10.1080/09638288.2019.1576782

Norris, T. (2019). *Porth's pathophysiology: Concepts of altered health states* (10th ed.). Philadelphia, PA: Lippincott Williams & Wilkins.

Risacher, S. L., McDonald, B. C., Tallman, E. F., West, J. D., Farlow, M. R., Univerzagt, F. W., et al. (2016). Association between anticholinergic medication use and cognition, brain metabolism, and brain atrophy in cognitively normal older adults. *Journal of the American Medical Association: Neurology, 73*(6), 721–732. doi:10.1001/jamaneurol.2016.0580

Rochon, P. (2018). Drug prescribing for older adults. *UpToDate.* Philadelphia, PA: Wolters Kluwer.

# Pharmacology and the Care of Pregnant or Lactating Women

## CLINICAL APPLICATION CASE STUDY

Lauren Ross is in the 35th week of pregnancy with her fourth child. During her weekly visit to the certified nurse midwife, her blood pressure is elevated, 164/112 mm Hg, on two consecutive readings taken 4 hours apart. The nurse midwife checks her urine for protein and determines that she is spilling protein in her urine. Ms. Ross has had mild epigastric pain and an unrelenting headache for the past 2 days. Also, her vaginal culture is positive for perinatal group B streptococcus. In addition, during her pregnancy, she has been taking the antidepressant escitalopram [Lexapro] 10 mg/day and has continued to smoke cigarettes. The nurse midwife admits her to the labor and delivery unit for observation.

## KEY TERMS

**Abortifacients:** drugs used to terminate pregnancy

**Eclampsia:** characterized by the onset of grand mal seizures; occurs in some women with preeclampsia

**Galactagogues:** a category of herbs known to induce lactation or stimulate the production of breast milk in postpartal women

**Organogenesis:** formation of organs during embryonic development

**Oxytocics:** drugs that initiate uterine contractions, thus inducing childbirth

**Preeclampsia:** pregnancy-associated hypertension with proteinuria and/or manifestations of end-organ failure

**Preterm labor:** uterine contractions with cervical changes before 37 weeks of gestation, resulting in birth

**Prostaglandins:** chemical mediators, such as uterotonics, that help initiate uterine contractions

**Teratogenic:** causing abnormal embryonic or fetal development

**Tocolytics:** drugs used to stop preterm labor

**Uterotonics:** drugs to control postpartum bleeding

## INTRODUCTION

Drug use before and during pregnancy and lactation requires special consideration. Women of childbearing age may become pregnant, and they may ingest drugs that may cause fetal harm before they know they are pregnant. In general, pregnant or lactating women should avoid or minimize the use of medications whenever possible. This chapter discusses drugs related to pregnancy and lactation, including infertility drugs, vaccines, tocolytics (drugs used to stop preterm labor), oxytocics (drugs used to initiate uterine contractions), uterotonics (drugs used to stop postpartum hemorrhage), and selected teratogenic drugs (agents causing abnormal embryonic or fetal development). Description of many of these drugs appears elsewhere in the text.

## DRUG THERAPY FOR INFERTILITY

Infertility applies to (1) women younger than age 35 years who have been unable to conceive after at least 12 months of regular sexual intercourse without the use of contraception as well as (2) those older than age 35 years old after 6 months of regular intercourse without the use of contraception. In women, the most common cause is an ovulation disorder. Other causes include blocked fallopian tubes or tubal abnormalities, endometriosis, pelvic adhesions, hormonal imbalances, and advanced female age. In men, causes include absence of sperm, declining sperm counts, testicular abnormalities, and ejaculatory dysfunction. Factors such as implantation, uterine and hormonal environment, and embryo integrity may also play a role. They are critical to fetal viability and a normally progressing pregnancy.

Drug therapy is an integral part of treating infertility. Drugs prescribed for a woman experiencing infertility increase follicular maturation and promote ovulation. It is necessary to take the total dose at the same time each day to enhance effects of a particular medication. Also, coitus every other day enhances fertility due to increased sperm counts.

Table 6.1 presents the routes and dosage ranges for the infertility drugs.

### Clomiphene Citrate

Ⓟ **Clomiphene citrate** is an ovarian stimulator and selective estrogen receptor modulator. This drug increases the amount of follicle-stimulating hormone (FSH) and luteinizing hormone (LH) secreted by the pituitary gland, thus inducing ovulation for women who have infrequent or absent menstrual periods. Health care providers use it for the treatment of ovulatory failure in women who have tried to become pregnant but have failed. Ovulation occurs 5 to 10 days after the course of clomiphene treatment has been completed. Prior to beginning the drug regimen, the nurse instructs the woman about taking her basal temperature 5 to 10 days following administration. An incremental rise in temperature is an indication that ovulation has recently occurred.

Clomiphene is a mixture of zuclomiphene and enclomiphene. Metabolized by the liver, the drug has a half-life of 5 days. It is excreted in the feces and urine.

Possible adverse effects of clomiphene include ovarian enlargement, hot flashes, breast pain and tenderness, and uterine bleeding. Some women have reported visual disturbances, abdominal discomfort, and headaches. Contraindications include liver disease, thyroid or adrenal disease, intracranial lesions, ovarian cysts, and abnormal uterine bleeding.

### Menotropin

Ⓟ **Menotropin** (Menopur) is a gonadotropin given to women who have been diagnosed with anovulation. The drug stimulates FSH and LH to promote the development and maturation of ovarian follicles. Administration is subcutaneous, given in alternating sides of the abdomen. Following its administration, the woman receives human chorionic gonadotropin (hCG) (see later discussion). Menotropin is well absorbed and excreted in the urine.

During menotropin therapy, it is necessary to monitor both hCG and serum estradiol measurements. The adverse effects and contraindications of menotropin are similar to those of clomiphene citrate.

### Follitropins

Ⓟ **Follitropin alfa** (Gonal-F, Gonal-F RFF) and follitropin beta (Follistim AQ) are drugs used to induce ovulation and thus promote fertility. Administration is subcutaneous, in calibrated syringes provided by the manufacturer. It is important that the drugs not be shaken before administration. After receiving follitropins, as with menotropins, women should also receive hCG (see later discussion)—1 day after the last dose of follitropin.

The adverse effects of the follitropins are similar to those of clomiphene. Contraindications include hypersensitivity to follitropins, as well as the presence of tumors in the ovary, breast, uterus, pituitary gland, or hypothalamus. It is necessary to monitor serum estradiol levels to determine the medication response.

### Human Chorionic Gonadotropin

Ⓟ **Human chorionic gonadotropin** (Pregnyl), or hCG, is a human formulation of hCG that is derived from the urine of pregnant women. It is used as a replacement for LH to

### TABLE 6.1
## DRUGS AT A GLANCE: Infertility Drugs*

| Drug | Routes and Dosage Ranges |
|---|---|
| Ⓟ **Clomiphene citrate** (🍁 Clomid, Serophene) | 50 mg PO once daily for 5 d; begin on the 5th day of the cycle if progestin-induced bleeding is scheduled or spontaneous uterine bleeding occurs prior to therapy; therapy may be initiated at any time if there has been no recent uterine bleeding; subsequent doses may be increased to 100 mg once daily for 5 d only if ovulation does not occur at the initial dose; max dosage: 100 mg PO once daily for 5 d for six cycles; discontinue if ovulation does not occur after three courses of treatment or if ovulatory responses occur but pregnancy is not achieved |
| Ⓟ **Menotropin** (Menopur; 🍁 Menopur, Repronex) | 225 IU sub-Q once beginning on cycle day 2 or 3; dosage adjustments may occur once every 2 d or by >150 IU; max daily dose should not exceed 450 IU and dosing should not extend beyond 20 d |
| Ⓟ **Follitropin alfa** (Gonal-F, Gonal-F RFF; 🍁 Gonal-F, Gonal- F Pen) | 75 IU sub-Q daily; dose adjustment up to 37.5 IU after 14 d; if necessary, it can be increased every 7 d (max dosage: 300 IU); if response to follitropin is appropriate, hCG is given 1 d following the last dose; do not exceed 35 d of treatment |
| Follitropin beta (Follistim AQ; 🍁 Puregon) | 50 IU (cartridge) or 75 IU (vials) sub-Q or IM for the first 7 d; increase by 25–50 IU at weekly intervals; if response to follitropin is appropriate, hCG is given 1 d following the last dose |
| Ⓟ **Human chorionic gonadotropin (hCG)** (Pregnyl; 🍁 Pregnyl) | 5000–10,000 units IM 1 d following menotropins or follitropins |
| Ⓟ **Leuprolide** (Eligard, Lupron Depot; 🍁 Eligard, Lupron, Lupron Depot) | 3.75 mg IM every 28 d for up to 24 mo or 11.25 mg every 3 mo for up to 24 mo |

*Pregnancy category of all infertility drugs is X.

stimulate ovulation following administration of menotropin or follitropin.

Adverse effects of hCG include arterial thrombosis, edema, depression, rupture of ovarian cysts, and ovarian hyperstimulation. Contraindications include neoplasms or known hypersensitivity to the hormone.

## Leuprolide

Ⓟ **Leuprolide** (Eligard, Lupron Depot) is a gonadotropin-releasing hormone analogue that has an unlabeled use in the treatment of infertility. Administered subcutaneously or intramuscularly, it prevents premature ovulation and enhances the production of a larger quantity of quality eggs.

Potential adverse effects of leuprolide include hot flashes, headache, depression, insomnia, and vaginitis.

## NCLEX Success

1. A couple has been trying to conceive for the past 8 months without success. Which of the following medications is the first drug of choice?

   A. leuprolide
   B. human chorionic gonadotropin
   C. follitropin beta
   D. clomiphene citrate

2. A woman diagnosed with anovulation receives a prescription for menotropin to be administered subcutaneously. When providing education about medication administration, the nurse should teach the woman to:

   A. massage the area prior to administering the drug
   B. administer the drug at a 90-degree angle
   C. alternate the sides of the abdomen for the injection sites
   D. take human chorionic gonadotropin before the menotropin

## DRUGS USED IN PREGNANCY

During pregnancy, mother and fetus undergo physiologic changes that influence drug effects. In pregnant women, physiologic changes alter drug pharmacokinetics (Table 6.2). In general, drug effects are less predictable because plasma volume expansion decreases plasma drug concentrations, and increased metabolism by the liver and increased elimination by the kidneys shorten the duration of drug actions and effects.

### Maternal–Placental–Fetal Circulation

Drugs ingested by the pregnant woman reach the fetus through the maternal–placental–fetal circulation, which is completed about the 3rd week after conception. On the maternal side,

### TABLE 6.2

### Pregnancy: Physiologic and Pharmacokinetic Changes

| Physiologic Change | Pharmacokinetic Change |
|---|---|
| Increased plasma and subsequent blood volume, up to 50% in a normal pregnancy<br>Increased cardiac output (30%–50%) and increased blood flow to the uterus, kidneys, skin, and breasts | After it is absorbed into the bloodstream, a drug (especially if water soluble) is distributed and "diluted" more than in the nonpregnant state. Drug dosage requirements may increase. However, this effect may be offset by other pharmacokinetic changes of pregnancy |
| Increased weight (average 25 lb) and body fat | Drugs (especially fat-soluble ones) are distributed more widely Drugs that are distributed to fatty tissues stay in the body longer because they are slowly released from storage sites into the bloodstream |
| Changes in protein binding, decreased serum albumin. Also, many plasma protein–binding sites are occupied by hormones and other endogenous substances that increase during pregnancy | The decreased capacity for drug binding leaves more free drug available for therapeutic or adverse effects on the mother and for placental transfer to the fetus. Thus, a given dose of a drug may produce greater effects than it would in the nonpregnant state |
| During most of a pregnancy, increased renal blood flow and glomerular filtration rate secondary to increased cardiac output | Increased excretion of drugs by the kidneys, especially those excreted primarily unchanged in the urine (e.g., lithium, penicillins) |
| In late pregnancy, renal blood flow may decrease when the woman assumes a supine position, secondary to the increased size and weight of the uterus | Decreased renal blood flow may result in delayed excretion and prolonged effects of renally excreted drugs |
| Increased hormones (e.g., estrogen, progesterone) induce drug-metabolizing enzymes in the liver | Increased metabolism and clearance of many drugs |

arterial blood pressure carries blood and drugs to the placenta. In the placenta, maternal and fetal blood are separated by a few thin layers of membrane, which drugs can readily cross.

 *Concept Mastery Alert*

Maternal arterial blood pressure delivers blood and drugs to the placenta. Diffusion takes place in the placenta.

Placental transfer begins about the 5th week after conception. After drugs enter the fetal circulation, relatively large amounts are pharmacologically active because the fetus has low levels of serum albumin and thus low levels of drug binding. Most drug molecules are transported to the fetal liver, where they are metabolized. Metabolism occurs slowly because the liver is immature in quantity and quality of drug-metabolizing enzymes. Drugs metabolized by the fetal liver are excreted by fetal kidneys into amniotic fluid. Excretion also is slow and inefficient due to immature development of fetal kidneys. Other drug molecules are transported directly to the heart, which then distributes them to the brain and coronary arteries. Drugs enter the fetal brain easily because the blood–brain barrier is poorly developed. Approximately half of the drug-containing blood is then transported through the umbilical arteries to the placenta, where it reenters the maternal circulation. The mother can metabolize and excrete some drug molecules for the fetus.

## Drug Effects on the Fetus

Drug effects are determined mainly by the type and amount of drug, duration of exposure, and level of fetal growth and development during exposure. The fetus is sensitive to drug effects because it is small, has few plasma proteins that can bind drug molecules, and has a weak capacity for metabolizing and excreting drugs. In addition, the fetus is exposed to any drugs circulating in maternal

blood. Molecular size, weight, and lipid solubility determine which substances (chemicals, drugs, and antibodies) are readily absorbed into the fetal circulation from the maternal circulation. When drugs are taken on a regular schedule, fetal blood usually contains 50% to 100% of the amount in maternal blood. This means that any drug that stimulates or depresses the central nervous, cardiovascular, respiratory, or other body system in the mother has the potential to stimulate or depress those systems in the fetus. In some cases, fetotoxicity occurs. Drugs that may be **teratogenic** (causing abnormal embryonic or fetal development) are a major concern. Drug-induced teratogenicity is most likely to occur when drugs are taken during the first 3 months of pregnancy, during **organogenesis** (formation of embryonic organs during the first 3–8 weeks after conception) (Fig. 6.1). Malformations that occur during the pre-embryonic period (1st and 2nd week of pregnancy postconception) rarely result in a viable fetus (fetal stage starts after completion of week 8 of embryonic life). During the embryonic and fetal stages, teratogenic insult and timing result in the targeting of specific organ growth during organogenesis and subsequent maturation and refinement of an organ's physiologic purpose. For drugs taken during the second and third trimesters, adverse effects are usually manifested in the neonate (birth to 1 month) or infant (1 month to 1 year) as growth retardation, respiratory problems, infection, or bleeding. It should be emphasized, however, that drugs taken at any time during pregnancy can affect the baby's brain because brain development continues throughout pregnancy and after birth.

 *Concept Mastery Alert*

Drugs that are potentially harmful to a fetus are considered *teratogenic*. Potentially teratogenic substances include alcohol, morphine, cocaine, salicylates, coumarin anticoagulants, sedatives, tetracyclines, thiazides, tobacco smoke, and large doses of vitamin K.

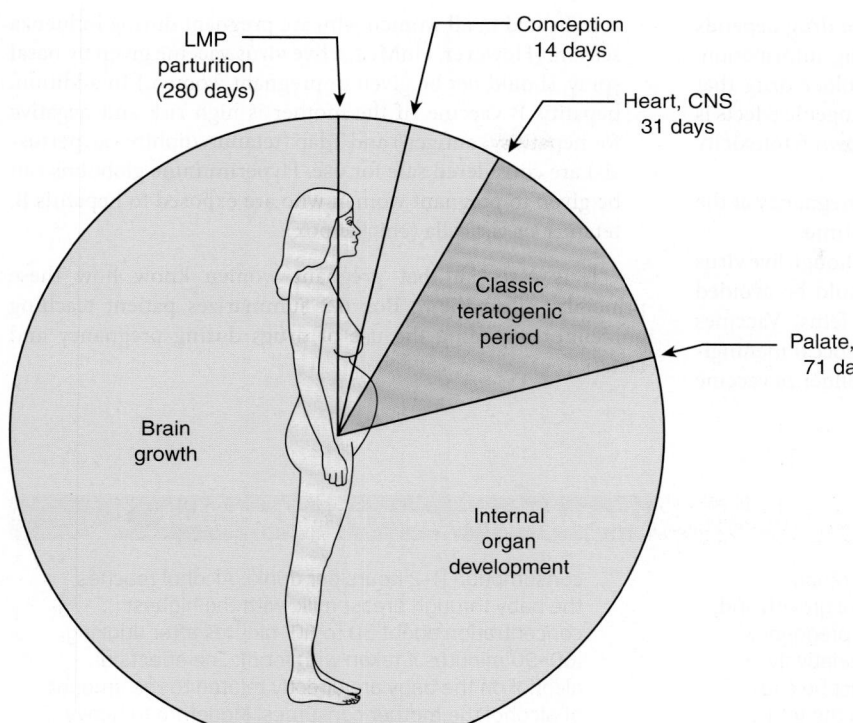

**Figure 6.1.** The gestational clock showing the classic teratogenic risk assessment. (Adapted from Niebyl, J. (1999). Drugs and related areas in pregnancy. In J. Sciarra (Ed.), *Obstetrics and gynecology*. Philadelphia, PA: Lippincott Williams & Wilkins.)

For 40 years, the U.S. Food and Drug Administration required manufacturers to assign pregnancy categories identifying potential risk for causing birth defects. Health care professionals sometimes made the wrong decisions about drugs based on these somewhat simplistic categories. The new system includes pregnancy information, risk summary, and clinical considerations, as well as data that should allow for better-informed prescribing decisions (see Chap. 2). Labeling changes for prescription drugs will be phased in gradually; therefore, the Drugs at a Glance tables in this edition provide the available pregnancy category for each listed drug. Box 6.1 is a list of teratogenic drugs.

## Principles of Drug Therapy in Pregnancy

Before administering a drug to a pregnant woman, it is the responsibility and obligation of all health care providers, including nurses, to conduct a risk–benefit assessment—a comprehensive analytic comparison of the benefits to the mother and the risks to the fetus. Inclusion of family in a decision regarding drug exposure during pregnancy and lactation to obtain informed consent is critical. Ideally, the risk to the fetus should be small compared with the potential maternal benefit. It is necessary to consider the consequences with and without drug therapy. Important factors are gestational age; drug route, dosage, and concentration; and duration of exposure.

General guidelines for drug therapy in pregnancy include the following:

- Pregnant women should take no drugs, regardless of their pregnancy risk category. It is essential that no drug be used during pregnancy unless it is clearly needed and the potential

benefit to the mother outweighs the risk of potential harm to the fetus.
- However, although the teratogenicity of many drugs is unknown, most medications required by pregnant women can be used safely, and most children are born healthy.

| BOX 6.1 | *Selected Teratogenic Drugs* |
|---|---|

**Risk Category D**

- Angiotensin-converting enzyme (ACE) inhibitors (captopril and others) (second and third trimesters)
- Angiotensin II receptor blockers (ARBs; losartan and others)
- Antibacterials (tetracycline, tigecycline)
- Antiepileptics (carbamazepine, valproate–category X for migraine prophylaxis)
- Antineoplastics (ibritumomab, idarubicin, ifosfamide, irinotecan)
- Antithyroid agents (propylthiouracil)
- Benzodiazepine (alprazolam, diazepam, lorazepam)
- Bisphosphonates (pamidronate, zoledronic acid)
- Opioid analgesics (with prolonged use or high doses at term)

**Risk Category X**

- Anticoagulant (warfarin)
- Antineoplastics (methotrexate)
- Antiviral (ribavirin)
- Benzodiazepine (temazepam, triazolam)
- Female sex hormones (estrogens, injectable progestins, oral contraceptives)
- Male sex hormones (androgens, anabolic steroids)
- Retinoids (acitretin, isotretinoin, and several topical preparations)
- Statin cholesterol-lowering drugs (atorvastatin, others)

- When drug therapy is necessary, the choice of drug depends on the stage of pregnancy and available drug information. During the first trimester, for example, an older drug that has not been associated with fetotoxic or teratogenic effects is usually preferred over a newer drug of unknown fetotoxicity or teratogenicity.
- It is important to give any drug used during pregnancy at the lowest effective dose for the shortest possible time.
- Some immunizations are safe in pregnancy, although live virus vaccines (e.g., measles, mumps, rubella) should be avoided because of possible harmful effects to the fetus. Vaccines against pneumococcal pneumonia, meningococcal meningitis, and hepatitis A can be used if indicated. Influenza vaccine is indicated in all women who are pregnant during influenza season. (However, FluMist, a live virus vaccine given by nasal spray, should *not* be given to pregnant women.) In addition, hepatitis B vaccine (if the mother is high risk and negative for hepatitis B antigen) and Tdap (tetanus, diphtheria, pertussis) are considered safe for use. Hyperimmune globulins can be given to pregnant women who are exposed to hepatitis B, tetanus, or varicella (chickenpox).

It is essential that pregnant women know how these principles affect them. Box 6.2 summarizes patient teaching guidelines regarding the use of drugs during pregnancy and lactation.

---

**BOX 6.2**  *Patient Teaching Guidelines: Drug Use During Pregnancy and Lactation*

- Any systemic drug ingested by a pregnant woman reaches the fetus and may interfere with fetal growth and development. For most drugs, safety during pregnancy has not been established, and all drugs are relatively contraindicated. Therefore, any drug use must be cautious and minimal to avoid potential harm to the fetus.
- Avoid drugs when possible and use them very cautiously when necessary. If women who are sexually active and not using effective contraception take any drugs, there is a high risk that potentially harmful agents may be ingested before pregnancy is suspected or confirmed. It is estimated that 50% or more of pregnancies are unplanned.
- Lifestyle or nontherapeutic drugs associated with problems during pregnancy include alcohol, caffeine, and cigarette smoking. Women should completely avoid alcohol when trying to conceive and throughout pregnancy; no amount is considered safe. Caffeine intake should be limited to no more than 200 to 300 mg of caffeine per day; excessive intake should be avoided. Women who smoke should quit if possible during pregnancy to avoid the effects of nicotine, carbon monoxide, and other chemicals on the fetus.
- Herbal supplements should be used with caution; their effects during pregnancy are unknown.
- Measures to prevent the need for drug therapy include a healthful lifestyle (adequate nutrition, exercise, rest, and sleep; avoiding alcohol; and cigarette smoking) and avoiding infection (personal hygiene, avoiding contact with people known to have infections, maintaining indicated immunizations).
- Inform any health care provider from whom treatment is sought if there is a possibility of pregnancy.
- Many drugs are excreted in breast milk to some extent and reach the nursing infant. The infant's health care provider should be informed about medications taken by the nursing mother and consulted about potential drug effects on the infant. Before taking over-the-counter medications, consult a health care provider. With regard to nontherapeutic drugs, recommendations include the following:
  - Alcohol should be used in moderation, and nursing should be withheld temporarily after alcohol consumption (1–2 hours per drink). Alcohol reaches the baby through breast milk, with the highest concentration about 30 to 60 minutes after drinking (60–90 minutes if taken with food). The effects of alcohol on the baby are directly related to the amount of alcohol the mother consumes. Moderate to heavy drinking (two or more drinks per day) can interfere with the ability to breast-feed, harm the baby's motor development, and slow the baby's weight gain. If you plan to drink (e.g., wine with dinner), you can avoid breast-feeding for a few hours (until the alcohol has time to leave your system), or you can pump her milk before drinking alcohol and give it to the baby after you have had the alcohol. (You can also pump and discard the milk that is most affected by the ingested alcohol.)
- Caffeine is considered compatible with breast-feeding. However, large amounts should be avoided because infants may be jittery and have difficulty sleeping.
- Cigarette smoking is not an absolute contraindication but should be strongly discouraged. Nicotine and an active metabolite are concentrated in milk, and the amounts reaching the infant are proportional to the number of cigarettes smoked by the mother. Ideally, the mother who smokes would stop. If unable (or unwilling) to stop, the woman should decrease the number of cigarettes as much as possible, avoid smoking before nursing, and avoid smoking (or allowing other people to smoke) in the same room with the infant. The risk of sudden infant death syndrome (SIDS) is greater when smoking or when the baby is around secondhand (passive) smoke. Maternal smoking and passive smoke exposure may also increase respiratory and ear infections in infants.
- Most drugs of abuse (e.g., cocaine, heroin, marijuana, methamphetamine, phencyclidine) are contraindicated. Mothers with opioid dependence who are enrolled in a supervised methadone maintenance program may be allowed to breast-feed.

## NCLEX Success

3. A woman with a seizure disorder has been taking phenytoin since she was 6 years old. She has recently married and wants to start a family. She understands the risk related to the use of phenytoin during pregnancy. What should the nurse advise the woman about pregnancy?

    A. She should discuss her concerns with her gynecologist and neurologist.
    B. She should stop the phenytoin and take folic acid.
    C. She should begin to take prenatal vitamins.
    D. She should consult a genetic counselor about her seizure disorder.

4. The nurse is providing immunization education to a pregnant woman. She should receive which of the following vaccines during cooler seasonal temperatures?

    A. rubella
    B. mumps
    C. influenza
    D. tetanus

### Unfolding Patient Stories: Danielle Young Bear • Part 1

**Danielle Young Bear** is a 32-year-old construction worker who made a clinic appointment for back pain and spasms. The provider has ordered cyclobenzaprine and ibuprofen. While the nurse is providing education on the medications, the patient states that she is pregnant. What drug exposure risks during pregnancy should the nurse consider? (Danielle Young Bear's story continues in Chap. 16.)

Care for Danielle and other patients in a realistic virtual environment: **vSim** *for Nursing* (thepoint.lww.com/vSimPharm). Practice documenting these patients' care in DocuCare (thepoint.lww.com/DocuCareEHR).

## FETAL THERAPEUTICS

Although the major concern about drugs ingested during pregnancy is adverse effects on the fetus, a few drugs are given to the mother for therapeutic effects on the fetus. These include digoxin for fetal tachycardia or heart failure, levothyroxine for hypothyroidism, penicillin for exposure to maternal syphilis and group B *Streptococcus* (GBS), and prenatal betamethasone to promote surfactant production, thus improving fetal lung function and decreasing respiratory distress syndrome in preterm infants. Also, pregnant women who are rhesus factor (Rh) negative receive Rh immune globulin (RhoGAM) for antenatal and postpartal prevention of sensitization to the Rh factor and hemolytic disease of the newborn.

## MATERNAL THERAPEUTICS

Thus far, the main emphasis on drug use during pregnancy has related to actual or potential adverse effects on the fetus. Despite the general principle that drug use should be avoided whenever possible, pregnant women may require drug therapy for immunizations, various illnesses, increased nutritional needs, pregnancy-associated problems, chronic disease processes, treatment of preterm labor, induction of labor, pain management during labor, and prevention of postpartum hemorrhage.

To meet the increased nutritional needs of pregnancy, health care providers order prenatal vitamins and mineral supplements for pregnant women. Folic acid supplementation is especially important to prevent neural tube birth defects, primarily spina bifida. Such abnormalities occur early in pregnancy, often before a woman realizes she is pregnant. For this reason, it is recommended that all women of childbearing potential ingest 400 or 600 mcg of folic acid daily, either from food and/or a supplement.

The use of natural herbs as a supplement and as treatment for common ailments has greatly increased in popularity. Although herbs are natural, some may be poisonous. Not all herbs are safe for consumption during pregnancy and lactation. Box 6.3 summarizes information on the use of herbs in pregnancy.

### Clinical Application 6.1

- What issues relating to teratogenic substances are of concern in Ms. Ross' pregnancy?

## Management of Pregnancy-Associated Symptoms

### Anemias

Two types of anemia are common during pregnancy. One is physiologic anemia (often defined as a hemoglobin below 11 g/dL or hematocrit below 33%), which results from expanded blood volume. The second is iron deficiency anemia, which is often related to long-term nutritional deficiencies.

Experts recommend an increase in iron consumption to about 30 mg/d. This is readily met by most prenatal vitamins and is adequate for nonanemic women. Women with iron deficiency anemia should receive additional iron supplementation of 60 to 200 mg/d until anemia is corrected.

### Constipation

Elevated progesterone levels cause smooth muscle relaxation and decrease peristalsis leading to constipation. Preferred treatment is to increase exercise and intake of fluids and high-fiber foods. If a laxative is required, a bulk-producing agent such as psyllium (Metamucil) is the most physiologic for the mother and safest for the fetus because it is not absorbed systemically. A stool softener such as docusate (Colace) or an occasional saline laxative (milk of magnesia) may also be used.

BOX 6.3     *Use of Herbs During Pregnancy*

- Some herbs may contain ingredients that are contraindicated in pregnancy and lactation. Many herbs can cause miscarriage, preterm birth, and uterine contractions, which induce labor.
- As remedies, herbs are not subjected to rigorous testing and evaluation because they are not prescription drugs. Consequently, the quality and strength of such supplements may vary significantly, reducing safety for use during pregnancy and lactation.
- The U.S. Food and Drug Administration urges pregnant and lactating women to discuss the use of herbs or essential oils with their health care providers. Many women may take herbal supplements without informing their obstetricians or nurse midwives, thus complicating and increasing the likelihood of drug interactions with herbal supplements.
- In an effort to make herbal supplements safe, some organizations specializing in herbal remedies have performed extensive testing and evaluations on herbs to devise a

safety rating scale for the general population as well as pregnant and breast-feeding women. However, the safety ratings can often be controversial and vague. For instance, some herbs may be safe when used orally in amounts found in food but considered unsafe or contraindicated when used in medicinal or concentrated amounts, especially in pregnancy.
- The following herbal supplements may be unsafe during pregnancy: black cohosh, blue cohosh, dong quai, ephedra, goldenseal, passion flower, pau d'arco, pennyroyal, roman chamomile, saw palmetto, and yohimbe.
- The following herbal supplements are likely to be safe during pregnancy:
Red raspberry leaf—helps tone uterus, increase milk production, decrease nausea, and ease labor pains
Peppermint leaf—relieve nausea, vomiting, and flatulence
Ginger root—relieve nausea and vomiting
Slippery elm bark—decreases nausea and relieves heartburn
Oats and oat straw—reduces anxiety and restlessness.

Mineral oil should be avoided because it interferes with absorption of fat-soluble vitamins. Reduced absorption of vitamin K can lead to bleeding in newborns. Castor oil, all strong laxatives, and excessive amounts of any laxative should be avoided because they can cause uterine contractions and initiate labor.

### Gastroesophageal Reflux Disease

Gastroesophageal reflux disease (GERD), of which heartburn (pyrosis) is the main symptom, is very common in pregnant women, especially as gestation increases. Hormonal changes relax the lower esophageal sphincter, and the growing fetus increases abdominal pressure. These developments allow gastric acid to pass into the esophagus and cause discomfort and esophagitis. In addition, GERD may trigger asthma attacks in pregnant women with asthma.

Nonpharmacologic interventions include eating small meals; not eating for 2 to 3 hours before bedtime; avoiding caffeine, gas-producing foods, and constipation; and sitting in an upright position. For patients who do not obtain adequate relief with these measures, drug therapy may be needed. Antacids may be used if necessary. Because little systemic absorption occurs, the drugs are unlikely to harm the fetus if used in recommended doses. A histamine ($H_2$) receptor antagonist such as ranitidine (Zantac) may also be effective. Proton pump inhibitors such as esomeprazole (Nexium) are thought to be safe, but some clinicians reserve them for patients for whom $H_2$ blockers are ineffective.

### Gestational Diabetes Mellitus

Gestational diabetes mellitus (GDM) is glucose intolerance that first occurs during pregnancy. Women with risk factors (obesity; age older than 25 years; family history of diabetes; being Hispanic, Native American, Asian, or African American; previous pregnancy loss; fetal anomalies; or large baby) may be screened as early as the first prenatal visit. If early testing is not performed, universal screening may be done between 24 and 28 weeks of gestation because of the maternal peripheral

resistance of insulin due to hormones after the 24th week. The criterion for a diagnosis of GDM is based on the results of two or more elevated levels of the 100-g oral glucose tolerance test: fasting plasma glucose level of more than 95 mg/dL, 1-hour glucose level of more than 180 mg/dL, 2-hour glucose level of more than 155 mg/dL, and 3-hour glucose level of more than 140 mg/dL.

Women with GDM are at higher risk for complications of pregnancy and possible fetal harm. Poor glycemic control, primarily hyperglycemia in early gestation resulting in fetal hyperinsulinemia, increases the likelihood of structural defects in the fetus, particularly during organogenesis. Congenital deformities in the fetus often involve the heart and the central nervous system (CNS), leading to multiorgan malformations. Hyperinsulinemia increases the amount of growth factor causing macrosomia. Additionally, hyperinsulinemia interferes with the production of surfactant, which contributes to fetal lung maturity. Lack of surfactant results in respiratory distress syndrome in the neonate. Infants of mothers with GDM who had been under close diabetic monitoring during pregnancy may have complications of hypoglycemia, hyperbilirubinemia, hypocalcemia, and polycythemia.

The goal of treatment during pregnancy is to keep blood glucose levels as near normal as possible because even mild hyperglycemia can be detrimental to the fetus; it stimulates the fetal pancreas to secrete high levels of insulin.

Insulin (see Chap. 41) does not cross the placenta and has a long history of safe usage. Thus, it is the drug of choice for treatment of diabetes during pregnancy. For women who are unable or unwilling to take insulin, oral antidiabetic agents such as metformin or glyburide may be reasonable alternatives.

When the pregnancy ends, blood glucose levels usually return to a normal range within a few weeks. Women may breast-feed, and hypoglycemics are safe during lactation. Up to two-thirds of women with gestational diabetes will have gestational diabetes in a subsequent pregnancy and 50% to 70% will develop type 2 diabetes within 15 to 25 years.

## NCLEX Success

**5. A nurse knows that teaching was successful when expectant parents give which of the following rationales for administering folic acid supplements?**

   A. prevent hydrocele
   B. increase absorption
   C. prevent neural tube deformity
   D. decrease blood glucose

**6. A nurse is providing prenatal teaching in the obstetric clinic. Which of the following herbal supplements helps in the prevention of nausea and vomiting?**

   A. St. John's wort
   B. ginger
   C. black cohosh
   D. garlic

### Nausea and Vomiting

Nausea and vomiting often occur during early pregnancy due to high levels of hCG and estrogen. Low blood sugar, as well as magnesium deficiency, can exacerbate nausea and vomiting. Intractable vomiting with subsequent weight loss and its effect on fetal growth and development must be assessed when considering antiemetic drug therapy.

Pregnant women may require antiemetic medications, especially if nausea and vomiting are severe and threaten maternal and fetal nutritional or metabolic status (hyperemesis gravidarum). Treatment with an antihistamine ($H_1$ antagonists) such as meclizine; dopamine antagonists such as metoclopramide (Reglan), promethazine (Promethegan), or prochlorperazine (Compro); and serotonin antagonists such as ondansetron (Zofran) are used as part of the initial approach to care. If drug therapy is unsuccessful in controlling nausea and vomiting, or weight loss and electrolyte imbalance persists, total parenteral nutrition may be necessary until oral fluids are tolerated.

### Hypertensive Disorders in Pregnancy

Hypertensive disorders in pregnancy include preeclampsia and eclampsia, conditions that endanger the lives of mother and fetus. **Preeclampsia** is manifested by hypertension and proteinuria, or hypertension and significant end-organ dysfunction with or without proteinuria after 20 weeks of gestation in a previously normotensive woman. Preeclampsia most often occurs during a first pregnancy, but it may affect women with chronic hypertension, diabetes mellitus, or multiple fetuses.

Management of hypertension in pregnancy varies. Outpatient observation, with frequent monitoring of mother and fetus, may be sufficient. Antihypertensive therapy is recommended for women with severe hypertension (systolic blood pressure greater than 160 mm Hg or diastolic blood pressure greater than 110 mm Hg). Drug therapy for severe preeclampsia includes oral nifedipine (Procardia) (see Chap. 28), intravenous (IV) hydralazine or labetalol (Trandate) (see Chap. 26) for blood pressure control, as well as magnesium sulfate (see Chap. 53) for the prevention of seizures.

### ! QSEN Alert: Safety

Magnesium sulfate is considered a high-alert medication and requires special precautions for administration and monitoring because of potentially severe adverse effects.

Safety measures include a unit protocol that standardizes drug concentration, flow rate, type of infusion pump, and frequency and type of maternal–fetal assessment data to be documented (serum magnesium levels, respiratory status, reflexes, uterine activity, urine output, fetal heart rate). This therapy reduces perinatal deaths and severe maternal hypertension.

If not effectively treated, preeclampsia may progress to **eclampsia**, which is characterized by potentially fatal seizures. Maternal complications can occur in up to 70% of women with eclampsia including hemolysis, elevated liver enzymes, and low platelets (HELLP) syndrome and disseminated intravascular coagulation, cardiopulmonary arrest, and perinatal death.

Overdoses of magnesium sulfate may lead to hypotension, muscle paralysis, respiratory depression, and cardiac arrest. Close monitoring for signs of hypermagnesemia is necessary, and serum levels may be drawn in women who have clinical signs of magnesium toxicity (Table 6.3). Calcium gluconate, the antidote for magnesium sulfate, should be readily available for use if hypermagnesemia occurs. Administration is slow IV push over 2 to 5 minutes. Neonates born to mothers who received magnesium sulfate require assessment for hypermagnesemia and respiratory depression at birth.

### Clinical Application 6.2

- What assessments reveal that Ms. Ross is at risk for preeclampsia?
- Why would administration of antiepileptic drugs be appropriate for Ms. Ross?
- The protein in Lauren's 24-hour urine collection is 500 mg. Her blood pressure continues to be high, with evidence of hyperreflexia (3+ reflexes). A magnesium sulfate drip is initiated with a loading dose of 4 g over 20 minutes per infusion pump. Oxytocin (Pitocin) infusion is started to induce labor. What are critical nursing assessments in this situation?

### TABLE 6.3

#### Magnesium Levels With Associated Signs and Symptoms of Toxicity*

| Magnesium Value (mEq/L) | Signs and Symptoms |
|---|---|
| 8–12 | Loss of deep tendon reflexes |
| 15 | Respiratory distress |
| 5–10 | Electrocardiographic changes |
| 25 | Cardiac arrest |

*Normal adult values for magnesium, 1.5 to 2 mEq/L; therapeutic serum magnesium level, 4 to 7 mEq/L.

# Management of Selected Infections in Pregnancy

## Group B Streptococcus

An estimated 25% of pregnant women are infected with GBS. Although rarely serious in adults, GBS can cause sepsis, meningitis, and pneumonia in the newborn if the mother does not receive intrapartum antibiotic prophylaxis. Potential maternal outcomes include urinary tract infection (UTI), chorioamnionitis, postcesarean wound infection, and postpartum endometritis.

Because of the potentially serious consequences of infection with GBS, pregnant women should have a rectovaginal culture at 35 to 37 weeks of gestation. A positive culture indicates infection that should be treated with an intravenous antibiotic that is effective against GBS. Penicillin (see Chap. 18) is the drug of choice, but alternative antibiotics can be prescribed for women with a penicillin allergy.

> ### Clinical Application 6.3
>
> - Explain the risk associated with perinatal GBS.

## Human Immunodeficiency Virus

Human immunodeficiency virus (HIV) infection in pregnant women requires antiretroviral drug therapy for the mother. This helps prevent transmission to the fetus/newborn. Almost all HIV infections are transmitted perinatally, either in utero, during labor and delivery, or in breast milk. The goal of treatment is to reduce the viral load as much as possible, which reduces the risk of transmission to the fetus/newborn. Antiretroviral drug therapy for the pregnant woman reduces perinatal transmission to less than 1% to 2%. In general, highly active antiretroviral therapy, or HAART, is safe, with recommended dosage the same as for nonpregnant women (see Chap. 23).

When labor starts, the HIV-positive pregnant woman should receive IV zidovudine. The dosage is 2 mg/kg infused over 1 hour and then 1 mg/kg/h, until the umbilical cord is clamped.

## Urinary Tract Infections

UTIs commonly occur during pregnancy and may include asymptomatic bacteriuria, cystitis, and pyelonephritis. Asymptomatic bacteriuria should be treated in pregnant women because of its association with cystitis and pyelonephritis. If untreated, symptomatic cystitis occurs in approximately 30% to 40% of pregnant women. Asymptomatic bacteriuria and UTIs are also associated with increased preterm births and infants with low birth weights. Hospitalization and intravenous antibiotics may be needed for management of pyelonephritis.

## Influenza

Influenza poses a substantial risk for pregnant women and their fetuses. Serious complications include bacterial pneumonia and dehydration, which can be fatal. Pregnant women are more likely to be hospitalized with influenza-related complications than nonpregnant women. All women who are pregnant or might be pregnant during the influenza season should receive the inactivated influenza vaccine. The influenza vaccine provides immunity to the fetus because the vaccine crosses the placenta. The immunity protects infants until they are old enough to be vaccinated.

## Tetanus, Diphtheria, and Pertussis

The tetanus–diphtheria–pertussis (Tdap) vaccine, licensed in 2005, is the first vaccine for adolescents and adults that protects against all three diseases—tetanus, diphtheria, and pertussis. A single dose of the Tdap vaccine is recommended for all pregnant women (in each pregnancy). If not given during pregnancy, it may be administered immediately postpartum. Administration of the Tdap, rather than the tetanus–diphtheria–toxoid vaccine (Td), is preferable because the prevalence of pertussis in the United States has been increasing.

## NCLEX Success

7. A woman has been diagnosed with gestational diabetes. What effect does maternal hyperglycemia have on the fetus?

   A. It results in fetal hyperinsulinemia.
   B. It produces seizures in the newborn.
   C. It increases the mother's risk of preterm labor.
   D. It decreases the birth weight.

8. A woman is receiving intravenous (IV) magnesium sulfate to control symptoms of preeclampsia. Which of the following signs or symptoms indicates a need for the administration of IV calcium gluconate?

   A. urine ketosis
   B. respiratory rate of 36 breaths/min
   C. anuria
   D. loss of deep tendon reflexes

9. A pregnant woman is discussing immunizations recommended during pregnancy with her provider. Which of the following vaccines is recommended during each pregnancy?

   A. tetanus-diphtheria-pertussis
   B. tetanus-diphtheria
   C. live attenuated influenza vaccine
   D. measles, mumps, and rubella

# DRUGS THAT ALTER UTERINE MOTILITY: TOCOLYTICS

Drugs given to reduce the strength and frequency of uterine contractions, thus helping inhibit labor and maintain the pregnancy, are called **tocolytics**. Uterine contractions with cervical changes before 37 weeks of gestation are considered **preterm labor**. Preterm labor may occur spontaneously, or premature rupture of membranes, infection, preeclampsia, multiple gestation, cigarette smoking, or alcohol may precipitate it. Drug therapy is most effective when the cervix is minimally dilated and amniotic membranes are intact. Tocolytics do not reduce the number of preterm births, but they may postpone birth long enough to reduce problems associated with prematurity (e.g., respiratory distress, bleeding in the brain, infant death)

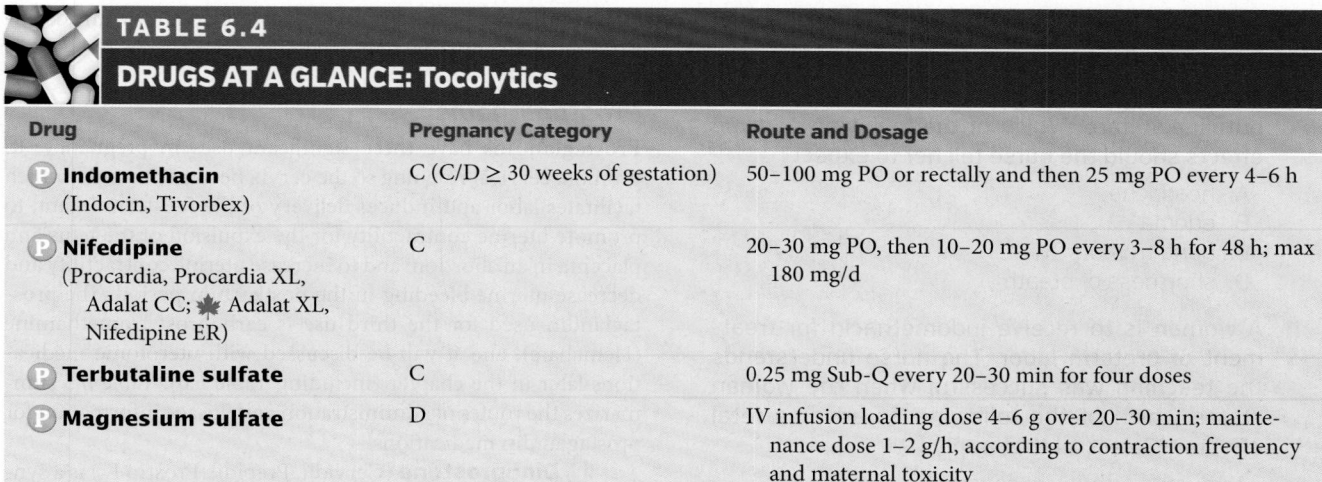

| Drug | Pregnancy Category | Route and Dosage |
|---|---|---|
| P **Indomethacin** (Indocin, Tivorbex) | C (C/D ≥ 30 weeks of gestation) | 50–100 mg PO or rectally and then 25 mg PO every 4–6 h |
| P **Nifedipine** (Procardia, Procardia XL, Adalat CC; ✿ Adalat XL, Nifedipine ER) | C | 20–30 mg PO, then 10–20 mg PO every 3–8 h for 48 h; max 180 mg/d |
| P **Terbutaline sulfate** | C | 0.25 mg Sub-Q every 20–30 min for four doses |
| P **Magnesium sulfate** | D | IV infusion loading dose 4–6 g over 20–30 min; maintenance dose 1–2 g/h, according to contraction frequency and maternal toxicity |

and allow for neuroprotection (reduce likelihood of cerebral palsy). The goal of treatment is to delay birth long enough for antenatal administration of a corticosteroid such as betamethasone (Celestone Soluspan) to the mother to improve pulmonary maturity and function in fetal lungs by the increased production of surfactant. First-line tocolytics include nonsteroidal anti-inflammatory drugs (NSAIDs), calcium channel blockers, and beta-agonists. Magnesium sulfate may also be used as a tocolytic and for its neuroprotective effects. Table 6.4 presents route and dosage information for the tocolytics.

---

**! QSEN Alert: Evidence-Based Practice**

Cigarette smoking during pregnancy is the most modifiable risk factor associated with adverse pregnancy outcomes, including preterm birth, neonatal growth restriction, and sudden infant death syndrome. In addition, smoking and exposure to secondhand smoke increase the risk of infertility, placental abruption, preterm premature rupture of membranes, and placenta previa. Pregnant women should be asked regularly about tobacco usage, including cigarettes, smokeless tobacco, and e-cigarettes and provided pregnancy-tailored counseling on cessation. A common strategy for smoking cessation is the "5 As": ask about and document smoking status, advise mothers who smoke to stop smoking and avoid secondhand smoke, assess the mother's readiness to quit smoking, assist the mother who wants to quit, and arrange for proper smoking cessation strategies. Nicotine replacement and bupropion are reasonable drug options that may be added to cessation counseling for pregnant or breast-feeding women who are otherwise unable to quit. Reinforcing success and providing ongoing support increase maternal success with smoking cessation.

---

## Nonsteroidal Anti-inflammatory Drugs

The NSAID P **indomethacin** (Indocin, Tivorbex) acts as a tocolytic by inhibiting uterine prostaglandins that initiate the uterine contractions of normal labor. Maternal adverse effects include nausea and vomiting, heartburn, headache, dizziness, and increased bleeding problems. Fetal adverse effects include constriction of the ductus arteriosus and oligohydramnios (decreased amniotic fluid). Because of these concerns, administration is not recommended after 32 weeks of gestation and for longer than 48 hours. There is a **BLACK BOX WARNING ◆** for this NSAID because of the increased risk of adverse cardiovascular events and gastrointestinal (GI) bleeding.

## Nifedipine

P **Nifedipine** (Procardia, Procardia XL, Adalat CC) is a calcium channel blocking drug that decreases uterine contractions and lowers blood pressure by blocking calcium movement into muscle cells. A common adverse effect is maternal hypotension, which may reduce blood flow between the placenta and the uterus and thus compromise the fetus. Prolonged events of this nature can lead to adverse fetal outcomes, and severe adverse reactions have occurred when nifedipine is used in conjunction with IV magnesium sulfate. Women with cardiovascular disease or who are hemodynamically unstable should not receive nifedipine.

## Terbutaline Sulfate

P **Terbutaline sulfate** is a beta-adrenergic agent that inhibits uterine contractions by reducing intracellular calcium levels. Adverse maternal effects may include tachycardia and palpitations, tremors, hypokalemia, hyperglycemia, and pulmonary edema. Terbutaline sulfate crosses the placenta, producing fetal tachycardia and neonatal hypoglycemia. Contraindications include hyperthyroidism and diabetes, as well as placenta previa or placental abruption. There is a **BLACK BOX WARNING ◆** advising against prolonged administration (longer than 48–72 hours) because of the potential for serious maternal heart problems and death.

## Magnesium Sulfate

P **Magnesium sulfate**, which has neuromuscular blocking activity, has long been given intravenously to help prevent preterm birth. This agent also offers neuroprotective properties to the neonate when administered before 32 weeks of gestation. Adjuvant use includes treatment for severe preeclampsia and eclampsia. Guidelines for administration of the drug are the same in tocolysis as in hypertension in pregnancy. In women with renal insufficiency, it is necessary to decrease the dosage or use an alternative treatment. Contraindications include myasthenia gravis.

## NCLEX Success

10. A woman experiencing preterm labor receives terbutaline sulfate. Which of the following adverse effects should the nurse tell her to expect?

    A. headache
    B. edema
    C. hand tremors
    D. shortness of breath

11. A woman is to receive indomethacin for treatment of preterm labor. The nurse understands the teaching was successful when the woman states which of the following as adverse fetal effects? [Select all that apply.]

    A. ductus arteriosus constriction
    B. polyhydramnios
    C. oligohydramnios
    D. ductus venosus constriction

12. A woman is admitted to the labor and delivery unit in preterm labor. The woman was diagnosed with hyperthyroidism 3 years ago. Which tocolytic is contraindicated?

    A. magnesium sulfate
    B. terbutaline sulfate
    C. nifedipine
    D. indomethacin

## DRUGS USED DURING LABOR AND DELIVERY AT TERM

Labor usually begins spontaneously and proceeds through delivery of the newborn and placenta. If labor does not occur spontaneously, it may be induced using an oxytocic, a drug that stimulates uterine contractions. Drugs often used during labor, delivery, and the immediate postpartum period include prostaglandins as well.

## Labor Induction

Common reasons for labor induction include postterm pregnancy, intrauterine growth restriction, maternal hypertension or diabetes, and premature rupture of membranes. Labor can also be initiated for the termination of a pregnancy with administration of an **abortifacient** drug.

### Prostaglandins

**Prostaglandins** have three significant uses in pregnancy: to promote cervical ripening so the cervix becomes thinner, which facilitates labor and induces delivery of the full-term infant; to promote uterine contractility for the expulsion of the fetus and placenta in an abortion; and to increase uterine contractility and decrease uterine bleeding in the postpartum period. The prostaglandin used for the third use is carboprost tromethamine (Hemabate), and it will be discussed with uterotonic medications later in the chapter (including Table 6.6). Table 6.5 summarizes the routes of administration and dosage information for prostaglandin medications.

Ⓟ **Dinoprostone** (Cervidil, Prepidil, Prostin E$_2$) is a synthetic prostaglandin E$_2$ that stimulates uterine contractions, such as the ones in labor. The drug is available as an endocervical gel, a vaginal insert, and a vaginal suppository. The first two forms enhance cervical ripening so the fetus can pass easily through the birth canal. The vaginal suppository is an abortifacient.

Adverse effects of dinoprostone include back pain, abnormal uterine contractions, GI upset, diarrhea, and fever. Contraindications include hypersensitivity to prostaglandins, as well as previous cesarean section, uterine surgery, cephalopelvic disproportion, fetal distress, and vaginal bleeding. Administration to patients with asthma, glaucoma, or ruptured membranes warrants caution. Oxytocin may be initiated 30 minutes after removal of the Cervidil vaginal insert or 6 to 12 hours after final dose of Prepidil endocervical gel. A **BLACK BOX WARNING ◆** indicates that the medication should be used only with strict adherence to the recommended dosages and by medically trained personnel who can provide immediate care if needed.

Ⓟ **Misoprostol** (Cytotec), a synthetic prostaglandin E$_1$, inhibits gastric acid secretion and increases bicarbonate to protect the lining of the stomach. An unlabeled use of the drug is to increase cervical ripening and induce labor. If the course of treatment changes and oxytocin is to be given, it is essential to wait 4 hours from the last administration of misoprostol before starting oxytocin. The nurse assesses for hyperstimulation of the uterus and monitors for a nonreassuring fetal heart rate. There is a **BLACK BOX WARNING ◆** related to the risk of uterine rupture and induced abortion if administered for gastric ulcer prevention in an unknown pregnant woman. Contraindications include prior cesarean section or uterine surgery.

## TABLE 6.5

### DRUGS AT A GLANCE: Prostaglandins

| Drug | Pregnancy Category | Routes and Dosages |
|---|---|---|
| Ⓟ **Dinoprostone** (Cervidil, Prepidil, Prostin E$_2$; 🍁 Cervidil, Prepidil, Prostin E$_2$) | C | 0.5 mg inserted into cervical canal; repeated every 6 h; max dose 1.5 mg in 24 h; 10 mg vaginal insert placed in posterior fornix of vagina; remove in 12 h; not for VBAC |
| Ⓟ **Misoprostol** (Cytotec) | X | Intravaginally 25 mcg (1/4 of a 100-mcg tablet) every 3–6 h; not for VBAC; for postpartum hemorrhage, 600–1000 mg rectally, 600–1000 mg orally, or 800 mg sublingual |

VBAC, vaginal birth after cesarean.

| TABLE 6.6 | | |
|---|---|---|
| **DRUGS AT A GLANCE: Oxytocics and Uterotonics** | | |
| Drug | Pregnancy Category | Routes and Dosage |
| Ⓟ **Oxytocin** (Pitocin, 🍁 Oxytocin for injection) | X | Induction/augmentation: IV by infusion pump, 0.5–1 milliunits/min, in 30–60 min intervals gradually increased by 1–2 milliunits/min until desired contractions<br>Postpartum hemorrhage: infusion of 30 units in 500 mL of IV fluids; 10–40 units added to 1000 mL of IV fluids infused at a bolus rate; 10 units IM after delivery of placenta |
| Ⓟ **Methylergonovine maleate** (Methergine) | C | 0.2 mg IM after delivery of the placenta or neonate's anterior shoulder, or during postpartum; may be repeated every 2–4 h<br>0.2 mg PO 3–4 times daily; max 7 d |
| Ⓟ **Carboprost tromethamine** (Hemabate, 🍁 Hemabate) | C | 250 mcg IM every 15–90 min, depending on uterine response; max 8 doses |

## Oxytocics

Ⓟ **Oxytocin** (Pitocin), a synthetic form of oxytocin, is the most commonly used **oxytocic** drug. Use of this manufactured hormone induces labor or augments weak, irregular uterine contractions during labor. Physiologic doses produce a rhythmic uterine contraction–relaxation pattern that approximates the normal labor process. It also activates oxytocin and is contraindicated in the presence of fetal distress or unfavorable fetal positions and presentations, a hypertonic uterus, cephalopelvic disproportion, and obstetrical emergencies where surgical intervention is favored such as prolapse of the umbilical cord or placenta previa. Table 6.6 summarizes the dosage and route of administration for oxytocin.

> ❗ **QSEN Alert: Safety**
>
> Oxytocin is considered a high-alert medication and requires special precautions for administration and monitoring because of potentially severe adverse effects.

Maternal adverse effects include cardiac dysrhythmias, hypertension, nausea, vomiting, excessive uterine stimulation, and water intoxication. Close monitoring of uterine activity and fetal response is essential. If a labor and delivery nurse is not available to monitor the fetal–maternal effects of oxytocin, it is necessary to suspend the infusion. There is a **BLACK BOX WARNING** ◆ regarding the appropriate use of the medication for medical, rather than elective induction of labor.

## NCLEX Success

13. A woman is admitted to labor and delivery for labor induction due to postterm pregnancy. Labor has not begun on its own, and the cervix is unfavorable. Which of the following medications promotes cervical ripening?
    A. dinoprostone
    B. nifedipine
    C. naproxen sodium
    D. oxytocin

14. The certified nurse midwife administers misoprostol in the woman's vagina to increase cervical ripening. The cervix ripens, but the contractions are not significant for the fetus to pass through the birth canal, and oxytocin is ordered. Which of the following is most important with regard to the administration of oxytocin?
    A. Begin the oxytocin immediately.
    B. Begin the oxytocin in 2 hours.
    C. Begin the oxytocin in 4 hours.
    D. Begin the oxytocin in 8 hours.

## Pain Management

During early labor, pain occurs with uterine contractions. During later stages of labor, pain occurs with perineal stretching.

### Analgesics

Intravenous systemic analgesics are commonly used to control pain during labor and delivery. These medications include opioids such as morphine and meperidine (Demerol), synthetic opioids such as fentanyl (Sublimaze), and opioid-antagonists such as butorphanol and nalbuphine (see Chap. 49). They may prolong labor and cause sedation and respiratory depression in the mother. These medications also cross the placenta and may result in alterations in fetal heart rate patterns and neonatal respiratory depression. If neonatal respiratory depression occurs, naloxone (Narcan) can be given.

Regional analgesia may be more effective than IV analgesics for pain management. Epidural analgesia involves administration of an opioid such as fentanyl, and an anesthetic such as ropivacaine or bupivacaine, through a catheter placed in the epidural space. With regional anesthesia, the mother is alert and comfortable. The neonate is rarely depressed. For a cesarean section, spinal anesthesia is commonly used due to its rapid onset of effect using anesthetics like with epidural administration. A long-acting form of morphine, Duramorph, or other opioid medication can also be added to the spinal anesthesia to provide pain relief for approximately 24 hours. Possible adverse effects include maternal hypotension and urinary retention (bladder distention). No significant effects on the fetus or neonate have been reported.

## Anesthetics

Local anesthetics are less commonly used to control discomfort and pain due to their short duration. They are injected by physicians for regional anesthesia in the pelvic area. Bupivacaine (see Chap. 50) is commonly used. Fetal bradycardia may briefly occur after administration but is usually not significant.

### Clinical Application 6.4

- An oxytocin (Pitocin) infusion begins to induce Ms. Ross' labor after her fetus is treated with betamethasone (Celestone Soluspan) to promote lung maturity. What effect might magnesium sulfate have on her labor progress?

## Uterotonics for Postpartum Hemorrhage

**Uterotonics** are drugs used to stop postpartum hemorrhage. After delivery of the placenta, oxytocin is the drug of choice for prevention or control of postpartum uterine bleeding. It is delivered IV through a bolus rate using an infusion pump. The drug reduces uterine bleeding by contracting the uterine muscle. It also plays a role in the letdown of breast milk to the nipples during lactation.

In the event of postpartum hemorrhage, other drugs (uterotonics) may be indicated for immediate use, such as **carboprost tromethamine** (Hemabate). This drug is a prostaglandin $F_2$ alpha agent that stimulates the uterus to contract. Contraindications include known allergy to prostaglandins, acute pelvic inflammatory disease, and active pulmonary, hepatic, renal, or cardiac disease. Caution is warranted in asthma; hypertension; hypotension; anemia; uterine abnormalities; and diseases of the heart, kidneys, or liver. The use of antiemetic and antidiarrheal drugs reduces GI upset. Adequate hydration during administration and throughout the postpartum phase is necessary. There is a **BLACK BOX WARNING ◆** that the medication should be used only with strict adherence to the recommended dosages and by medically trained personnel who can provide immediate care if needed. Table 6.6 provides route and dosage information for carboprost.

**Methylergonovine** (Methergine) is an oxytocic drug that increases the strength, duration, and frequency of the uterine contractions. Indications for use include the treatment of postpartum atony and hemorrhage as well as for uterine stimulation during the second stage of labor after delivery of the anterior shoulder. Contraindications include known allergy to methylergonovine and hypertension. It is important to monitor patients for hypertension, headache, dizziness, palpitations, and GI upset. Table 6.6 provides route and dosage information for methylergonovine.

Misoprostol (Cytotec), which is used for cervical ripening, may also be used for the management of postpartum hemorrhage.

### Clinical Application 6.5

- Why is Ms. Ross at high risk for postpartum hemorrhage?
- What preventive measure is taken immediately after delivery of the placenta?

# LACTATION

## Lactation Induction

Metoclopramide (Reglan) stimulates the hormone prolactin after delivery, thus inducing lactation. The galactagogue, or lactation inducing, effect of this drug is considered an off-label use of metoclopramide. The recommended dose is 10 to 15 mg two to three times a day for 7 to 14 days. Higher doses of the drug in the postpartum period have been associated with depression, and use in women with a history of depression warrants caution.

The herbs fenugreek, goat's rue, milk thistle, blessed thistle, and fennel seeds are just some herbal **galactagogues** thought to induce lactation or stimulate the production of breast milk in postpartum women.

## Drug Use During Lactation

Antidepressants such as selective serotonin reuptake inhibitors (SSRIs) and serotonin and norepinephrine reuptake inhibitors (SNRIs) disturb the serotonin balance and are first-line choices for pharmacologic management of depression in lactating women. Although antidepressants have been detected in human milk, the amount is very low to undetectable. For mothers with severe depression, the benefits often outweigh the risks, and pharmacologic treatment is recommended.

Box 6.4 presents a list of medications that are contraindicated during lactation. For a summary of patient teaching guidelines regarding the use of drugs during lactation, as well as pregnancy, see Box 6.2.

| BOX 6.4 | *Selected Drugs That Are Contraindicated or Not Recommended During Lactation* |
|---|---|

Angiotensin-converting enzyme (ACE) inhibitors (e.g., captopril, others)
Angiotensin receptor blockers (ARBs; e.g., losartan, others)
Antibacterials (tigecycline, sulfamethoxazole/trimethoprim during newborn period)
Antidepressants (amitriptyline, bupropion, citalopram, fluoxetine, venlafaxine)
Antiepileptics (lamotrigine, topiramate, zonisamide)
Antifungals (itraconazole, terbinafine)
Antihistamines (clemastine)
Antimanic agent (lithium)
Antipsychotics (clozapine, olanzapine, risperidone, others)
Antivirals (famciclovir)
Benzodiazepine antianxiety and sedative/hypnotic drugs (alprazolam, diazepam, triazolam, others)
Beta-adrenergic blockers (metoprolol, others)
Diuretics (hydrochlorothiazide)
Nonbenzodiazepine sedative/hypnotics (ramelteon)
Opioid analgesics (codeine, hydromorphone)
Proton pump inhibitors (esomeprazole, omeprazole, others)
Retinoids (isotretinoin)
Statin cholesterol-lowering drugs (atorvastatin, simvastatin, others)

## Lactation and Birth Control

Exclusive breast-feeding (no formula supplementation) causes a woman to have an absence of menstrual periods. The potential for ovulation is reduced but does not offer total protection against pregnancy. The use of birth control during lactation is safe for the newborn. The concern is related to the quantity of milk production due to the presence of additional hormones in the maternal system.

Progesterone (progestin)-only contraceptives are the contraceptive of choice because they are unlikely to cause a decrease in milk production. These include several types: the "mini-pill," implant (Nexplanon), injection (Depo-Provera), and intrauterine devices (Kyleena, Liletta, Mirena, Skyla). These are good choices for exclusively breast-feeding mothers because of the already decreased fertility with continuous lactation. Estrogen-containing contraceptives such as the vaginal ring (NuvaRing) and the transdermal patch (Xulane) have been associated with decreasing breast milk production.

## THE NURSING PROCESS

A concept map outlines the nursing process related to drug therapy considerations in this chapter. Additional nursing implications related to the disease process should also be considered in care decisions.

**Assessment**
- Assess each female patient of childbearing age for possible pregnancy.
- If the patient is known to be pregnant, assess for gestational age; use of prescription, over-the-counter, herbal, nontherapeutic, and illegal drugs; and acute or chronic health problems.
- For labor (preterm, spontaneous, or induced), assess for length of gestation, uterine contractions, vaginal bleeding or discharge, cervical dilatation, fetal heart rate patterns, maternal vital signs, and length of labor.

**Outcomes of Therapy**

The patient will
- Avoid unnecessary drug ingestion.
- Use nonpharmacologic measures when possible.
- Obtain optimal care during pregnancy, labor and delivery, and the postpartum period.
- Avoid behaviors that may lead to complications of pregnancy and labor and delivery.
- Breastfeed safely and successfully, if desired.

**Nursing Interventions**
- Use nondrug measures to prevent or minimize the need for drug therapy during pregnancy.
- Promote/provide optimal prenatal care.
- Assist women with chronic health problems to manage the disorder effectively and decrease risks of harm to self and baby.
- Help patients and families cope with complications of pregnancy and newborn attachment.

**Evaluation**
- Observe and interview actions taken to promote reproductive and general health and compliance with instructions for promoting and maintaining a healthy pregnancy and exclusive breastfeeding.
- Interview regarding ingestion of therapeutic and nontherapeutic drugs during pre-pregnancy, pregnancy, and lactating states.
- Observe and interview regarding health status of mother and neonate.

## KEY CONCEPTS

- Regardless of the designated pregnancy risk category or presumed safety, no drug should be used during pregnancy unless it is clearly needed and potential benefit to the mother outweighs the risk of potential harm to the fetus.
- A folic acid supplement is recommended for women who may become pregnant and during pregnancy to prevent neural tube defects, especially if a woman is epileptic.
- Depression immediately postpartum ("baby blues") may occur but should not extend past 14 days after birth. Counseling is recommended, with possible antidepressant therapy.
- The American Academy of Pediatrics (AAP) supports breast-feeding as optimal nutrition, and not a lifestyle choice, for infants during the 1st year of life and does not recommend stopping maternal drug therapy unless necessary.
- Prostaglandins promote cervical ripening to facilitate labor and delivery.

- There is a **BLACK BOX WARNING** ◆ associated with the tocolytics terbutaline sulfate and indomethacin, the prostaglandin agents dinoprostone, misoprostol, and carboprost tromethamine, as well as the oxytocic medication oxytocin.
- Oxytocin induces labor or augments weak, irregular uterine contractions during labor.
- Uterotonic agents prevent or control postpartum hemorrhage.
- Most systemic drugs taken by the mother reach the infant in breast milk. For some, the amount of drug is too small to cause significant effects; for others, effects on the nursing infant are unknown or potentially adverse.
- Most over-the-counter and prescription drugs should be taken only with physician approval during breast-feeding.
- Women with HIV infection should not breast-feed. The virus can be transmitted to the nursing infant.

## CLINICAL REASONING CASE STUDY

| | |
|---|---|
| **Meet the Patient** | Jessica and Michael Joseph have been trying to get pregnant for the last year without success. They have an appointment with Jessica's gynecologist to discuss their difficulties in becoming pregnant. Trina Johnson, DNP, FNP-C, RN is the nurse practitioner who will be seeing them initially. Upon examination there is no evidence of infertility in either Jessica or Michael. Dr. Johnson prescribes clomiphene citrate 50 mg PO once daily for 5 days. Jessica is to begin the administration of clomiphene citrate on the 5th day of the cycle. Dr. Johnson also instructs Jessica and Michael on the measurement of the basal temperature.<br><br>• What is clomiphene citrate?<br>• Why has Dr. Johnson prescribed clomiphene citrate?<br>• What is the action of clomiphene citrate?<br>• What is the rationale for educating Jessica and Michael on how to assess basal temperature? |
| **Assessing Drug Information** | • Clomiphene citrate (Serophene [DSC]) is an ovulation stimulator; selective estrogen receptor modulator.<br>• The mechanism of action of clomiphene citrate is at the level of the hypothalamus to occupy the cell surface and intracellular estrogen receptors for longer duration then estrogen. This action then interferes with receptor recycling to deplete the intracellular estrogen receptors and inhibit estrogen negative feedback. This inhibition increases GnRH secretion and the release of FSH and LH. As a result, growth of the ovarian follicle occurs followed by follicular rupture.<br>• Ovulation occurs in 5–10 days after the course of treatment is completed.<br>• The rise in the basal temperature is predictive of ovulation. |
| **Nursing Actions** | • Instruct Jessica and Michael on the administration of clomiphene citrate.<br>　• On the fifth day of her cycle, Jessica should begin taking 50 mg of clomiphene citrate once daily for 5 days.<br>　• Ovulation should occur 5–10 days after the course of clomiphene citrate.<br>• Instruct Jessica on the assessment of basal temperature.<br>　• Purchase a basal thermometer (available at drug stores).<br>　• Begin assessing and recording basal temperature the day following the completion of the course of clomiphene citrate.<br>　• The basal temperature is the temperature at rest. Jessica should take her temperature at the same time every morning prior to rising.<br>• Instruct Jessica that the body temperature dips slightly before the ovary releases the egg, then rises 24 hours after the egg is released and stays up for several days (e.g., 97° before ovulation and 97.6–98.6° after ovulation). |

*Visit* thePoint® *at* **http://thePoint.lww.com/Frandsen12e** *for answers to NCLEX Success questions (in Appendix A), answers to Clinical Application Case Studies (in Appendix B), and more!*

## REFERENCES AND RESOURCES

American College of Obstetricians and Gynecologists. (2018). ACOG committee opinion #751. *Obstetrics & Gynecology, 132*(3), e131–e137.

American Pregnancy Association. (2017). *Herbs and pregnancy.* Retrieved September 17, 2018, from http://americanpregnancy.org/pregnancy-health/herbs-and-pregnancy/

Anawalt, B. D., & Page, S. T. (2017). Causes of male infertility. *UpToDate.* Lexi Comp, Inc.

Auerbach, M., & Landy, H. L. (2018). Anemia in pregnancy. *UpToDate.* Lexi Comp, Inc.

August, P. (2018). Management of hypertension in pregnant and postpartum women. *UpToDate.* Lexi Comp Inc.

August, P., & Sibai, B. M. (2018). Preeclampsia: clinical features and diagnosis. *UpToDate.* Lexi Comp Inc.

Barss, V. A. (2018). Immunizations during pregnancy. *UpToDate.* Lexi Comp Inc.

Briggs, G. G., Freeman, R. K., Towers, C. V., & Forinash, A. B. (2017). *Drugs in pregnancy and lactation* (11th ed.). Philadelphia, PA: Wolters Kluwer Health/Lippincott Williams & Wilkins.

Brodribb, W. (2018). ABM clinical protocol #9: Use of galactagogues in initiating or augmenting maternal milk production, second revision 2018. *Breastfeeding Medicine, 13*(5), 307–314.

Brucker, M. C., & King, T. L. (2017). The 2015 US food and drug administration pregnancy and lactation labeling rule. *Journal of Midwifery & Women's Health, 62*(3), 308–316.

Durnwald, C. (2018). Diabetes mellitus in pregnancy: screening and diagnosis. *UpToDate.* Lexi Comp, Inc.

Durnwald, C. (2018). Gestational diabetes mellitus: glycemic control and maternal prognosis. *UpToDate.* Lexi Comp, Inc.

Garner, C. D. (2018). Nutrition in pregnancy. *UpToDate.* Lexi Comp, Inc.

Hooton, T. M., & Gupta, K. (2017). Urinary tract infections and asymptomatic bacteriuria in pregnancy. *UpToDate.* Lexi Comp, Inc.

Jamieson, D. J., & Rasmussen, S. A. (2018). Influenza and pregnancy. *UpToDate.* Lexi Comp, Inc.

Karch, A. M. (2019). *Lippincott pocket drug guide for nurses.* Philadelphia, PA: Wolters Kluwer Health/Lippincott Williams & Wilkins.

Kuohung, W., & Hornstein, M. (2017). Overview of infertility. *UpToDate.* Lexi Comp, Inc.

Kuohung, W., & Hornstein, M. (2017). Causes of female infertility. *UpToDate.* Lexi Comp, Inc.

Lockwood, C. L., & Magriples, U. (2018). Prenatal care: Patient education, health promotion, and safety of commonly used drugs. *UpToDate.* Lexi Comp, Inc.

Mattson, S., & Smith, J. E. (2016). *Core curriculum for maternal-newborn nursing* (5th ed.). Missouri: Elsevier Saunders.

Norwitz, E. R. (2018). Preeclampsia: Management and prognosis. *UpToDate.* Lexi Comp Inc.

Ricci, S. S. (2017). *Essentials of maternity, newborn, and women's health nursing* (4th ed.). Philadelphia, PA: Wolters Kluwer Health/Lippincott Williams & Wilkins.

Rodriguez-Thompson, D. (2018). Cigarette and tobacco products in pregnancy: Impact on pregnancy and the neonate. *UpToDate.* Lexi Comp Inc.

Rodriguez-Thompson, D. (2018). Cigarette smoking in pregnancy: Cessation strategies and treatment options. *UpToDate.* Lexi Comp Inc.

Simhan, H. N., & Caritis, S. (2017). Inhibition of acute preterm labor. *UpToDate.* Lexi Comp Inc.

Smith, J. A., & Fox, K. A. (2018). Treatment and outcome of nausea and vomiting of pregnancy. *UpToDate.* Lexi Comp Inc.

Sriraman, N. K., Melvin, K., Meltzer-Brody, S.; & Academy of Breastfeeding Medicine. (2015). ABM clinical protocol #18: Use of antidepressants in breastfeeding mothers. *Breastfeeding Medicine, 10*(6), 290–299.

Tasnif, Y., Morado, J., & Herbert, M. F. (2016). Pregnancy-related pharmacokinetic changes. *Clinical Pharmacology & Therapeutics, 100*(1), 53–62.

UpToDate. (2019). *Drug information.* Lexi-Comp, Inc.

Wambach, K., & Riordan, J. (2016). *Breastfeeding and human lactation* (5th ed.). Burlington, MA: Jones & Bartlett, LLC.

# Pharmacology and Women's Health

## LEARNING OBJECTIVES

*After studying this chapter, you should be able to:*

1. Identify the mechanisms of action of endogenous estrogens and progesterone.
2. Describe the fundamental workings of the menstrual cycle.
3. Identify the signs and symptoms associated with common reproductive health problems experienced by women.
4. Identify the prototype drug for the estrogens, progestins, and estrogen–progestin combinations.
5. Describe the estrogens in terms of action, use, contraindications, adverse effects, and nursing implications.
6. Describe the progestins in terms of action, use, contraindications, adverse effects, and nursing implications.
7. Describe the estrogen–progestin combinations in terms of action, use, contraindications, adverse effects, and nursing implications.
8. Evaluate the benefits and risks associated with postmenopausal hormone replacement therapy.
9. Implement the nursing process in patients taking estrogens, progestins, and estrogen–progestin combinations.

## CLINICAL APPLICATION CASE STUDY

Paula Bigelow, a 52-year-old woman, has been complaining of vaginal dryness, hot flashes, and night sweats for the past 6 months. She reports that her last normal menstrual period was over 1 year ago.

## KEY TERMS

**Estrogen:** hormone produced primarily by the ovaries and secondarily by the adrenal cortex that promotes growth of specific body cells and development of most female secondary sexual characteristics

**Menopause:** permanent end of menstrual periods, which usually occurs in women 48 to 55 years of age

**Progesterone:** hormone produced in the ovaries and adrenal cortex that prepares the lining of the uterus for pregnancy

**Progestin:** synthetic form of progesterone that is similar to the hormone produced naturally by the body most often used in combination with an estrogen in contraceptive products

# INTRODUCTION

This chapter focuses on drug therapy in women's health care. **Estrogen** and **progesterone** are female sex hormones produced primarily by the ovaries and secondarily by the adrenal cortex in nonpregnant women. Small amounts of estrogens are also synthesized in the liver, kidney, brain, skeletal muscle, testes, and adipose tissue. In normal premenopausal women, estrogen synthesis in adipose tissue may be a significant source of the hormone. Some evidence indicates that a minimum body weight (about 105 lb) and fat content (16%–24%) are required for initiation and maintenance of the menstrual cycle. The observation that women with anorexia nervosa, chronic disease, or malnutrition, as well as women who engage in long-distance running, usually have amenorrhea supports this view. With anorexia nervosa, regaining weight and body mass usually reestablishes normal menstrual patterns.

As with other steroid hormones, estrogen and progesterone are synthesized from cholesterol. The ovaries and adrenal glands can manufacture cholesterol or extract it from the blood. Through a series of chemical reactions, cholesterol is converted to progesterone and then to androgens, testosterone, and androstenedione. The ovaries use these male sex hormones to produce estrogens. After formation, the hormones are secreted into the bloodstream in response to stimulation by the anterior pituitary gonadotropic hormones, follicle-stimulating hormone (FSH), and luteinizing hormone (LH). In the bloodstream, the hormones combine with serum proteins and are transported to target tissues, where they enter body cells. They cross cell membranes easily because of their steroid structure and lipid solubility. Inside the cells, the hormones bind to estrogen or progesterone receptors and regulate intracellular protein synthesis. Estrogen can enhance target-tissue responses to progesterone by increasing progesterone receptors. Progesterone seems to inhibit tissue responses to estrogen by decreasing estrogen receptors.

# OVERVIEW OF REPRODUCTION IN WOMEN

To adequately understand the pharmacologic effects of estrogens and **progestins** (synthetic progesterone), it is important to understand the physiology of female reproductive hormones and the menstrual cycle.

## Physiology

### Estrogens

The main function of the estrogens is to promote growth in tissues related to reproduction and sexual characteristics in women. Estrogens also have specific effects on other body tissues (Box 7.1). Three ovarian estrogens (estradiol, estrone, and estriol, known as endogenous estrogens) are secreted in significant amounts.

| BOX 7.1 | *Effects of Endogenous Estrogens* |
|---|---|

**Breasts**

- Stimulate growth at puberty by causing deposition of fat, formation of connective tissue, and construction of ducts. These ducts become part of the milk-producing apparatus after additional stimulation by progesterone.

**Sexual Organs**

- Enlarge the fallopian tubes, uterus, vagina, and external genitalia at puberty, when estrogen secretion increases greatly
- Cause the endometrial lining of the uterus to proliferate and develop glands that later nourish the implanted ovum when pregnancy occurs
- Increase resistance of the epithelial lining of the vagina to trauma and infection

**Skeleton**

- Stimulate skeletal growth so that, beginning at puberty, height increases rapidly for several years. Estrogen then causes the epiphyses to unite with the shafts of the long bones, and linear growth is halted. This effect of estrogen is stronger than the similar effect of testosterone in the male. Consequently, women stop growing in height several years earlier than do men and on the average are shorter than men.
- Conserve calcium and phosphorus for healthy bones and teeth. This action promotes bone formation and decreases bone loss.
- Broaden the pelvis in preparation for childbirth

**Skin and Subcutaneous Tissue**

- Increase vascularity in the skin. This leads to greater skin warmth and likelihood of bleeding in women.
- Cause deposition of fat in subcutaneous tissue, especially in the breasts, thighs, and buttocks, which produces the characteristic female figure.

**Anterior Pituitary Gland**

- Decrease pituitary secretion of follicle-stimulating hormone and increase secretion of luteinizing hormone when blood levels are sufficiently high (negative feedback mechanism)

**Metabolism**

- Affect metabolism of both reproductive and nonreproductive tissues. Estrogen receptors are found in female reproductive organs, breast tissue, bone, brain, liver, heart, and blood vessels. They are also found in various tissues in men.
- Increase protein anabolism, bone growth, and epiphyseal closure in young girls
- Decrease bone resorption
- Increase sodium and water retention, serum triglycerides, and high-density lipoproteins (HDLs or "good" cholesterol)
- Decrease low-density lipoproteins (LDLs or "bad" cholesterol)
- Increase the amount of cholesterol in bile and thereby increase gallstone formation

**Blood Coagulation**

- Enhance coagulation by increasing blood levels of several clotting factors, including prothrombin and factors VII, IX, and X, and probably increase platelet aggregation

Estradiol is the major estrogen because it exerts more estrogenic activity than the other two estrogens combined.

In nonpregnant women, between puberty and menopause (permanent end of menstrual periods), estrogens are secreted in a monthly cycle called the menstrual cycle. During the first half of the cycle, before ovulation, estrogens are secreted in progressively larger amounts. During the second half of the cycle, estrogens and progesterone are secreted in increasing amounts until 2 to 3 days before the onset of menstruation. At that time, secretion of both hormones decreases abruptly. When the endometrial lining of the uterus loses its hormonal stimulation, it is discharged vaginally as menstrual flow.

During pregnancy, the placenta in conjunction with the fetus produces large amounts of estrogen causing enlargement of the uterus and breasts, growth of glandular tissue in the breasts, and relaxation of ligaments and joints in the pelvis. All these changes are necessary for the growth and birth of the fetus.

Finally, estrogens are deactivated in the liver and readily excreted through the kidneys. Metabolites are also formed in the gastrointestinal (GI) tract, brain, skin, and other steroid target tissues. Most of the conjugates are excreted in urine, and some are excreted in bile and recirculated to the liver or excreted in feces.

## Progesterone

In general, progesterone has different effects on lipid metabolism compared with estrogen. That is, progesterones decrease high-density lipoprotein (HDL) cholesterol and increase low-density lipoprotein (LDL) cholesterol, both of which increase the risk of cardiovascular disease. Physiologic progesterone increases insulin levels but does not usually impair glucose tolerance. However, long-term administration of potent synthetic exogenous progestins, such as norgestrel, may decrease glucose tolerance and make diabetes mellitus more difficult to control. Like estrogen, progesterone is metabolized in the liver.

In nonpregnant women, progesterone is secreted by the corpus luteum during the last half of the menstrual cycle, which occurs after ovulation. This hormone continues the changes in the endometrial lining of the uterus begun by estrogens during the first half of the menstrual cycle. These changes provide for implantation and nourishment of a fertilized ovum. When fertilization does not take place, the estrogen and progesterone levels decrease and menstruation occurs.

If the ovum is fertilized, progesterone acts to maintain the pregnancy. The corpus luteum produces progesterone during the first few weeks of gestation. Then, the placenta produces the progesterone needed to maintain the endometrial lining of the uterus. In addition to its effects on the uterus, progesterone prepares the breasts for lactation by promoting development of milk-producing cells. Milk is not secreted, however, until the

cells are further stimulated by prolactin from the anterior pituitary gland. Progesterone also may help maintain pregnancy by decreasing uterine contractility. This, in turn, decreases the risk of spontaneous abortion.

## *Menstrual Cycle*

The menstrual cycle consists of the follicular phase (days 1–14) and the luteal phase (days 15–28). Hormones in the hypothalamus, pituitary gland, and ovary regulate this cycle. The usual length of a complete menstrual cycle is 28 days, and the first day of menstrual bleeding is day 1.

Figure 7.1 shows how the hormones interact in this cycle. Initially, the hypothalamus releases gonadotropin-releasing hormone (GnRH), which causes the anterior pituitary gland to produce FSH in the follicular phase of the cycle. FSH results in the maturing of ovarian follicles, which in turn produce estrogens. Increasing estrogen levels result in the continued maturation of the ovarian follicle and increasing growth of the endometrium. A negative feedback system responds to the increasing amounts of estrogen by decreasing the amount of FSH. At midcycle (typically day 14 of a 28-day menstrual cycle), the anterior pituitary gland releases LH, resulting in the rupture of the ovarian follicle and the development of the corpus luteum. This process is ovulation. The corpus luteum releases progesterone and estrogen, which causes the endometrial lining to continue to increase in thickness and

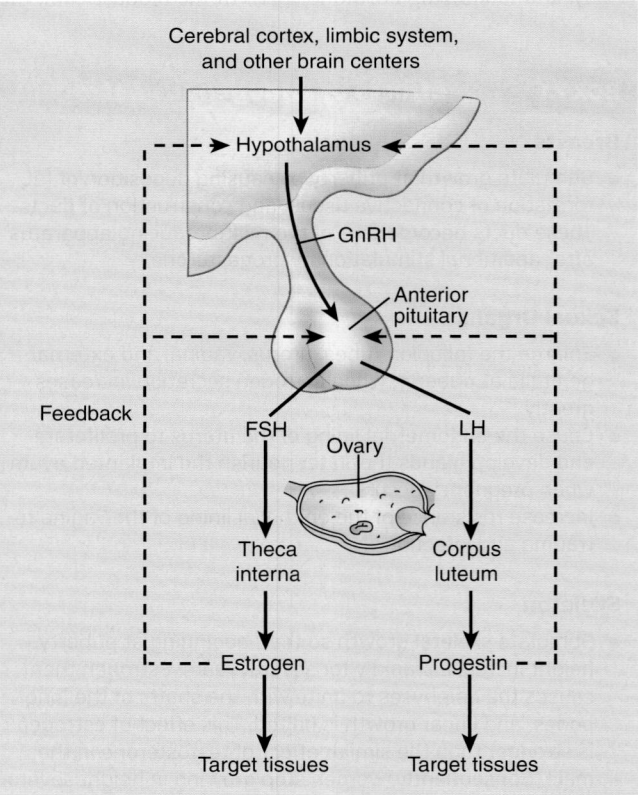

**Figure 7.1.** Hypothalamic–pituitary feedback control of estrogen and progesterone levels in the female. The *dashed line* represents negative feedback. [Reprinted with permission from Norris, T. L. (2019). *Porth's Pathophysiology: Concepts of Altered Health States* (10th ed., Fig. 44.5, p. 1273). Philadelphia, PA: Wolters Kluwer Health | Lippincott Williams & Wilkins.]

vascularity. If fertilization of the ovum does not occur, the corpus luteum atrophies, resulting in the reduced production of estrogen and progesterone. As estrogen and progesterone levels continue to decrease, the endometrium begins to regress, causing menstruation and the beginning of another menstrual cycle.

# COMMON REPRODUCTIVE HEALTH PROBLEMS IN WOMEN

Deficiencies in endogenous sex hormones result in the absence of normal sexual development. In women with deficiencies of these hormones, primary sex organ maturity will not occur and secondary sexual characteristics will not develop; normal growth and development of the adolescent will not occur, and reproduction is not possible. Assuming that the sexual organs and reproductive system are mature, endogenous sex hormone levels that drop after puberty will result in decreased secondary sexual characteristics. The ability to reproduce and carry a pregnancy to term is reduced.

In addition, normal and aberrant changes in hormone levels across the life span can lead to conditions associated with the reproductive system. The etiology, related pathophysiology, and clinical manifestations are briefly discussed in the following sections. Drug therapy may be helpful.

## Premenstrual Syndrome

Premenstrual syndrome (PMS) is characterized by physical, emotional, and behavioral symptoms that occur during the luteal phase or the last half of the menstrual cycle and resolve with menses. The term PMS is used for those women who experience these symptoms at a severe level that interferes with activities of daily living and personal relationships.

Perhaps as many as 90% of menstruating women experience at least one symptom of PMS before the onset of menses, and an estimated 30% to 40% of women seek treatment for the condition. Clinical manifestations include the following symptoms:

- Physical: bloating, abdominal pain, headache, back pain, and breast tenderness
- Emotional: agitation, irritability, anxiety, and depression
- Behavioral: outbursts of anger, confusion, social withdrawal, and oversensitivity to insignificant events

A more severe variant of PMS is premenstrual dysphoric disorder (PMDD), which now appears in the *Diagnostic and Statistical Manual of Mental Health Disorders* (American Psychiatric Association (APA), 2013). It is estimated that 3% to 8% of women in their reproductive years experience PMDD. Women with PMDD experience extreme symptoms that interfere greatly with work, school, social activities, and relationships. It is important to distinguish PMDD from other medical and psychiatric conditions.

The exact cause of PMS and PMDD is not known but is probably multifactorial. Although a hormonal abnormality has not been confirmed, evidence suggests an association with variation in the normal cyclical changes of reproductive hormones. The symptoms relate to progesterone production by the ovary. The corpus luteum produces metabolites of progesterone that bind to a neurosteroid-binding site on the gamma-aminobutyric acid (GABA) receptor. This changes the receptor, making it resistant to further activation and decreases central GABA-mediated inhibition. Neurotransmitters, particularly serotonin, are also associated with symptoms.

## Endometriosis

Endometriosis is one of the most common gynecologic problems in the United States, affecting an estimated 11% of women. Risk factors include family history of endometriosis, increasing age, short menstrual cycles with longer flow, young menarche, high-fat diet, and few or no pregnancies.

Chronic pelvic pain is a classic symptom of endometriosis. Other characteristic indications include menorrhagia, dysmenorrhea, dyspareunia, fatigue, and abdominal pain. Infertility is also associated with endometriosis, especially in severe cases.

The presence of endometrial tissue outside the uterine cavity is characteristic. This tissue can be attached to the ovaries, the fallopian tubes, the outside of the uterus, the bowels, and the retrovaginal septum. Experts suspect that the lesions originate through retrograde endometrial tissue loss during menses, coelomic metaplasia, and lymphatic spread. Endogenous sex hormones stimulate these lesions through proliferative, secretory, and menstrual breakdown phases. This bleeding outside the uterus can result in pain and the development of pelvic adhesions.

## Menopause

Menopause is a normal physiologic response to deficiencies of endogenous sex hormones. Perimenopause is the transitional period before menopause and typically occurs 2 to 8 years before menopause. Menopause is the absence of menses for 1 year, with the average age at 51.

Because of the insufficient levels of circulating estrogen, secondary sexual characteristics diminish. As a result, there is a decrease in skin elasticity, body hair, and breast and subcutaneous tissue. The uterus and ovaries decrease in size, and the vagina becomes atrophic. Dyspareunia, urinary stress incontinence, and urinary tract infections may occur because of these hormone changes. Decreased estrogen results in vasomotor symptoms of "hot flushes" or "hot flashes," and night sweats may occur. Palpitations, headaches, and dizziness may be present. In addition, postmenopausal women may exhibit insomnia, irritability, anxiety, and depression.

A reduction in the number of ovarian follicles (~100 per ovary) is the major contributing factor to menopause. Due to a reduction in the number of ovarian follicles, the secretion of inhibin B decreases, which causes an increase in FSH, and estradiol levels decrease. The hypothalamus and pituitary gland produce increased levels of GnRH, FSH, and LH in an attempt to stimulate the ovaries to produce estrogen and progesterone. The decreasing endogenous sex hormone levels result in a myriad of physical, psychological, and somatic symptoms. Long-term estrogen deficiency causes an imbalance in bone remodeling, which may lead to osteoporosis. Cardiovascular risk factors increase as total cholesterol and LDL increase and HDL decreases.

## Drug Therapy

### Premenstrual Syndrome

Antidepressants have proven effective in the treatment of PMS and PMDD, and a selective serotonin reuptake inhibitor (SSRI) or a serotonin and norepinephrine reuptake inhibitor (SNRI) may be ordered. Oral contraceptives containing drospirenone or any progestin provide additional options but are generally considered second-line therapy. If anxiety or insomnia are the main symptoms, a benzodiazepine such as alprazolam (Xanax) may be useful, but monitoring is necessary because drug dependency may develop.

### Endometriosis

Drug therapy to manage the symptoms of endometriosis includes the use of nonsteroidal anti-inflammatory agents; hormonal contraceptives, including a low-dose oral contraceptive and a hormonal intrauterine device; and GnRH agonists. No data support one treatment or treatment combination over another. The treatment choice is based on symptom severity, response to treatment, contraceptive needs, and cost.

### Menopause

Hormone replacement therapy (HRT) with estrogen is the most effective treatment available for relief of menopausal symptoms, most importantly vasomotor symptoms. The U.S. Food and Drug Administration (FDA) recommends the use of HRT only in women with symptoms severe enough to warrant its use, at the lowest dose and for the shortest duration possible, to ease the menopausal transition. Although alternate drug therapies are available, none are as effective as estrogen. The combination of the selective estrogen receptor modulator bazedoxifene (Duavee) with conjugated estrogens (Premarin) is available in the United States for the treatment of postmenopausal vasomotor symptoms and the prevention of osteoporosis. This fixed-dose combination drug is appropriate for women who have an intact uterus who do not require a progestin. (Estrogen is discussed in detail later in the chapter.)

### Other Drug Therapy That Alters the Reproductive Cycle

Women may take exogenous estrogens and progestins at various stages in the reproductive cycle. When exogenous estrogens and progestins are administered for therapeutic purposes, they produce the same effects as endogenous hormones. Multiple preparations of estrogens and progestins are available for various purposes and in several forms. Clinical indications, routes of administration, and dosages are presented in the Drugs at a Glance tables.

### NCLEX Success

1. The effects of endogenous estrogen are multifaceted. Which of the following statements is associated with the effects of endogenous estrogen?
   A. It decreases protein anabolism, bone growth, and epiphyseal closure in young girls.
   B. It increases low-density lipoproteins.
   C. It decreases vascularity in the skin.
   D. It promotes bone formation and decreases bone loss.

2. Once an ovum is fertilized, what hormone works to maintain pregnancy?
   A. estrogen
   B. progesterone
   C. follicle-stimulating hormone
   D. luteinizing hormone

## ESTROGENS

Exogenous estrogens are used to treat women's health disorders when endogenous estrogen levels are low or absent. **Conjugated estrogen** (Premarin), the prototype estrogen, is the most commonly used oral estrogen.

## Pharmacokinetics

Conjugated estrogen and some synthetic derivatives of natural estrogens (e.g., ethinyl estradiol, the most widely used synthetic steroidal estrogen) are chemically modified to be effective with oral administration. After oral administration, these estrogens are well absorbed and are released slowly over several hours. Degradation occurs very slowly in the liver, allowing for high intrinsic potency. Ethinyl estradiol reaches peak plasma levels within 2 hours. It is 98% bound to plasma proteins, and its half-life varies from 6 to 20 hours. Extensive first-pass metabolism occurs in the liver, where further metabolism and conjugation occur; excretion of the conjugates is in bile and urine.

Transdermal estradiol patches (e.g., Climara, Menostar, Vivelle-Dot) allow for absorption of estrogen through the skin to the bloodstream. The transdermal route bypasses the liver; thus, the amount of estrogen received is less. With this route, patients experience less nausea and vomiting than with the oral route. Serum levels produced through transdermal application more closely mimic premenopausal estrogen levels compared with serum levels with oral estrogens. This form of estrogen reaches peak plasma levels within 4 hours, and its half-life is approximately 4 hours.

## Action

Estrogens circulate in the bloodstream to target cells, where they enter cells and combine with receptor proteins in cell cytoplasm. After transport of the estrogen–receptor complex to the cell nucleus, this complex interacts with DNA to produce RNA and new DNA. These substances stimulate cell reproduction and production of various proteins. Estrogen primarily influences the reproductive system, although it also affects the skeletal, metabolic, and coagulation systems, as well as the skin and subcutaneous tissues.

Hormonal contraceptives that include estrogen act by several mechanisms. First, they inhibit hypothalamic secretion of GnRH, which inhibits pituitary secretion of FSH and LH. When these gonadotropic hormones are absent, ovulation and therefore conception cannot occur. Second, the drugs produce cervical mucus that resists penetration of spermatozoa into the upper reproductive tract. Third, the drugs interfere with endometrial maturation and reception of ova that are released and fertilized. These overlapping mechanisms make the drugs highly effective in preventing pregnancy.

## Use

Indications for use of exogenous estrogens include the following:

- As a component in birth control pills and other contraceptive preparations. Females 12 to 45 years of age use an estrogen, combined with a progestin, widely to control fertility. If pregnancy does occur, estrogens are contraindicated because their use during pregnancy has been associated with the occurrence of vaginal cancer in female offspring and possible harmful effects on male offspring. Use of birth control pills also includes treatment of menstrual disorders such as amenorrhea and dysmenorrhea.

Birth control pills can be used in specified combinations as emergency contraception (EC). At least 26 birth control pills can be used for EC. It is recommended that the first dose of EC be taken within 120 hours of unprotected intercourse followed by a second dose of birth control pills 12 hours later.

- Menopause. Health care providers prescribe estrogens to relieve symptoms of estrogen deficiency (e.g., atrophic vaginitis and vasomotor instability, which produces "hot flashes" or "hot flushes") and to prevent or treat osteoporosis. Such use is usually called estrogen replacement therapy (ERT). When prescribers order estrogen for women with an intact uterus, they also order a progestin to prevent unwanted thickening of the lining of the uterus and to decrease the risk of cancer of the uterus, a possible result of using estrogen alone. Both drug therapies are commonly referred to as HRT or menopausal hormone therapy (MHT), terms used to describe the administration of one or more female hormones during menopause.
- As a replacement therapy in deficiency states. Deficiency states usually result from hypofunction of the pituitary gland or the ovaries and may occur anytime during the life cycle. For example, in adolescent girls with delayed sexual development, health care providers may prescribe estrogen to produce the changes that normally occur at puberty. In women of reproductive age (~12–45 years of age), prescribers may order an estrogen occasionally for menstrual disorders, including amenorrhea and abnormal uterine bleeding due to estrogen deficiency.

Other uses of estrogens involve the treatment of moderate to severe vasomotor and atrophic symptoms associated with menopause, prevention of postmenopausal osteoporosis, and palliative treatment for metastatic breast carcinoma and advanced androgen-dependent prostatic cancer. Treatment of abnormal uterine bleeding caused by hormonal imbalance, in the absence of organic pathology, requires an intravenous injection. Table 7.1 presents dosage information for the various estrogens.

The short-term use (1–2 years) of estrogens (sometimes synthetic) in postmenopausal women may be indicated for management of menopausal symptoms. Note that the long-term use of estrogen-only therapy and estrogen–progestin combinations is no longer recommended for most women because of potentially serious adverse effects.

### Use in Children

There is little information about the effects of estrogens in children, and the drugs are not generally indicated for use in the pediatric age group. Because estrogens cause epiphyseal closure, caution is warranted with their use before completion of bone growth and attainment of adult height. When it is necessary to give hormonal contraceptives to adolescent girls, they should receive the smallest effective doses; this is also true in other populations.

 **QSEN Alert: Safety**

Women who take a daily dose of a conjugated estrogen and medroxyprogesterone acetate regimen need education regarding the importance of breast self-examinations and recommendations for clinical breast examinations and mammography screening. It is essential that nurses teach patients to notify their health care providers if a breast lump is detected, because HRT must be discontinued until diagnostic procedures are complete.

### Use in Patients With Renal Impairment

Estrogen use has been associated with fluid retention and dilated kidneys, especially when used in higher doses. Therefore, patients with renal impairment require close evaluation and management, and advanced impairment may be a contraindication.

### Use in Patients With Hepatic Impairment

Impaired liver function may lead to impaired estrogen metabolism, with resultant accumulation and adverse effects.

### Use in Patients With Critical Illness

Patients should avoid taking estrogen during a critical illness that results in limited mobility. There is an increased risk of thromboembolic disorders, such as thrombophlebitis, deep vein thrombosis, and pulmonary embolism.

### Use in Patients Receiving Home Care

Patients usually self-administer estrogens. Home care nurses may encounter patients or family members who take an estrogen when visiting the home for another reason. It may be necessary to teach or assist patients to take the drugs as prescribed. In addition, patients may need encouragement to keep appointments for follow-up supervision and blood pressure monitoring. In families that include postmenopausal women, home care nurses may need to teach about nonhormonal strategies for preventing osteoporosis and cardiovascular disease.

## Adverse Effects

The most serious adverse effect of estrogen use is the increased risk of thromboembolic conditions such as thrombophlebitis, pulmonary embolism, cerebrovascular thrombosis, and coronary thrombosis. Estrogens promote blood clotting by stimulating hepatic production of four clotting factors (II, VII, IX, X). Thromboembolic disorders are most likely to occur in women older than 35 years of age who take oral contraceptives and smoke cigarettes, postmenopausal women taking long-term estrogen and progestin therapy, and men or women who receive large doses of estrogens for cancer treatment.

Other adverse effects of conjugated estrogens include menstrual disorders, such as breakthrough bleeding, dysmenorrhea, and amenorrhea due to the hormonal imbalance that may occur with estrogen use. GI upset, such as nausea, vomiting, abdominal cramps, and bloating, may occur. Nausea is most commonly associated with early estrogen use (within the first 1–2 weeks) and usually subsides. Sometimes, when high doses

### TABLE 7.1

## DRUGS AT A GLANCE: Estrogens

| Drug | Pregnancy Category | Menopausal Symptoms | Female Hypogonadism | Prevention of Osteoporosis | Other |
|---|---|---|---|---|---|
| ⓟ **Conjugated estrogens, equine** (Premarin; ✳ Premarin, C.E.S., Congest) | X | PO 0.3–1.25 mg daily for 21 d followed by 7 d without the drug | PO 2.5–7.5 mg daily in divided doses, cyclically 20 d on and 10 d off the drug | PO 0.625 mg daily for 21 d and then 7 d without the drug | Dysfunctional uterine bleeding: IM or IV for emergency use, 25 mg, repeated in 6–12 h if necessary  Atrophic vaginitis: topical, 2.4 g of vaginal cream inserted daily |
| Esterified estrogens (Menest; ✳ Estragyn) | X | PO 0.3–1.25 mg daily | PO 2.5–7.5 mg daily in divided doses, cyclically 20 d on and 10 d off the drug | | Breast cancer (inoperable, progressing): PO 10 mg three times a day for at least 3 mo in selected postmenopausal women |
| Estradiol cypionate (Depo-Estradiol) | X | IM 1–5 mg every 3–4 wk | | | |
| Estradiol, micronized (Estrace, Estring, Vagifem; ✳ Estrace, Estring, Vagifem), vaginal tablet, or vaginal cream (Estring, vaginal ring) | X | PO 0.5–2 mg daily for 3 wk and then 1 wk off or daily Monday through Friday, none on Saturday or Sunday as prescribed | | PO 0.5 mg daily for 23 d and no drug for 5 d each month | Atrophic vaginitis: Cream, 2–4 g daily for 2 wk, then 1–2 g daily for 2 wk, then 1 g one to three times weekly; vaginal ring (Estring), 1 every 3 mo |
| Estradiol transdermal system Alora, Climara, Menostar, Vivelle-Dot EstroGel, Elestrin, Divigel, Evamist; ✳ Climara, Depo-Estradiol, Estradot, Menostar, Oesclim) | X | Climara: 0.025–0.1 mg/d topically to skin every week. Menostar: 0.014 mg/d applied topically each week. Vivelle-Dot: 0.025–0.1 mg/d topically to skin two times per week. Estrasorb (topical lotion; 1.74 g/pouch): two pouches applied topically to legs every day. Estrogel (topical gel; 1.25 g/pump): one pump applied topically every day. Evamist (topical spray; 1.53 mg/spray): one spray applied topically everyday | | Climara: 0.025–0.1 mg/d topically to skin every week. Menostar: 0.014 mg/d applied topically each week. Vivelle-Dot: 0.025–0.1 mg/d topically to skin two times per week | |
| Estropipate (Ogen 5) | X | PO 0.625–5 mg daily, cyclically | PO 1.25–7.5 mg daily for 3 wk, followed by a rest period of 8–10 d. Repeat as needed. | PO 0.625 mg daily for 25 d and no drug for 6 d each month | Ovarian failure: same dosage as for female hypogonadism Atrophic vaginitis: topical, 1–2 g vaginal cream daily |

of estrogens are used, nausea and vomiting are severe enough to require administration of antiemetic drugs. Gallbladder disease is common with estrogen use. Postmenopausal women who take estrogen are two to four times more likely than those who do not to require surgery for gallbladder disease. Central nervous system adverse reactions such as migraine headache, dizziness, and mental depression may be caused or aggravated in some women (the mechanism of action is unknown.) Edema and weight gain may occur due to fluid retention.

Cancer may be a consequence of estrogen use. When estrogens are used alone in postmenopausal women, they cause endometrial hyperplasia and may cause endometrial cancer. Women with an intact uterus should also be given a progestin, which opposes the effects of estrogen on the endometrium. Opinions differ regarding estrogens as a cause of breast cancer. Most studies indicate little risk; a few indicate some risk, especially with high doses for prolonged periods (i.e., 10 years or longer). However, estrogens do stimulate growth in breast cancers that have estrogen receptors.

The FDA has issued a **BLACK BOX WARNING ◆** regarding estrogen use; supervised use at the lowest dose for the shortest duration should be prescribed. Estrogens are associated with the following:

- An increased risk of endometrial cancer. Estrogens should not be used alone in women with an intact uterus.
- An increased risk of thromboembolic events such as myocardial infarction, stroke, deep vein thrombosis, and pulmonary embolism. Estrogens (with or without progestins) should not be used for the prevention of cardiovascular disease.
- An increased risk of dementia in postmenopausal women. Estrogens should not be used for the prevention of dementia.
- An increased risk of breast cancer development in women taking estrogen–progestin combinations.

## Contraindications

Estrogens have a wide variety of effects on body tissues and a number of reported adverse reactions. Therefore, the list of contraindications is long. It is important to avoid using estrogens in the following situations:

- Known or suspected pregnancy, because teratogenic effects capable of interfering with the normal development of the fetus may result
- Thromboembolic disorders, such as thrombophlebitis, deep vein thrombosis, or pulmonary embolism
- Known or suspected cancers of breast or genital tissues, because the drugs may stimulate tumor growth. An exception is the use of estrogens for treatment of metastatic breast cancer in women at least 5 years postmenopause.
- Undiagnosed vaginal or uterine bleeding
- Fibroid tumors of the uterus
- Active liver disease, including liver cancer and impaired liver function
- History of cerebrovascular disease, coronary artery disease, thrombophlebitis, hypertension, or conditions predisposing to these disease processes
- Tobacco use. Women who smoke cigarettes have a greater risk of thromboembolic disorders if they take estrogen supplements, possibly because of increased platelet aggregation

with estrogen ingestion and cigarette smoking. In addition, estrogen increases hepatic production of blood-clotting factors. The FDA has issued a **BLACK BOX WARNING ◆** regarding the risk for serious cardiovascular events resulting from the use of oral contraceptives in women who smoke. The risk increases with age; thus, oral contraceptives should not be use in women over the age of 35 who smoke.

- Family history of breast or reproductive system cancer

## Nursing Implications

An important nursing implication associated with estrogen use is the identification of those factors that result in the contraindication of estrogen use in high-risk women. Identification of these at-risk women can be accomplished through the completion of a thorough medical and social history. This history should assess for menopausal symptoms, cardiovascular disease (hypertension, hyperlipidemia, and cerebrovascular risk), gynecologic history (menstrual history, last menstrual period, and age at menopause), cancer history, and history of smoking. It is also necessary to obtain a family history relating to menopause, osteoporosis, cardiovascular disease, cerebral vascular disease, and cognitive disease, as well as allergy status. In the careful screening of any high-risk woman, the nurse assesses blood pressure, weight, height, pregnancy status, and lipid values. A clinical breast examination with a mammogram and pelvic examination are essential.

### Preventing Interactions

Several drugs interact with estrogens, decreasing their effect (Box 7.2). With corticosteroids and estrogen, increased therapeutic effects and a risk of toxicity of the corticosteroids occur. Use of ropinirole with estrogen may require a dosage adjustment of the estrogen. Estrogens have a decreased effect on tamoxifen, sulfonylurea antidiabetic drugs, and anticoagulants, especially warfarin. St. John's wort increases the breakdown of estrogen, which may decrease the effectiveness of birth control pills.

### Administering the Medication

Choice of preparation depends on the reason for use, desired route of administration, and duration of action. Although dosage needs vary with women and the health conditions for which the drugs are prescribed, a general rule is to use the smallest effective dose for the shortest effective time. Estrogens are often given cyclically. In one regimen, the drug is taken for 3 weeks and then omitted for 1 week; in another, it is omitted the first 5 days of the month. These regimens more closely resemble

---

**BOX 7.2**      *Drug Interactions: Estrogens*

**Drugs That Decrease the Effects of Estrogen**

- Anticonvulsants, such as carbamazepine, oxcarbazepine, phenytoin, and topiramate
  *Induce enzymes that accelerate the metabolism of estrogens*
- Barbiturates, rifampin, ritonavir, and tetracyclines
  *Induce enzymes that accelerate inactivation of estrogens*

normal secretion of estrogen and avoid prolonged stimulation of body tissues. It is necessary to give naturally occurring, nonconjugated estrogens (estradiol, estrone) intramuscularly because they are rapidly metabolized if administered orally. Administration of nonsteroidal synthetic preparations is usually oral or topical. Women may take estrogen with food or at bedtime to decrease nausea, a common adverse reaction.

Transdermal estradiol (e.g., Climara, Menostar, Vivelle-Dot) allows for absorption of estrogen through the skin to the bloodstream. Depending on the preparation, patients apply the patches weekly or biweekly. The total amount of drug absorbed and the resulting plasma drug concentrations from transdermal estrogen can increase during exposure to heat. The nurse should ensure that patients are advised to avoid prolonged sun exposure in the area of the patch.

### Assessing for Therapeutic Effects

The therapeutic effects of estrogen vary depending on the reason for use. When treatment of menopausal symptoms is the goal, it is essential to assess for the decrease in hot flashes, vaginal dryness, and night sweats. When amenorrhea is the target, the occurrence of menstruation indicates that the hormone is working. When female hypogonadism is the treatment goal, the occurrence of menstruation and the presence of breast enlargement, axillary and pubic hair, and other secondary sexual characteristics indicate proper actions of the medication. When prevention of osteoporosis is the objective, the therapeutic effect includes the absence of bone fractures.

### Assessing for Adverse Effects

The nurse assesses for the adverse effects of estrogen through the use of a history and physical examination. A careful assessment with each visit regarding the new onset of abdominal pain, chest pain, headache, vision change, and leg pain is essential in the early recognition of a potential blood clot. The nurse should ensure that blood pressure, glucose, lipid panel, pelvic examination (with Papanicolaou [Pap] smear), and mammography are monitored routinely based on the age of the patient.

### Patient Teaching

Box 7.3 presents patient teaching guidelines for estrogens.

### NCLEX Success

3. A nurse practitioner prescribes estrogen replacement therapy to relieve severe menopausal symptoms of hot flashes or flushes, which are the result of
   A. insufficient gonadotropin secretion
   B. vasomotor instability
   C. high levels of estrogen
   D. decreased progesterone

4. Hormone therapy is indicated for
   A. treatment of osteoporosis
   B. relief of vasomotor symptoms
   C. cardiovascular disease prevention
   D. endometrial cancer treatment

## PROGESTINS

Progestins are used for a range of contraceptive and noncontraceptive purposes either alone or in combination with estrogens. The choice of preparation varies with use. Ⓟ **Medroxyprogesterone acetate** (Provera), a synthetic progestin and a progesterone derivative, is the prototype progestin.

**BOX 7.3** **Patient Teaching Guidelines for Estrogens, Progestins, and Estrogen–Progestin Combinations**

- Take your weight weekly, and report sudden weight gain to your health care provider. [Such weight gain may be due to fluid retention and edema.]
- Report any unusual vaginal bleeding immediately to your health care provider.
- Discuss the increased thromboembolic risk associated with smoking while using estrogens or progestins.
- Know the warning signs that may occur if a thromboembolism should develop—think ACHES [[severe] abdominal pain, chest pain, headache, eye changes, severe leg pain]. Seek medical attention immediately if such symptoms occur.

- If taking estrogen for long periods, have a physical examination at least annually. Have your blood pressure checked, as well as a breast and pelvic examination. Adverse conditions may occur when these drugs are taken for long periods. Your health care provider needs to monitor for adverse drug effects such as high blood pressure, gallbladder disease, and blood-clotting disorders.
- If taking these medications for contraception, use a backup birth control method, and call your health care provider if you fail to take medications as prescribed or if an intrauterine device or a subdermal implant comes out of its own accord.

## Pharmacokinetics

Oral administration of medroxyprogesterone acetate and other progestins results in rapid absorption, and the drug can reach a maximum concentration in 1 to 2 hours. During the first 6 hours, half-life is about 2 to 3 hours; thereafter, half-life extends to 8 to 9 hours. Prompt degradation occurs in the liver, and metabolites are excreted primarily in the urine. Rapid absorption is also a characteristic of intramuscular progestins, which have a half-life of just a few minutes. Long-acting forms can maintain effective concentrations for 3 to 6 months; maximum concentrations can be achieved in 24 hours with a half-life of about 10 weeks. Gel preparations have sustained-release properties, and absorption is prolonged with half-lives of 1 to 2 days.

## Action

Medroxyprogesterone acetate and other progestins diffuse freely into cells, where they bind to progesterone receptors. The progestins act primarily on the endometrial lining of the uterus by changing it from a proliferative endometrium into a secretory endometrium. They also suppress the release of pituitary hormones, which inhibit ovulation. Finally, they inhibit spontaneous uterine contractions.

## Use

Progestins have both noncontraceptive and contraceptive uses, as part of estrogen–progestin combinations or as progestin-only preparations. Progestin-only pills are one option for women who cannot or prefer not to use estrogen-containing contraceptives. Implantable intrauterine devices (IUDs) or subdermal implants are types of long-acting reversible contraceptives. Health care providers use progestins to prevent hyperplasia of the endometrial lining of the uterus in women taking endogenous estrogen. In addition, progestins suppress ovarian function in dysmenorrhea, endometriosis, endometrial cancer, and uterine bleeding. These uses of progestins are extensions of the physiologic actions of progesterone on the neuroendocrine control of ovarian function and on the endometrium.

Progestin-only preparations are administered by a variety of routes. Etonogestrel (Nexplanon), a progestin-only preparation, is dispensed in a 4-mm rod implanted subdermally in the inner upper arm for long-acting reversible contraception. In addition, the progestin levonorgestrel is used as an EC. The EC is most effective if taken within 72 hours of unprotected intercourse but may be taken up to 120 hours after unprotected intercourse. Two-dose regimens for EC are equally as effective. Table 7.2 presents dosage information for the progestins.

**TABLE 7.2**

## DRUGS AT A GLANCE: Progestins

| Drug | Pregnancy Category | Routes and Dosage Ranges for Various Indications | | | |
|---|---|---|---|---|---|
| | | **Menstrual Disorders** | **Endometriosis** | **Cancer** | **Contraception** |
| P **Medroxyprogesterone acetate** (Provera, Depo-Provera, Depo-SubQ Provera 104; ✹ Depo-Provera, Provera) | X | Dysfunctional uterine bleeding: PO 2.5–10 mg daily for 5–10 d, beginning on 16th or 21st day of cycle | SubQ 104 mg/ 0.65 mL every 3 mo | Endometrial: IM 400–1000 mg weekly until improvement and then 400 mg mo | Depo-Provera 150 mg IM every 12 wk. Depo-SubQ Provera 104 mg IM every 12 wk |
| Etonogestrel (Nexplanon) (Subdermal implant) | X | | | | 68 mg in a 4-mm rod implanted subdermally. Daily release of etonogestrel is 60–70 mcg initially and gradually reduces to 25–30 mcg over 3 y |
| Levonorgestrel (Next Choice, New Day, Take Action) | X | | | | Emergency contraception:Two-dose regimen PO 0.75 mg, dose repeated in 12 hSingle dose regimen PO 1.5 mg; most effective when taken within 72 h of unprotected intercourse but may be taken up to 120 h after unprotected intercourse |

**TABLE 7.2**

# DRUGS AT A GLANCE: Progestins (Continued)

| Drug | Pregnancy Category | Routes and Dosage Ranges for Various Indications | | | |
| --- | --- | --- | --- | --- | --- |
| | | Menstrual Disorders | Endometriosis | Cancer | Contraception |
| Megestrol acetate (Megace ES; ✿ Megace OS, Megestrol) | X | | | Endometrial: PO 40–320 mg daily in 4 divided doses for at least 2 mo<br>Breast: PO 160 mg daily in 4 divided doses for at least 2 mo<br>Cachexia with HIV: PO initially 800 mg/d; normal range 400–800 mg/d (suspension only) or 625 mg/d ES suspension | |
| Progesterone (Crinone, Endometrin; ✿ Crinone, Endometrin; [vaginal gel], Prometrium) | X | Amenorrhea and dysfunctional uterine bleeding: IM 5–10 mg for 6–8 consecutive days<br>Secondary amenorrhea: 4% gel, 45 mg every other day<br>Other infertility: 90 mg vaginally daily in women requiring progesterone supplementation | | | |
| Depot medroxyprogesterone acetate IM (Depo-Provera, Provera; ✿ Depo-Provera, Provera) | X | | | | |
| Depot medroxyprogesterone acetate SubQ (Depo-SubQ Provera) | X | | | | |
| Levonorgestrel-releasing intrauterine device (Mirena, Kyleena; ✿ Jaydess, Kyleena, Mirena) | X | | | | Provides contraception for 5 y |
| Levonorgestrel-releasing intrauterine device (Liletta, Skyla) | X | | | | Provides contraception for 3 y |

**QSEN Alert: Safety**

The *etonogestrel implant* is one the most effective contraceptives available. It has an efficacy equal to or better than that of sterilization but without the risks of invasive surgery.

For approximately 20 to 25 years, postmenopausal women with an intact uterus took progestins in combination with estrogen for long-term HRT. In HRT, the purpose of a progestin is to prevent endometrial cancer, which can occur with unopposed estrogenic stimulation. However, as previously stated, this combination currently is not recommended for long-term use because evidence has indicated that the adverse effects outweigh the beneficial effects.

**QSEN Alert: Evidence-Based Practice**

Two large-scale randomized controlled trials, the Heart and Estrogen/Progestin Replacement Study [HERS] and the Women's Health Initiative [WHI], have disputed the cardioprotective effects of postmenopausal estrogen use. The U.S. Preventive Services Task Force [USPSTF] has reviewed the literature to update evidence about the benefits and harms of using HRT in postmenopausal women. The USPSTF has identified that there is moderate or high certainty that postmenopausal estrogen use has no net benefit for the primary prevention of chronic medical conditions and has recommend against the use [Grossman, et al., 2017]. This recommendation does not apply to women using HRT to treat menopausal symptoms or for women younger than 50 years who have had surgical menopause.

### Use in Children

Progestins are not intended for use in children.

### Use in Patients With Renal Impairment

Progestin metabolites are predominately excreted in urine. Therefore, patients with renal impairment require close evaluation and management, and advanced renal impairment may contraindicate progestin use.

### Use in Patients With Hepatic Impairment

Metabolism of progestins occurs primarily in the liver. Therefore, impaired liver function or liver disease prohibits use.

### Use in Patients With Critical Illness

Due to the increased risk of thromboembolic disorders, such as thrombophlebitis, deep vein thrombosis, and pulmonary embolism associated with the use of progestins, critical illness resulting in extended bed rest may increase the risk of using the drug. It may be less beneficial.

## Adverse Effects

The most significant risk associated with progestins is an increased risk of cardiovascular complications, such as stroke, heart attack, hypertension, thromboembolic and thrombotic disease, thrombophlebitis, retinal thrombosis, and pulmonary embolism. Other adverse effects include the following:

- Irregular vaginal bleeding (common; decreases during the first year of use). Amenorrhea may occur.
- Weight gain and fluid retention (common)
- Ophthalmic disorders, such as sudden, partial, or complete loss of vision
- An increased risk of migraines and mental depression
- Possible skin conditions, such as rash, acne, alopecia, and hirsutism
- GI upset, with nausea and vomiting
- Bone loss. A **BLACK BOX WARNING** ◆ stipulates that some forms of medroxyprogesterone acetate cause calcium loss in bones, leading to weak bones and possible bone breakage.

Nurses should be aware that the FDA has recognized some of these problems and issued a **BLACK BOX WARNING** ◆ for the progestins, stating that the drugs:

- Should not be used in pregnancy
- Should not be used in combination with estrogen for the prevention of cardiovascular disease or dementia
- Are associated with an increased risk of thromboembolic events, such as myocardial infarction, stroke, deep vein thrombosis, and pulmonary embolism in women taking estrogen–progestin combination therapy
- Are associated with an increased risk of dementia in postmenopausal women

## Contraindications

Contraindications to progestins include allergies to the drugs, pregnancy or suspected pregnancy, and breast-feeding. Other contraindications are a history of active cardiovascular disease; thrombophlebitis; thromboembolic disorders; cerebral hemorrhage; renal disease; hepatic disease; and carcinoma of the breast, ovaries, or endometrium. A final contraindication is undiagnosed vaginal bleeding. A history of depression warrants caution.

## Nursing Implications

Nursing implications associated with progestins are very similar to those associated with estrogens. The following information is essential in the identification of those women for whom progestin therapy is contraindicated:

- Assessment of medical and social history. The nurse assesses for menopausal symptoms, cardiovascular disease (hypertension, hyperlipidemia, and cerebral vascular risk), gynecologic history (menstrual history, last menstrual period, and age at menopause), cancer history, and history of smoking.
- Assessment of family history of menopause, osteoporosis, cardiovascular disease, cerebrovascular disease, cognitive disease, and allergy status
- Assessment of blood pressure, weight, height, with lipid panel, clinical breast examination with age-appropriate mammogram, pelvic examination, and Pap smear

### Preventing Interactions

Progestin use often alters liver function and endocrine function tests. It is essential that health care providers be aware that progestins are being used when laboratory testing is indicated. No reports of drug–drug, drug–food, or drug–herb interactions concerning progestin have appeared.

## Administering the Medication

Progestins can be administered through a variety of routes. Oral, intramuscular, subcutaneous, intravaginal, intrauterine, and subdermal and transdermal preparations of the drug are available. To reduce the GI effects of the oral preparations, it is necessary to take them with food or at bedtime. For treatment of dysfunctional uterine bleeding and amenorrhea, cyclic administration of the drug is often warranted.

## Assessing for Therapeutic Effects

When given for menstrual disorders, such as abnormal uterine bleeding, amenorrhea, dysmenorrhea, premenstrual discomforts, and endometriosis, the nurse observes for relief of symptoms.

### Clinical Application 7.3

- Mrs. Bigelow has been taking Prempro 0.625/ 2.5 mg every day for 1 month. She calls the office when you are on duty. She is complaining of left leg pain and swelling that have been occurring off and on for 4 days. What is the nursing intervention?

## Assessing for Adverse Effects

The nurse observes for breakthrough bleeding and provides reassurance to affected women. He or she assesses for irregular vaginal bleeding, which is a major reason that some women do not want to take progestin-only contraceptives. The nurse ensures that lipid panels are assessed, because decreased HDL and increased LDL cholesterol may occur with progestin use. These changes in LDL and HDL levels increase the risk of cardiovascular disease and may lead to discontinuation of the progestin. In women with a history of depression, discontinuation of the drug is essential at the first sign or indication of recurring depression.

## Patient Teaching

Box 7.3 presents patient teaching guidelines for progestins. Women who have an intact uterus should take both estrogen and progestin; the progestin component (e.g., Provera) prevents endometrial cancer, an adverse effect of estrogen-only therapy. Posthysterectomy, women should take estrogen-only medications. Combined estrogen–progestin therapy may increase blood sugar levels in women with diabetes. This effect is attributed to progestin and is unlikely to occur with estrogen-only therapy. Women with diabetes should report increased blood glucose levels. Take progestins with food or at bedtime to decrease nausea, a common adverse reaction. Patients should take their weight weekly and report sudden weight gain, which may result from fluid retention and edema. Patients should report any unusual vaginal bleeding.

### NCLEX Success

5. Progesterone is a progestin concerned almost entirely with reproduction. In nonpregnant women, progesterone is secreted by which of the following?
   A. corpus luteum
   B. hypothalamus
   C. anterior pituitary
   D. adrenal cortex

6. Postmenopausal women with an intact uterus taking estrogen for hormone replacement therapy require progestin because
   A. progestins enhance the effects of estrogen
   B. combination therapy provides osteoporosis prevention
   C. progestin opposes the effects of estrogen on the endometrium
   D. uterine cancer is increased

# ESTROGEN–PROGESTIN COMBINATIONS

The most effective and widely used contraceptives are estrogen–progestin combinations. For contraception, the prototype hormonal combination is ethinyl estradiol–norethindrone (Ortho-Novum). For HRT, the prototype drug is **conjugated estrogen–medroxyprogesterone** (Prempro).

Several varieties of progestins are part of combined oral contraceptives. The progestin component may determine the choice of a combination contraceptive product. Progestins have progestational, estrogenic, and androgenic qualities. These qualities vary depending on the type of the progestin and are an important consideration in the management of the adverse effects associated with hormonal contraceptives. Progestational qualities have an influence on the suppression of ovulation and reduction in menstrual bleeding. Estrogenic qualities may be associated with headache, breast tenderness, or fluid retention. Androgenic qualities are often associated with acne or hirsutism (unwanted female hair growth). Progestins with minimal androgenic activity are desogestrel and norgestimate; those with intermediate activity include norethindrone and ethynodiol, and those with high androgenic effects include norgestrel.

## Pharmacokinetics

Absorption of ethinyl estradiol is good with oral administration, and it reaches peak plasma levels within 2 hours. It is 98% bound to plasma proteins, and its half-life varies from 6 to 20 hours. The estrogen undergoes extensive first-pass metabolism, additional metabolism, and conjugation in the liver; the conjugates are then excreted in bile and urine.

## Action

The estrogen component of combined oral contraceptives prevents pregnancy by inhibiting ovulation; it prevents the formation of the follicle by suppressing FSH and LH and stabilizing the endometrium. The progestin component thins the endometrium, slows sperm transport, thickens cervical mucus, and suppresses the LH surge.

## Use

The primary use of estrogen–progestin contraceptives is to prevent pregnancy. Four different types of hormonal contraceptives are common: monophasic contraceptives, which contain fixed amounts of both estrogen and progestin components; biphasics, which contain either fixed amounts of estrogen and varied amounts of progestin; triphasics, which contain three different doses of estrogen and progestin; and quadriphasics, which contain four different doses of estrogen and progestin (Table 7.3).

## TABLE 7.3

## Estrogen–Progestin Combinations Used as Contraceptives

| Trade Names | Pregnancy Category | Estrogen | Progestin |
|---|---|---|---|
| **Monophasics** | | | |
| Aviane-28, Delyla, Falmina, Lessina-28, Orsythia, Vienva | X | Ethinyl estradiol 20 mcg | Levonorgestrel 0.1 mg |
| Altavera, Kurvelo, Levora, Marlissa, Portia-28, Seasonique; 🍁 Aviane-28, Portia, Seasonale, Seasonique | X | Ethinyl estradiol 30 mcg | Levonorgestrel 0.15 mg |
| Lo Loestrin Fe | X | Ethinyl estradiol 10 mcg | Norethindrone 1.0 mg |
| Junel Fe 1/20, Loestrin 1/20, Loestrin Fe 1/20, Microgestin Fe 1/20; 🍁 Minestrin | X | Ethinyl estradiol 20 mcg | Norethindrone 1.0 mg |
| Junel Fe 1.5/30, Junel 21 1.5/30, Loestrin 21 1.5/30, Loestrin Fe 1.5/30, Microgestin Fe 1.5/30; 🍁 Loestrin 1.5/30 | X | Ethinyl estradiol 30 mcg | Norethindrone 1.5 mg |
| **Ortho-Novum 1/35,** Nortrel 1/35, Ortho-Novum 1/35 Brevicon 1/35, Ortho 1/35; 🍁 Select 1/35 | X | Ethinyl estradiol 35 mcg | Norethindrone 1.0 mg |
| Alyacen, Aranelle, Balziva-28 | X | Ethinyl estradiol 35 mcg | Norethindrone 0.4 mg |
| Necon 0.5/35, Nortrel 0.5/35 | X | Ethinyl estradiol 35 mcg | Norethindrone 0.5 mg |
| Cryselle, Elinest, Low-Ogestrel | X | Ethinyl estradiol 30 mcg | Norgestrel 0.3 mg |
| Ogestrel | X | Ethinyl estradiol 50 mcg | Norgestrel 0.5 mg |
| Kelnor 1/35, Zovia 1/35E | X | Ethinyl estradiol 35 mcg | Ethynodiol diacetate 1.0 mg |
| Kelnor 1/50 | X | Ethinyl estradiol 50 mcg | Ethynodiol diacetate 1.0 mg |
| Apri; 🍁 Apri, Freya, Linessa, Marvelon | X | Ethinyl estradiol 30 mcg | Desogestrel 0.15 mg |
| Yasmin, Syeda, Zarah; 🍁 Mya, Yasmin (all also approved for PMDD) | X | Ethinyl estradiol 30 mcg | Drospirenone 3.0 mg |
| Gianvi, Yaz, Nikki; 🍁 Yaz, Zamine (all also approved for PMDD) | X | Ethinyl estradiol 20 mcg | Drospirenone 3.0 mg |
| Beyaz, Safyral; 🍁 Yaz Plus (all also approved for PMDD) | X | Ethinyl estradiol 20 mcg | Drospirenone 3.0 mg and 0.45 mg levomefolate calcium |
| Estarylla, Ortho-Cyclen, Sprintec, Tri-Cyclen; 🍁 Cyclen, Tri-Cyclen, Tricira Lo | X | Ethinyl estradiol 35 mcg | Norgestimate 0.25 mg |
| **Extended-Cycle Monophasics** | | | |
| Amethyst (taken continuously for 1 y) | X | Ethinyl estradiol 20 mcg | Levonorgestrel 0.09 mg |
| Altavera, Chateal, Kurvelo, Quasense, Seasonique; 🍁 Seasonale (taken continuously for 84 d, then low-dose estrogen pills for 7 d) | X | Ethinyl estradiol 30 mcg | Levonorgestrel 0.15 mg |
| LoSeasonique, Lutera, Orsythia, Sronyx (taken continuously for 84 d, then low-dose estrogen pills for 7 d) | X | Ethinyl estradiol 20 | Levonorgestrel 0.10 mg |
| **Biphasics** | | | |
| Kariva | X | Ethinyl estradiol 20/10 mcg | Desogestrel 0.15 mg |
| **Triphasics** | | | |
| Velivet, Caziant, Cyclessa; 🍁 Marvelon, Apri, Freya | X | Ethinyl estradiol 25 mcg | Desogestrel 0.1/0.125/0.15 mg |
| Necon 7/7/7, Dasetta 7/7/7 | X | Ethinyl estradiol 35 mcg | Norethindrone 0.5/0.75/1.0 mg |
| Aranelle, Leena, Tri-Norinyl; 🍁 Lolo, Brevicon | X | Ethinyl estradiol 35 mcg | Norethindrone 0.5/1.0/0.5 mg |
| Estrostep Fe, Tri-Legest Fe | X | Ethinyl estradiol 20/30/35 mcg | Norethindrone 1.0 mg |

### TABLE 7.3

## Estrogen–Progestin Combinations Used as Contraceptives (Continued)

| Trade Names | Pregnancy Category | Estrogen | Progestin |
|---|---|---|---|
| Ortho Tri-Cyclen, T Tri-Sprintec | X | Ethinyl estradiol 35 mcg | Norgestimate 0.18/0.215/0.25 mg |
| Ortho Tri-Cyclen Lo Tri-Lo-Sprintec; ❋ Tri-Cyclen Lo | X | Ethinyl estradiol 25 mcg | Norgestimate 0.18/0.215/0.25 mg |
| Enpresse, Lutera, Sronyx, Trivora-28 | X | Ethinyl estradiol 30/40/30 mcg | Levonorgestrel 0.05/0.075/ 0.125 mg |
| Quadriphasic | | | |
| Natazia | X | Estradiol valerate 3/2/2/1 mg | Dienogest 0.0/2.0/3.0/0.0 mg |
| **Extended-Cycle Quadriphasic** | | | |
| Quartette (taken 91 d, repeat) | X | Ethinyl estradiol 20/25/30/10 mcg | Levonorgestrel 0.15/0.15/0.15/0 |
| Ortho Evra transdermal patch (Xulane; ❋ Evra) | X | Ethinyl estradiol 750 mcg | Norelgestromin 6 mg |
| NuvaRing vaginal insert (NuvaRing vaginal insert; ❋ NuvaRing) | X | Ethinyl estradiol 2.7 mg | Etonogestrel 11.7 mg |

Biphasic, triphasic, and quadriphasic preparations mimic normal variations of hormone secretion, decrease the total dosage of hormones, and may decrease adverse effects. These contraceptives are dispensed in containers with color-coded tablets that must be taken in the correct sequence. Dispensers with 28 tablets contain 7 inactive or placebo tablets of a third color. Several combination products and alternative dosage forms are available to help individualize treatment and promote adherence.

Health care providers also use oral contraceptive preparations to treat menstrual disorders (e.g., amenorrhea, dysmenorrhea). The FDA has approved some oral contraceptives for the treatment of acne, such as Ortho Tri-Cyclen, Estrostep, and Yaz. Prescribers order Yaz and Beyaz for treatment of PMDD. Continuous-dosing oral contraceptives, which include Seasonale and Seasonique, are useful in the treatment of menorrhagia, metrorrhagia, endometriosis, and PMS. Such continuous-dosing oral contraceptives provide birth control protection for 3 consecutive months while suppressing ovarian function and reducing uterine bleeding; withdrawal bleeding occurs only four times per year.

Table 7.4 presents dosage information for noncontraceptive estrogen–progestin combinations.

### Use in Patients With Renal Impairment

Oral contraceptives are associated with fluid retention and dilated kidneys as a result of increased renin–angiotensin–aldosterone system activity. This alteration in the renal system occurs especially when the contraceptives are used in higher doses; therefore, patients with renal impairment require close evaluation and management. Severe renal impairment may be a contraindication to oral contraceptive use.

### Use in Patients With Hepatic Impairment

Due to the metabolism of combined oral contraceptives in the liver, hepatic impairment is an absolute contraindication for use. In addition, women who have had jaundice during pregnancy have an increased risk of recurrence if they take estrogen-containing contraceptives. Any patient in whom jaundice develops when taking estrogen should stop taking the drug. Because jaundice may indicate liver damage, the cause warrants investigation.

### Use in Patients With Critical Illness

Oral contraceptive use during a critical illness that results in limited mobility is contraindicated. There is an increased risk of thromboembolic disorders, such as thrombophlebitis, deep vein thrombosis, and pulmonary embolism.

### Use in Patients Receiving Home Care

Patients usually self-administer oral contraceptives. Home care nurses may encounter patients or family members taking one of the drugs when visiting the home for another reason. It may be necessary to teach or assist patients to take the drugs as prescribed. In addition, patients may need encouragement to keep appointments for follow-up supervision and blood pressure monitoring. When visiting families that include adolescent girls or young women, home care nurses may need to teach about birth control measures, adverse reactions, and adverse effects.

## Adverse Effects

Adverse effects of oral contraceptives may include the GI effects of nausea and vomiting. Taking the drugs with food or at bedtime minimizes nausea. Cardiovascular effects of thromboembolism, myocardial infarction, stroke, and hypertension may also occur. Earlier oral contraceptives, which contained larger amounts of estrogen than those currently used, did cause these problems, and they are much less common in most people who take low-dose preparations. However, for women 35 years of age and older who smoke, there is an increased risk of myocardial infarction and other cardiovascular disorders, even with low-dose pills. Also, gallbladder disease is more likely in

**TABLE 7.4**

## DRUGS AT A GLANCE: Estrogen–Progestin Combinations Used for Noncontraceptive Purposes

| Drug | Pregnancy Category | Routes and Dosage Ranges for Various Indications | | |
|---|---|---|---|---|
| | | **Menopausal Symptoms** | **Female Hypogonadism** | **Prevention of Osteoporosis** |
| P **Conjugated estrogens/ medroxyprogesterone acetate** (Prempro, Premphase; ✿ Premplus) | X | PO 0.3/1.5 mg–0.625/2.5 mg daily | | PO 0.3/1.5 mg–0.625/ 2.5 mg daily |
| Conjugated estrogens/medroxyproges-terone acetate (Premphase) | X | PO 0.625/5.0 mg daily | | PO 0.625/5.0 mg daily |
| Estradiol/norethindrone (Activella, Amabelz; ✿ Activelle, Estalis) | X | PO 0.05 mg/0.1 every day; PO 1 mg/0.5 mg every day | | PO 0.05 mg/0.1 every day; 1 mg/0.5 mg every day |
| Ethinyl estradiol/norethindrone acetate (FemHRT, Balziva, Briellyn, Cyclafem, Junel, Larin; ✿ FemHRT Brevicon, Minestrin, Synphasic) | X | PO 2.5 mcg/0.5 mg every day; PO 5 mcg/1 mg every day | | PO 2.5 mcg/0.5 mg every day; PO 5 mcg/1 mg every day |
| Estradiol/drospirenone (Angeliq; ✿ Angeliq) | X | PO 5 mcg/1 mg every day | | PO 5 mcg/1 mg every day |
| Estradiol/levonorgestrel (Climara Pro; ✿ Climara Pro) | X | Transdermal 0.045 mg/0.015 weekly | | |
| Estradiol/norethindrone (CombiPatch; ✿ Activelle, Estalis) | X | Transdermal 0.05 mg/0.14 mg twice a week; transdermal 0.05 mg/0.25 mg twice a week | | |

women who use oral contraceptives or estrogen–progestin HRT than in those who do not take hormones. Researchers attribute this to increased concentration of cholesterol in bile acids, which leads to decreased solubility and increased precipitation of stones. Finally, edema, weight gain, and headache are other adverse effects that may be associated with combined oral contraceptives.

The FDA has issued the following **BLACK BOX WARNING ◆** regarding the use of oral contraceptives:

- Cigarette smoking increases the risk of cardiovascular adverse effects, especially in women older than 35 years of age.
- Possibility of broken bones and osteoporosis, especially after menopause, from loss of stored calcium from bones with the use of Depo-Provera and Depo-SubQ Provera. There is a greater risk of bone loss with long-term use.
- Risks of thromboembolic events increase with use of the Ortho Evra transdermal patch due to the higher levels of estrogen that are circulated into the blood.

 **QSEN Alert: Evidence-Based Practice**

Several studies have examined the risk of venous thrombo-embolism with newer hormone contraceptives. The results have been conflicting. No large prospective randomized studies have compared varying amounts of estrogen and progestin or routes of administration with the risk of venous thromboembolism. Findings from a 2015 systematic review

of the literature revealed a low, overall increased risk of venous thromboembolic events with hormone contraceptive use in young women (1–5/10,000 woman-years). There was insufficient evidence to suggest that the contraceptive patch or vaginal ring has differences in venous thromboembolic events compared to oral contraceptives. The review reported that evidence suggests that tobacco use, age (older than 35 years), hypertension, obesity, and presence of hereditary thrombophilia increase the risk of venous thromboembolic events (American Society of Reproductive Health, 2017). Providing appropriate health education regarding the adverse thromboembolic effects associated with hormonal contraception is essential. In women 35 years of age or older, it is important to obtain a careful health history to assess for cardiovascular risk factors. Careful assessment and monitoring of blood pressure are essential, and elevations warrant discontinuation of hormonal contraception. Finally, hormonal contraception is contraindicated in women 35 years of age or older who use tobacco products.

## Contraindications

Despite the decreased estrogen dosage, combined oral contraceptives are associated with several contraindications. These include cigarette smoking, age of 35 years and older, a history of thromboembolic problems, and concurrent cirrhosis or active viral hepatitis, diabetes mellitus, hypertension, or migraine with aura. When estrogen is contraindicated, it is permissible to use a progestin-only contraceptive.

Yasmin, Yaz, and Beyaz contain the progestin drospirenone, which increases serum potassium. Therefore, contraindications to these oral contraceptives include renal, liver, or adrenal insufficiency; use of potassium-sparing diuretics, potassium supplements, angiotensin-converting enzyme inhibitors, angiotensin II receptor agonists, and heparin; and continuous, long-term use of nonsteroidal anti-inflammatory drugs.

## Nursing Implications

It is necessary to assess each patient's need and desire for contraception, as well as her willingness to comply with the prescribed regimen. Assessment includes determining a patient's knowledge about birth control, both pharmacologic and non-pharmacologic, and identifying patients in whom hormonal contraceptives are contraindicated or who are at increased risk for adverse drug effects. Adherence involves the willingness to take the drugs as prescribed and to have breast and pelvic examinations and blood pressure measurements every 6 to 12 months. The goal of effective oral contraceptive use is the prevention of pregnancy with the lowest effective dose of hormones.

### Preventing Interactions

Several medications may reduce the effectiveness of oral contraceptives (i.e., increase the likelihood of pregnancy; Box 7.4). These include medications for tuberculosis and HIV as well as anticonvulsants. (Box 7.2 lists specific drug–drug interactions that decrease the effectiveness of estrogen.) Patients should notify all health care providers who prescribe medications that they are taking a birth control pill. Use of an additional or alternative method of birth control is necessary (1) if a dose is missed or (2) if the oral contraceptive cannot be taken because of illness or infection.

---

**!** **QSEN Alert: Safety**

It is essential to add a different method of birth control while taking certain medications for the remainder of that reproductive cycle.

---

 **BOX 7.4** **Drug Interactions: Oral Contraceptives**

**Drugs That Decrease the Effects of Oral Contraceptives**

- Anticonvulsants, such as carbamazepine, hydantoins (ethotoin, mephenytoin, phenytoin), and succinimides
  *Induce hepatic cytochrome P450, resulting in increased metabolism*
- Barbiturates such as phenobarbital, primidone, griseofulvin
  *Increase metabolism*
- Benzodiazepines, rifampin, St. John's wort
  *Activate the hepatic enzyme cytochrome P450, resulting in increased metabolism*
- Topiramate
  *Decreases contraceptive efficacy and increases breakthrough bleeding*

As previously mentioned, St. John's wort increases the breakdown of estrogen, which can decrease the effectiveness of birth control pills.

### Administering the Medication

Numerous preparations are available, with different components and different doses of components, so that a preparation can be chosen to meet individual needs. Most oral contraceptives contain an estrogen and a progestin. The estrogen dose is usually 30 to 35 mcg. Smaller amounts (e.g., 20 mcg) may be adequate for small or underweight women; larger amounts (e.g., 50 mcg) may be needed for large or overweight women. Effects of estrogen components are similar when prescribed in equipotent doses, but progestins differ in progestogenic, estrogenic, antiestrogenic, and androgenic activity. Consequently, adverse effects may differ to some extent, and a patient may be able to tolerate one contraceptive better than another.

---

 **Clinical Application 7.4**

- Mrs. Bigelow has her FSH level measured, as ordered by her health care provider, and the levels are within normal range. After completion of her history, physical examination, and diagnostic tests, her health care provider begins her on hormonal contraceptives for menstrual regulation. She is on the second cycle of pills when she calls complaining of irregular bleeding on the pills and requests a new pill. What is the nurse's best response?

---

### Assessing for Therapeutic Effects

When taken correctly, estrogen–progestin contraceptive preparations are nearly 100% effective in preventing pregnancy. Therapeutic effects of oral contraceptives include the prevention of pregnancy with regulation of menses with shorter, lighter flow and reduction in ovarian cyst formation. Improvements in hemoglobin may occur due to decreased menstrual flow or if women are taking oral contraceptives with added iron.

### Assessing for Adverse Effects

It is very important to monitor for adverse drug effects such as high blood pressure, gallbladder disease, and blood-clotting disorders, which may be associated with oral contraceptive use. The assessment of weight, blood pressure, regularity of menses (occurring only on the withdrawal pills), absence of chest pain, abdominal pain, headache, vision changes, and leg pain indicates an absence of adverse effects of the oral contraceptives.

### Patient Teaching

It is essential that women seek information about the use of oral contraceptives. The nurse should be sure that women understand that oral contraceptives are very effective at preventing pregnancy but *do not* prevent transmission of sexually transmitted diseases (e.g., human immunodeficiency virus [HIV], *Chlamydia*, gonorrhea). Box 7.3 presents teaching guidelines for patients taking contraceptives.

## Unfolding Patient Stories: Rachel Heidebrink • Part 1

Rachel Heidebrink, a 22-year-old, is diagnosed with a pulmonary embolism following left hip surgery for a fractured left greater trochanter sustained during a motorcycle accident. The patient is on an oral estrogen–progestin combination for contraception. What actions should the nurse take when considering the diagnosis and adverse effects of the medication? (Rachel Heidebrink's story continues in Chapter 9.)

Care for Rachel and other patients in a realistic virtual environment: *vSim for Nursing* (thepoint.lww.com/vSimPharm). Practice documenting these patients' care in DocuCare (thepoint.lww.com/DocuCareEHR).

## NCLEX Success

7. Patient teaching for a woman who will be using the transdermal patch Ortho Evra should include which of the following? (Select all that apply.)

   A. Apply to skin daily.
   B. Apply to clean and dry skin.
   C. Apply the patch on the same day of the week each week for 3 weeks.
   D. Apply the patch the first day of the menstrual cycle initially.
   E. Use a backup method for birth control the first 2 weeks of using the patch.
   F. Use a backup method for birth control the first 3 weeks of using the patch.

8. The nurse is preparing a presentation of the risk factors of oral contraceptives. What factor is an absolute contraindication?

   A. bulimia
   B. cigarette smoking at age 33
   C. body mass index (BMI) of 23
   D. history of thromboembolism

9. When oral contraceptives are contraindicated in women with liver disease, what other birth control option would be safe?

   A. Ortho Evra (contraceptive patch)
   B. Depo-Provera (injectable progestin)
   C. barrier method (condoms)
   D. Nexplanon (subdermal implant)

10. After patient teaching of the warning signs associated with combination hormonal contraception, what statement would result in the nurse providing additional education?

    A. "Breakthrough bleeding is a sign of a uterine abnormality."
    B. "I should immediately go to the emergency department if I get a sudden, severe headache that is not relieved with rest or analgesic."
    C. "Severe leg pain and swelling should immediately be reported."
    D. "Cardiovascular problems are the most severe adverse effect associated with oral contraceptives."

## THE NURSING PROCESS

A concept map outlines the nursing process related to drug therapy considerations in this chapter. Additional nursing implications related to the disease process should also be considered in care decisions.

**Assessment**
- Obtain a thorough patient history relating to general and gynecologic health, social particulars, and family health.
- Obtain a history of drug and food allergies.
- Obtain baseline height, weight, body mass index, and blood pressure.
- Document the last menstrual period (rule out pregnancy).

**Outcomes of Therapy**

The patient will
- Choose the birth control method with minimal risks and most benefit.
- Report an understanding of the dosing schedule, risks, benefits, and warning signs of the method selected.
- Self-administer oral, transdermal, topical, or vaginal medications as prescribed.
- Report adverse effects of the birth control method.
- Report an understanding of the risks, benefits, and warning signs associated with hormonal replacement therapy.
- Report an understanding of the nonpharmacologic and pharmacologic choices of HRT.
- Choose the method of HRT with minimal risks and most benefits.
- Report adverse effects of the HRT.

**Nursing Interventions**
- Provide health teaching regarding various birth control methods with the risks and benefits.
- Identify and discuss any contraindications to birth control options.
- Encourage the patient to participate in choosing the birth control method.
- Provide instruction regarding the use of method chosen.
- Obtain written informed consents, which imply that the patient is making an informed decision regarding the birth control method and is aware of the risks and benefits.
- Review typical menopausal changes.
- Identify and discuss any contraindications to HRT.
- Provide health teaching regarding the nonpharmacologic and pharmacologic methods available for menopause, including risks, benefits, and warning signs.

**Evaluation**
- Provide a follow-up visit to assess the effectiveness of the hormone therapy.
- Observe and interview regarding compliance with instructions for drug therapy.
- Assess for side effects, adverse effects, and changes in the patient's health status.

## KEY CONCEPTS

- When exogenous estrogens and progestins are administered for therapeutic purposes, they produce the same effects as endogenous hormones.
- Oral contraceptives are very effective at preventing pregnancy, but they do not prevent transmission of sexually transmitted diseases.
- Cigarette smoking in women who use oral contraceptives increases risks of blood clots in the legs, lungs, heart, or brain.

- Because estrogens cause epiphyseal closure, caution is necessary when used in children before completion of bone growth and attainment of adult height.
- When estrogens are used alone in postmenopausal women, they cause endometrial hyperplasia and may cause endometrial cancer. Women with an intact uterus should also be given a progestin, which opposes the effects of estrogen on the endometrium.

- The FDA has issued a **BLACK BOX WARNING** ◆ that estrogens increase the risk of developing cancer of the uterus. The warning instructs women who take estrogens with or without progestins that there is an increased risk of dementia, myocardial infarctions, strokes, breast cancer, and blood clots. In addition, a **BLACK BOX WARNING** ◆ warns that estrogens and progestins should not be used in pregnancy.
- A **BLACK BOX WARNING** ◆ outlines the concern of the use of Depo-Provera and Depo-SubQ Provera being associated with the loss of stored calcium from bones, which increases the risk of broken bones and osteoporosis, especially after menopause. There is a greater risk of bone loss with long-term use.
- The FDA has issued a **BLACK BOX WARNING** ◆ regarding the risk for serious cardiovascular events from the use of oral contraceptives in women who smoke. As the risk increases with age, oral contraceptives should not be used in women over the age of 35 who smoke.

## CLINICAL REASONING CASE STUDY

**Meet the Patient**

Julie Campbell is a 35-year-old college student who presents to student health services requesting oral contraceptives to prevent unwanted pregnancy. Julie's medical history reveals that she is taking hydrochlorothiazide 25 mg orally every day for "fluid retention." She is a cigarette smoker (a half a pack per day for 10 years).

- What is the best nursing intervention regarding contraception in this case?
- Julie tells the nurse practitioner that other options for birth control are not desirable and that taking the pill is her preferred method. What information can the nurse provide to have her reconsider?

**Assessing Drug Information**

- An alternate form of birth control is recommended in Julie's case.
  - Oral contraceptives are contraindicated in women older than 35 years of age who smoke cigarettes because of an increased risk of thromboembolic disorders.
  - Some birth control pills are associated with fluid and water retention, which may increase risk of hypertension and other health concerns in someone prone to fluid retention.

**Nursing Actions**

- Educate Julie about the importance of smoking cessation and encourage ways to stop smoking, including smoking cessation programs or peer support groups, trigger avoidance, physical activity, and relaxation techniques.
- Provide alternate birth control options and provide teaching regarding the method(s) selected.
- Inform Julie that once she quits smoking she should discuss the safe use of birth control pills with her nurse practitioner.

Visit thePoint® at **http://thePoint.lww.com/Frandsen12e** for answers to NCLEX Success questions (in Appendix A), answers to Clinical Application Case Studies (in Appendix B), and more!

## REFERENCES AND RESOURCES

American Psychiatric Association. (2013). *Diagnostic and statistical manual of mental disorders* (5th ed.). Arlington, VA: American Psychiatric Publishing.

American Society of Reproductive Health. (2017). Combined hormonal contraception and the risk of venous thromboembolism: A guideline. *Fertility and Sterility, 107*(1), 43–51.

Boardman, H., Hartley, L., Eisinga, A., Main, C., & Figuls, M. R. (2016). Cochrane corner: Oral hormone therapy and cardiovascular outcomes in post-menopausal women. *Heart, 102*(1), 9–11.

di Scalea, L., & Pearlstein T. (2017). Premenstrual dysphoric disorder. *Psychiatric Clinics of North America, 40*(20), 201–216. doi: 10.1016/j.psc.2017.01.002

Grossman, D. C., Curry, S. J., Barry, M. J., Davidson, K. W., & Doubeni, C. A., et al. (2017). Menopausal hormone therapy for the primary prevention of chronic conditions: US Preventive Services Task Force recommendation statement. *JAMA, 318*(22), 2224–2233. doi: 10.1001/jama.2017.18261

Karch, A. (2019). *Focus on nursing pharmacology* (8th ed.). Philadelphia, PA: Lippincott Williams & Wilkins.

Norris, T. L. (2019). *Porth's Pathophysiology: Concepts of altered health states* (10th ed.). Philadelphia, PA: Wolters Kluwer.

Reid, R. L. (2017). *Premenstrual syndrome.* Retrieved from http://www.ncbi.nlm.nih.gov/books/NBK279045/

Ricci, S. S. (2016). *Essentials of maternity, newborn, and women's health nursing.* Philadelphia, PA: Lippincott Williams & Wilkins.

Trussell, J., Raymond, E. G., & Cleland, K. (2018). *Emergency contraception: a last chance to prevent unintended pregnancy.* Retrieved from http://ec.princeton.edu/questions/ec-review.pdf

Yonkers, K. A., & Simoni, M. K. (2018). Premenstrual disorders. *American Journal of Gynecology, 18*(1), 68–74, doi: 10.1016/j.ajog.2017.05.045

# Pharmacology and Men's Health

## LEARNING OBJECTIVES

*After studying this chapter, you should be able to:*

1. Discuss male reproductive problems in terms of etiology, pathophysiology, and clinical manifestations.
2. Describe the androgens in terms of prototype, mechanism of action, indications for use, major adverse effects, and nursing implications.
3. Identify potential consequences of abusing androgens and anabolic steroids.
4. Discuss the phosphodiesterase type 5 inhibitors in terms of prototype, mechanism of action, indications for use, major adverse effects, and nursing implications.
5. Describe the 5-alpha reductase inhibitors in terms of prototype, mechanism of action, indications for use, major adverse effects, and nursing implications.
6. Describe the alpha-adrenergic blockers in terms of prototype, mechanism of action, indications for use, major adverse effects, and nursing implications.
7. Implement the nursing process for men who have reproductive disorders.

## CLINICAL APPLICATION CASE STUDY

Phillip Johnson, a 52-year-old veterinarian, is seen in the clinic for hypertension control. He has a one-pack per day history of cigarette smoking and has begun walking to reduce his weight. For 5 years, he has been taking hydrochlorothiazide and atenolol to lower his blood pressure, which is well controlled. He has no other chronic health problems.

However, Mr. Johnson reports significant erectile dysfunction that has progressed over the past 9 months. This has significantly distressed him and his wife and has caused considerable marital discord.

## KEY TERMS

**Anabolic steroids:** synthetic drugs with increased anabolic activity and decreased androgenic activity compared with testosterone

**Androgen:** male sex hormones, primarily testosterone, secreted by the testes in men, the ovaries in women, and the adrenal cortex in both men and women

**Benign prostatic hypertrophy:** benign enlargement of the prostate gland; also known as benign prostatic hyperplasia

**Corpora cavernosa:** major erectile tissue of the penis

**Erectile dysfunction:** difficulty in initiating or maintaining penile erection that is satisfactory for sexual relations

**Erectogenic:** capable of causing an erection

**Ergogenic:** increase in muscular work capacity caused by drugs that enhance athletic performance

**Leydig cells:** cells in the testes that control androgen secretion

**Testosterone:** male sex hormone; secreted by the Leydig cells in the testes

# INTRODUCTION

This chapter explores the drugs used to manage disorders and conditions that affect men's reproductive health. To understand the drugs discussed in this chapter, it is necessary to understand the regulation of male reproductive function as well as recognize the main disorders of male reproduction.

# OVERVIEW OF REPRODUCTIVE HEALTH PROBLEMS IN MEN

**Androgens** are male sex hormones secreted by the testes in men, the ovaries in women, and the adrenal cortex in both men and women. Like the female sex hormones, the naturally occurring male sex hormones are steroids synthesized from cholesterol, which is why they are called **anabolic steroids**. The sex organs and adrenal glands can produce cholesterol or remove it from the blood. Cholesterol then undergoes a series of conversions to progesterone, androgenic prehormones, and **testosterone**. The androgens produced by the ovaries have little androgenic activity and are used mainly as precursor substances for the production of naturally occurring estrogens. The adrenal glands produce several androgens, including androstenedione and dehydroepiandrosterone (DHEA). Androstenedione and DHEA are weak androgens with little masculinizing effect that are mainly converted to estrogens.

Testosterone is normally the only important androgen. This male sex hormone has several effects on body tissues (Box 8.1). Certain cells in the testes, called **Leydig cells**, secrete testosterone in response to stimulation by luteinizing hormone (LH) from the anterior pituitary gland. The increased production of

---

| BOX 8.1 | *Effects of Testosterone on Body Tissues* |
|---|---|

### Fetal Development

Large amounts of chorionic gonadotropin are produced by the placenta during pregnancy. Chorionic gonadotropin is similar to luteinizing hormone (LH) from the anterior pituitary gland. It promotes development of the interstitial or Leydig cells in fetal testes, which then secrete testosterone. Testosterone production begins in the 2nd month of fetal life. When present, testosterone promotes development of male sexual characteristics (e.g., penis, scrotum, prostate gland, seminal vesicles, and seminiferous tubules) and suppresses development of female sexual characteristics. In the absence of testosterone, the fetus develops female sexual characteristics.

Testosterone also provides the stimulus for the descent of the testes into the scrotum. This normally occurs after the 7th month of pregnancy, when the fetal testes are secreting relatively large amounts of testosterone. If the testes do not descend before birth, administration of testosterone or gonadotropic hormone, which stimulates testosterone secretion, produces descent in most cases.

### Adult Development

Little testosterone is secreted in boys until 11 to 13 years of age. At the onset of puberty, testosterone secretion increases rapidly and remains at a relatively high level until about 50 years of age, after which it gradually declines.

The testosterone secreted at puberty acts as a growth hormone to produce enlargement of the penis, testes, and scrotum until approximately 20 years of age. The prostate gland, seminal vesicles, seminiferous tubules, and vas deferens also increase in size and functional ability. Under the combined influence of testosterone and follicle-stimulating hormone (FSH) from the anterior pituitary gland, sperm

production is initiated and maintained throughout the man's reproductive life. It affects various parts of the body.

- Skin. Testosterone increases skin thickness and activity of the sebaceous glands. Acne in the male adolescent is attributed to the increased production of testosterone.
- Voice. The larynx enlarges and deepens the voice of the adult man.
- Hair. Testosterone produces the distribution of hair growth on the face, limbs, and trunk typical of the adult man. In men with a genetic trait toward baldness, large amounts of testosterone cause alopecia (baldness) of the scalp.
- Skeletal muscles. Testosterone is largely responsible for the larger, more powerful muscles of men. This characteristic is caused by the effects of testosterone on protein metabolism. Testosterone helps the body retain nitrogen, form new amino acids, and build new muscle protein. At the same time, it slows the loss of nitrogen and amino acids formed by the constant breakdown of body tissues. Overall, testosterone increases protein anabolism (buildup) and decreases protein catabolism (breakdown).
- Bone. Testosterone makes bones thicker and longer. After puberty, more protein and calcium are deposited and retained in bone matrix. This causes a rapid rate of bone growth. The height of a male adolescent increases rapidly for a time and then stops as epiphyseal closure occurs. This happens when the cartilage at the end of the long bones in the arms and legs becomes bone. Further lengthening of the bones is then prevented.

### Anterior Pituitary Function

- High blood levels of testosterone decrease secretion of FSH and LH from the anterior pituitary gland. This, in turn, decreases testosterone production.

testosterone results in the changes associated with puberty in the adolescent male. The main functions of testosterone concern the development of male sexual characteristics, reproduction, and metabolism. Testosterone is necessary for normal sperm development.

About 97% of the testosterone secreted by the testes binds to plasma albumin or to sex hormone–binding globulin and circulates in the blood for 30 minutes to several hours. The bound testosterone is either transferred to the tissues or broken down into inactive products that are excreted. Much of the testosterone that transfers to tissues undergoes intracellular conversion to dihydrotestosterone (DHT), which combines with receptor proteins in the cytoplasm. A series of actions stimulates production of proteins. Almost all effects of testosterone result from the increased formation of proteins throughout the body, especially in the cells of target organs and tissues responsible for development of male sexual characteristics.

The portion of testosterone that does not become attached to tissues is converted into androsterone and DHEA by the liver. These are conjugated with glucuronic or sulfuric acid and excreted in the bile or urine.

# Etiology

## Androgen Deficiency

Lack of sufficient testosterone can result in congenital or acquired hypogonadism in the male. Causes include genetic diseases, head or testicular trauma, alkylating agents, tumors, and radiation injury.

- Primary hypogonadism results from a testicular disorder. Common diseases that can cause primary hypogonadism are mumps, testicular inflammation, and trauma.
- Secondary hypogonadism results from a problem in the hypothalamus or the pituitary gland, areas of the brain that signal the testicles to produce testosterone. A lack of production of gonadotropin-releasing hormone from the hypothalamus or a deficiency of FSH and LH from the anterior pituitary may result from thyroid disorders, Cushing's syndrome, or estrogen-secreting tumors. Chronic diseases (e.g., metabolic syndrome, diabetes) can lead to secondary hypogonadism.

## Erectile Dysfunction

**Erectile dysfunction** (ED) is defined as difficulty initiating or maintaining penile erection that is satisfactory for sexual relations. The condition affects more than 50% of men between 40 and 70 years of age. Incidence and prevalence increase with age. ED is common in men with systemic disorders such as hypertension, ischemic heart disease, and diabetes mellitus and is associated with thyroid conditions, prostate cancer, and spinal cord injuries. There appears to be a link between cardiovascular disease and ED. Cardiovascular disease enhances the risk of developing ED; conversely, some experts believe that ED is a powerful predictor of coronary artery disease, especially in men older than 60 years of age. ED and cardiovascular disease share many risk factors, and the pathophysiology of both conditions is mediated through endothelial dysfunction. In addition, a number of drugs (antidepressants, antihypertensive agents, antipsychotics, diuretics, histamine receptor antagonists) and lifestyle factors (alcohol, tobacco, or cocaine use, obesity) have been known to cause the condition. Low testosterone levels rarely lead to ED but may reduce a man's sex drive. Psychologic factors may also play a role, and these include sexual performance anxiety, relationship conflicts, and cultural and religious taboos.

## Benign Prostatic Hypertrophy

**Benign prostatic hypertrophy** (BPH), also known as benign prostatic hyperplasia, is benign enlargement of the prostate gland. More than 50% of men in their 60s and as many as 90% in their 70s and 80s have some symptoms of BPH. Part of the male reproductive system, the prostate is normally a walnut-sized gland composed of two lobes enclosed by an outer layer of tissue. This gland produces part of the seminal fluid that nourishes and transports sperm. The prostate is located in front of the rectum and below the bladder, where urine is stored, and it surrounds the urethra, the canal through which urine passes out of the body.

It is thought that BPH is a normal element of the male aging process. Causes include changes in hormone balance and cell growth. Testosterone undergoes reduction to form the more potent androgen DHT, which has greater affinity for androgen receptors than testosterone. During the formation and growth of an embryo, DHT plays a critical role in the formation of the male external genitalia, whereas in the adult, DHT acts as the primary androgen in the prostate and in hair follicles.

# Pathophysiology

## Androgen Deficiency

- Hypogonadism results from dysfunction of the hypothalamus, the anterior pituitary, or the gonads. Chapter 43 describes the role of the hypothalamic–pituitary–adrenal axis. Primary hypogonadism involves pathology of either Leydig cells or the seminiferous tubules, or both. Injury to Leydig cells results in decreased testosterone production, whereas seminiferous tubule dysfunction results in decreased or absent spermatogenesis. The majority of the conditions causing testicular injury predominantly involve tubules. Gonadotropins are elevated due to loss of negative feedback.
- Secondary hypogonadism involves decreased or incorrectly normal gonadotropin levels, leading to decreased testicular stimulation, spermatogenesis, and androgen production and, if prolonged, testicular atrophy.

## Erectile Dysfunction

The process of achieving penile erection involves the integration of psychological, neurologic, and vascular processes, which combine to initiate a physiologic response within the penile vasculature. Stimulation of penile shaft results in the secretion of nitric oxide, which causes the relaxation of the smooth muscles of the **corpora cavernosa** (the main erectile tissue of the penis). This results in increased blood flow into the sinusoids of the corpora cavernosa with subsequent filling, which obstructs venous outflow from the penis by compression of the veins against the tunica albuginea, resulting in penile erection. Additionally, adequate levels of testosterone and an intact pituitary gland are required.

## Benign Prostatic Hypertrophy

The prostate contains stromal and epithelial tissue. Stromal tissue is smooth muscle tissue that contracts around the urethra when activated and is regulated by alpha$_1$-adrenergic receptors. Epithelial tissue is the glandular portion of the prostate and is under the control of androgens, primarily testosterone. The enzyme 5-alpha reductase converts testosterone to DHT, its active metabolite, in epithelial tissue.

The prostate undergoes two main growth periods, first in puberty, when the prostate doubles in size, and second in early adulthood, at about 25 years of age, when the gland begins another growth phase that often results years later in BPH. A surrounding layer of tissue limits overgrowth of the epithelial or glandular tissue of the prostate, causing the gland to put pressure against the urethra. In addition, the bladder wall becomes thicker and more easily irritated; it contracts even when it contains small amounts of urine, leading to more frequent urination. At some point, the bladder weakens and loses the capacity to empty, and urine is retained in the bladder. The narrowing of the urethra and partial emptying of the bladder cause many of the problems associated with BPH.

## Clinical Manifestations

### Androgen Deficiency

Signs and symptoms of androgen deficiency in adult males include ED, infertility, decreased beard and body hair growth, decreased muscle mass, breast development (gynecomastia), and loss of bone mass (osteoporosis). Hypogonadism can also cause mental and emotional changes. As testosterone decreases, some men may experience symptoms similar to those of menopause in women, including fatigue, decreased sex drive, difficulty concentrating, and hot flashes.

To confirm a diagnosis of hypogonadism, it is necessary to perform laboratory tests. Serum testosterone is decreased. To determine the cause, it is also necessary to measure hormone levels in the serum: FSH, LH, prolactin, thyroid hormone, and estradiol. If normal or elevated FSH and LH serum levels are present with a low testosterone level and the testes are nonresponsive to hormonal stimulation, a primary hypogonadism is present. If FSH and LH are low along with the testosterone level, a secondary hypogonadism is present.

### Erectile Dysfunction

The main clinical manifestation of ED is the consistent inability to attain or maintain an erection satisfactory for sexual activity. An associated symptom may be reduced sexual desire.

### Benign Prostatic Hypertrophy

Clinical manifestations of BPH result from the obstruction of the urethra from the enlargement of the prostate gland, causing reduction in outflow of urine. Rarely do symptoms occur in men younger than 40 years of age. Men may experience urinary frequency, hesitancy, urgency, dribbling, and decrease force of the urinary stream. Nocturia, postvoid leakage, urinary stones, or infection can also occur.

On physical examination, a midline mass above the symphysis pubis, which likely represents an incompletely emptied bladder, may be visible. On digital rectal examination,

**TABLE 8.1**

### Drugs Administered for Maintenance of Male Reproductive Health

| Drug Class | Prototype | Other Drugs in the Class |
|---|---|---|
| Androgens | Testosterone | Testolactone Fluoxymesterone Methyltestosterone (Android, Testred) Danazol* |
| Phosphodiesterase type 5 inhibitors | Sildenafil (Viagra, Revatio) | Avanafil (Stendra) Tadalafil (Cialis) Vardenafil (Levitra) |
| Prostaglandins | | Alprostadil (Caverject aqueous, Caverject powder, Edex powder, Muse) |
| 5-Alpha reductase inhibitors | Finasteride (Proscar) | Dutasteride (Avodart) |
| Alpha$_1$-adrenergic blockers | Tamsulosin (Flomax) | Alfuzosin (Uroxatral) Doxazosin (Cardura) Silodosin (Rapaflo) Terazosin |

*Used in women.

rubbery enlargement of the prostate is present. Excretory urography may indicate emptying and filling defects in the bladder, urinary tract obstruction, calculi or tumors, and hydronephrosis.

## Drug Therapy

Table 8.1 outlines the drugs used to maintain male reproductive health, which include the androgens and anabolic steroids, the phosphodiesterase type 5 (PDE5) inhibitors and prostaglandins, and the 5-alpha reductase inhibitors and the alpha$_1$-adrenergic inhibitors.

## ANDROGENS AND ANABOLIC STEROIDS

When clinicians use male sex hormones or androgens from exogenous sources for therapeutic purposes, the effects are the same as those of naturally occurring hormones. These effects include inhibition of endogenous sex hormones and sperm formation through negative feedback of pituitary LH and FSH. Anabolic steroids are synthetic drugs with increased anabolic activity and decreased androgenic activity compared with endogenous testosterone. They were developed during attempts to modify testosterone so that its tissue-building and growth-stimulating effects could be retained while the drug's masculinizing effects could be eliminated or reduced.

Prescribers may order male sex hormones for women to antagonize or reduce the effects of female sex hormones. Thus, administration of androgenic or anabolic steroids to women causes suppression of menstruation and atrophy of the endometrial lining of the uterus.

Several dosage forms of androgens are available. They differ mainly in route of administration and pharmacokinetics.  **Testosterone** is the prototype.

## Pharmacokinetics

Like endogenous testosterone, the drug molecules are highly bound (98%) to plasma proteins and serum half-life varies (e.g., 8 days for intramuscular [IM] testosterone cypionate, 9 hours for oral fluoxymesterone). Testosterone is extensively metabolized in its first pass through the liver, so that nearly half of a dose is lost before it reaches the systemic circulation. About 90% of a dose is excreted in urine as conjugates of testosterone and its metabolites; the remainder is excreted in feces.

## Action

Like other steroid drugs, testosterone penetrates the cell membrane and binds to receptor proteins in the cell cytoplasm. The steroid–receptor complex is then transported to the nucleus, where it activates ribonucleic acid (RNA) and deoxyribonucleic acid (DNA) production and stimulates cellular synthesis of protein.

## Use

With testosterone, the most clear-cut indication for use is to treat androgen deficiency states (e.g., hypogonadism, cryptorchidism, impotence, oligospermia) in boys and men. In postpubertal men who become androgen deficient, the hormone reestablishes and maintains masculine characteristics and functions. Table 8.2 gives route and dosage information for testosterone and other androgens and anabolic steroids.

### Use in Children

The main indication for use of testosterone in children is for boys with established sex hormone deficiencies; the hormone stimulates the development of masculine characteristics.

> **! QSEN Alert: Safety**
>
> Because testosterone can cause epiphyseal closure, it is essential to examine a child's hands and wrists using radiography every 6 months to detect bone maturation and to check that there is no loss of height if receiving testosterone therapy.

## TABLE 8.2
### DRUGS AT A GLANCE: Androgens

| Drug | Pregnancy Category | Routes and Dosage Ranges | |
|---|---|---|---|
| | | **Hypogonadism** | **Other** |
| **Testosterone cypionate** (Depo-Testosterone; ✿ Andriol, Androderm, Axiron, Testim) | X | 50–200 mg IM every 2–4 wk | |
| **Testosterone enanthate** (Xyosted; ✿ Andriol, Androderm, Axiron, Testim) | X | 50–200 mg IM every 2–4 wk | |
| **Testosterone gel** (AndroGel 1%; ✿ AndroGel) | X | Apply 5 g (50 mg of drug) once daily in morning to skin of shoulders and upper arms or abdomen | |
| **Testosterone pellets** | X | 150–80 mg sub-Q every 3–6 mo | Delayed puberty: lower dosage range sub-Q, for a limited duration (e.g., every 3 mo for 2–3 doses) |
| **Testosterone transdermal systems** (Androderm; ✿ Andriol, Androderm, AndroGel, Axiron) | | Apply two systems (dose of 5 mg) nightly to back, abdomen, upper arm, or thigh | |
| Testolactone | C | | Breast cancer: 250 mg PO four times daily |
| Fluoxymesterone | X | 5–20 mg PO daily | |
| Methyltestosterone (Android, Testred) | X | | Cryptorchidism: 30 mg PO daily; buccal tablets, 15 mg PO daily |
| Danazol (✿ Cyclomen) | X | | Endometriosis: 800 mg PO daily in two divided doses for 3–9 mo  Fibrocystic breast disease: 100–400 mg PO daily in two divided doses for 3–6 mo |

Stimulation of skeletal growth should continue for approximately 6 months after testosterone therapy stops. If premature puberty occurs (e.g., precocious sexual development, enlarged penis), it is necessary to stop the drug. Testosterones may cause or aggravate acne. Scrupulous skin care and other antiacne treatment may be necessary, especially in adolescent boys.

### Use in Older Adults

In older adults with hypertension and other cardiovascular disorders, the sodium and water retention associated with testosterone may aggravate these conditions. Also, in men, the drugs may increase prostate size and interfere with urination, increase risk of prostatic cancer, and cause excessive sexual stimulation and priapism.

## Adverse Effects

Common adverse effects from testosterone include acne, change in sex drive, hair loss, headache, bitter taste or mouth irritation, or gum tenderness. Additionally, hypercalcemia, jaundice, and edema may occur. Virilizing or masculinizing effects may vary. In adult men with adequate secretion of testosterone, adverse effects include priapism, increased sexual desire, reduced sperm count, and prostate enlargement. In prepubertal boys, adverse effects may involve premature development of sex organs and secondary sexual characteristics, such as enlargement of the penis and pubic hair. Priapism may occur. In women, adverse effects include hirsutism, deepening of the voice, and menstrual irregularities.

## Contraindications

Contraindications to testosterone include pregnancy (because of possible masculinizing effects on a female fetus), preexisting liver disease, and disorders of the prostate. (Men with an enlarged prostate may have additional enlargement, and men with prostate cancer may experience tumor growth.)

## Nursing Implications

### Preventing Interactions

Some medications and herbs interact with testosterone, decreasing its effects (Box 8.2). Androgens may increase effects of cyclosporine and warfarin, apparently by slowing their metabolism and increasing their concentrations in the blood. If possible, people should avoid using these combinations. If they are necessary, the nurse monitors serum creatinine and cyclosporine levels (for cyclosporine) and prothrombin time or international

---

**BOX 8.2**  **Drug Interactions: Testosterone**

**Drugs That Decrease the Effects of Testosterone**
- Barbiturates
  *Increase enzyme induction and rate of metabolism*
- Calcitonin
  *Decreases calcium retention, thus antagonizing the calcium-retaining effects of androgens*

---

normalized ratio (INR) (for warfarin). Androgens also increase the effects of sulfonylureas. If possible, people should avoid using sulfonylureas concurrently.

**Concept Mastery Alert**

Concurrent use of androgens with sulfonylureas is to be avoided if possible because androgens increase the effect of sulfonylureas. If simultaneous use is required, smaller sulfonylurea doses may be necessary, and blood glucose levels are to be monitored closely. Patients are to be assessed for signs of hypoglycemia.

### Administering the Medication

Naturally occurring androgens are given by injection because they are metabolized rapidly by the liver if given orally. Some esters of testosterone have been modified to slow the rate of metabolism and thus prolong action. For example, IM testosterone cypionate and testosterone enanthate have slow onsets of action and last 2 to 4 weeks. As a result of first-pass metabolism, doses as high as 400 mg/d may be needed to produce adequate blood levels for full replacement therapy.

Several transdermal formulations of testosterone are available. They have a rapid onset of action and last approximately 24 hours. A topical gel (a 10-g dose delivers 100 mg) produces normal serum testosterone levels within 4 hours after application, and absorption of testosterone into the blood continues for 24 hours. Steady-state serum concentrations occur by the 2nd or 3rd day of use. When the gel is discontinued, serum testosterone levels remain in the normal range for 24 to 48 hours but decrease to pretreatment levels within about 5 days.

### Assessing for Therapeutic and Adverse Effects

The nurse assesses for return of sex hormone levels, development of masculine characteristics in boys, and return of libido in adult males.

The nurse should assess for adverse effects, including hypersensitivity reaction, changes in sexual drive or masculinization, hair loss, changes in taste, oral irritation, and/or gum tenderness. The nurse also monitors serum calcium and observes for signs of hypercalcemia (e.g., kidney stones, polyuria, abdominal pain, nausea, vomiting, depression).

### Patient Teaching

Box 8.3 presents patient teaching information for androgens.

## Other Drugs in the Class

Danazol is a synthetic testosterone with weak androgenic activity. Clinicians may use the drug in women to prevent or treat endometriosis or fibrocystic breast disease. Danazol is seldom prescribed continuously beyond 6 months because it produces the same androgenic adverse effects as other androgens, which are particularly of concern in females. Although some drug literature still lists metastatic breast cancer and some types of anemia as indications for use of androgens, newer drugs have largely replaced them for these purposes.

## BOX 8.3 — *Patient Teaching Guidelines for Androgens*

**General Considerations**

- Take the drugs only if prescribed and as prescribed. Use by athletes for body building is inappropriate and, if not prescribed by a licensed prescriber, is illegal.
- Continue medical supervision as long as the drugs are being taken.
- Weigh self once or twice weekly and record the amount. An increase may indicate fluid retention and edema.
- Practice frequent and thorough skin cleansing to decrease acne, which is most likely to occur in women and children.
- Keep all appointments for laboratory testing and follow-up care.
- As with all drugs, keep these medications in the original container, tightly closed, and out of reach of children.

**Self-Administration**

- Take oral preparations before or with meals, in divided doses.
- For buccal preparations, adhere to the following guidelines:

- Take in divided doses.
- Place the tablet between the cheek and gum and allow to dissolve (do not swallow).
- Avoid eating, drinking, or smoking while the tablet is in place.
- For transdermal systems, adhere to the following guidelines:
  - Apply two Androderm systems nightly to clean, dry skin on the back, abdomen, upper arm, or thigh. Do not apply to the scrotum. Rotate sites, with 7 days between applications to a site. Press firmly into place for adherence.
  - Apply the prescribed amount of gel to clean, dry, intact skin of the shoulders and upper arms or the abdomen (do not apply to the genital area), once daily, preferably in the morning. Wash hands after application and allow sites to dry before dressing. After application, wait at least 1 hour and preferably 4 to 6 hours before showering or swimming.

In breast cancer, androgens are second-line hormonal agents, after antiestrogens (e.g., tamoxifen). In anemia associated with renal failure, synthetic erythropoietin is more effective and more likely to be used. Administration of danazol is oral, and metabolism occurs in the liver. The route of excretion is unknown. A **BLACK BOX WARNING** ◆ issued by the U.S. Food and Drug Administration (FDA) states that danazol is contraindicated in pregnancy and that a pregnancy test should be administered prior to the start of therapy. In addition, a nonhormonal method of contraception should be used during treatment. The warning also states that use of the drug is associated with the risk of a thromboembolic event and/or intracranial hypertension.

Fluoxymesterone is an anabolic steroid with strong androgenic properties used in the treatment of hypogonadism, delayed male puberty, and breast cancers in women. This drug is often abused to increase athletic performance.

Methyltestosterone is a synthetic formulation of testosterone that can be used in adolescent males with delayed puberty to produce puberty. The drug is less extensively metabolized by the liver and more suitable for oral administration.

Testolactone, a derivative of progesterone, is an antineoplastic agent used to treat advanced breast cancer. The drug blocks the production of estrogen, which reduces the growth of breast cancers that are activated by estrogen. It does not seem to have the masculinizing effects of testosterone.

## Abuse of Androgens and Anabolic Steroids

Drugs used to enhance athletic performance are termed **ergogenic** (causing an increase in muscular work capacity). Androgens and anabolic steroids are widely abused in attempts to enhance muscle development, muscle strength, and athletic performance.

### ! QSEN Alert: Safety

Because of their abuse potential, androgens and anabolic steroids are Schedule III controlled substances.

Although nonprescription sales of the drugs are illegal, they apparently are easily obtained.

Athletes are considered a high-risk group because some start taking the drugs as early as middle school and continue for years. The use of performance-enhancing drugs in nonathletes is also on the rise to improve performance outside of sports. The number of teens taking anabolic steroids is thought to be small in comparison with the number using marijuana, amphetamines, and other illegal drugs. However, the number is increasing, and long-term effects may be as serious as the effects that occur with use of other illegal drugs. Although steroids have a reputation for being dangerous to adult athletes, such as body builders and football players, they are considered even more dangerous for teens because teens are still growing.

### ! QSEN Alert: Safety

Anabolic steroids can stop bone growth and damage the heart, kidneys, and liver of adolescents.

In addition to those who take steroids to enhance athletic performance, some males take the drugs to produce a more muscular appearance and impress females. Steroid abusers usually take massive doses and often take several drugs or combine injectable and oral drugs for maximum effects. The large doses produce potentially serious adverse effects in several body tissues:

- Cardiovascular disorders include hypertension, decreased high-density blood lipoproteins, and increased low-density lipoproteins, all of which promote heart attacks and strokes.

- Liver disorders include benign and malignant neoplasms, cholestatic hepatitis and jaundice, and peliosis hepatis, a disorder in which blood-filled cysts develop in the liver and may lead to hemorrhage or liver failure.
- Central nervous system disorders include aggression, hostility, combativeness, and dependence characterized by preoccupation with drug use, inability to stop taking the drugs, and withdrawal symptoms similar to those that occur with alcohol, cocaine, and narcotics. In some cases, psychosis may develop.
- Reproductive system disorders include decreased testicular function (e.g., decreased secretion of endogenous testosterone, decreased formation of sperm), testicular atrophy, and impotence in men. They include amenorrhea in women.
- Metabolic disorders include atherosclerosis-promoting changes in cholesterol metabolism and retention of fluids, with edema and other imbalances. Fluid and electrolyte retention contribute to the increased weight associated with drug use.
- Dermatologic disorders include moderate to severe acne in both sexes, depending on drug dosage.

Many of these adverse effects persist several months after the drugs are stopped and may be irreversible.

Androstenedione and DHEA, androgens produced by the adrenal cortex, are also available as over-the-counter (OTC) dietary supplements. They are marketed as safe, natural, alternative androgens for building muscles. These products, which have weak androgenic activity, act mainly as precursors for the production of sex hormones. Androstenedione, for example, may be converted to testosterone by way of an enzyme found in most body tissues. However, it may also be converted to estrogens, and the testosterone that is produced may be further converted to estrogen (estradiol).

DHEA is available alone as oral capsules or tablets and in a topical cream with vitamins and herbs. Contraindications to DHEA include prostate cancer or BPH as well as estrogen-responsive breast or uterine cancer, because DHEA may stimulate growth of the cancerous tissues. It is important that patients older than 40 years of age be aggressively screened for hormonally sensitive cancers before taking DHEA.

Adverse effects of DHEA include aggressiveness, hirsutism, insomnia, and irritability. Whether large doses of the OTC products can produce some of the serious adverse effects associated with standard anabolic steroids is unknown.

## NCLEX Success

1. The most clear-cut therapeutic indication for use of male sex hormones is which of the following?
   A. to treat androgen deficiency states in boys and men
   B. for bodybuilding purposes
   C. to treat metastatic breast cancer
   D. to treat anemia associated with renal failure

2. Four patients in an endocrine clinic are ordered to begin androgen therapy. The nurse reviews each patient's current medications and identifies which patient as able to begin androgen therapy without the risk of a known drug interaction?
   A. patient 1, taking cyclosporine
   B. patient 2, taking warfarin
   C. patient 3, taking sulfonylureas
   D. patient 4, taking heparin

3. A 19-year-old female athlete presents for her first prenatal visit and tells the nurse she has been on androgen therapy to improve her distance running. She asks the nurse if she can continue taking the androgens to maintain her "competitive edge." The nurse should instruct her that she
   A. can continue taking androgens, because the drugs pose no risk to the fetus
   B. can continue taking androgens, but a higher dose will be required due to increased drug metabolism during pregnancy
   C. can continue taking androgens until the third trimester, when they must be discontinued because androgens cause an increased risk of premature rupture of membranes
   D. must stop taking androgens immediately, because they pose a risk to the fetus; she should discuss this with her health care provider at today's visit

4. Which of the following statements by a male patient taking transdermal androgens indicates that teaching has been adequate? (Select all that apply.)
   A. "I need to weigh myself once or twice weekly and record the amount"
   B. "I should wash my face and body thoroughly to decrease the risk of acne"
   C. "The patch systems should be applied nightly to skin on my back, abdomen, upper arm, or thigh"
   D. "I should apply the patch systems in the morning to the same site each and every day"

### *Clinical Application 8.1*

- Mr. Johnson asks a nurse if he can take the "little blue pill that will improve his lovemaking" (sildenafil). How should the nurse respond?

## PHOSPHODIESTERASE TYPE 5 INHIBITORS

Prescribers commonly order PDE5 inhibitors as the first-line treatment for ED. These drugs do not cause an erection but help maintain the erection resulting from sexual stimuli by enhancing the vasodilatory effect of endogenous nitric oxide, increasing blood flow to the penis. The prototype PDE5 inhibitor is **sildenafil** (Viagra).

## TABLE 8.3

## DRUGS AT A GLANCE: Phosphodiesterase Type 5 Inhibitors

| Drug | Pregnancy Category | Routes and Dosage Ranges (Adult Males) |
|---|---|---|
| Sildenafil (Viagra, Revatio; GD-Sildenafil, Jamp-Sildenafil, Viagra) | B | Erectile dysfunction (Viagra): PO 25–100 mg 1 h before sexual activity; reduce dose with age older than 65 y, concurrent use of CYP3A4 inhibitors,* and renal or hepatic impairment |
| Avanafil (Stendra) | C | PO 100–200 mg 30 min before anticipated sexual activity, reduced dose with age older than 65 y, hepatic impairment, and concurrent use of CYP3A4 inhibitors* |
| Tadalafil (Cialis; Adcirca, Cialis) | B | PO 2.5–20 mg 2 h or more before anticipated sexual activity, PO 2.5–5 mg once daily, reduced dose with age older than 65 y, renal or hepatic impairment, and concurrent use of CYP3A4 inhibitors* |
| Vardenafil (Levitra; Levitra, Staxyn) | B | PO 5–20 mg 1 h before sexual activity, reduced dose with age older than 65 y, hepatic impairment, and concurrent use of CYP3A4 inhibitors* |

*CYP3A4 inhibitors include azole antifungals, erythromycin, and saquinavir.

## Pharmacokinetics

Sildenafil is significantly protein bound and is rapidly absorbed by the oral route. The drug is metabolized in the liver and is primarily excreted in the feces and to a lesser extent by the kidneys. The onset of action is 20 to 60 minutes, with a duration of up to 4 hours.

## Action

Sildenafil improves erectile function by inhibiting the enzyme responsible for the breakdown of cyclic guanosine monophosphate (cGMP), a vasodilatory neurotransmitter in corporal tissues of the penis. This causes a vasodilatory effect in the smooth muscle of the corpus cavernosum that allows for a harder and longer-lasting erection.

## Use

Sildenafil is used for the treatment of ED in men healthy enough for sexual activity. The FDA has also approved the drug for the treatment of pulmonary arterial hypertension in men. The drug should not be administered to women and children. Table 8.3 gives route and dosage information for sildenafil and other PDE5 inhibitors.

### Use in Patients With Hepatic Impairment

Caution is warranted with the use of sildenafil with hepatic impairment. Patients with cirrhosis or other significant liver dysfunction should start with a lower dose to minimize worsening of the hepatic impairment.

## Adverse Effects

Adverse reactions to sildenafil commonly include headache, facial flushing, dyspepsia, nasal congestion, and dizziness. Rarely, clinicians have reported nonarteritic ischemic optic neuropathy (NAION) due to obstruction of blood flow to the optic nerve, resulting in irreversible loss of vision in one or both eyes, as well as sudden permanent hearing loss accompanied by

dizziness and tinnitus. Priapism is rare and usually associated with excessive dosing or concurrent use with another **erectogenic** drug (capable of causing an erection).

## Contraindications

Contraindications to sildenafil include a known hypersensitivity to the drug.

### QSEN Alert: Safety

Prescribers should not order it for men who also take organic nitrates, commonly used to treat angina, because the sildenafil–nitrate combination can cause severe hypotension resulting in dizziness, syncope, heart attack, or stroke.

Also, men who are not healthy enough to engage in sexual activity should not take sildenafil.

## Nursing Implications

### Preventing Interactions

Sildenafil, like other PDE5 inhibitors, is primarily metabolized by the cytochrome P450 (CYP) enzyme CYP3A4. Many medications and herbs interact with sildenafil, increasing or decreasing its effects (Boxes 8.4 and 8.5).

**BOX 8.4**  *Drug Interactions: Sildenafil*

**Drugs That Increase the Effects of Sildenafil**
- Alcohol
  *Increases the risk of orthostatic hypotension, tachycardia, dizziness, and headache*
- Alpha-adrenergic blockers, antihypertensive drugs, cytochrome P450 3A4 inhibitors (e.g., azole antifungals, erythromycin, saquinavir, protease inhibitors)
  *Increase risk of hypotension*

## BOX 8.5 — Herb and Dietary Interactions: Sildenafil

**Herbs and Foods That Increase the Effects of Sildenafil**
- Grapefruit juice, saw palmetto, yohimbine

**Herbs and Foods That Decrease the Effects of Sildenafil**
- Fatty food

### Administering the Medication

Administration is generally oral. It is important not to take sildenafil more than once in a 24-hour period. A recent high-fat meal may delay drug action.

 **QSEN Alert: Evidence-Based Practice**

Sexuality is a significant quality-of-life consideration for all individuals. Age-related changes, chronic disease, treatment protocols, and concurrent health conditions can increase the risk of sexual dysfunction in men. In a prospective study of 161 men receiving orchiectomy and radiation therapy for early-stage testicular cancer, researchers explored the short-term effects of treatment on body image and sexual dysfunction (Wortel et al., 2015). Although the cancer itself is not associated with sexual dysfunction, treatment is associated with sexual dysfunction in about one third of patients. Findings demonstrated that more than 60% of the patients reported change in their body image following orchiectomy that was associated with sexual dysfunction. Six months after treatment, more than 20% of men reported a reduction of sexual activity, interest, and pleasure. Because testicular cancer (the most common cancer in men between the ages of 20 and 34 years) often affects men of reproductive age who are sexually active, the nurse should assess for the presence of body image disturbance and sexual dysfunction early in treatment to explore the impact, if present, on quality of life.

### Assessing for Therapeutic and Adverse Effects

The nurse should assess that the patient reports the ability to initiate or maintain a penile erection for satisfactory sexual relations. Additionally, the nurse assesses for signs of adverse effects, including headache, facial flushing, dyspepsia, nasal congestion, and dizziness. Patients with symptoms of NAION or sudden decrease or loss of hearing should discontinue sildenafil and seek immediate medical care. Although rare, persistent priapism requires prompt medical treatment to avoid permanent penile damage. Because ED is a strong predictor of coronary artery disease, it is recommended that a cardiovascular assessment be completed in a noncardiac patient who presents with ED.

### Patient Teaching

Box 8.6 contains patient teaching guidelines for sildenafil and other drugs for ED.

## Other Drugs in the Class

Three other FDA-approved PDE5 inhibitors have similar effectiveness and safety profiles. Avanafil (Stendra), the newest PDE5 inhibitor, is a fast-acting and highly selective member of the class. The drug reaches its peak in 30 minutes, with a duration of 6 hours. Meals do not affect absorption rate or peak levels. Absorption and metabolism of the drug occurs in the liver through the CYP450 system. Excretion takes place in the feces through the bile. Adverse effects, common to other PDE5 inhibitors, include headache, flushing of the face, nasal congestion, and back pain.

Tadalafil (Cialis) has a longer half-life, which gives men the option of taking the drug up to 12 hours before sexual intercourse or as a lower dose, once-a-day daily medication. The drug reaches its peak in 2 hours, with a duration of 24 to 36 hours. Meals do not affect absorption rate or peak levels. Adverse effects, which may linger because of in this longer-acting drug, include back and muscle pain.

Vardenafil (Levitra) has a time to peak effect of 1 hour and a duration of action of 4 hours. As with sildenafil, a high-fat meal delays absorption and reduces peak levels. The drug is available in an oral disintegrating tablet.

 **QSEN Alert: Safety**

Vardenafil is the only PDE5 inhibitor that prolongs the QT interval and should not be used with other drugs with similar effect, particularly class I and II antidysrhythmics (see Chap. 27).

Like sildenafil, vardenafil reduces blood pressure and to a lesser degree increases the risk of light sensitivity, blurred vision, and loss of blue–green color discrimination.

## BOX 8.6 — Patient Teaching Guidelines for Sildenafil and Other Drugs Used to Treat Erectile Dysfunction

**General Considerations**
- Take the drugs only as prescribed.
- Keep appointments for laboratory testing and follow-up care.
- As with all drugs, keep these medications in the original container, tightly closed, and out of reach of children.

**Self-Administration**
- Do not take any phosphodiesterase type 5 (PDE5) inhibitor with nitrates because a serious and potentially life-threatening drop in blood pressure may occur.
- Do not take sildenafil more than once a day.
- Avoid consuming a high-fat meal before taking sildenafil or vardenafil.
- Seek immediate medical attention for an erection lasting 4 hours or longer.
- Do not use intraurethral alprostadil without using a condom if your partner is pregnant.
- If symptoms of nonarteritic ischemic optic neuropathy or a sudden decrease or loss of hearing occurs while taking PDE5 inhibitors, discontinue the drug and seek medical attention.

| BOX 8.7 | *Adjuvant Medications Used to Treat Erectile Dysfunction: Alprostadil* |

**Intracavernosal Injection (Caverject Aqueous, Caverject Powder, Edex Powder)**

- Injection may occur along the dorsolateral aspect of the proximal third of the penis, avoiding visible veins.
- It is necessary to rotate injection sites from one side of the penis to the other and change injection site with each dose.
- Self-injection may occur no more than three times per week and only once in 24 hours.
- To determine dose adequate for achieving satisfactory erection without causing priapism, it is important to have an initial injection in provider's office.

**Intraurethral Administration (Muse)**

- Prior to introducing pellet into urethra, it is important to void; residual urine in urethra aids in dispersing the medication.
- Intraurethral administration may occur no more than two times in 24 hours.
- To determine dose adequate for achieving satisfactory erection without causing priapism, the patient should visit the provider.

# ADJUVANT MEDICATIONS USED TO TREAT ERECTILE DYSFUNCTION

Clinicians consider adjuvant drugs second-line therapy in the management of ED and generally reserve them for patients who manifest insufficient response to or adverse effects from PDE5 inhibitors. Alprostadil is a synthetic enzyme that causes relaxation of cavernosal smooth muscle and dilation of cavernosal arterioles leading to increased penile blood flow. It is a prostaglandin, specifically a prostaglandin $E_1$.

Administration of alprostadil occurs in two ways: either as an injection into the penis or as a pellet inserted into it (via the urethral opening at the end of the penis). Box 8.7 presents notes about administering the drug. Intracavernosal alprostadil (Caverject) relaxes trabecular smooth muscle and dilates cavernosal arteries, resulting in penile engorgement and reduced venous outflow. Intraurethral alprostadil (Muse) is less efficacious than the intracavernosal drug (60% or less). Administration by either route can produce dose–response improvements in frequency of an erection sufficient for intercourse. The onset of action is immediate following injection, and erection should not last longer than 1 hour with proper dosing (determined in a provider's office).

Intracavernosal injection of alprostadil is associated with a burning sensation, prolonged erection, and priapism, and long-term use is associated with penile fibrosis. Caution is warranted in patients concurrently receiving anticoagulants due to risk of bleeding and in patients at risk for priapism (e.g., sickle cell anemia or trait, multiple myeloma, leukemia). Intraurethral use of the drug is associated with penile pain and minor urethral bleeding. Experts do not recommend alprostadil for concurrent use with other vasoactive agents.

## *Clinical Application 8.2*

- After an evaluation, the nurse practitioner suspects that Mr. Johnson's erectile dysfunction may result from the combination of obesity and antihypertensive medications. He receives a prescription for lisinopril, an angiotensin-converting enzyme inhibitor, which he will take along with hydrochlorothiazide. What patient teaching guidelines should the nurse discuss with Mr. Johnson and his wife?

# DRUGS FOR BENIGN PROSTATIC HYPERTROPHY

The 5-alpha reductase inhibitors and the $alpha_1$-adrenergic blockers are the two major drug classes used to treat BPH. Each class works differently to enhance urination in males, and both classes of drugs can be prescribed simultaneously for management of BPH. Each class will be discussed separately.

## 5-ALPHA REDUCTASE INHIBITORS

**Finasteride** (Proscar), the prototype 5-alpha reductase inhibitor, represents this drug class and is used to treat BPH. The other drug in the class and used to treat BPH is dutasteride (Avodart).

### Pharmacokinetics

Finasteride is well absorbed as an oral drug. It is 90% bound to plasma proteins. The onset of action is rapid, with a duration of 5 to 7 days. The half-life is 5 to 7 hours. Finasteride may take 3 to 6 months to reach maximum effects. The drug crosses the blood–brain barrier and has been found in semen.

### Action

Finasteride acts by inhibiting 5-alpha reductase, the enzyme responsible for converting testosterone to 5-alpha DHT, one of its active metabolites. This inhibits the metabolism of testosterone, causing decreased proliferation of prostatic cells, which reduces the enlargement of the prostate gland and mechanical obstruction to the urethra.

### Use

Prescribers order finasteride mainly to treat BPH. However, the drug is also available in smaller doses as Propecia, which is indicated for the prevention of male pattern baldness. Table 8.4 gives route and dosage information for finasteride.

#### Use in Older Adults

Older adults are prone to the hypotensive and hypothermic adverse effects from the vasodilation produced by finasteride.

## TABLE 8.4

### DRUGS AT A GLANCE: 5-Alpha Reductase Inhibitors

| Drug | Pregnancy Category | Routes and Dosage Ranges [Adult Males] |
|------|:---:|---|
| Ⓟ **Finasteride** (Proscar; 🍁 PMS-Finasteride, Propecia, Proscar) | X | PO 5 mg/d to max of 5 mg/d |
| Dutasteride (Avodart; 🍁 ACT-Dutasteride, Apo-Dutasteride, Avodart) | X | PO 5 mg/d |

### Use in Renal or Hepatic Impairment

Caution is necessary when administering finasteride to patients with renal or hepatic impairment.

## Adverse Effects and Contraindications

Adverse effects of finasteride include various sexual dysfunctions, such as impotence, gynecomastia, reduced libido, and ejaculatory disorders. Dysfunction is usually transient. The drug may decrease sperm production, adversely affecting fertility.

Contraindications include known sensitivity to finasteride. Children and women, particularly those who are pregnant or lactating, should not take the drug.

## Nursing Implications

### Preventing Interactions

Concurrent use of finasteride has led to few drug and herb interactions. Use of the drug with testosterone reduces the effects of both finasteride and testosterone. Anticholinergics may decrease the effects of finasteride. The herb saw palmetto may increase the effects of the drug.

### Administering the Medication

People may take finasteride once a day around the same time each day, without regard to food.

### ❗ QSEN Alert: Safety

Pregnant caregivers, nurses, or pharmacists should not handle the crushed drug, which can be absorbed and harmful to a male fetus.

### Assessing for Therapeutic Effects

The nurse assesses for improved urinary function with patient voiding in sufficient amounts with no palpable bladder distention. Patients should report less urinary frequency, hesitancy, urgency, dribbling, nocturia, and an improved force of the urinary stream.

### Assessing for Adverse Effects

The nurse should take a thorough sexual history in patients taking finasteride, including information regarding the presence of impotence, infertility, gynecomastia, reduced libido, and ejaculatory disorders, such as decreased volume of ejaculate. The effect of the drug on sexual dysfunction may be difficult to assess in older males who report these disorders with increasing age and other health conditions.

### Patient Teaching

Box 8.8 presents patient teaching guidelines for finasteride and other drugs used to treat BPH.

---

### BOX 8.8    *Patient Teaching Guidelines for Treatment of Benign Prostatic Hypertrophy*

**General Considerations**

- Take finasteride as prescribed, and note that maximum benefit from the medication is achieved in 6 to 12 months.
- Make sure to keep appointments for laboratory testing and follow-up care.
- Keep these medications in the original container, tightly closed, protected from light, and out of reach of children.
- Report a sulfa allergy before beginning tamsulosin therapy; a cross-allergic reaction has been reported.
- Seek medical care immediately if you are unable to void, if you pass bloody urine, or if you develop a fever.

**Self-Administration**

- Take oral preparations without regard to meals.
- Do not take other prescription or OTC medications without consulting your health care provider.

- Be careful when changing positions because dizziness may occur when standing up.
- If you are a woman of childbearing age and are sexually active, use a barrier contraceptive to prevent pregnancy.
- Take terazosin at bedtime to reduce the adverse effects.
- Note that a decrease in libido and volume of ejaculate may occur; this is usually reversible when the drug is stopped.
- If you are having surgery, including dental surgery, tell the surgeon or dentist that you are taking tamsulosin. If you need to have eye surgery at any time during or after your treatment, be sure to tell your surgeon that you are taking or have taken tamsulosin.
- Do not drive a car, operate machinery, or perform dangerous tasks until you know how tamsulosin affects you. This medication may make you drowsy or dizzy.

**QSEN Alert: Safety**

Pregnant women should not handle broken or crushed finasteride or dutasteride because the drugs could have negative effects on a male fetus.

 **QSEN Alert: Safety**

People taking a 5-alpha reductase inhibitor should avoid donating blood because the blood could be administered to a pregnant woman.

## Other Drugs in the Class

Dutasteride (Avodart) is the only other 5-alpha reductase inhibitor and has a stronger ability than finasteride to reduce the levels of DHT, causing the prostate to decrease in size. Symptoms may improve after 3 months of therapy. However, it may take 6 months or longer to determine the full benefit of the drug. Women who are pregnant or may become pregnant should not handle dutasteride capsules for fear of causing birth defects in male fetuses. A combination of the dutasteride and tamsulosin is available under the trade name of Jalyn. Women should not use Jalyn.

## ALPHA₁-ADRENERGIC BLOCKERS

The alpha₁-adrenergic blockers are recommended over the PDE5 inhibitors for initial monotherapy for the treatment of BPH. Alpha₁-adrenergic blockers provide immediate therapeutic benefits, while PDE5 inhibitors require long-term treatment (6–12 months) before symptom improvement.

Ⓟ **Tamsulosin** (Flomax) is the prototype of the anti-BPH drugs. Other drugs in the class are used to treat hypertension (see Chap. 26), nasal congestion (see Chap. 31), and ophthalmic hyperemia (see Chap. 59).

## Pharmacokinetics

Tamsulosin is well absorbed and is highly protein bound. The drug is extensively metabolized by the cytochrome P450 enzyme system, mainly by CYP3A4 and CYP2D6. It is excreted by the kidneys.

## Action

Tamsulosin works by relaxing the muscles in the prostate and bladder neck, enhancing the ability to urinate. Blockage of alpha₁-adrenergic receptors decreases vascular smooth muscle contraction, influencing the activity of genitourinary smooth muscle.

## Use

Prescribers order tamsulosin to improve urination and reduce complications in men with BPH. Table 8.5 contains route and dosage information for tamsulosin and other alpha₁-adrenergic receptor blockers used to treat BPH.

## Adverse Effects

Tamsulosin may cause adverse effects, including postural hypotension, weakness, sleepiness, difficulty falling or staying asleep, stuffy or runny nose, sore throat, and blurred vision. The drug may also lead to abnormal ejaculation due to inhibition of alpha₁ₐ-adrenergic receptors on the vas deferens.

## Contraindications

Contraindications to tamsulosin include a known hypersensitivity to the drug.

 **QSEN Alert: Safety**

Evidence shows that a complication during cataract surgery may occur in patients taking tamsulosin. This problem is associated with the drug's effect on alpha₁ blockade of the dilator muscle of the iris, limiting dilation of the eye. It is important that patients are instructed to inform health care providers of taking tamsulosin prior to eye surgery because specific surgical procedures can be used to minimize risk.

## Nursing Implications

### Preventing Interactions

The cytochrome P450 enzyme system is essential for the metabolism of many medications, including tamsulosin. Thus, the

 **TABLE 8.5**

**DRUGS AT A GLANCE: Alpha₁-Adrenergic Blockers**

| Drug | Pregnancy Category | Routes and Dosage Ranges [Adult Males] |
|---|---|---|
| Ⓟ **Tamsulosin** (Flomax; 🍁 APO-Tamsulosin CR, Flomax CR, Teva-Tamsulosin) | B | PO 0.4 mg 30 min after a meal to max of 0.8 mg/d |
| Alfuzosin (Uroxatral; 🍁 Apo-Alfuzosin, Sandoz-Alfuzosin, Teva-Alfuzosin PR, Xatral) | B | PO 10 mg/d to max of 10 mg/d |
| Doxazosin (Cardura; 🍁 Apo-Doxazosin, Cardura-1-4) Doxazosin XL (Cardura XL) | C | PO 1–8 mg/d to max of 8 mg/d PO extended release: 4–8 mg/d to max of 8 mg/d |
| Silodosin (Rapaflo; 🍁 Rapaflo) | B | PO 8 mg/d |
| Terazosin (🍁 Apo-Terazosin, Dom-Terazosin, Hytrin) | C | PO start with 1 mg at bedtime to 1–5 mg/d to max of 20 mg/d |

## BOX 8.9 *Drug Interactions: Tamsulosin*

**Drugs That Increase the Effects of Tamsulosin**
- Cimetidine
  *Decreases clearance*
- Other alpha blocker medications (e.g., alfuzosin, doxazosin, prazosin, terazosin); anticoagulants (e.g., warfarin); and phosphodiesterase type 5 inhibitors (e.g., avanafil, sildenafil, tadalafil, vardenafil)
  *Increase the risk of orthostatic hypotension*

risk for drug interactions exists with tamsulosin, increasing its effects (Box 8.9).

### Administering the Medication

Patients should take tamsulosin 30 minutes after eating at the same mealtime daily because fasting alters bioavailability and peak concentration. They should swallow capsules intact; it is essential not to open, crush, or chew the capsules.

### Assessing for Therapeutic Effects

The nurse assesses for improved urinary function demonstrated by decreased urinary frequency, hesitancy, urgency, dribbling, nocturia, and improved force of the urinary stream. The patient should report a decrease in the pain associated with BPH as tamsulosin relaxes the smooth muscle in the bladder neck and the prostate, decreasing the resistance to urinary flow.

### Assessing for Adverse Effects

The nurse assesses for orthostatic hypotension, difficulty with sleep, blurred vision, nasal congestion, sore throat, weakness, headache, sleepiness, difficulty falling or staying asleep, stuffy or runny nose, sore throat, and blurred vision.

### Patient Teaching

Box 8.8 contains patient education guidelines for tamsulosin and other drugs used to treat BPH.

## Other Drugs in the Class

Alfuzosin (Uroxatral) is classed as a nonreceptor subtype selective alpha$_1$-adrenergic blocker also used to treat BPH. The drug is able to be uroselective due to accumulation of drug in prostatic tissue. It has a strong safety profile and is well tolerated.

Doxazosin (Cardura) is effective and widely used as a treatment for symptoms associated with BPH. The drug has a rapid onset of action (1–2 weeks). Maximal plasma concentrations are achieved within 1 to 4 hours. With the longer 22-hour half-life of doxazosin, the drug can be taken in the morning or evening, with no difference in the incidence of adverse effects. However, it generally needs to be initiated at bedtime to reduce the postural lightheadedness experienced soon after starting the drug. Major adverse effects include hypotension, dizziness, headache, nasal congestion, and fatigue. Sexual dysfunction is not commonly associated with drug use.

Silodosin (Rapaflo), the newest selective alpha$_1$-adrenergic receptor blocker, produces similar short-term symptom reduction as other drugs in the class but causes greater risk of adverse effects, including sexual side effects (i.e., abnormal ejaculation). Patients should take the drug with meals.

Terazosin has an efficacy profile similar to doxazosin, as well as a similar adverse effect profile. The drug's main variation is a shorter 12-hour half-life, which may be attributed to the increased incidence of hypotension, headache, dizziness, nasal congestion, and fatigue if the drug is administered in the morning. Consequently, experts recommend that terazosin be given at bedtime.

The combination of a 5-alpha reductase inhibitor and an alpha$_1$-adrenergic blocker may be more effective in men with large prostates when monotherapy has been ineffective.

## NCLEX Success

5. In which of the following men would the use of sildenafil be contraindicated?
   A. 52-year-old with type 1 diabetes
   B. 58-year-old with unstable angina
   C. 69-year-old with asthma
   D. 74-year-old with cirrhosis

6. A 63-year-old man begins to take dutasteride for benign prostatic hypertrophy. He asks the nurse how long he will need to take the medication. The man needs to take drug for how long?
   A. for 2 years
   B. indefinitely
   C. for 2 weeks
   D. until his prostate is normal

7. Finasteride is most effective
   A. if started early in the development of prostatic hypertrophy
   B. for improvement of erectile dysfunction
   C. when prostatic hypertrophy is advanced
   D. to decrease the risk of prostate cancer

8. A 66-year-old man recently diagnosed with benign prostatic hypertrophy is started on tamsulosin 0.4 mg PO daily. Which of the following if stated by the patient indicates that patient teaching has been successful? (Select all that apply.)
   A. "I should swallow the capsule whole and not chew it."
   B. "The best time to take the medication is in the morning before breakfast."
   C. "This medication should make it easier for me to urinate and the dribbling of urine should improve."
   D. "I can take this medication even with my allergy to penicillin."
   E. "I should change positions slowly after taking tamsulosin as it could lower my blood pressure."

# THE NURSING PROCESS

A concept map outlines the nursing process related to drug therapy considerations in this chapter. Additional nursing implications related to the disease process should also be considered in care decisions.

### Assessment

- Periodic monitoring is needed throughout drug therapy.
  - Assess for conditions in which the drugs are used (e.g., deficiency states, erectile dysfunction [ED], benign prostatic hypertrophy [BPH]).
  - Assess attitude toward taking male sex hormones or drugs to improve sexual function or urinary flow.
  - Assess willingness to adhere to instructions for taking the drugs and follow-up procedures.
  - Assess for conditions that increase risks of adverse effects or are contraindications (e.g., pregnancy, renal or liver disease, concurrent drugs).
- With androgens, check laboratory reports of liver function tests, serum electrolyte levels, and serum lipid levels. Assess weight and blood pressure regularly. For children, check radiograph examination reports of bone growth status initially and approximately every 6 months while androgens are being taken.
- With ED, assess risk factors for the development of the condition and current drugs.
- With BPH, assess urinary function, urine stream caliber and force, any symptoms of urinary hesitancy, and difficulty starting urination.

### Outcomes of Therapy

The patient will
- Use the drugs only as directed.
- Avoid preventable adverse drug effects.
- Adhere to monitoring and follow-up procedures.
- Develop prevention and self-care measures to avoid ED (e.g., limitation or avoidance of alcohol and other drugs, smoking cessation, regular exercise and rest, stress reduction) or support interventions to decrease symptoms of BPH.
- Report healthy sexual functioning or improved urinary patterns of elimination based on cause of drug therapy.
- Avoid preventable complications with concomitant nitrate use in patients taking sildenafil.

### Nursing Interventions

- Assist patients to use the drugs correctly (see Boxes 8.3, 8.6, and 8.8). Consider psychological counseling and therapy, as indicated. Demonstrate problem-solving skills regarding solutions to problems that occur.
- With androgen use, assist patient to reduce sodium intake if edema develops and record weight and blood pressure at regular intervals. Participate in school or community programs to inform children, parents, coaches, athletic trainers, and others of the risks of inappropriate use of androgens, anabolic steroids, and related dietary supplements.
- With ED, consider lifestyle modification and review of medication profile.
- With BPH, report any changes of urinary function, urine stream caliber and force, any symptoms of urinary hesitancy, or difficulty starting urination.

### Evaluation

- Interview and observe for relief of symptoms and compliance with instructions for drugs prescribed.
- Interview and observe for adherence with instructions for taking prescribed drugs.
  Interview and observe for therapeutic and adverse drug effects.
- With androgen use, observe athletes and other males for increased weight and behavioral changes that may indicate drug abuse with androgens.
- With BPH, observe for adequate urinary elimination.

## KEY CONCEPTS

- The main functions of testosterone are related to the development of male sexual characteristics, reproduction, and metabolism.
- Androgens and anabolic steroids are used to enhance athletic performance and are termed ergogenic (causing an increase in muscular work capacity); they are widely abused in attempts to enhance muscle development, muscle strength, and athletic performance.
- Because of their abuse potential, androgens and anabolic steroids are classified as Schedule III controlled substances.
- Because androgens cause premature epiphyseal closure, boys with established deficiency states receiving androgens should undergo radiographic examination every 6 months to detect bone maturation and prevent loss of adult height.
- A **BLACK BOX WARNING** ◆ issued by the FDA states that danazol is contraindicated in pregnancy and that a

pregnancy test should be administered prior to the start of therapy. In addition, a nonhormonal method of contraception should be used during therapy. The warning also reports the risk of a thromboembolic event and/or intracranial hypertension is associated with the use of the drug.
- PDE5 inhibitors are successful in the treatment of ED.
- PDE5 inhibitors should not be prescribed for men who also take organic nitrates because the drug combination can cause severe hypotension resulting in dizziness, syncope, heart attack, or stroke.
- BPH is an enlargement of the prostate that occurs with increasing frequency with age.
- The combination of a 5-alpha reductase inhibitor and an alpha₁-adrenergic blocker is more effective in men with large prostates when monotherapy has been ineffective.

## CLINICAL REASONING CASE STUDY

**Meet the Patient**

George Thompson, a 63-year-old man, presents with complaints of urinary frequency, nocturia, a feeling of incomplete emptying, and significant difficulties initiating a urine stream. He visits the occupational health nurse where he works. The nurse refers him to a urologist. He receives a diagnosis of benign prostatic hypertrophy and urinary tract infection. His urologist prescribes tamsulosin (Flomax) 0.4 mg/day PO and trimethoprim–sulfamethoxazole (Bactrim DS) 1 tablet PO every 12 hours for 10 days. Following his visit to the urologist, he sees his occupational health nurse and receives patient teaching related to his new medications.

One week after beginning his therapy with tamsulosin and trimethoprim–sulfamethoxazole, Mr. Thompson has his annual appointment with his ophthalmologist. He is diagnosed with bilateral cataracts. His ophthalmologist reviews his medications prior to scheduling his cataract surgery.

- What is the nurse's responsibility regarding Mr. Thompson's use of these medications?
- What is the action of tamsulosin?
- What patient teaching should you provide to Mr. Thompson related to the administration of tamsulosin?
- Why is it important for all health care providers to review each patient's medications before enacting any changes in medical care?

**Assessing Drug Information**

- Tamsulosin (Flomax) is an alpha₁-adrenergic blocker that works by relaxing the muscles in the prostate and bladder neck, enhancing the ability to urinate.
- Sulfamethoxazole with trimethoprim is a broad spectrum anti-infective agent that is effective in treating complicated urinary tract infections. The combination of the two medications inhibits the enzyme to prevent the bacterial synthesis of essential nucleic acids and proteins.
- When caring for patients, each health care provider must review the patient's medical history and prescribed medications. Because Mr. Thompson is taking tamsulosin, he is at risk for floppy iris syndrome if the cataract surgery is performed. The ophthalmologist may discontinue the tamsulosin; additionally, alterations in the cataract surgery may be needed.

**Nursing Actions**

- When more than one prescriber is providing medical care to a patient, the nurse may be the one who identifies drug interactions. It is important for all health care providers to review the patient's medications to determine any drug to drug interactions.
- Instruct Mr. Thompson that the first dose of tamsulosin may cause orthostatic hypotension. He should take his first five doses at bedtime.
- Instruct Mr. Thompson to use caution when changing positions. He should go from lying to sitting then standing with a pause of a minute between position changes.
- When administering sulfamethoxazole–trimethoprim, Mr. Thompson should take it with a full glass of water.
- Mr. Thompson should maintain an adequate fluid intake of 1500 mL/day while taking sulfamethoxazole–trimethoprim.

*Visit* thePoint® *at* **http://thePoint.lww.com/Frandsen12e** *for answers to NCLEX Success questions (in Appendix A), answers to Clinical Application Case Studies (in Appendix B), and more!*

## REFERENCES AND RESOURCES

Doumas, M., Lazaridis, A. Katsiki, N., & Athyros, V. (2015). PDE-5 inhibitors: Clinical points. *Current Drug Targets, 16*(5), 420–426.

Guyton, A. C., & Hall, J. E. (2015). *Textbook of medical physiology* (13th ed.). Philadelphia, PA: Elsevier.

Hatzimouratidis, K., Salonia, A., Adaikan, G., Buvat, J., Carrier, S., El-Meliegy, A., et al. (2016). Pharmacotherapy for erectile dysfunction: Recommendations from the Fourth International Consultation for Sexual Medicine (ICSM 2015). *The Journal of Sexual Medicine, 13*(4), 465–488. doi:10.1016/j.jsxm.2016.01.016

Hinkle, J. H., & Cheever, K. H. (2017). *Brunner & Suddarth's textbook of medical-surgical nursing* (14th ed.). Philadelphia, PA: Lippincott Williams & Wilkins.

Jung, J. H., Kim, J., MacDonald, R., Reddy, B., Kim, M. H., & Dahm, P. (2017). Silodosin for the treatment of lower urinary tract symptoms in men with benign prostatic hyperplasia. *Cochrane Database of Systematic Reviews,* (11), CD012615. doi:10.1002/14651858. CD012615.pub2

Karch, A. (2017). *Focus on nursing pharmacology.* Philadelphia, PA: Lippincott Williams & Wilkins.

Kim, E. H., Larson, J. A., & Andriole, G. L. (2016). Management of benign prostatic hyperplasia. *Annual Review of Medicine, 67*(1), 137–151.

Lepor, H. (2016). Alpha-blockers for the treatment of benign prostatic hyperplasia. *Urologic Clinics, 43*(3), 311–323.

Matsui, H., Sopko, N. A., Hannan, J. L., & Bivalacqua, T. J. (2015). Pathophysiology of erectile dysfunction. *Current Drug Targets, 16*(5), 411–419.

Momaya, A., Fawal, M., & Estes, R. (2015). Performance-enhancing substances in sports: A review of the literature. *Sports Medicine, 45*(4), 517–531.

Norris, T. L. (2019). *Porth's Pathophysiology: Concepts of altered health status* (10th ed.). Philadelphia, PA: Lippincott Williams & Wilkins.

Verze, P., Margreiter, M., Esposito, K., Montorsi, P., & Mulhall, J. (2015). The link between cigarette smoking and erectile dysfunction: A systematic review. *European Urology Focus, 1*(1), 39–46.

Wortel, R.C., Ghidey Alemayehu, W., & Incrocci, L. (2015). Orchiectomy and radiotherapy for stage I-II testicular seminoma: A prospective evaluation of short-term effects on body image and sexual function. *Journal of Sexual Medicine 12*(1), 210–218.

Zhao, S., Wang, J., Gao R., & Yao, H. (2015). Erectile dysfunction and cardiovascular disease. *International Journal of Cardiology Metabolic & Endocrine, 9*, 10–11.

UpToDate. (2019). *Drug information.* Lexi-Comp, Inc.

# SECTION 3

# Drugs Affecting the Hematopoietic and Immune Systems

# Drug Therapy for Coagulation Disorders

## CLINICAL APPLICATION CASE STUDY

Andrew Oliver is a 45-year-old man who works as a mental health counselor. He presents to a small community emergency department with an acute anterior ST elevation myocardial infarction. Within 20 minutes of arrival, he receives alteplase by continuous intravenous (IV) infusion over 3 hours. He also simultaneously receives an IV bolus of heparin and is started on a heparin drip. You are the nurse assigned to his care.

## KEY TERMS

**Anticoagulants:** drugs that prevent formation of new clots and extension of clots already present; do not dissolve formed clots

**Antiplatelet drugs:** drugs that prevent one or more steps in the prothrombotic activity of platelets

**Embolus:** object that migrates through the circulation until it lodges in a blood vessel, causing occlusion; may be a thrombus, fat, air, amniotic fluid, a bit of tissue, or bacterial debris

**Essential thrombocythemia:** chronic blood disorder characterized by the overproduction of platelets by megakaryocytes in the absence of another cause

**Fibrinolysin:** enzyme that breaks down the fibrin meshwork that stabilizes blood clots; also referred to as plasmin

**Hemostasis:** prevention or stoppage of blood loss from an injured blood vessel and is the process that maintains the integrity of the vascular compartment

**Heparin-induced thrombocytopenia (HIT):** immune-mediated adverse effect that leads to thrombogenesis resulting in a decrease in platelet count associated with heparin administration in patients with detectable HIT antibodies

**Plasmin:** enzyme that breaks down the fibrin meshwork that stabilizes blood clots; also referred to as fibrinolysin

**Plasminogen:** inactive protein found in many body tissues and fluids

**Thrombogenesis:** formation of a blood clot

**Thrombolysis:** breakdown or dissolution of blood clots

**Thrombolytics:** drugs that dissolve blood clots

**Thrombosis:** formation of a blood clot

**Thrombus:** blood clot

## INTRODUCTION

Anticoagulant, antiplatelet, and thrombolytic drugs are used in the prevention and management of thrombotic and thromboembolic disorders. **Thrombogenesis** (or **thrombosis**), the formation of blood clots, is a normal body defense mechanism to prevent blood loss. Thus, this process may be lifesaving when it occurs as a response to hemorrhage; however, it may be life threatening when it occurs at other times, because the **thrombus**, or blood clot, can obstruct a blood vessel and block blood flow to tissues beyond the clot either at the site of clot formation or to another part of the body. To aid understanding of drug therapy for thrombotic disorders, normal hemostasis, endothelial functions in relation to blood clotting, platelet functions, blood coagulation, and characteristics of arterial and venous thrombosis are described.

## OVERVIEW OF COAGULATION DISORDERS

### Physiology

#### Hemostasis

**Hemostasis** is the process that maintains the integrity of the vascular compartment. It involves activation of several mechanisms, including vasoconstriction, formation of a platelet plug (a cluster of aggregated platelets), sequential activation of clotting factors in the blood (Fig. 9.1), and growth of fibrous tissue (fibrin) into the blood clot to make it more stable and to repair the tear (opening) in the damaged blood vessel. Overall, normal hemostasis is a complex process involving numerous interacting activators and inhibitors, including endothelial factors, platelets, and blood coagulation factors (Box 9.1).

#### Clot Lysis

When a blood clot is being formed, **plasminogen**, an inactive protein present in many body tissues and fluids, is bound to fibrin and becomes a component of the clot. After the outward

blood flow is stopped and the tear in the blood vessel is repaired, plasminogen is activated by plasminogen activator (produced by endothelial cells or the coagulation cascade) to produce plasmin. **Plasmin** (also called **fibrinolysin**) is an enzyme that breaks down the fibrin meshwork that stabilizes the clot; this fibrinolytic or thrombolytic action dissolves the clot.

### Etiology

Normally, thrombi are constantly being formed and dissolved, but the blood remains fluid and flow is not significantly obstructed. If the balance between thrombogenesis and **thrombolysis**, dissolution of blood clots, is upset, thrombotic or bleeding disorders ensue. Thrombosis may occur in both arteries and veins. Arterial thrombosis is usually associated with atherosclerotic plaque, hypertension, and turbulent blood flow. These conditions damage arterial endothelium and activate platelets to initiate the coagulation process. Arterial thrombi cause disease by obstructing blood flow. If the obstruction is incomplete or temporary, local tissue ischemia (deficient blood supply) occurs. If the obstruction is complete or prolonged, local tissue death (infarction) occurs.

Venous thrombosis is usually associated with venous stasis. When blood flows slowly, thrombin and other procoagulant substances present in the blood become concentrated in local areas and initiate the clotting process. With a normal rate of blood flow, these substances are rapidly removed from the blood, primarily by Kupffer's cells in the liver. A venous thrombus is less cohesive than an arterial thrombus, and an **embolus** can easily become detached and travel to other parts of the body. This embolus may be a thrombus, fat, air, amniotic fluid, tissue, or bacterial debris.

Venous thrombi cause disease by two mechanisms. First, thrombosis causes local congestion, edema, and perhaps inflammation by impairing normal outflow of venous blood (e.g., thrombophlebitis, deep vein thrombosis [DVT]). Second, embolization obstructs the blood supply when the embolus becomes lodged. The pulmonary arteries are common sites of embolization.

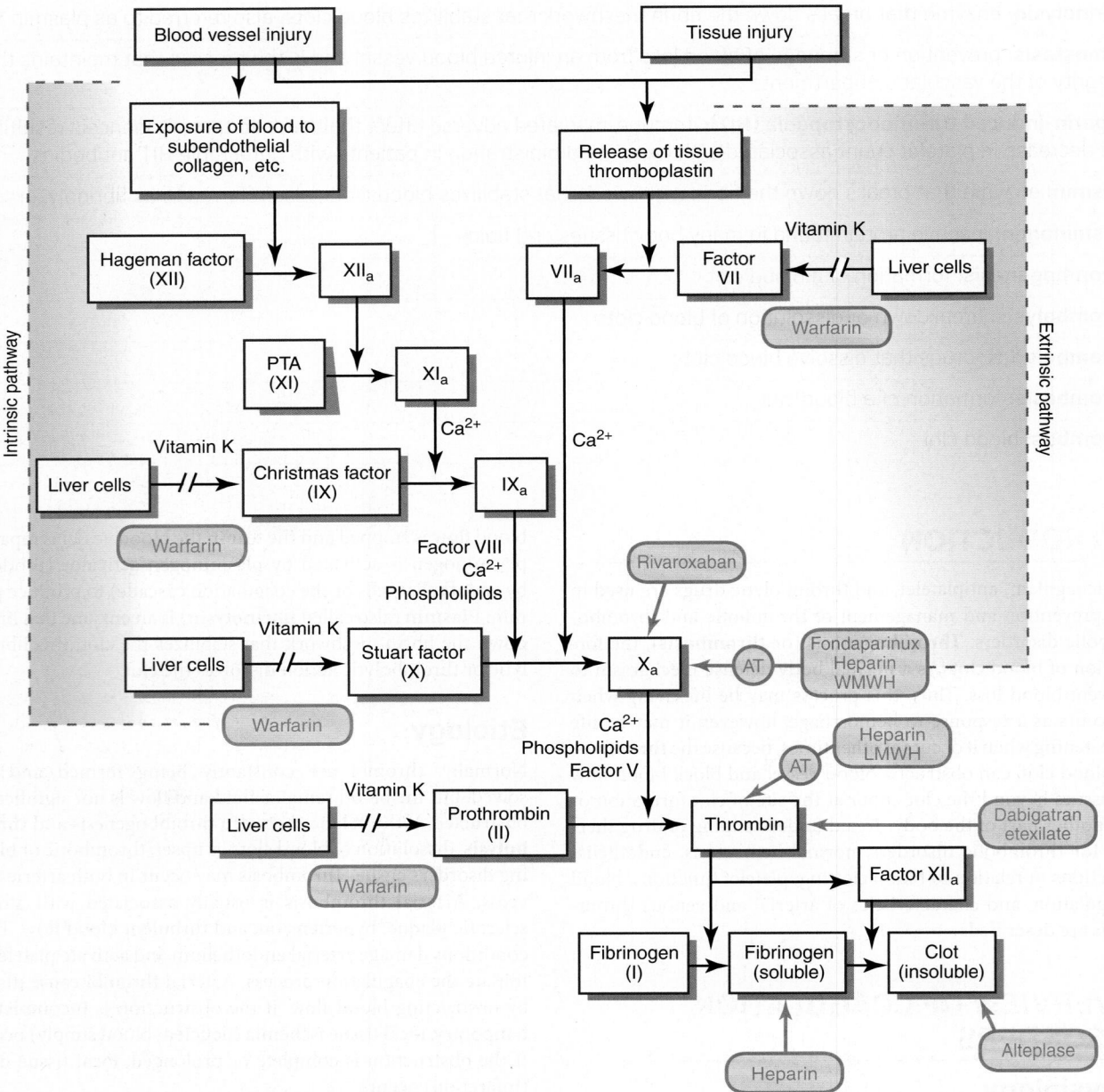

**Figure 9.1.** Details of the intrinsic and extrinsic clotting pathways. The sites of action of some of the drugs that can influence these processes are shown in *red*.

## Pathophysiology

Atherosclerosis is the basic disease process that often leads to pathologic thrombosis. Atherosclerosis begins with accumulation of lipid-filled macrophages (i.e., foam cells) on the inner lining of arteries. Foam cells develop in response to elevated blood lipid levels and eventually become fibrous plaques (i.e., foam cells covered by smooth muscle cells and connective tissue). Advanced atherosclerotic lesions also contain hemorrhages, ulcerations, and scar tissue.

Atherosclerosis can affect any organ or tissue but often involves the arteries supplying the heart, brain, and legs. Over time, plaque lesions become larger and extend farther into the lumen of

the artery. Eventually, a thrombus may develop at plaque sites and partially or completely occlude an artery. In coronary arteries, a thrombus may precipitate myocardial ischemia (angina or infarction) (see Chap. 28); in carotid or cerebral arteries, a thrombus may precipitate a stroke; in peripheral arteries, a thrombus may cause intermittent claudication (pain in the legs with exercise) or acute occlusion. Thus, serious impairment of blood flow may occur with a large atherosclerotic plaque or a relatively small plaque with superimposed vasospasm and thrombosis. Consequences and clinical manifestations of thrombi and emboli depend primarily on their location and size.

Thrombotic disorders occur much more often than bleeding disorders and are emphasized in this chapter. Bleeding

The blood vessels and blood normally maintain a balance between procoagulant and anticoagulant factors that favors anticoagulation and keeps the blood fluid. Injury to blood vessels and tissues causes complex reactions and interactions among vascular endothelial cells, platelets, and blood coagulation factors that shift the balance toward procoagulation and thrombosis.

### Endothelial Cells

Normal endothelium helps to prevent thrombosis by producing anticoagulant factors, inhibiting platelet reactivity, and inhibiting activation of the coagulation cascade. However, endothelium promotes thrombosis if the blood vessel wall is damaged, if function is altered, or when blood flow is altered or becomes static. After a blood clot is formed, the endothelium also induces its dissolution and restoration of blood flow.

### Platelets

The only known function of platelets is hemostasis. Platelets (also called thrombocytes) are produced in the bone marrow and released into the bloodstream, where they circulate for approximately 7 to 10 days before they are removed by the spleen. They contain no nuclei and therefore cannot repair or replicate themselves.

The cell membrane of a platelet contains a coat of glycoproteins that prevents the platelet from adhering to normal endothelium but allows it to adhere to damaged areas of endothelium and collagen in the blood vessel wall. Breakdown of the cell membrane releases arachidonic acid (which can be metabolized to produce thromboxane $A_2$) and allows leakage of platelet contents (e.g., thromboplastin and other clotting factors), which function to stop bleeding.

When platelets come in contact with a damaged vascular surface, they become activated and aggregate at a site of injury to help plug a hole in a torn blood vessel. Aggregated platelets release substances that recruit new platelets and stimulate additional aggregation. This activity helps the platelet plug become large enough to block blood flow out of a damaged blood vessel. If the opening is small, the platelet plug can stop blood loss. If the opening is large, a platelet plug and a blood clot are both required to stop the bleeding. Platelets usually disappear from a blood clot within 24 hours and are replaced by fibrin.

### Blood Coagulation

The blood coagulation process represented in Figure 9.1 normally causes hemostasis within 1 to 2 minutes. It involves sequential activation of clotting factors that are normally present in blood and tissues as inactive precursors and formation of a meshwork of fibrin strands that cements blood components together to form a stable, dense clot. Major phases include release of thromboplastin by disintegrating platelets and damaged tissue; conversion of prothrombin to thrombin, which requires thromboplastin and calcium ions; and conversion of fibrinogen to fibrin by thrombin.

Blood coagulation results from activation of the intrinsic or extrinsic coagulation pathway. Both pathways, which are activated when blood passes out of a blood vessel, are needed for normal hemostasis. The intrinsic pathway occurs in the vascular system; the extrinsic pathway occurs in the tissues. Although the pathways are initially separate, the terminal steps (i.e., activation of factor X and thrombin-induced formation of fibrin) are the same leading to the formation of thrombin, which then activates fibrinogen to form fibrin, and the clot is complete.

---

disorders may result from excessive amounts of drugs that inhibit clotting.

## Clinical Manifestations

Clinical manifestations of thrombosis vary depending on the size and location (arterial or venous system) of the thrombus. Symptoms are the result of decreased perfusion to an area due to the restriction or cessation of blood flow. Arterial blood clots in the cerebral, pulmonary, or cardiac system can produce a cerebrovascular accident, pulmonary embolism, or myocardial infarction, respectively. Venous blood clots may lead to DVT; classic symptoms include leg swelling and pain on palpation in the calf or thigh. However, half of all affected patients do not have any symptoms of DVT.

## Drug Therapy

Drugs given to prevent or treat thrombosis alter some aspect of the blood coagulation process (Table 9.1; see Fig. 9.1). Anticoagulant drugs, which prevent formation of new clots and extension of already existing clots, do not dissolve clots that have already formed. Widely used in thrombotic disorders, they are more effective in preventing venous thrombosis than arterial thrombosis. Antiplatelet drugs are used to prevent arterial thrombosis. Thrombolytic drugs are used to dissolve thrombi and limit tissue damage in selected thromboembolic disorders.

### ⚠ QSEN Alert: Teamwork and Collaboration

Both the American College of Cardiology and the American Heart Association recommend that hospitals establish multidisciplinary teams to develop institution-specific written protocols, based on established clinical practice guidelines, for the triage and management of patients who present with symptoms indicative of acute myocardial ischemia. Additionally, a team-based approach to patient assessment and preliminary management helps to ensure that a patient receives essential care within the ideal 10 minutes after presentation of first medical contact.

## ANTICOAGULANT DRUGS

There are four types of **anticoagulants**: heparins, vitamin K antagonists, direct thrombin inhibitors (DTIs), and direct factor Xa inhibitors.

## HEPARINS

 **Heparin** is a pharmaceutical preparation of the natural anticoagulant produced primarily by mast cells in pericapillary connective tissue, and it is the prototype anticoagulant. Endogenous heparin is found in various body tissues, most abundantly in the liver and lungs. Exogenous heparin is obtained from bovine lung or porcine intestinal mucosa and standardized in units of

## TABLE 9.1

## Drugs Administered for the Treatment of Coagulation Disorders

| Drug Class | Prototype(s) | Other Drugs in the Class |
|---|---|---|
| **Anticoagulant Drugs** | | |
| Heparins | Heparin | Dalteparin<br>Enoxaparin |
| Other anticoagulant drugs | | Fondaparinux |
| Vitamin K antagonists | Warfarin | |
| Direct thrombin inhibitors | Dabigatran etexilate | Argatroban<br>Bivalirudin<br>Desirudin |
| Direct factor Xa inhibitors | Rivaroxaban | Apixaban<br>Edoxaban |
| **Antiplatelet Drugs** | | |
| Adenosine diphosphate receptor antagonists | Clopidogrel | Prasugrel<br>Tirofiban<br>Cangrelor |
| Other antiplatelet drugs | | Abciximab<br>Anagrelide<br>Aspirin<br>Cilostazol<br>Dipyridamole<br>Eptifibatide<br>Vorapaxar |
| Thrombolytic drugs | Alteplase | Tenecteplase |
| Drugs used to control bleeding | | Aminocaproic acid<br>Idarucizumab<br>Protamine sulfate<br>Tranexamic acid<br>Vitamin K |

biologic activity. See later for a discussion of low-molecular-weight heparins (LMWHs).

## Pharmacokinetics

It is necessary to give heparin intravenously or subcutaneously, because the gastrointestinal (GI) tract does not absorb the drug. After IV injection, the drug acts immediately. After subcutaneous injection, heparin acts within 20 to 30 minutes. Metabolism takes place in the liver and the reticuloendothelial system. Excretion, primarily in the form of inactive metabolites, occurs in the urine. Hemodialysis does not remove it.

## Action

Heparin combines with antithrombin III (a natural anticoagulant in the blood) to inactivate clotting factors IX, X, XI, and XII; inhibit the conversion of prothrombin to thrombin; and prevent thrombus formation (see Fig. 9.1). After thrombosis has developed, heparin can inhibit additional coagulation by inactivating thrombin, preventing the conversion of fibrinogen to fibrin, and

inhibiting factor XIII (fibrin-stabilizing factor). Other effects include inhibition of factors V and VIII and platelet aggregation.

## Use

Prophylactically, patients at risk for certain disorders take low doses of heparin prophylactically to prevent DVT and pulmonary embolism. These disorders include the following:

- Major illnesses (e.g., acute myocardial infarction, heart failure, serious pulmonary infections, stroke)
- Major abdominal or thoracic surgery
- A history of thrombophlebitis or pulmonary embolism, including pregnant women
- Gynecologic surgery, especially in patients who have been taking estrogens or oral contraceptives or have other risk factors for DVT
- Restrictions such as bed rest or limited activity expected to last longer than 5 days

Therapeutically, patients receive heparin for management of acute thromboembolic disorders (e.g., DVT, thrombophlebitis, pulmonary embolism). In these conditions, the aim of therapy is to prevent further thrombus formation and embolization. Another use is in disseminated intravascular coagulation (DIC), a life-threatening condition characterized by widespread clotting, which depletes the blood of coagulation factors. The depletion of coagulation factors then produces widespread bleeding. The goal of heparin therapy in DIC is to prevent blood coagulation long enough for clotting factors to be replenished and thus be able to control hemorrhage. In addition, clinicians use heparin to prevent clotting during cardiac and vascular surgery, extracorporeal circulation, hemodialysis, and blood transfusions and in blood samples to be used in laboratory tests. Heparin does not cross the placental barrier and is not secreted in breast milk, making it the anticoagulant of choice for use during pregnancy and lactation.

Table 9.2 presents the dosage information for the heparins.

### Use in Children

Limited information about the use of anticoagulants in children is available. When children take heparin for systemic anticoagulation, weight is the basis for determination of dosage (~50 units/kg). It is essential to use extreme caution to ensure that the vial concentration of heparin is correct. Fatalities in infants involving heparin overdoses have occurred. In addition, premature infants should not take heparin solutions containing benzyl alcohol as a preservative; fatal reactions have resulted.

 **QSEN Alert: Technology**

Several major adverse events have resulted from the use of heparin, and it is classified as a high-alert drug. Nurses demonstrate consistent practice in administrating heparin by their heightened individual awareness of the risks and by advocating for systems to account for human error such as bar coding and "smart" pumps. Effective standardized practices to support safety and quality include special safeguards to reduce the risk of errors that may harm the patient.

### Use in Older Adults

Older adults often have atherosclerosis and thrombotic disorders, including myocardial infarction, thrombotic stroke, and peripheral

**TABLE 9.2**

## DRUGS AT A GLANCE: Anticoagulants

| Drug | Pregnancy Category | Indications for Use | Routes and Dosage Ranges (Adults, Unless Specified) |
|---|---|---|---|
| **Heparins** | | | |
| Ⓟ **Heparin** | C | Prevention and management of thromboembolic disorders (e.g., DVT, pulmonary embolism, atrial fibrillation with embolization) | Adults: IV injection, 5000 units initially, followed by 5000–10,000 units every 4–6 h, to a maximum dose of 25,000 units/d; IV infusion, 5000 units (loading dose), then 15–25 units/kg/h<br>DIC, IV injection, 50–100 units/kg every 4 h; IV infusion, 20,000–40,000 units/d at initial rate of 0.25 units/kg/min, then adjusted according to aPTT; Sub-Q 10,000–12,000 units every 8 h, or 14,000–20,000 units every 12 h<br>Low-dose prophylaxis, Sub-Q 5000 units 2 h before surgery, then every 12 h until discharged from hospital or fully ambulatory<br>Children: DIC, IV injection, 25–50 units/kg every 4 h; IV infusion, 50 units/kg initially, followed by 100 units/kg every 4 h or 20,000 units/m² over 24 h |
| Dalteparin (Fragmin; 🍁 Fragmin) | B | Prophylaxis of DVT in patients having abdominal or hip replacement surgery | Abdominal surgery, Sub-Q 2500 IU 1–2 h before surgery and then once daily for 5–10 d after surgery<br>Hip replacement surgery (3 options), Sub-Q 2500 IU within 2 h before surgery and the evening of surgery (4–8 h after surgery) and then 5000 IU once daily for 5–10 d; Sub-Q 2500 IU 4–8 h after surgery and then 5000 IU at least 6 h after postsurgical dose once daily for 5–10 d; Sub-Q 2500 IU within 2 h before surgery then Sub-Q 2500 IU 4–8 h after surgery and then 5000 IU once daily for 5–10 d |
| Enoxaparin (Lovenox; 🍁 Lovenox, Lovenox HP, Lovenox with Preservative) | B | Prevention and management of DVT and PE<br>Management of unstable angina, to prevent or treat myocardial infarction | DVT prophylaxis in patients having hip or knee replacement surgery, Sub-Q 30 mg twice daily, with first dose within 12–24 h after surgery and continued until risk of DVT diminished or until adequately anticoagulated on warfarin<br>Abdominal surgery, Sub-Q 40 mg once daily with first dose given 2 h before surgery, for 7–10 d<br>DVT/PE management, outpatients, Sub-Q 1 mg/kg every 12 h; inpatients, 1 mg/kg every 12 h or 1.5 mg/kg every 24 h<br>Moderate to high risk of thromboembolic disorders, Sub-Q 40 mg once daily; continue for length of hospital stay or until patient is fully ambulatory and risk of VTE has diminished<br>Non–ST elevation acute coronary syndromes, 1 mg/kg every 12 h in conjunction with recommended antiplatelet (i.e., PO aspirin 100–325 mg once daily) ST elevation myocardial infarction between 15 min before or 30 min after fibrinolytic therapy, <75 y single IV bolus of 30 mg plus 1 mg/kg Sub-Q every 12 h with first Sub-Q dose given with IV bolus (max dose 100 mg for first 2 doses only); ≥75 y no IV bolus, Sub-Q 0.75 mg/kg every 12 h (maximum 75 mg for first 2 doses only) |
| Fondaparinux (Arixtra; 🍁 Arixtra) | B | Prevention of DVT following hip fracture surgery or knee or hip replacement<br>Treatment of acute DVT or PE | Sub-Q 2.5 mg daily, with first dose 6–8 h after surgery and continuing for 5–9 d<br><50 kg, sub-Q 5 mg once daily<br>50–100 kg, sub-Q 7.5 mg once daily<br>>100 kg, sub-Q 10 mg once daily |

(*Continued on page 156*)

**TABLE 9.2**

## DRUGS AT A GLANCE: Anticoagulants (Continued)

| Drug | Pregnancy Category | Indications for Use | Routes and Dosage Ranges (Adults, Unless Specified) |
|---|---|---|---|
| **Vitamin K Antagonist** | | | |
| Ⓟ **Warfarin** (Coumadin, Jantoven; ❁ Apo-Warfarin, Coumadin, Taro-Warfarin) | D | Long-term prevention or management of venous thromboembolic disorders, including DVT, PE, and embolization associated with atrial fibrillation and prosthetic heart valves. May also be used after myocardial infarction to decrease reinfarction, stroke, venous thromboembolism, and death | PO 2–5 mg/d for 2–3 d, then adjusted according to the INR; average maintenance daily dose, 2–5 mg |
| **Direct Thrombin Inhibitors** | | | |
| Ⓟ **Dabigatran etexilate** (Pradaxa; ❁ Pradaxa) | C | Decrease the risk of stroke and systemic embolism with nonvalvular atrial fibrillation | PO 150 mg twice daily; in severe renal failure 75 mg twice daily |
| Argatroban (Argatroban) | B | Thrombosis prophylaxis or management in heparin-induced thrombocytopenia; adjunct to PTCA | IV continuous infusion 2 mcg/kg/min |
| Bivalirudin (Angiomax; ❁ Angiomax) | B | Patients with unstable angina undergoing PTCA; acute coronary syndrome; used concomitantly with aspirin therapy | IV bolus dose of 0.75 mg/kg followed by 4-h infusion at rate of 1.75 mg/kg/min |
| Desirudin (Iprivask) | C | Prophylaxis of DVT in patients having hip replacement surgery | Sub-Q, 15 mg every 12 h; first dose should be given 5–15 min before surgery and may be administered for up to 12 d postsurgery |
| **Direct Factor Xa Inhibitors** | | | |
| Ⓟ **Rivaroxaban** (Xarelto; ❁ Xarelto) | C | Prophylaxis of DVT, which may lead to PE in patients having knee or hip replacement surgery<br>Treatment and secondary prevention of DVT<br>Stroke prevention in nonvalvular atrial fibrillation | PO 10 mg once daily; may be administered for up to 12 d postsurgery for knee replacement and 35 d postsurgery for hip replacement<br>PO 15 mg twice daily with food for 21 d; followed by 20 mg once daily with food<br>PO 20 mg once daily with evening meal with creatinine clearance >50 mL/min or 15 mg once daily with evening meal with creatinine clearance 15–50 mL/min |
| Apixaban (Eliquis; ❁ Eliquis) | B | Prophylaxis of DVT in patients having hip or knee replacement surgery<br>Stroke prevention with atrial fibrillation<br>Treatment of DVT and/or PE | PO 2.5 mg twice daily for 35 d with hip replacement; for 12 d for knee replacement.<br>5 mg twice daily or 2.5 mg twice daily with any two ≥80 y, body weight ≤60 kg, or serum creatinine ≥1.5 mg/dL<br>DVT and PE treatment: PO 10 mg twice daily for 7 d; followed by 5 mg twice daily |
| Edoxaban (Savaysa; ❁ Lixiana) | C | Prevention of venous thromboembolic disease and stroke prevention in patients with nonvalvular atrial fibrillation<br>Treatment of DVT and/or PE | Prevention: PO 60 mg d<br>Treatment: after 5 d of parenteral anticoagulant in hemodynamically stable patients:<br>≤60 kg, PO 30 mg once daily<br>>60 kg, PO 60 mg once daily |

aPTT, activated partial thromboplastin time; DIC, disseminated intravascular coagulation; DVT, deep vein thrombosis; INR, international normalized ratio; PE, pulmonary embolism; PTCA, percutaneous transluminal coronary angioplasty or atherectomy; sec, seconds.

arterial insufficiency, for which they receive an anticoagulant drug. They are more likely than younger adults to experience bleeding and other complications associated with this therapy. With standard heparin, general principles for safe and effective use apply. With LMWHs, elimination may be delayed in older adults with renal impairment, and the drugs should be used cautiously.

### Use in Patients With Renal Impairment

People with renal impairment may take heparin in usual dosages. However, the half-life of the drug may increase.

### Use in Patients With Hepatic Impairment

Likewise, people with hepatic impairment may take heparin in usual dosages. However, the half-life of the drug may increase or decrease.

### Use in Patients With Critical Illness

Heparin is often used in patients who are critically ill. However, the risk of bleeding is increased in the presence of other coexisting conditions. People who are critically ill have a high risk of DVT and pulmonary embolism, as well as a higher morbidity and mortality, including an increase in length of hospital stay, the need and duration of mechanical ventilation, and death. Effective prevention and treatment of thrombosis is necessary and typically includes LMWHs. In addition, it is essential to consider intermittent pneumatic compression devices and other measures to prevent DVT or pulmonary embolism.

### Use in Patients Receiving Home Care

Patients may take standard heparin at home using the subcutaneous route, and use of LMWHs for home management of venous thrombosis has become standard practice. Daily visits by a home care nurse may be necessary if the patient or a family member is unable or unwilling to inject the medication. It is essential to take platelet counts before therapy begins and every 2 to 3 days during heparin therapy. If the platelet count falls below 100,000 platelets per microliter of blood or to less than half the baseline value, it is necessary to discontinue the heparin.

## Adverse Effects

Hemorrhage is the major side effect of heparin therapy, hypersensitivity to the drug has occurred, and local irritation with subcutaneous injections of heparin can cause erythema and mild pain. **Heparin-induced thrombocytopenia (HIT)** (type II) is a potentially life-threatening complication of heparin administration, leading to a decrease in platelet count and detectable HIT antibodies. This condition occurs in 1% to 3% of people receiving heparin at therapeutic levels for 4 to 14 days, sometimes sooner in those who have previously received heparin. HIT is one of the most common immune-mediated adverse drug reactions. All patients exposed to any heparin at therapeutic or prophylactic doses or minute amounts in heparin flushes or on heparin-coated catheters, as well as those receiving LMWH, are at risk. If HIT occurs, it is necessary to discontinue all heparin and manage anticoagulation with a DTI such as argatroban.

## Contraindications

Contraindications include GI ulcerations (e.g., peptic ulcer disease, ulcerative colitis), intracranial bleeding, dissecting aortic

**BOX 9.2    Drug Interactions: Heparin**

**Drugs That Increase the Effects of Heparin**

- Alteplase, direct thrombin inhibitors, platelet inhibitors
  *Increase the risk of bleeding*
- Antithrombin
  *Increases pharmacologic effects*
- Cephalosporins
  *Lead to potential coagulopathies and risk of bleeding*
- Penicillins (parenteral)
  *Lead to altered platelet aggregation and increased risk of bleeding*
- Warfarin
  *May prolong and possibly invalidate the PT; if receiving both heparin and warfarin, draw blood for the PT at least 5 hours after the last IV heparin dose*

**Drugs That Decrease the Effects of Heparin**

- Antihistamines, digoxin, nicotine, nitroglycerin (IV), tetracycline
  *Decrease the anticoagulant effect*

IV, intravenous; PT, prothrombin time.

aneurysm, blood dyscrasias, severe kidney or liver disease, severe hypertension, polycythemia vera, and recent surgery of the eye, spinal cord, or brain. Caution is necessary in patients with hypertension, renal or hepatic disease, alcoholism, history of GI ulcerations, drainage tubes (e.g., nasogastric tubes, indwelling urinary catheters), threatened abortion, endocarditis, and any occupation with high risks of traumatic injury.

## Nursing Implications

### Preventing Interactions

Many medications interact with heparin, increasing or decreasing its effect (Box 9.2). Some herbs and foods increase the effects of the drug (Box 9.3). No herbs or foods that decrease the effects of heparin have been identified.

### Administering the Medication

Traditional anticoagulants have two major limitations: a narrow therapeutic window of adequate anticoagulation without bleeding and a highly variable individual dose–response that requires monitoring by laboratory testing. Prescribers use the activated partial thromboplastin time (aPTT), which is sensitive to changes in blood clotting factors, except factor VII, to regulate heparin dosage. Thus, normal or control values of aPTT indicate normal blood coagulation, and therapeutic values of adequate anticoagulation indicate low levels of clotting factors and delayed blood coagulation. During heparin therapy, the aPTT should be maintained at

**BOX 9.3    Herb and Dietary Interactions: Heparin**

**Herbs and Foods That Increase the Effects of Heparin**

- Chamomile, garlic, ginger, ginkgo, ginseng, high-dose vitamin E approximately 1.5 to 2.5 times the control or baseline value. The normal control value is 25 to 35 seconds; therefore, therapeutic values of adequate anticoagulation are 45 to 70 seconds, approximately. With continuous IV infusion, blood for the aPTT may be drawn at any time; with intermittent administration, blood for the aPTT should be drawn approximately 1 hour before a dose of heparin is scheduled. It is not necessary to monitor aPTT with low-dose standard heparin given subcutaneously for prophylaxis of thromboembolism or with the LMWHs (e.g., enoxaparin).

The nurse should be aware that heparin has disadvantages: parenteral injection is necessary, and the drug has a short duration of action, which means that there is a need for frequent administration.

### Assessing for Therapeutic Effects

The nurse assesses for the absence or reduction of signs and symptoms of thrombotic disorders (e.g., less edema and pain with DVT, less chest pain and respiratory difficulty with pulmonary embolism, absence of uncontrolled bleeding). It is also necessary to ensure that aPTT values are within the therapeutic range.

### Assessing for Adverse Effects

The nurse assesses the patient for signs of overt bleeding or HIT. Protamine sulfate, which is discussed in more detail later in the chapter, is an antidote for standard heparin and LMWHs. Protamine is typically given for bleeding that may not respond to merely withdrawing the heparin or when hemorrhaging is present.

### Patient Teaching

Education related to bleeding risk is essential for patients receiving heparin. The nurse reinforces instructions for safe use of the drug and related anticoagulants, reminding patients to obtain laboratory tests, and teaching how to observe for signs and symptoms of bleeding. Additional patient teaching guidelines for anticoagulants, including heparins, are outlined in Box 9.4.

---

**BOX 9.4**  *Patient Teaching Guidelines for Anticoagulants*

**General Considerations**

- Anticoagulant drugs are given to people who have had, or who are at risk of having, a heart attack, stroke, or other problems from blood clots. For home management of deep vein thrombosis, which usually occurs in the legs, you are likely to be given heparin injections for a few days, followed by warfarin for long-term therapy. These medications help prevent the blood clot from getting larger, traveling to your lungs, or recurring later.

- All anticoagulants can increase the risk of bleeding, so you need to take safety precautions to prevent injury.

- To help prevent blood clots from forming and decreasing blood flow through your arteries, you need to reduce risk factors that contribute to cardiovascular disease. This can be done by a low-fat, low-cholesterol diet (and medication if needed) to lower total cholesterol to below 200 mg/dL and low-density lipoprotein cholesterol to below 130 mg/dL; weight reduction if overweight; control of blood pressure if hypertensive; avoidance of smoking; stress reduction techniques; and regular exercise.

- To help maintain a steady level of anticoagulation with warfarin, do not change your intake of foods that are high in vitamin K, which decreases the effects of warfarin. These foods include broccoli, brussels sprouts, cabbage, cauliflower, chives, collard greens, kale, lettuce, mustard greens, peppers, spinach, tomatoes, turnips, and watercress.

- To help prevent blood clots from forming in your leg veins, avoid or minimize situations that slow blood circulation, such as wearing tight clothing, crossing the legs at the knees, prolonged sitting or standing, and bed rest. For example, on automobile trips, stop and walk around every 1 to 2 hours; on long plane trips, exercise your feet and legs at your seat and walk around when you can.

- Following instructions regarding these medications is extremely important. Too little medication increases your risk of problems from blood clot formation; too much medication can cause bleeding.

- While taking any of these medications, you need regular medical supervision and periodic blood tests. The blood

tests can help your health care provider regulate drug dosage and maintain your safety.

- Notify your health care provider if you suddenly stop tobacco smoking, because this may result in a reduced clearance of warfarin. A dosage change may be necessary.

- With enoxaparin, you need an injection, usually every 12 hours. You or someone close to you may be instructed in injecting the medication, or a visiting nurse may do the injections, if necessary.

- You need to take the drugs as directed. Avoid taking other drugs without the health care provider's knowledge and consent, inform any health care provider (including dentists) that you are taking an anticoagulant drug before any invasive diagnostic tests or treatments are begun, and keep all appointments for continuing care.

- With warfarin therapy, you need to avoid walking barefoot; avoid contact sports; use an electric razor; avoid injections when possible; and carry an identification card, necklace, or bracelet (e.g., MedicAlert) stating the name of the drug and the health care provider's name and telephone number.

- A routine blood test is necessary to ensure that your warfarin dose is appropriate. The results of this test determine your daily dose of warfarin. Once the warfarin dose stabilizes, the blood tests are done less often (e.g., every 2 weeks).

- Report any sign of bleeding (e.g., excessive bruising of the skin, blood in urine or stool). If superficial bleeding occurs, apply direct pressure to the site for 3 to 5 minutes or longer if necessary.

**Self-Administration**

- With enoxaparin, wash hands and cleanse the skin to prevent infection; inject deep under the skin, around the navel, upper thigh, or buttocks; and change the injection site daily. If excessive bruising occurs at the injection site, rubbing an ice cube over an area before the injection may be helpful.

- With warfarin as with all medications, take as prescribed. Because the prescriber may set a dosing schedule that could vary from one day to the next, do not rely on memory but keep a written record of the date and the amount of medication taken.

## Other Drugs in the Class

LMWHs are synthetic heparins, have smaller molecular structures, and efficiently inactivate factor Xa via antithrombin. The drugs are as effective as IV heparin in treating thrombotic disorders and provide a more predictable anticoagulant response at recommended doses. The drugs do not cross the placenta. Indications for their use include prevention or management of thromboembolic complications associated with surgery or ischemic complications of unstable angina and myocardial infarction. The currently available LMWHs, dalteparin (Fragmin) and enoxaparin (Lovenox), differ from standard heparin and each other and are not interchangeable.

LMWHs are typically given subcutaneously in fixed or weight-based dosing without monitoring of blood coagulation. These characteristics simplify outpatient anticoagulant therapy and safety. Enoxaparin may be administered intravenously in specific situations but should not be given intramuscularly. The drugs are also associated with less thrombocytopenia than is standard heparin. However, monitoring of platelet counts during therapy is necessary. With significant bleeding, protamine sulfate may be considered although it does not completely neutralize LMWHs; clinical bleeding may be reduced. The Institute for Safe Medication Practices (ISMP) classifies the LMWHs as high-alert drugs because there is a possible risk of significant harm when the drugs are used in error.

Fondaparinux (Arixtra) indirectly and selectively inhibits factor Xa by mechanisms identical to LMWHs but without affecting thrombin activity. As a synthetic pentasaccharide, the drug binds to antithrombin and is administered for prophylaxis of DVT in people undergoing hip or knee surgery. It is administered subcutaneously and has a longer half-life than LMWHs, necessitating only a once-daily dose. The ISMP classifies fondaparinux as a high-alert drug because there is a possible risk of significant harm when the drug is used in error. Fondaparinux has no effect on prothrombin time, aPTT, platelet aggregation, or bleeding time, so it does not require routine coagulation monitoring. As with other anticoagulants, bleeding is a concern particularly in patients with renal dysfunction, because fondaparinux is primarily eliminated by the kidneys. Currently, no agent for reversal of fondaparinux is available.

### Clinical Application 9.1

- To regulate the amount of heparin Mr. Oliver receives, his aPTT is measured. What is the therapeutic value for aPTT?

## VITAMIN K ANTAGONISTS

**Warfarin** (Coumadin) is the most commonly used oral anticoagulant and is the prototype vitamin K antagonist. Table 9.2 presents dosage information for warfarin.

## Pharmacokinetics

Warfarin is well absorbed after oral administration. Administration with food may delay the rate but not the extent of absorption. The drug is highly bound to plasma proteins (98%), mainly albumin.

Metabolism takes place in the liver. Excretion, primarily as inactive metabolites, occurs in the kidneys. Renal impairment does not affect drug metabolism but may decrease excretion of the drug.

## Action

Warfarin acts in the liver to prevent synthesis of vitamin K–dependent clotting factors (i.e., factors II, VII, IX, and X). Similar to vitamin K in structure, warfarin therefore acts as a competitive antagonist to hepatic use of vitamin K. Conversely, vitamin K serves as the antidote for warfarin. Warfarin has no effect on circulating clotting factors or on platelet function, so the anticoagulant effects do not occur for 3 to 5 days after warfarin is started because clotting factors already in the blood follow their normal pathway of elimination.

## Use

Warfarin is most useful in long-term prevention or management of venous thromboembolic disorders, including DVT, pulmonary embolism, and embolization associated with atrial fibrillation and prosthetic heart valves. In addition, warfarin therapy after myocardial infarction may decrease reinfarction, stroke, venous thromboembolism, and death. The smaller doses used now are equally effective as ones used formerly, with similar antithrombotic effects and decreased risks of bleeding.

### Use in Children

After cardiac surgery, children receive warfarin to prevent thromboembolism, but there are no established doses and guidelines for safe, effective use. Accurate drug administration, close monitoring of blood coagulation tests, safety measures to prevent trauma and bleeding, avoiding interacting drugs, and informing others in the child's environment (e.g., teachers, babysitters, health care providers) are necessary.

### Use in Older Adults

Warfarin metabolism may be altered in older adults. As patient age increases, a lower dose of warfarin is usually required to produce a therapeutic effect.

### Use in Patients With Hepatic Impairment

Warfarin is more likely to cause bleeding in patients with hepatic disease because of decreased synthesis of vitamin K and decreased plasma proteins. In addition, only the liver eliminates warfarin; thus, it may accumulate in people with hepatic impairment, and dosage adjustment may be necessary.

### Use in Patients With Critical Illness

Because the anticoagulant and antithrombotic effects of warfarin take several days to occur, patients who are critically ill require concurrent treatment with other anticoagulants, such as heparin or LMWHs. Heparin is usually continued until the international normalized ratio (INR) is the therapeutic range.

### Use in Patients Receiving Home Care

For prevention of DVT, warfarin is usually self-administered at home, with periodic office or clinic visits for blood tests and other follow-up care. For home management of DVT, warfarin may be self-administered, but a nurse usually visits, performs a fingerstick INR, and notifies the prescriber, who then prescribes the appropriate dose of warfarin. Precautions to decrease risks of bleeding are necessary. However, the risk of bleeding has decreased in recent years because lower doses of warfarin are now used. In addition, medical conditions other than anticoagulation may cause bleeding during warfarin therapy.

## Adverse Effects

The primary adverse effect associated with warfarin therapy is hemorrhage. Additionally, nausea, vomiting, abdominal pain, alopecia, urticaria, dizziness, and joint or muscle pain may occur.

## Contraindications

Contraindications to warfarin include GI ulcerations, blood disorders associated with bleeding, severe kidney or liver disease, severe hypertension, and recent surgery of the eye, spinal cord, or brain. Caution is warranted in patients with mild hypertension, renal or hepatic disease, alcoholism, history of GI ulcerations, drainage tubes (e.g., nasogastric tubes, indwelling urinary catheters), or occupations with high risks of traumatic injury. Warfarin, a pregnancy category X medication, is contraindicated during pregnancy because it crosses the placenta and may produce fatal fetal hemorrhage. The U.S. Food and Drug Administration (FDA) has issued a **BLACK BOX WARNING** ◆ for warfarin because of the risk of its causing major or fatal bleeding.

## Nursing Implications

### Preventing Interactions

Many medications and herbs interact with warfarin, increasing or decreasing its effect (Boxes 9.5 and 9.6).

### Administering the Medication

Vitamin K antagonists such as warfarin have a narrow therapeutic window of adequate anticoagulation without bleeding and a highly variable individual dose–response that requires monitoring by laboratory testing.

 **QSEN Alert: Safety**

When warfarin therapy begins, daily evaluation of INR is necessary until a stable daily dose is reached (the dose that maintains the prothrombin time [PT] and INR within therapeutic ranges and does not cause bleeding). A therapeutic PT value is approximately 1.5 times control, or 18 seconds. Thereafter, a patient's INR values require checking every 2 to 4 weeks for the duration of oral anticoagulant drug therapy. If a prescriber changes the warfarin dose, more frequent INR measurements are necessary until a stable daily dose is again established. The nurse should administer warfarin after ensuring that laboratory values are within therapeutic parameters.

 **QSEN Alert: Safety**

Institutions often have protocol for the therapeutic range of INR. In the absence of a protocol, the nurse holds the dose if the INR is above 3.0 and notifies the health care provider.

**BOX 9.5**  *Drug Interactions: Warfarin*

**Drugs That Increase the Effects of Warfarin**

- Acetaminophen (high dose), allopurinol, amiodarone
  *Increase the anticoagulant effect*
- Alteplase, androgens, aspirin and other nonsteroidal anti-inflammatory drugs, azithromycin, bismuth subsalicylate, carbamazepine, chloral hydrate, chloramphenicol, cimetidine, ciprofloxacin and other quinolone antibiotics, cisapride, clarithromycin, clofibrate, cotrimoxazole, direct thrombin inhibitors, heparin, macrolide antibiotics, omeprazole, pravastatin, propranolol, quinidine, ranitidine, ritonavir, sertraline, simvastatin, sulfinpyrazone, sulfonamide, tamoxifen, tetracyclines, thyroid hormones, tricyclic antidepressants, vancomycin, vitamin E
  *Increase the risk of bleeding*
- Antithrombin
  *Increases the pharmacologic effect*
- Cephalosporins
  *Result in potential coagulopathies and risk of bleeding*

**Drugs That Decrease the Effects of Warfarin**

- Chlordiazepoxide, haloperidol, intravenous lipid emulsions (contains soybean oil), isotretinoin, meprobamate, spironolactone
  *Cause effects by various mechanisms*
- Chlorthalidone
  *May diminish warfarin's ability to cause blood clots to form*
- Ethchlorvynol, trazodone
  *Cause effects by unknown mechanism*
- Etretinate
  *May induce anticoagulant's hepatic microsomal enzyme*

### Assessing for Therapeutic Effects

As with heparin, the nurse assesses for the absence or reduction of signs and symptoms of thrombotic disorders (e.g., less edema and pain with DVT, less chest pain and respiratory difficulty with pulmonary embolism, absence of uncontrolled bleeding, hematuria, or blood in the stools). It is also necessary to ensure that PT and INR values are within the therapeutic range.

**BOX 9.6**  *Herb and Dietary Interactions: Warfarin*

**Herbs and Foods That Increase the Effects of Warfarin**

- Angelica, cat's claw, chamomile, chondroitin, cranberry juice, feverfew, garlic, ginkgo, goldenseal, grape seed extract, green tea, psyllium, turmeric

**Herbs and Foods That Decrease the Effects of Warfarin**

- Ginseng, St. John's wort, vitamin K, foods high in vitamin K (broccoli, brussels sprouts, cabbage, cauliflower, chives, collard greens, kale, lettuce, mustard greens, peppers, spinach, tomatoes, turnips, and watercress)

### Assessing for Adverse Effects

The nurse assesses for signs of bleeding, including excessive bruising of the skin, bleeding from IV sites or the gum line, and blood in urine or stool. As previously stated, vitamin K is the antidote for warfarin and may be administered if the INR level is 5 or more and signs of bleeding are present. Additionally, prothrombin complex concentrate (PCC), human (Kcentra), is used for urgent warfarin reversal with major or life-threatening hemorrhage.

### Patient Teaching

The nurse reinforces instructions for safe use of warfarin, assists patients to obtain required laboratory tests, and teaches how to observe for signs and symptoms of bleeding. Additional patient teaching guidelines for anticoagulant medications, including vitamin K antagonists, are outlined in Box 9.4.

---

**Unfolding Patient Stories: Rachel Heidebrink • Part 2**

Think back to Chapter 7, where you met Rachel Heidebrink who underwent surgery for a hip fracture sustained in a motorcycle accident. She is diagnosed with a pulmonary embolism (PE) on postoperative day 1. How would the nurse explain the effect of heparin for the management of a PE and why the route of administration begins with an intravenous loading dose followed by a continuous infusion? What nursing assessments and interventions ensure the safe administration of intravenous heparin?

Care for Rachel and other patients in a realistic virtual environment: *vSim for Nursing* (thepoint.lww.com/vSimPharm). Practice documenting these patients' care in DocuCare (thepoint.lww.com/DocuCareEHR).

---

**Clinical Application 9.2**

- Mr. Oliver's prescriber adds warfarin to his treatment regimen. The order is for warfarin 5 mg PO daily and for evaluation of baseline PT and INR. The nurse administers the warfarin and order the blood work for the next morning. What therapeutic INR value indicates that the warfarin dosage is appropriate?

---

**NCLEX Success**

1. The nurse is reviewing the laboratory results of a hospitalized patient receiving intravenous heparin therapy for pulmonary embolism. The activated partial thromboplastin time (aPTT) is 38 seconds (control 28 seconds). The nurse should

   A. not give the next dose because the level is too high
   B. continue the present order because the level is appropriate
   C. notify the health care provider that the aPTT is low and anticipate orders to increase the dose
   D. request an order for warfarin now that the patient is heparinized

2. In explaining the use of warfarin to a female patient, the nurse is correct in telling her which of the following regarding warfarin? (Select all that apply.)

   A. Warfarin is a vitamin K antagonist.
   B. Warfarin does not cross the placenta.
   C. Warfarin is used for long-term anticoagulation therapy.
   D. Warfarin is metabolized by the liver.

3. In developing a safe plan of care, the nurse recognizes that which of the following agents is the antidote for heparin?

   A. protamine zinc
   B. vitamin K
   C. protamine sulfate
   D. vitamin D

4. Which of the following assessment findings are positive outcomes in a patient receiving warfarin for the management of pulmonary embolism? (Select all that apply.)

   A. report of absence of chest pain
   B. respiratory rate of 18/min with no use of accessory muscles
   C. absence of uncontrolled bleeding
   D. international normalized ratio serum level of 3.2
   E. prothrombin time serum level of 18 seconds
   F. presence of hematuria

## DIRECT THROMBIN INHIBITORS

DTIs have benefits compared with agents such as heparin and warfarin, including the inhibition of both circulating and clot-bound thrombin. Other advantages of DTIs include a more predictable dose–response anticoagulant effect, inhibition of thrombin-induced platelet aggregation, and the lack of production of immune-mediated thrombocytopenia. Heparin and warfarin are indirect inhibitors of thrombin. The DTIs exert their effect by interacting directly with the thrombin molecule without the need of a cofactor, such as heparin cofactor II or antithrombin. As such, they inhibit thrombin's ability to convert soluble fibrinogen to fibrin and to activate the fibrin-generating factors V, VIII, and IX. Because thrombin also stimulates platelets, DTIs also have antiplatelet activity.

Both parenteral and oral DTIs are available. The original prototype of the bivalent type, hirudin, is not commercially available; however, its discovery led to the development through recombinant technology of parenteral derivatives, bivalirudin, desirudin, argatroban, and one oral DTI, dabigatran. Lepirudin, another derivative, was discontinued and is no longer on the market. In this discussion, the only oral DTI, **dabigatran etexilate** (Pradaxa), serves as the prototype. Table 9.2 presents dosage information for the DTIs.

## Pharmacokinetics

Dabigatran etexilate is an inactive prodrug that is rapidly and hydrolyzed to dabigatran, its active form, in the body by plasma and hepatic esterases. The drug is excreted in the urine, and the systemic elimination is proportional to the glomerular filtration rate. Typically, the elimination half-life is 12 to 17 hours, which can be extended in the elderly and those with renal failure.

## Action

As an inactive prodrug, dabigatran etexilate lacks anticoagulant activity. With conversion to the active form in the body, dabigatran has been shown to specifically and reversibly inhibit both free and fibrin-bound thrombin, the key enzyme in the coagulation cascade, thereby inhibiting coagulation. DTIs have no known antagonists. Given orally, the drug peaks in 1 hour.

## Use

Dabigatran etexilate is used to prevent strokes and systemic embolization in individuals with nonvalvular atrial fibrillation. In addition, it is given for the treatment and prevention of deep venous thrombosis and pulmonary embolism. Therapeutic drug monitoring is not necessary.

### Use in Older Adults

Dabigatran etexilate is identified in the Beers Criteria as a potentially inappropriate medication; it should be used with caution in older adults who have a creatinine clearance less than 30 mL/min or those 75 years and older. However, no dosage adjustment of dabigatran etexilate is needed in elderly patients with normal renal function. But the risk of bleeding, a common side effect, increases with age.

### Use in Patients With Renal Impairment

Because dabigatran etexilate is cleared by the kidneys, it accumulates in patients with renal insufficiency, and dosage adjustments may be required based on creatinine clearance calculations. The use of the drug is not recommended in patients receiving hemodialysis.

### Adverse Effects

The most common adverse effects associated with the administration of dabigatran etexilate are bleeding, dyspepsia, abdominal pain, gastritis, and anemia.

 **QSEN Alert: Safety**

After reports of severe liver injury in patients treated with dabigatran etexilate, Health Canada, a federal agency focused on maintaining and enhancing the health of Canadians, is working with the drug's manufacturer to update safety information regarding the apparent link between the drug and liver injury.

## Contraindications

Contraindications include a known hypersensitivity to any of the components of dabigatran etexilate and in patients with active pathologic bleeding or with a mechanical prosthetic heart valve. Use in pregnancy and lactation requires caution.

## Nursing Implications

The ISMP classifies dabigatran etexilate as a high-alert drug because of the possible risk of significant harm that results when it is used in error.

**BOX 9.7**  *Drug Interactions: Dabigatran Etexilate*

**Drugs That Increase the Effects of Dabigatran Etexilate**
- Anticoagulants, apixaban, aspirin, antiplatelet agents (especially clopidogrel), collagenase, dasatinib, deferasirox, deoxycholic acid, edoxaban, hemin, limaprost, nonsteroidal anti-inflammatory agents, pentosan polysulfate sodium, prostacyclin analogues, salicylates, sugammadex, sulfinpyrazone, thrombolytics, tibolone, ticagrelor, vorapaxar
  *Increase the risk of bleeding*
- Amiodarone, clarithromycin, dronedarone, ketoconazole P-glycoprotein/ABCB1 inhibitors, quinidine, verapamil
  *May increase serum concentration*

**Drugs That Decrease the Effects of Dabigatran Etexilate**
- Antacids, atorvastatin, lumacaftor, P-glycoprotein/ABCB1 inducers, proton pump inhibitors
  *May decrease serum concentration*
- Estrogen derivatives, progestins
  *May decrease the anticoagulant effects*

### Preventing Interactions

Many medications interact with dabigatran etexilate, altering its effect (Boxes 9.7 and 9.8). No foods decrease the drug's bioavailability, although the drug's peak plasma concentration is delayed 2 hours if taken with food.

### Administering the Medication

The drug capsules should be administered intact with a full glass of water without regard to meals. If the capsules are open or chewed, absorption is increased, and the risk of adverse drug effects is enhanced.

### Assessing for Therapeutic Effects

The nurse assesses for the absence of signs and symptoms of thrombotic disorders, including HIT, and for laboratory values within normal range. A therapeutic range has not been established for tests of anticoagulant activity.

### Assessing for Adverse Effects

The most common adverse effect associated with the administration of dabigatran etexilate is bleeding; therefore, assessing for signs of bleeding is a priority. Additionally, the nurse assesses for other adverse effects, including GI and hematologic effects. The anticoagulant effects of dabigatran can be reversed by idarucizumab (Praxbind).

**BOX 9.8**  *Herb and Dietary Interactions: Dabigatran Etexilate*

**Herbs and Foods That Increase the Effects of Dabigatran Etexilate**
- Alfalfa, anise, bilberry, omega-3 fatty acids, vitamin E

## Patient Teaching

Patients need to understand that stopping the drug without provider instruction could increase the risk of blood clots. Patients should notify other health care providers about taking dabigatran etexilate, particularly with spinal or epidural procedures that increase the risk of bleeding around the spine, because paralysis may occur. Additional general patient teaching guidelines for anticoagulants, including the DTIs, are outlined in Box 9.4.

## Other Drugs in the Class

In comparison to heparin, which binds only circulating thrombin, DTIs such as bivalirudin and desirudin block circulating thrombin and clot-bound thrombin. Bivalirudin is given intravenously as a specific and reversible DTI approved for the treatment of patients with unstable angina undergoing percutaneous transluminal coronary angioplasty (PTCA), as an anticoagulant in patients undergoing PTCA, and as an alternative to heparin in patients with or at risk of developing HIT. Desirudin has been shown to be more effective than enoxaparin in preventing DVT following total hip replacement. Desirudin is administered subcutaneously, and highly protein bound drugs do not modify its effects.

Argatroban is indicated for HIT, is eliminated in the liver, and can be used in people with end-stage renal disease. Administered intravenously, argatroban is very short acting due to its reversible binding to thrombin.

## DIRECT FACTOR Xa INHIBITORS

Direct factor Xa inhibitors inactivate circulating and clot-bound factor Xa. Unlike fondaparinux, which acts indirectly, this class of drugs binds directly and, by doing so, inhibits the production of thrombin. These direct oral anticoagulants, along with dabigatran, are at least as effective as the vitamin K antagonists but are associated with less life-threatening bleeding. Currently, three orally acting direct factor Xa inhibitors are approved, rivaroxaban, apixaban, and edoxaban; no direct factor Xa inhibitors are available for intravenous infusion. **Rivaroxaban** serves as the prototype.

## Pharmacokinetics

Rivaroxaban is rapidly absorbed and is highly bound to protein. The drug undergoes partial metabolism by CYP3A4 (an isozyme of the cytochrome P-450 system) and is excreted in the urine (36% as unchanged drug) and feces (7% as unchanged drug). Peak plasma levels are reached in 2 to 4 hours, and the half-life is 5 to 9 hours.

## Actions

Rivaroxaban inhibits platelet activation and formation of fibrin clotting by inhibition of factor Xa in both intrinsic and extrinsic coagulation pathways.

## Use

Rivaroxaban is used in the treatment and secondary prevention of venous thromboembolism and in stroke prevention in patients with nonvalvular atrial fibrillation.

### Use in Children

The safety of rivaroxaban in children has not been established.

### Use in Older Adults

According to the Beers Criteria (see Chap. 5), dosage adjustment is indicated in older adults with creatinine clearance between 30 and 50 mL/min. Rivaroxaban is a potentially inappropriate medication in older adults with a creatinine clearance less than 30 mL/min because of increased risk of bleeding.

### Use in Patients With Renal Impairment

Rivaroxaban is metabolized in the kidney and the liver. Therefore, the drug should not be used in individuals with a creatinine clearance of less than 15 mL/min; with delayed excretion of the drug, there may be increased risk of bleeding.

### Use in Patients With Hepatic Impairment

Rivaroxaban should not be used in individuals with moderate to severe hepatic impairment.

### Use in Patients With Critical Illness

Individuals who are critically ill may have complications that may necessitate the use of rivaroxaban, including treatment and secondary prevention of venous thromboembolism and for stroke prevention in patients with atrial fibrillation. The critically ill have a high risk of DVT and pulmonary embolism, as well as an increased risk of bleeding in the presence of other coexisting conditions, particularly those involving the kidneys or liver.

### Use in Patients Receiving Home Care

Rivaroxaban for home use following knee or hip surgery for the prevention of venous thrombosis or management of nonvalvular atrial fibrillation has become common practice as the drug requires no INR monitoring. Additionally, rivaroxaban has fixed dosing schedule, a lower bleeding risk, and few drug interactions as compared to heparin. Regular home care by the nurse, particularly in the older adult, can enhance the safe use of the drug and recognition of signs and symptoms of bleeding before serious bleeding occurs.

### Adverse Effects

Bleeding is the most common adverse effect of rivaroxaban, and this risk increases if the drug is taken with other agents that alter hemostasis. Intracranial, gastric, and retinal bleeding has been reported. Additionally, the possibility of spinal or epidural hematoma exists in patients undergoing epidural anesthesia or spinal puncture with procedures or trauma that can lead to permanent paralysis. Dosage adjustment is recommended with anticipated procedures involving the spine.

## Contraindications

Contraindications to rivaroxaban include a known hypersensitivity to the drug. The drug appears unsafe during pregnancy; it is associated with pregnancy-related hemorrhage and risk to the fetus. Benefits of therapy in pregnancy should outweigh risks.

# Nursing Implications

## Preventing Interactions

Numerous drugs and some herbs are known to interact with rivaroxaban, increasing or decreasing its effect (Boxes 9.9 and 9.10).

## Administering the Medication

Rivaroxaban is generally given at a fixed dose. Although 10-mg tablets can be administered without regard to food, 15- and 20-mg tablets should be taken with food. The drug should be administered with the evening meal for nonvalvular atrial fibrillation.

## Assessing for Therapeutic Effects

The nurse should assess for absence of DVT or other unanticipated clotting. No routine monitoring of INR or other coagulation parameters is required.

## Assessing for Adverse Effects

As with all anticoagulants, the nurse should observe for signs of bleeding, for any change in baseline renal or hepatic function that could enhance the risk of bleeding, and for concurrent administration of drugs known to interact with rivaroxaban.

## Patient Teaching

Education related to bleeding risk is essential for patients receiving rivaroxaban. The nurse reinforces instructions for safe use of the drug and related anticoagulants and teaching how to observe for signs and symptoms of bleeding. Patients should notify other health care providers about taking rivaroxaban, particularly before spinal or epidural procedures that increase the risk of bleeding around the spine, because paralysis may occur. Additional patient teaching guidelines for anticoagulants, including rivaroxaban, are outlined in Box 9.4.

---

**BOX 9.9** **Drug Interactions: Rivaroxaban**

**Drugs That Increase the Effects of Rivaroxaban**
- Anticoagulants, apixaban, aspirin, antiplatelet agents, collagenase, dasatinib, edoxaban, hemin, ibrutinib, limaprost, nonsteroidal anti-inflammatory agents, pentosan polysulfate sodium, prostacyclin analogues, salicylates, sugammadex, thrombolytics, tibolone, tipranavir, vorapaxar, vitamin E
  *Increase the risk of bleeding*
- Clarithromycin, osimertinib
  *May increase serum concentration*

**Drugs That Decrease the Effects of Rivaroxaban**
- Bosentan, CYP3A4 inducers, deferasirox, estrogen derivatives, fusidic acid, nevirapine, progestins, siltuximab
  *May decrease serum concentration*
- Estrogen derivatives, progestins
  *May decrease the anticoagulant effects*

---

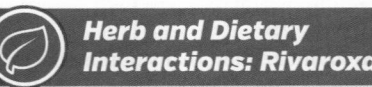

**BOX 9.10** **Herb and Dietary Interactions: Rivaroxaban**

**Herbs and Foods That Increase the Effects of Rivaroxaban**
- Alfalfa, anise, bilberry, grapefruit juice

**Herbs and Foods That Decrease the Effects of Rivaroxaban**
- St. John's wort

## Other Drugs in the Class

Apixaban (Eliquis) and edoxaban (Savaysa) are additional oral direct factor Xa inhibitors. A major advantage of these drugs is fixed dosing, less variability in drug effect for a given dose, and the lack of required monitoring. Although the overall risks of bleeding are similar to vitamin K antagonists, the risks for intracranial bleeding are less with the direct factor Xa inhibitors. These drugs carry the same risks in spinal or epidural procedures as rivaroxaban; the risk of paralysis may occur. As with rivaroxaban, and other anticoagulants, premature discontinuation of the direct factor Xa inhibitors without adequate alternative anticoagulation increases the risk of thrombosis. All drugs in the class pose a risk of hemorrhage and are classified as high-alert drugs by the ISMP because the drugs carry a heightened risk of causing significant patient harm when used in error. No drug that reverses the effects of the direct factor Xa inhibitors is currently available, and the drugs are not removed with dialysis. Should a patient experience hemorrhaging, oral activated charcoal may be given if the timing of administration would prove beneficial.

---

**QSEN Alert: Evidence-Based Practice**

Clinical practice guidelines for the treatment of acute venous thromboembolism, issued by the American College of Chest Physicians (2012), identify the direct oral thrombin and factor Xa inhibitors (apixaban, edoxaban, rivaroxaban, or dabigatran) as the preferred agents for long-term anticoagulation in patients who are not pregnant and do not have active cancer or severe renal insufficiency. This preference was based on randomized trials that consistently reported similar efficacy, a lower bleeding risk, and improved convenience when compared with warfarin.

## ANTIPLATELET DRUGS

**Antiplatelet drugs** prevent one or more steps in the prothrombotic activity of platelets. As described previously, platelet activity is very important in both physiologic hemostasis and pathologic thrombosis. Arterial thrombi, which are composed primarily of platelets, may form on top of atherosclerotic plaque and block blood flow in the artery. They may also form on heart walls and valves and embolize to other parts of the body.

Drugs used clinically for antiplatelet effects act by a variety of mechanisms to inhibit platelet activation, adhesion, aggregation, or procoagulant activity. These include drugs that block platelet receptors for thromboxane A₂, adenosine diphosphate (ADP), glycoprotein (GP) IIb/IIIa, and phosphodiesterase. Figure 9.2 describes the mechanism of action of some of the

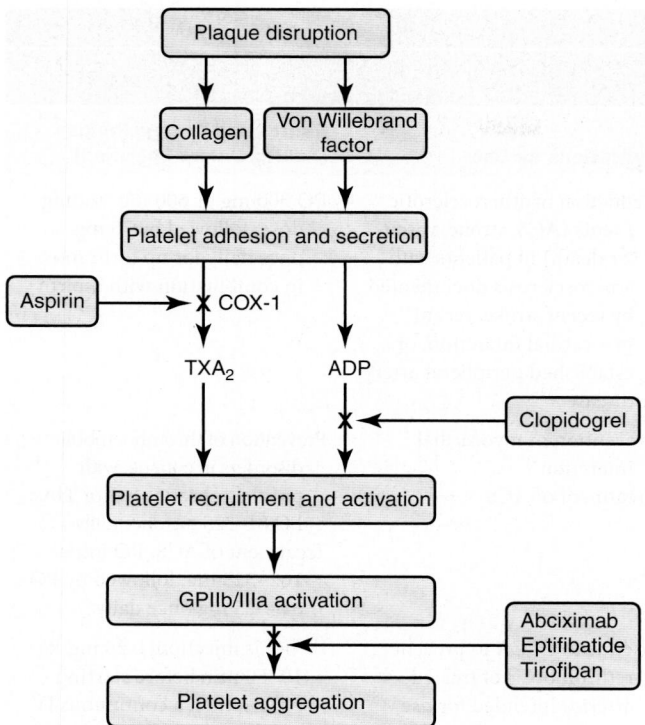

**Figure 9.2.** Details of the site of action of antiplatelet drugs on the process of platelet aggregation.

antiplatelet drugs. Aspirin, a cyclooxygenase inhibitor that has potent antiplatelet effects, is briefly discussed in this chapter and well described in Chapter 16.

## ADENOSINE DIPHOSPHATE RECEPTOR ANTAGONISTS

The antiplatelet drug **clopidogrel** (Plavix) is the prototype ADP receptor antagonist and is in a class of drugs called thienopyridines. Clopidogrel and the other ADP receptor antagonists, prasugrel, ticagrelor, and cangrelor have antiplatelet effects similar to aspirin and inhibit the ADP receptor on the surface of platelets. Clopidogrel has three shortcomings: delayed onset of action, irreversible inhibitory effects on platelets with no reversing agent or antidote, and significant individual variability in platelet response.

## Pharmacokinetics

Clopidogrel is rapidly absorbed after oral administration and undergoes extensive first-pass metabolism in the liver. Clopidogrel is a prodrug and is converted to its active form by hepatic CYP2C19 (an isozyme of the cytochrome P-450 system). To a lesser extent, activation of the drug also occurs via CYP3A4 enzymes. Platelet inhibition may occur 2 hours after a single dose, but the onset of action is slow, so that an initial loading dose is usually administered. The drug has a half-life of about 8 hours. The drug is excreted in the urine and feces.

## Action

Clopidogrel irreversibly blocks the ADP receptor on platelet cell surface. Effective dose-dependent prevention of platelet

aggregation can be seen within 2 hours of a single oral dose, but the onset of action is slow, so that a loading dose of 300 to 600 mg is usually administered. Platelet inhibition essentially lasts for the lifespan of the platelet (7–10 days). With repeated doses of 75 mg/d, maximum inhibition of platelet aggregation is achieved within 3 to 7 days. Platelet aggregation progressively returns to baseline about 5 days after discontinuing clopidogrel.

## Use

Indications for use include reduction of myocardial infarction, stroke, and vascular death in patients with atherosclerosis and in those after placement of coronary stents. Specific uses include prevention of vascular ischemic events in patients with symptomatic atherosclerosis or with acute coronary syndrome (ACS) (with or without ST-segment elevation). The absolute risk reduction from clopidogrel and other ADP receptor antagonists is greater in patients at higher cardiovascular risk, particularly in patients with ACSs or those who have had a coronary stent implanted. In ACS, clopidogrel is given with aspirin (dual antiplatelet therapy). Patients may also take clopidogrel in conjunction with aspirin to prevent thrombosis following placement of an intracoronary stent.

People with atrial fibrillation who are unable to take vitamin K antagonists take clopidogrel instead. Adding clopidogrel to aspirin in people with atrial fibrillation reduces the rate of major vascular events compared with aspirin alone but is associated with a greater risk of bleeding. Prescribers also order clopidogrel as an alternative antiplatelet drug for patients who cannot tolerate aspirin. Table 9.3 presents dosages for clopidogrel and other antiplatelet drugs.

### Use in Children

The safety and efficacy of clopidogrel in children have not been established.

### Use in Older Adults

Older adults are more likely than younger ones to experience bleeding and other complications of antiplatelet drugs. Clopidogrel is commonly used to prevent thrombotic stroke but can increase the risk of hemorrhagic stroke. A safe loading dose for clopidogrel in patients 75 years of age and older has not yet been established.

### Use in Patients With Hepatic Impairment

Because clopidogrel is metabolized in the liver, it may accumulate in people with hepatic impairment. Caution is necessary.

## Adverse Effects

The most common adverse effects associated with clopidogrel are pruritus, rash, purpura, and diarrhea. Thrombotic thrombocytopenic purpura, hemorrhage, and severe neutropenia have also occurred. People with variant forms of CYP2C19 may be poor or ultrarapid metabolizers of clopidogrel. Ultrarapid metabolizers of clopidogrel may have an increased risk of bleeding. With poor metabolizers, the benefits of the drug may not be adequate (see QSEN Safety Alert). The updated 2013 Clinical Pharmacogenetics Implementation Consortium Dosing Guidelines for clopidogrel recommend an alternative antiplatelet

**TABLE 9.3**

# DRUGS AT A GLANCE: Antiplatelets

| Drug | Pregnancy Category | Indications for Use | Routes and Dosage Ranges (Adults, Unless Specified) |
|---|---|---|---|
| **Ⓟ Clopidogrel** (Plavix; ❦ Plavix) | B | Reduction of atherosclerotic events (ACS, stroke, vascular death) in patients with atherosclerosis documented by recent stroke, recent myocardial infarction, or established peripheral artery disease | PO 300 mg or 600 mg loading dose; followed by 75 mg once daily for up to 12 mo in combination with aspirin |
| Aspirin (Ascriptin, Bayer, Ecotrin; ❦ Asaphen, Entrophen, Novasen, Praxis) | D (if full-dose aspirin is taken in the third trimester) | Prevention of myocardial infarction Treatment of ACS | Prevention of thromboembolic disorders in patients with prosthetic heart valves or TIAs: PO 81–325 mg once daily Treatment of ACS: PO initial 162–325 mg; followed by PO 81–325 mg once daily |
| Abciximab (ReoPro; ❦ ReoPro) | C | Used with PTCA to prevent rethrombosis of treated arteries Intended for use with aspirin and heparin | IV bolus injection, 0.25 mg/kg 10–60 min before starting PTCA, then a continuous IV infusion of 0.125 mcg/kg/min (max 10 mcg/min) for up to 12 h |
| Anagrelide (Agrylin; ❦ Agrylin) | C | Essential thrombocythemia, to reduce the elevated platelet count, the risk of thrombosis, and associated symptoms | PO 0.5 mg four times daily or 1 mg twice daily initially, then titrate to lowest dose effective in maintaining platelet count <600,000/mm$^3$ |
| Cangrelor (Kengreal) | C | | IV 30 mcg/kg bolus prior to PTCA followed immediately by an infusion of 4 mcg/kg/min continued at least for 2 h or for duration of the PTCA, whichever is longer |
| Cilostazol | C | Intermittent claudication, to increase walking distance (before leg pain occurs) | PO 100 mg twice daily, 30 min before or 2 h after breakfast and dinner; reduce to 50 mg twice daily with concurrent use of fluconazole, itraconazole, erythromycin, or diltiazem |
| Dipyridamole (❦ Persantine) | B | Prevention of thromboembolism after cardiac valve replacement, given with warfarin | PO 25–75 mg three times per day, 1 h before meals |
| Dipyridamole and aspirin (Aggrenox; ❦ Aggrenox) | D | Reduction of stroke risk in patients with previous TIA or thrombotic event | PO 1 capsule (200 mg extended-release dipyridamole/25 mg aspirin) twice daily |
| Eptifibatide (Integrilin; ❦ Integrilin, eptifibatide injection) | B | Acute coronary syndrome, including patients who are to be managed medically and those undergoing PTCA | IV bolus injection, 180 mcg/kg, followed by continuous infusion of 2 mcg/kg/min. See manufacturer's instructions for preparation and administration |

**TABLE 9.3**

## DRUGS AT A GLANCE: Antiplatelets [Continued]

| Drug | Pregnancy Category | Indications for Use | Routes and Dosage Ranges (Adults, Unless Specified) |
|---|---|---|---|
| Prasugrel (Effient; Effient) | B | Acute coronary syndrome | PO: Adults ≥60 kg: loading dose: 60 mg; maintenance dose: 10 mg once daily (in combination with aspirin 81–325 mg/d). |
| Tirofiban (Aggrastat; Aggrastat) | B | Acute coronary syndrome, with heparin, for patients who are to be managed medically or those undergoing PTCA<br>Acute myocardial infarction<br>Pulmonary embolism | IV infusion, loading dose: 25 mcg/kg over 5 min, then 0.15 mcg/kg/min for up to 18 h. Patients with renal impairment (creatinine clearance ≤60 mL/min) should receive the same loading dose followed by 0.075 mcg/kg/min for up to 18 h. See manufacturer's instructions for preparation and administration |
| Ticagrelor (Brilinta; Brilinta) | B | Reduction of thrombosis in patients with coronary artery disease | PO initial 180 mg as loading dose; followed by 90 mg twice daily, 12 h after loading dose in combination with aspirin |
| Vorapaxar (Zontivity; Zontivity) | B | Reduction of thrombosis in patients with history of myocardial infarction or with peripheral arterial disease | PO 2.08 mg once daily in combination with aspirin and/or clopidogrel |

ACS, acute coronary syndrome; PTCA, percutaneous transluminal coronary angioplasty or atherectomy; TIA, transient ischemic attack.

therapy (e.g., prasugrel, ticagrelor) for CYP2C19 poor or intermediate metabolizers if there are no contraindications.

### ! QSEN Alert: Safety

The FDA has issued a **BLACK BOX WARNING** ◆ concerning the use of clopidogrel in the 2% to 14% of the US population who are reduced metabolizers of the drug. As a result of genetic variations in CYP2C19 function, the drug may be less effective in altering platelet activity in these individuals. These "poor metabolizers" may remain at risk for heart attack, stroke, and cardiovascular death, and alternate dosing of the clopidogrel or the use of other antiplatelet drugs should be considered. Genomic testing is available to determine if a patient is a poor metabolizer, although it is not routinely recommended at this time.

## Contraindications

Contraindications to clopidogrel include hypersensitivity to the drug or any other component. It should not be used in patients with active bleeding in conditions such as intracranial hemorrhage or peptic ulcer disease. A category B medication, the drug requires cautious use in pregnant and lactating women.

## Nursing Implications

### Preventing Interactions

Many medications interact with clopidogrel, increasing or decreasing its effect (Box 9.11). Although certain herbs and foods increase the effects of clopidogrel, none seem to decrease the effects of the drug (Box 9.12).

### Administering the Medication

Patients take clopidogrel once daily without regard to food intake. As previously stated, although the drug may be effective 2 hours after a single dose, the onset of action is slow, and an initial loading dose is usually administered. The FDA has approved a 300-mg tablet as a loading dose for appropriate patients. The effect of the drug is apparent as soon as 2 hours after the 300-mg dose.

Clinicians have demonstrated that dual antiplatelet therapy with aspirin and clopidogrel reduces stent thrombosis following percutaneous coronary intervention. It is recommended that patients who receive implants with a bare-metal stent or a drug-eluting stent take dual antiplatelet therapy for at least 12 months. If well tolerated, dual antiplatelet therapy can be continued for another 18 months.

## BOX 9.11  *Drug Interactions: Clopidogrel*

**Drugs That Increase the Effects of Clopidogrel**
- Aspirin, nonsteroidal anti-inflammatory drugs, platelet inhibitors, thrombolytics
  *Increase the risk of bleeding*
- Atorvastatin
  *May affect antiplatelet activity*
- Barbiturates, carbamazepine, rifampin, rifapentine
  *Enhance antiplatelet effect*
- Rifabutin
  *May increase metabolism of clopidogrel*

**Drugs That Decrease the Effects of Clopidogrel**
- Amiodarone, dalfopristin, delavirdine, diltiazem, quinupristin, Vaprisol, zafirlukast
  *Affect CPY34A enzymes, which play a role in clopidogrel metabolism*
- Clarithromycin, erythromycin, ketoconazole, verapamil
  *Reduce antiplatelet activity*
- Omeprazole, lansoprazole
  *May lead to inadequate platelet response*
- Selective serotonin reuptake inhibitors
  *May increase the risk of bleeding*

## BOX 9.12  *Herb and Dietary Interactions: Clopidogrel*

**Herbs and Foods That Increase the Effects of Clopidogrel**
- Garlic, ginkgo biloba, ginger, green tea, horse chestnut, St. John's wort

### Assessing for Adverse Effects

The nurse assesses for common adverse effects, including pruritus, rash, purpura, and diarrhea; thrombotic thrombocytopenic purpura and hemorrhage; and severe neutropenia. No antidote exists for the effects of clopidogrel and the ADP receptor antagonist, prasugrel.

### Patient Teaching

The nurse instructs patients to take medication as directed and not to double the medication if a dose is missed. Additional patient teaching guidelines are outlined in Box 9.13.

## Other Drugs in the Class

Prasugrel (Effient) is an antiplatelet drug that has demonstrated improved cardiac outcome compared with clopidogrel for ACSs involving percutaneous coronary intervention. Also, this agent is used to reduce thrombotic cardiovascular events, including stent thrombosis. Although the drug requires hepatic conversion to an active metabolite, similar to clopidogrel, it is about 10 times more potent and has a more rapid onset of action, increasing the risk of bleeding. However, unlike clopidogrel, this activation is a rapid single-step process, and the TRITON-TIMI 38 trial demonstrated that individuals who are poor metabolizers

### Assessing for Therapeutic Effects

The nurse assesses for the absence of vascular ischemic events (e.g., pain, cyanosis, coolness of extremities). In addition, he or she ensures that hemoglobin and hematocrit levels are within normal limits.

## BOX 9.13  *Patient Teaching Guidelines for Antiplatelet Drugs*

**General Considerations**
- Antiplatelet drugs are given to people who have had, or who are at risk of having, a heart attack, stroke, or other problems from blood clots. For prevention of a heart attack or stroke, you are most likely to be given an antiplatelet drug (e.g., aspirin, clopidogrel).
- All antiplatelet drugs can increase your risk of bleeding, so you need to take safety precautions to prevent injury.
- Following instructions regarding these medications is extremely important. Too little medication increases your risk of problems from blood clot formation; too much medication can cause bleeding.
- While taking any of these medications, you need regular medical supervision and periodic blood tests. The blood tests can help your health care provider regulate drug dosage and maintain your safety.
- You need to take the drugs as directed, avoid taking other drugs without the health care provider's knowledge and consent, inform any health care provider (including dentists) that you are taking an antiplatelet

drug before any invasive diagnostic tests or treatments are begun, and keep all appointments for continuing care. This drug should be withheld 5 to 7 days prior to a planned surgical procedure.
- Report any sign of bleeding (e.g., excessive bruising of the skin, blood in urine or stool) to your health care provider. If superficial bleeding occurs, apply direct pressure to the site for 3 to 5 minutes or longer if necessary. In addition, notify your prescriber promptly if you develop fever, chills, or a sore throat.

**Self-Administration**
- Take aspirin with food or after meals, with 8 oz of water, to decrease stomach irritation. However, stomach upset is uncommon with the small doses used for antiplatelet effects. Do not crush or chew coated tablets (long-acting preparations).
- Take cilostazol 30 minutes before or 2 hours after morning and evening meals for better absorption and effectiveness.
- Take clopidogrel (Plavix) without regard to food.

of CYP2C19 had different clinical responses to prasugrel in comparison to clopidogrel.

Ticagrelor (Brilinta) and Cangrelor (Kengreal), the latest ADP receptor antagonists, differ from clopidogrel and prasugrel in that the receptor blockade they cause is reversible. Both ticagrelor and cangrelor are effective and relatively safe when compared to clopidogrel. These drugs are used to reduce the rate of cardiovascular death, myocardial infarction, and stroke in patients with a history of myocardial infarction or ACS.

Cangrelor, the only intravenous ADP receptor antagonist, is administrated as an adjunct to PTCA to prevent a myocardial infarction during the procedure. The drug is administered intravenously prior to PTCA and continued throughout the duration of the procedure. Should ongoing use of an ADP receptor antagonist be required postprocedure, an oral ADP receptor antagonist is initiated. Cangrelor may also be administered in patients requiring repeat coronary revascularization and stent thrombosis in patients not currently receiving an ADP receptor antagonist or a glycoprotein IIb/IIIa inhibitor. Platelet inhibition occurs within 2 minutes, and no antiplatelet effect is observed an hour after discontinuation because of the drug's short half-life.

Ticagrelor also decreases the rate of stent thrombosis in individuals requiring a stent for the treatment of ACS. The most recent data suggest that ticagrelor has broader applicability of use in individuals with ACS as compared to prasugrel. (However, prasugrel seems to be better tolerated.) Ticagrelor may be administered without regard to meals, and for patients unable to swallow the tablets whole, the drug may be crushed and mixed with water to create a suspension for oral or nasogastric use. Ample water should be given after a suspension is used. Adverse effects of ticagrelor include increased uric acid levels and dyspnea. The FDA has issued a **BLACK BOX WARNING ◆** regarding the use of ticagrelor; the drug increases the risk of bleeding, including significant and possibly fatal hemorrhage. If possible, bleeding should be managed without the discontinuing of ticagrelor because the risk of cardiovascular events increases if it is discontinued. The chances of hemostasis with platelet transfusion are not known and may be limited. However, with life-threatening or serious bleeding, platelet transfusion may be required.

## OTHER ANTIPLATELET DRUGS
### Thromboxane A₂ Inhibitors

Aspirin exerts pharmacologic actions by inhibiting synthesis of prostaglandins. In this instance, it acetylates cyclooxygenase, the enzyme in platelets that normally synthesizes thromboxane $A_2$, a prostaglandin product that causes platelet aggregation. Thus, aspirin prevents formation of thromboxane $A_2$, thromboxane $A_2$–induced platelet aggregation, and thrombus formation. A single dose of 300 to 600 mg or multiple doses of 30 mg (e.g., daily for several days) of the drug inhibit the cyclooxygenase in circulating platelets almost completely. These antithrombotic effects persist for the life of the platelet (7–10 days). Aspirin may be used long term for prevention of myocardial infarction or stroke and in patients with prosthetic heart valves. It is also used for the immediate treatment of suspected or actual acute

myocardial infarction, for transient ischemic attacks (TIAs), and for evolving thrombotic strokes. Adverse effects are uncommon with the small doses used for antiplatelet effects. However, there is an increased risk of bleeding, including hemorrhagic stroke. Because approximately 85% of strokes are thrombotic, the benefits of aspirin or other antiplatelet agents are thought to outweigh the risks of hemorrhagic strokes (~15%). No antidote exists for the effects of aspirin because it produces irreversible platelet effects; platelet transfusion may be required. Further discussion of aspirin is found in Chapter 16.

Nonsteroidal anti-inflammatory drugs (NSAIDs), including ibuprofen and many other aspirin-related drugs, inhibit cyclooxygenase reversibly. Their antiplatelet effects subside when the drugs are eliminated from the circulation and the drugs usually are not used for antiplatelet effects. However, patients who take an NSAID daily (e.g., for arthritis pain) may not need to take additional aspirin for antiplatelet effects. Acetaminophen does not affect platelets in usual doses (see Chap. 16).

## Glycoprotein IIb/IIIa Receptor Antagonists

Despite significant pharmacodynamics differences between the three GP IIb/IIa antagonists, no evidence to date suggests significant differences in clinical outcomes. Abciximab (ReoPro) is a monoclonal antibody that prevents the binding of fibrinogen, von Willebrand factor, and other molecules to GP IIb/IIIa receptors on activated platelets. This action inhibits platelet aggregation. This drug is used with PTCA or removal of atherosclerotic plaque to prevent rethrombosis of treated arteries. It is used with aspirin and heparin and is contraindicated in patients who have recently received an oral anticoagulant or IV dextran. Other contraindications include active bleeding, thrombocytopenia, history of a serious stroke, surgery or major trauma within the previous 6 weeks, uncontrolled hypertension, or hypersensitivity to drug components.

Eptifibatide (Integrilin) and tirofiban (Aggrastat) inhibit platelet aggregation by preventing activation of GP IIb/IIIa receptors on the platelet surface and the subsequent binding of fibrinogen and von Willebrand factor to platelets. Antiplatelet effects occur during drug infusion and stop when the drug is stopped. The drugs are indicated for ACS (e.g., unstable angina, myocardial infarction) in patients who are to be treated medically or by angioplasty or atherectomy. Drug half-life is approximately 2.5 hours for eptifibatide and 2 hours for tirofiban; the drugs are cleared mainly by renal excretion. With tirofiban, plasma clearance is approximately 25% lower in older adults and approximately 50% lower in patients with severe renal impairment (creatinine clearance less than 30 mL/min). The drugs are contraindicated in patients with hypersensitivity to any component of the products; current or previous bleeding (within previous 30 days); a history of thrombocytopenia after previous exposure to tirofiban; a history of stroke within 30 days or any history of hemorrhagic stroke; major surgery or severe physical trauma within the previous month; severe hypertension (systolic blood pressure greater than 180 mm Hg with tirofiban or greater than 200 mm Hg with eptifibatide, or diastolic blood pressure greater than 110 mm Hg with either drug); a history of intracranial hemorrhage, neoplasm, arteriovenous malformation, or aneurysm; a platelet count less than 100,000/mm³; serum creatinine 2 mg/dL or above (for the 180-mcg/kg bolus and the 2-mcg/kg/min infusion) or 4 mg/dL or above (for the 135-mcg/kg bolus and the 0.5-mcg/kg/min infusion); or dependency on dialysis (eptifibatide).

Bleeding is the most common adverse effect, with most major bleeding occurring at the arterial access site for cardiac catheterization. If bleeding occurs and cannot be controlled with pressure, the drug infusion and heparin should be discontinued. These drugs should be used cautiously if given with other drugs that affect hemostasis (e.g., warfarin, thrombolytics, other antiplatelet drugs).

## Phosphodiesterase-3 Enzyme Inhibitor

Cilostazol inhibits phosphodiesterase, an enzyme that metabolizes cyclic adenosine monophosphate (cAMP). This inhibition increases intracellular cAMP, which then inhibits platelet aggregation and produces vasodilation. The inhibition of platelet aggregation induced by various stimuli (e.g., thrombin, ADP, collagen, arachidonic acid, epinephrine, shear stress) is reversible. The drug is highly protein bound (95%–98%), mainly to albumin; extensively metabolized by hepatic cytochrome P-450 enzymes; and excreted in urine (74%) and feces. Cilostazol and its two active metabolites accumulate with chronic administration and reach steady state within a few days.

The drug is indicated for management of intermittent claudication. Symptoms usually improve within 2 to 4 weeks but may take as long as 12 weeks. The most common adverse effects are diarrhea and headache. The FDA has issued a **BLACK BOX WARNING** ◆ for the use of cilostazol because it is contraindicated in patients with heart failure of any severity.

## Other Agents

Anagrelide inhibits platelet aggregation induced by cAMP phosphodiesterase, ADP, and collagen. However, it is indicated only to reduce platelet counts for patients with **essential thrombocythemia** (a disorder characterized by excessive numbers of platelets). Doses to reduce platelet production are smaller than those required to inhibit platelet aggregation.

Dipyridamole inhibits platelet adhesion, but its mechanism of action is unclear. It is used for prevention of thromboembolism after cardiac valve replacement and is given with warfarin. The combination of dipyridamole and aspirin is indicated for prevention of stroke in those who have had stroke precursors (TIAs) or a previously completed thrombotic stroke.

### NCLEX Success

5. In developing a safe plan of care, the nurse should recognize that the antidote for warfarin is
    A. protamine zinc
    B. vitamin K
    C. protamine sulfate
    D. idarucizumab

6. The nurse explains to a patient that aspirin suppresses blood clotting by
    A. inactivating thrombin
    B. promoting fibrin degradation
    C. decreasing synthesis of clotting factors
    D. decreasing platelet aggregation

## THROMBOLYTIC DRUGS

The purpose of giving **thrombolytic** agents is to dissolve thrombi. These drugs stimulate conversion of plasminogen to plasmin, a proteolytic enzyme that breaks down fibrin, the framework of a thrombus. The main use of thrombolytic agents is for management of acute, severe thromboembolic disease, such as myocardial infarction, pulmonary embolism, and iliofemoral thrombosis.

The goal of thrombolytic therapy is to reestablish blood flow as quickly as possible and prevent or limit tissue damage. In coronary circulation, restoration of blood flow reduces morbidity and mortality by limiting myocardial infarction size. In cerebral circulation, rapid thrombus dissolution minimizes neuronal death and brain infarction that produce irreversible brain injury. For people with massive pulmonary embolism, the goal of fibrinolytic therapy is to restore pulmonary artery perfusion. Drugs with shorter half-lives increase the risk of rethrombosis or infarction. Anticoagulant drugs, such as heparin and warfarin, and antiplatelet agents are given following thrombolytic therapy to decrease reformation of a thrombus. Thrombolytic drugs are also used to dissolve clots in arterial or venous cannulas or catheters. **Alteplase** is the prototype recombinant tissue plasminogen activator (rtPA). However, tenecteplase is the thrombolytic of choice in the United States and Canada; it is just as effective as alteplase but results in a decreased risk of noncerebral bleeding.

## Pharmacokinetics

Administration of alteplase is by IV infusion. Metabolism occurs predominately in the liver. Following discontinuation of the infusion, more than 50% of the drug is cleared, with more than 80% clearance within 10 minutes. Excretion takes place in the urine. Whether alteplase crosses the placenta or is excreted into breast milk is unknown.

## Action

Alteplase is a protein that lyses unwanted fibrin blood clots by catalyzing the conversion of plasminogen to plasmin.

## Use

Indications for alteplase include lysis of acute coronary arterial thromboembolism associated with evolving transmural myocardial infarction or acute pulmonary thromboembolism. Clinicians also considered it as first-line therapy for the treatment of acute ischemic stroke in selected people.

Table 9.4 presents dosage information for alteplase and other thrombolytic drugs.

| TABLE 9.4 |
|---|
| **DRUGS AT A GLANCE: Thrombolytics** |

| Drug | Pregnancy Category | Indications for Use | Routes and Dosage Ranges (Adults, Unless Specified) |
|---|---|---|---|
| ℗ **Alteplase** (Activase, Cathflo Activase;  Activase rtPA, Cathflo Activase) | C | Acute ischemic stroke<br>Acute myocardial infarction<br>Acute PE | Ischemic stroke:<br>IV infusion, 0.9 mg/kg total dose administered (not to exceed 90 mg), with 10% of the total dose administered as an initial IV loading dose over 1 min, and the remainder administered over 60 min<br>Myocardial infarction or PE:<br>IV infusion, 100 mg over 3 h (1st h, 60 mg with a bolus of 6–10 mg over 1–2 min initially; 2nd h, 20 mg; 3rd h, 20 mg)<br>Myocardial infarction: accelerated IV infusion, 100 mg total dosage administered as a 15-mg IV bolus, followed by 50 mg IV infused over 30 min, and then 35 mg IV infused over the next 60 min.<br>IV infusion, 100 mg over 3 h (1st h, 60 mg with a bolus of 6–10 mg over 1–2 min initially; 2nd h, 20 mg; 3rd h, 20 mg) |
| Tenecteplase (TNKase;  TNKase) | C | Acute myocardial infarction | IV bolus dose based on weight, 30 mg (for <60 kg) not to exceed 50 mg (>90 kg) |

PE, pulmonary embolism.

## Use in Older Adults

Caution is warranted in older patients (65–80 years of age). Alteplase is not recommended in people older than 80 years of age.

### Use in Patients With Hepatic Impairment

Caution is necessary in patients with significant hepatic impairment.

## Adverse Effects

As with other anticoagulants and antiplatelet agents, bleeding is the main adverse effect of alteplase. To minimize this risk, it is important to select recipients carefully, avoid invasive procedures when possible, and omit anticoagulant or antiplatelet drugs (except for aspirin) while thrombolytics are being given. The major risk of rtPA therapy is symptomatic brain hemorrhage, and when rtPA treatment is chosen, the prescriber should obtain informed consent signed by the stroke patient or family member. There is a 3% mortality rate and a 6% to 8% risk of symptomatic hemorrhage associated with its use. In rtPA overdose, aminocaproic acid serves as an antidote.

## Contraindications

Due to an increased risk of bleeding, alteplase is contraindicated in patients with uncontrolled severe hypertension, aneurysm, arteriovenous malformation, known coagulopathy or internal bleeding, intracranial or intraspinal surgery or trauma within the past 3 months, intracranial mass, recent major surgery, or current use of oral anticoagulants. Alteplase can increase the risk of cerebral embolism in people with atrial fibrillation or atrial flutter.

## Nursing Implications

Only experienced personnel in an emergency department, a critical care unit, or diagnostic/interventional setting with cardiac and other monitoring devices in place should perform thrombolytic therapy. It is necessary to minimize intramuscular injections in patients who are receiving systemic thrombolytic therapy, because bleeding, bruising, or hematomas may develop.

The nurse assesses patients for cardiac dysrhythmias, including sinus bradycardia, premature ventricular contractions, and ventricular tachycardia resulting from reperfusion following coronary thrombolysis. He or she must promptly identify and report any evidence of bleeding.

# Preventing Interactions

Many medications and herbs interact with alteplase, increasing its effect (Boxes 9.14 and 9.15). No herbs or foods appear to decrease its effect.

## *Administering the Medication*

Before a thrombolytic agent is begun, it is essential to check INR, aPTT, platelet count, and fibrinogen to establish baseline values and to determine whether a blood coagulation disorder is present. Two or three hours after thrombolytic therapy is started, the nurse must ensure that the fibrinogen level is measured to determine that fibrinolysis is occurring. Alternatively, he or she can check INR or aPTT for increased values because the breakdown products of fibrin exert anticoagulant effects. During and following alteplase administration, the nurse monitors blood pressure frequently and ensures that it is well controlled. The ISMP lists alteplase as a high-alert drug because of its potential risk of causing significant harm when used in error.

Administration is IV as a bolus injection or infusion. The nurse administers all infusions using an IV infusion device. It is necessary to reconstitute alteplase as indicated and not to shake it.

## *Assessing for Therapeutic Effects*

The goal is to minimize total ischemic time and restore blood flow. Therapeutic effects include the following:

- For cardiac revascularization—stabilization of the patient, reversal of symptoms, stabilization of cardiac rhythm, decrease of the ST-segment elevations by 50% of the initial height, and absence of bleeding complications
- For cerebral revascularization—stabilization of the patient, reversal of symptoms, normal mentation, and absence of bleeding complications

## *Assessing for Adverse Effects*

The nurse assesses for evidence of bleeding. In addition, it is necessary to determine that the condition leading to initiation of thrombolytic therapy is reversed and that there is a return of function. If bleeding does occur, it is most likely from a venipuncture or invasive procedure site, and local pressure may control it. If bleeding cannot be controlled or involves a vital organ, it is necessary to stop the thrombolytic drug and replace fibrinogen with whole blood plasma or cryoprecipitate. Giving aminocaproic acid or tranexamic acid may also be appropriate. When the drugs are used in acute myocardial infarction, cardiac dysrhythmias may occur when blood flow is reestablished. Therefore, antidysrhythmic drugs should be readily available.

---

**BOX 9.14** **Drug Interactions: Alteplase**

**Drugs That Increase the Effects of Alteplase**
- Aspirin or other salicylates, abciximab, cilostazol, clopidogrel, dalteparin, dipyridamole, enoxaparin, eptifibatide, fondaparinux, heparin, nonsteroidal anti-inflammatory drugs, tinzaparin, tirofiban, warfarin
  *Increase the risk of bleeding*

---

**BOX 9.15**  *Herb and Dietary Interactions: Alteplase*

**Herbs and Foods That Increase the Effects of Alteplase**
- Cat's claw, dong quai, evening primrose, feverfew, garlic, ginkgo, ginseng, green tea, horse chestnut, red clover

---

## *Patient Teaching*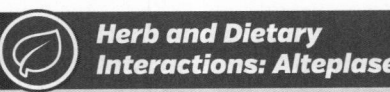

The nurse instructs patients and significant others regarding the purpose of the drug, the underlying condition, and the increased risk of bleeding. Patients should take special care brushing their teeth to reduce bleeding at the gum line. Discharge planning emphasizes managing the complications of the underlying disease (myocardial infarction or stroke) and seeking timely professional help if symptoms recur.

# Other Drugs in the Class

All of the available agents are effective with recommended uses. Thus, the choice of a thrombolytic agent depends mainly on risks of adverse effects and costs. All of the drugs may cause bleeding. Tenecteplase (TNKase) is the other rtPA drug used mainly in acute myocardial infarction to dissolve clots obstructing coronary arteries and reestablish perfusion of tissues beyond the thrombotic area. The most common adverse effect is bleeding, which may be internal (e.g., intracranial, GI, genitourinary) or external (e.g., venous or arterial puncture sites, surgical incisions). Tenecteplase causes less noncerebral bleeding than alteplase, is easier to administer, and lacks antigenicity.

Streptokinase, the original thrombolytic enzyme, and urokinase, a naturally occurring product, are no longer available in the United States. These drugs have been removed from the market because they were not fibrin specific, which enhanced the risk of bleeding. In addition, reteplase has also been removed from the market, but attempts by the manufacturer to seek new drug approval from the FDA are ongoing.

---

**Clinical Application 9.3**

- Before providing care for Mr. Oliver, the nurse reviews his chart (medical diagnosis and medication orders).
- What is the main reason why patients such as Mr. Oliver receive alteplase and heparin?
- What laboratory values should be obtained before a thrombolytic is administered?
- For what adverse effects should the nurse monitor?
- What nursing assessments and patient care goals are necessary in this case?

---

# DRUGS USED TO CONTROL BLEEDING

Anticoagulant, antiplatelet, and thrombolytic drugs profoundly affect hemostasis, and their major adverse effect is bleeding. As a result, systemic hemostatic agents (antidotes) may be needed to prevent or treat significant bleeding episodes. Antidotes should be used cautiously because overuse can increase risks of recurrent thrombotic disorders. Table 9.5 presents the dosage information for the drugs used to control bleeding.

## Reversal of Heparin and Low-Molecular-Weight Heparins

Protamine sulfate is an antidote for standard heparin and LMWHs. Because heparin is an acid and protamine sulfate is a base, protamine neutralizes heparin activity. Protamine dosage depends on the amount of heparin administered during the previous 4 hours. Each milligram of protamine neutralizes approximately 100 units of heparin or dalteparin and 1 mg of enoxaparin. The FDA has issued a **BLACK BOX WARNING ◆** with the use of protamine sulfate because of the risk of severe hypotension, cardiovascular collapse, noncardiogenic pulmonary edema, catastrophic pulmonary vasoconstriction, and pulmonary hypertension with its use. A single dose should not exceed 50 mg because of the risk of severe hypotension, cardiovascular collapse, noncardiogenic pulmonary edema, catastrophic pulmonary vasoconstriction, and pulmonary hypertension with its use. The drug is given by slow IV infusion over at least 10 minutes (to prevent or minimize adverse effects of hypotension, bradycardia, and dyspnea). Its effects occur

## TABLE 9.5

### DRUGS AT A GLANCE: Drugs Used to Control Bleeding

| Drug | Pregnancy Category | Indications for Use | Dosage (Adults, Unless Specified) |
|---|---|---|---|
| Aminocaproic acid (Amicar) | C | Control bleeding caused by overdoses of thrombolytic agents or bleeding disorders caused by hyperfibrinolysis (e.g., cardiac surgery, blood disorders, hepatic cirrhosis, prostatectomy, neoplastic disorders); antidote for tPA | PO, IV infusion, 5 g initially, followed by 1.0 to 1.25 g/h for 8 h or until bleeding is controlled; maximum dose, 30 g/24 h |
| Idarucizumab (Praxbind; 🍁 Praxbind) | Unknown; approved in 2015 | Antidote for dabigatran etexilate (Pradaxa) Control life-threatening bleeding with overdosage of dabigatran Prevention or decrease of bleeding if emergency surgery is required | IV 5 g, administered as two separate 2.5 g doses no more than 15 min apart |
| Protamine sulfate | C | Treatment of heparin overdosage | Depends on the amount of heparin given within the previous 4 h |
| Prothrombin complex concentrate, human (Kcentra; 🍁 Beriplex P/N, Octaplex) | C | Urgent reversal of warfarin overdosage in adults with acute major bleeding or in need of urgent surgery | Individualize dosing based on patient's current predose INR value and body weight INR 2 to <4: 25 units/kg; not to exceed 2500 units INR 4–6: 35 units/kg; not to exceed 3500 units INR >6: 50 units/kg; not to exceed 5000 units Administer vitamin K concurrently to maintain vitamin K–dependent clotting factor levels once the effects of prothrombin complex concentrate have diminished |
| Tranexamic acid (Cyklokapron, Lysteda; 🍁 Cyklokapron, GD-Tranexamic Acid, Tranexamic Acid Injection BP) | B | Control bleeding caused by overdoses of thrombolytic agents Prevent or decrease bleeding from tooth extraction in patients with hemophilia | PO 25 mg/kg 3–4 times daily, starting 1 d before surgery, or IV 10 mg/kg immediately before surgery, followed by 25 mg/kg PO 3–4 times daily for 2–8 d |
| Vitamin K (Mephyton; 🍁 AquaMEPHYTON, Konakion, Mephyton) | C | Antidote for warfarin overdosage | PO 2.5–10 mg (rarely up to 25–50 mg) in a single dose, may repeat 12–48 h if needed, or IV, Sub-Q 2.5–10 mg (rarely up to 25–50 mg) in a single dose, measure INR after 6–8 h. Repeat dose if needed |

immediately and last for approximately 2 hours. A second dose may be required because heparin activity lasts approximately 4 hours. Severe hypotensive and anaphylactoid reactions may result from protamine administration. Thus, the drug should be given in settings with equipment and personnel for resuscitation and management of anaphylactic shock.

## Reversal of Vitamin K Antagonists

Vitamin K (Mephyton) is an antidote for warfarin overdosage. An oral dose of 10 to 20 mg usually stops minor bleeding and returns the INR to a normal range within 24 hours. INR serum levels less than 5 with no significant bleeding may be managed with withholding of the warfarin based on protocols; INR levels greater than 5 may require the use of oral vitamin K. Decisions about management of a patient with an INR above the therapeutic range are based on the degree of elevation of the INR serum level, the clinical status of the patient with regard to bleeding, thrombogenic potential, as well as risk factors such as age and presence of concurrent disease.

Urgent reversal of warfarin overdosage in adults with acute major bleeding or in need of emergent surgery can be accomplished with PCC (Kcentra). The drug, collected from pooled human plasma, contains therapeutic levels of all four vitamin K–dependent coagulation factors (II, VII, IX, and X) and the antithrombotic proteins C and S. Dosing is based on the most current predose INR value and body weight. The drug should be administered concurrently with vitamin K to maintain factor levels once the effects of PCC have diminished. Resumption of anticoagulation should occur once the risk of thromboembolism outweighs the risk of acute bleeding. Unlike plasma, PCC does not require blood group typing or thawing, so it can be administered more quickly than frozen plasma and at recommended doses is administered in a significantly lower volume than plasma.

The FDA has issued a **BLACK BOX WARNING** ◆ with the use of PCC because reversal of an anticoagulant state in patients being treated with vitamin K–antagonist therapy may predispose the patient to a thromboembolic complication. Benefits of reversal must be weighed against potential risk of a subsequent thromboembolic event.

## Reversal of Oral Direct Thrombin Inhibitors

Idarucizumab (Praxbind), a humanized monoclonal antibody fragment, is the antidote for dabigatran, currently the only oral DTI. The drug reverses the anticoagulant effects of dabigatran for uncontrolled or life-threatening bleeding or for emergency surgery or procedures. In adults, the drug is given intravenously, administered as two separate doses no more than 15 minutes apart. The drug's half-life is about 45 minutes in individuals with normal renal function and the duration of the effect is about 24 hours. However, if coagulation parameters reelevate within

12 hours of administration, a second dose may be considered. Reversing the effects of dabigatran will subject a patient to an elevated risk of thrombosis, so it is necessary to resume anticoagulant therapy after 24 hours of administering idarucizumab, as appropriate.

## Reversal of Thrombolytic Agents

Aminocaproic acid (Amicar) and tranexamic acid (Cyklokapron) are used to stop bleeding caused by overdoses of thrombolytic agents. Aminocaproic acid also may be used in other bleeding disorders caused by hyperfibrinolysis (e.g., in cardiac surgery, blood disorders, hepatic cirrhosis, prostatectomy, neoplastic disorders). Tranexamic acid also is used for short periods (2–8 days) in patients with hemophilia to prevent or decrease bleeding from tooth extraction or menorrhagia.

Depending on the indication for administration, aminocaproic acid may be infused as a loading dose over 15 to 60 minutes to reduce the risk of hypotension and dysrhythmias with a rapid bolus. A continuous infusion may be required. Tranexamic acid can be administered orally or intravenously. Tablets should be swallowed whole. A rapid IV bolus can be given, but the drug is usually administered diluted and administered intravenously over 5 to 30 minutes. Dosage of the drug should be reduced in the presence of moderate or severe renal impairment.

## NCLEX Success

7. Clopidogrel is indicated for which of the following?
   A. reduction of myocardial infarction, stroke, and vascular death in patients with atherosclerosis
   B. adjunctive therapy to warfarin for deep vein thrombosis
   C. heparin-induced thrombocytopenia
   D. patients in whom bleeding is a consideration

8. A patient who received a copy of her genomic testing and is classed as a "poor metabolizer" of clopidogrel asks the nurse what it means. The nurse, understanding the variant response to CYP2C19, would be most correct in stating which of the following?
   A. "You metabolize the medication different than some individuals and may not receive the same benefit from drug therapy."
   B. "You lack the CPY2C19 isozyme, so you will not need to take clopidogrel."
   C. "You will be prescribed less of the medication than is normally necessary."
   D. "You are at a higher risk of bleeding from the drug, so you must be extra careful."

## THE NURSING PROCESS

A concept map outlines the nursing process related to drug therapy considerations in this chapter. Additional nursing implications related to the disease process should also be considered in care decisions.

**Assessment**

- Assess risk factors, history, or disease associated with thromboembolism, such as smoking, immobility, obesity, oral contraceptives, recent surgery, prosthetic heart valve, atrial fibrillation,  and heart failure.
- Assess for signs and symptoms of thrombotic and thromboembolic disorders, such as  DVT, pulmonary embolism, and disseminated intravascular coagulation (DIC).

**Outcomes of Therapy**

The patient will
- Receive or take anticoagulant and antiplatelet drugs correctly.
- Be monitored closely for therapeutic and adverse drug effects, especially when drug therapy is started and when changes are made in drugs or dosages.
- Use nondrug measures to decrease venous stasis and prevent thromboembolic disorders. Act to prevent trauma from falls and other injuries.
- Avoid or report adverse drug reactions.
- Verbalize or demonstrate knowledge of safe management of anticoagulant drug therapy.
- Keep follow-up appointments for tests of blood coagulation and drug dosage regulation.
- Avoid preventable bleeding episodes.

**Nursing Interventions**

- For patients who cannot ambulate safely because of weakness, sedation, or other conditions, keep the call light within reach, keep bed rails elevated, and assist in ambulation. Provide an electric razor for shaving.
- Avoid intramuscular injections, venipunctures, and arterial punctures when possible. Avoid inserting nasogastric tubes or indwelling urinary catheters if possible.
- See additional patient teaching guidelines in text.

**Evaluation**

- Interview and observe for relief of symptoms and compliance with instructions for which anticoagulants are prescribed.
- Interview and observe for accurate drug administration.
- Observe for signs and symptoms of thromboembolic disorders or bleeding.
- Evaluate blood coagulation tests for therapeutic ranges.
- Observe and interview regarding adverse drug effects.

## KEY CONCEPTS

- Anticoagulant drugs are given to prevent formation of new clots and extension of clots already present.
- Antiplatelet drugs are used to prevent arterial thrombosis.
- Thrombolytic agents are used to dissolve thrombi and limit tissue damage in selected thromboembolic disorders.
- Heparin is the anticoagulant of choice in acute venous thromboembolic disorders because the anticoagulant effect begins immediately with IV administration.
- When anticoagulation is required during pregnancy, heparin is used because it does not cross the placenta.
- Currently available LMWHs (dalteparin, enoxaparin) differ from standard heparin and each other and are not interchangeable.
- During heparin therapy, the aPTT should be maintained at approximately 1.5 to 2.5 times the control or baseline value.
- Monitoring of aPTT is not necessary with low-dose standard heparin given subcutaneously for prophylaxis of thromboembolism or with the LMWHs.
- Protamine sulfate is the antidote for standard heparin and LMWHs.
- The FDA has issued a **BLACK BOX WARNING ◆** with the use of protamine sulfate because of the risk of severe hypotension, cardiovascular collapse, noncardiogenic pulmonary edema, catastrophic pulmonary vasoconstriction, and pulmonary hypertension with its use.
- Warfarin dosage is regulated according to the INR (derived from prothrombin time [PT]), for which a therapeutic value is between 2.0 and 3.0 in most conditions; a therapeutic PT value is approximately 1.5 times the control, or 18 seconds.
- Vitamin K (Mephyton) and prothrombin complex concentrate can reverse the effects of warfarin.
- The FDA has issued a **BLACK BOX WARNING ◆** with warfarin because of its risk of causing major or fatal bleeding.
- The FDA has issued a **BLACK BOX WARNING ◆** with the use of prothrombin complex concentrate because reversal of an anticoagulant state in patients being treated with vitamin K antagonist therapy may predispose the patient to a thromboembolic complication.
- Aspirin has long been the most widely used antiplatelet drug for prevention of myocardial reinfarction and arterial thrombosis in patients with TIAs and prosthetic heart valves. However, clopidogrel may be more effective than aspirin.
- No antidote exists for the effects of aspirin or the adenosine diphosphate receptor antagonists because both produce irreversible platelet effects; platelet transfusion may be required.
- The FDA has issued a **BLACK BOX WARNING ◆** with the use of clopidogrel in people who are reduced metabolizers of the drug; these people may remain at risk for heart attack, stroke, and cardiovascular death because of the drug's reduced effect on platelet function.
- The FDA has issued a **BLACK BOX WARNING ◆** with the use of cilostazol as it is contraindicated in patients with heart failure of any severity.
- The FDA has issued a **BLACK BOX WARNING ◆** with the use of ticagrelor as it increases the risk of bleeding, including significant and possibly fatal hemorrhage.
- When the thrombolytic agents are used in acute myocardial infarction, cardiac dysrhythmias may likely occur when blood flow is reestablished; antidysrhythmic drugs should be readily available.

## CLINICAL REASONING CASE STUDY

**Meet the Patient**

Jane Carter, a 67-year-old retired college faculty member, has a history of TIAs and takes clopidogrel (Plavix) because she cannot tolerate aspirin. She presents for a routine clinic visit. Her complete blood count (CBC) results are as follows: white blood cells 3000 cells/mcL, red blood cells 4.2 to 5.4 million cells/mcL, hemoglobin 12 to 16 g/dL, hematocrit 42%, platelets 100,000/mm³.

- What are the benefits of clopidogrel in patients with a history of TIA?
- How would you interpret her CBC results?
- Given Ms. Carter's laboratory results, what adverse effects would you need to observe for and instruct her about?

**Assessing Drug Information**

- Clopidogrel is an adenosine diphosphate (ADP) receptor antagonist with antiplatelet effects similar to aspirin. The drug inhibits the ADP receptor on the surface of platelets, preventing platelets from clumping together as part of a blood clot.
- Clopidogrel produces irreversible platelet inhibition for the lifespan of the platelet (7–10 days) and has no reversing agent or antidote.
- Clopidogrel is indicated for prevention of thrombotic stroke in people who have had stroke precursor events (e.g., TIAs) or a completed thrombotic stroke. This antiplatelet drug is considered a second-line drug for patients who cannot take aspirin.
- Clopidogrel is a prodrug and is converted to its active form by hepatic CYP2C19 (an isozyme of the cytochrome P450 system). People with variant forms of CYP2C19 may be poor or ultrarapid metabolizers of clopidogrel. Ultrarapid metabolizers of clopidogrel may have an increased risk of bleeding. With poor metabolizers, the benefits of the drug may not be adequate.
- The most common adverse effects associated with clopidogrel are bleeding, pruritus, rash, purpura, and diarrhea.

**Nursing Actions**

- Ms. Carter has neutropenia and thrombocytopenia. Her red blood cell count and hemoglobin/hematocrit are within normal limits.
- She has an increased risk of bleeding and infection. The nurse observes for bleeding and instructs the patient about the risk of bleeding, including gastrointestinal and cerebral bleeding. Nosebleeds, bleeding at the gum line, petechiae, or other episodes of bleeding may indicate signs of adverse effects and should be reported promptly. Instruction on reducing the risk and recognizing signs of infection should occur.
- The nurse instructs Ms. Carter to take the medication as directed and not to double the medication if a dose is missed. Additional patient teaching guidelines are outlined in Box 9.11.

Visit thePoint® at **http://thePoint.lww.com/Frandsen12e** *for answers to NCLEX Success questions (in Appendix A), answers to Clinical Application Case Studies (in Appendix B), and more!*

## REFERENCES AND RESOURCES

Baglin, T., Hillarp, A., Tripodi, A., Elalamy, I., Bueller, H., & Ageno, W. (2013). Measuring oral direct inhibitors of thrombin and factor Xa: A recommendation from the Subcommittee on Control of Anticoagulation of the Scientific and Standardization Committee of the International Society on Thrombosis and Haemostasis. *Journal of Thrombosis and Haemostasis, 11*(4), 756–760.

Callaway, C. W., Donnino, M. W., Fink, E. L., Geocadin, R. G., Golan, E., Kern, K. B., et al. (2015). Post-cardiac arrest care: 2015 American Heart Association guidelines update for cardiopulmonary resuscitation and emergency cardiovascular care. *Circulation, 132,* S465–S482.

Guyatt, G. H., Akl, E. A., Crowther, M., Gutterman, D. D., & Schuünemann, H. J. (2012). Executive summary: Antithrombotic Therapy and Prevention of Thrombosis, 9th ed: American College of Chest Physicians Evidence-Based Clinical Practice Guidelines. *Chest, 141*(2 Suppl), 7–47.

Karch, A. M. (2019). *2019 Lippincott's pocket drug guide for nurses.* Philadelphia, PA: Lippincott Williams & Wilkins.

Lansberg, M. G., O'Donnell, M. J., Khatri, P., Lang, E. S., Nguyen-Huynh, M. N., Schwartz, N. E., et al. (2012). Antithrombotic and thrombolytic therapy for ischemic stroke: Antithrombotic Therapy and Prevention of Thrombosis, 9th ed: American College of Chest Physicians Evidence-Based Clinical Practice Guidelines. *Chest, 141*(2 Suppl), e601S–e636S.

Levy, J. H., Ageno, W., Chan, N. C., Crowther, M., Verhamme, P., & Weitz, J. I. and for the Subcommittee on Control of Anticoagulation. (2015). When and how to use antidotes for the reversal of direct oral anticoagulants:

Guidance from the SSC of the ISTH. *Journal of Thrombosis and Haemostasis, 14*(3), 63-627. https://doi.org/10.1111/jth.13227

Norris, T. L. (2019). *Porth's pathophysiology: Concepts of altered health states* (10th ed.). Philadelphia, PA: Lippincott Williams & Wilkins.

Pollack, C. V., Reilly, P. A., Eikelboom, J., Glund S., Verhamme, P., Bernstein, R. A., et al. (2015). Idarucizumab for dabigatran reversal. *New England Journal of Medicine, 373,* 511–520.

Powers, W. J., Rabinstein, A. A., Ackerson, T., Adeoye, O. M., Bambakidis, N. C., Becker, K., et al. on behalf of the American Heart Association Stroke Council. (2018). 2018 Guidelines for the Early Management of Patients With Acute Ischemic Stroke: A Guideline for Healthcare Professionals From the American Heart Association/American Stroke Association. *Stroke, 49,* e46–e110. doi:10.1161/STR.0000000000000158

Smith, E. E., Kent, D. M., Bulsara, K. R., Leung, L. Y., Lichtman, J. H., Reeves, M. J., et al. (2018). Effect of dysphagia screening strategies on clinical outcomes after stroke: A systematic review for the 2018 guidelines for the early management of patients with acute ischemic stroke: a guideline for healthcare professionals from the American Heart Association/American Stroke Association. *Stroke, 49,* e123–e128. doi:10.1161/STR.0000000000000159

Tomaselli, G. F., Mahaffey, K. W., Cuker, A., Dobesh, P. P., Doherty, J. U., Eikelboom, J. W., et al.; Writing Committee. (2017). 2017 ACC Expert Consensus Decision Pathway on Management of Bleeding in Patients on Oral Anticoagulants: A Report of the American College of Cardiology Task Force on Expert Consensus Decision Pathways. *Journal of the American College of Cardiology, 70,* 3042–3067. doi:10.1016/j.jacc.2017.09.1085

UpToDate. (2019). *Drug information.* Lexi-Comp, Inc.

Weitz, J. I. (2015). Anticoagulation therapy in 2015: Where we are and where we are going. *Journal of Thrombosis and Thrombolysis, 39,* 264–272.

# Drug Therapy for Dyslipidemia

## LEARNING OBJECTIVES

*After studying this chapter, you should be able to:*

1. Recognize the role of dyslipidemia in atherosclerotic cardiovascular disease.
2. Identify sources and functions of cholesterol and triglycerides.
3. Educate patients regarding lifestyle modification strategies to prevent or reduce dyslipidemia.
4. Identify the prototype drug from each drug class used to treat dyslipidemia.
5. Describe the classes of dyslipidemic drugs in terms of their mechanism of action, indications for use, major adverse effects, and nursing implications.
6. Implement the nursing process in the care of patients with dyslipidemia.

## CLINICAL APPLICATION CASE STUDY

Edward Watkins, a 62-year-old man, has had elevated cholesterol and triglyceride levels at his two previous visits to the nurse practitioner. He has tried diet modification and increasing exercise; however, he remains overweight and his lipid values remain elevated. His latest laboratory findings at this visit are total serum cholesterol 239 mg/dL, low-density lipoprotein (LDL) cholesterol 162 mg/dL, high-density lipoprotein cholesterol 40 mg/dL, and triglycerides 220 mg/dL. His nurse practitioner decides to prescribe atorvastatin 10 mg PO once daily and gemfibrozil 600 mg PO twice a day.

## KEY TERMS

**Central adiposity:** accumulation of abdominal fat, resulting in an increased waist circumference

**Cholesterol:** component of cell membrane that is produced and processed in the liver; a fat essential for the formation of steroid hormones that is produced in cells and taken in by dietary sources

**Dyslipidemia:** abnormal lipid levels in the blood; associated with atherosclerosis and its many pathophysiologic effects (e.g., myocardial ischemia and infarction, stroke, peripheral arterial occlusive disease)

**Lipoproteins:** specific proteins in plasma that transport blood lipids; contain cholesterol, phospholipid, and triglyceride bound to protein. They vary in density and amounts of lipid and protein

**Metabolic syndrome:** cluster of several cardiovascular risk factors linked with obesity: increased waist circumference, elevated triglycerides, reduced high-density lipoprotein cholesterol, elevated blood pressure, and elevated fasting glucose

# INTRODUCTION

Elevated blood lipids are a major risk factor for atherosclerosis and cardiovascular disorders such as coronary artery disease and stroke. Therapeutic lifestyle changes (including dietary modification, physical activity, and smoking cessation) have been the cornerstone of population-based interventions to manage dyslipidemia. However, making the commitment is often insufficient to achieve recommended treatment targets. When lifestyle changes alone do not reduce blood lipids, dyslipidemic drugs are used in the management of patients with elevated blood lipids. Several organizations have released guidelines for the treatment of dyslipidemia and have placed different emphasis on the importance of targeting individual blood lipid levels (i.e., total cholesterol, low-density lipoprotein [LDL] cholesterol, high-density lipoprotein [HDL] cholesterol, triglycerides) and benchmark levels of cardiac risk to improve morbidity and mortality. Guidelines from 2013 for treatment of dyslipidemia released by the American College of Cardiology and the American Heart Association (ACC/AHA) updated the previous Adult Treatment Panel III recommendations of the National Cholesterol Education Program (NCEP). The recent 2018 ACC/AHA guidelines recommend using a lower-risk benchmark and standards for individuals who take dyslipidemic drugs and provide a calculator for a 10-year risk estimate for myocardial infarction or stroke. In these guidelines, treatment considerations to manage cardiovascular risk are more meaningful than targeting optimization of blood lipid levels. The U.S. Preventive Services Task Force recommends using statins to prevent cardiovascular disease.

Dyslipidemic drugs are used to decrease blood lipids, prevent or delay the development of atherosclerotic plaque, promote the regression of existing atherosclerotic plaque, and reduce morbidity and mortality from atherosclerotic cardiovascular disease (ASCVD). To understand the clinical use of these drugs, it is necessary to understand characteristics of blood lipids, metabolic syndrome, and types of blood lipid disorders.

# OVERVIEW OF DYSLIPIDEMIA

## Etiology

Blood lipids, which include **cholesterol**, phospholipids, and triglycerides, are derived from the diet or synthesized by the liver and intestine. Most cholesterol is found in body cells, where it is a component of cell membranes and performs other essential functions. In cells of the adrenal glands, ovaries, and testes, cholesterol is required for the synthesis of steroid hormones (e.g., cortisol, estrogen, progesterone, testosterone). In liver cells, cholesterol is used to form cholic acid, which is conjugated with other substances to form bile salts; these salts promote absorption and digestion of fats. In addition, a small amount of cholesterol is found in blood serum. Serum cholesterol is the portion of total body cholesterol involved in formation of atherosclerotic plaques. Unless a person has a genetic disorder of lipid metabolism, the amount of cholesterol in the blood is strongly related to dietary intake of saturated fat. Phospholipids are essential components of cell membranes, and triglycerides provide energy for cellular metabolism.

Blood lipids are transported in plasma by specific proteins called **lipoproteins**. Each lipoprotein contains cholesterol, phospholipid, and triglyceride bound to protein. The lipoproteins vary in density and amounts of lipid and protein. Density is determined mainly by the amount of protein, which is denser than fat. Thus, density increases as the proportion of protein increases. The lipoproteins are differentiated according to these properties, which can be measured in the laboratory. For example, HDL cholesterol contains larger amounts of protein and smaller amounts of lipid; LDL cholesterol contains less protein and larger amounts of lipid. Other plasma lipoproteins are chylomicrons and very-low-density lipoproteins (VLDLs). Additional characteristics of lipoproteins are described in Box 10.1.

## Pathophysiology

Abnormal lipid levels in the blood, or **dyslipidemia** (also called hyperlipidemia because blood levels of lipoproteins accompany increased blood lipid levels), is associated with atherosclerosis and its many pathophysiologic effects (e.g., myocardial ischemia and infarction, stroke, peripheral arterial occlusive disease). Ischemic heart disease has a high rate of morbidity and mortality. Elevated total cholesterol and LDL cholesterol and reduced HDL cholesterol are the abnormalities that are major risk factors for coronary artery disease. Elevated triglycerides also play a role in cardiovascular disease. For example, high blood levels reflect excessive caloric intake (excessive dietary fats are stored in adipose tissue; excessive proteins and carbohydrates are converted to triglycerides and also stored in adipose tissue) and obesity. High caloric intake also increases the conversion of VLDL to LDL cholesterol, and high dietary intake of triglycerides and saturated fat decreases the activity of LDL receptors and increases synthesis of cholesterol. Very high triglyceride levels are associated with acute pancreatitis.

Dyslipidemia may be primary (i.e., genetic or familial) or secondary to dietary habits, other diseases (e.g., diabetes mellitus, alcoholism, hypothyroidism, obesity, obstructive liver disease), and medications (e.g., beta-adrenergic blockers, cyclosporine, oral estrogens, glucocorticoids, sertraline, thiazide diuretics, anti–human immunodeficiency virus [HIV] protease inhibitors).

**Metabolic syndrome** is a group of cardiovascular risk factors linked with obesity. In 2001, the Third Report of the NCEP Expert Panel on Detection, Evaluation, and Treatment of High Blood Cholesterol in Adults (NCEP III) clustered several elements of metabolic syndrome: **central adiposity** (increased waist circumference), elevated triglycerides, reduced HDL cholesterol, elevated blood pressure, and elevated fasting glucose. Questions have been raised as to whether the metabolic syndrome, as currently defined, describes any unique pathophysiology and whether metabolic syndrome confers additional risk beyond its individual components. Although the syndrome is associated with a doubling of cardiovascular disease risk, much of this increase is the sum of its individual components. This chapter specifically addresses management of components of metabolic syndrome related to dyslipidemia; additional discussion of other factors is found in Chapters 28 and 41.

| BOX 10.1 | *Types of Lipoproteins* |
|---|---|

**Chylomicrons**, the largest lipoprotein molecules, are synthesized in the wall of the small intestine. They carry recently ingested dietary cholesterol and triglycerides that have been absorbed from the gastrointestinal tract. Hyperchylomicronemia normally occurs after a fatty meal, reaches peak levels in 3 to 4 hours, and subsides within 12 to 14 hours. Chylomicrons carry triglycerides to fat and muscle cells, where the enzyme lipoprotein lipase breaks down the molecule and releases fatty acids to be used for energy or stored as fat. This process leaves a remnant containing cholesterol, which is then transported to the liver. Thus, chylomicrons transport triglycerides to peripheral tissues and cholesterol to the liver.

**Low-density lipoprotein (LDL) cholesterol**, sometimes called "bad cholesterol," transports approximately 75% of serum cholesterol and carries it to peripheral tissues and the liver. LDL cholesterol is removed from the circulation by receptor and nonreceptor mechanisms. The receptor mechanism involves the binding of LDL cholesterol to receptors on cell surface membranes. The bound LDL molecule is then engulfed into the cell, where it is broken down by enzymes and releases free cholesterol into the cytoplasm.

Most LDL cholesterol receptors are located in the liver. However, nonhepatic tissues (e.g., adrenal glands, smooth muscle cells, endothelial cells, and lymphoid cells) also have receptors by which they obtain the cholesterol needed for building cell membranes and synthesizing hormones. These cells can regulate their cholesterol intake by adding or removing LDL receptors.

Approximately two thirds of the LDL cholesterol is removed from the bloodstream by the receptor-dependent mechanism. The number of LDL receptors on cell membranes determines the amount of LDL degradation (i.e., the more receptors on cells, the more LDL is broken down). Conditions that decrease the number or function of receptors (e.g., high dietary intake of cholesterol, saturated fat, or calories) increase blood levels of LDL.

The remaining one third is removed by mechanisms that do not involve receptors. Nonreceptor uptake occurs in various cells, especially when levels of circulating LDL cholesterol are high. For example, macrophage cells in arterial walls can attach LDL, thereby promoting accumulation of cholesterol and the development of atherosclerosis. The amount of LDL cholesterol removed by nonreceptor mechanisms is increased with inadequate numbers of receptors or excessive amounts of LDL cholesterol.

A high serum level of LDL cholesterol is atherogenic and a strong risk factor for coronary heart disease. The body normally attempts to compensate for high serum levels by inhibiting hepatic synthesis of cholesterol and cellular synthesis of new LDL receptors.

**Very-low-density lipoprotein (VLDL)** contains approximately 75% triglycerides and 25% cholesterol. It transports endogenous triglycerides (those synthesized in the liver and intestine, not those derived exogenously, from food) to fat and muscle cells. There, as with chylomicrons, lipoprotein lipase breaks down the molecule and releases fatty acids to be used for energy or stored as fat. The removal of triglycerides from VLDL leaves a cholesterol-rich remnant, which returns to the liver. Then the cholesterol is secreted into the intestine, mostly as bile acids, or it is used to form more VLDL and recirculated.

**High-density lipoprotein (HDL) cholesterol**, often referred to as "good cholesterol," is a small but very important lipoprotein. It is synthesized in the liver and intestine, and some is derived from the enzymatic breakdown of chylomicrons and VLDL. It contains moderate amounts of cholesterol. However, this cholesterol is transported from blood vessel walls to the liver for catabolism and excretion. This reverse transport of cholesterol has protective effects against coronary heart disease.

The mechanisms by which HDL cholesterol exerts protective effects are unknown. Possible mechanisms include clearing cholesterol from atheromatous plaque, increasing excretion of cholesterol so less is available for reuse in the formation of LDL cholesterol, and inhibiting cellular uptake of LDL cholesterol. Regular exercise and moderate alcohol consumption are associated with increased levels of HDL cholesterol; obesity, diabetes mellitus, genetic factors, smoking, and some medications (e.g., steroids and beta-adrenergic blockers) are associated with decreased levels. HDL cholesterol levels are not directly affected by diet.

## Clinical Manifestations

A lipid profile consists of a total cholesterol, HDL cholesterol, LDL cholesterol, and triglycerides. For accurate interpretation, blood samples for laboratory testing of triglycerides should be drawn after the patient has fasted for 12 hours. Fasting does not appear to be required for cholesterol testing. However, since triglycerides require fasting, and guidelines for interpreting nonfasting levels for evaluating cardiovascular risk have not been established; therefore, fasting is recommended prior to tests for a lipid profile. Normal lipid levels in adults and children are outlined in Table 10.1. Of the types of dyslipidemias most often described, hypercholesterolemia is usually emphasized; however, hypertriglyceridemia is also associated with most types of hyperlipoproteinemia.

In the past, the total cholesterol-to-HDL cholesterol ratio has been used to predict the risk of developing atherosclerosis (total cholesterol value divided by the value of the HDL cholesterol). Currently, the ACC/AHA recommendations do not target fixed LDL and HDL cholesterol goals but focus on calculating and reducing cardiovascular risk.

## Screening

Evidence indicates that atherosclerotic lesions can begin in childhood, and recommendations from the National Heart, Lung, and Blood Institute (2012) support selective screening of children with a fasting lipid profile at age 2 who have a family history (first-degree relatives) of premature ASCVD (by age 55 in males or by age 65 in females), have a parent with dyslipidemia, have any other risk factors or high-risk conditions, or have no available family history. If a new family history is identified or a high-risk condition develops as a child grows, a fasting lipid profile is advised. Recommendations indicate that universal lipid screening should begin between ages 9 and 11.

**TABLE 10.1**

## Plasma Cholesterol and Triglyceride Levels in Adults and Children

| | Adults | Children (>3 Years of Age) |
|---|---|---|
| Total serum cholesterol (mg/dL) | Desirable = <200<br>Borderline = 200–239<br>Undesirable = 240 or above | Desirable = <170<br>Borderline = 170–199<br>Undesirable = 200 or above |
| LDL cholesterol (mg/dL) | Desirable = <130<br>Borderline = 130–159<br>Undesirable = 160 or above | Desirable = 110–129<br>Undesirable = >130 or above |
| HDL cholesterol (mg/dL) | Desirable = 40 or above*<br>Undesirable = <40 | Desirable level = >45<br>Borderline = 35–45<br>Undesirable = <35 |
| Triglycerides (mg/dL) | Desirable = <150<br>Borderline = 150–199<br>Undesirable = 200 or above | Desirable = <125<br>Undesirable = >125 or above |

*If the HDL cholesterol level is 60 mg/dL or above, one risk factor for coronary heart disease can be subtracted in adults when calculating risk.

In the absence of risk factors for ASCVD, middle-aged adults should be screened for dyslipidemia at least every 1 to 2 years. With known ASCVD risk and increasing age, frequency of testing should be based on current treatment guidelines, individual clinical circumstances, and the provider's best judgment.

## Management

Overall, the most effective blood lipid profile for prevention or management of arteriosclerotic cardiovascular disease and its sequelae is high HDL cholesterol, low LDL cholesterol, and low total cholesterol; a low triglyceride level is also desirable (see Table 10.1). Treatment goals for patients with lipid abnormalities should be personalized by levels of risk. Therapeutic lifestyle changes are recommended to lower serum cholesterol levels for all age groups, particularly in patients who already have cardiovascular disease or diabetes mellitus.

### Lifestyle Changes

Primary prevention of cardiovascular risk factors associated with dyslipidemia should begin in all healthy children older than 2 years and continue for life. The previously mentioned 2018 guidelines of the ACC/AHA support their 2013 evidence-based recommendations regarding the importance of lifestyle management in the treatment of dyslipidemia. Strategies that promote risk reduction of lifestyle factors include an emphasis on balanced nutrition and exercise. In normal children and adolescents or those with dyslipidemia older than age 2, the use of the evidence-based Cardiovascular Health Integrated Lifestyle Diet, or CHILD 1, is recommended. Within appropriate age-, sex-, and activity-based requirements for growth and nutrition, intake of total fat can be safely limited to 25% to 30% of total calories, saturated fat intake to 8% to 10% of calories, and dietary cholesterol to 300 mg. High dietary fiber intake from foods (not supplements) is encouraged.

In adults, modification of total fat intake is recommended. Intake of total fat can be safely limited to 25% to 30% of total calories, saturated fat intake to 7% of calories, and dietary

cholesterol to 200 mg with only enough calories to reach or maintain a healthy weight. LDL cholesterol–lowering macronutrients should be increased in the diet and include 2 g/day of plant stanols/sterols (e.g., margarine spreads [Benecol], stanol-fortified orange juice, cereals, granola bars) and 10 to 25 g/day of soluble fiber (e.g., psyllium preparations, oat bran, pectin, fruits, and vegetables). If patient is overweight or obese, a reduced-calorie diet consisting of fruits and vegetables (five or more servings/day), grains (six or more servings/day, one third of those as whole grains), fish, and lean meats is recommended. Additional focus on managing modifiable risk factors such as hypertension, diabetes, obesity, and cigarette smoking further reduces dyslipidemia and the development of ASCVD.

In children older than 5 years of age, 1 hour of daily moderate to vigorous activity is recommended. There is no evidence that increasing physical activity in normal children is harmful. In adults, an increase in physical activity, including an emphasis on regular moderate-intensity aerobic exercise (usually 30 minutes at least three times weekly), will promote enhanced cardiovascular health and promote weight loss. In addition to aerobic activity, muscle-strengthening activity is recommended at least 2 days a week.

Support for patients who smoke in their cessation efforts is critical. In addition to numerous other benefits, HDL levels are higher in nonsmokers. If the patient is perimenopausal, hormone replacement therapy can raise HDL and lower LDL.

Box 10.2 identifies some herbs and foods reported to have an effect on serum cholesterol and triglyceride levels.

### Clinical Application 10.1

- What is the purpose of attempting weight reduction and increasing activity for Mr. Watkins before starting dyslipidemic medications?
- How would the nurse interpret the current laboratory values of Mr. Watkins?

| BOX 10.2 | *Herbs and Foods Reported to Have Evidence-Based Effects on Cholesterol and Triglyceride Levels* |
|---|---|

**Flaxseed**

- Low-density lipoprotein (LDL) cholesterol: decreased with flaxseed and flaxseed lignans; no apparent decrease with flaxseed oil
- Triglycerides: no apparent effect
- Absorption of all medications may be decreased when taken with flax, resulting in a less than therapeutic effect.

**Garlic**

- LDL cholesterol: no significant effect
- Triglycerides: no significant effect
- Bleeding may be increased when garlic is combined with anticoagulants, and insulin doses may need to be decreased as a result of the hypoglycemic effect of garlic.

**Red Yeast Rice**

- Total and LDL cholesterol: decreased
- Triglycerides: no significant effect
- Dosage standardization is a concern, and information about long-term safety is unavailable.

**Soy**

- LDL cholesterol: benefit at most small
- Triglycerides: no significant effect
- Intake of soy proteins may have other beneficial vascular effects.

## NCLEX Success

1. The primary focus for prevention and management of metabolic syndrome and its sequelae is

    A. elevated high-density lipoprotein (HDL) cholesterol, depressed low-density lipoprotein (LDL) cholesterol, and low total cholesterol
    B. low HDL cholesterol, low LDL cholesterol, and low total cholesterol
    C. low triglycerides
    D. high HDL cholesterol, low LDL cholesterol, and low triglycerides

2. A person with type 1 diabetes mellitus and hypertension has the following lipid profile: total serum cholesterol 288 mg/dL, low-density lipoprotein (LDL) cholesterol 200 mg/dL, high-density lipoprotein (HDL) cholesterol 48 mg/dL, and triglycerides 200 mg/dL. How would you evaluate the results of the lipid profile? (Select all that apply.)

    A. LDL cholesterol is elevated.
    B. HDL cholesterol is within normal limits.
    C. Triglyceride level is elevated.
    D. Total cholesterol is within normal limits.

3. A 48-year-old man visits his health care provider for his annual checkup. He is otherwise in good health, but assessment findings reveal the new onset of a slight increase in blood pressure and a total serum cholesterol of 240 mg/dL. What can the nurse anticipate as the preferred treatment for this patient?

    A. a low-lipid diet and an exercise program
    B. a low-lipid diet and a cholesterol synthesis inhibitor
    C. an exercise program and a fibrate
    D. a low-lipid diet and an exercise program

### Drug Therapy

Clinical data suggest that drug therapy may be efficacious even for those with mild to moderate elevations of LDL cholesterol, particularly with preexisting cardiovascular disease. Dyslipidemic drugs act by altering the production, absorption, metabolism, or removal of lipids and lipoproteins. Depending on cardiovascular risk, drug therapy is initiated after 6 months of dietary and other lifestyle changes fail to decrease dyslipidemia to an acceptable level. It is also recommended for patients with signs and symptoms of coronary heart disease, a strong family history of coronary heart disease or dyslipidemia, or other risk factors for atherosclerotic vascular disease (e.g., hypertension, diabetes mellitus, cigarette smoking). Although several dyslipidemic drugs are available, none is effective in all types of dyslipidemia, so drug selection is based on the type of dyslipidemia and its severity. To lower cholesterol using a single drug, a statin is preferred. To lower cholesterol and triglycerides, a statin, a cholesterol absorption inhibitor, gemfibrozil, or a fibrate may be used. To lower triglycerides, gemfibrozil, ezetimibe, or a cholesterol absorption inhibitor may be given. Alternatively, in specific clinical situations (triglyceride level greater than 500 mg/dL), the vitamin niacin may be used. Categories of drugs are described in upcoming sections. Table 10.2 and the Drugs at a Glance tables list individual drugs used in the treatment of dyslipidemia. Figure 10.1 shows the sites of action of dyslipidemic drugs.

## HMG-COA REDUCTASE INHIBITORS

**Atorvastatin** (Lipitor), one of the most widely used drugs in the United States, is the prototype of the class of drugs called the hydroxymethylglutaryl-coenzyme A (HMG-CoA) reductase inhibitors or statins. By decreasing production of cholesterol, the statins decrease total serum cholesterol, LDL cholesterol, VLDL cholesterol, and triglycerides. They reduce LDL cholesterol within 2 weeks and reach maximal effects in approximately 4 to 6 weeks. HDL cholesterol levels remain unchanged or may increase.

The most commonly prescribed statin, atorvastatin, is useful for treating dyslipidemia and is an overall tool in the primary prevention of cardiovascular disease. Several clinical trials have supported the beneficial effects of statins in women with coronary artery disease. In addition, studies have suggested that atorvastatin may possess some benefits that other statins do not. Research has focused on multiple outcomes, including intimal thickness, results of imaging studies, mortality, incidence of stroke, and progression of lesions, but there continue to be questions about the benefit profiles of individual statin drugs.

**TABLE 10.2**

## Drugs Administered for the Treatment of Dyslipidemia

| Drug Class | Prototype | Other Drugs in the Class |
|---|---|---|
| HMG-CoA reductase inhibitors (statins) | Atorvastatin (Lipitor) | Fluvastatin (Lescol)<br>Lovastatin (Altoprev)<br>Pitavastatin (Livalo)<br>Pravastatin (Pravachol)<br>Rosuvastatin (Crestor)<br>Simvastatin (Zocor) |
| Bile acid sequestrants | Cholestyramine (Prevalite, Questran) | Colesevelam (Welchol)<br>Colestipol (Colestid) |
| Fibrates | Fenofibrate (Tricor) | Gemfibrozil (Lopid) |
| Cholesterol absorption inhibitor | Ezetimibe (Zetia) | |
| PCSK9 inhibitors | Alirocumab (Praluent) | Evolocumab (Repatha) |
| Miscellaneous dyslipidemic agent | | Niacin |

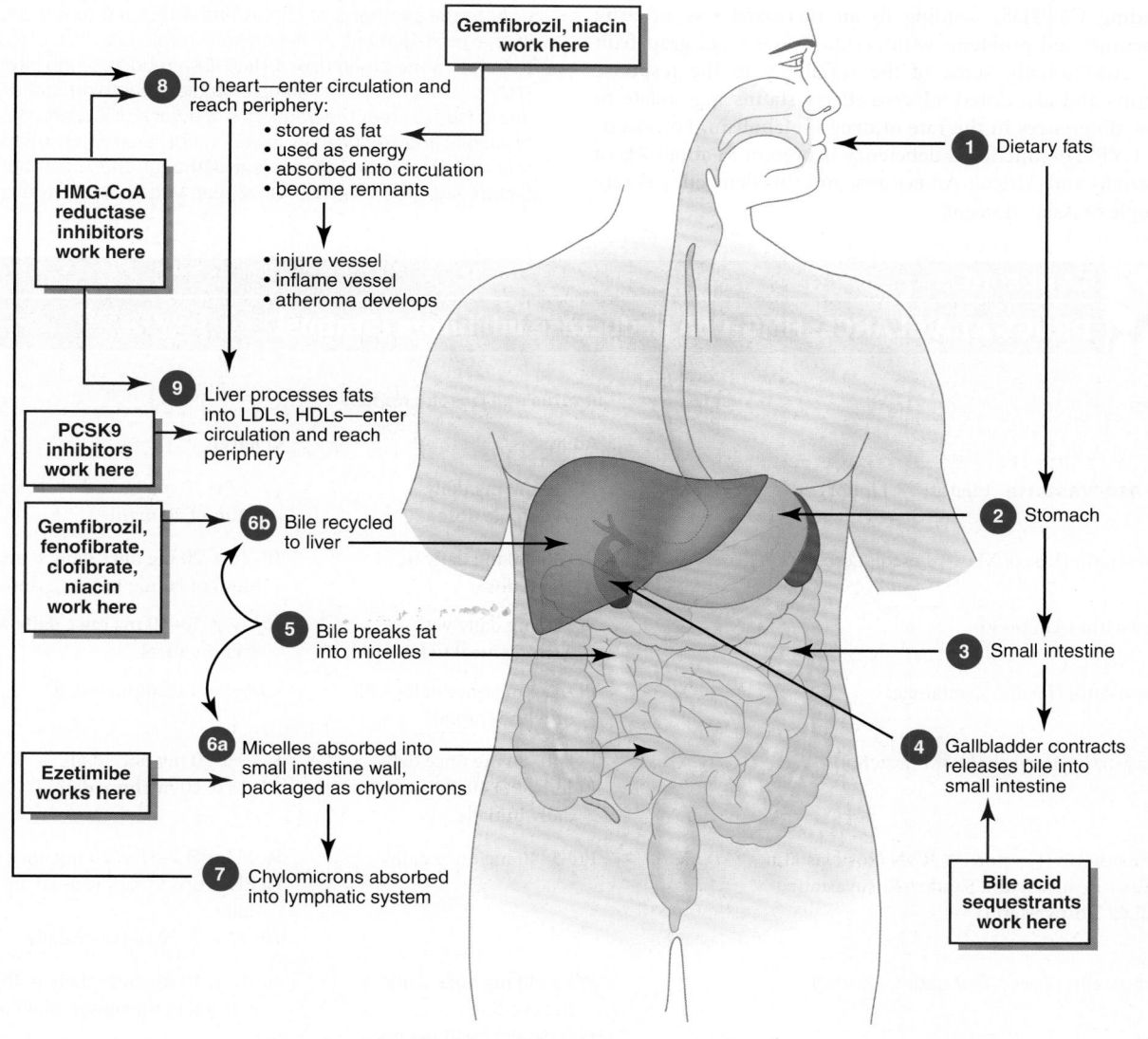

**Figure 10.1.** Sites of action of dyslipidemic drugs.

**QSEN Alert: Safety**

Atorvastatin demonstrates the most favorable benefit:cost ratio of the four commonly used statin drugs, particularly in younger adults with low or medium cardiovascular risk.

## Pharmacokinetics

Atorvastatin is rapidly absorbed following oral administration and undergoes extensive first-pass metabolism by the liver, which results in low levels of drug available for general circulation. Peak effect occurs in 1 to 2 hours. Food decreases the rate and extent of absorption. Metabolism occurs in the liver, with 80% to 85% of drug metabolites excreted in feces and the remaining products excreted in urine.

## Action

The statins inhibit an enzyme (HMG-CoA reductase) required for hepatic synthesis of cholesterol. In part, metabolism involves one or more hepatic cytochrome P450 enzymes (including CYP2D6), leading to an increased risk of drug interactions and problems with certain foods (e.g., grapefruit juice). Additionally, some of the variability in the response to statins and associated adverse effects statins may relate to genetic differences in the rate of drug metabolism. For example, a CYP2D6 functional deficiency is present in about 7% of Caucasians and African Americans, and this deficiency is rare in people of Asian descent.

## Use

Atorvastatin and the other statins are indicated for the treatment of hypercholesterolemia and reducing cardiovascular events in people with multiple risk factors. The statins are the most powerful drug class for reduction of LDL cholesterol. They result in an 18% to 55% decrease in LDL levels, as well as a 5% to 15% increase in HDL levels and a 7% to 30% decrease in triglycerides.

Table 10.3 presents dosage information for atorvastatin and other statins.

**QSEN Alert: Evidence-Based Practice**

Over the past century, evidence has shown that LDLs are the major risk factor for arteriosclerotic cardiovascular disease. In fact, in every mammalian species ever studied, elevated plasma LDL levels produce atherosclerosis (Goldstein & Brown, 2015). At any level of LDL, the likelihood of a myocardial infarction is increased in the presence of known cardiovascular risk factors, such as cigarette smoking and hypertension (see Chap. 28). Researchers linked the contribution of the compound 3-hydroxy-3-methylglutarate attached to coenzyme A (HMG-CoA) to the synthesis of cholesterol, which led to a revolution in the management of hypercholesterolemia. This discovery then led to the broad use of HMG-CoA reductase inhibitors, or statins. Evidence from multiple studies regarding statins has demonstrated that the frequency of myocardial infarctions can be significantly reduced by lowering LDL even when inflammation and risk factors are present. Although these contributory factors are important, they all require LDL to initiate the lesion.

 **TABLE 10.3**

## DRUGS AT A GLANCE: HMG-CoA Reductase Inhibitors (Statins)

| Drug | Pregnancy Category | Routes and Dosage Ranges | |
|---|---|---|---|
| | | **Adults** | **Children** |
| Ⓟ **Atorvastatin** (Lipitor; ✹ Lipitor) | X | PO 10–80 mg daily in a single dose | *10–17 y*: 10 mg once daily to maximum of 20 mg/d |
| Fluvastatin (Lescol XL; ✹ Lescol, Lescol XL) | X | PO 40–80 mg daily in 1 or 2 doses | *10–16 y*: 20 mg once daily to maximum of 80 mg in 1 or 2 doses |
| Lovastatin (Altoprev) | X | PO 20 mg daily with evening meal to 80 mg/d | *10–17 y*: 10–40 mg once daily with evening meal |
| Pitavastatin (Livalo; Zypitamag) | X | PO 1–4 mg once daily with or without food | *<18 y*: not recommended |
| Pravastatin (Pravachol; ✹ Pravachol) | X | PO 40–80 mg once daily Elderly, PO 40–80 mg once daily initially | *8–13 y*: 20 mg once daily *14–18 y*: 40 mg once daily |
| Rosuvastatin (Crestor; ✹ RAN-Rosuvastatin, Riva-Rosuvastatin, Sandoz-Rosuvastatin, Teva-Rosuvastatin) | X | PO 5–40 mg once daily | HoFH: *PO 7–17 y*: 20 mg once daily HeFH: *PO 8 to <10 y*: 5–10 mg once daily *10–17 y*: 5–20 mg once daily |
| Simvastatin (Zocor, FloLipid; ✹ Zocor) | X | PO 5–40 mg once daily in the evening Elderly, PO 5–40 mg once daily in the evening | *10–17 y*: 10 mg once daily in the evening to maximum of 40 mg/d |

HeFH, heterozygous familial hypercholesterolemia; HoFH, homozygous familial hypercholesterolemia.

## Use in Children

Statins are now considered first-line therapy in the treatment of dyslipidemia in children. As with adults, management of children with dyslipidemia focuses on lifestyle modifications.

## Use in Older Adults

As in younger adults, diet, exercise, and weight control should be tried first to reduce cholesterol levels. When drug therapy is required, statins are effective for lowering LDL cholesterol and usually are well tolerated by older adults.

## Use in Patients With Renal Impairment

In renal impairment, plasma levels are not affected, and dosage reductions are not necessary.

## Use in Patients With Hepatic Impairment

Atorvastatin and other statins, which are metabolized in the liver, may accumulate in patients with impaired hepatic function. Thus, they are contraindicated in patients with active liver disease or unexplained elevations of serum aspartate aminotransferase or alanine aminotransferase. These drugs should be used cautiously, in reduced dosages, for patients who ingest substantial amounts of alcohol or who have a history of liver disease.

## Use in Patients Receiving Home Care

Because liver enzymes may be elevated during atorvastatin use, patients need liver function tests and repeat lipid profile testing on a routine basis. Increasing availability of home cholesterol-monitoring devices will require additional patient teaching about technique and interpretation of the results. Patients should notify their health care provider if unexplained muscle pain or tenderness occurs.

# Adverse Effects

Statins are usually well tolerated; the most common adverse effects (nausea, constipation, diarrhea, abdominal cramps or pain, headache, skin rash) are usually mild and transient. Hepatic dysfunction has been a source of concern, although the actual risk appears to be small. Myopathies are important adverse effects and can range from discreet muscle pain to rhabdomyolysis. Statins can injure muscle tissue, resulting in muscle ache, pain, or weakness. Factors that increase the risk of rhabdomyolysis include advanced age, frail or small body frame, high dosage of statins, concomitant use of drugs that interfere with CPY3A4 including fibrates, hypothyroidism, and multiple systemic diseases such as renal insufficiency secondary to diabetic nephropathy.

### QSEN Alert: Safety

When women of childbearing age are treated with drug therapy for dyslipidemia, adequate patient education is critical to minimize complications associated with pregnancy. The absolute risk of teratogenicity with the use of statins appears to be relatively small; however, the use of birth control measures with statin use is essential in sexually active women. Careful consideration should be given if potential benefits warrant use of the drug class in pregnant women despite potential risks. The nurse advocates in the patient's care.

# Contraindications

Statins are potentially teratogenic (pregnancy category X). Careful consideration is necessary if potential benefits warrant use of these drugs in pregnant women. Additional contraindications include lactation, because the drugs are secreted in breast milk, and hypersensitivity to statins.

# Nursing Implications

The statins are the most effective dyslipidemic agents for improving clinical outcomes when used for primary and secondary prevention of cardiovascular disease. The choice and use of statins are based on a number of factors, including the degree of dyslipidemia, a specific drug's actions, drug interactions, the presence of renal or liver impairment, and cost.

## Preventing Interactions

Many medications and herbs interact with atorvastatin, increasing or decreasing its effect (Boxes 10.3 and 10.4).

## Administering the Medication

Because the bulk of cholesterol synthesis appears to occur at night, administration of statins normally takes place in the evening or at bedtime. However, atorvastatin has a long half-life, and evidence suggests that the drug can be given without regard to time of day. There is no definitive global recommendation for the entire class; thus, the timing of administration of statins should be based on manufacturer recommendations.

**BOX 10.3 — Drug Interactions: Atorvastatin**

**Drugs That Increase the Effects of Atorvastatin**
- Magnesium- and aluminum-containing antacids
  *Interfere with absorption; administer atorvastatin 2 hours before or after antacids.*
- Amiodarone and colchicine
  *Decrease metabolism*
- Azole antifungals
  *Increase the risk of myopathy; it is recommended that statin therapy be interrupted temporarily if systemic azole antifungals are needed.*
- Cyclosporine, CYP3A inhibitors, diltiazem, fibric acid derivatives, niacin, and verapamil
  *Increase the risk of severe myopathy or rhabdomyolysis*
- Erythromycin, macrolide antibiotics, nefazodone, and protease inhibitors
  *Decrease elimination*

**Drugs That Decrease the Effects of Atorvastatin**
- Cholestyramine
  *Decreases rate of bioavailability; administer atorvastatin at least 4 hours after this bile acid sequestrant.*
- Colestipol
  *Decreases plasma levels*

**BOX 10.4** *Herb and Dietary Interactions: Atorvastatin*

**Herbs and Foods That Increase the Effects of Atorvastatin**
- Grapefruit juice, pomegranate juice, red yeast rice, sitostanol, and vitamin $B_3$

**Herbs and Foods That May Decrease the Effects of Atorvastatin**
- Fibers such as oat bran and pectin

## Assessing for Therapeutic Effects

The nurse monitors lipid response to therapy, looking for decreased levels of total serum cholesterol, LDL cholesterol, and triglycerides, as well as increased levels of HDL cholesterol. Effects occur in 1 to 2 weeks, with maximum effects in 4 to 6 weeks.

## Assessing for Adverse Effects

Common adverse effects include nausea, diarrhea, abdominal pain, dyspepsia, and elevated liver function tests. The nurse monitors for signs or symptoms of muscle pain or weakness, mainly during the first months of therapy and when dosages are adjusted upward. If unexplained severe muscle symptoms, fatigue, or cola-colored urine develop, the statin should be held and the prescriber notified to address the possibility of rhabdomyolysis.

### Patient Teaching

Women of childbearing age should receive contraceptive counseling to enhance awareness of the risks associated with statin use. In addition, education should focus on the importance of monitoring liver function on a regular basis. Liver function tests are recommended before starting a statin, at 12 weeks after starting the drug, at every increase in dose, and then periodically. The nurse monitors patients with increased serum aminotransferases until the abnormal values resolve. If the increases are more than three times the upper limit of normal levels and persist, it is necessary to reduce the dose or change the drug.

The general teaching guidelines presented in Box 10.5 are a good resource.

## Other Drugs in the Class

Table 10.3 lists the other statins. Absorption following oral administration varies depending on the drug. Lovastatin and pravastatin are poorly absorbed, and fluvastatin has the highest rate of absorption. Most of the statins undergo extensive first-pass metabolism by the liver, which results in low levels of drug available for general circulation.

Patients may take pravastatin or simvastatin with or without food in the evening. They may take fluvastatin on an empty stomach or at bedtime. It is important to avoid taking them with grapefruit juice. Note that concurrent use of cimetidine, ranitidine, and omeprazole increases the effects of fluvastatin.

**BOX 10.5** *Patient Teaching Guidelines for Dyslipidemic Drugs*

- As you probably know, heart and blood vessel disease causes a great deal of illness and many deaths. The basic problem is usually atherosclerosis, in which the arteries are partly blocked by cholesterol deposits. Cholesterol, a waxy substance made in the liver, is necessary for normal body functioning. However, excessive amounts in the blood increase the likelihood of having a heart attack, stroke, or leg pain from inadequate blood flow. One type of cholesterol (LDL or "bad") attaches to artery walls, where it can enlarge over time and block blood flow. The other type (high-density lipoprotein [HDL] or "good") carries cholesterol away from the artery and back to the liver, where it can be broken down. Thus, the healthiest blood cholesterol levels in adults are low total cholesterol (less than 200 mg/dL), low LDL (less than 130 mg/dL), and high HDL (greater than 35 mg/dL). High levels of blood triglycerides, another type of fat, are also unhealthy.

- Dyslipidemic drugs are given to lower high concentrations of fats (total cholesterol, LDL cholesterol, and triglycerides) in your blood. The goal of management is to prevent heart attack, stroke, and peripheral arterial disease. If you already have heart and blood vessel disease, the drugs can improve your symptoms, activity level, and quality of life.

- Eating a low-fat diet can help. This is often the first step in treating high cholesterol or triglyceride levels and

may be prescribed for 6 months or longer before drug therapy is begun. When drug therapy is prescribed, the diet should be continued. An important part is reducing the amount of saturated fat (from meats, dairy products). In addition, eating a bowl of oat cereal daily can help lower cholesterol by 5% to 10%. Diet counseling by a dietitian or nutritionist can be helpful in developing guidelines that fit your needs and lifestyle. Overeating or gaining weight may decrease or cancel the lipid-lowering effects of the drugs.

- Make other lifestyle changes to help improve cholesterol levels that include regular aerobic exercise (raises HDL), losing weight (raises HDL, lowers LDL, lowers triglycerides), and not smoking (HDL levels are higher in nonsmokers).

- As an adult, have measurements of total cholesterol and HDL cholesterol at least once ever every 5 years. People with a personal or family history of dyslipidemia or other risk factors for cardiovascular disease should be tested more often.

- Techniques for home monitoring of cholesterol levels are improving and are more available for self-use. You may receive instructions about performing self-monitoring and reporting your results to your health care provider.

# BILE ACID SEQUESTRANTS

**Cholestyramine** (Prevalite, Questran), the prototype bile acid sequestrant, has the ability to reduce LDL cholesterol. It has little or no effect on HDL cholesterol and either no effect or an increased effect on triglyceride levels. There is no evidence that cholestyramine can be used as monotherapy, but it can play a role as an add-on drug with statins in combination therapy.

## Pharmacokinetics

Cholestyramine is not absorbed when taken orally. Therefore, the drug is excreted in feces essentially unchanged.

## Action

Cholestyramine binds bile acids in the intestinal lumen, causing the bile acids to be excreted in feces, preventing recirculation to the liver. Loss of bile acids stimulates hepatic synthesis of more bile acids from cholesterol. As more hepatic cholesterol is used to produce bile acids, more serum cholesterol moves into the liver to replenish the supply, thereby lowering serum cholesterol (primarily LDL). LDL cholesterol levels decrease within a week of starting cholestyramine and other bile acid sequestrants and reach maximal reductions within a month. When the drugs are stopped, pretreatment LDL cholesterol levels return within a month.

## Use

Cholestyramine reduces LDL cholesterol levels (15%–30%) and also produces a minimal elevation in HDL cholesterol (3%–5%). Table 10.4 presents dosage information for cholestyramine and other bile acid sequestrants.

### Use in Children

Cholestyramine and other bile acid sequestrants are safe and moderately effective in children and adolescents ages 6 to 18 years and decrease both total cholesterol and LDL cholesterol levels. A modest elevation in triglyceride levels has been reported. Children do not tolerate the reported gastrointestinal (GI) adverse effects well.

### Use in Older Adults

Cholestyramine and other bile acid sequestrants are effective in older adults, although these individuals do not tolerate the adverse effects well.

## TABLE 10.4

### DRUGS AT A GLANCE: Bile Acid Sequestrants

| Drug | Pregnancy Category | Routes and Dosage Ranges | |
|---|---|---|---|
| | | **Adults** | **Children** |
| **Cholestyramine** (Prevalite, Questran, Questran Light; ❋ Olestyr, PMS-Cholestyramine, Questran, Novo-Cholamine) | C | PO tablets, 4 g once or twice daily initially, gradually increased at monthly intervals to 8–16 g daily in 2 divided doses. Maximum daily dose, 24 g. PO powder, 4 g 1–6 times daily | 240 mg/kg/d in 3 divided doses |
| Colesevelam (Welchol; ❋ Lodalis) | B | PO 3.75 g daily in 1 or 2 doses with meals. Maximum daily dose, 4.375 g | |
| Colestipol (Colestid, Colestid Flavored; ❋ Colestid) | C | PO tablets, 2 g once or twice daily initially, gradually increased at 1- to 2-mo intervals, up to 16 g daily. PO granules, 5 g daily initially, gradually increased at 1- to 2-mo intervals, up to 30 g daily in single or divided doses | |

### Use in Patients With Renal Impairment

Extended use of cholestyramine in patients with renal impairment requires caution because the drug releases chloride. This effect can increase the risk of hyperchloremic metabolic acidosis.

### Use in Patients With Hepatic Impairment

Cholestyramine can further raise serum cholesterol. Therefore, its use in people with primary biliary cirrhosis warrants caution.

## Adverse Effects

Cholestyramine is not absorbed systemically, so the main adverse effects are GI ones (abdominal fullness, flatulence, diarrhea, and constipation). Constipation is especially common, and a bowel program may be necessary to control this problem.

## Contraindications

Cholestyramine is contraindicated in people with complete biliary obstruction, because bile is not secreted into the intestine. The drug can bind with vitamin K; thus, use in individuals with any coagulopathy requires caution.

## Nursing Implications

### Preventing Interactions

Cholestyramine may decrease absorption of many oral medications (e.g., digoxin, folic acid, glipizide, propranolol, tetracyclines, thiazide diuretics, thyroid hormones, fat-soluble vitamins, and warfarin). Apparently, no drugs significantly affect cholestyramine. Herbs and foods that increase the effects of cholestyramine include fibers such as oat bran and pectin. No herbs and foods seem to decrease the effects of cholestyramine.

In a patient who is taking cholestyramine in addition to other drugs, dosage of the interactive drug may need to be changed when the bile acid sequestrant is added or withdrawn. Also, because cholestyramine binds bile acids, cholestyramine may interfere with normal fat digestion and absorption and therefore may prevent absorption of the fat-soluble vitamins A, D, E, and K.

### Administering the Medication

It is necessary to mix cholestyramine powder with water or other fluids, soups, cereals, or fruits such as applesauce and to follow with more fluid. The nurse ensures that the drug is not taken in a dry form. It is essential that cholestyramine not be given with other drugs; to minimize altered absorption, people should take the other drugs 1 hour before or 4 to 6 hours after cholestyramine.

### Assessing for Therapeutic Effects

The nurse observes for decreased levels of total serum cholesterol, LDL cholesterol, and triglycerides and increased levels of HDL cholesterol. Maximum effects occur in approximately 1 month.

### Assessing for Adverse Effects

The most common adverse effect is constipation. Other conditions relate to GI effects: abdominal discomfort or pain, nausea, vomiting, flatulence, diarrhea, anorexia, and steatorrhea.

Increased bleeding tendencies may result from vitamin K malabsorption.

### Patient Teaching

The nurse assesses the adequacy of levels of fat-soluble vitamins A, D, E, and K; supplementation may be required. Good dental hygiene is important because holding the mixture in the mouth can damage the teeth. Some products may contain aspartame or sugar, so caution is necessary in patients with phenylketonuria or diabetes mellitus.

Also, the nurse teaches patients that these drugs are used mainly to reduce LDL cholesterol further in those who are already taking a statin drug. The inhibition of cholesterol synthesis by a statin drug makes bile acid–binding drugs more effective. In addition, the combination increases HDL cholesterol and can further reduce the risk of cardiovascular disorders. Box 10.5 contains additional patient teaching information.

## Other Drugs in the Class

In patients with elevated LDL cholesterol, colesevelam (Welchol) and colestipol (Colestid) may be used along with diet modifications to reduce serum cholesterol. Colesevelam is also used as an adjunct agent to improve glycemic control in adults with type 2 diabetes mellitus (see Chap. 41). Like cholestyramine, colesevelam and colestipol are not absorbed systemically but may interfere with absorption of fat-soluble vitamins A, D, E, and K. These drugs are not expected to be excreted in breast milk, but they may affect vitamin levels in nursing infants. Some products may contain phenylalanine. Patients who take the granular form of colestipol should not swallow the granules dry. Patients who take the tablet form of either drug should swallow tablets whole, without cutting, crushing, or chewing. The adverse effects profile and interactions are similar for all bile acid sequestrants.

> ### Clinical Application 10.2
>
> - Why is the combination of atorvastatin and gemfibrozil prescribed for Mr. Watkins?
> - A nurse is counseling Mr. Watkins about his medication. He asks when he will need to have his laboratory work completed. What is the nurse's response?
> - When educating Mr. Watkins about his new medication, the nurse teaches him about common adverse effects. What should be included in teaching about the adverse effects of atorvastatin? What signs and symptoms of complications does the nurse discuss with him?

## FIBRATES

Fibrates are derivatives of fibric acid and are similar to endogenous fatty acids. The first fibrate to be developed, clofibrate, has essentially been replaced by other fibrates and is not discussed. Therefore, **fenofibrate** (Tricor) serves as the prototype in this discussion.

## Pharmacokinetics

Fenofibrate is administered orally and is highly protein bound, primarily to albumin. Time to peak effect is 6 to 8 hours. Metabolism occurs in the liver and excretion is by urinary elimination.

## Action

Fenofibrate and other fibrates increase the oxidation of fatty acids in liver and muscle tissue. Thus, they decrease hepatic production of triglycerides, decrease VLDL cholesterol, and increase HDL cholesterol.

## Use

Fibrates are the most effective drugs for reducing serum triglyceride values, and their main indication for use is high serum triglycerides (greater than 500 mg/dL); they may result in a 20% to 50% decrease in triglyceride levels. They are also helpful for patients with low HDL cholesterol levels (10%–20% increase). Additionally, fibrates are the drug of choice for hypertriglyceridemia associated with diabetes, gout, gastritis, or ulcer disease. There are no specific recommendations for use of these drugs in patients who are critically ill; drug interactions and adverse effects may restrict their use in critical illness.

Table 10.5 presents dosage information for the fibrates.

### Use in Children

Published studies of the use of fenofibrate and other fibrates in children are limited. Thus, the safety and efficacy of fibrates in children are unclear.

### Use in Older Adults

Caution is warranted with dosage determination. For fenofibrate, lower starting dosages are recommended (67 mg/day).

### Use in Patients With Renal Impairment

As previously stated, fibrates are excreted mainly by the kidneys; therefore, they accumulate in the serum of patients with renal impairment. Fenofibrate is contraindicated in patients with severe renal impairment, and the recommended starting dose is 67 mg/day in patients with a creatinine clearance of less than 50 mL/minute. It is necessary to evaluate the effects of this dose effects on renal function and to check triglyceride levels before increasing this dose. Fibrates may cause a reversible elevated serum creatinine. Patients with diabetes mellitus require close monitoring because renal disease is a serious complication in this population.

### Use in Patients With Hepatic Impairment

Fibrates may cause hepatotoxicity. Abnormal elevations of serum aminotransferases have occurred with both gemfibrozil and fenofibrate, but they usually subside after the drug is discontinued. Contraindications to fenofibrate include severe hepatic impairment, including primary biliary cirrhosis, and persistent elevations in liver function tests and preexisting gallbladder disease. In addition, hepatitis (hepatocellular, chronic active, and cholestatic) has reportedly occurred after use of fenofibrate from a few weeks to several years. It is necessary to monitor liver function during the first year of drug administration. Discontinuation of the drug is warranted if elevated enzyme levels persist at more than three times the normal limit.

### Use in Patients Receiving Home Care

Because liver enzyme tests are recommended, patients who are housebound may need assistance in obtaining blood tests (e.g., lipids, liver function tests). The nurse advises patients to notify their health care provider if unexplained muscle pain or tenderness occurs. Increasing availability of home cholesterol-monitoring devices will require additional patient teaching about technique and interpretation of the results.

## Adverse Effects

The main adverse effects are GI discomfort and diarrhea, which may occur less often with fenofibrate than with other fibrates. Fibrates may also increase cholesterol concentration in the biliary tract and formation of gallstones.

### TABLE 10.5

### DRUGS AT A GLANCE: Fibrates

| Drug | Pregnancy Category | Routes and Dosage Ranges | |
|---|---|---|---|
| | | **Adults** | **Children** |
| ℗ **Fenofibrate** (Antara, Fenoglide, Fibricor, Lipofen, Tricor, Triglide, Trilipix; ✳ Lipidil EZ, Lipidil Supra) | C | Antara (micronized) 30–90 mg once daily<br>Fenofibrate (micronized) PO 43–130 once daily with meals<br>Fenoglide 40–120 mg once daily<br>Fibricor 35–105 mg once daily<br>Tricor 48–145 mg once daily<br>Triglide 160 mg once daily<br>Trilipix 45–135 mg once daily | Fenofibrate (micronized) PO 67 mg/d/20 kg body weight with meals |
| Gemfibrozil (Lopid) | C | PO 1200 mg daily, in 2 divided doses, 30 min before morning and evening meals | Safety and efficacy data limited |

**Drugs That Increase the Effects of Fenofibrate**
- Statins
  *Increase the risk of severe myopathy or rhabdomyolysis*
- Cyclosporine
  *Mechanism for increase is unknown.*

**Drugs That Decrease the Effects of Fenofibrate**
- Bile acid sequestrant drugs
  *Decrease absorption; to avoid, take fenofibrate about 1 hour before or 4 to 6 hours after the bile acid sequestrant.*

## Contraindications

Contraindications include a hypersensitivity to fibrates, hepatic or (severe) renal impairment, preexisting gallbladder disease, primary biliary cirrhosis, or persistent liver function abnormalities of unknown origin.

## Nursing Implications

### Preventing Interactions

Fenofibrate and other fibric acid derivatives may enhance the hypoprothrombinemic effect of warfarin-type oral anticoagulants, increasing the risk of bleeding. Patients receiving warfarin concurrently require a substantially decreased dosage of warfarin because fibrates displace warfarin from binding sites on serum albumin. Other drug–drug interactions are outlined in Box 10.6. No herbal interactions have been identified.

### Administering the Medication

It is necessary to give fenofibrate with food to increase drug absorption.

### Assessing for Therapeutic Effects

The nurse assesses for decreased levels of total serum cholesterol, LDL cholesterol, and triglycerides and increased levels of HDL cholesterol. With fibrates, effects occur in approximately 1 month.

### Assessing for Adverse Effects

GI disturbances as well as elevated liver function tests are common. Reportedly, hypersensitivity reactions, myopathy, rhabdomyolysis, blood dyscrasias, hepatotoxicity, cholelithiasis, cholestatic jaundice, pancreatitis, and reduced libido also occur,

although these effects are rare. Risk of myopathy increases with concomitant use of statins.

### Patient Teaching

The nurse instructs patients to report signs and symptoms of adverse effects to the health care provider. Throughout drug therapy, patients should have periodic blood tests. See Box 10.5 for general patient teaching information.

## Other Drugs in the Class

It is necessary to give gemfibrozil on an empty stomach, about 30 minutes before the morning and evening meal.

## CHOLESTEROL ABSORPTION INHIBITOR

**Ezetimibe** (Zetia) is the prototype of the newest class of dyslipidemic drugs, which act in the small intestine to inhibit absorption of cholesterol and decrease the delivery of intestinal cholesterol to the liver, resulting in reduced hepatic cholesterol stores and increased clearance of cholesterol from the blood. This distinct mechanism is complementary to that of HMG-CoA reductase inhibitors, producing synergistic cholesterol-lowering effects when these drugs are used in combination. Ezetimibe reduces total cholesterol and triglycerides and increases HDL cholesterol.

## Pharmacokinetics

Ezetimibe is significantly protein bound, is metabolized in the small intestine and liver, and is excreted predominately in feces. The time to peak effect is 4 to 12 hours.

## Action

Ezetimibe blocks biliary and dietary cholesterol absorption at the brush border of the intestine without affecting absorption of fat-soluble vitamins and triglycerides.

## Use

Ezetimibe is used together with dietary management for treatment of primary dyslipidemia. The drug may result in a 14% to 17% decrease in LDL levels. It can be used as monotherapy on in combination with a statin. When given as monotherapy (without a statin), ezetimibe does not require dosage reduction in geriatric patients. Table 10.6 presents dosage information for the drug.

| TABLE 10.6 | | | |
|---|---|---|---|
| **DRUGS AT A GLANCE: Cholesterol Absorption Inhibitor (Ezetimibe)** | | | |
| **Drug** | **Pregnancy Category** | **Routes and Dosage Ranges** | |
| | | **Adults** | **Children** |
| Ⓟ **Ezetimibe** (Zetia; ✦ Ezetrol) | C | PO 10 mg once daily | *<10 y:* not recommended *≥10 y:* PO 10 mg once daily |

### Use in Children

Safety and efficacy in children younger than 10 years of age have not been established.

### Use in Patients With Hepatic Impairment

Dosage adjustment of ezetimibe is necessary in patients with mild hepatic impairment. The drug is not recommended in patients with moderate to severe hepatic impairment.

## Adverse Effects

The most common adverse effects of ezetimibe include headache, diarrhea, hypersensitivity reactions such as rash, and nausea.

## Contraindications

Contraindications include pregnancy and lactation. Additional contraindications are hypersensitivity to ezetimibe or concomitant use with a statin in people with active hepatic disease.

## Nursing Implications

The nurse instructs patients to maintain a low-cholesterol diet during ezetimibe therapy. Patients should report side effects to their health care providers.

### Preventing Interactions

Some medications interact with ezetimibe, increasing or decreasing its effect (Box 10.7). Apparently, no herbs interact with this drug.

### Administering the Medication

Ezetimibe may be administered with or without food. The patient takes the drug:

- At the same time each day
- At night if used in combination with a statin (ezetimibe may be given at the same time as a statin)
- Either 2 hours before or 4 hours after bile sequestrants to prevent altered absorption

### Assessing for Therapeutic Effects

The nurse monitors lipid response to therapy with ezetimibe. Desired results include decreases in total cholesterol, LDL cholesterol, and triglycerides, with increases in HDL cholesterol. A therapeutic response occurs within 2 weeks of initiation of therapy and lasts as long as the drug is continued.

**BOX 10.7**  *Drug Interactions: Ezetimibe*

**Drugs That Increase the Effects of Ezetimibe**
- Cyclosporine
  *Increases blood levels*

**Drugs That Decrease the Effects of Ezetimibe**
- Bile acid sequestrant drugs
  *Mechanism for decrease is unknown.*

### Assessing for Adverse Effects

The nurse observes for headache, dizziness, fatigue, diarrhea, and abdominal pain.

### Patient Teaching

The nurse instructs patients to report signs and symptoms of adverse effects to the health care provider. Throughout drug therapy, patients should have periodic blood tests. See Box 10.5 for general patient information.

## PCSK9 INHIBITORS

PCSK9 inhibitors are fully humanized monoclonal antibodies that inactivate a protein in the liver called proprotein convertase subtilisin/kexin 9 (PCSK9) that regulates the life span of the cholesterol clearing receptors on the liver. The inhibition of PCSK9 significantly lowers LDL cholesterol levels. **Alirocumab** (Praluent) serves as the prototype of this class of drugs.

## Pharmacokinetics

Alirocumab is administered subcutaneously every 2 to 4 weeks, and at recommended dosages, median times to maximum serum concentrations are 3 to 7 days. Following subcutaneous injection, the drug is distributed primarily in the circulatory system. As a protein, the drug degrades to small peptides and individual amino acids. At low concentrations, the drug is eliminated through binding to the PCSK9 receptors; at higher concentrations, it is eliminated principally through nonsaturable proteolysis.

## Action

Unlike statins that lower cholesterol by inhibiting the synthesis of cholesterol, the PCSK9 inhibitors promote modulation of the receptor that clears cholesterol, thereby prolonging the receptor activity and promoting the clearance of cholesterol.

## Use

Alirocumab is indicated in adults with ASCVD or familial hypercholesterolemia who require additional lowering of LDL cholesterol when diet and maximally tolerated statin therapy have not produced the desired therapeutic response. The ability of alirocumab to reduce the outcomes of a myocardial infarction or cerebrovascular accident has not been determined, although clinical trials are ongoing. Early results suggest that cardiovascular events could be decreased with PCSK9 inhibitors. Table 10.7 presents dosage information for the alirocumab and the other PCSK9 inhibitors. These drugs may result in a 60% to 70% reduction in LDL levels.

### Use in Children

Safety and efficacy in children and adolescents have not been established.

### Use in Older Adults

There is no reported need for adjustments in drug dosage in older adults.

| TABLE 10.7 | | | |
|---|---|---|---|
| **DRUGS AT A GLANCE: PCSK9 Inhibitors** | | | |
| **Drug** | **Pregnancy Category** | **Routes and Dosage Ranges** | |
| | | **Adults** | **Children** |
| Ⓟ **Alirocumab** (Praluent; ✷ Praluent) | None; approved in 2015 | Sub-Q: 75–150 mg every 2 wk | Safety and efficacy not established |
| Evolocumab (Repatha, Repatha Pushtronex System, Repatha SureClick; ✷ Repatha) | None; approved in 2015 | Sub-Q: 140 mg every 2 wk or 420 mg once monthly | *13–17 y*: refer to adult dosing |

## Use in Patients With Renal Impairment

No adjustment to dosage is required in patients with mild to moderate renal impairment. No data are available for use in individuals with severe renal impairment.

## Use in Patients With Hepatic Impairment

No adjustment to dosage is required in patients with mild to moderate hepatic impairment. No data are available for use in individuals with severe hepatic impairment.

## Use in Patients Receiving Home Care

Patients who are housebound may need assistance in obtaining serum lipid blood tests or instructed on home-monitoring techniques. The nurse advises patients to notify their health care provider if adverse effects occur or if they become pregnant. Patients should be advised to seek emergency treatment should signs of an allergic reaction occur. Patients should be supported to maximize lifestyle modification, including diet, exercise, and smoking cessation, to reduce cholesterol while taking alirocumab.

## Adverse Effects

Alirocumab appears to be well tolerated, with injection site reactions the most common adverse effect. In addition, nasopharyngitis, itching, influenza, muscle pain, diarrhea, and serious allergic reactions have been reported with use of the drug.

## Contraindications

Contraindications include known hypersensitivity to the drug or a component to the formulation. Limited information is available regarding additional contraindications.

## Nursing Implications

### Preventing Interactions

No interactions have been reported that increase or decrease the therapeutic or adverse effects of the drug.

### Administering the Medication

The drug should be administered by subcutaneous injection into the upper arm, abdomen, or thigh. The injection site should be rotated with each injection, and other drugs should not be given at the same injection site at the same time. The prefilled syringe or pen should be warmed to room temperature for 30 to 40 minutes before use. Note that it may take 20 seconds to inject the drug subcutaneously.

### Assessing for Therapeutic Effects

The nurse monitors lipid response to therapy, looking for decreased levels of LDL cholesterol. Maximum effects begin in approximately 1 week; monitoring should occur within 4 to 8 weeks of initiation or dosage adjustment.

### Assessing for Adverse Effects

The nurse should determine that no injection site reactions are present. In addition, it is necessary to observe that the patient manifests no signs or symptoms of influenza, cough, muscle pain, diarrhea, or allergic reaction to the drug.

### Patient Teaching

Patients (and providers) need to read patient information and instructions each time the patient administers alirocumab in case new information is available. The nurse provides guidance to patients and caregivers regarding the proper subcutaneous injection technique, including aseptic technique and how to use the prefilled syringe or pen correctly. Patient instruction regarding discarding needles and syringes in a puncture-resistant disposal container is necessary. Women should notify their health care provider if they become pregnant while taking alirocumab. Box 10.5 contains general patient teaching information.

## Other Drugs in the Class

The only other drug currently approved as a PCSK9 inhibitor is evolocumab (Repatha). To date, the indications and drug profile of evolocumab appear similar to alirocumab. As further clinical trials proceed, the benefit of one drug over another in the class may be identified. Because evolocumab is administered as a 420-mg dose, three separate 140-mg injections consecutively within a 30-minute period must be administered. Both drugs in the class are expensive, possibly limiting use in patients who might benefit from a PCSK9 inhibitor.

## MISCELLANEOUS DYSLIPIDEMIC AGENT

Niacin (nicotinic acid) is a vitamin that is no longer recommended as a dyslipidemic agent except in patients with high triglyceride levels (greater than 500 mg/dL) who have not been able to achieve the desired response or do not tolerate other drug therapy. For decreasing LDL cholesterol, other drugs (evolocumab or ezetimibe) are more effective when added to statin therapy. Although niacin does significantly increase HDL cholesterol, there is no evidence that the increase leads to improved patient outcomes. Serious concerns have been raised about the safety and efficacy of this vitamin in combination with statin therapy. Some formulations of sustained-release over-the-counter (OTC) niacin have been associated with an increased risk of hepatotoxicity. Niacin also increases blood glucose, causing possible problems with glucose control for people with diabetes. Poor tolerability often limits the use of niacin; the high doses required for dyslipidemic effects result in adverse effects. Niacin commonly causes skin flushing, pruritus, and gastric irritation, and it may lead to tachycardia, hypotension, dizziness, hyperglycemia, hyperuricemia, elevated liver aminotransferases, and hepatitis.

Nicotinamide, another common form of niacin, does not have the lipid-lowering properties of nicotinic acid. OTC preparations of niacin are not federally regulated in the United States, and preparations that are marketed as causing "no flush" may have no free nicotinic acid and are therefore ineffective in treating dyslipidemia. Table 10.8 presents dosage information for this oral drug.

## COMBINATION THERAPY USED TO TREAT DYSLIPIDEMIA

When monotherapy is not effective in attaining target LDL cholesterol levels, combination therapies with lipid-lowering drugs that have different mechanisms of action are recommended. In general, the drug combinations that are most effective in reducing total and LDL cholesterol are (1) a statin with a cholesterol absorption inhibitor or a bile acid sequestrant or (2) niacin with a bile acid sequestrant. When a goal of therapy is to increase the level of HDL cholesterol, a fibrate, cholesterol absorption inhibitor, or niacin may be used. However, because niacin is no longer recommended except in specific situations, drug therapy may be more successful and better controlled with administration of individual drugs in combination. However, a fibrate–statin combination should be avoided because of increased risks of severe myopathy, and a niacin–statin combination increases the risks of hepatotoxicity. Adverse reactions from combination statin and cholesterol absorption inhibitor therapy are reported to be similar to those from statins alone. Combination preparations are not intended for initial therapy. The adverse effects and contraindications associated with individual drugs also apply when they are used in combination. All combinations, like individual preparations, should be used in conjunction with a cholesterol-reducing diet.

## NCLEX Success

6. John Jones, a 47-year-old teacher, now takes cholestyramine, and the nurse teaches him about the medication and its use. The nurse should be concerned if, after the teaching session, Mr. Jones states

   A. "I should take the medicine with a full glass of water when I take my other medications"
   B. "I am taking this medication to decrease my LDL cholesterol level"
   C. "I should swallow the tablets whole"
   D. "I may need to supplement my intake of the fat-soluble vitamins A, D, E, and K"

7. Karen James, a 32-year-old accountant with type 1 diabetes mellitus, is taking gemfibrozil to reduce her serum triglyceride level. She asks why she could not take niacin, as her husband does. The nurse responds

   A. "Either drug reduces triglycerides. Why don't you ask your nurse practitioner if the drug therapy could be changed?"
   B. "Gemfibrozil is the only drug recommended for use to lower cholesterol"
   C. "Niacin therapy is not recommended for use in women"
   D. "Niacin increases blood glucose levels and is not preferred for people with diabetes"

8. The nurse practitioner adds cholestyramine to statin therapy in a patient with markedly elevated serum levels of LDL cholesterol. Which of the following if stated by the patient indicates that patient teaching has been successful? [Select all that apply.]

   A. "I need to mix the powder with water or other fluids before I take it."
   B. "I should wait 1 hour after I eat to take the medication."
   C. "I need to maintain good oral hygiene as the medication can damage my teeth."
   D. "If I notice an increased bleeding tendency, I need to notify the nurse practitioner."
   E. "I might have some GI effects, including constipation or abdominal pain."

| **TABLE 10.8** | | | |
|---|---|---|---|
| **DRUGS AT A GLANCE: Miscellaneous Dyslipidemic Agent (Niacin)** | | | |
| **Drug*** | **Pregnancy Category** | **Routes and Dosage Ranges** | |
| | | **Adults** | **Children** |
| Niacin (immediate release) (Niacor, Niaspan, Slo-Niacin; ✱ Niaspan, Niaspan FCT, Niodan) | C | PO 1–6 g daily, in 3 or 4 divided doses, with or just after meals | PO 55–87 mg/kg/d, in 3 or 4 divided doses, with or just after meals |

*Do not substitute the immediate-release for the extended-release preparation.

## THE NURSING PROCESS

A concept map outlines the nursing process related to drug therapy considerations in this chapter. Additional nursing implications related to the disease process should also be considered in care decisions.

**Assessment**
- Assess risk factors, history, or disease associated with atherosclerotic vascular disease, such as smoking, immobility, obesity, hypertension, or diabetes mellitus; signs and symptoms of an elevated serum cholesterol (>200 mg/100 mL) or triglycerides (>150 mg/100 mL); or both.

**Outcomes of Therapy**

The patient will
- Take lipid-lowering drugs as prescribed, decrease dietary intake of saturated fats and cholesterol, lose weight if obese and maintain the lower weight, have periodic measurements of blood lipids, avoid preventable adverse drug effects, receive positive reinforcement for efforts to lower blood lipid levels, and report feeling less anxious and more in control as risks of atherosclerotic cardiovascular disease are decreased.
- Begin primary prevention strategies in childhood with healthful eating habits (e.g., avoiding excessive fats, meat, and dairy products; obtaining adequate amounts of all nutrients, including dietary fiber; avoiding obesity), exercise, and avoiding cigarette smoking.

**Nursing Interventions**
- Help patients control risk factors. Weight loss often reduces blood lipids and lipoproteins to a normal range.
- Support measures to increase blood flow to tissues, including exercise, limiting time with legs in dependent position, and use of compression hose; provide appropriate teaching related to drug therapy (see Box 10.5).
- The most effective measures for preventing dyslipidemia and atherosclerosis are those related to a healthful lifestyle (e.g., diet low in cholesterol and saturated fats, weight control, exercise). Refer patients to a nutritionist. Overeating or gaining weight may decrease or cancel the lipid-lowering effects of the drugs.
- Secure counseling for smoking cessation for those who smoke, with patient understanding of the harm of exposure to second-hand smoke.
- Encourage adult patients to have their serum cholesterol level measured at least once every 5 years or as instructed by their health care provider. Adults and children with a personal or family history of dyslipidemia or other risk factors should be tested more often.
- Help patients and family members understand the desirability of lowering high blood lipid levels before serious cardiovascular diseases develop.

**Evaluation**
- Observe for decreased blood levels of total and LDL cholesterol and triglycerides with drug therapy; observe for increased levels of HDL cholesterol.
- Observe and interview regarding compliance with instructions for drug, diet, exercise, and other therapeutic and behavioral modification measures.
- Observe and interview regarding adverse drug effects.
- Validate the patient's ability to identify foods high and low in cholesterol and saturated fats.

## KEY CONCEPTS

- New treatment guidelines for cholesterol are focused on reducing arteriosclerotic cardiovascular disease and not on a specific serum lipid profile.
- Unless a person has a genetic disorder of lipid metabolism, the amount of cholesterol in the blood is strongly related to dietary intake of saturated fat.
- For accurate interpretation of a patient's lipid profile, blood samples for laboratory testing of triglycerides

should be drawn after the patient has fasted for 12 hours. Recommendations for fasting for cholesterol testing vary but are typically drawn as part of a lipid profile in a fasting state.

- Strong emphasis is placed on lifestyle changes (i.e., low-fat diet, regular aerobic exercise, losing weight, and smoking cessation) that can help improve total and LDL cholesterol levels and reduce the risk of ASCVD.

- The HMG-CoA reductase inhibitors (statins) are the most effective dyslipidemic agents for improving clinical outcomes when used for primary and secondary prevention of ASCVD.
- Take lovastatin with food; take fluvastatin or simvastatin in the evening, with or without food; atorvastatin, rosuvastatin, and pravastatin can be taken with or without food and without regard to time of day.
- Skin flushing may occur with niacin; preparations that are marketed as causing "no flush" may have no free nicotinic acid and are therefore ineffective in treating dyslipidemia.

- Fibrates are the most effective drugs for reducing serum triglyceride levels. Statins, niacin, and omega-3 fatty acids also reduce serum triglycerides.
- It is necessary to give fenofibrate and other fibrates with food to increase drug absorption.
- Niacin is no longer recommended for treatment of dyslipidemia except in people with high triglyceride levels (greater than 500 mg/dL) who have not been able to achieve the desired response or do not tolerate other drug therapy.

## CLINICAL REASONING CASE STUDY

**Meet the Patient**

Jason Smith, age 8, is seen in the pediatrician's office with the following fasting serum lipid profile: total serum cholesterol 278 mg/dL, low-density lipoprotein (LDL) cholesterol 210 mg/dL, high-density lipoprotein (HDL) cholesterol 38 mg/dL, and triglycerides 175 mg/dL. His paternal grandfather had a myocardial infarction at age 46, and his father was recently diagnosed with dyslipidemia. The boy has no history of diabetes mellitus, hypertension, or contact with second-hand smoke. He is in the 55th percentile in weight on a children's growth chart. He is started on pravastatin (Pravachol) 20 mg once daily.

- What is the goal of treatment of dyslipidemia in children?
- What are the main nonpharmacologic measures to decrease total and LDL cholesterol and serum triglycerides and increase HDL cholesterol in children?
- What improvement in Jason's laboratory values will indicate to the nurse that pravastatin is effective?
- What additional patient teaching information would you need to provide to Jason's parents?

**Assessing Drug Information**

- Pravastatin is recommended for children Jason's age and older for the reduction of LDL cholesterol and triglycerides. The drug also increases HDL cholesterol.
- Jason's parents should observe for adverse effects including dizziness, fatigue, headache, myalgia, nausea, vomiting, diarrhea, and cough.

**Nursing Actions**

- The primary goal of dyslipidemia treatment in children is to reduce the risk of arteriosclerotic cardiovascular disease.
- Changes in Jason's lab values that would indicate that pravastatin is effective include a decrease in LDL cholesterol and triglycerides level and an increase in HDL cholesterol level. Desirable laboratory values for lipid profile in children >3 years of age include LDL cholesterol level 110–129 mg/dL, triglycerides < 125 mg/dL, and HDL > 45 mg/dL.)
- Educate Jason and his parents to take lipid-lowering drugs as prescribed, keep appointments for periodic measurements of blood lipids, avoid preventable adverse drug effects, and provide positive reinforcement for efforts to lower blood lipid levels.
- Support primary prevention strategies with healthful eating habits (e.g., avoiding excessive fats, meat, and dairy products; obtaining adequate amounts of all nutrients, including dietary fiber; avoiding obesity).
- Reinforce the importance of avoiding cigarette smoking, including second-hand smoke.
- Encourage at least 1 hour of daily moderate to vigorous activity; family activities may increase consistent participation.
- Provide appropriate teaching related to drug therapy and risk factor modification (see Box 10.5).

Visit thePoint® at **http://thePoint.lww.com/Frandsen12e** *for answers to NCLEX Success questions (in Appendix A), answers to Clinical Application Case Studies (in Appendix B), and more!*

## REFERENCES AND RESOURCES

American Academy of Pediatrics. (1992). National Cholesterol Education Program: Report of the expert panel on blood cholesterol levels in children and adolescents. *Pediatrics, 89,* 525–584.

Bibbins-Domingo, K., Grossman, D. C., Curry, S. J., Davidson, K. W., Epling, J. W., Garcia, F. A. R., et al. (2016). Statin use for the primary prevention of cardiovascular disease in adults: US Preventive Services Task Force recommendation statement. *Journal of the American Medical Association, 316*(19), 1997–2007. doi:10.1001/jama.2016.15450

Goldstein, J. L., & Brown, M. S. (2015). A century of cholesterol and coronaries: From plaques to genes to statins. *Cell, 161*(1), 161–172.

Grundy, S. M., Stone, N. J., Bailey, A. L., Beam, C., Birtcher, K. K., Blumenthal, R. S., et al. (2019). 2018 AHA/ACC/AACVPR/AAPA/ABC/ACPM/ADA/AGS/APhA/ASPC/NLA/PCNA guideline on the management of blood cholesterol: A report of the American College of Cardiology/American Heart Association Task Force on Clinical Practice Guidelines. *Circulation, 139,* e1082–e1143. doi:10.1161/CIR.0000000000000625

Hendrani, A. D., Adesiyun, T., Quispe, R., Jones, S. R., Stone, N. J., Blumenthal, R. S., et al. (2016). Dyslipidemia management in primary prevention of cardiovascular disease: Current guidelines and strategies. *World Journal of Cardiology, 8*(2), 201–210.

National Heart, Lung, and Blood Institute. (2012). *Expert panel on integrated guidelines for cardiovascular health and risk reduction in children and adolescents* (NIH Publication No. 12-7486). Bethesda, MD: National Institutes of Health.

National Institutes of Health Expert Panel. (2001). *Third report of the National Cholesterol Education Program (NCEP) Expert Panel on detection, evaluation, and treatment of high blood cholesterol in adults (Adult Treatment Panel III)* (NIH Publication No. 01-3670). Bethesda, MD: National Institutes of Health.

Norris, T.L. (2019). *Porth's Pathophysiology: Concepts of altered health states* (10th ed.). Philadelphia, PA: Wolters Kluwer.

Pagidipati, N. J., & Granger, C. B. (2017). Guideline: The USPSTF recommends low- to moderate-dose statins to prevent CVD in selected adults 40 to 75 years of age. *Annals of Internal Medicine, 166*(6), JC26. doi:10.7326/ACPJC-2017-166-6-026

Robinson, J. G., Farnier, M., Krempf, M., Bergeron, J., Luc, G., Averna, M., et al. (2015). Efficacy and safety of alirocumab in reducing lipids and cardiovascular events. *New England Journal of Medicine, 372*, 1489–1499.

Shipman, K. E., Strange, R. C., & Ramachandran, S. (2016). Use of fibrates in the metabolic syndrome: A review. *World Journal of Diabetes, 7*(5), 74–88.

Stone, N. J., Robinson, J. G., Lichtenstein, A. H., Bairey Mertz, C. N., Blum, C. B., Lloyd-Jones, D. M., et al. (2014). 2013 ACC/AHA guideline on the treatment of blood cholesterol to reduce atherosclerotic cardiovascular risk in adults: A report of the American College of Cardiology/American Heart Association Task Force on practice guidelines. *Circulation, 129*, S1–S45.

UpToDate. (2016a). *Intensity of lipid lowering therapy in secondary prevention of cardiovascular disease*. Lexi Comp, Inc.

UpToDate. (2016b). *Lipid lowering with drugs other than statins and fibrates*. Lexi Comp, Inc.

UpToDate. (2019). *Drug information*. Lexi-Comp, Inc.

Yebyo, H.G., Aschmann, H. E., & Puhan, M. A. (2019). Finding the balance between benefits and harms when using statins for primary prevention of cardiovascular disease: A modeling study. *Annals of Internal Medicine, 170*(1), 1–10. doi:10.7326/M18-1279

# Drug Therapy for Hematopoietic Disorders

## LEARNING OBJECTIVES

*After studying this chapter, you should be able to:*

1. Briefly describe hematopoietic and immune functions.
2. Identify common clinical manifestations of inadequate erythropoiesis and diminished host defense mechanisms.
3. Discuss characteristics of erythropoiesis-stimulating agents in terms of the prototype, mechanism of action, indications for use, adverse effects, principles of therapy, and nursing implications.
4. Describe the characteristics of colony-stimulating factors in terms of the prototype, mechanism of action, indications for use, adverse effects, principles of therapy, and nursing implications.
5. Discuss interferons in terms of the prototype, mechanism of action, indications for use, adverse effects, principles of therapy, and nursing implications.
6. Implement the nursing process in the care of patients who take drugs to enhance hematopoietic and immune system function.

## CLINICAL APPLICATION CASE STUDY

Alice Paul is a 76-year-old woman who is being treated with chemotherapy for inoperable liver cancer. She receives a combination chemotherapy regimen every 6 weeks. She is in the oncologist's office for routine laboratory work 10 days after chemotherapy and complains of severe fatigue. The results of her blood work are as follows: hemoglobin 10.9 g/dL, hematocrit 32%, white blood cell (WBC) count 2000 cells/mm$^3$, absolute neutrophil count (ANC) 800 cells/mm$^3$, and platelet count 120,000/μL.

## KEY TERMS

**Biologic response modifiers:** intrinsic and extrinsic substances in the body that enhance the body's response to infection; for example, interferons, monoclonal antibodies, interleukin-2, and types of colony-stimulating factors

**Cytokines:** small proteins released by cells that specifically affect cell-to-cell communication; these include colony-stimulating factors, interleukins, and interferons

**Erythropoiesis:** production of red blood cells

**Erythropoietin:** hormone secreted by the kidneys that stimulates bone marrow production of red blood cells

**Hematopoiesis:** formation of blood cells

**Immunocompetence:** normal immune system function

**Immunodeficiency:** inadequate or impaired immune function

**Immunostimulants:** drugs that stimulate immune function to fight infection and disease

**Neutropenia:** low neutrophil count

**Pegylation:** process of modifying a protein drug by treatment with polyethylene glycol

## INTRODUCTION

Adequate blood cell production, or **hematopoiesis**, and normal immune system function, or **immunocompetence**, are vital processes in the human body's ability to fight harmful invaders. Inadequate or impaired hematopoiesis or immune function (**immunodeficiency**) leads to high risks of infection and cancer. Efforts to enhance a person's own body systems to fight disease include the development of drugs to stimulate hematopoiesis and immune function. People take these drugs to restore normal function or to increase the ability of the immune system to eliminate potentially harmful invaders. This chapter discusses several drugs that affect hematopoietic function and the immune system.

## OVERVIEW OF HEMATOPOIESIS AND IMMUNE FUNCTION

Hematopoietic and immune blood cells originate in bone marrow in stem cells, which are often called pluripotent stem cells because they are capable of becoming different types of cells. As these stem cells reproduce, some cells are exactly like the original cells and are retained in the bone marrow to maintain a continuing supply. However, most reproduced stem cells differentiate to form other types of cells. The early offspring are committed to become a particular type of cell, and a committed stem cell that produces a cell type in a specific cell line is called a colony-forming unit (CFU). Figure 11.1 illustrates the process of hematopoiesis in red and white cells. Hematopoietic growth factors or **cytokines** control the reproduction, growth, and differentiation of stem cells and CFUs. They also initiate the processes required to produce fully mature cells. Overall, cytokines are involved in numerous physiologic responses, including hematopoiesis, cellular proliferation and differentiation, inflammation, wound healing, and cellular and humoral immunity.

## Physiology

### *Hematopoietic Cytokines*

To understand the effects of drug therapy to enhance hematopoiesis or immune function, it is necessary to appreciate the physiologic effects of the endogenous hematopoietic cytokines. The following section discusses the three major groups of cytokines, and it briefly considers **erythropoiesis** and immune function as well.

Hematopoietic cytokines are diverse substances produced mainly by bone marrow and WBCs. They regulate many cellular activities by acting as chemical messengers among cells and as growth factors for blood cells. Cytokines act by binding to receptors on target cells. After binding, the cytokine–receptor complexes trigger signal transduction pathways that alter gene expression in the target cells.

Several factors affect cytokine actions and functions. First, cytokines affect any cells they encounter that have cytokine receptors and are able to respond; they do not act in response to specific antigens. However, cytokine receptors are often

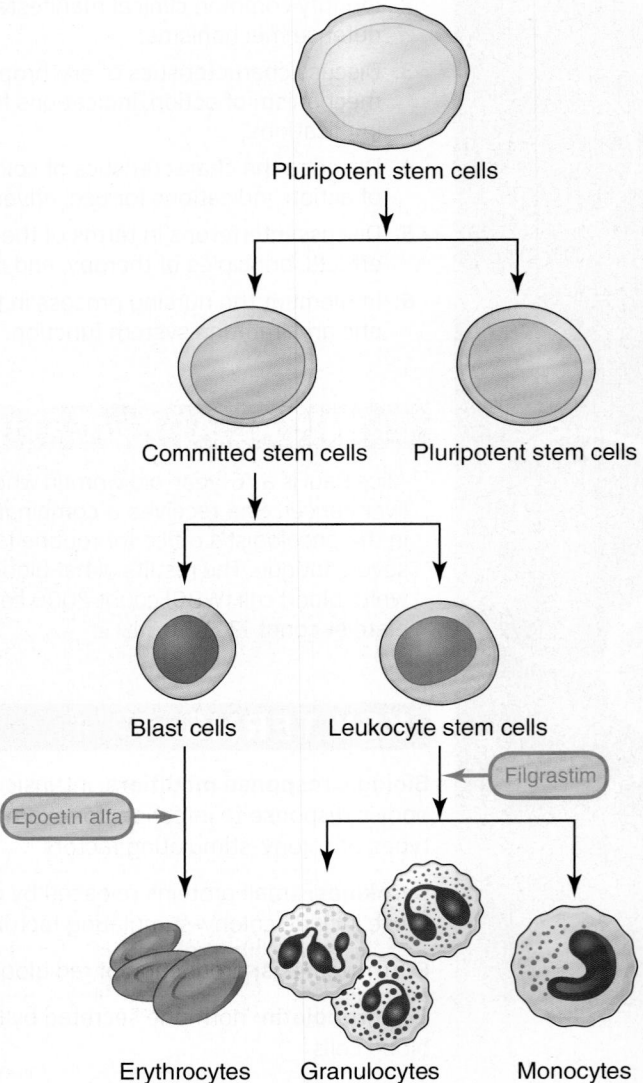

**Figure 11.1.** Hematopoietic and immune blood cell development. Formation, development, and differentiation of erythrocytes and leukocytes, with the site of effects of selected prototype drugs.

expressed on a cell only after that cell has interacted with an antigen, so that cytokine activation is limited to antigen-activated lymphocytes. Second, researchers have determined the actions of most cytokines in laboratories by analyzing the effects of recombinant cytokines, often at nonphysiologic concentrations, and then adding them individually to in vitro systems. Within the human body, however, cytokines rarely, if ever, act alone. Several cytokines, which may have synergistic or antagonistic effects on each other, may affect a target cell. Third, cytokines often induce the synthesis of other cytokines. The resulting interactions may profoundly alter physiologic responses. Fourth, proteins that act as cytokine antagonists are found in the bloodstream and other extracellular fluids. These proteins may bind directly to a cytokine and inhibit its activity or bind to a cytokine receptor but fail to activate the cell.

### Colony-Stimulating Factors

The name *colony-stimulating factor* (CSF) comes from the cluster pattern derived when hemopoietic stem cells are cultured. There are various types of CSFs based on the different types of colonies that grow in the presence of different factors. For example, the substance found to stimulate formation of colonies of granulocytes is called granulocyte colony-stimulating factor (G-CSF), and for macrophages, it is called macrophage colony-stimulating factor (M-CSF). The exposure of pluripotent (progenitor) cells to CSFs controls the production, growth, and differentiation of specific blood cell types. CSFs pertinent to this discussion include those related to the production of red blood cells (RBCs) and leukocyte stem cells.

### Interferons

Interferons are cytokines that communicate between cells to trigger the immune system in response to pathogens, including viruses, bacteria, parasites, and tumor cells. They "interfere" with the ability of viruses in infected cells to replicate and spread to uninfected cells. Interferons also inhibit reproduction and growth of other cells, including tumor cells, and activate natural killer (NK) cells and macrophages. In addition, they enhance communication between cells when antigens or tumors are identified.

These antiproliferative and immunomodulatory activities are important in normal host defense mechanisms. Symptoms of infections, such as fever, muscle pain, and flulike symptoms, also result from the production of interferons and other cytokines.

### Interleukins

Interleukins (ILs) initially received their name because scientists thought they were produced by and acted only on leukocytes. However, body cells other than leukocytes can produce these cytokines, and they can act on nonhematopoietic cells. The majority of ILs are synthesized by helper CD4 T lymphocytes, in addition to monocytes, macrophages, and endothelial cells. They are responsible for activating B and T lymphocytes as well as hematopoietic cells. Researchers have characterized 36 ILs and identified more. Especially important ILs are IL-3 (stimulates growth of stem cell precursors of all blood cells), IL-2 (stimulates T and B lymphocytes), IL-12 (stimulates hematopoietic cells and lymphocytes), and IL-11 (stimulates platelets and other cells). ILs may act only in combination with another

factor, may be suppressive rather than stimulatory (e.g., IL-10), or may involve a specific function (e.g., IL-8 mainly promotes movement of leukocytes into injured tissues as part of the inflammatory response).

### Erythropoiesis

**Erythropoietin**, a hormone secreted by the kidneys, stimulates bone marrow production of RBCs, or erythropoiesis. The hormone travels through the circulation to the bone marrow, where it stimulates red cell differentiation, maturation, and proliferation. The major signal for erythropoietin production is a decreased oxygen level detected by the proximal tubule cells in the kidneys. Conditions that trigger erythropoietin production include hemorrhage, anemia, chronic obstructive pulmonary disease, and high altitude. Erythropoietin also promotes the production of hemoglobin, necessary for a functioning erythrocyte.

Parameters used to measure erythropoiesis include RBC count, hemoglobin concentration and hematocrit, and mean corpuscular volume. In addition, the reticulocyte count quantitatively measures the bone marrow's production of new RBCs.

### Immune Function

Immune cells are WBCs that circulate in the blood and lymphatic vessels or reside in lymphoid tissues. These cells are present in virtually all body tissues, and their ability to circulate throughout the body and to migrate between blood and lymphoid tissues makes them a major component of host defenses. The cells are activated by exposure to antigens (e.g., viruses, bacteria, parasites). Although all WBCs play a role in phagocytic and immune processes, neutrophils, monocytes, and lymphocytes are especially important.

Cytokines also provide defense support to the immune system. These protein substances secreted by specific cells of the immune system carry signals locally between cells and thus have an effect on the interactions between them. The cytokines include the CSFs, interferons, and ILs, as well as cell signal molecules, such as tumor necrosis factor (see previous discussion).

## Clinical Manifestations

As RBCs or WBCs decrease, conditions related to inadequate hematopoiesis or poor immune function develop. Clinical manifestations of inadequate erythropoiesis include anemia. This results in a decrease in the oxygen-carrying capacity of blood and consequently a decreased oxygen availability to the tissues. A compensatory increase in heart rate and cardiac output initially increases cardiac output, offsetting the lower oxygen-carrying capacity of the blood. However, the oxygen demand becomes greater than the supply, and clinical manifestations are directly attributable to tissue hypoxia. Muscle weakness and easy fatigability are common. In severe anemia, the skin is usually pale to a waxy pallor, and cyanosis is typically absent. Headache, irritability, light-headedness, slowed thought processes, and depression are common central nervous system effects. (However, children appear to have a remarkable ability to function quite well with low hemoglobin levels.)

Clinical manifestations of diminished host defense mechanisms demonstrate decreased resistance to infections, including frequent colds and flu symptoms, recurring parasitic infections, and opportunistic infections. Complete blood (cell) count (CBC) measurements include **neutropenia** (low neutrophil count). Specifically, the ANC is the number of neutrophils in the blood, which can be used as a direct measurement of a person's ability to combat infection. The ANC is determined by multiplying the total number of WBCs by the percentage of neutrophils.

## Drug Therapy

The drugs described in this chapter stimulate the production of either erythrocytes or leukocytes. Hematopoietic growth factors enhance the erythrocyte production and oxygen-carrying capability. **Immunostimulants** are drugs that enhance immune function; they help a person fight disease. Health care providers use these drugs to restore normal function or to increase the ability of the immune system to eliminate potentially harmful invaders. Available drugs include erythropoiesis-stimulating agents (ESAs), CSFs, and several interferons. The following sections and Table 11.1 describe these drugs, which are the primary focus of this chapter. The section on *Adjuvant Medications* briefly discusses two ILs. Other chapters also discuss drugs with immunostimulant properties. These include traditional immunizing agents (see Chap. 12); levamisole, which restores functions of macrophages and T cells and is used with fluorouracil in the treatment of intestinal cancer (see Chap. 14); and antiviral drugs used in the treatment of acquired immunodeficiency syndrome (AIDS; see Chap. 23).

Most hematopoietic and immunostimulant drugs are synthetic versions of endogenous cytokines. Manufacturers use molecular biology–associated techniques to delineate the type and sequence of amino acids and to identify the genes responsible for producing the substances. Technicians then insert these genes into bacteria (usually *Escherichia coli*) or yeasts capable of producing the substances exogenously. Exogenous drug preparations have the same mechanisms of action as the endogenous products. Thus, CSFs bind to receptors on the cell surfaces of immature blood cells in the bone marrow and increase the number, maturity, and functional ability of the cells.

In cancer, the exact mechanisms by which interferons and ILs exert antineoplastic effects are unknown. However, their immunostimulant effects are thought to enhance activities of immune cells (i.e., NK cells, T cells, B cells, and macrophages),

induce tumor cell antigens (which make tumor cells more easily recognized by immune cells), or alter the expression of oncogenes (genes that can cause a normal cell to change to a cancer cell).

All these drugs may produce adverse effects so that patients may not feel better when taking the drug. The combination of injections and adverse effects may lead to nonadherence in taking the drugs as prescribed.

## ERYTHROPOIESIS-STIMULATING AGENTS

The hematopoietic growth factor Ⓟ **epoetin alfa** (Epogen, Procrit) is the prototype recombinant form of human erythropoietin that helps the body produce more RBCs. The clinical benefit of treatment of anemia with an ESA is to reduce the need and cost of blood transfusions, lessen the risk of infectious diseases from transfusions, and potentially enhance the overall quality of life as anemia is relieved. Although ESAs have been used to treat anemia associated with a variety of conditions, evidence indicates that the patients who benefit consistently from ESAs are prescribed epoetin alfa or another ESA for chemotherapy-associated anemia or those with anemia due to chronic kidney disease.

## Pharmacokinetics

Both subcutaneous and intravenous (IV) administrations lead to good absorption (digestive enzymes would destroy the drug if it were given orally). The distribution is unknown, and metabolism occurs in the plasma. Excretion of a small amount occurs in the kidneys. The onset of action is 11 to 14 days. Whether the drug crosses the placenta or is excreted in breast milk is not known.

## Action

Epoetin alfa induces erythropoiesis by stimulating erythroid progenitor cells. This causes the release of reticulocytes from the bone marrow, leading to an increase in hemoglobin and hematocrit levels.

### TABLE 11.1

### Drugs Administered for Hematopoiesis and Immunostimulation

| Drug Class | Prototype[s] | Other Drugs in the Class |
|---|---|---|
| Erythropoiesis-stimulating agents | Epoetin alfa (Epogen, Procrit) | Darbepoetin alfa (Aranesp)<br>Epoetin beta (Mircera) |
| Colony-stimulating factors | Filgrastim (G-CSF) (Neupogen) | Pegfilgrastim (G-CSF) (Neulasta)<br>Sargramostim (GM-CSF) (Leukine) |
| Interferons | Interferon alfa 2b (Intron A) | Peginterferon alfa-2a (Pegasys)<br>Interferon alfa n3 (Alferon N)<br>Interferon beta 1a (Avonex, Rebif)<br>Interferon beta 1b (Betaseron)<br>Interferon gamma 1b (Actimmune) |

G-CSF, granulocyte colony-stimulating factor; GM-CSF, granulocyte–macrophage colony-stimulating factor.

## Use

Experts recommend epoetin alfa as a treatment option for cancer patients with chemotherapy-associated anemia who have a hemoglobin level that has decreased below 10 g/dL. Another use for the drug is in the prevention and treatment of anemia associated with chronic kidney disease.

Clinical practice guidelines for use of ESAs from the American Society of Hematology and the American Society of Clinical Oncology (Rizzo et al., 2010) advise that ESAs should be administered at the smallest possible dose that increases hemoglobin to the lowest acceptable level to avoid blood transfusions. The U.S. Food and Drug Administration (FDA) has issued a **BLACK BOX WARNING ◆** directing prescribers that treatment of anemia with an ESA in patients with cancer who are not receiving chemotherapy offers no benefit and may cause serious harm.

Table 11.2 presents route and dosage information for the ESAs.

### Use in Children

The basis for epoetin alfa dosing in children is body weight and hemoglobin level.

>  **QSEN Alert: Safety**
>
> Premature infants should not receive epoetin alfa from multidose vials because they contain benzyl alcohol, which can be fatal. Single-dose vials do not contain benzyl alcohol.

### Use in Older Adults

In general, hematopoietic drugs have the same uses and responses in older adults as in younger adults. However, older adults may be at greater risk of adverse effects, especially if large doses are used or if hemoglobin is increased quickly or raised above acceptable limits.

### Use in Patients With Critical Illness

Patients with cancer may receive epoetin alfa to manage anemia induced by chemotherapy that depresses bone marrow function. Patients with chronic kidney disease may also benefit from an ESA because they have reduced production of erythropoietin by the kidney and shortened red cell survival. In addition, they may be critically ill and could benefit from stabilizing hemoglobin levels. However, they are more susceptible to venous thrombosis and may respond more unfavorably to adverse reactions, such as hypertension, nausea, vomiting, and diarrhea.

### Use in Patients Receiving Home Care

Patients often take epoetin alfa in the home, whether self-administered or given by a caregiver. The home health nurse may need to teach patients or caregivers how to accurately administer the drug and provide assistance in obtaining appropriate laboratory tests (e.g., CBC, platelet count, tests of renal or hepatic function) to monitor the responses to the drug.

## Adverse Effects

The most common adverse effect of epoetin alfa is hypertension; raising the hemoglobin slowly minimizes this. Other adverse effects include nausea, vomiting, diarrhea, and arthralgias.

>  **QSEN Alert: Safety**
>
> Epoetin alfa increases risks of myocardial infarction and stroke, especially if it is used to achieve hemoglobin levels greater than 12 g/dL.

Injection of epoetin alfa increases the risk of thrombus formation. The FDA has issued a **BLACK BOX WARNING ◆** advising prescribers to avoid using ESAs in patients with hemoglobin values of 12 g/dL or above. In addition, serious adverse cardiovascular reactions and stroke have been reported in controlled trials when ESAs are administered to patients with chronic kidney disease to target hemoglobin levels greater than 11 g/dL. Epoetin alfa should be administered at the lowest dose effective in raising hemoglobin levels sufficiently to avoid the need for blood transfusion. Regular monitoring of hemoglobin is necessary until the level stabilizes.

## Contraindications

Contraindications to epoetin alfa include known hypersensitivity to the drug or to albumin (or other cell-derived products from mammals). In addition, people with uncontrolled hypertension should not take epoetin alfa because it may further increase blood pressure.

| **TABLE 11.2** | | |
|---|---|---|
| **DRUGS AT A GLANCE: Erythropoiesis-Stimulating Agents** | | |
| **Drug** | **Pregnancy Category** | **Routes and Dosage Ranges** |
| Ⓟ **Epoetin alfa** (Epogen, Procrit; 🍁 Eprex) | C | Cancer chemotherapy: Adults, 150–300 units/kg sub-Q three times weekly 1 mo to 12 y, 600 units/kg IV, sub-Q once a week<br>Chronic kidney disease: Adults, 50–100 units/kg IV, sub-Q three times weekly to achieve or maintain hemoglobin level of no more than 12 g/dL 1 mo to 12 y, 50 units/kg IV, sub-Q three times a week |
| Darbepoetin alfa (Aranesp; 🍁 Aranesp) | C | Adults: Sub-Q, IV 0.45 mcg/kg once weekly, adjusted to achieve and maintain hemoglobin level no more than 12 g/dL |
| **Epoetin beta** (Mircera) | C | Chronic kidney disease (on dialysis): Adults, IV (preferred) 0.6 mcg/kg once every 2 wk adjusted to achieve or maintain hemoglobin level of no more than 11 g/dL<br>Chronic kidney disease (not on dialysis): Adults, IV, sub-Q 0.6 mcg/kg once every 2 wk adjusted to achieve or maintain hemoglobin level of no more than 10 g/dL |

# Nursing Implications

## Preventing Interactions

No significant interactions with drugs or herbs with epoetin alfa have been reported.

## Administering the Medication

For patients with chronic kidney disease on hemodialysis, the nurse gives epoetin alfa by bolus injection at the end of dialysis. For other patients with an IV line, IV administration is appropriate. For patients without an IV line or who are ambulatory, subcutaneous administration is suitable. The nurse ensures that the remainder of a multidose vial is discarded 21 days after opening.

 **QSEN Alert: Safety**

A multidose vial of epoetin alfa is not appropriate for use in children because of the risk of medication error.

## Assessing for Therapeutic Effects

The nurse observes for increased RBCs, hemoglobin, and hematocrit; increased energy and exercise capacity; and improved quality of life. Therapeutic effects depend on the dose and the patient's underlying condition. The goal is usually to achieve and maintain a hemoglobin level of no more than 12 g/dL. With epoetin alfa, it is necessary to measure iron stores (transferrin saturation and serum ferritin) before and periodically during treatment. The nurse ensures that hemoglobin levels are measured twice weekly until stabilized and maintenance drug doses are established.

## Assessing for Adverse Effects

The nurse ascertains that blood pressure remains within a safe range and also assesses for nausea, vomiting, diarrhea, or joint pain. Because there is an increased risk of myocardial infarction and stroke, assessment of mental status changes and chest pain or decreased cardiac perfusion is necessary.

 **QSEN Alert: Safety**

In addition, it is important to assess for signs of deep vein thrombus formation (e.g., swelling, pain, and redness of the affected limb) in patients taking epoetin alfa.

## Patient Teaching

 **QSEN Alert: Safety**

Epoetin alfa is not effective unless sufficient iron is present; therefore, patient teaching may need to emphasize the importance of taking an iron supplement.

Box 11.1 presents additional patient teaching guidelines for this drug.

# Other Drugs in the Class

Darbepoetin alfa (Aranesp) is another ESA used in the prevention or treatment of anemia associated with several conditions, including chronic kidney disease and myelosuppressive (depressed bone marrow function) anticancer chemotherapy. Epoetin alfa and darbepoetin are similarly effective in achieving and maintaining target hemoglobin levels. Darbepoetin is a relatively long-acting agent compared to epoetin alfa's shorter-acting duration. The absorption of this drug is slow via the subcutaneous route, and in kidney disease, peak plasma levels occur in adults in about 48 hours (36 hours in children). In cancer, the time to peak plasma levels is 74 hours (49 hours in children). Hemoglobin levels increase after 2 to 6 weeks of therapy with darbepoetin. Studies indicate that a patient with cancer-related anemia and hemoglobin of 10 g/dL or less feels better and requires fewer blood transfusions with use of the drug. No significant interactions have reportedly occurred with this drug.

Epoetin beta (Mircera) is used in the treatment of anemia associated with chronic kidney disease in adults—whether or not they require dialysis. The FDA has issued a **BLACK BOX WARNING**  for epoetin beta, reporting that it is not indicated and is not recommended for treatment of chemotherapy-induced anemia. Researchers terminated a study because more deaths occurred in patients taking epoetin beta than in those taking another ESA. This drug is also not indicated as a substitute for RBC transfusions in patients who need immediate correction of anemia. The adverse effects profile for epoetin beta is similar to that of other ESAs, with hypertension being the most common effect. As with all ESAs, an adequate intake of iron is required for drug effectiveness, and an iron supplement is usually necessary.

*Clinical Application 11.1*

- What is the significance of Mrs. Paul's laboratory results?

 **QSEN Alert: Evidence-Based Practice**

Researchers designed a prospective, observational registry study to evaluate the safety of darbepoetin alfa in children 16 years of age or younger with anemia and chronic kidney disease (Schaefer et al., 2016). Over a period of up to 2 years, dosage patterns, frequency of adverse events, transfusions requirements, and hemoglobin concentrations were observed in 319 children. Nearly half of the children were on dialysis (with a comparable number on hemodialysis vs. peritoneal dialysis). During the study period, hemoglobin concentration rose slightly in the initial 3 months and remained stable, as did the darbepoetin alfa dose. Some children (15%) required transfusions. Hypertension (48.6%) and seizures (17.2%) were the most frequently encountered adverse effects. Findings indicated that darbepoetin alfa was effective in treating anemia in these patients. However, the noninterventional design of the study may limit the degree generalizability to standard management.

# NCLEX Success

1. Patients with chronic kidney disease benefit from epoetin alfa because the drug

   A. metabolizes the hormone that interferes with red blood cell (RBC) production

   B. neutralizes accumulating waste products in the kidney that destroy circulating RBCs

   C. replaces erythropoietin no longer produced in the proximal tubules of the kidney

   D. increases the kidney's excretion of toxic substances that decrease RBC production

**BOX 11.1**  *Patient Teaching Guidelines for Hematopoietic Drugs and Immunostimulants*

**General Considerations**

- Help your body maintain immune mechanisms and other defenses by healthy lifestyle habits, such as a nutritious diet, adequate rest and sleep, and avoidance of tobacco and alcohol.
- Practice meticulous personal hygiene and avoid people and circumstances in which you are exposed to infection.
- Keep appointments with health care providers for follow-up care, blood tests, and so forth.
- Inform any other physician, dentist, or health care provider about your condition and the medications you are taking.
- It is possible to administer several of these medications at home, even though they are given by injection. If you are going to self-inject a medication at home, allow sufficient time to learn and practice the techniques under the supervision of a health care provider. Correct preparation and injection are necessary to increase beneficial effects and decrease adverse effects. Be sure to dispose of needles and syringes properly.
- With interferons, report the occurrence of depression or thoughts of suicide, dizziness, hives, itching, chest tightness, cough, difficulty breathing or wheezing, or visual problems. These symptoms may require that the drug be stopped or the dosage reduced. In addition, avoid pregnancy (use effective contraceptive methods), avoid prolonged exposure to sunlight, wear protective clothing, and use sunscreens.

**Self- or Caregiver Administration**

- Take the drugs as prescribed. Although this is important with all medications, it is especially important with these. Obtaining beneficial effects and decreasing adverse effects depend largely on how the drugs are taken.
- Use correct techniques to prepare and inject the medications. Instructions for mixing the drugs should be followed exactly.
  - With epoetin alfa, follow these instructions:
    - Do not freeze or shake the drug vial.

- Obtain appropriate laboratory tests to monitor the responses to the drug.
- Take an iron supplement, if instructed, to ensure absorption of the drug.
- Consume foods that contain vitamin C (e.g., fruit juice, strawberries, cantaloupe) to increase the absorption of iron.
- With filgrastim, follow these instructions:
  - Take acetaminophen (e.g., Tylenol, others), if desired, to decrease bone pain.
  - Notify your prescriber if pain is not relieved, especially if taking high-dose IV therapy, because opioids may be necessary.
  - Recognize that dosage modification may be necessary if your WBC count is greater than 100,000 cells/mm³.
- With interferons, follow these instructions:
  - Store the drug in the refrigerator.
  - Do not freeze or shake the drug vial.
  - Do not change brands (changes in dosage may result).
  - Take at bedtime to reduce some common adverse effects (e.g., flulike symptoms such as fever, headache, fatigue, anorexia, nausea, and vomiting).
  - Take acetaminophen (e.g., Tylenol, others), if desired, to prevent or decrease fever and headache.
  - Maintain a fluid intake of 2 to 3 quarts daily.
- With ILs, follow these instructions:
  - Store the drug in the refrigerator.
  - Do not freeze or shake the drug vial.
  - Do not use if solution is discolored or if it contains particles.
  - Do not breast-feed while taking this drug.
  - Take acetaminophen (e.g., Tylenol, others), if desired, to prevent or decrease fever and headache.
  - Maintain a fluid intake of 2 to 3 quarts daily.
  - Report any of the following to your prescriber: shortness of breath, edema, chest pain, unusual fatigue or weakness, and irregular heartbeat.

2. The expected outcome of administering epoetin alfa or darbepoetin alfa to a patient with chronic kidney disease is
   A. decreased bleeding
   B. increased white blood cell production
   C. increased red blood cell production
   D. improved renal function

3. The nurse who is administering epoetin alfa knows that most patients who take epoetin alfa or darbepoetin alfa also need to take
   A. iron
   B. potassium
   C. antacids
   D. analgesics

# GRANULOCYTE COLONY-STIMULATING FACTORS

The drug ⓟ **filgrastim** (Neupogen) is the prototype G-CSF used to stimulate blood cell production by the bone marrow in patients with bone marrow transplantation or chemotherapy-induced neutropenia. This drug can help prevent infection by reducing the incidence, severity, and duration of neutropenia associated with several chemotherapy regimens. Health care providers also use it to collect stem cells for transplantation. Experts believe that filgrastim promotes the growth of arterioles around blocked areas in coronary arteries. It may be more effective than drugs that stimulate capillary growth, because arterioles are larger and can carry more blood.

# Pharmacokinetics

Filgrastim is completely absorbed. The duration of action of the drug is 4 days. It is systemically degraded, and the nature of its excretion is unknown. There is no evidence of drug accumulation over a period of 11 to 20 days. Filgrastim crosses the placenta and may enter breast milk.

# Action

Filgrastim stimulates the production, maturation, and activation of neutrophils within bone marrow.

# Use

Indications for filgrastim include (1) preventing infection in patients with neutropenia induced by cancer chemotherapy or bone marrow transplantation or (2) mobilizing stem cells from bone marrow to peripheral blood, where they can be collected and reinfused after chemotherapy that depresses bone marrow function. Most patients who take the drug have fewer days of fever, infection, and antimicrobial drug therapy. In addition, by promoting bone marrow recovery after a course of cytotoxic antineoplastic drugs, it also may allow higher doses or more timely administration of subsequent antitumor drugs. Table 11.3 presents route and dosage information for the CSFs.

## Use in Children

The therapeutic and adverse effects of filgrastim in children are similar to those in adults. In clinical trials, filgrastim produced a greater incidence of subclinical spleen enlargement in children than in adults, but whether this affects growth and development or has other long-term consequences is unknown.

## Use in Older Adults

In general, filgrastim has the same uses and responses in older adults as in younger adults. Older adults may be at greater risk for adverse effects, especially if large doses are used. Older adults are more likely to develop infections (including reactivation of tuberculosis and herpes zoster) and less able to recover from them. Therefore, older adults need protective measures, such as rigorous personal hygiene; good nutrition; adequate exercise, rest, and sleep; minimal exposure to potential pathogens, when possible; and appropriate immunizations (e.g., influenza, pneumonia, tetanus). When an infection develops in older adults, signs and symptoms (e.g., fever, drainage) may be absent or less pronounced than in younger adults.

## Use in Patients With Renal Impairment

Little information about the use of filgrastim in patients with renal impairment is available. Authorities recommend that patients with preexisting impairment have renal function tests every 2 weeks.

## Use in Patients With Hepatic Impairment

Close monitoring may be necessary, because the dose, regimen, or timing of administration may need to be altered with hepatic impairment.

## TABLE 11.3

### DRUGS AT A GLANCE: Colony-Stimulating Factors

| Drug | Pregnancy Category | Routes and Dosage Ranges (Adults) |
|---|---|---|
| Ⓟ **Filgrastim** (G-CSF) (Neupogen, Granix, Zarxio, Nivestym; 🍁 Neupogen, Grastofil) | C | Myelosuppressive chemotherapy: 5 mg/kg/d sub-Q injection, IV infusion over 15–30 min, or continuous sub-Q or IV infusion, up to 2 wk until ANC reaches 10,000/mm³ <br> Bone marrow transplantation: 10 mcg/kg/d IV infusion initially at least 24 h after chemotherapy and >24 h after bone marrow infusion, then titrated according to neutrophil count (5 mcg/kg/d if ANC over 1000/mm³ for 3 consecutive days; stop drug if over 1000/mm³ for 3 d; if ANC drops below 1000/mm³, restart filgrastim at 5 mcg/kg/d; if ANC drops below 1000/mm³ during 5 mcg/kg/d dose, increase to 10 mcg/kg/d). Collection of peripheral stem cells: 10 mcg/kg/d sub-Q for 6–7 d, with collection on the last 3 d of drug administration. <br> Severe, chronic neutropenia: 5 or 6 mcg/kg sub-Q, once or twice daily, depending on clinical response and ANC |
| Pegfilgrastim (G-CSF) (Neulasta, Neulasta Onpro, Fulphila, Udenyca; 🍁 Neulasta) | C | 6 mg sub-Q once per chemotherapy cycle; do not give between 14 d before and 24 h after cytotoxic chemotherapy |
| Sargramostim (GM-CSF) (Leukine; 🍁 Leukine) | C | Acute myeloid leukemia: Adults ≥55 y 250 mcg/m²/d IV infusion over 4 h, starting on day 11 or 4 d following induction chemotherapy after bone marrow infusion for maximum of 42 d <br> Bone marrow reconstitution: 250 mcg/m²/d IV infusion over 2 h, starting 2–4 h after bone marrow infusion and continuing for 21 d <br> Graft failure or delay: 250 mcg/m²/d IV infusion over 2 h for 14 d; course of treatment may be repeated after 7 d of therapy if engraftment has not occurred <br> Mobilization of stem cells: 250 mcg/m²/d sub-Q or IV over 24 h |

ANC, absolute neutrophil count; G-CSF, granulocyte colony-stimulating factor; GM-CSF, granulocyte–macrophage colony-stimulating factor.

### Use in Patients With Critical Illness

Critically ill patients may be given filgrastim to restore, promote, or accelerate bone marrow function.

> **QSEN Alert: Safety**
>
> Patients should not receive filgrastim within 24 hours before or 24 hours after cytotoxic chemotherapy because it may act as a growth factor for any tumor, particularly of the myeloid type.

Patients in a hospital setting are most vulnerable to infection, particularly nosocomial organisms, especially if their neutrophil count falls below 500/mm.[3]

### Use in Patients Receiving Home Care

The home care nurse needs to assess patients who take filgrastim while at home for sign of an infection and to teach them measures to reduce exposure to infection. The nurse also needs to assess for accurate administration of the drug as well as for ability of the patient to obtain appropriate laboratory tests (e.g., CBC, platelet count, tests of renal or hepatic function) (see Box 11.1).

## Adverse Effects and Contraindications

The most common adverse effects of filgrastim are drowsiness, fatigue, flulike symptoms, nausea, and bone pain. Contraindications include a known sensitivity to the drug and *E. coli*–derived proteins.

## Nursing Implications

### Preventing Interactions

No medications reportedly increase or decrease the effects of filgrastim. Likewise, no herbs or foods appear to increase or decrease the drug's effects.

### Administering the Medication

The nurse administers filgrastim by subcutaneous or IV injection according to indication per the manufacturer's recommendation:

- For cancer chemotherapy: subcutaneous bolus injection, IV infusion over 15 to 30 minutes, or continuous subcutaneous or IV infusion
- For bone marrow transplantation: IV infusion over 4 hours or by continuous IV or subcutaneous infusion
- For collection of stem cells: as a bolus or a continuous infusion
- For chronic neutropenia: subcutaneous injection

It is important not to shake a vial of filgrastim and to use it only once.

### Assessing for Therapeutic Effects

The nurse assesses for a decreased incidence of infection and a maintenance of the ANC within a target range of 1500 to 10,000 cells/mm[3].

### Assessing for Adverse Effects

The nurse observes for drowsiness, fatigue, flulike symptoms, nausea, and bone pain. In addition, it is necessary to assess for erythema at subcutaneous injection sites.

> **QSEN Alert: Safety**
>
> The nurse should check the ANC and report to the prescriber if it is 10,000 cells/mm³ or greater.

### Patient Teaching

The nurse teaches the patient and family about accurate drug preparation and injection techniques as well as proper disposal of needles and syringes. Box 11.1 contains additional patient teaching guidelines.

## Other Drugs in the Class

Pegfilgrastim (Neulasta), which stays in the body longer and can be given less often than filgrastim, is another CSF, a G-CSF. (Conjugation of filgrastim with polyethylene glycol produces pegfilgrastim.) Uses for pegfilgrastim include prevention of infection in neutropenia induced by cancer chemotherapy as well as treatment of bone marrow transplantation for Hodgkin's disease, non-Hodgkin's lymphoma, or acute lymphoblastic leukemia. It is important to note that after transplantation, it takes 2 to 4 weeks for the engrafted bone marrow cells to mature and begin producing blood cells. During this time, patients have virtually no functioning granulocytes and are at high risk for infection. Pegfilgrastim helps reduce the incidence, severity, and duration of neutropenia associated with several chemotherapy regimens and restore, promote, or accelerate bone marrow function.

Most patients who take pegfilgrastim, like those who take filgrastim, have fewer days of fever, infection, and antimicrobial drug therapy. The drug also may allow higher doses or more timely administration of subsequent antitumor drugs by promoting bone marrow recovery after a course of cytotoxic antineoplastic drugs. Patients should not take it 14 days before and 24 hours after cytotoxic chemotherapy. As with filgrastim, the most common adverse effects are drowsiness, fatigue, flulike symptoms, nausea, and bone pain. Additionally, lithium may potentially cause a drug interaction with pegfilgrastim; lithium increases the production of WBCs, increasing the risk of a stroke or heart attack.

Sargramostim (Leukine) is a granulocyte–macrophage CSF (GM-CSF) used to treat patients who undergo bone marrow transplantation for Hodgkin's disease, non-Hodgkin's lymphoma, or acute lymphoblastic leukemia. As with pegfilgrastim, it takes 2 to 4 weeks after transplantation for the engrafted bone marrow cells to mature and begin producing blood cells. During this time, there are essentially no functioning granulocytes, and there is a high risk of infection. Sargramostim promotes engraftment and function of the transplanted bone marrow, thereby decreasing the risk of infection. If the graft is successful, the granulocyte count starts to rise in approximately 2 weeks.

Health care providers also use sargramostim in stem cell transplantation to stimulate the movement of hematopoietic stem cells from the bone marrow to circulating blood, where they can be readily collected. Indications for use are after bone marrow transplantation to promote bone marrow function or to treat graft failure or delayed function. Transplantation of large numbers of stem cells can lead to more rapid engraftment and recovery, with less risk of transplant failure and complications. When giving sargramostim to patients with cancer who have had bone marrow transplantation, it is necessary to start the drug 2 to 4 hours after the bone marrow infusion and at least 24 hours after the last dose of antineoplastic chemotherapy or 12 hours after the last radiotherapy treatment. The nurse should ensure that CBCs are performed twice weekly during therapy; the neutrophil count should not exceed approximately 20,000/mm$^3$.

In some patients with preexisting renal impairment, sargramostim increases serum creatinine. Values decline to baseline levels when the drug is stopped or its dosage reduced. With preexisting hepatic impairment, sargramostim also can increase serum bilirubin and liver enzymes. Values return to baseline when the drug is stopped or its dosage reduced.

Corticosteroids and lithium are known to increase effects of sargramostim. These drugs have myeloproliferative (bone marrow–stimulating) effects of their own, which may add to those of sargramostim.

Adverse effects occur more often with sargramostim than filgrastim and include bone pain, fever, headache, muscle aches, generalized maculopapular skin rash, and fluid retention (peripheral edema, pleural effusion, pericardial effusion). Bone pain occurs in approximately 33% to 50% of patients. Other effects occur in more than 10% of patients. Pleural and pericardial effusions are more likely at doses greater than 20 mcg/kg/d.

## NCLEX Success

4. Which of the following adverse effects should the nurse discuss with a patient receiving filgrastim?
   A. fatigue
   B. bleeding
   C. headache
   D. bone pain

5. The nurse is administering filgrastim to a patient who has received a bone marrow transplant. Which laboratory parameter should the nurse monitor to determine if the drug is effective?
   A. hemoglobin
   B. basophils
   C. hematocrit
   D. neutrophils

6. The nurse is caring for a patient who is undergoing chemotherapy for cancer. The physician orders filgrastim. The nurse explains to the patient that an expected outcome after the administration of filgrastim is
   A. fewer infections
   B. decreased anemia
   C. longer life expectancy
   D. less nausea and vomiting

# INTERFERONS

Interferons, called alfa, beta, or gamma, according to specific characteristics, are **biologic response modifiers** that bind to specific cell surface receptors and alter intracellular activities. In viral infections, these immunostimulants induce enzymes that inhibit protein synthesis and degrade viral RNA. As a result, viruses are less able to enter uninfected cells, reproduce, and release new viruses. In addition to their antiviral effects, interferons also have antiproliferative and immunoregulatory activities. They can increase expression of major histocompatibility complex molecules, augment the activity of NK cells, increase the effectiveness of antigen-presenting cells in inducing the proliferation of cytotoxic T cells, aid the attachment of cytotoxic T cells to target cells, and inhibit angiogenesis (formation of blood vessels). (The recent development of more effective drugs has replaced the interferons as the standard of treatment for certain conditions.)

Synthetically produced interferons have the same capabilities as endogenous interferons. Thus, indications include treatment of viral infections and certain cancers (for specific details, see *Use*). ⓟ **Interferon alfa 2b** (Intron A) is the prototype for this class of drugs and is a product of recombinant DNA technology using *E. coli*.

## Pharmacokinetics

Interferon alfa 2b is about 80% absorbed and widely distributed but does not cross the blood–brain barrier. There is minimal hepatic metabolism. Excretion is primarily renal. Peak onset of action is 3 to 12 hours. The elimination half-life is approximately 2 to 3 hours.

## Action

Interferon alfa 2b has both antiviral and antineoplastic activities. It exerts its cellular activities by binding to specific membrane receptors on the cell surface enhancing immune response, inhibiting viral replication in virus-infected cells. The drug enhances the overall function of the immune system by increasing phagocytic activity of macrophages and monocytes, which augments cytotoxicity against cancer cells. Additionally, it suppresses the growth and reproduction of similar cells by cell division.

## Use

Indications for use of interferon alfa 2b in adults 18 years of age and older include hairy cell leukemia, chronic hepatitis B and C, AIDS-related Kaposi's sarcoma, genital warts, malignant melanoma, lymphoma (follicular), and condylomata. Table 11.4 presents route and dosage information for the interferons.

### Use in Children

Interferons are used in children for the treatment of hemangiomas and for chronic hepatitis C. The drug is administered subcutaneously.

- For hemangiomas, the usual daily dose is 3 million units/m$^2$ once.
- For chronic hepatitis C, the usual dose is 3 to 5 million units/m$^2$ three times/week for children 3 years of age or more and adolescents.

Multidose vials should not be used in children because they contain benzyl alcohol, which could increase the risk of neurologic complications.

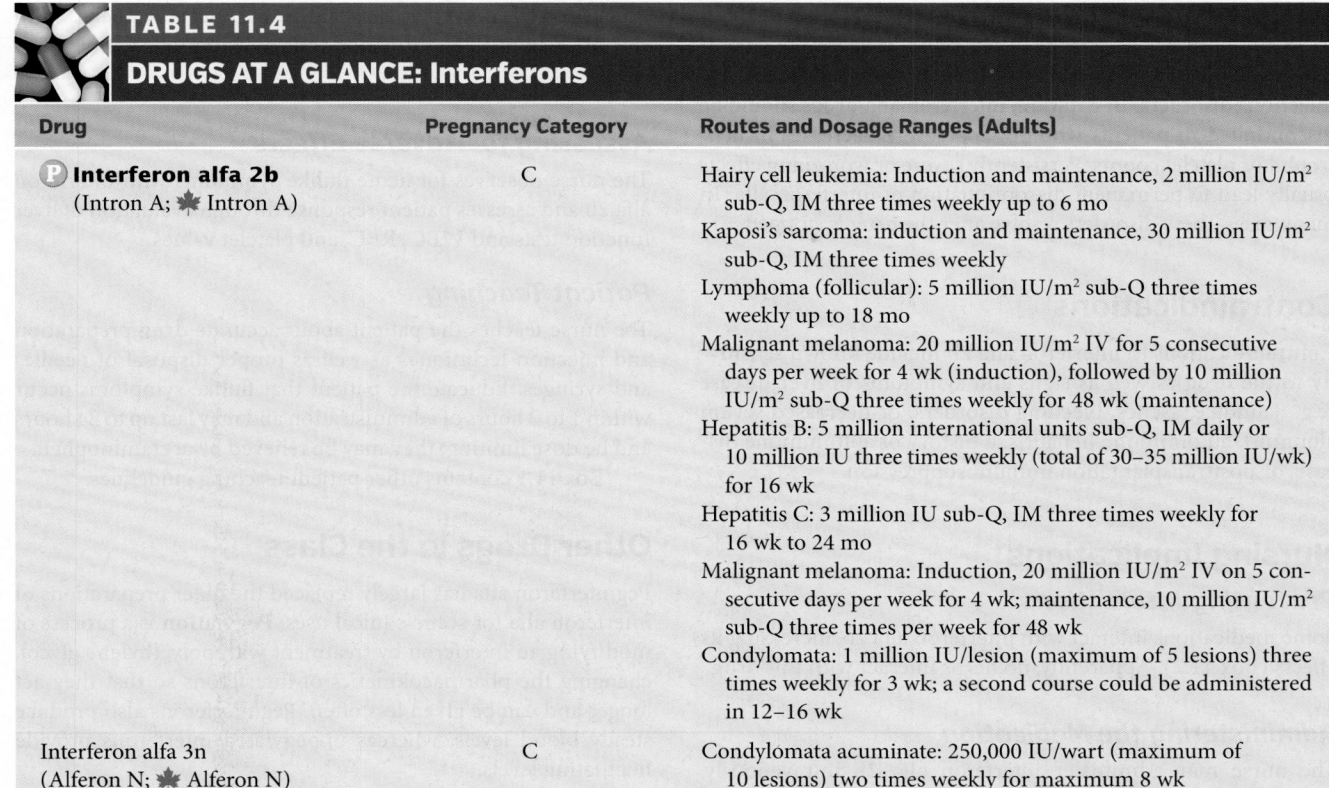

| Drug | Pregnancy Category | Routes and Dosage Ranges (Adults) |
|---|---|---|
| **Ⓟ Interferon alfa 2b**<br>(Intron A; ❋ Intron A) | C | Hairy cell leukemia: Induction and maintenance, 2 million $IU/m^2$ sub-Q, IM three times weekly up to 6 mo<br>Kaposi's sarcoma: induction and maintenance, 30 million $IU/m^2$ sub-Q, IM three times weekly<br>Lymphoma (follicular): 5 million $IU/m^2$ sub-Q three times weekly up to 18 mo<br>Malignant melanoma: 20 million $IU/m^2$ IV for 5 consecutive days per week for 4 wk (induction), followed by 10 million $IU/m^2$ sub-Q three times weekly for 48 wk (maintenance)<br>Hepatitis B: 5 million international units sub-Q, IM daily or 10 million IU three times weekly (total of 30–35 million IU/wk) for 16 wk<br>Hepatitis C: 3 million IU sub-Q, IM three times weekly for 16 wk to 24 mo<br>Malignant melanoma: Induction, 20 million $IU/m^2$ IV on 5 consecutive days per week for 4 wk; maintenance, 10 million $IU/m^2$ sub-Q three times per week for 48 wk<br>Condylomata: 1 million IU/lesion (maximum of 5 lesions) three times weekly for 3 wk; a second course could be administered in 12–16 wk |
| Interferon alfa 3n<br>(Alferon N; ❋ Alferon N) | C | Condylomata acuminate: 250,000 IU/wart (maximum of 10 lesions) two times weekly for maximum 8 wk |
| Peginterferon alfa 2a<br>(Pegasys, Pegasys ProClick; ❋ Pegasys) | C | Chronic hepatitis B: Sub-Q, 180 mcg (1 mL) once weekly for 48 wk<br>Chronic hepatitis C: Sub-Q, 180 mcg once weekly for 24 wk for viral genotypes 2 and 3; for 48 wk for viral strains 1 and 4 |
| Peginterferon alfa 2b<br>(PegIntron, Sylatron; ❋ PegIntron) | C | 1 mcg sub-Q once weekly for 1 y |
| Interferon beta 1a<br>(Avonex, Rebif; Rebif Rebidose ❋ Avonex, Rebif) | C | Avonex, 30 mcg IM once per week<br>Rebif, 8.8 mcg sub-Q for 2 wk, then 22 mcg for 2 wk, and then 44 mcg; give all doses three times weekly, with at least 48 h between doses |
| Interferon beta 1b<br>(Betaseron, Extavia; ❋ Betaseron, Extavia) | C | 0.25 mg sub-Q every other day |
| Interferon gamma 1b<br>(Actimmune) | C | 50 $mcg/m^2$ sub-Q three times weekly; max dose 50 $mcg/m^2$ |

### Use in Patients With Hepatic Impairment

Hepatic enzymes may become elevated during treatment, especially in people with preexisting liver disease. Such an increase may require discontinuing the drug. Known hepatic impairment is a contraindication.

### Use in Patients Receiving Home Care

The interferon is often self-administered or given by a caregiver to chronically ill patients. The home care nurse may need to teach patients or caregivers accurate drug preparation and injection techniques as well as proper disposal of needles and syringes. It may also be necessary to provide assistance in obtaining appropriate laboratory tests (e.g., CBC, platelet count, tests of renal or hepatic function) to monitor patients' responses to the medications.

## Adverse Effects

In the majority of patients, flulike symptoms (e.g., fever, chills, fatigue, muscle aches, headache, tachycardia) develop within 2 hours of administration of interferon alfa 2b and last up to 24 hours. Other symptoms include chest pain and alopecia. Adverse hematologic effects include neutropenia, anemia, and thrombocytopenia.

The FDA has issued a **BLACK BOX WARNING** ◆ for all interferon alfa products because they can cause or aggravate fatal or life-threatening neuropsychiatric, ischemic, autoimmune, and infectious disorders. In addition, interferon alfa drugs should be discontinued in patients who develop severe decreases in neutrophil or platelet counts. Persistently severe or worsening effects usually lead to permanent discontinuation of interferon alfa. In many cases, these disorders resolve after the drug is stopped.

## Contraindications

Contraindications to interferon alfa 2b include known sensitivity to the drug as well as signs and symptoms of liver disease (e.g., jaundice, ascites, bleeding disorders, or decreased serum albumin), autoimmune hepatitis, a history of autoimmune disease, or posttransplantation immunosuppression.

## Nursing Implications

### Preventing Interactions

Some medications interact with interferon alfa 2b, increasing its effects (Box 11.2). Apparently, no herbs interact with this drug.

### Administering the Medication

The nurse may administer interferon alfa 2b intravenously, subcutaneously, intramuscularly, or intralesionally, as ordered. Administration is three times weekly, on a regular schedule (e.g., Monday, Wednesday, and Friday), at about the same time of day, at least 48 hours apart, per manufacturer's recommendation. To treat condylomata intralesionally, it is important to inject the drug into the base of each wart with a small-gauge needle. For large warts, injections may occur at several points per the manufacturer's recommendation.

### Assessing for Therapeutic Effects

With parenteral interferons, the nurse observes for improvement in signs and symptoms. With hairy cell leukemia, hematologic tests may improve within 2 months, but optimal effects may require 6 months of drug therapy. With Kaposi's sarcoma,

skin lesions may resolve or stabilize over several weeks. With chronic hepatitis, liver function tests may improve within a few weeks.

### Assessing for Adverse Effects

The nurse observes for acute flulike symptoms with interferon alfa 2b and assesses patient response through evaluation of liver function tests and WBC, RBC, and platelet values.

### Patient Teaching

The nurse teaches the patient about accurate drug preparation and injection techniques as well as proper disposal of needles and syringes. Educate the patient that flulike symptoms occur within 1 to 2 hours of administration and may last up to 24 hours and be dose limiting; they may be relieved by acetaminophen.

Box 11.1 contains other patient teaching guidelines.

## Other Drugs in the Class

Peginterferon alfa has largely replaced the older preparations of interferon alfa for some clinical uses. **Pegylation** is a process of modifying an interferon by treatment with polyethylene glycol, changing the pharmacokinetics of interferons so that they act longer and can be given less often. Peginterferons also produce steady blood levels, whereas unpegylated interferons provide fluctuating levels.

Peginterferon alfa has largely replaced the older preparations of interferon alfa for some clinical uses. Pegylation is a process of modifying an interferon by treatment with polyethylene glycol, changing the pharmacokinetics of interferons so that they act longer and can be given less often. Peginterferons also produce steady blood levels, whereas unpegylated interferons provide fluctuating levels.

Peginterferon alfa-2a (Pegasys), in combination with ribavirin, with or without an antihepaciviral, is recommended only for certain genotypes of chronic hepatitis C, particularly in settings where newer interferon-free regimens are not accessible because of cost. Interferon alfa 3n (Alferon N) is used to treat condylomata acuminata (genital warts) in adults. Its side-effect profile, particularly the flulike symptoms, is similar to that of other interferons.

Interferon beta 1a (Avonex, Rebif) and interferon beta 1b (Betaseron) are used for multiple sclerosis, an autoimmune neurologic disorder in which the drug slows progression of neurologic dysfunction, prolongs remissions, and reduces the severity of relapses. Flulike symptoms are common adverse effects.

Interferon gamma 1b (Actimmune) is used to treat chronic granulomatous disease, which involves impaired phagocytosis of ingested microbes and frequent infections. Drug therapy reduces the incidence and severity of infections.

---

**BOX 11.2**   *Drug Interactions: Interferon Alfa 2b*

**Drugs That Increase the Effects of Interferon Alfa 2b**

- Bowel-cleansing phosphate and sulfate preparations, iopamidol, metrizamide, and other iodinated contrast media
  *Increase the risk of seizure activity*
- Clozapine
  *Increases the risk and/or severity of hematologic toxicity*
- Deferiprone, zidovudine
  *Increase the risk of severe bone marrow toxicity*
- Leflunomide
  *Increases the risk of infections*

---

**!   QSEN Alert: Safety**

A pregnancy if the mother or the father is taking ribavirin may result in a child with birth defects. Therefore, patient teaching must include the use of birth control measures to prevent pregnancy during treatment and for at least 6 months after stopping the drug.

# ADJUVANT MEDICATIONS USED TO STIMULATE THE IMMUNE SYSTEM: INTERLEUKINS

Note that ILs are listed as high-alert medications by the Institute for Safe Medication Practices because the drug class has heightened risk of causing significant patient harm when used in error.

Aldesleukin (Proleukin) is a recombinant DNA version of IL-2. It activates cellular immunity, produces tumor necrosis factor (IL-1) and interferon gamma, and inhibits tumor growth. Its uses include treatment of metastatic kidney cancer and metastatic melanoma skin cancer. The FDA has issued a **BLACK BOX WARNING** ◆ for aldesleukin, citing numerous concerns. Only patients with normal cardiac and pulmonary functions should receive the drug, and administration should occur in a hospital setting with critical care expertise and beds under supervision of an oncologist. Aldesleukin administration has been associated with capillary leak syndrome, which is characterized by a loss of vascular tone and extravasation of plasma proteins and fluid into the extravascular space. This results in hypotension and reduced organ perfusion that may be severe and can result in death. Development of moderate to severe lethargy should be a sign to withhold the drug. Finally, aldesleukin is associated with impaired neutrophil count with an increased risk of sepsis and bacterial endocarditis. Because few nurses are likely to give this drug, this chapter omits details about administration and patient monitoring.

Oprelvekin (Neumega) is recombinant IL-11, which stimulates platelet production. This drug is used to prevent severe thrombocytopenia and reduce the need for platelet transfusions in adults with nonmyeloid cancer receiving myelosuppressive chemotherapy and who are at high risk for thrombocytopenia. The drug should be discontinued at least 2 days prior to the next planned chemotherapy cycle. The FDA has issued a **BLACK BOX WARNING** ◆ for oprelvekin because of the risk for allergic or hypersensitivity reactions, including anaphylaxis. The drug should be permanently discontinued in any patient developing an allergic or hypersensitivity reaction. Subcutaneous injections of the drug should be rotated among sites. The patient should be educated regarding signs of a hypersensitivity reaction, including wheezing; chest tightness; rash; itching; fever; and swelling of face, lips, tongue, or throat. Dilutional anemia, severe fluid overload, and dysrhythmias have been reported.

## Clinical Application 11.2

- Mrs. Paul has a great risk of infection, with a low WBC count and low ANC. What should the nurse teach the patient about preventing infection?

## NCLEX Success

7. Mrs. Thomas, a 60-year-old woman with cancer who started on interferon alfa 2b today, calls the clinic and reports that she has been having fever, chills, fatigue, and muscle aches since she has returned home. For relief of these symptoms, the nurse reinforces and says that the patient should take

   A. aspirin
   B. codeine
   C. ibuprofen
   D. acetaminophen

8. Interferons may be used to treat

   A. most types of cancer
   B. chronic hepatitis C
   C. chronic anemia
   D. mental depression

9. Which of the following, if expressed by a patient taking interleukins, indicate that patient teaching was successful? (Select all that apply.)

   A. "I should store the medication in the refrigerator."
   B. "I should not use the medication if it is discolored."
   C. "I need to drink additional fluids while taking the medication."
   D. "I need to shake the medication to mix it well before taking."
   E. "I should not take acetaminophen if I have a fever or headache."
   F. "Shortness of breath and edema are side effects that I will need to learn to live with."

## Clinical Application 11.3

- Epoetin alfa is prescribed for Mrs. Paul's anemia. What dietary considerations should the nurse communicate to Mrs. Paul?

## THE NURSING PROCESS

A concept map outlines the nursing process related to drug therapy considerations in this chapter. Additional nursing implications related to the disease process should also be considered in care decisions.

**Assessment**

- Assess the patient's status in relation to conditions for which hematopoietic and immunostimulant drugs are used (e.g., infection, neutropenia, cancer).
- Assess nutritional status and functional abilities.
- Assess adequacy of support systems and coping mechanisms.
- Assess baseline values of laboratory and other diagnostic test reports to aid monitoring of responses to hematopoietic and immunostimulant drug therapy.

**Outcomes of Therapy**

The patient will
- Participate in interventions to prevent or decrease infection.
- Remain afebrile during immunostimulant therapy.
- Experience increased immunocompetence as indicated by increased white blood cell (WBC) count (if initially leukopenic) or tumor regression.
- Experience relief or reduction of disease symptoms.
- Maintain nutritional level, appropriate appetite, and functional level of independence as able.
- Learn to self-administer medications accurately when indicated.

**Nursing Interventions**

- Support patient and others to practice and promote good hand hygiene techniques and sterile technique and to avoid contact with infected people.
- Encourage patients to participate in self-care and decision-making when feasible and engage with family members and significant others when feasible.
- Promote adequate nutrition, rest, sleep, and exercise.
- Inform patients about diagnostic test results, planned changes in therapeutic regimens, and evidence of progress.
- Use isolation procedures when indicated, usually when the neutrophil count is less than 500/mm$^3$.
- Monitor the complete blood (cell) count (CBC) and other diagnostic test reports for normal or abnormal values, reporting test results to prescribers when indicated. It is essential that darbepoetin and epoetin be stopped when the hemoglobin level approaches 12 g/dL and filgrastim and sargramostim be stopped when WBC counts normalize.
- Schedule drug administration, diagnostic tests, and other elements of care to conserve patients' energy.
- Assist patients or caregivers in learning how to prepare and inject darbepoetin alfa, epoetin alfa, filgrastim, or an interferon, when indicated.

**Evaluation**

- Compare current CBC reports with baseline values for changes toward normal levels (e.g., WBC count 5000–10,000/mm$^3$).
- Compare weight and nutritional status with baseline values for maintenance or improvement.
- Observe and interview for decreased numbers or severity of disease symptoms and signs of infection.
- Observe for increased energy and ability to participate in ADLs.
- Observe and interview outpatients regarding adherence to follow-up care.
- Observe and interview regarding the mental and emotional status of the patient and family members.

## KEY CONCEPTS

- Patients with anemia associated with chronic kidney disease or bone marrow–damaging chemotherapy may take epoetin alfa and darbepoetin to increase their RBC count. It is important to rule out other medical conditions causing anemia prior to starting an ESA.
- The FDA has issued a **BLACK BOX WARNING ◆** advising prescribers to avoid using ESAs in patients with hemoglobin values of 12 g/dL or above. In addition, serious adverse cardiovascular reactions and stroke have been reported in controlled trials when an ESA is administered to patients with chronic kidney disease to target hemoglobin levels greater than 11 g/dL.
- The FDA has issued a **BLACK BOX WARNING ◆** directing prescribers that treatment of anemia with an ESA in patients with cancer who are not receiving chemotherapy offers no benefit and may cause serious harm. In addition, it is important to prescribe these drugs at the lowest dose effective in raising hemoglobin levels just enough to avoid the need for blood transfusion; the nurse helps ensure that hemoglobin levels are monitored regularly until they stabilize.
- The FDA has issued a **BLACK BOX WARNING ◆** for epoetin beta, citing that the drug is not indicated or recommended for treatment of chemotherapy-induced anemia.
- Adverse effects of epoetin alfa, darbepoetin, and epoetin beta include increased risks of hypertension, myocardial infarction, and stroke, especially when used to increase hemoglobin above 12 g/dL.
- Filgrastim and other CSFs are used to increase WBCs and decrease risks of infection in patients with or at high risk of severe neutropenia.
- Interferons are used mainly for viral hepatitis and certain types of cancer.
- The FDA has issued a **BLACK BOX WARNING ◆** for all interferon alfa products because they can cause or aggravate fatal or life-threatening neuropsychiatric, ischemic, autoimmune, and infectious disorders.
- Some interferons, as well as filgrastim, are conjugated with polyethylene glycol, in a process called pegylation, to prolong drug actions.
- With the advent of BCR-ABL TKIs, interferon alfa 2a is no longer the preferred initial treatment of choice for patients with chronic myeloid leukemia who are not candidates for hematopoietic cell transplantation.
- The FDA has issued a **BLACK BOX WARNING ◆** for aldesleukin, citing numerous concerns. Only patients with normal cardiac and pulmonary functions should receive the drug, and administration should occur in a hospital setting with critical care expertise and beds under supervision of an oncologist.
- The FDA has issued a **BLACK BOX WARNING ◆** for oprelvekin because of the risk of allergic or hypersensitivity reactions, including anaphylaxis.

## CLINICAL REASONING CASE STUDY

| | |
|---|---|
| **Meet the Patient** | John Renault, a 51-year-old man who has been diagnosed with Hodgkin's disease, has completed a course of antineoplastic chemotherapy. He is currently in the hospital for a bone marrow transplant. His physician prescribes filgrastim (Neupogen), a colony-stimulating factor (CSF).<br><br>• As a nurse, discuss the plan of care and provide Mr. Renault with necessary drug information.<br>• Mr. Renault receives the bone marrow transplant and questions the need for the CSF, stating, "I have new bone marrow now. Won't that make all the bone cells I need?" How should the nurse respond? |
| **Assessing Drug Information** | • Colony-stimulating factors, such as filgrastim, are used to restore or accelerate bone marrow function (production, maturation, and activation of neutrophils) in patients undergoing a bone marrow transplant.<br>• In addition, the drug can help prevent infection by reducing the incidence, severity, and duration of neutropenia associated with several chemotherapy regimens.<br>• The most common adverse effects of filgrastim are drowsiness, fatigue, flulike symptoms, nausea, and bone pain. The drug may cause erythema at subcutaneous injection sites. |
| **Nursing Actions** | • The plan of care should include assessment of the patient's absolute neutrophil count (ANC); Mr. Renault is most vulnerable to infection if the count falls below 500/mm³. At this level, isolation procedures should be used. It is necessary to assess the complete blood count and platelet counts twice weekly during therapy. If the ANC exceeds 10,000/mm³, discontinuation of therapy is necessary.<br>• The nurse ensures that everyone who encounters the patient uses proper hand hygiene. It is important to use sterile technique for all injections, intravenous site care, wound dressing changes, and any other invasive diagnostic or therapeutic measures. Also, the nurse teaches Mr. Renault and his family members about drug preparation, subcutaneous injection techniques, and disposal of needles and syringes so that drug administration can occur at home.<br>• The nurse should explain that, after a bone marrow transplant, it typically takes 2 to 4 weeks for the new bone marrow cells to mature and begin producing blood cells. During this time, Mr. Renault will have virtually no functioning granulocytes and will be at high risk for infection.<br>• The nurse should observe for infection with the goal of maintaining the ANC within a target range of 1500 to 10,000 cells/mm³ and should report an ANC count of 10,000 cells/mm³ or greater.<br>• The filgrastim is needed to promote the functioning of the transplanted bone marrow and can reduce the incidence and severity of infections while Mr. Renault is neutropenic.<br>• Box 11.1 contains additional patient teaching guidelines related to filgrastim. In addition, the nurse should provide patient teaching related to care following bone marrow transplantation. |

*Visit the*Point® *at* **http://thePoint.lww.com/Frandsen12e** *for answers to NCLEX Success questions (in Appendix A), answers to Clinical Application Case Studies (in Appendix B), and more!*

## REFERENCES AND RESOURCES

American Association for the Study of Liver Diseases/Infectious Diseases Society of America. *Recommendations for testing, managing, and treating hepatitis C.* Retrieved December 24, 2018, from http://www.hcvguidelines.org

DiPiro, J. T., Talbert, R. L., Yee, G. C., Matzke, G. R., Wells, B. G., & Posey, L. M. (Eds.). (2016). *Pharmacotherapy: A pathophysiologic approach* (10th ed.). New York: McGraw-Hill Education.

Elliott, S. (2011). Erythropoiesis-stimulating agents. *Cancer Treatment Research, 157,* 55–74.

French, C. J., Glassford, N. J., Gantner, D., Higgins, A. M., Cooper, D. J., Nichol, A., et al. (2017). Erythropoiesis-stimulating agents in critically ill trauma patients: A systematic review and meta-analysis. *Annals of Surgery, 265*(1), 54–62.

Hinkle, J. L., & Cheever, K. H. (Eds.). (2017). *Brunner & Suddarth's textbook of medical-surgical nursing* (14th ed.). Philadelphia, PA: Lippincott Williams & Wilkins.

Joint Panel from the American Association of the Study of Liver Diseases and the Infectious Diseases Society of America. (2014). *Recommendations for testing, managing, and treating hepatitis C.* Retrieved May 2, 2016, from http://www.hcvguidelines.org

Karch, A. M. (2018). *2019 Lippincott's pocket drug guide for nurses.* Philadelphia, PA: Lippincott Williams & Wilkins.

Norris, T. L. (2018). *Porth's pathophysiology: Concepts of altered health states* (10th ed.). Philadelphia, PA: Lippincott Williams & Wilkins.

Papadakis, M. A., & McPhee, S. J. (2018). *Current medical diagnosis and treatment 2019* (58th ed.). New York: McGraw-Hill Education.

Rizzo, J. D., Brouwers, M., Hurley, P., Seidenfeld, J., Arcasoy, M. O., Spivak, J. L., et al. (2010). American Society of Hematology/American Society of Clinical Oncology clinical practice guideline update on the use of epoetin and darbepoetin in adult patients with cancer. *Blood, 116*(20), 4045–4059.

Schaefer, F., Hoppe, B., Jungraithmayr, T., Klaus, G., Pape, L., Farouk, M., et al. (2016). Safety and usage of darbepoetin alfa in children with chronic kidney disease: prospective registry study. *Pediatric Nephrology, 31*(3), 443–453.

Trotta, F., Belleudi, V., Fusco, D., Amato, L., Mecozzi, A., Mayer, F., et al. (2017). Comparative effectiveness and safety of erythropoiesis-stimulating agents (biosimilars vs originators) in clinical practice: A population-based cohort study in Italy. *British Medical Journal Open, 7,* e011637. doi:10.1136/bmjopen-2016-011637

UpToDate. (2019). *Drug information.* Lexi-Comp, Inc.

# Drug Therapy: Immunizations

## LEARNING OBJECTIVES

*After studying this chapter, you should be able to:*

1. Describe the types of immunity and the agents that produce them.
2. Identify immunizations recommended for children and adolescents.
3. Identify immunizations recommended for adults.
4. Identify authoritative sources for immunization information.
5. Be able to teach parents (and their children) about the importance of immunizations to public health.
6. Be able to teach people about recommended immunizations and record keeping.

## CLINICAL APPLICATION CASE STUDY

Cynthia Williams, a 26-year-old college student, brings her 15-month-old son Riley to a family practice clinic for a well-child visit. Mrs. Williams says that Riley has had his previous immunizations at the county health department every 2 months until the age of 6 months but that he has not had any immunizations since then.

## KEY TERMS

**Active immunity:** antigenic immune response with antibody formation to an infection through administration of a vaccine or toxoid or through natural exposure to the disease

**Antigenicity:** ability of an antigen to bind specifically with certain products to promote better antibody formation

**Immunization:** bolstering a person's immune system by inducing antibody formation, thereby providing active protection against a specific infectious disease

**Passive immunity:** temporary state of immunity produced in a person who is susceptible to an infectious organism by administering serum containing antibodies to the disease

**Toxoids:** altered bacterial toxins that are administered to stimulate antitoxin production and protect against the harmful effects of the toxin

**Vaccines:** microorganisms or components of microorganisms that are administered to stimulate antibody production against the microorganism prior to a natural infection

# INTRODUCTION

**Immunization**, which involves bolstering a person's immune system by inducing antibody formation, thereby providing active protection against a specific infectious disease, has greatly improved human health and life expectancy. Immunizations are one of the key factors in reducing mortality and improving life expectancy in the United States over the past century. The past 55 years of immunization have led to the elimination or near elimination of several vaccine-preventable diseases in the United States. Sustaining a well-developed vaccine delivery system and adequate surveillance of disease and of vaccine coverage can continue to significantly decrease the incidence of deaths, disabilities, and illness. The nurse plays a pivotal role in this process of assessing, teaching, administering immunizations, and evaluating patients who have received them for adverse effects.

# OVERVIEW OF IMMUNIZATION

## Types of Immunity

There are two main types of immunity. **Active immunity** results from administering a dead or weakened microorganism or piece of the microorganism to a person. The person's immune system responds by producing immunoglobulins (antibodies) specific for that microorganism, providing protection against disease with later exposure. **Passive immunity** results from parenteral administration of immune serum containing disease-specific antibodies to a nonimmune person. Passive immunity is only temporary, and the person still needs a vaccine against a specific disease to develop antibodies that provide long-term immunity. Preparations used for immunization are biologic products prepared by pharmaceutical companies and are regulated by the U.S. Food and Drug Administration (FDA). The widespread use of these products in the United States has dramatically decreased the incidence of many infectious diseases, such as polio, influenza, pneumococcal disease, and hepatitis B.

## Kinds of Immunizing Agents

### Agents for Active Immunity

The biologic products used for active immunity are vaccines and toxoids. For maximum effectiveness, both of these products must be given before exposure to the pathogenic microorganism. Administration by the recommended route helps ensure the desired immunologic response.

**Vaccines** are suspensions of microorganisms or their antigenic products that have been killed (inactivated) or attenuated (weakened or reduced in virulence) so they can induce antibody formation while preventing infection altogether or causing only a very mild form of it. Many vaccines produce long-lasting immunity. Attenuated live vaccines produce active immunity, usually lifelong, that is similar to that produced by natural infection. There is a small risk that live vaccines may produce disease in people with severely impaired immune function, but this risk is very low with new vaccines developed using recombinant DNA technology.

**Toxoids** are bacterial toxins or products that have been modified to destroy toxicity while retaining antigenic properties (i.e., ability to induce antibody formation). Immunization with toxoids is not permanent, and scheduled repeat doses (boosters) are required to maintain immunity.

Additional components, such as aluminum or calcium phosphate, are added to some vaccines and toxoids, to slow absorption and increase **antigenicity** (ability of an antigen to bind specifically with certain products to promote better antibody formation). Products containing aluminum can only be given intramuscularly because greater tissue irritation occurs with subcutaneous injections of the immunizing agent.

In general, vaccines and toxoids are quite safe, and risks of the diseases they prevent are significantly greater than the risks of the vaccines. However, risks and benefits of vaccination are always considered individually, because no vaccine is completely effective or completely safe. People may still develop a disease after being immunized against it, but symptoms are usually less severe, and complications are fewer than if they had not been immunized. Adverse vaccine effects are usually mild and of short duration. The FDA evaluates vaccine safety before and after a vaccine is marketed; however, some adverse effects become apparent only after a vaccine is used in a large population.

### Agents for Passive Immunity

Immune serums are the biologic products used for passive immunity. They act rapidly to provide temporary immunity lasting about 1 to 3 months in people exposed to or experiencing an infectious disease. The goal of therapy is to prevent or modify the disease process (i.e., decrease the incidence and severity of symptoms).

Immune globulin (IG) products are made from the serum of people with high concentrations of the specific antibody or immunoglobulin required. These products may consist of whole serum or only contain the immunoglobulin portion of serum in which the specific antibodies are concentrated. Immunoglobulin fractions are preferred over whole serum because they are more likely to be effective in disease prevention. All plasma used to prepare these products is screened for hepatitis B surface antigen. Hyperimmune serums are available for cytomegalovirus, hepatitis B, rabies, rubella, tetanus, and varicella zoster (shingles).

**BLACK BOX WARNING ◆** IG products can increase a patient's risk for the development of thrombosis. Risk factors that can contribute to thrombosis with IG include increased age, prolonged immobilization, hypercoagulability, past history of venous or arterial thrombosis, the use of estrogens, indwelling central vascular catheters, hyperviscosity, and cardiovascular disease. Administer the minimum dose for patients at risk for thrombosis, and monitor for signs and symptoms of thrombosis or hyperviscosity. The patient should be well hydrated.

# INDIVIDUAL IMMUNIZING AGENTS

Box 12.1 provides information about current recommendations for immunizations. Table 12.1 lists vaccines and toxoids that are used routinely in the United States, and Table 12.2 lists immune serums that are used regularly in this country.

| BOX 12.1 | *Recommended Immunizations by Age Group* |
|---|---|

### Healthy Children and Adolescents (0–18 years)

- Rotavirus vaccine (either RV1 [Rotarix] or RV5 [RotaTeq]) to protect infants against rotavirus gastroenteritis. With Rotarix, a two-dose series at 2 and 4 months is recommended; for RotaTeq, a three-dose series is recommended at 2, 4, and 6 months. (If any dose in the series is either RotaTeq or unknown, default to 3-dose series.) Catch-up vaccination: Do not start the series on or after age 15 months; the maximum age for the final doses is 8 months.
- A five-dose series of DTaP at ages 2, 4, 6, and 15 through 18 months and 4 through 6 years. Tdap booster is recommended at age 11 or 5 years after the last Td immunization. Boostrix is used for people 10 to 18 years of age, and Adacel is used for people 11 to 64 years of age.
- Four-dose series of pneumococcal vaccine (PCV13, Prevnar) for healthy young children, at 2, 4, and 6 months and at age 12 through 15 months.
- Two-dose series of chickenpox vaccine (e.g., Varivax), with the first dose at 12 to 15 months and the second dose at 4 to 6 years of age. Chickenpox vaccine is also recommended for adolescents who have never had chickenpox or been vaccinated previously with a single dose; two doses of vaccine are required for full immunity.
- *Haemophilus influenzae* type b (Hib) conjugate vaccine–at 6 weeks (minimum age) for PRP-T [ACTHIB, DTaP–IPV/ Hib [Pentacel], Hib–MenCY [MenHibri]], and PRP–OMP [PedvaxHIB or COMVAX], and at 12 months for PRP-T [Hiberix]. A two- or three-dose Hib vaccine primary series and a booster dose (dose 3 or 4 depending on vaccine used in primary series) is administered at age 12 through 15 months to complete a full Hib series.
- A combined two-dose series vaccine for measles, mumps, rubella, and chickenpox (ProQuad) for children first dose at ages 12 through 15 months and the second dose at 4 to 6 years. Another vaccine combination (Pentacel), which contains diphtheria, tetanus, pertussis, polio, and *H. influenzae* type b (Hib), can be used for primary immunization in infancy as well as for booster doses. Combination vaccines are recommended for use in children who need multiple vaccines at a single visit.
- Hepatitis A vaccination for all children in the United States, with the first of two doses between 1 and 2 years of age and a second dose at least 6 months after the first dose. A hepatitis B (Hep B) monovalent vaccine should be given to all newborns within 24 hours of birth, with the second dose at age 1 to 2 months and the third dose at least 8 weeks after second dose and at least 16 weeks after first dose.

- Annual flu vaccination for all children older than 6 months of age. Infants younger than 2 years of age and all children with underlying medical conditions should receive the trivalent inactive vaccine (TIV).
- Human papillomavirus (HPV) vaccine (Gardasil) for all adolescents 11 or 12 years of age (can be given as early as 9 years) or up to 26 years of age if not received earlier. Bivalent HPV2 vaccine (Cervarix) and nine-valent HPV 9 vaccine (Gardasil 9) can be given to females 9 through 26 years of age. All vaccines are most effective if given before the person becomes sexually active.
- Meningococcal vaccine administration at 11 or 12 years of age with a booster dose at age 16 years. If not received earlier, two doses at least 8 weeks apart are recommended for adolescents up to age 21. Two serogroup B meningococcal (MenB) vaccines are recommended in patients between 16 and 23 years of age for short-term protection against meningitis are recommended, with a preference for administration between 16 and 18 years of age.

### Adults

- Chickenpox vaccine for nonpregnant adults who never had the disease or vaccine; a second dose of vaccine for adults who previously received a single dose.
- HPV vaccine in women up to age 26 years, men up to age 21 years, and men 22 to 26 years who have sex with men, if not previously received.
- Tdap vaccine once in adults who have not received it as an adolescent and then a Td (tetanus, diphtheria) booster every 10 years. In addition, women should have the Tdap vaccine each time they are pregnant, preferably at 27 through 36 weeks of pregnancy. Tdap booster vaccine (e.g., Adacel) once is necessary for all adults younger than 65 years of age, especially health professionals and those who have close contact with infants (less than 1 year of age).
- Annual flu vaccination for all adults. People with underlying medical conditions should receive TIV.
- Two serogroup B meningococcal (MenB) vaccines are recommended in adults up to age 23 for short-term protection against meningitis, if not previously received.
- The pneumococcal vaccine, PPSV23 (Pneumovax) for all adults older than 65 years or/and adults younger than 65 years with certain chronic health conditions. The maximum is two doses in a lifetime. The pneumococcal vaccine (PCV13) Prevnar is recommended for all adults older than 65 years and for adults younger than 65 years with immunocompromise who are at high risk for pneumococcal disease.
- Zoster vaccine (Zostavax) (to prevent herpes zoster [shingles]) in adults 60 years and older

## Use

Clinical indications for vaccines and toxoids include the following:

- Routine immunization of children against diphtheria, *Haemophilus influenzae* type b infection, hepatitis A and B, influenza, measles (rubeola), mumps, pertussis, pneumococcal infection, poliomyelitis, rotavirus, rubella (German measles), tetanus, and varicella (chickenpox)
- Postexposure prophylaxis with hepatitis A vaccine or IG effectively prevents infection with hepatitis A virus

(HAV) when administered within 2 weeks of exposure. Preexposure prophylaxis through the administration of hepatitis A vaccine or IG provides protection for unvaccinated persons traveling in high or intermediate HAV endemic areas.

- Routine immunization of adolescents and adults against diphtheria, tetanus, and pertussis; varicella, if immunity not established; as well as influenza annually
- Immunization of prepubertal girls or women of childbearing age against rubella

**TABLE 12.1**

## DRUGS AT A GLANCE: Vaccines and Toxoids for Active Immunity

| Name/Characteristics | Pregnancy Category | Indications for Use | Routes and Dosage Ranges | |
|---|---|---|---|---|
| | | | **Adults** | **Children** |
| **Vaccines** | | | | |
| ***H. influenzae* type b (Hib)** (ActHIB, PedvaxHIB, Pentacel, Hiberix; ✿ ActHIB, Hiberix) May be given at the same time as DTaP; measles, mumps, rubella (MMR); injected polio vaccine (IPV) | C | Routine immunization: ActHIB, Hiberix or Pentacel, 4-dose series 2, 4, 6, 12–15 mo PedvaxHIB, 3-dose series at 2, 4, 12–15 mo | Adults who are recipients of a successful hematopoietic stem cell transplant: revaccinate with a 3-dose regimen beginning 6–12 mo after the transplant, regardless of vaccination history. Doses should be administered ≥4 wk apart | 0.5 mL IM at 2, 4, and 12–15 mo of age Administer IM; shake well prior to administration; administered within 24 h of reconstitution |
| **Hepatitis A** (Havrix, VAQTA; ✿ Avaxim, HAVRIX, VAQTA) More than 90% effective within 4 wk after first dose; contraindicated during febrile illness, immunosuppression; Havrix and VAQTA are interchangeable | C | All children at age 1 y; workers in day care centers, laboratories, food-handling establishments; men who have sex with men; IV drug users; military personnel and travelers to areas where hepatitis A is endemic; community residents during an outbreak; people with chronic liver disease (e.g., hepatitis B or C, cirrhosis) or who receive transfusions for clotting disorders | Havrix (1440 units in 1 mL), 1 mL IM initially and 6–12 mo later (2 doses) VAQTA (50 units/mL), IM in deltoid, 1 mL initially and 6–12 mo later (2 doses) | Havrix (360 or 720 units in 0.5 mL), 1–18 y, 360 units IM initially, then 1 and 6–12 mo later (2 doses) VAQTA (25 units/0.5 mL), 25 units IM initially and 6–18 mo later |
| **Hepatitis B** (Engerix-B, Recombivax HB; ✿ Engerix-B, Recombivax HB) Approximately 96% effective in children and young adults and 88% in adults older than 40 y; duration of protection unknown; serum antibody levels can be obtained | C (contraindicated) | All infants and children up to age 18; people with occupational exposure to blood (health care and emergency workers); household contacts or sexual partners of people with hepatitis B infection; people with HIV, end-stage renal disease, on hemodialysis; people with multiple sexual partners; men who have sex with men; IV drug users; residents and staff of institutions for developmentally disabled people; residents of correctional facilities | 20 y and older Engerix-B, 1 mL IM initially, then 1 and 6 mo later (3 doses); predialysis and dialysis patients, 2 mL IM initially and 1, 2, and 6 mo later (4 doses) Recombivax HB, 1 mL IM initially and 1 and 6 mo later (3 doses); predialysis and dialysis patients, 1 mL IM initially and 1 and 6 mo later (3 doses) | Neonates to 19 y Engerix-B, 0.5 mL IM initially and 1 and 6 mo later (3 doses) Recombivax HB, 0.5 mL IM initially and 1 and 6 mo later (3 doses) |

**TABLE 12.1**

## DRUGS AT A GLANCE: Vaccines and Toxoids for Active Immunity (Continued)

| Name/Characteristics | Pregnancy Category | Indications for Use | Routes and Dosage Ranges | |
|---|---|---|---|---|
| | | | **Adults** | **Children** |
| **Human papillomavirus (HPV)** (Gardasil, Cervarix, Gardasil 9; ❋ Gardasil, Cervarix) Because HPV is a common sexually transmitted infection, the vaccine is most effective when taken before becoming sexually active. | B | Gardasil, prevention of diseases caused by HPV types 6, 11, 16, and 18 (cervical, vaginal, and vulvar cancer; genital warts) in people ages 9 to 26 Cervarix, prevention of HPV types 16 and 18; recommended for girls and women from ages 9 to 26 Gardasil 9, prevention of HPV types 6, 11, 16, 18, 31, 33, 45, 52, and 58; recommended for people from ages 9 to 26 | 0.5 mL IM initially, 2 mo after first dose, and 6 mo after first dose (3 doses) Gardasil 9, 0.5 mL IM initially and 6–12 mo after first dose (2 doses) | 9 y and older; same as adults Routine vaccination at 11–12 y 2-dose schedule, minimum interval between first and second doses is 5 mo 3-dose schedule, minimum interval between first and second doses is 4 wk; minimum interval between the second and third dose is 12 wk; minimum interval between first and third dose is 5 mo |
| **Influenza** (Afluria; Quadrivalent, Fluzone, Fluzone High-Dose; ❋ Agriflu, Fluzone, Fluzone High Dose, Agriflu, Fluad, Fluad Pediatric, Flulaval Tetra, Fluviral, Quadrivalent Influvac) Formulated annually to include current strains; provides protective antibody concentrations for about 6 mo | C | Annual immunization for all people older than 6 mo of age | 0.5 mL IM in a single dose; immunization, then 1 dose each season | 6–35 mo, 0.25 mL IM, 1 dose if previously vaccinated; 2 doses at least 1 mo apart if first vaccination 3–8 y, 0.5 mL IM, 1 dose if previously vaccinated 6 mo to 8 y, two IM doses of inactivated influenza vaccine (administered a minimum of 4 wk apart) if first vaccination 9 y and older, 0.5 mL IM in a single dose |
| **Measles, mumps, and rubella (MMR)** (M–M–R II; ❋ M–M–R II, Priorix) Preferred and more commonly used than single immunizing agents; contains live, attenuated viruses that cause measles, mumps, and rubella; protects more than 95% of recipients for many years | C | Immunization at 12–15 mo and a second dose at 4–6 y | 0.5 mL IM | Same as adults |
| **Meningococcal group B vaccine (MenB-fHBP)** (Bexsero, Trumenba; ❋ Trumenba) | B | Short-term protection against meningitis, with a preference for administration between ages 16 and 18 | ≤25 y (Bexsero) 0.5 mL IM as a 2-dose series at least 1 mo apart ≤25 y (Trumenba) 0.5 mL IM as a 2-dose series at least 1 mo apart; or 0.5 mL IM initially, then 1–2 and 6 mo as a 3-dose series | ≥10 y (Bexsero) same dose series as adults ≥10 y (Trumenba) same dose series as adults |

*(Continued on page 214)*

**TABLE 12.1**

# DRUGS AT A GLANCE: Vaccines and Toxoids for Active Immunity (Continued)

| Name/Characteristics | Pregnancy Category | Indications for Use | Routes and Dosage Ranges | |
|---|---|---|---|---|
| | | | **Adults** | **Children** |
| **Pneumococcal polyvalent** (Pneumovax 23; Pneumovax 23, Pneumo 23) Contains 23 strains of pneumococci, which cause most of the serious pneumococcal infections in the United States; protection begins about 3 wk after vaccination and lasts for years | C | Adults 65 y and older who are otherwise healthy; people ages 2 to 64 y who have chronic conditions that cause increased risk of pneumococcal infection (e.g., cardiovascular or respiratory disease; asthma, diabetes mellitus, Hodgkin's disease, multiple myeloma, cirrhosis, alcohol dependence, kidney disease, immunosuppression) or who smoke | 0.5 mL Sub-Q, IM as a single dose; may be repeated after 5 y if given before age 65 | Not recommended for children under 2 y 2 y and older, same dose as adults; may be repeated after 5 y |
| **Pneumococcal 13-valent** (Prevnar 13; Prevnar 13) Contains 13 *Streptococcus pneumoniae* antigens conjugated to a protein to increase antigenicity | C | All children up to age 6 y to prevent systemic pneumococcal infections (e.g., bacteremia, meningitis, pneumonia, otitis media) in young children | Adults 19 to <65 y with specified underlying medical conditions: IM 0.5 mL as a single IM dose Adults ≥ 65 y: IM 0.5 mL as a single dose | Birth–6 mo, 0.5 mL IM at 2, 4, 6, and 12–15 mo (4 doses) 7–11 mo, 0.5 mL IM initially, at least 4 wk later, and after 1 y birthday (3 doses) 12–23 mo, 0.5 mL IM initially and at least 2 mo later (2 doses) 24 mo to 9 y, 0.5 mL IM in a single dose |
| **Poliomyelitis, inactivated (IPV)** (IPOL; ✽ Imovax Polio) | C | Routine immunization of infants; immunization of adults not previously immunized and at risk for exposure (e.g., health care or laboratory workers) | 0.5 mL Sub-Q monthly for 2 doses, then a third dose 6–12 mo later Incompletely vaccinated: adults with at least 1 previous doses of OPV, <3 doses of IPV, or a combination of OPV and IPV equaling <3 doses, administer at least one 0.5 mL dose of IPV. Additional doses to complete the series may be given if time permits Completely vaccinated and at increased risk of exposure: one 0.5 mL dose | 0.5 mL Sub-Q at 2, 4, and 6–18 mo and 4–6 y of age (4 doses) or at 2 and 4 mo (2 doses) |

| TABLE 12.1 |
| --- |

**DRUGS AT A GLANCE: Vaccines and Toxoids for Active Immunity** (Continued)

| Name/Characteristics | Pregnancy Category | Indications for Use | Routes and Dosage Ranges | |
| --- | --- | --- | --- | --- |
| | | | **Adults** | **Children** |
| **Rabies vaccine** (Imovax Rabies, RabAvert; ❈ Imovax Rabies) Immunity develops in 7–10 d and lasts 1 y or longer | C | Preexposure immunization in people at high risk for exposure (e.g., veterinarians, animal handlers); postexposure prophylaxis in people who have been bitten by potentially rabid animals or who have skin scratches or abrasions exposed to animal saliva (e.g., animal licking of wound), urine, or blood | Preexposure, 1.0 mL IM for 3 doses, 1 mL on days 0, 7, and 21 or 28; then, booster doses (1 mL) every 2–5 y based on antibody titers Postexposure, 1 mL IM for immunocompetent 4 doses 1 mL on days 0, 3, 7, 14; immunocompromised IM 5 doses 1 mL each on days 0, 3, 7, 14, 28; in addition, patients should receive rabies immune globulin with the first dose (day 0). After the initial dose, other doses are given 3, 7, 14, and 28 d later | Same as adults |
| **Rotavirus** (RotaTeq; Rotarix; ❈ RotaTeq, Rotarix) Can be given with most other childhood vaccines; adverse effects are usually mild (e.g., diarrhea); a few cases of intussusception have been reported after administration of RotaTeq | C | Prevention of rotavirus gastroenteritis in infants between 6 and 32 wk of age | Individual doses administered orally | RotaTeq: Infants 6–32 wk of age: Oral 2 mL per dose for 3 dose, the first given at 6–12 wk of age, followed by subsequent doses at 4–10 wk intervals. Administer all doses by 32 wk of age Rotarix: Infants 6–24 wk of age: Oral 1 mL per dose for 2 doses, the first dose given at 6 wk of age, followed by the second dose given ≥4 wk later. The 2 series should be completely by 24 wk of age |
| **Varicella** (Varivax; ❈ Varilrix, Varivax III) Contains live, attenuated varicella virus; contraindicated in hematologic or lymphatic malignancy, immunosuppression, febrile illness, or pregnancy | C (contraindicated) | Immunization of children 12 mo and older; immunization of adults who have not had chickenpox | 0.5 mL Sub-Q, followed by a 2nd dose of 0.5 mL 4–8 wk after the first dose | 12–15 mo, 0.5 mL Sub-Q followed by a 2nd dose at 4–6 y of age |

(*Continued on page 216*)

**TABLE 12.1**

# DRUGS AT A GLANCE: Vaccines and Toxoids for Active Immunity (Continued)

| Name/Characteristics | Pregnancy Category | Indications for Use | Routes and Dosage Ranges | |
|---|---|---|---|---|
| | | | **Adults** | **Children** |
| **Zoster vaccine** (Shingrix; 🍁 Shingrix) Not indicated for prevention or treatment of chickenpox or treatment of shingles; duration of protection unknown | C (contraindicated) | Prevention of herpes zoster in adults 50 y and older | Adults ≥50 y: IM 0.5 mL administered as a 2-dose series at 0 and 2–6 mo If the primary series is delayed or interrupted, the series does not need to be restarted. If the interval between dose 1 and 2 is <4 wk, then the second dose should be repeated | |
| **Toxoids** | | | | |
| **Diphtheria, tetanus toxoids, and acellular pertussis (DTaP and Tdap)** (Adacel, Boostrix, Daptacel, Infannix; 🍁 Adacel, Boostrix) **(pediatric type) (DT)** Contains a larger amount of diphtheria antigen than "tetanus and diphtheria toxoids, adult type (Td)" | | Routine immunization of infants and children 6 y and younger in whom pertussis vaccine is contraindicated (those who have adverse reactions to initial doses of DTaP vaccine); not recommended for use in adults | | Infants and children 6 y and younger, 0.5 mL IM for 2 doses at least 4 wk apart, followed by a booster dose 1 y later and when the child starts school |
| **Tetanus and diphtheria toxoids (adult type) (Td)** (TDAX, Tenivac; 🍁 Td Absorbed) Contains a smaller amount of diphtheria antigen than "diphtheria and tetanus toxoids, pediatric type (DT)" | C | Primary immunization or booster doses in adults and children older than 6 y | Tenivac manufacturer labeling: patients previously not immunized should receive 2 primary doses of 0.5 mL each given at an interval of 8 wk; third (reinforcing) dose of 0.5 mL 6–8 mo later 0.5 mL IM for 2 doses, at least 4 wk apart, followed by a booster dose 6–12 mo later and every 10 y thereafter | Older than 6 y, same as adults |
| **Tetanus toxoid** Protects about 100% of recipients for 10 y or more; for primary immunization of infants and children 6 y of age or older, usually given in combination (e.g., DTaP or DT); for primary immunization of adults usually given or alone or combined with diphtheria toxoid (e.g., Td adult type) | C | Routine immunization of infants and young children; primary immunization of adults; prevention of tetanus in previously immunized people who sustain a potentially contaminated wound Prophylaxis, 0.5 mL IM if wound contaminated and no booster dose was received for 5 y; 0.5 mL if wound is clean and no booster dose was received for 10 y | Primary immunization in adults not previously immunized, 0.5 IM mL for 3 doses: initially, 4–8 wk later, then at 6–12 mo; then, 0.5-mL booster dose every 10 y | Same as adults |

**TABLE 12.2**

## DRUGS AT A GLANCE: Immune Serums for Passive Immunity

| Serum/Characteristics | Pregnancy Category | Indications for Use | Routes and Dosage Ranges |
|---|---|---|---|
| **CMV immune globulin, intravenous, human (CMV-IGIV)** (CytoGam; ✳ CytoGam)<br>Contains antibodies against CMV | C | Prevention of CMV infection in the heart, kidney, liver, lung, and pancreas transplant recipients | Posttransplantation: infusion, 150 mg/kg IV within 72 h; then 100–150 mg/kg at 2, 4, 6, and 8 wk; and then 50–100 mg/kg at 12 and 16 wk |
| **Hepatitis B immune globulin, human (HBIG)** (HepaGam B, Hyper HEP B S/D, Nabi-HB; ✳ Hyper HEP B S/D)<br>Solution of immunoglobulins that contains antibodies to HBsAg | C (contrain-dicated) | To prevent hepatitis after exposure; neonates born to HBsAg-positive or unknown-status mothers are given HBIG and the first dose of hepatitis B vaccine within 12 h of birth | Adults and children 0.06 mL/kg (usual adult dose, 3–5 mL) IM as soon as possible after exposure, preferably within 7 d; repeat dose in 1 mo |
| **Immune globulin (human) (IG; IGIM)** (Asceniv, Bivigam, Carimune NF, Gammagard, Hizentra, Privigen, Gamastan S/D, Hizentra, Privigen, Xembefy; ✳ Cutaquig, Cuvitru, Gamastan S/D, Gammagard S/D, Gamunex, Hizentra, IGIVnex, Iveegam Immuno, Octagam, Panzyga)<br>Given IM only; commonly called "gamma globulin"; obtained from pooled plasma of normal donors; consists primarily of IgG, which contains concentrated antibodies; produces adequate serum levels of IgG in 2–5 d | C | To decrease the severity of hepatitis A, measles, and varicella after exposure; to treat immunoglobulin deficiency | Adults and children<br>Exposure to hepatitis A: 0.02 mL/kg IM<br>Exposure to measles: 0.25 mL/kg IM within 6 d of exposure<br>Exposure to varicella: 0.6–1.2 mL/kg IM<br>Exposure to rubella (pregnant women only): 0.55 mL/kg IM<br>Immunoglobulin deficiency: 1.3 mL/kg IM initially and then 0.6 mL/kg every 3–4 wk |
| **Immune globulin intravenous (IGIV)** (Bivigam, Carimune NF, Gammagard, Hizentra, Privigen; ✳ Gamastan S/D, Hizentra, Privigen)<br>Given IV only; provides immediate antibodies; half-life about 3 wk; mechanism of action in ITP is unknown; **BLACK BOX WARNING ◆** —IGIV has been associated with thrombosis, renal dysfunction and failure, and death; it should be used cautiously in patients with renal impairment or at risk for developing the condition | C | Immunodeficiency syndrome; idiopathic thrombocytopenic purpura (ITP) | See manufacturers' instructions |
| **Rabies immune globulin (human) RIG** (HyperRAB S/D, Imogam Rabies HT; ✳ HyperRAB S/D, Imogam Rabies Pasteurized)<br>Gamma globulin obtained from plasma of people hyperimmunized with rabies vaccine; not useful in treatment of clinical rabies infection | C | Postexposure prevention of rabies, in conjunction with rabies vaccine | Adults and children 20 units/kg IM (half the dose may be injected around the wound) as soon as possible after possible exposure (e.g., animal bite) |
| **Rh₀(D) immune globulin (human)** (HYPERRHO S/D Full Dose, MICRhoGAM, RhoGAM, WinRho SDF; ✳ Hyperrho S/D Full Dose, HypRho-D, WinRho SDF)<br>Prepared from fractionated human plasma; a sterile concentrated solution of specific immunoglobulin (IgG) containing anti-Rh₀(D) | C | To prevent sensitization in a subsequent pregnancy to the Rh₀(D) factor in an Rh-negative mother who has given birth to an Rh-positive infant by an Rh-positive father | *Obstetric use*: Administer according to the manufacturer's labeling<br>Inject contents of 1 vial IM for every 15 mL fetal packed red cell volume within 72 h after delivery, miscarriage, or abortion. Consult package instructions for blood typing and drug administration procedures |

(*Continued on page 218*)

**TABLE 12.2**

**DRUGS AT A GLANCE: Immune Serums for Passive Immunity** (Continued)

| Serum/Characteristics | Pregnancy Category | Indications for Use | Routes and Dosage Ranges |
|---|---|---|---|
| **Tetanus immune globulin (human)** (HyperTET S/D;  HyperTET S/D) Solution of globulins from plasma of people hyperimmunized with tetanus toxoid Tetanus toxoid (Td) should also be given to initiate active immunization if minor wound and more than 10 y since Td, if major wound and more than 5 y since Td, or if Td primary immunization series was incomplete | C | To prevent tetanus in patients with wounds possibly contaminated ith *Clostridium tetani* and whose immunization history is uncertain or incomplete Treatment of tetanus infection | Adults and children Prophylaxis, 250 units IM as a single dose in conjunction with a tetanus toxoid containing vaccine Treatment of clinical disease, 3000–6000 units IM in a single dose |
| **Varicella-zoster immune globulin (human) (VZIG)** (VariZIG;  VariZIG) The globulin fraction of human plasma; antibodies last 1 mo or longer | C | Postexposure to chickenpox or shingles, to prevent or decrease severity of infections in children under 15 y of age who have not been immunized or who are immunodeficient because of illness or drug therapy Infants born to mothers who develop varicella 5 d before or 2 d after delivery and premature infants of <28 wk of gestation | IM 125 units/10 kg up to a maximum of 625 units within 48 h after exposure if possible; may be given up to 96 h after exposure. Minimal dose, 125 units |

CMV, cytomegalovirus; HBsAg, hepatitis B surface antigen; IgG, immunoglobulin G.

---

**! QSEN Alert: Safety**

Tetanus prophylaxis in wound management [CDC/ACIP] is as follows:

- Assess the type of wound and provide appropriate wound care.
- Clean wounds contaminated with dirt, feces, soil, and saliva; clean puncture wounds from crushing, tears, burns, and frostbite. Wounds containing necrotic or gangrenous area should be débrided.
- Tetanus toxoid: For children age less than 7 years, DTaP [DT if pertussis vaccine is contraindicated]; for children age ≥7 years and adults, Td is preferred to tetanus toxoid alone; Tdap may be preferred if the patient has not previously been vaccinated with Tdap or if tetanus vaccine is indicated for a pregnant woman.
- For patients with HIV or severe immunodeficiency with contaminated wounds, administer tetanus immunoglobulin regardless of history of tetanus immunization.

**! QSEN Alert: Safety**

Rubella during the first trimester of pregnancy is associated with a high incidence of birth defects in the newborn.

- Immunization of people at high risk for serious morbidity or mortality from a chronic condition. For example,

pneumococcal vaccine is recommended in people 65 years of age and older, as well as in people younger than 65 years of age with chronic diseases.
- Immunization of adults and children at high risk for a particular disease. For example, pneumococcal vaccine is recommended for people older than 2 years of age who have chronic respiratory disease or have had a splenectomy. Also, administration of quadrivalent human papillomavirus (HPV) vaccine is recommended in young adolescents to prevent genital warts and the risk of cervical cancer.

### Use in Children

Routine immunization of children has reduced the prevalence of many common childhood diseases (listed previously, e.g., diphtheria, measles [rubeola], mumps, pertussis, and varicella [chickenpox]), and immunization rates have increased in recent years. By 4 to 6 years of age, children should have received vaccinations against these diseases. Because some vaccines are administered more than once, a child may receive more than 20 injections by 2 years of age. Two strategies to increase immunizations are the use of combination vaccines and the administration of multiple vaccines (in separate syringes and at different sites) at one visit to a health care provider whenever feasible. Combination vaccines decrease the number of injections, and giving multiple vaccines at one visit decreases the number of visits to a health care provider. Several combination vaccines are now available (Box 12.2), and others continue to be developed.

---

**BOX 12.2** *Combination Vaccines Used for Routine Childhood Immunizations*

DTaP–IPV (Kinrix)
DTaP–Hep B–IPV (Pediarix)
DTaP–IPV–Hib (Pentacel)
DTaP–Hib (TriHIBit)
Hib–Hep B (Comvax)
Hep A–Hep B (Twinrix)
MMR–Var (ProQuad)

Studies indicate that these strategies are effective in improving rates of immunizations. Children's health care providers should implement the recommended childhood immunization schedule issued in January of each year by the Centers for Disease Control and Prevention (CDC). Also, they should refer to current guidelines about immunizations for children with chronic illnesses (e.g., asthma, heart disease, diabetes) or immunosuppression (e.g., from cancer, organ transplantation, or human immunodeficiency virus [HIV] infection).

## Use in Adolescents, Young Adults, and Middle-Aged Adults

Adolescents who received all primary immunizations as infants and young children should have a second dose of varicella (chickenpox) vaccine, hepatitis A and B vaccines (if not received earlier), a tetanus–diphtheria–pertussis booster (Tdap) between ages 11 and 18 years if 5 years have passed since a prior tetanus–diphtheria (Td) booster, as well as meningococcal vaccine at age 11 or 12 with a booster dose at age 16. Adolescents of both genders should receive two doses of the quadrivalent HPV vaccine if not received earlier. Young adults who are health care workers, sexually active, or belong to a high-risk group should receive varicella vaccine (or a second dose if they previously received a single dose), hepatitis A and hepatitis B vaccines if not previously received, and Tdap, as well as measles–mumps–rubella (MMR) if they are not pregnant and rubella titer is inadequate or if proof of immunization is unavailable. In addition, annual influenza vaccine is recommended for adolescents as well as children and infants older than 6 months of age. In adults ≤25 years of age, routine vaccination for meningococcal group B disease is recommended when there is increased risk of serogroup B meningococcal disease or during serogroup B meningococcal disease. Middle-aged adults should maintain immunizations against tetanus–diphtheria with one booster dose of Tdap and influenza vaccine annually. High-risk groups (e.g., those with chronic illness and health care providers) should receive the hepatitis B vaccine series (if not previously received). Middle-aged adults born after 1956 should have at least one dose of MMR vaccine unless they have had either the vaccine or each of the three diseases.

## Use in Older Adults

Older adults become more susceptible to some diseases, and influenza, pneumococcal infections, tetanus, and shingles can be especially serious in this population. The varicella-zoster virus, the same virus that causes chickenpox, can cause shingles later in life. An additional varicella vaccine to prevent zoster infections (shingles) is available for adults 60 years and older who have had chickenpox.

Recommended immunizations for older adults 65 years of age and older include a Td booster every 10 years, annual influenza vaccine, and a one-time administration of pneumococcal vaccine at 65 years of age. A second dose of pneumococcal vaccine may be given at 65 years if the first dose was given 5 years previously. As with younger adults, immunization for most other diseases is recommended for older adults at high risk for exposure due to occupation or travel.

> **⚠ QSEN Alert: Safety**
>
> The recommended influenza vaccine should ideally be administered in September or October. Earlier administration of the influenza vaccine in July or August will result in a decrease in immunity.

## Use in Patients With Specific Health Problems
### Use in Patients With Immunosuppression

Compared with healthy people who are immunocompetent, patients with immunosuppression usually have an adequate, but reduced, antibody response to immunization. They require individualized immunizations. In general, patients with diabetes mellitus or chronic pulmonary, renal, or hepatic disorders who are not receiving immunosuppressant drugs may receive both live attenuated and killed vaccines and toxoids to induce active immunity. However, they may need higher doses or more frequent administration to achieve adequate immunity. With hepatitis B vaccine, for example, larger initial doses may be required and booster doses may be needed later, if antibody concentrations fall.

Patients with active malignant disease may receive killed vaccines or toxoids but not live vaccines (an exception is people with leukemia who have not received chemotherapy for at least 3 months). When patients receive vaccines, it is important to give them at least 2 weeks before the start of chemotherapy or 3 months after chemotherapy is completed. Health care providers may give immune serum, which provides passive temporary immunity, to immunocompromised people who are exposed to an infectious disease, such a rubella or varicella, to reduce the risk of a person's developing a serious infection.

Patients receiving a systemic corticosteroid in high doses (e.g., prednisone 20 mg or equivalent daily) or for longer than 2 weeks should wait at least 3 months before being receiving a live-virus vaccine. Short-term use (less than 2 weeks) or low-to-moderate doses (less than 20 mg of prednisone daily) of corticosteroids are not contraindications to immunizations. In addition, long-term alternate-day therapy with short-acting agents, maintenance physiologic replacement doses, and the use of topical, inhaled, or intra-articular injections of corticosteroids are not contraindications.

Patients with HIV infection have less-than-optimal responses to immunizing agents because this viral infection produces major defects in both cell-mediated and humoral immunity. Live bacterial (bacillus Calmette–Guérin [BCG], oral typhoid) or viral (MMR, varicella) vaccines should not be given, because the bacteria or viruses may be able to reproduce and cause active infection. People with asymptomatic HIV infection should receive inactivated vaccines; those exposed to measles or varicella may be given immune globulin or varicella-zoster immune globulin for passive immunization.

For children with HIV infection, most routine immunizations (DtaP, inactivated polio vaccine, MMR, *H. influenzae* type b [Hib], influenza) are recommended. MMR is not recommended in children with severe immunosuppression from HIV. Varicella vaccine is recommended only for children with no evidence of immunosuppression. Pneumococcal vaccine is recommended for HIV-infected people older than 2 years of age.

### Use in Patients With Cancer

 **QSEN Alert: Safety**

Patients with active malignant disease should not receive live vaccines.

Although these patients may receive killed vaccines and toxoids, antibody production may be inadequate to provide immunity. When possible, patients should have needed immunizations 2 weeks before or 3 months after immunosuppressive radiation or chemotherapy treatments. For example, patients with Hodgkin's lymphoma who are older than 2 years of age should receive immunizations with pneumococcal and Hib vaccines 10 to 14 days before treatment is started. In addition, patients who have not received chemotherapy for 3 to 4 weeks may receive influenza vaccine and may have an adequate antibody response. Passive immunity with immunoglobulins may take the place of active immunity if there is an exposure to an active infection (e.g., varicella) during chemotherapy.

### *Clinical Application 12.1*

- Mrs. Williams asks if Riley, who is getting over a "cold" and has some clear nasal discharge, should wait before having his scheduled immunizations. What is the nurse's best response?
- Mrs. Williams reports the last time she had any immunizations was at 14 years of age. Based on her age and gender, what vaccines do authorities recommend?

## Adverse Effects

Mild reactions to vaccines, such as injection site soreness and redness, fever, and muscle aches, are common, whereas severe and serious reactions, such as anaphylaxis or serum sickness, are rare. Adverse reactions to individual immunizing agents include the following:

- DTaP: soreness, erythema, edema at injection sites, anorexia, nausea, severe fever, encephalopathy, and seizures
- Hib vaccine: pain and erythema at injection sites
- Hepatitis B vaccine: injection site soreness, erythema, induration, fever, and anaphylaxis
- Influenza vaccine: via injection—pain, induration, and erythema at injection sites and flulike symptoms such as chills, fever, malaise, muscle aches; via intranasal spray—runny nose, headache, cough, sore throat, and irritability in children
- MMR vaccine: mild symptoms of measles—cough, fever up to 39.4°C (102°F), headache, malaise, photophobia, skin rash, sore throat, febrile seizures, arthralgia (joint pain), and anaphylaxis in recipients who are allergic to eggs

- Pneumococcal vaccine: local effects—soreness, induration, and erythema at injection sites; systemic effects—chills, fever, headache, muscle aches, nausea, photophobia, and weakness
- Polio vaccine: soreness at injection sites, fever, and anaphylaxis
- Varicella vaccine: early effects—transient soreness or erythema at injection sites; late effect—a mild, maculopapular skin rash with a few lesions
- Immune globulin intravenous (IGIV): chills, dizziness, dyspnea, fever, flushing, headache, nausea, urticaria, vomiting, tightness in chest, pain in chest, hip, or back, renal dysfunction, acute kidney disease, and death

## Contraindications

Contraindications to most vaccines and toxoids include the following:

- Acute febrile illness
- Immunosuppressive drug therapy
- Immunodeficiency states such as congenital immunodeficiency or active HIV disease
- Hematologic cancers (leukemia or lymphoma) or generalized malignancy
- Pregnancy

### *Preventing Interactions*

Immunosuppressant drug therapy and interferon administration may interfere with vaccine response to live vaccines. Antiviral drugs may also interfere with the immune response to a live viral vaccine and should not be given 48 hours before and for 14 days after viral vaccine administration. Likewise, passive immunization with IG for exposure to a viral infection (e.g., measles, hepatitis A, varicella) can likewise interfere with active immunity, and it is necessary to delay administration of the viral vaccine for 2 to 6 months or more, depending on the person's immune status.

 **QSEN Alert: Safety**

Measles vaccine can interfere with the activity of meningococcal vaccine, and it is essential to separate these two vaccines by at least a month.

Measles vaccine can also interfere with the response to tuberculosis (TB) skin testing. Patients should have the TB skin test either simultaneously with the measles vaccine, or they should delay it for 4 to 6 weeks after the test.

 **QSEN Alert: Safety**

In addition, salicylates may increase the risk of Reye's syndrome with administration of the varicella vaccine.

### *Administering the Medication*

Following package insert instructions for storing, reconstituting, and safely administering combination vaccines is essential for effectiveness of all immunizations. To maintain effectiveness of vaccines and other biologic preparations, the nurse helps ensure that immunization products are stored properly. Most products require refrigeration at 2°C to 8°C (35.6°F–46.4°F). It is important to follow the manufacturer's instructions for storage strictly.

## BOX 12.3 *Administering Immunizing Agents*

Accurate administration includes the following:
- Reading the package insert and check the expiration date on all biologic products (e.g., vaccines, toxoids, human immune serums)
- Following instructions for administering each vaccine
- Checking the patient's temperature before giving a vaccine
- Giving intramuscular (IM) human immune serum globulin with an 18- to 20-gauge needle, preferably in the gluteal muscles. If the dose is 5 mL or more, divide it and inject it

into two or more IM sites. Follow manufacturer's instructions for preparation and administration of intravenous (IV) formulations.
- Having aqueous epinephrine 1:1000 readily available before administering any vaccine
- After administration of an immunizing agent in a clinic or office setting, having the patient stay in the area for at least 30 minutes
- Providing patients with a Vaccine Information Statement (VIS)

The nurse reconstitutes vaccines only with the supplied diluent and then uses them within the time frame recommended after reconstitution to maintain vaccine effectiveness.

Box 12.3 summarizes administration considerations for immunizations.

### Assessing for Therapeutic Effects

Most vaccines take about 2 weeks for full antibody response and protection against the disease. A fourfold increase in immunoglobulin titer levels indicates an adequate antibody response. It is necessary to obtain antibody titer levels during pregnancy to determine immunity to viral infections such as measles and rubella because the fetus may be affected by active maternal infection during the pregnancy.

### Assessing for Adverse Effects

Careful screening of people for contraindications and observing vaccine precautions minimize serious adverse vaccine events.

 **QSEN Alert: Safety**

By law, health care providers must report potentially serious adverse effects using the Vaccine Adverse Event Reporting System (VAERS).

The National Vaccine Injury Compensation Program, established in 1986 in the United States, covers injury, disability, or death that may occur due to vaccine administration in cases where significant adverse effects are linked directly to immunization.

 **QSEN Alert: Evidence-Based Practice**

The Global Health Security Agenda was developed in February 2014 to "prevent, detect, and effectively respond to infectious disease threats, whether naturally occurring or caused by accidental or intentional release of dangerous pathogens." One key objective is to improve the global community's capacity to prevent, detect, and respond to public health. Its surveillance of immunization laws across countries assists researchers to examine epidemiology data and provide a justification for immunization policies. This process assists in global health security (Ghedamu & Meier, 2019).

### Patient Teaching

The nurse ensures that the patient or parent receives current vaccine information about the benefits and risks of immunization—a Vaccine Information Statement (VIS)—for each vaccine

dose given. Current VIS forms for all recommended vaccines, along with indications, contraindications, and the timing of immunizations doses, are available for downloading at the CDC Web site (see "References and Resources"). Box 12.4 presents additional patient teaching information.

## NCLEX Success

1. A nurse is explaining to a parent how vaccines work. Vaccines provide which of the following?
   A. active immunity
   B. passive immunity
   C. innate immunity
   D. nonspecific immunity

2. The nurse is caring for a patient with severe immunosuppression. This condition is a contraindication to which of the following?
   A. all injectable immunizations
   B. the use of live bacterial or viral vaccines
   C. the use of immune globulins for passive immunity
   D. annual influenza vaccine

3. A child is receiving an immunization. The nurse should inform the parents that common aftereffects may include which of the following?
   A. skin rash and itching
   B. redness and soreness at the injection site
   C. muscle weakness and difficulty in walking
   D. nausea, vomiting, and diarrhea

## KEEPING UP-TO-DATE WITH IMMUNIZATION RECOMMENDATIONS

Recommendations regarding immunizations change periodically as additional information and new immunizing agents become available. Experts review and update vaccine recommendations in the United States on a frequent basis. Consequently, health care providers need to update their knowledge of vaccine recommendations at least annually. The best source of information for current recommendations is the CDC. The most current immunization schedules for all age groups are available at the CDC Web site (see "References and Resources" for Web site addresses). The main source of CDC recommendations is the Advisory Committee on Immunization

## BOX 12.4 — *Patient Teaching Guidelines for Immunizations*

- Appropriate vaccinations should be maintained for adults as well as for children. Consult the [Centers for Disease Control and Prevention] Web site or a health care provider for current information because recommendations for particular groups may change.

- Maintain immunization records for yourself and all members of your family. This is important because immunizations are often obtained at different places and over a period of many years. Written, accurate, up-to-date records help to prevent diseases and reduce unnecessary immunizations.

- If a health care provider recommends an immunization and you do not know whether you have had the immunization or the disease, it is probably safer to be immunized than to risk having the disease. Immunization after a previous immunization or after having the disease usually is not harmful.

- Most vaccines can cause fever and soreness at the site of injection. Acetaminophen [e.g., Tylenol] can

be taken two to three times daily for 24 to 48 hours if needed to decrease fever and discomfort. Routine premedication with acetaminophen is not recommended. Lower antibody levels may occur, and it may not be necessary.

- Women of childbearing age who receive a rubella [German measles] or a varicella [chickenpox] immunization must avoid becoming pregnant [i.e., use effective contraception] for 3 months afterward.

- If skin lesions develop after receiving live varicella vaccine [to prevent chickenpox], avoid skin contact with newborns, pregnant women, and anyone whose immune system is impaired. Skin lesions from a newly immunized person may transmit the vaccine virus to susceptible close contacts.

- After receiving a vaccine, stay in the area for approximately 30 minutes. If an allergic reaction is going to occur, it will usually do so within that time.

Practices, which consists of experts appointed to advise the CDC on strategies to eliminate vaccine-preventable diseases. Information on vaccines needed for travel to foreign countries (e.g., Japanese encephalitis, typhoid, yellow fever) is also available at the CDC Web site and is frequently updated.

Other sources of information about immunizations include the American Academy of Pediatrics and the American Academy of Family Physicians. Local health departments may also be a source of information about immunizations, whether routine or necessary for foreign travel. Immunization sources can also provide information on new vaccine releases, vaccine availability, and usage of specific vaccines.

### Clinical Application 12.2

- Mrs. Williams does not have a personal immunization record for Riley. When administering the immunizations, the nurse records Riley's immunization information on both the clinic record and on a personal immunization record. Is there any way that the nurse can obtain Riley's previous vaccine record?

## Unfolding Patient Stories: Juan Carlos • Part 1

Juan Carlos, a 52-year-old Hispanic male with diabetes mellitus type 2, hypertension, and hyperlipidemia, is seen at the clinic for his annual checkup. According to age and health status, what vaccinations are recommended for him? What factors should the nurse consider if Juan's immunizations are not up-to-date? How would the nurse intervene when cultural factors, past experiences, or apprehension cause a reluctance to receive vaccinations? (Juan Carlos' story continues in Chapter 41.)

Care for Juan and other patients in a realistic virtual environment: *vSim for Nursing* (thepoint.lww.com/vSimPharm). Practice documenting these patients' care in DocuCare (thepoint.lww.com/DocuCareEHR).

## NCLEX Success

4. A nurse is caring for a 74-year-old man. The nurse recognizes that he would most likely to have a decreased immune response to the influenza vaccine if he is taking which of the following medications?

   A. levothyroxine
   B. prednisone
   C. metoprolol
   D. lovastatin

5. A nurse is preparing to administer an unfamiliar vaccine. To obtain current information and provide patient teaching about vaccine recommendations and contraindications, it is best to do which of the following?

   A. Ask a coworker about the vaccine [when and how it should be administered].
   B. Use a drug guide to look up the vaccine information.
   C. Access an Internet search engine to find vaccine information.
   D. Obtain vaccine information and a Vaccine Information Statement [VIS] from the Centers for Disease Control and Prevention [CDC] Web site.

## THE NURSING PROCESS

A concept map outlines the nursing process related to drug therapy considerations in this chapter. Additional nursing implications related to the disease process should also be considered in care decisions.

**Assessment**

- Determine the patient's previous history of diseases for which immunizing agents are available (e.g., measles, influenza).
- Ask the patient about previous immunization history and any adverse effects experienced.
- Determine whether the patient has any conditions that contraindicate administration of immunizing agents (e.g., malignancy, pregnancy, immunosuppressive drug therapy).
- For pregnant women not known to be immunized against rubella, a serum antibody titer should be measured to determine resistance or susceptibility to the disease.
- For patients with wounds, assess the type of wound and determine how, when, and where it was sustained. Such information may reveal whether tetanus immunization is needed.
- For patients exposed to infectious diseases, assess the extent of exposure (e.g., household or brief, casual contact) and when it occurred.

**Outcomes of Therapy**

The patient will
- Avoid diseases for which immunizations are available and recommended.
- Obtain recommended immunizations for self and children.
- Keep immunization appointments and maintain immunization records.

**Nursing Interventions**

- Provide information about the availability of immunizing agents.
- Assist patients in developing a system to maintain immunization records for themselves and their children.
- For someone exposed to rubeola, administration of measles vaccine within 48 hours can help prevent the disease.
- For someone with a puncture wound or a dirty wound, administration of tetanus immune globulin will prevent tetanus, a life-threatening disease.
- For someone with an animal bite, wash the wound immediately with large amounts of soap and water, then seek prompt health care. Administration of rabies immune globulin and vaccine may be needed to prevent rabies, a life-threatening disease.
- Explain to the patient that contracting rubella or undergoing rubella immunization during pregnancy, especially during the first trimester, may cause severe birth defects in the infant.

**Evaluation**

- Appraise patient's knowledge of and compliance with immunization schedules
- Check immunization records when indicated.
- Interview and observe for adverse drug effects following administration of immunizing agents.

## KEY CONCEPTS

- Many infectious diseases can be prevented by immunizations.
- Immunizations are needed for all age groups.
- Children in the United States are much more likely to receive recommended immunizations than are adolescents and adults.
- Active immunity is achieved through administration of a vaccine or toxoid or through natural exposure to the disease.
- Passive immunity is a temporary state of immunity produced in a person who is susceptible to an infectious organism by administering serum containing antibodies to the disease.
- Women of childbearing age who receive a rubella (German measles) or a varicella (chickenpox) immunization must avoid becoming pregnant (i.e., use effective contraception) for 3 months after they receive the vaccine.

- A **BLACK BOX WARNING** ◆ exists for IGIV because it has been associated with thrombosis, renal dysfunction, kidney disease, and death.
- Health care providers who provide or participate in immunizations need to keep their knowledge base current with annual updates regarding recommendations from the CDC.
- Health care providers need to assess and inform patients about recommended immunizations.
- A patient or parent must receive a VIS for each recommended vaccines, along with indications, contraindications, and the timing of immunizations doses with each vaccine dose.
- New immunizing products continue to be developed.

## CLINICAL REASONING CASE STUDY

**Meet the Patient**

Deborah Little is a 22-year-old mother of 6-month-old twin girls. She has brought the girls into the pediatric clinic for well-child checkups and immunizations. She is questioning the need for the immunizations, stating that she does not understand why some require multiple doses. She states that she is concerned that "all of these shots will be traumatic for the girls."

- What is the difference between vaccines and toxoids? Why are booster doses necessary?
- What strategies will increase the likelihood that Ms. Little will complete the required immunizations for her daughters?

**Assessing Drug Information**

- Vaccines are made from microorganisms or their products that have been killed or weakened. They cause antibody formation while preventing or causing a very mild form of the disease. Many vaccines result in lifelong immunity.
- Toxoids are made from bacterial toxins or products that have been altered so that they are no longer toxic while retaining the ability to induce the formation of antibodies. Toxoids do not produce permanent immunity; thus, repeat or booster doses are necessary for immunity to be maintained.

**Nursing Actions**

- Acknowledge Ms. Little's concern about the large number of immunizations required for her daughters.
- Emphasize the benefit of immunizations in preventing many childhood diseases.
- Explain that combination vaccines will be used whenever possible to reduce the number of injections for the children. The development of combination vaccines increases the likelihood of compliance with the recommended immunization schedules.
- Inform Ms. Little that efforts will be made to complete the required immunizations in as few office visits as possible. The administration of multiple immunizations for different diseases during the same office visit also means that more patients are likely to have all their immunizations.
- Furnish Ms. Little with a Vaccine Information Statement for each recommended vaccine, along with indications, contraindications, and the timing of immunization doses with each vaccine dose.
- Consider preemptive analgesia to prevent unmitigated pain with injections.
- Provide appropriate teaching related to immunization (see Box 12.4).

---

*Visit* **the Point** *at* **http://thePoint.lww.com/Frandsen12e** *for answers to NCLEX Success questions (in Appendix A), answers to Clinical Application Case Studies (in Appendix B), and more!*

## REFERENCES AND RESOURCES

American Academy of Pediatrics (AAP). Homepage. Retrieved from http://www.aap.org

Centers for Disease Control and Prevention. Recommendations and guidelines: Advisory Committee on Immunization Practices (ACIP). Retrieved from https://www.cdc.gov/vaccines/hcp/acip-recs/

Centers for Disease Control and Prevention. Travelers' health. Retrieved from http://www.cdc.gov/travel

Centers for Disease Control and Prevention. (2019). Tetanus. Retrieved from https://www.cdc.gov/tetanus/clinicians.html#wound-management

Centers for Disease Control and Prevention. Vaccines and immunizations. Immunization schedules. Retrieved from http://www.cdc.gov/vaccines/recs/schedules

Ghedamu, T. S. & Meier, B. M. (2019). Assessing national public health law to prevent infectious disease outbreaks. Immunization law as a basis for global health security. *Journal of Law, Medicine, and Ethics, 47*, 412–426.

Meites, E., Szilagyi, P. G., Chesson, H. W., Unger, E. R., Romero, J. R., & Markowitz, L. E. (2019). Human Papillomavirus vaccination for adults: Updated recommendations of the advisory committee on immunization practices. *Morbidity and Mortality Weekly Report, 68*(32), 698–702.

Nelson, N. P., Link-Gelles, R., Hofmeister, M. G., Romero, J. R., Moore, K. L., Ward, J. W., et al. (2018). Update: Recommendations of the advisory committee on immunization practices for use of hepatitis A vaccine for postexposure prophylaxis and for preexposure prophylaxis for international travel. *Morbidity and Mortality Weekly Report, 67*(43), 1216–1220.

Norris, T. L. (2019). *Porth's pathophysiology: Concepts of altered health states* (10th ed.). Philadelphia, PA: Wolters Kluwer.

UpToDate. (2019). *Drug Information.* Lexi-Comp, Inc.

Vaccine Adverse Event Reporting System (VAERS). Homepage. Retrieved from http://www.vaers.hhs.gov

# 13

# Drug Therapy to Decrease Immunity

## LEARNING OBJECTIVES

*After studying this chapter, you should be able to:*

1. Describe the allergic and immune disorders as well as organ transplantation in terms of etiology, pathophysiology, and clinical manifestations.
2. Discuss characteristics and uses of major immunosuppressant drugs in autoimmune disorders and organ transplantation.
3. Describe the cytotoxic immunosuppressant agents in terms of prototype, action, use, adverse effects, contraindications, and nursing implications.
4. Discuss the conventional antirejection agents in terms of prototype, action, use, adverse effects, contraindications, and nursing implications.
5. Describe the adjuvant drugs in terms of prototypes, indications and contraindications for use, major adverse effects, and administration.
6. Implement the nursing process in the care of patients receiving immunosuppressant drugs.

## CLINICAL APPLICATION CASE STUDY

Sam Jones, a 35-year-old mechanic with type 1 diabetes mellitus and end-stage renal disease, received a renal transplant from a living donor 2 years ago. To prevent organ rejection, he is currently taking cyclosporine, mycophenolate mofetil, and prednisone daily. He has monthly appointments at the nephrology clinic and has serum trough levels for cyclosporine measured before each visit. A month ago, Mr. Jones was hospitalized and received four infusions of muromonab-CD3 for an acute organ rejection reaction.

## KEY TERMS

**Autoantigens:** protein complexes on a person's own tissue that stimulate an abnormal immune reaction

**Autoimmune disorder:** conditions associated with an abnormal immune response to self-antigens (autoantigens) on body tissue, resulting in ongoing inflammation and damage to body tissues

**Checkpoint therapy:** immunologic checkpoint blockade that uses monoclonal antibodies to either activate or antagonize immunologic pathways

**Cytotoxic:** causing cell death

**Graft rejection reaction:** activated immunologic response by the recipient to graft donor organ cells resulting in graft tissue damage and loss of graft organ function

**Graft versus host disease:** complication of bone marrow or stem cell transplantation where activated T cells in donor bone marrow attack host tissues producing inflammatory changes in the skin, liver, and gastrointestinal tract; also can occur infrequently with a blood transfusion

**Immunosuppression:** suppression of the immune system

**Monoclonal antibody:** immunoglobulin therapeutically replicated in laboratory cells to react with a specific cell antigen altering the immune response to that antigen

**Murine antibodies:** immunoglobulins created in mouse cells for use as therapeutic treatment for human diseases

**Polyclonal antibodies:** mixtures of antibodies [immunoglobulin A [IgA], plus IgD, IgE, IgG, and IgM] produced by several clones of B lymphocytes

# INTRODUCTION

The immune response, normally a protective process, recognizes and destroys potentially harmful outside substances, helping the body defend itself against disease. However, disease processes can also develop when the immune system perceives a harmless substance, such as an antigen or the person's own body tissues, as foreign and tries to eliminate them. This inappropriate activation of the immune response is a major factor in allergic conditions (e.g., allergic asthma) and autoimmune disorders (e.g., rheumatoid arthritis, Crohn's disease, psoriasis). **Autoimmune disorders** occur when a person's immune system loses its ability to differentiate self from nonself. As a result, an immune response against host tissues occurs.

An appropriate, but undesirable, immune response also occurs when foreign tissue from another organism is transplanted into the body. With transplant therapy, if the immune response is not suppressed, a **graft rejection reaction** occurs, where the body reacts to the implanted cells as with other antigens and attempts to destroy the foreign tissue. Although numerous advances have been made in transplantation technology, the ability to modulate the immune response remains a major factor in determining the success or failure of transplant therapy.

Immunosuppressant drugs are used to decrease an undesirable immune response by interfering with the production or function of immune cells and cytokines that contribute to tissue inflammation and damage. Drugs used therapeutically as immunosuppressants constitute a diverse group, some of which also are used for other purposes. Drug groups that are used to reduce the immune response include corticosteroids (see Chap. 17) and some **cytotoxic** (causing cell death) antineoplastic drugs (see Chap. 14). Health care providers use these drugs, discussed here in relation to their effects in modulating the body's response to autoimmune disorders or organ transplantation, to treat inflammatory autoimmune disorders or to prevent or treat transplant rejection reactions. The nursing management of patients receiving these drugs is the main focus of this chapter. To aid in the understanding of immunosuppressant drugs, descriptions of selected inflammatory autoimmune disorders, tissue transplantation, and rejection reactions appear below.

# OVERVIEW OF ALTERED IMMUNE FUNCTION

## Etiology

In healthy people, the immune system's ability to inherently differentiate between cell surface proteins on its own cells (called self-antigens or **autoantigens**) and antigens on foreign cells provides protection against disease. However, in people who have received an organ transplant, this protective mechanism must be altered to avoid damage to the transplant and organ rejection. Drug therapy to suppress the body's ability to recognize self from nonself is a major part of transplantation protocols.

Tissue and organ transplantation involves replacing diseased host tissue with healthy donor tissue. The goal of such treatment is to save and enhance the quality of the recipient's life. Skin grafts and kidney and liver transplants are more commonly performed; heart, lung, intestine, and pancreas transplants are increasing in frequency. The use of biologic agents, which stimulate the production of hematopoietic stem cells from bone marrow and mobilize them into circulating blood (see Chap. 11), has helped improve the availability of stem cells for transplant, reducing the need for bone marrow transplants.

Although many factors affect graft survival, including the degree of matching between donor tissues and recipient tissues, drug-induced **immunosuppression** is a major part of transplantation protocols. The goal is to provide adequate immunosuppression while minimizing adverse effects on normal body tissue. If immunosuppression is inadequate, a graft rejection reaction will occur with solid organ transplantation, and **graft versus host disease** (GVHD) will develop with bone marrow/stem cell transplantation. If immunosuppressive drug therapy is excessive, serious infection may occur, some malignancies such as lymphomas and skin cancers may develop, and organ damage related to the proliferation of activated lymphocytes in normal body cells may result.

## Pathophysiology

After self-antigens develop, the tissue containing them is perceived as foreign and antigenic, triggering an inappropriate immune response that may involve T lymphocytes in direct destruction of tissue, as well as the production of proinflammatory cytokines, chemical messengers that attract and activate phagocytes contributing to the inflammatory immune process. Stimulation of B lymphocytes to produce antibodies leads to further inflammation and tissue damage.

Knowledge about the role of inflammatory cells and cytokines in the immune response to tissue injury continues to expand. This has led to the development of biologic agents that can modulate inflammatory cytokine production by activated lymphocytes. Cytokines act as messengers between different types of lymphocytes to increase or decrease the immune response, modifying the production and activity of different white blood cells. Attachment of an antigen to an antigen-presenting cell activates macrophages to produce interleukin-1 (IL-1) and T cells to produce IL-2. Lymphocyte activation by IL-1 causes the activated lymphocytes and other immune cells to produce more IL-2 receptors, amplifying the immune response. IL-2 activates production and promotes the activity of cytotoxic T cells, macrophages, natural killer (NK) cells, and B lymphocytes. Hence, decreasing IL-2 production induces lymphocyte apoptosis, reducing the numbers of T lymphocytes available to participate in an immune response.

Another inflammatory mediator mediating the inflammatory process of autoimmune disease is tumor necrosis factor (TNF)-alpha, a cytokine that plays a major role in the response to infection. Functions of TNF include activation of monocytes, macrophages, and cytotoxic T cells; enhancement of NK cell functions; increased leukocyte movement into areas of tissue injury; increased phagocytosis by neutrophils; and stimulation of B and T lymphocytes. Although TNF can be beneficial in helping to fight infection, an excessive TNF response has been associated with the pathogenesis of autoimmune disorders. Overproduction of cytokines, such as IL-2 and TNF, contributes to prolonged tissue inflammation and damage in autoimmune disease.

In addition to the factors that activate an immune response, there are also factors that prevent the immune system from "turning off" an abnormal immune or inflammatory process. One of these factors may be a decrease in the number of suppressor T cells, which help modulate the immune response. Another factor may be inadequate amounts of anti-inflammatory cytokines (e.g., IL-10) to modulate the immune reaction.

A transplant rejection reaction occurs when the host's immune system is stimulated to destroy the transplanted organ. The immune cells of the transplant recipient attach to the donor cells of the transplanted organ and react against the antigens in the donor organ. The rejection process involves T and B lymphocytes, antibodies, multiple cytokines, and inflammatory mediators. In most cases, T-cell activation and proliferation are more important initially in the rejection reaction than B-cell activation and the presence of active antibodies. Studies have shown that the activation of T cells is a very tightly regulated process comprising many receptor interactions. Typically, during an organ rejection reaction, helper T cells become activated by donor antigen attachment to an antigen-presenting cell; the activated helper T cells then stimulate B cells to produce antibodies, leading to a delayed hypersensitivity reaction weeks or months later. The antibodies injure the transplanted organ by activating complement, producing antigen–antibody complexes or causing antibody-mediated tissue destruction.

This reaction can destroy the solid organ graft within 2 weeks if the recipient's immune system is not adequately suppressed by immunosuppressant drugs. Immunosuppressive drug therapy begins either immediately before or at the time of the transplant procedure to prevent antibody formation. Scientists are increasingly recognizing the role of the immune system in rejection. Current research is ongoing on new protocols that involve gradually reducing the dosage of conventional antirejection drugs to the minimal dose necessary to prevent rejection. In addition, researchers continue to study a subset of individuals who manifest a pattern of gene expression that allows tolerance of the transplanted organ when antirejection drugs are stopped.

# Clinical Manifestations

## Allergic Disorders

Allergic asthma is characterized by increased production of IgE in response to inhaled allergens. The IgE–allergen complexes trigger inflammation, producing airway edema and increasing mucus production. People use immunosuppressants to reduce the airway edema and excessive vascular permeability that accompany this type of asthma (see Chap. 33).

## Immune Disorders

Crohn's disease is a chronic, recurrent, inflammatory bowel disorder that can affect any area of the gastrointestinal (GI) tract. The chronic inflammation is attributed to a mixture of inflammatory mediators (e.g., IL-1 and IL-6, TNF-alpha) produced by overactivated macrophages in the lining of the bowel, which contribute to GI ulceration, bleeding, and diarrhea. The goal of treatment is to decrease inflammation and promote healing of bowel lesions.

Psoriasis, a hyperproliferative skin disorder, is characterized by an abnormal overproduction of skin cells, forming plaque lesions. Activated T lymphocytes producing cytokines are believed to stimulate the abnormal growth of the affected skin cells with accompanying inflammation from tissue infiltration of neutrophils and monocytes. Some medications (e.g., beta-adrenergic blockers, lithium) may precipitate or aggravate psoriasis.

Psoriatic arthritis is a type of arthritis associated with psoriasis that is similar to rheumatoid arthritis. It may be characterized by extensive and disabling joint damage, especially in the hand and finger joints.

Rheumatoid arthritis occurs when an abnormal immune response leads to chronic inflammation and damage of joint cartilage and bone. It is thought to involve the activation of T lymphocytes, release of inflammatory cytokines, and formation of antibodies in the joint tissue as well as other organs. Research in recent years has delineated the roles of TNF-alpha and IL-1 in the pathophysiology of rheumatoid arthritis. Symptoms may include fatigue, loss of energy, lack of appetite, low-grade fever, muscle and joint aches, and stiffness. Joints frequently become red, swollen, painful, and tender.

## Rejection Reactions With Solid Organ Transplantation

Rejection reactions may be either acute or chronic. Acute reactions may occur from 10 days to a few months after transplantation and mainly involve cellular immunity and proliferation of T lymphocytes. Characteristics include signs of organ failure and inflammation of blood vessels, leading to arterial narrowing or obliteration. Treatment with immunosuppressant drugs is usually effective in ensuring short-term survival of the transplant but does not prevent chronic rejection. Chronic reactions, which occur after months or years of normal function, are caused by both cellular and humoral immunity and do not respond to increasing immunosuppressive drug therapy. Characteristics include fibrosis of blood vessels and progressive failure of the transplanted organ.

Rejection reactions produce both general manifestations of inflammation and specific organ manifestations, depending on the organ involved. With renal transplantation, for example, acute rejection reactions produce fever, flank tenderness over the graft organ site, and symptoms of renal failure (e.g., increased serum creatinine, decreased urine output, edema, weight gain, hypertension). Chronic renal rejection reactions are characterized by a gradual increase in serum creatinine levels over 4 to 6 months. Along with observing for symptoms of decline in organ function, periodic organ tissue biopsies are often required to diagnose a chronic organ rejection process.

### Bone Marrow/Stem Cell Transplantation and Graft Versus Host Disease

With bone marrow/stem cell transplantation, the donor marrow or stem cells, which contain T lymphocytes, develop an active immune response against antigens on the host's tissues, producing GVHD. Tissue damage is produced directly by the action of cytotoxic T cells and indirectly through the release of inflammatory mediators (e.g., complement) and cytokines (e.g., TNF-alpha and ILs).

Acute GVHD occurs in 30% to 50% of patients, usually within 6 weeks of transplant. Signs and symptoms include delayed recovery of blood cell production in the bone marrow, skin rash, liver dysfunction (indicated by increased alkaline phosphatase, aminotransferases, and bilirubin), and diarrhea. The skin reaction is usually a pruritic maculopapular rash that begins on the palms and soles and may progress to cover the entire body. Liver involvement can lead to bleeding disorders and the development of hepatic encephalopathy.

Chronic GVHD occurs when symptoms persist or occur 100 days or more after transplantation. It is characterized by abnormal humoral and cellular immunity, severe skin disorders, and liver disease. Chronic GVHD appears to be an autoimmune disorder in which activated donor T cells continue to respond to the recipient's surface proteins as if they are foreign antigens.

## Drug Therapy

Immunosuppressant drugs compose several groups of pharmacologic agents, with often overlapping mechanisms and sites of action (Table 13.1; Fig. 13.1). Older groups of immunosuppressant drugs often depress the immune system of the recipient nonspecifically. Therapeutic use of these drugs increases the risk of serious infections with bacteria, viruses, fungi, or protozoa. In addition, most cytotoxic immunosuppressant drugs that slow the proliferation of activated lymphocytes also produce damage to rapidly dividing cells in other tissues (e.g., mucosal cells, intestinal cells, hematopoietic stem cells).

As a result, serious, life-threatening complications can occur with the use of immunosuppressant agents. For example, patients with autoimmune disorders or organ transplants, who are receiving long-term immunosuppressant drug therapy, are at increased risk for serious infections, cancer (especially lymphoma), hypertension, renal and hepatic disease, and metabolic bone disease. The Institute for Safe Medication Practices considers immunosuppressants to be members of a high-alert drug class in community health care because these drugs have a heightened risk of causing significant patient harm when used in error. The U.S. Food and Drug Administration (FDA) has issued numerous black box warnings for these drugs.

Newer drug groups modify the immune response more specifically in response to excessive levels of cytokines and T-cell activity that cause tissue damaging inflammation and autoimmune reactions. These drugs, called immunomodulators or biologic response modifiers, are part of the growing number of drugs with more specific immunosuppressive actions that have been developed through monoclonal antibody cloning technology. Most are used in combination with older immunosuppressants for synergistic effects with lower doses that minimize drug toxicities, whereas some are replacing the older, nonspecific immunosuppressants.

Immunosuppressants discussed here are cytotoxic immunosuppressant agents, conventional antirejection agents, and adjuvant medications, including antibody preparations, cytokine inhibitors, and corticosteroids.

## CYTOTOXIC IMMUNOSUPPRESSIVE AGENTS

Cytotoxic immunosuppressive drugs damage or kill dividing cells, such as immunologically competent lymphocytes. Health care providers use these drugs primarily in cancer chemotherapy (see Chap. 14). However, in smaller doses, some cytotoxic drugs also exhibit immunosuppressive activities and are useful in the treatment of autoimmune disorders and the prevention of rejection reactions in organ transplantation. For many years, azathioprine was the drug selected to induce immunosuppression and prevent rejection reactions to transplanted organs. Now, Ⓟ **mycophenolate mofetil** (CellCept), the prototype in this discussion, has essentially replaced it. Corticosteroids are combined with immunosuppressant agents as a front-line therapy for the treatment of clinical GVHD. It is unclear how the mechanism of action of the two drug classes provides prophylactic effects. Methylprednisolone possesses a 6-alpha-methyl group that blocks the specific binding of the corticosteroid to transcortin. Transcortin is a protein that transports steroids in the plasma. Methylprednisolone is bound to albumin. The lack of transcortin binding leads to a greater penetration of the cytotoxic immunosuppressive agent into the bronchial alveolar fluids, providing a greater therapeutic advantage in treating pulmonary inflammation.

Mycophenolate plus cyclosporine or tacrolimus is effective in the prevention of acute GVHD and is associated with a reduction in mucositis and an increase in blood forming cells that facilitate transplant recovery.

**TABLE 13.1**

## Drugs Administered to Suppress Immunity

| Drug Class | Prototype(s) | Other Drugs in the Class |
|---|---|---|
| **Cytotoxic Immunosuppressive Agents** | | |
| | Mycophenolate mofetil IV (CellCept) | Azathioprine (Azasan, Imuran) |
| | Mycophenolate sodium PO (Myfortic) | Leflunomide (Arava) |
| | | Methotrexate (Otrexup, Rasuvo, Trexall, Xatmep) |
| **Conventional Antirejection Agents** | | |
| | Cyclosporine | Everolimus (Zortress, Afinitor) |
| | | Sirolimus (Rapamune) |
| | | Tacrolimus (Prograf) |
| **Janus Associated Kinase Inhibitor** | | |
| | Ruxolitinib (Jakafi) | |
| **Adjuvant Medications Used to Suppress Immune Function** | | |
| Antibody preparations | Muromonab-CD3 (Orthoclone OKT3) | *Monoclonal* |
| | | Alemtuzumab (Campath, Lemtrada) |
| | | Basiliximab (Simulect) |
| | | Bevacizumab (Avastin, Mvasi) |
| | | Cetuximab (Erbitux) |
| | | Ipilimumab (Yervoy) |
| | | Nivolumab (Opdivo) |
| | | Omalizumab (Xolair) |
| | | Panitumumab (Vectibix) |
| | | Rituximab (Rituxan, Truxima) |
| | | Trastuzumab (Herceptin, Kanjinti, Ogivri) |
| | | *Polyclonal* |
| | | Antithymocyte globulin (Atgam, Thymoglobulin) |
| | | Others |
| Tumor necrosis factor-alpha–blocking agents | Infliximab (Remicade, Inflectra, Renflexis) | Adalimumab (Humira, Humira Pediatric Crohn's Start, Humira Pen) |
| | | Certolizumab (Cimzia, Cimzia Prefilled, Cimzia Starter Kit) |
| | | Etanercept (Enbrel, Enbrel Mini, Enbrel SureClick) |
| | | Golimumab (Simponi, Simponi Aria) |
| | | Leflunomide (Arava) |
| Interleukin-blocking agents | Anakinra (Kineret) | Alefacept (Amevive) |
| | | Tocilizumab (Actemra, Actemra ACTPen) |
| | | Ustekinumab (Stelara) |
| | | Ixekizumab (Taltz) |
| Fusion protein inhibitors | Abatacept (Orencia, Orencia ClickJect) | Belatacept (Nulojix) |

## Pharmacokinetics

Mycophenolate mofetil is a prodrug that, after oral or intravenous (IV) administration, is rapidly broken down to mycophenolic acid, the active component. Metabolism to an active metabolite occurs in the liver, finally resulting in inactive metabolites. Excretion takes place in the urine.

## Action

Mycophenolate is an antimetabolite agent that interferes with the production of cellular deoxyribonucleic acid (DNA) and ribonucleic acid (RNA) and thus blocks cellular reproduction, growth, and development. As its active component, mycophenolic acid inhibits an enzyme needed for DNA synthesis and reduces the proliferation of lymphocytes.

## Use

Uses of mycophenolate mofetil include the prophylaxis of organ rejection after cardiac, hepatic, and renal transplants, as well as immunosuppression after other solid organ transplant procedures involving the lung, pancreas, and small intestine. Mycophenolate sodium (Myfortic), an oral formulation, has received FDA approval for use after kidney transplant to prevent organ rejection. Table 13.2 gives route and dosage information

**Figure 13.1.** Activity of immunosuppressant drugs. Available immunosuppressants inhibit the immune response by blocking that response at various sites.

### TABLE 13.2

## DRUGS AT A GLANCE: Cytotoxic Immunosuppressive Agents

| Drug | Pregnancy Category | Routes and Dosage Ranges | |
|---|---|---|---|
| | | **Adults** | **Children** |
| Ⓟ **Mycophenolate mofetil** (CellCept, CellCept IV, Myfortic; 🍁 ACH-Mycophenolate, APO-Mycophenolate, CellCept, CellCept IV) | D | Renal transplantation: PO, IV 1 g twice daily<br>Cardiac and hepatic transplantation: PO, IV 1.5 g twice daily<br>Extended-release tablets (Myfortic), PO 720 mg twice daily | Safety and efficacy not established |
| Azathioprine (Azasan, Imuran; 🍁 Apo-Azathioprine, Imuran) | D | PO, IV 3–5 mg/kg/d initially; may be able to decrease to 1–3 mg/kg/d | Safety and efficacy not established |
| Leflunomide (Arava; 🍁 ACCEL-Leflunomide, APO-Leflunomide, Arava) | X | PO 100 mg once daily for 3 d, then 20 mg once daily | Not recommended for children younger than 18 y of age |
| Methotrexate (Otrexup, Rasuvo, Trexall, Xatmep; 🍁 JAMP-Methotrexate, Metoject) | X | PO 7.5 mg/wk as single dose, or 2.5 mg every 12 h for 3 doses once weekly | Safe for children 2–16 y of age with juvenile rheumatoid arthritis |

for mycophenolate and other cytotoxic immunosuppressant agents.

## Use in Children

Children 3 months of age and older undergoing renal transplantation have taken mycophenolate. Those who experience postoperative delayed graft function do not require dosage adjustments. Children with impaired renal function taking mycophenolate warrant close observation for adverse effects.

## Use in Older Adults

Mycophenolate has similar therapeutic and adverse effects in older adults compared with younger adults. However, because older adults often have multiple disorders and decreased organ function, it is especially important that drug choices, dosages, and monitoring tests be individualized.

## Use in Patients With Renal Impairment

Mycophenolate produces higher plasma levels in renal transplant recipients with severe renal impairment than in patients with less severe renal impairment (and in healthy volunteers). It is important to avoid doses higher than 1 g twice a day in these patients.

## Use in Patients With Hepatic Impairment

Liver impairment may interfere with metabolism, increasing drug half-life.

## Use in Patients Receiving Home Care

With patients who are taking mycophenolate and other immunosuppressant drugs, a major role of the home care nurse is to assess the environment for potential sources of infection, assist patients and other members of the household to understand the patient's susceptibility to infection, and teach ways to decrease risks of infection. Although infections often develop from the patient's own body flora or reactivation of a latent infection, other potential sources include people with infections, caregivers, water or soil around live plants, and raw fruits and vegetables. Attention to environmental cleansing as well as good personal and hand hygiene is required with immunosuppressant therapy. In addition, the nurse may need to assist with setting up a medication schedule and scheduling clinic visits for monitoring and follow-up care.

The home care nurse also assesses the patient's ability to safely self-administer the medications as prescribed, monitors for adverse drug effects, and observes for signs of drug toxicity. Drug interactions with drugs from multiple prescribers as well as drug–nutrient and drug–herbal interactions can all have an impact on the patient's response to immunosuppressant drug therapy.

## Adverse Effects

Common GI adverse effects of mycophenolate include nausea, vomiting, and diarrhea. The most serious risks associated with the use of this drug and some other immunosuppressant drugs are infection and increased risk of malignancy. Latent infections with the tuberculosis bacillus or hepatitis B virus may become active infections during immunosuppressant therapy.

## Contraindications

Use of cytotoxic immunosuppressant drugs is not recommended during pregnancy or lactation. The FDA has issued a **BLACK BOX WARNING**  for mycophenolate mofetil regarding the risk of fetal loss and malformations. Women of childbearing age must use contraception. A negative pregnancy test for such women is required prior to starting therapy. Contraceptive counseling for patients of both sexes is recommended prior to treatment and for several months after stopping treatment.

## Nursing Implications

### Preventing Interactions

Several drugs can increase and decrease the effects of mycophenolate, increasing or decreasing its effects (Box 13.1). Herbal preparations such as alfalfa, echinacea, ginseng, and bee venom, which potentially stimulate immune function, may interfere with mycophenolate and other immunosuppressant drug activity; thus, it is necessary to avoid them during therapy.

### Administering the Medication

> **! QSEN Alert: Safety**
>
> It is necessary to handle immunosuppressant drugs such as mycophenolate with care to avoid direct contact with skin or mucous membranes. Such contacts have produced teratogenic effects in animals. Patients should swallow oral tablets or capsules whole, without crushing or altering them, and they should avoid inhaling the powder from the capsules. Caregivers should use caution to avoid direct contact when handling the drug.

For best absorption, it is important to take oral mycophenolate on an empty stomach. To ensure correct dosing, it is important to measure the oral solution carefully using an accurate measuring device.

### Assessing for Therapeutic Effects

After organ transplant, the absence of signs and symptoms of a rejection reaction is evidence of the therapeutic effects of mycophenolate immunosuppressive therapy. (Inflammatory changes in the organ tissue along with laboratory evidence of organ impairment usually accompany acute rejection reactions.) Periodic organ tissue biopsy is used to evaluate for signs of chronic rejection reaction.

> **BOX 13.1**  **Drug Interactions: Mycophenolate Mofetil**
>
> **Drugs That Increase the Effects of Mycophenolate Mofetil**
> - Acyclovir, ganciclovir, probenecid, and salicylates
>   *Decrease excretion*
>
> **Drugs That Decrease the Effects of Mycophenolate Mofetil**
> - Antacids containing magnesium, aluminum, and calcium; cholestyramine
>   *Decrease absorption as drug binds with mycophenolate*

## Assessing for Adverse Effects

A primary focus for nursing assessment is evidence of signs of infection, including fever, chills, sore throat, headache, swollen glands, cough, and urinary burning or frequency. Following organ transplant surgery, patients often take prophylactic antimicrobials for the first 3 to 6 months to prevent opportunistic infections. Wound healing may be slower during cytotoxic drug therapy with suppression of the normal inflammatory response.

Nursing care includes assessment of GI symptoms, oral intake, elimination pattern, fluid and electrolyte balance, and weight changes. Skin assessment for signs of rash, bruising, petechiae, and color changes such as pallor or jaundice of the skin or sclera offers important clues to allergic or hematologic complications and hepatotoxicity. Laboratory monitoring of the complete blood count (CBC), renal function tests, and liver function tests performed prior to therapy and periodically during treatment limits the potential for bone marrow suppression and potential hepatotoxicity.

### Clinical Application 13.1

- At his office visit, Mr. Jones tells the nurse that he has been regularly attending his son's Little League baseball games at a local park. What self-care measures related to his long-term need for immunosuppressive drug therapy should the nurse recommend?

## Patient Teaching

The nurse should advise patients not to donate blood during and for 6 weeks after treatment. Individuals of reproductive age should receive counseling regarding pregnancy prevention and planning and the importance of consulting a health care provider if there is a possibility of pregnancy. Men should not donate sperm during therapy or for at least 90 days following mycophenolate discontinuation. Female partners of male patients should use highly effective contraception during and for 3 months after treatment.

Box 13.2 lists additional patient teaching guidelines for the cytotoxic immunosuppressant drugs.

### ! QSEN Alert: Safety

Mixing with orange or apple juice improves taste; do not use grapefruit juice because it inhibits the metabolism of cyclosporine.

## Other Drugs in the Class

Health care providers have long used methotrexate (Otrexup, Rasuvo, Trexall, Xatmep) for the treatment of cancer (higher doses), as well as for the treatment of autoimmune disorders, such as severe rheumatoid arthritis, juvenile rheumatoid arthritis, and severe psoriasis (lower doses). The use of methotrexate in

combination with cyclosporine is the most widely used regimen in the prevention of GVHD after bone marrow transplantation.

Excretion of methotrexate is mainly in the urine, so the drug's half-life is prolonged in patients with renal impairment, with risks of accumulation to toxic levels and additional renal damage. However, the risks are less with the small doses used for treatment of rheumatoid arthritis than for the high doses used in cancer chemotherapy. To decrease these risks, it is important to document adequate renal function using the drug. Patients should be well hydrated.

The lower doses of methotrexate used for autoimmune disorders and transplant therapy reduce the incidence and severity of adverse effects. Oral mucositis can occur with methotrexate therapy, interfering with nutritional intake and contributing to the risk of infection. However, even in the low doses used in rheumatoid arthritis and psoriasis, methotrexate may cause hepatotoxicity. Prior to and during therapy, monitoring the CBC, renal function, and liver function is essential. Liver function tests help guide methotrexate dosage. In general, dosage reduction is warranted if bilirubin is between 3 and 5 mg/dL, or aspartate aminotransferase (AST) is above 180 International Units per liter, and the drug should be omitted if bilirubin is above 5 mg/dL. Many clinicians recommend serial liver biopsies for patients on long-term, low-dose methotrexate.

Administration of methotrexate is weekly for rheumatoid arthritis or psoriasis, and patients should keep an accurate record of the date and time of each dose. To reduce gastric upset, they may take the drug with food. However, daily dosing for cytotoxic immunosuppressants should be consistent with regard to time and food (i.e., at the same time of day, with the same meal).

### ! QSEN Alert: Safety

It is necessary to follow individual manufacturer's instructions for reconstituting and administering IV preparations of methotrexate—in consultation with a pharmacist as needed.

Leflunomide (Arava), an anti-inflammatory immunosuppressant, is useful only in the treatment of adults with rheumatoid arthritis. Authorities do not recommend the drug for children younger than 18 years of age. Contraindications include the presence of active hepatitis B or C infection or if the alanine aminotransferase (ALT) level is greater than two times normal. With leflunomide, hepatotoxicity is a concern; hence, it is essential to obtain liver function tests before starting therapy. Also, patients should have renal function tests, as well as liver function tests, every month for the first 6 months then every 6 to 8 weeks thereafter. The FDA has issued a **BLACK BOX WARNING ◆** for leflunomide regarding the risk of fetal loss and malformations. Women of childbearing age must use contraception. A negative pregnancy test for such women of childbearing age is necessary prior to starting therapy. Contraceptive counseling for both genders is recommended prior to treatment and for several months after stopping treatment.

Azathioprine (Azasan, Imuran) is occasionally part of a maintenance immunosuppressive regimen following transplant, although cyclosporine or tacrolimus is used more commonly.

BOX 13.2  *Patient Teaching Guidelines for Cytotoxic Immunosuppressant Drugs and Antirejection Drugs*

### General Considerations

- People taking medications that suppress the immune system are at high risk for development of infections. As a result, patients, caregivers, and others in the patient's environment need to wash their hands often and thoroughly, practice meticulous personal hygiene (e.g., take good care of the mouth, gums, and skin), avoid contact with infected people, and practice other methods of preventing infection.

- Understand that lifelong drug treatment to prevent potential organ rejection is required after transplant therapy. Obtain complete instructions about all the medications used to prevent rejection, including the purpose and activity of the drug; dose; route of administration (e.g., oral, injection); frequency and timing, potential adverse effects, and their management; and signs of complications and drug toxicity. Poor adherence and missed medication doses are an important cause of organ rejection and need for a subsequent transplant.

- Report adverse drug effects (e.g., signs or symptoms of infection such as sore throat or fever, decreased urine output if taking cyclosporine, easy bruising or bleeding if taking methotrexate) to a health care provider. If you have had a transplant, know the signs of transplant rejection.

- Try to maintain healthy lifestyle habits, such as a nutritious diet, adequate rest and sleep, and avoiding tobacco and alcohol. These measures enhance immune mechanisms and other body defenses.

- Carry identification that lists the drugs being taken; the dosage; the prescriber's name, address, and telephone number; and instructions for emergency treatment. Use of a MedicAlert bracelet is recommended in case of an accident or other emergency situation.

- Inform all health care providers that you are taking immunosuppressant drugs.

- Maintain regular supervision by a health care provider. This is extremely important for evaluating health status, evaluating drug responses and indications for dosage change, detecting adverse drug reactions, and having blood tests or other monitoring tests when indicated.

- Take no other drugs, prescription or nonprescription, without notifying the prescriber who is managing immunosuppressant therapy. Immunosuppressant drugs may influence reactions to other drugs, and other drugs may influence reactions to the immunosuppressants. Thus, taking other drugs may decrease therapeutic effects or increase adverse effects. In addition, some vaccinations should be avoided while taking immunosuppressant drugs.

- People of reproductive capability who are sexually active should practice effective contraceptive techniques during immunosuppressive drug therapy. With methotrexate, use contraception during and for at least 3 months (men) or one ovulatory cycle (women) after stopping the drug. With mycophenolate, effective contraception should be continued for 6 weeks after the drug is stopped. With sirolimus, effective contraception must be used before, during, and for 12 weeks after drug therapy.

- Wear protective clothing and use sunscreens to decrease exposure of skin to sunlight and risks of skin cancers. Also, methotrexate and sirolimus increase sensitivity to sunlight and may increase sunburn. Have cancer screening for early detection if you take immunosuppressant drugs.

### Self-Administration

- Follow instructions about taking the drugs. This is vital to achieving beneficial effects and decreasing adverse effects. If unable to take a medication, report to the prescriber or other health care provider; do not stop unless advised to do so. For transplant recipients, missed doses may lead to transplant rejection; for patients with autoimmune diseases, missed doses may lead to acute flare-ups of symptoms. Take medications at approximately the same time each day to maintain consistent drug levels in the blood.

- With cyclosporine oral solution, use the same solution consistently. The available cyclosporine solutions (Neoral, Gengraf, Sandimmune) are not equivalent and cannot be used interchangeably. If a change in formulation is necessary, the dispensing pharmacy should consult the prescriber.

- Measure oral cyclosporine solution with the dosing syringe provided; add to orange or apple juice that is at room temperature (avoid grapefruit juice) into a glass container, stir well, and drink at once (do not allow diluted solution to stand before drinking). Rinse the glass with more juice to ensure the total dose is taken. Do not rinse the dosing syringe with water or other cleaning agents. Take on a consistent schedule with regard to time of day and meals.

  These are the manufacturer's recommendations.

  The amount of fluid should be large enough to increase palatability, especially for children, but small enough to be consumed quickly. Rinsing ensures the entire dose is taken.

- Take mycophenolate on an empty stomach; food decreases drug absorption by approximately 40%. Do not crush mycophenolate tablets and do not open or crush the capsules.

- Take sirolimus consistently with or without food; do not mix or take the drug with grapefruit juice. Grapefruit juice inhibits metabolism and increases adverse effects. If also taking cyclosporine, take the sirolimus 4 hours after a dose of cyclosporine.

- If taking the oral solution, use the syringe that comes with the medication to measure and withdraw the dose from the bottle. Empty the dose into a glass or plastic container with at least 2 oz (1/4 cup or 60 mL) of water or orange juice. *Do not use any other liquid to dilute the drug.* Stir the mixture vigorously, and drink it immediately. Refill the container with at least 4 oz (1/2 cup or 120 mL) of water or orange juice, stir vigorously, and drink at once.

- Take tacrolimus with food to decrease stomach upset.

- If giving or taking an injected drug, be sure you understand how to mix and inject the medication correctly. With etanercept, for example, rotate injection sites, give a new injection at least 1 inch from a previous injection site, and do not inject the medication into areas where the skin is tender, bruised, red, or hard. When possible, practice the required techniques and perform at least the first injection under supervision of a qualified health care professional.

Health care providers use azathioprine after organ transplant in children, as well as treatment of psoriasis, psoriatic arthritis, systemic lupus erythematosus, immune thrombocytopenia, inflammatory bowel disease, and other inflammatory disorders, but safety data are limited. Contraindications include pregnancy and lactation, and extreme caution is essential with hepatic disease or hepatic impairment. Drug metabolism occurs in the liver and erythrocytes. Researchers have reported genetic variation in the rate of metabolism.

Adverse effects of azathioprine include bone marrow suppression with neutropenia, thrombocytopenia, and anemia; hepatotoxicity with increased risk of posttransplant venoocclusive liver disease; GI upset, nausea, vomiting, and diarrhea; fever and muscle aches; and skin rash. It is necessary to obtain baseline liver function tests and a pregnancy test prior to therapy. Lower doses are required in the presence of renal disease to prevent drug toxicities such as myelosuppression and hepatotoxicity. Patients should have CBCs and liver function tests on a set schedule. Azathioprine has a high potential for toxicity, so regular assessments for adverse effects are critical. The FDA has issued a **BLACK BOX WARNING** ◆ for chronic immunosuppression with azathioprine because the drug increases risk of malignancy.

# CONVENTIONAL ANTIREJECTION AGENTS

Ⓟ **Cyclosporine** (Neoral, Gengraf, Sandimmune), the first antirejection drug used to prevent transplant rejection reactions, is the prototype antirejection agent. Cyclosporine and related drugs are fungal metabolites with strong immunosuppressive effects. By selectively inhibiting proliferation of helper T cells and expression of cytokines, these antirejection drugs reduce the activity of other immune cells involved in graft rejection. Consequently, they are widely used in transplant therapy to prevent or reduce the graft rejection response.

## Pharmacokinetics

Absorption of cyclosporine is highly variable. After oral administration, absorption is rather poor. The drug is highly bound to plasma proteins, and approximately 50% is distributed in erythrocytes, so drug levels in whole blood are higher than those in plasma. Peak plasma levels occur 4 to 5 hours after a dose. Metabolism of cyclosporine involves the CYP3A4 liver enzyme system, and elimination occurs mainly in the bile.

## Action

Cyclosporine inhibits calcineurin, a protein needed for the synthesis of IL-2 and the subsequent proliferation of T cells and B cells. The drug binds with calcineurin on T lymphocytes and interferes with the production of IL-2. As previously described, activated T cells produce a cytokine, IL-2, which, in turn, inhibits signaling through the T-cell receptor. This action activates other lymphocytes, amplifying the immune response and producing the damaging inflammatory changes in tissue that occur with organ rejection and autoimmune disease.

## Use

Health care providers use cyclosporine to prevent rejection reactions and prolong graft survival after solid organ transplantation (e.g., kidney, liver, heart, lung) or to treat chronic rejection in patients previously treated with other immunosuppressive agents. The drug inhibits both cellular and humoral immunity but affects T lymphocytes significantly more than B lymphocytes. With cyclosporine-induced deprivation of IL-2, T cells stimulated by the graft antigen are unable to multiple and differentiate, and graft organ destruction is inhibited. In addition to its use in solid organ transplantation, cyclosporine is useful in the prevention and treatment of GVHD, a complication of bone marrow transplantation. In GVHD, T lymphocytes from the transplanted marrow of the donor mount an immune response against the tissues of the recipient. Cyclosporine may inhibit donor T-cell activity, reducing the risk of GVHD. Other indications for use include treatment of psoriasis and rheumatoid arthritis.

Cyclosporine dosing is weight based in both adults and children, with higher doses given immediately before and after the transplant and then tapered over several months to minimize adverse effects and avoid excessive immunosuppression. Table 13.3 outlines the routes and dosages for cyclosporine and related drugs.

### Use in Children

Children as young as 6 months of age may receive cyclosporine in its oral form. Experience with this drug indicates that children require relatively high doses because they metabolize the drug rapidly.

### Use in Older Adults

Due to an increased incidence of infection and a greater risk of malignancy, it is necessary to monitor older adults carefully during antirejection drug therapy. Doses are individualized, considering age, function, and concurrent conditions. More frequent assessment and therapeutic blood level monitoring are essential in older adults after organ transplantation because of the increased risk of organ toxicity.

### Use in Patients With Renal Impairment

Patients with solid organ transplants commonly use cyclosporine, but the risk of nephrotoxicity increases as a result. Clinical studies have demonstrated that this nephrotoxicity is dose related. To reduce toxicity and increase efficacy, attention must be given to dosage, other adverse effects, and potential drug interactions. Monitoring serum blood levels can help reduce this risk, and nephrotoxicity usually subsides after decreasing the dosage or stopping the drug. In kidney transplant recipients, when serum creatinine and blood urea nitrogen (BUN) levels remain elevated, an evaluation of the patient and tissue biopsy is often necessary to differentiate cyclosporine-induced nephrotoxicity from a transplant rejection reaction.

| **TABLE 13.3** | | | |
| --- | --- | --- | --- |
| **DRUGS AT A GLANCE: Conventional Antirejection Agents** | | | |
| **Drug** | **Pregnancy Category** | **Routes and Dosage Ranges** | |
| | | **Adults** | **Children** |
| Ⓟ **Cyclosporine** (Sandimmune, Gengraf, Neoral; ✻ Apo-Cyclosporine, Neoral) | C | Sandimmune: PO 15 mg/kg 4–12 h before transplantation, then 15 mg/kg once daily for 1–2 wk, and then decrease by 5% per week to a maintenance dose of 5–10 mg/kg/d; IV 5–6 mg/kg infused over 2–6 h<br>Neoral/Gengraf: PO, the first dose in patients with new transplants is the same as the first oral dose of Sandimmune; later doses are titrated according to cyclosporine blood levels | Same as in adults with caution |
| Everolimus (Zortress, Afinitor, Afinitor Disperz; ✻ Afinitor, Afinitor Disperz) | D | Zortress/Afinitor: PO 10-mg tablet once daily | 1 y of age or older: Afinitor Disperz PO tablet for oral suspension, 4.5 mg/m² once daily. Tablets are not interchangeable. |
| Sirolimus (Rapamune; ✻ Rapamune) | C | PO 6 mg as soon after kidney transplantation as possible, then 2 mg daily | Older than 13 y of age: PO 3 mg/m² as loading dose, then 1 mg/m² daily |
| Tacrolimus (Prograf, Astagraf XL, Envarsus XR; ✻ Advagraf, Envarsus, Prograf, Sandoz Tacrolimus) | C | IV infusion, 25–50 mcg/kg/d, starting 6 h after transplantation or later, until the patient can tolerate oral drug; PO 150–200 mcg/kg/d, in 2 divided doses every 12 h, with the first dose 8–12 h after stopping the IV infusion | IV 50–100 mcg/kg/d; PO 200–300 mcg/kg/d |

### Use in Patients With Hepatic Impairment

With cyclosporine, it is important to check serum bilirubin and liver enzymes prior to and during treatment. Clinical trials have shown that cyclosporine is associated with mild elevations of serum bilirubin, often without elevated ALT or alkaline phosphatase. These complications are now less frequent, possibly because dosing and monitoring of cyclosporine levels have become more precise.

### Use in Patients With Critical Illness

Use of immunosuppressants during critical illness requires individualized risk versus benefit decision-making. It is necessary to balance the need to prevent transplant organ rejection against the risk of infection and associated drug toxicities, which may lead to loss of the engrafted organ.

### Use in Patients Receiving Home Care

Survival rates are now longer in transplant recipients, and multiple organ transplants and retransplants occur. Thus, there are challenges in managing chronic rejection and minimizing drug toxicities in the home setting. Promoting correct medication use is critical to maintaining therapeutic blood levels after

transplantation and preventing organ rejection. Due to the variable bioavailability of cyclosporine when taken orally, patients should consistently take the drug at the same time each day. In addition to monitoring medication use, the home care nurse provides self-care teaching, monitors for sources of infection, obtains and monitors blood work, and implements health maintenance measures.

## Adverse Effects

Nephrotoxicity, hirsutism, gingival hypertrophy, hypertension, and hyperlipidemia are significant adverse effects of cyclosporine. The FDA has issued a **BLACK BOX WARNING ◆** for cyclosporine regarding risks of hypertension and nephrotoxicity. After solid organ transplantation, with the need to continue lifelong immunosuppression to avoid graft rejection, serious infection is an ongoing concern.

As previously stated, transplant recipients are living longer, and this has led to the recognition that there are long-term adverse effects associated with immunosuppressant drug therapy. As a consequence of long-term survival and chronic immunosuppression, patients have an increased risk of developing a malignancy. The incidence of malignancy is unknown, but after 10 years of immunosuppression, authorities often estimate it to be 20% or more. The most common malignancies in transplant recipients are skin cancers and lymphomas, and solid organ tumors may also occur. Regular screening tests for breast, cervical, colon, and prostate cancer, along with annual skin examinations, are recommended. The FDA has issued a **BLACK BOX WARNING** ◆ limiting all long-term use of antirejection drugs to prescribers experienced in transplant therapy because of the increased risk of infections and certain malignancies such as lymphoma and skin cancer.

## Contraindications

Contraindications to cyclosporine include the combined use of antirejection drugs that have the same mechanism of action and toxicities (e.g., tacrolimus and cyclosporine). Prescribers usually avoid such use after organ transplant.

## Nursing Implications

### Preventing Interactions

Numerous potential drug interactions affect the blood levels of cyclosporine, increasing or decreasing its effects (Box 13.3). Because these drugs are metabolized mainly by CYP3A4 enzymes and have a low therapeutic index, any drugs that increase or decrease levels of these enzymes have the potential to alter blood levels of cyclosporine. The herb St. John's wort may reduce this drug's therapeutic effects.

### Administering the Medication

It is necessary to initiate antirejection drugs several hours prior to the transplant procedure. Administration is by IV infusion only until the patient can take the drug by the oral route. The risk of a severe allergic reaction is significantly higher following IV administration. Dilution of an oral cyclosporine solution should follow package instructions.

To improve bioavailability, cyclosporine preparations were once prepared in alcohol and olive oil for oral administration and in alcohol and castor oil for IV administration. Anaphylactic reactions, attributed to the castor oil, have occurred with the IV formulation. Neoral and Gengraf are oral microemulsion formulations that are better absorbed than oral Sandimmune.

**BOX 13.3** **Drug Interactions: Cyclosporine**

**Drugs That Increase the Effects of Cyclosporine**
- Aminoglycoside antibiotics and amphotericin B
  *Increase nephrotoxic effects*
- Azithromycin, fluconazole, and related antifungals; macrolide antibiotics
  *Increase blood levels and toxic effects*

**Drugs That Decrease the Effects of Cyclosporine**
- Carbamazepine, phenytoin, and rifampin
  *Decreases therapeutic effects*

These different drug formulations are not equivalent in their absorption and cannot be used interchangeably.

### Assessing for Therapeutic Effects

The nurse assesses therapeutic effects by monitoring for organ function and signs of rejection with solid organ transplants, assessing serum blood levels, and monitoring and managing adverse drug effects. Cyclosporine has a very narrow therapeutic index; therefore, prescribers use serum drug levels to regulate cyclosporine dosing, and close monitoring is necessary. They use blood levels measured 2 hours after a dose for dosage adjustments. Subtherapeutic levels may lead to organ transplant rejection, whereas high levels increase adverse effects.

### Assessing for Adverse Effects

Acute nephrotoxicity can occur, progressing to chronic nephrotoxicity and kidney failure. It is essential to monitor renal function tests (serum creatinine and BUN) and urine protein throughout cyclosporine therapy. To check for hepatotoxicity, it is necessary to conduct liver function tests (bilirubin, ALT, and AST) regularly. Periodic monitoring of fasting lipid levels (cholesterol, high- and low-density lipoproteins, and triglycerides) should also occur.

### Patient Teaching

Box 13.2 presents patient teaching information for the conventional antirejection drugs.

## Other Drugs in the Class

Everolimus (Zortress, Afinitor) reduces T-cell activation to decrease the immune response after kidney transplant and rejection. This drug, generally combined with cyclosporine and prednisone, allows lower posttransplant doses of both cyclosporine and the steroid; this minimizes adverse effects. Everolimus is available only as an oral formulation, and patients should take the drug consistently, with or without food, to maintain consistent therapeutic blood levels. It has been associated with an increased incidence of angioedema, early kidney graft thrombosis, delayed wound healing, elevated lipid levels, new-onset diabetes, and an increased risk of nephrotoxicity and proteinuria when combined with cyclosporine. It is necessary to obtain therapeutic blood levels of both cyclosporine and everolimus to minimize the risks of renal toxicity when the drugs are used concurrently.

**QSEN Alert: Safety**

Use of an alcohol-free dexamethasone mouthwash prior to administration of everolimus will reduce the incidence and severity of stomatitis. Instruct the patient to swish and spit the mouthwash before taking the drug.

Sirolimus is an immunosuppressant used to prevent organ rejection in kidney transplants. Often, it is given concomitantly with a corticosteroid and cyclosporine. Sirolimus may have synergistic effects with cyclosporine because it has a different mechanism of action, and prescribers may order both drugs in combination. However, because the two drugs are metabolized by the same liver CYP3A4 enzymes, cyclosporine can increase blood levels of sirolimus, potentially to toxic levels. Consequently, it is essential that the drugs not be given at the same time; patients should take sirolimus 4 hours after a dose of cyclosporine.

Extensive metabolism of sirolimus occurs in the liver, and the drug may accumulate in the presence of hepatic impairment. If this occurs, reducing the maintenance dose by 35% may be warranted; changing the loading dose is not necessary. Monitoring using serum drug levels in patients who are likely to have altered drug metabolism due to age, concurrent disease, or other drugs is important. Use of sirolimus in children after renal transplant to reduce the risk of nephropathy from cyclosporine or tacrolimus allows these other drugs to be given at lower doses or discontinued. Contraindications to use of sirolimus include recent lung and liver transplantation due to an increased incidence of delayed healing and graft failure in the transplanted organs. The FDA has issued a **BLACK BOX WARNING ◆** that use of sirolimus in lung and liver transplant patients has been associated with increased morbidity and mortality.

Tacrolimus is similar to cyclosporine in its mechanisms of action, pharmacokinetic characteristics, and adverse effects. It prevents transplant rejection by inhibiting proliferation of T lymphocytes. Some transplant centers now use tacrolimus rather than cyclosporine, mainly because cyclosporine is given with corticosteroids. Using tacrolimus may allow corticosteroids to be reduced or stopped, thereby decreasing the adverse effects of long-term corticosteroid therapy. Tacrolimus, like cyclosporine, is not well absorbed orally, so it is necessary to give higher oral doses than IV doses to obtain similar blood levels. With IV administration, onset of action is rapid, but with oral administration, onset varies. It is essential that patients take the oral drug on a consistent time schedule because its bioavailability may vary. Dosing of tacrolimus is individualized according to clinical response, adverse effects, and serum blood levels.

Metabolism of tacrolimus takes place in the liver and intestine, and excretion of the several metabolites occurs in bile and urine. Dosage reduction is necessary with impaired liver or renal function. It is essential to give the drug at the lowest effective dose because it may cause nephrotoxicity.

### Clinical Application 13.2

- Mr. Jones calls the nephrology clinic to report shortness of breath and fatigue. Despite a decrease in appetite, he reports his weight has increased by 2 kg over the last week. The nurse recognizes that he is most likely experiencing which adverse effects from one of his immunosuppressant medications?

## JANUS ASSOCIATED KINASE INHIBITOR

Ⓟ **Ruxolitinib** (Jakafi) is classified as a Janus kinase inhibitor that is administered orally for acute treatment to prevent GVHD. It is also an antineoplastic agent used to treat polycythemia vera.

### Pharmacokinetics

The onset of action is approximately 1.5 weeks or 1 to 11 days. With chronic GVHD, the median time is 3 weeks. Ruxolitinib is rapidly absorbed. The protein binding is 97% to albumin. Metabolism is in the liver with the CYP3A4 isoenzyme (it is also metabolized minimally by CYP2C9). The half-life is approximately 3 hours, with a peak of action in 1 to 2 hours. It is excreted primarily in the kidneys and 22% in the feces.

### Action

Ruxolitinib selectively inhibits Janus-associated kinases, mediating the signals of cytokine and growth factors that are responsible for hematopoiesis and immune function.

### Use

Ruxolitinib is used for acute treatment of steroid-refractory acute GVHD in adult and pediatric patients. It is also used to treat polycythemia vera and myelofibrosis in adults. Table 13.4 outlines the routes and dosages for ruxolitinib.

### TABLE 13.4

### DRUGS AT A GLANCE: Janus-Associated Kinase Inhibitor

| Drug | Pregnancy Category | Routes and Dosage Ranges | |
|---|---|---|---|
| | | Adults | Children |
| Ⓟ **Ruxolitinib** (Jakafi; ✹ Jakafi) | Ruxolitinib is not recommended during pregnancy | PO 5 mg twice daily; increase dose to 10 mg twice daily after at least 3 d of treatment if ANC and platelets are not decreased by >50% compared to first day of ruxolitinib therapy | Children ≥12 years: PO 5 mg twice daily; consider increasing the dose to 10 mg twice daily after at least 3 d of treatment if ANC and platelets are not decreased by >50% compared to first day of ruxolitinib therapy |

## Adverse Effects

The central nervous system adverse effects include dizziness, headache, fatigue, and insomnia. Increased serum cholesterol is noted, as well as hypertriglyceridemia. Hematologic adverse effects include anemia, thrombocytopenia, and neutropenia. In postmarketing administration, the rate of hepatitis B exacerbation was reported.

## Contraindications

There are no manufacturer's labeling that indicate contraindications. The intake of grapefruit juice will increase the effect of ruxolitinib, and patients should be instructed to eliminate it from the diet.

## Nursing Implications

### Preventing Interactions

Immunosuppressant and corticosteroid agents interact with ruxolitinib. In addition, chemotherapeutic agents will increase immune suppression.

### Administering the Medication

Ruxolitinib is administered orally without regard to food intake. For patients who have an inability to swallow, it can be administered through a nasogastric tube measuring 8 French or larger. The tablet should be suspended in 40 mL of water, stirred for 10 minutes, and administered within 6 hours of dispersion. Administer with the appropriate size syringe, and flush the NG tube with 75 mL of water. Administration is the same for pediatric patients. Do not administer with grapefruit juice due to increase of serum drug levels or potential toxicity. Prior to initiation of ruxolitinib therapy, the patient should be assessed for tuberculosis. A tuberculin skin test should be evaluated before therapy is started; if the test is positive, the medication should not be given. The administration of this drug in a patient with a positive tuberculin test will decrease the immune response and increase the patient's risk of the development of active tuberculosis.

### Assessing for Therapeutic and Adverse Effects

The CBC should be assessed at baseline and every 2 to 4 weeks. In patients with stage 3 to 4 liver GVHD, the CBC may be assessed more frequently. In addition, lipid levels should be monitored every 8 to 12 weeks. Perform period skin assessments to assess for the development of skin infections.

## ADJUVANT MEDICATIONS USED TO SUPPRESS IMMUNE FUNCTION

A significant number of adjuvant medications are used as immunosuppressants. Table 13.5 summarizes indications for use and dosages for these drugs.

## Corticosteroids

Corticosteroids are potent anti-inflammatory agents that suppress the systemic immune response. Chapters 17 and 33 contain information about specific agents, including effects of therapeutic doses of corticosteroids. Used in a wide variety of inflammatory and allergic disorders, pharmacologic doses of corticosteroids block the production of IL-1, relieving signs and symptoms of inflammation by decreasing the accumulation of lymphocytes and macrophages and reducing levels of other cell-damaging cytokines. Corticosteroids, used in pharmacologic doses, suppress inflammation by suppressing activation and growth of lymphoid T cells and decreasing the formation and function of antibodies by B cells. For patients with transplanted tissues, corticosteroids are usually given with other agents to prevent acute graft rejection. Increasingly, in autoimmune disease, health care providers use biologic response modifiers, combined with a cytotoxic immunosuppressant (or alone), as primary therapy. These disease-modifying anti-inflammatory drugs, known as DMARDs, more specifically address the underlying autoimmune tissue process and can slow the destructive changes. Currently, prescribers order corticosteroids for episodic use during acute exacerbations of autoimmune disease and then taper or discontinue them as soon as possible.

The important adverse effects of corticosteroids have led many transplant centers to try to minimize or eliminate the use of these drugs as part of chronic immunosuppressive therapy when possible. Methods such as gradually tapering doses after transplant to no more than 10 mg daily in adults and using alternate-day therapy in children are strategies used to minimize the long-term adverse effects of corticosteroids.

## Antibody Preparations

Antibody (immunoglobulin) preparations are produced in the laboratory or derived from animals injected with human lymphoid tissue to stimulate an immune response. Health care providers use such preparations in inflammatory autoimmune disorders, transplantation rejection reactions, and cancer treatment to block cell receptors that are part of the abnormal inflammation or cell proliferation process. The antibodies produced may be monoclonal or polyclonal. This section discusses several drugs.

**Monoclonal antibodies** originate from a single B-cell source. The isolation and cloning of individual B lymphocytes result in the production of biologically identical antibody molecules. To produce a monoclonal antibody, the human antigen to which the desired antibody will respond is first injected into a mouse or hamster. The animal mounts an immune response in which its B lymphocytes are stimulated to produce a specific antibody against that antigen. These B lymphocytes are then recovered from the spleen of the animal and fused with immortal myeloma cells (a cell line that can live forever in culture). This produces an antibody-secreting hybridoma, a cellular "antibody factory" able to produce large amounts of the desired identical antibody. The antibodies can then be isolated from the culture and prepared for clinical use. Because the antibodies are proteins and would be destroyed if taken orally, immunoglobulins must always be given by parenteral injection.

Because monoclonal antibodies are derived from one single cell line or clone, it is possible to design them to suppress the specific components of the immune system that cause tissue damage in particular disorders. These antibodies are able to block cellular growth receptors or inhibit proinflammatory

**TABLE 13.5**

## DRUGS AT A GLANCE: Adjuvant Medications Used as Immunosuppressants

| Drug | Pregnancy Category | Routes and Dosage Ranges | |
|---|---|---|---|
| | | **Adults** | **Children** |
| **Antibody Preparations** | | | |
| **Monoclonal Antibodies** | | | |
| Ⓟ **Muromonab-CD3** (Orthoclone OKT3; Orthoclone OKT3) | C | 5 mg bolus IV injection once daily for 10–14 d | By weight, IV ≤30 kg, 2.5 mg/d for 10–14 d >30 kg, 5 mg/d for 10–14 d; may increase 2.5-mg/d increments if needed |
| Alemtuzumab (Campath, Lemtrada; 🍁 Lemtrada, MabCampath) | C | Campath (IV): progressively increase to a maintenance of 30 mg per dose three times weekly on alternate days for a total duration of therapy of up to 12 wk Lemtrada (IV): 12 mg daily for 5 consecutive days (total 60 mg), followed 12 mo later by 12 mg daily for 3 consecutive days (total 36 mg); total duration of therapy, 24 mo | Safety and efficacy not established |
| Basiliximab (Simulect; 🍁 Simulect) | B | 20 mg IV within 2 h before transplantation and 20 mg 4 d after transplantation (total of 2 doses) | 2–15 y, IV 12 mg/m² up to a maximum of 20 mg for 2 doses, as for adults |
| Bevacizumab (Avastin Mvasi; 🍁 Avastin, Mvasi, Zirabev) | | Varies with disease process and concurrent chemotherapy IV: 5–15 mg/kg every 2–3 wk until disease progression or unacceptable toxicity | Safety and efficacy not established |
| Cetuximab (Erbitux; 🍁 Erbitux) | | IV, initial loading dose, 400 mg/m² infused over 120 min; maintenance dose, 250 mg/m² infused over 60 min weekly until disease progression or unacceptable toxicity | Safety and efficacy not established |
| Ipilimumab (Yervoy; 🍁 Yervoy) | C | IV, melanoma (unresectable or metastatic) 3 mg/kg every 3 wk for maximum of 4 doses; melanoma (adjuvant therapy) IV, 10 mg/kg every 3 wk for 4 doses, followed by 10 mg/kg every 12 wk for up to 3 y | Safety and efficacy not established |
| Nivolumab (Opdivo; 🍁 Opdivo) | May cause fetal harm in pregnancy; women should not breast feed | IV, 240 mg once every 2 wk or 480 mg every 4 wk until disease progression or unacceptable toxicity | Children ≥12 years or older IV <40 kg: 3 mg/kg once every 2 wk until disease progression or unacceptable toxicity |
| Panitumumab (Vectibix; 🍁 Vectibix) | May cause fetal harm in pregnancy; women should not breast feed | IV, colorectal cancer 6 mg/kg every 14 d as a single agent or in combination with fluorouracil, leucovorin, and irinotecan | Safety and efficacy not established |
| Omalizumab (Xolair; 🍁 Xolair) | B | 150–375 mg sub-Q every 2–4 wk based on body weight and pretreatment total serum IgE levels | ≥12 y: sub-Q; refer to adult dosing. |

(*Continued on page 240*)

**TABLE 13.5**

## DRUGS AT A GLANCE: Adjuvant Medications Used as Immunosuppressants
(Continued)

| Drug | Pregnancy Category | Routes and Dosage Ranges | |
|---|---|---|---|
| | | **Adults** | **Children** |
| Rituximab (Rituxan, Truxima; ❋ Rituxan) | C | Varies with disease process and combination regimens; IV infusion: usual starting dose 375 mg/m²; additional cycles may vary | Autoimmune hemolytic anemia: infants ≥4 mo, children, and adolescents; IV infusion, 375 mg/m² once weekly for 2–4 doses<br>Chronic ITP: children and adolescents; IV infusion, 375 mg/m² once weekly for 4 doses<br>Posttransplant lymphoproliferative disorder: infants ≥11 mo, children, and adolescents; IV infusion, 375 mg/m² once weekly for 3–4 doses |
| Trastuzumab (Herceptin, Kanjinti, Ogivri; ❋ Herceptin) | D | Varies with concurrent chemotherapy; IV, initial loading dose, 4 mg/kg infused over 90 min, followed by; maintenance dose, 2 mg/kg infused over 30 min weekly for total of 12–18 wk | Safety and efficacy not established |
| **Polyclonal Antibodies** | | | |
| Antithymocyte globulin (Atgam, equine; Thymoglobulin, rabbit; ❋ Thymoglobulin) | C | Atgam, IV: 15 mg/kg/d for 14 d, then every other day for 14 d (total of 21 doses)<br>Thymoglobulin, 1.5 mg/kg/d IV for 7–14 d | Atgam: renal transplant rejection; children and adolescents; IV, 10 to 15 mg/kg once daily for 14 d, up to total of 21 doses in 28 d, if needed<br>Aplastic anemia: IV, 10 to 20 mg/kg once daily for 8 to 14 d; up to total of 21 doses in 28 d, if needed |
| **Tumor Necrosis Factor-Alpha–Blocking Agents** | | | |
| Infliximab (Remicade, Inflectra, Renflexis; ❋ Inflectra, Remicade, Remsima, Renflexis) | B | IV infusion, 3–5 mg/kg initially, 2 and 6 wk later, then every 8 wk | ≥6 y: same as adults |
| Adalimumab (Humira, Humira Pediatric Crohn's Start, Humira Pen; ❋ Humira) | B | Sub-Q 160 mg every other week then 80 mg/d 15 then 40 mg every other week beginning day 29 | ≥6 y: <40 kg, sub-Q 80 mg every other week then 40 day 15; >40 kg, sub-Q 160 mg then 40 mg/d 15; 40 mg beginning week |
| Certolizumab (Cimzia, Cimzia Prefilled, Cimzia Starter Kit; ❋ Cimzia) | B | Sub-Q 400 mg every 2 wk for 3 doses then every 4 wk | Safety and efficacy not established |
| Etanercept (Enbrel, Enbrel Mini, Enbrel SureClick; ❋ Enbrel, Brenzys, Erelzi) | B | Sub-Q 25 mg twice weekly, 72–96 h apart | ≥2 y, 4–17 y, sub-Q 0.8 mg/kg once weekly up to a maximum of 50 mg per dose |

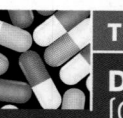

**TABLE 13.5**

## DRUGS AT A GLANCE: Adjuvant Medications Used as Immunosuppressants
(Continued)

| Drug | Pregnancy Category | Routes and Dosage Ranges | |
|---|---|---|---|
| | | **Adults** | **Children** |
| Golimumab (Simponi, Simponi Aria; ✹ Simponi, Simponi IV) | Use of this medication should be individualized to optimize maternal disease and pregnancy outcomes | IV, ankylosing spondylitis, psoriatic arthritis, rheumatoid arthritis 2 mg/kg at weeks 0, 4, and every 8 wk Sub-Q, ulcerative colitis 200 mg at week 0 then 100 mg at week 2, followed by 100 mg every 4 weeks | Safety and efficacy not established |
| Leflunomide (Arava; ✹ Arava, Mylan-Leflunomide) | B | Sub-Q: 50 mg once a month IV: 2 mg/kg at weeks 0, 4, and then every 8 wk thereafter | Safety and efficacy not established |
| | | **Adults** | **Children** |
| **Interleukin-Blocking Agents** | | | |
| Anakinra (Kineret; ✹ Kineret) | B | 100 mg sub-Q once daily | Safety and efficacy not established |
| Alefacept (Amevive) | B | 15 mg IM once weekly for 12 wk; 7.5 mg IV once weekly for 12 wk | Safety and efficacy not established |
| Ixekizumab (Taltz; ✹ Taltz) | Unknown; approved in 2016 | 160 mg (two 80 mg injections) sub-Q at week 0, followed by 80 mg at weeks 2, 4, 6, 8, 10, and 12, then 80 mg every 4 wk | Safety and efficacy not established |
| Tocilizumab (Actemra, Actemra ACTPen; ✹ Actemra) (given with or without methotrexate) | C | 8 mg/kg IV, diluted in 100 mL normal saline infused over 1 h every 4 wk | <25 kg, IV: 8 mg/kg dilute in 50 mL normal saline infused over 1 h every 2–4 wk |
| Ustekinumab (Stelara; ✹ Stelara) | B | Sub-Q by weight <100 kg, 45-mg dose >100 kg, 90-mg dose Initial dose repeated in 4 wk, then every 12 wk thereafter | Children ≥12 y may be dosed by weight but FDA approval not received |
| **Fusion Protein Inhibitors** | | | |
| Abatacept (Orencia, Orencia ClickJect; ✹ Orencia) | B | IV, according to body weight, initially at 2 and 4 wk after initial dose, then every 4 wk; weight below 60 kg, 500 mg; 60–100 kg, 750 mg; above 100 kg, 1000 mg | IV, according to body weight, initially at 2 and 4 wk after initial dose, then every 4 wk; <75 kg, 10 mg/kg; 75–100 kg, 750 mg; more than 100 kg, 1000 mg |
| Belatacept (Nulojix) | C | IV infusion over 30 min; initially 10 mg/kg before transplant; repeated in 96 h and then at weeks 2, 4, 8, and 12; 5 mg/kg at week 16 and every 4 wk thereafter | Safety and efficacy not established |

cytokines that mediate inflammatory tissue damage associated with autoimmune disorders or transplant organ rejection. The generic names of drugs of the monoclonal antibodies end in "-mab," which identifies their origin and classification.

Older animal-derived IgA preparations (e.g., antithymocyte globulin [ATG], muromonab-CD3) are themselves antigenic. They usually elicit human antibodies against the animal cells within 2 weeks; hence, their use is appropriate only for short periods. Newer mouse-derived **murine antibodies** (e.g., basiliximab) are humanized, have parts of human antibodies added by recombinant DNA technology, and are less likely to elicit an immune response. However, because antibodies are proteins, there is a risk of hypersensitivity reactions with administration of all biologic antibody products.

**Polyclonal antibodies** are mixtures of antibodies (IgA, IgD, IgE, IgG, and IgM) produced by several clones of B lymphocytes.

Polyclonal immune globulin preparations contain a mixture of immunoglobulins. Each lymphocyte clone produces structurally and functionally different antibodies, even though a single antigen induces the humoral immune response.

## Monoclonal Antibodies

Immunoglobulin monoclonal antibodies, known as mAbs, were first developed in 1985. This classification of drugs is used to treat immunologic diseases. They also reverse drug effects and treat cancer. As of 2017, approximately 500 mAbs have been developed. The action of mAbs is to modulate immunity, destroy cells, and neutralize infectious agents. The monoclonal antibodies (mAbs) recruit proteins and immune cells to kill target cells. Some act through sequestration of plasma proteins or drugs, others block the physiologic interaction with the ligand receptors.

Monoclonal antibodies represent several drug classes that mimic the antibodies produced by the body as part of the immune response to invaders. When a monoclonal antibody attaches to a cell, it can make the cancer cell more visible to the immune system, block growth signals, stop new blood vessels from growing, deliver radiation or chemotherapy to cancer cells, or block the inflammatory process and subsequent destructive changes. The use of antibodies and other techniques to circumvent the defenses that tumors use to suppress the immune system is known as **checkpoint therapy**.

The original monoclonal antibody prototype is Ⓟ **muromonab-CD3** (Orthoclone OKT3). It acts against an antigenic receptor called CD3, which is found on the surface membrane of most T cells in blood and body tissues. CD indicates clusters of differentiation or groups of cells with the same surface markers (antigenic receptors). The drug's name derives from its source (murine or mouse cells) and its action (monoclonal antibody against the CD3 antigen). The CD3 molecule is associated with the antigen recognition structure of T cells and is essential for T-cell activation. Muromonab-CD3 binds with its antigen (CD3) and therefore blocks all known functions of T cells containing the CD3 molecule. Because rejection reactions are mainly T-cell–mediated immune responses against antigenic engrafted tissues, the drug's ability to suppress such reactions accounts for its therapeutic effects in treating renal, cardiac, and hepatic transplant rejection.

Basiliximab (Simulect) is a humanized IgG monoclonal antibody that acts as IL-2 receptor antagonist. By binding to IL-2 receptors on the surface of activated lymphocytes, it inhibits lymphocyte proliferation and cytokine production, critical components of the cellular immune response involved in rejection reactions. Uses include prevention of rejection of kidney transplants. Prescribers order the drug to be given in combination with cyclosporine and a corticosteroid. Common adverse effects include constipation, diarrhea, edema, fever, headache, hypertension, infection, nausea, and vomiting.

Alemtuzumab (Campath, Lemtrada) is a humanized monoclonal IgG antibody that binds to CD52, a protein present on the surface of mature T and B cells. Health care providers use Campath to treat B-cell chronic lymphocytic leukemia, and the drug is available in the United States only through a restricted distribution program. Lemtrada is available for the treatment of relapsing forms of multiple sclerosis (MS).

The FDA recommends that, because of its safety profile, Lemtrada be used to treat MS after inadequate response to least two

drugs. After treatment with alemtuzumab, these CD52-bearing T and B lymphocytes are targeted for destruction, which are believed to be the key mediators of the inflammatory process that causes MS. The FDA has issued a **BLACK BOX WARNING** ◆ for alemtuzumab because of numerous risks associated with the development of serious and sometimes fatal autoimmune conditions (Lemtrada), bone marrow suppression (Campath), life-threatening infusion reactions (Campath, Lemtrada), and the development of malignancies, including thyroid cancer, melanoma, and lymphoproliferative disorders (Lemtrada). Prescribers may order antiemetics with alemtuzumab to prevent associated nausea and vomiting. In addition, antihistamines and/or antipyretics may also be warranted. Concurrent antiviral drug prophylaxis is necessary.

Bevacizumab (Avastin) is a humanized monoclonal antibody that is classified as a vascular endothelial growth factor receptor inhibitor. This drug blocks growth signals and may prevent tumors from developing blood supplies, thus keeping them small. In a tumor that has already developed a blood vessel network, bevacizumab could cause the vessels to die and tumors to shrink. This drug is useful for (1) first- or second-line treatment with standard chemotherapy agents to treat certain metastatic or recurrent lung, renal, ovarian, and colorectal cancers and for (2) treatment of glioblastoma multiforme. The FDA has issued a **BLACK BOX WARNING** ◆ for bevacizumab because GI perforation has occurred in patients receiving the drug. It should be permanently discontinued if GI perforation occurs.

Cetuximab (Erbitux) and panitumumab (Vectibix) are epidermal growth factor receptor (EGFR) inhibitors. These drugs are useful as monotherapy or in combination with select standard chemotherapy agents to treat certain recurring metastatic colorectal cancers. They attach to EGFRs on cancer cells that accept a certain growth signal; blocking this signal may slow or stop the cancer from growing. Only certain patients with genetic mutations (wild-type KRAS) benefit from treatment; those with colorectal tumors harboring a KRAS mutation demonstrate little or no positive effect from treatment. According to Mortara et al. (2018), vitamin D supplementation with cetuximab may improve cetuximab antibody-dependent cell-mediated cytotoxicity in patients being treated for colon cancer.

Prior to the administration of cetuximab, the patient should receive an $H_1$ antagonist, such as diphenhydramine, IV 30 to 60 minutes prior to the first dose and subsequently based on assessment for skin rash or hypersensitivity reaction. Panitumumab must be administered with an infusion pump through a low protein-binding 0.2 or 0.22 μm in-line filter. Doses ≤1000 mg are infused over 1 hour. Doses greater than 1000 mg should be infused over 90 minutes. During the infusion, the patient should be assessed for allergic skin reactions and hypersensitivity.

---

### ❗ QSEN Alert: Evidence-Based Practice

Lung cancer is a leading cause of death throughout the world. The research team of Tang, Ramis-Cabrer, Wang, and Barreiro (2019) hypothesized that the biologic mechanisms of immunomodulators will reduce tumor burden in lung cancer. The researchers found that mice with cancer had significant reduction in tumor area and weight when treated with monoclonal antibodies. Immunomodulators elicited a reduction in tumor burden. The tumor proliferation and increased oxidative stress with apoptosis resulted.

Ipilimumab (Yervoy) is a recombinant human IgG immunoglobulin monoclonal antibody that uses immunologic checkpoint blockade (checkpoint therapy) to bind to cytotoxic T-lymphocyte–associated antigen 4, antagonizing the immunosuppressive receptor and thereby enhancing T-cell activation and proliferation. The drug is useful in the treatment of unresectable or metastatic melanoma or as an adjuvant treatment for cutaneous melanoma with regional lymph node involvement. In melanoma, the drug may also indirectly mediate T-cell immune responses against tumors. Ipilimumab was the first treatment to demonstrate enhanced survival from melanoma. The FDA has issued a **BLACK BOX WARNING ◆** for ipilimumab because severe and fatal immune-mediated adverse effects, such as enterocolitis, dermatitis, neuropathy, and endocrinopathy, may occur.

### ! QSEN Alert: Safety

In 2019, Health Canada concluded that there may be a link between the use of nivolumab and ipilimumab, alone or in combination, and the development of hemophagocytic lymphohistiocytosis.

Nivolumab [Opdivo] is an immunoglobulin monoclonal antibody that inhibits cell death of the PD-1 activity to block the ligands PD-L1 and PD-L2 from binding. This action inhibits the immune response. Nivolumab is administered for the treatment of metastatic colorectal, head and neck, and hepatocellular cancer, and Hodgkin lymphoma. It is also administered as adjunctive therapy for melanoma. Adrenal insufficiency may require hormone replacement with corticosteroid therapy.

Omalizumab (Xolair) is a humanized monoclonal antibody that selectively binds to human IgE, reducing sensitivity to inhaled or ingested allergens. IgE is commonly involved in type I hypersensitivity reactions that manifest the most prevalent allergic responses. The drug is used to treat allergic asthma not relieved by inhaled corticosteroids. Chapter 33 contains a further discussion of omalizumab, including dosage, route, and frequency of administration. Because of the risk of anaphylaxis, the FDA has issued a **BLACK BOX WARNING ◆** for omalizumab. Administration should occur only in a health care setting under direct medical supervision by provider who can initiate treatment of life-threatening anaphylaxis.

Rituximab (Rituxan) is a monoclonal antibody directed against the protein CD20 antigen on the surface of B cells. The drug destroys B cells, so it is effective in treating diseases that are distinguished by overactive, dysfunctional, or extremely numerous B cells. This includes autoimmune disorders and cancers of the white blood cells, such as leukemias and lymphomas. When rituximab attaches to this protein on the B cells, it makes the cells more visible to the immune system, which can then attack.

Ibritumomab (Zevalin), which is approved for non-Hodgkin's lymphoma, combines a monoclonal antibody with radioactive particles. The drug attaches to receptors on cancerous blood cells and delivers a low level of radiation over a longer period of time helping to protect most of the surrounding healthy cells.

Trastuzumab (Herceptin) is approved as an adjuvant for the treatment of early-stage breast cancer and gastric metastatic cancer that is human epidermal growth factor receptor 2 (HER2) positive. The drug contains an antibody that attaches to the HER2 receptors on cancer cells. The cancer cells then ingest the antibody, which releases a few molecules of chemotherapy, damaging the cancer cells. Chapter 14 contains a further discussion of trastuzumab. The FDA has issued a **BLACK BOX WARNING ◆** for trastuzumab because its use can result in subclinical and clinical cardiac failure. The risk is increased with anthracycline-containing chemotherapy. Left ventricular function should be assessed with the administration of trastuzumab. The patient should also be assessed within 24 hours of administration for pulmonary toxicity. Monitor the patient for dyspnea and hypotension. The medication should be discontinued with signs and symptoms of anaphylaxis, angioedema, interstitial pneumonitis, or acute respiratory distress syndrome.

### Polyclonal Antibodies

ATG (Atgam, Thymoglobulin) is a nonspecific immune globulin preparation used for immunosuppression. Health care providers use ATG equine (Atgam), which is obtained from horse serum, to treat rejection reactions after kidney transplants and aplastic anemia in patients who are not considered candidates for bone marrow transplantation. They also use ATG rabbit (Thymoglobulin) to treat these rejection reactions. ATG contains antibodies that destroy lymphoid tissues and decrease the number of circulating T cells, thereby suppressing acute cellular and humoral immune responses. In addition to its high concentration of antibodies against T lymphocytes, the preparation contains low concentrations of antibodies against other blood cells.

With Atgam, it is necessary that potential recipients have skin tests before administration to determine if they are allergic to horse serum. Because there is a high risk of anaphylactic reactions in recipients previously sensitized to horse serum, patients with positive skin tests require desensitization before drug therapy is begun. It is essential that emergency equipment for airway and allergy management be immediately available when ATG is administered. The FDA has issued a **BLACK BOX WARNING ◆** for ATG urging that its use be restricted to experienced prescribers.

## Cytokine Inhibitors

Two major cytokines in chronic, inflammatory autoimmune disorders are TNF-alpha and IL-1. Knowledge of the role of these cytokines in autoimmune disease along with advances in monoclonal antibody production has led to the development of biologic agents directed against TNF and IL-1. Several monoclonal cytokine-inhibiting antibodies, which either block receptors for or reduce production of these cytokines, are used therapeutically in disorders such as rheumatoid arthritis, Crohn's disease, and psoriasis to suppress inflammation and promote tissue healing.

### Tumor Necrosis Factor-Alpha–Blocking Agents

The TNF-alpha–blocking agents act more rapidly than cytotoxic immunosuppressants (e.g., methotrexate) for autoimmune disorders and greatly improve the quality of life for patients with rheumatoid arthritis and Crohn's disease. However, their use is also associated with significant risks of serious infections, especially with opportunistic organisms. Tuberculosis characterized by increased extrapulmonary and/or disseminated disease may occur. Other serious infections include pneumococcal infections, necrotizing fasciitis, *Pneumocystis* pneumonia, and systemic fungal infections such as aspergillosis and cryptococcosis.

Ⓟ **Infliximab** (Remicade) is a humanized IgG monoclonal antibody used to treat rheumatoid arthritis and Crohn's disease. The drug inhibits TNF-alpha from binding to its receptors and thus neutralizes its actions. Its ability to neutralize TNF-alpha accounts for its anti-inflammatory effects. Adverse effects of infliximab include formation of autoimmune antibodies and hypersensitivity reactions. Infections reportedly developed in approximately 21% of patients in clinical trials. In addition, dyspnea, hypotension, and urticaria have occurred.

It is important (1) to administer infliximab in settings in which personnel and supplies (e.g., epinephrine, antihistamines, corticosteroids) are available for treatment of hypersensitivity reactions and (2) to discontinue the drug if severe reactions occur. The drug may aggravate heart failure.

Adalimumab (Humira) is a recombinant monoclonal antibody that binds to TNF-alpha receptor sites and prevents endogenous TNF-alpha from binding to the sites and exerting its injurious effects. Used to treat moderate to severe rheumatoid arthritis, the drug reduces the elevated levels of TNF-alpha in synovial fluid that are thought responsible for pain and joint destruction. Common adverse effects include injection site reactions, upper respiratory tract infections, headache, nausea, and skin rash.

Certolizumab (Cimzia), a TNF-alpha monoclonal antibody, has recently received approval for treating refractory Crohn's disease. As with the other TNF-alpha blockers, risk of infection and allergic reactions are the major adverse effects of this drug. In addition, caution is advised when using certolizumab in patients with heart failure. Other common adverse effects include upper respiratory or bladder infection, rash, GI upset, headache, and injection site reactions.

Etanercept (Enbrel) is a synthetic TNF receptor that binds with TNF and prevents it from binding with its "normal" receptors on cell surfaces. This action inhibits TNF activity in inflammatory and immune responses. The drug is indicated for the treatment of moderate to severe rheumatoid arthritis in adults and children. In this condition, the TNF increases in joint synovial fluid are considered important in joint inflammation and destruction. Etanercept may be effective in combination with methotrexate in patients who do not respond adequately to methotrexate alone. Common adverse effects include headache, injection site reactions, and infections.

Limited information is available about the use of many of the newer immunosuppressants in children. The FDA has approved three TNF-alpha blockers—etanercept, infliximab, and adalimumab—for use in children 4 to 17 years of age who have severe juvenile rheumatoid arthritis that has not responded to conventional therapy.

### Interleukin-Blocking Agents

Ⓟ **Anakinra** (Kineret) is a recombinant IL-receptor antagonist. The drug binds to the IL-1 receptor and thereby blocks the inflammatory effects of IL-1. Indications for use include moderate to severe rheumatoid arthritis in adults. It may be used alone or in combination with cytotoxic immunomodulators but not with TNF-alpha–blocking agents or the fusion protein inhibitor abatacept because of increased risk of infection when these biologic agents are combined. Common adverse effects include headache, injection site reactions (redness, bruising, inflammation, pain), infection, nausea, diarrhea, decreased white blood cells, sinusitis, and flulike symptoms.

Alefacept (Amevive) is a monoclonal antibody used to treat moderate to severe psoriasis. This drug binds to receptors on the surface of T lymphocytes, preventing the receptors from interacting with particular antigens, and thereby inhibiting activation of T lymphocytes. Common adverse effects include lymphopenia and injection site reactions (e.g., edema, inflammation, pain).

Tocilizumab (Actemra), a humanized monoclonal antibody that blocks IL-6 receptors, recently received approval for use in adults and children with severe rheumatoid arthritis that has not responded to conventional immunosuppressants. IL-6, an inflammatory cytokine, is found in higher than normal concentrations in joints of patients with rheumatoid arthritis and contributes to chronic inflammation and joint destruction in the disorder. Tocilizumab may be combined with methotrexate. Common adverse effects include upper respiratory infection, hyperlipidemia, hypertension, leukopenia, and elevated liver enzymes. Screening for tuberculosis prior to treatment and monitoring of lipid levels and liver enzymes every 3 months during therapy is recommended.

Ustekinumab (Stelara) is a monoclonal antibody used to treat psoriasis. It blocks IL-12 and IL-23, reducing the inflammatory response and overactivity of T cells. Common adverse effects include headache, infection, lymphocytosis, and a first-dose reaction characterized by chills, fever, muscle aches, and nausea.

Ixekizumab (Taltz) is another monoclonal antibody used to treat adults with moderate to severe plaque psoriasis who are candidates for systemic therapy or phototherapy. This humanized IgG4 monoclonal antibody selectively binds with the IL-17A cytokine and inhibits its interaction with the IL-17 receptor. Ixekizumab inhibits the release of proinflammatory cytokines and chemokines.

## Fusion Protein Inhibitors

Ⓟ **Abatacept** (Orencia) is a fusion protein inhibitor synthesized from an IgG antibody fused to a cell protein that binds to antigen-presenting molecules. This action prevents the activation of T lymphocytes and the production of inflammatory cytokines. It inhibits activation of T lymphocytes in synovial membranes of joints affected by rheumatoid arthritis and decreases inflammation and structural joint destruction. Abatacept may be used alone or with other antirheumatoid arthritis drugs except anakinra and TNF-alpha–blocking agents. Common adverse effects include dizziness, headache, infections, and nausea. Evidence does not suggest the need for dose adjustment in the presence of liver or renal disease.

Belatacept (Nulojix), a fusion protein inhibitor, is approved for use in the prevention of acute organ rejection after kidney transplantation. The drug binds to a receptor protein on antigen-presenting cells and inhibits the costimulatory signal required for T-cell activation. This prevents T-cell activation and cytokine production, thus reducing the risk of transplant organ rejection. There is an increased risk of lymphoma in people who develop Epstein-Barr virus infection during belatacept therapy. Because of that risk, the FDA has issued a ◼ **BLACK BOX WARNING** ◆ that limits belatacept use to people who test positive for Epstein-Barr virus prior to transplant. Authorities do not recommend the drug for use after liver transplant because of increased risk of graft loss and associated mortality. Adverse effects include anemia, peripheral edema, hypertension, vomiting, diarrhea, constipation, fever, bladder and kidney infection, and leukopenia.

## Clinical Application 13.3

- What are the specific teaching points to be covered with Mr. Jones regarding proper self-administration of his medication (cyclosporine, mycophenolate, and prednisone)?

## NCLEX Success

3. The nurse should instruct the patient taking cyclosporine or tacrolimus that toxic levels of the drug may be reached if taken with which of the following beverages that inhibit metabolism of the drugs?

   A. orange juice
   B. coffee
   C. grapefruit juice
   D. milk

4. A nurse is caring for a patient who is taking immunosuppressant drugs. The most critical information to teach the patient is ways to do which of the following?

   A. to decrease infection
   B. to avoid weight gain
   C. to maintain a good fluid intake
   D. to increase rest and decrease exercise

5. A patient in an outpatient clinic is taking mycophenolate after a kidney transplant. Which of the following over-the-counter products is likely to interfere with the activity of this immunosuppressant?

   A. diphenhydramine, used for itchy mosquito bites
   B. acetaminophen, used for a tension headache
   C. magnesium/aluminum hydroxide, used for heartburn
   D. benzocaine/dextromethorphan throat lozenges, used for throat irritation

6. A woman is taking leflunomide for rheumatoid arthritis, and her provider monitors her laboratory results on a regular basis. Which of the following laboratory findings indicates that the patient is experiencing an adverse effect?

   A. increased red blood cell count
   B. decreased creatinine
   C. increased white blood cell count
   D. decreased liver enzymes

7. Monoclonal antibodies are engineered to specifically target a certain antigen, such as one found on cancer cells. Which of the following actions by monoclonal antibodies have demonstrated effectiveness in cancer therapy? (Select all that apply.)

   A. Make the cancer cell more visible to the immune system.
   B. Block growth signals.
   C. Increase growth of new blood vessels.
   D. Deliver radiation or chemotherapy to cancer cells.

# THE NURSING PROCESS

A concept map outlines the nursing process related to drug therapy considerations in this chapter. Additional nursing implications related to the disease process should also be considered in care decisions.

## Assessment

- Assess for signs and symptoms of current infection or factors predisposing patients to potential infection, environmental factors that predispose to infection, nutritional status, and baseline values of laboratory and other diagnostic test results to aid monitoring of responses to immunosuppressant drug therapy.
- Assess adequacy of support systems for transplant recipients and autoimmune conditions.
- Assess patients after transplant for surgical wound healing, signs of organ rejection, and adverse effects of immunosuppressant drugs.
- Assess patients with autoimmune disorders (e.g., rheumatoid arthritis, Crohn's disease) for manifestations of the disease process and responses to drug therapy.

## Outcomes of Therapy

The patient will

- Receive appropriate care before and after tissue or organ transplantation, including prevention or early recognition and treatment of rejection reactions.
- Verbalize essential information about immunosuppressant drugs and take according to treatment plan.
- Participate in interventions to prevent infection while immunosuppressed.
- Recognize adverse drug effects and seek treatment promptly.
- Keep appointments for follow-up care.
- Maintain diagnostic test values within acceptable limits.
- Demonstrate appropriate coping strategies in self and support systems.

## Nursing Interventions

- Support patient and others to practice and promote good hand hygiene techniques and sterile technique and to avoid contact with infected people.
- Encourage patients to participate in self-care and decision-making when feasible and engage with family members and significant others when feasible.
- Use protective isolation techniques according to institutional policies after transplantation and/or when the neutrophil count is less than 500 per mm$^3$.
- Teach patient to report fever and other signs of infection immediately.
- Assist patient to maintain adequate nutrition, rest, sleep, and exercise patterns.
- Inform patient about diagnostic test results, changes in therapeutic regimen, and evidence of progress.
- Monitor renal function (creatinine, BUN), liver function (serum bilirubin, AST, ALT, alkaline phosphatase, albumin), CBC, and other diagnostic test results related to organ function throughout drug therapy.
- Consult multidisciplinary health care team members on the patient's behalf when indicated.
- Assist patients in learning strategies to manage day-to-day activities during long-term immunosuppression.

## Evaluation

- Interview and observe for accurate drug administration.
- Interview and observe for personal hygiene practices and infection-avoiding maneuvers.
- Interview and observe for therapeutic and adverse drug effects with each patient contact.
- Compare current CBC and other reports with baseline values for acceptable levels, according to the patient's condition.
- Observe and assess outpatients regarding ability to comply and cope with follow-up care.
- Observe and assess outpatients regarding ability to recognize adverse effects that require prompt medical intervention.
- Interview and observe for organ function and absence of rejection reactions in posttransplantation patients.

## KEY CONCEPTS

- Immunosuppressants are used to decrease the immune response in allergic and autoimmune disorders and to avoid graft rejection after transplantation.

- With current treatments, most transplant patients must continue to take immunosuppressive drugs the rest of their lives.

- When caring for patients who are taking immunosuppressant drugs, it is critical for the home care nurse to assess the environment for potential sources of infection, assist patients and other members of the household to understand the patient's susceptibility to infection, and teach ways to decrease risks of infection.

- Mycophenolate mofetil is used for prophylaxis of organ rejection after cardiac, hepatic, and renal transplants, as well as immunosuppression after transplant procedures involving the lung, pancreas, and small intestine.

- The FDA has issued a **BLACK BOX WARNING** ◆ for mycophenolate mofetil regarding the risk of fetal loss and malformations. Women of childbearing age must use contraception.

- The FDA has issued a **BLACK BOX WARNING** ◆ for leflunomide, another cytotoxic immunosuppressant, regarding the risk of fetal loss and malformations. Women of childbearing age must use contraception.

- The FDA has issued a **BLACK BOX WARNING** ◆ for chronic immunosuppression with azathioprine as the drug increases risk of malignancy.

- Cyclosporine and tacrolimus, immunosuppressants widely used in organ transplantation, often cause nephrotoxicity and are subject to numerous drug interactions (enzyme-inhibiting drugs increase blood levels and enzyme-inducing drugs decrease blood levels).

- The FDA has issued a **BLACK BOX WARNING** ◆ for cyclosporine regarding the risk of hypertension and associated nephrotoxicity.

- The FDA has issued a **BLACK BOX WARNING** ◆ that use of sirolimus in lung and liver transplant patients has been associated with increased morbidity and mortality.

- Immunosuppressant drugs greatly increase risks of infection and some kinds of cancer such as lymphoma and skin cancer.

- The FDA has issued a **BLACK BOX WARNING** ◆ limiting all antirejection drugs use to prescribers experienced in transplant therapy, because of the increased risk of infection as well as malignancies such as lymphoma and skin cancer with their long-term use.

- Recognizing pharmacogenomic differences and integration of a new generation of technology has personalized immunologic drug regimens that maximize therapeutic effects and minimize adverse drug effects.

- Immunoglobulins (e.g., ATG, muromonab-CD3) are often used to prevent and suppress an acute rejection reaction after transplant therapy.

- The FDA has issued a **BLACK BOX WARNING** ◆ for ATG, urging that its use be restricted to experienced prescribers.

- Newer monoclonal antibody therapies have more specific effects on specific immune system receptors and may cause fewer or less severe adverse effects than traditional drugs.

- The FDA has issued a **BLACK BOX WARNING** ◆ for trastuzumab because its use can result in subclinical and clinical cardiac failure. The risk is increased with anthracycline-containing chemotherapy.

- Due to the risk of anaphylaxis, the FDA has issued a **BLACK BOX WARNING** ◆ for omalizumab. The drug should only be administered to patients in a health care setting under direct medical supervision by provider who can initiate treatment of life-threatening anaphylaxis should the need arise.

- The FDA has issued a **BLACK BOX WARNING** ◆ that limits belatacept use to people who test positive for Epstein-Barr virus prior to transplant due to the significant risk of lymphoma with an initial Epstein-Barr virus infection during belatacept therapy.

- The FDA has issued a **BLACK BOX WARNING** ◆ because GI perforation has occurred in patients receiving bevacizumab. The drug should be permanently discontinued if GI perforation occurs.

- The FDA has issued a **BLACK BOX WARNING** ◆ for alemtuzumab's numerous associated effects: the development of serious and sometimes fatal autoimmune conditions (Lemtrada), bone marrow suppression (Campath), life-threatening infusion reactions (Campath, Lemtrada), and the development of malignancies, including thyroid cancer, melanoma, and lymphoproliferative disorders (Lemtrada) with its use.

- The FDA has issued a **BLACK BOX WARNING** ◆ for ipilimumab because of possible severe and fatal immune-mediated adverse effects, such as enterocolitis, dermatitis, neuropathy, and endocrinopathy.

## CLINICAL REASONING CASE STUDY

**Meet the Patient**

Angelique Nieves is a 31-year-old elementary school teacher who has been diagnosed with rheumatoid arthritis. She is currently taking methotrexate for this condition but has continued to experience significant joint pain, particularly in her hands. She tells the nurse during her office visit today that her pain and joint stiffness are making it difficult for her to work and to care for her two young children. Her primary care provider has prescribed etanercept (Enbrel) to be given in addition to the methotrexate.

- Ms. Nieves asks the nurse to explain how the etanercept and methotrexate work and asks why she is to continue taking the methotrexate when it has not helped. How should the nurse respond?
- What nursing assessments and interventions should the nurse implement to reduce Ms. Nieves' risk of infection?
- What additional precautions should the nurse take to minimize adverse effects from Ms. Nieves' medications?

**Assessing Drug Information**

- Methotrexate inhibits the production and function of immune cells, thus diminishing the body's attack on its own tissues.
- Etanercept inhibits tumor necrosis factor (TNF), a cytokine, a substance that is produced by the immune system. In rheumatoid arthritis, TNF is increased in the synovial fluid in the joints, and experts believe that it plays an important role in inflammation and destruction of joints.
- Common adverse effects of etanercept include headache, injection site reaction, and infection.
- Common adverse effects of methotrexate include nausea, vomiting, diarrhea, gastric ulcers, and gastrointestinal bleeding. Risk of infection are significant; specific risks include tuberculosis, pneumococcal infections, necrotizing fasciitis, Pneumocystis pneumonia, and systemic fungal infections.
- Prescribers may add etanercept to methotrexate in patients with rheumatoid arthritis who do not respond to methotrexate alone.

**Nursing Actions**

- Recognize that prior to beginning etanercept, the nurse should:
  - Administer a tuberculin test and the pneumococcal vaccine.
  - Administer the meningococcal vaccine, if ordered.
  - Educate about importance of taking trimethoprim–sulfamethoxazole (TMP–SMZ) to prevent infection, if ordered.
  - Instruct on importance of notifying provider and beginning prescriptions for antibiotics immediately if fever or symptoms of upper respiratory infection occur.
- Educate about the importance of avoiding contact with people who are ill and maintaining conscientious handwashing and personal hygiene.
- Encourage a healthy lifestyle, including adequate rest, diet, and exercise, to strengthen Ms. Nieves' resistance to infection.
- Encourage outdoor sunscreen to protect from the increased sensitivity to sunlight from methotrexate.
- Monitor regular complete blood count values to detect anemia, neutropenia, and thrombocytopenia, and periodic monitoring of liver function tests.
- Reinforce the importance of contraceptive measures during and for at least one ovulatory cycle after stopping methotrexate because of the risk of fetal abnormalities with pregnancy.
- Provide additional teaching related to drug therapy and risk factor modification (see Box 13.2).

---

*Visit* thePoint® *at* **http://thePoint.lww.com/Frandsen12e** *for answers to NCLEX Success questions (in Appendix A), answers to Clinical Application Case Studies (in Appendix B), and more!*

## REFERENCES AND RESOURCES

Chao, N. J. (2019a). Overview of immunosuppressive agents used for prevention and treatment of graft-versus-host disease. *UpToDate.* Wolters Kluwer.

Chao, N. J. (2019b). Prevention of acute graft-versus-host disease. *UpToDate.* Wolters Kluwer.

Hinkle, J. L., & Cheever, K. H. (2018). *Brunner and Suddarth's textbook of medical-surgical nursing* (14th ed.). Philadelphia, PA: Wolters Kluwer.

Manis, J. P. (2019). Overview of therapeutic monoclonal antibodies. *UpToDate.* Wolters Kluwer.

Mortara, L., Bariboldi, M. B., Bosi, A., Pinotti, G., Guasti, L., Squizzato, A., et al. (2018). Vitamin D deficiency has a negative impact on cetuximab-medicated cellular cytotoxicity against human colon carcinoma cells. *Targeted Oncology, 13,* 657–665. doi:10.1007/s11523-018-0586-x

Sussman, N. L. & Vierling, J. M. (2019). Liver transplantation in adults: Overview of immunosuppression. *UpToDate.* Wolters Kluwer.

Tang, J., Ramis-Cabrer, D., Wang, X., & Barreiro, E. (2019). Immunotherapy with monoclonal antibodies in lung cancer of mice: oxidative stress and other biological events. *Cancers, 11,* 1–16. doi:10.3390/cancers11091301

UpToDate. (2019). *Drug Information.* Lexi-Comp, Inc.

# 14

# Drug Therapy for the Treatment of Cancer

## LEARNING OBJECTIVES

*After studying this chapter, you should be able to:*

1. Describe the etiology of cancer development.
2. Describe the major types of antineoplastic drugs in terms of mechanism of action, indications for use, and the nursing process.
3. Discuss adverse effects of cytotoxic antineoplastic drugs and their prevention or management.
4. Apply patient education regarding the administration of some anticancer drugs.
5. Understand how to implement assessment and nursing interventions in the care of patients undergoing drug therapy for cancer, including how to teach and promote efforts to prevent cancer.

## CLINICAL APPLICATION CASE STUDY

Annette D'Angelo is a 64-year-old retired schoolteacher. Six months ago, she had her annual gynecologic visit and received a clean bill of health. Recently, she noticed abdominal bloating and felt extremely full after meals. She went to the emergency department with nausea and vomiting, and the physician diagnosed a bowel obstruction. In surgery, Ms. D'Angelo had a total hysterectomy and salpingo-oophorectomy with bowel resection. It turns out that she has stage III epithelial carcinoma of the ovary and fallopian tube, and she will require chemotherapy and radiation therapy.

## KEY TERMS

**Alopecia:** hair loss

**Cell cycle:** series of intracellular events occurring from one cell division to the next

**Chemotherapy:** in oncology, the treatment of cancer with an antineoplastic drug or with a combination of such drugs typically given in cycles

**Mucositis:** inflammation of mucous membranes

**Mutation:** structural change in the genetic material of a cell

**Myelosuppression:** bone marrow depression

**Neutropenia:** low neutrophil count

**Oncogenes:** genes that have the potential to cause a normal cell to become cancerous

**Palliation:** alleviation of pain and symptoms without expecting to eliminate the cause

**Protooncogenes:** genes that have the potential to change into active oncogenes

**Remission:** period when symptoms of a disease have subsided ["remitted"]

**Thrombocytopenia:** low platelet count

**Tumor lysis syndrome:** life-threatening condition that occurs when large numbers of cancer cells are killed or damaged simultaneously and release their intracellular contents into the bloodstream

**Tumor suppressor genes (also called antioncogenes):** genes that inhibit unrestrained cell growth; when inactivated, mutant abnormal cells may be allowed to proliferate

## INTRODUCTION

The term *cancer* is used to describe many disease processes with the common characteristics of uncontrolled cell growth, invasiveness, and metastasis as a result of intracellular genetic changes that allow new cells to grow in an unregulated manner. Oncology is the study of cancer and its treatment. Drugs used in oncologic disorders include cytotoxic medications that kill, damage, or slow the growth of cancer cells as well as those that prevent or treat adverse drug effects. **Chemotherapy** is a major treatment modality for cancer, along with surgery and radiation therapy. Chu and DeVita (2019) have stated that chemotherapy for the treatment of cancer is used in four main clinical settings:

1. Primary induction treatment for advanced disease, which involves administration to patients who have cancer with no other effective approach to treatment.
2. Neoadjuvant treatment for localized disease, which involves the use of surgery and radiation as well as chemotherapy. Neoadjuvant chemotherapy is the administration of systemic therapy before surgery. The goal of this therapy is to reduce the morbidity and mortality and ultimately increase the chances for complete resection of the cancer.
3. Adjuvant treatment, which involves surgery and/or radiation.
4. Direct instillation of chemotherapy in the affected region of the body.

Major groups of anticancer drugs include traditional cytotoxic agents (e.g., alkylating agents, antimetabolites, antitumor antibiotics, plant alkaloids), newer cytotoxic "biologic targeted therapies" (e.g., monoclonal antibodies, growth factor inhibitors), and hormone inhibitors, which are not cytotoxic. In addition, several drugs play a role in ameliorating the adverse effects of cytotoxic drugs (e.g., cytoprotectants), including some immunostimulants.

This chapter describes the characteristics of cancer etiology, pathophysiology, clinical manifestations, and the drugs used in the treatment of this disease. A nurse who has additional training in chemotherapy use administers these drugs. The focus of this chapter is on the nursing management of patients receiving the medication and not on dosing and administration of individual drugs. The general considerations for chemotherapy management are outlined for each major drug group.

## OVERVIEW OF CANCER

### Etiology

Normal cells reproduce in response to a need for tissue growth or repair and stop reproduction in response to growth regulation signals. The normal **cell cycle** is the interval between the "birth" of a cell and its subsequent division into two daughter cells. This cycle involves the orderly stages of growth as well as protein, deoxyribonucleic acid (DNA), and ribonucleic acid (RNA) synthesis (Fig. 14.1). Newly formed daughter cells may then enter the resting phase ($G_0$) or proceed through the reproductive cycle to form more new cells. Normal cells regulated by normal growth genes are well differentiated in appearance and function, and they have a characteristic life span.

In contrast, malignant cells have lost the normal genetic regulation that controls cell growth, invading normal tissues and taking blood and nutrients away from these tissues. In hyperplasia, these cells grow in an uncontrolled fashion without regard to growth regulation signals (e.g., contact with other cells) that stop the growth of normal cells. In dysplasia, a buildup of extra

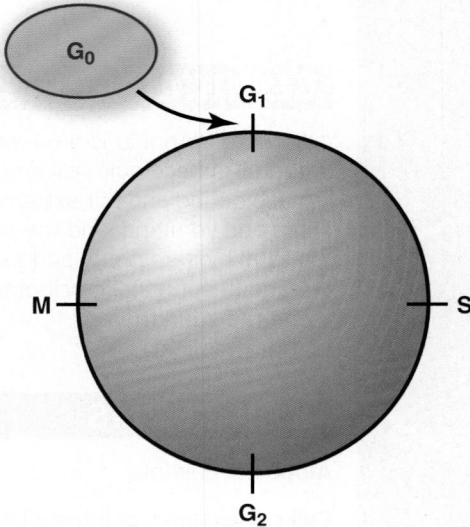

**Figure 14.1.** Normal cell cycle. The normal cell cycle (the interval between the birth of a cell and its division into two daughter cells) involves several phases. During the resting phase ($G_0$), cells perform all usual functions except replication–that is, they are not dividing but are capable of doing so when stimulated. Different types of cells spend different lengths of time in this phase, after which they either reenter the cell cycle and differentiate or die. During the first active phase ($G_1$), ribonucleic acid (RNA) and enzymes required for production of deoxyribonucleic acid (DNA) are developed. During the next phase (S), DNA is synthesized for chromosomes. During $G_2$, RNA is synthesized, and the mitotic spindle is formed. Mitosis occurs in the final phase (M). The resulting two daughter cells may then enter the resting phase ($G_0$) or proceed through the reproductive cycle.

cells changes how the tissue is organized. Also, malignant cells are undifferentiated, having lost the structural and functional characteristics of the cells from which they originated. In addition, they lack cell adhesion; hence, as well as invading normal tissue, malignant cells enter blood and lymph vessels, circulate through the body, and can produce additional neoplasms at sites distant from the primary tumor.

A malignant cell develops from a damaged normal cell, beginning with a random **mutation** (abnormal structural change in the genetic material of a cell) that occurs in conjunction with acquired damage to genes that regulate normal cell growth. Usually, body defenses (e.g., an immune response) destroy a mutated cell if the DNA damage cannot be repaired by normal cell enzymes. However, if the mutated cell eludes destruction by the immune system and additional mutations develop without repair or apoptosis (programmed cell death) during succeeding cell divisions, malignant transformation may occur. Underlying the failure to repair or destroy these abnormal cells is damage to genes that regulate cell growth; the cells have lost their ability to effectively regulate cell growth. Additional changes allow cells with progressively more malignant characteristics to survive despite their abnormalities. It often takes years for malignant cells to be able to grow into a clinically detectable neoplasm.

Cancer is a heterogeneous disease and has multiple causes, such as environmental factors (tobacco) and genetic factors that may combine to contribute to the progression of malignancy. Tumor cells develop in epithelial, connective, lymph, or nerve tissue. Genetic causes of cancer include mutation of genes, abnormal activation of genes that regulate cell growth and mitosis, and damage to **tumor suppressor genes**.

## Pathophysiology

Abnormal genes, called **oncogenes**, which are involved in cancer growth, are mutations of normal growth-regulating genes, called **protooncogenes**, which are present in all body cells. When protooncogenes are exposed to carcinogens and genetically altered to become oncogenes, they may stimulate cell growth continuously, allowing abnormal, disordered, and unregulated cell replication (Fig. 14.2). The unregulated cell growth and proliferation promoted by oncogenes contribute to neoplastic transformation of the cell. Tumors of the breast, colon, lung, and bone have all been linked to activation of oncogenes.

Tumor suppressor genes (antioncogenes) normally function to inhibit inappropriate cellular growth and proliferation. Abnormal tumor suppressor genes (i.e., absent, damaged, mutated, or inactivated) may be inherited or result from exposure to carcinogens. When a tumor suppressor gene inside a cell is inactivated, abnormal cells can begin unregulated cell growth. One tumor suppressor gene, p53, is present in virtually all normal tissues. When cellular DNA is damaged, the p53 gene allows time for DNA repair and restricts proliferation of cells with abnormal DNA. Mutations of the p53 gene, a common genetic change in cancer, are associated with more than 90% of small cell lung cancers and more than 50% of breast and colon cancers. Mutant p53 proteins can also form complexes with normal p53 proteins and inactivate the function of the normal suppressor gene.

Thus, activation of oncogenes and inactivation of antioncogenes probably both play roles in cancer development. Multiple genetic abnormalities are characteristic of cancer cells

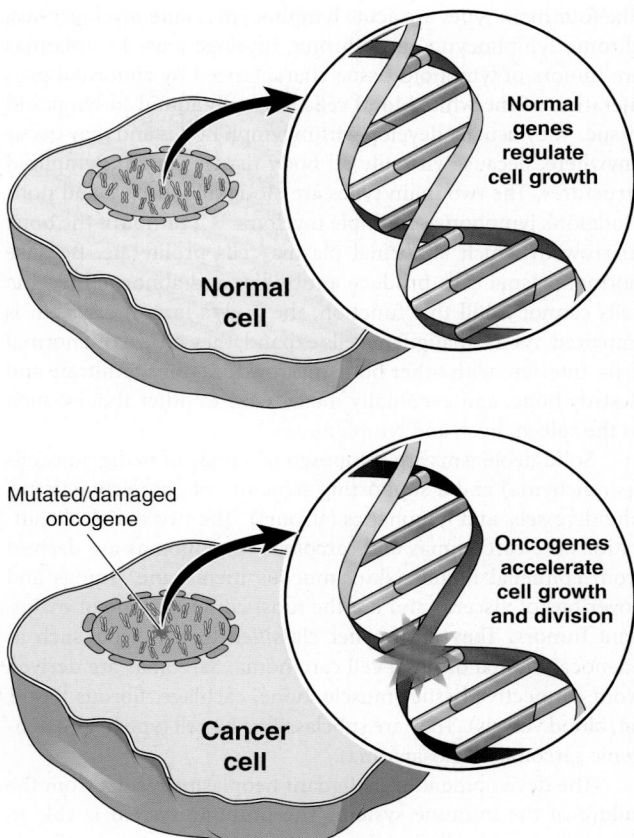

**Figure 14.2.** A mutated oncogene is a cancer cell. It is irregularly shaped and possesses a break in the DNA, leading to the loss of differentiation and rapid cell growth.

and may occur concurrently or sequentially. Overall, evidence indicates that neoplastic transformation is a progressive process involving both a series of cellular mutations and damage to growth-regulating genes, which allows abnormal cells to replicate without normal immune destruction. Malignancy probably results from a combination of genetic and environmental factors experienced over a person's lifetime, including random cell mutations, exposure to carcinogens, and host genetic or tissue characteristics that increase susceptibility to cancer development.

Once a cancer develops, factors influencing its continued growth include blood and nutrient supply, immune response, and hormonal stimulation (e.g., in tumors of the breast, uterus, ovary, and prostate). Malignant tumors are able to form new blood vessels, a process called angiogenesis, to support their growth and escape immune destruction as a result of their similarity to other normal cells.

### Types of Malignant Neoplasms

Malignant neoplasms are classified according to the type of tissue involved and other characteristics. With the exception of the acute leukemias, they are considered chronic diseases.

Hematologic malignancies involve the bone marrow and lymphoid tissues; they include leukemias, lymphomas, and multiple myeloma. Leukemias are cancers of the bone marrow characterized by overproduction of abnormal white blood cells.

The four main types are acute lymphocytic, acute myelogenous, chronic lymphocytic, and chronic myelogenous. Lymphomas are tumors of lymphoid tissue characterized by abnormal proliferation of the white blood cells normally found in lymphoid tissue. They usually develop within lymph nodes and may occur anywhere, because virtually all body tissues contain lymphoid structures. The two main types are Hodgkin's disease and non-Hodgkin's lymphoma. Multiple myeloma is a tumor of the bone marrow in which abnormal plasma cells proliferate. Because normal plasma cells produce antibodies and abnormal plasma cells cannot fulfill this function, the body's immune system is impaired. As the malignant cells expand, they crowd out normal cells, interfere with other bone marrow functions, infiltrate and destroy bone, and eventually metastasize to other tissues, such as the spleen, liver, and lymph nodes.

Solid neoplasms are composed of a mass of malignant cells (parenchyma) and a supporting structure of connective tissue, blood vessels, and lymphatics (stroma). The two major classifications are carcinomas and sarcomas. Carcinomas are derived from epithelial tissues (skin, mucous membrane, linings and coverings of viscera) and are the most common type of malignant tumors. They are further classified by cell type, such as adenocarcinoma or basal cell carcinoma. Sarcomas are derived from connective tissue (muscle, bone, cartilage, fibrous tissue, fat, blood vessels). They are subclassified by cell type (e.g., osteogenic sarcoma, angiosarcoma).

The development of malignant neoplasms results from the failure of the immune system. The immune system is able to detect abnormal cells and destroy them. In the event a patient is immunocompromised, the risk of malignant neoplasm growth increases (Hinkle & Cheever, 2018).

### Grading and Staging of Malignant Neoplasms

When a malignant neoplasm is identified, it is further "graded" according to the degree of malignancy and "staged" according to tissue involvement. Grades 1 and 2 are similar to the normal tissue of origin and show cellular differentiation. Grades 3 and 4 are unlike the normal tissue of origin, less differentiated, and more malignant. Staging indicates whether the neoplasm is localized or metastasized and which organs are involved. These characteristics assist in treatment decision making. For example, localized tumors are usually amenable to surgery, radiation, or chemotherapy combined with radiation (concurrent) therapy, whereas metastatic disease requires systemic chemotherapy.

## Clinical Manifestations

Clinical manifestations vary according to the location and extent of the disease process. There are few effects initially. However, local effects occur as the tumor grows; it becomes large enough to cause pressure, distort or affect blood supply in surrounding tissues, interfere with organ function, or obstruct ducts and organ outlets. Systemic conditions such as cachexia, anorexia, and weight loss result from the effects of the growing tumor's increasing overall metabolic demands and altering glucose utilization at the cellular level. Other symptoms and signs may include anemia, malnutrition, pain, immunosuppression, infection, hemorrhagic tendencies, thromboembolism, and hypercalcemia, as well as various symptoms related to impaired function of affected organs and tissues.

## Drug Therapy

Chemotherapy is most often used to indicate the use of traditional cytotoxic antineoplastic drugs for the treatment of cancer. Except for hormone inhibitors that slow the growth of cancer cells stimulated by hormones, the purpose of all antineoplastic drugs is to damage or kill cancer cells (i.e., be cytotoxic). The goal of treatment with cytotoxic antineoplastic drugs is cure, **remission** (period when symptoms of a disease have subsided), or **palliation** (alleviation of pain and symptoms without expecting to eliminate the cause). In hematologic malignancies such as leukemias, drug therapy is the treatment of choice because the disease is disseminated and must be treated systemically rather than locally, with surgery or radiation. In solid tumors, drug therapy may be used, before (neoadjuvant) or after (adjuvant) surgery or radiation therapy and when there is metastasis that is not surgically resectable.

Antineoplastic drugs are also sometimes used in the treatment of nonmalignant conditions. For example, smaller doses of methotrexate are used as an immunosuppressant for treating the inflammation of rheumatoid arthritis and psoriasis.

Traditional chemotherapeutic drugs share common general characteristics (Box 14.1). Most chemotherapy regimens contain a combination of drugs with actions at different places in the cell cycle process of cell growth and replication (Fig. 14.3), destroying a greater number of cancer cells and reducing the risk of the emergence of drug resistance. Drug resistance may emerge when (1) cancer cells overexpress target genes that prevent the drugs being absorbed by the malignant cells, (2) tumor cells are able to inactivate the drug, or (3) apoptosis that occurs in tumor cells is defective. Oncologists order many newer drugs for use after initial cytotoxic drug therapy to prevent drug resistance from affecting the tumor response.

When administering chemotherapy agents, the prescriber will calculate the dosages utilizing the body surface area method. Chemotherapy administration usually occurs in cycles, depending on the type of cancer and which drugs are used. Cyclic administration involves taking the drugs for a specific period, with a recovery period following each treatment cycle. The recovery period allows time for the patient to produce new, healthy cells to replace the normal rapidly dividing cells that have been affected by the drugs. Chemotherapy is often continued as long as it is effective and does not produce unacceptable toxicity or until there is no longer any evidence of malignancy. Table 14.1 outlines the drugs used in cancer treatment.

## CYTOTOXIC ANTINEOPLASTIC DRUGS USED TO TREAT CANCER

The consequences of inappropriate or erroneous chemotherapy may be fatal for patients (from the disease or from the treatment); thus, medical oncologists experienced in use of cancer drugs manage chemotherapy regimens.

> ### ! QSEN Alert: Safety
>
> Because of the toxicity of these drugs, nurses who administer intravenous (IV) cytotoxic chemotherapy receive special training and are certified in handling and administering the chemotherapy drugs safely and accurately.

| BOX 14.1 | *Characteristics of Cytotoxic Antineoplastic Drugs* |
|---|---|

- Most of these drugs kill malignant cells by interfering with cell replication, with the supply and use of nutrients (e.g., amino acids, purines, pyrimidines), or with the genetic materials in the cell nucleus (DNA or RNA).
- The drugs act during the cell's reproductive cycle. Some, called cell cycle specific, act mainly during specific phases such as DNA synthesis or formation of the mitotic spindle. Others act during any phase of the cell cycle and are called cell cycle nonspecific.
- The drugs are most active against rapidly dividing cells, both normal and malignant. Commonly damaged normal cells are those of the bone marrow, the lining of the gastrointestinal tract, and the hair follicles. Healthy cells usually recover fairly soon. However, malignant cells have lost normal genetic growth regulation and continue to actively divide in an unregulated way; thus, more of them are susceptible to the effects of cytotoxic drugs.
- Each drug dose kills a specific percentage of cells. To achieve a cure, all malignant cells must be killed or reduced to a small number that can be killed by the person's immune system.
- Most cytotoxic antineoplastic drugs are potential teratogens, and women should not become pregnant during

drug therapy and for several months after the therapy stops.
- Weight-based dosing is used to individualize dosing with all cytotoxic drugs due to their potential to cause significant toxicities to normal cells as well as cancer cells.
- Oncologists combine various cytotoxic drugs with different cell cycle activities and different organ toxicities in treatment plans called "regimens" to more effectively kill the cancer cells while minimizing damage to normal tissues.
- Most cytotoxic drugs are water soluble rather than lipid soluble; thus, they do not cross cell membranes readily and must be administered by intravenous injection or infusion.
- Many of the cytotoxic drugs are prodrugs that are metabolized by liver enzymes to active metabolites, which then have cytotoxic activity affecting protein, DNA, or RNA synthesis or cell division.
- Because cytotoxic drugs are primarily metabolized in the liver and then excreted in urine, they can also have toxic effects on the liver and kidney, especially at higher doses.
- Many cytotoxic antineoplastic drugs have U.S. Food and Drug Administration (FDA)-issued **BLACK BOX WARNING ◆** about potentially serious adverse effects, and all have special precautions for safe usage.

This chapter focuses on the overall nursing considerations for caring for patients receiving chemotherapy, not the administration of particular drugs. Therefore, information is not presented in a prototype format.

## Pharmacokinetics

Most cytotoxic drugs are water soluble rather than lipid soluble and require administration by IV injection or infusion. Some, such as cyclophosphamide, are better absorbed and are available as oral formulations. A few, such as methotrexate, are also given intrathecally. The nitrosoureas (e.g., carmustine, lomustine) are unique in being lipid soluble and able to cross the blood–brain barrier; hence, they are widely used in the treatment of brain tumors. Carmustine is also formulated as a dissolving wafer, which can be implanted in the brain tissue at the time of surgical tumor resection.

Liposomal preparations of some cytotoxic drugs (e.g., doxorubicin) use a lipid membrane to encase the drug molecules.

Liposomal preparations can increase drug concentration in malignant tissues that are more permeable, allowing the lipid vesicle to more easily concentrate in the tumor, while lowering the concentration in normal tissues that are less permeable, thereby increasing effectiveness and decreasing toxicity (e.g., cardiotoxicity).

## Action

Cytotoxic antineoplastic drugs are usually classified in terms of their mechanisms of action (alkylating agents, antimetabolites) or their sources (plant alkaloids, antibiotics).

### Alkylating Drugs

Alkylating drugs include nitrogen mustard derivatives, nitrosoureas, platinum compounds, and triazenes. Before these drugs are administered, it is important to assess liver function.

- Nitrogen mustard derivatives are cell cycle–nonspecific agents, causing cross-linking of DNA and RNA and interfering with subsequent cell division. These agents exert biologic activity by covalently binding to macromolecules of DNA, RNA, and proteins. This activity interrupts the cell's DNA ability to replicate and transcribe leading to cell death or impairing cell function (Clowse & McCune, 2019). The most widely used alkylating drug, a nitrogen mustard derivative, is ⓟ **cyclophosphamide** (Cytoxan). This prodrug begins to act when it is converted metabolically. Cyclophosphamide prevents cell division through the cross-linking of DNA strands, resulting in decreased DNA synthesis.
- Nitrosoureas are highly lipid-soluble agents that interfere with DNA replication and RNA synthesis, and they may inhibit essential enzymatic reactions in cancer cells. Carmustine and lomustine are both cell cycle nonspecific. These features allow them to enter the brain and cerebrospinal fluid more readily

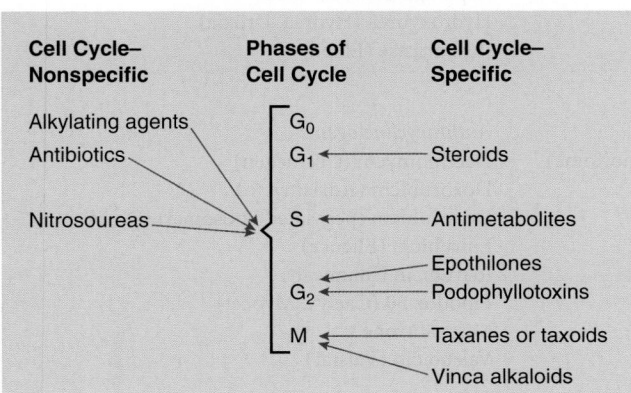

**Figure 14.3.** Cell cycle effects of cytotoxic antineoplastic drugs.

**TABLE 14.1**

## Drugs Administered for the Treatment of Cancer

| Drug Class | Prototype(s) | Other Drugs in the Class |
|---|---|---|
| **Alkylating Drugs** | | |
| | Cyclophosphamide (Cytoxan) (nitrogen mustard derivative) | *Nitrogen mustard derivatives*<br>Altretamine (Hexalen)<br>Bendamustine (Bendeka, Treanda)<br>Busulfan (Busulfex, Myleran)<br>Chlorambucil (Leukeran)<br>Estramustine (Emcyt)<br>Ifosfamide (Ifex)<br>Mechlorethamine hydrochloride (Valchlor)<br>Melphalan (Evomela, Alkeran)<br>*Nitrosoureas*<br>Carmustine (BiCNU, Gliadel)<br>Lomustine (Gleostine)<br>Procarbazine (Matulane)<br>Streptozocin (Zanosar)<br>Thiotepa (Tepadina)<br>*Platinum compounds*<br>Carboplatin<br>Cisplatin<br>Oxaliplatin (Eloxatin)<br>*Triazene*<br>Dacarbazine |
| **Antimetabolites** | | |
| | *Antifolate*<br>Methotrexate (Otrexup, Rasuvo)<br>*Purine antagonist*<br>Mercaptopurine (Purinethol, Purixan)<br>*Pyrimidine*<br>Fluorouracil (5-FU; Adrucil) | *Antifolate*<br>Pemetrexed (Alimta)<br>Pralatrexate (Folotyn)<br>*Purine antagonist*<br>Cladribine (Mavenclad)<br>Clofarabine (Clolar)<br>Cytarabine (Cytosar)<br>Thioguanine (Tabloid)<br>*Pyrimidine*<br>Azacitidine (Vidaza)<br>Capecitabine (Xeloda)<br>Decitabine (Dacogen)<br>Floxuridine<br>Gemcitabine (Gemzar)<br>Nelarabine (Arranon)<br>*Miscellaneous*<br>Asparaginase (Erwinaze)<br>Hydroxyurea (Hydrea, Droxia)<br>Rasburicase (Elitek) |
| **Antitumor Antibiotics** | | |
| | Daunorubicin (Cerubidine)<br>Daunorubicin (liposomal) (DaunoXome) (anthracycline agents) | *Anthracycline agents*<br>Dactinomycin (Cosmegen)<br>Doxorubicin (Adriamycin)<br>Doxorubicin (pegylated liposomal) (Doxil)<br>Epirubicin (Ellence)<br>Idarubicin (Idamycin)<br>Lipodox 50 (Caelyx, Myocet)<br>Mitoxantrone<br>Valrubicin (Valstar) |
| | Bleomycin (Blenoxane)/D (polypeptide antibiotic) | *Polypeptide antibiotics*<br>Mitomycin (Mitosol)<br>Pentostatin (Nipent) |

**TABLE 14.1**

## Drugs Administered for the Treatment of Cancer (Continued)

| Drug Class | Prototype(s) | Other Drugs in the Class |
|---|---|---|
| **Plant Alkaloids** | | |
| | Vincristine sulfate (Vincasar PFS) | *Camptothecins*<br>Irinotecan (Camptosar)<br>Topotecan (Hycamtin)<br>*Podophyllotoxins*<br>Etoposide (Toposar)<br>(VePesid)<br>Teniposide (Vumon)<br>*Taxanes*<br>Cabazitaxel (Jevtana)<br>Docetaxel (Docefrez, Taxotere)<br>Paclitaxel (nanoparticle albumin bound) (Abraxane)<br>Paclitaxel (conventional) (Apo-Paclitaxel)<br>*Vinca alkaloids*<br>Vincristine (liposomal) (Marqibo)<br>Vinblastine<br>Vinorelbine (Navelbine) |
| **Antimicrotubules** | | |
| Epothilone B analogs | | Eribulin mesylate (Halaven)<br>Ixabepilone (Ixempra kit) |
| **Biologic Antineoplastic Drugs** | | |
| Monoclonal antibodies | Alemtuzumab (Campath, Lemtrada) | Bevacizumab (Avastin)<br>Blinatumomab (Blincyto)<br>Cetuximab (Erbitux)<br>Dinutuximab (Unituxin)<br>Ibritumomab tiuxetan (Zevalin, Tiuxetan)<br>Ipilimumab (Yervoy)<br>Nivolumab (Opdivo)<br>Obinutuzumab (Gazyva)<br>Ofatumumab (Arzerra)<br>Panitumumab (Vectibix)<br>Pertuzumab (Perjeta)<br>Rituximab (Rituxan)<br>Tositumomab (Bexxar)<br>Trastuzumab (Herceptin) |
| Growth factor and tyrosine kinase inhibitors | Erlotinib (Tarceva) | Afatinib (Gilotrif)<br>Axitinib (Inlyta)<br>Bosutinib (Bosulif)<br>Cabozantinib (Cabometyx, Cometriq)<br>Ceritinib (Zykadia)<br>Dabrafenib (Tafinlar)<br>Dasatinib (Sprycel)<br>Everolimus (Afinitor Disperz, Zortress)<br>Ibrutinib (Imbruvica)<br>Imatinib (Gleevec)<br>Lapatinib (Tykerb)<br>Lenvatinib (Lenvima)<br>Nilotinib (Tasigna)<br>Palbociclib (Ibrance)<br>Pazopanib (Votrient)<br>Ponatinib (Iclusig)<br>Regorafenib (Stivarga)<br>Sorafenib (NexAVAR)<br>Sunitinib (Sutent)<br>Temsirolimus (Torisel)<br>Trametinib (Mekinist) |

*(Continued on page 256)*

**TABLE 14.1**

**Drugs Administered for the Treatment of Cancer** (Continued)

| Drug Class | Prototype(s) | Other Drugs in the Class |
| --- | --- | --- |
| Proteasome inhibitor | Bortezomib (Velcade) | Carfilzomib (Kyprolis) Ixazomib (Ninlaro) |
| **Antineoplastic Hormone Inhibitors** | | |
| | *Antiestrogens* Tamoxifen (Soltamox) *Aromatase inhibitors* Anastrozole (Arimidex) *Antiandrogens* Flutamide (Eulexin) | Fulvestrant (Faslodex) Toremifene (Fareston) Exemestane (Aromasin) Letrozole (Femara) Abiraterone (Zytiga) Bicalutamide (Casodex) Enzalutamide (Xtandi) Nilutamide (Nilandron) |
| | *Gonadotropin-releasing hormone agonists* Leuprolide acetate (Eligard, Lupron Depot) | Goserelin (Zoladex) Triptorelin (Trelstar, Trelstar Mixject) |
| **Cytoprotectant Drugs** (see Chap. 11) | | Amifostine (Ethyol) Dexrazoxane (Zinecard) Epoetin alfa (Epogen, Procrit, Retacrit) Filgrastim (Neupogen, Zarxio) Leucovorin Mesna (Mesnex) Oprelvekin (Neumega) Palifermin (Kepivance) Sargramostim (Leukine) |

than other antineoplastic drugs, which make them useful for treating lymphomas and brain tumors.

- Platinum compounds are cell cycle–nonspecific agents that are effective throughout the life cycle of the cell. **Ⓟ Carboplatin** is the prototype of the platinum compound chemotherapy agents. They cross-link with DNA, inhibiting DNA, RNA, and protein synthesis. Cisplatin is the most widely used of the platinum compounds.
- Triazene compounds are cell cycle–nonspecific agents with antitumor and mutagenic properties. They interfere with DNA replication, RNA transcription, and protein synthesis. The drugs are effective for metastatic malignant melanoma, Hodgkin's disease, and various sarcomas. The most widely used drug in the class is **Ⓟ dacarbazine**.

## Antimetabolites

Antimetabolites are drugs that are similar to metabolites or nutrients needed by cells for reproduction. Folate antagonists, purine antagonists, pyrimidine analogs, and miscellaneous antimetabolites are commonly prescribed individually or in combination with other chemotherapy agents.

- Folate antagonists such as **Ⓟ methotrexate** (Otrexup, Rasuvo) interfere with DNA synthesis, repair, and cellular replication, thus inhibiting the formation of folates.
- Purine antagonists such as **Ⓟ mercaptopurine** (Purinethol, Purixan) inhibit DNA and RNA synthesis. This action occurs in the S phase of the cell cycle.
- Pyrimidine analogs such as **Ⓟ fluorouracil** also affect DNA and RNA synthesis. The incorporation of fluorouracil into the tumor cell RNA, replacing uracil, means that cell growth is then affected.

Miscellaneous antimetabolites include asparaginase, hydroxyurea, and rasburicase. Asparaginase reduces the asparagine source that provides the destructive action of leukemia cells, thus inhibiting cell function. Hydroxyurea stops the cell cycle at the $G_1$/S phase and reduces $G_1$ phase to stop DNA repair. Rasburicase converts uric acid to allantoin: uric acid is increased in some malignancies.

These drugs are all most effective against rapidly growing tumors. Individual drugs vary in their effectiveness with different kinds of cancer.

## Antitumor Antibiotics

Two types of antitumor antibiotics are noted as anthracycline agents and polypeptide agents. **Ⓟ Daunorubicin** binds to DNA so that DNA and RNA transcription is blocked. They are active in all phases of the cell cycle, and their cytotoxic effects are similar to those of the alkylating agents. **Ⓟ Bleomycin** inhibits DNA, RNA, and protein synthesis in susceptible cells, preventing cell division. Mitomycin (Mitosol) causes DNA cross-linking and inhibits DNA synthesis.

## Plant Alkaloids

Plant alkaloids include several types of drugs.

- Camptothecins (also called DNA topoisomerase inhibitors) inhibit an enzyme required for DNA replication and repair.
- Podophyllotoxins, etoposide, and teniposide act by delaying the transit of cells from the S phase and can arrest cells in the late S phase or early $G_2$ phase of the cell cycle and prevent mitosis. These medications are topoisomerase II inhibitors, which cause DNA strand breakage.
- Taxanes are antimicrotubular agents that promote microtubule assembly and inhibit the weakening of microtubules.

They inhibit depolymerization of microtubules, stopping the cell cycle and the tumor cell proliferation.

- Vinca alkaloids are also antimicrotubular agents, with ⓟ **vincristine sulfate** as the prototype. Liposomal vincristine (Marqibo), vinblastine, and vinorelbine (Navelbine) are the other drugs in the class. They are cell cycle–specific agents that interfere with cell mitosis. Despite having similar structures, they have different antineoplastic activities and adverse effects.

> ⓘ **QSEN Alert: Safety**
>
> Vincristine is only administered intravenously and the syringe should be labeled clearly "IV use only."
>
> - Prepacked syringes should be labeled "Do not remove covering until it is to be administered."
> - Vincristine is contraindicated in patients with demyelinating Charcot-Marie-Tooth syndrome.
> - There is a risk of dyspnea if vincristine is administered with mitomycin C.
> - Gastrointestinal (GI) toxicity and necrosis can occur if vincristine is administered with mitomycin C.

## Use

Researchers have found that certain combinations of cytotoxic drugs with different cytotoxic activities in the cell cycle and different organ toxicities are most effective in certain types of cancer. Hence, concurrent administration of multiple drugs based on the patient's type of malignancy may be necessary. However, when both cytotoxic and hormone inhibitor drug therapies are required, concurrent administration is not appropriate, because hormone antagonists decrease malignant cell growth and cytotoxic agents are most effective when the cells are actively dividing. Patients with breast cancer usually receive a hormone-inhibiting drug before a cytotoxic drug in metastatic disease and after chemotherapy when used for adjuvant treatment.

It is important to use weight-based dosing to individualize dosing of all cytotoxic drugs to minimize toxicity of normal cells. In addition, some cytotoxic drugs have a cumulative maximum dose that can be given for cancer treatment without risk of irreversible vital organ damage (e.g., heart failure with doxorubicin, pulmonary fibrosis with carmustine and bleomycin). Table 14.2 provides route and dosage information for some cytotoxic antineoplastic drugs.

### TABLE 14.2

### DRUGS AT A GLANCE: Cytotoxic Antineoplastic Drugs

| Drug/Pregnancy Category | Routes and Dosage Ranges* | Clinical Uses | Adverse Effects |
|---|---|---|---|
| **Alkylating Drugs** | | | |
| *Nitrogen Mustard Derivatives* | | | |
| ⓟ **Cyclophosphamide** (Cytoxan; ✿ Procytox)/D | Induction therapy, PO 1–5 mg/kg/d; IV 40–50 mg/kg in divided doses over 2–5 d or 10–15 mg/kg every 7–10 d or 3–5 mg/kg twice weekly Maintenance therapy, PO 1–5 mg/kg daily | Hodgkin's disease; non-Hodgkin's lymphomas; leukemias; cancer of head and neck, breast, lung, or ovary; multiple myeloma; neuroblastoma | Bone marrow depression, nausea, vomiting, alopecia, hemorrhagic cystitis, hypersensitivity reactions, secondary leukemia, or bladder cancer |
| Altretamine (Hexalen) | PO 260 mg/m²/d for 14 or 21 consecutive days in a 28-d cycle (administer total daily dose in 4 divided doses, due to high emetic potential) Temporarily hold for 14 d or longer and resume dose at 200 mg/m²/d if platelet count is <75,000/mm³ or WBC < 2000/mm³ | Cancer of the ovary | Bone marrow suppression: leukopenia and thrombocytopenia **BLACK BOX WARNING ◆** — Neurotoxicity: ataxia, vertigo, mood disorder, and disorders of consciousness |
| Bendamustine (Belrapzo, Bendeka, Treanda; ✿ Treanda)/D | IV 100 mg/m² on days 1 and 2 of a 21-d treatment cycle up to 8 cycles | Chronic lymphocytic leukemia, Hodgkin's lymphoma, and multiple myeloma | Peripheral edema, fatigue, skin rash, weight loss, and lymphocytopenia |
| Busulfan (Busulfex, Myleran; ✿ Busulfex, Myleran)/D | 60 mg/kg or 1.8 mg/m²/d; usual range 4–8 mg/d; titrate dose to maintain WBC ≥ 15,000/mm³ | Chronic lymphocytic leukemia | Edema, tachycardia, hypertension, thrombosis, hepatic venoocclusive disease, nausea, vomiting, stomatitis, hypomagnesemia, hyperglycemia, hypocalcemia, hypophosphatemia, neutropenia, and thrombocytopenia |

*(Continued on page 258)*

**TABLE 14.2**

**DRUGS AT A GLANCE: Cytotoxic Antineoplastic Drugs** (Continued)

| Drug/Pregnancy Category | Routes and Dosage Ranges* | Clinical Uses | Adverse Effects |
|---|---|---|---|
| Chlorambucil (Leukeran; ❦ Leukeran)/D | US labeling: PO 1 mg/kg/d for 3–6 wk or 0.4 mg/kg pulsed doses administered intermittently, biweekly, or monthly (increased by 0.1 mg/kg/dose until response or toxicity is seen) Canadian labeling: 0.15 mg/kg/d until WBC is 10,000/mm³, interrupt treatment for 4 wk, then may resume at 0.1 mg/kg/dose until response or toxicity is seen | Chronic lymphocytic leukemia, Hodgkin's and non-Hodgkin's lymphomas | Bone marrow depression, hepatotoxicity, and secondary leukemia |
| Estramustine (Emcyt; ❦ Emcyt)/D | PO 140 mg (1 h before or 2 h after meals). Do not administer with milk | | Edema, nausea, vomiting, leukopenia, thrombocytopenia, and increased bilirubin |
| Ifosfamide (Ifex; ❦ Ifex)/D | IV 1.2 g/m²/d for 5 consecutive days. Repeat every 3 wk or after white blood cell and platelet counts return to normal after a dose | Germ cell testicular cancer | Bone marrow depression, hemorrhagic cystitis, nausea and vomiting, alopecia, CNS depression, and seizures |
| Mechlorethamine hydrochloride (Valchlor)/D | MOPP regimen: 6 mg/m² on days 1 and 8 of a 28-d treatment cycle for 6–8 cycles Stanford V regimen: 6 mg/m² as a single dose on day 1 in weeks 1, 5, and 9 Malignant effusion: 0.4 mg/kg as a single dose | Hodgkin's lymphoma Malignant effusion | Drowsiness, encephalopathy with high doses, alopecia, agranulocytosis, granulocytopenia, hemolytic anemia, secondary leukemia, and thrombocytopenia |
| Melphalan (Alkeran, Evomela; ❦ Alkeran)/D | PO 6 mg/d for 2–3 wk, then 28 drug-free days, then 2 mg daily IV 16 mg/m² every 2 wk for 4 doses and then every 4 wk | Multiple myeloma and ovarian cancer | Bone marrow depression, nausea and vomiting, and hypersensitivity reactions |
| **Nitrosoureas** | | | |
| Ⓟ **Carmustine** (BiCNU, Gliadel; ❦ BiCNU)/D | IV 150–200 mg/m² every 6 wk Wafer, implanted in brain after tumor resection | Hodgkin's disease, non-Hodgkin's lymphomas, multiple myeloma, and brain tumors | Bone marrow depression, nausea, and vomiting |
| Lomustine (Gleostine; ❦ CeeNU)/D | PO 130 mg/m² every 6 wk | Hodgkin's disease and brain tumors | Nausea and vomiting and bone marrow depression |
| Procarbazine (Matulane; ❦ Matulane)/D | PO 100 mg/m² days 1–7 every 21 d | Hodgkin's lymphoma | Edema, flushing, alopecia, diaphoresis, hepatic insufficiency, jaundice, hypersensitivity, herpes virus, hearing loss, polyuria, and arthralgia |
| Streptozocin (Zanosar; ❦ Zanosar)/D | Daily schedule: 500 mg/m² for 6 d every 6 wk Weekly schedule: 1000 mg/m² once weekly; if therapeutic response not achieved after 2 wk may increase dose to 1500 mg/m² weekly | Pancreatic islet carcinoma metastasis | Glucose intolerance, bone marrow suppression, extravasation of tissue, and increased lactate dehydrogenase |
| Thiotepa (Tepadina; ❦ Tepadina)/D | Bladder cancer: intravesical: 60 mg in 30–60 mL NS retained for 2 h once weekly for 4 wk Intercavity: 0.6–0.8 mg/kg Ovarian and breast cancer: IV 0.3–0.4 mg/kg every 1–4 wk | Bladder cancer Breast cancer Ovarian cancer | Dizziness, fatigue, alopecia, contact dermatitis, anemia, bleeding, leukopenia, thrombocytopenia, dysuria, urinary retention, and asthma |

### TABLE 14.2

## DRUGS AT A GLANCE: Cytotoxic Antineoplastic Drugs (Continued)

| Drug/Pregnancy Category | Routes and Dosage Ranges* | Clinical Uses | Adverse Effects |
|---|---|---|---|
| **Platinum Compounds** | | | |
| Ⓟ **Carboplatin**/D | IV infusion 360 mg/m² on day 1 every 4 wk | Palliation of ovarian cancer and endometrial cancer | Bone marrow depression, nausea and vomiting, and nephrotoxicity |
| Cisplatin/D | IV 100 mg/m² once every 4 wk | Advanced carcinomas of testes, bladder, and ovary | Nausea, vomiting, anaphylaxis, nephrotoxicity, bone marrow depression, ototoxicity, and peripheral neuropathy |
| Oxaliplatin (Eloxatin)/D | IV infusion 85 mg/m² every 2 wk | Advanced colon cancer (with 5-fluorouracil and leucovorin) | Anaphylaxis, anemia, increased risk of bleeding or infection, and cold-induced acute neurotoxicities |
| **Triazene** | | | |
| Ⓟ **Dacarbazine**/D | Hodgkin's lymphoma: 375 mg/m² on days 1 and 15 every 4 wk  Metastatic malignant melanoma: 250 mg/m² over 30 min once daily on days 1–5 every 3 wk | Hodgkin's lymphoma  Metastatic malignant melanoma | Infusion site pain  Alopecia  Nausea and vomiting  Severe myelosuppression |
| **Antimetabolites** | | | |
| *Miscellaneous* | | | |
| Asparaginase (Erwinaze)/D | IM or IV 25,000 units/m² three times/wk (Mon., Wed., and Fri.) for 6 doses | Acute lymphocytic leukemia | Hypersensitivity reactions, including anaphylaxis |
| Hydroxyurea (Hydrea, Droxia, Siklos; ✳ Apo-Hydroxyurea, Mylan-Hydroxyurea, Hydrea)/D | PO 15 mg/kg/d as a single dose; if blood counts are acceptable, may increase by 5 mg/kg/d  Droxia (sickle cell anemia): 15 mg/kg/d as a single dose orally: monitor blood counts every 2 wk  Canadian labeling: PO 20–30 mg/kg daily  Solid tumors: 80 mg/kg as a single dose every 3rd day | Chronic myelogenous leukemia (CML), melanoma, ovarian cancer, and head and neck cancer  Sickle cell anemia | Bone marrow depression, nausea, vomiting, and peripheral neuritis |
| Rasburicase (Elitek; ✳ Fasturtec)/D | 0.2 mg/kg/d for up to 5 d | Secondary tumor lysis | Peripheral edema, headache, rash, hypophosphatemia, nausea, and vomiting |
| *Antifolates* | | | |
| Ⓟ **Methotrexate** (Otrexup, Rasuvo, Rheumatrex, Trexall, Xatmep; ✳ JAMP-Methotrexate, Metoject, PMS-Methotrexate, RATIO-Methotrexate sodium)/D | Intrathecal: 15 mg/d one of early intensification phase. Repeat in 4 wk  CNS prophylaxis: 15 mg/d on days 1, 8, 15, 22, and 29  PO 20 mg/m² on days 36, 43, 50, 57, and 64  Choriocarcinoma: PO, IM 15 mg/m² daily for 5 d | Leukemias; non-Hodgkin's lymphomas; osteosarcoma; choriocarcinoma of testes; cancers of breast, lung, head, and neck | Bone marrow depression, nausea, vomiting, mucositis, diarrhea, fever, and alopecia |
| Pemetrexed (Alimta; ✳ Alimta, Taro-Pemetrexed)/D | IV 500 mg/m² on day 1 of each 21-d cycle (in combination with cisplatin) | Malignant pleural mesothelioma; non–small cell lung cancer | Fatigue, rash, nausea, anorexia, anemia, stomatitis, and pharyngitis |
| *Purines* | | | |
| Ⓟ **Mercaptopurine** (Purixan; ✳ Purinethol)/D | PO 1.5–2.5 mg/kg/d (100–200 mg for average adult) | Acute and chronic leukemias | Bone marrow depression, nausea, vomiting, and mucositis |

*(Continued on page 260)*

**TABLE 14.2**

**DRUGS AT A GLANCE: Cytotoxic Antineoplastic Drugs** (Continued)

| Drug/Pregnancy Category | Routes and Dosage Ranges* | Clinical Uses | Adverse Effects |
|---|---|---|---|
| Cladribine (Mavenclad; 🍁 Mavenclad)/D | IV infusion 0.09 mg/kg/d for 7 consecutive days | Hairy cell leukemia | Bone marrow depression, nausea, and vomiting |
| Clofarabine (Clolar; 🍁 Clolar)/D | 52 mg/m²/d for 5 d every 2–6 wk CrCl 30–60 reduce dose by 50% | Acute lymphocytic leukemia | Tachycardia, nausea, vomiting, thrombocytopenia, anemia, leukopenia, neutropenia, and somnolence |
| Cytarabine (Cytosar; 🍁 Cytosar)/D | IV 100 mg/m²/d continuous infusion for 7 d or 200 mg/m²/d continuous infusion (as 100 mg/m² over 12 h every 12 h) for 7 d | Acute myeloid leukemia | Bone marrow depression, nausea, vomiting, anaphylaxis, mucositis, and diarrhea |
| Thioguanine (🍁 Lanvis)/D | PO 2 mg/kg/d. May increase to 3 mg/kg/d if no response after 4 wk | Acute myelogenous (non-lymphocytic) leukemia | Hyperuricemia, fluid retention, splenomegaly, stomatitis, anemia, ascites, and esophageal varices |

*Pyrimidines*

| Drug/Pregnancy Category | Routes and Dosage Ranges* | Clinical Uses | Adverse Effects |
|---|---|---|---|
| Ⓟ **Fluorouracil** (5-FU) (Adrucil)/D | IV: dosage is depended on cancer staging and cancer type. Topical: apply to skin cancer lesion two times per day for 2–6 wk | Carcinomas of the breast, colon, stomach, and pancreas; solar keratoses and basal cell carcinoma | Bone marrow depression, nausea, vomiting, and mucositis; pain, pruritus, and burning at site of application |
| Azacitidine (Vidaza; 🍁 NAT-Azacitidine, REDDY-Azacitidine, Vidaza)/D | Sub-Q, initial cycle: 75 mg/m²/d for 7 d and then every 4 wk; dose can be increased to 100 mg/m²/d. Treatment for a minimum of 6 cycles | Acute myeloid leukemia Myeloid dysplastic syndrome | Chest pain, peripheral edema, nausea, vomiting, and bone marrow depression |
| Capecitabine (Xeloda; 🍁 ACH-Capecitabine, SANDOZ Capecitabine, TARO-Capecitabine, TELVA-Capecitabine, Xeloda)/D | PO 1250 mg/m² twice daily for 2 wk, every 21 d (can be given in combination with docetaxel) | Breast, colon, esophageal, gastric, pancreas, and ovarian cancer | Diarrhea, edema, vomiting, and hyperbilirubinemia |
| Decitabine (Dacogen)/D | 15 mg/m² over 3 h every 8 h for 3 d (134 mg/m²/cycle) every 6 wk for at least 4 cycles | Acute myeloid leukemia Myeloid dysplastic syndrome | Chest pain, peripheral edema, nausea, vomiting, bone marrow depression, diarrhea, and hyperbilirubinemia |
| Floxuridine | 0.5 g administered as a continuous hepatic intra-arterial infusion with an infusion pump | Colorectal cancer Hepatic metastasis | Diarrhea, stomatitis, bone marrow depression, cholecystitis, jaundice |
| Gemcitabine (Gemzar, Infugem; 🍁 ACT Gemcitabine)/fetal harm if administered during pregnancy | IV 1250 mg/m² on days 1 and 8 of 21 day cycle; given with paclitaxel | Breast cancer Ovarian cancer | Fever, flulike symptoms, headache, cough, myelosuppression, alopecia |
| Nelarabine (Arranon; 🍁 Atriance)/fetal harm if administered during pregnancy | IV 1500 mg/m² on days 1, 3, and 5 repeated every 21 d | T-cell leukemia Lymphoma | Dizziness, headache, paresthesia, somnolence, constipation, thrombocytopenia |

**Antitumor Antibiotics**

| Drug/Pregnancy Category | Routes and Dosage Ranges* | Clinical Uses | Adverse Effects |
|---|---|---|---|
| Ⓟ **Bleomycin**/D | IV, IM, sub-Q 0.25–0.5 units/kg once or twice weekly | Squamous cell carcinoma, Hodgkin's and non-Hodgkin's lymphomas, and testicular carcinoma | Pulmonary toxicity, mucositis, alopecia, nausea, vomiting, hypersensitivity reactions, and hypotension |

**TABLE 14.2**

## DRUGS AT A GLANCE: Cytotoxic Antineoplastic Drugs (Continued)

| Drug/Pregnancy Category | Routes and Dosage Ranges* | Clinical Uses | Adverse Effects |
|---|---|---|---|
| Ⓟ **Daunorubicin** (Cerubidine; 🍁 Cerubidine)/D | IV <60 y 45 mg/m² daily for 3 d ≥60 y 30 mg/m² daily for 3 d After course in each age group, then administer days 1 and 2 in combination with cytarabine | Acute leukemias and lymphomas | Cardiac failure, alopecia, red urine discoloration, bone marrow depression, and hyperuricemia |
| Daunorubicin liposomal (DaunoXome)/D | IV infusion 40 mg/m² every 2 wk | AIDS-related Kaposi's sarcoma | Bone marrow depression, nausea, and vomiting |
| Dactinomycin (Cosmegen; 🍁 Cosmegen)/D | IV 15 mcg/kg/d for 5 d and repeated every 2–4 wk | Rhabdomyosarcoma, Wilms' tumor, choriocarcinoma, testicular carcinoma, and Ewing's sarcoma | Bone marrow depression, nausea, and vomiting. Extravasation may lead to tissue necrosis |
| Doxorubicin conventional (Doxorubicin; 🍁 Doxorubicin PFS)/D | Adults, IV 60–75 mg/m² every 21 d Children, IV 30 mg/m² daily for 3 d, repeated every 4 wk | Acute leukemias; lymphomas; carcinomas of breast, lung, and ovary | Bone marrow depression, alopecia, mucositis, gastrointestinal (GI) upset, and cardiomyopathy. Extravasation may lead to tissue necrosis |
| Doxorubicin (pegylated liposomal) (Doxil, Lipodox; 🍁 Caelyx)/D | IV infusion 20 mg/m², once every 3 wk | AIDS-related Kaposi's sarcoma and multiple myeloma | Bone marrow depression, nausea, vomiting, fever, and alopecia |
| Epirubicin (Ellence; 🍁 PMS-Epirubicin)/D | IV infusion 100–120 mg/m² every 3–4 wk | Breast cancer | Cardiotoxicity, decreased left ventricular ejection fraction, atrioventricular block, and bradycardia |
| Idarubicin (Idamycin PFS)/D | IV injection 12 mg/m²/d for 3 d, with cytarabine | Acute myeloid leukemia | Congestive heart failure, headache, alopecia, nausea, vomiting, dark yellow urine, seizure, and peripheral neuropathy |
| Mitomycin (Mutamycin)/D | IV 20 mg/m² every 6–8 wk | Metastatic carcinomas of stomach and pancreas | Bone marrow depression, nausea, and vomiting. Extravasation may lead to tissue necrosis |
| Mitoxantrone/D | IV infusion 12 mg/m² on days 1–3, for induction of remission in leukemia | Acute nonlymphocytic leukemia and prostate cancer | Bone marrow depression, heart failure, and nausea |
| Pentostatin (Nipent; Nipent)/D | IV 4 mg/m² every other week | Hairy cell leukemia unresponsive to interferon alfa | Bone marrow depression, hepatotoxicity, nausea, and vomiting |
| Valrubicin (Valtaxin)/D | Intravesically 800 mg once weekly for 6 wk | Bladder cancer | Dysuria, urgency, frequency, bladder spasms, and hematuria |
| **Plant Alkaloids** | | | |
| *Camptothecins* | | | |
| Irinotecan (🍁 Camptosar)/D | IV infusion 125 mg/m² over 90 min on days 1, 8, 15, and 22 of a 6-wk treatment cycle (may adjust upward to 150 mg/m²) | Metastatic cancer of colon or rectum | Bone marrow depression and diarrhea |
| Topotecan (Hycamtin; 🍁 Hycamtin, ACT Topotecan, PMS-Topotecan)/D | IV infusion 1.5 mg/m² daily for 5 consecutive days every 21 d | Advanced ovarian cancer and small cell lung cancer | Bone marrow depression, nausea, vomiting, and diarrhea |

*(Continued on page 262)*

**TABLE 14.2**

# DRUGS AT A GLANCE: Cytotoxic Antineoplastic Drugs (Continued)

| Drug/Pregnancy Category | Routes and Dosage Ranges* | Clinical Uses | Adverse Effects |
|---|---|---|---|
| *Podophyllotoxins* | | | |
| Etoposide (Toposar; ✹ VePesid, GEN-Etoposide)/D | IV 50–100 mg/m²/d for 5 d PO 100–200 mg/m²/d for 5 d. Administer daily doses >200 mg in 2 divided doses | Small cell lung cancer and testicular cancer Non-Hodgkin's lymphoma, non–small cell lung cancer, small cell lung cancer, and testicular cancer | Bone marrow depression, allergic reactions, nausea, vomiting, and alopecia |
| Teniposide (✹ Vumon)/D | IV infusion 165 mg/m² twice weekly for 8–9 doses Down syndrome patients with leukemia: administer first course dose at one half the recommendation | Acute lymphocytic leukemia in children | Bone marrow depression, allergic reactions, nausea, vomiting, and alopecia |
| *Antimicrotubule/Taxane Derivatives* | | | |
| Cabazitaxel (Jevtana; ✹ Jevtana)/D | Premedicate with IV diphenhydramine 25 mg, dexamethasone 8 mg, and ranitidine 50 mg 30 min before cabazitaxel IV 25 mg/m² once every 3 wk (in combination with prednisone) | Prostate cancer | Fatigue, diarrhea, bone marrow depression, alopecia, mucosal inflammation, febrile neutropenia, and increased AST, ALT, and bilirubin |
| Docetaxel (✹ Taxotere)/D | IV infusion 60–100 mg/m² every 3 wk | Advanced breast cancer and non–small cell lung cancer | Bone marrow depression, nausea, vomiting, hypersensitivity reactions, and peripheral neuropathy |
| Paclitaxel (nanoparticle albumin bound) (Abraxane)/D | Breast cancer: IV 260 mg/m² every 3 wk Non–small cell lung cancer: IV 100 mg/m² on days 1, 8, and 15 of each 21-d cycle (in combination with carboplatin) Pancreatic adenocarcinoma: IV 125 mg/m² on days 1, 8, and 15 of a 28-d cycle (in combination with gemcitabine) | Metastatic breast cancer, locally and advanced or metastatic non–small cell lung cancer, and metastatic pancreatic adenocarcinoma | ECG abnormality, peripheral edema, peripheral neuropathy, alopecia, nausea, vomiting, bone marrow depression, oral candidiasis, keratitis, and increased serum creatinine |
| Paclitaxel (conventional) (✹ Apo-Paclitaxel)/D | Premedicate with PO dexamethasone 20 mg at 12 and 6 h prior to the dose, IV diphenhydramine 50 mg 30–60 min prior to dose, and IV famotidine Breast cancer: 175 mg/m² over 3 h every 3 wk for 4 cycles (administer sequentially following an anthracycline-containing regimen) Non–small cell lung cancer: IV 135 mg/m² over 24 h every 3 wk with cisplatin Ovarian: 135 or 175 mg/m² 3 h every 3 wk (if previously untreated, combine with cisplatin) | Breast cancer, non–small cell lung cancer, and ovarian cancer | ECG abnormality, peripheral edema, peripheral neuropathy, alopecia, nausea, vomiting, bone marrow depression, and increased serum creatinine |
| *Antimicrotubule/Vinca Alkaloid* | | | |
| Ⓟ **Vincristine sulfate** (Vincasar PFS) | Adults: IV 1.4 mg/m² weekly Children: IV 2 mg/m² weekly | Hodgkin's and other lymphomas, acute leukemia, neuroblastoma, and Wilms' tumor | Peripheral neuropathy. Extravasation may lead to tissue necrosis |
| Vincristine (liposomal) (Marqibo) | IV 2.25 mg/m² once every 7 d | Philadelphia chromosome–negative acute lymphoblastic leukemia | Fever, fatigue, nausea, diarrhea, anorexia, bone marrow depression, cardiac arrest, mental status changes, and weakness |

**TABLE 14.2**

**DRUGS AT A GLANCE: Cytotoxic Antineoplastic Drugs** (Continued)

| Drug/Pregnancy Category | Routes and Dosage Ranges* | Clinical Uses | Adverse Effects |
|---|---|---|---|
| Vinblastine | Adults: IV 3.7–11.1 mg/m² (average 5.5–7.4 mg/m²) weekly<br>Children: IV 2.5–7.5 mg/m² weekly | Metastatic testicular carcinoma, Hodgkin's disease, and choriocarcinoma | Bone marrow depression, nausea, and vomiting. Extravasation may lead to tissue necrosis |
| Vinorelbine (Navelbine) | IV injection 30 mg/m² once weekly | Non–small cell lung cancer | Bone marrow depression and peripheral neuropathy. Extravasation may lead to tissue necrosis |
| *Antimicrotubule: Epothilone B Analog* | | | |
| Eribulin mesylate (Halaven; ✿ Halaven)/ fetal harm if administered during pregnancy | IV ¼ mg/m² on days 1 and 8 of a 21-d treatment cycle | Breast cancer and liposarcoma | Fatigue, weight loss, constipation, nausea, vomiting, weakness, dyspnea, fever, cough, and increased ALT |
| Ixabepilone (Ixempra kit)/adverse pregnancy events in animal studies; use contraception in women of childbearing age | IV infusion 40 mg/m² over 3 h, every 3 wk | Advanced breast cancer | Bone marrow suppression, peripheral neuropathy, nausea, vomiting, diarrhea, mucositis, and hypersensitivity |

*Dosages may vary significantly or change often, according to use in different types of cancer and in different combinations.
AIDS, acquired immunodeficiency syndrome; ALT, alanine aminotransferase; AST, aspartate aminotransferase; CNS, central nervous system; ECG, electrocardiogram; WBC, white blood (cell) count.

## Use in Children

Children are at risk for certain types of malignancies, including acute leukemias, lymphomas, brain tumors, Wilms' tumor, and sarcomas of muscle and bone. In recent years, there have been rapid advances in cancer care for children and high cure rates for many pediatric malignancies. Many of the advances have resulted from the systematic enrollment of children in well-designed clinical trials.

Pediatric oncologists should design, order, and supervise chemotherapy for children. To determine dosage of cytotoxic drugs, prescribers should use body surface area, because this takes overall size into account. Special efforts are necessary to maintain nutrition, organ function, psychological support, growth and development, and other aspects of health status during and after therapy. Most chemotherapy agents cause significant nausea and vomiting. In 1997, a chemotherapy drug–related table was developed, ranking agents in terms of intensity of emetic adverse effects for adults. In 2016, the Multinational Association of Supportive Care in Cancer updated these emetic risk groups. In addition, guidelines for prevention of nausea and vomiting in children receiving high emetic chemotherapy can be accessed at http://www.mascc.org/antiemetic-guidelines.

Children who are receiving chemotherapy associated with a high risk of vomiting or retching should receive emetic prophylaxis with 5-hydroxytryptamine receptor antagonists (5-HT₃RAs) (granisetron, ondansetron, tropisetron, or palonosetron), dexamethasone, and aprepitant. It should be noted that dexamethasone is contraindicated in some pediatric protocols such as those for leukemia or brain tumors because of the possible interference with apoptosis, fungal infections, or the distribution of chemotherapy across the blood–brain barrier (Roila et al., 2016).

Both nurses and physicians need to be aware of the emetic level of the agents administered. The administration of two or more drugs with moderate to high emetic response will require stronger antiemetic therapy. The 5-HT₃RAs have proven effective in the prevention and treatment of chemotherapy-induced nausea and vomiting (CINV), particularly in the acute phase or first 24 hours after chemotherapy has been administered. Aprepitant, a neurokinin-1 receptor antagonist, is more effective in the delayed phase (after 24 hours) (Di Lorenzo, 2019).

Alternative and complementary therapy for the treatment of CINV may help. This includes ginger or other herbal supplements for functional dyspepsia or other motility disorders. Hypnotherapy may be beneficial for children who experience anticipatory nausea and vomiting prior to the administration of chemotherapy.

Long-term follow-up care is important for childhood cancer survivors because they have an increased risk of health problems. For example, children who receive an anthracycline drug (e.g., doxorubicin) are at increased risk for cardiotoxic effects (e.g., heart failure) during treatment or after receiving the drug. Efforts to reduce cardiotoxicity include using alternative drugs (if effective), giving smaller cumulative doses of the anthracycline and observing patients closely so that early manifestations can be recognized and treated before heart problems occur. In addition, after successful cytotoxic chemotherapy, children are at increased risk for developing cancers in later life (e.g., leukemia) (LaCasce & Ng, 2019). In addition, long-term survivors of Hodgkin's lymphoma may develop an impairment in the growth of soft tissues or bones, thyroid dysfunction, gonadal dysfunction, cardiopulmonary toxicity, second malignancies, or the impairment of overall health (McClain & Kamdar, 2019).

## Use in Older Adults

Increasing age is a risk factor for development of cancer, and the number of new cancer cases is about 10 times greater in people 65 years of age and older. Although elderly people are more likely to have chronic cardiovascular, renal, and other disorders (comorbidities) that increase their risks of serious adverse effects, age alone should not be the reason for denying them the potential benefits of traditional cytotoxic chemotherapy. However, it is important to consider several factors when treating older adults for cancer. Physiologic age-related changes that may add to the challenge of managing cancer include decreased renal function, reduced hepatic blood flow, and diminished cardiac reserve. For example, older adults are more sensitive to the neurotoxic effects of vincristine and need reduced dosages of some drugs (e.g., cyclophosphamide, methotrexate) if they have impaired renal function. Therefore, it is necessary to monitor creatinine clearance (CrCl), because serum creatinine is not a reliable indicator of renal function in older adults due to decreased muscle mass. Also, it is important to assess for signs and symptoms of toxicity of chemotherapy agents with regard to diminished metabolism and elimination of drugs. In the event a patient suffers from liver metastasis, drug metabolism will be greatly affected. Most antineoplastic drugs are metabolized by the liver; thus, decreased liver blood flow and decreased liver size can lead to accumulation of drug due to decreased clearance, resulting in increased toxicity in the elderly adult.

In addition, psychosocial issues that may affect treatment include access to care, financial and transportation issues, functional status, need for independence, and social support.

## Use in Patients With Renal Impairment

Some antineoplastic drugs are nephrotoxic (e.g., cisplatin, methotrexate), and the kidneys play a large role in their excretion. The presence of impaired renal function increases the risk of further impairment or accumulation of toxic drug levels. Thus, it is necessary to monitor renal function carefully during therapy and reduce drug dosages according to CrCl levels. The following paragraphs describe the renal effects of selected cytotoxic chemotherapy drugs and precautions to reduce nephrotoxicity.

The alkylating drugs may be nephrotoxic. These effects usually subside when the drug is stopped. For example, cisplatin, an alkylating agent, has multiple active metabolites that are renally excreted, causing renal tubular damage. When a patient already has significant renal dysfunction, oncologists avoid using this drug.

The antimetabolites may also be nephrotoxic. Methotrexate use in patients with impaired renal function may lead to accumulation of toxic amounts or additional renal damage. Evaluation of the patient's renal status should take place before and during methotrexate therapy. If significant renal impairment occurs, it is necessary to discontinue the drug or to reduce the dosage until renal function improves. In patients who receive high doses of methotrexate for treatment of osteosarcoma, the drug may cause renal damage resulting in acute renal failure. Nephrotoxicity is attributed to precipitation of methotrexate and a metabolite in renal tubules. Reducing renal impairment involves monitoring renal function closely, ensuring adequate hydration, alkalinizing the urine, and measuring serum drug levels. With mercaptopurine, dosage reduction is necessary to prevent nephrotoxicity. With irinotecan, dosage reduction is necessary in patients with moderate renal impairment (CrCl, 20–39 mL/minute).

Caution is warranted with many other drugs when used in patients with renal impairment. Cytarabine is detoxified mainly by the liver. However, patients with renal impairment may have more central nervous system–related adverse effects, and dosage reduction may be necessary. Gemcitabine has resulted in mild proteinuria and hematuria during clinical trials, and hemolytic–uremic syndrome has been reported in a few patients. Signs of this syndrome may include anemia, elevated bilirubin and reticulocyte counts, and renal failure. If this condition occurs, it is essential to stop gemcitabine immediately; hemodialysis may be required. Bleomycin is rarely associated with nephrotoxicity, but its elimination half-life is prolonged in patients with a CrCl of less than 35 mL/minute. Asparaginase often increases blood urea nitrogen; acute renal failure and fatal renal insufficiency have been reported. Procarbazine may cause more severe adverse effects if given to patients with impaired renal function. Hospitalization is recommended for the first course of treatment.

## Use in Patients With Hepatic Impairment

Some antineoplastic drugs are hepatotoxic, and the liver is the site of the metabolism of many. Patients with metastatic cancer often have impaired liver function, and their risk of further impairment or accumulation of toxic drug levels increases. It is necessary to monitor hepatic function with most drugs. However, abnormal values for the usual liver function tests (e.g., serum aspartate aminotransferase [AST] and alanine aminotransferase [ALT], bilirubin, alkaline phosphatase) may indicate liver injury but do not indicate decreased ability to metabolize drugs. Dosage reduction may be necessary in some cases. The following paragraphs describe the hepatic effects of selected cytotoxic chemotherapy drugs and precautions to reduce hepatotoxicity.

Alkylating drugs may lead to hepatotoxicity.

Antimetabolites also have hepatotoxic effects. Methotrexate may cause acute hepatotoxicity (increased serum ALT and AST, hepatitis) as well as chronic hepatotoxicity (fibrosis and cirrhosis). Chronic toxicity is potentially fatal. It is more likely to occur after prolonged use (e.g., 2 years or longer) and after a total dose of at least 1.5 g. It is essential that liver function tests be closely monitored in patients with preexisting liver damage or impaired hepatic function. Gemcitabine has increased serum ALT and AST in most patients during clinical trials. Mercaptopurine causes hepatotoxicity, especially with higher doses (above 2.5 mg/kg/d) and in combination with doxorubicin. Encephalopathy and fatal liver necrosis have occurred. It is essential to stop the drug if signs of hepatotoxicity (e.g., jaundice, hepatomegaly) occur. Serum aminotransferases, alkaline phosphatase, and bilirubin should be monitored weekly initially and then monthly.

Antitumor antibiotics may be hepatotoxic as well. Daunorubicin (liposomal formulation) requires dosage reduction according to serum bilirubin (e.g., bilirubin 1.2–3 mg/dL, three fourths the normal dose; bilirubin above 3 mg/dL, one half the normal dose). Doxorubicin toxicity increases with impaired hepatic function. It is necessary to perform liver function tests before drug administration and to reduce the dosage of both regular and liposomal formulations according to the serum bilirubin. Idarubicin is not appropriate for patients with a serum bilirubin above 5 mg/dL.

Some plant alkaloids have hepatic effects. Irinotecan may cause abnormal liver function tests in patients with liver metastases. Paclitaxel may cause more toxicity in patients with impaired hepatic function. Hospitalization is recommended for the first course of therapy. Topotecan is cleared from plasma more slowly in patients with hepatic impairment. Vinblastine and vincristine may cause more toxicity with hepatic impairment, and dosage should be reduced 50% for patients with a direct serum bilirubin value above 3 mg/dL.

Asparaginase is hepatotoxic in most patients; it may increase preexisting hepatic impairment and hepatotoxicity of other medications. Signs of liver impairment, which usually subside when the drug is discontinued, include (1) increased AST, ALT, alkaline phosphatase, and bilirubin and (2) decreased serum albumin, cholesterol, and plasma fibrinogen. Procarbazine may cause increased hepatotoxicity in cases of impaired hepatic function.

### Use in Patients With Critical Illness

Cytotoxic drug treatment is often significantly dose reduced or discontinued in the setting of critical illness when there is compromised perfusion to the liver and kidneys, which can increase toxicity. However, palliative chemotherapy, which can alleviate pain or obstruction in critically ill patients with advanced cancer, is used on a case-by-case basis with consideration of therapeutic benefits versus the risks of treatment toxicities.

### Use in Home Care

Although administration of cytotoxic drug therapy occurs most frequently in a clinic or hospital setting, people often self-administer oral cytotoxic drugs, and some give themselves IV infusions at home. All cytotoxic drugs are hazardous substances and require special handling and disposal, according to safety guidelines, in the home. The home care nurse may be involved in a wide range of activities associated with antineoplastic drug therapy, including administering the anticancer drugs, administering other drugs to prevent or manage adverse effects, and assessing patient and family responses to therapy.

 **QSEN Alert: Evidence-Based Practice**

Patients who have undergone hematopoietic stem cell transplantation require more intense chemotherapy than the bone marrow is able to tolerate. As a result, many of these patients require drug therapy to prevent CINV. Nakagaki, Barras, Curley, Butler, and Kennedy (2017) conducted a randomized open-label prospective study to evaluate the effectiveness of olanzapine, infused ondansetron, and palonosetron for the treatment of breakthrough CINV. In the study, patients received either ondansetron (32-mg infusion over 24 hours), olanzapine (10-mg wafer once daily) plus ondansetron 8 mg IV three times per day, or a single dose of palonosetron 0.25 mg IV instead of ondansetron. Metoclopramide 10 mg orally was administered as a rescue method for nausea. The study results showed that olanzapine is an effective treatment for breakthrough CINV in hematopoietic stem cell transplantation. Palonosetron was effective in treating nausea for 24 hours.

In addition, a major nursing role involves teaching about the disease process, management of pain and other symptoms, information about the specific anticancer drugs being given, prevention or management of adverse drug effects, preventing infection, maintaining adequate food and fluid intake, and self-care measures. Referral to palliative care early in the disease trajectory has resulted in improved quality of life, cost of care, and even survival in patients with metastatic cancer.

## Adverse Effects

Common adverse effects of the cytotoxic chemotherapy agents include **alopecia** (hair loss), anemia, bleeding, fatigue, **mucositis** (inflammation and erosion of oral mucous membranes), nausea and vomiting, **neutropenia** (low neutrophil count), **myelosuppression** (bone marrow depression), and **thrombocytopenia** (low platelet count). The dose-limiting toxicity for most of the cytotoxic drugs is myelosuppression.

The administration of irinotecan may cause diarrhea. Early forms of diarrhea may be associated with cholinergic symptoms. The administration of atropine can prevent these cholinergic symptoms. Loperamide should be administered with late forms of diarrhea, which is life threatening.

**Clinical Application 14.1**

Ms. D'Angelo has recovered from her surgery and will begin chemotherapy to treat her cancer. She is scheduled to receive paclitaxel IV 175 mg/m² over 3 hours every 3 weeks. What patient teaching will you provide to Ms. D'Angelo?

 **QSEN Alert: Safety**

When cytotoxic drugs are combined, it is essential to monitor the complete blood (cell) count (CBC) before and after each treatment to allow time for bone marrow recovery before the next treatment.

Other problems may include damage to the heart, liver, lungs, kidneys, or nerves. In general, adverse effects depend on the specific drugs used and the patient's health status. Baseline liver and kidney function testing is necessary before all cytotoxic drug treatment, and the presence of preexisting disease may contraindicate use of a drug that is associated with serious liver or renal toxicity. Box 14.2 describes the adverse effects of treatment with antineoplastic drugs.

With treatment of leukemias and lymphomas, a serious, life-threatening adverse effect called **tumor lysis syndrome** may occur. This condition develops when large numbers of cancer cells are killed or damaged simultaneously and release their intracellular contents into the bloodstream. As a result, hyperkalemia, hyperphosphatemia, hyperuricemia, hypomagnesemia, hypocalcemia, and acidosis develop. Signs and symptoms depend on the severity of the metabolic imbalances but may include GI upset, fatigue, altered mental status, hypertension, muscle cramps, paresthesias (numbness and tingling), tetany, seizures, electrocardiographic changes (e.g., dysrhythmias), cardiac arrest, reduced urine output, and acute renal failure. To

| **BOX 14.2** | *Complications of Chemotherapy and Their Management* |

Complications of anticancer drug therapy range from minor to life-threatening. Vigilant efforts toward prevention or early detection and treatment are needed.

- **Nausea** and **vomiting** commonly occur and are treated with antiemetics (see Chap. 38). With traditional cytotoxic chemotherapy, the drugs are most effective when started before drug administration and continued on a regular schedule for 24 to 48 hours afterward. An effective regimen is a serotonin receptor antagonist (e.g., ondansetron) and a corticosteroid (e.g., dexamethasone), given orally or intravenously. Other measures include a benzodiazepine (e.g., lorazepam) for anticipatory nausea and vomiting and limiting oral intake for a few hours. Guidelines have not been developed for managing nausea and vomiting with the biologic antineoplastic drugs.
- **Anorexia** interferes with nutrition. Well-balanced meals, with foods the patient is able and willing to eat, and nutritional supplements, to increase intake of protein and calories, are helpful.
- **Fatigue** is often caused or aggravated by anemia and can be treated with administration of erythropoietin. Alternating periods of activity and rest and an adequate diet may also be helpful.
- **Alopecia** (hair loss) occurs with cyclophosphamide, doxorubicin, methotrexate, and vincristine. Counsel patients taking these drugs that hair loss is temporary and that hair may grow back a different color and texture; suggest the purchase of wigs, hats, and scarves before hair loss is expected to occur; and instruct women to use a mild shampoo and avoid rollers, permanent waves, hair coloring, and other treatments that damage the hair.
- **Mucositis** (also called stomatitis) often occurs with the antimetabolites, antibiotics, plant alkaloids, and growth factor/tyrosine kinase inhibitors. It usually lasts 7 to 10 days and may interfere with nutrition; lead to oral ulcerations, infections, and bleeding; and cause pain. Nurse or patient interventions to minimize or treat this mucositis include the following:
  - Brush the teeth after meals and at bedtime with a soft toothbrush and floss once daily. Stop brushing and flossing if the platelet count drops below 20,000/mm$^3$ because gingival bleeding is likely. Teeth may then be cleaned with soft, sponge-tipped or cotton-tipped applicators.
  - Rinse the mouth several times daily, especially before meals (to decrease unpleasant taste and increase appetite) and after meals (to remove food particles that promote growth of microorganisms). One suggested solution is 1 tsp of table salt and 1 tsp of baking soda in 1 quart of water. Commercial mouthwashes are not recommended, because their alcohol content causes drying of oral mucous membranes.
  - Encourage the patient to drink fluids. Systemic dehydration and local dryness of the oral mucosa contribute to the development and progression of mucositis. Pain and soreness contribute to dehydration. Fluids usually tolerated include tea, carbonated beverages, ices (e.g., popsicles), and plain gelatin desserts. Fruit juices may be diluted with water, ginger ale, Sprite, or 7 Up to decrease pain, burning, and further tissue irritation. Drinking fluids through a straw may be more comfortable, because this decreases contact of fluids with painful ulcerations.
  - Encourage the patient to eat soft, bland, cold, nonacidic foods. Although individual tolerances vary, it is usually better to avoid highly spiced or rough foods.
  - Remove dentures entirely or for at least 8 hours daily because they may irritate oral mucosa.
  - Inspect the mouth daily for signs of inflammation and lesions.
  - Give medications for pain. Local anesthetic solutions, such as viscous lidocaine, can be taken a few minutes before meals. Because the mouth and throat are anesthetized, swallowing and detecting the temperature of hot foods may be difficult, and aspiration or burns may occur. Doses should not exceed 15 mL every 3 hours or 120 mL in 24 hours. If systemic analgesics are used, they should be taken 30 to 60 minutes before eating.
  - For oral infections resulting from mucositis, local or systemic antimicrobial drugs are used. Fungal infections with *Candida albicans* can be treated with antifungal tablets, suspensions, or lozenges. Severe infections may require systemic antibiotics, depending on the causative organism as identified by cultures of mouth lesions.
- **Infection** is common because the disease and its treatment lower host resistance to infection.
  - If fever occurs, especially in a neutropenic patient, possible sources of infection are usually cultured, and antibiotics are started immediately.
  - Severe neutropenia can be prevented or its extent and duration minimized by administering filgrastim or sargramostim to stimulate the bone marrow to produce leukocytes. A protective environment may be needed to decrease exposure to pathogens.
  - Instruct the patient to avoid exposure to infection by avoiding crowds, anyone with a known infection, and contact with fresh flowers, soil, animals, or animal excrement. Frequent and thorough hand hygiene by the patient and everyone involved in his or her care is necessary to reduce exposure to pathogenic microorganisms.
  - The patient should take a bath daily and put on clean clothes. In addition, the perineal area should be washed with soap and water after each urination or defecation.
  - When venous access devices are used, take care to prevent them from becoming sources of infection. For implanted catheters, inspect and cleanse around exit sites according to agency policies and procedures. Use strict sterile technique when changing dressings or flushing the catheters. For peripheral intravenous lines, the same principles of care apply, except that sites should be changed every 3 days or if signs of phlebitis occur.
  - Avoid indwelling urinary catheters when possible. When they are necessary, cleanse the perineal area with soap and water at least once daily and provide sufficient fluids to ensure an adequate urine output.
  - Help the patient maintain a well-balanced diet. Oral hygiene and analgesics before meals may increase food intake. High-protein, high-calorie foods and fluids can be given between meals. Nutritional supplements can

| **BOX 14.2** | **Complications of Chemotherapy and Their Management** (Continued) |
|---|---|

be taken with or between meals. Provide fluids with high nutritional value (e.g., milkshakes or nutritional supplements) if the patient can tolerate them and has an adequate intake of water and other fluids.

- **Bleeding** may be caused by thrombocytopenia and may occur spontaneously or with minor trauma. Precautions should be instituted if the platelet count drops to 50,000/mm³ or below. Measures to avoid bleeding include giving oprelvekin to stimulate platelet production and prevent thrombocytopenia; avoiding trauma, including venipuncture and injections, when possible; using an electric razor for shaving; checking skin, urine, and stool for blood; and, for platelet counts less than 20,000/mm³, stop brushing and flossing the teeth.
- **Extravasation.** Several drugs (called vesicants) cause severe inflammation, pain, ulceration, and tissue necrosis if they leak into soft tissues around veins. Thus, efforts are needed to prevent extravasation or to minimize tissue damage if it occurs.
  - Identify patients at risk for extravasation, including those who are unable to communicate (e.g., sedated patients, infants), have vascular impairment (e.g., from multiple attempts at venipuncture), or have obstructed venous drainage after axillary node surgery.
  - Be especially cautious with the anthracyclines (e.g., doxorubicin) and the vinca alkaloids (e.g., vincristine). Choose peripheral IV sites carefully, avoiding veins that are small or located in an edematous extremity or near a joint. Inject the drugs slowly (1–2 mL at a time) into the tubing of a rapidly flowing IV infusion, for rapid dilution and detection of extravasation. Observe the venipuncture site for swelling and ask the patient about pain or burning. After a drug has been injected, continue the rapid flow rate of the IV fluid for 2 to 5 minutes to flush the vein.

- If using a central IV line, do not give the drug unless patency is indicated by a blood return. Using a central line does not eliminate the risk of extravasation.
- When extravasation occurs, the drug should be stopped immediately. Techniques to decrease tissue damage include aspirating the drug (about 5 mL of blood, if able) through the IV catheter before it is removed, elevating the involved extremity, and applying warm (with dacarbazine, etoposide, vinblastine, and vincristine) or cold (with daunorubicin and doxorubicin) compresses. Nurses involved in cytotoxic chemotherapy must know the procedure to be followed if extravasation occurs so that it can be instituted immediately.
- **Hyperuricemia** from rapid breakdown of malignant cells can lead to kidney damage. Risks of nephropathy can be decreased by high fluid intake, high urine output, alkalinizing the urine with sodium bicarbonate, and giving allopurinol to inhibit uric acid formation.
- **Hand–foot syndrome** (also called palmar–plantar erythrodysesthesia or erythema) is a sunburn type of skin reaction with redness, tenderness, and possibly peeling, numbness, and tingling of palms and soles. It is associated with some traditional cytotoxic drugs (e.g., capecitabine, doxorubicin, fluorouracil) and some growth factor/tyrosine kinase inhibitors (e.g., lapatinib, sorafenib, sunitinib). It is attributed to leakage of drug from capillaries into the palms and soles; heat and friction increase leakage. Management efforts involve decreasing heat and friction (e.g., minimizing exposure of hands and feet to hot water), avoiding increased pressure (e.g., from long walks, squeezing small implements in cooking, gardening), or applying ice packs for 15 or 20 minutes at a time. Acetaminophen may be taken for discomfort.

prevent or minimize tumor lysis syndrome, aggressive hydration with IV normal saline, alkalinization with IV sodium bicarbonate, and administration of allopurinol (e.g., 300 mg daily for adults and 10 mg/kg/d for children) to reduce uric acid levels are necessary. Treatment of hyperkalemia may include IV dextrose and regular insulin (to drive potassium into cells) or Kayexalate to eliminate potassium in feces. Treatment of hyperphosphatemia may include administration of aluminum hydroxide or another phosphate-binding agent. Maintenance of urine pH of 7 or higher prevents renal failure due to precipitation of uric acid crystals in the kidneys. Hemodialysis may be necessary if the other measures are ineffective in maintaining urinary elimination.

## Contraindications

There are several contraindications to the use of cytotoxic antineoplastic drugs.

- Generally, pregnancy and lactation preclude their use.
- Myelosuppression may be a factor.

 **QSEN Alert: Safety**

Use of the cytotoxic agents that cause bone marrow suppression is not appropriate in people with a white blood count less than 2000 cells/mm³, a neutrophil count less than 1500 cells/mm³, and/or platelet count less than 50,000/mm³.

Hematologic monitoring prior to and after each treatment is necessary to limit the risk of infection and serious bleeding.

- The taxanes, paclitaxel, and docetaxel can produce severe peripheral neuropathy involving the sensory nerve fibers. It is called a dying-back process, affecting the distal nerve and then the Schwann cells and neuronal cells (Lee, 2019). In the event severe neuropathy or the neutrophil count is less than 500 mm³ for 1 week or longer, hematopoietic growth factor (granulocyte colony-stimulating factor) should be initiated.
- As previously stated, specific cytotoxic drugs may lead to certain adverse effects, and these drugs may be contraindicated in individual patients. Severe hepatic or renal impairment is also a contraindication to the use of specific cytotoxic agents that cause significant toxicities to the liver and kidney, respectively.

# Nursing Implications

The nurse should be aware that each antineoplastic drug is used in the schedule, route, and dosage judged to be most effective for a particular type of cancer. With combinations of drugs, it is necessary to adhere to the recommended schedule precisely because safety and effectiveness may be schedule dependent.

## Preventing Interactions

Interactions involving changes in hepatic metabolism are the most common reason for cytotoxic drug interactions. Cytochrome P450 (CYP) 3A4 enzymes in the liver metabolize a number of cytotoxic drugs, including taxanes, vinca alkaloids, and irinotecan. Drugs that inhibit these enzymes such as the azole antifungals, erythromycins, and protease inhibitors may increase blood levels and toxicities of a cytotoxic drug. CYP3A4 enzyme inducers, on the other hand (e.g., carbamazepine, griseofulvin, phenytoin, St. John's wort), can decrease blood levels and cytotoxic drug effects. In addition, use of noncancer drugs that have the same toxicities can cause drug interactions. Antimicrobials with renal toxicity, such as amphotericin B and aminoglycosides, can increase the nephrotoxicity of cisplatin and carboplatin. The chemotherapy nurse and a pharmacist should evaluate the potential for drug interactions.

## Administering the Medication

A certified chemotherapy nurse administers IV cytotoxic drugs. He or she verifies free flow of IV fluid into the vein and assesses adequate blood return. Peripheral infusion of cytotoxic drugs occurs through a newly initiated IV catheter in a large, upper extremity vein. Whenever possible, veins of the antecubital fossa, wrist, dorsum of the hand, and the arm where an axillary lymph node dissection has been performed are ones to avoid. Insertion of an indwelling central venous catheter is often appropriate for patients who have poor peripheral venous access, who require many doses of chemotherapy, or who require continuous infusions. When multiple drugs are given, administration of the drug most likely to cause venous irritation takes place first. Some of the cytotoxic drugs given by IV infusion are potential tissue irritants or vesicants and cause tissue necrosis if they leak outside the vein into surrounding tissue (extravasation).

### Clinical Application 14.2

Mrs. D'Angelo returns to the infusion center for her next paclitaxel infusion. She reports that she has developed mouth pain. Candidiasis and mucositis are apparent. The drug of choice to treat oral candidiasis is oral fluconazole. What effect will fluconazole have on today's infusion of paclitaxel?

Established infusion guidelines aid nurses who administer these drugs and increase the safety of both patients and nurses. These guidelines include the following:

- Ensure appropriate orders (e.g., be sure the prescriber is qualified to write chemotherapy orders; do not accept verbal or telephone orders).
- Do not give injectable drugs unless certified to administer chemotherapy.

**QSEN Alert: Safety**

Check all IV drug preparations for appropriate dilution, dosage that corresponds to the prescriber's order, absence of precipitates, expiration dates, and so forth.

**QSEN Alert: Safety**

Avoid direct contact with solutions for injection by wearing gloves, face shields, and protective clothing (e.g., disposable, liquid-impermeable gowns).

- If handling a powdered form of a drug, avoid inhaling the powder.
- Do not prepare the drugs in eating areas (to decrease risk of oral ingestion).
- Ensure adequate hydration before and after administration, frequent voiding, and use of a protective medication (e.g., mesna) to help prevent hemorrhagic cystitis.

**QSEN Alert: Safety**

Dispose of contaminated materials (e.g., needles, syringes, ampules, vials, IV tubing, and bags) in puncture-proof containers labeled "Warning: Hazardous Material."

**QSEN Alert: Safety**

Wear gloves when handling patients' clothing, bed linens, or excreta. Blood and body fluids are contaminated with drugs or metabolites for about 3 to 5 days after a dose.

**QSEN Alert: Safety**

Wash hands thoroughly after exposure or potential exposure and after removing gloves.

## Assessing for Therapeutic Effects

The nurse helps evaluate treatment effects by assessing for:

- Absence of or reduction in tumor size on physical examination, radiograph, computed tomography scan, magnetic resonance imaging scan, or bone scan
- Laboratory testing, which demonstrates decrease in malignant cells, normalization of serum chemistry levels, and decrease in abnormal tumor serum (tumor marker) protein levels
- Improved functional status, appetite, weight gain, and energy
- Decrease in cancer-related symptoms (e.g., pain, fatigue, dyspnea, cough, anorexia, nausea, vomiting)

## Assessing for Adverse Effects

The nurse assesses for the many adverse effects the cytotoxic drugs have on body tissues. Box 14.2 summarizes common adverse effects of these drugs and their management.

## Patient Teaching

Box 14.3 presents patient teaching guidelines for anticancer drugs.

## BOX 14.3  *Patient Teaching Guidelines for Drugs Used for the Treatment of Cancer*

- There are many different chemotherapy drugs, and the ones used for a particular patient depend on the type of malignancy, its location, and other factors. Some are taken orally at home; many are given intravenously, in outpatient clinics, by nurses who are specially trained to administer the medications and monitor your condition. The medications are usually given in cycles such as every few weeks.

- The goal of chemotherapy is to be as effective as possible with tolerable side effects. Particular side effects vary with the medications used; some increase risks of infection, and some cause anemia, nausea, or hair loss. All of these can be managed effectively, and several medications can help prevent or minimize side effects. In addition, some helpful activities are listed below.

- Keep all appointments for chemotherapy, blood tests, and checkups. This is extremely important. Chemotherapy effectiveness depends on its being given on time; blood tests help to determine when the drugs should be given and how the drugs affect your body tissues.

- Do everything you can to avoid infection, such as avoiding other people who have infections and washing your hands frequently and thoroughly. If you have a fever, chills, sore throat, or cough, notify your oncologist.

- Try to maintain or improve your intake of nutritious food and fluids; this will help you feel better and maintain your weight at a more optimal level to promote healing. A dietitian can be helpful in designing a diet to meet your needs and preferences.

- If your chemotherapy may cause bleeding, decrease the likelihood by shaving with an electric razor, avoiding aspirin and other nonsteroidal anti-inflammatory drugs (including over-the-counter Advil, Aleve, and others), and avoiding injections, cuts, and other injuries when possible. If you notice excessive bruising, bleeding gums when you brush your teeth, or blood in your urine or bowel movement, notify your oncologist immediately.

- If hair loss is expected with the medications you take, use wigs, scarves, and hats. Purchase them before starting chemotherapy, if possible. Hair loss is temporary; your hair will grow back!

- Inform any other physician, dentist, or health care provider that you are taking chemotherapy before any diagnostic test or treatment begins. Some procedures may be contraindicated or require special precautions.

- If you are of childbearing age, use effective contraceptive measures during and a few months after chemotherapy.

- For medications taken at home, instructions for taking the drugs should be followed exactly for the most beneficial effects.

- Although specific instructions vary depending on the drugs you are taking, the following are a few precautions with some commonly used drugs:
  - With cyclophosphamide, take the tablets on an empty stomach. If severe stomach upset occurs, take with food. Also, drink 2 or 3 quarts of fluid daily, if possible, and urinate often, especially at bedtime. If blood is seen in the urine or signs of cystitis occur (e.g., burning with urination), report to a health care provider. The drug is irritating to the bladder lining and may cause cystitis. High fluid intake and frequent emptying of the bladder help to decrease bladder damage.
  - With doxorubicin, the urine may turn red for 1 to 2 days after drug administration. This discoloration is harmless; it does not indicate bleeding. Also, report to a health care provider if you have edema, shortness of breath, and excessive fatigue. Doxorubicin may need to be stopped if these symptoms occur.
  - With fluorouracil, drink plenty of liquids while taking.
  - With methotrexate, avoid alcohol, aspirin, and prolonged exposure to sunlight.
  - With oxaliplatin, avoid exposure to cold during, and for 3 to 5 days after, drug administration. This helps prevent or minimize nerve damage that may cause numbness, tingling, and pain in the throat or hands. Swallowing and daily activities that require hand grasping may be impaired.
  - With vincristine, eat high-fiber foods, such as whole cereal grains, if you are able, to prevent constipation. Also, try to maintain a high fluid intake. A stool softener or bulk laxative may be prescribed for daily use.

## NCLEX Success

1. A male patient is being treated for Hodgkin's lymphoma with vincristine. He also takes phenytoin daily in the morning for a seizure disorder. How will these two medications interact?
   A. Vincristine, when combined with phenytoin, will increase sedation.
   B. Phenytoin and vincristine are metabolized by CYP3A4, increasing vincristine toxicity.
   C. Phenytoin administered with vincristine will decrease cytotoxic drug effects.
   D. Vincristine will increase the patient's risk of having a seizure.

2. For a patient receiving a cytotoxic drug that will likely result in bone marrow depression, which of the following teaching considerations should be the priority for the nurse with the patient and family members or caregivers?
   A. Wash hands often, and avoid people with colds, flu, or other infections.
   B. Do not expect fatigue and weakness, which are uncommon.
   C. Expect gastrointestinal upset. More nausea and vomiting may occur when the blood cell counts are low.
   D. Take acetaminophen for fever.

3. In explaining antineoplastic therapy to a family member of a patient who is to receive treatment with a cytotoxic drug, which of the following explanations is most accurate?

   A. Antineoplastic therapy damages both malignant and nonmalignant cells.
   B. It causes few adverse effects.
   C. It stimulates growth of cancer cells.
   D. It must be given daily.

4. A female patient with chronic lymphocytic leukemia is beginning to receive an oral cyclophosphamide. Which of the following instructions is most accurate? [Select all that apply.]

   A. Administer the drug with food only with gastric upset.
   B. Take the drug on an empty stomach.
   C. Take the drug at bedtime.
   D. Administer the drug 1 hour before a meal or 2 hours afterward.

## ADJUVANT MEDICATIONS USED TO TREAT CANCER

### Biologic Antineoplastic Drugs

Two factors promoting carcinogenesis are (1) failure of the immune system to eliminate mutant and malignant cells and (2) failure of growth-regulating processes to control the proliferation of premalignant and malignant cells. Biologic agents target cellular differences between the malignant and normal cells. By doing this, they stimulate the immune system to fight cancer cells and inhibit their growth and proliferation.

Treatment of cancer with biologic agents continues to expand, as more of these agents are designed to interact with proteins overexpressed on the surface of cancer cells. The ability to test individual tumor tissues for the presence of altered cell surface proteins and growth factors has become feasible. Thus, these drugs inhibit malignant cell growth and in some cases stimulate the immune system to destroy tumor cells. Biologic drugs are useful both alone and combined with cytotoxic drug treatment, reducing the adverse effects of traditional cytotoxic chemotherapy. Others, such as imatinib, which is used for chronic myeloid leukemia (it targets the tyrosine kinase enzyme involved in leukemia cell growth), are effective as monotherapy treatment for malignancy.

Biologic antineoplastic drugs include immunotherapy drugs and drugs that "target" biologic processes of malignant cells. Some immunologic anticancer drugs are discussed in Chapter 11 (e.g., interferon alfa for acquired immunodeficiency syndrome [AIDS]-related Kaposi's sarcoma, selected leukemias, malignant melanoma, and non-Hodgkin's lymphoma and interleukin-2 for renal cell carcinoma). Newer biologic agents (targeted therapies) are commonly used to treat lung, colorectal, breast, and hematologic malignancies in older adults. Table 14.3 presents the route and dosage information of biologic agents used in cancer treatment plus the use and adverse effects information for the currently approved biologic antineoplastic drugs—the monoclonal antibodies, tyrosine kinase inhibitors, and proteasome inhibitors.

### Monoclonal Antibodies

Monoclonal antibodies, which may be used alone or in combination with traditional cytotoxic antineoplastic drugs and other treatment modalities, have become an integral part of treatment plans for a variety of cancers. Metabolic pathways for

## TABLE 14.3

### DRUGS AT A GLANCE: Biologic Antineoplastic Drugs

| Drug/Pregnancy Category | Routes and Dosage Ranges | Clinical Uses | Adverse Effects |
|---|---|---|---|
| **Monoclonal Antibodies** | | | |
| ℗ **Alemtuzumab** (Campath; ✳ Lemtrada, MabCampath)/C | IV infusion, initially, 3 mg/d as a 2-h infusion. Increase to 10 mg/d and then to 30 mg/d as tolerated maintenance and 30 mg/d three times weekly on alternate days for up to 12 wk | B-cell chronic lymphocytic leukemia | Allergic infusion reactions (dyspnea, fever, chills, skin rash), immunosuppression, hypotension, hypertension, peripheral edema, nausea, vomiting, diarrhea, and mucositis |
| Bevacizumab (Avastin; ✳ Avastin)/C | IV infusion 5 mg/kg once every 14 d until disease progression is detected | Breast, cervical, colorectal, and renal cell cancer; refractory glioblastoma, non–small cell lung cancer, epithelial ovarian, fallopian, primary peritoneal cancer, and endometrial cancer | Heart failure, hemorrhage, hypertension, diarrhea, leukopenia, pain, dyspnea, dermatitis, stomatitis, and vomiting |

**TABLE 14.3**

## DRUGS AT A GLANCE: Biologic Antineoplastic Drugs [Continued]

| Drug/Pregnancy Category | Routes and Dosage Ranges | Clinical Uses | Adverse Effects |
|---|---|---|---|
| Blinatumomab (Blincyto; 🍁 Blincyto)/D | Premedicate with dexamethasone 20 mg IV 1 h prior to the first dose of each cycle, prior to first dose of each cycle<br>Cycle 1: IV 9 mcg daily administered as a continuous infusion on days 1–7 followed by 28 mcg daily as a continuous infusion on days 8–28 of a 6-wk treatment cycle<br>Cycles 2–5: 28 mcg daily administered as a continuous infusion on days 1–28 of a 6-wk cycle | Acute lymphoblastic leukemia (B-cell precursor), Philadelphia chromosome negative | Peripheral edema, neurotoxicity, skin rash, hypokalemia, hypomagnesemia, hyperglycemia, nausea, constipation, infection, bone marrow depression, and hypersensitivity |
| Cetuximab (Erbitux; 🍁 Erbitux)/C | IV infusion, initially, 400 mg/m² over 2 h; maintenance, 250 mg/m² over 1 h once weekly | Metastatic colorectal cancer and head and neck squamous cell cancer | Anemia, leukopenia, infusion reaction, nausea, diarrhea, stomatitis, vomiting, dyspnea, and fever |
| Dinutuximab (Unituxin)/D | Children: premedicate with IV morphine 50 mcg/kg, diphenhydramine 0.5–1 mg/kg/dose and acetaminophen 10–15 mg/kg/dose prior to infusion<br>IV 17.5 mg/m² d for 4 consecutive days for a maximum of 5 cycles (in combination with sargramostim, isotretinoin) | Neuroblastoma | Hypotension, pain, urticarial, proteinuria, increased ALT and AST, vomiting, diarrhea, bone marrow depression, increased serum creatinine, and fever |
| Ibritumomab tiuxetan (Zevalin; 🍁 Zevalin)/D | Premedicate with PO acetaminophen 650 mg and diphenhydramine 50 mg<br>Administer with rituximab<br>IV 250 mg/m² at 50 mL per hour on day 1; days 7, 8, 9 250 mg/m² at 100 mL/h Y-90 3.2 mg/2 L | Non-Hodgkin's lymphoma | Severe or fatal infusion reaction and severe bone marrow depression |
| Ipilimumab (Yervoy; 🍁 Yervoy)/D | IV 3 mg/kg every 3 wk for a maximum of 4 doses | Melanoma, unresectable or metastatic | Anemia, diarrhea, decreased hemoglobin, weight loss, and increased ALT and AST |
| Nivolumab (Opdivo; 🍁 Opdivo)/D | IV 3 mg/kg once every 2 wk | Hodgkin's lymphoma, melanoma, non–small cell lung cancer, and renal cell cancer | Peripheral edema, malaise, skin rash, hyponatremia, hyperkalemia, increased TSH, hypocalcemia, increased serum cholesterol, diarrhea, and increased creatinine |
| Obinutuzumab (Gazyva; 🍁 Gazyva)/D | Premedicate with acetaminophen, antihistamine, and glucocorticoid 30–60 min prior to treatment<br>IV 100 mg on day 1 followed by 900 mg on day 2 and followed by 1000 mg weekly for 2 doses (days 8 and 15)<br>Cycle 2–6: 1000 mg on day 1 every 28 d for 5 doses | Chronic lymphocytic leukemia and follicular lymphoma | Hypophosphatemia, hypocalcemia, hyperkalemia, hyponatremia, hypoalbuminemia, hypokalemia, bone marrow depression, increased AST and ALT, musculoskeletal pain, and increased serum creatinine |
| Ofatumumab (Arzerra; 🍁 Arzerra)/D | Premedicate with acetaminophen, antihistamine, and corticosteroid 30–120 min prior to treatment<br>IV cycle 1 (cycle is 28 d): 300 mg on day 1; followed by 1000 mg on day 8<br>Subsequent cycles: 1000 mg on day 1 every 28 d; continue for at least 3 cycles | Chronic lymphocytic leukemia | Fatigue, skin rash, diarrhea, nausea, bone marrow depression, infection, pneumonia, and infusion reaction |

*(Continued on page 272)*

**TABLE 14.3**

# DRUGS AT A GLANCE: Biologic Antineoplastic Drugs (Continued)

| Drug/Pregnancy Category | Routes and Dosage Ranges | Clinical Uses | Adverse Effects |
|---|---|---|---|
| Panitumumab (Vectibix; ❋ Vectibix)/C | IV infusion, 6 mg/kg over 60 min every 14 d. Doses over 1000 mg should be given over 90 min | Metastatic colorectal cancer | Infusion reactions, skin rash, pulmonary fibrosis, nausea, vomiting, and diarrhea; **90% of patients receiving panitumumab have developed severe dermatologic adverse effects** |
| Pertuzumab (Perjeta; ❋ Perjeta)/D | IV 840 mg over 60 min followed by a maintenance dose of 420 mg over 30–60 min every 3 wk for 3–6 cycles; may be administered | Metastatic breast cancer | Bone marrow depression, alopecia, upper respiratory infection, fatigue, weakness, diarrhea, nausea, and vomiting; **possible decreased left ventricular ejection fraction and congestive heart failure; evaluate cardiac function prior and during treatment** |
| Rituximab (Rituxan; ❋ Rituxan, Rituxan SC)/C | IV infusion 375 mg/m² once weekly for 4–8 doses<br>Chronic lymphocytic leukemia: IV 375 mg/m² given on the day prior to fludarabine/cyclophosphamide then 500 mg/m² on day 1 every 28 d of a cycles 2–6 | Non-Hodgkin's lymphoma and chronic lymphocytic leukemia | Hypersensitivity reactions, peripheral edema, fever, rash, fatigue, nausea, diarrhea, weight gain, bone marrow depression, cough, and increased ALT |
| Tositumomab (iodine 131–tositumomab) (Bexxar; ❋ Bexxar)/X | IV infusion over 60 min. If administered with iodine 131, infuse over 20 min | Non-Hodgkin's lymphoma | Fever, chills, nausea, vomiting, skin rash, headache, cough, infection, and pain |
| Trastuzumab (Herceptin; ❋ Herceptin)/D | IV infusion 4 mg/kg initially and then 2 mg/kg once weekly | Metastatic breast cancer | Cardiotoxicity (dyspnea, edema, heart failure) |
| **Kinase Inhibitors** | | | |
| ⓟ **Erlotinib** (Tarceva; ❋ Tarceva, APO-Tarceva, PMS-Erlotinib; Teva-Erlotinib)/D | Non–small cell lung: PO 150 mg once daily<br>Pancreatic: PO 100 mg once daily | Non–small cell lung cancer and pancreatic cancer | Dyspnea, edema, thrombosis, fatigue, alopecia, skin rash, increased ALT and AST, bone marrow depression, and infection |
| Afatinib (Gilotrif; ❋ Gilotrif)/D | PO 40 mg once daily | Non–small cell lung cancer, metastatic | Acne, weight loss, hypokalemia, increased ALT and AST, epistaxis, cystitis, and conjunctivitis |
| Axitinib (Inlyta; ❋ Inlyta)/D | PO 5 mg twice | Renal cell cancer | Hypertension, fatigue, voice disorder, headache, palmar–plantar erythrodysesthesia, skin rash, decreased serum bicarbonate, proteinuria, increased AST and ALT, and increased alkaline phosphatase |
| Bosutinib (Bosulif; ❋ Bosulif)/D | PO 500 mg once daily | Philadelphia chromosome-positive chronic myelogenous leukemia | Edema, fatigue, headache, hypophosphatemia, bone marrow depression, increased ALT and AST, arthralgia, cough, dyspnea, and fever |
| Cabozantinib (Cabometyx, Cometriq; ❋ Cabometyx)/D | Renal cancer: PO 60 mg once daily<br>Thyroid cancer (medullary, metastatic): PO 140 mg once daily (do not exceed 180 mg) | Renal cell cancer<br>Metastatic medullary thyroid cancer | GI perforation, hypertension, fatigue, voice disorder, headache, palmar–plantar erythrodysesthesia, skin rash, decreased serum bicarbonate, proteinuria, increased AST and ALT, and increased alkaline phosphatase |

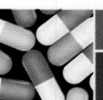

**TABLE 14.3**

## DRUGS AT A GLANCE: Biologic Antineoplastic Drugs (Continued)

| Drug/Pregnancy Category | Routes and Dosage Ranges | Clinical Uses | Adverse Effects |
|---|---|---|---|
| Ceritinib (Zykadia; ❋ Zykadia)/D | PO 750 mg once daily | Non–small cell lung cancer | Nausea, vomiting, skin rash, fatigue, diarrhea, decreased hemoglobin, and increased AST and ALT |
| Dabrafenib (Tafinlar; ❋ Tafinlar)/D | PO 150 mg every 12 h | Metastatic melanoma | Peripheral edema, rash, alopecia, hyperglycemia, hypophosphatemia, bone marrow depression, increased AST and ALT, and increased alkaline phosphatase |
| Dasatinib (Sprycel); ❋ Sprycel/D | PO 100–140 mg daily | Chronic myelogenous leukemia and acute lymphoblastic leukemia | Anemia, diarrhea, dyspnea, edema, fever, infection, nausea, pain, and skin rash |
| Everolimus (Afinitor, Afinitor Disperz, Zortress; ❋ Afinitor Disperz)/D | PO 10 mg daily | Breast, neuroendocrine tumors, lung, pancreatic, and renal cancer | Fatigue, edema, hypertension, diabetes mellitus, and increased serum creatinine |
| Ibrutinib (Imbruvica; ❋ Imbruvica)/D | PO 420 mg once daily | Chronic lymphocytic leukemia | Edema, fatigue, increased uric acid, infection, urinary tract infection, arthropathy, fever, atrial fibrillation, and increased serum creatinine |
| Imatinib (Gleevec) (Apo-Imatinib; ❋ ACT-Imatinib, Gleevec, Teva-Imatinib)/D | Adults: PO 400–800 mg/d Children: 3 y and older, PO 260–340 mg/m²/d | Philadelphia chromosome-positive chronic myeloid leukemia and gastrointestinal stromal tumors | Dyspnea, edema, heart failure, hemorrhage, nausea, vomiting, diarrhea, neutropenia, and thrombocytopenia |
| Lapatinib (Tykerb; ❋ Tykerb)/D | PO 1250 mg (5 tablets) once daily on days 1–21, with capecitabine PO 2000 mg/m²/d (in 2 doses, 12 h apart) on days 1–14 in a repeating 21-d cycle | Advanced breast cancer | Diarrhea, dyspnea, insomnia, nausea, vomiting, and stomatitis |
| Lenvatinib (Lenvima; ❋ Lenvima)/D | Renal cell carcinoma: PO 18 mg once daily in combination with everolimus Thyroid cancer: 24 mg once daily | Renal cell carcinoma and thyroid cancer | Hypertension, fatigue, headache, voice disorder, increased thyroid-stimulating hormone, proteinuria, hemorrhage, arthralgia, renal insufficiency, and cough |
| Nilotinib (Tasigna; ❋ Tasigna)/D | PO 400 mg BID | Chronic myeloid leukemia | QT prolongation, peripheral edema, hyperglycemia, pruritus, night sweats, nausea, vomiting, neutropenia, increased ALT and AST, and limb pain |
| Palbociclib (Ibrance; ❋ Ibrance)/D | PO 125 mg once daily for 21 d, followed by a 7-d rest | Breast cancer | Bone marrow depression, fatigue, peripheral neuropathy, nausea, vomiting, and alopecia |
| Pazopanib (Votrient; ❋ Votrient)/D | PO 800 mg once daily | Renal cell carcinoma and soft tissue sarcoma | Hypertension, edema, cardiac insufficiency, QT prolongation, hair discoloration, increased ALT and AST, and diarrhea |
| Ponatinib (Iclusig; ❋Iclusig)/D | PO 45 mg once daily | Philadelphia chromosome-positive, acute lymphoblastic leukemia, and chronic myeloid leukemia | Bone marrow depression, increased ALT and AST, fever, urinary tract infection, hypertension, peripheral edema, congestive heart failure, and arterial ischemia; **monitor for evidence of arterial occlusion, heart failure, hepatotoxicity, and venous thromboembolism** |

*(Continued on page 274)*

**TABLE 14.3**

## DRUGS AT A GLANCE: Biologic Antineoplastic Drugs (Continued)

| Drug/Pregnancy Category | Routes and Dosage Ranges | Clinical Uses | Adverse Effects |
|---|---|---|---|
| Regorafenib (Stivarga; ✹ Stivarga)/D | PO 160 mg daily for the first 21 d of a 28-d schedule | Colorectal cancer and locally advanced, unresectable, or metastatic gastrointestinal stromal tumor | Hypertension, fatigue, alopecia, headache, palmar–plantar erythrodysesthesia, skin rash, decreased serum bicarbonate, proteinuria, increased AST and ALT, and bone marrow depression |
| Sorafenib (NexAVAR; ✹ NexAVAR)/D | PO 400 mg twice daily | Hepatocellular cancer, renal cell cancer, and thyroid cancer | Hypertension, fatigue, voice disorder, peripheral sensory neuropathy, hypoalbuminemia, hypophosphatemia, increased thyroid-stimulating hormone, hypocalcemia, bone marrow depression, increased ALT and AST, myalgia, limb pain, dyspnea, and cough |
| Sunitinib (Sutent; ✹ Sutent)/D | Pancreatic neuroendocrine tumor: 37.5 mg once daily<br>Gastrointestinal stromal tumor and renal cell cancer: 50 mg once daily for 4 wk of a 6-wk treatment cycle (4 wk on, 2 wk off) | Pancreatic neuroendocrine tumor, gastrointestinal stromal tumor, and renal cell cancer | Hypertension, decreased left ventricular ejection fraction, peripheral edema, chest pain, fatigue, mouth pain, skin discoloration, increased uric acid, and increased AST and ALT, serum alkaline phosphatase, and serum bilirubin |
| Temsirolimus (Torisel; ✹ Torisel)/D | IV 25 mg once daily | Renal cell carcinoma | Edema, chest pain, headache, insomnia, hyperglycemia, hypercholesterolemia, hypophosphatemia, bone marrow depression, increased alkaline phosphatase, increased serum AST, mucositis, nausea, vomiting, dyspnea, and cough |
| Trametinib (Mekinist; ✹ Mekinist)/C | PO 2 mg once daily | Melanoma | Hypertension, cardiomyopathy, decreased left ventricular ejection fraction, dermatitis, rash, palmar–plantar erythrodysesthesia, hypoalbuminemia, diarrhea, stomatitis, abdominal pain, increased ALT and AST, and hematuria |
| ***Proteasome Inhibitors*** | | | |
| Ⓟ **Bortezomib** (Velcade; Velcade, ✹ ACT Bortezomib, PMS-Bortezomib)/D | IV injection, 1.5 mg/m², twice weekly for 2 wk, followed by a 10-d rest period | Multiple myeloma | Edema, nausea, vomiting, diarrhea, anemia, neutropenia, thrombocytopenia, and peripheral neuropathy |
| Carfilzomib (Kyprolis; ✹ Kyprolis)/D | Cycle 1: IV 20 mg/m² over 10 min on days 1 and 2. If tolerated, increase dose to 27 mg/m² over 10 min on days 8, 9, and 16 of a 28-d cycle<br>Cycle 2–12: IV 27 mg/m² over 10 min on days 1, 2, 8, 9, 15, and 16 of a 28-d treatment cycle<br>Cycle 13 and beyond: 56 mg/m² over 30 min on days 1, 2, 15, and 16 of a 28-d treatment cycle. Continue until disease progression or unacceptable toxicity | Multiple myeloma | Edema, hypertension, chest wall pain, fatigue, insomnia, peripheral neuropathy, hypokalemia, hypomagnesemia, nausea, vomiting, increased AST and creatinine, and bone marrow depression |
| Ixazomib (Ninlaro; ✹ Ninlaro)/D | PO 4 mg once weekly on days 1, 8, and 15 d of a 28-d cycle in combination with lenalidomide and dexamethasone | Multiple myeloma | Peripheral edema, peripheral neuropathy, skin rash, diarrhea, constipation, nausea, vomiting, bone marrow depression, eye disease, and upper respiratory tract infection |

ALT, alanine aminotransferase; AST, aspartate aminotransferase; TSH, thyroid-stimulating hormone.

many of the monoclonal antibodies are incompletely identified, but experts believe that the drugs are processed mainly in the reticuloendothelial system.

The monoclonal antibodies act in various ways:

- Ⓟ **Alemtuzumab** (Campath, Lemtrada), blinatumomab (Blincyto), ipilimumab (Yervoy), and rituximab (Rituxan) bind to an antigen on both normal T and B lymphocytes and malignant lymphoid cells to activate antibody- and complement-mediated cytotoxicity. The malignant lymphoid cells are more susceptible to immune destruction, and the normal lymphocytes can later repopulate in the bloodstream.
- Obinutuzumab (Gazyva) and ofatumumab (Arzerra) are monoclonal antibodies that bind to the antigen CD20 to activate an antibody-dependent response, causing tumor cell death.
- Bevacizumab (Avastin), cetuximab (Erbitux), ibritumomab (Zevalin), and trastuzumab (Herceptin) all bind to growth factor receptors found on blood vessels, colorectal cancer cells, and breast cancer cells, respectively, to prevent intracellular growth factors from becoming activated and stimulating cell growth. In addition, cetuximab binds to the epidermal growth factor (EGF) receptor to block the binding of EGF. The blockage prevents the phosphorylation and activation of receptor-associated kinases and apoptosis results.
- Panitumumab (Vectibix) is a recombinant human immunoglobulin G2 that binds to the EGF receptor, which inhibits the binding of EGF. EGF blocks phosphorylation and tyrosine kinase activation to stop cell growth and proliferation. Pertuzumab (Perjeta) has a similar action, but it targets the human epidermal growth factor receptor 2 protein (HER2). It is combined with trastuzumab for a greater human epididymis 2, or HE2, inhibition.
- Dinutuximab (Unituxin) is administered to children who have been diagnosed with a neuroblastoma. This monoclonal antibody binds to the disialoganglioside GD2, which is abundant or highly expressed in a neuroblastoma. The binding to GD2 allows for cell lysis and complement-dependent cytotoxicity.
- Like ibritumomab, the tositumomab radioconjugate (Bexxar) is a monoclonal antibody conjugated with a radioisotope that targets receptors on B lymphocytes.
- Nivolumab (Opdivo) is a G4 monoclonal antibody. Monoclonal antibodies are used in cancer treatment. Nivolumab inhibits cell death by binding with programmed death receptor 1 (PD-1), thus blocking its L1 and L2 ligands. The negative PD-1 receptor signaling then disrupts the T-cell cytotoxic response. By blocking the T-cell cytotoxic response, tumor-specific T cells enter the tumor to induce programmed tumor cell death.
- Catumaxomab is a tumor-targeted treatment with antigen-binding properties that moves T cells and antigen-presenting cells to the tumor and produces an antitumor immune response. It has the potential to decrease the symptoms of ovarian cancer.

Fewer adverse effects are associated with monoclonal antibody therapy than those of cytotoxic drugs. However, although some adverse effects are rare, they are serious (e.g., heart failure, bleeding problems, electrolyte imbalances) and vary depending on the drug.

Significant drug interactions with the monoclonal antibodies are few. Enzymes in the liver do not metabolize the monoclonal antibodies; hence, they do not compete with other drugs

for these enzymes. However, when combined with cytotoxic agents in the same treatment regimen, dosage reductions are often advisable.

Administration of monoclonal antibodies is by IV infusion because all preparations would be destroyed by GI enzymes if taken orally. The infusion occurs over a given period, generally 90 to 120 minutes initially, in a monitored health care setting. Premedication may be necessary, and frequent observation of the patient for signs of a hypersensitivity infusion reaction is important. In cases of acute hypersensitivity (urticaria, hypotension, dyspnea, wheezing), it is essential that the infusion be stopped and emergency measures implemented promptly (oxygen, epinephrine, bronchodilators, IV diphenhydramine, and dexamethasone). Mild infusion reactions require slowing or temporarily stopping the infusion and administering IV diphenhydramine 50 mg and acetaminophen 650 to 1000 mg orally.

> **! QSEN Alert: Safety**
>
> When tositumomab radioconjugate (Bexxar) is given, radiation safety precautions (careful body fluid precautions, good handwashing, and limiting intimate contact time) are necessary for a week after dosing.

> **Clinical Application 14.3**
>
> Ms. D'Angelo's oncologist has determined that she requires a different medication because of the adverse effects of paclitaxel. She will be started on bevacizumab and topotecan, on a platinum-free regimen. What are the actions of bevacizumab and topotecan?

### Growth Factor and Tyrosine Kinase Inhibitors

Growth factors such as EGF (which stimulates the growth of epithelial cells in the skin and other organs) and platelet-derived growth factor (which stimulates the proliferation of vascular smooth muscle and endothelial cells) bind to transcellular membrane receptors and initiate intracellular events that result in cell growth. EGF, which is normally produced in the kidneys and salivary glands, is found in almost all body fluids. When EGF binds to the external portion of the EGF receptor, also called the tyrosine kinase receptor, it sends signals to intracellular kinase enzymes stimulating cell proliferation and angiogenesis. Intracellular tyrosine kinases play an important role in the proliferation and differentiation of cells; thus, blocking these receptors can decrease intracellular protein synthesis and lead to cell death (Fig. 14.4).

Ⓟ **Erlotinib** (Tarceva) is a growth inhibitor that blocks the tyrosine kinase portion of the EGF receptor, inhibiting cell proliferation and inducing cell death. The action and use of other EGF inhibitors that are similar to erlotinib are described further. Axitinib inhibits the vascular endothelial receptors to promote cell death in renal cancer tumor growth. Bosutinib, dasatinib, and imatinib inhibit the kinase BCR-ABL and the proto-oncogene c-KIT. Both of these growth factors are significant in the development of chronic myelogenous leukemia.

**Figure 14.4.** Actions of selected biologic targeted drugs. These drugs prevent epidermal growth factor (EGF) from combining with its receptors and thereby prevent or decrease cell growth. Cetuximab and trastuzumab bind with the extracellular portion of the EGF receptor. Erlotinib blocks the intracellular (tyrosine kinase) portion of the EGF receptor.

Cabozantinib (Cometriq) slows the advancement of medullary thyroid cancer. Cabozantinib (Cabometyx) is effective in treating advanced renal cell carcinoma. Both of these drugs are strong CYP3A4 inhibitors and inducers. It may require 2 to 3 days to adjust the dosage when administered with another medication that is metabolized by CYP3A4. The U.S. Food and Drug Administration (FDA) has issued a **BLACK BOX WARNING ◆** for Cometriq because it may cause GI perforation. Therefore, it is important to instruct the patient about the signs and symptoms of this condition. Ceritinib is an inhibitor of anaplastic lymphoma kinase, which is active in the pathogenesis of non–small cell lung cancer. The patient will require a 5-HT₃RA to prevent nausea and vomiting. Dabrafenib is commonly administered with trametinib to inhibit the mitogen-activated protein kinase pathway leading to oncogene homolog B1 (BRAF) V600 melanoma cell death. BRAF V600 is a mutation of metastatic melanoma. Ibrutinib irreversibly inhibits Bruton's tyrosine kinase (BTK), which is a factor of the B-cell receptor that is integral in the survival of cancerous B cells. Ibrutinib decreases B-cell proliferation through the inhibition of BTK. Mechanistic target of rapamycin (mTOR) is another type of kinase inhibitor. Everolimus is a macrolide immunosuppressant in this subclass of kinase inhibitors. Its action decreases the lipoma volume in renal angiomyolipomas. Temsirolimus, another mTOR inhibitor, binds to the protein FKBP-12, halting the $G_1$ phase of the tumor cell in the treatment of renal carcinoma.

Lapatinib, another kinase inhibitor, is an oral agent administered for advanced and metastatic breast cancer. Some breast tumors have a strong expression of HER2, and this drug affects the expression of the EGF (ErbB1) and HER2.

Lenvatinib is a tyrosine kinase inhibitor used to treat advanced renal cell cancer and thyroid cancer. It is a vascular endothelial growth factor (VEGF) inhibitor. It blocks the VEGF receptors 1, 2, and 3; fibroblast growth factor receptors 1, 2, 3, and 4; platelet-derived growth factor receptor (PDGFR); KIT; and RET to slow the rate of cancer advancement. Pazopanib inhibits the same factors as lenvatinib along with fibroblast growth factor receptor, interleukin-2 receptor–inducible T-cell kinase, leukocyte-specific protein tyrosine kinase, and transmembrane glycoprotein receptor tyrosine kinase to treat renal cell carcinoma or soft tissue sarcoma. Nilotinib targets BCR-ABL kinase, c-KIT, and PDGFR in the treatment of chronic myeloid leukemia. The action of this medication has a stronger effect than imatinib. Prior to the administration of nilotinib, a patient should have a baseline ECG and another 7 days after the first dose. The FDA has issued a **BLACK BOX WARNING ◆** for nilotinib alerting patients who take the drug that they may be prone to the development of a prolonged QT interval. Nilotinib should not be administered to patients with hypokalemia or hypomagnesemia. It is also a strong inhibitor of CYP3A4. Also, it is important to instruct the patient to take the medication 1 hour before a meal or 2 hours after a meal. In addition, the patient should not consume grapefruit or grapefruit juice.

The drugs pazopanib, ponatinib, regorafenib, sorafenib, and sunitinib are kinase inhibitors with multiple targets. They reduce tumor growth by various actions to block tumor angiogenesis. They are BCR-ABL inhibitors used to treat acute lymphoblastic leukemia and chronic myeloid leukemia.

Common adverse effects of the tyrosine kinase inhibitors include leukopenia, thrombocytopenia, skin rashes, and diarrhea. Skin care, maintaining adequate hydration and nutrition, and monitoring for signs of dehydration and electrolyte imbalances are priorities with use of these antineoplastic drugs.

With the tyrosine kinase inhibitors, drugs also metabolized by the CYP3A4 liver enzyme system may affect tyrosine kinase inhibitors. Enzyme inhibitors (azole antifungals, erythromycin, protease inhibitors) and grapefruit juice may increase blood levels, whereas CYP3A4 enzyme inducers (rifampin, carbamazepine, phenytoin, St. John's wort) may decrease blood levels. An increase or decrease in dosage may be necessary with concurrent administration of inducers or inhibitors, respectively.

Self-administration of the oral tyrosine kinase inhibitors generally occurs in the home setting.

>  **QSEN Alert: Safety**
>
> It is essential that these drugs be handled as hazardous substances and stored securely in the original labeled container. No crushing or cutting of tablets should occur. If the patient is unable to swallow the oral formulation whole or has a feeding tube, it is necessary to dissolve the tablet in water in accordance with individual manufacturer's instructions and ingest it immediately.

### Proteasome Inhibitors

Proteasomes are enzyme complexes in the cytoplasm and nucleus of all body cells, both normal and malignant. These enzymes regulate intracellular protein activity. Ⓟ **Bortezomib** (Velcade) inhibits proteasomes, affecting multiple proteins within cells. Experts believe it has multiple mechanisms of cytotoxicity (e.g., preventing formation of new blood vessels in tumors and accelerating death of malignant cells). The drug is moderately protein bound (83%) and is metabolized by several CYP450 enzyme systems in the liver. Administration leads to cell cycle arrest, delayed tumor growth, and cell death. With bortezomib, which can cause myelosuppression, it is necessary to determine the blood cell count at baseline and periodically during therapy.

Other proteasome inhibitors include the following:

- Carfilzomib (Kyprolis), which inhibits chymotrypsin activity of the 20S proteasome. This action stops the cell cycle, leading to apoptosis.
- Ixazomib (Ninlaro), which inhibits chymotrypsin activity of beta-5 subunit of the 20S proteasome. This action also interrupts the cell cycle, leading to apoptosis.

## Antineoplastic Hormone Inhibitor Drugs

The main hormonal agents used in the treatment of cancer are the corticosteroids (see Chap. 17) and drugs that block the production of activity of estrogens and androgens. Pharmacologic doses of corticosteroids suppress lymphocyte production, causing lymphocyte apoptosis and regression of lymphoid tissue. Other uses for these drugs include treatment of the complications of cancer, including nausea and vomiting, intracerebral edema from brain metastases, and hypercalcemia. However, adverse effects may occur. Chronic use of oral glucocorticoids during the maintenance phase of leukemia

treatment can contribute to the development of long-term adverse effects such as osteoporosis, myopathy, hypertension, glucose intolerance, cataracts, and decreased growth rate in children. Hence, intermittent long-term therapy with glucocorticoids is generally used to maximize cytotoxic effects on lymphoid tissue while minimizing adverse long-term consequences. Prednisone and dexamethasone are the preparations most commonly used for cancer treatment. Sex hormone–blocking drugs are used mainly to control tumor growth and relieve symptoms. They are not cytotoxic, and adverse effects are usually mild.

Sex hormones act as growth factors in some malignancies (e.g., estrogens in breast cancer, testosterone in prostate cancer). Surgical removal of the ovaries or testes, which produce hormones, or therapy with hormone receptor–blocking drugs may be effective in decreasing hormonal stimulation and slowing the growth of hormone-dependent cancers. Removal of the ovaries is most likely in premenopausal women with breast cancer and the testes in men with prostate cancer. Currently used drugs interfere with hormone production or hormone action at the cellular level (Fig. 14.5).

The main hormone inhibitor drugs are the antiestrogens, aromatase inhibitors, antiandrogens, and gonadotropin-releasing hormone (GnRH) analogs. Chapter 7 and Table 14.4 describe these drugs.

### Antiestrogens

Ⓟ **Tamoxifen** (Soltamox) and toremifene (Fareston) are selective estrogen receptor modulators (SERMs) used in the treatment of breast cancer. One estrogen receptor antagonist, fulvestrant (Faslodex), may also be useful. These drugs, which bind to estrogen receptors in both normal and malignant cells, are effective only in the treatment of tumors with estrogen receptors. SERMs block some estrogen receptors while activating others (increasing bone mineral density and improving lipid levels). Fulvestrant is a pure estrogen antagonist, blocking all estrogen receptors. In breast cancer, all of these drugs compete with estrogen for receptor binding sites and thereby decrease estrogen-mediated growth stimulation of malignant cells.

Tamoxifen is an antiestrogen that has been widely used to prevent recurrence of breast cancer after surgical excision in women ages 40 and older and to treat metastatic breast cancer in postmenopausal women with estrogen receptor–positive disease. It is usually necessary to take the drug for 2 to 5 years to prevent tumor recurrence. Some studies indicate greater effectiveness when an aromatase inhibitor (see below) is used instead of tamoxifen after 2 to 5 years of therapy. Although both antiestrogens and aromatase inhibitors block the growth of breast tumors that respond to estrogen, their mechanisms of action are different. Tamoxifen inhibits the ability of breast cancer cells to use estrogen for growth by blocking receptors, whereas an aromatase inhibitor inhibits the production of estrogen in the ovaries, fat, muscle, and other tissues.

>  **QSEN Alert: Safety**
>
> Sexually active premenopausal women who take tamoxifen should use effective nonhormonal barrier contraception during therapy and for 2 months after the drug is discontinued.

**Figure 14.5.** Actions of hormone inhibitor drugs. Drugs used to treat breast cancer block the production of estrogens (e.g., gonadotropin hormone–releasing hormone [GnRH] analogs, aromatase inhibitors) or prevent estrogens from binding to receptors in breast cancer cells (antiestrogens). Drugs used to treat prostate cancer block the production of androgens (e.g., GnRH analogs) or prevent DHT, the active from of testosterone, from binding to receptors in prostate cancer cells (antiandrogens). FSH, follicle-stimulating hormone; LH, luteinizing hormone.

## TABLE 14.4

## DRUGS AT A GLANCE: Antineoplastic Hormone Inhibitor Drugs

| Drug/Pregnancy Category | Routes and Dosage Ranges | Clinical Uses | Adverse Effects |
|---|---|---|---|
| **Antiestrogens** | | | |
| Ⓟ **Tamoxifen** (Soltamox; ✿ Apo-Tamox, Mylan-Tamoxifen, Nolvadex-D, Teva-Tamoxifen, PMS-Tamoxifen)/D | PO 20 mg daily for 5 y (premenopausal) PO 20 mg daily for 2–3 y (postmenopausal) | Breast cancer, after surgery or radiation; prophylaxis in high-risk women; and treatment of metastatic disease | Hot flashes, nausea, vomiting, vaginal discharge, and risk of endometrial cancer in women who have not had a hysterectomy |
| Fulvestrant (Faslodex; ✿ Faslodex, TEVA-Fulvestrant)/D | IM 250 mg once monthly (one 5-mL or two 2.5-mL injections) | Advanced breast cancer in postmenopausal women | GI upset, hot flashes, and injection site reactions |

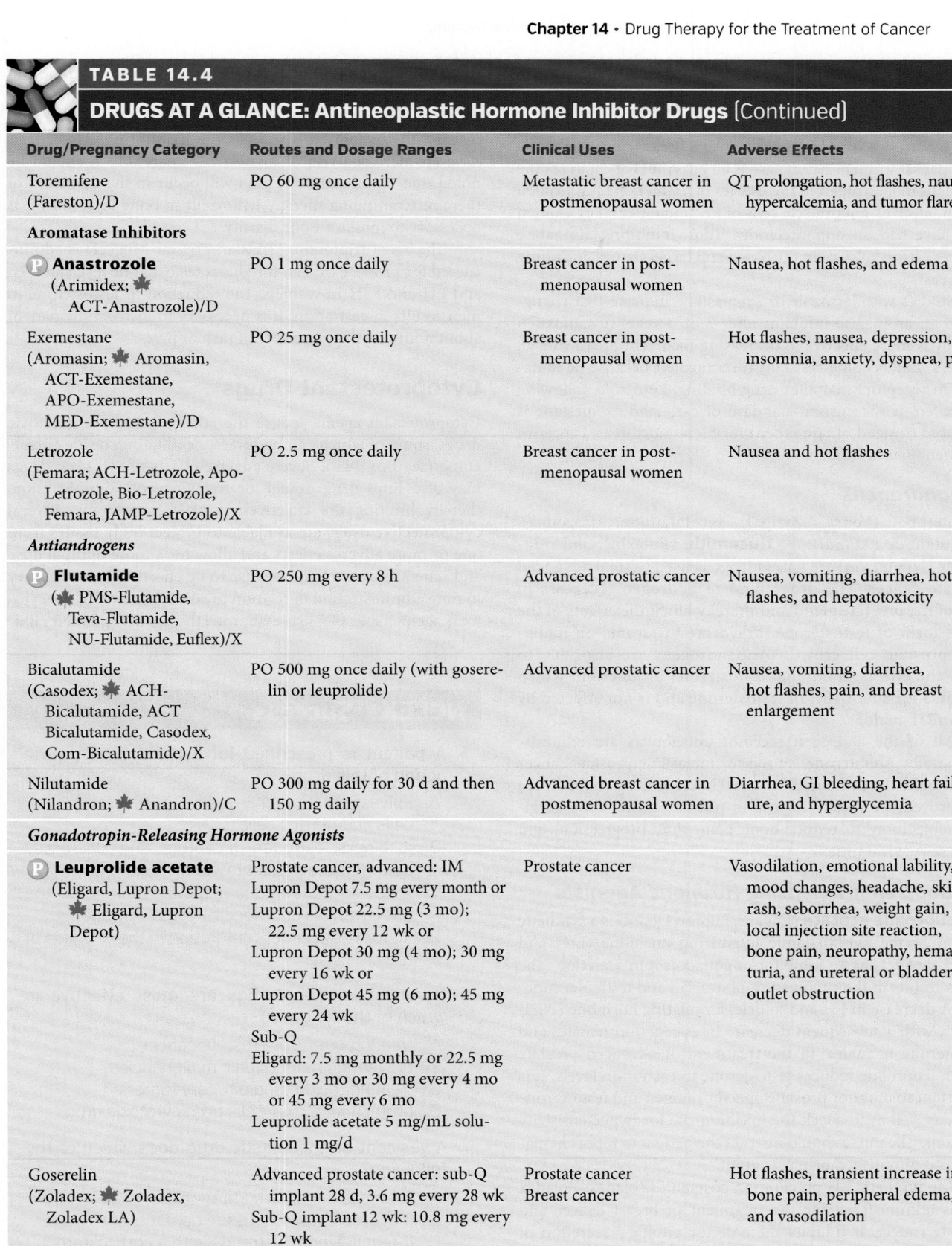

### TABLE 14.4
### DRUGS AT A GLANCE: Antineoplastic Hormone Inhibitor Drugs (Continued)

| Drug/Pregnancy Category | Routes and Dosage Ranges | Clinical Uses | Adverse Effects |
|---|---|---|---|
| Toremifene (Fareston)/D | PO 60 mg once daily | Metastatic breast cancer in postmenopausal women | QT prolongation, hot flashes, nausea, hypercalcemia, and tumor flare |
| **Aromatase Inhibitors** | | | |
| Ⓟ **Anastrozole** (Arimidex; ✹ ACT-Anastrozole)/D | PO 1 mg once daily | Breast cancer in post-menopausal women | Nausea, hot flashes, and edema |
| Exemestane (Aromasin; ✹ Aromasin, ACT-Exemestane, APO-Exemestane, MED-Exemestane)/D | PO 25 mg once daily | Breast cancer in post-menopausal women | Hot flashes, nausea, depression, insomnia, anxiety, dyspnea, pain |
| Letrozole (Femara; ACH-Letrozole, Apo-Letrozole, Bio-Letrozole, Femara, JAMP-Letrozole)/X | PO 2.5 mg once daily | Breast cancer in post-menopausal women | Nausea and hot flashes |
| *Antiandrogens* | | | |
| Ⓟ **Flutamide** (✹ PMS-Flutamide, Teva-Flutamide, NU-Flutamide, Euflex)/X | PO 250 mg every 8 h | Advanced prostatic cancer | Nausea, vomiting, diarrhea, hot flashes, and hepatotoxicity |
| Bicalutamide (Casodex; ✹ ACH-Bicalutamide, ACT Bicalutamide, Casodex, Com-Bicalutamide)/X | PO 500 mg once daily (with goserelin or leuprolide) | Advanced prostatic cancer | Nausea, vomiting, diarrhea, hot flashes, pain, and breast enlargement |
| Nilutamide (Nilandron; ✹ Anandron)/C | PO 300 mg daily for 30 d and then 150 mg daily | Advanced breast cancer in postmenopausal women | Diarrhea, GI bleeding, heart failure, and hyperglycemia |
| *Gonadotropin-Releasing Hormone Agonists* | | | |
| Ⓟ **Leuprolide acetate** (Eligard, Lupron Depot; ✹ Eligard, Lupron Depot) | Prostate cancer, advanced: IM Lupron Depot 7.5 mg every month or Lupron Depot 22.5 mg (3 mo); 22.5 mg every 12 wk or Lupron Depot 30 mg (4 mo); 30 mg every 16 wk or Lupron Depot 45 mg (6 mo); 45 mg every 24 wk Sub-Q Eligard: 7.5 mg monthly or 22.5 mg every 3 mo or 30 mg every 4 mo or 45 mg every 6 mo Leuprolide acetate 5 mg/mL solution 1 mg/d | Prostate cancer | Vasodilation, emotional lability, mood changes, headache, skin rash, seborrhea, weight gain, local injection site reaction, bone pain, neuropathy, hematuria, and ureteral or bladder outlet obstruction |
| Goserelin (Zoladex; ✹ Zoladex, Zoladex LA) | Advanced prostate cancer: sub-Q implant 28 d, 3.6 mg every 28 wk Sub-Q implant 12 wk: 10.8 mg every 12 wk Canadian labeling: same as above Breast cancer: sub-Q 3.6 mg every 28 d | Prostate cancer Breast cancer | Hot flashes, transient increase in bone pain, peripheral edema, and vasodilation |
| Triptorelin (Trelstar, Trelstar Mixject; ✹ Decapeptyl, Trelstar) | IM 3.75 mg every 4 wk or 11.25 mg every 12 wk or 22.5 mg every 24 wk | Advanced prostatic cancer | Increased serum glucose, decreased hemoglobin and red blood cells, increased serum alkaline, musculoskeletal pain, and increased blood urea nitrogen |

## Aromatase Inhibitors

Ⓟ **Anastrozole** (Arimidex), exemestane (Aromasin), and letrozole (Femara) are aromatase inhibitors used to prevent or treat recurrence of estrogen-responsive breast cancer in postmenopausal women. Aromatase is an enzyme that catalyzes the production of estrogen in the ovaries of premenopausal women and in fat, liver, and muscle cells of postmenopausal or women who have had an oophorectomy. Thus, inhibiting aromatase reduces estrogen levels in the blood and target tissues, including the breast.

Studies with letrozole or exemestane indicate that changing to an aromatase inhibitor after 2 or 3 years of tamoxifen therapy is more effective in decreasing recurrent breast cancer. Tumors may become resistant to tamoxifen because of mutations in receptors that alter drug binding. Letrozole, following tamoxifen, is the current standard of care, and exemestane is also used (instead of tamoxifen) for metastatic breast cancer in postmenopausal women.

## Antiandrogens

Abiraterone (Yonsa, Zytiga), bicalutamide (Casodex), enzalutamide (Xtandi), Ⓟ **flutamide** (Eulexin), and nilutamide (Nilandron) are antiandrogens used to treat advanced prostate cancer. The drugs bind to androgen receptors in cells of the prostate gland and thereby block the effects of the active form of testosterone, dihydrotestosterone, on malignant prostate cell growth. Antiandrogens are also able to block the effects of adrenal testosterone production, which accounts for about 10% of testosterone and is not affected by the GnRH analogs.

All of the androgen receptor antagonists are administered orally. Abiraterone is used for metastatic prostate cancer and should be combined with a GnRH analog. Nilutamide is approved specifically for use in prostate cancer after surgical orchiectomy to reduce bone pain, slow progression, and increase survival time.

## Gonadotropin-Releasing Hormone Agonists

Ⓟ **Leuprolide acetate** (Eligard, Lupron Depot) is a synthetic version of the hypothalamic luteinizing hormone (LH) and GnRH that acts as an inhibitor of gonadotropin secretion. The action results in the suppression of ovarian and testicular function. A decrease in LH and follicle-stimulating hormone (FSH) results, with a subsequent decrease in estrogen in females and testosterone in males. In the treatment of advanced prostate cancer, leuprolide reduces testosterone to castration levels. It is important to monitor prostate-specific antigen and testosterone levels, as well as to check the injection site for hypersensitivity reactions. The nurse should instruct the patient to report hematuria and diminished urinary output.

The synthetic LH preparation goserelin (Zoladex, Zoladex LA) is administered for the treatment of breast cancer and prostate cancer. It inhibits the anterior pituitary secretion of gonadotropin. In the initial phase of treatment, the levels of LH and FSH are increased, and a sustained suppression of the pituitary gonadotropins results. The ultimate effect of goserelin will result in an inhibition of GnRH. Long-term administration to males decreases serum testosterone at or below castration levels. Goserelin raises blood glucose levels, so it is important to instruct the patient on blood glucose monitoring. Also, males have an increased risk of myocardial infarction. It should be noted that significant bone pain will occur in the first week of therapy. Continuing therapy will result in bone loss; thus, it is necessary to monitor bone density.

The agent triptorelin (Trelstar, Trelstar Mixject) is administered for prostate cancer. It reduces testosterone levels in men and LH and FSH in women. The reduction in testosterone in men results in castration. It is necessary to instruct the patient about notifying the prescriber of rash or hives.

# Cytoprotectant Drugs

Cytoprotectant agents reduce the adverse effects of cytotoxic drugs, some of which can be severe, debilitating, or life-threatening (see Box 14.2). Severe adverse effects of cytotoxic drugs may also limit drug dosage or frequency of administration, thereby limiting the effectiveness of chemotherapy. Several cytoprotective drugs are available to protect body tissues from one or more adverse effects and allow for a more optimal dose and schedule of cytotoxic agents. To be effective, it is necessary to time administration in relation to administration of the cytotoxic agent. Table 14.5 lists cytoprotective agents and their clinical uses.

## NCLEX Success

5. **A patient is prescribed fulvestrant. What is the action of this drug?**
   A. Fulvestrant is highly cytotoxic to both cancer cells and normal cells.
   B. It blocks estrogen receptors and decreases estrogen-mediated growth stimulation.
   C. It boosts the immune response to increase the effectiveness of other chemotherapy agents.
   D. It stops cancer cell maturation in the $G_1$ phase of the cell cycle.

6. **Hormone inhibitor drugs are most effective in which of the following?**
   A. treating breast or prostate cancer
   B. preventing hematologic malignancies
   C. treating thyroid and pituitary tumors
   D. protecting normal cells from cytotoxic drugs

7. **A vesicant antineoplastic drug does which of the following?**
   A. It causes minor skin irritation.
   B. It causes extensive tissue damage.
   C. It requires administration with a corticosteroid.
   D. It requires deep intramuscular injection if diluted with normal saline.

**TABLE 14.5**

## DRUGS AT A GLANCE: Cytoprotectant Drugs

| Drug/Pregnancy Category | Routes and Dosage Ranges | Clinical Use |
|---|---|---|
| Amifostine (Ethyol)/C | IV infusion 910 mg/m² once daily within 30 min of starting chemotherapy | Reduction of cisplatin-induced renal toxicity |
| Dexrazoxane (Zinecard; ✹ Zinecard)/C | IV 10 times the amount of doxorubicin (e.g., dexrazoxane 500 mg/m² per doxorubicin 50 mg/m²) and then give doxorubicin within 30 min of completing dexrazoxane dose | Reduction of doxorubicin-induced cardiomyopathy in women with metastatic breast cancer who have received a cumulative dose of 300 mg/m² and need additional doxorubicin |
| Epoetin alfa (Epogen, Procrit, Retacrit; ✹ Eprex)/C | Sub-Q 150–300 units/kg three times weekly, adjusted to maintain desired hematocrit | Treatment of chemotherapy-induced anemia |
| Filgrastim (Granix, Neupogen, Nivestym, Zarxio; ✹ Grastofil, Neupogen)/C | Sub-Q, IV 5 mcg/kg/d, at least 24 h after cytotoxic chemotherapy, up to 2 wk or an absolute neutrophil count of 10,000/mm³ | Treatment of chemotherapy-induced neutropenia |
| Leucovorin (✹ Lederle Leucovorin)/C | "Rescue," PO, IV, IM 15 mg every 6 h for 10 doses, starting 24 h after methotrexate begun<br>Colorectal cancer, IV 20 mg/m² or 200 mg/m², followed by 5-fluorouracil, daily for 5 d, repeated every 28 d | "Rescue" after high-dose methotrexate for osteosarcoma<br>Advanced colorectal cancer, with 5-fluorouracil |
| Mesna (Mesnex; ✹ Uromitexan)/B | IV, 20% of ifosfamide dose for 3 doses (at time of ifosfamide dose, then 4 h and 8 h after ifosfamide dose) | Prevention of cyclophosphamide and ifosfamide-induced hemorrhagic cystitis |
| Oprelvekin (Neumega)/C | Sub-Q 50 mcg/kg once daily, usually for 10–21 d | Prevention of thrombocytopenia |
| Palifermin (Kepivance; ✹ Kepivance)/C | IV bolus, 60 mcg/kg daily for 6 total doses 3 consecutive days before and 3 d after high-dose chemotherapy (4th dose at least 1 d before stem cell infusion) | Prevent oral mucositis in hematologic malignancies before stem cell transplant |
| Sargramostim (Leukine)/C | IV infusion, 250 mcg/m²/d until absolute neutrophil count is above 1500/mm³ for 3 d, up to 42 d | Myeloid reconstitution after bone marrow transplant; to decrease chemotherapy-induced neutropenia |

## THE NURSING PROCESS

A concept map outlines the nursing process related to drug therapy considerations in this chapter. Additional nursing implications related to the disease process should also be considered in care decisions.

**Assessment**

- Assess the patient's condition before chemotherapy is started and often during treatment. Useful information includes the type, grade, and stage of the tumor, as well as the signs and symptoms of cancer. General manifestations include anemia, malnutrition, weight loss, pain, and infection. Specific manifestations depend on the organs affected.
- Assess for other diseases and organ dysfunctions (e.g., cardiac, pulmonary, renal, hepatic) that can influence individual response to chemotherapy.
- Assess emotional status, coping mechanisms, family relationships, financial resources, and social support mechanisms. Anxiety and depression are common features during cancer diagnosis and treatment.
- Assess laboratory test results before chemotherapy to establish baseline data and during chemotherapy to monitor drug effects.
  - **Blood tests for tumor markers** (tumor-specific antigens on cell surfaces). Alpha-fetoprotein is a fetal antigen normally present during intrauterine and early postnatal life but absent in adulthood. Increased amounts may indicate hepatic or testicular cancer. Carcinoembryonic antigen (CEA) is secreted by several types of malignant cells (e.g., colorectal cancer). A rising level may indicate tumor progression; levels that are elevated before surgery and disappear after surgery indicate adequate tumor excision. If CEA levels rise later, it probably indicates tumor recurrence. With chemotherapy, falling CEA levels indicate effectiveness. Other tumor markers are immunoglobulins (elevated levels may indicate multiple myeloma) and prostate-specific antigens (elevated levels may indicate prostatic cancer).
  - **CBC** to check for anemia, leukopenia, and thrombocytopenia because most cytotoxic antineoplastic drugs cause bone marrow depression. It is necessary to perform a CBC and white blood cell differential before each cycle of chemotherapy to determine dosage and frequency of drug administration, to monitor bone marrow function so fatal bone marrow depression does not occur, and to assist in planning nursing care. For example, the patient is very susceptible to infection when the leukocyte count is low, and bleeding is likely when the platelet count is low.
  - **Other tests.** These include tests of kidney and liver function, serum calcium, uric acid, and others, depending on the organs affected by the cancer or its treatment.

**Outcomes of Therapy**

The patient will
- Receive assistance in coping with the diagnosis of cancer.
- Experience reduced anxiety and fear.
- Receive chemotherapy accurately and safely.
- Experience reduction of tumor size, shift towards normal laboratory values, or other therapeutic effects of chemotherapy.
- Experience minimal bleeding, infection, nausea and vomiting, and other consequences of chemotherapy.
- Maintain adequate food and fluid intake and body weight.

**Nursing Interventions**

- Strengthen host defenses by promoting a healthful lifestyle (e.g., good nutrition, adequate rest and exercise, stress management techniques, avoiding or minimizing alcohol and tobacco use).
- For patients receiving cytotoxic anticancer drugs, try to prevent or minimize the incidence and severity of adverse reactions.
- Provide supportive care to patients and families. Physiologic care includes pain management, comfort measures, and assistance with nutrition, hygiene, ambulation, and other activities of daily living as needed. Psychological care includes allowing family members or significant others to be with the patient and participate in care when desired and keeping patients and families informed.

**Evaluation**

- Monitor drug administration for accuracy.
- Observe and interview for therapeutic effects of chemotherapy.
- Compare current laboratory reports with baseline values for changes toward normal values.
- Compare weight and nutritional status with baseline values for maintenance or improvement.
- Observe and interview for adverse drug effects and interventions to prevent or manage them.
- Observe and interview for effective pain management and other symptom control.

## KEY CONCEPTS

- Traditional cytotoxic antineoplastic drugs are nonselective in their effect on proliferating cells; therefore, bone marrow toxicity is a common adverse effect of many cytotoxic drugs. These drugs kill the same fraction of cells with each cycle of chemotherapy treatment; repeated cycles of cytotoxic drugs potentially lower the number of cancer cells to a level where a person's immune responses are able to take over and destroy the remaining cancer cells.

- Cytoprotectant agents protect body tissues from one or more adverse effects of cytotoxic drugs and allow for a more optimal dose and schedule of cytotoxic agents.

- Biologic targeted antineoplastic agents are designed to specifically attack a target that is expressed exclusively, or disproportionally, by the cancer cell.

- The FDA has issued a **BLACK BOX WARNING** ◆ for cabozantinib (Cometriq) because it may cause GI perforation.

- The FDA has issued a **BLACK BOX WARNING** ◆ for nilotinib indicating that patients who take the drug may be prone to the development of a prolonged QT interval.

- Hormonal therapies that block the effects of estrogen (in an estrogen-responsive tumor) and androgen (in an androgen-responsive tumor), respectively, are essential in the treatment of breast and advanced prostate cancers.

- GnRH agonist analogs decrease the release of FSH and LH by down-regulating receptor response, thus inhibiting the release of LH and FSH. This action blocks the production of ovarian estrogen in women to postmenopausal levels and testicular testosterone in men to castration levels.

- Cancer in older adults presents a unique challenge, due in part to the presence of comorbidities and the physical, biologic, and physiologic changes that occur with normal aging. Until recently, older adults were excluded from participating in clinical trials.

## CLINICAL REASONING CASE STUDY

**Meet the Patient**

Trevor Fox, a 42-year-old man with a history of mild renal insufficiency, has been diagnosed with Hodgkin's disease. He has completed a course of radiation therapy and is preparing to begin adjuvant chemotherapy, with a drug regimen that includes doxorubicin, bleomycin, vinblastine, and dacarbazine.

- Mr. Fox asks the nurse why he has to take so many different chemotherapeutic drugs. How should the nurse respond?
- Discuss the major adverse effects of chemotherapy that Mr. Fox may expect. What nursing interventions may mitigate these effects?

**Assessing Drug Information**

- Combination drug therapy is used in cancer treatment because it is more effective, less toxic, and less likely to cause drug resistance.
- The adverse effect of bone marrow suppression can result in blood counts reaching the lowest point 7 to 14 days after drug administration and increasing back to normal after 21 days.
- Chemotherapy agents commonly cause nausea and vomiting.
- Pulmonary toxicity is a complication of bleomycin.
- Cardiotoxicity, a life-threatening complication, may result from use of doxorubicin.
- There is a potential for severe allergic reaction with hypotension with the administration of bleomycin. A test dose of 1 to 2 mg of bleomycin should be administered subcutaneously prior to giving the first full dose to avoid this complication.

**Nursing Actions**

- Educate Mr. Fox about the adverse effects of all medications.
- Educate Mr. Fox about the bone marrow depression and its effect in increasing the chance of acquiring an infection.
- In order to reduce his exposure to infection, educate Mr. Fox to practice strict hand hygiene and to avoid crowds, people with known infection, and fresh flowers, soil, and animals.
- Anemia may occur, and Mr. Fox should monitor for fatigue, using rest periods as needed.
- Nausea and vomiting are common adverse effects, and Mr. Fox should receive scheduled doses of antiemetics. Educate him about the use of antiemetic agents.
- Pulmonary toxicity is a complication of bleomycin. Educate Mr. Fox to be alert for the development of a cough and dyspnea and to report these conditions to his health care provider.
- Cardiotoxicity is a life-threatening complication that may result from use of doxorubicin. The nurse should monitor Mr. Fox for signs of heart failure, including dyspnea, edema, and fatigue. Dysrhythmias may also occur, along with electrocardiographic changes. Perform a thorough cardiac assessment for Mr. Fox on a regular basis.
- There is a potential for severe allergic reaction with hypotension with the administration of bleomycin. Administer a test dose of 1 to 2 mg of bleomycin subcutaneously to Mr. Fox prior to giving the first full dose to avoid this complication.
- Additional patient teaching information can be found in Box 14.3.

> *Visit* thePoint® *at* **http://thePoint.lww.com/Frandsen12e**
> *for answers to NCLEX Success questions (in Appendix A), answers to Clinical Application Case Studies (in Appendix B), and more!*

## REFERENCES AND RESOURCES

Chu, E., & DeVita, V. T. (2019). *Physicians' cancer chemotherapy drug manual 2019*. Burlington, MA: Jones & Bartlett Learning.

Clowse, M. B., & McCune, W. J. (2019). General toxicity of cyclophosphamide in rheumatic disease. In: *UpToDate*. Waltham, MA.

Di Lorenzo, C. (2019). Approach to the infant or child with nausea and vomiting. In: *UpToDate*. Waltham, MA.

Hesketh, P. J. (2019). Prevention and treatment of chemotherapy-induced nausea and vomiting in adults. In: *UpToDate*. Waltham, MA.

Hinkle, J. L., & Cheever, K. H. (2018). *Brunner & Suddarth's textbook of medical-surgical nursing* (14th ed.). Philadelphia, PA: Lippincott Williams & Wilkins.

Konstantinopoulos, P. A., & Bristow, R. E. (2019). Neoadjuvant chemotherapy for new diagnosed advanced ovarian cancer. In: *UpToDate*. Waltham, MA.

LaCasce, A. S. & Ng, A. H. (2019). Second malignancies after treatment of classic Hodgkin lymphoma. In: *UpToDate*. Waltham, MA.

Lee, E. Q. (2019). Overview of neurologic complications of non-platinum chemotherapy. In: *UpToDate*. Waltham, MA.

McClain, K. L., & Kamdar, K. (2019). Overview of Hodgkin lymphoma in children and adolescents. In: *UpToDate*. Waltham, MA.

Nakagaki, M., Barras, M., Curley, C., Butler, J. P., & Kennedy, G. A. (2017). A randomized trial of olanzapine versus palonosetron versus infused ondansetron for the treatment of breakthrough chemotherapy-induced nausea and vomiting in patient undergoing hematopoietic stem cell transplantation. *Supportive Care in Cancer, 25*, 607–613 doi:10.1007/s00520-016-3445-2

National Cancer Institute. (2016). *What is cancer?* Retrieved June 5, 2019, from http://www.cancer.gov/about-cancer/understanding/what-is-cancer#differences-cancer-cells-normal-cells

Norris, T. L. (2019). *Porth's pathophysiology: Concepts of altered health states* (10th ed.). Philadelphia, PA: Wolters Kluwer.

Pritchard, K. I. (2019). Adjuvant endocrine therapy for non-metastatic, hormone receptor-positive breast cancer. In: *UpToDate*. Waltham, MA.

Roila, F., et al. (2016). 2016 MASCC and ESMO guideline update for the prevention of chemotherapy- and radiotherapy-induced nausea and vomiting of nausea and vomiting in advanced cancer patients. *Annals of Oncology, 27*, v119–v133.

UpToDate. (2019). *Drug information*. Lexi-Comp, Inc.

# Drugs Affecting Inflammation and Infection

# Inflammation, Infection, and the Use of Antimicrobial Agents

## LEARNING OBJECTIVES

*After studying this chapter, you should be able to:*

1. Identify the common etiologies of inflammation.
2. Discuss the pathophysiology of inflammation.
3. Describe, in general, the groups of drugs used to treat inflammation.
4. Identify the common pathogens and methods of infection control.
5. Discuss the pathophysiology of infection.
6. Discuss ways to minimize emergence of drug-resistant microorganisms.
7. Discuss ways to increase the benefits and decrease the risk associated with antimicrobial drug therapy.
8. Know how to apply the nursing process to the care of the patient who is receiving antimicrobial therapy.

## CLINICAL APPLICATION CASE STUDY

Alisa Warren is a 25-year-old woman with early-onset rheumatoid arthritis who works as a social worker in a pediatric hospital. She has a heavy caseload, and her lunch often consists of a soda, chips, and a sweet roll from the snack machine. She and her husband spend most evenings watching movies and television because her pain prevents her from participating in many activities. Recently, her practitioner prescribed methylprednisolone, a corticosteroid, to help manage the inflammation associated with the arthritis.

## KEY TERMS

**Antibacterial:** ability to kill bacteria or interfere with the ability of bacteria to grow and replicate

**Antibiotic:** drug that has the ability to kill or inhibit bacterial growth and replication

**Antibiotic resistance:** ability of certain bacteria to survive and multiply in the presence of antibiotics

**Anti-infective:** agent or substance with antibacterial, antiviral, and antifungal properties

**Anti-inflammatory agent:** drug indicated when the inflammatory response is inappropriate, abnormal, or persistent or destroys tissue

**Antimicrobial agent:** drug used to prevent or treat infections caused by pathogenic (disease-producing) microorganisms such as bacteria, fungi, viruses, and parasites

**Bacteria:** single-celled microorganisms that do not have nuclei and reproduce by fission or splitting

**Bactericidal:** agent that kills bacteria

**Bacteriostatic:** agent that inhibits bacterial growth and replication

**Broad spectrum:** effective against a wide range of bacteria

**Colonization:** presence and growth of microorganisms on host tissues

**Community-acquired infection:** infection caused by microorganisms that originated in a setting outside of a health care facility

**Community-acquired pneumonia:** pneumonia contracted by a person outside of a health care facility

**Detection of antigens:** technique to identify pathogens that uses features of culture and serology but reduces the time required for diagnosis

**Fungi:** plantlike microorganisms that live as parasites on living tissue or as saprophytes on decaying organic matter

**Health care–associated pneumonia:** pneumonia that has been acquired in other health care facilities, such as nursing homes

**Hospital-acquired infection:** infection acquired from microorganisms in hospitals and other health care facilities

**Inflammation:** immunologic response to allergy, infection, or injury that increases the migration of leukocytes and blood flow to assist in repairing tissues

**Opportunistic:** microorganisms in normal flora that become pathogenic under conditions that are favorable for their (over)growth

**Penicillin-binding proteins:** proteins in bacteria that serve as target sites for penicillin to bind

**Serology:** method of identifying infectious agents by measuring the antibody level (titer) in the serum of an infected host

**Susceptibility:** vulnerability of the bacteria to an antibiotic's effects

**Viruses:** intracellular parasites that survive only in living tissues

# INTRODUCTION

This chapter is an introduction to the pathophysiologic effects of **inflammation** and infection. Readers should note that the format of this chapter is different from previous chapters. This chapter presents an overview of the anti-inflammatory and antimicrobial therapy to allow an understanding of a broad classification of the drugs involved and their impact on decreasing inflammation associated with infection and the infective process.

To help prevent inflammation caused by allergy, injury, or infection, the nurse should be familiar with **anti-inflammatory agents**. The anti-inflammatory agents administered to reduce the inflammatory process include aspirin, nonsteroidal anti-inflammatory drugs (NSAIDs), and corticosteroids. These drugs are indicated when the inflammatory response is inappropriate, abnormal, or persistent or in the presence of tissue destruction. Health care providers use medicines known as **antimicrobial agents** to prevent or treat infections caused by pathogenic (disease-producing) microorganisms such as **bacteria**, **fungi**, **viruses**, and parasites. They treat inflammation resulting from infectious processes with antimicrobial drugs.

Most microorganisms live in equilibrium with the human host and do not cause disease; however, even beneficial bacteria may cause infections in certain conditions. When the balance is upset and infection occurs, characteristics of the infecting microorganisms and the adequacy of host defense mechanisms

are major factors in determining the severity of the infection and the person's ability to recover. In addition, overuse of antimicrobial agents may lead to serious infections caused by drug-resistant microorganisms. To help prevent infectious diseases and participate effectively in antimicrobial drug therapy, the nurse must be knowledgeable about microorganisms, host responses to microorganisms, and antimicrobial drugs.

## OVERVIEW OF INFLAMMATION

To adequately understand the pharmacologic treatment of inflammation, it is important to understand the causes, pathophysiology, and clinical manifestations of inflammation. This will make it easier to understand the drug therapy associated with the treatment of inflammation, as addressed in Chapters 16 and 17.

### Etiology

Inflammation is the cellular response of the body to tissue damage and injury. The cells and tissues of the body are killed or injured by chemical, physical, or infectious agents. The body's autoimmune response can also produce an inflammatory process. The immunologic response of the body produces increased migration of leukocytes and flow of blood to the cells and tissues affected to help repair the tissues.

# Pathophysiology

There are two types of inflammation. Acute inflammation is the immediate response to injury of local tissues. The body responds by attempting to remove the offending agent to limit the amount of damage to the tissues affected. Chronic inflammation occurs over longer periods, even years. An acute inflammatory response may become chronic.

## *Acute Inflammation*

The process of acute inflammation occurs in three stages. The first stage is the vascular stage; notable changes occur in the small blood vessels at the site of the cellular and tissue injury. At the time of the injury, vasoconstriction results, followed by vasodilation of the capillaries and venules to increase capillary blood flow, increasing temperature and redness at the site. The body then increases protein exudates into the extravascular spaces. As protein exudates occupy the extravascular spaces, the capillary osmotic pressure diminishes and the interstitial osmotic pressure increases, resulting in increasing amounts of fluid in the tissue spaces causing swelling, pain, and diminished function or mobility. In the event that the inflammation is caused by an infectious agent, the localizing effects increase the risk of the spread of infection (Fig. 15.1).

The second stage of acute inflammation is also known as the cellular stage. At this time, there is an influx of leukocytes, primarily neutrophils, to the injury site. As the leukocytes invade, there is a slowing of the blood flow and margination, which is the adhesion of the leukocytes to the wall of the blood vessels. The leukocytes then transmigrate from the vascular space to the extravascular tissue. They travel to the tissue injury site by chemotaxis (Fig. 15.2).

The third stage involves opsonization, which facilitates phagocytosis. During opsonization, a substance coats the foreign antigens, producing inflammation. This inflammation makes the antigens more susceptible to the macrophages and leukocytes, thus increasing phagocytic activity. The two opsonins are complement factor C3b and antibodies (Fig. 15.3).

## *Chronic Inflammation*

There are two kinds of chronic inflammation. Nonspecific chronic inflammation is a diffuse accumulation of macrophages and lymphocytes in the area of tissue destruction, yielding fibroblast proliferation and scarring. Granulomatous chronic inflammation generates 1- to 2-mm granulomas made up of macrophages surrounded by lymphocytes. The granulomatous process results from foreign bodies that have not been controlled by the acute inflammatory process.

# Clinical Manifestations

In acute inflammation, pain, redness, and swelling are apparent. Breaks in the integumentary system result in the drainage of exudate. In the event of a viral or bacterial infection associated with the inflammation, fever and general malaise sometimes occur. In chronic inflammation, tissue destruction and scarring may develop. The development of scarring replaces the connective or parenchymal tissue, resulting in diminished mobility or function. As previously stated, granulomas may occur because of an uncontrolled acute inflammatory process.

**Figure 15.1.** Stage 1: vascular stage. The vascular stage of acute inflammation, which is characterized by changes in the small blood vessels at the site of injury. It begins with vasoconstriction followed rapidly by vasodilation. Vasodilation results in an increase in capillary blood flow, causing heat and redness, which are two of the cardinal signs of inflammation. This is accompanied by an increase in vascular permeability with outpouring of protein-rich fluid (exudate) into the extravascular spaces. The loss of proteins reduces the capillary osmotic pressure and increases the interstitial osmotic pressure. This, coupled with an increase in capillary pressure, causes a marked outflow of fluid and its accumulation in the tissue spaces, producing the swelling, pain, and impaired function that represent the other cardinal signs of acute inflammation. As fluid moves out of the vessels, stagnation of flow and clotting of blood occur. This aids in localizing the spread of infectious microorganisms.

# Drug Therapy

Aspirin, NSAIDs, and corticosteroids are administered to decrease inflammation (see Chaps. 16 and 17). Aspirin and NSAIDs block the synthesis of prostaglandin in the central and peripheral nervous systems. The anti-inflammatory response produced by the administration of corticosteroids occurs through the inhibition of interleukin-1, cytokines, and the tumor necrosis factor. Corticosteroids also impair phagocytosis

Blood flow

**Figure 15.2.** Stage 2: leukocyte margination, adhesion, and transmigration. The cellular stage of acute inflammation involves the delivery of leukocytes, mainly neutrophil, to the site of injury so they can perform their normal functions of host defense. The delivery and activation of leukocytes can be divided into the following steps: adhesion and margination, transmigration, and chemotaxis. The recruitment of leukocytes to the precapillary venules, where they exit the circulation, is facilitated by the slowing of blood flow and margination along the vessel surface. Leukocyte adhesion and transmigration from the vascular space into the extravascular tissue is facilitated by adhesion molecules on the leukocyte and endothelial surfaces. After extravasation, leukocytes migrate in the tissues toward the site of injury by chemotaxis, or locomotion oriented along a chemical gradient.

by preventing phagocytic cells from leaving the bloodstream. They decrease the amount of lymphocytes, fibroblasts, and collagen needed for tissue repair.

### Clinical Application 15.1

- Now that Ms. Warren has been given a corticosteroid to decrease the inflammation of her joints, what is she at risk for developing?

## OVERVIEW OF MICROORGANISMS

Infections occur when microorganisms invade a host, attach to host cell receptors, and multiply in sufficient numbers to cause injury. The infection stimulates the body's immune response. In many instances, this immune response is sufficient to contain an infection. However, most microorganisms have characteristics that allow them to adapt to ensure their survival, and these adaptations help protect them from normal body defense mechanisms.

Antimicrobial drugs are an important intervention to treat infections that could otherwise cause significant injury and harm to the human host. To understand antimicrobial drug use, it is important to have a basic understanding of the microorganisms they target. The following sections provide information about microorganisms and how they interact with human hosts.

Microorganisms that cause infectious disease include bacteria, viruses, fungi, and parasites. Bacteria are single-celled microorganisms without nuclei that reproduce by fission or

**Figure 15.3.** Stage 3: opsonization and phagocytosis. Once at the site of injury, the products generated by tissue injury trigger a number of leukocyte responses, including phagocytosis and cell killing. Opsonization of microbes (1) by complement factor C3b and antibody facilitates recognition by neutrophil C3b and the antibody Fc receptor. Receptor activation (2) triggers intracellular signaling and actin assembly in the neutrophil, leading to formation of pseudopods that enclose the microbe within a phagosome. The phagosome (3) then fuses with an intracellular lysosome to form a phagolysosome into which lysosomal enzymes and oxygen radicals (4) are released to kill and degrade the microbe.

splitting. They are classified according to whether they are aerobic (require oxygen) or anaerobic (cannot live in the presence of oxygen), their ability to retain Gram's stain (gram positive) or to reject Gram's stain (gram negative), and their shape (e.g., cocci, rods). **Antibiotics** are antimicrobial drugs used to treat bacterial infections. Viruses are intracellular parasites that survive only in living tissues. They are officially classified according to their structure but are more commonly described according to origin and the disorders or symptoms they produce. Human pathogens include adenoviruses, herpesviruses, and retroviruses (see Chap. 23). Fungi are plantlike microorganisms that live as parasites on living tissue or as saprophytes on decaying organic matter. Approximately 50 species are pathogenic in humans (see Chap. 24). Parasites are microorganisms in the animal kingdom that infect other animals. Parasites that infect human hosts include arthropods, protozoa, and helminths (see Chap. 25).

# Etiology

## Normal Flora

**Colonization** is the presence and growth of microorganisms. The microorganisms do not necessarily cause tissue injury or elicit an immune response in the human body. The human body also has sterile areas, in which microorganisms do not live. Sterile areas that do not communicate directly with the external environment include organs such as the heart and liver, the musculoskeletal system, and body fluids such as urine. Areas typically populated by microorganisms include the skin, upper respiratory tract, and colon.

Normal skin flora includes staphylococci, streptococci, diphtheroids, and transient environmental microorganisms. The upper respiratory tract contains staphylococci, streptococci, pneumococci, and diphtheroids, as well as *Haemophilus influenzae*. The external genitalia contain skin organisms, and the vagina contains lactobacilli, *Candida*, and *Bacteroides*. The colon contains *Escherichia coli*, *Klebsiella*, *Enterobacter*, *Proteus*, *Pseudomonas*, *Bacteroides*, clostridia, lactobacilli, streptococci, and staphylococci.

Normal flora protects the human host in a variety of ways. For example, normal bowel flora synthesizes vitamin K and vitamin B complex. The intestinal flora also plays a role in digestion. Furthermore, by competing with potential pathogens for nutrients and by preventing adhesion and growth of pathogens, beneficial microorganisms interfere with the ability of potential pathogens to cause infections.

In certain instances, normal flora can become pathogenic. For example, microorganisms that are part of the normal flora and nonpathogenic in one area of the body may be pathogenic in other parts of the body; for example, *E. coli* is part of the normal intestinal flora, but it is a common cause of urinary tract infections.

## Host Defense Mechanisms

Although the numbers and virulence of microorganisms help determine whether a person acquires an infection, another major factor is the host's ability to defend itself against the would-be invaders.

Major defense mechanisms of the human body are intact skin and mucous membranes, various **anti-infective** secretions, mechanical movements, phagocytic cells, and the immune and inflammatory processes. The skin prevents penetration of foreign particles, and its secretions and normal bacterial flora inhibit growth of pathogenic microorganisms. Secretions of the gastrointestinal, respiratory, and genitourinary tracts (e.g., gastric acid, mucus) kill, trap, or inhibit growth of microorganisms. Coughing, swallowing, and peristalsis help remove foreign particles and pathogens trapped in mucus, as does the movement of cilia. Phagocytic cells in various organs and tissues engulf and digest pathogens and cellular debris. The immune system produces lymphocytes and antibodies. The inflammatory process is the body's response to injury by microorganisms, foreign particles, chemical agents, or physical irritation of tissues. Inflammation localizes, destroys, dilutes, or removes the injurious agents so tissue healing can occur (see previous discussion).

Many factors impair host defense mechanisms and predispose to infection by disease-producing microorganisms. These factors include the following:

- Breaks in the skin and mucous membranes related to trauma, inflammation, open lesions, or insertion of prosthetic devices, tubes, and catheters for diagnostic or therapeutic purposes
- Impaired blood supply
- Neutropenia and other blood disorders
- Malnutrition
- Poor personal hygiene
- Suppression of normal bacterial flora by antimicrobial drugs
- Suppression of the immune system and the inflammatory response by immunosuppressive drugs, cytotoxic antineoplastic drugs, and adrenal corticosteroids
- Diabetes mellitus and other chronic diseases
- Advanced age

---

**! QSEN Alert: Evidence-Based Practice**

Understanding and applying the principles of hand hygiene is critical for nurses in caring for their patients and themselves. The study by Zivich, Gancz, and Aiello [2018] provides occupational health nurses with evidence to educate their employees on the importance of hand hygiene. The researchers reviewed current literature concerning the effects of hand hygiene on infectious disease prevention in nonclinical office-based workplaces. The literature review revealed that hand hygiene interventions reduced self-reported illnesses. In addition, the authors found that minimal hand hygiene reduced the incidence of employee illness.

---

**Clinical Application 15.2**

- Which alteration in Ms. Warren's defense mechanisms places her at risk for the development of an infection?
- What intervention is primary in preventing the transmission of infection?

## NCLEX  Success

1. A college student is seen in the campus health center with a sore throat. Examination of the throat reveals redness and swelling but no sign of infection. Which of the following is an accurate description of the inflammatory process?

   A. A granuloma will develop if the inflammation is unresolved.
   B. The student is not at risk for the development of an infection.
   C. There is an influx of leukocytes to the throat.
   D. Scarring will result from phagocytic action.

2. A sputum specimen report from the laboratory states, "Contamination with typical oral flora." Which interpretation is correct?

   A. Bacteria in the mouth are growing in the lungs.
   B. The normal flora has become pathogenic.
   C. The patient has a pulmonary infection.
   D. The sputum from the lungs has mixed with bacteria in the mouth.

# Pathophysiology

Infection begins with colonization by microorganisms. Infectious disease occurs when growth of microbial pathogens results in injury and is accompanied by clinical signs and symptoms indicative of an infection. Box 15.1 describes common bacterial pathogens of humans. Accurate assessment and documentation of symptoms can aid in early detection and diagnosis of infectious disease.

## Opportunistic Pathogens

**Opportunistic** microorganisms are usually normal endogenous or environmental flora and nonpathogenic. However, they become pathogens in hosts whose defense mechanisms are impaired. Opportunistic infections are likely to occur in people with severe burns, cancer, human immunodeficiency virus (HIV) infection, indwelling intravenous or urinary catheters, and antibiotic or corticosteroid drug therapy. Opportunistic bacterial infections, often caused by drug-resistant microorganisms, are usually serious and may be life threatening. Fungi of the *Candida* genus, especially *Candida albicans*, may cause life-threatening bloodstream or deep tissue infections, such as abdominal abscesses. Viral infections may cause fatal

## BOX 15.1    *Common Bacterial Pathogens*

### Gram-Positive Bacteria

#### Staphylococci

*Staphylococcus aureus* bacteria are part of the normal microbial flora of the skin and upper respiratory tract and also are common pathogens. Some people carry (are colonized with) *S. aureus* in the anterior nares. The bacteria are spread mainly by direct contact with people who are infected or who are carriers. The hands of health care workers are considered a major source of indirect spread and hospital-acquired infections. The bacteria also survive on inanimate surfaces for long periods of time.

*S. aureus* organisms can cause skin infections such as boils and carbuncles. When burns or surgical wounds become contaminated with *S. aureus*, they often produce endotoxins that destroy erythrocytes, leukocytes, platelets, fibroblasts, and other human cells. These bacteria may also cause infections of the respiratory tract and urinary tract. Also, when many strains are ingested, they produce enterotoxins that cause food poisoning. The enterotoxins survive heating at temperatures high enough to kill the bacteria, so reheating foods does not prevent food poisoning.

High-risk groups for staphylococcal infections include newborns, older adults, and people who are malnourished or obese or who have diabetes. In children, staphylococcal infections of the respiratory tract are most common in those younger than 2 years of age. In adults, staphylococcal pneumonia often occurs in people with chronic lung disease or as a secondary bacterial infection after influenza. The influenza virus destroys the ciliated epithelium of the respiratory tract and thereby aids bacterial invasion.

*Staphylococcus* species, non-*aureus* (SSNA) describes a group of bacteria that are also part of the normal microbial flora of the skin and mucosal surfaces and are increasingly common pathogens. The most common member of this group involved in infections is *Staphylococcus epidermidis*.

Infections due to SSNA are often associated with the use of treatment devices such as intravascular catheters, prosthetic heart valves, cardiac pacemakers, orthopedic prostheses, cerebrospinal fluid shunts, and peritoneal catheters. SSNA infections include endocarditis, bacteremia, and other serious infections and are especially hazardous to immunocompromised patients. Treatment usually requires removal of any infected medical device as well as appropriate antibiotic therapy.

#### Streptococci

Certain streptococci are part of the normal microbial flora of the throat and nasopharynx in many healthy people. These bacteria do not usually cause disease unless the mucosal barrier is damaged by trauma, previous infection, or surgical manipulation. Such damage allows the bacteria to enter the bloodstream and gain access to other parts of the body where they colonize and then cause an infection.

*Streptococcus pneumoniae* bacteria, often called "pneumococci," are common bacterial pathogens. They cause pneumonia, sinusitis, otitis media, and meningitis. Pneumococcal pneumonia usually develops when the mechanisms that normally expel inhaled microorganisms (i.e., the mucociliary blanket and cough reflex) are impaired by viral infection, smoking, immobility, or other insults. When *S. pneumoniae* reach the alveoli, they proliferate, cause acute inflammation, and spread rapidly to involve one or more lobes. Alveoli fill with proteinaceous fluid, neutrophils, and bacteria. Older adults have high rates of illness and death from pneumococcal pneumonia, which can often be prevented by pneumococcal vaccine (see Chap. 12). Pneumococcal sinusitis and otitis media usually follow a viral illness, such as the common cold. The viral infection injures the protective ciliated epithelium and fills the air spaces with nutrient-rich tissue fluid, in which the pneumococci thrive. *S. pneumoniae* is a common pathogen in bacterial sinusitis. In young children, upper respiratory tract infections may be complicated by acute

| **BOX 15.1** | *Common Bacterial Pathogens* (Continued) |

sinusitis. Many children have repeated episodes of pneumococcal otitis media by 6 years of age. Recurrent otitis media during early childhood may result in reduced hearing acuity. Pneumococcal meningitis may develop from sinus or middle ear infections or an injury that allows pneumococcal bacteria from the nasopharynx to enter the meninges. *S. pneumoniae* infection is a common cause of bacterial meningitis in adults. Other potential secondary complications include septicemia, endocarditis, pericarditis, and empyema.

*Streptococcus pyogenes* (beta-hemolytic streptococcus) bacteria are often part of the normal flora of the skin and oropharynx that may become pathogenic in other body regions. The bacteria spread from person to person by direct contact with oral or respiratory secretions. They cause severe streptococcal pharyngitis ("strep throat"), scarlet fever, and rheumatic fever. Endocarditis and glomerulonephritis may occur as sequelae following untreated or inadequately treated streptococcal pharyngitis.

### Enterococci

Enterococci are normal flora in the human intestine but are also found in soil, food, water, and animals. Although the genus *Enterococcus* contains approximately 12 species, the main pathogens are *Enterococcus faecalis* and *Enterococcus faecium*. Most enterococcal infections occur in hospitalized patients, especially those in critical care units. Risk factors for hospital-acquired infections include serious underlying disease, prior surgery, renal impairment, and the presence of urinary or vascular catheters. These bacteria, especially *E. faecalis*, are usually secondary invaders in urinary tract or wound infections. Enterococci may also cause endocarditis. This serious infection occurs most often in people with underlying heart disease, such as an injured valve. When the bacteria reach a heart valve, they multiply and release emboli of foreign particles into the bloodstream. Symptoms of endocarditis include fever, heart murmurs, enlarged spleen, and anemia. This infection is diagnosed by isolating enterococci from blood cultures. If not treated promptly and appropriately, enterococcal endocarditis may be fatal.

### Gram-Negative Bacteria

#### Bacteroides

*Bacteroides* are anaerobic bacteria normally found in the digestive, respiratory, and genital tracts. They are the most common bacteria in the colon. *Bacteroides fragilis*, the major human pathogen, causes intra-abdominal and pelvic abscesses (e.g., after surgery or trauma that allows fecal contamination of these tissues), brain abscesses (e.g., from bacteremia or spread from a middle ear or sinus infection), and bacteremia, which may spread the bacteria throughout the body.

#### Escherichia coli

*E. coli* inhabit the intestinal tract of humans. They are normally nonpathogenic in the intestinal tract where they serve a beneficial role by synthesizing vitamins and by competitively discouraging growth of potential pathogens. In other parts of the body, however, they act as pathogens.

*E. coli* cause most urinary tract infections. They also cause pneumonia and sepsis in immunocompromised hosts and meningitis and sepsis in newborns. *E. coli* pneumonia often occurs in debilitated patients after colonization of the oropharynx. In healthy people, the normal gram-positive

bacteria of oral cavities attach to material that coats the surface of oral mucosa and prevents transient *E. coli* from establishing residence. Debilitated or severely ill people produce an enzyme that destroys the material that allows gram-positive flora to adhere to oral mucosa. This allows *E. coli* (and other gram-negative enteric bacteria) to compete successfully with the normal gram-positive flora and colonize the oropharynx. Then, droplets of the oral flora are aspirated into the respiratory tract, where impaired protective mechanisms allow survival of the aspirated bacteria.

*E. coli* also cause enteric gram-negative sepsis, which is acquired from the normal enteric bacterial flora. When *E. coli* and other gram-negative bacteria reach the bloodstream of healthy people, host defenses eliminate the organisms; however, when the organisms reach the bloodstream of people with severe illnesses or immunocompromised status, the host is unable to mount adequate defenses and sepsis occurs. In newborns, *E. coli* are the most common gram-negative bacteria causing hospital-acquired septic shock and meningitis.

*E. coli* often cause diarrhea and dysentery. One strain, called *O157:H7*, causes hemorrhagic colitis, a disease characterized by severe abdominal cramps, copious bloody diarrhea, and hemolytic uremic syndrome (hemolytic anemia, thrombocytopenia, and acute renal failure). Hemolytic uremic syndrome occurs most often in children. The main reservoir of this strain is the intestinal tract of animals, especially cattle, and several epidemics have been associated with ingestion of undercooked ground beef. Other sources include contaminated water and milk and person-to-person spread.

#### Klebsiella

*Klebsiella* bacteria, which are normal bowel flora, may infect the respiratory tract, urinary tract, bloodstream, burn wounds, and meninges, most often as opportunistic infections in debilitated persons. *Klebsiella pneumoniae* are a common cause of pneumonia, especially in people with pulmonary disease, bacteremia, and sepsis.

### Proteus

*Proteus* bacteria are normally found in the intestinal tract and in decaying matter. They most often cause urinary tract and wound infections but may infect any tissue, especially in debilitated people. Infection often occurs with antibiotic therapy, which decreases drug-sensitive bacteria and allows drug-resistant *Proteus* bacteria to proliferate.

### Pseudomonas

*Pseudomonas* bacteria are found in water, soil, skin, and intestines. They are found in the stools of some healthy people and possibly 50% of inpatients. *Pseudomonas aeruginosa*, the species most often associated with human disease, can cause infections of the respiratory tract, urinary tract, wounds, burns, meninges, eyes, and ears. Because of its resistance to many antibiotics, it can cause severe infections in people receiving antibiotic therapy for burns, wounds, and cystic fibrosis. *P. aeruginosa* colonizes the respiratory tract of most patients with cystic fibrosis and infects approximately 25% of burn patients. Infection is more likely to occur in hosts who are very young or very old or who have an impaired immune system. Sources of infection include catheterization of the urinary tract, trauma or procedures involving the brain or spinal cord, and contamination of respiratory ventilators.

| BOX 15.1 | *Common Bacterial Pathogens* (Continued) |
|---|---|

### Serratia

*Serratia marcescens* bacteria are found in infected people, water, milk, feces, and soil. They cause serious hospital-acquired infections of the urinary tract, respiratory tract, skin, burn wounds, and bloodstream. They also may cause hospital epidemics and produce drug-resistant strains. High-risk patients include newborns, the debilitated, and the immunosuppressed.

### Salmonella

Approximately 1400 *Salmonella* species have been identified; several are pathogenic to humans. The bacteria cause gastroenteritis, typhoid fever, septicemia, and a severe, sometimes fatal type of food poisoning. The primary reservoir is the intestinal tract of many animals. Humans become infected through ingestion of contaminated water or food. Water becomes polluted by introduction of feces from any

animal excreting salmonellae. Infection via food usually results from ingestion of contaminated meat or by hands transferring organisms from an infected source. In the United States, undercooked poultry and eggs are common sources.

*Salmonella* enterocolitis is a common cause of foodborne outbreaks of gastroenteritis. Diarrhea usually begins several hours after ingesting contaminated food and may continue for several days, along with nausea, vomiting, headache, and abdominal pain.

### Shigella

*Shigella* species cause gastrointestinal problems ranging from mild diarrhea to severe bacillary dysentery. Humans, who seem to be the only natural hosts, become infected after ingestion of contaminated food or water. Effects of shigellosis are attributed to loss of fluids, electrolytes, and nutrients and to the ulceration that occurs in the colon wall.

---

pneumonia in people with renal or cardiac disorders, in those with HIV infection, and in those who have received bone marrow transplants.

### Clinical Application 15.3

- Although Ms. Warren realizes that she has an increased risk of infection, she enjoys her work. What factors other than the administration of corticosteroid medications place her at risk for contracting an infection?
- What teaching can a nurse provide to decrease Ms. Warren's risk of infection?

## Laboratory Identification of Pathogens

Laboratory tests of infected fluids or tissues can identify the pathogen that is responsible for an infection. Bacteria and fungi can be differentiated by simple microscopy. In this test, a specimen is applied to a slide and examined under a microscope. Various dyes, such as Gram's stain, and solutions, such as potassium hydroxide, are often applied to help differentiate or further classify microorganisms.

In some cases, there are insufficient microbes in a specimen to identify a causative organism. To obtain a sufficient amount of microbes, laboratory personnel resort to culturing microorganisms from a specimen sample. Culture involves growing a microorganism in the laboratory. Identification of some microorganisms (e.g., intracellular pathogens such as chlamydiae and viruses) requires different techniques. Serology identifies infectious agents indirectly by measuring the antibody level (titer) in the serum of an infected host. A tentative diagnosis can be made if the antibody level against a specific pathogen rises during the acute phase of the disease and falls during convalescence. The **detection of antigens** is a technique to identify pathogens that uses features of culture and serology but reduces the time required for diagnosis. Microbial deoxyribonucleic acid (DNA) and ribonucleic acid can also be

used to identify pathogenic microorganisms. Examples of these tests include DNA probe hybridization and polymerase chain reaction, which can detect whether DNA for a specific organism is present in a sample.

## Community-Acquired Versus Hospital-Acquired Infections

Infections are often categorized as community acquired or hospital acquired. **Community-acquired infections** are infections caused by microorganisms that originated in a community setting outside of a health care facility. One type of common community-acquired infection is **community-acquired pneumonia** (CAP), which is an infection of the lung parenchyma, in which the patient does not acquire the infection in a health care facility. Globally, CAP is the leading cause of morbidity and mortality. In contrast, **hospital-acquired infections** are infections acquired from microorganisms in hospitals and other health care facilities. A hospital-acquired pneumonia is contracted in the hospital. The categorization of **health care–associated pneumonia** is no longer used because it was overly sensitive and led to increased, inappropriately broad antibiotic use. Ventilator-associated pneumonia is pneumonia that is acquired ≥48 hours after endotracheal intubation. As a general rule, community-acquired infections are less severe and easier to treat. Hospital-acquired infections are usually more severe and difficult to manage because they are often caused by microorganisms that are less susceptible to the effects of antimicrobial drugs. These microorganisms are discussed in the next section.

## Antibiotic-Resistant Microorganisms

**Antibiotic resistance** is the ability of certain bacteria to survive and multiply despite antibiotic therapy. Bacteria that have this ability to live in the presence of antibiotics are said to be antibiotic resistant.

Infections that are often associated with high rates of resistance include lower respiratory tract infections and those infections associated with cystic fibrosis or osteomyelitis.

These infections are often difficult to treat because they tend to recur, involve multiple or resistant organisms, or, in the case of osteomyelitis, involve anatomic locations where antibiotics do not penetrate well. The increasing prevalence of antibiotic-resistant bacteria is a major public health concern (Box 15.2). Infections caused by antibiotic-resistant organisms often require more toxic and expensive drugs, leading to prolonged illness or hospitalization and increased mortality rates.

Interestingly, antibiotic overuse can contribute to antibiotic resistance. Resistant organisms are especially likely to emerge in critical care units and large hospitals where seriously ill patients often require extensive antibiotic therapy. The constant presence of antibiotics provides an environment conducive to the survival of the fittest bacteria, which is facilitated by killing of microorganisms that might ordinarily serve to keep these bacteria in check. Furthermore, because pathogenic microorganisms are often spread by contaminated

---

| BOX 15.2 | *Antibiotic-Resistant Staphylococci, Streptococci, and Enterococci* |

### Methicillin-Resistant and Vancomycin-Intermediate/Vancomycin-Resistant *Staphylococcus* Species

Penicillin-resistant staphylococci developed in the early days of penicillin use because these bacteria produced beta-lactamase enzymes (penicillinases) that destroyed penicillin. Methicillin was one of five drugs developed to resist the action of beta-lactamase enzymes; however, eventually, strains of *Staphylococcus aureus* became resistant to these drugs as well. The mechanism of resistance in methicillin-resistant *Staphylococcus aureus* (MRSA) is alteration of penicillin-binding proteins (PBPs). PBPs, the target sites of penicillins and other beta-lactam antibiotics, are proteins required for maintaining integrity of bacterial cell walls. Beta-lactam antibiotics bind to these PBPs and produce defective bacterial cell walls, which kill the bacteria. MRSA have an additional altered PBP. Methicillin cannot bind effectively to this PBP, and so it is unable to inhibit bacterial cell wall synthesis except with very high drug concentrations. Consequently, minimum inhibitory concentrations (MICs) of methicillin increased to high levels that were difficult to achieve.

The term "MRSA" is commonly used but misleading because the bacteria are widely resistant to many antibiotics other than just methicillin. MRSA frequently colonize nasal passages of health care workers and are increasing as a cause of hospital-acquired infections, especially in critical care units. In addition, the incidence of methicillin-resistant *Staphylococcus epidermidis* (MRSE, often reported as methicillin-resistant *Staphylococcus* species, non-*aureus* [SSNA]) isolates is increasing.

A major reason for concern about infections caused by MRSA and MRSE is that bacteria are now developing resistance to vancomycin, an antibiotic previously used extensively to treat or prevent infections caused by *S. aureus*, *S. epidermidis*, and enterococci. Options to treat these infections are limited, and measures to reduce the incidence and prevent spread of methicillin- and vancomycin-resistant organisms are of paramount importance.

### Penicillin-Resistant *Streptococcus pneumoniae* (Pneumococci)

Penicillin has long been the drug of choice for treating pneumococcal infections caused by *S. pneumoniae* (e.g., CAP, bacteremia, meningitis, and otitis media). However, penicillin-resistant strains and multidrug-resistant strains are being identified with increasing frequency. Risk factors for the development of resistant strains include frequent antibiotic use and prophylactic use of antibiotics. After resistant strains have developed, they spread to other people, especially in areas where people are in close contact such as in children's daycare centers and in hospital settings.

*S. pneumoniae* are thought to develop resistance to penicillin by decreasing the ability of their PBPs to bind with penicillin. Bacteria displaying high-level penicillin resistance may also be cross-resistant to drugs from the same or similar antibiotic classes. To decrease the spread of resistant *S. pneumoniae*, the Centers for Disease Control and Prevention (CDC) has proposed:

- Improved surveillance to delineate prevalence by geographic area and assist clinicians in choosing appropriate antimicrobial therapy.
- Rational use of antibiotics to reduce exposures to drug-resistant pneumococci. For example, prophylactic antibiotic therapy for otitis media may increase colonization and infection of young children with drug-resistant organisms.
- Pneumococcal vaccination for people older than 2 years of age with increased risk of pneumococcal infection and for all people older than 65 years of age.

### Vancomycin-Resistant Enterococci

Enterococci are a component of normal intestinal flora that can act as pathogens if they infect other areas of the body. Vancomycin is an antibiotic that was commonly used to treat these bacteria; however, in large part to the widespread use of vancomycin to treat other drug-resistant staphylococcal infections such as MRSA and MRSE, vancomycin-resistant *Enterococcus* (VRE) have emerged. Additionally, some strains of enterococci have developed additional resistance to other antibiotics. The incidence of multi-drug-resistant enterococci and VRE has increased in recent years.

To decrease the spread of VRE, the CDC recommends limiting the use of vancomycin. Specific recommendations include avoiding or minimizing its use in routine surgical prophylaxis, empiric therapy for febrile patients with neutropenia (unless the prevalence of MRSA or MRSE is high), systemic or local prophylaxis for intravascular catheter infection or colonization, selective decontamination of the gastrointestinal tract, eradication of MRSA colonization, primary treatment of antibiotic-associated colitis, and routine prophylaxis for very low-birth-weight infants or patients on continuous ambulatory peritoneal dialysis. Thorough hand hygiene and environmental cleaning are also important, because VRE can survive for long periods on hands, gloves, stethoscopes, and environmental surfaces. Personnel must remove or change gloves after contact with patients known to be colonized or infected with VRE. Ideally, designated stethoscopes are restricted for use only with VRE-infected patients. If stethoscopes must be used for both VRE-infected and uninfected patients, it is important to thoroughly clean stethoscopes between patients.

hands or objects, patients in critical care units are more at risk for infection with antibiotic-resistant organisms resulting from person-to-person transmission by health care workers or equipment.

Resistant organisms and the antibiotics to which they develop resistance vary in geographic areas, communities, and hospitals according to the use of particular antibiotics. Nationally, resistant bacterial strains of major concern include penicillin-resistant *Streptococcus pneumoniae*, MRSA and MRSE, VRE, extended-spectrum beta-lactamase (ESBL)-producing gram-negative bacilli, and multidrug-resistant tuberculosis (MDR-TB). All of these organisms are resistant to multiple antibiotics. A CAP caused by drug-resistant *S. pneumoniae* is difficult to treat. Risk factors associated with this CAP are age of 65 years or older and a history of immunosuppressive illness or therapy, alcoholism, and medical comorbidities. Use of beta-lactam, macrolide, or fluoroquinolone therapy in the past 3 to 6 months increases the prevalence of *S. pneumoniae* CAP. Drug-resistant organisms are described in Box 15.2, and MDR-TB is discussed in Chapter 22. Viruses and fungi also develop resistance to antimicrobial drugs, as discussed in Chapters 23 and 24, respectively.

---

> ! **QSEN Alert: Safety**
>
> It is essential to monitor patients receiving antibiotics closely for evidence of improvement. A failure to improve within 24 to 36 hours could indicate antibiotic resistance.

---

**NCLEX Success**

3. When a woman who is taking an antibiotic develops a thick, white, curdlike vaginal discharge with pruritus, the nurse suspects that the patient has a vaginal yeast infection. What would explain this development?
   A. A drug for a fungal infection should have been prescribed instead of a drug for bacterial infection.
   B. The antibiotic has altered the normal vaginal environment.
   C. The antibiotic that was prescribed was not effective.
   D. Yeast infections are side effects of antibiotics.

4. A health care worker has nasal colonization of methicillin-resistant *Staphylococcus aureus* (MRSA). Which interpretation of this finding by the nurse is correct?
   A. The health care worker has a nasal infection caused by MRSA.
   B. The health care worker poses a danger to patients.
   C. The health care worker is immune to MRSA.
   D. The health care worker produces beta-lactamase.

---

> **Clinical Application 15.4**
>
> • Despite taking care to prevent an infection, Ms. Warren becomes ill and develops a fever with other signs and symptoms of an infection. The family nurse practitioner asks her what infectious illnesses her assigned patients have had and whether she has had direct contact with these patients. The nurse also asks if any of her friends or family members have been ill. What rationale underlies the nurse's questions?

---

## Mechanisms of Antibiotic Resistance in Bacteria

Bacterial resistance to antimicrobial drugs may be either intrinsic or acquired.

The five main processes of intrinsic mechanisms of resistance are outlined below:

1. Bacteria may inactivate the antibiotic. For example, some bacteria produce enzymes that change the chemical structure of certain antibiotics, thus rendering them ineffective.
2. Bacteria may modify target sites for the antibiotic. For example, **penicillin-binding proteins** (PBPs) are bacterial proteins that function in cell wall synthesis. Penicillin typically binds to these bacterial proteins. By altering the PBPs, the bacteria prevent the antibiotic from recognizing and engaging this target.
3. Bacteria may alter metabolic pathways or substitute the usual enzymes needed to carry out activities involved with growth and reproduction. In doing this, bacteria develop resistance to antibiotics that exert their effect by interfering with enzymes needed for growth and reproduction.
4. Bacteria may alter their cell wall structure to reduce permeability. This confers resistance to antibiotics that must enter the bacterial cell to attach to a target.
5. Some bacteria have the ability to pump drug molecules out of the cell (efflux). By removing the antibiotic, the bacteria prevent the antibiotic from engaging the target site and exerting an effect.

The mechanisms of acquired resistance include genetic alterations. The three processes of acquired resistance are as follows:

1. In gene transfer, bacteria are in close approximation to then transfer to genetic content. For example, bacteria with inherent mechanisms for antibiotic resistance may transfer genetic content material that confers this antibiotic resistance to other species of bacteria. When these genetically altered bacteria replicate, the resistance is passed on to subsequent generations of bacteria.
2. In transfer mutations, the mutations often develop during bacterial replication. If the mutation provides antibiotic resistance, the mutated bacteria can continue to multiply and thus produce billions of copies of resistant microorganisms.
3. Selective pressure, or natural selection, refers to the survival of the fittest bacteria. When antibiotic therapy is initially begun, the weakest bacteria are killed first while the strongest bacteria,

which are best able to withstand the effects of antibiotic therapy, remain. If antibiotic therapy is stopped prematurely before these more resistant microorganisms are overcome, the more resistant organisms predominate. These mechanisms explain why, when a new antibiotic is used, resistance may rapidly appear and be disseminated to multiple bacteria.

## Clinical Manifestations

The clinical manifestations of infections are outlined in Box 15.2.

## Drug Therapy

Several terms are used to describe drugs that are used to treat infections caused by microorganisms. Anti-infective, like antimicrobial, is a general descriptive term that designates agents with **antibacterial**, antiviral, and antifungal properties. Antibacterial is a term that designates agents that kill bacteria or interfere with the ability of bacteria to grow and replicate. An antibiotic is a drug that has the ability to kill or inhibit bacterial growth and replication; therefore, an antibiotic is an antibacterial drug. Antibiotics are used to treat bacterial infections.

Both antiviral and antifungal drugs are agents that have the ability to destroy or inhibit the replication of viruses or fungi, respectively. Antiviral drugs are used to treat viral infections, and antifungal drugs are used to treat fungal infections.

Additional terms are used to describe the properties of antibacterial drugs. **Broad-spectrum** antibiotics are antibacterial drugs that are effective against a wide range of bacteria (e.g., both gram-positive and gram-negative bacteria), whereas narrow-spectrum antibiotics are those that are effective against a limited range or a specific type of bacteria. Generally, a narrow-spectrum antibiotic is preferred over a broad-spectrum antibiotic when possible because broad-spectrum drugs are more likely to kill some normal flora, which disrupts the microbial balance. As a result, the patient is at greater risk for an opportunistic infection when taking a broad-spectrum antibiotic. The action of an antibacterial drug is usually described as **bactericidal** (kills the bacteria) or **bacteriostatic** (inhibits growth of the bacteria). Whether a drug is bactericidal or bacteriostatic often depends on its concentration at the infection site and the sensitivity of the bacteria to the drug. Because successful treatment with bacteriostatic antibiotics depends on the ability of the host's immune system to eliminate the inhibited bacteria, bactericidal drugs are preferred in serious infections, especially in people with impaired immune function.

Antimicrobials are among the most frequently used drugs worldwide. Their success in saving lives and decreasing severity and duration of infectious diseases has encouraged their extensive use. Unfortunately, these same attributes have led to antibiotic overuse, misuse, or abuse. Inappropriate use of antibiotics is responsible for unnecessary adverse drug effects, emergence of drug-resistant microorganisms, and increases in health care costs. All health care professionals should note that the goal of treatment with antibiotics is to eradicate the causative microorganism and return the host to full physiologic functioning. This differs from the goal of most drug therapy, which is to relieve signs and symptoms rather than cure the underlying disorder.

Guidelines to promote more appropriate use of antimicrobial drugs include the following:

- Avoid the use of antibacterial drugs to treat viral infections; antibacterial drugs are ineffective in viral infections.
- Give antibacterial drugs only when a significant bacterial infection is diagnosed or strongly suspected or when there is an established indication for prophylaxis.
- Use a narrow-spectrum antibacterial drug instead of a broad-spectrum drug, whenever possible, in order to decrease the risk of a superinfection.
- Collect specimens (e.g., sputum, urine) for culture and Gram's stain before giving the first dose of an antibiotic. For best results, specimens must be collected accurately and taken directly to the laboratory. If analysis is delayed, contaminants may overgrow pathogenic microorganisms.
- Minimize antimicrobial drug therapy for fever unless other clinical manifestations or laboratory data indicate infection.
- Follow recommendations of the CDC for prevention and treatment of infections, especially those caused by drug-resistant organisms (e.g., gonorrhea, penicillin-resistant streptococcal infections, MRSA, VRE, MDR-TB).
- Consult infectious disease physicians, infection control nurses, and infectious disease pharmacists about local patterns of drug-resistant organisms and treatment of complicated infections.

Box 15.3 presents patient teaching guidelines for antimicrobials.

### Empiric Therapy

Because laboratory tests used to definitively identify causative organisms and to determine **susceptibility** to antibiotics usually require 48 to 72 hours, the prescriber usually initiates treatment with an antimicrobial drug that is likely to be effective. Drug therapy undertaken prior to obtaining a definite diagnosis is called empiric therapy. This empiric therapy is based on an informed estimate of the most likely pathogen(s) given the patient's signs and symptoms and the site of infection, as well as knowledge of communicable diseases currently infecting other people in the community. For example, urinary tract infections are often caused by *E. coli*; thus, an antibiotic that is effective against this microorganism is indicated.

### Culture and Sensitivity Studies

Culture identifies the causative microorganism. The sensitivity is the laboratory test to determine the susceptibility of an antimicrobial agent in the treatment of the causative microorganism. Once a specific microorganism is identified by laboratory culture, it is important to determine susceptibility, which is the vulnerability of the bacteria to the effects of an antibiotic. Susceptibility tests determine which drugs are likely to be effective against the organism. Laboratory reports indicate whether the organism is susceptible (S) or resistant (R) to the tested drugs. It is then possible to "match the drug to the bug."

 *Concept Mastery Alert*

Culturing bacteria helps identify the causative organism. To determine which antibiotic agents would be effective for the causative organism, a susceptibility test is performed.

## BOX 15.3 | *Patient Teaching Guidelines for Antimicrobial Drugs*

### General Considerations

- Wash hands often and thoroughly, especially before preparing food or eating and after exposure to body secretions (e.g., urine, feces, sputum, nasal secretions). This is probably the most effective way to prevent infection and to avoid spreading an infection to others.
- Eat a balanced diet and get adequate fluid intake, rest, and exercise. This helps the body fight infection, prevents further infection, and increases the effectiveness of antimicrobial drugs by optimizing body processes.
- Take all prescribed doses of an antimicrobial drug. This prevents recurrence of the infection. Also, stopping antimicrobial drugs when symptoms are relieved can lead to the development of antibiotic-resistant microorganisms that cause infections that are more severe and harder to treat.
- Report any problems that occur when taking an antimicrobial drug. This allows identification of important adverse effects that can be managed through interventions or through substitution by another equally effective antimicrobial drug.
- Discard all discontinued antimicrobial drugs. This is important because antimicrobial drugs are carefully selected to treat specific illnesses, so taking inadequate amounts of an inappropriate drug can cause greater harm than benefit.
- Report any other drugs being taken to the prescriber. This is necessary in order to avoid drug interactions that could have harmful consequences.
- Report any drug allergies to all health care providers and wear a medical identification emblem that lists allergens. This is necessary to ensure that the antimicrobial drug ordered is safe.

- Notify the prescriber if you are pregnant. This is important because some antimicrobial drugs can cause problems for the developing fetus.
- Be aware that antibiotics are not indicated for treatment of viral infections. If an antibiotic is not indicated, taking it may result in more harm than good.

### Self-Administration

- Take antimicrobial drugs at evenly spaced intervals around the clock, unless instructed otherwise. This helps maintain adequate blood levels.
- Ask if the antimicrobial drug can be taken with food. This is important because food may decrease drug absorption for some oral antimicrobials; therefore, these are taken on an empty stomach, approximately 1 hour before or 2 hours after meals.
- Store most liquid preparations in the refrigerator, check expiration dates, and discard any that remains after all prescribed doses have been taken. This is important to ensure that the medicine remains stable and is evenly dispersed in solution.
- Take the medications with a full glass of water. This helps tablets and capsules to dissolve better in the stomach and decreases stomach irritation.
- Report nausea, vomiting, diarrhea, skin rash, recurrence of symptoms for which the antimicrobial drug was prescribed, or signs of new infection (e.g., fever, cough, sore mouth, drainage) to a health care professional. These problems may indicate adverse effects of the drug, lack of therapeutic response to the drug, or another infection. Any of these requires evaluation and may indicate changes in drug therapy.

---

One indication of susceptibility is the minimum inhibitory concentration (MIC). The MIC is the lowest concentration of an antibiotic that prevents visible growth of microorganisms. Some laboratories report MIC instead of, or in addition to, S or R.

Susceptible organisms have low or moderate MICs that can be attained by giving usual doses of an antimicrobial agent. For the drug to be effective, its serum and tissue concentrations should usually exceed the MIC of an organism for a certain period. By how much and for how long drug concentrations need to exceed the MIC depend on the drug class and the bacterial species. Some antibiotics may be given for shorter lengths of time as a result of a postantibiotic effect, a persistent effect of an antimicrobial on bacterial growth after brief exposure of the organisms to a drug.

Resistant organisms have high MICs and may require higher concentrations of drug than can be achieved in the body. In some cases, the minimum bactericidal concentration (MBC) is reported, indicating no growth of the organism in the presence of a particular antibiotic. The MBC is especially desirable for infected hosts with impaired immune functions.

A patient's response to antimicrobial therapy cannot always be correlated with the MIC of an infecting pathogen. Thus,

reports of drug susceptibility testing must be applied in the context of the site of infection, the characteristics of the drug, and the clinical status of the patient.

## NCLEX Success

5. **When a patient fails to respond to an antibiotic, the nurse suspects antibiotic resistance. Which mechanism of resistance does the nurse recognize as an example of acquired antibiotic resistance?**

   A. Alterations are made in the bacterial cell wall structure to make it less permeable.

   B. Bacteria exchange genetic content that transfers resistance from one bacterial strain to another.

   C. Efflux is used to extrude bacteria from within the bacterial cell.

   D. Metabolic pathways are altered so bacteria targeting a specific enzyme of the metabolic pathway are ineffective.

6. A patient who is taking an antibiotic for an infection shows no signs of improvement. When a laboratory report indicates that the causative organism is not susceptible to the prescribed antibiotic, what is the priority nursing intervention? (Select all that apply.)
   A. Notify the pharmacist to provide a different antibiotic.
   B. Notify the prescriber of the culture report.
   C. Stop the current antibiotic and use the susceptible antibiotic.
   D. Inform the patient that the antibiotic is ineffective.
   E. Notify the prescriber of the sensitivity report.

7. What is the best action a nurse can take to prevent infection?
   A. Instruct patients with respiratory illnesses on proper pulmonary hygiene.
   B. Recommend influenza and pneumococcal vaccines to patients older than 65 years of age.
   C. Teach a patient the importance of adequate nutrition and rest.
   D. Wash hands before and after each patient contact.

## Patterns of Antibiotic Resistance

Over time, patterns of antibiotic resistance change in the community and in health care facilities; therefore, continuing efforts must be made to identify which antibiotics are most effective. Bacteria that are resistant to certain antibiotics are typically susceptible to others. Infectious disease specialists and laboratory personnel are helpful resources to identify resistance patterns and trends in these instances, and this information may be considered when deciding empiric therapy.

## Ability to Penetrate Infected Tissues

Several antimicrobials are effective in urinary tract infections because they concentrate in the urine. However, the choice of an effective antimicrobial drug may be limited in infections of the brain, eyes, gallbladder, or prostate gland because many drugs are unable to reach therapeutic concentrations in these tissues. For infection in these areas, the prescriber will consider the ability of the drug to penetrate the affected region rather than deciding therapy based solely on susceptibility testing.

## Toxicity and Risk-to-Benefit Ratio

In general, the least toxic drug is used; however, for serious infections, drugs with an increased risk of toxicity may be necessary. In these instances, the prescriber will weigh the benefits of treatment versus the risks of adverse effects when determining therapy.

## Cost

It is always necessary to take the cost of the medication into account. If a less expensive drug is likely to be effective in a given infection, it is recommended instead of a more expensive agent. For hospitals and nursing homes, personnel costs relating to preparation and administration are also important to consider. For example, for the patient who cannot swallow tablets, a liquid preparation may be less expensive to prepare than a tablet that needs to be crushed.

## Combination Therapy

Antimicrobial drugs are often used in combination. Indications for combination therapy may include the following:

- Infections caused by multiple microorganisms (e.g., abdominal and pelvic infections).
- Hospital-acquired infections, which may be caused by many different organisms.
- Serious infections in which a combination of antimicrobial drugs is synergistic.
- Likely emergence of drug-resistant organisms if a single drug is used (e.g., in tuberculosis).
- Fever or other signs of infection in patients whose immune system is suppressed. Combinations of antibacterial plus antiviral and/or antifungal drugs may be needed.
- Implement isolation procedures appropriately, when indicated.
- To prevent spread of respiratory infections, teach patients to cough into the bend of their elbow instead of covering their mouth or nose with hands or tissues. Advise patients to avoid crowds when they are ill.
- To prevent the likelihood that patients will acquire infections, advise them to avoid crowds during influenza season (approximately November through February) and when other communicable diseases are spreading through the local community. Recommend an annual influenza vaccine and pneumococcal vaccine (see Chap. 12) to high-risk populations (e.g., people with chronic diseases such as diabetes and heart, lung, or renal problems; older adults; health care personnel who are likely to be exposed).
- Assist or instruct patients at risk about pulmonary hygiene measures to prevent accumulation or promote removal of respiratory secretions. These measures include ambulating, turning, coughing and deep breathing exercises, and incentive spirometry.
- Use sterile technique when changing any dressing. If a wound is not infected, sterile technique helps prevent infection. If the wound is already infected, sterile technique avoids introducing new bacteria. Remove dressings with clean gloves, discard them in a moisture-proof bag, and wash hands before putting on sterile gloves to apply the new dressing.
- To minimize the spread of infections, adhere to current established guidelines published by the CDC for isolation precautions to prevent transmission of infectious agents in health care settings. The Standard Precautions for All Patient Care and Transmission-Based Precautions are available at https://www.cdc.gov/infectioncontrol/basics/standard-precautions.html and https://www.cdc.gov/infectioncontrol/basics/transmission-based-precautions.html.
- For patients with infections, monitor temperature for increased or decreased fever and monitor the WBC count for changes.
- For patients receiving antimicrobial therapy, maintain an adequate fluid intake to assist with renal clearance to decrease drug toxicity.
- Assist the patient with hand hygiene, maintaining nutrition and fluid balance, getting adequate rest, and handling secretions correctly. These measures help the body to fight the infection, prevent further infection, and enhance the effectiveness of antimicrobial medications.
- Assist patients in using antimicrobial drugs safely and effectively.
- Instruct patient on all aspects of medication administration.

## THE NURSING PROCESS

A concept map outlines the nursing process related to drug therapy considerations in this chapter. Additional nursing implications related to the disease process should also be considered in care decisions.

**Assessment**

- Assess for inflammation and infection.
- Understand that the general signs and symptoms of infection are the same as for inflammation. Local signs of inflammation include redness, heat, edema, and pain; systemic signs include fever and leukocytosis.
- Assess for signs and symptoms of inflammation. Inflammation is the normal response to any injury; infection requires the presence of a microorganism. The two often occur together. Inflammation may weaken the tissue, allowing microorganisms to invade and cause infection. Infection (tissue injury by microorganisms) stimulates inflammation.
- Assess for the presence of factors that increase the risk of infection.
- Assess culture and sensitivity reports for appropriate antibacterial therapy.
- Assess for drug allergies. If the patient has allergies, assess for specific signs and symptoms.
- Assess baseline renal and hepatic function.

**Outcomes of Therapy**

The patient will
- Adhere to anti-inflammatory medication regimen as ordered.
- Receive antimicrobial drugs accurately when given by health care providers or caregivers.
- Take drugs as prescribed and for the length of time prescribed when self-administered as an outpatient.
- Experience decreased inflammation, fever, white blood cell (WBC) count, and other signs and symptoms of infection.
- Be monitored regularly for therapeutic and adverse drug effects.
- Receive prompt recognition and treatment of potentially serious adverse effects.
- Verbalize and practice measures to prevent future infections.
- Be safeguarded against hospital-acquired infections by health care providers.

**Evaluation**

- Evaluate the patient's adherence to medication administration.
- Evaluate for adverse drug effects.
- Evaluate for decreasing signs and symptoms of infection and inflammation.
- Evaluate patient's understanding of patient teaching regarding antimicrobial medications and anti-inflammatory agents.

## KEY CONCEPTS

- Inflammation is the cellular response of the body to injury by chemicals, physical trauma, or infectious agent.
- Aspirin, NSAIDs, and corticosteroids are administered to decrease inflammation.
- Aspirin and NSAIDs block the synthesis of prostaglandin in the central and peripheral nervous system.
- Corticosteroids inhibit interleukin-1, cytokines, and the tumor necrosis factor.
- Normal flora has a beneficial role in the human host but can become pathogenic if they invade a normally sterile part of the body or if environmental controls fail to limit their growth.
- Infection occurs when growth of microbial pathogens causes injury to host tissues.
- Opportunistic infections occur when harmless microorganisms in normal flora become pathogenic under conditions that are favorable for their overgrowth.

- Community-acquired infections are infections caused by microorganisms from a community setting outside of a health care facility, whereas hospital-acquired infections are infections acquired from microorganisms in hospitals and other health care facilities.
- Hospitals and other health care facilities are places where there is an increased prevalence of antibiotic-resistant bacteria, which are increasing in prevalence, are associated with prolonged illness and hospitalization and increased mortality rates, and have become a public concern.
- Bacterial mechanisms of antibiotic resistance include inactivation of an antibiotic, modification of target cells for antibiotics, alteration of metabolic pathways, alteration of bacterial cell wall structure, and efflux. These mechanisms may be passed to other classes of bacteria through gene transfer.

- Human defenses against infection include intact skin and mucous membranes, secretions that inhibit bacterial growth, mechanical movements such as coughing, and immune and inflammatory responses; when defenses are compromised, the risk of infection increases.
- Antimicrobial drugs are an important intervention to treat infections that could otherwise cause significant injury and harm to the human host.
- Antibacterial drugs are a type of antimicrobial drug that is used to treat bacterial infections; these are commonly called antibiotics.
- Antibiotics are generally not indicated for viral infections, fungal infections, and other infections not caused by bacteria.
- Broad-spectrum antibiotics are effective against a wide range of bacteria. Narrow-spectrum antibiotics are effective against a limited range of bacteria.
- Bactericidal antibiotics kill bacteria, and bacteriostatic antibiotics inhibit bacterial growth and reproduction.
- Antibiotics exert an effect by inhibiting bacterial metabolism, inhibiting cell wall synthesis, inhibiting protein synthesis, or inhibiting nucleic acid function or synthesis.
- Decisions regarding antimicrobial selection are based on several factors, including the causative organism, site of infection, risk-to-benefit ratio, and cost.
- Combination therapy is used to treat multiple microorganisms.

## CLINICAL REASONING CASE STUDY

**Meet the Patient**

James Kujawa, a 3-year-old boy, has streptococcal pharyngitis (strep throat). His pediatrician has prescribed amoxicillin 125 mg twice a day for 7 days. Amoxicillin elixir is 125 mg/5 mL. You are providing patient teaching to the parents. They are to administer 5 mL every 8 hours.

- What is the action of amoxicillin?
- The mother states she does not know what milliliters are. How will you instruct her on the medication administration?
- You instruct the parents on the importance of finishing the entire amount of medication and to never skip a dose. What is the purpose of this teaching?
- The mother asks if she can give the medication to the child's sister to prevent "strep throat." What patient teaching will need to be implemented with the mother?
- The parents return in 1 week and state the child was feeling better after 3 days so they stopped the medication. What is the child at risk for developing?

**Assessing Drug Information**

- Amoxicillin is a broad-spectrum semi-synthetic aminopenicillin. It inhibits the final step of bacterial cell wall synthesis. It binds to specific penicillin binding proteins in the cell wall of the rapidly multiplying bacteria.
- Monitor for the development of rash with the administration of the first few doses of amoxicillin.
- Store amoxicillin elixir in the refrigerator and out of James' reach.
- Finish the entire prescription in the 7 days it has been prescribed to prevent the development of future superinfections.

**Nursing Actions**

- Instruct the parents that a teaspoon measuring spoon is equal to 5 mL.
- James' parents could also use a 5-mL syringe provided by the nurse or pharmacist. They should fill the syringe to the 5 mL mark, then place the elixir in James' cheek, allowing him to swallow it slowly.
- Instruct James' parents to observe for development of a rash with the administration of the first few doses. If a rash develops they should notify the pediatrician.
- Reinforce the importance of finishing the entire prescription. Not completing the course of treatment creates a scenario that contributes to bacterial resistance. It may also lead to additional problems because the streptococcal strain that causes strep throat may cause cardiac or renal problems if not adequately treated.
- Stress that antibiotics are not indicated for prevention of strep throat in healthy people with competent immune systems.

Visit thePoint® at **http://thePoint.lww.com/Frandsen12e** for answers to NCLEX Success questions (in Appendix A), answers to Clinical Application Case Studies (in Appendix B), and more!

## REFERENCES AND RESOURCES

Centers for Disease Control and Prevention. (2019). *Standard precautions for all patient care.* Retrieved from https://www.cdc.gov/infectioncontrol/basics/standard-precautions.html

Centers for Disease Control and Prevention. (2019). *Transmission-based precautions.* Retrieved from https://www.cdc.gov/infection-control/basics/transmission-based-precautions.html

Norris, T. L. (2019). *Porth's pathophysiology: Concepts of altered health states.* Philadelphia, PA: Lippincott Williams & Wilkins.

Ramirez, J. A. (2019). Antibiotic studies for the treatment of community-acquired pneumonia in adults. In *UpToDate.* Waltham, MA.

Turbett, S. E., & Pierce, V. M. (2019). Overview of antibacterial susceptibility testing. In *UpToDate.* Waltham, MA.

Zivich, P. N., Gancz, A. S., & Aiello, A. E. (2018). Effect of hand hygiene on infectious diseases in the office workplace: A systemic review. *American Journal of Infection Control, 46,* 448–455. doi:10.1016/j.ajic.2017.10.006

# Drug Therapy to Decrease Pain, Fever, and Inflammation

## LEARNING OBJECTIVES

*After studying this chapter, you should be able to:*

1. Discuss the role of prostaglandins in the etiology of pain, fever, and inflammation.
2. Identify the major manifestations of fever and inflammation.
3. Understand the pathophysiology of osteoarthritis.
4. Understand the pathophysiology of gout.
5. Identify the prototype and describe the action, use, adverse effects, contraindications, and nursing implications for the salicylates.
6. Identify the action, use, adverse effects, contraindications, and nursing implications for acetaminophen.
7. Identify the prototype and describe the action, use, adverse effects, contraindications, and nursing implications for the propionic acid derivatives.
8. Identify the prototype and describe the action, use, adverse effects, contraindications, and nursing implications for the oxicam derivatives.
9. Identify the prototype and describe the action, use, adverse effects, contraindications, and nursing implications of the acetic acid derivatives.
10. Identify the prototype and describe the action, use, adverse effects, contraindications, and nursing implications of the selective COX-2 inhibitors.
11. Identify the prototype and describe the action, use, adverse effects, contraindications, and nursing implications for the mitotic agent.
12. Identify the prototype and describe the action, use, adverse effects, contraindications, and nursing implications for uricosuric medications.
13. Know how to implement the nursing process in the care of patients undergoing drug therapy for pain, fever, and inflammation.

## CLINICAL APPLICATION CASE STUDY

Audrey Mason is a 72-year-old retired physical education teacher and housewife, who is being seen by her primary care provider for bilateral hip and knee pain. She has been taking a minimum of eight 325-mg aspirins per day without pain relief. Her physician orders x-rays of her hips and knees, which reveal osteoarthritis in both joints. She begins taking ibuprofen [Motrin] 600 mg three times per day. In addition, she receives a diagnosis of degenerative joint disease related to osteoarthritis and a referral to an orthopedic surgeon. The surgeon schedules Mrs. Mason for a right total knee replacement in 1 month. Because she is 40 lb overweight, the surgeon places her on a calorie-reduction diet.

## KEY TERMS

**Antiprostaglandin:** drug that inhibits the synthesis of prostaglandins

**Antipyretic:** drug that has the ability to lower body temperature

**Arachidonic acid:** phospholipid released in the cell membrane in response to cellular injury

**Cyclooxygenase:** enzyme that produces prostaglandins from arachidonic acids

**Hyperuricemia:** elevated levels of uric acid in the blood resulting from accelerated generation of uric acid through purine metabolism or impaired renal excretion of uric acid

**Nonsteroidal anti-inflammatory drug (NSAID):** medication that inhibits the synthesis of prostaglandins; used to prevent and treat mild to moderate pain and inflammation

**Prostaglandin:** chemical mediator found in most body tissues; helps regulate many cell functions and participate in the inflammatory response as well as initiate uterine contractions in labor

**Pyrogen:** fever-producing agent

**Reye's syndrome:** potentially fatal disease characterized by encephalopathy and fatty liver accumulations; associated with the use of aspirin and NSAIDs after viral infections such as chickenpox or influenza in children and adolescents

**Salicylism:** toxic effects of a salicylate drug; may occur with an acute overdose or with chronic use of therapeutic doses, especially the higher doses taken for anti-inflammatory effects

**Tophi:** deposits of uric acid crystals in the joints, kidneys, and soft tissues

**Uricosuric:** drug that increases urinary excretion of uric acid

## INTRODUCTION

This chapter provides an introduction to the pharmacologic care of the patient who is experiencing pain, fever, or inflammation. The pharmacologic agents administered for inflammation can also diminish fever and relieve pain. Acetaminophen also decreases fever and relieves pain, but it does not reduce inflammation. Other topics of discussion will be osteoarthritis and gout. This will allow the nurse to apply knowledge of disease that produces inflammation and the related administration of anti-inflammatory agents to reduce pain. The drugs discussed in this chapter include aspirin (acetylsalicylic acid), acetaminophen, and the **nonsteroidal anti-inflammatory drugs** (NSAIDs), as well as those drugs used to prevent or treat gout.

It is important to note that aspirin, acetaminophen, and NSAIDs can also be called **antiprostaglandins** because they inhibit the synthesis of prostaglandins. **Prostaglandins** are chemical mediators found in most body tissues; they help regulate many cell functions and participate in the inflammatory response. They are formed when cellular injury occurs and phospholipids in cell membranes respond by releasing **arachidonic acid**. Cyclooxygenase (COX) enzymes then metabolize arachidonic acid to produce prostaglandins, which act briefly in the area where they are produced and are then inactivated. The enzyme COX-1 is normally synthesized continuously and is present in all tissues and cell types, especially in platelets and endothelial cells as well as in the gastrointestinal (GI) tract and the kidneys. Prostaglandins produced by COX-1 are important in numerous homeostatic functions and have protective effects on the stomach and kidneys. In the stomach, prostaglan-

dins decrease gastric acid secretion, increase mucus secretion, and regulate blood circulation. In the kidneys, they help maintain adequate blood flow and function. In the cardiovascular system, they help regulate vascular tone (i.e., vasoconstriction and vasodilation) and platelet function. Drug-induced inhibition of these prostaglandins results in the adverse effects associated with aspirin and related nonselective NSAIDs, especially gastric irritation, ulceration, and bleeding. Inhibition of COX-1 activity in platelets may be more responsible for GI bleeding than inhibition of COX-1 activity in gastric mucosa.

 *Concept Mastery Alert*

COX-1 enzymes are continuously present in all tissues, not just at the time of inflammation. They secrete a cyto-protective mucus.

COX-2 is also normally present in several tissues (e.g., brain, bone, kidneys, GI tract, female reproductive system). However, it is thought to occur in small amounts or to be inactive until stimulated by pain and inflammation. In inflamed tissues, COX-2 is induced by inflammatory chemical mediators such as interleukin-1 (IL-1) and tumor necrosis factor alpha (TNF-alpha). In the GI tract, trauma and *Helicobacter pylori* infection, a common cause of peptic ulcer disease, also induce COX-2. Overall, prostaglandins produced by COX-2 are associated with pain and other signs of inflammation. Inhibition of COX-2 results in the therapeutic effects of analgesia and anti-inflammatory activity. The COX-2 inhibitor drugs are NSAIDs designed to selectively inhibit COX-2 and relieve pain and

*[handwritten margin note: heart kidneys Prostaglandins Stomach]*

inflammation with fewer adverse effects than those that inhibit both COX-1 and COX-2, especially stomach damage. However, with long-term use, adverse effects still occur in the GI, renal, and cardiovascular systems.

As indicated in Table 16.1 and Figure 16.1, prostaglandins exert various and opposing effects in different body tissues.

## OVERVIEW OF PAIN, FEVER, AND INFLAMMATION

To adequately understand the administration of aspirin, acetaminophen, and NSAIDs, it is important to understand the role prostaglandins play in mediating pain, fever, and inflammation.

### Pain

Pain is the sensation of discomfort, hurt, or distress. It is a common human ailment and may occur with tissue injury and inflammation. Prostaglandins sensitize pain receptors and increase the pain associated with other chemical mediators of inflammation and immunity, such as bradykinin, histamine, and leukotriene (Box 16.1).

### Fever

Fever is an elevation of body temperature above the normal range. Body temperature is controlled by a regulating center in the hypothalamus. Normally, there is a balance between heat production and heat loss so that a constant body temperature is maintained. When there is excessive heat production, mechanisms to increase heat loss are activated. As a result, blood vessels dilate, more blood flows through the skin, sweating occurs, and body temperature usually stays within normal range.

Fever occurs when the set point of the hypothalamus is raised in response to the presence of **pyrogens** (fever-producing agents). Endogenous pyrogens include cytokines such as IL-1, IL-6, and tumor necrosis factor (see Box 16.1). Exogenous pyrogens include bacteria and their toxins or other by-products. The upward adjustment of the hypothalamic set point in response to the presence of a pyrogen is mediated by prostaglandin $E_2$ (see Table 16.1). The body responds to the higher hypothalamic set point by vasoconstriction of blood vessels and shivering, raising the core body temperature to the higher set point. Fever may accompany conditions such as dehydration, inflammation, infectious processes, some drug use, brain injury, or diseases involving the hypothalamus.

### Inflammation

Inflammation is the normal body response to tissue damage from any source, and it may occur in any tissue or organ. It is an attempt by the body to remove the damaging agent and repair the damaged tissue. The signs and symptoms of inflammation are the work of a variety of chemical mediators (see Box 16.1). Prostaglandin $E_2$ and others induce inflammation and also enhance the effects of other mediators of the inflammatory response. Local manifestations are redness, heat, edema, and pain. Redness and heat result from vasodilation and increased blood supply. Edema results from leakage of blood plasma into the area. Pain occurs when pain receptors on nerve endings are stimulated by heat, edema, and pressure; chemicals released by the damaged cells; and prostaglandins. Systemic manifestations include leukocytosis, increased erythrocyte sedimentation rate, fever, headache, loss of appetite, lethargy or malaise, and weakness. Both local and systemic manifestations vary according to the cause and extent of tissue damage. In addition, inflammation may be acute or chronic. See Chapter 15 for more information.

Inflammation may be a component of virtually any illness. Inflammatory conditions affecting organs or systems are often named by adding the suffix "itis" to the involved organ or system (e.g., hepatitis). Current research findings suggest that inflammation may be important in the pathology of disorders

## TABLE 16.1

### Prostaglandins

| Prostaglandin | Locations | Effects |
|---|---|---|
| PGD$_2$ | Airways, brain, mast cells | Bronchoconstriction |
| PGE$_2$ | Brain, kidneys, vascular smooth muscle, platelets | Bronchodilation<br>Gastroprotection<br>Increased activity of the GI smooth muscle<br>Increased sensitivity to pain<br>Increased body temperature<br>Vasodilation |
| PGF$_2$ | Airways, eyes, uterus, vascular smooth muscle | Bronchoconstriction<br>Increased activity of the GI smooth muscle<br>Increased uterine contraction (e.g., menstrual cramps) |
| PGI$_2$ (prostacyclin) | Brain, endothelium, kidneys, platelets | Decreased platelet aggregation<br>Gastroprotection<br>Vasodilation |
| PGA$_2$ (thromboxane A$_2$) | Kidneys, macrophages, platelets, vascular smooth muscle | Increased platelet aggregation<br>Vasoconstriction |

GI, gastrointestinal.

**Figure 16.1.** Metabolic pathways for arachidonic acid result in production of physiologic and pathologic (i.e., inflammatory) prostaglandins. Nonselective and selective nonsteroidal anti-inflammatory drugs (NSAIDs) inhibit production of prostaglandins by inhibiting steps in the arachidonic acid pathway. GI, gastrointestinal.

---

*Chemical Mediators of Inflammation and Immunity*

**Bradykinin** is a kinin in body fluids that becomes physiologically active with tissue injury. When tissue cells are damaged, white blood cells (WBCs) increase in the area and ingest damaged cells to remove them from the area. When the WBCs die, they release enzymes that activate kinins. The activated kinins increase and prolong the vasodilation and increased vascular permeability caused by histamine. They also cause pain by stimulating nerve endings for pain in the area. Thus, bradykinin may aggravate and prolong the erythema, heat, and pain of local inflammatory reactions. It also increases mucous gland secretion.

**Complement** is a group of plasma proteins essential to normal inflammatory and immunologic processes. More specifically, complement destroys cell membranes of body cells (e.g., red blood cells, lymphocytes, platelets) and pathogenic microorganisms (e.g., bacteria, viruses). The system is initiated by an antigen–antibody reaction or by tissue injury. Components of the system (called C1 through C9) are activated in a cascade type of reaction in which each

component becomes a proteolytic enzyme that splits the next component in the series. Activation yields products with profound inflammatory effects. C3a and C5a, also called anaphylatoxins, act mainly by liberating histamine from mast cells and platelets, and their effects are therefore similar to those of histamine. C3a causes or increases smooth muscle contraction, vasodilation, vascular permeability, degranulation of mast cells and basophils, and secretion of lysosomal enzymes by leukocytes. C5a performs the same functions as C3a and also promotes movement of WBCs into the injured area (chemotaxis). In addition, it activates the lipoxygenase pathway of arachidonic acid metabolism in neutrophils and macrophages, thereby inducing formation of leukotrienes and other substances that increase vascular permeability and chemotaxis.

In the immune response, the complement system breaks down antigen–antibody complexes, especially those in which the antigen is a microbial agent. It enables the body to produce inflammation and localize an infective agent. More

BOX 16.1    *Chemical Mediators of Inflammation and Immunity* (Continued)

specific reactions include increased vascular permeability, chemotaxis, and opsonization (coating a microbe or other antigen so it can be more readily phagocytized).

**Cytokines** may act on the cells that produce them, on surrounding cells, or on distant cells if sufficient amounts reach the bloodstream. Thus, cytokines act locally and systemically to produce inflammatory and immune responses, including increased vascular permeability and chemotaxis of macrophages, neutrophils, and basophils. Two major types of cytokines are interleukins (produced by leukocytes) and interferons (produced by T lymphocytes or fibroblasts). IL-1 mediates several inflammatory responses, including fever; IL-2 (also called T-cell growth factor) is required for the growth and function of T lymphocytes. Interferons are cytokines that protect nearby cells from invasion by intracellular microorganisms, such as viruses and rickettsiae. They also limit the growth of some cancer cells.

**Histamine** is formed (from the amino acid histidine) and stored in most body tissue, with high concentrations in mast cells, basophils, and platelets. Mast cells, which are abundant in skin and connective tissue, release histamine into the vascular system in response to stimuli (e.g., antigen–antibody reaction, tissue injury, and some drugs). After it is released, histamine is highly vasoactive, causing vasodilation (increasing blood flow to the area and producing hypotension) and increasing permeability of capillaries and venules (producing edema). Other effects include contracting smooth muscles in the bronchi (producing bronchoconstriction and respiratory distress), GI tract, and uterus; stimulating salivary, gastric, bronchial, and intestinal secretions; stimulating sensory nerve endings to cause pain and itching; and stimulating movement of eosinophils into injured tissue. Histamine is the first chemical mediator released in the inflammatory response and immediate hypersensitivity reactions (anaphylaxis).

When histamine is released from mast cells and basophils, it diffuses rapidly into other tissues. It then acts on target tissues through both histamine-1 (H$_1$) and histamine-2 (H$_2$) receptors. H$_1$ receptors are located mainly on smooth muscle cells in blood vessels and the respiratory and GI tracts. When histamine binds with these receptors, resulting events include contraction of smooth muscle, increased vascular permeability, production of nasal mucus, stimulation

of sensory nerves, pruritus, and dilation of capillaries in the skin. H$_2$ receptors are also located in the airways, GI tract, and other tissues. When histamine binds to these receptors, there is increased secretion of gastric acid by parietal cells in the stomach mucosal lining, increased mucus secretion and bronchodilation in the airways, contraction of esophageal muscles, tachycardia, inhibition of lymphocyte function, and degranulation of basophils (with additional release of histamine and other mediators) in the bloodstream. In allergic reactions, both types of receptors mediate hypotension (in anaphylaxis), skin flushing, and headache. The peak effects of histamine occur within 1 to 2 minutes of its release and may last as long as 10 minutes, after which it is inactivated by histaminase (produced by eosinophils) or *N*-methyltransferase.

**Leukotrienes**, like prostaglandins, are derived from arachidonic acid metabolism. Leukotrienes, identified as LTB$_4$, LTC$_4$, LTD$_4$, and LTE$_4$, mediate inflammation and immune responses. LTB$_4$ plays a role in chemotaxis, mediating the aggregation of leukocytes at sites of injury. LTC$_4$, LTD$_4$, and LTE$_4$ produce smooth muscle contractility, bronchospasm, and increased vascular permeability.

**Nitric oxide** (NO) is synthesized by a variety of cells by the enzyme NO synthase from the amino acid arginine. It readily diffuses across cell membranes, where it reacts with a wide variety of molecules and is inactivated. NO inhibits aggregation of platelets, preventing formation of blood clots. NO relaxes smooth muscles in blood vessels, producing vasodilation. It inhibits inflammation in the walls of blood vessels. NO also plays a role in protecting against invading microbes. Helper T lymphocytes, active in the inflammatory response, secrete NO. NO also enhances the killing of phagocytized microbes within the lysosomes of cells.

**Platelet-activating factor** (PAF), like prostaglandins and leukotrienes, is derived from arachidonic acid metabolism and has multiple inflammatory activities. It is produced by mast cells, neutrophils, monocytes, and platelets. Because these cells are widely distributed, PAF effects can occur in virtually every organ and tissue. Besides causing platelet aggregation, PAF activates neutrophils, attracts eosinophils, increases vascular permeability, causes vasodilation, and causes IL-1 and TNF-alpha to be released. PAF, IL-1, and TNF-alpha can induce each other's release.

(not previously identified as inflammatory conditions) such as heart disease and Alzheimer's disease. Anti-inflammatory drugs are indicated when the inflammatory response is inappropriate, abnormal, or persistent or destroys tissue.

Table 16.2 lists the medications administered in the reduction of pain, fever, and inflammation.

## SPECIFIC CONDITIONS

### OSTEOARTHRITIS

Osteoarthritis produces inflammation and degeneration of joints. To adequately understand the pharmacologic treatment of osteoarthritis, it is important to understand the etiology, pathophysiology, and clinical manifestations of the disease.

## Etiology

Aging plays a significant role in the destruction of joints. The degeneration of the articular cartilage begins at approximately 30 years of age and peaks between 50 and 60 years. Primary osteoarthritis occurs without a history of an injury or disease. Secondary osteoarthritis results from a previous injury or the presence of an inflammatory process. Other factors that contribute to the development of osteoarthritis include obesity, repetitive use of a joint, and congenital predisposition.

## Pathophysiology

The articular cartilage is the smooth weight-bearing surface at the ends of long bones. The main function of cartilage is to absorb shock and decrease friction during movement and weight-bearing

## TABLE 16.2

## Medications Administered for Pain, Fever, and Inflammation

| Drug Class | Prototype | Other Drugs in the Class |
|---|---|---|
| Salicylate | Aspirin (acetylsalicylic acid) | Choline magnesium trisalicylate<br>Salsalate<br>Magnesium salicylate (Doans Pills) |
| Nonnarcotic analgesic antipyretic | Acetaminophen (Tylenol, paracetamol) | |
| **Nonsteroidal anti-inflammatory drugs (NSAIDs)** | | |
| Propionic acid derivatives | Ibuprofen (Motrin) | Diflunisal<br>Fenoprofen (Fenortho, Nalfon)<br>Flurbiprofen<br>Ketoprofen<br>Meclofenamate sodium<br>Mefenamic acid<br>Nabumetone<br>Naproxen sodium (Aleve, Anaprox)<br>Oxaprozin (Daypro)<br>Tolmetin sodium |
| Oxicam derivatives | Meloxicam (Mobic) | Piroxicam (Feldene) |
| Acetic acid derivatives | Indomethacin (Indocin, Tivorbex) | Diclofenac potassium (Cambia, Zorvolex)<br>Etodolac (Lodine)<br>Ketorolac<br>Nabumetone<br>Sulindac |
| Selective COX-2 inhibitor | Celecoxib (CeleBREX) | |

COX-2, cyclooxygenase-2.

activities. The cartilage transmits the load down to the subchondral bone, dissipating the mechanical stress at the joint. Along with the synovial fluid in the joint, the articular cartilage reduces friction when the joint moves. Osteoarthritis is the degradation of the cartilage, bone, and synovium. Repetitive movement of a joint causes the articular cartilage to be worn down, leading to joint failure. Chondrocytes develop in the joint with the release of enzymes, causing the joint to degenerate. Progressively, the articular cartilage is lost, and inflammation develops in the synovial fluid.

## Clinical Manifestations

Osteoarthritis produces joint pain, stiffness, and instability, possibly with some degree of immobility. The joints commonly affected by osteoarthritis are the carpometacarpal joint (the distal joint of the hand) and metatarsophalangeal joint of the feet, knees, hips, and cervical or lumbar vertebrae. The pain experienced by the patient is related to the inflammation of the synovium. As the synovial fluid increases, the joint capsule becomes stretched and causes irritation to the nerve endings of the periosteum. Joint stiffness is most common on arising, especially on awaking in the morning, and decreases with movement. An impaired joint can limit mobility and cause structural changes.

## Drug Therapy

Medications used in the treatment of osteoarthritis include aspirin, acetaminophen, and NSAIDs (see Table 16.2). As previously mentioned, all of these medications produce an analgesic effect

and reduce fever. However, only aspirin and the NSAIDs reduce inflammation. As the medications are discussed, their properties will be explained in detail, identifying their use and implications for administration. See Figure 16.2.

### Clinical Application 16.1

- In an education session with Mrs. Mason, the nurse employed by Mrs. Mason's insurance provider is instructing her about the pathophysiology of osteoarthritis. What information should the nurse provide?
- What is the rationale for placing Mrs. Mason on a calorie-reduction diet?

### NCLEX Success

1. A man arrives in the emergency department with a swollen right ankle from a fall. He is complaining of pain and limited mobility. What factor is contributing to the pain in the right ankle? (Select all that apply.)
   A. blocking of cyclooxygenase-1 (COX-1)
   B. blocking of COX-1 and COX-2
   C. release of prostaglandin $E_2$
   D. release of cytochrome P450
   E. release of arachidonic acid

**Figure 16.2.** Tissue injury and the action of nonsteroidal anti-inflammatory agents.

2. A home care nurse is visiting an 88-year-old man, who is taking acetaminophen for arthritic pain in his knees. Which of the following patient teaching statements is most appropriate to implement?

 A. "Acetaminophen will only relieve pain but not the inflammation from arthritis."
 B. "Acetaminophen is appropriate for the treatment of inflammation from arthritis."
 C. "Your primary health care provider should consider a prescription of Vicodin (acetaminophen/hydrocodone)."
 D. "The acetaminophen should be administered on an empty stomach."

3. A patient is admitted to the emergency department with dehydration. Which of the following assessments of the patient's vital signs does the nurse expect to assess?

 A. elevated blood pressure
 B. diminished pulse
 C. diminished respirations
 D. elevated temperature

# GOUT

Gout is an arthritic condition characterized by an overproduction of uric acid or an inability to excrete uric acid, resulting in **hyperuricemia**. Not all patients with hyperuricemia will develop symptoms of gout; in those patients who do have inflammation, it is caused by uric acid crystal deposits in the synovial joint lining. The joint then becomes enlarged due to the infiltration of neutrophils, monocytes, and leukocytes (Becker & Gaffo, 2020). Uric acid is a by-product of purine metabolism. Hyperuricemia occurs when the serum uric acid level exceeds 6.8 mg/dL, the saturation point at which urate crystallizes in biologic fluids at normal body temperature.

There are three stages of gout. Acute gouty arthritis or gouty attack, the first stage, is characterized by hyperuricemia, pain, and swelling of one joint. The pain usually begins at night and persists for 10 days. The most commonly affected joint is the great toe. Intercritical gout, the second stage, is characterized by a symptom-free period of several years followed by the recurrence of symptoms. Chronic tophaceous gout, the third stage, is characterized by the presence of solid deposits of urate crystals, known as **tophi**, in the joints and elsewhere (Fig. 16.3). In the kidneys, urate deposits may form renal calculi or cause other damage (Becker & Perez-Ruiz, 2020). After the first attack of acute gouty arthritis, up to 10 years may pass before permanent damage to the joints and kidneys occurs.

The treatment of gout involves the administration of NSAIDs and corticosteroids (see Chap. 17) to reduce inflammation as well as **uricosuric** agents to increase the elimination of uric acid. Table 16.3 lists the antigout medications and uricosuric agents. These drugs will be discussed later in this chapter.

> **! QSEN Alert: Evidence-Based Practice**
>
> Ma, Chen, Zhao, and Zhai (2018) conducted a meta-analysis to assess the use of naproxen role in reducing the occurrence of heterotropic ossification after hip surgery. The study included 269 patients. The results of the study indicated that naproxen decreased the occurrence of heterotopic ossification without increasing complications of hip surgery.

**Figure 16.3.** **A.** Gouty tophi projections. **B.** Tophi: Jelly-like projections under the skin.

**TABLE 16.3**

**Medications Administered for Gout**

| Drug Class | Prototype | Other Drugs in the Class |
|---|---|---|
| Mitotic agent | Colchicine (Colcrys, Mitigare) | |
| Uricosuric | Allopurinol (Zyloprim) | Febuxostat (Uloric) Pegloticase (Krystexxa) Probenecid Rasburicase (Elitek) |

## SALICYLATES

The salicylates, of which aspirin is the prototype, relieve pain by acting both centrally and peripherally to block the transmission of pain impulses. They act peripherally to prevent the sensation of pain receptors to various chemical substances released by damaged cells. These **antipyretic** agents also reduce fever by acting on the hypothalamus to decrease its response to pyrogens and resetting the body temperature at a lower level. In addition, these drugs diminish inflammation by preventing prostaglandins from increasing the pain and edema produced by other substances released by damaged cells.

Aspirin and other salicylates also have the ability to suppress platelet aggregation. Low-dose aspirin is indicated for patients who have experienced an ischemic stroke, transient ischemic attack, angina, and acute myocardial infarction (or any myocardial infarction), reducing the risk of death and/or a recurrent event (level A recommendations). This indication stems from its antiplatelet activity and resultant effects on blood coagulation (i.e., decreased clot formation). Low-dose aspirin, 75 to 81 mg/day, is used for primary prevention of myocardial infarction or stroke in healthy adults. High-dose aspirin, 4 to 8 g/day, is effective in reducing inflammation in rheumatoid disorders.

## Pharmacokinetics

Aspirin is administered orally or rectally with an onset of action of 5 to 30 minutes orally and 1 to 2 hours rectally. The oral preparation peaks in 15 to 120 minutes, and the duration of action is 3 to 6 hours. The rectal preparation peaks in 4 to 5 hours, and the duration of action is 6 to 8 hours. The drug is metabolized in the liver and has a half-life of 15 minutes to 12 hours. Excretion takes place in the urine. The drug crosses the placenta and enters the breast milk.

## Action

The ability of aspirin to inhibit prostaglandins produces the inflammatory effects needed for analgesia and antirheumatic effects. Its antipyretic effects are less well understood. Authorities believe that the drug acts on the thermoregulatory center of the hypothalamus, thus blocking the effects of the endogenous pyrogens and inhibiting the synthesis of prostaglandins. Aspirin also has antiplatelet effects. At low doses, it blocks the synthesis of thromboxane $A_2$ to inhibit platelet aggregation; this lasts for the life of the platelet.

## Use

As an analgesic agent, aspirin is used to relieve mild to moderate pain. As an antipyretic agent, it is used only in adults (see "Use in Children"). As an anti-inflammatory agent, it is used to decrease inflammation in patients with osteoarthritis, juvenile rheumatoid arthritis, and spondyloarthropathies. In addition, aspirin is used for its antiplatelet effects to reduce the risk of transient ischemic attacks and cerebrovascular accidents as well as the risk of death from myocardial infarction. Aspirin, 625 mg, is given to patients who have undergone coronary artery bypass grafting 6 hours after the procedure and daily for 1 year afterward. Table 16.4 presents specific dosage information for aspirin and other salicylates. In the event a woman is pregnant and diagnosed with polycythemia vera, which is uncommon in women of childbearing age, she will require a low-dose aspirin regimen throughout pregnancy despite known adverse effects to the fetus.

### Use in Children

Aspirin is not recommended because of its association with Reye's syndrome, a life-threatening illness characterized by encephalopathy, hepatic damage, and other serious problems. This syndrome usually occurs after a viral infection, such as influenza or chickenpox, during which aspirin was given for fever.

### Use in Older Adults

Aspirin is safe in therapeutic doses for analgesic and antipyretic use. In addition, it is usually safe in the low doses prescribed for prevention of myocardial infarctions and cerebrovascular accidents.

### Use in Patients With Renal Impairment

Aspirin is nephrotoxic in high doses, and protein binding of aspirin is reduced in patients with renal failure, which means that blood levels of the active drug are higher than they would be otherwise. Aspirin can also decrease the blood flow in the kidneys by inhibiting the synthesis of prostaglandins that dilate renal blood vessels. When renal blood flow is normal, these prostaglandins have limited activity. However, when renal blood flow is decreased, synthesis of these prostaglandins is increased, and they protect the kidneys from ischemia and hypoxia by antagonizing the vasoconstrictive effects of angiotensin II, norepinephrine, and other substances. Thus, in patients who depend on prostaglandins to maintain an adequate renal blood flow, the prostaglandin-blocking effects of aspirin result in constriction of renal arteries and arterioles, decreased renal blood flow, decreased glomerular filtration rate, and retention of salt and water.

## Adverse Effects

GI adverse effects of aspirin include nausea, dyspepsia, heartburn, and epigastric discomfort. Decreased platelet aggregation results in GI blood loss and hemorrhage. In addition, petechiae and bruising may also occur. Aspirin toxicity occurs at levels above 300 mcg/mL. Acute toxicity results in respiratory alkalosis, hyperpnea, tachypnea, hemorrhage, confusion, pulmonary edema, seizures, tetany, metabolic acidosis, fever,

**TABLE 16.4**

**DRUGS AT A GLANCE: Salicylates**

| Drug | Pregnancy Category | Routes and Dosage Ranges | |
|---|---|---|---|
| | | **Adults** | **Children** |
| Ⓟ **Aspirin** (acetylsalicylic acid; 🍁 Asaphen) | D | Pain, fever: PO 325–650 mg every 4 h PRN; usually single dose, 650 mg<br>Osteoarthritis or rheumatoid arthritis: PO 2–6 g/d in divided doses<br>Acute rheumatic fever: PO 5–8 g/d, in divided doses<br>Prophylaxis of myocardial infarction, transient ischemic attack, and cerebrovascular accident: PO 81–325 mg/d<br>Transient ischemic attack: PO 1300 mg/d in divided doses (650 mg twice a day or 325 mg four times a day)<br>Acute myocardial infarction: PO 162–325 mg or rectal suppository 600 mg<br>Pregnant women with polycythemia vera: PO 75 mg daily during pregnancy | **Do not administer to children with chickenpox or influenza.**<br>**Recommended daily doses by weight:**<br>24–35 lb (10.6–15.9 kg), 162 mg; 36–47 lb (16–21.4 kg), 243 mg; 48–59 lb (21.5–26.8 kg), 324 mg; 60–71 lb (26.9–32.3 kg), 405 mg; 72–95 lb (32.4–43.2 kg), 486 mg; 96 lb or above (43.3 kg or above), 648 mg<br>Pain, fever: PO 10–15 mg/kg every 4 h, up to 60–80 mg/kg/d<br>Juvenile rheumatoid arthritis: PO 90–130 mg/kg/d, divided doses, every 6–8 h; target plasma salicylate level, 150–300 mg/mL<br>Acute rheumatic fever: PO 100 mg/kg/d, divided doses, for 2 wk, then 75 mg/kg/d for 4–6 wk |
| Choline magnesium trisalicylate | C | Arthritis: PO 1.5–2.5 g/d in divided doses; do not exceed 4.5 g/d<br>Pain or fever: PO 2–3 g/d in divided doses | PO 217.5–652.5 mg every 4 h as needed |
| Magnesium salicylate (Doans Pills) | C | PO 650 mg three to four times per day | Older than 2 y of age: PO 50–75 mg/kg/d divided in 4–6 doses (maximum: 3.6 g/d) |
| Salsalate | C | Osteoarthritis or rheumatoid arthritis: PO 20 mg/d or 10 mg twice daily | Dosage not established |

coma, and cardiovascular collapse. Renal and respiratory failure occurs with doses of 20 to 25 g in adults and 4 g in children. **Salicylism**, toxicity due to salicylates that may be associated with chronic use, is characterized by dizziness, tinnitus, difficulty hearing, and mental confusion.

## Contraindications

Aspirin is contraindicated in patients with a known sensitivity to aspirin; in those who are allergic to tartrazine, due to a cross-sensitivity; and in those with a known risk of bleeding. The U.S. Food and Drug Administration (FDA) has issued a **BLACK BOX WARNING ◆** stating that children or teenagers should not take aspirin to treat chickenpox or flulike symptoms because of the risk of Reye's syndrome. This condition is a potentially fatal disease characterized by encephalopathy and fatty liver accumulations. It is associated with the use of aspirin and NSAIDs in children and adolescents after viral infections such as chickenpox or influenza.

Aspirin should be administered cautiously to patients with impaired renal function. It is a salicylate that crosses the placenta entering the fetal circulation placing the fetus at risk for adverse effects such as intrauterine growth retardation, salicylate toxicity, increased risk of bleeding, and neonatal acidosis.

Low birth weight, increased intracranial bleeding, and stillbirth have been reported in infants of mothers who took aspirin late in pregnancy.

## Nursing Implications

### Preventing Interactions

Medications and herbs interact with aspirin, increasing or decreasing its effects (Boxes 16.2 and 16.3).

### Administering the Medication

Aspirin should be taken with a full glass of water or other fluid and with food or just following food. Administering the medication with food decreases gastric irritation. Although the crushing of tablets or capsules results in faster absorption, this action destroys the long-acting feature and increases the risk of adverse effects and toxicity.

The dose of aspirin given depends mainly on the condition being treated. Low doses (325 mg initially and 75–81 mg daily) are used for the drug's antiplatelet effects in preventing arterial thrombotic disorders such as myocardial infarction and stroke. Because aspirin is highly protein bound, lower-than-average doses are needed for patients with low serum albumin levels,

## BOX 16.2 — *Drug Interactions: Aspirin*

### Drugs That Increase the Effects of Aspirin

- Acidifying agents [e.g., vitamin C]
  *Acidify urine and thereby decrease the urinary excretion rate of salicylates*
- Anticoagulants, oral
  *Increase the risk of bleeding; patients taking anticoagulants should not take aspirin*
- Angiotensin-converting enzyme inhibitors, beta-adrenergic blockers
  *Decreased antihypertensive effects*
- Codeine, hydrocodone, and oxycodone
  *Have additive analgesic effects due to mechanism of action*
- Corticosteroids
  *Have additive gastric irritation and possible ulcerogenic effects*

### Drugs That Decrease the Effects of Aspirin

- Alkalinizing agents [e.g., sodium bicarbonate]
  *Increase the rate of renal excretion*
- Ibuprofen
  *Competes with aspirin for COX-1 inhibition*
  *Negates the cardioprotective benefits of low-dose aspirin*
- Misoprostol
  *Prevents aspirin-induced gastric ulcers*

*low dose· antiplatelet*

because a larger proportion of each dose is free to exert pharmacologic activity. Larger doses are needed for anti-inflammatory effects (maximum daily dosage, 8000 mg) than for analgesic and antipyretic effects (325–650 mg every 4 hours). In general, patients taking low-dose aspirin to prevent myocardial infarction or stroke should continue to take the aspirin if their prescribers order a COX-2–inhibiting NSAID because the COX-2 inhibitors have little effect on platelet function.

## Assessing for Therapeutic Effects

When administering aspirin, the nurse assesses for the therapeutic effects of the drug. If aspirin is given for pain, the nurse uses a pain scale to assess the intensity of the patient's pain, which should decrease. If the drug is given for fever, the nurse records the patient's temperature every 2 to 4 hours and should see a reduction in temperature. If the drug is given for inflammation, the nurse assesses for signs of inflammation, which should decrease. Patients receiving aspirin as a preventive agent for myocardial infarction or transient ischemic attack should be without chest pain or confusion.

## BOX 16.3 — *Herb and Dietary Interactions: Aspirin*

### Herbs and Foods That Increase the Effects of Aspirin

- Alcohol
- Ginkgo

*Herbs*

## Assessing for Adverse Effects

The nurse assesses the patient for bleeding tendencies, GI irritation, nausea, vomiting, and diarrhea, which all may result from aspirin use. The nurse assesses the skin for signs of decreased coagulation. The nurse performs a thorough pulmonary and integumentary assessment, looking for signs of hypersensitivity to aspirin, including dyspnea, bronchospasm, and rash.

### Toxicity: Recognition and Management

Salicylate intoxication (salicylism) may occur with an acute overdose or with chronic use of therapeutic doses, especially the higher doses taken for anti-inflammatory effects. Chronic ingestion of large doses saturates a major metabolic pathway, thereby slowing drug elimination, prolonging the serum half-life, and causing drug accumulation. The therapeutic serum level of salicylate is 100 to 300 mcg/mL for the treatment of arthritis and rheumatic fever. Toxicity occurs at levels above 300 mcg/mL.

As previously stated, salicylism is characterized by dizziness, tinnitus, difficulty hearing, and mental confusion. Additional manifestations include nausea, vomiting, fever, fluid and electrolyte deficiencies, visual changes, drowsiness, hyperventilation, and other conditions. Severe central nervous system (CNS) dysfunction (e.g., delirium, stupor, coma, seizures) indicates life-threatening toxicity.

### Treatment of Overdose

In mild salicylate toxicity, stopping the drug or reducing the dose is usually sufficient. In severe salicylate overdose, treatment is symptomatic and aimed at preventing further absorption from the GI tract, increasing urinary excretion, and correcting fluid, electrolyte, and acid–base imbalances. When the drug may still be in the GI tract, gastric lavage and activated charcoal help reduce absorption. Intravenous (IV) sodium bicarbonate produces an alkaline urine in which salicylates are more rapidly excreted, and hemodialysis effectively removes salicylates from the blood. IV fluids are indicated when high fever or dehydration is present. The specific content of IV fluids depends on the serum electrolyte and acid–base status.

### Patient Teaching

Box 16.4 presents patient teaching guidelines for aspirin.

## Other Drugs in the Class

Choline magnesium trisalicylate, a weak inhibitor of COX-1 and COX-2, provides a decrease in the formation of prostaglandins, producing antipyretic, analgesic, and anti-inflammatory effects. The primary use of choline magnesium trisalicylate is in the management of acute shoulder pain. Other uses are the relief of osteoarthritis, rheumatoid arthritis, and juvenile idiopathic arthritis.

Magnesium salicylate is a less potent prostaglandin than aspirin. It can cause acid–base imbalances. As with all salicylates, the patient should be taught the risk of GI bleed. The drug is well observed and peaks in 20 minutes.

## BOX 16.4 — *Patient Teaching Guidelines for Aspirin*

- Keep aspirin out of the reach of children.
- Use the drug as directed, and do not overadminister the medication due to the risk of toxicity.
- Take the medication with food or after meals to prevent stomach upset.
- Do not crush or chew enteric-coated or sustained-release tablets.
- Aspirin is as effective as more costly medication.
- Watch for bleeding, ringing in the ears, or diminished hearing.
- Understand that fever is one way the body fights infection. Taking the medication for fever is not usually recommended unless the fever is high or is accompanied by other symptoms.
- Avoid aspirin for approximately 2 weeks before and after major surgery or dental procedures to decrease the risk of excessive bleeding. If pregnant, do not take aspirin for approximately 2 weeks before the estimated delivery date.
- Inform a health care provider if you have ever had an allergic reaction [e.g., asthma, difficulty breathing, hives], severe GI symptoms [e.g., ulcer, bleeding], or rash or other skin disorder after taking aspirin.
- Avoid and minimize ingestion of alcohol due to gastric irritation and risk of bleeding.
- Use aspirin cautiously with patients on a low-sodium diet; one aspirin tablet contains 553 mg of sodium.

Salsalate is a salicylate with antipyretic, analgesic, antirheumatic, and anti-inflammatory properties. It is indicated for relief of pain and fever as well as treatment of rheumatic fever, rheumatoid arthritis, and osteoarthritis. It is absorbed in the small intestine rather than in the stomach and is reported to cause fewer GI adverse effects than aspirin. Onset, peak, and duration of action are similar to aspirin. The drug is metabolized in the liver and excreted in the urine.

### Clinical Application 16.2

- Mrs. Mason is taking eight 325-mg aspirin tablets per day without adequate pain relief. She is at risk for what adverse effects associated with aspirin?

## NCLEX Success

4. A nurse is teaching a child care class to prospective grandparents. Which of the following medications is contraindicated in children?

   A. ibuprofen
   B. acetaminophen
   C. amoxicillin
   D. aspirin

5. An automobile worker visits an occupational health nurse. He has pain in his right hand due to repetitive movements, for which he has been taking aspirin 650 mg every 2 hours. Which of the following symptoms is indicative of salicylate toxicity?

   A. ringing in the ears
   B. halos around lights
   C. edema
   D. dysrhythmia

6. A physician tells a patient to take aspirin for back pain. It is most important to instruct the patient to

   A. take the medication on an empty stomach to enhance absorption
   B. take the medication after a meal to prevent gastric irritation
   C. crush the enteric-coated tablet for increased effectiveness
   D. take the medication 2 hours after a meal to enhance absorption

## NONNARCOTIC ANALGESIC ANTIPYRETIC: ACETAMINOPHEN

**Acetaminophen** (also called APAP, an abbreviation of *N*-acetyl-*p*-aminophenol) is a nonprescription drug commonly used as an aspirin substitute because it does not cause nausea, vomiting, or GI bleeding and it does not interfere with blood clotting. It is equivalent to aspirin in analgesic and antipyretic effects; however, it does not have the anti-inflammatory activity of aspirin.

### Pharmacokinetics

Acetaminophen is well absorbed with oral administration, and peak plasma concentrations are reached within 30 to 120 minutes. Duration of action is 3 to 4 hours. Acetaminophen is metabolized in the liver (Fig. 16.4). Approximately 94% is excreted in the urine as nontoxic glucuronate and sulfate conjugates, and 2% is excreted unchanged. The remaining 4% is metabolized by cytochrome P450 enzymes to a toxic metabolite, which is normally inactivated by conjugation with glutathione and excreted in the urine. With usual therapeutic doses, a sufficient amount of glutathione is available in the liver to detoxify acetaminophen.

### Action

To reduce fever, acetaminophen acts directly on the hypothalamus to increase vasodilation and sweating. To diminish pain, it acts via an unknown mechanism of action.

### Use

Acetaminophen is used to reduce fever and decrease minor pain. The drug is sometimes given to children and patients at risk for seizures who are receiving the diphtheria, pertussis, and tetanus

**Figure 16.4.** Metabolic pathway for acetaminophen. CYP450, cytochrome P450.

immunization to reduce pain and fever; this is an unlabeled use. Table 16.5 presents specific dosage for acetaminophen.

### Use in Children

Acetaminophen is usually the drug of choice for pain or fever in children. Children seem less susceptible to liver toxicity than adults, apparently because they form less of the toxic metabolite during metabolism of acetaminophen. However, there is a risk of overdose and hepatotoxicity because acetaminophen is a very common ingredient in over-the-counter (OTC) cold, flu, fever, and pain remedies. An overdose can occur with large doses of one product or smaller amounts of several different products. In addition, toxicity has occurred when parents or caregivers have given the liquid concentration intended for children to infants. The concentrations are different and cannot be given interchangeably. It is necessary to measure infant doses using a dropper and child doses using a teaspoon. The nurse should caution parents and caregivers to ask pediatricians for written instructions on giving acetaminophen to their children, to read the labels of all drug products very carefully, and to avoid giving children acetaminophen from multiple sources.

Ibuprofen also has antipyretic properties (see subsequent discussion). Alternating acetaminophen and ibuprofen every 4 hours over a 3-day period to control fever in young children (6–36 months of age) has been shown to be more effective than monotherapy with either agent.

### Use in Older Adults

The American Geriatrics Society recommends acetaminophen be the initial consideration for treatment of middle to moderate pain of musculoskeletal origin (level B). Acetaminophen is usually safe in recommended doses unless liver damage is present or the person is a chronic alcohol abuser.

### Use in Patients With Renal Impairment

Acetaminophen is normally metabolized in the liver to metabolites that are excreted by the kidneys, and these metabolites may accumulate in patients with renal failure.

| Drug | Pregnancy Category | Routes and Dosage Ranges | |
|---|---|---|---|
| | | **Adults** | **Children** |
| Ⓟ **Acetaminophen** (Tylenol; 🍁 Abenol, Apo-Acetaminophen, Atasol, Novo-Gesic) | B | PO or rectal suppository: 325–650 mg every 4–6 h<br>Extended release: 1300 mg every 8 h<br>IV injection: Ofirmev 1000 mg administered in a 100-mL vial over 15 min | Recommended doses by age:<br>PO, 0–3 mo, 40 mg; 4–11 mo, 80 mg; 12–23 mo, 120 mg; 2–3 y, 160 mg; 4–5 y, 240 mg; 6–8 y, 320 mg; 9–10 y, 400 mg; 11 y, 480 mg<br>Rectal: 3–11 mo, 80 mg every 6 h; 12–36 mo, 80 mg every 4 h; 3–6 y, 120 mg every 4–6 h; 6–12 y, 325 mg every 4–6 h |

**TABLE 16.5**

**DRUGS AT A GLANCE: Acetaminophen**

In addition, acetaminophen is nephrotoxic in overdose because it forms a metabolite that attacks kidney cells and may cause necrosis.

### Use in Patient With Hepatic Impairment

Acetaminophen can cause fatal liver necrosis in overdose because it forms a metabolite that can destroy liver cells. The hepatotoxic metabolite is formed more rapidly when drug-metabolizing enzymes in the liver have been stimulated by ingestion of alcohol, cigarette smoking, and drugs such as anti-seizure medications and others. Thus, patients who consume large quantities of alcohol, smoke, and take antiseizure medications are at high risk for hepatotoxicity with usual therapeutic doses.

### Use in Patients Receiving Home Care

Home care nurses are responsible for monitoring patients' use of acetaminophen. The drug does have hepatic and renal adverse effects.

## Adverse Effects

Hepatotoxicity and renal failure are the most common adverse effects of acetaminophen. Hypersensitivity reactions marked by rash and fever may occur in patients who have developed an allergy to the drug. Myocardial damage may develop in patients when doses of 5 to 8 g/day are ingested over several weeks or when 4 g/day have been ingested over 1 year.

## Contraindications

Contraindications to acetaminophen use include known hypersensitivity to the drug. Caution is necessary with administration in impaired hepatic and renal function. The drug crosses the placenta and enters the breast milk; therefore, caution is also required in pregnancy and lactation.

## Nursing Implications

### Preventing Interactions

Medications and herbs interact with acetaminophen, increasing or decreasing its effects (Boxes 16.5 and 16.6). It is important to be aware of the interaction of herbal supplements with acetaminophen. Although they do not increase or decrease the effects of acetaminophen, they do place the patient at risk for adverse effects.

---

**BOX 16.5**  **Drug Interactions: Acetaminophen**

**Drugs That Increase the Effects of Acetaminophen**
- Carbamazepine, phenytoin, and rifampin
  *Increase the risk of hepatotoxicity*

**Drugs That Decrease the Effects of Acetaminophen**
- Carbamazepine, phenytoin, and rifampin
  *Delay absorption*

---

**BOX 16.6**  **Herb and Dietary Interactions: Acetaminophen**

**Herbs That Increase the Effects of Acetaminophen**
- Willow and meadow root
- Ginkgo

---

### Administering the Medication

Acetaminophen is administered orally or by rectal suppository. It is important that the recommended dosage not be exceeded. Acetaminophen should be given with food to reduce GI upset. The recommended maximum daily dose of acetaminophen is 4 g for adults; additional amounts constitute an overdose. Ingestion of an overdose may be accidental or intentional. One contributing factor may be that some people think the drug is so safe that they can take any amount without harm. Another may be that people take the drug in several formulations without calculating or realizing that they are taking potentially harmful amounts. Numerous brand names of acetaminophen are available OTC, and acetaminophen is an ingredient in many prescription and OTC combination products (e.g., oxycodone and acetaminophen [Percocet], as well as OTC cold, flu, headache, and sinus remedies). The FDA also recommends limiting the duration of use (5 days or less in children, 10 days or less in adults, and 3 days in both adults and children when used to reduce fever) unless directed by a physician.

**! QSEN Alert: Safety**

For chronic alcohol abusers, short-term ingestion of usual therapeutic doses of acetaminophen may cause hepatotoxicity, and it is recommended that these persons ingest no more than 2 g daily. The FDA has issued a warning advising people who ingest three or more alcoholic drinks daily to avoid acetaminophen or to ask a physician before taking even small doses.

**! QSEN Alert: Safety**

Acetaminophen administered during pregnancy increases the risk of attention deficit hyperactivity disorder in children.

### Assessing for Therapeutic Effects

When administering acetaminophen as an antipyretic agent, the nurse assesses for reduced fever. The nurse records the patient's temperature every 2 to 4 hours. When administering the drug as an analgesic, the nurse assesses for decreased pain.

### Assessing for Adverse Effects

The most common and severe adverse effect associated with acetaminophen use is hepatotoxicity and hepatic failure. The nurse assesses for jaundice. It is also important to assess urinary output, blood urea nitrogen, and creatinine because of the risk of renal toxicity. In addition, it is critical to assess for a rash or fever because these are the first signs of a hypersensitivity reaction. The nurse assesses a patient who has a past history of myocardial damage and takes acetaminophen daily for chest pain and dyspnea. If the patient develops a rash, he or she should stop taking the drug.

### Toxicity: Recognition and Management

Acetaminophen poisoning may occur with a single large dose (possibly as little as 6 g, but usually 10–15 g) or with chronic ingestion of excessive doses (5–8 g/day for several weeks or 3–4 g/day for 1 year). Potentially fatal hepatotoxicity is the main concern and is most likely with doses of 20 g or more. Metabolism of acetaminophen produces a toxic metabolite that is normally inactivated by combining with glutathione. In overdose situations, the supply of glutathione is depleted and the toxic metabolite accumulates and directly damages liver cells (see Fig. 16.1). Acute renal failure may also occur.

Early symptoms (12–24 hours after ingestion) of toxicity are nonspecific (e.g., anorexia, nausea, vomiting, diaphoresis) and may not be considered serious or important enough to report or seek treatment. At 24 to 48 hours, symptoms may subside, but tests of liver function (e.g., aspartate aminotransferase, alanine aminotransferase, bilirubin, prothrombin time) begin to show increased levels. Later manifestations may include jaundice, vomiting, and CNS stimulation with excitement and delirium, followed by vascular collapse, coma, and death. Peak hepatotoxicity occurs in 3 to 4 days; recovery in nonfatal overdoses occurs in 7 to 8 days.

It is important to obtain plasma acetaminophen levels when an overdose is known or suspected, preferably within 4 hours after ingestion and every 24 hours for several days. Minimal hepatotoxicity is associated with plasma levels of less than 120 mcg/mL at 4 hours after ingestion or less than 30 mcg/mL at 12 hours after ingestion. With blood levels greater than 300 mcg/mL at 4 hours after ingestion, about 90% of patients develop liver damage.

### Treatment of Overdose

Gastric lavage is recommended if acetaminophen overdose is detected within 4 hours after ingestion, and activated charcoal can be given to inhibit absorption. In addition, the specific antidote is acetylcysteine (Acetadote), a mucolytic agent given by inhalation in respiratory disorders. Acetylcysteine may be given orally or intravenously (dosages are listed with other antidotes in Chap. 2). The drug supplies cysteine, a precursor substance required for the synthesis of glutathione. The synthesized glutathione combines with a toxic metabolite and decreases hepatotoxicity. Acetylcysteine is most beneficial if given within 8 hours of acetaminophen ingestion but may be helpful within 36 hours. It does not reverse damage that has already occurred.

### *Patient Teaching*

Box 16.7 presents patient teaching guidelines for acetaminophen.

---

**BOX 16.7** *Patient Teaching Guidelines for Acetaminophen*

- Do not exceed the recommended dosage, and do not take any other medications containing acetaminophen.
- Inform the health care provider of the development of a rash or fever.
- For better absorption, chew "chewable" tablets and do not swallow them whole.

---

7. A toddler is running a fever of 103°F. Which of the following medications is alternated to treat the fever?
   A. aspirin and acetaminophen
   B. acetaminophen and ibuprofen
   C. naproxen sodium and ibuprofen
   D. aspirin and ibuprofen

8. Which of the following medications is contraindicated with acetaminophen?
   A. oxycodone with acetaminophen
   B. furosemide
   C. phenytoin
   D. ampicillin

*Carb*
*Phen*
*Rif*

# NONSTEROIDAL ANTI-INFLAMMATORY DRUGS

As discussed in the introduction to this chapter, the mechanism of action of NSAIDs involves the blocking of COX enzymes. These drugs are classified into two types, or "generations." First-generation NSAIDs block both COX-1 and COX-2, and second-generation NSAIDs block only COX-2. Both first- and second-generation NSAIDs have the potential to cause serious cardiovascular thrombotic events. All NSAIDs are contraindicated in the setting of coronary artery bypass graft surgery. The nonsteroidal anti-inflammatory agents ibuprofen and indomethacin are used initially in treating patent ductus arteriosus.

## PROPIONIC ACID DERIVATIVES

The propionic acid derivatives are NSAIDs that inhibit prostaglandin synthesis in both the central and peripheral nervous systems. The prototype is  **ibuprofen** (Motrin, Advil).

### Pharmacokinetics

Ibuprofen is 80% absorbed in the GI tract. Its onset of action is 1 hour, producing antipyretic effects, reaching a peak in 1 to 2 hours. The duration of action is 6 to 8 hours. Ibuprofen is metabolized in the liver and eliminated in the urine. A small amount of the medication is eliminated in biliary excretion.

### Action

Ibuprofen blocks prostaglandin synthesis and modulates T-cell production. It inhibits the inflammatory cells by the process of chemotaxis to destroy the cells of inflammation. A first-generation NSAID, it blocks COX-1 and COX-2 but is more selective with COX-1.

### Use

Ibuprofen is used to relieve mild to moderate pain, including dysmenorrhea (painful menstruation). It is also used to treat inflammation related to rheumatoid arthritis and osteoarthritis. In addition, it is effective in reducing fever. During initial attacks of acute gout, NSAIDs such as ibuprofen may be administered. Table 16.6 gives dosage information for ibuprofen and the other propionic acid derivatives.

## Use in Children

Ibuprofen is recommended for reduction of fever for children older than 6 months of age. As previously stated, it can be alternated with acetaminophen to reduce fever. In addition, it is FDA approved for the treatment of patent ductus arteriosus in neonates who do not respond to conventional medical treatment.

## Use in Older Adults

Ibuprofen is relatively safe in therapeutic doses for occasional use as an analgesic or antipyretic in older people. The incidence of musculoskeletal disorders such as osteoarthritis is higher in older adults. However, the nurse should ensure that older adults taking ibuprofen on a long-term basis are evaluated for GI blood loss, renal dysfunction, edema, hypertension, and drug–drug or drug–drug disease interactions. A gastroprotective agent is recommended for patients at risk for upper GI bleeding.

## Use in Patients With Renal Impairment

Ibuprofen can cause or aggravate renal impairment even though it is eliminated mainly by hepatic metabolism. By inhibiting

## TABLE 16.6

## DRUGS AT A GLANCE: Propionic Acid Derivatives

| Drug | Pregnancy Category | Routes and Dosage Ranges | |
|---|---|---|---|
| | | **Adults** | **Children** |
| Ⓟ **Ibuprofen** (Motrin, Advil) | B, D in the third trimester | Osteoarthritis, rheumatoid arthritis: PO 300–600 mg three or four times per day; maximum, 3200 mg/d<br>Pain, dysmenorrhea: PO 400 mg every 4–6 h PRN; max 3200 mg/dL<br>V 400–800 mg every 6 h<br>Migraine: PO 400 mg at onset of headache | 6 mo to 12 y: fever, initial temperature 39.2°C (102.5°F) or less, PO 5 mg/kg every 6–8 h; initial temperature above 39.2°C (102.5°F), PO 5–10 mg/kg every 6–8 h; max dose 40 mg/kg/d<br>Juvenile arthritis: PO 20–40 mg/kg/d, in three or four divided doses |
| Diflunisal | C | Osteoarthritis and rheumatoid arthritis: PO 500–1000 mg/d in two divided doses, increased to a maximum of 1500 mg/d if necessary<br>Pain: PO 500–1000 mg initially and then 250–500 mg every 8–12 h | Not recommended for children <12 y of age |
| Fenoprofen (Fenortho, Nalfon) | Birth defects have been reported in utero | Osteoarthritis and rheumatoid arthritis: PO 400–600 mg three to four times per day; maximum dose 3200 mg/d<br>Pain: 200 mg every 4–6 h as needed | Dosage not established |
| Flurbiprofen (✳ Teva-Flurbiprofen) | C (ophthalmic) | Osteoarthritis, rheumatoid arthritis: PO 200–300 mg/d in two, three, or four divided doses<br>Inhibition of intraoperative miosis: 1 drop every 30 min, beginning 2 h before surgery (total of four drops) | Dosage not established |
| Ketoprofen (✳ Anafen, Ketoprofen E) | C | Pain, dysmenorrhea: PO 25–50 mg every 6–8 h PRN<br>Osteoarthritis, rheumatoid arthritis: PO 150–300 mg/d in three or four divided doses<br>Extended release: 200 mg once daily<br>Maximum: 300 mg/d for regular formulation; 200 mg/d for extended release; 100–150 mg/d for patients with impaired renal function | Do not give to children <16 y unless directed by a physician |
| Meclofenamate sodium | C | Inflammatory disease: PO 200–400 mg/d in 3–4 divided doses; maximum 400 mg/d<br>Dysmenorrhea: PO 100 mg three times per day starting at the onset of menstrual flow | Dosage not established |

*(Continued on page 316)*

### TABLE 16.6

### DRUGS AT A GLANCE: Propionic Acid Derivatives (Continued)

| Drug | Pregnancy Category | Routes and Dosage Ranges | |
|------|--------------------|--------------------------|---|
| | | **Adults** | **Children** |
| Mefenamic acid (✸ DOM-Mefenamic acid, PMS-Mefenamic acid, Ponstan) | Birth defects have been reported in utero | Pain: PO 500 mg and then 250 mg every 6 h not to exceed 1-wk administration<br>Dysmenorrhea: PO 500 mg beginning at the onset of menstrual bleeding followed by 250 mg every 6 h. Do not exceed 3 d | Adolescents ≥14 y same as adult dosing |
| Nabumetone (✸ Mylan-Nabumetone) | Birth defects have been reported in utero | Arthritis: PO Initial 1000 mg as a single dose; adjust dose according to the patient response up to 2000 mg/d 1–2 divided doses<br>Patients <50-kg dose should be <1000 mg/d | Dosage not established |
| Naproxen sodium (Aleve, Naprosyn, ✸ Anaprox, Apo-Napro-Na) | C | Naproxen: PO 250–500 mg twice daily<br>Gout: PO 750 mg initially and then 250 mg every 8 h until symptoms subside<br>Max: 1250 mg/d<br>Naproxen sodium, pain, dysmenorrhea, acute tendonitis; bursitis, PO 550 mg every 12 h or 275 mg every 6–8 h<br>Maximum: 1375 mg/d<br>OA, RA, AS: PO 275–550 mg twice a day<br>Acute gout: PO 825 mg initially and then 275 mg every 8 h until symptoms subside<br>Controlled release (Naprelan): 750–1000 mg once daily | Juvenile arthritis (naproxen only): PO 10 mg/kg/d in two divided doses. Oral suspension (125 mg/5 mL) twice daily according to weight: 13 kg (29 lb), 2.5 mL; 25 kg (55 lb), 5 mL; 39 kg (84 lb), 7.5 mL<br>OTC preparation not recommended for children <12 y |
| Oxaprozin (Daypro; ✸ Apo-Oxaprozin) | C | PO 600–1200 mg once daily<br>Max: 1800 mg/d or 26 mg/kg/d, whichever is lower, in divided doses | 6–16 y<br>22–31 kg: 600 mg once daily<br>32–54 kg: 900 mg once daily<br>≥55 kg: 1200 mg once daily |
| Tolmetin sodium | Birth defects have been reported in utero | Osteoarthritis and rheumatoid arthritis: PO 400 mg initially three times per day, adjust dose according to patient response after 102 weeks; maintenance 600–1800 mg/d in three divided doses | Juvenile idiopathic/rheumatoid arthritis: Children ≤2 y and adolescents <50 kg: PO 15–30 mg/kg/d in 3–4 divided doses; maximum dose 15–30 mg/kg/d in 3–4 divided doses or 1800 mg/d<br>Adolescents ≥50 kg, PO 200–600 mg every 8 h; maximum daily dose, 30 mg/kg/d, 1800 mg/d |

prostaglandins that dilate renal blood vessels, it can decrease the blood flow in the kidneys. When renal blood flow is normal, the activity of these prostaglandins is limited. However, when renal blood flow is decreased, synthesis of these prostaglandins is increased, and they protect the kidneys from ischemia and hypoxia by antagonizing the vasoconstrictive effects of angiotensin II, norepinephrine, and other substances. Thus, in patients who depend on prostaglandins to maintain an adequate renal blood flow, the prostaglandin-blocking effects of ibuprofen result in constriction of renal arteries and arterioles, decreased renal blood flow, decreased glomerular filtration rate, and retention of salt and water. Ibuprofen can also cause kidney damage by other mechanisms, including a hypersensitivity reaction that leads to acute renal failure, manifested by proteinuria, hematuria, and pyuria. Biopsy reports usually indicate inflammatory reactions such as glomerulonephritis or interstitial nephritis.

People at highest risk from the use of ibuprofen and related drugs are those with preexisting renal impairment, those older than 50 years of age, those taking diuretics, and those with hypertension, diabetes, or heart failure. Measures to prevent or minimize renal damage include avoiding nephrotoxic drugs when possible, treating the disorders that increase risk of renal damage, stopping the ibuprofen if renal impairment occurs, monitoring renal function, reducing dosage, and maintaining hydration.

### Use in Patients With Hepatic Impairment

Ibuprofen is metabolized in the liver, requiring that the dosage of the medication be decreased in patients with hepatic problems. The maximum daily dosage of ibuprofen in patients with hepatitis is 2 g.

### Use in Patients With Critical Illness

The FDA has issued a **BLACK BOX WARNING** ◆ stating that ibuprofen is contraindicated for the treatment of perioperative pain after coronary artery bypass graft.

### Use in Patients Receiving Home Care

It is important for the home care nurse to instruct the patient about all aspects of administration of ibuprofen. Because the medication is available in OTC preparations with many trade names, patients may not realize that they are taking an ibuprofen-containing drug. Overdosing may occur.

## Adverse Effects

The GI adverse effects of ibuprofen are many: dry mouth, gingival hyperplasia, dyspepsia, heartburn, nausea, epigastric pain, constipation, and GI ulceration with occult blood loss. The genitourinary effects include nephrotoxicity, elevated blood urea nitrogen and creatinine, and edema. The respiratory adverse effects include dyspnea, bronchospasm, hemoptysis, and pharyngitis. In addition, anaphylactic reactions may also occur. The FDA has issued a **BLACK BOX WARNING** ◆ stating that NSAIDs cause an increased risk of serious cardiovascular thrombotic events, including stroke or myocardial infarction.

## Contraindications

Ibuprofen is contraindicated in patients with a known allergy to NSAIDs and salicylates. Allergic reactions are more common in patients with rhinitis, asthma, chronic urticaria, and nasal polyps (Nursing, 2019).

## Nursing Implications

### Preventing Interactions

Medications and herbs interact with ibuprofen, increasing or decreasing its effects (Boxes 16.8 and 16.9).

### Administering the Medication

Ibuprofen is administered orally, and the total daily dose should not exceed 3200 mg. When administered intravenously, it should

**BOX 16.9** **Herb and Dietary Interactions: Ibuprofen**

**Herbs and Foods That Increase the Effects of Ibuprofen**
- Alcohol
- Garlic, ginger, and ginkgo
- Feverfew

be diluted in a concentration of 4 mg/mL or less using 0.9% sodium chloride, 5% dextrose, or lactated Ringer's. The dilution remains stable for 24 hours. Prior to the administration of the IV preparation, the patient should be well hydrated. Researchers have reported that the rapid infusion of ibuprofen intravenously was safe and effective in treating pain. The maximum total serum amount of IV ibuprofen was twice that of oral ibuprofen.

### Assessing for Therapeutic Effects

When ibuprofen is administered for pain, the nurse assesses for pain. The patient should report diminished pain on a pain scale. When the drug is administered for fever, the nurse records the patient's temperature every 2 to 4 hours. Reduced fever should occur. When the drug is administered for inflammation, the nurse notes anti-inflammatory effects, particularly in the joints related to arthritis. Decreased inflammation should occur.

### Assessing Adverse Effects

The nurse assesses the patient for dyspepsia or GI bleeding, including hemoptysis or melena. He or she also assesses complete blood count and clotting times for signs of anticoagulation. In addition, the nurse assesses for signs and symptoms of hypersensitivity to ibuprofen, including rash and bronchospasm.

### Patient Teaching

Box 16.10 presents patient teaching guidelines for ibuprofen.

## Other Drugs in the Class

Several other propionic acid derivatives are available.

- Diflunisal has the same action as the prototype drug ibuprofen. The onset of action is approximately 1 hour, with the maximum effect in 2 to 3 hours. The duration of action is 8 to 12 hours. It is 99% protein bound. Adequate albumin levels for drug distribution are important. The drug half-life is 8 to 12 hours. The half-life is prolonged in patients with

**BOX 16.8** **Drug Interactions: Ibuprofen**

**Drugs That Increase the Effects of Ibuprofen**
- Anticoagulants
  *Increase the risk of bleeding*
- Codeine, oxycodone, and hydrocodone
  *Have an additive analgesic effect*
- Corticosteroids
  *Have additive gastric irritant and possible ulcerogenic effects*

**BOX 16.10** **Patient Teaching Guidelines for Ibuprofen**

- Take this drug with food or liquid to decrease gastric irritation.
- Drink 2 to 3 quarts of fluid daily when taking this drug regularly.
- Report any signs of bleeding (e.g., nosebleed, vomiting blood, bruising, blood in the urine or stool), difficulty breathing, severe stomach upset, swelling, or weight gain to your health care provider.

renal impairment. Diflunisal is extensively metabolized to glucuronide conjugates.

- Fenoprofen has the same action as ibuprofen. It has a rapid onset of action and reaches a full benefit in 2 to 3 weeks. It reaches its peak serum effect in 2 hours with a 3-hour half-life. Fenoprofen peak serum level is decreased when administered with food. However, it is important to administer with food to decrease stomach upset.
- Flurbiprofen is 99% protein bound to albumin, and it is important that the patient is well hydrated when administering this protein-bound medication. Flurbiprofen also inhibits chemotaxis and neutrophil aggregation to decrease inflammatory cytokines. The medication is rapidly absorbed and metabolized by CYP2C9. The elderly are at greater risk for GI bleeding.
- Ketoprofen has the same actions as flurbiprofen.
- Meclofenamate sodium inhibits prostaglandin synthesis. It is used for inflammatory disease processes and dysmenorrhea. It is also used in palliative care to enhance analgesic and anti-inflammatory action. The Beers Criteria has identified mefenamic acid as an inappropriate medication in patients 65 years or older due to risk of GI bleed.
- Mefenamic acid is administered for pain related to menstruation or mild to moderate pain.
- Nabumetone is similar to other NSAID preparations. Patients without prior exposure to anaphylactic reactions from aspirin may experience allergic reactions. Patients with bronchial asthma, aspirin intolerance, or rhinitis are at increased risk.
- Naproxen (Naprosyn) is an NSAID used to treat mild to moderate pain related to primary dysmenorrhea. It metabolized by CYP1A2 and CYP2C9.
- Oxaprozin (Daypro) is similar to the other drugs in the class.
- Tolmetin sodium is used to treat juvenile idiopathic/rheumatoid arthritis in children 2 years and older. As with other NSAIDs, there is an increased risk of GI bleed in patients 65 years and older. Elevations in the hepatic enzymes have been reported with the administration of tolmetin sodium.

### Clinical Application 16.3

- When teaching to Mrs. Mason about ibuprofen, what is it necessary to say about the action of the medication?
- What are the adverse reactions of ibuprofen?
- What specific patient teaching should be provided to Mrs. Mason?

## OXICAM DERIVATIVES

Oxicam derivatives are another type of NSAID. The prototype is **meloxicam** (Mobic).

### Pharmacokinetics

Meloxicam is metabolized by the liver and excreted in the feces and urine. The onset of action is 1 hour, and peak serum concentrations occur in 5 to 6 hours. The drug crosses the placenta and enters breast milk.

### Action

Meloxicam is a COX-1 and COX-2 inhibitor, producing anti-inflammatory, analgesic, and antipyretic effects. It is more selective for COX-2 inhibition in the brain, kidney, ovary, uterus, cartilage, bone, and sites of inflammation.

### Use

Meloxicam is administered for the treatment of osteoarthritis and rheumatoid arthritis. It is used in children 2 years of age and older for relief of signs and symptoms of pauciarticular or polyarticular juvenile rheumatoid arthritis. Table 16.7 gives the dosage information for meloxicam and a related drug.

#### Use in Patients With Renal Impairment

Likewise, the dosage of meloxicam does not require adjustment in mild to moderate renal impairment. The use of the drug in patients with creatinine clearance less than 20 mL/min has not been studied and is not recommended in these patients. Patients undergoing hemodialysis should receive a maximum of 7.5 mg/day.

#### Use in Patients With Hepatic Impairment

The use of meloxicam in patients with hepatic impairment has not adequately been studied. The dosage of the drug does not appear to be necessary in patients with mild to moderate hepatic impairment.

### Adverse Effects

Meloxicam is associated with several adverse effects. Respiratory effects include dyspnea, hemoptysis, bronchospasm, pharyngitis, and rhinitis. Hematologic effects consist of bleeding, platelet inhibition, and decreased hemoglobin and hematocrit, along

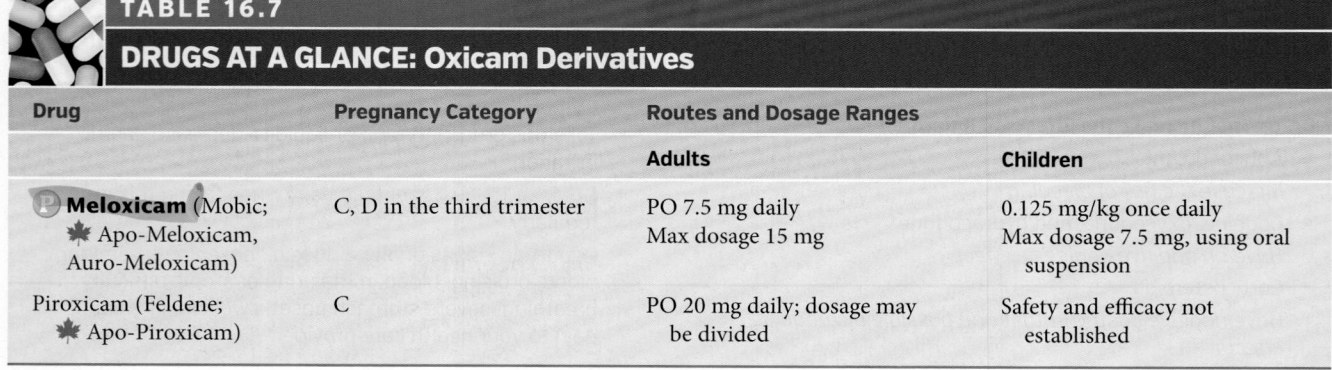

| TABLE 16.7 | | | |
|---|---|---|---|
| **DRUGS AT A GLANCE: Oxicam Derivatives** | | | |
| **Drug** | **Pregnancy Category** | **Routes and Dosage Ranges** | |
| | | **Adults** | **Children** |
| **Meloxicam** (Mobic; Apo-Meloxicam, Auro-Meloxicam) | C, D in the third trimester | PO 7.5 mg daily<br>Max dosage 15 mg | 0.125 mg/kg once daily<br>Max dosage 7.5 mg, using oral suspension |
| Piroxicam (Feldene; Apo-Piroxicam) | C | PO 20 mg daily; dosage may be divided | Safety and efficacy not established |

with bone marrow depression and edema. GI effects include nausea, dyspepsia, diarrhea, vomiting, and diarrhea. The FDA has issued a **BLACK BOX WARNING ◆** stating that patients who take meloxicam are at risk for cardiovascular events and GI bleeding. In addition, headache, dizziness, drowsiness, and insomnia may occur.

## Contraindications

Meloxicam should not be administered to patients with a known aspirin allergy. It is also contraindicated postoperatively in patients who have just undergone coronary artery bypass surgery.

## Nursing Implications

### Preventing Interactions

Some medications interact with meloxicam, increasing its effects (Box 16.11). As with all NSAIDs, alcohol, garlic, ginseng, and ginger increase the risk of bleeding. Giving meloxicam with lithium increases the risk of lithium toxicity.

### Administering the Medication

Administration of meloxicam with food or fluids reduces gastric irritation. It is necessary to shake the oral suspension gently before use.

### Assessing for Therapeutic Effects

When giving meloxicam for pain, the nurse assesses the pain level using a pain scale to determine that analgesic effects are attained. When giving it for fever, the nurse records the patient's temperature every 2 to 4 hours to check for diminished body temperature. When giving it for inflammation, the nurse assesses for diminished redness and swelling.

### Assessing for Adverse Effects

The nurse assesses the patient for signs and symptoms of hypersensitivity reactions such as shortness of breath and bronchospasm. It is also necessary to assess for hemoptysis as well as blood in the stool or urine. In addition, the nurse must assess for signs and symptoms of cardiovascular events.

### Patient Teaching

Box 16.12 presents patient teaching guidelines for meloxicam.

## Other Drugs in the Class

Piroxicam (Feldene) is similar to meloxicam in terms of pharmacokinetics. It is metabolized predominantly by CYP2C9. Patients who are poor CYP2C9 metabolizers have reduced metabolism and increased serum levels.

---

**BOX 16.11    Drug Interactions: Meloxicam**

**Drugs That Increase the Effects of Meloxicam**
- Angiotensin-converting enzyme inhibitors and diuretics
  *Increase the risk of renal failure*
- Aspirin and anticoagulants
  *Increase the risk of gastrointestinal bleeding*

---

**BOX 16.12    Patient Teaching Guidelines for Meloxicam**

- Take these drugs with food to decrease gastric irritation.
- Take only the prescribed dose.
- Do not operate machinery until you know how these drugs affect you. Dizziness and drowsiness may occur.
- Report sore throat, dyspnea, edema, and tarry stools to your health care provider.

---

**NCLEX    Success**

9. A child who is diagnosed with pneumonia is taking ibuprofen for a fever. The nurse observes a rash. Which of the following reactions does the nurse suspect?
   A. thromboembolism
   B. streptococcal reaction
   C. hypersensitivity
   D. viral infection

10. A prescriber in an orthopedic care practice orders meloxicam for the treatment of osteoarthritis. Which of the following medications when combined with meloxicam places the patient at greatest risk?
    A. antimicrobials
    B. lithium
    C. selective serotonin inhibitors
    D. hydrochlorothiazide

## ACETIC ACID DERIVATIVES

The prototype NSAID of the acetic acid derivative group is **indomethacin** (Indocin, Tivorbex). The acetic acid derivatives have strong anti-inflammatory effects and more severe adverse effects than the propionic acid derivatives.

## Pharmacokinetics

With oral administration of indomethacin, the onset of action is 30 minutes, with a peak in 1 to 2 hours and a duration of action of 4 to 6 hours. With IV administration, onset of action is immediate, with an unknown peak and a duration of action of 15 to 30 minutes. The drug is metabolized in the liver and has a half-life of 4.5 to 6 hours. It is excreted by the kidneys. Indomethacin has the ability to cross the placenta and enter the breast milk.

## Action

Indomethacin provides anti-inflammatory, analgesic, and antipyretic activities by inhibiting the prostaglandin synthesis. The exact mechanism is unknown, but it inhibits COX-1 and COX-2. It is mainly a selective COX-1 inhibitor.

# Use

Indomethacin is administered to relieve pain associated with rheumatoid arthritis, osteoarthritis, ankylosing spondylitis, bursitis, tendonitis, and gouty arthritis. During initial attacks of acute gout, the drug may be given. Parenteral, but not oral, administration is used to produce closure of patent ductus arteriosus in premature infants who weigh 500 to 1750 g. Table 16.8 gives dosage information for indomethacin and the other acetic acid derivatives.

## Use in Children

The safety and efficacy of indomethacin have not been established in children. As previously stated, the FDA has approved IV indomethacin for treatment of patent ductus arteriosus in premature infants. (The ductus arteriosus joins the pulmonary artery to the aorta in the fetal circulation. When it fails to close at the time of birth, blood is shunted from the aorta to the pulmonary artery, causing severe cardiopulmonary problems.) If anuria or oliguria occurs after premature infants receive the IV form, no further doses should be given. If the ductus reopens, the drug is repeated in 12 to 24 hours. Indications that the ductus has reopened would be the signs and symptoms of heart failure such as dyspnea and a heart murmur. The reader should note that oral administration for closure of patent ductus arteriosus in premature infants is an unlabeled use of the drug.

## Use in Older Adults

The Beers Criteria indicate that indomethacin is inappropriate in the geriatric population and is associated with a high risk of

---

### TABLE 16.8

## DRUGS AT A GLANCE: Acetic Acid Derivatives

| Drug | Pregnancy Category | Routes and Dosage Ranges | |
|---|---|---|---|
| | | **Adults** | **Children** |
| ⓟ **Indomethacin** (Indocin, Tivorbex; 🍁 Apo-Indomethacin, Sandoz-Indomethacin) | B, D in the third trimester | PO, rectal suppository: 75 mg/d initially, increased by 25 mg/d at weekly intervals to a maximum of 150–200 mg/d, if necessary<br>Acute gouty arthritis, acute painful shoulder: PO 75–150 mg/d in three or four divided doses until pain and inflammation are controlled (e.g., 3–5 d for gout; 7–14 d for painful shoulder), then discontinued | In special circumstances, such as juvenile rheumatoid arthritis, children older than 2 y of age may receive the drug Initial dose is 2 mg/kg/d in divided doses, not to exceed 4 mg/kg/d<br>Premature infants with patent ductus arteriosus: IV 0.1–0.25 mg/kg every 12 h for a total of three doses |
| Diclofenac potassium (Cambia, Zorvolex; 🍁 Apo-Diclo, Apo-Diclo SR Voltaren, Voltaren XR, Cambia, Zipsor) | C, D in the third trimester | Osteoarthritis: PO 100–150 mg/d in divided doses (e.g., 50 mg two or three times or 75 mg twice or 100 mg once daily)<br>Rheumatoid arthritis: PO 150–200 mg/d in two, three, or four divided doses<br>Ankylosing spondylitis: PO 100–125 mg/d in four or five divided doses (e.g., 25 mg four or five times daily)<br>Pain, dysmenorrhea: (diclofenac potassium only) PO 50 mg three times daily<br>Acute migraine: 50-mg packet mixed in 30–60 mL water as a single dose at the onset of a headache (Cambia)<br>Mild to moderate pain: 25 mg liquid capsule PO four times daily<br>Actinic keratosis topical: cover lesion with gel and smooth into skin; do not cover with dressing (Solaraze)<br>Transdermal patch: apply to the most painful area two times daily (Flector)<br>Ophthalmic: 1 drop to the affected eye starting 24 h after cataract surgery for 2 wk | Dosage not established<br>Off-label use: juvenile idiopathic arthritis in children ≥3 y<br>2–3 mg/kg/d in divided doses |
| Etodolac (Lodine; 🍁 Taro-Etodolac) | C | Pain: 200–400 mg PO every 6–8 h<br>Osteoarthritis: 600–1200 mg/d PO in 2–4 divided doses<br>Rheumatoid arthritis: 500 mg PO twice daily | PO extended release<br>20–30 mg: 400 mg once daily<br>31–45 kg: 600 mg once daily<br>46–80 kg 800 mg once daily<br>>60 kg: 1000 mg once daily |

**TABLE 16.8**

**DRUGS AT A GLANCE: Acetic Acid Derivatives** (Continued)

| Drug | Pregnancy Category | Routes and Dosage Ranges | |
|---|---|---|---|
| | | **Adults** | **Children** |
| Ketorolac | C, D in the third trimester | Single dose: IV 30 mg, IM 60 mg<br>Multiple dose: IM or IV 30 mg every 6 h PRN to a maximum of 120 mg/d<br>PO 20 mg as the first dose for patients who received 60 mg IM or 30 mg IV as a single dose or 30 mg in a multiple dose followed by 10 mg every 4–6 h to a maximum of 40 mg/d<br>Older adults (>65 y), those with renal impairment, those with weight <50 kg (110 lb; IV, IM 15 mg every 6 h to a maximum of 60 mg/d)<br>Itching from allergic conjunctivitis: ophthalmic<br>Acular PF: for cataract surgery, 1 drop every four times daily after surgery and continue for 2 wk<br>Acular LS: 1 drop four times daily PRN for burning and stinging for up to 4 d after surgery<br>Pain and photophobia: use for 3 d | Use one single-dose injection 1 mg/kg IM up to a maximum of 30 mg or 0.5 mg/kg IV up to a maximum of 15 mg |
| Nabumetone (Relafen DS) (Apo-Nabumetone, Mylan-Nabumetone, Teva-Nabumetone) | C, D in the third trimester | PO 1000–2000 mg/d in one or two doses | Dosage not established |
| Sulindac (✽ Apo-Sulin, Teva-Sulindac) | C | PO 150–200 mg twice a day; maximum, 400 mg/d<br>Acute gout, acute painful shoulder: PO 200 mg twice a day until pain and inflammation subside (e.g., 7–14 d), then reduce dosage or discontinue | Dosage not established |

severity. When an older adult must take indomethacin, it is necessary to use the lowest recommended dose and frequency.

### Use in Patients With Renal Impairment
Caution is also required with administration of indomethacin to patients with renal impairment. (Severe renal impairment is a contraindication.)

### Use in Patients With Hepatic Impairment
Caution is necessary with administration of indomethacin to patients with hepatic impairment. Dosage reduction is appropriate.

## Adverse Effects
Indomethacin and all acetic acid derivatives result in a risk of GI bleeding and bleeding ulcer. Abdominal pain, distention, vomiting, and transient ileus may occur. CNS adverse effects include headache, dizziness, somnolence, and insomnia. Patients are at risk for renal impairment and decreased clotting time.

With IV preparations, the most severe respiratory adverse effect is pulmonary hemorrhage.

## Contraindications
Indomethacin should not be administered to patients with a known history of salicylate hypersensitivity. Patients with a past history of GI bleeding should not take the drug. It should not be administered postoperatively to patients who have just had a coronary artery bypass graft. The parenteral formulations are contraindicated in infection, bleeding, thrombocytopenia, coagulation defects, and necrotizing enterocolitis. As stated earlier, indomethacin is contraindicated in severe renal impairment.

## Nursing Implications
### Preventing Interactions
Certain drugs interact with indomethacin (Box 16.13). The administration of alcohol, feverfew, garlic, ginger, and ginkgo also increases the bleeding potential.

## BOX 16.13 — *Drug Interactions: Indomethacin*

**Drugs That Increase the Effects of Indomethacin**

- Phenytoin, salicylates, sulfonamides, and sulfonylureas
  *Result in displacement of protein-binding activities*
- Salicylates, anticoagulants, and lithium
  *Increase the risk of bleeding*

### Administering the Medication

It is important to administer oral indomethacin after meals or with an antacid to decrease GI irritation. Patients with gouty arthritis should not take the sustained-release preparation. Patients with a history of proctitis or rectal bleeding should not use rectal suppositories. IV administration requires dilution of 1 mg with 1 mL of sterile water or normal saline. It is necessary to administer the dose over 5 to 10 seconds. Good IV access is imperative to prevent extravasation of the drug into the tissues. Storage of the oral preparation of indomethacin in a light-protected container is essential.

### Assessing for Therapeutic Effects

Before administering indomethacin, it is important to assess patients for salicylate allergy, which can cause bronchospasm, dyspnea, and rash. After the drug has had time to work, it is imperative to assess for diminished pain and inflammation. The nurse observes the patient's mobility in response to diminished inflammation. When administering indomethacin for gout, inflammation is generally relieved in 24 to 36 hours.

### Assessing for Adverse Effects

A careful assessment of the cardiac and CNS effects is imperative. The nurse assesses for bleeding, vomiting, and abdominal pain. The FDA has issued a **BLACK BOX WARNING ◆** for indomethacin, stating that an increased risk of adverse cardiovascular thrombotic effects, including myocardial infarction and cerebrovascular accident, has been noted with the drug. Because of the risk of hypersensitivity, the nurse assesses for dyspnea, bronchospasm, and hemoptysis. In addition, if the patient complains of abdominal pain that is indicative of transient ileus, the nurse notifies the physician immediately.

### ! QSEN Alert: Safety

Assessment for GI pain, rapid pulse, and diaphoresis is essential in patients who receive ketorolac. These symptoms are indicative of GI perforation.

### Patient Teaching

Box 16.14 lists patient teaching guidelines for indomethacin.

## Other Drugs in the Class

Several other acetic acid derivatives deserve mention.

Diclofenac reversibly inhibits COX-1 and COX-2 to produce an anti-inflammatory response. It is readily absorbed by the GI tract, with 50% to 60% reaching the systemic circulation.

## BOX 16.14 — *Patient Teaching Guidelines for Indomethacin*

- If you are the parents or another member of a family of an infant being treated for patent ductus arteriosus, be sure you receive and understand the action, adverse effects, and therapeutic effects of indomethacin, as well as its administration guidelines.
- Administer the oral preparation with food or immediately after a meal.
- If necessary, take the medication with an antacid to decrease gastric irritation.
- Report adverse effects such as chest pain, weakness, or disorientation to your health care provider.
- Do not operate machinery due to dizziness or somnolence.
- Report sore throat, fever, rash, weight gain, or tarry stools to your health care provider.

The nonsteroidal effects are well distributed to the synovial fluid and easily pass into the breast milk. The drug is more than 99% bound to albumin and undergoes first-pass metabolism. Two thirds of elimination of diclofenac is in the urine, and one third is in the feces. The half-life of the transdermal preparation is 12 hours, whereas that of the oral preparation is 1 to 2 hours. Diclofenac is used to relieve the inflammatory symptoms of rheumatoid arthritis, osteoarthritis, and ankylosing spondylitis. The transdermal formulation is administered to relieve acute pain. The topical preparation is used to treat actinic keratosis. In addition, there is an ophthalmic preparation administered to relieve photosensitivity following refractive surgery.

Etodolac possesses the same mechanism of action as diclofenac. It undergoes metabolism in the liver to hydroxylated metabolites and etodolac glucuronide, and the hydroxylated metabolites then undergo further glucuronidation. The drug reportedly causes less gastric irritation, especially in older adults at high risk for GI bleeding.

Ketorolac, an injectable NSAID often used for pain, is contraindicated in patients at risk for excessive bleeding. Thus, this drug should not be administered during labor and delivery, before or during any major surgery, with suspected or confirmed cerebrovascular bleeding, or to patients who are currently taking aspirin or other NSAIDs. The FDA has issued a **BLACK BOX WARNING ◆** for ketorolac; the drug places the patient at risk for GI irritation, inflammation, ulceration, bleeding, and perforation. Parenteral ketorolac reportedly compares with morphine and other opioids in analgesic effectiveness for moderate or severe pain. However, its use is limited to 5 days because it increases the risk of bleeding. Hematomas and wound bleeding have been reported with postoperative use. An intranasal form of ketorolac is currently in phase III drug testing trials and shows promise in relieving postsurgical pain and in reducing the amount of other analgesics (e.g., morphine) required in the postoperative period.

Nabumetone is administered for rheumatoid and osteoarthritis. It blocks prostaglandin synthesis through the inhibition of COX. Prior to administering nabumetone, a baseline hemoglobin and hematocrit should be assessed. The patient should be instructed to report any signs or symptoms of abdominal pain or black tarry stools.

Sulindac is used for inflammatory disorders, including ankylosing spondylitis and acute painful shoulder due to bursitis or tendonitis. The therapeutic response of sulindac is usually noted in 1 week. The drug is 90% absorbed and 98% bound to albumin.

# SELECTIVE COX-2 INHIBITOR: CELECOXIB

**Celecoxib** (CeleBREX) is the only selective COX-2 inhibitor on the market in the United States. The selective COX-2 inhibitors etoricoxib and parecoxib, which are available in the United Kingdom and other countries, are currently under review by the FDA. COX-2 inhibitors were designed to selectively block production of prostaglandins associated with pain and inflammation without blocking those associated with protective effects on gastric mucosa, renal function, and platelet aggregation. Thus, they produce less gastric irritation and renal impairment than aspirin and other NSAIDs.

## Pharmacokinetics

Celecoxib, which is administered orally, has a slow onset of action. The drug reaches its peak in 3 hours. It is highly protein bound (97%), and the serum half-life is 11 hours. It is metabolized by the cytochrome P450 enzymes in the liver to inactive metabolites that are then excreted in the urine. A small amount is excreted unchanged in the urine. Celecoxib crosses the placenta and enters the breast milk.

## Action

COX-2 is activated with inflammation. Celecoxib inhibits the COX-2 enzyme to decrease inflammation. It does not affect the COX-1 enzyme, thus protecting the lining of the GI tract and not inhibiting clotting factors.

## Use

Celecoxib is administered for acute and long-term treatment of juvenile rheumatoid arthritis, rheumatoid arthritis, osteoarthritis, and ankylosing spondylitis. It is used to treat acute pain and primary dysmenorrhea. In addition, the drug is given in familial adenomatous polyposis to reduce the number of colorectal polyps. Unlabeled uses include the treatment of acute pain, ankylosing spondylitis, juvenile idiopathic arthritis, osteoarthritis, primary dysmenorrhea, and rheumatoid arthritis. Table 16.9 presents specific dosage and pregnancy information for celecoxib.

### Use in Children

Celecoxib is recommended only for children aged 2 and older to treat juvenile rheumatoid arthritis. In children, the median peak serum concentration is 3 hours. The range of peak serum concentration is 3 to 6.2 hours.

### Use in Patients With Renal Impairment

In patients with significant renal impairment, celecoxib should not be administered.

### Use in Patients With Hepatic Impairment

In patients with hepatic impairment, the dosage of celecoxib should be reduced by 50%.

## Adverse Effects

The CNS adverse reactions of celecoxib include headache, dizziness, somnolence, and insomnia. Some patients have noted ophthalmic changes with administration of the drug. Patients taking celecoxib are at increased risk for myocardial infarction and cerebrovascular accident. The FDA has issued a **BLACK BOX WARNING** ◆ for celecoxib concerning its cardiac and vascular risks. Dermatologic adverse effects include rash, pruritus, sweating, dry mucous membranes, and stomatitis.

Dyspepsia and GI bleeding can occur with the administration of prolonged high doses of celecoxib, but the risk is not as profound as the COX-1 and COX-2 inhibitors. Anaphylactic reactions can also occur if the patient is allergic to celecoxib or has an aspirin or NSAID-related allergy.

## Contraindications

Celecoxib is contraindicated in patients who have a known allergy to sulfonamides, NSAIDs, and aspirin. It is also contraindicated in patients with renal impairment. It should not be administered to patients with perioperative pain or to those who have just undergone coronary artery bypass graft surgery.

| TABLE 16.9 |
|---|
| **DRUGS AT A GLANCE: Celecoxib** |

| Drug | Pregnancy Category | Routes and Dosage Ranges | |
|---|---|---|---|
| | | **Adults** | **Children** |
| **Celecoxib** (CeleBREX; ❀ ACT Celecoxib, AG-Celecoxib) | C up to 30 wk D after 30 wk | PO 100 mg two times daily may be increased to 200 mg/d two times daily<br>Acute pain, dysmenorrhea: 400 mg and then 200 mg two times daily<br>Familial adenomatous polyposis: 400 mg two times daily<br>Ankylosing spondylitis: 200 mg/d after 6 wk, a trial of 400 mg/d may be tried for 6 wk; if no effect is seen, another therapy is recommended | Children older than 2 y of age PO 10 or 25 kg or less: 50-mg capsule BID<br>More than 25 kg: 100-mg capsule BID |

# Nursing Implications

## Preventing Interactions

The administration of anticoagulants or aspirin with celecoxib increases the risk of bleeding. Patients taking lithium and celecoxib are at risk for lithium toxicity. Celecoxib combined with alcohol or smoking increases the patient's risk of GI bleeding.

## Administering the Medication

When administering celecoxib, the nurse should be certain to administer it 2 hours before or after an antacid to ensure absorption. Prior to administering celecoxib, assess the patient for allergic reactions to NSAIDs. It is necessary to store the medication in a light-protected container.

## Assessing for Therapeutic Effects

The nurse assesses for diminished pain and swelling associated with inflammation. The nurse assesses joints for redness, heat, and stiffness. Mobility should increase with the administration of celecoxib.

## Assess for Adverse Effects

The nurse assesses the patient for signs and symptoms of chest pain, shortness of breath, confusion, or numbness of the extremities. These symptoms are indicative of cardiac event such as myocardial infarction or cerebrovascular accident. Also, it is necessary to assess for dyspepsia, GI irritation, and GI bleeding. In addition, the nurse assesses for CNS depression and ophthalmic changes. Finally, he or she assesses for anaphylactic reactions, including sore throat, itching, weight gain, and edema.

## Patient Teaching

Box 16.15 patient teaching guidelines for celecoxib.

---

**BOX 16.15** *Patient Teaching Guidelines for Celecoxib*

- Administer the medication with food or meals to prevent gastric upset.
- Take the medication as prescribed.
- Do not operate machinery if you have central nervous system depression.
- Report sore throat, rash, itching, weight gain, swelling of feet and ankles, and changes in vision to your health care provider.

---

# ANTIGOUT MEDICATION

## MITOTIC AGENT: COLCHICINE

**Colchicine** (Colcrys, Mitigare), the prototype agent for the treatment and prevention of gout, is the most commonly administered antigout medication.

---

**! QSEN Alert: Safety**

Colchicine has a narrow therapeutic index. The drug accumulates leading to severe and potentially fatal adverse effects.

---

## Pharmacokinetics

Colchicine is absorbed rapidly in the GI tract, with a slow onset of action; it reaches its peak in 1 to 2 hours. The drug is metabolized in the liver and has a half-life of 26 to 31 hours. It is primarily eliminated in the feces, with a smaller amount excreted in the urine. Colchicine crosses the placenta and enters the breast milk.

## Action

Colchicine inhibits the migration of WBCs into the body tissues containing urate crystals. The phagocytic action of the drug decreases the inflammatory reaction to the urate crystals deposited in the tissues.

## Use

Colchicine is administered for the treatment and prophylaxis of acute gout in adults. An off-label use of colchicine is ordered for patients with acute or recurrent pericarditis. Table 16.10 gives the dosage and pregnancy information for this drug.

### Use in Children

Colchicine is only administered to children 4 years of age and older to treat familial Mediterranean fever.

### Use in Older Adults

Colchicine is administered cautiously in older adults, and the dosage should be reduced by half in people 70 years of age and older.

---

**NCLEX Success**

11. A newborn infant has been treated with parenteral indomethacin for treatment of patent ductus arteriosus. Which of the following symptoms would be indicative of a reopening of the ductus arteriosus in 12 hours after the original dosage?
    - A. dyspnea
    - B. pain
    - C. elevated creatinine level
    - D. hepatic failure

12. A 76-year-old woman is taking celecoxib for arthritic pain in her back. When administering celecoxib, which of the following patient teaching points is most important?
    - A. Any chest pain should be reported to the prescriber immediately.
    - B. Celecoxib can be administered with warfarin.
    - C. Increased mobility should be reported to the prescriber.
    - D. Celecoxib can be administered with aspirin during periods of infection.

| TABLE 16.10 | | | |
|---|---|---|---|
| **DRUGS AT A GLANCE: Colchicine** | | | |
| **Drug** | **Pregnancy Category** | **Routes and Dosage Ranges** | |
| | | **Adults** | **Children** |
| Ⓟ **Colchicine** (Colcrys, Mitigare; ✵ JAMP-Colchicine, PMS-Colchicine, Sandoz Colchicine) | C | Acute gout: PO 1.2 mg at the first sign of gout flare  Prophylaxis of gout flares: PO 0.6 mg/d to a maximum of 1.2 mg/d | Safety and efficacy not established |

### Use in Patients With Renal Impairment

For mild to moderate renal impairment, a regular dosage of colchicine is administered. If the creatinine clearance is less than 30 mL/min, a dosage adjusted is not necessary, but the drug should not be given more often than once every 2 weeks. For patients on dialysis, 0.6 mg is given as a single dose no more than once every 2 weeks.

### Use in Patients With Hepatic Impairment

In mild to moderate hepatic impairment, colchicine should be administered cautiously. The patient should be assessed closely for adverse effects. In severe hepatic impairment, the dosage should be the same, but the drug should not be given more often than once every 2 weeks.

### Adverse Effects

GI adverse effects are the most common due to the absorption and elimination in the GI tract. These GI conditions include nausea, vomiting, and abdominal pain and dyspepsia. Hematologic adverse effects such as bone marrow depression and aplastic anemia may occur. Hepatotoxicity is also an adverse effect of colchicine. Other adverse effects include peripheral neuropathy, alopecia, rash, purpura, dermatoses, myopathy, muscle pain, and weakness.

## Contraindications

Colchicine is contraindicated in patients who have a known hypersensitivity to the medication. It should not be administered concurrently with cyclosporines or ranolazine or with a strong to moderate CYP3A4 inhibitor in the presence of hepatic or renal impairment. It is administered cautiously in pregnancy or in the presence of renal or hepatic impairment.

## Nursing Implications

### Preventing Interactions

Several medications, when combined with colchicine, result in toxicity and severe adverse effects. These agents increase the serum level of colchicine and the risk of toxicity. They are atazanavir, clarithromycin, indinavir, itraconazole, ketoconazole, nefazodone, nelfinavir, ritonavir, saquinavir, telithromycin, diltiazem, erythromycin, fluconazole, and verapamil. In addition, colchicine should not be combined with grapefruit juice or alcohol. It also decreases cyanocobalamin (vitamin $B_{12}$) absorption.

### Administering the Medication

It is necessary to administer colchicine with food to reduce gastric distress.

### Assess for Therapeutic Effects

Therapeutic effects occur within 24 to 48 hours after oral administration. The nurse assesses for decreased pain, swelling, and inflammation of affected joints. Edema may not decrease for several days.

### Assess for Adverse Effects

The nurse assesses for severe GI adverse effects such as vomiting and diarrhea, which may lead to an alteration in fluid and electrolytes with dehydration. The nurse also assesses for numbness, tingling, or muscle weakness. In addition, it is important to assess for bone marrow depression. The nurse also monitors liver enzymes.

## Patient Teaching

Box 16.16 presents patient teaching guidelines for the mitotic agent colchicine.

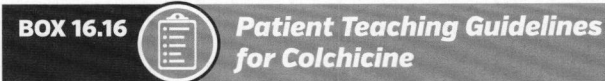

**BOX 16.16  Patient Teaching Guidelines for Colchicine**

- Take colchicine as prescribed and at the onset of acute gouty symptoms.
- For acute gouty flare-ups, take one dose and the second dose 1 hour later.
- Do not drink grapefruit juice or alcohol.
- GI adverse effects are common with colchicine; call your prescriber if the abdominal pain is too severe.
- Report severe diarrhea and muscle weakness to your health care provider.
- Understand that the resulting bone marrow depression may cause fatigue, increased risk of bleeding, or increased risk of infection.
- See your primary health provider with persistent gouty attacks.
- Follow a low-purine diet by avoiding beer, alcohol, organ and game meats, sardines, anchovies, scallops, asparagus, spinach, and peas.

# URICOSURIC AGENTS

Several uricosuric agents are used to reduce serum uric acid levels. **Allopurinol** (Zyloprim), a xanthine oxidase inhibitor, is the prototype uricosuric drug.

## Pharmacokinetics

Allopurinol is absorbed in the GI tract, with an onset of action of 24 to 48 hours and a peak of action of 2 to 6 hours. The drug's half-life is 1 to 3 hours. It is metabolized as an active metabolite oxypurinol and is eliminated slowly in the urine. It is also excreted in the breast milk.

## Action

Allopurinol inhibits the enzyme that is responsible for the conversion of purines to uric acid. This action reduces the purines to uric acid and thus reduces the uric acid production to decrease the serum and urinary uric acid levels. The result of this action is the reduction of the symptoms of gout.

## Use

Allopurinol and uricosuric agents are administered for the management of the signs and symptoms of primary and secondary gout or stages of gout. It is also given in acute and chronic tophaceous gout to reduce uric acid concentrations. Other indications include leukemia, lymphoma, and malignancies that result in elevated serum uric acid levels. Table 16.11 gives the specific dosage information and the pregnancy categories for these drugs.

### Use in Children

Allopurinol is not routinely administered to children, except to those with hyperuricemia secondary to cancer and

| | TABLE 16.11 | | | |
|---|---|---|---|---|
| | **DRUGS AT A GLANCE: Uricosuric Agents** | | | |
| **Drug** | **Pregnancy Category** | **Routes and Dosage Ranges** | | |
| | | **Adults** | | **Children** |
| **Allopurinol** (Zyloprim, Aloprim; Apo-Allopurinol, Apo-Allopurinol A) | C | Gout and hyperuricemia: PO 100–800 mg/k/d in divided doses, depending on the severity of the disease (200–300 mg/d is the usual dose) Maintenance: establish dose that maintains serum uric acid levels within normal limits Hyperuricemia: PO 200–300 mg/d; adjust the dose based on urate levels Prevention of uric acid nephropathy in certain malignancies: PO 600–800 mg/d for 203 d with a high fluid intake; maintenance dose as above Recurrent calcium oxalate stones: PO 200–300 mg/d; adjust dose based on 24-h urinary urate determinations Parenteral administration: IV 200–400 mg/m²/d as a continuous infusion or at 6-, 8-, or 1-h intervals Dosage based on creatinine clearance: 140 mL/min—400 mg 120 mL/min—350 mg 100 mL/min—300 mg 80 mL/min—250 mg 60 mL/min—200 mg 40 mL/min—150 mg | | Secondary hyperuricemia associated with various malignancies: 6–10 y, PO 300 mg/d; adjust dose based on serum uric acid levels <6 y: PO 150 mg/d; adjust dose after 48 h of treatment based on serum uric acid level Parenteral: 200 mg/m²/d IV as continuous infusion or at 6-, 8-, or 12-intervals |
| Febuxostat (Uloric; Uloric, MAR-Febuxostat) | C | PO 40 mg/d; if serum uric acid level is not <6 mg/dL in 2 wk, dosage should be increased to 80 mg/d | | Safety and efficacy not established |
| Pegloticase (Krystexxa) | C | IV 8 mg every 2 wk | | Safety and efficacy not established |
| Probenecid | B | PO 0.25 g BID for 1 wk; then 0.5 g BID; maintenance, continue dosage that maintains the normal serum uric acid levels. When no attacks occur for 6 mo or longer, decrease the dose to 0.5 g every 6 mo | | Safety and efficacy not established |
| Rasburicase (Elitek; Fasturtec) | C | Hyperuricemia associated with malignancy IV 0.2 mg/kg once daily for up to 5 d (use beyond 5 d or more than one course is not recommended) | | IV 0.2 mg/kg once daily for up to 5 d (use beyond 5 d or more than one course is not recommended) |

chemotherapy treatment. When administering allopurinol intravenously, it is essential to ensure that the child is hydrated to maintain a neutral or slightly alkaline urine output.

### Use in Older Adults

Allopurinol may be used in geriatric patients. The initial dose is 100 mg/day, which can be increased until the desired uric acid level is obtained. It is necessary to maintain fluid intake to produce a urine output of at least 2000 mL/day. The dosage should be reduced in the event of diminished renal function.

### Use in Patients With Renal Impairment

The dosage of allopurinol is reduced based on the patient's creatinine clearance. See Table 16.11 for the specific dosage information.

### Use in Patients With Hepatic Impairment

Allopurinol is administered cautiously in patients with hepatic impairment. The dosage does not need to be adjusted, but it is important to monitor liver function.

## Adverse Effects

Allopurinol has several adverse effects. CNS adverse effects include drowsiness, headache, and vertigo. Hematologic adverse effects are agranulocytosis, aplastic anemia, and bone marrow depression. The most common GI effects are nausea, vomiting, diarrhea, abdominal pain, and indigestion. Hepatotoxicity and renal insufficiency are risk factors with the use of allopurinol.

## Contraindications

Patients with a known hypersensitivity to allopurinol should not take allopurinol. Also, patients with a family history or history of idiopathic hemochromatosis should not receive the drug.

## Nursing Implications

### Preventing Interactions

Several medications, including azathioprine, mercaptopurine, cyclophosphamide, cyclosporine, and thiazide diuretics, increase the risk of uricosuric-associated toxicity. The administration of ampicillin and amoxicillin with allopurinol increases the risk of developing a rash. Anticoagulation effects are increased when combined with warfarin and aspirin. Alcohol combined with allopurinol decreases the excretion of uric acid.

### Administering the Medication

It is necessary to administer allopurinol after meals to ensure absorption.

### Assess for Therapeutic Effects

The nurse assesses for decreased pain, inflammation, and joint swelling. In patients with tophi (see Fig. 16.2), it is important to assess for increased joint mobility and decrease in tophi prominence. It is vital to assess serum uric acid levels. The normal serum uric acid level is 3.0 to 7.0 mg/dL.

---

**BOX 16.17** 📋 *Patient Teaching Guidelines for Allopurinol*

- Take fluid to yield at least 2000 mL of urine output per day.
- Report decreased urine output or cloudy urine, which could be indicative of uric acid stone formation, to your health care provider.
- Report any rashes or skin eruptions to your health care provider.
- Do not drive or operate machinery until the central nervous system effects are known.
- Maintain appointments for serum uric acid levels, liver enzymes, and creatinine clearance to be drawn.

---

### Assess for Adverse Effects

The nurse assesses for diminished urine output or cloudy urine, which may be indicative of the development of uric acid kidney stones. It is also important to assess for GI effects such as nausea, vomiting, diarrhea, and abdominal pain. The nurse assesses for bruising, bleeding, and anemia. Finally, the nurse assesses aspartate aminotransferase and alanine aminotransferase levels for hepatotoxicity and creatinine clearance for renal insufficiency.

### Patient Teaching

Box 16.17 presents patient teaching guidelines for the uricosuric medications, including allopurinol.

## Other Drugs in the Class

Febuxostat (Uloric) is the first medication for the treatment of gout to be developed in 40 years. A chemically engineered nonpurine agent, it selectively inhibits xanthine oxidase. Clinical studies have indicated that it is more effective in lowering serum uric acid levels than allopurinol. The most common adverse effect is hepatotoxicity. It is also necessary to assess patients who take febuxostat for the development of cardiovascular events such as myocardial infarction.

Pegloticase (Krystexxa) is a uric acid–specific uricosuric medication. Prior to the IV administration of pegloticase, all other antihyperuricemic medications should be discontinued. The patient should be premedicated with corticosteroids and antihistamines. Pegloticase has a high rate of anaphylactic reactions. It is important to observe the patient carefully for rash, wheezing, and bronchospasm.

Rasburicase (Elitek) has the ability to enzymatically degrade uric acid. It is administered for hyperuricemia associated with malignancy. Rasburicase can result in methemoglobinemia. Methemoglobin is a transformation product of oxyhemoglobin, which then enters the circulating blood.

---

❗ **QSEN Alert: Safety**

In Canada, a safety alert was issued for febuxostat in which data suggested a link between a drug reaction and rash with eosinophilia and systemic symptoms. In addition, many patients who experienced serious skin reaction with febuxostat also reported similar skin reaction while using allopurinol. Each patient who receives febuxostat should be assessed for the development of a rash. The nurse should inform the physician if a rash develops and suggest that a complete blood count be obtained.

Probenecid increases the urinary excretion of uric acid. This uricosuric action means that it can be used therapeutically to treat hyperuricemia and gout. It is not effective in acute attacks of gouty arthritis but prevents hyperuricemia and tophi associated with chronic gout. Probenecid may cause acute gout until serum uric acid levels are within the normal range; concomitant administration of colchicine prevents this effect. (Probenecid also is used with penicillin, most often in treating sexually transmitted diseases. It increases blood levels and prolongs the action of penicillin by decreasing the rate of urinary excretion.)

## Unfolding Patient Stories: Danielle Young Bear • Part 2

Recall Danielle Young Bear, the 32-year-old construction worker you met in Chapter 6, who is being seen at the clinic for lower back pain that was not relieved with treatment from a traditional Native American healer using herbal medicine and burning aromatic plants. What questions can the nurse ask Danielle to identify her cultural health beliefs on how she perceives and manages pain? Because she requests a nonnarcotic, inexpensive medication, compare and contrast the actions and side effects of acetaminophen, aspirin, and ibuprofen for managing pain and inflammation.

Care for Danielle and other patients in a realistic virtual environment: *vSim for Nursing* (thepoint.lww.com/vSimPharm). Practice documenting these patients' care in DocuCare (thepoint.lww.com/DocuCareEHR).

## NCLEX Success

13. A patient is being treated with colchicine for acute gouty flare-up. Which of the following statements indicates the need for increased patient education?

    A. "I am going to stop taking the colchicine because of the diarrhea I am having."
    B. "The gastrointestinal effects are difficult to deal with, but I know they will decrease my gouty symptoms."
    C. "I will continue my colchicine just as it has been prescribed for me."
    D. "The diarrhea I am experiencing can result in dehydration. If I have lethargy, I will call my prescriber."

14. A man with an acute gouty flare-up is taking allopurinol. Which of the following subjective statements indicates that he has developed uric acid kidney stones?

    A. "I have pain in my right toe and left elbow."
    B. "I am dizzy and feel like I am going to faint."
    C. "I am urinating every hour–approximately 8 oz."
    D. "I have excruciating pain in my lower abdomen."

15. A man is taking allopurinol for acute gout. He has also been receiving anticoagulant therapy since having a myocardial infarction. What is the priority assessment?

    A. diminished pain in the inflamed joint
    B. adherence to the medication regimen
    C. bleeding
    D. abdominal pain

## THE NURSING PROCESS

A concept map outlines the nursing process related to drug therapy considerations in this chapter. Additional nursing implications related to the disease process should also be considered in care decisions.

**Assessment**
- Assess for signs and symptoms of pain, site of pain, type and duration of pain, and factors that relieve or increase pain.
- Assess for limitation in activity or mobility.
- In patients with gout assess for abdominal pain, joint pain, redness, swelling, and limitation in mobility.
- Assess for fever (thermometer readings above 99.6°F or 37.3°C). Signs and symptoms include hot, dry skin, flushed face, reduced urine output, and dehydration.
- Assess the use of OTC analgesic, antipyretic, or anti-inflammatory agents.
- Assess for allergic reactions to aspirin or NSAIDs.
- Assess for history of peptic ulcer disease, GI bleeding, hepatic and renal disease.

**Outcomes of Therapy**

The patient will
- Experience relief of discomfort with minimal adverse drug effects.
- Experience increased mobility and activity tolerance.
- Inform health care providers if taking aspirin, an NSAID, or acetaminophen regularly.
- Self-administer the drugs safely.
- Avoid overuse of the drugs.

**Nursing Interventions**
- Implement measures to prevent or minimize pain, fever, and inflammation.
- Treat the disease processes (e.g., infection, arthritis) or circumstances (e.g., impaired blood supply, lack of physical activity, poor positioning or body alignment) thought to be causing pain, fever, or inflammation.
- Treat pain as soon as possible; early treatment may prevent severe pain and anxiety and allow the use of milder analgesic drugs. Use distraction, relaxation techniques, or other nonpharmacologic techniques along with drug therapy, when appropriate.
- With acute musculoskeletal injuries (e.g., sprains), think RICE: Rest, Ice, Compression, Elevation to decrease pain, swelling, and inflammation. Cold therapy should be applied for 20 minutes every 3 to 4 hours for 48 hours.
- Assist patients to drink 2 to 3 L of fluid daily when taking an NSAID regularly. This strategy decreases gastric irritation and helps to maintain good kidney function. With long-term use of aspirin, fluids help prevent precipitation of salicylate crystals in the urinary tract. With antigout drugs, fluids help prevent precipitation of urate crystals and formation of urate kidney stones. Fluid intake is especially important initially when serum uric acid levels are high and large amounts of uric acid are being excreted.
- Provide appropriate teaching for any drug therapy.

**Evaluation**
- Interview and observe regarding relief of symptoms.
- Interview and observe regarding mobility and activity levels.
- Interview and observe regarding safe, effective use of the drugs.
- Select drugs appropriately.

## KEY CONCEPTS

- Aspirin, other NSAIDs, and acetaminophen inhibit COX enzymes, which are required for prostaglandin formation.
- Aspirin and other nonselective NSAIDs inhibit both COX-1 and COX-2. The COX-2 inhibitor, celecoxib, is more selective for the COX-2 enzyme. The exact mechanism of action of acetaminophen is unclear.
- The FDA has issued a **BLACK BOX WARNING** ◆ for aspirin stating that children or teenagers should not take aspirin to treat chickenpox or flulike symptoms because of the risk of Reye's syndrome.
- Prostaglandins produced by COX-1 are important in regulating homeostasis and are associated with platelet aggregation and protective effects on the stomach and kidneys. Drug-induced inhibition results in gastric ulceration, renal dysfunction, and diminished blood clotting.
- Prostaglandins produced by COX-2 are associated with pain and inflammation. Drug-induced inhibition results in therapeutic effects of analgesia and anti-inflammatory activity.
- People with hypersensitivity to aspirin should not take NSAIDs due to the risk of cross-sensitivity to other antiprostaglandin drugs.
- The use of gastroprotective drugs such as antacids, $H_2$ blockers, and proton pump inhibitors may be indicated to prevent upper GI bleeding with chronic use of aspirin and other nonselective NSAIDs.
- Acetaminophen is the drug of choice for fever in children. Acetaminophen and ibuprofen may be alternated in the treatment of children with fever.
- The major drawback of acetaminophen use is the potentially fatal liver damage with overdose. Acetylcysteine is the specific antidote to acetaminophen overdose.
- The FDA has issued a **BLACK BOX WARNING** ◆ stating that ibuprofen is contraindicated for the treatment of perioperative pain after coronary artery bypass graft.

- The FDA has issued a **BLACK BOX WARNING** ◆ stating that nonsteroidal anti-inflammatory drugs cause an increased risk of serious cardiovascular thrombotic events, including stroke or myocardial infarction.
- A **BLACK BOX WARNING** ◆ states that patients who take meloxicam are at risk for cardiovascular events and GI bleeding.
- Another **BLACK BOX WARNING** ◆ reports that an increased risk for adverse cardiovascular thrombotic effects, including myocardial infarction and cerebrovascular accident, may occur with indomethacin.
- The FDA has issued a **BLACK BOX WARNING** ◆ stating that patients who take meloxicam are at risk for cardiovascular events and GI bleeding.
- Drugs related to indomethacin are etodolac, ketorolac (Toradol), and nabumetone. Etodolac reportedly causes less gastric irritation, especially in older adults at high risk for GI bleeding.
- The FDA has issued a **BLACK BOX WARNING** ◆ for ketorolac; this drug places the patient at risk for GI irritation, inflammation, ulceration, bleeding, and perforation.
- The FDA has issued a **BLACK BOX WARNING** ◆ for celecoxib concerning its cardiac and vascular risks.
- Allopurinol, which inhibits the synthesis of uric acid, is the drug of choice for people with gout due to "overproduction" of uric acid.
- Colchicine is the only antigout drug with anti-inflammatory effects; it is useful for treating acute attacks.
- Febuxostat, probenecid, and sulfinpyrazone are uricosuric drugs effective in treating people with gout who "underexcrete" uric acid.
- During treatment for gout, the nurse encourages patients to increase fluid intake to 2000 mL/day to prevent renal calculi.

## CLINICAL REASONING CASE STUDY

**Meet the Patient**

Oleatha Sousa, a 76-year-old woman, is seen by her neurosurgeon for severe low back pain radiating down her left leg. Magnetic resonance imaging reveals spinal stenosis. She has refused epidural injections, and her physician prescribes celecoxib (Celebrex) 100 mg orally twice a day.

• What drug information regarding celecoxib will the nurse provide?
• What adverse effects should the nurse provide?

**Assessing Drug Information**

• Celecoxib is a COX-2 only inhibitor. All other NSAIDs inhibit COX-1 and COX-2.
• Celecoxib and all NSAIDs have a **BLACK BOX WARNING** ◆ stating that an increased risk of adverse cardiovascular thrombotic effects, including myocardial infarction and cerebrovascular accident, can result from these medications.
• Celecoxib only inhibits COX-2, thus decreasing inflammation. The other NSAIDs decrease platelet aggregation, increasing the risk of bleeding.
• Adverse effects of NSAIDs include gastric irritation and bleeding.
• Adverse effects of celecoxib include dizziness, somnolence, and insomnia. Some patients note ophthalmic changes. Dermatologic adverse effects include rash, pruritus, sweating, dry mucous membranes, and stomatitis. Diminished pain and increased mobility may also occur.

**Nursing Actions**

• Instruct Mrs. Sousa about the action of the celecoxib.
• Reinforce that drug interactions are a possibility. Mrs. Sousa should not take other NSAIDs or aspirin.
• Instruct Mrs. Sousa that it is safe to take acetaminophen.
• Instruct Mrs. Sousa that celecoxib can alter visual acuity and cause dizziness. She should use caution when changing positions or ambulating.
• Encourage Mrs. Sousa to drink 2 to 3 quarts of fluid daily.
• Instruct Mrs. Sousa to seek medical attention if she experiences chest pain, shortness of breath, sudden weakness, confusion, slurred speech, or any signs and symptoms of myocardial infarction or stroke.
• Instruct Mrs. Sousa to report abdominal pain, tarry stools, or upper gastrointestinal distress.

---

*Visit* thePoint® *at* **http://thePoint.lww.com/Frandsen12e** *for answers to NCLEX Success questions (in Appendix A), answers to Clinical Application Case Studies (in Appendix B), and more!*

## REFERENCES AND RESOURCES

Anonymous. (2019). *Nursing 2019 drug handbook*. Philadelphia, PA: Lippincott Williams & Wilkins.

Becker, M., & Gaffo, A. L. (2020). Treatment of gout flares. In *UpToDate*. Wolters Kluwer.

Becker, M. A., & Perez-Ruiz, F. (2020). Pharmacologic urate-lowering therapy and treatment of tophi in patients with gout. In *UpToDate*. Wolters Kluwer.

Hinkle, J. H., & Cheever, K. H. (2017). *Brunner & Suddarth's textbook of medical-surgical nursing* (14th ed.). Philadelphia, PA: Lippincott Williams & Wilkins.

Karch, A. M. (2019). *2019 Lippincott Pocket Drug drug guide for nurses*. Philadelphia, PA: Lippincott Williams & Wilkins.

Ma, R., Chen, G. H., Zhao, L. J., & Zhai, X. C. (2018). Efficacy of naproxen prophylaxis for the prevention of heterotrophic ossification after hip surgery: A meta analysis. *Journal of Orthopaedic Surgery and Research, 13*(1), 1.

Norris, T. L. (2019). *Porth's pathophysiology: Concepts of altered health states* (10th ed.). Philadelphia, PA: Lippincott Williams & Wilkins.

UpToDate. (2019). *Drug information*. Lexi-Comp, Inc.

# Drug Therapy With Corticosteroids

## LEARNING OBJECTIVES

*After studying this chapter, you should be able to:*

1. Understand the physiologic effects of endogenous corticosteroids.
2. Identify the pathophysiology of adrenal cortex disorders.
3. Describe the action and the clinical indications for use of exogenous corticosteroids.
4. Understand the contraindications and adverse effects of corticosteroids as well as the nursing implications of their use.
5. Analyze how other drugs and substances as well as other factors may affect the need for corticosteroids.
6. Apply the nursing process when a patient is administered a corticosteroid.

## CLINICAL APPLICATION CASE STUDY

Emma Mae Thompson is a 65-year-old woman who lives alone. Since she was 15 years old, she has smoked one pack of unfiltered cigarettes per day. When she was diagnosed with chronic obstructive pulmonary disease (COPD) 5 years ago, she quit smoking. She takes albuterol sulfate one inhalation per nebulizer every 12 hours and beclomethasone dipropionate 160 mcg every 12 hours. Recently, she was treated for pneumonia. Mrs. Thompson's physician prescribes prednisone orally in a tapering dose, according to the following schedule:

Day 1: 10 mg before breakfast, 5 mg before lunch, 5 mg before supper, 10 mg at bedtime
Day 2: 5 mg before breakfast, 5 mg before lunch, 5 mg before supper, 10 mg at bedtime
Day 3: 5 mg before breakfast, 5 mg before lunch, 5 mg before supper, 5 mg at bedtime
Day 4: 5 mg before breakfast, 5 mg before supper, 5 mg at bedtime
Day 5: 5 mg before breakfast, 5 mg at bedtime
Day 6: 5 mg before breakfast

## KEY TERMS

**Addison's disease:** primary adrenocortical insufficiency with inadequate production of cortisol and aldosterone

**Addisonian crisis:** condition that mimics hypovolemic and septic shock; also known as adrenocortical insufficiency

**Aldosterone:** mineralocorticoid hormone secreted by the adrenal cortex to increase sodium reabsorption by the kidneys and indirectly regulate blood levels of potassium, sodium, and bicarbonate; also regulates pH, blood volume, and blood pressure

**Corticosteroid:** steroid hormone produced by the adrenal cortex; examples include androgens, glucocorticoids, and mineralocorticoids

**Cortisol:** the main glucocorticoid secreted as part of the body's response to stress

**Cushing's disease:** adrenocortical hyperfunction; may result from excessive corticotropin or primary adrenal tumor

**Glucocorticoid:** adrenal cortical hormone that protects the body against stress and affects protein and carbohydrate metabolism

**Immunosuppression:** suppression of the immune system

**Mineralocorticoid:** steroid hormone released by the adrenal cortex to promote sodium and water retention and potassium excretion

**Negative feedback mechanism:** when the output of a system affects the stimulus for the system (e.g., hormone secretion produces an effect that shuts off the stimulus for further hormone secretion)

**Steroid:** lipid-soluble hormone produced by the gonadal organs or the adrenal cortex

# INTRODUCTION

This chapter provides an introduction to the **corticosteroids**, also known as the **glucocorticoids** or **steroids**. These lipid-soluble hormones are produced by the gonadal organs or the adrenal cortex, part of the adrenal glands. These hormones affect almost all body organs and are extremely important in maintaining homeostasis when secreted in normal amounts. Disease results from inadequate or excessive secretion. Exogenous corticosteroids are used as drugs in a variety of disorders. Their use must be closely monitored, because they have profound therapeutic and adverse effects. To understand the effects of corticosteroids used as drugs (exogenous corticosteroids), it is necessary to understand the physiologic effects and other characteristics of the endogenous hormones.

# PHYSIOLOGY OF ENDOGENOUS CORTICOSTEROIDS

Corticosteroid secretion is controlled by the hypothalamus, the anterior pituitary, and adrenal cortex (the hypothalamic–pituitary–adrenal, or HPA, axis). Various stimuli (e.g., low plasma levels of corticosteroids, pain, anxiety, trauma, illness, being placed under anesthesia) activate the system. These stimuli cause the hypothalamus of the brain to secrete corticotropin-releasing hormone or factor (known as CRH or CRF), which stimulates the anterior pituitary gland to secrete corticotropin, and corticotropin then stimulates the adrenal cortex to secrete corticosteroids.

The rate of corticosteroid secretion is usually maintained within relatively narrow limits but changes according to need. When plasma corticosteroid levels rise to an adequate level, secretion of corticosteroids slows or stops. The mechanism by which the hypothalamus and anterior pituitary "learn" that no more corticosteroids are needed is called a **negative feedback mechanism** (Fig. 17.1).

This negative feedback mechanism is normally very important, but it does not work during stress responses. The stress response activates the sympathetic nervous system (SNS) to produce more epinephrine and norepinephrine and the adrenal cortex to produce as much as 10 times the normal amount of **cortisol**. The synergistic interaction of these hormones increases the person's ability to respond to stress. However, the increased SNS activity continues to stimulate cortisol

production (the main glucocorticoid secreted as part of the body's response to stress) and overrules the negative feedback mechanism. Excessive and prolonged corticosteroid secretion damages body tissues.

Corticosteroids are secreted directly into the bloodstream. Cortisol is approximately 90% bound to plasma proteins, and this high degree of protein binding slows cortisol movement out of the plasma, so that it has a relatively long plasma half-life of 60 to 90 minutes. The remaining 10% is unbound and biologically active. In contrast, **aldosterone** is only 60% bound to plasma proteins and has a short half-life of 20 minutes. In general, protein binding functions as a storage area from which the hormones are released as needed. This promotes more consistent blood levels and more uniform distribution to the tissues.

The adrenal cortex produces approximately 30 steroid hormones, which are divided into glucocorticoids, **mineralocorticoids**, and adrenal sex hormones. Chemically, all corticosteroids are derived from cholesterol and have similar chemical structures. However, despite their similarities, slight differences cause them to have different functions.

## Glucocorticoids

Although the term "corticosteroids" actually refers to all secretions of the adrenal cortex, it is most often used to designate the glucocorticoids, which are important in metabolic, inflammatory, and immune processes. Glucocorticoids include cortisol, corticosterone, and cortisone. Cortisol accounts for at least 95% of glucocorticoid activity; corticosterone and cortisone account for a small amount of activity. Glucocorticoids are secreted cyclically, with the largest amount being produced in the early morning and the smallest amount during the evening hours (in people with a normal day–night schedule). At the cellular level, glucocorticoids account for most of the characteristics and physiologic effects of the corticosteroids (Box 17.1). The chronic use of the glucocorticoids will produce adverse effects that include suppression of the hypothalamic–pituitary–adrenal axis, Cushing's disease, increased susceptibility to infections, and mental status changes.

## Mineralocorticoids

Mineralocorticoids are a class of steroids that play a vital role in the maintenance of fluid and electrolyte balance through their influence on salt and water metabolism. Aldosterone is

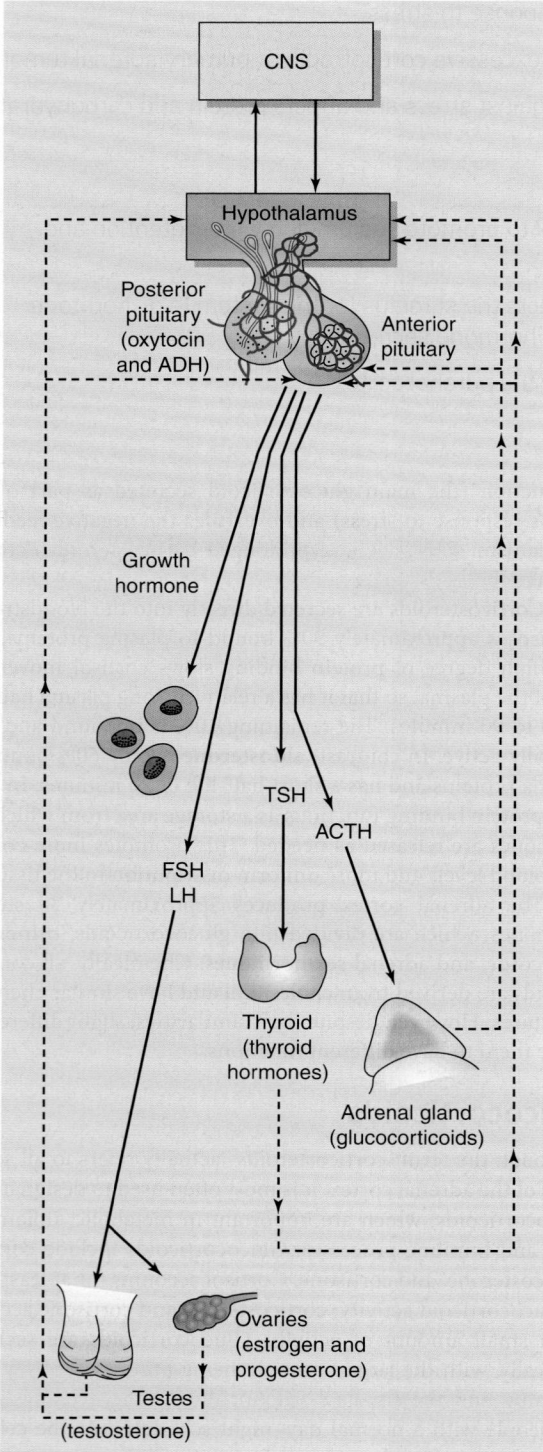

**Figure 17.1.** Control of hormone production by the hypothalamic–pituitary target cell feedback mechanism. Hormone levels from the target glands regulate the release of hormones from the anterior pituitary through a negative feedback system. The *dashed line* represents feedback control. ACTH, adrenocorticotropic hormone; ADH, antidiuretic hormone; CNS, central nervous system; FSH, follicle-stimulating hormone; LH, luteinizing hormone; TSH, thyroid-stimulating hormone. [From Norris, T. L. (2019). *Porth's pathophysiology: Concepts of altered health states* (10th ed., Fig. 40.3, p. 1183). Philadelphia, PA: Wolters Kluwer Health | Lippincott Williams & Wilkins.]

the main mineralocorticoid and is responsible for approximately 90% of mineralocorticoid activity. Characteristics and physiologic effects of mineralocorticoids are summarized in Box 17.2.

## Adrenal Sex Hormones

The adrenal cortex secretes male (androgens) and female (estrogens and progesterone) sex hormones. Compared with the effect of hormones produced by the testes and ovaries, the adrenal sex hormones have an insignificant effect on normal body function. Adrenal androgens, secreted continuously in small quantities by both sexes, are responsible for most of the physiologic effects exerted by the adrenal sex hormones. They increase protein synthesis (anabolism), which increases the mass and strength of muscle and bone tissue; they affect development of male secondary sex characteristics; and they increase hair growth and libido in women. Excessive secretion of adrenal androgens in women causes masculinizing effects (e.g., hirsutism, acne, breast atrophy, deepening of the voice, amenorrhea). Female sex hormones are secreted in small amounts and normally exert few physiologic effects. Excessive secretion may produce feminizing effects in men (e.g., breast enlargement, decreased hair growth, voice changes).

## PATHOPHYSIOLOGY OF ADRENAL CORTEX DISORDERS

Disorders of the adrenal cortex involve increased or decreased production of corticosteroids, especially cortisol as the primary glucocorticoid and aldosterone as the primary mineralocorticoid. These disorders include the following:

- **Primary adrenocortical insufficiency (Addison's disease)** is associated with destruction of the adrenal cortex by disorders such as tuberculosis, cancer, or hemorrhage; with atrophy of the adrenal cortex caused by autoimmune disease or prolonged administration of exogenous corticosteroids; and with surgical excision of the adrenal glands. In primary adrenocortical insufficiency, there is inadequate production of both cortisol and aldosterone.
- **Secondary adrenocortical insufficiency**, produced by inadequate secretion of corticotropin, is most often caused by prolonged administration of corticosteroids. This condition is largely a glucocorticoid deficiency; mineralocorticoid secretion is not significantly impaired.
- **Congenital adrenogenital syndromes and adrenal hyperplasia** result from deficiencies in one or more enzymes required for cortisol production. Low plasma levels of cortisol result in excessive corticotropin secretion, which then leads to excessive adrenal secretion of androgens and hyperplasia (abnormal increase in number of cells).
- **Androgen-producing tumors** of the adrenal cortex, which are usually benign, produce masculinizing effects.
- **Adrenocortical hyperfunction (Cushing's disease)** may result from excessive corticotropin or a primary adrenal tumor. Adrenal tumors may be benign or malignant. Benign tumors often produce one corticosteroid normally secreted by the adrenal cortex, but malignant tumors often secrete several corticosteroids.

| BOX 17.1 | *Effects of Glucocorticoids on Body Processes and Systems* |

## Carbohydrate Metabolism

- ↑ Formation of glucose (gluconeogenesis) by breaking down protein into amino acids. The amino acids are then transported to the liver, where they are acted on by enzymes that convert them to glucose. The glucose is then returned to the circulation for use by body tissues or storage in the liver as glycogen.
- ↓ Cellular use of glucose, especially in muscle cells. This is attributed to a ↓ effect of insulin on the proteins that normally transport glucose into cells and by ↓ numbers and functional capacity of insulin receptors.
- Both the ↑ production and ↓ use of glucose promote higher levels of glucose in the blood (hyperglycemia) and may lead to diabetes mellitus. These actions also increase the amount of glucose stored as glycogen in the liver, skeletal muscles, and other tissues.

## Protein Metabolism

- Breakdown of protein into amino acids (catabolic effect); ↑ rate of amino acid transport to the liver and conversion to glucose
- ↓ Rate of new protein formation from dietary and other amino acids (antianabolic effect)
- The combination of ↑ breakdown of cell protein and ↓ protein synthesis leads to protein depletion in virtually all body cells except those of the liver. Thus, glycogen stores in the body are ↑ and protein stores are ↓.

## Lipid Metabolism

- ↑ Breakdown of adipose tissue into fatty acids; the fatty acids are transported in the plasma and used as a source of energy by body cells.
- ↑ Oxidation of fatty acids within body cells

## Inflammatory and Immune Responses

- ↓ Inflammatory response. Inflammation is the normal bodily response to tissue damage and involves three stages. First, a large amount of plasma-like fluid leaks out of capillaries into the damaged area and becomes clotted. Second, leukocytes migrate into the area. Third, tissue healing occurs, largely by growth of fibrous scar tissue. Normal or physiologic amounts of glucocorticoids probably do not significantly affect inflammation and healing, but large amounts of glucocorticoids inhibit all three stages of the inflammatory process.
- More specifically, corticosteroids stabilize lysosomal membranes (and thereby prevent the release of inflammatory proteolytic enzymes); ↓ capillary permeability (and thereby ↓ leakage of fluid and proteins into the damaged tissue); ↓ the accumulation of neutrophils and macrophages at sites of inflammation (and thereby impair phagocytosis of pathogenic microorganisms and waste products of cellular metabolism); and ↓ production of inflammatory chemicals, such as interleukin-1, prostaglandins, and leukotrienes, by injured cells.

- ↓ Immune response. The immune system normally protects the body from foreign invaders, and several immune responses overlap inflammatory responses, including phagocytosis. In addition, the immune response stimulates the production of antibodies and activated lymphocytes to destroy the foreign substance. Glucocorticoids impair protein synthesis, including the production of antibodies; ↓ the numbers of circulating lymphocytes, eosinophils, and macrophages; and ↓ amounts of lymphoid tissue. These effects help account for the immunosuppressive and antiallergic actions of the glucocorticoids.

## Cardiovascular System

- Help regulate arterial blood pressure by modifying vascular smooth muscle tone by modifying myocardial contractility and by stimulating renal mineralocorticoid and glucocorticoid receptors
- ↑ The response of vascular smooth muscle to the pressor effects of catecholamines and other vasoconstrictive agents

## Nervous System

- Physiologic amounts help to *maintain normal nerve excitability*; pharmacologic amounts ↓ nerve excitability, slow activity in the cerebral cortex, and alter brain wave patterns.
- ↓ Secretion of CRH by the hypothalamus and of corticotropin by the anterior pituitary gland. This results in suppression of further glucocorticoid secretion by the adrenal cortex (negative feedback system).

## Musculoskeletal System

- Maintain muscle strength when present in physiologic amounts but cause muscle atrophy (from protein breakdown) when present in excessive amounts.
- ↓ Bone formation and growth and ↑ bone breakdown. Glucocorticoids also ↓ intestinal absorption and ↑ renal excretion of calcium. These effects contribute to bone demineralization (osteoporosis) in adults and to ↓ linear growth in children.

## Respiratory System

- Maintain open airways. Glucocorticoids do not have direct bronchodilating effects but help maintain and restore responsiveness to the bronchodilating effects of endogenous catecholamines, such as epinephrine.
- Stabilize mast cells and other cells to inhibit the release of bronchoconstrictive and inflammatory substances, such as histamine.

## Gastrointestinal System

- ↓ Viscosity of gastric mucus. This effect may ↓ protective properties of the mucus and contribute to the development of peptic ulcer disease.

↑, increase/increased; ↓, decrease/decreased.

| BOX 17.2 | *Effects of Mineralocorticoids on Body Processes and Systems* |

- The overall physiologic effects are to conserve sodium and water and eliminate potassium. Aldosterone increases sodium reabsorption from kidney tubules, and water is reabsorbed along with the sodium. When sodium is conserved, another cation must be excreted to maintain electrical neutrality of body fluids; thus, potassium is excreted. This is the only potent mechanism for controlling the concentration of potassium ions in extracellular fluids.
- Secretion of aldosterone is controlled by several factors, most of which are related to kidney function. In general, secretion is increased when the potassium level of

extracellular fluid is high, the sodium level of extracellular fluid is low, the renin–angiotensin system of the kidneys is activated, or the anterior pituitary gland secretes corticotropin.
- Inadequate secretion of aldosterone causes hyperkalemia, hyponatremia, and extracellular fluid volume deficit (dehydration). Hypotension and shock may result from decreased cardiac output. Absence of mineralocorticoids causes death.
- Excessive secretion of aldosterone produces hypokalemia, hypernatremia, and extracellular fluid volume excess (water intoxication). Edema and hypertension may result.

- **Hyperaldosteronism** is a rare disorder caused by adenoma (a benign tissue from glandular tissue) or hyperplasia of the adrenal cortex cells that produce aldosterone. It is characterized by hypokalemia, hypernatremia, hypertension, thirst, and polyuria.

# DRUG THERAPY WITH EXOGENOUS CORTICOSTEROIDS

Exogenous corticosteroids, or glucocorticoids, are administered to treat disorders of the adrenal cortex or endocrine system. The administration of corticosteroids decreases the inflammatory symptoms and alters the immune response produced by

nonendocrine disorders. People once viewed hydrocortisone, a short-acting corticosteroid and an exogenous equivalent of endogenous cortisol, as the prototype corticosteroid drug. Now, they consider 🔵 **prednisone**, an intermediate-acting corticosteroid, to be the prototype corticosteroid. Table 17.1 lists the glucocorticoids and mineralocorticoids.

## Pharmacokinetics

The rate of absorption of corticosteroids depends on the route of administration. Oral administration results in rapid absorption by the gastrointestinal (GI) tract, with rapid distribution to the intestines, muscles, liver, and kidneys. The corticosteroid is metabolized

| **TABLE 17.1** | | |
|---|---|---|
| **Adrenal Corticosteroid Drugs** | | |
| **Drug Class** | **Prototype** | **Other Drugs in the Class** |
| Glucocorticoid | Prednisone (Deltasone, predniSONE, Intensol, Rayos) | Beclomethasone (QVAR RediHaler, Beconase AQ, QNASL) |
| | | Betamethasone (betamethasone acetate and sodium phosphate) (Celestone, Soluspan, Pod-Care 100C, ReadySharp Betamethasone) |
| | | Budesonide (Rhinocort Allergy, Entocort EC, Uceris) |
| | | Cortisone acetate |
| | | Dexamethasone (Decadron, Dexamethasone Intensol, DexPak) |
| | | Flunisolide |
| | | Fluticasone (Arnuity Ellipta, Flovent Diskus, Flovent HFA); fluticasone topical (Cutivate) |
| | | Hydrocortisone (Ala Cort, Ala Scalp, Anucort, Anusol, Colocort, Cortef, Cortenema, Cortifoam, Nutracort, Solu-Cortef) |
| | | Methylprednisolone (Depo-Medrol, Medrol, P-Care D40, P-Care D80, SOLU-Medrol) |
| | | Mometasone (Asmanex, Asmanex HFA, Sinuva, Elocon, Nasonex) |
| | | Prednisolone (Pred Forte, Pred Mild) |
| | | Triamcinolone (Kenalog, Oracort, Triderm) Triamcinolone (nasal) acetonide (GoodSense Nasal Allergy Spray, Nasacort Allergy; Nasacort Allergy (all over-the-counter) Triamcinolone (systemic; intralesional) (Kenalog, Kenalog 80, P-Care K40, P-Care K80, Pod-Care 100K, Pro-C-Dure 5, Pro-C-Dure 6, Zilretta) Triamcinolone (topical) (Trianex, Triderm) |
| Mineralocorticoid | Fludrocortisone | |

by the liver by cytochrome P-450 3A4 enzymes, and the medication is conjugated to inactive metabolites. About 25% of the metabolites are excreted in the bile and then in the feces. The other 75%, which enter the circulation, are excreted in the kidneys. Plasma binding affects metabolism of corticosteroids, which means that patients with serum albumin levels less than 3.5 g/dL are prone to increased effects of corticosteroids and symptoms of hypercorticism.

The administration of exogenous corticosteroids suppresses the HPA axis. As a result, secretion of corticotropin decreases, causing atrophy of the adrenal cortex and decreased production of endogenous adrenal corticosteroids.

## Action

Like endogenous glucocorticoids, exogenous corticosteroids act at the cellular level by binding to drug receptors in target tissues. The lipid-soluble drugs easily diffuse through the cell membranes of target cells. Inside the cell, they bind with receptors in intracellular cytoplasm. The drug–receptor complex then moves to the cell nucleus, where it interacts with DNA to stimulate or suppress gene transcription.

Corticosteroids can increase or decrease the transcription of many genes to alter the synthesis of proteins. These proteins regulate many physiologic effects, such as the transportation of proteins. Metabolic effects do not occur for at least 45 to 60 minutes because of the time required for protein synthesis. Several hours or days may be needed for full production of proteins.

Because the genes vary in different types of body cells, corticosteroid effects also vary, depending on the specific cells being targeted. For example, supraphysiologic concentrations of glucocorticoids induce the synthesis of lipolytic and proteolytic enzymes and other specific proteins in various tissues. Overall, corticosteroids have multiple mechanisms of action and effects (Fig. 17.2), including the following:

- **Inhibiting arachidonic acid metabolism.** Normally, when a body cell is injured or activated by various stimuli, the enzyme phospholipase $A_2$ causes the phospholipids in cell membranes to release arachidonic acid. Free arachidonic acid is then metabolized to produce proinflammatory prostaglandins (see Chap. 16) and leukotrienes. At sites of tissue injury or inflammation, corticosteroids induce the synthesis of proteins that suppress the activation of phospholipase $A_2$.

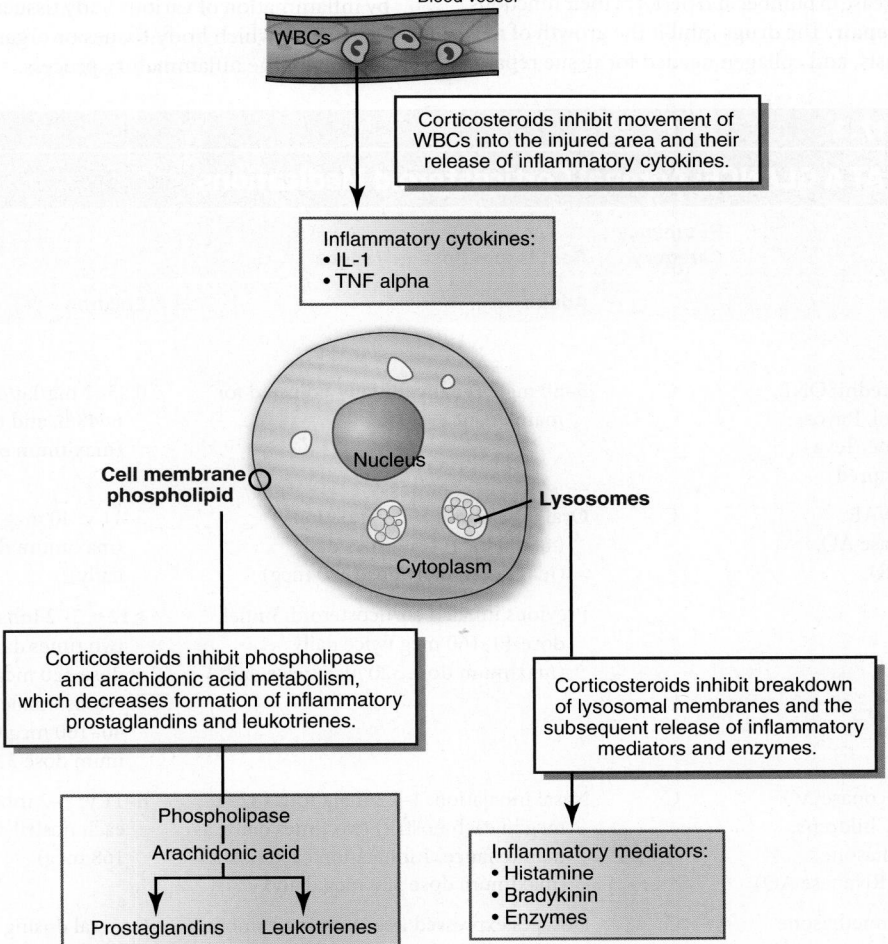

**Figure 17.2.** Inflammatory processes and anti-inflammatory actions of corticosteroids. Cellular responses to injury include the following: phospholipid in the cell membrane is acted on by phospholipase to release arachidonic acid, metabolism of arachidonic acid produces the inflammatory mediators prostaglandins and leukotrienes, lysosomal membrane breaks down and releases inflammatory chemicals (e.g., histamine, bradykinin, intracellular digestive enzymes), and white blood cells (WBCs) are drawn to the area and release inflammatory cytokines (e.g., interleukin-1 [IL-1] alpha). Overall, corticosteroid drugs act to inhibit the release, formation, or activation of various inflammatory mediators. TNF, tumor necrosis factor.

This action, in turn, decreases the release of arachidonic acid and the formation of prostaglandins and leukotrienes.

- **Strengthening or stabilizing biologic membranes.** Two biologic membranes are especially important in inflammatory processes. Stabilization of cell membranes inhibits the release of arachidonic acid and production of prostaglandins and leukotrienes, as described above. Stabilization of lysosomal membranes inhibits release of bradykinin, histamine, enzymes, and perhaps other substances from lysosomes. (Lysosomes are intracellular structures that contain inflammatory chemical mediators and enzymes that destroy cellular debris and phagocytized pathogens.) This reduces capillary permeability and thus prevents leakage of fluid into the injured area and development of edema. It also reduces the chemicals that normally cause vasodilation and tissue irritation.
- **Inhibiting the production of interleukin-1, tumor necrosis factor, and other cytokines.** This action also contributes to the anti-inflammatory and immunosuppressant effects of corticosteroids.
- **Impairing phagocytosis.** The drugs inhibit the ability of phagocytic cells to leave the bloodstream and move into the injured or inflamed tissue.
- **Impairing lymphocytes.** The drugs inhibit the ability of these immune cells to increase in number and perform their functions.
- **Inhibiting tissue repair.** The drugs inhibit the growth of new capillaries, fibroblasts, and collagen needed for tissue repair.

## Use

Corticosteroids are administered to control symptoms but do not cure underlying disease processes. They are extensively used to treat many different disorders. Except for replacement therapy in deficiency states, the use of corticosteroids is largely empiric. Because the drugs affect virtually every aspect of inflammatory and immune responses, they are used in the treatment of a broad spectrum of diseases with an inflammatory or immunologic component.

Table 17.2 presents information about routes of administration and dosage ranges.

### General Indications

The corticosteroids discussed in this chapter are used to treat potentially serious or disabling disorders, including the following:

- Allergic or hypersensitivity disorders, such as allergic reactions to drugs, serum and blood transfusions, and dermatoses with an allergic component
- Collagen disorders, such as systemic lupus erythematosus, scleroderma, and periarteritis nodosa. Collagen is the basic structural protein of connective tissue, tendons, cartilage, and bone, and it is therefore present in almost all body tissues and organ systems. The collagen disorders are characterized by inflammation of various body tissues. Signs and symptoms depend on which body tissues or organs are affected and the severity of the inflammatory process.

### TABLE 17.2

### DRUGS AT A GLANCE: Adrenal Corticosteroid Medications

| Drug | Pregnancy Category | Routes and Dosage Ranges | |
|------|---------|------------------------|----------|
| | | **Adults** | **Children** |
| Glucocorticoids | | | |
| **Prednisone** (predniSONE, Deltasone, Intensol, Rayos; ❀ Apo-Prednisone, Teva-PredniSONE, Winpred) | C | 5–60 mg PO daily initially, adjusted for maintenance | 0.25–2 mg/kg/dose PO every 6–48 h, and then 1–2 mg/kg/24 h (maximum 60 mg/24 h) |
| Beclomethasone (QVAR RediHaler, Beconase AQ, QNASL; ❀ QVAR) | C | Oral inhalation: 1–2 inhalations (40–80 mcg) two times daily (maximum daily dose 320 mcg) | 5–11 y: 40 mcg twice daily (maximum dose 80 mg twice daily) |
| | | Previous inhaled corticosteroid: Initial dose 40–160 mcg twice daily (maximum dose 320 mcg twice daily) | ≥12 y: 1–2 inhalations (40–80 mcg) two times daily (maximum daily dose 320 mcg) |
| | | | Previous inhaled corticosteroid: 40–160 mcg twice daily (maximum dose 320 mcg) |
| Beclomethasone (Beconase AQ, QNASL, QNASL Children's; ❀ Apo-Beclomethasone, Mylan-Beclo AQ, Rivanase AQ) | C | Nasal inhalation: 1–2 inhalations (42–84 mcg in each nostril) two times daily; as maintenance, 1 inhalation each nostril (maximum dose 320 mcg daily) | 6–11 y: 1–2 inhalations (42–84 mcg) each nostril daily (maximum dose 168 mcg) |
| Betamethasone (betamethasone acetate and sodium phosphate) (Celestone, Soluspan, Pod-Care 100C, ReadySharp Betamethasone; ❀ Celestone, Soluspan) | C | Dosages expressed as a combined amount of betamethasone sodium phosphate and betamethasone acetate; 1 mg equivalent to betamethasone sodium phosphate 0.5 mg and betamethasone acetate 0.5 mg<br>Initial dose 0.25–9 mg/d IM (based on the severity of disease and patient response | General dosing for treatment of inflammatory and allergic conditions: 0.02–0.3 mg/kg/d |

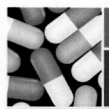
| Drug | Pregnancy Category | Routes and Dosage Ranges | |
|---|---|---|---|
| | | **Adults** | **Children** |
| Betamethasone acetate and sodium phosphate (Celestone Soluspan; Betaject, Celestone Soluspan) | | 0.25–9 mg IM daily; 0.25–2 mL intra-articular injection | |
| Budesonide (Pulmicort Flexhaler; ✹ Pulmicort Nebuamp, Pulmicort Turbuhaler, TEVA-Budesonide) | C | Oral inhalation: 360 mcg twice daily; maximum dose 720 mcg twice daily<br>Maintenance: 200–400 mcg twice daily or 400 mcg once daily | *National Asthma Education and Prevention Program* (*NAEPP 2007*): 5–11 y<br>Low dose: 180–400 mcg/d<br>Medium dose: >400–800 mcg/d<br>High dose: >800 mcg/d<br>Children ≥12 y: Refer to adult dosing. |
| Budesonide (Rhinocort Allergy; ✹ Mylan-Budesonide AQ, Rhinocort Aqua, Rhinocort Turbuhaler) | C | Nasal inhalation: One spray (32 mcg) in each nostril once daily or twice daily | 6–11 y: one spray in each nostril once daily (total dose 64 mcg/d)<br>≥12 y: Refer to adult dosing. |
| Budesonide (Entocort EC; ✹ Cortiment, Entocort) | C | Oral capsule<br>Crohn's disease or ulcerative colitis: 9 mg PO once daily in the morning, for up to 8 wk | Children ≥ 8 y and adolescents ≤ 17 y (weighing >25 kg) 9 mg daily in the morning for up to 8 wk and then 6 mg once daily for 2 wk |
| Budesonide (Uceris; ✹ Entocort) | C | Rectal foam (Uceris)<br>Initial: 2 mg twice daily for 2 wk<br>Maintenance: 2 mg once daily for 4 wk<br>Rectal enema (Entocort): initial 2 mg (one enema) once daily at night prior to bedtime for 4 wk | |
| Cortisone acetate | C | PO 25–300 mg daily, individualized for condition and response<br>Physiologic replacement: PO 25–35 mg/d | |
| Dexamethasone (Decadron, Dexamethasone Intensol, DexPak; ✹ Apo-Dexamethasone, Dexamethasone Omega Unidose) | C | 0.75–9 mg PO daily in 2–4 doses; higher range for serious diseases | 0.08–0.3 mg/kg/d |
| Flunisolide | C | Oral inhalation: 2 inhalations (160 mcg) twice daily<br>Maximum dose: 320 mcg twice daily | 6–11 y: 80 mcg twice daily<br>Maximum dose: 160 mcg twice daily<br>≥12 y: Refer to adult dosing. |
| Flunisolide (Apo-Flunisolide, Nasalide, Rhinalar) | C | Nasal inhalation: 2 sprays in each nostril twice daily; maximum daily dose 8 sprays in each nostril | 6–14 y: 1 spray in each nostril three times daily or 2 sprays in each nostril two times daily; maximum daily dose 4 sprays in each nostril |
| Fluticasone (Arnuity Ellipta, Flovent Diskus, Flovent HFA) | C | Oral inhalation: Arnuity Ellipta: 100 mcg once daily; maximum 100 mcg once daily<br>Flovent HFA: 2 inhalations (88 mcg) two times daily (maximum daily dose 440 mcg inhaled two times daily) | <12 y: Not recommended |
| Fluticasone (Flonase Allergy Relief OTC; ✹ Apo-Fluticasone, RATIO- Flonase, TEVA-Fluticasone) | C | Nasal inhalation: 200 mcg daily initially (2 sprays each nostril once daily or 1 spray each nostril twice daily). After a few days, reduce dosage to 100 mcg daily (1 spray each nostril once daily) for maintenance therapy. | 4–11 y: 100 mcg daily (1 spray per nostril once daily). *Do not use more than 2 mo per year.*<br>≥12 y: Refer to adult dosing. |
| Fluticasone topical (Cutivate; ✹ Cutivate) | C | Apply a thin film to affected area one to two times daily | ≥3 mo: Refer to adult dosing. |

*(Continued on page 340)*

**TABLE 17.2**

## DRUGS AT A GLANCE: Adrenal Corticosteroid Medications (Continued)

| Drug | Pregnancy Category | Routes and Dosage Ranges | |
|---|---|---|---|
| | | **Adults** | **Children** |
| Hydrocortisone (Ala Cort, Ala Scalp, Anucort, Anusol, Colocort, Cortef, Cortenema, Cortifoam, Nutracort, Solu-Cortef; ✿ Barriere-HC, Cortenema, Cortifoam, Emo Cort, Hyderm, Hydroval, NOVO-Hydrocort, Prevex HC, SANDOZ Hydrocortisone, Sama HC) | C | Apply sparingly to skin two to four times daily | Same as adults |
| Hydrocortisone (A-Hydrocort, Cortef, Solu-Cortef; Cortef, Solu-Cortef) | C | Anti-inflammatory or immunosuppression IM, IV: initial 100–500 mg/dose at intervals of 2, 4, or 6 h PO: initial 20–240 mg/d Multiple sclerosis IM, IV: 800 mg/d for 1 wk, followed by 320 mg every other day for 1 mo PO: 200 mg/d for 1 wk, followed by 80 mg every other day for 1 mo *For adrenal insufficiency, see* Chapter 45 | PO: 2.5–10 mg/kg/d or 75–300 mg/m²/d in 3–4 divided doses IM, IV: 0.56–8 mg/kg/d |
| Hydrocortisone (Cortenema; Cortenema) | C | 100 mg enema rectally every night for 21 d or until optimal response | |
| Hydrocortisone acetate (Cortifoam; Cortifoam) | C | 1 applicator rectally one to two times per day for 2–3 wk and then once every 2–3 d if needed | |
| Methylprednisolone (Depo-Medrol, Medrol, P-Care D40, P-Care D80, SOLU-Medrol; ✿ Depo-Medrol, Medrol, SOLU-Medrol, Uni-MED) | C | 4–48 mg daily PO initially, gradually reduced to lowest effective level 10–40 mg IM or IV initially, adjusted to condition and response Acute respiratory distress syndrome Early severe: (day 1–6 of onset) IV loading dose of 1 mg/kg over 30 min; followed by a slow taper <br>• Days 1–14: 1 mg/kg/d in divided doses or as a continuous infusion <br>• Days 15–21: 0.5 mg/kg/d in divided doses or as a continuous infusion <br>• Days 22–25: 0.25 mg/kg/d in divided doses or as a continuous infusion <br>• Days 26–28: 0.125 mg/kg/d in divided doses or as a continuous infusion <br>Late persistent (day 7–14 of onset) IV loading dose of 2 mg/kg over 30 minutes, followed by a slow taper <br>• Days 1–14: 2 mg/kg/d in divided doses or as a continuous infusion <br>• Days 15–21: 1 mg/kg/d in divided doses or as a continuous infusion <br>• Days 22–25: 0.5 mg/kg/d in divided doses or as a continuous infusion <br>• Days 26–28: 0.25 mg/kg/d in divided doses or as a continuous infusion <br>• Days 29–30: 0.125 mg bolus over 30 minutes | Infants and children: Not <0.5 mg/kg/24 h IM or IV |

**TABLE 17.2**

**DRUGS AT A GLANCE: Adrenal Corticosteroid Medications** (Continued)

| Drug | Pregnancy Category | Routes and Dosage Ranges | |
|---|---|---|---|
| | | **Adults** | **Children** |
| Methylprednisolone acetate (Depo-Medrol) | C | 40–120 mg IM once daily | |
| Mometasone (Asmanex, Asmanex HFA, Nasonex, Sinuva, Elocon; ✹ Asmanex Twisthaler, Apo-Mometasone, Mosaspray, Nasonex, SANDOZ Mometasone, Elocon PMS, TARO-Mometasone, TEVA-Mometasone) | C | Oral inhalation<br>• Low-dose therapy: 110–220 mcg/d<br>• Medium-dose therapy: >220–440 mcg/d<br>• High-dose therapy: >440 mcg/d<br>2 sprays (100 mcg/spray) in each nostril once daily (200 mcg/d)<br>Topical cream applied sparingly to affected area<br>Topical lotion applied, a few drops to affected area | Oral inhalation<br>Children 4–11 years: 110 mcg inhaler in the evening<br>2–11 y: 1 spray (50 mcg) in each nostril once daily (100 mcg/d)<br>>12 y: same as adults<br>Children >2 y to adolescents<br>Topical cream applied sparingly to affected area<br>Topical lotion applied a few drops to affected area |
| Prednisolone (Millipred, Millipred DP, Millipred DP 12-Day, Pediapred; ✹ Pediapred, PMS-Prednisolone) | C | 5–60 mg PO daily initially, adjusted for maintenance | 0.1–2 mg/kg/d PO in divided doses |
| Prednisolone (Pred Forte, Pred Mild; ✹ Diopred, Minims Prednisolone, PMS-Prednisolone, Sod Phos Fort, Pred Forte, SANDOZ Prednisolone, TEVA-Prednisolone) | C | 1–2 drops in conjunctival sac two to four times per day; during the initial 24–48 h, the dosing frequency may be increased if necessary. If signs and symptoms fail to improve after 2 days, reevaluate. Do not discontinue therapy prematurely; withdraw therapy with gradual tapering of dose in chronic conditions. | Ophthalmic inflammation in children is an off-label use.<br>Prednisone acetate: 1% instill 1–2 drops into conjunctival sac three to six times daily. |
| Triamcinolone acetonide (GoodSense Nasal Allergy Spray, Nasacort Allergy; Nasacort Allergy) (all over-the-counter; ✹ Apo-Triamcinolone AQ, Nasacort AQ) | C | Nasal inhalation: 2 sprays (110 mcg) in each nostril once daily (total dose 220 mcg/d); may increase to maximal daily dose of 440 mcg if indicated | 2–6 y: 1 spray (55 mcg) in each nostril once daily<br>≥6 y: 2 sprays (110 mcg) in each nostril once daily (220 mcg/d) initially; reduce to 1 spray per nostril once daily (110 mcg/d) |
| Triamcinolone (Kenalog, Kenalog 80, P-Care K40, P-Care K80, Pod-Care 100K, Pro-C-Dure 5, Pro-C-Dure 6, Zilretta; ✹ Kenalog-10, Kenalog-40) | C | Intralesional: 1 mg initial dose; dose varies due to disease and lesion to be treated; may be treated weekly or less frequently<br>Intra-articular: 2–20 mg every 3–4 wk as needed | Lowest possible dose to control disease |
| Triamcinolone (Trianex, Triderm; ✹ Aristocort, Aristocort R, Oracort, Triaderm) | C | Apply a thin film to affected areas two to four times per day. | 0.25%–0.5%: Apply a thin film. |
| Mineralocorticoid | | | |
| Fludrocortisone (Florinef; ✹ Florinef) | C | Chronic adrenocortical insufficiency: 0.1 mg PO daily<br>Salt-losing adrenogenital syndromes: 0.1–0.2 mg daily | 0.05–0.1 mg PO daily |

• Dermatologic disorders that may be treated with systemic corticosteroids include acute contact dermatitis, erythema multiforme, herpes zoster (prophylaxis of postherpetic neuralgia), lichen planus, pemphigus, skin rashes caused by drugs, and toxic epidermal necrolysis. Corticosteroid preparations that are applied topically in dermatologic disorders are discussed in Chapter 61.

• Endocrine disorders, such as adrenocortical insufficiency and congenital adrenal hyperplasia (see Chap. 45 for additional information). Corticosteroids are given to replace or substitute for the natural hormones (both glucocorticoids and mineralocorticoids) in cases of insufficiency and to suppress corticotropin when excess secretion causes adrenal hyperplasia. These conditions are rare and account for a small percentage of corticosteroid use.

- GI disorders, such as ulcerative colitis and regional enteritis (Crohn's disease)
- Hematologic disorders, such as idiopathic thrombocytopenic purpura or acquired hemolytic anemia
- Hepatic disorders characterized by edema, such as cirrhosis and ascites
- Neoplastic disease, such as acute and chronic leukemias, Hodgkin's disease, other lymphomas, and multiple myeloma (see later discussion)
- Neurologic conditions, such as cerebral edema, brain tumor, acute spinal cord injury (see later discussion), and myasthenia gravis
- Ophthalmic disorders, such as optic neuritis, sympathetic ophthalmia, and chorioretinitis. Corticosteroid preparations that are applied topically in ophthalmologic disorders are discussed in Chapter 59.
- Organ or tissue transplants and grafts (e.g., kidney, heart, bone marrow). Corticosteroids suppress cellular and humoral immune responses (see Chap. 13) and help prevent rejection of transplanted tissue. Drug therapy is usually continued as long as the transplanted tissue is in place.
- Renal disorders characterized by edema, such as the nephrotic syndrome
- Respiratory disorders, such as asthma, status asthmaticus, COPD, and inflammatory disorders of nasal mucosa (rhinitis)
- Rheumatic disorders, such as ankylosing spondylitis, acute and chronic bursitis, acute gouty arthritis, rheumatoid arthritis, and osteoarthritis
- Shock. Corticosteroids are clearly indicated only for shock resulting from **addisonian crisis** (also known as adrenal or adrenocortical insufficiency), which may mimic hypovolemic or septic shock. The use of corticosteroids in septic shock has been highly controversial, and randomized studies and meta-analyses have indicated that corticosteroids are not beneficial in treating septic shock. However, more recent small studies indicate possible clinical usefulness in septic shock, because this form of shock may be associated with relative adrenal insufficiency. In anaphylactic shock resulting from an allergic reaction, corticosteroids may increase or restore cardiovascular responsiveness to adrenergic drugs.

## Clinical Application 17.1

- What is the purpose of administering prednisone to Mrs. Thompson?
- What is the purpose of tapering the dose?
- Could prednisone be discontinued without tapering the dose?

## NCLEX Success

1. A woman is experiencing periods of increased anxiety and panic attacks over her illness and that of her family members. Epinephrine and norepinephrine are released. What glucocorticoid is released by the adrenal cortex in response to stress?

    A. insulin
    B. glucose
    C. thyroid hormone
    D. cortisol

2. A boy has contracted a rash caused by poison ivy over a large portion of his arms and legs following a camping trip. His health care provider has prescribed oral prednisone, which is to be administered in a tapering dose over the next 10 days. What effect does the medication have on the rash?

    A. It decreases the accumulation of neutrophils and macrophages at the site, thus reducing inflammation.
    B. It eliminates the itching associated with the allergy.
    C. It increases the white blood cell count to assist in healing.
    D. It increases the protein metabolism to allow for the rejuvenation of tissue.

3. A patient is receiving prednisone 10 mg orally every day to reduce symptoms of Crohn's disease. Which of the following effects is associated with daily administration of prednisone?

    A. atrophy of the adrenal cortex
    B. decreased serum glucose
    C. weight loss
    D. fluid volume deficit

4. A patient with chronic obstructive pulmonary disease is being administered a corticosteroid by nebulizer. What effect does the corticosteroid have?

    A. decrease in blood pressure
    B. decrease in mucus secretion
    C. decrease in edema
    D. increase in immunity

5. A patient is admitted to the emergency department in anaphylactic shock following numerous bee stings. The prescriber orders parenteral administration of corticosteroids. What effect is expected from the administration of these agents?

    A. decreased heart rate and blood pressure
    B. increased circulation to the lower extremities
    C. increased or restored cardiovascular responsiveness
    D. decreased production of aldosterone

## Specific Uses

### Allergic Rhinitis

Allergic rhinitis (also called seasonal rhinitis, hay fever, and perennial rhinitis) is a common problem for which corticosteroids are given by nasal spray, once or twice daily. The drugs decrease mucus secretion and inflammation. Therapeutic effects usually occur within a few days with regular use. Systemic adverse effects are minimal with recommended doses but may occur with higher doses, including adrenocortical insufficiency from HPA suppression.

### Arthritis

Corticosteroids are the most effective drugs for rapid relief of the pain, edema, and restricted mobility associated with acute episodes of joint inflammation. They are usually given on a short-term basis. When inflammation is limited to three or fewer joints, the preferred route of drug administration is by injection directly into the joint. Intra-articular injections relieve symptoms in approximately 2 to 8 weeks, and several formulations are available for this route. However, corticosteroids do not prevent disease progression and joint destruction. As a general rule, a joint should not be injected more often than three times yearly because of risks of infection and damage to intra-articular structures from the injections and from overuse when pain is relieved.

### Asthma

Corticosteroids are commonly used in the treatment of asthma because of their anti-inflammatory effects. In addition, corticosteroids increase the effects of adrenergic bronchodilators to prevent or treat bronchoconstriction and bronchospasm. The drugs increase the number of beta-adrenergic receptors and increase or restore responsiveness of beta receptors to beta-adrenergic bronchodilating drugs. Research indicates that responsiveness to beta-adrenergic bronchodilators increases within 2 hours and that numbers of beta receptors increase within 4 hours.

In acute asthma or status asthmaticus unrelieved by inhaled beta-adrenergic bronchodilators, high doses of systemic corticosteroids are given orally or intravenously along with bronchodilators for approximately 5 to 10 days. Although these high doses suppress the HPA axis, the suppression lasts for only 1 to 3 days, and other serious adverse effects are avoided. Thus, systemic corticosteroids are used for short-term therapy, as needed, and not for long-term treatment. People who regularly use inhaled corticosteroids also require high doses of systemic drugs during acute attacks because aerosols are not effective. As soon as acute symptoms subside, it is necessary to taper the dose; people should take the lowest effective maintenance dose or discontinue the drug. In chronic asthma, inhaled corticosteroids are the drugs of first choice. This recommendation evolved from increased knowledge about the importance of inflammation in the pathophysiology of asthma and the development of aerosol corticosteroids that are effective with minimal adverse effects.

Inhaled drugs may be given alone or with systemic drugs. In general, inhaled corticosteroids can replace oral drugs when daily dosage of the oral drug has been tapered to 10 to 15 mg of prednisone or the equivalent. When a patient is being switched from an oral to an inhaled corticosteroid, the inhaled drug should be started during tapering of the oral drug, approximately 1 or 2 weeks before discontinuing or reaching the lowest anticipated dose of the oral drug. When a patient requires a systemic corticosteroid, coadministration of an aerosol allows smaller doses of the systemic corticosteroid. Although the inhaled drugs can cause suppression of the HPA axis and adrenocortical function, especially at higher doses, they are much less likely to do so than systemic drugs. However, the U.S. Food and Drug Administration (FDA) has issued a **BLACK BOX WARNING** ◆ for people who are transferred from systemically active corticosteroids to flunisolide inhaler because deaths have occurred from adrenal insufficiency.

> **!** **QSEN Alert: Evidence-Based Practice**
>
> Mohammad et al. [2018] conducted a study to assess the effect of adjunctive perioperative corticosteroids during the perioperative phase following knee arthroplasty. A meta-analysis was conducted to determine the analgesic and safety effects of perioperative corticosteroid use and patient response. They examined 14 randomized controlled trials that included 1396 knee arthroplasties. The mean dose of oral prednisone was 50 to 75 mg. The administration of systemic corticosteroids demonstrates statistical significance with modest pain reduction at 12 to 24 hours.

### Cancer

Corticosteroids are commonly used in the treatment of lymphomas, lymphocytic leukemias, and multiple myeloma. In these disorders, corticosteroids inhibit cell reproduction and are cytotoxic to lymphocytes. In addition to their anticancer effects in hematologic malignancies, corticosteroids are beneficial in treatment of several signs and symptoms that often accompany cancer, although the mechanisms of action are unknown and drug/dosage regimens vary widely. Corticosteroids are used to treat anorexia, nausea and vomiting, cerebral edema and inflammation associated with brain metastases or radiation of the head, spinal cord compression, pain and edema related to pressure on nerves or bone metastases, graft versus host disease after bone marrow transplantation, and other disorders that occur in patients with cancer. Patients tend to feel better when taking corticosteroids, although the basic disease process may be unchanged. *Feel better only.*

#### Primary Central Nervous System Lymphomas

Formerly considered rare tumors of older adults, central nervous system (CNS) lymphomas are being diagnosed more frequently in younger patients. They are usually associated with chronic **immunosuppression** (suppression of the immune system) caused by immunosuppressant drugs or acquired immunodeficiency syndrome (AIDS). Many of these lymphomas are very sensitive to corticosteroids, and therapy is indicated when the diagnosis is established.

#### Other Central Nervous System Tumors

Corticosteroid therapy may be useful in both supportive and definitive treatment of brain and spinal cord tumors, and neurologic signs and symptoms often improve dramatically within 24 to 48 hours. Corticosteroids help relieve symptoms by controlling edema around the tumor, at operative sites, and at sites receiving radiation therapy. Some patients no longer require corticosteroids after surgical or radiation therapy, whereas others require continued therapy to manage neurologic symptoms. Adverse effects of long-term corticosteroid therapy may include mental changes ranging from mild agitation to psychosis and steroid myopathy (muscle weakness and atrophy) that may be confused with tumor progression. Mental symptoms usually improve if the drug dosage is reduced and resolve if the drug is discontinued; steroid myopathy may persist for weeks or months.

### Chemotherapy-Induced Emesis

Corticosteroids have strong antiemetic effects; the mechanism is unknown. One effective regimen is a combination of an oral or intravenous (IV) dose of dexamethasone (10–20 mg) and a serotonin antagonist or metoclopramide given immediately before the chemotherapeutic drug. This regimen is the treatment of choice for chemotherapy with cisplatin, which is a strongly emetic drug.

### Postoperative Nausea and Vomiting

Postoperative nausea and vomiting is a common complication during recovery from anesthesia. It is most common in women; there is also a high risk in children. Nausea and vomiting occur due to a variety of factors. For example, anxiety and fear play a role in their development. Stimulation of the vestibular system will induce nausea and vomiting. The high cortical centers communicate with the central pattern generator in the medulla. The antiemetic regimen to prevent postoperative nausea and vomiting includes the application of a scopolamine patch 2 hours prior to the induction of anesthesia, dexamethasone 4 to 8 mg IV after anesthetic induction, and ondansetron 4 mg IV at the conclusion of the surgery.

### Chronic Obstructive Pulmonary Disease

Corticosteroids are more helpful in acute exacerbations of COPD than in stable disease. However, oral corticosteroids may improve pulmonary function and symptoms in some patients. As in asthma and rhinitis, the drugs decrease mucus secretion and inflammation. Lymphocytes are involved in the inflammatory response in both asthma and COPD. In patients with COPD, the CD8 cell numbers increase and lead to secretion of proinflammatory cytokines and cytotoxic molecules. The administration of the medication roflumilast, a phosphodiesterase 4 inhibitor, and corticosteroids decreases the degradation cyclic adenosine monophosphate to decrease the inflammatory activity (Ferguson & Make, 2019; Stoller, 2019). Note that inhaled corticosteroids can also be used. Although they produce minimal adverse effects, their effectiveness in COPD has not been clearly demonstrated.

### Inflammatory Bowel Disease

Patients who suffer from Crohn's disease or ulcerative colitis often require periodic corticosteroid therapy. In moderate Crohn's disease, oral prednisone, 40 mg daily, is usually given until symptoms subside. With severe disease, patients often require hospitalization, IV fluids for hydration, and parenteral corticosteroids until symptoms subside. Budesonide may be used for Crohn's disease. It inhibits protein synthesis, thus decreasing the formation of inflammatory cytokines. The oral capsule dissolves in the small intestine and acts locally before being absorbed into the bloodstream and transported to the liver for metabolism. It has fewer adverse effects than systemic corticosteroids but is also less effective and more expensive. The topical formulation is available in foam or enema to be administered in the proximal and splenic flexure to reduce colonic inflammation (Peppercorn & Cheifetz, 2019).

In ulcerative colitis, corticosteroids are usually used when aminosalicylates (e.g., mesalamine) are not effective or when symptoms are more severe. Initially, hydrocortisone enemas may be effective. If they are not, oral prednisone (20–60 mg daily) may be given until symptoms subside. In severe disease, oral prednisone may be required initially. After remission of symptoms is achieved, the dose can be tapered by 2.5 to 5 mg/day each week to a dose of 20 mg. Then, tapering may be slowed to 2.5 to 5 mg/day every other week. As in Crohn's disease, patients with severe ulcerative colitis often require hospitalization and parenteral corticosteroids. One regimen uses IV hydrocortisone 300 mg/day or the equivalent dose of another drug. When the patient's condition improves, oral prednisone can replace the IV corticosteroid.

### Spinal Cord Injury

High-dose corticosteroid therapy to treat spinal cord injury is a common practice in clinical settings, although controversy exists regarding its use. Data suggest that methylprednisolone may be effective in acute spinal cord injury when given in high doses within 8 hours of the injury. Methylprednisolone improves neurologic recovery, although it does not improve mortality, and its use is unlikely to result in normal neurologic function. In addition, severe adverse outcomes, including wound and systemic infections, GI hemorrhage, and pneumonia, have been reported.

### Septic Shock

During critical illness, the body induces a state of absolute or relative adrenal insufficiency. The patient's illness affects cortisol levels and the function of the HPA activation, resulting in increased levels of cortisol. The impairment of HPA results in adrenocortical hyporesponsiveness and resistance to glucocorticoids. In patients with refractory shock with a blood pressure less than 90 mm Hg for more than 1 hour following fluid resuscitation and administration of vasopressor medication, hydrocortisone less than 400 mg/day in divided doses is recommended (Kaufman, 2019).

> **! QSEN Alert: Evidence-Based Practice**
>
> Lin et al. (2019) conducted a meta-analysis to assess the evidence and latest clinical practice guidelines on the use of corticosteroids in sepsis. The objective of the study was to evaluate whether the administration of corticosteroids reduced the mortality of adult patients with sepsis. The meta-analysis revealed that a long course of low-dose corticosteroid treatment marginally improved the 28-day mortality rate in patients with septic shock and vasopressor-dependent septic shock. Early administration of hydrocortisone and fludrocortisone in a continuous infusion or bolus dosing is important for an improved prognosis. One adverse effect of the treatment is the development of hyperglycemia and hypernatremia.

## Prevention of Acute Adrenocortical Insufficiency

Suppression of the HPA axis may occur with corticosteroid therapy and may lead to life-threatening inability to increase cortisol secretion when needed to cope with stress. It is most likely to occur with abrupt withdrawal of systemic corticosteroid drugs. The risk of HPA suppression is high with systemic drugs given for more than a few days, although patients vary in degree and duration of suppression with comparable doses, and the minimum dose and duration of therapy that cause suppression are unknown.

When corticosteroids are given for replacement therapy, adrenal insufficiency is lifelong, and drug administration must be continued (see Chap. 45). When the drugs are given for purposes other than replacement and then discontinued, the HPA axis usually recovers within several weeks to months, but recovery may take a year. Several strategies have been developed to minimize HPA suppression and risks of acute adrenal insufficiency, including the following:

- Administering a systemic corticosteroid during high-stress situations (e.g., moderate or severe illness, trauma, surgery) to patients who have received pharmacologic doses for 2 weeks within the previous year or who receive long-term systemic therapy (i.e., are steroid dependent)
- Giving short courses of systemic therapy for acute disorders, such as asthma attacks, and then decreasing the dose or stopping the drug within a few days
- Gradually tapering the dose of any systemic corticosteroid. Although specific guidelines for tapering dosage have not been developed, higher doses and longer durations of administration in general require slower tapering, possibly over several weeks. The goal of tapering may be to stop the drug or to decrease the dosage to the lowest effective amount.
- Using local rather than systemic therapy when possible, alone or in combination with low doses of systemic drugs. Numerous preparations are available for local application, including aerosols for oral or nasal inhalation; formulations for topical application to the skin, eyes, and ears; and drugs for intra-articular injections.
- Using alternate-day therapy (ADT), which involves titrating the daily dose to the lowest effective maintenance level and then giving a double dose every other day

## *Use in Special Populations*

### Use in Children

Corticosteroids are used for the same conditions in children as in adults; a common indication is for treatment of asthma. With severe asthma, continual corticosteroid therapy may be required. For children with asthma, evidence indicates that with inhaled corticosteroids, starting with a moderate dose of the drug is comparable with starting with a high dose and titrating down. A concern with children is growth retardation, which can occur short term with small doses and administration by inhalation. Many children have a growth spurt when the corticosteroid is discontinued. Adult stature does not appear to be affected by inhaled corticosteroid therapy during childhood.

 *Concept Mastery Alert*

Because of the potential for growth retardation, it is important to assess the growth pattern—height and weight—for a child receiving long-term therapy with systemic corticosteroids.

Parents and prescribers can monitor drug effects by recording height and weight weekly. ADT is less likely to impair normal growth and development than daily administration. In addition, for both systemic and inhaled corticosteroids, each child's dose should be titrated to the lowest effective amount.

### Use in Older Adults

Corticosteroids are used for the same conditions in older adults as in younger ones. Older adults are especially likely to have conditions that are aggravated by the drugs (e.g., heart failure, hypertension, diabetes mellitus, arthritis, osteoporosis, increased susceptibility to infection, concomitant drug therapy that increases risks of GI ulceration, and bleeding). Adverse effects such as mania, depression, psychosis, and delirium are extremely common in older patients treated with corticosteroids. Consequently, it is important to consider risk–benefit ratios of systemic corticosteroid therapy carefully, especially for long-term therapy.

When used, lower doses are usually indicated because of decreased muscle mass, plasma volume, hepatic metabolism, and renal excretion in older adults. In addition, therapeutic and adverse responses should be monitored regularly by a health care provider (e.g., blood pressure, serum electrolytes, and blood glucose levels at least every 6 months). As in other populations, adverse effects are less likely to occur with oral or nasal inhalations than with oral drugs.

**! QSEN Alert: Safety**

When caring for a patient with COPD and a history of heart failure who takes a tapering dose of prednisone, it is necessary to instruct the patient to check his or her weight daily. The patient should also assess his or her extremities for edema. If the patient's weight increases, edema is evident, and shortness of breath develops, the patient should notify his or her primary health provider.

### Use in Patients With Renal Impairment

It is necessary to use systemic corticosteroids with caution because of slowed excretion, with possible accumulation and signs and symptoms of hypercorticism. In renal transplantation, use of corticosteroids, along with other immunosuppressive drugs, to prevent or treat rejection reactions, is extensive. In these patients, as in others, adverse effects of systemic corticosteroids may include infections, hypertension, glucose intolerance, obesity, cosmetic changes, bone loss, growth retardation in children, cataracts, pancreatitis, peptic ulcerations, and psychiatric disturbances. Prescribers should keep doses to a minimum, and eventually, withdrawal of drugs may be necessary in some patients.

## Use in Patients With Hepatic Impairment

Metabolism of corticosteroids is slowed by severe hepatic disease, and corticosteroids may accumulate and cause signs and symptoms of hypercorticism. In addition, patients with liver disease should take prednisolone rather than prednisone. Liver metabolism of prednisone is required to convert it to its active form, prednisolone.

## Use in Patients With Critical Illness

Use of corticosteroids in the treatment of serious illness has been extensive, with much empiric usage.

### Adrenal Insufficiency

Adrenal insufficiency is the most clear-cut indication for use of a corticosteroid, and even a slight impairment of the adrenal response during severe illness can be lethal if corticosteroid therapy is not instituted. Adrenal insufficiency is covered in depth in Chapter 45.

### Acute Respiratory Failure in Chronic Obstructive Pulmonary Disease

Some studies of patients with COPD have found that the parenteral administration of methylprednisolone may be effective for the treatment of acute respiratory failure. However, if other medications do not produce adequate bronchodilation, IV corticosteroid therapy is a reasonable treatment choice in the first 72 hours of the illness. The nurse assesses the patient for pulmonary infection because corticosteroid therapy places the patient at increased risk for pulmonary infection.

### Acute Respiratory Distress Syndrome

Although corticosteroids have been widely used in the past to assist in the treatment of patients with acute respiratory distress syndrome (ARDS), the current literature indicates that the benefits of corticosteroid therapy are uncertain. Studies examining the benefit of corticosteroid therapy revealed that improved gas exchange decreased the number of days patients with ARDS were on mechanically assisted ventilation (Siegel, 2019). The studies reviewed by Siegel revealed the importance of monitoring individual patients who are administered corticosteroids for signs and symptoms of infection.

### Acquired Immunodeficiency Syndrome

Health care providers are increasingly recognizing adrenal insufficiency in patients with AIDS, who require assessment and treatment for the condition, if indicated. Corticosteroids improve survival and decrease risks of respiratory failure with pneumocystosis, a common cause of death in patients with AIDS. The recommended regimen is prednisone 40 mg twice daily for 5 days, then 40 mg once daily for 5 days, and then 20 mg daily until completion of treatment for pneumocystosis. The effect of corticosteroids on risks of other opportunistic infections or neoplasms is unknown.

## Use in Patients Receiving Home Care

Corticosteroids are extensively used in the home setting, by all age groups, for a wide variety of disorders, and by most routes of administration. Because of potentially serious adverse effects, especially with oral drugs, it is extremely important that these drugs be used as prescribed. A major responsibility of home care nurses is to teach, demonstrate, supervise, monitor, or do whatever is needed to facilitate correct use. In addition, home care nurses must teach patients and caregivers interventions to minimize adverse effects of these drugs.

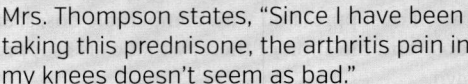

**Clinical Application 17.2**

Mrs. Thompson states, "Since I have been taking this prednisone, the arthritis pain in my knees doesn't seem as bad."

- Why has her arthritic pain in her knees decreased with the administration of oral prednisone?
- What patient teaching is specific to the administration of prednisone?

# NCLEX   Success

6. A patient is taking fluticasone 440 mcg inhaled two times per day. The patient is being seen in the pulmonary clinic and says, "I have been very congested and it has been hard to breathe, so for the past 10 days, I have been using my inhaler four times per day." The nurse should assess the patient for which of the following systemic adverse effects?

   A. hypoglycemia
   B. hypercalcemia
   C. anxiety
   D. hypothalamic–pituitary–adrenal (HPA) suppression

7. A liver transplant patient is receiving corticosteroids. These drugs are important to the care of this patient because they

   A. prevent thrombocytopenia
   B. increase immunity
   C. prevent tissue rejection
   D. decrease inflammation

8. A cancer patient asks the nurse why he is being given a corticosteroid before his chemotherapy. Which of the following is the nurse's best response?

   A. It will prevent the development of anemia related to the chemotherapy.
   B. It will prevent the development of hiccups, which is associated with chemotherapy.
   C. It will prevent nausea and vomiting that occur with chemotherapy.
   D. It will boost your immune system and prevent infection.

9. When administering long-term systemic corticosteroid medications, which of the following dosing schedules is recommended?

   A. alternate-day therapy
   B. once daily at noon
   C. weekly therapy
   D. nightly therapy

## Adverse Effects

Administration of more than 5 mg daily of corticosteroids results in adverse reactions. Possible adverse effects include the following:

- **Adrenocortical insufficiency:** fainting, weakness, anorexia, nausea, vomiting, hypotension, shock, and death (if untreated)
- **Adrenocortical excess**
- **Cushingoid features:** "moon face" and buffalo hump due to the redistribution of fat
- **CNS effects:** vertigo, headache, paresthesias, insomnia, and seizures
- **Cardiovascular symptoms:** hypotension, shock, hypertension, heart failure, thromboembolism, thrombophlebitis, fat embolism, and cardiac dysrhythmias
- **Diminished immunity:** increased susceptibility to infection
- **Endocrine effects:** diabetes mellitus, hyperglycemia, and hypercholesterolemia; diminished $T_3$ and $T_4$ levels, resulting in hypothyroidism; and reduced growth because of altered synthesis of DNA
- **Fluid and electrolyte effects:** fluid retention, hypokalemia, and hypocalcemia
- **Integumentary effects:** reddened skin, thinner skin, stretch marks, skin tears, and delayed wound healing
- **Musculoskeletal effects:** hypocalcemia, which places the patient at risk for osteoporosis and fracture development, and serum hypocalcemia, which increases the release parathyroid hormone, increasing the loss of calcium from bone
- **Ocular effects:** cataracts and glaucoma
- **Reproductive effects:** amenorrhea or irregular menstrual cycles

> **⚠ QSEN Alert: Patient-Centered Care**
>
> There is evidence that the administration of corticosteroids to patients receiving chemotherapy may result in hiccups. Health care providers must be cognizant of the effect of oral steroids can have on the development of hiccups.

## Contraindications

Corticosteroids are contraindicated in patients who experience allergic response to the medications. Patients with systemic fungal infections should not receive corticosteroids. Other contraindications include amebiasis, hepatitis B, vaccinia, varicella, and antibiotic-resistant infections. Also, patients who have been diagnosed with immunosuppression should not take corticosteroids. Patients receiving corticosteroids should not receive live virus vaccines, because of the risk of contracting the virus.

Caution is necessary when administering corticosteroids to patients with kidney disease, liver disease, hypothyroidism, recent GI surgery, peptic ulcer and inflammatory bowel disease, heart failure, thrombophlebitis, and diabetes mellitus.

 *caution*

## Nursing Implications

Many factors have an effect on drug dosage, such as the specific drug to be given, the desired route of administration, the reason for use, expected adverse effects, and patient characteristics. In general, the patient should take the smallest effective dose for the shortest effective time. It is necessary to individualize the dosage according to the severity of the disorder being treated, whether the disease is acute or chronic, and the patient's response to drug therapy. The calculation of corticosteroid dosages should be based on the severity of disease rather than the child's weight. If life-threatening disease is present, patients usually receive high doses until acute symptoms subside. Gradual dose reduction follows, until a maintenance dose is determined or the drug is discontinued. If life-threatening disease is not present, patients may still receive relatively high doses initially and then lower ones. Gradual reduction (tapering) over several days is necessary. With long-term corticosteroid therapy, periodic attempts to reduce dosage are desirable to decrease adverse effects. One way is to reduce the dose gradually until symptoms worsen, indicating the minimally effective dose.

Prescribers order physiologic doses (~15–20 mg of hydrocortisone or its equivalent daily) to replace or substitute for endogenous adrenocortical hormone. They usually order pharmacologic doses (supraphysiologic amounts) for anti-inflammatory, antiallergic, antistress, and immunosuppressive effects.

Compared with hydrocortisone, newer corticosteroids are more potent on a weight basis but are equipotent in anti-inflammatory effects when given in equivalent doses. Statements of equivalency with hydrocortisone are helpful in evaluating new drugs, comparing different drugs, and changing drugs or dosages. However, dosage equivalents apply only to drugs given orally or intravenously.

### Preventing Interactions

Many medications increase or decrease the therapeutic effects of corticosteroids. Herbal interactions with corticosteroids are most often related to changes in sodium and potassium (Box 17.3). Licorice increases the effects of corticosteroids, which may potentiate its effects; cautious use of licorice with corticosteroids is necessary.

### Administering the Medication

Corticosteroids can be given by several different routes to produce local or systemic effects, depending on the clinical problem. If feasible, these drugs should be given locally rather than systemically to prevent or decrease systemic toxicity. In recent years, several formulations have been developed for oral inhalation in the treatment of asthma and for nasal inhalation in the treatment of allergic rhinitis. When these drugs must be given systemically, the oral route is preferred. Parenteral administration is indicated only for patients who are seriously ill or unable to take oral medications. For intramuscular (IM) or IV injections, sodium phosphate or sodium succinate salts are used because they are most soluble in water. For intra-articular or intralesional injections, acetate salts are used because they have low solubility in water and provide prolonged local action.

Scheduling of drug administration is more important with corticosteroids than with most other drug classes. Most adverse effects occur with long-term administration of high doses. A major adverse reaction is suppression of the HPA axis and subsequent loss of adrenocortical function. Certain schedules are often recommended to prevent or minimize HPA suppression.

BOX 17.3 *Drug Interactions:*
*Corticosteroids*

**Drugs That Increase the Effects of Corticosteroids**

- Estrogens, oral contraceptives, ketoconazole, macrolide antibiotics (e.g., erythromycin)

  *Increase the effects of corticosteroids by inhibiting the enzymes that normally metabolize corticosteroids in the liver.*

- Diuretics (e.g., furosemide and thiazides)

  *Increase hypokalemia.*

**Drugs That Decrease the Effects of Corticosteroids**

- Antacids and cholestyramine

  *Decrease the absorption of corticosteroids.*

- Carbamazepine, phenytoin, rifampin

  *Induce microsomal enzymes in the liver and increase the rate at which corticosteroids are metabolized or deactivated.*

Corticosteroids can be given in relatively large, divided doses for approximately 48 to 72 hours in acute situations until the condition has been brought under control. After acute symptoms subside or 48 to 72 hours have passed, the dosage is tapered so that a slightly smaller dose is given each day until the drug can be discontinued completely (total period of use: ~1 week). Such a regimen may be useful in allergic reactions, contact dermatitis, exacerbations of chronic conditions (e.g., bronchial asthma), and stressful situations such as surgery.

Daily administration is required in cases of chronic adrenocortical insufficiency. The entire daily dose can be taken each morning, between 6:00 and 9:00 AM. This schedule simulates normal endogenous corticosteroid secretion.

### Stress Dosage Therapy

As previously stated, long-term use of pharmacologic doses (e.g., more than 5 mg of prednisone daily) of corticosteroids produces adverse reactions. For this reason, such corticosteroid therapy should be reserved for life-threatening conditions or severe, disabling symptoms that do not respond to treatment with more benign drugs or other measures. For people receiving chronic corticosteroid therapy, dosage must be increased during periods of stress or illness. Some common sources of stress for most people include surgery and anesthesia, infections, anxiety, and extremes of temperature. Note that events that are stressful for one patient may not be stressful for another. Some guidelines for corticosteroid dosage during stress include the following:

- During minor or relatively mild illness (e.g., viral upper respiratory infection, any febrile illness, strenuous exercise, gastroenteritis with vomiting and diarrhea, minor surgery), doubling the daily maintenance dose is usually adequate. After the stress period is over, it is appropriate to reduce the dosage abruptly to the usual maintenance dose.

- During major stress or severe illness, even larger doses are necessary. For example, a patient undergoing abdominal surgery may require 300 to 400 mg of hydrocortisone on the day of surgery. Gradual dose reduction to usual maintenance doses within approximately 5 days is sufficient if

postoperative recovery is uncomplicated. As a general rule, it is better to administer excessive doses temporarily than to risk inadequate doses and adrenal insufficiency. The patient also may require sodium chloride and fluid replacement, antibiotic therapy if infection is present, and supportive measures if shock occurs.

- During acute stress situations of short duration, such as traumatic injury or invasive diagnostic tests (e.g., angiography), a single dose of approximately 100 mg of hydrocortisone immediately after the injury or before the diagnostic test is usually sufficient.

- Many chronic diseases that require long-term corticosteroid therapy are characterized by exacerbations and remissions. It is usually necessary to increase the dosage of corticosteroids during acute flare-ups of disease symptoms but can then decrease the dosage gradually to maintenance levels.

### Alternate-Day Therapy

ADT, in which a double dose is taken every other morning, is usually preferred for other chronic conditions. This schedule allows rest periods so that adverse effects are decreased while anti-inflammatory effects continue. ADT seems to be as effective as more frequent administration in most patients with bronchial asthma, ulcerative colitis, and other conditions for which long-term corticosteroid therapy is prescribed. ADT is used only for maintenance therapy (i.e., clinical signs and symptoms are controlled initially with more frequent drug administration). ADT can be started after symptoms have subsided and stabilized.

Intermediate-acting glucocorticoids (e.g., prednisone, prednisolone, methylprednisolone) are the drugs of choice for ADT. Long-acting drugs (e.g., betamethasone, dexamethasone) are not recommended because of their prolonged suppression of adrenocortical function.

ADT has other advantages. It probably decreases susceptibility to infection and does not retard growth in children, as do other schedules.

ADT is not usually indicated in patients who have previously received corticosteroids on a long-term basis. First, these patients already have maximal HPA suppression, so a major advantage of ADT is lost. Second, if these patients begin ADT, recurrence of symptoms and considerable discomfort may occur on days when drugs are omitted. Patients with severe disease and very painful or disabling symptoms also may experience severe discomfort with ADT.

### Assessing for Therapeutic Effects

The goal of corticosteroid therapy is usually to reduce symptoms to a tolerable level. Total suppression of symptoms may require excessively large doses and produce excessive adverse effects. Because systemic corticosteroids can cause serious adverse reactions, indications for their clinical use should be as clear-cut as possible. Therapeutic effects depend largely on the reason for use.

Prescribers order hydrocortisone for the treatment of Addison's disease. Following the parenteral administration of the medication, the nurse monitors the patient for activity tolerance, ability to move in bed, and restoration of fluid balance. Decreases in weakness, weight loss and anorexia, nausea and vomiting, hyperpigmentation, hypotension, hyponatremia, and hyperkalemia should be evident.

Prednisone is the drug of choice for nonendocrine disorders in which anti-inflammatory, antiallergic, antistress, and immunosuppressive effects are desired. The nurse assesses the patient for diminished inflammation. Inhaled corticosteroids also reduce inflammation and allergic responses and do not lead to the serious adverse effects of systemic corticosteroids.

Health care providers consider dexamethasone (parenteral or oral) the corticosteroid of choice for cerebral edema associated with brain tumors, craniotomy, or head injury, because it is thought to penetrate the blood–brain barrier more readily and achieve higher concentrations in cerebrospinal fluids and tissues. It also has minimal sodium- and water-retaining properties. With brain tumors, the drug is more effective in metastatic lesions and glioblastomas than astrocytomas and meningiomas. The therapeutic response to the medication is decreased intracranial pressure.

In patients treated for rheumatoid arthritis with corticosteroid agents, the nurse assesses for decreased pain and edema in the joints, increased mobility, and increased ability to perform activities of daily living.

Organ transplant recipients administered corticosteroids to prevent rejection of the transplanted tissues should have absence of signs and symptoms of rejections.

## Assessing for Adverse Effects

It is necessary to assess patients for a variety of adverse effects, which may affect every body tissue and organ. The nurse assesses patients with adrenocortical insufficiency for fainting, weakness, anorexia, nausea, vomiting, hypotension, and shock. He or she assesses patients with adrenocortical excess for "moon face," "buffalo hump," diabetes mellitus, nervousness, euphoria, anxiety, and behavioral changes.

Adrenocortical excess also leads to the musculoskeletal conditions, such as osteoporosis, fractures, muscle weakness and atrophy, and growth retardation in children. Cardiovascular effects include fluid and electrolyte changes, with fluid retention, edema, hypertension, heart failure, hypernatremia, hypokalemia, and metabolic acidosis. Ocular changes include increased intraocular pressure, glaucoma, and cataracts. The nurse assesses for increased susceptibility to infection and changes to the skin, including redness, thinning, stretch marks, and tissue injury. Women may experience menstrual irregularities, acne, and excessive facial hair.

## Patient Teaching

Box 17.4 identifies patient teaching guidelines for corticosteroids.

---

**BOX 17.4**  *Patient Teaching Guidelines for Long-Term Corticosteroid Therapy*

### General Considerations

- Realize that in most instances, corticosteroids are used to relieve symptoms; they do not cure the underlying disease process. However, they can improve comfort and quality of life.
- When taking an oral corticosteroid (e.g., prednisone) for longer than 2 weeks, take the drug as directed. This is extremely important. Missing a dose or two, stopping the drug, changing the amount or time of administration, taking extra drug (except as specifically directed during stress situations), or any other alterations may result in complications. Some complications are relatively minor; several are serious, even life threatening. When these drugs are being discontinued, the dosage is gradually reduced over several weeks. They must not be stopped abruptly.
- Wear a special medical alert bracelet or tag or carry an identification card stating the drug being taken; the dosage; the prescriber's name, address, and telephone number; and instructions for emergency treatment. If an accident or emergency situation occurs, health care providers must know about corticosteroid drug therapy to give additional amounts during the stress of the emergency.
- Report to all health care providers consulted that corticosteroid drugs are being taken or have been taken within the past year. Current or previous corticosteroid therapy can influence treatment measures, and such knowledge increases the ability to provide appropriate treatment.

- Maintain regular medical supervision. This is extremely important so that the prescriber can detect adverse reactions, evaluate disease status, and evaluate drug response and indications for dosage change, as well as other responsibilities that can be carried out only with personal contact between the prescriber and the patient. Periodic blood tests, x-ray studies, and other tests may be performed during long-term corticosteroid therapy.
- Take no other drugs, prescription or nonprescription, without notifying the prescriber who is supervising corticosteroid therapy. Corticosteroid drugs influence reactions to other drugs, and some other drugs interact with corticosteroids to either increase or decrease their effects. Thus, taking other drugs can decrease the expected therapeutic benefits or increase the incidence or severity of adverse effects.
- Avoid exposure to infection when possible. Avoid crowds and people known to have an infection. Also, wash hands frequently and thoroughly. These drugs increase the likelihood of infection, so preventive measures are necessary. Also, if infection does occur, healing is likely to be slow.
- Practice safety measures to avoid accidents (e.g., falls and possible fractures due to osteoporosis, cuts or other injuries because of delayed wound healing, soft tissue trauma because of increased tendency to bruise easily).
- Weigh frequently when starting corticosteroid therapy and at least weekly during long-term maintenance. An initial weight gain is likely to occur and is usually attributed to increased appetite. Later weight gains may be caused by fluid retention.

**BOX 17.4** **_Patient Teaching Guidelines for Long-Term Corticosteroid Therapy_** [Continued]

- Ask the prescriber about the amount and kind of activity or exercise needed. As a general rule, being as active as possible helps prevent or delay osteoporosis, a common adverse effect. However, increased activity may not be desirable for everyone. A patient with rheumatoid arthritis, for example, may become too active when drug therapy relieves joint pain and increases mobility.

- Follow instructions for other measures used in treatment of the particular condition (e.g., other drugs and physical therapy for rheumatoid arthritis). Such measures may allow smaller doses of corticosteroids and decrease adverse effects.

- Understand that the dosage may need to be temporarily increased with illness, surgery, or other stressful situations because corticosteroids impair the ability to respond to stress. Clarify with the prescriber predictable sources of stress and the amount of drug to be taken if the stress cannot be avoided.

- In addition to stressful situations, report sore throat, fever, or other signs of infection; weight gain of 5 lb or more in a week; or swelling in the ankles or elsewhere. These symptoms may indicate adverse drug effects, and changes in corticosteroid therapy may be indicated.

- Realize that muscle weakness and fatigue or disease symptoms may occur when drug dosage is reduced, withdrawn, or omitted (e.g., the nondrug day of alternate-day therapy). Although these symptoms may cause some discomfort, they should be tolerated if possible rather than increasing the corticosteroid dose. If severe, of course, dosage or time of administration may have to be changed.

- Understand that dietary changes may be helpful in reducing some adverse effects of corticosteroid therapy. Decreasing salt intake (e.g., by not adding table salt to foods and avoiding obviously salty foods, such as many snack foods and prepared sandwich meats) may help decrease swelling. Eating high-potassium foods, such as citrus fruits and juices or bananas, may help prevent potassium loss. An adequate intake of calcium, protein, and vitamin D (meat and dairy products are good sources) may help to prevent or delay osteoporosis. Vitamin C (e.g., from citrus fruits) may help to prevent excessive bruising.

- Do not object when your prescriber reduces your dose of oral corticosteroid, with the goal of stopping the drug entirely or continuing with a smaller dose. Long-term therapy should be used only when necessary because of the potential for serious adverse effects, and the lowest effective dose should be given.

- Understand that with local applications of corticosteroids, there is usually little systemic absorption and few adverse effects, compared with oral or injected drugs. When effective in relieving symptoms, it is better to use a local than a systemic corticosteroid. In some instances, combined systemic and local application allows administration of a lesser dose of the systemic drug.

- Commonly used local applications are applied topically for skin disorders, by oral inhalation for asthma, and by nasal inhalation for allergic rhinitis. Although long-term use is usually well tolerated, systemic toxicity can occur if excess corticosteroid is inhaled or if occlusive dressings are used over skin lesions. Thus, a corticosteroid for local application must be applied correctly and not overused.

- Know that corticosteroids are not the same as the steroids often abused by athletes and body builders. Those are anabolic steroids derived from testosterone, the male sex hormone.

**Self- or Caregiver Administration**

- Take an oral corticosteroid with a meal or snack to decrease GI upset.

- If taking the medication once a day or every other day, take before 9:00 AM; if taking multiple doses, take at evenly spaced intervals throughout the day.

- Report to the prescriber if unable to take a dose orally because of vomiting or some other problem. In some circumstances, the dose may need to be given by injection.

- If taking an oral corticosteroid in tapering doses, be sure to follow instructions exactly to avoid adverse effects.

- When applying a corticosteroid to skin lesions, do not apply more often than ordered and do not cover with an occlusive dressing unless specifically instructed to do so.

- With an intranasal corticosteroid, use on a regular basis (usually once or twice daily) for the best anti-inflammatory effects.

- With an oral inhalation corticosteroid, use on a regular schedule for anti-inflammatory effects. The drugs are _not_ effective in relieving acute asthma attacks or shortness of breath and should not be used "as needed" for that purpose. Use metered-dose inhalers as follows (unless instructed otherwise by a health care provider):

1. Shake canister thoroughly.
2. Place canister between lips (both open and pursed lips have been recommended) or outside lips.
3. Exhale completely.
4. Activate canister while taking a slow, deep breath.
5. Hold breath for 10 seconds or as long as possible.
6. Wait at least 1 minute before taking additional inhalations.
7. Rinse mouth after inhalations to decrease the incidence of oral thrush (a fungal infection).
8. Rinse mouthpiece at least once per day.

## Clinical Application 17.3

The home care nurse is visiting
Mrs. Thompson. She says, "I am having
itching in my vaginal area, and drinking
citrus juices is painful." During the assessment, the
nurse notices white patches in her mouth.

- What are the white patches in Mrs. Thompson's mouth?
- Why has she developed itching in the vaginal area?
- What is the cause of these symptoms?

## NCLEX Success

10. A child is taking long-term systemic corticosteroids. What factor influences the child's diminished growth?
    A. hypokalemia
    B. fluid retention
    C. altered DNA synthesis
    D. increase in parathyroid hormone

11. A woman is being treated with long-term corticosteroid therapy. Her husband has just received a diagnosis of terminal cancer. How is his diagnosis likely to affect her treatment?
    A. She may need to have her dose of corticosteroid increased because of the stress.
    B. She may need a decrease in corticosteroids because of the increase in cortisol.
    C. She may need to be changed to a different corticosteroid because of the stress.
    D. She may be switched to a parenteral form of corticosteroid.

12. A patient diagnosed with Addison's disease is taking exogenous corticosteroids. The nurse should assess the patient for which of the following adverse effects?
    A. hyperglycemia
    B. hyperkalemia
    C. hypercalcemia
    D. hypermagnesemia

13. Which of the following psychosocial changes are most likely to occur with the administration of corticosteroids?
    A. lethargy
    B. malaise
    C. ataxia
    D. euphoria

14. A patient is taking systemic corticosteroids. Which of the following nursing interventions is most important to implement?
    A. Assess for signs and symptoms of adrenocortical excess.
    B. Hold the corticosteroid before surgery or diagnostic testing.
    C. Assess for fluid volume deficit.
    D. Decrease the intake of vitamin C.

## THE NURSING PROCESS

A concept map outlines the nursing process related to drug therapy considerations in this chapter. Additional nursing implications related to the disease process should also be considered in care decisions.

**Assessment**

With the initiation of corticosteroid therapy:
- For a patient receiving short-term corticosteroid therapy, assess the extent and severity of symptoms. This will be a baseline to evaluate the effectiveness of corticosteroid therapy.
- For a patient receiving long-term systemic corticosteroid therapy:
  - Assess for such conditions as diabetes mellitus, tuberculosis, and peptic ulcer disease, because corticosteroids may result in the development or exacerbation of these disorders. If one of these conditions is present, it is essential that corticosteroid therapy be altered and other medications given concomitantly.
  - Assess for signs and symptoms of infection. If acute infection is present, treatment with appropriate antibiotics either before corticosteroid drugs are started or concomitantly with corticosteroid therapy is necessary.
  - Assess for infection-related symptoms, which should decrease.
  - Assess for wound healing because corticosteroids impair healing.
- With previous or current corticosteroid therapy:
  - If corticosteroids have been prescribed in the past, assess the patient's past response to corticosteroids.
  - Assess the patient for significant sources of stress, such as hospitalization, diagnostic testing, infection, illness, and psychosocial problems.
  - Assess the type of systemic corticosteroid medication the patient is taking, the dosage and schedule of administration, the purpose for which the medication has been prescribed, and the length of time to be administered.
  - If the patient undergoes anesthesia and surgery, expect that he or she will commonly require higher doses of corticosteroids for several days. Specific regimens vary according to the type of anesthesia, surgical procedure, patient condition, prescriber preference, and other variables.
  - Expect that a patient undergoing an invasive diagnostic test may be given one extra dose of corticosteroid.
  - Assess for acute adrenal insufficiency.
  - Assess for signs and symptoms of adrenocortical excess and adverse drug effects.
  - Assess for signs and symptoms of the disease for which long-term corticosteroid therapy is given.

**Outcomes of Therapy**

The patient will
- Administer the drug correctly, and understand the adverse effects, including risk of infection.
- See a health care provider regularly to monitor for therapeutic and adverse drug effects.
- Seek the health care provider for strategies to cope with body image changes.
- Verbalize or demonstrate essential drug information.

**Nursing Interventions**

- Instruct the patient on the effects of steroid therapy.
- Assess for diminished inflammation.
- Assess for infection.
- Instruct on good handwashing.
- Instruct on the adverse effects of steroid therapy.
- Encourage activity to slow demineralization of bone.
- Instruct the patient to avoid stress and exposure to extreme temperatures.
- Instruct the patient to eat a diet high in protein, calcium, and vitamin D.
- Reverse or protective isolation is sometimes indicated for organ transplant patients receiving corticosteroid.
- Because long-term corticosteroid therapy weakens the skin and bones, there are risks of skin damage and fractures with even minor trauma; use care during ADLs and procedures.

**Evaluation**

- Interview and observe for relief of symptoms for which corticosteroids were prescribed.
- Interview and observe for accurate drug administration.
- Interview and observe for adverse drug effects on a regular basis.

## KEY CONCEPTS

- The most frequently desired pharmacologic effects of exogenous corticosteroids are anti-inflammatory, immunosuppressive, antiallergic, and antistress functions.
- Mineralocorticoid and androgenic effects of exogenous corticosteroids are usually considered adverse reactions.
- Daily administration of corticosteroids and mineralocorticoids is required in cases of chronic adrenocortical insufficiency (Addison's disease).
- Adrenocortical hyperfunction (Cushing's disease) may result from excessive corticotropin or a primary adrenal tumor.
- Strategies to minimize HPA suppression and risks of acute adrenal insufficiency include (1) administering a systemic corticosteroid during high-stress situations to patients who receive long-term systemic therapy (i.e., are steroid dependent); (2) giving short courses of systemic therapy for acute disorders; (3) gradually tapering the dose of any systemic corticosteroid; (4) using local rather than systemic therapy when possible, alone or in combination with low doses of systemic drugs; and (5) using ADT.
- Adverse effects of systemic corticosteroids may include infections, hypertension, glucose intolerance, obesity, cosmetic changes, bone loss, growth retardation in children, cataracts, pancreatitis, peptic ulcerations, and psychiatric disturbances.
- A **BLACK BOX WARNING** ◆ has been issued by the FDA for people who switch from a systemically active corticosteroid to a flunisolide inhaler; deaths have been reported from adrenal insufficiency.

## CLINICAL REASONING CASE STUDY

**Meet the Patient**

Milton Finnicairo, a 48-year-old patient, is admitted to hospice. He has an aggressive form of brain cancer with metastasis. He is having nausea and vomiting at least five times per day. He is also complaining of increasing headaches and pain on the right side of the head near the temporal lobe. The hospice physician has prescribed dexamethasone sodium phosphate 16 mg intramuscular every morning. You are the hospice nurse providing care to Mr. Finnicairo and his family.

- Why has dexamethasone sodium phosphate been ordered for this patient?
- What is the action of dexamethasone?
- How will you teach Mr. Finnicairo's family to administer his daily injection of dexamethasone?

**Assessing Drug Information**

- Dexamethasone sodium phosphate is a long-acting adrenocorticoid that produces anti-inflammatory effects.
- Dexamethasone sodium phosphate IM reduces the increased intracranial pressure related to the neoplasm of the brain. It penetrates the blood–brain barrier to achieve a higher concentration in the cerebrospinal fluid and tissues.
- Dexamethasone sodium phosphate is more effective in metastatic lesions and glioblastomas than astrocytomas and meningiomas.
- Dexamethasone enters the target cells and binds to specific receptors. It initiates complex reactions to inhibit phagocytosis and lysosomal enzyme relief to decrease inflammation and cause immunosuppression.

**Nursing Actions**

- The hospice nurse should assess Mr. Finnicairo's relief of pain, nausea, and vomiting after the administration of dexamethasone sodium phosphate.
- Instruct Mr. Finnicairo's family to utilize good handwashing which will protect him from infection.
- Instruct Mr. Finnicairo and his family about the action and use of dexamethasone sodium phosphate.
- Instruct Mr. Finnicairo's family on the intramuscular administration of dexamethasone sodium phosphate 16 mg/1 mL.
  - Perform hand hygiene.
  - Cleanse the vial stopper with alcohol.
  - Draw back on the syringe to the desired amount.
  - Instill the air into the top of the vial.
  - Invert the vial and draw up 1 mL.
  - Select the site in the deltoid or vastus lateralis. (Instruct on the identification of the deltoid site by locating the upper arm landmark and placing four fingers across the deltoid muscle, with the first finger on the acromion process. The deltoid is 2 inches below the acromion process. The vastus lateralis is the anterior lateral aspect of the thigh, located by dividing the area between the greater trochanter of the femur and the lateral femoral condyle into thirds and selecting the middle third.)
  - Cleanse the site identified with an alcohol swab in a circular motion.
  - Remove the needle cover.
  - Inject using the Z-track technique.
  - Aspirate before injecting.
  - Be certain to rotate sites.

*Visit* thePoint® *at* **http://thePoint.lww.com/Frandsen12e** *for answers to NCLEX Success questions (in Appendix A), answers to Clinical Application Case Studies (in Appendix B), and more!*

## REFERENCES AND RESOURCES

Feinleib, J., Kwan, L. H., & Yamani, A. (2019). Postoperative nausea and vomiting. In *UpToDate*. Lexi-Comp Inc.

Ferguson, G. T., & Make, B. (2019). Management of refractory chronic obstructive pulmonary disease. In *UpToDate*. Lexi-Comp Inc.

Hesketh, P. J. (2019). Prevention and treatment of chemotherapy-induced nausea and vomiting in adults. In *UpToDate*. Lexi-Comp Inc.

Hinkle, J. H., & Cheever, K. H. (2018). *Brunner & Suddarth's textbook of medical-surgical nursing* (14th ed.). Philadelphia, PA: Lippincott Williams & Wilkins.

Karch, A. M. (2019). *2019 Lippincott's nursing drug guide*. Philadelphia, PA: Lippincott Williams & Wilkins.

Kaufman, D. A. (2019). Glucocorticoid therapy in septic shock. In *UpToDate*. Lexi-Comp Inc.

Lin, L. L., Gu, H. Y., Luo, J., Wang, L., Zhang, C., Niu, U. M., et al. (2019). Impact and beneficial critical points of clinical outcome in corticosteroid management of adult patients with sepsis: Meta-analysis an grade assessment. *Frontiers in Pharmacology, 10*, 1–31. doi:10.3389/fphar.2019.01101

Mohammad, H. R., Hamilton, T. W., Strickland, L., Trivella, M., Murray, D., & Pandit, H. (2018). Perioperative adjuvant corticosteroids for postoperative analgesia in knee arthroplasty: A meta-analysis of 1,396 knees. *Acta Orthopaedica, 89*(1), 71–76. doi:10.1080/17453674.2017.139409

Nieman, L. K. (2019). Pharmacologic use of glucocorticoids. In *UpToDate*. Lexi-Comp Inc.

Norris, T. L. (2019). *Porth's Pathophysiology: Concepts of altered health status* (10th ed.). Philadelphia, PA: Lippincott Williams & Wilkins.

Peppercorn, M. A., & Cheifetz, A. S. (2019). Budesonide in the treatment of inflammatory bowel disease in adults. In *UpToDate*. Lexi-Comp Inc.

Siegel, M. (2019). Acute respiratory distress syndrome: Supportive care and oxygenation in adults. In *UpToDate*. Lexi-Comp Inc.

Stoller, J. K. (2019). Management of exacerbations of chronic obstructive pulmonary disease. In *UpToDate*. Lexi-Comp Inc.

UpToDate. (2019). *Drug Information*. Lexi-Comp, Inc.

# Drug Therapy With Beta-Lactam Antibacterial Agents

## LEARNING OBJECTIVES

*After studying this chapter, you should be able to:*

1. Describe general characteristics of beta-lactam antibiotics.
2. Discuss the penicillins in relation to effectiveness, safety, spectrum of antibacterial activity, mechanism of action, indications for use, administration, observation of patient response, and teaching of patients.
3. Recognize the importance of questioning patients about allergies before the initial dose of all drugs, especially penicillins.
4. Describe characteristics of beta-lactamase inhibitor drugs.
5. Give the rationale for combining a penicillin and a beta-lactamase inhibitor drug.
6. Discuss the cephalosporins in relation to effectiveness, safety, spectrum of antibacterial activity, mechanism of action, indications for use, administration, observation of patient response, and teaching of patients.
7. Discuss the carbapenems in relation to effectiveness, safety, spectrum of antibacterial activity, mechanism of action, indications for use, administration, observation of patient response, and teaching of patients.
8. Discuss the one monobactam drug in relation to effectiveness, safety, spectrum of antibacterial activity, mechanism of action, indications for use, administration, observation of patient response, and teaching of patients.
9. Implement the nursing process when caring for patients receiving beta-lactam antibacterials.

## CLINICAL APPLICATION CASE STUDY

Paul O'Brian, a 55-year-old professional musician who travels frequently, has no known drug allergies. He is being scheduled for the placement of a new cardiac pacemaker tomorrow. The physician orders that cefazolin be administered "on call" for the procedure (1 g IV).

## KEY TERMS

**Beta-lactamase:** enzyme produced by some bacteria that attacks the beta-lactam ring, rendering the drug ineffective and leading to a resistance to beta-lactam antibiotics

**Cross-allergenicity:** allergy to a drug of another class with a similar chemical structure

**Extended-spectrum:** bactericidal activity against a wide range of bacteria

**Superinfection:** infection after a previous infection; typically caused by microorganisms that are resistant to the antibiotics used previously

# INTRODUCTION

This chapter will discuss the pharmacologic care of the patient who is receiving a drug in the antibiotic class of beta-lactam antibacterials, specifically the penicillins, cephalosporins, carbapenems, and monobactams. Beta-lactam antibacterial drugs inhibit synthesis of bacterial cell walls by binding to proteins (penicillin-binding proteins; see Chap. 15) in bacterial cell membranes. This binding produces a defective cell wall that allows leakage of the intracellular contents, destroying the microorganisms. Beta-lactam antibacterial drugs are typically considered bactericidal.

Beta-lactam antibacterials derive their name from the beta-lactam ring that is part of their chemical structure. An intact beta-lactam ring is essential for the antibacterial activity of these drugs. Several gram-positive and gram-negative bacteria produce **beta-lactamases**, which are enzymes that disrupt

the beta-lactam ring and inactivate the beta-lactam antibacterial drugs. This is the major mechanism by which microorganisms acquire resistance to these drugs. Penicillinase and cephalosporinase are beta-lactamase enzymes that act on penicillins and cephalosporins to render them resistant and ineffective. Patients receive beta-lactamase inhibitors concurrently with the beta-lactam antibacterial drugs to overcome this resistance.

Although a beta-lactam ring is common to all beta-lactam antibiotics, the characteristics of these drugs vary widely because of differences in their chemical structures. Because of these differences, the range of activity to particular bacteria is also different. The drugs may also differ in the routes of administration, susceptibility to beta-lactamase enzymes, and adverse effects. Table 18.1 lists the various types of beta-lactam antibiotics.

## TABLE 18.1

## Beta-Lactamase Antibacterials Administered for the Treatment of Infection

| Drug Class | Prototype | Other Drugs in the Class |
|---|---|---|
| Penicillins | Ⓟ **Ampicillin** (Principen) | Amoxicillin (Amoxil, Larotid) |
| | | Carbenicillin indanyl sodium (Geocillin) |
| | | Penicillin G benzathine (Bicillin LA) |
| | | Penicillin G procaine |
| | | Penicillin V (Penicillin VK) |
| | | Dicloxacillin |
| | | Nafcillin |
| | | Oxacillin (Bactocill) |
| | | Piperacillin |
| | | Ampicillin–sulbactam (Unasyn) |
| | | Amoxicillin–clavulanate (Augmentin) |
| | | Piperacillin/tazobactam |
| Cephalosporins | Ⓟ **Cefazolin** (Ancef) | Cefadroxil |
| | | Cephalexin (Keflex) |
| | | Cefaclor |
| | | Cefotetan |
| | | Cefoxitin |
| | | Cefprozil |
| | | Cefuroxime |
| | | Cefdinir |
| | | Cefditoren |
| | | Cefixime |
| | | Cefotaxime |
| | | Cefpodoxime |
| | | Ceftazidime (Fortaz) |
| | | Ceftibuten |
| | | Ceftriaxone |
| | | Cefepime (Maxipime) |
| | | Ceftaroline (Teflaro) |
| | | Ceftolozane–tazobactam (Zerbaxa) |
| | | Ceftazidime–avibactam (Avycaz) |
| Carbapenems | Ⓟ **Imipenem–cilastatin** (Primaxin) | Ertapenem (Invanz) |
| | | Meropenem (Merrem) |
| | | Doripenem |
| | | Meropenem–vaborbactam (Vabomere) |
| Monobactam | Ⓟ **Aztreonam** (Azactam) | |

# PENICILLINS

The penicillins are effective and safe, and they are among the most commonly prescribed antibacterials. The first antibiotic developed was penicillin, which was derived from the *Penicillium* mold. When penicillin was introduced, it was effective against many organisms. It was once necessary to give the drug parenterally because it was destroyed by gastric acid, and injections were painful. With extensive use, strains of drug-resistant staphylococci appeared. Scientists developed semisynthetic derivatives, formed by adding side chains to the penicillin nucleus, to increase gastric acid stability, beta-lactamase stability, and antimicrobial spectrum of activity, especially against gram-negative microorganisms. As a class, penicillins usually are more effective in treating infections caused by gram-positive bacteria than those caused by gram-negative bacteria. However, their clinical usefulness varies significantly according to the subgroup or individual drug and microbial patterns of resistance.

**Ampicillin** (Principen) is the prototype penicillin.

## Pharmacokinetics

After absorption, ampicillin is widely distributed. Penetration into the cerebrospinal fluid (CSF) occurs only with inflamed meninges. The kidneys rapidly excrete ampicillin, largely as unchanged drug, and it produces high drug concentrations in the urine. It is present in breast milk, and the volume of distribution increases during pregnancy, when the half-life, generally 1 to 2 hours, is decreased.

## Action

Ampicillin, like all penicillins, inhibits bacterial cell wall synthesis by binding to one or multiple penicillin-binding proteins.

## Use

Clinical indications for use of ampicillin include bacterial infections caused by susceptible microorganisms. Health care providers use the drug in the treatment or prophylaxis of infective endocarditis. The drug's broad spectrum is often useful in skin, soft tissue, respiratory, gastrointestinal (GI), and genitourinary infections. The broad-spectrum coverage of ampicillin extends its activity against gram-negative bacilli. Note that the incidence of resistance among streptococci, staphylococci, and other microorganisms continues to increase.

Table 18.2 provides route and dosage information for the individual penicillins.

### TABLE 18.2
### DRUGS AT A GLANCE: Penicillins

| Drug | Pregnancy Category | Routes and Dosage Ranges | |
|---|---|---|---|
| | | **Adults** | **Children** |
| **Penicillins G and V** | | | |
| These drugs remain effective for a limited number of uses. They are the drugs of choice for the treatment of streptococcal pharyngitis, for prevention of recurrent attacks in patients who have had previous acute rheumatic fever due to group A streptococcus and for treatment of neurosyphilis. | | | |
| Penicillin G benzathine (Pfizerpen; ❋ Crystapen) | B | IM 1.2–2.4 million units in a single dose Prophylaxis of recurrent rheumatic fever, IM 1.2 million units every 3–4 wk Treatment of syphilis, IM 2.4 million units (1.2 million units in each buttock) as a single dose | IM 25,000–50,000 units/kg (max 2.4 million units) Prophylaxis of recurrent rheumatic fever, 25,000–50,000 units/kg times one dose q 3–4 wk (maximum 1.2 million units) |
| Penicillin G procaine | B | IV, IM 600,000–4.8 million units daily in 1 or 2 doses | IM 25,000–50,000 units/kg/d in divided doses every 12–24 h |
| Penicillin V (❋ Apo-Pen VK, Novo-Pen-VK, Nu-Pen-VK) | B | PO 125–500 mg every 6–8 h | PO 125–250 mg twice daily |
| **Penicillinase-Resistant (Antistaphylococcal) Penicillins** | | | |
| Penicillinase-resistant penicillins are the drugs of choice for methicillin-susceptible *Staphylococcus aureus*. Although called "methicillin resistant," these staphylococcal microorganisms are also resistant to other antistaphylococcal penicillins. | | | |
| Dicloxacillin | B | PO 125–1000 mg every 6 h | Not recommended in newborns ≤40 kg: 12.5–100 mg/kg/d divided every 6 h ≥40 kg: 125–500 mg every 6 h |
| Nafcillin | B | IM 500 mg every 4–6 h IV 500 mg–2 g every 4–6 h; max daily dose 18 g for serious infections | IM 25 mg/kg every 12 h IV 50–200 mg/kg/d in divided doses every 4–6 h |

*(Continued on page 358)*

**TABLE 18.2**

# DRUGS AT A GLANCE: Penicillins [Continued]

| Drug | Pregnancy Category | Routes and Dosage Ranges | |
|---|---|---|---|
| | | **Adults** | **Children** |
| Oxacillin (Bactocill) | B | IM, IV 250–2000 mg every 4–6 h | ≤40 kg: IM, IV 100–200 mg/kg/d in divided doses every 6 h<br>>40 kg: same as adults |

**Aminopenicillins**

The aminopenicillins are drugs of choice for prevention of bacterial endocarditis due to procedures that produce transient bacteremia. Ampicillin is excreted mainly by the kidneys; thus, it is useful in some urinary tract infections (UTIs). Because some is excreted in bile, it is useful in biliary tract infections not caused by biliary obstruction. It is used in the treatment of bronchitis, sinusitis, and otitis media.

| Drug | Pregnancy Category | Adults | Children |
|---|---|---|---|
| Ⓟ **Ampicillin** (❋ Ampicillin for Injection, Apo-Ampi, Novo-Ampicillin, Nu-Ampi) | B | PO, IM, IV 250–500 mg every 6 h. In severe infections, doses up to 2 g every 4 h may be given IV | Infants/children: PO 50–100 mg/kg/d in divided doses every 6 h (max dose 2–4 g/d)<br>IM, IV 100–400 mg/kg/d in divided doses every 6 h (max dose 12 g/d) |
| Amoxicillin (Amoxil, Larotid; ❋ Apo-Amoxi, Mylan-Amoxicillin, Novamoxin, NPR-Amoxicillin, Nu-Amoxi, PHL-Amoxicillin, Pro-Amox-250, Pro-Amox-500) | B | PO 250–500 mg every 8 h or 500–875 mg every 12 h | 3 mo or more: PO 20–30 mg/kg/d in divided doses every 12 h<br>More than 3 mo: 20–50 mg/kg/d in divided doses every 8–12 h |
| Piperacillin (❋ Piperacillin for injection) | B | IM, IV 200–300 mg/kg/d in divided doses every q4–6 h. IM injections should not exceed 2 g/injection and use should be reserved for uncomplicated infections. Usual adult dosage, 3–4 g every 4–6 h; max daily dose 24 g | Infants/children/adolescents (non–FDA approved)<br>≥12 y IV 200–300 mg/kg/d in divided doses every 4–6 h; max daily dose 24 g/d |

**Penicillin–Beta-Lactamase Inhibitor Combinations**

The beta-lactamase inhibitors display negligible antimicrobial activity but contain the beta-lactam ring. Coadministered with beta-lactam antibiotics, the inhibitors' sole function is to bind with the beta-lactamases (enzymes that degrade the beta-lactam ring) to prevent inactivation of the beta-lactam antibiotics.

| Drug | Pregnancy Category | Adults | Children |
|---|---|---|---|
| Ampicillin–sulbactam (Unasyn) | B | IM, IV 1.5–3 g q6h Maximum dose of 4 g/d of sulbactam | 1 y or older: IV 100–400 mg/kg/d in divided doses q6h (max 8 g ampicillin/d; 12 g Unasyn)<br>Doses up to 300 mg/kg/d may be given for severe infections in infants older than 1 mo of age |
| Amoxicillin–clavulanate (Augmentin, Augmentin XR; ❋ Amoxi-Clav, Apo-Amoxi-Clav, Clavulin, Novo-Clavamoxin, ratio-Aclavulanate) | B | PO 250–1000 mg every 8 h or 875 mg every 12 h | ≥40 kg: same as adults<br><40 kg: 20–90 mg/kg/d in divided doses every 8–12 h |
| Piperacillin/tazobactam (Zosyn; ❋ AJ-PIP/TAZ, piperacillin, and tazobactam for injection) | B | IV 2.25–4.5 g every 6–8 h | ≥40 kg: same as adults<br>IV 80–100 mg/kg/d based on piperacillin component every 8 h |

### Use in Children

Ampicillin and other penicillins are widely used to treat infections in children and are generally safe. However, caution is necessary in neonates because immature kidney function slows drug elimination. Dosage should be based on age, weight, severity of the infection being treated, and renal function. Specialized pediatric dosing references provide guidance to dosing based on age and weight.

### Use in Older Adults

Ampicillin and other penicillins are relatively safe in older adults. However, decreased renal function, other disease processes, and concurrent drug therapies increase the risks of adverse effects. Prior to the administration of any antibiotics, it is important to verify if the dosage should be adjusted based on the patient's creatinine clearance. Elderly patients are susceptible to **superinfections** (infections after a previous infection, typically caused by microorganisms that are resistant to the antibiotics used earlier) when given any anti-infective agent.

### Use in Patients With Renal Impairment

Because ampicillin is excreted primarily by the kidneys, it is important to use caution with renal impairment.

### Use in Patients With Hepatic Impairment

Ampicillin can be used in patients with hepatic impairment, as can almost all the penicillins. Caution is necessary when using amoxicillin–clavulanate (Augmentin) in patients with hepatic injury or destruction. No specific recommendations for dosage adjustment are available. Development of cholestatic jaundice and hepatic dysfunction with previous use of the drug are contraindications. Cholestatic liver impairment usually subsides when the drug is stopped.

### Use in Patients With Critical Illness

The use of ampicillin in the people who are critically ill is not nearly as great as it once was, primarily because resistance to the drug has emerged and other broad-spectrum agents are available. Patients frequently take other beta-lactam agents concomitantly with other antimicrobial drugs because critically ill patients often have multiple organisms that cause infections. The **extended-spectrum** drugs (e.g., piperacillin, which is a derivative of ampicillin) and penicillin–beta-lactamase inhibitor combinations (e.g., Zosyn), which have bactericidal activity against a wide range of bacteria, are most likely to be used in critical care units for the treatment of respiratory diseases such as pneumonia, blood, or other infections. Through chemical modification, these extended-spectrum drugs affect additional types of bacteria, typically gram-negative bacteria. With cephalosporins, third- and fourth-generation drugs are commonly used and are usually given by intermittent intravenous (IV) infusions every 8 or 12 hours. Blood levels of penicillins need to be maintained above the minimum inhibitory concentration (MIC) of the microorganisms causing the infection. Thus, continuous or extended infusions may be of benefit with serious infections, especially those caused by relatively resistant organisms such as *Pseudomonas* or *Acinetobacter*. It is necessary to monitor function of the kidneys, liver, and other organs in critically ill patients and to reduce drug dosages when indicated.

### Use in Patients Receiving Home Care

When using oral beta-lactam antibiotics such as ampicillin, the home care nurse mainly needs to teach patients about accurate administration of the drug and observation for therapeutic and adverse effects. With using liquid suspensions for children, it is necessary to shake to resuspend the medication and measure with a measuring spoon or calibrated device to ensure safe dosing. Household spoons should not be used because they vary widely in capacity and may lead to incorrect dosing.

## Adverse Effects

The most common adverse effects of ampicillin are hypersensitivity reactions, including rash and/or anaphylactoid reactions. Commonly reported GI adverse effects include abdominal pain, diarrhea, gastritis, and nausea and vomiting. Nephropathy, such as interstitial nephritis, although infrequent, has occurred with all penicillins. It is most often associated with high doses of parenteral penicillins and is attributed to hypersensitivity reactions.

In addition, high doses of penicillin G irritate the central nervous system (CNS). The adverse effects related to CNS toxicity include confusion, lethargy, twitching, dysphagia, seizures, and coma. The penicillinase-resistant penicillins may result in hepatotoxicity. The extended-spectrum penicillins may lead to hypokalemia and hypernatremia.

Note that the Food and Drug Administration (FDA) has issued a **BLACK BOX WARNING ◆** to alert health care providers that inadvertent IV administration of penicillin G benzathine may result in cardiopulmonary arrest and death. Long-acting repository forms have additives that decrease their solubility in tissue fluids and delay their absorption.

## Contraindications

Contraindications include hypersensitivity or allergic reactions to any penicillin formulation. An allergic reaction to one penicillin means the patient is allergic to all drugs of the penicillin class. The potential for **cross-allergenicity**, also referred to as cross-sensitivity, is the allergy to a drug of another class with a similar chemical structure. The cephalosporins and carbapenems each possess the characteristic bicyclic core structure. This chemical unit is thought to be most responsible for beta-lactam hypersensitivity. Recent data suggest that the incidence is less than 1%, lower than previously thought.

## Nursing Implications

### Preventing Interactions

Many medications and herbs interact with ampicillin, increasing or decreasing its effects (Boxes 18.1 and 18.2). In addition, ampicillin inhibits the renal tubular secretion of methotrexate, which may lead to prolonged and higher drug concentrations of methotrexate.

Penicillins are often given concomitantly with aminoglycosides for serious infections, such as those caused by *Pseudomonas aeruginosa*. These drugs should not be admixed in a syringe,

## BOX 18.1 Drug Interactions: Ampicillin

**Drugs That Increase the Effects of Ampicillin**

- Allopurinol

  *Increases the incidence of skin rash*
- Clavulanic acid

  *Overcomes resistance in bacteria that secrete beta-lactamase*
- Probenecid

  *Inhibits the renal tubular secretion*
- Uricosuric drugs

  *Block renal excretion*

**Drugs That Decrease the Effects of Ampicillin**

- Chloroquine

  *Decreases the serum concentration*
- Fusidic acid

  *Diminishes the therapeutic effect*
- Tetracycline derivatives

  *Diminish the therapeutic effect*

given in an IV solution, or administered via Y-site, because the penicillin inactivates the aminoglycoside. If feasible, dose separation is ideal.

### Administering the Medication

It is necessary to give oral ampicillin, like most oral penicillins, on an empty stomach, approximately 1 hour before or 2 hours after a meal. Patients should take the oral drug with a full glass of water, preferably to promote absorption and decrease inactivation, which may occur in an acidic environment. If need be, they may take it with food; however, the absorption rate decreases with food. Oral suspensions of the drug are stable for 7 days at room temperature and 14 days when refrigerated.

When diluted with 0.9% sodium chloride, ampicillin is stable for 8 hours for concentrations up to 30 mg/mL. It is stable for only 1 hour when diluted with dextrose-containing solutions for concentrations of 10 to 20 mg/mL. It is necessary to give IV penicillins for the full, prescribed course of treatment to prevent complications such as rheumatic fever, endocarditis, and glomerulonephritis. IV concentrations should not exceed 30 mg/mL.

### Assessing for Therapeutic Effects

It is not necessary to obtain drug levels when administering ampicillin or any of the antimicrobials in the penicillin class. When administering ampicillin, it is recommended that serum creatinine and blood urea nitrogen (BUN) be monitored.

## BOX 18.2 Herb and Dietary Interactions: Ampicillin

**Herbs and Foods That Decrease the Effects of Ampicillin**

- Food

  *Decreases absorption*

   Food w/ GI upset is OK
- Khat

  *Decreases absorption*

### Assessing for Adverse Effects

The nurse carefully assesses the characteristics of a rash, if present. It is necessary to distinguish, if possible, a hypersensitivity reaction from a nonallergic ampicillin rash.

### Patient Teaching

The nurse instructs patients to take oral penicillins for the full, prescribed course of treatment to prevent complications. Box 18.3 outlines patient teaching guidelines for ampicillin and other oral penicillins.

## Other Drugs in the Class

### Antistaphylococcal Penicillins and Aminopenicillins

The choice of a beta-lactam antibacterial depends on the organism causing the infection, severity of the infection, and other factors. Penicillin G or the aminopenicillin amoxicillin is the drug of choice in many infections. Other aminopenicillins are indicated

## BOX 18.3 Patient Teaching Guidelines for Oral Penicillins

**General Considerations**

- Do not take any penicillin if you have ever had an allergic reaction to penicillin in which you had difficulty breathing, swelling, or skin rash. However, some people call a minor stomach upset an allergic reaction, which is incorrect, and they are not given penicillin when that is the best antibiotic in a given situation.
- Complete the full course of drug treatment for greater effectiveness and prevention of secondary infection with drug-resistant bacteria.
- Follow instructions carefully about how much of the drug you are supposed to take and how often you are supposed to take it. Drug effectiveness depends on maintaining adequate blood levels. Penicillins often need more frequent administration than some other antibiotics, because they are rapidly excreted by the kidneys.

**Self- Or Caregiver Administration**

- Take most penicillins on an empty stomach, 1 hour before or 2 hours after a meal. Penicillin V, amoxicillin, and Augmentin can be taken with food. [Take Augmentin with meals to increase absorption and decrease GI upset.]
- Take each dose with a full glass of water; do not take with orange juice or with other acidic fluids [they may destroy the drug].
- Take at even intervals, preferably around the clock.
- Shake liquid penicillins well, so they are mixed thoroughly, and measure the dose accurately.
- Discard liquid penicillin after 1 week if it is stored at room temperature or after 2 weeks if it is refrigerated. Liquid forms deteriorate and should not be taken after their expiration dates.
- Report skin rash, hives, itching, severe diarrhea, shortness of breath, fever, sore throat, black tongue, or any unusual bleeding to your health care provider. These symptoms may indicate an allergy to penicillin.

in *Pseudomonas* infections. Antistaphylococcal penicillin is indicated in staphylococcal infections; the antistaphylococcal drugs of choice are nafcillin for IV use and dicloxacillin for oral use.

Proper administration of penicillins is important. With intramuscular (IM) penicillins, it is necessary to inject them deep into large muscle masses to decrease tissue irritation. With IV penicillins, it is necessary to usually first dilute reconstituted penicillins in 50 to 100 mL of 5% dextrose or 0.9% sodium chloride injection and infuse them over 30 to 60 minutes to minimize vascular irritation and phlebitis. It should be noted that ticarcillin may cause decreased platelet aggregation.

### Penicillin–Beta-Lactamase Inhibitor Combinations

Beta-lactamase inhibitors are drugs with a beta-lactam structure but minimal antibacterial activity. They bind with and inactivate the beta-lactamase enzymes produced by many bacteria (e.g., *Escherichia coli*; *Klebsiella*, *Enterobacter*, and *Bacteroides* species; *Staphylococcus aureus*). When combined with a penicillin, the beta-lactamase inhibitor protects the penicillin from destruction by the enzymes and extends the penicillin's spectrum of antimicrobial activity. Thus, the combination drug may be effective in infections caused by bacteria that are resistant to a beta-lactam antibiotic alone.

Clavulanate, sulbactam, and tazobactam are the beta-lactamase inhibitors available in combinations with penicillins.

- Ampicillin–sulbactam is available as Unasyn, in vials with 1 g of ampicillin and 0.5 g of sulbactam or 2 g of ampicillin and 1 g of sulbactam.
- Amoxicillin and clavulanate is marketed as Augmentin, in 250-, 500-, and 875-mg tablets, each of which contains 125 mg of clavulanate.

> **! QSEN Alert: Safety**
>
> Two 250-mg tablets are not equivalent to one 500-mg tablet.
>
> - Augmentin is also available as 1000-mg extended-release tablets containing 62.5 mg of clavulanate. In addition, a chewable formulation is available as 200 mg of amoxicillin and 28.5 mg of clavulanate, as well as 400 mg of amoxicillin and 57 mg of clavulanate.
> - Piperacillin/tazobactam is marketed as Zosyn, an IV formulation. Patients with sepsis may require loading doses of 3.375 to 4.5 g over 30 minutes.

### NCLEX Success

1. A nurse is preparing to administer the first dose of piperacillin/tazobactam to a patient in an infusion clinic. The nurse should take which of the following precautions?

   A. Ask the patient about past allergic reactions to penicillins.
   B. Ask the patient about past allergic reactions to aminoglycosides.
   C. Mix the piperacillin/tazobactam with lidocaine to reduce pain of infusion.
   D. Instruct the patient to eat a snack to decrease stomach upset from piperacillin/tazobactam.

2. A woman is to receive amoxicillin–clavulanate 500 mg PO every 8 hours for bronchitis. The nurse retrieves two 250-mg tablets from the medication cart. This is incorrect for which of the following reasons?

   A. The amount of sulbactam in amoxicillin–clavulanate 250 mg is 62.5 mg per tablet, twice the intended amount.
   B. This provides twice the intended dose of clavulanate.
   C. The 250-mg tablets have less absorption than the 500-mg tablets.
   D. Administration of amoxicillin–clavulanate is only intravenous, so selecting tablets means that the wrong drug is being administered.

## CEPHALOSPORINS

Cephalosporins are a widely used group of drugs derived from a fungus and closely related chemically to the penicillins. Although technically cefoxitin and cefotetan are not cephalosporins, they are categorized with the cephalosporins because of their similarities to the group. Cephalosporins are broad-spectrum agents with activity against both gram-positive and gram-negative bacteria. Compared with penicillins, these drugs are generally less active against gram-positive organisms but more active against gram-negative ones.

## Classification

Cephalosporins are classified into five subgroups, or "generations," based on their pharmacology and spectrum of activity.

### First-Generation Cephalosporins

The first cephalosporin, cephalothin, is no longer available for clinical use. However, it may be used to determine susceptibility to first-generation cephalosporins, which have essentially the same spectrum of antimicrobial activity. In general, first-generation cephalosporins have strong activity against gram-positive bacteria and poor activity against gram-negative bacteria. Therefore, these drugs are effective against streptococci, staphylococci (except methicillin-resistant *Staphylococcus aureus* [MRSA]), *Shigella*, *E. coli*, *Proteus mirabilis*, and *Bacteroides* species (except *Bacteroides fragilis*). They are not effective against *Enterobacter*, *Pseudomonas*, and *Serratia* species.

Often, health care providers use first-generation cephalosporins for surgical prophylaxis, especially with prosthetic implants, because gram-positive organisms such as staphylococci cause most infections of surgical sites. Prescribers may also order them for treatment of infections caused by susceptible organisms in body sites where drug penetration and host defenses are adequate.

**Cefazolin,** the prototype cephalosporin, is the drug of choice for surgical prophylaxis in most surgical procedures. Some advantages of cefazolin over other first-generation cephalosporins include less frequent dosing, higher blood levels after parenteral administration, and increased gram-positive coverage.

## Second-Generation Cephalosporins

Second-generation cephalosporins are more active against some gram-negative organisms and somewhat less active against gram-positive cocci than the first-generation agents. Thus, they may be effective in infections resistant to other antibiotics, including infections caused by *Haemophilus influenzae*, *Klebsiella* species, *E. coli*, and some strains of *Proteus*. Because each of these drugs has a different antimicrobial spectrum, susceptibility tests must be performed for each drug rather than for the entire group, as may be done with first-generation drugs. Cefoxitin (Mefoxin) and cefotetan (Cefotan), for example, are active against *B. fragilis*, an anaerobic organism resistant to most drugs.

Often, other uses for second-generation cephalosporins also include surgical prophylaxis, especially for gynecologic and colorectal surgery. In the past, prescribers ordered the drugs for treatment of intra-abdominal infections such as pelvic inflammatory disease, diverticulitis, and other infections caused by organisms inhabiting pelvic and colorectal areas (perhaps caused by penetrating wounds of the abdomen). This practice is no longer recommended because of the increasing resistance of *Bacteroides* species to these agents.

## Third-Generation Cephalosporins

Third-generation cephalosporins further extend the spectrum of activity against gram-negative organisms. In addition to activity against the usual enteric pathogens (e.g., *E. coli*, *Proteus*, and *Klebsiella* species), they are also active against several strains resistant to other antibiotics and to first- and second-generation cephalosporins. Thus, they may be useful in infections caused by unusual strains of enteric organisms such as the group Enterobacteriaceae (which includes *Citrobacter*, *Serratia*, *Enterobacter*, *P. mirabilis*, and *E. coli*). Another difference is the ability of third-generation cephalosporins to penetrate inflamed meninges to reach therapeutic concentrations in CSF. Thus, they may be useful in meningeal infections caused by common pathogens, including *H. influenzae*, *Neisseria meningitidis*, and *Streptococcus pneumoniae*. Although some of the drugs are active against *Pseudomonas* organisms, drug-resistant strains may emerge when a cephalosporin is used alone for treatment of pseudomonal infection.

Overall, cephalosporins gain gram-negative activity and lose gram-positive activity as they move from the first to the third generation. The second- and third-generation drugs are more active against gram-negative organisms because they are more resistant to the beta-lactamase enzymes (cephalosporinases) produced by some bacteria to inactivate cephalosporins.

## Fourth-Generation Cephalosporins

Fourth-generation cephalosporins have a greater spectrum of antimicrobial activity and greater stability against breakdown by beta-lactamase enzymes compared with third-generation drugs. Cefepime, the first fourth-generation cephalosporin to be developed, is active against both gram-positive and gram-negative organisms. With gram-positive organisms, it is active against streptococci and staphylococci (except for methicillin-resistant staphylococci). With gram-negative organisms, its activity against *P. aeruginosa* is similar to that of ceftazidime, and its activity against Enterobacteriaceae is greater than that

of third-generation cephalosporins. Moreover, cefepime retains activity against strains of Enterobacteriaceae and *P. aeruginosa* that have acquired resistance to third-generation agents.

## Fifth-Generation Cephalosporins

Ceftaroline (Teflaro) is an IV cephalosporin used for the treatment of community-acquired pneumonia and skin infections. It is the first cephalosporin to be considered active against resistant gram-positive organisms, such as MRSA, vancomycin-resistant *S. aureus* (VRSA), vancomycin-insensitive *S. aureus* (VISA), and heteroresistant VISA. Because ceftaroline retains activity against VISA and VRSA, it is often used off-label in vancomycin failures.

# Pharmacokinetics

After the cephalosporins are absorbed, they achieve therapeutic concentrations in most body fluids and tissues, with maximum concentrations in the liver and kidneys. However, many cephalosporins do not reach therapeutic levels in the CSF. Most third-generation cephalosporins achieve more consistent CSF penetration in those patients with inflamed meninges.

Cefazolin is distributed into most body tissues and crosses the placenta. The onset of action is rapid with both IV and IM administration. The drug peaks at the end of IV infusion and within 1 to 2 hours with IM injection. The duration of action is 6 to 12 hours. The drug, which is largely excreted unchanged via the kidneys, concentrates in the urine. Thus, metabolism is not hepatic. Therefore, no dosage adjustments are necessary with hepatic impairment.

# Action

Cefazolin inhibits the third and last step of bacterial wall synthesis by binding to one or more penicillin-binding proteins.

# Use

Cefazolin is a frequently used parenteral agent. It reaches a higher serum concentration, is more protein bound, and has a slower rate of elimination than other first-generation drugs. These factors prolong serum half-life, which means that cefazolin can be given less frequently.

Clinical indications for the use of the cephalosporins include surgical prophylaxis and treatment of infections of the respiratory tract, skin and soft tissues, bones and joints, urinary tract, brain and spinal cord, and bloodstream (septicemia). In infections caused by MRSA, cephalosporins are not clinically effective even if in vitro testing indicates susceptibility (except for the newest cephalosporin, ceftaroline). Infections caused by *Neisseria gonorrhoeae*, at one time susceptible to penicillin, are now treated with a third-generation cephalosporin such as ceftriaxone.

Table 18.3 provides important route and dosage information about cephalosporins.

## Use in Children

As with penicillins, cefazolin and other cephalosporins are extensively used to treat infections in children and are commonly safe. They should be used cautiously in neonates because immature kidney function slows their elimination. Dosage should be based on age, weight, severity of the infection, and renal function.

## TABLE 18.3

## DRUGS AT A GLANCE: Cephalosporins

| Drug | Pregnancy Category | Characteristics/Indications | Routes and Dosage Ranges | |
|---|---|---|---|---|
| | | | **Adults** | **Children** |
| **First Generation** | | | | |
| **Cefazolin** (Ancef; cefazolin for injection) | B | Active against streptococci, staphylococci, *Neisseria, Salmonella, Shigella, Escherichia, Klebsiella, Listeria, Bacillus, Haemophilus influenzae, Corynebacterium diphtheriae, Proteus mirabilis,* and *Bacteroides* (except *B. fragilis*) | IM, IV 1–2 g every 8 h (max dose 12 g/d) | IM, IV 25–100 mg/kg/d in divided doses every 6–8 h (max dose 6 g/d) |
| Cefadroxil ( Apo-Cefadroxil, PRO-Cefadroxil, Teva-Cefadroxil) | B | Active against streptococci such as *Streptococcus pyogenes,* staphylococci, *Escherichia, P. mirabilis,* and *Klebsiella*<br>Prosthetic joint infection: active against *Staphylococcus* (oxacillin susceptible) | PO 1 g/d in a single or 2 divided doses for 10 d<br>Prosthetic joint infection: 500 mg every 12 h | PO 30 mg/kg/d in a single dose or divided every 12 h |
| Cephalexin (Keflex; Apo-Cephalex, Dom-Cephalexin, Keflex, PMS Cephalexin, Teva-Cephalexin) | B | Active against streptococci such as *Streptococcus pyogenes, Staphylococcus aureus, P. mirabilis, Klebsiella pneumoniae, H. influenzae,* and *Moraxella catarrhalis* | PO 250–500 mg every 6–8 h | >1 y to <15 y: PO 25–100 mg/kg/d in divided doses every 6–8 h (maximum dose: 4 g/d) |
| **Second Generation** | | | | |
| Cefaclor ( Apo-Cefaclor, Ceclor, Novo-Cefaclor) | B | Active against streptococci and staphylococci | PO 200–500 mg every 8 h | PO 20–40 mg/kg/d in divided doses every 8–12 h for 7 d |
| Cefotetan (Cefotan) | B | Effective against most organisms except *Pseudomonas*<br>Highly resistant to beta-lactamase enzymes | IV, IM 1–6 g/d in divided doses every 12 h<br>Surgical prophylaxis, IV 1–2 g 30–60 min before surgery | IV, IM 20–40 mg/kg every 12 h (max 6 g/d) |
| Cefoxitin (Mefoxin; cefoxitin for injection) | B | The first cephamycin (derived from a different fungus than cephalosporins)<br>Possible major clinical use: stems from increased activity against *B. fragilis,* an organism resistant to most other antimicrobial drugs | IV 1–2 g every 6–8 h<br>Surgical prophylaxis, IV 1 or 2 g 30–60 min before surgery | IV 80–160 mg/kg/d in divided doses every 4–6 h. Do not exceed 12 g/d |
| Cefprozil ( Apo-Cefprozil, Auro-Cefprozil) | B | | PO 500 mg every 24 h for 10 d (administer >10 d for *Streptococcus pyogenes*) | Otitis media: PO ≥6 mo PO 7.5 mg/kg/dose<br>Tonsillitis: 2–12 y PO 7.5 mg/kg/dose every 12 h (maximum dose 1000 mg/d) |

*(Continued on page 364)*

**TABLE 18.3**

## DRUGS AT A GLANCE: Cephalosporins [Continued]

| Drug | Pregnancy Category | Characteristics/Indications | Routes and Dosage Ranges | |
|---|---|---|---|---|
| | | | **Adults** | **Children** |
| Cefuroxime (Zinacef; ❋ Apo-Cefuroxime, Auro-Cefuroxime, Ceftin, cefuroxime for injection, PRO-Cefuroxime) | B | Similar to other second-generation cephalosporins<br>Penetrates CSF in the presence of inflamed meninges | PO 250–500 mg every 12 h for 10 d<br>IV, IM 500 mg–1.5 g every 6–8 h<br>Surgical prophylaxis, IV 1.5 g 30–60 min before initial skin incision | PO 20–30 mg/kg/d in two divided doses for 10 d<br>IV, IM 75–150 mg/kg/d in divided doses every 6–8 h (max dose 6 g/d) |
| **Third Generation** | | | | |
| Cefdinir | B | Active against *H. influenzae*, *Streptococcus pneumoniae*, and *S. pyogenes* | PO 300 mg twice/d for 5–10 d or 600 g daily for 10 d | PO 7–14 mg/kg twice/d for 5–10 d |
| Cefditoren | B | Active against *Streptococcus pneumoniae*, *S. pyogenes*, and *M. catarrhalis* | PO 200–400 mg/d twice daily for 10 d | >12 y: refer to adult dosing |
| Cefixime (Suprax; ❋ Auro-Cefixime, Suprax) | B | Active against *Escherichia*, *P. mirabilis*, *H. influenzae*, *Streptococcus pneumoniae*, and *Klebsiella* | PO 400 mg daily in divided doses every 12–24 h | PO 8 mg/kg divided doses every 12–24 h |
| Cefotaxime (❋ cefotaxime sodium for injection, Claforan) | B | Activity against most gram-positive and gram-negative bacteria, including several strains resistant to other antibiotics<br>Recommended for serious infections caused by susceptible microorganisms | IV, IM 1–2 g every 4–12 h; max dose, 12 g/d | IV, IM >50 kg: same as adults<br><50 kg to 12 y and age >1 mo: IV, IM 50–180 mg/kg/d, in divided doses every 6–8 h |
| Cefpodoxime | B | Active against *Streptococcus pyogenes*, *H. influenzae*, *K. pneumoniae*, *Staphylococcus aureus*, *P. mirabilis*, and *Staphylococcus saprophyticus* | PO 100–400 mg every 12 h for 10 d | PO ≥2 mo to <12 y 10 mg/kg/d divided every 12 h<br>≥12 y 100–400 mg every 12 h |
| Ceftazidime (Fortaz, Tazicef; ❋ ceftazidime for injection, Fortaz) | B | Active against gram-positive and gram-negative organisms<br>Especially effective against gram-negative organisms, including *P. aeruginosa* and other bacterial strains resistant to aminoglycosides<br>Indicated for serious infections caused by susceptible organisms | IV, IM 500–2000 mg every 8–12 h<br>Cystic fibrosis: 90–150 mg/kg/d | Mild infections: IM, IV 30–50 mg/kg/d divided every 8 h (maximum dose: 3000 mg/d)<br>Severe infections: 200 mg/kg/d divided every 8 h (maximum dose 6 g/d) |
| Ceftibuten | B | Active against *Streptococcus pneumoniae*, *S. pyogenes*, and *M. catarrhalis* | PO 400 mg daily for 10 d | 6 mo to <12 y 9 mg/kg/dose for 10 d (maximum dose 400 mg/d)<br>≥12 y: refer to adult dosing |

**TABLE 18.3**

## DRUGS AT A GLANCE: Cephalosporins (Continued)

| Drug | Pregnancy Category | Characteristics/Indications | Routes and Dosage Ranges | |
|---|---|---|---|---|
| | | | **Adults** | **Children** |
| Ceftriaxone (✱ ceftriaxone for injection) | B | First third-generation cephalosporin approved for once-daily dosing<br>Antibacterial activity against most gram-positive and gram-negative bacteria, including several strains resistant to other antibiotics | IV, IM 1–2 g every 12–24 h | Infants/children IM, IV 50–100 mg/kg/d in 1–2 divided doses (max dose 4 g/d)<br>Meningitis, IV, IM 100 mg/kg/d, not to exceed 4 g daily, in divided doses every 12 h |
| **Fourth Generation** | | | | |
| Cefepime (Maxipime) | B | Indicated for use in sepsis; in severe infections of the lower respiratory and urinary tract, skin and soft tissue, and female reproductive tract; and in febrile neutropenic patients<br>May be used as monotherapy for all infections caused by susceptible organisms. Higher doses should be used for serious infections due to *P. aeruginosa* | IV 1–2 g every 8–12 h<br>IM 0.5–1 g every 12 h | IM, IV 50 mg/kg every 8–12 h, not to exceed recommended adult dose |
| **Fifth Generation** | | | | |
| Ceftaroline (Teflaro) | B | Active against *Streptococcus pyogenes, S. agalactiae, S. pneumoniae, H. influenzae, K. pneumoniae, Klebsiella oxytoca, Staphylococcus aureus* (including methicillin-susceptible and methicillin-resistant isolates), *P. mirabilis, Staphylococcus saprophyticus,* and *Escherichia coli* | Community-acquired pneumonia: IV 600 mg every 12 h for 5–7 d<br>Skin infection: IV 600 mg every 12 h for 5–14 d | IV ≥ 2 mo to <2 y: 8 mg/kg/dose every 8 h for 5–14 d<br>≥2 y to <18 y: 12 mg/kg/dose every 8 h for 5–14 d |
| **Cephalosporin–Beta-Lactamase Inhibitor Combinations** | | | | |
| Ceftolozane–tazobactam (Zerbaxa) | B | For treatment of intra-abdominal infections caused by *Enterobacter cloacae, Escherichia coli, Klebsiella oxytoca, K. pneumoniae, P. aeruginosa, B. fragilis, Streptococcus anginosus, S. constellatus,* and *S. salivarius* | IV 1.5 g every 8 h for 4–14 d | |
| Ceftazidime–avibactam (Avycaz) | No category; adverse events fetal events have been documented in animal studies | Active against *Enterobacter cloacae, Escherichia coli, K. oxytoca, K. pneumoniae, P. aeruginosa, Enterobacter aerogenes,* and *Proteus* | IV 2.5 g every 8 h for 5–14 d<br>Intra-abdominal infections: combine with metronidazole | |

**QSEN Alert: Safety**

Specialized pediatric dosing references can provide guidance for dosing of most cephalosporins based on the child's age and weight.

## Use in Older Adults

As with penicillins, cefazolin and other cephalosporins are relatively safe, although decreased renal function, other disease processes, and concurrent drug therapies increase the risks of adverse effects in older adults.

## Use in Patients With Renal Impairment

Cefazolin and all other parenteral cephalosporins, except ceftriaxone, require dosage adjustment in patients with renal impairment. Usual doses may produce high and prolonged serum drug levels, and therefore, a lower dose or an increased period between doses is necessary. Cefazolin is moderately dialyzable, and the normal dose or a supplemental dose should be administered after dialysis.

## Use in Patients With Critical Illness

Some cephalosporins are used in surgical prophylaxis. The particular drug depends largely on the type of organism likely to be encountered in the operative area. First-generation cephalosporins, mainly cefazolin, are used for procedures associated with gram-positive postoperative infections because of activity against streptococci and methicillin-susceptible staphylococci. Second-generation cephalosporins, mainly cefotetan and cefoxitin, are often used for abdominal procedures, especially gynecologic and colorectal surgery, in which enteric gram-negative postoperative infections may occur. Third-generation cephalosporins should not be used for surgical prophylaxis because they are less active against staphylococci than cefazolin, and the gram-negative organisms they are most useful against are rarely encountered in elective surgery. Additionally, fourth- and fifth-generation cephalosporins are not typically used for surgical prophylaxis. Widespread usage for prophylaxis promotes emergence of drug-resistant organisms.

 **QSEN Alert: Patient-Centered Care**

When used perioperatively, cephalosporins should be given within 60 minutes before the first skin incision is made so the drug has time to reach therapeutic serum and tissue concentrations.

A single dose is usually sufficient, although repeat doses are necessary in patients undergoing a surgical procedure exceeding 2 to 4 hours or procedures involving major blood loss. (Postoperative doses are no longer recommended [cardiac procedures may be an exception]. If cephalosporins are used, they should generally not be given more than 24 hours after surgery.) Blood levels need to be maintained above the MIC of the microorganisms causing the infection being treated for at least 40% to 50% of the dosing interval. Continuous or extended infusion strategies may be of benefit with serious infections, especially those caused by relatively resistant organisms such as *Pseudomonas* or *Acinetobacter*.

 **QSEN Alert: Evidence-Based Practice**

Patients with hematological malignancy who have undergone hematopoietic cell transplantation are prone to the development of multidrug-resistant *Pseudomonas aeruginosa*. These patients are prone to increased risk of morbidity and mortality. Ceftolozane–tazobactam is a good option for the treatment of multidrug-resistant *P. aeruginosa*. Hakki and Lewis [2018] conducted a study to report the use of ceftolozane–tazobactam for invasive multidrug-resistant *P. aeruginosa* in patients who have been diagnosed with hematologic malignancy and have undergone hematopoietic cell transplantation. Treatment was successful while on ceftolozane–tazobactam. No participants died while on ceftolozane–tazobactam, and all patients remained alive 30 days following discontinuation of the drug combination.

## Use in Patients Receiving Home Care

With cefazolin, as well as with oral agents such as cephalexin and cefprozil, the home care nurse mainly needs to teach patients about accurate administration and observation for therapeutic and adverse effects. With cefazolin or other parenteral cephalosporins, the nurse should teach the patient and family how to administer the drug and not to use the drug if (1) it is cloudy or discolored or if (2) the vial is damaged. It is important to keep needles and syringes out of the reach of children and pets and dispose of them properly.

 **QSEN Alert: Patient-Centered Care**

With liquid suspensions for children, shaking to resuspend the medication and measuring with a measuring spoon or calibrated device to ensure safe dosing are necessary. Parents or caregivers should not use household spoons because they vary widely in capacity and may lead to incorrect dosing.

## Adverse Effects

Adverse effects to cefazolin and the other cephalosporins are similar to those of most other antibiotics: abdominal pain, diarrhea, gastritis, nausea, and vomiting. Primarily, effects of particular importance are hypersensitivity reactions and superinfections.

## Contraindications

A contraindication to the use of a cephalosporin is a previous severe anaphylactic reaction to a penicillin. Because cephalosporins are chemically similar to penicillins, there is a risk of cross-sensitivity. However, incidence of cross-sensitivity is low, especially in patients who have had delayed reactions (e.g., skin rash) to penicillins. Another contraindication is cephalosporin allergy. Immediate allergic reactions with anaphylaxis, bronchospasm, and urticaria occur less often than delayed reactions with skin rash, drug fever, and eosinophilia.

## Nursing Implications

### Preventing Interactions

Cephalosporins have been associated with a decrease in prothrombin activity, which may be due to depletion of vitamin K in the gut flora. It is necessary to monitor patients previously stabilized on anticoagulants. Box 18.4 outlines drug–drug

**BOX 18.4** ⬭ *Drug Interactions: Cephalosporins*

**Drugs That Increase the Effects of Cephalosporins**

- Aminoglycosides
  *Increase the risk of nephrotoxicity*
- Entecavir
  *Leads to competitive inhibition of transporters in renal tubules*
- Furosemide
  *Increases the risk of nephrotoxicity*
- Nimodipine
  *Increases the risk of nephrotoxicity*
- Vancomycin
  *Increases the risk of nephrotoxicity*

interactions. There are no identified herbal interactions. However, each gram of cefazolin has 46 mg (2 mEq) of sodium, which may have a negative effect on patients with heart failure.

### Administering the Medication

To prevent complications, it is essential to administer cefazolin and other cephalosporins for the full, prescribed course of treatment.

---

**❗ QSEN Alert: Safety**

It is important to avoid giving cephalosporins to people with life-threatening allergic reactions to penicillin (anaphylaxis, laryngeal swelling, angioedema, or hives).

---

The nurse should not mix ceftriaxone and IV solutions of calcium-containing salts or administer these drugs simultaneously, because of the potential for ceftriaxone–calcium precipitation. It is possible to minimize adverse effects by administering most oral cephalosporins with food or milk.

### Assessing for Therapeutic Effects

Drug levels are not required when administering cefazolin or any of the cephalosporins. If the patient is experiencing renal impairment, monitoring of serum creatinine and BUN is recommended, because adjustment for renal dysfunction may be necessary.

### Assessing for Adverse Effects

The nurse carefully evaluates any rash. If possible, it is necessary to distinguish a hypersensitivity reaction from a nonallergic cefazolin rash.

### Patient Teaching

The nurse instructs patients that cephalosporins, like all antibiotics, should be given for the full, prescribed course of treatment to prevent complications. Box 18.5 outlines patient teaching guidelines.

## Other Drugs in the Class

As previously described, cephalosporins are grouped into generations by their antimicrobial properties. Each newer generation of cephalosporins has significantly greater gram-negative antimicrobial properties than the preceding generation, with decreased activity against gram-positive organisms. Fourth-generation cephalosporins, however, have true broad-spectrum activity acting against some gram-positive and many gram-negative organisms, including greater stability against degradation by beta-lactamase enzymes and anti-*Pseudomonas* activity. Fifth-generation cephalosporins have a gram-negative spectrum similar to the third-generation cephalosporins as well as anti-MRSA activity.

---

**BOX 18.5** 📋 *Patient Teaching Guidelines for Oral Cephalosporins*

**General Considerations**

- Inform your physician if you have ever had a severe allergic reaction to penicillin in which you had difficulty breathing, swelling, or skin rash. A small number of people are allergic to both penicillins and cephalosporins because the drugs are somewhat similar in their chemical structures.
- Also, inform your physician if you have had a previous allergic reaction to a cephalosporin (e.g., Keflex). If you are not sure whether a new prescription is a cephalosporin, ask the pharmacist before having the prescription filled.
- Complete the full course of drug treatment for greater effectiveness and prevention of secondary infection with drug-resistant bacteria.
- Follow instructions about dosing frequency; effectiveness depends on maintaining adequate blood levels.

**Self- Or Caregiver Administration**

- Take most oral drugs with food or milk to prevent stomach upset.

- Take cefpodoxime and cefuroxime (Zinacef) with food to increase absorption.
- Do not take cefaclor, cefdinir, or cefpodoxime with antacids containing aluminum or magnesium (e.g., Maalox, Mylanta) or with Pepcid, Tagamet, or Zantac. These drugs decrease absorption of these antibiotics and make them less effective. If necessary to take one of the drugs, take it 2 hours before or 2 hours after a dose of these antibiotics.
- Shake liquid preparations well to mix thoroughly and measure the dose accurately.
- Report the occurrence of diarrhea, especially if it is severe or contains blood, pus, or mucus. Cephalosporins can cause antibiotic-associated colitis and the drug may need to be stopped.
- Inform your health care provider if you are breast-feeding. These drugs enter breast milk.

Cefotetan may cause ~~hypoprothrombinemia~~ (by killing intestinal bacteria that normally produce vitamin K or a chemical structure that prevents activation of prothrombin) or platelet dysfunction. Treatment of bleeding may involve giving vitamin K but does not restore normal platelet function or normal bacterial flora in the intestines.

### Cephalosporin–Beta-Lactamase Inhibitor Combinations

Two cephalosporin–beta-lactamase combinations are available in the United States. Ceftolozane–tazobactam has broad-spectrum capabilities against aerobic and facultative gram-negative bacilli; it is effective against extended-spectrum Enterobacteriaceae. The primary use of this drug combination is treatment of infections resulting from multidrug-resistant *P. aeruginosa*. It is also used to treat complicated intra-abdominal infections and urinary tract infections caused by *E. coli*, *Klebsiella*, *Proteus*, and *P. aeruginosa*. Ceftolozane binds to one or more penicillin-binding proteins to inhibit the final step of peptidoglycan synthesis to interrupt bacterial cell wall synthesis. Tazobactam covalently binds to plasmid-mediated and chromosomal bacterial beta-lactamases. It also irreversibly inhibits beta-lactamases, including penicillinases and cephalosporinases. Ceftolozane is not metabolized, whereas tazobactam is hydrolyzed to an inactive metabolite. Both are excreted largely unchanged in the urine. Ceftolozane–tazobactam is administered intravenously over 60 minutes. If combined with probenecid, the serum concentration of ceftolozane–tazobactam is increased. Like most cephalosporin antibiotics, there is a risk of cross-reactivity with penicillin allergies. The drug is otherwise well tolerated.

Ceftazidime–avibactam, which is effective against carbapenem-resistant Enterobacteriaceae (CRE), is indicated for intra-abdominal infections and urinary tract infections, including pyelonephritis. This drug combination is frequently used off-label to treat pneumonia, bacteremia, or other infections due to CRE. The mechanism of action of this drug is similar to that of other beta-lactam antibiotics. The avibactam component functions as a beta-lactamase inhibitor, which like tazobactam inhibits the degradation of the ceftazidime by plasmid-mediated beta-lactamases.

---

### NCLEX Success

3. A cardiac surgeon orders cefazolin 1 g IV "on call" to the operating room for a patient scheduled for a heart valve replacement. The surgery is scheduled for 7:00 AM the next morning. What is the rationale for giving the antibiotic at 6:30 AM? The last dose was administered more than 8 hours ago.
   A. The cefazolin must be given 60 minutes before the procedure for legal reasons.
   B. The cefazolin must be given within 60 minutes before the first skin incision to reach therapeutic concentrations.
   C. The cefazolin trough level will be checked at 6:00 AM, which would allow the level to come back before administration of the "on call" dose.
   D. The last dose was administered yesterday.

4. Which of the following classes of cephalosporins have the best activity against gram-positive organisms?
   A. first-generation cephalosporins
   B. second-generation cephalosporins
   C. third-generation cephalosporins
   D. fourth-generation cephalosporins

---

### Clinical Application 18.1

The nurse asks Mr. O'Brian if he has had an allergy to penicillin or cephalosporins. He denies any known allergies to drugs.
- Why is cefazolin the drug of choice for his cardiac pacemaker procedure?
- Before administrating this medication, what factors should the nurse assess?
- Why did the nurse ask the patient about a penicillin allergy with the administration of a cephalosporin?

---

## CARBAPENEMS

Carbapenems are broad-spectrum, bactericidal beta-lactam antimicrobials. The group consists of four drugs. 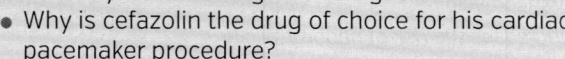 **Imipenem–cilastatin (Primaxin)** is the prototype.

### Pharmacokinetics

Imipenem–cilastatin, which is given parenterally, is distributed in most body fluids and body tissues. The drug has a rapid onset of action and peaks at the end of the infusion, and its duration is 6 to 8 hours. An enzyme (dehydropeptidase) in renal tubules rapidly breaks down the imipenem component; therefore, the drug reaches only low concentrations in the urine. However, the cilastatin inhibits the destruction of imipenem, increasing the urinary concentration of imipenem and reducing its potential renal toxicity. Recommended doses indicate the amount of imipenem; the solution contains an equivalent amount of cilastatin. (The drugs are available only in the combined form.)

### Action

Like other beta-lactam drugs, imipenem–cilastatin and the other carbapenems ~~inhibit synthesis of bacterial cell walls~~ by binding with penicillin-binding proteins.

### Use

Imipenem–cilastatin is effective in infections caused by a wide range of bacteria, including penicillinase-producing staphylococci, *E. coli*, *Proteus* species, *Enterobacter–Klebsiella–Serratia* species, *P. aeruginosa*, and *Enterococcus faecalis*. Its main use is in the treatment of infections caused by organisms resistant to other drugs. Considered to ~~be a very broad-spectrum antibiotic,~~ imipenem–cilastatin covers a range of gram-negative and gram-positive aerobes and anaerobes. It is used to treat infections of the lower respiratory tract, urinary tract, intra-abdominal

## TABLE 18.4

## DRUGS AT A GLANCE: Carbapenems

| Drug | Pregnancy Category | Routes and Dosage Ranges | |
|---|---|---|---|
| | | **Adults** | **Children** |
| Imipenem–cilastatin (Primaxin; ✽ imipenem and cilastatin for injection) | C | IV 250–1000 mg every 6–8 h based on imipenem component (max dose 4 g/d) IM 500–750 mg every 12 h | >3 mo: noncentral nervous system infections IV 15–25 mg/kg every 6 h (max dose 4 g/d) |
| Ertapenem (Invanz; ✽ Invanz) | B | IV, IM 1 g once daily | 3 mo–12 y: IV, IM 15 mg/kg twice daily (max dose 1 g/d) |
| Meropenem (Merrem; ✽ Meropenem for injection) | B | IV 1.5–6 g/d in divided doses every 8 h | ≥3 mo: 10–40 mg/kg in divided doses every 8 h (max dose 6 g/d) |
| Doripenem | B | IV 500 mg every 8 h | Safety and efficacy not yet established |
| **Carbapenem–Beta-Lactamase Inhibitor Combinations** | | | |
| Meropenem–vaborbactam (Vabomere; ✽ Vabomere) | B | IV 4 g every 8 h | Safety and efficacy not yet established |

infections, bone and joints, and skin and skin structures. It can also be used to treat polymicrobial infections (caused by multiple microorganisms), bacterial septicemia, and endocarditis.

Table 18.4 gives specific route and dosage information for carbapenems.

### Use in Children

Use of imipenem–cilastatin is appropriate in children. However, children with CNS infections should not receive the drug because of the risk of seizures. Caution is warranted in neonates with all carbapenems because immature kidney function slows the elimination of these drugs. Dosages are calculated based on age, weight, severity of infection, and renal function. Specialized pediatric dosing references can provide guidance to dosing of most carbapenems based on the child's age and weight.

### Use in Older Adults

Imipenem–cilastatin and other carbapenems are relatively safe, although decreased renal function, other disease processes, and concurrent drug therapies increase the risks of adverse effects in older adults. Lower doses may be necessary in the elderly, depending on renal function and severity of infection.

### Use in Patients With Renal Impairment

It is necessary to reduce the dosage of imipenem–cilastatin and all other carbapenems in most patients with renal impairment, and caution is warranted in patients with creatinine clearance ≤20 mL/min because of the increased risk of seizures. Patients with severe renal impairment (≤5 mL/min) should not receive imipenem–cilastatin unless hemodialysis is initiated within 48 hours.

### Use in Patients With Hepatic Impairment

Imipenem–cilastatin may cause abnormalities in liver function test results (i.e., elevated alanine and aspartate aminotransferases,

alkaline phosphatase), but hepatitis and jaundice rarely occur. There are no specific recommendations or guidelines for dosage adjustment in patients with hepatic impairment.

### Use in Patients With Critical Illness

Imipenem–cilastatin is typically used for illnesses that are considered critical. It has a broad spectrum of activity and less resistant patterns than the penicillins and cephalosporins. Carbapenems generally resist cleavage by most beta-lactamases. Carbapenem-resistant strains of *P. aeruginosa* are arising due to the altered permeability to this class of drugs and specific changes that occur on the protein outer membranes.

### Use in Patients Receiving Home Care

The need for frequent dosing means that imipenem–cilastatin is not typically given in the home setting. However, basic principles of IV care are an important component in administering this medication at home. Potential for secondary infections is a concern.

## Adverse Effects

Adverse effects, including the risk of cross-sensitivity in patients with penicillin hypersensitivity and gastric disturbances, are similar to those of other beta-lactam antibiotics. In addition, there have been reports of CNS toxicity, including seizures. Seizures are more likely in patients with a preexisting seizure disorder or when recommended doses are exceeded; however, they have occurred in other patients as well.

## Contraindications

Contraindications to imipenem–cilastatin include a hypersensitivity to carbapenems. There is a potential for cross-reactivity with patients that have a severe penicillin allergy due to the common beta-lactam ring. Patients with severe shock or atrioventricular block should not receive the IM formulation (containing lidocaine).

## Nursing Implications

### Preventing Interactions

Box 18.6 outlines drug–drug interactions with imipenem–cilastatin. There are no herbal interactions. All carbapenems may decrease the serum concentrations of divalproex. The drug may cause positive Coombs test results.

### Administering the Medication

It is important to avoid administering imipenem–cilastatin and the other carbapenems to people with life-threatening allergic reactions to penicillin (anaphylaxis, laryngeal swelling angioedema, or hives). In addition, IM administration of imipenem–cilastatin is not recommended for people with severe or life-threatening infections such as endocarditis, shock, or septicemia. To prepare imipenem–cilastatin for IM injection, lidocaine, a local anesthetic, is added to decrease pain. The solution is contraindicated in people allergic to this type of local anesthetic. The IM formulation is not for IV use.

### Assessing for Therapeutic Effects

Drug levels are not required when administering imipenem–cilastatin or any of the carbapenems. It is recommended that serum creatinine and BUN be monitored instead.

### Assessing for Adverse Effects

The nurse carefully assesses any rash. It is necessary to distinguish, if possible, a hypersensitivity reaction from a nonallergic imipenem–cilastatin rash.

### Patient Teaching

Imipenem–cilastatin and the other carbapenems are typically used for illnesses that are considered critical. Therefore, patient teaching guidelines focus on instructing the patient and family about the purpose of the drug and the importance of reporting adverse effects.

## Other Drugs in the Class

Other carbapenems are available. They include:

- Ertapenem is administered for catheter-related infections of the blood and hospital-acquired ventilator-associated pneumonia (VAP) in patients with multiple drug-resistant organisms. It has no activity against *Acinetobacter*, *Pseudomonas*, and *Enterococcus*.

---

**BOX 18.6** **Drug Interactions: Imipenem–Cilastatin**

**Drugs That Increase the Effects of Imipenem–Cilastatin**

- Cyclosporine
  *May increase central nervous system effects*
- Ganciclovir
  *May lead to generalized seizures*
- Probenecid
  *Increases drug level and half-life*

---

- Meropenem has an overall spectrum of activity similar to that of imipenem, although meropenem is less active against gram-positive bacteria. The drug is often given in the treatment of febrile neutropenia, which frequently occurs in patients with hematologic malignancies and in cancer patients who take chemotherapeutic drugs that cause bone marrow suppression.
- Doripenem is similar to ertapenem and meropenem. It is administered for complicated intra-abdominal with bacteriostatic and bactericidal effects. It is well distributed to body tissues, particularly the peritoneum and retroperitoneum.

## MONOBACTAMS

Currently, the only monobactam available for use is **Aztreonam** (Azactam), which serves as the prototype of this class. Aztreonam is active against aerobic gram-negative bacteria, including Enterobacteriaceae and *P. aeruginosa*, and many strains that are resistant to multiple antibiotics. The coverage is similar to that of the aminoglycosides, but the drug does not cause kidney damage or hearing loss. Because gram-positive and anaerobic bacteria are resistant to aztreonam, the drug's ability to preserve normal gram-positive and anaerobic flora may be an advantage compared with other antimicrobial agents.

## Pharmacokinetics

Aztreonam, which is given parenterally, is distributed in most body fluids and tissues, including the lungs, liver, kidney, bone, uterus, intestine, sputum, bile, pleural fluid, and synovial fluids. In addition, the drug also crosses the placenta and is excreted in breast milk. It is stable in the presence of beta-lactamase enzymes. Peak action occurs in 1 hour, with a duration of 4 to 12 hours; the onset of action depends on the organism and dose. Aztreonam is metabolized in the liver to inactive metabolites, which are excreted in the urine.

## Action

Like other beta-lactam drugs, aztreonam inhibits synthesis of bacterial cell walls by binding with penicillin-binding proteins. However, aztreonam, because of its monobactam structure, has limited cross-allergenicity between itself and other beta-lactam antibiotics. It is generally considered safe to administer aztreonam to patients with a penicillin allergy.

## Use

Aztreonam is effective in infections caused by *N. gonorrhoeae*, *H. influenzae*, and most *Enterobacter–Klebsiella–Serratia* species, and it is often active against *P. aeruginosa*. Although it is often considered to have similar coverage to aminoglycosides, extended-spectrum penicillins, and third-generation cephalosporins, aztreonam lacks gram-positive coverage. Also, anaerobes are not susceptible to aztreonam. Indications for use include infections of the urinary tract, skin and skin structures, and lower respiratory tract. Other indications include intra-abdominal and gynecologic infections as well as gram-negative septicemia. The FDA considers aztreonam solution for inhalation as an orphan drug for control of gram-negative bacteria in the respiratory tracts of patients diagnosed with cystic fibrosis.

**TABLE 18.5**

## DRUGS AT A GLANCE: Aztreonam

| Drug | Pregnancy Category | Routes and Dosage Ranges | |
|---|---|---|---|
| | | **Adults** | **Children** |
| Aztreonam (Azactam) | B | For urinary tract infection: IM, IV 0.5–1 g every 8–12 h<br>For moderate systemic infection: IM, IV 1 g every 8–12 h or IV 2 g every 8–12 h<br>For meningitis: IV 2 g every 6–8 h | IM, IV 30 mg/kg every 6–8 h |

It should be noted that aztreonam may cause an elevation in hepatic enzymes; however, on discontinuation of the drug, most enzymes return to pretherapy levels. There are no specific recommendations or guidelines for dosage adjustment in patients with hepatic impairment.

Table 18.5 presents general route and dosage information for aztreonam.

### Use in Children

Aztreonam can be used in children older than 1 month of age. Some adverse effects occur more frequently in children. This increased incidence could result from the severity of the illness being treated or the higher doses that are typically administered in pediatrics. Dosages should be based on age, weight, severity of infection, and renal function.

### Use in Older Adults

Aztreonam is relatively safe, although decreased renal function, other disease processes, and concurrent drug therapies increase the risks of adverse effects in older adults.

### Use in Patients With Renal Impairment

It is necessary to reduce the dosage of aztreonam in patients with renal impairment. Aztreonam is moderately dialyzable, and patients with life-threatening infections should receive a supplemental dose after each hemodialysis session.

### Use in Patients With Critical Illness

Aztreonam is used for some critical illnesses. However, use typically is reserved for those patients with a severe penicillin allergy. Monotherapy with aztreonam may lead to resistant *P. aeruginosa* infections. Often, combination therapy is recommended.

### Use in Patients Receiving Home Care

The need for frequent dosing means that aztreonam is not typically given in the home setting. However, basic principles of IV care are an important component in administering this medication at home. Potential for secondary infections is a concern.

## Adverse Effects

In general, adverse effects of aztreonam are similar to those of other beta-lactam antibiotics, including possible hypersensitivity reactions. The most common adverse effects include rash, diarrhea, nausea, vomiting, and localized thrombophlebitis.

Prolonged use may cause fungal or bacterial superinfections. *Clostridium difficile*–associated diarrhea and pseudomembranous colitis should be concerns with extended use.

## Contraindications

Contraindications to aztreonam include a hypersensitivity to any component of aztreonam.

## Nursing Implications

### Preventing Interactions

Box 18.7 outlines drug–drug interactions for aztreonam. As yet, there are no identified herb or food interactions. Aztreonam and aminoglycosides, when used in combination, can demonstrate synergistic effects against some strains of organisms, specifically *P. aeruginosa* and some Enterobacteriaceae. This synergy has also been seen with other beta-lactam antibiotics. There is a potential for false-positive reactions in urine glucose tests using Benedict's solution, Clinitest, or Fehling's solution.

### Administering the Medication

Aztreonam may be administered intravenously or intramuscularly.

### Assessing for Therapeutic Effects

Drug levels are not required when administering aztreonam. Monitoring of serum creatinine, BUN, and liver function tests is recommended in patients taking aztreonam.

### Assessing for Adverse Effects

The nurse carefully assesses any rash. It is important to distinguish a hypersensitivity reaction from a nonallergic aztreonam rash, if possible.

**BOX 18.7**    **Drug Interactions: Aztreonam**

**Drugs That Increase the Effects of Aztreonam**
- Aminoglycosides
  *Increase the risk of nephrotoxicity*
- Furosemide
  *May increase serum levels*

**Drugs That Decrease the Effects of Aztreonam**
- Cefoxitin
  *Induces the production of beta-lactamases*
- Chloramphenicol
  *May antagonize bactericidal activity*

## Patient Teaching

Aztreonam is typically used for illnesses that are considered critical. Therefore, patient teaching guidelines focus on instructing the patient and family about the purpose of the drug and importance of reporting adverse effects.

## NCLEX Success

5. In acute renal failure, doses of which of the following antibiotics must be reduced? (Select all that apply.)
   A. nafcillin
   B. cefazolin
   C. meropenem
   D. aztreonam

6. A nurse working in the neurointensive care unit is caring for a patient with a head injury who has been experiencing seizures and now has pneumonia caused by *Pseudomonas aeruginosa*. The physician has prescribed imipenem 1 g IV every 6 hours plus gentamicin for the pneumonia. Before administering the antibiotics, the nurse should do which of the following?
   A. Avoid mixing the imipenem and gentamicin in the same IV bag to prevent inactivation of the gentamicin.
   B. Remind the physician of the patient's seizures and inquire whether a different antibiotic might be safer.
   C. Suggest to the physician that imipenem is used to treat gram-positive infections and will not be effective in this patient.
   D. Set the infusion pump to deliver the imipenem over 15 minutes.

## THE NURSING PROCESS

A concept map outlines the nursing process related to drug therapy considerations in this chapter. Additional nursing implications related to the disease process should also be considered in care decisions.

**Assessment**
- With all beta-lactam anti-infective agents (penicillins, cephalosporins, carbapenem, aztreonam), ask the patient if he or she has experienced a skin rash, hives, swelling, or difficulty breathing when the drug has been administered in the past.

**Outcomes of Therapy**
The patient will
- Take oral beta-lactam antibacterials as directed.
- Receive parenteral beta-lactam drugs by appropriate techniques to minimize tissue irritation.
- Receive prompt and appropriate treatment if hypersensitivity reactions occur.

**Nursing Interventions**
- After giving a penicillin parenterally in an outpatient setting, keep the patient in the area for at least 30 minutes. Anaphylactic reactions are more likely to occur with parenteral than oral use and within a few minutes after injection.
- In any patient care setting, keep emergency equipment and supplies readily available.
- Monitor patient response to beta-lactam drugs.
- Monitor dosages of beta-lactam drugs for patients with impaired renal function.
- Provide patient teaching regarding drug therapy (see Boxes 18-3 and 18-5).

**Evaluation**
- Observe for improvement in signs of infection.
- Interview and observe for adverse drug effects.

## KEY CONCEPTS

- Beta-lactam antibiotics include penicillins, cephalosporins, carbapenems, and monobactams.
- The choice of a beta-lactam antibacterial depends on the organism causing the infection, the severity of the infection, and other factors.
- Several gram-positive and gram-negative bacteria produce beta-lactamases, which are enzymes that disrupt the beta-lactam ring and inactivate these drugs. This is the major mechanism by which microorganisms acquire resistance to beta-lactam antibiotics.
- As a class, penicillins usually are more effective in infections caused by gram-positive bacteria than those caused by gram-negative bacteria.
- In the rare instance in which penicillin is considered essential, a skin test may be helpful in assessing hypersensitivity.
- Metabolic and electrolyte imbalances may occur in patients receiving penicillins who have renal impairment or congestive heart failure: hyperkalemia is most likely to occur with large IV doses of penicillin G potassium.

- A **BLACK BOX WARNING** ◆ alerts health care providers that inadvertent IV administration of penicillin G benzathine may result in cardiopulmonary arrest and death. Long-acting repository forms have additives that decrease their solubility in tissue fluids and delay their absorption.
- Cephalosporins are classified into five subgroups, or "generations," based on their pharmacology and spectrum of activity.
- Ceftaroline (Teflaro) is the first cephalosporin to be considered active against resistant gram-positive organisms, such as MRSA, VRSA, and VISA.
- Cephalosporins are closely related chemically to the penicillin, and cross-sensitivity should be anticipated.
- Because of its monobactam structure, aztreonam has limited cross-allergenicity between itself and other beta-lactam antibiotics and is generally considered safe to use in patients who are allergic to penicillin.

## CLINICAL REASONING CASE STUDY

**Meet the Patient**

Aliyah Lympus, a 10-year-old girl, has had a sore throat and cough for the past week. She says that during the night her chest began to hurt, particularly when she took a deep breath. Her mother reports that her daughter has had a fever for 3 days ranging from 100°F to 103°F. Currently, it is 102.6°F. Aliyah has rales in the lower lobes bilaterally, shortness of breath, and inspiratory retractions. The diagnosis is community-acquired pneumonia. She is admitted to the pediatric infectious disease division of St. Vincent's Children's Hospital. The pediatric nurse practitioner has ordered ceftaroline IV 400 mg every 8 hours.

- What assessments should be implemented when administering ceftaroline?
- What is the action of ceftaroline?
- What are the adverse effects of ceftaroline?
- What patient teaching should be provided to Aliyah and her parents?

**Assessing Drug Information**

- Ceftaroline is a bacteriocidal anti-infective agent that binds to the penicillin-binding proteins. It binds to one or more of the penicillin-binding proteins located on the cell wall. It inhibits the third and final stage of cell wall synthesis.
- Ceftaroline is used to treat community-acquired pneumonia.
- Ceftaroline adverse effects include; rash, hypersensitivity, phlebitis, constipation, diarrhea, nausea, vomiting, elevated AST or ALT, hypokalemia.

**Nursing Actions**

- Prior to administering ceftaroline, ask if Aliyah has ever had a reaction to a penicillin or cephalosporin anti-infective agent.
- Reconstitute the drug with 20 mL of sterile water and dilute in 50 mL of IV 5 dextrose with normal saline.
- Assess the drug for particulate matter. If solution is clear light yellow, then administer ceftaroline over 60 minutes.
- Assess the patient's response to the medication. Assess for hypersensitivity, seizures, bradycardia, neutropenia, thrombocytopenia, hyperkalemia, and hypokalemia.
- Assess for signs and symptoms of watery or bloody diarrhea.
- Monitor for anemia.
- Assess the girl's complete blood cell count and direct Coombs test for drug-induced hemolytic anemia.
- Instruct Aliyah and her parents to report frequent watery stools or bloody diarrhea.
- Instruct Aliyah to eat yogurt to enhance the development of normal flora in the gastrointestinal tract.

*Visit* thePoint® *at* **http://thePoint.lww.com/Frandsen12e** *for answers to NCLEX Success questions (in Appendix A), answers to Clinical Application Case Studies (in Appendix B), and more!*

## REFERENCES AND RESOURCES

Hakki, M., & Lewis, J. S. (2018). Ceftolozane-tazobactam therapy for multi-drug resistant *Pseudomonas aeruginosa* infections in patients with hematologic malignancies and hematopoietic-cell transplant recipients. *Infection, 46*, 431–434. doi:10.1007/s15010-018-1125-5

Hinkle, J. L., & Cheever, K. H. (2017). *Brunner & Suddarth's textbook of medical-surgical nursing* (14th ed.). Philadelphia, PA: Wolters Kluwer Health/Lippincott Williams & Wilkins.

Karch, A. M. (2019). *2019 Lippincott's pocket drug for nurses.* Philadelphia, PA: Lippincott Williams & Wilkins.

Letourneau, A. (2009). Penicillin, antistaphylococcal penicillins, and broad-spectrum penicillins. *UpToDate.* Waltham, MA.

Letourneau, A. (2019). Cephalosporins. *UpToDate.* Waltham, MA.

Norris, T. L. (2019). *Porth's pathophysiology: Concepts of altered health states* (10th ed.). Philadelphia, PA: Lippincott Williams & Wilkins.

Nursing 2019. (2019). *Drug handbook.* Philadelphia, PA: Wolters Kluwer Health/Lippincott Williams & Wilkins.

UpToDate. (2019). *Drug information.* Lexi-Comp, Inc.

# Drug Therapy With Aminoglycosides and Fluoroquinolones

## LEARNING OBJECTIVES

*After studying this chapter, you should be able to:*

1. State the rationale for the increasing use of single daily doses of aminoglycosides.
2. Discuss the importance of measuring serum drug levels during aminoglycoside therapy.
3. Describe measures to decrease nephrotoxicity and ototoxicity with aminoglycosides.
4. Identify characteristics of aminoglycosides and fluoroquinolones in relation to effectiveness, safety, spectrum of antimicrobial activity, indications for use, administration, and observation of patient responses.
5. Recognize factors influencing selection and dosage of aminoglycosides and fluoroquinolones.
6. Describe characteristics, uses, adverse effects, and nursing process implications of fluoroquinolones.
7. Discuss principles of using aminoglycosides and fluoroquinolones in renal impairment and critical illness.
8. Recognize the importance of the judicious use of aminoglycosides and the fluoroquinolones to decrease the rate of antibiotic resistance.
9. Implement the nursing process in the care of patients receiving aminoglycosides and fluoroquinolones.

## CLINICAL APPLICATION CASE STUDY

Edward Louis, an 84-year-old man, has a history of prostatitis and recurrent bacterial urinary tract infections. He is complaining of a fever, hesitancy, and dysuria. He is started on ciprofloxacin (Cipro) 500 mg orally every 12 hours, after exhausting all alternate drug treatment options. What patient education should the nurse provide?

## KEY TERMS

**Concentration-dependent bactericidal effect:** relation of bactericidal ability of a drug to its concentration the greater the concentration of the drug, the faster and the more extensive the killing of the bacteria. The goal is to maximize concentration of the drug

**Extended-interval dosing:** dosing regimen that provides once-daily administration of an aminoglycoside with demonstrated decreased nephrotoxicity and ototoxicity while maintaining therapeutic efficacy also called pulse dosing

**Ototoxicity:** adverse effects on the structures of the ear, especially the cochlea and auditory nerve

**Postantibiotic effect:** persistent effect of an antimicrobial on bacterial growth after brief exposure of the organisms to a drug

# INTRODUCTION

Health care practitioners have used the aminoglycosides to treat serious aerobic gram-negative infections extensively for many years. However, increasing rates of antibiotic resistance, which limit therapeutic options, have become a growing concern. Select aminoglycosides have shown stability in the face of the emergence of resistance. The quinolones are also older drugs originally used only for the treatment of urinary tract infections (see Chap. 20). Synthesis of the quinolones involves adding a fluorine molecule to the quinolone structure. This addition increases drug activity against gram-negative microorganisms, broadens the antimicrobial spectrum to include several other microorganisms, and allows the use of the drugs in treating systemic infections. General characteristics, mechanisms of action, indications for and contraindications to use, nursing process implications, and principles of therapy for the aminoglycosides and the fluoroquinolones are described in this chapter. Individual drugs and the prototype drugs, with routes of administration and dosage ranges, are presented in Table 19.1 and the Drugs at a Glance tables.

> **! QSEN Alert: Teamwork and Collaboration**
>
> Reducing the risks for health care–associated infections and antimicrobial-resistant organisms requires a comprehensive and persistent effort by multiple members of the health care team. This includes procedures to prevent the spread of infection from patient to patient or staff to patient, as well as measures to reduce the overall use of antimicrobial agents. These efforts should be an absolute priority for hospitals and health care workers, with the resources and coordination provided to create change and protect patients.

# AMINOGLYCOSIDES

Aminoglycosides are bactericidal agents with similar pharmacologic, antimicrobial, and toxicologic characteristics. They are frequently used for the treatment of serious infections caused by gram-negative aerobic microorganisms such as *Pseudomonas* and *Proteus* species, *Escherichia coli*, and *Klebsiella*, *Enterobacter*, and *Serratia* species as well as mycobacteria. Less commonly, aminoglycosides (in combination with other agents) have also

been used in the treatment of select gram-positive infections. The drugs are not effective against gram-negative anaerobes. Aminoglycosides have shown relative stability against the development of resistant organisms compared with other antibiotic classes. Despite their relatively broad spectrum of activity of aminoglycosides, widespread clinical use is limited because of the availability of other less toxic agents with comparable effectiveness that do not require serum drug concentration monitoring.  **Gentamicin**, the most widely used aminoglycoside, is the prototype. Patients often receive gentamicin in combination with other antibiotics for serious systemic infections in the clinical setting. Gentamicin and other aminoglycosides are typically not used as monotherapy because they demonstrate inadequate clinical effectiveness at most sites except in the treatment of lower urinary tract infections.

Maintenance doses are based on serum drug concentrations. Peak serum concentrations should be determined 30 to 60 minutes after drug administration (5–8 mcg/mL for gentamicin and tobramycin; 20–30 mcg/mL for amikacin). Measurement of both peak and trough levels helps maintain therapeutic serum levels without excessive toxicity. For gentamicin and tobramycin, peak levels above 10 to 12 mcg/mL and trough levels above 2 mcg/mL for prolonged periods have been associated with nephrotoxicity. For accuracy, it is necessary to draw blood samples at the correct times and to document the timing of drug administration and blood sampling accurately, based on institutional recommendations.

## Pharmacokinetics

Gentamicin is poorly absorbed from the gastrointestinal (GI) tract. Thus, when given orally, the drug exerts local effects in the GI tract. It is rapidly and completely absorbed from intramuscular (IM) injection sites and reaches peak effects in 30 to 90 minutes if circulatory status is proficient. After intravenous (IV) administration, the peak effect occurs 30 minutes after a 30-minute infusion. Plasma half-life is 2 to 4 hours in patients with normal renal function. The volume of distribution is increased by edema, ascites, and fluid overload, and it is decreased with dehydration.

After parenteral administration, gentamicin is widely distributed in extracellular fluid and reaches therapeutic levels in blood, urine, bone, inflamed joints, and pleural and ascitic fluids. Gentamicin accumulates in high concentrations in the proximal renal tubules of the kidney, potentially leading to acute tubular necrosis. This damage to the kidney is termed nephrotoxicity. Gentamicin also accumulates in high concentrations in the inner ear, damaging sensory cells in the cochlea (disrupting hearing) and the vestibular apparatus (disturbing balance). This damage to the inner ear is termed **ototoxicity**. Gentamicin is poorly distributed in the central nervous system, intraocular fluids, and respiratory tract secretions.

## Action

Aminoglycosides penetrate the cell walls of susceptible bacteria and bind irreversibly to 30S and 50S ribosomal subunits, intracellular structures that synthesize proteins. As a result, the bacteria cell membrane becomes defective and cannot synthesize the proteins necessary for their function and replication.

**TABLE 19.1**

## Drug Therapy With Aminoglycosides and Fluoroquinolones

| Drug Class | Prototype(s) | Other Drugs in the Class |
|---|---|---|
| Aminoglycosides | Gentamicin | Amikacin<br>Neomycin<br>Paromomycin<br>Plazomicin<br>Streptomycin<br>Tobramycin |
| Fluoroquinolones | Ciprofloxacin (Cipro) | Levofloxacin<br>Moxifloxacin (Avelox)<br>Ofloxacin<br>Delafloxacin (Baxdela) |

# Use

The major clinical use of gentamicin (most commonly with other antibacterial agents) is empiric therapy for serious infections caused by susceptible aerobic gram-negative organisms. Treatment of infections such as septicemia, respiratory tract infections, urinary tract infections, intra-abdominal infections, and osteomyelitis often involves gentamicin. In pseudomonal infections, patients may receive gentamicin concurrently with an antipseudomonal penicillin (e.g., piperacillin/tazobactam) for synergistic therapeutic effects. The penicillin-induced breakdown of the bacterial cell wall makes it easier for gentamicin to reach its site of action inside the bacterial cell. Researchers have demonstrated decreased mortality from combination antibiotic therapy in treatment of infections due to *Pseudomonas aeruginosa* and other multidrug-resistant gram-negative bacilli. Once a bacterial species has been identified and its susceptibilities to alternate agents are known, aminoglycosides are usually discontinued in favor of less toxic antibiotics in the completion of a treatment course.

Table 19.2 presents dosage information for gentamicin and the other aminoglycosides.

## Use in Children

Caution is necessary when using gentamicin and other aminoglycosides in children. Individualization of the dose is extremely critical because of the low therapeutic index of the drug. Larger individual doses or more frequent dosing intervals may be necessary in certain clinical situations. For instance, in the acute pulmonary exacerbations of cystic fibrosis, optimizing antibiotic dosing can improve the ability of regaining lung function following exacerbations. Initial doses of gentamicin in neonates and children are based on age. Serum levels should be obtained to assess the pharmacokinetic parameters to establish the frequency and dose of subsequent doses. It should be noted that the risk of nephrotoxicity and ototoxicity may be increased in neonates because of their immature renal function.

## Use in Older Adults

As in children, individualized dosing of gentamicin is critical in older adults because of the low therapeutic index of the drug. Decreased renal function, other disease processes, and concurrent drug therapies increase the adverse effects in older adults, specifically aminoglycoside-induced nephrotoxicity and ototoxicity. Monitoring of renal function during treatment with gentamicin, as well as other aminoglycosides, is extremely important. Prolonged therapy (longer than 1 week) increases the risk of toxicity and should be avoided when possible.

## Use in Patients With Renal Impairment

With impaired renal function, a reduction in dosage of aminoglycosides is essential. Gentamicin may accumulate in the serum and tissues of patients being treated with higher doses and for longer periods. Methods of adjusting dosage include lengthening the time between doses or reducing doses. For specific recommendations on adjusting aminoglycoside doses for renal impairment, nurses and other health care practitioners should consult references. In urinary tract infections, smaller doses can be used than in systemic infections because the aminoglycosides reach high concentrations in the urine.

## Use in Patients With Hepatic Impairment

Gentamicin is appropriate for use in patients with hepatic impairment. No adjustment in dosage or frequency is indicated. However, it is necessary to continue to monitor plasma concentrations. Gentamicin should be used with caution in severe hepatic disease, such as cirrhosis, because of the possibility of precipitating hepatorenal syndrome.

## Use in Patients With Critical Illness

Primary uses for gentamicin (in combination with other antibacterial agents) include serious infections caused by aerobic gram-negative bacilli that result in septicemia, nosocomial respiratory infections, complicated urinary tract infections and intra-abdominal infections, and osteomyelitis. Patients should not take gentamicin as monotherapy. Serious infections caused by *Serratia*, *Pseudomonas*, *Citrobacter*, *Acinetobacter*, and *Enterobacter* species warrant its use in combination with piperacillin/tazobactam, cefepime, meropenem, or imipenem–cilastatin. However, once susceptibilities to the identified organism are determined, prescribers usually discontinue aminoglycosides if a less toxic antibiotic may be used to complete the typical course of treatment. Because patients who are critically ill are at high risk for development of nephrotoxicity and ototoxicity with aminoglycosides, it is essential to follow guidelines for safe drug usage strictly.

## Use in Patients Receiving Home Care

Administration of gentamicin does not typically occur in the home setting. However, instruction about IV care is essential for caregivers who are giving this medication at home. Potential for secondary infections is of concern.

# Adverse Effects

Gentamicin and other aminoglycosides result in similar adverse reactions. A **BLACK BOX WARNING ◆** issued by the U.S. Food and Drug Administration (FDA) alerts health care professionals that these drugs are nephrotoxic and ototoxic and must be used very cautiously in the presence of renal impairment.

Nephrotoxicity, a well-known adverse reaction associated with aminoglycoside therapy, occurs more frequently in patients with a history of renal impairment. Extended duration of treatment with gentamicin may also contribute to nephrotoxicity. In most cases, nephrotoxicity is reversible on discontinuation of the drug. Ototoxicity (auditory or vestibular) may develop after extended use and may not be reversible. Dizziness, vertigo, tinnitus, and hearing loss may be signs of ototoxicity and damage to the eighth cranial nerve. Peripheral nephropathy, including numbness, skin tingling, and muscle twitching, also occurs. Therefore, the use of gentamicin in patients with myasthenia gravis and other neuromuscular disorders warrants extreme caution, because increased muscle weakness may occur.

> **! QSEN Alert: Safety**
>
> Aminoglycosides can cause fetal harm when administered to pregnant women. Although serious adverse effects have not been reported for all aminoglycosides, several accounts of irreversible congenial deafness in children whose mothers had taken streptomycin during pregnancy have been documented.

## TABLE 19.2

## DRUGS AT A GLANCE: Aminoglycosides

| Drug | Pregnancy Category | Characteristics | Routes and Dosage Ranges | |
|---|---|---|---|---|
| | | | **Adults** | **Children** |
| **Gentamicin** (Gentamicin Injection) | D | Effective against several gram-negative organisms, although some strains have become resistant<br>Acts synergistically with antipseudomonal penicillins against *P. aeruginosa* and with ampicillin or vancomycin against enterococci | Conventional dosing: IM, IV 1–2.5 mg/kg/dose every 8–24 h depending on renal function ODA dosing: 4–7 mg/kg/dose once daily | *<5 y*: IM, IV 2.5 mg/kg/dose every 8 h<br>*≥5 y*: IM, IV 2–2.5 mg/kg/dose every 8 h |
| Amikacin (Amikin) | D | Retains a broader spectrum of antibacterial activity than other aminoglycosides because it resists degradation by most enzymes that inactivate gentamicin and tobramycin<br>Major clinical use is in infections caused by organisms resistant to other aminoglycosides (e.g., *Pseudomonas, Proteus, E. coli, Klebsiella, Enterobacter, Serratia*), whether community or hospital acquired | IM, IV 15–20 mg/kg every 24 h<br>Renal dosing: 5–7.5 mg/kg/dose every 8–24 h | *Older children*: Same as adults<br>*Neonates*: IM, IV 10 mg/kg initially and then 7.5 mg/kg every 12 h |
| Neomycin | D | Given orally or topically to prepare GI tract for surgery. Although poorly absorbed from the GI tract, toxic levels may accumulate in the presence of renal failure<br>Used topically, often in combination with other drugs, to treat infections of the eye, ear, and skin (burns, wounds, ulcers, dermatoses)<br>When used for wound or bladder irrigations, systemic absorption may occur if the area is large or if drug concentration exceeds 0.1% | PO, suppression of intestinal bacteria (with erythromycin 1 g) 1 g given at 1 PM, 2 PM, and 11 PM the day before an 8 AM surgery; hepatic coma, 4–12 g daily in divided doses every 4–6 h for 5–6 d | |
| Paromomycin (Humatin) | C | Effective in the treatment of acute and chronic intestinal amebiasis | PO: 25–35 mg/kg/d divided every 8 h for 5–10 d | PO: 25–35 mg/kg/d divided every 8 h for 5–10 d |
| Plazomicin (Zemdri) | Not assigned 2018 | Used for the treatment of complicated urinary tract infections and pyelonephritis caused by *Escherichia coli, Klebsiella pneumoniae, Proteus mirabilis*, and *Enterobacter cloacae* in patients who have limited or no other treatment options | IV: 15 mg/kg once daily for 4–7 d infused over 30 min; continue with appropriate oral drug therapy for a combined total of 7–10 d | Has not been evaluated in children |
| Streptomycin (Streptomycin) | D | May be used in a 4- to 6-drug regimen for treatment of multidrug-resistant tuberculosis | IM 15/kg/d or 1–2 g/d | IM 20–40 mg/kg/d in 2 divided doses, every 12 h (maximum dose 1 g/d) |
| Tobramycin (Tobramycin) | D | Similar to gentamicin in antibacterial spectrum, but may be more active against *Pseudomonas* organisms<br>Often used with other antibiotics for septicemia and infections of burn wounds, other soft tissues, bone, the urinary tract, and the central nervous system | Conventional dosing: IM, IV 1–2.5 mg/kg/dose every 8–24 h depending on renal function ODA dosing: 4–7 mg/kg/dose once daily | *<5 y*: IM, IV 2.5 mg/kg/dose every 8 h<br>*≥5 y*: 2–2.5 mg/kg/dose every 8 h |

GI, gastrointestinal; IM, intramuscular; IV, intravenous; ODA, once-daily aminoglycoside.

## Contraindications

Contraindications include a hypersensitivity to aminoglycosides. Prescribers generally reserve aminoglycosides are for infections that have not responded to less toxic drugs.

## Nursing Implications

Dosage of aminoglycosides must be carefully monitored based on serum concentrations. Two major dosing schedules are used: one involving multiple daily doses (conventional dosing) and one involving **extended-interval dosing** (once-daily dosing or once-daily aminoglycosides [ODA]). The use of ODA dosing, unless contraindicated, has replaced the common multiple daily dosing in many people. The ODA method uses higher doses (e.g., 4–7 mg/kg) to produce high initial drug concentrations, with no repeat dosing until the serum concentration is quite low (typically 24 hours later). The rationale for this dosing approach is a potential increase in efficacy with a reduced incidence of nephrotoxicity. Most patients can be successfully treated using ODA. However, ODA is not appropriate for certain people. In general, the following circumstances contraindicate its use: age of 3 months or less and pregnancy or postpartum status. Extended-interval dosing of children older than 3 months may be a reasonable alternative in some situations and in patients in some age groups. The ODA dosing practice evolved from increased knowledge about the **concentration-dependent bactericidal effects** and **postantibiotic effects** of aminoglycosides. Concentration-dependent bactericidal effects mean that a large dose of aminoglycosides, with high peak serum concentrations, kills more microorganisms. Postantibiotic effects mean that aminoglycosides continue killing microorganisms even at low serum concentrations. Monitoring of random level (12-hour) serum evaluation in a single-dosing regimen replaces traditional peak and trough serum monitoring.

With the multiple-dose regimen, a patient receives an initial loading dose, based on patient weight and the desired peak serum concentration, to achieve therapeutic serum concentrations rapidly. If the patient is obese, adjusted body weight should be used because aminoglycosides are not significantly distributed in body fat. In patients with normal renal function, recommended loading doses for selected aminoglycosides are the following:

- Gentamicin: 1 to 2.5 mg/kg
- Tobramycin: 1 to 2.5 mg/kg
- Amikacin: 5 to 7.5 mg/kg

Prescribers adjust dosages according to serum drug levels and creatinine clearance (CrCl). With conventional dosing, it is necessary to take gentamicin peak levels 30 minutes after the end of a 30-minute IV infusion or 1 hour after IM injection. The nurse ensures that trough levels are obtained immediately before the next dose is given. With ODA dosing, it is necessary to obtain a 12-hour random gentamicin level 12 hours after the start of the infusion.

### Preventing Interactions

Many medications interact with gentamicin, increasing or decreasing its effects (Box 19.1). When patients who are taking agents that may lead to nephrotoxicity receive gentamicin,

**BOX 19.1**    **Drug Interactions: Gentamicin**

**Drugs That Increase the Effects of Gentamicin**

- Acyclovir, amphotericin B, carboplatin and cisplatin, cephalosporins, cyclosporine, ganciclovir, pamidronate, salicylates, and vancomycin
  *Increase the risk of nephrotoxicity*
- Arbekacin, loop diuretics
  *Increase the risk of nephrotoxicity and ototoxicity*

**Drugs That Decrease the Effects of Gentamicin**

- Penicillins
  *Decrease serum concentrations*

careful monitoring and caution are necessary. Caution is also warranted when administering diphenhydramine and chlorpheniramine with gentamicin, because gentamicin may mask symptoms of ototoxicity. In addition, ginger may increase the effect of gentamicin by masking these effects. No herbs or foods appear to increase the effect of the drug.

The nurse should not mix penicillins and aminoglycosides in a syringe or IV solution or administer them via a Y-site, because the penicillin inactivates the aminoglycoside. If feasible, dose separation is ideal.

### Administering the Medication

The nurse uses only the IV route of administration if possible, because IM injections may be erratic. If gentamicin is used concomitantly with a penicillin-class agent, it is necessary to administer the penicillin 1 hour before or after the gentamicin infusion. Gentamicin is available in an ophthalmic preparation, and concurrent administration of other ophthalmics should be spaced 10 minutes before or after the gentamicin preparation.

**QSEN Alert: Safety**

The nurse demonstrates consistent practice in administering antibiotics that require peak and trough levels by checking, prior to administration, for the latest values and next order for peak and trough levels. Effective standardized practices help ensure safety and quality and reduce harm to the patient.

### Assessing for Therapeutic Effects

The nurse assesses for response to drug therapy and ensures that signs and symptoms of the infection are resolving. These infections may include septicemia, respiratory tract infections, urinary tract infections, intra-abdominal infections, and osteomyelitis. It is important to observe for return to baseline vital signs and normalization of white blood count. The nurse assesses for absence of local signs of infection.

### Assessing for Adverse Effects

Monitoring of gentamicin serum concentrations is crucial for both effectiveness and the avoidance of toxicity. Serum concentrations should be evaluated when the patient has received three or four doses for a conventional dosing regimen.

Once the desired peak and trough have been achieved, periodic monitoring is necessary.

In addition, monitoring of renal function is essential in aminoglycoside therapy. It is necessary to discontinue treatment if signs of nephrotoxicity occur. In addition, patients with vertigo or tinnitus may demonstrate signs of vestibular injury, and ototoxicity should be a consideration. It is also necessary to discontinue treatment if signs of ototoxicity occur. Other adverse effects to assess for include edema, skin itching, reddening of skin, and possible rash.

### Patient Teaching

Patient teaching guidelines are outlined in Box 19.2.

## Other Drugs in the Class

Of the other aminoglycosides, tobramycin and amikacin are the most frequently administered by IM or IV routes and carry the same risks of ototoxicity and nephrotoxicity as gentamicin. A **BLACK BOX WARNING** ◆ exists for these drugs; neuromuscular blockage and respiratory paralysis have been reported following their use. The aminoglycosides are poorly absorbed from the GI tract. Thus, when given orally, they exert local effects on the GI tract.

In addition, streptomycin, neomycin, plazomicin, and paromomycin are used in specific situations. Specifically, neomycin is given orally to prepare the GI tract for surgery. It is not recommended for use in infants and children. Tobramycin and amikacin, which are most frequently administered by IM or IV routes, are similar to gentamicin against *Pseudomonas* organisms. Amikacin retains a broader spectrum of antibacterial activity because it resists degradation by most enzymes that inactivate gentamicin and tobramycin. Plazomicin (Zemdri) is reserved for use in adults with complicated urinary tract infections, including pyelonephritis due to *E. coli, Klebsiella pneumoniae, Enterobacter cloacae,* and *Proteus mirabilis,* who have limited or no other treatment options. Paromomycin is used in adults and children for the treatment of acute and chronic intestinal amebiasis. The drug acts directly on ameba and has antibacterial activity against normal and pathogenic organisms in the GI tract. Paromomycin interferes with bacterial protein synthesis. Prolonged use may result in fungal or bacterial superinfection, including *Clostridium difficile*-associated diarrhea

and pseudomembranous colitis. The drug is also administered as adjunct therapy in patients with hepatic coma. It should be administered orally with meals.

### NCLEX Success

1. A critically ill patient is receiving gentamicin 1.5 mg/kg intravenously every 8 hours. The patient has recently stopped making urine, and the most recent laboratory results indicate that the patient's creatinine level has risen from a normal value of 0.8 to 3.6 mg/dL. At the next scheduled time for administration of gentamicin, the nurse should

    A. administer half the prescribed dose
    B. hold the gentamicin and notify the provider
    C. administer gentamicin as prescribed
    D. draw a blood sample for testing the gentamicin trough level before the dose and then administer as prescribed

2. A physician writes an order for gentamicin 7 mg/kg intravenously every 24 hours and ampicillin 500 mg intravenously every 6 hours. The patient has a diagnosis of endocarditis. This is not an ideal antibiotic regimen for endocarditis because

    A. it is best to use multiple daily dosing of gentamicin for endocarditis
    B. the addition of gentamicin to ampicillin increases the risk of treatment failure in endocarditis
    C. the appropriate single daily dose of gentamicin is 15 mg/kg once daily
    D. streptomycin is the recommended aminoglycoside for use in endocarditis

## FLUOROQUINOLONES

Fluoroquinolones are synthetic drugs with activity against gram-negative and some gram-positive organisms. **Ciprofloxacin** (Cipro) is the prototype. Newer fluoroquinolones have been developed with a broader spectrum of activity that provides improved coverage of gram-positive organisms and, in one case, anaerobes. Although the oral administration of fluoroquinolones has allowed ambulatory treatment of infections that previously required parenteral therapy and hospitalization, the extensive use of these antibiotics has led to antimicrobial resistance to the drug class.

## Pharmacokinetics

Ciprofloxacin is well absorbed from the upper GI tract, like all quinolones; it achieves 70% bioavailability. Once absorbed, it achieves therapeutic concentrations in most body fluids. With immediate-release ciprofloxacin, concentrations peak in 30 minutes to 2 hours. Ciprofloxacin is partially metabolized in the liver; it forms four metabolites, which have limited activity. Hepatic conversion of ciprofloxacin to active metabolites is 10% to 20% of ciprofloxacin elimination. The kidneys are the main route of elimination, and approximately 30% to 60% of an oral dose is excreted unchanged in the urine. Additional excretion is achieved via the feces.

## Action

Fluoroquinolones are bactericidal agents that cause cell death. Ciprofloxacin acts by interfering with enzymes required for synthesis of bacterial DNA and therefore necessary for bacterial growth and replication.

## Use

Ciprofloxacin is the most potent fluoroquinolone against gram-negative bacteria. Like most fluoroquinolones, it is indicated for various infections caused by aerobic gram-negative and other microorganisms. Fluoroquinolones may be used to treat infections of the respiratory, genitourinary, and GI tracts, as well as infections of the bones, joints, skin, and soft tissues. The Centers for Disease Control and Prevention (CDC) no longer recommends the use of fluoroquinolones for gonococcal disease because resistance to this antimicrobial has developed. The 2015 Sexually Transmitted Diseases Treatment Guidelines, issued by the CDC, recommend dual treatment with ceftriaxone and azithromycin as the only regimen for treatment of gonorrhea. It is necessary to consult the CDC website on sexually transmitted diseases for the most current recommendations regarding gonococcal susceptibility.

Ciprofloxacin has multiple indications and can be used for acute sinusitis, lower respiratory infections, pneumonia, skin and soft tissue infections, prostatitis, and urinary tract infections. The FDA has recommended that use of quinolones be limited to complicated infections in patients for whom there are no alternate treatment options. Currently, ciprofloxacin is also recommended as first-line treatment for suspected *Bacillus anthracis* infections (anthrax) until culture and susceptibility results are available. The drug class also shows promise in the treatment of pulmonary tuberculosis. Table 19.3 presents important information about the fluoroquinolones.

### Use in Children

Ciprofloxacin, and other fluoroquinolones, is not a routinely used first-line therapy in children. However, risk–benefit analysis may indicate that fluoroquinolones are a reasonable alternative in some situations. Some animal studies have demonstrated the development of an arthritic sensation with erosions of the cartilage of the weight-bearing joints, but evidence suggests that this adverse event may not be found in humans. There is developing evidence that in some children, particularly those with cystic fibrosis, the benefit of using quinolones outweighs the small risk of joint toxicity. Ciprofloxacin has been approved for use in children with complicated urinary tract infections and pyelonephritis from *E. coli*. The drug is recommended in children for the prophylaxis and treatment of anthrax exposure.

### Use in Older Adults

Ciprofloxacin use in older adults necessitates close monitoring. Decreased renal function, other disease processes, and concurrent drug therapies increase the risks of adverse effects in older adults. In older adults with normal renal function, fluoroquinolones should be accompanied by an adequate fluid intake and urine output to prevent drug crystals from forming in the urinary tract. In addition, urinary alkalinizing agents should be avoided because drug crystals form more readily in alkaline urine. In older adults with impaired renal function, a common condition in this population, caution and reduced dosages are warranted.

## TABLE 19.3

## DRUGS AT A GLANCE: Fluoroquinolones

| Drug | Pregnancy Category | Characteristics | Routes and Dosage Ranges for Adults |
|---|---|---|---|
| Ⓟ **Ciprofloxacin** (Cipro; ✱ Cipro) | C | Effective in respiratory tract, urinary tract, gastrointestinal tract, and skin and soft tissue infections<br>Used as one of 4–6 drugs in treatment of multidrug-resistant tuberculosis<br>Used to treat anthrax infections | PO 250–750 mg every 12 h<br>UTI/pyelonephritis: extended-release tablets 500 mg–1 g every 24 h<br>IV 200–400 mg every 12 h |
| Delafloxacin (Baxdela) | Not assigned 2017 | Treatment of acute bacterial infections of skin and skin structure | PO 450 mg every 12 h for 5–14 d<br>IV 300 mg every 12 h for 5–14 d |
| Levofloxacin (✱ Levaquin) | C | Indicated for treatment of bronchitis, cystitis, pneumonia, sinusitis, skin and skin structure infections, and pyelonephritis | PO, IV 250–750 mg once daily. Infuse 250–500 mg IV dose slowly over 60 min. Infuse 750 mg IV dose over 90 min |
| Moxifloxacin (Avelox; ✱ Avelox) | C | Indicated for community-acquired pneumonia, sinusitis, bronchitis, skin and soft tissue infections, and intra-abdominal infections | PO, IV 400 mg once daily. Infuse IV dose slowly over 60 min |
| Ofloxacin (✱ Apo-Oflox) | C | See ciprofloxacin, above | PO 200–400 mg every 12 h for 3–10 d |

CDC, Centers for Disease Control and Prevention; UTI, urinary tract infection; IV, intravenous.

### Use in Patients With Renal Impairment

Ciprofloxacin requires a dose adjustment in renal impairment because usual doses may produce high and prolonged serum drug levels. However, even in renal failure, moxifloxacin (Avelox) does not require a dose adjustment. Reported renal effects include azotemia, crystalluria, hematuria, interstitial nephritis, nephropathy, and renal failure. Crystalluria rarely occurs in acidic urine but may occur in alkaline urine. Guidelines for reducing nephrotoxicity include using lower dosages, having longer intervals between doses, receiving adequate hydration, and avoiding substances that alkalinize the urine.

 **QSEN Alert: Evidence-Based Practice**

In December 2018, the U.S. Food and Drug Administration (FDA) issued a warning recommending that fluoroquinolones be avoided in patients with known aortic aneurysms or those with risk factors for aneurysm (Food and Drug Administration, 2018). This warning is based on observational studies suggesting the existence of an association between aortic aneurysm or dissection and systemic use of fluoroquinolones given by mouth or injection. However, the causal link of fluoroquinolones in the development of aortic aneurysms and dissection is unclear. The FDA recommends that fluoroquinolones be prescribed to these patients only when no other treatment options are available. Patients should be instructed to seek immediate medical treatment in an emergency department or by calling 911 for any symptoms associated with aortic aneurysm, including sudden, severe, and constant pain in the stomach, chest, or back.

### Use in Patients With Hepatic Impairment

It appears that dosage adjustment is not necessary in hepatic impairment. However, ciprofloxacin should be used with caution in patients with hepatic disease such as cirrhosis.

### Use in Patients With Critical Illness

Ciprofloxacin is commonly used in the critical care setting because of its broad spectrum of coverage. However, resistance is emerging because of overuse of the fluoroquinolones. The rate of resistance in *P. aeruginosa* is increasing due to the increased use of this drug class. Most resistance to fluoroquinolone activity appears most frequent in methicillin-resistant strains of *P. aeruginosa* and *Staphylococcus aureus*. In the United States, increases in fluoroquinolone resistance with enteric bacteria in the critical care setting are often associated with resistance to other antimicrobials.

Most activity of the fluoroquinolones is against aerobic gram-negative organisms, especially *Enterobacteriaceae*, *Moraxella catarrhalis*, *Haemophilus*, and *Neisseria* species. Levofloxacin and moxifloxacin have increased potency against gram-positive infections, and moxifloxacin has activity against anaerobic organisms. Some fluoroquinolones, including ciprofloxacin, ofloxacin, moxifloxacin, and levofloxacin, provide atypical pneumonia coverage as well.

### Use in Patients Receiving Home Care

Ciprofloxacin is given in the home setting, as are other fluoroquinolones. The drug may be given with food to help minimize GI upset. Patients should space out ciprofloxacin administration 4 to 6 hours with any of the following: antacids, multivitamins, sucralfate, or other products containing calcium, iron, or zinc. Absorption of ciprofloxacin may be impaired when these substances are administered together with ciprofloxacin, resulting in a decreased antibiotic effect. Administration of the oral suspension of ciprofloxacin via feeding tubes should not occur, because the oil-based formulation tends to adhere to the feeding tube. The frequent use of fluoroquinolones in the community setting has contributed to overall resistance to *P. aeruginosa*.

## Adverse Effects

Ciprofloxacin is generally well tolerated. The most frequent adverse effects are GI side effects and include nausea, vomiting, and abdominal discomfort. Some patients experience dizziness and mild headache. Allergic and skin reactions have occurred. Photosensitivity can occur while taking ciprofloxacin with exposure to direct or indirect sunlight, and artificial light or sunlamps may also precipitate photosensitivity reactions. Tendon rupture and tendinitis are serious concerns with the fluoroquinolones.

The FDA has expanded the current **BLACK BOX WARNING ◆** for fluoroquinolones, alerting health professionals not only to the increased disabling risk of tendinitis and tendon rupture but also to the significant risk of peripheral neuropathy, central nervous system and cardiac effects, and dermatologic and hypersensitivity reactions. The risk is greater for people older than 60 years of age; those with heart, kidney, and lung transplants; and those taking corticosteroid medications. Adverse effects can occur up to weeks after beginning fluoroquinolones and may potentially be permanent. Discontinuation of the fluoroquinolone is necessary with the development of adverse effects. In addition, a **BLACK BOX WARNING ◆** exists for fluoroquinolones, including ciprofloxacin, because the drug class may exacerbate muscle weakness in persons with myasthenia gravis; its use should be avoided in patients with this condition. QT interval prolongation may occur, and the degree of severity varies by agent.

## Contraindications

Contraindications include hypersensitivity and concurrent use of tizanidine. Current data have shown that ciprofloxacin crosses the placenta and is found in amniotic fluid and cord blood. Ciprofloxacin is recommended for the prophylaxis and treatment of pregnant women with anthrax exposure. Fluoroquinolones should be used in pregnant women for the treatment of other infections only if safer, effective drug therapy is not available.

## Nursing Implications

### Preventing Interactions

Many medications interact with ciprofloxacin, increasing or decreasing its effects (Box 19.3). Fluoroquinolones have the potential to prolong the QT interval and may increase the risks of torsade de pointes and sudden death. Patients should not receive drugs such as the antidysrhythmic amiodarone,

## BOX 19.3 — Drug Interactions: Ciprofloxacin

**Drugs That Increase the Effects of Ciprofloxacin**

- Fosphenytoin, ivabradine
  *Possibly prolong QT interval*
- Angiotensin-converting enzyme inhibitors, angiotensin II receptor blockers, spironolactone
  *May enhance the dysrhythmogenic effect*
- Probenecid
  *May decrease excretion*

**Drugs That Decrease the Effects of Ciprofloxacin**

- Aluminum-, calcium-, iron-, and magnesium-containing products, sucralfate, quinapril (contains magnesium)
  *Impair absorption*
- Didanosine, quinapril
  *Decrease serum concentrations*

## BOX 19.4 — Herb and Dietary Interactions: Ciprofloxacin

**Herbs and Foods That Alter the Effects of Ciprofloxacin**

- Aluminum-, magnesium-, calcium-, and iron-containing herbs and foods
- Dairy products
- Dong quai
- Enteral feedings
- St. John's wort

which prolong the QT interval, in conjunction with fluoroquinolones. Ciprofloxacin reduces theophylline clearance by 30%. Reportedly, fatal reactions have occurred after concurrent use of ciprofloxacin and theophylline.

Herbs and foods also interact with ciprofloxacin (Box 19.4). Ciprofloxacin can chelate with cations, and drugs containing iron, multivitamins, calcium, magnesium, aluminum salt, and sucralfate may significantly reduce the absorption of ciprofloxacin. Therefore, patients should take oral ciprofloxacin 2 hours before or 6 hours after such agents. Patients should also avoid taking oral ciprofloxacin with dairy products or other calcium-containing foods. In addition, patients should not take didanosine and ciprofloxacin simultaneously. Enteral feedings should be discontinued for 1 to 2 hours prior to and after ciprofloxacin administration; enteral feedings decrease drug absorption by more than 30%.

The nurse should also watch for severe hypoglycemia, which has developed in patients receiving concomitant glyburide and fluoroquinolones, including ciprofloxacin. Although most cases have affected patients with diabetes, severe cases of hyperglycemia have occurred in patients not previously diagnosed with the disease.

### Clinical Application 19.1

- Mr. Louis returns to the clinic for a repeat urine culture and sensitivity on day 7 of antibiotic therapy. What assessment findings, if found by the nurse, indicate that treatment with ciprofloxacin has been successful?

### Administering the Medication

Severe hypersensitivity reactions have occurred with the administration of fluoroquinolones. The nurse should discontinue the antibiotic immediately if skin rash or other signs or symptoms of hypersensitivity occur. To reduce the risk of irritation to the veins causing burning, swelling, and pain, the

nurse administers the IV formulation over 60 minutes through a verified patent IV line. If administration through a nasogastric tube is necessary, the nurse crushes immediate-release tablets and mixes them with water. Enteral feedings reduce the serum concentration of ciprofloxacin, and the nurse gives tube feedings 1 hour before and 2 hours after administering the drug. Patients should take fluoroquinolones, like all antibiotics, for the full prescribed course of treatment to prevent complications.

### Assessing for Therapeutic Effects

Assessing for factors that increase the risk of adverse effects is important, for example, impaired renal function, inadequate fluid intake, concomitant use of multivitamins or antacids, or frequent exposure to sunlight in the usual activities of daily living.

It is not necessary to take drug levels when administering ciprofloxacin or any of the fluoroquinolones. Serum creatinine and blood urea nitrogen (BUN) are recommended values to monitor when administering ciprofloxacin.

### Assessing for Adverse Effects

The nurse assesses adverse effects, such as nausea, diarrhea, vomiting, abdominal pain, headache, increased liver enzymes, and injection site reactions. It may be necessary to stop ciprofloxacin therapy if a harmful effect is severe enough. Any rash warrants careful evaluation, and if a hypersensitivity reaction occurs, the nurse discontinues the drug immediately and notifies the prescriber.

### Patient Teaching

Patient teaching guidelines are outlined in Box 19.5.

## Other Drugs in the Class

Other systemic fluoroquinolones include levofloxacin, moxifloxacin, delafloxacin, and ofloxacin. The mechanism of action, adverse effects profile, and interactions of these agents are similar to those of ciprofloxacin. Differences exist among individual fluoroquinolones with regard to effectiveness in killing various bacterial species. Levofloxacin, moxifloxacin, and ofloxacin are effective in the treatment of community-acquired pneumonia, acute exacerbation of chronic bronchitis, acute bacterial sinusitis, and skin and skin structure infections. Delafloxacin is used for the treatment of acute bacterial skin and skin structure infections. Levofloxacin is also used to treat postexposure inhalational

## BOX 19.5    *Patient Teaching Guidelines for the Fluoroquinolones*

### General Considerations

- Avoid exposure to sunlight during and for several days after taking one of these drugs. Stop taking the drug, and notify the prescribing prescriber if skin burning, redness, swelling, rash, or itching occurs. Sunscreen lotions do not prevent photosensitivity reactions.
- Be very careful if driving or doing other tasks requiring alertness or physical coordination. These drugs may cause dizziness or light-headedness.
- If receiving a fluoroquinolone antibiotic in the home care setting, make sure to administer it at regular intervals.
- Put all needles and syringes in a "sharps" container.

### Self-administration

- Take norfloxacin (Noroxin), levofloxacin solution, and ofloxacin 1 hour before or 2 hours after meals on an empty stomach. Ciprofloxacin (Cipro) may be taken with food to decrease gastrointestinal upset. Levofloxacin tablets and moxifloxacin (Avelox) can be taken with or without regard to meals.
- Drink 2 to 3 quarts of fluid daily if you are able. This helps prevent kidney problems.
- Do not take antacids containing magnesium or aluminum (e.g., Mylanta or Maalox); any products containing iron, magnesium, calcium (e.g., Tums), or zinc (e.g., multivitamins); or sucralfate or buffered didanosine preparations at the same time or for several hours before or after a dose of the fluoroquinolone. (Consult product-specific information for individual drug recommendations.)

---

anthrax and prophylaxis and treatment of plague due to *Yersinia pestis*. Levofloxacin and ofloxacin are useful in the treatment of cystitis and urinary tract infection. Ofloxacin also is prescribed for urethral and cervical gonorrhea, urethritis and cervicitis due to *Chlamydia trachomatis*, and other infections of the urethra and cervix, including pelvic inflammatory disease.

### Clinical Application 19.2

- At the clinic visit, Mr. Louis reports that he is experiencing a moderate amount of ringing in his ears and asks if he has an ear infection. How does the nurse respond?

### Unfolding Patient Stories: Harry Hadley • Part 1

Harry Hadley was diagnosed 3 days ago with cellulitis in his right lower leg caused by a feral cat bite. A wound culture was obtained and oral amoxicillin was started. His infection has worsened, and he is admitted to the hospital for treatment with intravenous vancomycin. Culture results are positive for MRSA. How would the nurse respond when Mr. Hadley questions why he was prescribed the amoxicillin 3 days ago instead of vancomycin? What are the spectra of organism coverage for amoxicillin and vancomycin? What drug resistance concerns should the nurse consider? Describe how the nurse evaluates wound culture and sensitivity findings and how the test determines the most effective anti-infective medication. (Harry Hadley's story continues in Chap. 61.)

Care for Harry and other patients in a realistic virtual environment: **vSim** *for Nursing* (thepoint.lww.com/vSim-Pharm). Practice documenting these patients' care in DocuCare (thepoint.lww.com/DocuCareEHR).

## NCLEX  Success

3. A patient from a nursing home arrives at the emergency department with acute pyelonephritis. The provider prescribes ciprofloxacin 500 mg PO twice daily. The patient has a history of seizures and bradycardia. The nurse should

   A. counsel the patient's caregiver to avoid administering the ciprofloxacin with the patient's anticonvulsant
   B. ask the provider to check blood levels of the patient's anticonvulsant(s) before giving the first dose of ciprofloxacin
   C. call the patient's seizure and dysrhythmia history to the provider's attention and inquire whether another type of antibiotic might be selected
   D. counsel the patient's caregiver to discontinue the ciprofloxacin after the patient's fever is gone

4. A nurse reading a patient's chart notices that the patient is scheduled to receive ciprofloxacin 500 mg PO at 9:00 AM. The medication administration record also indicates that Maalox 30 mL PO and hydrochlorothiazide 25 mg PO are due at 9:00 AM. The nurse should

   A. administer all the medications as scheduled
   B. hold the Maalox until 11:00 AM
   C. ask the provider to discontinue hydrochlorothiazide because of increased risk of ototoxicity
   D. administer the Maalox and ciprofloxacin but hold the hydrochlorothiazide

5. An outpatient has just received a prescription for ciprofloxacin 500 mg PO twice daily for acute bronchitis. The nurse should teach the patient

   A. not to take ciprofloxacin with a meal
   B. to restrict fluid intake to avoid fluid overload
   C. to take ciprofloxacin with an antacid (e.g., Tums) to decrease the chance of stomach upset
   D. to avoid prolonged exposure to sunlight

**THE NURSING PROCESS**

A concept map outlines the nursing process related to drug therapy considerations in this chapter. Additional nursing implications related to the disease process should also be considered in care decisions.

**Assessment**

With aminoglycosides, assess for the presence of factors that predispose the patient to nephrotoxicity or ototoxicity.
- Check laboratory reports of renal function (e.g., serum creatinine, CrCl, BUN) for abnormal values.
- Assess for impairment of balance or hearing, including audiometry reports if available.
- Analyze current medications for drugs that interact with aminoglycosides, increasing the risk of nephrotoxicity or ototoxicity.

With fluoroquinolones, assess for the presence of factors that increase risks of adverse drug effects (e.g., impaired renal function, inadequate fluid intake, concomitant use of multivitamins or antacids, frequent or prolonged exposure to sunlight in usual activities of daily living).
- Assess laboratory tests (e.g., complete blood counts, tests of renal and hepatic function) for abnormal values.

**Outcomes of Therapy**

The patient will
- Receive aminoglycoside dosages that are individualized by age, weight, renal function, and serum drug levels.
- Have serum aminoglycoside levels monitored when indicated.
- Have renal function tests performed regularly during aminoglycoside and fluoroquinolone therapy.
- Receive adequate hydration during aminoglycoside and fluoroquinolone therapy.
- Be regularly monitored for adverse drug effects.

**Nursing Interventions**

- With aminoglycosides, weigh patients accurately (dosage is based on total body weight for nonobese patients and adjusted body weight for obese patients) and monitor laboratory reports of BUN, serum creatinine levels, serum drug levels, and urinalysis for abnormal values.
- Force fluids to at least 2000 to 3000 mL daily if not contraindicated. Keeping the patient well hydrated reduces risks of nephrotoxicity with aminoglycosides and crystalluria with fluoroquinolones.
- Avoid concurrent use of other nephrotoxic drugs when possible.
- Provide appropriate teaching (see Boxes 19.2 and 19.5).

**Evaluation**

- Interview and observe for improvement in the infection being treated.
- Interview and observe for adverse drug effects.

**KEY CONCEPTS**

- The choice of aminoglycoside depends on local susceptibility patterns and specific organisms causing an infection.
- The major clinical use of parenteral aminoglycosides is to treat serious systemic infections caused by susceptible aerobic gram-negative organisms.
- A **BLACK BOX WARNING** ◆ alerts health care professionals that aminoglycosides are nephrotoxic and ototoxic and require very cautious use in the presence of renal impairment.
- A **BLACK BOX WARNING** ◆ reports that aminoglycosides can cause fetal harm when administered to a pregnant woman.
- A **BLACK BOX WARNING** ◆ exists for all aminoglycosides because neuromuscular blockage and respiratory paralysis have been reported following its use.

- Neomycin may be given to suppress intestinal bacteria before bowel surgery and to treat hepatic coma.
- Multiple-dose regimens (conventional dosing) of aminoglycosides must be carefully monitored with evaluation of peak and trough serum levels. Once-daily regimens are monitored with random level (12-hour) serum evaluation.
- Drugs reach higher concentrations in the kidneys and inner ears than in other body tissues; this is a major factor in nephrotoxicity and ototoxicity.
- Fluoroquinolones are associated with hyperglycemia and hypoglycemia, and older patients may be more at risk for these glucose disturbances.

- The FDA has issued a **BLACK BOX WARNING** ◆ for fluoroquinolones, related to concern for exacerbation of muscle weakness in persons with fluoroquinolone use in patients with myasthenia gravis.
- The FDA has expanded a **BLACK BOX WARNING** ◆ for fluoroquinolones, alerting health professionals not only to the increased disabling risk of tendinitis and tendon rupture but also to the significant risk of peripheral neuropathy, central nervous system and cardiac effects, and dermatologic and hypersensitivity reactions.
- Fluoroquinolones should be discontinued immediately if a skin rash or other signs or symptoms of hypersensitivity occur, and the prescriber should be notified.

## CLINICAL REASONING CASE STUDY

**Meet the Patient**

Mr. Sokolov, a 72-year-old retired teacher with a previous history of *P. aeruginosa* pneumonia, presents with difficulty breathing. A chest x-ray shows pneumonia. His white blood cell count is elevated, and he is running a fever. He is admitted to the hospital and started on IV antibiotics—gentamicin (Garamycin) and piperacillin and tazobactam for injection (Zosyn).

- What is the reason for giving an aminoglycoside and an antipseudomonal penicillin in the treatment of serious infections caused by *P. aeruginosa*?
- Why should an aminoglycoside and an antipseudomonal penicillin not be combined in a syringe or IV fluid for administration?
- How would you assess Mr. Sokolov for nephrotoxicity or ototoxicity?
- Which patient assessment findings and laboratory test results need to be monitored regularly for a patient receiving a systemic aminoglycoside?

**Assessing Drug Information**

- Gentamicin (in combination with other antibacterial agents) is primarily used for serious infections caused by aerobic gram-negative bacilli. Gentamicin should not be used as monotherapy for serious infections. Aminoglycosides and antipseudomonal penicillins exhibit synergistic activity when used together.
- It is important not to mix an aminoglycoside and a penicillin in a syringe or IV solution or administer them via a Y-site, because the penicillin inactivates the aminoglycoside. If feasible, dose separation is ideal. With concomitant use of gentamicin and a penicillin-class agent, it is necessary to administer the penicillin 1 hour before or after the gentamicin infusion.

**Nursing Actions**

- Assess Mr. Sokolov for improvement in clinical status related to bacterial infection.
- Monitor renal function and concomitant medications that might exacerbate nephrotoxicity or ototoxicity.
- Observe for adverse effects indicating nephrotoxicity (changes in renal function tests) or ototoxicity (dizziness, vertigo, tinnitus, and hearing loss).
- Monitor renal function for increasing serum blood urea nitrogen (BUN) and creatinine.
- Monitor the aminoglycoside serum concentration once the patient has received three or four doses of a conventional dosing regimen. Periodic monitoring is necessary once desired peak and trough levels are achieved. If the patient is receiving an extended-dosing aminoglycoside regimen, the use of a published nomogram that extrapolates the desired dosing interval from a single specimen can be used. Alternate monitoring can be accomplished with two specimens—one at 60 minutes after the infusion and the second 6 to 12 hours after the first or second dose.

Visit **thePoint**® at **http://thePoint.lww.com/Frandsen12e** for answers to NCLEX Success questions (in Appendix A), answers to Clinical Application Case Studies (in Appendix B), and more!

## REFERENCES AND RESOURCES

Bader, M. S., Loeb, M., & Brooks, A. A. (2017). An update on the management of urinary tract infections in the era of antimicrobial resistance. *Postgraduate Medicine, 129*(2), 242–258, doi: 10.1080/00325481.2017.1246055.

Centers for Disease Control and Prevention. Sexually Transmitted Diseases (STDs) Web site. Retrieved from http://www.cdc.gov/std

Food and Drug Administration. (2018). Fluoroquinolone Antibiotics: Safety Communication—Increased Risk of Ruptures or Tears in the Aorta Blood Vessel in Certain Patients [Posted 12/20/2018]. Retrieved from https://www.fda.gov/Safety/MedWatch/SafetyInformation/SafetyAlertsforHumanMedicalProducts/ucm628960.htm?utm_campaign=FDA%20MedWatch%20-%20Fluoroquinolone%20Antibiotics&utm_medium=email&utm_source=Eloqua. Accessed on May 03, 2019.

Hinkle, J. H., & Cheever, K. H. (2017). *Brunner & Suddarth's textbook of medical-surgical nursing* (14th ed.). Philadelphia, PA: Lippincott Williams & Wilkins.

Karch, A. M. (2019). *Lippincott's pocket guide for nurses.* Philadelphia, PA: Lippincott Williams & Wilkins.

Norris, T. L. (2019). *Porth's pathophysiology: Concepts of altered health states* (10th ed.). Philadelphia, PA: Lippincott Williams & Wilkins.

Schindler, B.D., Buensalido, J. A. L., & Kaatz, G.W. (2017) Fluoroquinolone resistance in bacteria. In: D. Mayers, J. Sobel, M. Ouellette, K. Kaye, & D. Marchaim (Eds.), *Antimicrobial Drug Resistance* (2nd ed., pp. 245–263). Cham, Switzerland: Springer. doi.org/10.1007/978-3-319-46718-4_16.

Stankowicz, M. S., Ibrahim, J., & Brown, D. L. (2015). Once-daily aminoglycoside dosing: An update on current literature. *American Journal of Health-System Pharmacy, 72*(16), 1357–1364.

UpToDate. (2019). *Drug information.* Lexi-Comp, Inc.

Workowski, K. A., & Bolan, G. A. (2015). Centers for Disease Control and Prevention. Sexually transmitted diseases treatment guidelines. *Morbidity and Mortality Weekly Report Recommendations Report, 64,* 1–137.

# Drug Therapy With Tetracyclines, Sulfonamides, and Urinary Antiseptics

## LEARNING OBJECTIVES

*After studying this chapter, you should be able to:*

1. Identify the prototype and describe the characteristics, action, use, adverse effects, contraindications, and nursing implications of the tetracyclines.
2. Identify the prototype and describe the characteristics, action, use, adverse effects, contraindications, and nursing implications of the sulfonamides.
3. Identify the prototype and describe the action, use, adverse effects, contraindications, and nursing implications for the adjuvant urinary antiseptic agents used in the treatment of urinary tract infections.
4. Implement the nursing process in the care of patients being treated with tetracyclines, sulfonamides, or urinary antiseptics.

## CLINICAL APPLICATION CASE STUDY

Karen Parsons is a 19-year-old college student. She comes to the health clinic with complaints of urinary frequency and burning on urination. Her medication history includes ongoing, long-term treatment of acne with a tetracycline. She takes 250 mg of the drug orally daily. The physician diagnoses her with a urinary tract infection and prescribes trimethoprim–sulfamethoxazole (Bactrim) DS (160/800 mg), one tablet orally twice daily for 3 days.

## KEY TERMS

**Antimicrobial resistance:** microbial resistance to drugs once successfully used to destroy microorganisms

**Crystalluria:** presence of crystals in the urine, indicating renal irritation

# INTRODUCTION

This chapter introduces the pharmacologic management of the patient experiencing an infection that is treated with tetracyclines or sulfonamides. These older, broad-spectrum, bacteriostatic drugs are rarely used for systemic infections because of **antimicrobial resistance** and the development of more effective or less toxic drugs. Such resistance occurs when the microbe develops resistance mechanisms to drugs once successfully used to destroy the microorganism. This discussion also introduces the urinary antiseptic agents administered for urinary tract infections (UTIs). Table 20.1 lists the drugs discussed in this chapter. The Drugs at a Glance tables present information about routes of administration and dosage ranges for both prototypes and other related drugs.

# TETRACYCLINES

The tetracyclines are antibiotics, derived from chlortetracycline, that have been used to treat serious, life-threatening infections. The drugs in this class have similar pharmacologic properties. Tetracyclines are effective against both gram-negative and gram-positive microorganisms, but the older drugs are usually not drugs of choice. Like all antibiotic classes, the antimicrobial activities of tetracyclines are subject to both class-specific and intrinsic antibiotic-resistance mechanisms. However, resistant bacteria infrequently inactivate tetracyclines biologically or alter the drugs chemically, as with many other antibiotics. Rather, resistance develops primarily as the result of the bacteria's preventing accumulation of the drug inside the cell. Researchers have made chemical modifications that have resulted in semisynthetic drugs with activity against specific drug-resistant organisms.

Prescribers still order tetracyclines for bacterial infections caused by *Brucella* and *Vibrio cholerae*. The drugs also remain effective against *Rickettsiae*, chlamydia, some Protozoa, spirochetes, and others (see "Use" of tetracyclines). **Tetracycline hydrochloride** is the prototype of this class.

## Pharmacokinetics

Administration of tetracycline is oral, and the stomach absorbs 75% of the medication. Its peak of action is 2 to 4 hours. Tetracycline is widely distributed to the tissues, with 65% of the drug protein bound. It has the ability to cross the placenta and enter breast milk. Elimination of 50% to 60% of the drug occurs in the urine within 72 hours. Its half-life in patients with normal renal function is 8 to 11 hours.

## Action

Tetracycline penetrates microbial cells by passive diffusion and an active transport system. Intracellularly, it binds to the 30S ribosomes and possibly the 50S ribosomes and inhibits microbial protein synthesis. In patients with acne, it suppresses the growth of *Propionibacterium acnes* with sebaceous follicles, reducing the free fatty acid content in the sebum.

## Use

Tetracycline is effective for treating *Mycoplasma*, *Chlamydia*, and *Rickettsia*. Health care providers administer it for the treatment of chronic bronchitis, gonorrhea, and syphilis in patients with a known allergy to penicillin. Combined with other drugs, it may be effective in the eradication of *Helicobacter pylori*, thus reducing the risk of duodenal ulcers. Tetracycline is also useful in treating small animal bites and Lyme disease. In addition, it may be useful as adjunctive therapy for acute intestinal amebiasis and acne vulgaris. Finally, prescribers order tetracycline when penicillin is contraindicated to treat infections caused by *Klebsiella*, *Neisseria gonorrhoeae*, *Treponema pallidum*, *Listeria monocytogenes*, *Clostridium*, *Bacillus anthracis*, *Fusobacterium fusiforme*, and *Actinomyces*.

Table 20.2 provides useful information about tetracycline and related drugs.

### Use in Children

Children younger than 8 years of age should not take tetracyclines (except for doxycycline) because of their effects on

---

### TABLE 20.1

## Drug Therapy With Tetracyclines, Sulfonamides, and Urinary Antiseptics

| Drug Class | Prototype(s) | Other Drugs in the Class |
|---|---|---|
| Tetracyclines | **Tetracycline** (Achromycin V) | Demeclocycline hydrochloride<br>Doxycycline (Vibramycin, Oracea, Monodox)<br>Minocycline hydrochloride (Minocin, Dynacin, Solodyn, Ximino)<br>Eravacycline (Xerava)<br>Omadacycline (Nuzyra)<br>Sarecycline (Seysara)<br>Tigecycline (Tygacil) |
| Sulfonamides | **Trimethoprim–sulfamethoxazole** (Bactrim, Septra, others) | Mafenide acetate (Sulfamylon)<br>Sulfadiazine (Microsulfon)<br>Silver sulfadiazine (Silvadene)<br>Sulfasalazine (Azulfidine) |
| Urinary Antiseptics | **Nitrofurantoin** (Macrobid) | Phenazopyridine hydrochloride (Azo-Standard, Pyridium)<br>Trimethoprim (Primsol, Proloprim) |

**TABLE 20.2**

## DRUGS AT A GLANCE: Tetracyclines

| Drug | Pregnancy Category | Routes and Dosage Ranges | |
|---|---|---|---|
| | | **Adults** | **Children** |
| **Tetracycline hydrochloride** (Achromycin V; ✲ Apo-Tetra, Nu-Tetra) | D | 250–500 mg PO every 6 h | Older than 8 y: 25–50 mg/kg/d PO in four divided doses |
| Demeclocycline hydrochloride (Declomycin) | D | 150 mg PO every 6 h or 300 mg every 12 h | Older than 8 y: 8–12 mg/kg/d PO in two to four divided doses |
| Doxycycline (Vibramycin, Oracea, Monodox; ✲ Apprilon, Vibramycin) | D | 100–200 mg/d PO/IV, in one to two divided doses. | Older than 8 y: weight <45 kg: 2–5 mg/kg/d PO/IV in one to two divided doses (max dose 200 mg/d)<br>Weight ≥45 kg: same as adults |
| Eravacycline (Xerava) | None, approved in 2018 | IV: 1 mg/kg every 12 h for 4–14 d | Not recommended for children |
| Minocycline hydrochloride (Minocin, Dynacin, Solodyn, Ximino; ✲ Dom Minocycline, Sandoz Minocycline) | D | 200 mg PO initially, then 100 mg every 12 h (max dose 400 mg/d)<br>200 mg IV initially, followed by 100 mg every 12 h<br>Acne:<br>45–54 kg: 45 mg PO daily<br>55–77 kg: 65 mg PO daily<br>78–102 kg: 90 mg PO daily<br>103–125 kg: 115 mg PO daily<br>126–136 kg: 135 mg PO daily | Older than 8 y: 4 mg/kg PO initially, then 2 mg/kg every 12 h; 4 mg/kg IV, followed by 2 mg/kg every 12 h (max dose 400 mg/d) |
| Omadacycline (Nuzyra) | None, approved in 2018 | Pneumonia, community-acquired IV: loading dose infuse 200 mg over 60 min or 100 mg over 30 min through a dedicated IV line; in no dedicated line, flush with NS or D5W before and after infusion of drug; maintenance dose: IV: 100 mg once daily or PO 300 mg once daily for 7–14 d<br>Skin and skin structure infections: loading dose infuse 200 mg over 60 min or 100 mg over 30 min through a dedicated IV line; in no dedicated line, flush with NS or D5W before and after infusion of drug or PO 450 mg once daily on days 1 and 2; maintenance dose: IV: 100 mg once daily or PO 300 mg once daily for 7–14 d | Not recommended for children |
| Sarecycline (Seysara) | None, approved in 2018 | Weight-based<br>33–54 kg: PO 60 mg once daily<br>55–84 kg: PO 100 mg once daily<br>85–136 kg: PO 150 mg once daily | ≥9 y: same as adults |
| Tigecycline (Tygacil; ✲ Tygacil) | D | Community-acquired pneumonia: IV 100 mg initially; 50 mg maintenance dose every 12 h for 7–14 d<br>Intra-abdominal infections: IV 100 mg initially; 50 mg maintenance dose every 12 h for 5–14 d<br>Skin and skin structure infections: IV 100 mg initially; 50 mg maintenance dose every 12 h for 5–14 d | 8–11 y: IV 1.2–2.0 mg/kg/dose every 2 h up to 50 mg/dose<br>≥12 y: IV 50 mg every 12 h |

*Children > 8 yo* (handwritten annotation)

teeth and bones. In teeth, the drugs interfere with enamel development and may cause a permanent yellow, gray, or brown discoloration. In bone, the drugs form a stable compound in bone-forming tissue and may interfere with bone growth.

### Use in Older Adults

A major concern with the use of tetracyclines is renal impairment, which commonly occurs in older adults. It is also necessary to monitor hepatic function in elderly patients during the administration of these drugs.

### Use in Patients With Renal Impairment

Patients with renal impairment should not take tetracyclines. High concentrations of these drugs inhibit protein synthesis in human cells. This antianabolic effect increases tissue breakdown (catabolism) and the amount of waste products to be excreted by the kidneys. Normally functioning kidneys can handle the increased workload, but when renal function is impaired, the body retains these waste products. This leads to azotemia, increased blood urea nitrogen (BUN), hyperphosphatemia, hyperkalemia, and acidosis. If a tetracycline is necessary because of an organism's sensitivity or a patient's inability to take other antimicrobial drugs, administration of doxycycline or minocycline is necessary.

### Use in Patients With Hepatic Impairment

The development of hepatotoxicity is rare, but caution is warranted when the medication is administered to patients with known hepatotoxicity. Tetracycline is generally contraindicated in pregnancy because it may cause fatal hepatic necrosis in the mother (as well as interfere with bone and tooth development in the fetus). However, there are some disorders where the benefit to the mother may outweigh the risk of hepatic dysfunction; these include rickettsial infections, ehrlichiosis, inhalational anthrax, and malaria.

## Adverse Effects

Several adverse effects may occur following the administration of tetracycline. These include the following:

- Hypersensitivity such as rash, urticaria, serum sickness, or anaphylaxis. Maculopapular and erythematous rashes may also occur.
- Central nervous system (CNS) conditions such as intracranial hypertension (most severe CNS effect).
- Gastrointestinal (GI) conditions such as flatulence, diarrhea, nausea, vomiting, and epigastric distress (commonly reported). Esophagitis, pancreatitis, and staphylococcal enterocolitis may also occur.
- Superinfections:
  - Candidal: sore throat; white patches on the oral mucosa; or a black, furry tongue
  - GI: pseudomembranous colitis
- Other conditions such as increased pigmentation, photosensitivity reactions, azotemia, renal and hepatic toxicity, as well as retardation of bone growth. Discoloration of the teeth and enamel hypoplasia may occur in children younger than 8 years of age.

## Contraindications

Contraindications to tetracycline include renal failure and known hypersensitivity to the drug. Other contraindications are young age (less than 8 years) and pregnancy; as previously stated, the drug causes permanent discoloration of teeth, defects in tooth enamel, and retardation of bone growth. Women who are breast-feeding should not take the drug because they secrete it into their breast milk. Possible hepatotoxicity may also be a problem.

## Nursing Implications

### Preventing Interactions

Many medications interact with tetracycline hydrochloride, increasing or decreasing its effects (Box 20.1). Tetracycline also affects the action of several drugs. Administering oral anticoagulants with tetracycline enhances the effect of vitamin K. Digoxin combined with tetracycline leads to increased digoxin absorption, resulting in digoxin toxicity. Giving penicillins with tetracycline interferes with the bactericidal effects of the penicillins. The combination of oral contraceptives and tetracycline results in diminished contraceptive effects. Some women need to use an additional form of birth control.

Foods that affect the action of tetracycline include dairy products, which decrease the absorption of the antibiotic.

### Administering the Medication

It is important to obtain a culture and sensitivity prior to beginning therapy with tetracycline. Administration of the drug is oral. The medication is most effective when taken on an empty stomach. Patients should take the medication 1 hour before meals or 2 hours after meals. It is important not to take it with dairy products, antacids, or iron supplements. The combination of tetracycline with metallic ions such as aluminum, calcium, iron, or magnesium inhibits tetracycline absorption. If the patient has consumed dairy products or antacids, it is necessary to withhold tetracycline for 2 hours.

**QSEN Alert: Safety**

Tetracycline should never be used after the expiration date. The administration of outdated tetracycline causes severe kidney damage.

**BOX 20.1** **Drug Interactions: Tetracycline**

**Drugs that Increase the Effects of Tetracycline**
- Methoxyflurane
  *Increases the risk of nephrotoxicity*

**Drugs that Decrease the Effects of Tetracycline**
- Aluminum, antacids, bismuth subsalicylate, didanosine, ferrous sulfate, calcium, kaolin, laxatives, magnesium, pectin, zinc
  *Decrease antibiotic absorption*

## Assessing for Therapeutic Effects

The nurse assesses for decreased signs and symptoms of the infection for which the medication is being administered. He or she checks for decreased pain and fever.

## Assessing for Adverse Effects

The nurse assesses for GI irritation, nausea, epigastric distress, diarrhea, and vomiting. He or she also assesses for rash, anaphylaxis, and serum sickness. If a patient is exposed to sunlight, it is necessary to assess for sunburn or photosensitivity reactions. In addition, the nurse checks the patient's complete blood count for anemia and signs and symptoms of superinfection.

## Patient Teaching

Box 20.2 identifies patient teaching guidelines for tetracycline.

# Other Drugs in the Class

Demeclocycline hydrochloride is useful in the treatment of bacterial infections such as acne, pertussis, and UTIs caused by gram-positive or gram-negative organisms. An unlabeled use is for the treatment of chronic syndrome of inappropriate secretion of antidiuretic hormone. When administering demeclocycline, it is important to monitor the patient's BUN. Increases in the BUN are secondary to antianabolic effects. Demeclocycline is the tetracycline most likely to cause photosensitivity.

Doxycycline (Vibramycin), one of the most active tetracyclines, is used most often clinically because it possesses advantages over traditional tetracyclines and minocycline. The drug is less likely to cause photosensitivity and causes less tooth discoloration and bony growth retardation (it binds calcium to a lesser extent than tetracycline); thus, it is the only tetracycline recommended for use in children younger than 8 years of age. Also,

doxycycline is one of the drugs (along with ciprofloxacin; see Chap. 19) recommended by the Centers for Disease Control and Prevention (CDC) for the treatment of *B. anthracis* (anthrax). People with inhalational anthrax should receive a multidrug regimen of either doxycycline or ciprofloxacin concurrently with at least one more recommended drug for 60 days following exposure. After susceptibility testing and clinical improvement, the regimen may be altered. The drug is also useful for infections with *Chlamydia trachomatis* and in respiratory tract infections due to *Mycoplasma pneumoniae*. In addition, doxycycline is effective in treating gonorrhea in patients who are allergic to penicillin. The oral form of doxycycline, which is well absorbed in the GI tract, reaches serum levels equivalent to those obtained with parenteral administration. It is highly lipid soluble, reaching therapeutic levels in the cerebrospinal fluid, eye, and prostate gland. It can be administered in smaller doses and less frequently than other tetracyclines because of its long serum half-life of 18 hours. Excretion occurs in the kidneys; however, authorities consider the drug safe for patients with impaired renal function. Doxycycline is incompatible with allopurinol, barbiturates, erythromycin lactobionate, heparin, meropenem, nafcillin, penicillin, piperacillin, sulfonamides, and riboflavin.

Parenteral administration of doxycycline requires mixing with lactated Ringer's or dextrose 5% and lactated Ringer's. Slow infusion is necessary. The minimum infusion period is 1 hour. Complete infusion should occur in 12 hours.

Eravacycline (Xerava), an intravenous agent, has shown promise in the treatment of serious infections caused by a broad range of aerobic and anaerobic gram-negative and gram-positive bacteria. It is approved for use in the treatment of complicated intra-abdominal infections caused by *S. aureus*, *Escherichia coli*, *Klebsiella pneumoniae*, *Klebsiella oxytoca*, *Enterococcus faecalis*, *Enterococcus faecium*, and others, even in patients with infections caused by extended-spectrum beta-lactamase–producing organisms. However, the drug is not indicated for the treatment of complicated UTIs in adults.

Minocycline hydrochloride (Minocin) is a semisynthetic tetracycline derivative used to treat a variety of bacterial infections, including UTIs, respiratory infections, skin infections, and severe acne. The drug is also useful in the treatment of rickettsial infections and as an adjunct to amebicides in the management of acute intestinal amebiasis. Oral absorption is good; foods and fluids affect absorption of minocycline less than other tetracyclines. Distribution in most body fluids and tissues is extensive, but penetration to the CNS is poor. From 55% to 96% of the drug is protein bound, and metabolism occurs in the liver. Excretion takes place in the urine and feces.

Intravenous (IV) administration of minocycline requires slow infusion. Prolonged IV administration of minocycline may be associated with thrombophlebitis. The drug is stable in all IV solutions but is incompatible with calcium-containing solutions.

Omadacycline (Nuzyra), which is available both orally and intravenously, has been successful in the treatment of community-acquired pneumonia and bacterial skin and skin structure infections. Susceptible bacteria include methicillin-resistant *Staphylococcus aureus* (MRSA), vancomycin-resistant *Enterococci*, penicillin-resistant *S. pneumoniae*, *Haemophilus influenzae*, and *E. coli*.

Sarecycline (Seysara) is used to treat acne vulgaris in patients who are at least 9 years of age. The drug is similar to

---

**BOX 20.2**  *Patient Teaching Guidelines for Tetracycline*

- Take tetracycline around the clock because it inhibits bacteria rather than kill the bacteria.
- Avoid sunlamps, tanning beds, and intense or prolonged exposure to sunlight.
- Wear sunscreen and protective clothing when in the sun.
- Report severe nausea, vomiting, diarrhea, skin rash, or perineal itching to your health care provider. These symptoms may indicate a need to change or stop the drug.
- Take the drug on an empty stomach, at least 1 hour before or 2 hours after meals.
- Do not take the drug with or within 2 hours of taking dairy products, antacids, or iron supplements.
- If you must take an antacid, take it at least 2 hours before or 4 hours after tetracycline.
- Take each dose with 8 oz of water.
- If you are taking an oral contraceptive, use another form of birth control for the duration of therapy. The effectiveness of oral contraceptives is decreased when combined with tetracycline.
- Never take outdated tetracycline due to the risk of severe reactions.

tetracycline in terms of adverse-effect profile. It can be administered without regard to food but should be taken with adequate fluids to reduce the risk of esophageal irritation and ulceration. In addition, it should not be given at the same time as any iron-containing preparations (i.e., aluminum, calcium, or magnesium antacids).

Tigecycline (Tygacil), an intravenous tetracycline, is derived from minocycline and is administered intravenously. The drug is useful in the treatment of community-acquired bacterial pneumonia, complicated skin and skin structure infections, and complicated intra-abdominal infections. Because tigecycline is not affected by the two major mechanisms of tetracycline resistance, it may have activity against tetracycline-resistant organisms. The drug has a broad spectrum of coverage and has bacteriostatic activity against many gram-positive pathogens including MRSA, vancomycin-resistant *Enterococcus,* and penicillin-resistant *Streptococcus pneumoniae*; some gram-negative organisms (important exceptions are *Proteus*, *Pseudomonas*, *Providencia*, and *Morganella* species); anaerobes; and atypical species. The U.S. Food and Drug Administration (FDA) has issued a **BLACK BOX WARNING ◆** because of the increased risk of mortality in patients treated with tigecycline compared with other drugs used to treat serious infections.

## Clinical Application 20.1

A nurse at the college health center is interviewing Ms. Parsons about her recent health history, and the nurse inquires about her sexual activity. Ms. Parsons replies that she has a new boyfriend with whom she has had sexual intercourse every day for the past 5 days. She says she is taking oral contraceptives. The nurse also gathers information regarding Ms. Parsons's sunbathing practices (the college is on the Gulf Coast). Ms. Parsons reports that she has been going to the beach daily.

- Based on the information gathered in the interview regarding the fact Ms. Parsons is sexually active, what should the nurse instruct her about related to the tetracycline she is taking?
- What teaching should the nurse at the health center provide related to the administration of tetracycline?
- Based on the fact that Ms. Parsons has been going to the beach daily, what is she at risk for developing?

## NCLEX Success

1. A patient is admitted to the emergency department following opening an envelope containing a substance that experts have identified as anthrax. Which of the following medications is likely to be administered?

   A. tetracycline
   B. doxycycline
   C. amoxicillin–clavulanic acid combination
   D. neomycin

2. A patient receiving tetracycline should receive the following instruction regarding the medication?

   A. Take tetracycline with food.
   B. Take tetracycline in combination with antacids.
   C. Take the first dose and then obtain a test known as culture and sensitivity.
   D. Take tetracycline with a full glass of water.

3. Which of the following foods should not be taken with tetracycline?

   A. orange juice with calcium
   B. cranberry juice cocktail
   C. tomato juice
   D. lemonade

4. A man is receiving treatment for a *Mycoplasma pneumoniae* infection. He says that drinking orange juice hurts his mouth. What priority assessment should the nurse make?

   A. Assess the patient's fecal output for signs and symptoms of diarrhea.
   B. Assess the patient's mouth for signs of candidal infection.
   C. Assess the patient's lung sounds for rales or rhonchi.
   D. Assess the patient's intake and output.

5. Which laboratory value should the nurse assess in patients who are receiving demeclocycline?

   A. blood urea nitrogen
   B. aspartate aminotransferase
   C. alanine aminotransferase
   D. creatinine

## SULFONAMIDES

Sulfonamides are bacteriostatic drugs that were once effective against a wide range of gram-positive and gram-negative bacteria. However, increasing resistance is making them less useful. It is important to document susceptibility with culture and sensitivity testing, but sulfonamides may be active against *Streptococcus pyogenes*, some staphylococcal strains, *H. influenzae*, *Nocardia*, *C. trachomatis*, and toxoplasmosis. The **trimethoprim–sulfamethoxazole** (TMP-SMZ) combination (Bactrim, Septra) is useful in UTIs due to *Enterobacteriaceae* and *Pneumocystis jirovecii* infection (in high doses), and it serves as the prototype. The combination of drugs demonstrates synergistic antimicrobial activity that is greater than the dose of either drug used alone. Other drugs in the class vary in extent of systemic absorption and clinical indications. Some sulfonamides are well absorbed and can be used in systemic infections; others are poorly absorbed and have more local effects. Table 20.3 summarizes key information about sulfonamides.

## Pharmacokinetics

TMP-SMZ is rapidly and nearly completely absorbed in the GI tract, and the half-life of the medication is 6 to 11 hours. It enters the extracellular spaces, crosses the placental and

## TABLE 20.3

## DRUGS AT A GLANCE: Sulfonamides

| Drug | Pregnancy Category | Routes and Dosage Ranges | |
|---|---|---|---|
| | | **Adults** | **Children** |
| **Trimethoprim–sulfamethoxazole** (Bactrim, Septra, others; ✦Apo-Sulfatrim) | C | UTI: one double-strength tablet PO twice daily for 3 d | UTI and otitis media: PO 8-mg/kg trimethoprim and 40-mg/kg sulfamethoxazole in two divided doses every 12 h for 10 d |
| Mafenide acetate (Sulfamylon) | C | Topical application to burned area, once or twice daily, in a thin layer | Same as adults |
| Sulfadiazine (Microsulfon) | C; D (last trimester) | 2–8 g PO daily in divided doses every 6 h | >2 y 100–200 mg/kg/d PO in divided doses every 6 h<br>Neonate: 50 mg/kg every 12 h for 12 mo |
| Silver sulfadiazine (Silvadene; ✦Dermazine, Flamazine) | B | Cover burned area with cream one to two times daily | Same as adults |
| Sulfasalazine (Azulfidine; ✦PMS-Sulfasalazine, Salazopyrin) | B | Ulcerative colitis: 3–4 g PO daily in four divided doses initially; 2 g daily in divided doses for maintenance; max dose, 4 g<br>Rheumatoid arthritis: maintenance, 2 g PO daily in divided doses, every 12 h | 30–60 mg/kg/d PO in two to six divided doses initially, followed by 30 mg/kg/d in four divided doses; max daily dose, 2 g |
| Combination drug in which the dosage is based on trimethoprim component | D (last trimester) | Shigellosis: same dose as above for 5 d<br>Severe UTI: IV 8–10 mg (trimethoprim component)/kg/d in two to four divided doses, up to 14 d<br>*P. jirovecii* pneumonia: IV 15–20 mg (trimethoprim component)/kg/d in three or four divided doses, every 6–8 h up to 21 d; IV doses should be given over 60–90 min | Shigellosis: same dose as above for 5 d<br>Severe UTI: IV 8–10 mg (trimethoprim component)/kg in two to four divided doses, every 6–8 h or every 12 h, up to 14 d<br>*P. jirovecii* pneumonia: IV 15–20 mg (trimethoprim component)/kg/d in three or four divided doses, every 6–8 h up to 21 d |

blood–brain barriers, and appears in small amounts in breast milk. Metabolism occurs in the liver, and excretion takes place in the kidneys as metabolites and unchanged drug.

## Action

TMP-SMZ and other sulfonamides act as antimetabolites of para-aminobenzoic acid (PABA), which microorganisms require to produce folic acid. In turn, folic acid is necessary for the production of bacterial intracellular proteins. Sulfonamides enter into the reaction instead of PABA, compete for the enzyme involved, and cause formation of nonfunctional derivatives of folic acid. Thus, sulfonamides halt multiplication of new bacteria but do not kill mature, fully formed bacteria. With the exception of the topical sulfonamides used in burn therapy, the presence of pus, serum, or necrotic tissue interferes with sulfonamide action because these materials contain PABA. Some bacteria can change their metabolic pathways to use precursors or other forms of folic acid and thereby develop resistance to the antibacterial action of sulfonamides. After resistance to one sulfonamide develops, cross-resistance to others is common.

## Use

TMP-SMZ acts by inhibiting bacterial synthesis of essential nucleic acids and proteins. Uses include the treatment of *P. jirovecii* pneumonitis, severe UTIs, *Shigella enteritis*, and *Enterobacteriaceae*. Other organisms treated with TMP-SMZ are *Viridans streptococcus*, *Staphylococcus epidermidis*, *Salmonella*, *Klebsiella*, *Nocardia*, and *Pseudomonas*.

 **QSEN Alert: Evidence-Based Practice**

With increasing rates of MRSA in both health care environments and the community, TMP-SMZ has been suggested as a treatment option. However, drug is currently not recommended for the treatment of bacteremia or pneumonia caused by MRSA.

Paul and colleagues (2015) completed a randomized control trial to assess the effectiveness of TMP-SMZ for the treatment of staphylococcal infections. Hospitalized adults with severe MRSA infections (252) were randomly placed in two groups, one that received TMP-SMZ to treat the MRSA infection and one that received vancomycin, the current standard treatment of MRSA. Researchers assessed patient outcomes, including clinical treatment failure or persistent bacteremia at day 7, persistence of fever, persistence of hypotension, and non-improving Sequential Organ Failure Assessment score. They also identified a primary safety outcome of all-cause mortality at 30 days. Findings indicated that TMP-SMZ was not a valuable alternative for the treatment of MRSA infections compared to vancomycin. The difference was particularly marked for patients with bacteremia. Adverse event rates were similar for TMP-SMZ and vancomycin. The authors concluded that TMP-SMZ should not be used for the treatment of severe MRSA infections but that further research is necessary because these findings are inconsistent with other studies.

### Use in Children

Children younger than 2 months of age should not receive TMP-SMZ and other systemic sulfonamides. If a fetus or young infant receives a sulfonamide by placental transfer, in breast milk, or by direct administration, the drug displaces bilirubin from binding sites on albumin. As a result, bilirubin may accumulate in the bloodstream (hyperbilirubinemia) and CNS (kernicterus), resulting in life-threatening toxicity.

### Use in Older Adults

TMP-SMZ may cause renal impairment. Therefore, when administering the drug to older adults, it is important to assess the patient's renal function. Older people are also at greater risk of hyperkalemia due to the effects of aging on renal function.

### Use in Patients With Renal Impairment

Patients with renal impairment should probably avoid taking TMP-SMZ and other systemic sulfonamides if other effective drugs are available. Acute renal failure has occurred when the drugs or their metabolites precipitated in renal tubules and caused obstruction. Preventive measures include intake of 1.5 to 3 L of fluid daily to reduce the formation of crystals and stones in the urinary tract.

### Use in Patients With Hepatic Impairment

Metabolism of TMP-SMZ occurs in the liver. Thus, patients with altered liver function should be given with caution.

## Adverse Effects

TMP-SMZ has several adverse effects. These include the following:

- GI effects: abdominal pain, nausea, vomiting, diarrhea, anorexia, and pancreatitis
- Hematologic effects: aplastic anemia, agranulocytosis, eosinophilia, thrombocytopenia, and leukopenia
- Dermatologic effects: pruritus, urticaria, Stevens-Johnson syndrome, and skin photosensitivity
- Renal effects: increased BUN and serum creatinine, renal failure, and interstitial nephritis

## Contraindications

Contraindications include a known hypersensitivity to any sulfa drug, trimethoprim, TMP-SMZ, or any other of the sulfonamides, salicylates, or megaloblastic anemia related to folate

deficiency. The drug is also contraindicated in infants less than 2 months of age.

## Nursing Implications

Culture and sensitivity testing should be completed prior to administering the drug. When administering TMP-SMZ, it is important to monitor potassium level as hyperkalemia may result particularly in the older adult and individuals with renal impairment or hypoaldosteronism. The drug should be discontinued at the first sign of a rash.

### Preventing Interactions

Trimethoprim and sulfamethoxazole both inhibit specific cytochrome P450 enzymes, leading to concurrent multiple drug and herb interactions, increasing or decreasing the effects of TMP-SMZ (Boxes 20.3 and 20.4). The drug inhibits warfarin metabolism and is associated with a threefold increased risk of GI bleeding when compared with other antibiotics. Other interactions include sulfonylureas (hypoglycemia), anticonvulsants (toxicity), and methotrexate (pancytopenia).

### Administering the Medication

In general, TMP-SMZ is commonly administered orally, with or without food. It is important to take it with a full glass of water. In patients with severe pneumonia caused by *P. jirovecii*, the drug is administered parenterally.

---

> **(!) QSEN Alert: Safety**
>
> When administering TMP-SMZ parenterally, it is important that the medication be diluted and administered over 60 to 90 minutes. The drug has variable stability in normal saline. The drug should not be administered intramuscularly.

---

**BOX 20.3**  *Drug Interactions: TMP-SMZ*

**Drugs that Increase the Effects of TMP-SMZ**

- Alkalinizing agents such as sodium bicarbonate
  *Increase the rate of urinary excretion, raising the levels of sulfonamides in the urinary tract and increasing effectiveness in urinary tract infections*
- Methenamine compounds such as urinary acidifiers
  *Increase the risk of nephrotoxicity*
- Salicylates, nonsteroidal anti-inflammatory agents, oral anticoagulants, phenytoin, methotrexate
  *Increase the risk of nephrotoxicity by displacing sulfonamides from plasma protein binding sites*
- Sulfonylureas
  *Increase hypoglycemic reactions*

---

**BOX 20.4**  *Herb and Dietary Interactions: TMP-SMZ*

**Herbs and Foods that Increase the Effects of TMP-SMZ**

- Garlic, ginseng, ginger, St. John's wort

It is essential that the parenteral TMP-SMZ drug combination not be mixed with other drugs and that IV lines be flushed to remove any residual drug prior to administration.

### Assessing for Therapeutic Effects

If the patient is taking TMP-SMZ for treatment of a UTI, the nurse assesses for decreased symptoms of this infection, such as the elimination of pain when voiding, cloudy urine, and fever. If the patient is taking TMP-SMZ for treatment of *Pneumocystis* pneumonia, it is necessary to assess for resolution of symptoms including nonproductive cough, shortness of breath, or fever. If the drug is given for prophylaxis of pneumocystosis, the nurse observes for development of symptoms.

### Assessing for Adverse Effects

The nurse assesses the patient's intake and output. If the intake is greater than the output, assessment of renal function is necessary. The nurse also assesses for hyperkalemia, anemia, and changes in the complete blood count that are indicative of blood dyscrasias. In addition, it is necessary to assess for signs and symptoms of superinfection or hypersensitivity reactions. Septra, an IV form of TMP-SMZ, contains sodium metabisulfite, which has the potential to produce allergic reactions in some patients. It is necessary to assess for hives, skin redness, itching, wheezing, shortness of breath, and possible anaphylaxis.

### Patient Teaching

Box 20.5 identifies patient teaching guidelines for TMP-SMZ.

## Other Drugs in the Class

Mafenide (Sulfamylon) is a topical anti-infective agent administered for bacteriostatic treatment of gram-negative and gram-positive organisms such as *Pseudomonas aeruginosa* and other anaerobes that may be associated with second- and third-degree burns. Topical application with sterile gloved hands follows cleansing of the burn site. The drug is absorbed rapidly, reaching its peak in 2 to 4 hours. It is inactivated in the blood to a weak carbonic anhydrase inhibitor and eliminated by the kidneys. Close monitoring of the patient's fluid and electrolyte status is necessary. Metabolic acidosis is a possibility. The nurse attempts to assess for signs and symptoms of allergic reaction; however, it is difficult to determine whether the reaction is due to allergy or severe burns.

Sulfadiazine (Microsulfon) is a short-acting sulfonamide that interferes with bacterial utilization of PABA. It inhibits folic acid biosynthesis that is required for the bacteria's growth. It is used in combination with pyrimethamine for the treatment of cerebral toxoplasmosis and chloroquine-resistant malaria. When this medication is used, it is imperative that the patient maintains a fluid intake that allows for an output of 1500 mL of urine in 24 hours. Combination with pyrimethamine decreases the development of **crystalluria** (precipitation of drug crystals in the urine) and stone formation. It is important to instruct the patient to consume fluids liberally and report any symptoms of blood dyscrasias, such as pallor, fever, or sore throat.

Silver sulfadiazine (Silvadene), a silver salt, has bactericidal effects on the bacterial cell wall and cell membrane that inhibit folic acid synthesis. It has antimicrobial activity against bacteria and yeast. This medication is indicated for the treatment of second- and third-degree burns. It is effective against *Pseudomonas, E. coli, Klebsiella, Proteus, Staphylococcus,* and *Streptococcus.* Topical application with sterile gloved hands one to two times per day follows cleansing of the burn site in a whirlpool bath or spot cleansing. With large burn areas and prolonged use, patients may absorb significant amounts of silver sulfadiazine systemically. It is necessary to monitor for adverse effects of sulfonamides. Contraindications include pregnancy and age less than 1 month.

Sulfasalazine (Azulfidine) is used for ulcerative colitis and rheumatoid arthritis. The bacteriostatic action of the medication occurs in the intestine, where the intestinal flora converts the drug to two metabolites, one of which acts as an anti-inflammatory agent. It reduces *Clostridium* and *E. coli* in the stools. Sulfasalazine is contraindicated in patients who have an allergy to salicylates. The nurse instructs patients that taking this drug may make their urine yellow-orange.

---

**BOX 20.5**  **Patient Teaching Guidelines for TMP-SMZ**

- Take TMP-SMZ with 8 oz of water.
- Take the drug before or after meals.
- Drink a minimum of 2 to 3 L of fluid per day.
- The effectiveness of oral contraceptives is decreased when combined with TMP-SMZ.
- Avoid sunlamps, tanning beds, and intense or prolonged exposure to sunlight.
- When in the sun, wear sunscreen and protective clothing.
- Do not take any over-the-counter medications without the prescriber's knowledge.
- Inform your dentist or prescriber that you are taking a sulfonamide. Changes in laboratory values may occur as a result of taking the drug.
- If you have diabetes, be sure to monitor your blood sugar values. Reduced blood sugar levels can occur.

---

### Clinical Application 20.2

- What aspects of patient teaching should the nurse at the college health center provide to Ms. Parsons regarding the administration of sulfamethoxazole and trimethoprim?
- The nurse should tell Ms. Parsons about which adverse effects?

### NCLEX Success

6. A woman develops a urinary tract infection following the delivery of an infant. The nurse practitioner is considering prescribing trimethoprim–sulfamethoxazole. What assessment is necessary to make?

   A. if the woman is breast-feeding
   B. if the woman has been treated with the medication in the past
   C. if anyone in her family has a known allergy to the drug
   D. if she is experiencing hematuria

7. When administering a sulfonamide, which of the following interventions is most effective in decreasing crystalluria?

    A. administering 8 oz of cranberry juice
    B. providing a full liquid diet during the course of drug therapy
    C. inserting a Foley catheter for the measurement of an accurate intake and output
    D. providing a minimum of 1500 mL of fluid per day

8. A physician has ordered trimethoprim-sulfamethoxazole (TMP-SMZ) for a woman with a urinary tract infection. The nurse has asked the patient about whether she takes any over-the-counter medications. The patient reports that she regularly takes St. John's wort as a mood elevator. Which of the following patient teaching interventions is most important?

    A. Taking St. John's wort and TMP-SMZ results in no known interactions.
    B. TMP-SMZ combined with St. John's wort leads to an increased therapeutic effect of the TMP-SMZ.
    C. TMP-SMZ has a decreased effect when given with St. John's wort.
    D. When given in combination, TMP-SMZ and St. John's wort result in manic tendencies.

9. A nurse is applying silver sulfadiazine (Silvadene) to a child's burns. Which of the following nursing interventions is most important when applying the medication?

    A. providing pain medication
    B. using sterile gloves
    C. giving the child a bath
    D. teaching the parent to apply the medication

10. A physician has ordered intravenous sulfamethoxazole with trimethoprim. How should the nurse administer the medication?

    A. in 500 mL of 0.45% normal saline
    B. in 150 mL of 10% dextrose and water
    C. in 125 mL of 5% dextrose and water
    D. in 125 mL of 5% dextrose and 0.45% normal saline

# ADJUVANT MEDICATIONS USED TO TREAT URINARY TRACT INFECTIONS: URINARY ANTISEPTICS

The adjuvant medications used to treat UTIs are trimethoprim and the urinary antiseptic agents. Urinary antiseptics may be bactericidal for sensitive organisms in the urinary tract because these drugs are concentrated in renal tubules and reach high levels in urine. They are not used in systemic infections because they do not attain therapeutic plasma levels. The adjuvant medications include nitrofurantoin, phenazopyridine, and trimethoprim. Table 20.4 provides dosage information for the adjuvant urinary tract agents administered as adjunctive therapy for UTIs.

## Nitrofurantoin

**Nitrofurantoin** (Macrobid, Macrodantin) is an anti-infective agent that is administered for the treatment and prophylaxis of UTIs. The drug is effective for UTIs caused by *E. coli*, *S. aureus*, *Enterobacter*, *Enterococcus*, and *Klebsiella*. Administration of nitrofurantoin with food aids in absorption and decreases the onset of adverse effects. The two formulations differ with regard to the size of crystals in the preparation. Older adults should not take the medication because of the risk of renal, pulmonary, and hepatic toxicities. Contraindications include renal insufficiency as well as pregnancy—in the first trimester, there is a risk of fetal malformations, and between week 38 and delivery, there is a risk of hemolytic anemia. Other significant adverse effects of nitrofurantoin include (1) nonspecific ST- and T-wave changes and bundle branch block and (2) CNS changes such as fever, malaise, depression, headache, lethargy, and vertigo. In addition, the nurse should inform patients that the drug may cause the urine to turn brown.

Although few drugs interact with nitrofurantoin, magnesium-containing antacids may reduce absorption and subsequent urinary secretion. Concurrent use of fluconazole may lead to hepatic and pulmonary toxicities.

## Phenazopyridine

Phenazopyridine hydrochloride (Azo-Standard, Pyridium) is a urinary analgesic that is administered to provide pain relief related to burning, urgency, frequency, and irritation of the lower urinary tract mucosa. The pain is a result of infection, trauma, cystoscopic examinations, surgery, or catheter insertion. Phenazopyridine, an azo dye, is a drug that acts directly on the urinary tract mucosa to provide analgesia. Metabolism occurs in the liver. It is necessary to administer the medication with food to decrease GI distress. The nurse should tell the patient that his or her urine will turn reddish orange. The FDA has issued a **BLACK BOX WARNING ◆** cautioning that if the patient's skin turns yellow, it is important to report this to the health care provider immediately. This is a sign that phenazopyridine is accumulating in the patient's system. It is also necessary to report a sore throat, fever, bruising, or bleeding. Contraindications to phenazopyridine include renal insufficiency and hepatitis.

## Trimethoprim

Trimethoprim (Primsol) is a folate antagonist that is a urinary tract anti-infective. Most commonly administered in combination with sulfamethoxazole or as an adjuvant agent with the sulfonamides (see Sulfonamides), it is also given singly. Prescribers order it for susceptible infections and UTIs. The CDC has recommended that trimethoprim be used (unlabeled use) in the

## TABLE 20.4

## DRUGS AT A GLANCE: Adjuvant Drugs for Urinary Tract Infections/Urinary Antiseptics

| Drug | Pregnancy Category | Routes and Dosage Ranges | |
|---|---|---|---|
| | | **Adults** | **Children** |
| **Nitrofurantoin** (Macrobid; ✳ Macrodantin, Macrobid) | B | Macrobid: 100 mg every 12 h for 7 d<br>Macrodantin: 100 mg PO two times daily for 5 d<br>Prophylaxis of recurrent urinary tract infection (UTI) in women Macrodantin: 50–100 mg PO at bedtime | Children older than 12 y: dual-release capsules: 100 mg every 12 h for 7 d<br>Children 1 mo and older: macrocrystal capsules, 5–7 mg/kg/d PO in four divided doses for 7 d |
| Phenazopyridine hydrochloride (Azo-Standard, Pyridium; ✳ Pyridium) | B | 100–200 mg PO three times daily after meals | 6–12 y: 12 mg/kg/d PO, in three divided doses after meals for 2 d |
| Trimethoprim (Primsol, Proloprim) | C | 100 mg PO every 12 h for 10 d or 200 mg every 24 h for 10 d | 4–6 mg/kg/d in divided doses every 12 h<br>Otitis media: Children ≥10 mg/kg/d PO in divided doses every 12 h for 10 d |

treatment of *P. jirovecii* pneumonia. This drug inhibits folic acid reduction to tetrahydrofolate, thus interfering with the bacterial cell growth. Contraindications include a known folate deficiency, fragile X syndrome, and a creatinine clearance less than 15 mL/minutes. Patient teaching should include taking the entire course of medication even if symptoms improve; having a sufficient fluid intake (2000–3000 mL/24 hours); and reporting symptoms such as sore throat, fever, bruising, or rash to the health care provider. Rash and pruritus are the most common adverse effects. There also have been occasional reports of nausea, vomiting, thrombocytopenia, and leukopenia.

## NCLEX Success

11. A nurse practitioner has prescribed nitrofurantoin for a woman with a urinary tract infection. Which of the following cardiovascular adverse effects is this patient at risk for developing?

A. inverted T wave
B. widened QRS
C. premature ventricular contraction (PVC)
D. bundle branch block

12. A man has had a urinary tract infection, and a prescriber orders phenazopyridine. Which of the following adverse effects should he report immediately to his health care provider? (Select all that apply.)

A. yellowing of the skin
B. edema
C. bruising
D. malaise
E. sore throat
F. fever

## Clinical Application 20.3

In addition to the sulfamethoxazole with trimethoprim, Ms. Parsons receives a prescription for phenazopyridine 200 mg three times per day.

● What patient teaching related to the administration of phenazopyridine does the nurse provide to Ms. Parsons?
● The nurse should teach Ms. Parsons that phenazopyridine will affect her urine in what way?
● What other patient teaching should Ms. Parsons receive?

## THE NURSING PROCESS

A concept map outlining the nursing process related to drug therapy considerations in this chapter is found in the map below. General aspects of the nursing process in antimicrobial drug therapy, described in Chapter 15, apply to the patient receiving tetracyclines, sulfonamides, and urinary antiseptics. Additional nursing implications related to the disease process should also be considered in care decisions.

### Assessment

- With tetracyclines, assess for conditions in which the drugs must be used cautiously or are contraindicated, such as impaired renal or hepatic function.
- With sulfonamides, assess for signs and symptoms of disorders for which the drugs are used:
  - For UTIs, assess urinalysis reports for white blood cell and bacteria counts; urine culture reports for type of bacteria; and symptoms of dysuria, frequency, and urgency of urination.
  - For burns, assess the size of the wound, amount and type of drainage, presence of edema, and amount of eschar.
  - Ask patients specifically if they have ever taken a sulfonamide and, if so, whether they had an allergic reaction.
- With urinary antiseptics, assess for signs and symptoms of UTI.

### Outcomes of Therapy

The patient will
- Receive or self-administer the drugs as directed.
- Experience relief of signs and symptoms of infection being treated.
- Receive prompt and appropriate treatment if adverse effects occur.

### Nursing Interventions

- During tetracycline therapy for systemic infections, monitor laboratory tests of renal function for abnormal values.
- During sulfonamide therapy, encourage sufficient fluids to produce a urine output of at least 1500 mL daily. A high fluid intake decreases the risk of crystalluria.
- Avoid urinary catheterization when possible. If catheterization is necessary, use sterile technique. The urinary tract is normally sterile except for the lower third of the urethra.
  - A single catheterization may cause infection. With indwelling catheters, bacteria colonize the bladder and produce infection within 2 to 3 weeks, even with meticulous care.
  - When indwelling catheters must be used, measures to decrease UTI include using a closed drainage system; keeping the perineal area clean; forcing fluids, if not contraindicated, to maintain a dilute urine; and removing the catheter as soon as possible. Do not disconnect the system and irrigate the catheter unless obstruction is suspected. Never raise the urinary drainage bag above bladder level.
- Force fluids in anyone with a UTI unless contraindicated. Bacteria do not multiply as rapidly in dilute urine. In addition, emptying the bladder frequently allows it to refill with uninfected urine. This decreases the bacterial population of the bladder.
- Teach women to cleanse themselves from the urethral area toward the rectum after voiding or defecating to avoid contamination of the urethral area with bacteria from the vagina and rectum. Also, voiding after sexual intercourse helps cleanse the lower urethra and prevent UTI.
- Provide additional teaching related to any drug therapy (see Boxes 20.2 and 20.5).

### Evaluation

- Interview and observe for administering medications as prescribed.
- Interview and observe for improvement in the infection being treated.
- Interview and observe for adverse drug effects.

## KEY CONCEPTS

- Tetracyclines are effective against both gram-positive and gram-negative organisms. However, many of these organisms have developed resistance to the older tetracyclines.
- Chemical modifications of tetracyclines have introduced semi-synthetic drugs in the classes that have activity against specific drug-resistant organisms, including MRSA, vancomycin-resistant *Enterococcus*, and penicillin-resistant *S. pneumoniae*.
- Unlike many other antibiotics, tetracyclines are infrequently inactivated biologically or altered chemically by resistant bacteria.
- Demeclocycline hydrochloride is used to treat bacterial infections such as acne, pertussis, and urinary tract infections.
- Doxycycline (Vibramycin) (or ciprofloxacin) is recommended for the treatment of *B. anthracis*.
- Minocycline hydrochloride (Minocin) is a semisynthetic tetracycline derivative used to treat mucopurulent cervicitis, *M. pneumoniae*, *Rickettsia*, and *Chlamydia*.
- The FDA has issued a **BLACK BOX WARNING ◆** because of the increased risk of mortality in patients treated with tigecycline compared with other drugs used to treat serious infections.
- Sulfonamides are bacteriostatic against a wide range of gram-positive and gram-negative bacteria, although increasing resistance is making them less useful.
- Mafenide (Sulfamylon) is a topical anti-infective agent applied to second- and third-degree burns that when inactivated in the blood becomes a weak carbonic anhydrase inhibitor.
- Silver sulfadiazine (Silvadene) is a silver salt that provides bactericidal effects on the bacterial cell wall and cell membrane to inhibit folic acid synthesis.
- Trimethoprim–sulfamethoxazole (TMP-SMZ; Bactrim, Septra) is a combination of anti-infective sulfonamide and trimethoprim. (Trimethoprim is a synthetic anti-infective agent.)
- Sulfasalazine (Azulfidine) is contraindicated in people who are allergic to salicylates.
- Both tetracyclines (except doxycycline) and sulfonamides are contraindicated in patients with renal failure.
- Urinary antiseptics may be bactericidal for sensitive organisms in the urinary tract because these drugs are concentrated in renal tubules and reach high levels in urine but are not used in systemic infections because they do not attain therapeutic plasma levels.
- The FDA has issued a **BLACK BOX WARNING ◆** for phenazopyridine cautioning that if the patient's skin turns yellow, it is important to discontinue the drug and notify the health care provider immediately because this is a sign that phenazopyridine is accumulating in the patient's system.

## CLINICAL REASONING CASE STUDY

**Meet the Patient**

Jake Purcell is a home care patient with an indwelling catheter. His wife has been the primary caregiver for her husband for many years. Previously, he received treatment for a urinary tract infection with trimethoprim. Last evening he began running a fever of 102.5°F orally. His urine is cloudy with streaks of blood. A urine specimen is sent to the laboratory for culture and sensitivity. Following collection of the culture, a nurse practitioner prescribes trimethoprim and sulfamethoxazole. After 48 hours, the culture reveals that his urine is growing *Klebsiella* and *Escherichia coli* (*E. coli*). The nurse practitioner discontinues the sulfamethoxazole and trimethoprim. He then prescribes nitrofurantoin (Furadantin).

- What is the action of trimethoprim and sulfamethoxazole?
- What are the adverse effects of trimethoprim and sulfamethoxazole?
- Will trimethoprim and sulfamethoxazole be effective against *Klebsiella* and *E. coli*?
- What medication will be effective for the treatment of a UTI caused by *Klebsiella* and *E. coli*?
- What is the action of nitrofurantoin?
- What patient teaching should be provided to Mr. Purcell's wife?

**Assessing Drug Information**

- Sulfamethoxazole with trimethoprim is a broad spectrum anti-infective agent that is effective in treating complicated urinary tract infections. The combination of the two medications inhibits the enzyme to prevent the bacterial synthesis of essential nucleic acids and proteins.
- The adverse effects of sulfamethoxazole and trimethoprim are: toxic epidermal necrolysis, also known as Stevens-Johnson syndrome, pseudomembranous enterocolitis, agranulocytosis, thrombocytopenia, and allergic myocarditis.
- Trimethoprim and sulfamethoxazole is not effective for the treatment of a urinary tract infection caused by *Klebsiella* and *E. coli*. It is administered for the treatment of *P. jiroveci* pneumonitis, severe UTIs, *Salmonella enteritidis*, and Enterobacteriaceae.
- Nitrofurantoin (Macrodantin, Macrobid) is effective for the treatment of a UTI caused by *Klebsiella* and *E. coli*.
- Nitrofurantoin interferes with several bacterial enzyme systems. It is soluble in urine and is most active in acidic urine.

**Nursing Actions**

- The home care nurse should review catheter care with Mrs. Purcell.
- The home care nurse instructs Mrs. Purcell to increase Mr. Purcell's fluid intake to 1500 mL/day.
- At the start of sulfamethoxazole and trimethoprim, the home care nurse instructs Mrs. Purcell to examine Mr. Purcell's skin for any signs of redness, burning, or skin sloughing. This is indicative of epidermal necrolysis. If found, she is instructed to call the nurse practitioner immediately.
- When Mr. Purcell is switched to nitrofurantoin, Mrs. Purcell is instructed to monitor Mr. Purcell's intake and output and to report any change in the intake and output ratio.
- The home care nurse should assess Mr. Purcell's pulmonary function. An acute pulmonary sensitivity reaction can occur in the first week of therapy. The home care nurse informs Mrs. Purcell to call the home care nurse or prescriber if Mr. Purcell develops any shortness of breath or difficulty breathing.
- Instruct Mrs. Purcell that Mr. Purcell's urine will turn brown and that it is a normal reaction.
- When administering nitrofurantoin, Mr. Purcell does not need to consume the large amounts of fluid as he would with sulfamethoxazole and trimethoprim.

---

Visit **thePoint** at **http://thePoint.lww.com/Frandsen12e** *for answers to NCLEX Success questions (in Appendix A), answers to Clinical Application Case Studies (in Appendix B), and more!*

## REFERENCES AND RESOURCES

Hinkle, J. H., & Cheever, K. H. (2017). *Brunner & Suddarth's textbook of medical-surgical nursing* (14th ed.). Philadelphia, PA: Lippincott Williams & Wilkins.

Karch, A. (2017). *Focus on nursing pharmacology.* Philadelphia, PA: Lippincott Williams & Wilkins.

May, D. B. (2019a). *Tetracyclines.* UpToDate. Lexi-Comp, Inc.

May, D. B. (2019b). *Trimethoprim-sulfamethoxazole: An overview.* UpToDate. Lexi-Comp, Inc.

Norris, T. L. (2019). *Porth's pathophysiology: Concepts of altered health states* (10th ed.). Philadelphia, PA: Wolters Kluwer.

Paul, M., Bishara, J., Yahav, D., Goldberg, E., Neuberger, A. Ghanem-Zoubi, N., et al. (2015). Trimethoprim-sulfamethoxazole versus vancomycin for severe infections caused by methicillin resistant *Staphylococcus aureus*: Randomized controlled trial. *British Medical Journal, 350,* h2219. doi:https://doi.org/10.1136/bmj.h2219

UpToDate. (2019). *Drug information.* Lexi-Comp, Inc.

# Drug Therapy With Macrolides and Miscellaneous Anti-infective Agents

## LEARNING OBJECTIVES

*After studying this chapter, you should be able to:*

1. Describe the characteristics and specific uses of macrolide anti-infective agents.
2. Identify the prototype and describe the action, use, adverse effects, contraindications, and nursing implications of macrolides.
3. Describe the action, use, adverse effects, contraindications, and nursing implications of miscellaneous anti-infective agents.
4. Implement the nursing process in the care of patients being treated with macrolides and miscellaneous anti-infective agents.

## CLINICAL APPLICATION CASE STUDY

Juro Nikki, a 65-year-old man, has had chronic obstructive pulmonary disease for a number of years. He presents to the physician's office with a respiratory tract infection. He begins taking azithromycin, 500 mg for one dose and then 250 mg, orally daily for 4 days.

## KEY TERMS

**Glycylcyclines:** class of anti-infective agents that are structurally related to the tetracyclines and share many of the same properties; used for the treatment of complicated skin and skin structure infections caused by methicillin-resistant *Staphylococcus aureus* and vancomycin-sensitive *Enterococcus faecalis*, as well as treatment of complicated intra-abdominal infections

**Gray syndrome:** dangerous condition that occurs in newborns who are given chloramphenicol; may lead to fatalities

**Lincosamides:** similar to macrolides in their mechanism of action and antimicrobial spectrum

**Lipopeptides:** a new class of antibiotics that kills gram-positive bacteria by inhibiting synthesis of bacterial proteins, DNA, and RNA

**Methicillin-resistant *Staphylococcus aureus*:** microorganisms resistant to broad-spectrum antibiotics such as penicillin and erythromycin; frequently colonizes nasal passages of health care workers and is increasing as a cause of infection in health care facilities

**Methicillin-sensitive *Staphylococcus aureus*:** methicillin-susceptible strains of *Staphylococcus aureus*

***Mycobacterium avium* complex:** caused by atypical mycobacteria; opportunistic infection that occurs mainly in people with advanced human immunodeficiency virus infection

**Oxazolidinones:** newer class of antibiotics; active against aerobic gram-positive bacteria by inhibiting protein synthesis

**Red man syndrome:** adverse reaction when dalbavancin or vancomycin is administered too quickly; characterized by hypotension, flushing, and skin rash

**Staphylococcal species nonaureus:** other strains of antibiotic-resistant staphylococci

**Streptogramins:** class of antibacterial drugs; produced by *Streptomyces graminofaciens* bacteria

**Vancomycin-resistant enterococci:** pathogenic bacteria that are resistant to vancomycin

**Vancomycin-resistant *Enterococcus faecium*:** *Enterococcus faecium* that is resistant to vancomycin

## INTRODUCTION

The drugs described in this chapter are heterogeneous in their antimicrobial spectra, characteristics, and clinical uses. Some are used often, and some are used only in specific circumstances. The drugs to be described in the following sections include the macrolides and miscellaneous anti-infective agents. The Drugs at a Glance tables present information about individual drugs and the prototype drugs, with routes of administration and dosage ranges.

## MACROLIDES

The macrolides, which include erythromycin as well as azithromycin, clarithromycin, and fidaxomicin, have similar antibacterial spectra and mechanisms of action. Macrolides are widely distributed into body tissues and fluids and may be bacteriostatic or bactericidal, depending on drug concentration in infected tissues. They are effective against gram-positive cocci, including group A streptococci, pneumococci, and most staphylococci. They are also effective against species of *Corynebacterium*, *Treponema*, *Legionella*, *Chlamydia*, *Neisseria*, and *Mycoplasma* as well as some anaerobic species of genera such as *Bacteroides* and *Clostridia*.

The prototype macrolide is **erythromycin.** This drug is now used less often because of microbial resistance, numerous drug interactions, and the development of newer macrolides. Compared with erythromycin, the other drugs in the class, such as azithromycin, clarithromycin, and fidaxomicin, have enhanced antibacterial activity, require less frequent administration, and cause less nausea, vomiting, and diarrhea (see Other Drugs in the Class). Erythromycin is available in several preparations. Ophthalmic and topical preparations are discussed in Chapters 59 and 61, respectively.

## Pharmacokinetics

The oral preparation of erythromycin has an onset of action in 1 to 2 hours and reaches its peak in 1 to 4 hours. The intravenous (IV) preparation has a more rapid onset of action, reaching a peak of action in less than 1 hour. Both the oral and parenteral forms cross the placenta and enter the breast milk. Erythromycin is metabolized in the liver by the cytochrome P-450 3A4 (CYP3A4) isoenzymes and is absorbed in the small intestine. It is excreted mainly in bile; approximately 20% is excreted in urine. Depending on the specific salt formulation used, food can have a variable effect on the absorption of oral erythromycin.

## Action

Erythromycin enters the microbial cells and reversibly binds to the 50S subunits of ribosomes, thereby inhibiting microbial protein synthesis and leading to cell death. The medication has bacteriostatic or bacteriocidal activity against susceptible bacteria.

## Use

Erythromycin is useful in the following ways:

- As a penicillin substitute in patients who are allergic to penicillin
- For prevention of rheumatic fever, gonorrhea, syphilis, pertussis, and chlamydial conjunctivitis in newborns (ophthalmic ointment)
- For treatment of other infections (e.g., Legionnaires disease, genitourinary infections caused by *Chlamydia trachomatis*, intestinal amebiasis caused by *Entamoeba histolytica*)

The drug is administered for upper respiratory infections caused by group A beta-hemolytic streptococci. It is used with sulfonamides for upper respiratory infections caused by *Haemophilus influenzae*. Prophylactically, erythromycin is administered to prevent alpha-hemolytic streptococcal endocarditis before dental or other procedures in patients who have valvular heart disease and are allergic to penicillin. Table 21.1 provides route and dosage information for erythromycin and other macrolides.

### Use in Patients With Hepatic Impairment

Using erythromycin warrants caution in patients with hepatic impairment (and perhaps it should not be given at all), because it is metabolized in the liver to an active metabolite that is excreted in the bile. Avoiding the drug or dosage reduction may be necessary in hepatic failure. It has also been associated with cholestatic hepatitis.

### Use in Patients With Critical Illness

Erythromycin is seldom used in critical care settings, partly because broader-spectrum bactericidal drugs are usually

## TABLE 21.1

## DRUGS AT A GLANCE: Macrolides

| Drug | Pregnancy Category | Routes and Dosage Ranges | |
|---|---|---|---|
| | | **Adults** | **Children** |
| **Erythromycin**  Erythromycin stearate Erythromycin lactobionate (E.E.S. 400, EES Granules, Ery-Tab, EryPed 200 or 400, Erythrocin) | B | 250–500 mg PO every 6–12 h  Severe infections: up to 4 g daily in divided doses  Lactobionate: 15–20 mg/kg/d IV in divided doses q6h or 500 mg–1 g q6h or may be given as a continuous infusion over 24 h (max dose 4 g/d)  Severe infections: up to 4 g daily in divided doses | PO 30–50 mg/kg/d PO in divided doses every 6–12 h  Lactobionate: 15–50 mg/kg/d IV in divided doses every 6 h, not to exceed 4 g/d |
| Azithromycin (Zithromax, Zithromax Tri-Pak, Zithromax Z-Pak; ❋ Azithromycin, Apo-Azithromycin Z, Azithromycin for Injection, Dom-Azithromycin, Novo-Azithromycin, PRO-Azithromycin, Zithromax) | B | Respiratory and skin infections: 500 mg PO as a single dose on day 1 and then 250 mg once daily for 2–5 d  Extended-release suspension (Zmax): 2 g as a single dose; PO 1 g as a single dose  Nongonococcal urethritis and cervicitis caused by *C. trachomatis*: 1 g as a single dose  MAC: prevention, 1200 mg PO once per week; treatment, 600 mg PO once daily; secondary prophylaxis, 500–600 mg daily in combination with ethambutol  Bacterial sinusitis: Tri-Pak 500 mg PO daily for 3 d, or Zmax extended-release formula 2 g PO as a single dose  CAP: IV 500 mg daily for at least 2 d followed by 500 mg PO daily for total of 7–10 d treatment | 6 mo to 2 y, otitis media: 1-d regimen: PO 30 mg/kg as a single dose (maximum dosage 1500 mg); 3-d regimen PO 10 mg/kg once daily for 3 d (maximum dosage 500 mg)  3-d regimen, pharyngitis/tonsillitis: PO 12 mg/kg (not to exceed 500 mg) once daily for 2–5 d |
| Clarithromycin (❋ ACT-Clarithromycin XL, APO-Clarithromycin, APO-Clarithromycin XL, Biaxin, Biaxin BID, Dom-Clarithromycin, PMS Clarithromycin) | C | PO 250–500 mg q12h or 1000 mg daily for 7–14 d  Prevention/treatment of MAC: 500 mg PO q12h or 1000 mg XL daily; discontinue when CD4 count is >100 cells/mm³  Chronic maintenance: 500 mg daily plus ethambutol  Bronchitis and CAP (extended-release): PO 250 mg every 12 h or 1000 mg daily for 7 d  Acute maxillary sinusitis: PO 1000 mg daily for 14 d | PO 7.5 mg/kg, not to exceed 500 mg every 12 h  Prevention/treatment of MAC: same as above |
| Fidaxomicin (Dificid; ❋ Dificid) | B | *C. difficile* diarrhea: PO 200 mg BID for 10 d | Safety and efficacy not established |

CAP, community-acquired pneumonia; MAC, *Mycobacterium avium* complex.

needed in critically ill patients and partly because it inhibits liver metabolism and slows elimination of several other drugs. For a critically ill patient who needs a macrolide antibiotic, one of the newer macrolides is preferred because the newer drugs have activity against several groups of microorganisms and fewer effects on the metabolism of other drugs.

## Adverse Effects

Erythromycin may result in several adverse effects. Gastrointestinal (GI) effects include nausea, vomiting, diarrhea, cramping, anorexia, hepatotoxicity, and pseudomembranous colitis. If fever and jaundice occur after 1 to 2 weeks of drug administration, they subside after the drug is discontinued. Central nervous system (CNS) effects are reversible hearing loss, confusion, lability of emotions, and alterations in thought processes. Cardiac effects, with the IV form of the drug, include possible ventricular dysrhythmias. Allergic reactions include redness of the skin, rash, bronchospasm, or anaphylaxis.

## Contraindications

Contraindications to erythromycin include a known hypersensitivity reaction to the drug or any macrolide. As previously stated, hepatic insufficiency requires careful use. The U.S. Food and Drug Administration (FDA) has issued a **BLACK BOX WARNING** ◆ regarding erythromycin estolate, a Canadian preparation of erythromycin; administration to patients with known liver disease warrants caution. Women who are breast-feeding should not take erythromycin because the drug is concentrated in the breast milk. This can alter the bowel flora of the infant and interfere with fever assessments. Also, people should not take erythromycin if they are concurrently using drugs highly dependent on CYP3A4 liver enzymes for metabolism.

## Nursing Implications

### Preventing Interactions

Many medications interact with erythromycin, increasing or decreasing its effects (Box 21.1). Also, both grapefruit juice and St. John's wort decrease absorption of the antibiotic.

In addition, as stated previously, the CYP3A4 isoenzymes in the liver metabolize erythromycin. The drug interacts with other drugs metabolized by the same isoenzyme and interferes with the elimination of several drugs. As a result, the affected drugs are eliminated more slowly, their serum levels are increased, and they are more likely to cause adverse effects and toxicity unless the erythromycin dosage is reduced. In combination with potent inhibitors of CYP3A4 (e.g., fluconazole, diltiazem), erythromycin increases the risk of sudden cardiac death.

---

**BOX 21.1** — **Drug Interactions: Erythromycin**

**Drugs That Increase the Effects of Erythromycin**

- Chloramphenicol
  *Increases effectiveness against strains of resistant Staphylococcus aureus*
- Streptomycin
  *Increases effectiveness against Enterococcus in bacteremia, brain abscess, endocarditis, meningitis, and urinary tract infection*

**Drugs That Decrease the Effects of Erythromycin**

- Antacids, calcium, magnesium, aluminum, zinc
  *Decrease antibiotic absorption*
- Etravirine, lincosamide antibiotics
  *Decrease serum concentration of erythromycin*
- Ethanol
  *Decreases absorption of erythromycin*

---

A partial list of other interacting drugs includes carbamazepine (Tegretol), cyclosporine (Sandimmune), digoxin (Lanoxin), disopyramide (Norpace), lopinavir/ritonavir (Kaletra), lovastatin, nevirapine (Viramune), pimozide (Orap), quinidine, rifampin (Rifadin), ritonavir (Norvir), simvastatin (Zocor), theophylline (Theochron), triazolam (Halcion), and warfarin (Coumadin). These drugs represent a variety of drug classes.

### Administering the Medication

It is necessary to take oral erythromycin according to manufacturer's instructions. Drinking 6 to 8 oz of water with the medication is important; adequate intake of water aids the absorption of the medication. It is necessary to take the drug on an empty stomach at evenly spaced intervals around the clock. Regular intervals help maintain therapeutic blood levels. People should not take erythromycin after taking antacids. Antacids decrease the absorption of both the tablet and suspension form of erythromycin.

The nurse may administer the IV administration preparation of erythromycin without regard to meals. It is important to consult the manufacturer's instructions for dissolving, diluting, and administering the parenteral form of erythromycin to achieve therapeutic effects. The IV formulation has limited stability in the solution. Also, instructions differ for intermittent and continuous infusions. The nurse infuses the medication in a peripheral or central IV site every 6 hours over 30 to 60 minutes.

### Assessing Therapeutic Effects

The nurse assesses for decreased pain, fever, and malaise. Both the local and systemic signs of the infection are decreased; the patient has decreased signs and symptoms of the specific infection for which erythromycin is being administered.

### Assessing for Adverse Effects

With erythromycin, it is important to assess the patient's hearing. The loss of hearing is reversible with the discontinuation of the medication. The nurse also assesses for nausea, vomiting, and diarrhea. These symptoms may be severe and result in an alteration in acid–base balance. In addition, the nurse assesses for superinfection, as noted, with the development of pseudomembranous colitis. It is important to assess the patient's psychosocial responses that are adverse effects of erythromycin, such as crying, laughing, and altered thought processes. Finally, the nurse assesses for skin rash, urticaria, edema, dermatitis, and bronchospasm. These symptoms are indicative of an allergic reaction to erythromycin.

When administering the IV form of the drug, the nurse assesses the infusion site for phlebitis.

### Patient Teaching

Box 21.2 identifies patient teaching guidelines for erythromycin.

## Other Drugs in the Class

The macrolides azithromycin and clarithromycin are active against the atypical mycobacteria that cause *Mycobacterium avium* **complex** (MAC) disease. MAC disease (see Chap. 22) is an opportunistic infection that occurs mainly in people with advanced human immunodeficiency virus (HIV)

## BOX 21.2 — *Patient Teaching Guidelines for Erythromycin*

- Take erythromycin around the clock because it inhibits bacteria; it does not kill them.
- Take erythromycin on an empty stomach, 1 hour before meals or 2 to 3 hours after meals.
- Do not drink grapefruit juice while taking erythromycin.
- Complete the full course of the prescription.
- Do not take with or within 2 hours of dairy products or antacids.
- Take each dose with 8 oz of water.
- Be aware that the effectiveness of oral contraceptives is decreased when combined with erythromycin.
- Adverse effects that you may experience include stomach cramping, gastrointestinal discomfort, labile emotions, crying, laughing, and abnormal thinking.
- Report severe or watery diarrhea, nausea, vomiting, dark urine, yellowing of the eyes or skin, loss of hearing, itching, and rash to your prescriber.

infection. *Helicobacter pylori*, a pathogen implicated in peptic ulcer disease, is also susceptible to treatment with azithromycin or clarithromycin as part of a combination regimen (see Chap. 37).

Azithromycin (Zithromax) is useful in the treatment of lower respiratory infections, pharyngitis, and tonsillitis caused by *Haemophilus ducreyi*, *H. influenzae*, *Moraxella catarrhalis*, and *Streptococcus pneumoniae*. Prescribers order the drug for children older than 6 months of age for otitis media. It is also effective for treatment of community-acquired pneumonia (CAP) caused by *S. pneumoniae* as well as for genital ulcer disease in men and pelvic inflammatory disease in women. As previously stated, people with advanced HIV take azithromycin for MAC.

The onset of action of azithromycin is rapid, with a peak in 2.5 to 3.2 hours. The duration of action is 24 hours. The medication is metabolized in the liver and is distributed extensively to the tissues, skin, lungs, sputum, tonsils, and cervix. A minimal amount enters the cerebrospinal fluid (CSF). Major elimination of the drug is in the bile, with only 6% of excretion in the urine. The mechanism of action is the inhibition of RNA-dependent protein synthesis at the chain elongation step; the drug binds to the 50S ribosomal subunit to block the involved transpeptide. The parenteral form of azithromycin is stable in 5% dextrose and water; 5% dextrose and lactated Ringer's solution, lactated Ringer's solution, normal saline; and all 5% dextrose and saline IV fluids.

The adverse effects of azithromycin are similar to those of erythromycin. Caution is necessary with azithromycin in patients who have gonorrhea, syphilis, pseudomembranous colitis, and hepatic and renal impairment, as well as in lactating women. Alfuzosin, amiodarone, and artemether combined with azithromycin can enhance QT elongations. Careful assessment of the cardiac status is crucial when these medications are combined. Close monitoring of the international normalized ratio (INR) and prothrombin time is necessary when azithromycin is administered with warfarin. Patients should

take the oral medication on an empty stomach, 2 hours before or after the administration of aluminum- or magnesium-containing antacids.

Clarithromycin is a macrolide administered for bronchitis, sinusitis, otitis media, MAC, peptic ulcer disease, pertussis, pharyngitis, tonsillitis, and pneumonia. Prescribers also order the drug for prophylactic use in patients with underlying cardiac conditions who are undergoing invasive procedures that predispose them to infective endocarditis. It is also useful in skin infections caused by *Staphylococcus aureus* and *Streptococcus pyogenes* as well as in duodenal ulcers caused by *H. pylori*.

Absorption of clarithromycin is rapid, and the serum half-life is 3 to 7 hours. The drug is 42% to 50% protein bound, and it is widely distributed to all body tissues except the CNS. The metabolism of the medication takes place partially in the liver with CYP3A4 and is converted to the active metabolite. Metabolism occurs in the liver, and elimination takes place in the urine, with 20% to 40% of the drug unchanged. (An additional 10% to 15% remains as the metabolite.) Clarithromycin binds to the 50S ribosome to inhibit protein synthesis. One of its metabolites is two times as active as the parent compound against certain organisms.

The adverse effects of clarithromycin are headache, rash, abnormal taste, nausea, vomiting, abdominal pain, and dyspepsia. People should not take the drug with ergot derivatives, pimozide, cisapride, astemizole, colchicine, or terfenadine because of the risk of increased levels of the medications and toxicity. Generally, people may take it with or without food; however, they should take the extended-release form on an empty stomach. As with the other macrolides, use of aluminum- or magnesium-containing antacids within 2 hours of administration of clarithromycin decreases absorption of the antibiotic.

Fidaxomicin (Dificid) is a macrolide antibiotic that is used to treat *Clostridium difficile*–associated diarrhea. The medication is able to block the RNA polymerase sigma subunit, leading to inhibited protein synthesis in *C. difficile* and eventual cell death. It is minimally absorbed and is widely distributed in the GI tract. Fidaxomicin is converted to a less effective metabolite, OP-118, and is primarily excreted in the feces. Administration is oral, for 10 days. No dosage adjustment is necessary in patients with altered renal or hepatic function. Researchers have observed no adverse effects in animal studies.

### Clinical Application 21.1

The home care nurse is visiting Mr. Nikki to assess his lung status and medication regimen. Along with azithromycin, Mr. Nikki is taking omeprazole 20 mg orally daily for gastric reflux and 30 mL of Maalox at night. Since his myocardial infarction 6 months ago, he has been also taking warfarin 2 mg orally daily.

- The nurse is educating Mr. Nikki about all aspects of azithromycin. Identify all aspects of patient teaching that he should receive.
- What instructions does the nurse provide regarding the other medications Mr. Nikki is taking?
- What laboratory tests are important to monitor during the administration of azithromycin?

## NCLEX Success

1. A patient is admitted to the critical care unit with a diagnosis of Legionnaires disease. Based on your knowledge of pharmacology, which medication is the drug of choice to treat the infection?

   A. azithromycin
   B. clarithromycin
   C. erythromycin
   D. vancomycin

2. The nurse instructs a patient on the administration of clarithromycin. Which of the following patient teaching instructions is appropriate?

   A. Take the medication on an empty stomach.
   B. Take the medication with a calcium supplement.
   C. Take the medication with a glass of milk.
   D. Take the medication with cheese.

3. A teenage boy receives a prescription for erythromycin for an upper respiratory tract infection. He complains that he cannot hear the teacher, who then sends him to the school nurse's office. After assessing the patient's hearing with a tuning fork, the nurse determines that his hearing is diminished. What is the most important nursing intervention?

   A. The nurse should notify the parents to call the physician; this is an adverse effect of erythromycin.
   B. The nurse should inform the parents of a physician who specializes in ear, nose, and throat surgery.
   C. The nurse should instruct the patient to stop taking the erythromycin and his hearing will improve.
   D. The nurse should call the physician and inform the patient of a change in antibiotics.

4. A parent of a high school student calls the school nurse regarding her daughter's crying. The parent states that this behavior is unusual for her daughter. Which of the following medications contributes to changes in behavior?

   A. metronidazole
   B. naproxen sodium
   C. vitamin C
   D. erythromycin

5. A man had rheumatic fever as a child. He has an appointment for a tooth extraction. His dentist prescribes which of the following medications prior to the extraction?

   A. chloramphenicol
   B. vancomycin
   C. clarithromycin
   D. digoxin

# MISCELLANEOUS ANTI-INFECTIVE AGENTS

The miscellaneous anti-infective agents have properties similar to those of other drug classes and may belong to new classes. To simplify the understanding of these medications, they are introduced in a summary format. The medications discussed in this section include chloramphenicol, clindamycin, dalbavancin, daptomycin, linezolid, metronidazole, oritavancin, quinupristin–dalfopristin, rifaximin, tedizolid, telavancin, tigecycline, and vancomycin. Table 21.2 summarizes route and dosage information for these antibacterial drugs.

### QSEN Alert: Patient-Centered Care

Prior to beginning therapy with anti-infective agents, it is necessary to review the prescriber's orders and culture the suspected site of infection. The culture and sensitivity report determines the anti-infective agent that is most effective in treating the infection.

This is particularly important before starting vancomycin, quinupristin–dalfopristin, daptomycin, or linezolid. These drugs have relatively narrow spectra of activity, and it is critical to determine appropriate indications for their use to decrease the likelihood of resistance.

## Chloramphenicol

Chloramphenicol is a broad-spectrum, bacteriostatic antibiotic that is active against most gram-positive and gram-negative bacteria, rickettsiae, chlamydiae, and treponemes. It acts by cand diffuses well into body tissues and fluids, including CSF, but low drug levels are obtained in urine. It is metabolized in the liver and excreted in the urine.

Chloramphenicol is rarely used now to treat infections because of the effectiveness and low toxicity of alternative drugs. However, it is still used in serious infections for which no adequate substitute drug is available. Specific infections include meningococcal, pneumococcal, or *Haemophilus pneumoniae* type b (Hib) meningitis in penicillin-allergic patients; anaerobic brain abscess; *Bacteroides fragilis* infections; and rickettsial infections and brucellosis when tetracyclines are contraindicated. In infections caused by **vancomycin-resistant enterococci** (VRE), pathogenic bacteria that are resistant to vancomycin, chloramphenicol is effective against some enterococcal strains.

Chloramphenicol is associated with several adverse effects. The FDA has issued a **BLACK BOX WARNING** ◆ reporting the development of serious and fatal blood dyscrasias with chloramphenicol use. Irreversible bone marrow depression, which may lead to aplastic anemia, may appear weeks or months after therapy. A dose-related reversible bone marrow depression usually responds to discontinuation of the drug. Monitoring with a complete blood count, platelet count, reticulocyte count, and serum iron test every 2 days is essential. Experts recommend that patients be hospitalized to facilitate close monitoring. In addition, periodic measurements of serum drug levels are recommended when possible. Therapeutic levels are 5 to 20 mcg/mL.

### TABLE 21.2

## DRUGS AT A GLANCE: Miscellaneous Anti-infective Agents

| Drug | Pregnancy Category | Routes and Dosage Ranges | |
|---|---|---|---|
| | | **Adults** | **Children** |
| Chloramphenicol (❋ Chloromycetin Succinate) | C | IV 50–100 mg/kg/d in divided doses every 6 h (max dose 4 g/d) | Meningitis (infants older than 30 d and children): 50–100 mg/kg/d in divided doses every 6 h<br>Other infections (infants older than 30 d and children): 50–75 mg/kg/d in divided doses every 6 h (max daily dose 4 g) |
| Clindamycin hydrochloride (Cleocin; ❋ Apo-Clindamycin, Ava-Clindamycin, Clindamycin-150 or 300, Dalacin C, Dalacin C Palmitate, Riva Clindamycin, Teva-Clindamycin) | B | PO 150–450 mg q6–8h (max dose 1.8 g/d)<br>1.2–2.7 g/d IM or IV 600–2700 mg in 2–4 divided doses; max dose: 4.8 g/d | PO 8–40 mg/kg/d in divided doses q6–8h; up to 20 mg/kg/d in severe infections<br>Neonates, 15–20 mg/kg/d in divided doses q6–8h<br>1 mo and older, IM, IV 20–40 mg/kg/d in divided doses q6–8h; up to 40 mg/kg/d in severe infections |
| Dalbavancin (Dalvance) | C | Skin infections: single-dose regimen, 1500 mg as a single dose<br>Two-dose regimen: 1000 mg as a single dose initially followed by 500 mg as a single dose 1 wk later<br>Reduced dose with renal impairment | Dosage and safety not established |
| Daptomycin (Cubicin, Cubicin RF; ❋ Cubicin, Cubicin RF) | B | Skin/soft tissue infections: 4 mg/kg IV q24h for 7–14 d<br>MSSA, MRSA, bacteremia, or right-sided endocarditis: 6 mg/kg/d for 2–6 wk | Safety and efficacy not established |
| Linezolid (Zyvox; ❋ Apo-Linezolid, Linezolid injection, Sandoz-Linezolid, Zyvoxam) | C | 400–600 mg PO or IV q12h for 10–28 d | ≤11 y: 10 mg/kg PO or IV q8h<br>≥12 y: refer to adult dosing |
| Metronidazole (Flagyl; ❋ APO-MetroNIDAZOLE, Auro-MetroNIDAZOLE, PMS-MetroNIDAZOLE) | B | Anaerobic bacterial infection: 500 mg PO, IV q6–8 h, not to exceed 4 g/d<br>Surgical prophylaxis and colorectal surgery: 500 mg IV infused over 30–60 min 0.5–1 h before surgery<br>C. difficile colitis: 250–500 mg PO q6–8 h for 10–14 d | Anaerobic infections (older than 7 d and weight 1200–2000 g): 15 mg/kg/d PO, IV in divided doses q12h<br>Anaerobic infections in children older than 7 d and weighing more than 2000 g: 30 mg/kg/d in divided doses q12h<br>≥1 mo, 15–35 mg/kg/d PO in divided doses q8h; 30 mg/kg/d IV in divided doses q6h |
| Oritavancin (Orbactiv) | B | Skin infections: IV 1200 mg as a single dose | Dosage and safety not established |
| Quinupristin–dalfopristin (Synercid; ❋ Synercid) | B | Skin and skin structure infections: 7.5 mg/kg IV over 60 min q12h<br>VREF bacteremia: 7.5 mg/kg IV over 60 min q8h | Same as adults<br>Shunt infection caused by VRE: 7.5 mg/kg/dose q8h |
| Rifaximin (Xifaxan; ❋ Zaxine) | C | 200 mg PO three times daily for 3 d | 12 y and older: same as adults |

(*Continued on page 408*)

| TABLE 21.2 | | | |
|---|---|---|---|
| **DRUGS AT A GLANCE: Miscellaneous Anti-infective Agents** (Continued) | | | |
| **Drug** | **Pregnancy Category** | **Routes and Dosage Ranges** | |
| | | **Adults** | **Children** |
| Tedizolid phosphate (Sivextro) | C | Bacterial skin infection: IV 200 mg once daily for 6 d | Dosage and safety not established |
| Telavancin (Vibativ; 🍁 Vibativ) | C | Skin infection: IV 10 mg/kg every 24 h for 1–2 wk<br>Ventilator-associated bacterial pneumonia: IV 10 mg/kg every 24 h for 1–3 wk (reduced dose in renal impairment) | Dosage and safety not established |
| Tigecycline (Tygacil; 🍁 Tygacil) | D | 100 mg IV single dose initially; maintenance dose 50 mg q12h for 5–14 d | Dosage and safety not established |
| Vancomycin (Firvanq, Vancocin, Vancocin HCl; 🍁 JAMP-Vancomycin, PMS Vancomycin, Vancocin) | B | Antibiotic-associated pseudo-membranous colitis: 100–500 mg PO q6h (PO dose not for treating systemic infections)<br>20–45 mg/kg/d IV in divided doses | Antibiotic-associated pseudomem-branous colitis: 40 PO mg/kg/d in divided doses q6–8h (PO dose not for treating systemic infections)<br>1 mo and older, 10–15 mg/kg IV q6h |

MRSA, methicillin-resistant *Staphylococcus aureus*; MSSA, methicillin-sensitive *Staphylococcus aureus*; VREF, vancomycin-resistant *Enterococcus faecium*.

Discontinuation of therapy should occur as soon as possible, and use of the drug for trivial infections or for prophylaxis of infections should not take place. Also, chloramphenicol concentrations may increase in patients with impaired renal function. Dose adjustments may be necessary. In addition, the patient may need an increase in dietary riboflavin, pyridoxine, and vitamin $B_{12}$. It is important to consult a dietician regarding dietary needs.

Neonates should not receive chloramphenicol because of the risk of **gray syndrome**, a dangerous condition that occurs in newborns. Symptoms of gray syndrome begin 3 to 4 days after the drug is administered. Infants present with abdominal distention, progressive pallid cyanosis, vasomotor collapse, irregular respirations, and death. If drug therapy is stopped within a few hours of symptom onset of gray syndrome, affected infants will recover. Infants are also at risk for gray syndrome if their mothers are receiving chloramphenicol and are breast-feeding.

When administering chloramphenicol, the nurse reconstitutes the drug in 50 to 100 mL of 5% dextrose and water and infuses it over 15 to 30 minutes. Chloramphenicol combined with rifampin or phenobarbital results in accelerated hepatic metabolism of chloramphenicol. *rifampin ↑*

## Clindamycin

Clindamycin hydrochloride (Cleocin), a **lincosamide**, is similar to the macrolides in its mechanism of action and antimicrobial spectrum. Bacteriostatic in usual doses, this drug is effective against gram-positive cocci, including group A streptococci, pneumococci, most staphylococci, and some anaerobes such as *Bacteroides* and *Clostridia*. Clindamycin enters microbial cells and attaches to 50S subunits of ribosomes, thereby inhibiting microbial protein synthesis.

Clindamycin is often used to treat infections caused by *B. fragilis*. Because these bacteria are usually mixed with gram-negative organisms from the gynecologic or GI tracts, prescribers usually order that clindamycin be given with another drug, such as an aminoglycoside or a fluoroquinolone, to treat mixed infections. The drug may be useful as a penicillin substitute in patients who are allergic to penicillin and who have serious streptococcal, staphylococcal, or pneumococcal infections in which the causative organism is susceptible to clindamycin (including prevention of perinatal group B streptococcal disease). A topical solution is useful in the treatment of acne, and a vaginal cream is available. Clindamycin does not reach therapeutic concentrations in the CNS and cannot be used for treating meningitis.

Clindamycin is well absorbed with oral administration and reaches peak plasma levels within 1 hour after a dose. It is widely distributed in body tissues and fluids, except CSF, and it crosses the placenta. It is highly bound (90%) to plasma proteins. It is metabolized in the liver, and the metabolites are excreted in the bile and urine.

Adverse effects associated with clindamycin are many. It may be necessary to reduce the dosage in patients with severe hepatic failure to prevent accumulation and toxic effects. The FDA has issued a **BLACK BOX WARNING ◆** for clindamycin regarding the potential of severe and possible fatal colitis. If diarrhea develops in a patient receiving clindamycin, discontinuation of the drug is essential. With severe and persistent diarrhea, it is critical to check the stools for white blood cells, blood, mucus, and the presence of *C. difficile* toxin. It may be necessary to perform sigmoidoscopy to more definitively determine whether the patient has pseudomembranous colitis. The appearance of lesions on sigmoidoscopy means that the clindamycin should be stopped immediately. Although pseudomembranous colitis may occur with any antibiotic, it has often been associated with clindamycin therapy. Other adverse effects of clindamycin include nausea and vomiting.

Neonates and infants should receive clindamycin only if the drug is clearly indicated, and then, monitoring of liver and kidney function is necessary. Diarrhea and pseudomembranous colitis may occur with topical clindamycin for treatment of acne. Clindamycin should be used cautiously in patients with liver impairment because it is excreted by the liver.

People should take oral clindamycin with a full glass of water to avoid esophageal irritation. It is important *not* to refrigerate the reconstituted oral solution. When administering clindamycin intramuscularly, the nurse gives no more than 600 mg in one injection. To avoid pain, induration, and abscess formation, it is necessary to administer the medication into the deep tissues. When administering clindamycin intravenously, the nurse dilutes 300 to 600 mg of the drug in 50 mL of IV fluid and gives it over 10 to 20 minutes, or he or she dilutes 900 mg in 50 to 100 mL and administers it over 20 minutes. The dilution of the medication in IV fluids decreases the risk of phlebitis. The patient is at risk for cardiac arrest if the medication is administered as a bolus. It is important that clindamycin not be administered with erythromycin; the combination decreases the effects of clindamycin.

## Dalbavancin

Dalbavancin (Dalvance) is a glycopeptide antibiotic. The drug binds to D-alanyl-D-alanine terminus in the nascent cell wall peptidoglycan, which prevents cross-linking and interferes with the cell wall synthesis. It has bactericidal action against *S. aureus* and *S. pyogenes* in skin and skin structure infections. Dalbavancin is 90% protein bound, primarily to albumin. It is excreted unchanged in the urine and as a hydroxyl metabolite in the feces. The drug possesses a half-life of 346 hours.

Administration of dalbavancin is by a single- or double-dose regimen. Infusion should be slow to prevent **red man syndrome**, an adverse reaction characterized by hypotension, flushing, and skin rash. The nurse must assess the patient's hydration level with the administration of the drug. In the presence of hepatic or renal insufficiency, it is recommended that a reduced dose of the drug be given. Assessment of bilirubin, aspartate aminotransferase, and alanine aminotransferase (ALT) levels is necessary throughout the course of treatment. Any elevation in ALT will require discontinuation of the drug.

## Daptomycin

Daptomycin (Cubicin) belongs to the **lipopeptide** class. It is a bactericidal agent effective only for gram-positive infections caused by *S. aureus* (including oxacillin-resistant strains), *S. pyogenes*, group B streptococci, and *Enterococcus faecalis* (vancomycin-susceptible strains only). In combination with gentamicin, daptomycin is synergistic in killing staphylococci and enterococci. Indications are limited to the treatment of complicated skin and skin structure infections caused by the above organisms.

Available only for IV administration, daptomycin reaches target concentrations by the third daily dose. The drug is excreted primarily by the kidneys. Its mechanism of action is unique. Daptomycin kills bacteria by inhibiting synthesis of bacterial proteins, DNA, and RNA.

The most common adverse effects of daptomycin are constipation, nausea, diarrhea, and vomiting. Adverse musculoskeletal effects have occurred, primarily at increased serum creatine kinase (CK) levels. These effects are usually asymptomatic, but it is necessary to discontinue the drug in patients who develop muscle pain or weakness. Unexplained increases in serum CK levels associated with symptoms of myopathy should prompt discontinuation of daptomycin. Also, if daptomycin is combined with "statin" cholesterol-lowering medications, the risk of musculoskeletal adverse effects is greater. If possible, concomitant use of these "statins" should be avoided. In addition, no information regarding use in children or during pregnancy and lactation is available.

When administering daptomycin intravenously, the nurse mixes the daptomycin with normal saline or lactated Ringer's solution and infuses it over 30 minutes. The drug is incompatible with dextrose-containing IV solutions.

## Linezolid

Linezolid (Zyvox) is a member of the **oxazolidinone** class, a newer class of antibiotics. It is active against aerobic gram-positive bacteria. The drug exhibits bactericidal activity against most staphylococci, enterococci, and streptococci. It is indicated for pneumonia (both community-acquired and nosocomial), complicated and uncomplicated skin and skin structure infections, and **vancomycin-resistant *Enterococcus faecium*** (VREF) infections. The drug is bacteriostatic against enterococci (including *E. faecalis* and *E. faecium*) and staphylococci (including methicillin-resistant strains) and bactericidal for most streptococci.

Linezolid acts by inhibiting protein synthesis by a unique mechanism. The drug binds to the bacterial 23S ribosomal RNA of the 50S subunit, thus preventing an essential component of the bacterial translation process. It is well absorbed orally, distributes widely, and undergoes hepatic elimination.

The FDA has issued a **BLACK BOX WARNING ◆** stating that linezolid should not be administered to patients who are currently taking selective serotonin reuptake inhibitors, serotonin–norepinephrine reuptake inhibitors, tricyclic antidepressants, or monoamine oxidase inhibitors. It is thought that linezolid inhibits the action of monoamine oxidase A, an enzyme responsible for breaking down serotonin in the brain. Thus, high levels of serotonin build up in the brain, causing toxicity. This buildup of serotonin is referred to as serotonin syndrome; affected patients present with muscle twitching, excessive sweating, shivering, shaking, fever, and diarrhea. The combination results in severe CNS reactions. It is necessary to discontinue the psychiatric agent prior to administration of the linezolid and closely monitor the patient for CNS adverse effects. The nurse assesses for mental status changes, muscle twitching, shivering, and lack of coordination.

Also, myelosuppression (bone marrow depression; e.g., anemia, leukopenia, pancytopenia, thrombocytopenia) is a serious adverse effect that may occur with prolonged linezolid therapy—longer than 2 weeks. Monitoring of the patient's complete blood count is necessary; if myelosuppression occurs, discontinuation of the drug is warranted. Myelosuppression usually improves with drug discontinuation. Pseudomembranous colitis may also occur. Mild cases usually resolve with drug discontinuation; moderate or severe cases may require fluid and electrolyte replacement and an antibacterial drug that is effective against *C. difficile* organisms. Hypertension may occur with the concomitant ingestion of linezolid and adrenergic drugs (e.g., dopamine, epinephrine), and therefore, it is necessary to monitor blood pressure and heart rate. In addition, oral linezolid causes symptomatic hypoglycemia.

The effects of linezolid in pregnant women and in children are largely unknown. Because linezolid is a weak monoamine oxidase inhibitor, patients should avoid food high in tyramine content (aged cheeses, fermented or air-dried meats, sauerkraut, soy sauce, tap beers, red wine) while taking the drug.

When administering the IV preparation of linezolid, the nurse infuses the drug over 30 to 120 minutes. It is important to infuse no other medications with linezolid sequentially and flush the line with 5% dextrose and water, normal saline, or lactated Ringer's solution.

## Metronidazole

Metronidazole (Flagyl) is effective against anaerobic bacteria, including gram-negative bacilli such as *Bacteroides*, gram-positive bacilli such as *Clostridia*, and some gram-positive cocci. The drug is also effective against protozoa that cause amebiasis, giardiasis, and trichomoniasis (see Chap. 25). It achieves therapeutic concentrations in body fluids and tissues and can be used to treat anaerobic brain abscesses. Metronidazole is eliminated by the liver and kidneys.

Clinical indications for metronidazole include prevention or treatment of anaerobic bacterial infections (e.g., in colorectal surgery, intra-abdominal infections) and treatment of *C. difficile* infections associated with pseudomembranous colitis. As part of a combination regimen, the drug is also useful in treatment of infections caused by *H. pylori*. It is contraindicated during the first trimester of pregnancy and must be used with caution in patients with CNS or blood disorders. The safety and efficacy of metronidazole have been established in children only for the treatment of amebiasis, although the drug is used for other infections in pediatric patients without reported unusual adverse effects.

Metronidazole has several adverse effects. Dermatologic effects are skin rash, pruritus, and thrombophlebitis at the infusion site. CNS effects include seizures, peripheral paresthesias, ataxia, confusion, dizziness, and headache. The most common GI effects are nausea, vomiting, diarrhea, and metallic taste. The nurse tells the patient that consumption of alcohol when taking metronidazole will produce a disulfiram reaction. This reaction results in symptoms of flushing, headache, nausea, vomiting, and chest and abdominal pain.

Prior to administering metronidazole, it is important to review the manufacturer's instructions for administration. Metronidazole requires specific techniques for preparation and administration.

## Oritavancin

Oritavancin is a glycopeptide used to treat acute bacterial skin and skin structure infections. The organisms that are susceptible to this anti-infective agent include several species of *Streptococcus* (*S. pyogenes*, *S. agalactiae*, *S. dysgalactiae*, *S. anginosus*) and *E. faecalis*. Oritavancin disrupts the bacterial cell wall membrane, leading to cell death. Significant adverse effects of oritavancin include tachycardia, hypersensitivity, headache, dizziness, and peripheral edema. Also, in the postmarketing phase of drug development, *C. difficile* diarrhea reportedly occurred.

## Quinupristin–Dalfopristin

Quinupristin–dalfopristin (Synercid) belongs to a class of antimicrobials referred to as **streptogramins**, produced by the bacterium *Streptomyces graminofaciens*. Both components are active antimicrobials that affect bacterial ribosomes to decrease protein synthesis. The combination is bacteriostatic against *E. faecium* (including vancomycin-resistant strains) and bactericidal against **methicillin-sensitive *Staphylococcus aureus*** (MSSA). It is not active against *E. faecalis*. Quinupristin–dalfopristin is indicated for skin and skin structure infections caused by *S. aureus* or group A *Streptococcus*. It is also used for treatment of patients with serious or life-threatening infections associated with VREF bacteremia. However, a **BLACK BOX WARNING ◆** reports that FDA approval for this use is based on the ability of quinupristin–dalfopristin to clear bacteria from the bloodstream rather than on its ability to cure the underlying infection. Further clinical studies are underway to verify the clinical benefits of the drug for curing VREF infections.

Quinupristin–dalfopristin undergoes biliary excretion and fecal elimination. The drug combination is a strong inhibitor of CYP3A4 enzymes and therefore interferes with the metabolism of drugs such as cyclosporine, antiretrovirals, carbamazepine, and many others. Toxicity may occur with the inhibited drugs.

When administering quinupristin–dalfopristin parenterally, the nurse mixes it in a minimum of 250 mL of 5% dextrose solution and infuses it over 60 minutes to decrease venous irritation. Medication toxicity may occur if it is administered in shorter infusion times. To decrease irritation, it may be necessary to use a central venous catheter for drug administration. The medication is not to be mixed with any other drug. The IV line should not be flushed with saline or heparin-containing solutions, which are incompatible with quinupristin–dalfopristin. The medication is compatible with anidulafungin, aztreonam, caspofungin, ciprofloxacin, fenoldopam, fluconazole, haloperidol, metoclopramide, and potassium chloride. When administering quinupristin–dalfopristin with these medications, the nurse must infuse them with 5% dextrose and water.

## Rifaximin

Rifaximin (Xifaxan) is a structural analog of rifampin. It is useful in infectious (traveler's) diarrhea caused by *Escherichia coli* but is not effective in diarrhea caused by *Campylobacter jejuni* (see Chap. 40). Whether rifaximin is effective to treat diarrhea caused by *Shigella* or *Salmonella* species is not known. Because of its very limited systemic absorption (97% eliminated in feces), health care providers cannot use rifaximin to treat systemic infections, including infections caused by invasive strains of *E. coli*. Therefore, diarrhea occurring with fever or bloody stools requires treatment with alternative agents. After treatment with rifaximin begins, patients reporting worsening or persistent diarrhea for longer than 24 to 48 hours, fever, or blood in the stool should receive therapy with an alternative agent. Patients may take rifaximin before or after meals.

Adverse effects of rifaximin are flatulence, headache, abdominal pain, nausea, constipation, and vomiting. Prolonged use of rifaximin may result in bacterial or fungal superinfection. The patient may develop *C. difficile* or pseudomembranous colitis more than 2 months after the discontinuation of antibiotic therapy.

## Tedizolid

Tedizolid (Sivextro) is an oxazolidinone antibiotic used for the treatment of acute bacterial skin and skin structure infections caused by *Enterococcus*, *Staphylococcus*, and *Streptococcus*. The organisms susceptible to the drug include gram-positive types of *S. aureus* (including **methicillin-resistant *Staphylococcus aureus*** [MRSA] and MSSA isolates), *S. pyogenes*, *S. agalactiae*, *S. anginosus*, and *E. faecalis*. Tedizolid binds the 50S ribosome, preventing the formation of the 70S initiation complex, which is essential for bacterial translation and inhibits protein synthesis. The oral form is well absorbed and 70% to 90% protein bound. Metabolism occurs in the liver, where the drug is converted to phosphatases. Most excretion is in the feces (82%), and the remainder (18%) is in the urine.

Administration is oral or IV. The IV form should be 0.8 mg/mL in normal saline. There is no need to adjust the dose for renal or hepatic impairment. The manufacturer's labeling does not identify any contraindications to this medication. Drug–drug interactions with monoamine oxidase inhibitors may occur.

## Telavancin

Telavancin (Vibativ) is a glycopeptide antibiotic that is administered for the treatment of complicated skin and skin structure infections caused by *E. faecalis* and certain species of *Streptococcus* (*S. pyogenes*, *S. agalactiae*, and *S. anginosus*). It is also administered for hospital-acquired and ventilator-associated bacterial pneumonia caused by *S. aureus*. The polymerization to telavancin blocks the polymerization and cross-linking of peptidoglycan. The drug then binds to D-alanine–D-alanine on the cell wall. Telavancin inhibits bacterial cell wall synthesis and also changes the cell's permeability.

Administration is IV; the dosage is 10 mg/kg every 24 hours for 1 to 2 weeks. Telavancin is administered parenterally over 60 minutes with a 5% dextrose solution, lactated Ringer's, or normal saline. The line should be flushed before and after the medication is infused. The drug's adverse effects include a metallic taste, nausea, vomiting, increased serum creatinine, pruritus, and diarrhea. A prolonged QT interval is apparent on an electrocardiogram. In a **BLACK BOX WARNING ◆**, the FDA has reported that patients who take telavancin have an increased creatinine clearance of 50 mL/minutes or less have an increased chance of mortality.

> **QSEN Alert: Safety**
>
> Women of childbearing age should have a serum pregnancy test prior to administration. Adverse outcome in the fetus can occur.

## Tigecycline

Tigecycline (Tygacil) is a **glycylcycline** anti-infective agent structurally related to the tetracyclines. Health care providers use it for CAP, complicated intra-abdominal infections, and skin or skin structure infections. The drug has both bactericidal and bacteriostatic properties. It is a derivative of minocycline but is not classified as a tetracycline. Tigecycline is effective in treating MRSA. The drug is distributed extensively to the tissues and is highly protein bound. The medication is metabolized in the liver and excreted in the feces and urine. It acts by binding to the 30S ribosome of susceptible bacteria to inhibit protein synthesis.

The nurse administers tigecycline intravenously over 30 to 60 minutes in a dedicated IV line or a Y-site connection. The medication is stable in normal saline, lactated Ringer's solution, and 5% dextrose and water. It is incompatible with amphotericin B, chlorpromazine, diazepam, methylprednisolone, sodium succinate, and voriconazole.

## Vancomycin

Vancomycin (Firvanq, Vancocin) is active only against gram-positive microorganisms. Parenteral vancomycin has been used extensively to treat infections caused by MRSA and methicillin-resistant **staphylococcal species nonaureus** (SSNA, including *Staphylococcus epidermidis*) as well as endocarditis caused by *Streptococcus viridans* (in patients allergic to or with infections resistant to penicillins and cephalosporins) or *E. faecalis* (with an aminoglycoside).

*S. pneumoniae* remain susceptible to vancomycin, although vancomycin-tolerant strains have been identified. Prophylactic use of the drug for gram-positive infections in patients who are at high risk for developing MRSA infections (e.g., those with diabetes, previous hospitalization, or MRSA in their nasal passages) and who require placement of long-term intravascular catheters and other invasive treatment or monitoring devices is extensive. Oral vancomycin is useful only to treat staphylococcal enterocolitis and pseudomembranous colitis caused by *C. difficile*.

Partly because of this widespread use, health care providers encounter VRE more often, especially in critical care units, and treatment options for infections caused by these organisms are limited. To decrease the spread of VRE, the Centers for Disease Control and Prevention (CDC) recommends limiting the use of vancomycin. Specific recommendations include avoiding or minimizing use in empiric treatment of febrile patients with neutropenia (unless the prevalence of MRSA or SSNA is high), in initial treatment for *C. difficile* colitis (metronidazole is preferred), and as prophylaxis for surgery, low birth weight infants, intravascular catheter colonization or infection, and peritoneal dialysis.

Vancomycin acts by inhibiting cell wall synthesis. Excretion of vancomycin occurs in the kidneys; it is necessary to reduce the dosage in the presence of renal impairment. In bacterial colitis, administration of vancomycin is oral because the drug is not absorbed from the GI tract and acts within the bowel lumen. Elimination of large amounts of vancomycin in the feces occurs after oral administration.

For systemic infections, administration of the drug is IV, and it reaches therapeutic plasma levels within 1 hour after infusion. It is very important to give IV infusions slowly, over 1 to 2 hours, to avoid an adverse reaction characterized by hypotension, flushing, and skin rash. This reaction, sometimes called red man syndrome, is attributed to histamine release. Close monitoring of serum drug levels of IV vancomycin is important. When administering IV vancomycin, the nurse dilutes 500-mg doses in 100 mL and 1-g doses in 200 mL of 0.9% NaCl or 5% dextrose injection and infuses it over at least 60 minutes.

---

### ⚠ QSEN Alert: Evidence-Based Practice

In a 2019 study of linezolid versus daptomycin treatment for periprosthetic joint infections, it was found that both linezolid and daptomycin are effective in treating gram-positive pathogens. Oe, et al., found that daptomycin provided higher clinical success rates and fewer adverse effects. The patients in the study group had higher red blood cell counts and decreased C-reactive protein levels. Thus, the effectiveness of linezolid and daptomycin are equivalent to control infections, but daptomycin had significant decreases in C-reactive protein and inflammation of the joint.

---

### *Clinical Application 21.2*

Mr. Nikko develops bloody diarrhea that is positive for *C. difficile* on culture. His prescriber now orders vancomycin 500 mg orally every 6 hours.
- What is the action of vancomycin?
- Why is vancomycin administered orally?

---

## NCLEX   Success

6. A nurse practitioner sees a 19-year-old college student in the student health center for severe diarrhea. The nurse diagnoses traveler's diarrhea based on the young woman's history; she had recently returned from Mexico. She receives a prescription for rifaximin 200 mg orally three times daily for 3 days. Four days later, she calls the office and reports to the nurse that she has a fever and that the diarrhea has not resolved. Which of the following is the most appropriate information to communicate to the student?

   A. Advise the student to return to the clinic for further tests and a different antibiotic.
   B. Call the pharmacy and authorize one refill of rifaximin.
   C. Advise the student that it takes up to 48 to 72 hours after the completion of treatment for the diarrhea to completely resolve.
   D. Tell the student to continue to drink plenty of fluids and report back in 24 hours.

7. A recent nursing graduate is preparing to administer vancomycin to a man intravenously. The nurse states the patient reported that he experienced flushing with his last dose of vancomycin. The nurse should

   A. infuse the vancomycin over 30 minutes to decrease the chance of a reaction
   B. hold the vancomycin dose until the physician's rounds the following morning
   C. dilute the vancomycin in 50 mL of normal saline solution and infuse over 60 minutes
   D. contact the physician, report the reaction, and request an order for diphenhydramine pretreatment

A concept map outlines the nursing process related to drug therapy considerations in this chapter. Additional nursing implications related to the disease process should also be considered in care decisions.

**Assessment**
- Assess for infections that macrolides and the designated miscellaneous drugs are used to prevent or treat.
- Assess each patient for signs and symptoms of the specific current infection.
- Assess culture and susceptibility reports when available.
- Assess each patient for risk factors that increase risks of infection (e.g., immunosuppression) or risks of adverse drug reactions (e.g., impaired renal or hepatic function).

**Outcomes of Therapy**
The patient will
- Take or receive macrolides and miscellaneous antimicrobials accurately, for the prescribed length of time.
- Experience decreased signs and symptoms of the infection being treated.
- Be monitored regularly for therapeutic and adverse drug effects.
- Verbalize and practice measures to prevent recurrent infection.

**Nursing Interventions**
- Use measures to prevent and minimize the spread of infection (see Chap. 15).
- Monitor for fever and other signs and symptoms of infection.
- Monitor laboratory reports for indications of the patient's response to drug therapy (e.g., white blood cell count, tests of renal function).
- Encourage fluid intake to decrease fever and maintain good urinary tract function.
- Provide foods and fluids with adequate nutrients to maintain or improve nutritional status, especially if febrile and hypermetabolic.
- Assist patients to prevent or minimize infections with streptococci, staphylococci, and other gram-positive organisms.
- Provide appropriate patient teaching for any drug therapy (see accompanying display).

**Evaluation**
- Interview and observe for improvement in the infection being treated.
- Interview and observe for adverse drug effects.

### KEY CONCEPTS

- Macrolides, which include erythromycin, azithromycin, clarithromycin, and fidaxomicin, inhibit microbial protein synthesis.
- The FDA has issued a **BLACK BOX WARNING ◆** concerning erythromycin estolate, a Canadian preparation of erythromycin; administration to patients with known liver disease warrants caution. The use of erythromycin concurrently with drugs highly dependent on CYP3A4 liver enzymes for metabolism is contraindicated.
- Erythromycin shares a similar antibacterial spectrum with penicillin, making it a good choice for patients with penicillin allergy.
- Chloramphenicol, which is effective against some strains of VRE, is rarely used because of possible blood dyscrasias.

- The FDA has issued a **BLACK BOX WARNING ◆** reporting serious and fatal blood dyscrasias with chloramphenicol administration.
- Clindamycin belongs to the lincosamide class of antimicrobials, similar to macrolides in its mechanism of action and antimicrobial spectrum.
- The FDA has issued a **BLACK BOX WARNING ◆** for clindamycin regarding the potential for severe and possible fatal colitis.
- Daptomycin belongs to the lipopeptide class of antibiotics, which kills gram-positive bacteria by inhibiting synthesis of bacterial proteins, DNA, and RNA.

- Linezolid belongs to the oxazolidinone class of antibiotics. It is effective against MRSA and VRE.
- A **BLACK BOX WARNING** ◆ states that linezolid is contraindicated with selective serotonin reuptake inhibitors, serotonin–norepinephrine reuptake inhibitors, tricyclic antidepressants, and monoamine oxidase inhibitors.
- Metronidazole is effective against infections with anaerobic bacteria and some protozoa.
- Quinupristin–dalfopristin belongs to the streptogramin class of antibiotics. It is indicated for VREF and MSSA.
- A **BLACK BOX WARNING** ◆ for quinupristin–dalfopristin reports that FDA approval for use in VREF bacteremia is based on the ability of the drug to clear bacteria from the bloodstream rather than its ability to cure the underlying infection.
- Rifaximin is prescribed for traveler's diarrhea caused by *E. coli* infection.
- A **BLACK BOX WARNING** ◆ for telavancin reports that patients with an increased creatinine clearance of 50 mL/minutes or less have an increased chance of mortality.
- Tigecycline is a glycylcycline anti-infective agent administered for CAP, complicated intra-abdominal infections, and skin or skin structure infections. It is distributed extensively to the tissues and is highly protein bound.
- Vancomycin is effective against gram-positive organisms only, including MRSA and SSNA.

## CLINICAL REASONING CASE STUDY

| **Meet the Patient** | Anastasia White is a 47-year-old woman who has been experiencing a persistent cough and has a temperature of 104.3. She calls her primary care provider and she prescribes erythromycin 500 mg PO every 12 hours. Two days later she still has a fever and is experiencing severe pain in the right side of her chest. She is seen by the nurse practitioner who orders a chest x-ray. The chest x-ray reveals a right lower lobe pneumonia. The NP prescribes azithromycin 500 mg the first day then 250 mg once daily for days 2 to 5.<br><br>• Why was erythromycin ineffective in treating Ms. White's cough and temperature?<br>• Why is azithromycin more effective?<br>• What is the action and adverse effects of azithromycin?<br>• What patient teaching should the nurse practitioner provide to Ms. White? |
|---|---|
| **Assessing Drug Information** | • Erythromycin is a macrolide antiinfective agent that has become less effective in treating respiratory infections, such as those caused by *Legionella* or *mycoplasma*, due to microbial resistance.<br>• Azithromycin is effective in treating community acquired pneumonia, caused by *H. influenzae, streptococcus pneumoniae* or *mycobacterium avium complex*.<br>• Azithromycin is not as microbial resistant as other medications in macrolide class.<br>• Azithromycin inhibits RNA-dependent protein synthesis at the chain elongation step. It then binds to the 50S ribosome subunit to block the transpeptide, thus preventing bacterial reproduction.<br>• Adverse effects of azithromycin include; hypersensitivity reactions, nausea, vomiting, superinfection, and QT prolongation. |
| **Nursing Actions** | • Instruct Ms. White to take azithromycin without regard to food. She should take the first dose of 2 tablets then 1 per day for 5 days.<br>• Assess Ms. White for reduction in chest pain and reduced temperature.<br>• Assess Ms. White for any adverse effects.<br>• Instruct Ms. White on the signs and symptoms of a hypersensitivity reaction, such as rash, dyspnea, or bronchospasm. |

Visit **thePoint**® at **http://thePoint.lww.com/Frandsen12e** for answers to NCLEX Success questions (in Appendix A), answers to Clinical Application Case Studies (in Appendix B), and more!

## REFERENCES AND RESOURCES

Hinkle, J. H., & Cheever, K. H. (2018). *Brunner & Suddarth's textbook of medical-surgical nursing* (14th ed.). Philadelphia, PA: Lippincott Williams & Wilkins.

Karch, A. M. (2019). *Lippincott's nursing drug guide*. Philadelphia, PA: Lippincott Williams & Wilkins.

Norris, T. (2019). *Porth's pathophysiology: Concepts of altered health states* (10th ed.). Philadelphia, PA: Lippincott Williams & Wilkins.

Oe, M. S. K., Hirata, M., Kawamura, H., Ueda, N., Nakamura, T., Iida, H., et al. (2019). Linezold versus daptomycin treatment for periprosthetic joint infections: a retrospective cohort study. *Journal of Orthopaedic Surgery and Research*, 34(114), 1–8. doi:10.1186-019-1375-7

UpToDate. (2019). *Drug information*. Lexi-Comp, Inc.

# Drug Therapy for Tuberculosis and *Mycobacterium Avium* Complex Disease

## LEARNING OBJECTIVES

*After studying this chapter, you should be able to:*

1. Describe the etiology and pathophysiology of tuberculosis and *Mycobacterium avium* complex.
2. Describe the characteristics of latent, active, and drug-resistant tuberculosis.
3. Describe drug therapy for tuberculosis, including the rationale for multiple-drug therapy.
4. List the action, uses, adverse effects, contraindications, and nursing implications of first-line antitubercular drugs.
5. Describe how second-line antitubercular drugs are added to drug regimens to treat multidrug-resistant tuberculosis.
6. Describe the drugs used to prevent or treat *Mycobacterium avium* complex.
7. Discuss ways to increase adherence to antitubercular drug therapy regimens.
8. Understand how to implement the nursing process in the care of patients undergoing drug therapy for tuberculosis.

## CLINICAL APPLICATION CASE STUDY

Jennifer Grant is a 27-year-old woman. While doing volunteer work in a foreign country, she is exposed to tuberculosis, and now she has a fever, productive cough, and night sweats. Her health care provider refers her to an infectious disease specialist at a local university hospital. Her sputum culture for acid-fast bacilli is positive for *Mycobacterium tuberculosis*, and her chest x-ray is consistent with tuberculosis. Ms. Grant is started on a once-daily regimen of isoniazid 300 mg for 6 months, rifampin 600 mg for 6 months, pyrazinamide 2000 mg for 2 months, and ethambutol 1200 mg for 2 months. She is an alert, cooperative patient. You are the nurse in the university hospital's infectious disease clinic where Ms. Grant is receiving follow-up care.

## KEY TERMS

**Directly observed therapy:** method of medication administration where a nurse (or responsible adult) observes a patient taking a dose of antitubercular drug; highly recommended when using intermittent regimens and for high-risk patients

**Extensively drug-resistant tuberculosis:** relatively rare type of multidrug-resistant tuberculosis that is resistant to isoniazid and rifampin plus resistant to any fluoroquinolone and at least one of three injectable second-line drugs (i.e., amikacin, kanamycin, or capreomycin)

**Hepatitis:** inflammation of the liver; usually caused by an infectious agent, toxin, or drug

**Jaundice:** yellow discoloration of the skin and of body tissues and fluids resulting from abnormally high levels of bilirubin in the blood; common symptom when drugs cause liver damage

**Multidrug-resistant tuberculosis:** tuberculosis that is resistant to at least one first-line antitubercular drug and at least isoniazid and rifampin

## INTRODUCTION

Tuberculosis (TB) is an infectious disease that usually affects the lungs but may involve the lymph nodes, pleurae, bones, joints, kidneys, and the gastrointestinal (GI) tract. TB, which commonly occurs in many parts of the world, affects one third of the world's population. According to the World Health Organization (2018a, 2018b), TB is among the top 10 causes of death in the world. In 2018, there were 10 million TB cases, with 1.3 million deaths related to the disease. **Multidrug-resistant tuberculosis** (MDR-TB) cases numbered approximately 558,000. Eight countries accounted for two thirds of new TB cases: India, China, Indonesia, the Philippines, Pakistan, Nigeria, Bangladesh, and South Africa. In 2018, there were 9029 reported cases in the United States. Since 2017, the rate of TB in the United States has fallen by 1.3%. However, TB remains a leading cause of death worldwide for people living with human immunodeficiency virus (HIV).

## OVERVIEW OF TUBERCULOSIS AND *MYCOBACTERIUM AVIUM* COMPLEX DISEASE

### Etiology

*M. tuberculosis*, the tubercle bacillus, is the cause of TB. In general, these bacilli multiply slowly, and they may lie dormant in the body for many years. *M. avium* and *Mycobacterium intracellulare*, which may also cause lung disease, are different types of mycobacteria that resemble each other so closely that they are usually grouped together as *Mycobacterium avium* complex (MAC). These atypical mycobacteria are found in water (including natural water sources, indoor water systems, pools, and hot tubs) and soil throughout the United States as well as in animals.

### Pathophysiology

There are four phases in the initiation and progression of TB.

1. **Transmission.** This occurs when an uninfected person inhales infected airborne droplets that are exhaled by an infected person. Major factors affecting transmission are the number of bacteria expelled by the infected person and the closeness and duration of the contact between the infected and the uninfected person.
2. **Primary infection.** Authorities estimate that 30% of people who are exposed to TB bacilli become infected and develop a mild, pneumonia-like illness that is often undiagnosed. The initial infection occurs about 2 to 10 weeks after exposure. Within approximately 6 months of exposure, macrophages encapsulate the bacilli in calcified tubercles. The macrophages

are unable to eliminate the bacteria completely. In the center of the calcified tubercle lies a caseous (cheesy) mass that contains small numbers of viable but dormant TB bacilli. The calcified tubercles, most commonly located in the upper lobes of the lungs, are visible on a chest radiograph.

3. **Latent TB infection.** The immune system is able to stop bacterial growth in most people who become infected with TB bacteria. The bacteria become inactive, although they remain alive in the body and can become active later. People with inactive or latent TB infection have no symptoms, do not feel sick, and do not spread TB to others. Active TB can develop years later if the latent infection is not effectively treated. In many people with latent TB, the infection remains inactive throughout their lives. In others, the TB bacteria become active and cause disease, usually when a person's immune system becomes weak as a result of disease, immunosuppressive drugs, or aging.
4. **Active TB.** About 5% to 10% of people develop active TB when they are first infected. People with latent TB develop active disease in two ways: further exposure to infected airborne droplets or reactivation of the latent TB because of weakened immune status. Although the lungs are the most common site for an active TB infection, the disease can spread to other parts of the body. Disseminated TB can infect the musculoskeletal system; the spine is the most common site, followed by the knees and hips. Other sites include the brain, liver, and kidneys.

Both new and reactivated infections of TB are more likely in people whose immune system is depressed by diseases such as HIV, diabetes mellitus, or cancer. Immunosuppression results from drugs used during cancer treatment and after organ transplantation. In people with both TB and HIV, TB progresses more rapidly, often involves extrapulmonary sites, is more severe, and is often fatal.

In addition to latent TB, a major concern among public health and infectious disease authorities is an increase in drug-resistant infections. Drug-resistant mutants of *M. tuberculosis* microorganisms may be present in any infected person. When infected people receive anti-TB drugs, the drugs do not kill or weaken the drug-resistant mutants. Instead, the resistant bacteria are able to reproduce in the presence of the drugs and to transmit the property of drug resistance to newly produced bacteria. Eventually, the majority of TB bacilli in the body are drug resistant. Once a drug-resistant strain of TB emerges, it can be transmitted to other people just like a drug-susceptible strain.

The emergence of drug-resistant TB organisms has long been attributed mainly to poor patient adherence to prescribed anti-TB drug therapy—that is, when previously infected patients do not take the drugs and doses prescribed for the length of time prescribed. However, drug-resistant strains can spread from one person to another, and there is increasing evidence that many drug-resistant infections are new infections, especially in people whose immune system is suppressed. Drug-resistant TB has been identified in many parts of the world, especially in India, China, and Russia, and is a major concern in HIV-infected people. Most cases in the United States occur in foreign-born people. Factors contributing to the development of drug-resistant disease include delayed diagnosis and delayed determination of drug susceptibility (which can take several weeks). In addition, some countries lack adequate laboratory facilities or do not test TB bacteria for susceptibility to second-line anti-TB drugs. These delays in effective treatment allow rapid disease progression and rapid transmission to others, especially to those with impaired immune systems. Important causes of drug-resistant TB include failure to properly complete a full course of TB treatment; prescription of the wrong treatment by a health care provider (wrong dose or length of time); lack of availability of drugs for proper treatment; and poor quality drugs. Additional risk factors include redevelopment of TB after past treatment; immigration from an area where drug-resistant TB is common; and spending time with someone known to have drug-resistant TB (CDC, 2020).

MDR-TB is TB that is resistant to at least isoniazid (INH) and rifampin (RIF), two of the most effective anti-TB drugs available. MDR-TB is associated with rapid progression, with 4 to 16 weeks from diagnosis to death, and a high death rate (50%–80%). It is also difficult and expensive to treat; most experts recommend 18 months of drug therapy. The cure rate is only about 50% or less for MDR-TB compared with a cure rate of 90% or more for drug-susceptible strains of TB. Authorities now describe some MDR-TB cases as **extensively drug-resistant tuberculosis** (XDR-TB), an even more worrisome threat to public health. XDR-TB is resistant to INH, RIF, any fluoroquinolone, and at least one of three injectable second-line drugs. Some cases of TB are resistant to six or seven drugs, and there are essentially no effective drugs for their treatment.

Experts believe that the organisms that cause MAC are transmitted by inhalation of droplets of contaminated water; there is no evidence of spread to humans from animals or other humans. MAC rarely causes significant disease in immunocompetent people but causes an opportunistic pulmonary infection in approximately 50% of patients with advanced HIV infection.

## Clinical Manifestations

The initial symptoms of TB are a low-grade temperature, weight loss, cough, fatigue, and night sweats. The cough may be nonproductive or productive. Pulmonary and systemic symptoms may be present for weeks to months. Hemoptysis may occur. Dyspnea and orthopnea become progressively worse as TB becomes more advanced. Symptoms are less pronounced in the elderly. Extrapulmonary TB occurs in 16% of US cases; it is more prevalent in patients with HIV disease (Hinkle & Cheever, 2018).

Symptoms of MAC include a productive cough, weight loss, hemoptysis, and fever. As the disease becomes disseminated through the body, chronic lung disease develops, and the bacteria are found in the blood, bone marrow, liver, lymph nodes, and other body tissues.

Box 22.1 gives information about the tuberculin skin test reactions and TB blood tests, which may be useful in diagnosis.

| BOX 22.1 | *Guidelines for Interpretation of Tests for Tuberculosis* |
|---|---|

**Mantoux Skin Test**

Intradermal injection of five tuberculin units of purified protein derived from *Mycobacterium tuberculosis*

**When to Use (General)**

- For people who are at high risk for acquiring tuberculosis (TB) because of exposure to someone with TB
- For people who are at high risk to progression from latent to active TB because of other medical conditions

**How to Interpret Results**

*Induration: 5 mm or More*

- Consider positive in:
  - HIV-infected persons
  - Recent contact with a person with TB
  - People with changes on chest radiograph consistent with prior TB
  - People with organ transplants
  - People who are immunosuppressed for other reasons (e.g., prednisone use)

*Induration: 10 mm or more*

- Consider positive in:
  - Recent immigrants from high-prevalence countries
  - Injectable drug users
  - Residents and employees of high-risk congregate settings (e.g., long-term care facilities or prisons)
  - Mycobacteriology laboratory personnel
  - People in high-risk clinical positions

- Children younger than 4 years of age
- Infants, children, and adolescents exposed to high-risk adults

*Induration: 15 mm or More*

- Consider positive in any person, including people with no known risk of TB

**False-Positive Reactions Possible**

- When a non-TB mycobacterial infection is present or when the patient has had previous bacillus Calmette-Guérin (BCG) vaccination (BCG, derived from *Mycobacterium bovis*, is used to vaccinate children against TB in many parts of the world.)

**False-Negative Reactions Possible**

- When the patient's weakened immune system is unable to react to the skin test
- When there has been a very recent TB infection (within 8–10 weeks of exposure)
- When live-virus vaccinations (e.g., measles or smallpox) have been given recently

**Blood Test**

Interferon gamma release assay (IGRA) measures the concentration of a substance (interferon gamma), which is released from white blood cells when the blood of a person infected with *M. tuberculosis* is mixed with antigens derived from *M. tuberculosis* (e.g., QuantiFERON-TB Gold)

*(Continued on page 418)*

| BOX 22.1 | *Guidelines for Interpretation of Tests for Tuberculosis* [Continued] |
|---|---|

**When to Use**

- The Centers for Disease Control and Prevention [CDC] states that this test can be used in place of tuberculin skin testing in all situations in which a tuberculin skin test is recommended.*[a]*

**How to Interpret Results**

- Positive: indicates a patient has been infected with TB
- Negative: indicates that infection with TB is unlikely
- Indeterminate: also possible

**Major Advantages**

- People need only a single visit for the test; results are available in 24 hours.
- People who have received previous BCG vaccinations do not have false-positive results.

*[a]*The IGRA does not determine whether there is latent TB or active disease.

| Clinical Application 22.1 |  |
|---|---|

- Identify the signs and symptoms of TB shown by Ms. Grant. Is her TB latent or active?

## Drug Therapy

Drugs are used to treat both latent TB and active TB. Patients with latent TB cannot spread the disease to others, but treatment of the latent disease prevents progression of the disease to an active state. It is particularly important to treat latent TB in those patients who are at high risk for progression to active TB. Treatment of active TB prevents worsening of the disease in the individual patient and prevents spread of the disease to others. *It is essential to initiate drug therapy promptly and to complete the entire course of treatment.*

Four treatment regimens have been approved for latent TB. Fewer drugs are necessary to treat latent TB because fewer mycobacterial organisms are present. The drugs used in the four treatment regimens are INH, RIF, and rifapentine (Table 22.1).

The U.S. Food and Drug Administration (FDA) has approved 10 drugs for the treatment of active TB. However, the

following discussion considers only the first-line anti-TB drugs, which are INH, RIF, and other rifamycins, ethambutol, and pyrazinamide. (Note that more drugs are necessary to treat active TB, because more mycobacterial organisms are present.) People with active TB need to take several drugs for 6 to 9 months.

*Use of multiple drugs to treat TB is necessary to prevent the development of drug-resistant TB.* TB regimens are modified for use with HIV, drug resistance, and pregnancy, as well as in children. Because drug susceptibility testing results can be delayed, treatment always begins empirically; it may be necessary to adjust the regimen when results are known (Table 22.2).

Second-line anti-TB drugs are also used in combination with other drugs when there is drug resistance to one of the first-line drugs or the patient is unable to tolerate use of a first-line drug. The second-line drugs are certain aminoglycoside antibiotics (amikacin, capreomycin sulfate [Capastat], kanamycin, and streptomycin); cycloserine (Seromycin); ethionamide (Trecator); para-aminosalicylic acid (Paser); and certain fluoroquinolones (most commonly used are moxifloxacin [Avelox] and levofloxacin [Levaquin]). Recently, two new anti-TB drugs have been developed (the first new anti-TB drugs in many years): bedaquiline (Sirturo) and delamanid (Deltyba). The FDA has licensed bedaquiline; delamanid has not yet been licensed

### TABLE 22.1

#### Treatment Regimens for Latent Tuberculosis

| Drugs | Duration | Interval | Minimum Dosage |
|---|---|---|---|
| Isoniazid | 9 mo | Daily (treatment for adults; persons living with HIV if antiretrovirals interact with RIF or RPT; children over age 2; pregnant women) | 270 doses |
| | | Twice weekly | 76 doses |
| Isoniazid | 6 mo | Daily | 180 doses |
| | | Twice weekly | 52 doses |
| Isoniazid and rifapentine | 3 mo | Once weekly<br>• Treatment for persons 2 y or older and patients with HIV/AIDS and receiving antiretroviral treatment<br>• Not recommended for children younger than 2 y of age; women who are pregnant or expect to become pregnant in the next 3 months; and patients with presumed infection with isoniazid- or rifampin- (RIF)-resistant TB. | 12 doses |
| RIF | 4 mo | Daily | 120 doses |
| INH and RIF | 3 mo | Daily | 90 doses |

HIV/AIDS, human immunodeficiency virus/acquired immunodeficiency syndrome.

**TABLE 22.2**

## Drug Regimens for Microbiologically Confirmed Pulmonary Tuberculosis Caused by Drug-Susceptible Organisms

| Regimen | Drug[a] | Intensive Phase — Interval and Dose[b] (Minimum Duration) | Drugs | Continuation Phase — Interval and Dose[b,c] (Minimum Duration) | Range of Total Doses | Comments[c,d] | Regimen Effectiveness |
|---|---|---|---|---|---|---|---|
| 1 | INH RIF PZA EMB | 7 d/wk for 56 doses (8 wk), or 5 d/wk for 40 doses (8 wk) | INH RIF | 7 d/wk for 126 doses (18 wk), or 5 d/wk for 90 doses (18 wk) | 182–130 | This is the preferred regimen for patients with newly diagnosed pulmonary tuberculosis | Greater |
| 2 | INH RIF PZA EMB | 7 d/wk for 56 doses (8 wk), or 5 d/wk for 40 doses (8 wk) | INH RIF | Three times weekly for 54 doses (18 wk) | 110–94 | Preferred alternative regimen in situations in which more frequent DOT during continuation phase is difficult to achieve | |
| 3 | INH RIF PZA EMB | Three times weekly for 24 doses (8 wk) | INH RIF | Three times weekly for 54 doses (18 wk) | 78 | Use regimen with caution in patients with HIV and/or cavitary disease. Missed doses can lead to treatment failure, relapse, and acquired drug resistance | |
| 4 | INH RIF PZA EMB | 7 d/wk for 14 doses then twice weekly for 12 doses[e] | INH RIF | Twice weekly for 36 doses (18 wk) | 62 | Do not use twice-weekly regimens in HIV-infected patients or patients with smear-positive and/or cavitary disease. If doses are missed, then therapy is equivalent to once weekly, which is inferior | Lesser |

DOT, directly observed therapy; EMB ethambutol; HIV, human immunodeficiency virus; INH, isoniazid; PZA, pyrazinamide; RIF, rifampin.

[a]Other combinations may be appropriate in certain circumstances; additional details are provided in the section "Recommended Treatment Regimens."

[b]When DOT is used, drugs may be given 5 days per week and the necessary number of doses adjusted accordingly. Although there are no studies that compare 5 with 7 daily doses, extensive experience indicates this would be an effective practice. DOT should be used when drugs are administered <7 days per week.

[c]Based on expert opinion, patients with cavitation on initial chest radiograph and positive cultures at completion of 2 months of therapy should receive a 7-month (31-week) continuation phase.

[d]Pyridoxine (vitamin B6), 25–50 mg/day, is given with INH to all persons at risk of neuropathy (eg, pregnant women; breastfeeding infants; persons with HIV; patients with diabetes, alcoholism, malnutrition, or chronic renal failure; or patients with advanced age). For patients with peripheral neuropathy, experts recommend increasing pyridoxine dose to 100 mg/day.

[e]See [426]. Alternatively, some US tuberculosis control programs have administered intensive-phase regimens 5 days per week for 15 doses (3 weeks), then twice weekly for 12 doses.

Used with permission from Nahid, P., Dorman, S. E., Alipanah, N., et al. (2016). Official American Thoracic Society/Centers for Disease Control and Prevention/Infectious Diseases Society of America clinical practice guidelines: Treatment of drug-susceptible tuberculosis. *Clinical Infectious Diseases*, 63(7), 853–867.

by the FDA but is conditionally approved in Europe (UpToDate, 2019). Second-line drugs also include other antibiotics (amoxicillin–clavulanate; imipenem–cilastatin; linezolid; meropenem).

Adequate drug therapy of patients with active TB usually produces improvement within 2 to 3 weeks, with decreased fever and cough, weight gain, improved well-being, and improved chest radiographs. Most patients have negative sputum cultures within 3 to 6 months. If the patient is symptomatic or if the culture is positive after 3 months, nonadherence or drug resistance must be considered. Cultures that are positive after 6 months often include drug-resistant organisms. The World Health Organization (2019) recommends the addition of medications when treating MDR-TB. Levofloxacin (or moxifloxacin),

bedaquiline, and linezolid are group A drugs to be added to the administration of group B drugs that include clofazimine and cycloserine (or terizidone). In the event the Group A or B regimens cannot be used, the following drugs may be added; ethambutol, delamanid, pyrazinamide, imipenem–cilastatin (or meropenem), amikacin (or streptomycin), ethionamide (or prothionamide), and *p*-aminosalicylic acid. The regimen for treating drug-resistant TB (resistant to single first-line agent) or MDR-TB (resistant to both INH and RIF) may include four to six drugs, including an injectable agent to which the organism is sensitive.

Diagnosis of drug-resistant TB is established by identification of the TB organism in sputum and by drug susceptibility testing showing resistance to one or more anti-TB drugs. Treatment of MDR-TB generally lasts 20 to 26 months. A shortened 9- to 12-month regimen is used for patients who are not pregnant, are infected with a TB organism susceptible to fluoroquinolones and injectable anti-TB drugs, and have no prior exposure to second-line agents (Schluger, Heysell, & Friedland, 2019). WHO prioritizes the use of oral agents over injectable agents. Evidence-based recommendations for the duration of treatment for XDR-TB are not available.

### Clinical Application 22.2

- Ms. Grant is taking INH, rifampin (RIF), pyrazinamide, and ethambutol. Why is she taking four drugs? How long will she continue to take these four drugs?

## ISONIAZID

**Isoniazid** (INH), the most commonly used anti-TB drug and the prototype, is bactericidal, relatively inexpensive, and nontoxic. Although use by itself for treatment of latent TB is appropriate, use with other anti-TB drugs is essential for treatment of active TB.

## Pharmacokinetics

INH is well absorbed from the GI tract, with peak serum concentrations occurring 1 to 2 hours after a 300-mg dose. Food slows absorption. The drug penetrates and reaches therapeutic concentrations in essentially all body fluids and cavities, including the cerebrospinal fluid (CSF). Its half-life is 1 to 4 hours.

It is acetylated in the liver to acetylisoniazid, which is excreted by the kidneys. Metabolism of INH is genetically determined; some people are "slow acetylators," and others are "rapid acetylators." A person's rate of acetylation affects response to INH. If the rate is slow, INH is more likely to accumulate to toxic concentrations, and the development of peripheral neuropathy is more likely. However, there is no significant difference in the clinical effectiveness of INH. Liver or kidney impairment may slow elimination.

## Action

INH is selective for mycobacteria, inhibiting formation of bacterial cell walls. The drug not only kills actively growing intracellular and extracellular organisms but also inhibits the growth of dormant organisms in macrophages and tuberculous lesions.

## Use

It is appropriate to use INH alone or in combination with other anti-TB drugs in the treatment of latent TB. However, it is essential that it *always* be given in combination with other anti-TB drugs in the treatment of active TB. Table 22.3 gives route of administration and dosage information for INH.

For the treatment of TB in pregnant women, the initial regimen should be INH, RIF, and ethambutol for 2 months, followed by INH and RIF for 7 months. Box 22.2 contains more information about the use of anti-TB drugs in pregnancy.

### Use in Children

Changing INH therapy from daily to twice weekly may be problematic for infants and toddlers because the increased medication volume can result in medication intolerance and vomiting.

| | | | TABLE 22.3 |
|---|---|---|---|
| | | | **DRUGS AT A GLANCE: Isoniazid** |

| Drug | Pregnancy Category | Routes and Dosage Ranges | |
|---|---|---|---|
| | | **Adults** | **Children** |
| **Isoniazid** (INH; DOM-Isoniazid, Isotamine, PDP-Isoniazid) | C | Oral (PO) or intramuscular (IM) <br> Latent tuberculosis (TB): 5 mg/kg once daily (maximum 300 mg/dose) for 9 mo (6 mo if cost reduction is necessary) OR 15 mg/kg twice weekly (maximum 900 mg/dose) for 9 mo <br> HIV disease: therapy for 9 mo <br> Interruption in treatment: therapy for 12 mo <br> Active TB: 5 mg/kg/d once daily (usually 300 mg/d) for 26 wk OR 5 mg/kg/d for 2 wk then 15 mg/kg/dose twice weekly (maximum 900 mg/dose) for 24 wk; when treating active TB, INH is part of a multidrug regimen <br> HIV disease: therapy for 9 mo <br> Extrapulmonary TB: same regimen as pulmonary TB <br> TB meningitis: therapy for 9–12 mo | Infants and children up to age 15, PO or IM <br> Latent TB: 10–20 mg/kg/d once daily (maximum 300 mg/dose) for 9 mo OR 20–40 mg/kg twice weekly (maximum 900 mg/dose) for 9 mo <br> Active TB: 10–15 mg/kg/d once daily (maximum 300 mg/d) for 26 wk OR 10–15 mg/kg/d once daily (maximum 300 mg/d) for 2 wk then 20–30 mg/kg/dose twice weekly (maximum 900 mg/dose) for 24 wk; when treating active TB, INH is part of a multidrug regimen <br> HIV disease: same regimen as active TB extended for 9 mo <br> Central nervous system or disseminated TB: therapy for 9–12 mo |

HIV, human immunodeficiency virus.

| **BOX 22.2** | *Treatment of Tuberculosis in Pregnancy* |
|---|---|

- Initial regimen: isoniazid (INH), rifampin (RIF), and ethambutol daily for 2 months followed by INH and RIF twice weekly for 7 months (total treatment 9 months).
  - INH: good safety record in pregnancy; breast-feeding should not be discouraged during treatment with INH; pregnant and breast-feeding women who are receiving INH should take vitamin $B_6$ (pyridoxine) supplementation, and their breast-fed infants should also receive pyridoxine.
  - RIF: good safety record in pregnancy; breast-feeding should not be discouraged during treatment.
- Ethambutol: may cause ophthalmic abnormalities in infants born to women receiving ethambutol; drug should be used in pregnancy if the benefits outweigh the risks.
- Pyrazinamide: not recommended; effect on fetus is unknown.
- Antituberculosis drugs contraindicated in pregnancy: streptomycin, kanamycin, amikacin, capreomycin, fluoroquinolones

Young children may need to remain on daily therapy for a longer time. INH suspension is sorbitol based and can cause GI distress or diarrhea. If a child is able to take soft foods, it may be necessary to crush INH tablets and mix them with semisolid foods.

INH therapy appears to be more effective in children than in adults, and the risk of INH-related **hepatitis** (inflammation of the liver) is minimal in infants, children, and adolescents, who generally tolerate the drug better than adults. Authorities do not recommend the routine administration of vitamin $B_6$ (pyridoxine) for children taking INH but stipulate that it be given to breast-feeding infants, children, and adolescents with vitamin $B_6$-deficient diets, as well as to children who experience paresthesias when taking INH.

## Use in Older Adults

Although INH is the drug of choice for treatment of latent TB, its use is controversial in older adults. Because risks of drug-induced hepatotoxicity are higher in this population, some clinicians believe patients with positive skin tests should have additional risk factors (e.g., recent skin test conversion, immunosuppression, and previous gastrectomy) before receiving INH.

## Use in Patients With Renal Impairment

In a patient with healthy kidneys, no adjustment in dosage is necessary with INH. However, because the drug is eliminated in the urine, severe renal impairment may affect elimination; caution is warranted when severe renal impairment is present.

## Use in Patients With Hepatic Impairment

Damage to the liver is a serious adverse effect of INH. This risk is compounded because INH is given concurrently with other anti-TB drugs that also can cause liver damage. The risk of INH-induced hepatitis worsens if the patient consumes alcohol daily or has chronic liver disease. The nurse assesses the patient monthly for symptoms of hepatitis (anorexia, nausea, fatigue, malaise, **jaundice** [yellowish discoloration of the skin and tissues]). The FDA has issued a **BLACK BOX WARNING ◆** for INH, stating that severe and sometimes fatal hepatitis may occur, usually within the first 3 months of treatment, although it may develop even after many months of therapy. Therefore, it is important that liver function tests be monitored and that the drug be discontinued if signs and symptoms of hepatotoxicity occur. Hepatitis and liver damage are more likely to occur in middle-aged and older adults. There is also an increased risk of fatal hepatitis associated with INH use in women, particularly black and Hispanic women, and in pregnancy during the postpartum period. The risk of hepatotoxicity is possible even in children who take INH. It is necessary to discontinue INH if serum bilirubin is ≥3 mg/dL or liver enzymes are greater than five times upper limit of normal and to defer use of INH for latent TB if patient has acute hepatic disease.

## Use in Patients With Critical Illness

TB is a common opportunistic infection in people with advanced HIV infection. It may develop from an initial infection or reactivation of latent TB.

## Use in Patients Receiving Home Care

If individual patients take INH and other anti-TB drugs for latent or active infection, the home care nurse needs to ensure that the patient takes the drugs as directed. The nurse may need to carry out **directly observed therapy (DOT)**, which involves observing the patient taking the anti-TB medication. The Centers for Disease Control and Prevention (CDC) highly recommends DOT when using intermittent regimens and for high-risk patients, such as those whose treatment has been interrupted or who often do not obtain necessary medication refills (Holzschuh et al., 2017). Another approach is video directly observed therapy (VDOT) using computers or smartphones. The nurse remotely observes the patient swallowing pills in real time, or the patient uses a smartphone application to record self swallowing each dose and sends the videos for review (Reichman & Lardizabal, 2020).

Other specific interventions vary widely and may include teaching about the importance of taking the drugs and the possible consequences of not taking them (i.e., spreading the disease to others, more severe disease, longer treatment regimens with more toxic drugs); monitoring for adverse drug effects (especially signs and symptoms of hepatotoxicity); assisting the patient to manage adverse effects or report them to the prescriber; assisting in obtaining the drugs; and keeping follow-up appointments for blood tests and chest radiographs.

> **!  QSEN Alert: Evidence-Based Practice**
>
> Alipanah et al. (2018) reviewed studies of adherence to multidrug treatment of both drug-susceptible tuberculosis and drug-resistant tuberculosis. Randomized controlled trials and prospective/retrospective cohort studies were included. The authors identified 7729 articles; of these, 129 met the inclusion criteria for their quantitative analysis. Seven approaches to patient adherence were studied: directly observed therapy (DOT) versus self-administered therapy (SAT); patient

education regarding disease process/risks/treatment adherence; incentives (such as a cash award for compliance) and enablers (such as transportation to a clinic); reminders given at clinic appointments; emotional/psychological support; digital health interventions (text messages or video observed therapy); and combinations of the above. Several interventions consistently showed associations with improved adherence and TB treatment outcomes. DOT was associated with better treatment outcomes than SAT, especially for TB patients living with HIV. DOT provided by a trained health worker rather than a family member was associated with a higher rate of adherence and a lower rate of treatment failure. DOT provided in the community (rather than in a clinic) was associated with higher rates of treatment completion sputum conversion by 2 months; there was also less treatment failure. Combining DOT or SAT with the other interventions improved outcomes. The authors encourage a patient-centered approach to TB treatment utilizing adherence interventions tailored to each individual. The expense of the above adherence interventions requires adaption in different settings and the marshalling of additional resources. Adherence interventions for patients undergoing treatment for MDR-TB require further study.

## Adverse Effects

Potentially serious adverse effects of INH include hepatotoxicity and peripheral neuropathy. Manifestations of hepatotoxicity are symptoms of hepatitis or elevated liver enzymes. Indications of peripheral neuropathy may include numbness and tingling in the hands and feet. Those at high risk for peripheral neuropathy include pregnant women; breast-feeding infants; and patients with HIV infection, diabetes, alcoholism, malnutrition, chronic renal failure, or advanced age. Preventing peripheral neuropathy requires concurrent administration of pyridoxine (vitamin B₆). Patients with risk factors should take 25 to 50 mg/day.

## Contraindications

Contraindications to INH include a hypersensitivity to the drug, acute hepatic disease, or INH-induced liver damage. Caution is warranted in elderly patients, as well as in those people with chronic non–INH-related liver disease or chronic alcoholism, in those with seizure disorders (especially if taking phenytoin), and in those with severe renal impairment.

### Clinical Application 22.3

● It is very important that the health department keep track of Ms. Grant's treatment to ensure that she takes her prescribed medications. Why is it essential that Ms. Grant take the full course of her therapy?

## Nursing Implications

### Preventing Interactions

Some drugs increase the effects of INH. RIF and pyrazinamide, frequently given in combination with INH, are hepatotoxic, and their administration with INH increases the risk of liver injury.

Alcohol increases the risk of hepatotoxicity even if alcohol use is stopped during INH therapy. INH increases the risks of toxicity associated with several drugs by inhibiting their metabolism and increasing their blood levels. These include benzodiazepines (diazepam and triazolam), carbamazepine, metoprolol, and phenytoin. Concurrent use should be avoided when possible or blood levels of the drug whose metabolism is inhibited should be monitored. INH may enhance the adverse hepatic effects of acetaminophen. Antacids and food slow the absorption of INH.

### Administering the Medication

Administration of INH is usually oral (PO), but an intramuscular (IM) form is also available. Regardless of the route, it is necessary to take liver enzymes prior to beginning administration and then monthly thereafter if risk factors for liver injury are present. Patients should take INH on an empty stomach, 1 hour before or 2 hours after a meal, with a full glass of water. Food delays absorption. However, people may take INH with food if it causes GI upset. Because INH is a weak monoamine oxidase inhibitor, a mild tyramine reaction is rare but possible. Consuming histamine-containing foods (skipjack, tuna, or tropical fish) with INH may cause a histamine reaction with headache, sweating, palpitations, itching, wheezing, and dyspnea.

Only patients who are unable to take the drug orally should receive INH parenterally. The nurse gives INH by deep injection into a large muscle mass at an approved site. It is necessary to rotate the site. Local pain and irritation may accompany the injection.

### Assessing for Therapeutic Effects

If the patient is being treated with INH for latent TB, the nurse observes for signs and symptoms of active disease, such as fever, productive cough, positive sputum cultures, night sweats, fatigue, and malaise. If the patient is being treated for active TB, the nurse observes for clinical improvement, such as a decrease in the following symptoms—cough, sputum production, fever, night sweats, and fatigue; the nurse should also see an increased appetite and weight as well as an increasing feeling of well-being. Follow-up sputum smears and sputum cultures should be negative for acid-fast bacilli. It is necessary to obtain sputum cultures monthly until two consecutive cultures are negative. The appearance of the chest radiograph should also improve.

### Assessing for Adverse Effects

The nurse frequently assesses for signs and symptoms of hepatotoxicity, including hepatitis (jaundice, anorexia, nausea, vomiting, and abdominal pain). The nurse reports their development to the health care provider promptly to prevent possible liver failure and death. Also, he or she must report any increase in liver enzymes or bilirubin immediately. In addition, the nurse assesses for signs and symptoms of peripheral neuropathy (tingling, numbness, and paresthesias of the extremities).

### Patient Teaching

Box 22.3 presents patient teaching guidelines for INH.

**BOX 22.3** · *Patient Teaching Guidelines for Isoniazid*

- If you have a positive tuberculin skin test and you are taking isoniazid (INH) to treat latent tuberculosis (TB), follow the drug regimen exactly or the length of time prescribed to prevent development of active TB. Treatment may last for months or years.
- If you are being treated for active TB, you should begin to feel better in about 2 to 3 weeks. If you do not, notify the health care provider who is managing the TB infection.
- When you take your INH every day, take the ordered dose of vitamin $B_6$ (pyridoxine) at the same time, so you do not forget to take your vitamin $B_6$. Vitamin $B_6$ helps prevent the adverse effects of leg numbness and tingling.
- Take INH on an empty stomach if possible, 1 hour before or 2 hours after a meal. If stomach upset occurs, take the drug with food.

- Take all other anti-TB drugs prescribed along with INH.
- Avoid alcoholic beverages while taking INH.
- INH can cause liver damage. Watch for the following signs and symptoms of liver damage (i.e., hepatitis): loss of appetite, nausea, yellowing of skin or eyes (jaundice), light-colored stools, dark urine, fatigue, and malaise. If such symptoms occur, stop taking INH and **immediately** report the symptoms to the health care provider who is managing the TB infection.
- If you begin to experience numbness, burning, or tingling of your arms or legs, notify the TB health care provider. These are the symptoms of another adverse effect of INH.
- The health care provider will order blood tests to check your liver function. Be sure to keep these appointments to have blood drawn. You may also need to have sputum cultures.

*Clinical Application 22.4*

- The nurse assesses Ms. Grant when she returns to the clinic for follow-up visits. For what adverse effects of INH does the nurse plan to monitor her?

**NCLEX　Success**

1. The nurse who is giving isoniazid (INH) anticipates an order for which one of the following vitamins, usually given with INH?

    A. vitamin $B_3$ (niacin)
    B. vitamin $B_6$ (pyridoxine)
    C. folic acid (folate)
    D. vitamin D (calcitriol)

2. The nurse should teach patients taking isoniazid to avoid alcohol because of the increased risk of

    A. central nervous system depression
    B. liver damage
    C. drug-resistant tuberculous organisms
    D. rapid drug metabolism

3. The nurse would assess a patient taking isoniazid for

    A. elevated levels of serum aspartate aminotransferase
    B. symptoms of hyperkalemia
    C. decreased urine output
    D. hearing loss

4. A patient is taking isoniazid. Which one of the following adverse effects does the nurse include in discharge teaching?

    A. numbness and tingling of extremities
    B. thirst and decreased urine output
    C. loose, watery bowel movements
    D. eye pain and visual disturbances

# RIFAMYCINS

Rifamycins are a class of drugs that is bactericidal for the treatment of intracellular and extracellular TB organisms. **Rifampin** (RIF; Rifadin) is the prototype rifamycin. RIF and INH are synergistic in combination, eliminating TB bacilli from sputum and producing clinical improvement faster than any other drug regimen, unless the causal bacteria are resistant to one or both drugs.

## Pharmacokinetics

RIF is well absorbed orally and diffuses well into body tissues and fluids, with highest concentrations occurring in the liver, lungs, gallbladder, and kidneys. Peak serum concentration occurs in 2 to 4 hours with PO administration and immediately with intravenous (IV) administration. The drug crosses the blood–brain barrier and enters the CSF. The drug is metabolized in the liver and excreted primarily in bile; a small amount is excreted in urine. Its elimination half-life is approximately 3 to 4 hours, depending on the dose. Because it is a strong inducer of drug-metabolizing enzymes, its half-life becomes shorter with continued use.

## Action

RIF is bactericidal for TB organisms. It kills mycobacteria by inhibiting synthesis of RNA and thereby causing production of defective, nonfunctional proteins.

## Use

Health care providers use RIF to treat susceptible TB infections. Patients use it alone for latent TB and in combination with other anti-TB drugs for active TB. For the use of RIF in pregnancy, see Box 22.2. Home care considerations with RIF and the other rifamycins are the same as for INH.

RIF has important uses other than in the treatment of TB, including prophylaxis for people exposed to meningococcal meningitis as well as in the treatment of MAC. An unlabeled use is in the treatment of leprosy, which is caused by *Mycobacterium leprae.* The drug also has several other unlabeled uses: treatment of prosthetic valve endocarditis due to methicillin-resistant *Staphylococcus aureus* (MRSA), prophylaxis for exposure to *Haemophilus influenzae* infections and *Neisseria meningitidis,* and treatment of certain staphylococcal infections (including MRSA) when combined with another antistaphylococcal antibiotic to prevent resistance.

Table 22.4 gives route and dosage information for RIF and the other rifamycins.

## Use in Children

*(handwritten: Rif ≠ INH)*

Children take RIF if their TB is INH resistant.

## Use in Patients With Hepatic Impairment

The half-life of RIF is prolonged with hepatic impairment, and liver damage is most likely to occur with preexisting liver disease or concurrent use of other hepatotoxic drugs. Monitoring for symptoms of hepatotoxicity at least monthly is necessary. It is important to measure liver enzymes before starting and periodically during RIF therapy. If signs of liver damage occur, it is essential to discontinue the drug, check the liver enzymes, and perform a medical evaluation. A dosage reduction to lower the risk of hepatotoxicity is necessary in at-risk patients.

## Use in Patients With Critical Illness

RIF interacts with many nonnucleoside reverse transcriptase inhibitors (NNRTIs) and protease inhibitors (PIs), generally reducing the effectiveness of these antiretroviral drugs. RIF decreases blood levels and therapeutic effects of the anti-HIV drugs. However, this effect is much less pronounced with rifabutin, another rifamycin (see *Other Drugs in the Class*).

## Adverse Effects

Adverse effects of RIF include GI upset, skin rashes, hepatotoxicity, and acute renal failure. The drug causes a harmless red–orange discoloration of urine, tears, sweat, and other body fluids. It may stain soft contact lenses permanently. Prolonged use may result in bacterial or fungal superinfections, including pseudomembranous colitis or *Clostridium difficile*–associated diarrhea.

*(handwritten: red orange, cdiff.)*

### TABLE 22.4
### Drugs At A Glance: Rifamycins

| Drug | Pregnancy Category | Routes and Dosage Ranges | |
|---|---|---|---|
| | | Adults | Children |
| **Rifampin** (RIF; Rifadin, Rifadin, Rofact) | C | Oral (PO) or intravenous (IV) Latent tuberculosis (TB): 10 mg/kg/d (maximum 600 mg/d) for 4 mo Active TB: 10 mg/kg/d (maximum 600 mg/d) OR 10 mg/kg twice weekly (maximum 600 mg); when treating active TB, RIF is part of a multidrug regime | Oral (PO) or IV Latent TB: 10–20 mg/kg/d once daily (maximum 600 mg/d) for 6 mo Active TB: 10–20 mg/kg/d (maximum 600 mg/d) OR 10–20 mg/kg twice weekly (maximum dose 600 mg); when treating active TB, RIF is part of a multidrug regimen |
| Rifapentine (Priftin) | C | Latent TB: once weekly for 3 mo in combination with isoniazid (maximum dose 900 mg) 25.1–32 kg: 600 mg 32.1–50 kg: 750 mg >50 kg: 900 mg Active TB: initial phase, 600 mg PO twice weekly with an interval of not <72 h between doses; continuation phase, 600 mg PO once weekly for 4 mo; when treating active TB, rifapentine is part of a multidrug regimen | Latent TB: Children 2–adolescence once weekly for 3 mo in combination with isoniazid (maximum dose 900 mg) 10–14 kg: 300 mg 14.1–25 kg: 450 mg 25.1–32 kg: 600 mg 32.1–50 kg: 750 mg >50 kg: 900 mg Active TB: children 12–adolescence refer to adult dosing |
| Rifabutin (Mycobutin; Mycobutin)* | B | Latent TB: 300 mg PO once daily for 4 mo Active TB: 300 mg PO once daily as part of a multidrug regimen Disseminated MAC in advanced HIV infection Prophylaxis: 300 mg PO once daily (150 mg twice daily if GI upset) Treatment: 300 mg PO once daily as adjunct therapy with clarithromycin or azithromycin (plus ethambutol) | Infants and children TB: 10–20 mg/kg PO once daily or intermittently two to three times/week (maximum dose 300 mg) MAC prophylaxis: (for patients 6 y or older), 300 mg PO once daily Treatment (add-on therapy for severe infection): 10–20 mg/kg PO once daily (maximum 300 mg) Adolescents, same as adult |

*Administered as alternative to rifampin.
GI, gastrointestinal; MAC, *Mycobacterium avium* complex.

# Contraindications

Contraindications to RIF include hypersensitivity to the drug (or other rifamycins). Caution is warranted in patients who have a history of liver disease, in those who are currently receiving medications known to cause harm to the liver (particularly pyrazinamide), in those with a history of alcoholism, or in those who are receiving treatment for HIV.

# Nursing Implications

## Preventing Interactions

RIF has many interactions with other drugs. It induces hepatic cytochrome P4503A4 enzymes and accelerates the metabolism of numerous other drugs, thereby decreasing their serum concentrations, half-lives, and therapeutic effects. Use of RIF requires careful review of the patient's drug regimen for potential interactions.

Drugs that RIF affects include antiretroviral drugs (NNRTIs and PIs), benzodiazepines, corticosteroids, cyclosporine, estrogens, fluconazole, methadone, metoprolol, phenytoin, propranolol, oral contraceptives, oral sulfonylureas, theophylline, verapamil, and warfarin. The following examples illustrate the effects of RIF on other drugs. RIF may decrease the serum concentration of the NNRTIs efavirenz and nevirapine. The anti-TB drug also decreases the serum concentration of the PI ritonavir. RIF interacts with warfarin; a decreased anticoagulant effect occurs approximately 5 to 8 days after RIF is started and lasts for 5 to 7 days after RIF is stopped. Close monitoring of the prothrombin time and INR is essential with an increase of the dosage of warfarin as necessary. In addition, RIF decreases the effectiveness of oral contraceptives, and women who use these contraceptives and take RIF should use another method of birth control. Finally, concurrent administration with RIF with methadone may precipitate signs and symptoms of opiate withdrawal unless methadone dosage is increased.

## Administering the Medication

PO administration involves taking RIF once, twice, or three times weekly, usually. Less frequent administration is more convenient, and patients are more likely follow such as treatment program. They should take the drug on an empty stomach, either 1 hour before or 2 hours after a meal. However, if patients are unable to tolerate it on an empty stomach, they may take it with a meal and a large glass of water. Food may delay or reduce the peak of action.

RIF is available for IV administration. The nurse reconstitutes the drug with 10 mL of sterile water to yield 60 mg/mL. He or she adds this to $D_5W$ 100 mL and infuses it over 30 minutes or adds this to $D_5W$ 500 mL and infuses it over 3 hours. The infusion rate should range from 30 minutes to 3 hours depending on the dose and volume of IV solution. The final concentration should not exceed 6 mg/mL.

## Assessing for Therapeutic Effects

If the patient is being treated with RIF for latent TB, the nurse observes for signs and symptoms of active disease. If the patient is being treated with the drug for active disease, the nurse observes for clinical improvement. Therapeutic effects are usually apparent with the first 2 to 3 weeks of drug therapy for active disease.

## Assessing for Adverse Effects

The nurse assesses for GI adverse effects such as anorexia, epigastric distress, abdominal cramps, nausea, vomiting, and diarrhea. Even pseudomembranous colitis is possible. The nurse observes for hypersensitivity reactions such as fever, tachycardia, anorexia, and malaise; flushing, itching, and rash may also occur. RIF can also produce a flulike syndrome of fever, chills, and muscle aches.

The patient taking RIF must be observed for signs and symptoms of hepatotoxicity—increased serum liver enzymes and bilirubin, jaundice, anorexia, abdominal pain, nausea, and vomiting. Observation for these adverse effects is crucial if the patient already has liver damage, has liver disease, or is taking another drug that also causes hepatotoxicity. Any symptoms of hepatotoxicity must be reported immediately to the health care provider to prevent further liver damage, liver failure, or death.

## Patient Teaching

Box 22.4 presents patient teaching guidelines for RIF and the rifamycins.

# Other Drugs in the Class

Rifapentine (Priftin) is a first-line drug used for the treatment of TB. This bactericidal drug is similar to RIF in effectiveness, adverse effects, and enzyme induction activity. Patients must use rifapentine with at least one other drug, such as INH, to which the causative bacteria are susceptible. They may take it, in combination with INH, in a 3-month regimen for the treatment of latent TB. The major advantage of rifapentine is that it can be used in combination with INH in a once-weekly dosing regimen during the 4-month continuation phase of treatment for active TB.

When taking rifapentine, mild GI adverse effects, such as nausea and vomiting, may occur. Another common adverse effect is hyperuricemia. Like RIF, rifapentine also produces orange discoloration of body fluids. Severe adverse effects include leukopenia, neutropenia, and thrombocytosis, as well as hepatotoxicity, which is rare. Contraindications include hypersensitivity to rifamycins. Caution is warranted in liver disease. Careful monitoring for liver damage is necessary.

Rifabutin (Mycobutin), a bactericidal rifamycin, is also a first-line drug for the treatment of TB. Other uses include treatment of MAC in people with advanced HIV disease and substituting for RIF in patients with HIV disease. Like rifapentine, rifabutin decreases blood levels and therapeutic effects of the anti-HIV drugs (as well as many other drugs). However, this effect is much less pronounced with rifabutin. Rifabutin has no advantage over RIF in the treatment of TB, but patients may take it concurrently with INH to patients who need prophylaxis against both *M. tuberculosis* and *M. avium*.

Like RIF and rifapentine, rifabutin causes a harmless red-orange discoloration of body fluids and permanent staining of soft contact lenses. Adverse effects include GI upset (nausea, vomiting, and diarrhea), hepatitis, muscular aches, neutropenia, skin rash, and uveitis (an eye disorder with inflammation, pain, and impaired vision).

- If you have a positive tuberculin skin test and you are receiving rifampin (RIF) or rifapentine to treat latent tuberculosis (TB), you should follow the drug regimen exactly for the length of time prescribed to prevent development of active TB. Treatment may last for months.
- If you are being treated for active TB, you should begin to feel better in about 2 to 3 weeks. If you do not, notify the health care provider who is managing the TB infection.
- Take RIF on an empty stomach, 1 hour before or 2 hours after a meal. If you cannot tolerate the drug on an empty stomach, take the drug with meals and with a full glass of water.
- If you are unable to swallow capsules, notify your prescriber and contact your pharmacists. RIF is available as an oral suspension.
- Take all other anti-TB drugs prescribed along with RIF.
- Avoid alcoholic beverages while taking RIF.
- RIF can cause liver damage. Watch for signs and symptoms of hepatitis: fever, loss of appetite, nausea, vomiting, yellowing of skin or eyes, light-colored stools, dark urine,

and malaise. If such symptoms occur, stop taking RIF immediately and promptly report the symptoms to the health care provider who is managing the TB infection.
- The health care provider will order blood tests to check on liver function throughout your RIF therapy. Keep all appointments.
- RIF causes a red–orange discoloration of tears, saliva, urine, and other body secretions. Although the discoloration is harmless, it may permanently stain soft contact lenses. Consult an eye care professional; you may need to refrain from wearing your soft contact lenses.
- RIF decreases the effectiveness of oral contraceptives. Use a barrier type of contraception during RIF therapy.
- If you are taking rifabutin, report the following symptoms of uveitis (sensitivity to light, excessive tears, or eye pain) to the health care provider as soon as possible.
- Ask a medical professional for information about any drugs that you take that may interact with RIF and the other rifamycins. Learn about those signs and symptoms that indicate drug ineffectiveness and that need to be reported to the health care provider.

**Clinical Application 22.5**

- The nurse teaches Ms. Grant about her medication. What adverse effect of RIF should the nurse include in patient teaching so that the patient does not become alarmed and stop taking the medication?

**NCLEX Success**

5. The nurse is caring for a patient who is taking isoniazid and rifampin. Which one of the following groups of symptoms is indicative of an adverse effect that is worsened by the combination of the two drugs?
   A. numbness and tingling of the extremities
   B. nausea, abdominal pain, and jaundice
   C. decreased urine output and elevated blood urea nitrogen
   D. dizziness and loss of hearing

6. A health care provider has prescribed rifampin for a patient who is being discharged to home. The nurse should include which one of the following in the discharge teaching?
   A. "You will have to measure your urine output while taking rifampin."
   B. "Rifampin increases the risk of having seizures or convulsions."
   C. "Ask your eye care provider about wearing your contact lenses."
   D. "There is no necessary follow-up blood work."

7. A patient with HIV is taking rifampin and a protease inhibitor. The nurse should assess the patient for what condition?
   A. a worsened allergic reaction to rifampin
   B. elevated blood urea nitrogen and serum creatinine
   C. drowsiness, lethargy, and decreased responsiveness
   D. increased viral load and decreased CD4 count

8. The nurse is reviewing a patient's medications and sees that the patient is receiving rifampin. The nurse's greatest concern about rifampin and its drug interactions is
   A. it decreases the metabolism of many other drugs
   B. it increases the metabolism of many other drugs
   C. it increases the risk for GI bleeding if given with warfarin
   D. it increases the risk of adverse effects from anti-seizure drugs

# ADJUVANT FIRST-LINE ANTITUBERCULAR DRUGS

Several other drugs are used to treat TB. Table 22.5 contains route and dosage information for these drugs.

## Pyrazinamide

Pyrazinamide is part of a multidrug anti-TB regimen used with INH, RIF, and ethambutol during the first 2 months, the initial phase, of treatment for active TB. This drug is bactericidal

**TABLE 22.5**

**DRUGS AT A GLANCE: Adjuvant First-Line Antitubercular Drugs***

| Drug | Pregnancy Category | Routes and Dosage Ranges† | |
|---|---|---|---|
| | | **Adults** | **Children** |
| Pyrazinamide (✹ PDP-Pyrazinamide; Tebrazid) | C | Active tuberculosis (TB): oral (PO) initial 2 mo phase follow with continuation phase of 4–7 additional months<br>Daily therapy (maximum dose 2000 mg regardless of weight)<br>40–55 kg: 1000 mg<br>56–75 kg: 1500 mg<br>76–90 kg: 2000 mg<br>Twice-weekly therapy (maximum dose 4000 mg regardless of weight)<br>40–55 kg: 2000 mg<br>56–75 kg: 3000 mg<br>76–90 kg: 4000 mg<br>Three times/week (maximum dose 3000 mg regardless of weight)<br>40–55 kg: 1500 mg<br>56–75 kg: 2500 mg<br>76–90 kg: 3000 mg<br>Part of a multidrug regimen | Active TB: PO initial 2 mo phase follow with continuation phase of 4–7 additional months<br>Daily therapy, 15–30 mg/kg/d (maximum 2 g/d)<br>Twice-weekly therapy, 50 mg/kg/dose once daily (maximum 2 g/d) |
| Ethambutol (Myambutol; ✹ Etibi) | C | Active TB<br>Initial dose, 15 mg/kg PO once daily (maximum 1.5 g); then suggested by lean body weight<br>Daily therapy, 15–25 mg/kg (maximum 1.6 g)<br>40–55 kg: 800 mg<br>56–75 kg: 1200 mg<br>76–90 kg: 1600 mg<br>Twice-weekly therapy, 50 mg/kg (maximum 4 g)<br>40–55 kg: 2000 mg<br>56–75 kg: 2800 mg<br>76–90 kg: 4000 mg<br>Disseminated MAC in advanced HIV infection: 15 mg/kg once daily; when treating MAC, ethambutol is given in combination with clarithromycin or azithromycin with/without rifabutin | Active TB<br>Children<br>Daily therapy, 15–20 mg/kg/d PO (maximum 1 g/d)<br>Twice weekly, 50 mg/kg PO (maximum 2.5 g/dose)<br>Adolescents 13 y of age or older, use adult dosage<br>MAC, secondary prophylaxis or treatment (if HIV exposed or infected)<br>Infants and children, 15–25 mg/kg/d once daily (maximum 2.5 g/d) with clarithromycin (or azithromycin) with or without rifabutin<br>Adolescents 13 y old or older, use adult dosages |

*When treating active TB, pyrazinamide and ethambutol are part of a multidrug regimen.
†Twice-weekly therapy should always be administered using directly observed therapy (DOT). For three times weekly therapy, consult the literature.
HIV, human immunodeficiency virus; MAC, *Mycobacterium avium* complex.

against actively growing mycobacteria in macrophages, but its exact mechanism of action is unknown. It is well absorbed from the GI tract and penetrates most body fluids and tissues, including macrophages containing tuberculous mycobacteria. It has a rapid onset and peaks in 2 hours. It is metabolized in the liver and excreted mainly by the kidneys. Its half-life is 9 to 10 hours.

The most common adverse effect of pyrazinamide is GI upset. Gout may also occur; pyrazinamide inhibits urate excretion, and this characteristic causes hyperuricemia in most patients and may cause acute attacks of gout. The most severe adverse effect is hepatotoxicity; a patient with preexisting liver impairment should not take the drug unless it is essential. Pyrazinamide enhances the hepatotoxic effect of RIF. The nurse

must assess patients without liver impairment for symptoms of liver dysfunction every 2 weeks during the usual 8 weeks of therapy. If such symptoms occur, measurement of liver enzymes is necessary. If significant liver damage is indicated, it is essential to discontinue the pyrazinamide.

Contraindications to pyrazinamide include a hypersensitivity to the drug pyrazinamide, severe preexisting hepatic damage, or acute attacks of gout. Caution is warranted in patients with a history of alcoholism.

## Ethambutol

Ethambutol (Myambutol) is a tuberculostatic drug that inhibits synthesis of RNA and thus interferes with mycobacterial protein metabolism. It may be a component in a four-drug regimen for initial treatment of active TB that may be caused by drug-resistant organisms. When culture and susceptibility reports become available (usually after several weeks), it may be appropriate to stop ethambutol if the causative organisms are susceptible to INH and RIF or continue it if the organisms are resistant to either INH or RIF and susceptible to ethambutol. To achieve therapeutic serum levels, patients should take the total daily dose of ethambutol at one time. Mycobacterial resistance to the drug develops slowly.

Ethambutol is well absorbed from the GI tract, even when given with food. The drug has a rapid onset, peaks in 2 to 4 hours, and lasts 20 to 24 hours. It is metabolized in the liver and excreted primarily by the kidneys. (Dosage reduction is necessary with impaired renal function.) The half-life is 3 to 4 hours.

 *Concept Mastery Alert*

It is important to educate a patient who has been pre-scribed ethambutol on the visual acuity adverse effect of the medication. Some patients taking this medication have developed optic neuritis, which is an inflammatory, demyelinating disorder of the optic nerve. A patient with optic neuritis will have a decrease in visual acuity and an inability to distinguish red from green. The patient teaching should include this information, and the patient should notify the prescriber promptly. Ethambutol should be discontinued if this disorder develops. The visual acuity should improve when the medication is discontinued.

## NCLEX Success

9. A male patient is receiving pyrazinamide. The nurse assesses him for which of the following?

   A. elevated liver enzymes and jaundice
   B. elevated white blood cell count and fever
   C. elevated cardiac troponin levels and chest pain
   D. elevated creatine kinase and muscle weakness

10. The nurse questions an order for pyrazinamide for a patient with

    A. active TB
    B. a recent heart attack
    C. an acute attack of gout
    D. a history of smoking

11. A patient who is receiving ethambutol comes into the clinic for a follow-up visit. Which finding on the assessment indicates a serious adverse reaction to the drug?

    A. a sputum culture that is negative for acid-fast bacilli
    B. changes in visual acuity
    C. poor appetite and GI upset
    D. dizziness and hearing loss

## FIRST-LINE DRUG COMBINATIONS USED TO TREAT TUBERCULOSIS

INH/RIF (Rifamate) and INH/RIF/pyrazinamide (Rifater) are combination products developed to increase convenience for patients and promote adherence to the prescribed drug therapy regimen for drug-susceptible TB. A tablet of Rifamate contains 150 mg of INH and 300 mg of RIF, and two tablets daily provide the recommended doses for a 6-month, short-course treatment regimen. A tablet of Rifater contains 150 mg of INH, 120 mg RIF, and 300 mg pyrazinamide and is FDA approved for the first 2 months of a 6-month, short-course treatment. Dosage depends on weight, with four tablets daily for patients weighing 44 kg or less, five tablets daily for those weighing 45 to 54 kg, and six tablets daily for those weighing 55 kg or more. Rifater not only reduces the number of pills a patient has to take each day but also prevents the patient from taking only one of the three medications, which can lead to MDR-TB.

## SECOND-LINE DRUGS USED TO TREAT TUBERCULOSIS

The second-line anti-TB drugs are indicated for treatment of the following infections:

- Strains of *M. tuberculosis* that are resistant to first-line drugs
- TB when the patient has a hypersensitivity or inability to tolerate a first-line drug
- MDR-TB and XDR-TB

The second-line drugs are always used in combination regimens with first-line drugs. In many cases, the second-line drugs are less effective than the first-line drugs. Second-line drugs often have more frequent and severe adverse effects, and they may be more expensive as well. Little research exists on the use of the second-line drugs to treat latent TB in people exposed to MDR-TB. Health care providers have gained experience in the use of combinations of first-line and second-line drugs in the treatment of MDR-TB and XDR-TB. Table 22.3 provides a summary of the first-line drugs and the different classes of second-line drugs.

### Clinical Application 22.6

- Ms. Grant completes her course of anti-TB therapy. However, her TB does not resolve. Susceptibility tests indicate that she has drug-resistant TB. What changes does her prescriber make to her drug regimen?

## DRUGS USED TO TREAT *MYCOBACTERIUM AVIUM* COMPLEX DISEASE

The main drugs used in treatment of MAC disease in patients with HIV are the macrolides azithromycin and clarithromycin (see Chap. 21) as well as ethambutol and rifabutin (described earlier in this chapter). Other drugs include amikacin, fluoroquinolones, and streptomycin. Treatment of MAC begins with twice-daily administration of clarithromycin 500 mg or azithromycin 500 to 600 mg once daily. A second drug is also used, either ethambutol or rifabutin. Ethambutol is preferable because its use is associated with a lower relapse rate. Also, rifabutin interacts with clarithromycin, decreasing clarithromycin levels. In patients who are severely immunocompromised, rifabutin or a fluoroquinolone (levofloxacin or moxifloxacin) may also be used as a third drug.

The U.S. Public Health Service and the Infectious Disease Society of America recommend at least 12 months of therapy. In some patients whose immune status improves with antiretroviral therapy, MAC treatment can be discontinued. However, the experts have not yet determined an exact timeline for discontinuing the anti-MAC drugs, and close follow-up is necessary to prevent relapse.

# SPECIAL STRATEGIES TO INCREASE ADHERENCE TO ANTITUBERCULAR DRUG REGIMENS

The complex drug regimens necessary to treat TB require special strategies to assist patients in adhering to their drug treatment plan. The combination of complex drug regimens administered over long periods of time and the risk of transmission of the disease to others if the patient does not adhere to the drug regimen presents the nurse with unique challenges. Strategies for successful drug treatment involve the nurse, the treating physician, the family and friends of the patient, public health departments, and the community as a whole. The nurse has a role in each of the following strategies.

- Supporting the use of short-course regimens, intermittent drug administration, and DOT. Shorter regimens and intermittent drug administration, if possible, make adherence easier for patients. Fixed-dose combinations of drugs are useful; they reduce the number of pills needed. The CDC and other experts strongly recommend DOT to ensure patient adherence. Incentives and enablers also prove useful. These include assistance with transportation to the health care provider for follow-up evaluations and tokens or food coupons given to patients each time they appear at the health care facility for treatment or follow-up.
- Educating patients, family members, and patient contacts. This may be especially important with treatment of latent TB. Most people are more motivated to take medications and schedule follow-up care when they have symptoms than when they feel well and have no symptoms. It is essential to

emphasize the importance of treatment for the future health of the individual person, significant others, and the community. In addition, the patient should receive information about common and potential adverse effects of drug therapy and what to do if they occur.
- Providing support services and resources. These require substantial financial resources and may include more workers to provide DOT at the patient's location, flexible clinic hours, and reduced waiting times and to assist patients with child care, transportation, or other social service needs that encourage them to initiate and continue treatment. Lack of these services (e.g., clinics far from patients' homes, with inconvenient hours, long waiting times, and unsupportive staff) may deter patients from seeking evaluation for a positive skin test, initiating treatment, or completing the prescribed treatment and follow-up care.
- Individualizing treatment regimens. Individualized treatment is necessary whenever possible to increase patient convenience and minimize disruption of usual activities of daily living.
- Promoting communication and continuity of care. With patients for whom English is not their first language, it is desirable to have a health care provider who speaks their language or who belongs to their ethnic group. This provider may be able to teach patients more effectively, elicit cooperation with treatment, administer DOT, and be a consistent support person.

## NCLEX Success

12. The nurse taking care of a patient with tuberculosis (TB) receives an order for levofloxacin. This drug may be used to treat
    A. latent TB
    B. active TB
    C. drug-resistant TB
    D. adverse effects of isoniazid

13. A female patient has not adhered to her drug regimen for tuberculosis. Which of the following is most effective to enhance adherence?
    A. explaining the importance of adherence
    B. having the patient's family administer the medication
    C. evaluating serum drug levels to determine adherence
    D. having nursing staff directly watch her take her medication

## THE NURSING PROCESS

A concept map outlines the nursing process related to drug therapy considerations in this chapter. Additional nursing implications related to the disease process should also be considered in care decisions.

### Assessment

- Assess for latent TB infection. Identify high-risk patients:
  - Close contacts of someone with active TB
  - Elderly or undernourished patients
  - Patients with AIDS, diabetes mellitus, silicosis, Hodgkin's disease, or leukemia
  - Alcoholics
  - Patients receiving immunosuppressive drugs
  - Immigrants from parts of the world where the disease is endemic
- Assess for active TB infection. For active disease, observe for fatigue, weight loss, anorexia, malaise, fever, and a productive cough. In early phases, however, there may be no symptoms. If available, check diagnostic test reports for indications of TB (chest radiograph, tuberculin skin test, or sputum smear and culture).
  - In children, initial signs and symptoms may occur within a few weeks after exposure, before skin tests become positive, and resemble those of bacterial pneumonia. In addition, indications of disease in lymph nodes, GI and urinary tracts, bone marrow, and meninges may be present.
  - In older adults, signs and symptoms of TB are often less prominent than in younger adults, or are similar to those in other respiratory disorders. Thus, an older adult is less likely to have a fever, a positive skin test, significant sputum production, hemoptysis, or night sweats. However, mental status changes and mortality are higher in older adults than in younger adults.
  - In patients with HIV infection, skin tests showing 5 mm of induration are considered positive. In addition, disease manifestations in patients with AIDS differ from those in people with undamaged immune systems. For example, malaise, weight loss, weakness, and fever are prominent. Other symptoms often resemble those of bacterial pneumonia, involve multiple lobes of the lungs, and involve extrapulmonary sites of infection.
- Assess candidates for anti-TB drug therapy for previous exposure and reaction to the primary drugs and for the current use of drugs that interact with the primary drugs.
- Assess for signs and symptoms of MAC disease, especially in patients with advanced HIV infection who have a CD4+ cell count of 50/mm$^3$ or less.

### Outcomes of Therapy

The patient will
- Adhere to the antituberculin medication regimen.
- Keep appointments for follow-up care.
- Report adverse drug effects.
- Act to prevent the spread of TB.

### Nursing Interventions

- Educate patients so that they understand the disease process and the necessity for long-term treatment and follow-up.
- Provide information about TB and its treatment through the use of written materials that are age appropriate, appropriate to the patient's educational background, and in the patient's own language.
- Teach the patient about measures to prevent the spread of TB.
- Teach the patient how to adhere to the multidrug regimen through correct administration of the drugs for the correct length of time.
- Teach the patient the signs and symptoms of adverse drug reactions and which need to be reported to the health care provider.
- Follow hospital policies and procedures regarding appropriate isolation techniques for hospitalized patients with TB.
- Follow public health policies set by the Centers for Disease Control regarding TB care.

### Evaluation

- Observe for improvement in signs and symptoms of TB and MAC disease.
- Interview and observe for adverse drug effects and check laboratory reports of hepatic and renal function (when available).
- Question the patient regarding compliance with instructions for taking anti-TB and anti-MAC drugs.

## KEY CONCEPTS

- TB is a worldwide problem. Although TB is not as extensive in the United States as it is in many other countries, the public health infrastructure for diagnosing and treating the disease needs to be maintained.
- MDR-TB and XDR-TB are of increasing concern.
- DOT is recommended to prevent inadequate drug therapy and development of drug-resistant TB organisms.
- INH is the treatment of choice for latent TB.
- The FDA has issued a **BLACK BOX WARNING ◆** for INH, stating that severe and sometimes fatal hepatitis may occur,

usually within the first 3 months of treatment, although it may develop even after many months of therapy.
- In drug-susceptible active TB, the treatment of choice is 2 months of INH, rifampin (RIF), pyrazinamide, and ethambutol, followed by 4 months of INH and RIF.
- In drug-resistant TB, there is no standardized treatment regimen; treatment must be individualized for each patient according to drug susceptibility reports. The second-line anti-TB drugs are used in the treatment of drug-resistant TB; typically, an injectable drug and a fluoroquinolone are added to the regimen.

## CLINICAL REASONING CASE STUDY

| | |
|---|---|
| **Meet the Patient** | Myeshia Hollingsworth was diagnosed with active tuberculosis. She has been prescribed isoniazid, ethambutol, rifampin, and pyrazinamide. She is to take 56 doses, each daily for 8 weeks.<br>• What is the action of isoniazid, ethambutol, rifampin, and pyrazinamide?<br>• Which of these medications are hepatotoxic?<br>• What patient teaching should the nurse provide to the patient to prevent hepatotoxicity?<br>• What tests does the healthcare provider order before therapy with these drugs to check for active liver disease?<br>• For what does the nurse assess at each follow-up visit? |
| **Assessing Drug Information** | • Isoniazid has selective activity for mycobacteria, inhibiting formation of the bacterial cell wall. It kills actively growing intracellular and extracellular organisms. It inhibits the growth of dormant organisms in macrophages and tuberculosis lesions.<br>• Ethambutol is a tuberculostatic drug that inhibits synthesis of RNA and thus interferes with mycobacterial protein synthesis.<br>• Rifampin is bactericidal for tuberculosis organisms.<br>• Pyrazinamide is a bactericidal agent against actively growing mycobacteria in macrophages; the exact mechanism of action is unknown.<br>• Isoniazid, rifampin, and ethambutol are all hepatotoxic. |
| **Nursing Actions** | • Assess the patient's history to discover conditions that put her at greater risk for hepatotoxicity, such as hepatitis, cirrhosis, or other disease processes that damage the liver.<br>• Assess the patient's liver enzyme levels (alanine and aspartate aminotransferase) prior to beginning the anti-TB drug regimen and as ordered by the physician. The levels may be monitored weekly, every other week, or monthly while the patient remains on the regimen.<br>• Assess the patient for signs and symptoms of jaundice, abdominal pain, dark urine, or clay-colored stools.<br>• Interview the patient and learn whether she consumes alcohol daily. If so, instruct her to refrain from alcoholic beverages while taking the anti-TB drugs.<br>• At each follow-up appointment, assess for conditions that indicate hepatotoxicity.<br>• Assess for early symptoms of hepatitis as evidenced by anorexia, nausea, fatigue, and malaise. In addition, assess for late symptoms of hepatitis as evidenced by jaundice, abdominal pain, ascites, or clay-colored stools.<br>• Instruct the patient to report any of these symptoms immediately to her primary care provider. |

*Visit* thePoint® *at* **http://thePoint.lww.com/Frandsen12e** *for answers to NCLEX Success questions (in Appendix A), answers to Clinical Application Case Studies (in Appendix B), and more!*

## REFERENCES AND RESOURCES

Alipanah, N., Jarlsberg, L., Miller, C., Lynn, N. N., Falzon, D., Jaramillo, E., et al. (2018). Adherence interventions and outcomes of tuberculosis treatment: A systematic review and meta-analysis of trials and observational studies. *PLoS Medicine, 15*(7), 1–44. Retrieved June 6, 2019, from CINAHL.

Centers for Disease Control and Prevention. (2020). *TB Risk Factors.* Retrieved from: https://www.cdc.gov/tb/topic/basics/risk.htm

Currier, J. S. (2019). *Mycobacterium avium* complex (MAC) infections in HIV-infected patients. In UpToDate. Retrieved June 4, 2019, from www.uptodate.com./contents/mycobacterim-avium-complex

Drew, R. H., & Sterling, T. R. (2019). Antituberculous drugs: An overview. In UpToDate. Retrieved May 30, 2019, from www-uptodate-com./contents/antituberculous-drugs-an-overview

Hinkle, J. L., & Cheever, K. H. (2018). *Brunner & Suddarth's textbook of medical-surgical nursing* (14th ed.). Philadelphia, PA: Wolters Kluwer Health/Lippincott Williams & Wilkins.

Holzschuh E. L., Province S., Johnson K., Wallis C., Shemwell C., Martin G., et al. (2017). Use of video directly observed therapy for treatment of latent tuberculosis infection-Johnson county, Kansas, 2015. *Morbidity and Mortality Weekly Report, 66*(14), 387–389.

Horsburgh, C. R. Jr. (2019). Treatment of latent tuberculosis infection in HIV-uninfected nonpregnant adults. In UpToDate. Lexi-Comp, Inc. Retrieved June 17, 2019, from www.uptodate.com

Nahid, P., Dorman, S. E., Alipanah, N., et al. (2016). Official American Thoracic Society/Centers for Disease Control and Prevention/Infectious Diseases Society of America clinical practice guidelines: Treatment of drug-susceptible tuberculosis. *Clinical Infectious Diseases, 63*(7), 853–867.

Norris, T. L. (2019). *Porth's pathophysiology: Concepts of altered health states* (10th ed.). Philadelphia, PA: Wolters Kluwer Health/Lippincott Williams & Wilkins.

Nursing 2019. (2019). *Drug handbook.* Philadelphia, PA: Wolters Kluwer Health/Lippincott Williams & Wilkins.

Reichman, L. B., & Lardizabal, A. A. (2020). Adherence to tuberculosis treatment. In UpToDate.

Schluger, N. W., Heysell, S. K., & Friedland. (2019). Treatment of drug-resistant pulmonary tuberculosis in adults. In UpToDate. Lexi-Comp, Inc. Retrieved June 4, 2019, from www.uptodate.com

Sterling, T. R. (2019). Treatment of drug-susceptible pulmonary tuberculosis in HIV-uninfected adults. In UpToDate. Lexi-Comp, Inc. Retrieved June 17, 2019, from www.uptodate.com

UpToDate. (2019). *Drug information.* Lexi-Comp, Inc.

World Health Organization. (2018a). Tuberculosis. Retrieved June 3, 2019, from http://www.who.int/news-room/fact-sheets/detail/tuberculosis.

World Health Organization. (2019). Global Tuberculosis Report 2019. Retrieved from https://www.who.int/news-room/fact-sheets/detail/tuberculosis

World Health Organization. (2019). *WHO consolidated guidelines on drug-resistant tuberculosis treatment.* Geneva: World Health Organization.

# Drug Therapy for Viral Infections

## LEARNING OBJECTIVES

*After studying this chapter, you should be able to:*

1. Identify the characteristics of viruses and common viral infections.
2. Identify the major clinical manifestations of common viral infections.
3. Identify the prototype and describe the action, use, adverse effects, contraindications, and nursing implications for antiviral agents administered for herpes simplex and varicella–zoster virus.
4. Identify the prototype and describe the action, use, adverse effects, contraindications, and nursing implications for antiviral agents administered for cytomegalovirus.
5. Identify the prototype and describe the action, use, adverse effects, contraindications, and nursing implications of drugs administered for respiratory syncytial virus.
6. Identify the prototypes and describe their action, use, adverse effects, contraindications, and nursing implications of drugs administered for influenza.
7. Identify the prototype and describe the action, use, adverse effects, contraindications, and nursing implications for the nucleoside analog antiviral agents administered for hepatitis.
8. Identify the prototype and describe the action, use, adverse effects, contraindications, and nursing implications for the nucleoside reverse transcriptase inhibitors administered for human immunodeficiency virus (HIV).
9. Identify the prototype and describe the action, use, adverse effects, contraindications, and nursing implications for the nonnucleoside reverse transcriptase inhibitors administered for HIV.
10. Identify the prototype and describe the action, use, adverse effects, contraindications, and nursing implications for the protease inhibitors administered for HIV.
11. Identify the prototype and describe the action, use, adverse effects, contraindications, and nursing implications for the integrase strand transfer inhibitors administered for HIV.
12. Identify the prototype and describe the action, use, adverse effects, contraindications, and nursing implications for fusion protein inhibitors administered for HIV.
13. Identify the prototype and describe the action, use, adverse effects, contraindications, and nursing implications for CCR5 antagonists administered for HIV.
14. Identify the combination medications administered for HIV; describe the action, use, adverse effects, contraindications, and nursing implications.
15. Implement the nursing process in the care of the patient undergoing drug therapy for viral infections.

## CLINICAL APPLICATION CASE STUDY

Ann Jackson is 30 years old. She calls her primary health care provider's office. She says that she has a cold sore under her nose on the right side. Since childhood, she has had outbreaks of this infection occasionally. Her physician orders valacyclovir 2000 mg orally once daily for 1 day.

## KEY TERMS

**Antiretroviral drugs:** antiviral medications used in the treatment of retroviral infections such as HIV

**Genital herpes:** a herpesvirus that appears on the genitals

**Hepatitis:** liver inflammation due to a virus; five different viruses cause viral hepatitis—hepatitis A, B, C, D, and G

**Herpesvirus:** any virus belonging to the family of the Herpesviridae

**Highly active antiretroviral therapy:** several combinations of antiretroviral drugs used at one time to treat HIV/AIDS

**Human immunodeficiency virus (HIV):** an infection caused by a retrovirus that infects the immune system, leading to acquired immunodeficiency syndrome (AIDS). There are two types of HIV virus, HIV-1 and HIV-2; most infections in the United States are caused by HIV-1, and infections with HIV-2 occur mainly in Africa.

**Immunocompetent:** having a normal immune response

**Retrovirus:** virus with an RNA genome that relies on reverse transcriptase to transform its genome from RNA to DNA (e.g., HIV)

**Viral load:** number of HIV RNA particles in the blood; does not measure viral levels in tissues, where viral reproduction may be continuing

## INTRODUCTION

Viruses cause pneumonia, hepatitis, acquired immunodeficiency syndrome (AIDS), and other disorders that affect most body systems. Many potentially pathogenic viral strains exist, including more than 150 that infect the human respiratory tract. Viral infections vary from mild, localized diseases with few symptoms to severe systemic illnesses and death. Viruses replicate in the host with the use of metabolic processes. Antiviral agents that possess a narrow spectrum of effect on the viral process have the ability to target the invading virus. This chapter describes general characteristics of viruses and viral infections. Box 23.1 provides more specific information about selected viral infections. The text then discusses antiviral agents.

## OVERVIEW OF VIRUSES AND VIRAL INFECTIONS

### Etiology

Viruses, the infectious agents that cause viral infections, are intracellular parasites that gain entry to human host cells by binding to receptors on cell membranes. Methods of spread of viral infections include secretions from infected people, ingestion of contaminated food or water, breaks in the skin or mucous membranes, sexual contact, pregnancy, breast-feeding, and organ transplantation. All human cells do not have receptors for all viruses; cells that lack receptors for a particular virus are resistant to infection by that virus. Thus, the locations and numbers of the receptors determine which host cells can be infected by a virus. For example, the mucous membranes lining the tracheobronchial tree have receptors for the influenza A virus; helper T lymphocytes and other white blood cells have CD4 molecules, which are the receptors for the HIV.

## Pathophysiology

Inside host cells, viruses use cellular metabolic activities for their own survival and replication. Viral replication involves dissolution of the protein coating and exposure of the genetic material (deoxyribonucleic acid [DNA] or ribonucleic acid [RNA]). With DNA viruses, the viral DNA enters the host cell's nucleus, where it becomes incorporated into the host cell's chromosomal DNA. Then, host cell genes are coded to produce new viruses. In addition, the viral DNA incorporated with host DNA is transmitted to the host's daughter cells during host cell mitosis and becomes part of the inherited genetic information of the host cell and its progeny. With RNA viruses (e.g., HIV), or retroviruses, viral RNA must be converted to DNA by an enzyme called reverse transcriptase before replication can occur. HIV is an infection caused by a retrovirus that infects the immune system, leading to AIDS.

After new viruses are formed, they are released from the infected cell either by budding and breaking off from the cell membrane (leaving the host cell intact) or by causing lysis of the cell. When the cell is destroyed, the viruses are released into the blood and surrounding tissues, from which they can transmit the viral infection to other host cells.

Viruses induce antibodies and immunity. Antibodies are proteins that defend against microbial or viral invasion. They are very specific (i.e., an antibody protects only against a specific virus or other antigen). For example, in a person who has had measles, antibody protection (immunity) develops against future infection by the measles virus, but immunity does not develop against other viral infections, such as chickenpox or hepatitis. People who are immunocompetent have intact immune systems. Most adults possess immunity to some viral diseases because they have become infected earlier in their lives. The primary infection remains latent in the tissue and is spread by blood and body fluids. Patients who are immunocompromised have impaired or weakened immune systems and may develop the infection because of decreased immunity.

| BOX 23.1 | *Selected Viral Infections* |
|---|---|

## Avian Influenza A (H5N1)

In recent years, the highly pathogenic H5N1 subtype of influenza A has been found in numerous countries. It occurs mainly in birds and poultry, but a few hundred human cases have been confirmed. Most human cases occur after exposure to infected poultry or surfaces contaminated with poultry droppings. Because human infection may cause respiratory failure and has a high mortality rate, the possibility that these viral strains might mutate so that they infect humans more easily is a major public health concern. This virus is considered the most likely cause of a future world-wide influenza epidemic.

## Coronaviruses

Corona viruses can cause one third of community-acquired upper respiratory tract infections in children and adults. The viruses may cause diarrhea in infants and children. These viral infections are classified as a family within the Nidovirales order. The viruses replicate using a set of messenger RNAs. There are four generations: alpha, beta, gamma, and delta.

### Severe Acute Respiratory Syndrome (SARS)

In 2003, the world experienced an outbreak of severe acute respiratory syndrome or SARS. This illness began in the Guangdong Province of China and spread to Hong Kong, Vietnam, Singapore, and Canada. There were 774 deaths and a case fatality rate of 9.6%. The clinical manifestations of SARS included fever, lower respiratory track illnesses with cough and shortness of breath, and lung infiltrates. Some patients developed acute respiratory distress syndrome. Older adults with chronic disease possessed a potential for poor prognosis. In addition, patients who were admitted with an elevated serum lactate dehydrogenase level possessed a greater risk for a poor prognosis.

The treatment regimen for SARS was supportive care to assist with pulmonary instability, high-dose glucocorticoids, and ribavirin. Antiretroviral agents lopinavir and ritonavir were administered. Remdesivir was an experimental antiretroviral agent that has activity against SARS.

### Middle East Respiratory Syndrome (MERS)

In 2012, two patients in the Middle East were diagnosed with a coronavirus called Middle East respiratory syndrome. The treatment for MERS COV includes ribavirin. The use of glucocorticoids delayed the clearance of the virus. The administration of interferon-alpha 2B (Chap. 11) and ribavirin resulted in a reduction in viral replication.

### COVID-19

In 2019, Wuhan, a city in the Hubei Province of China, saw an outbreak of pneumonia cases. By February 2020, the outbreak spread globally and was designated as COVID-19 by the World Health Organization (WHO). The spread of COVID-19 appears to be person to person by way of airborne droplets. This spread is similar to that of influenzae. The period of infectivity is unknown at the time this textbook went to press (July 2020). After the onset of symptoms, the viral RNA levels are elevated; thus, it is thought that viral transmission is more likely early in the viral disease. The incubation period is thought to be 14 days, but cases have developed in 4 to 5 days. Thus, the median incubation period is 4 days. The following comorbid conditions increase the severity of the illness: cardiovascular disease, diabetes mellitus, hypertension, chronic lung disease, and chronic kidney disease. Additional risk factors include severe obesity and liver disease. Older persons are also at greater risk for severe disease and death.

The clinical manifestations of COVID-19 include fever, fatigue, dry cough, anorexia, myalgia, dyspnea, and increased sputum production. COVID-19 testing is completed with a swab to test for SARS-CoV-2. A nasopharyngeal swab is used to collect secretions from deep within the upper respiratory tract. If the patient has a productive cough, an oropharyngeal swab should be used to collect sputum. If the patient is on mechanical ventilation, the patient should be tested by aspirating secretions from the lower respiratory tract.

Home care for patients with nonsevere infections includes antipyretics, analgesics, and adequate hydration. Good hand hygiene and disinfection of frequently touched surfaces is recommended. Also, the patient should wear a mask and isolate from other individuals in the home. The patient should quarantine for 2 weeks. The WHO and Centers for Disease Control and Prevention (CDC) recommend that glucocorticoids not be prescribed because they have been noted to increase the risk of mortality in patients with influenzae.

A number of investigational approaches are being explored to treat COVID-19. Remdesivir is a nucleoside analog that has in vitro activity against severe acute respiratory syndrome coronavirus-2.

Chloroquine/hydroxychloroquine studies in the treatment of SARS-CoV-2 are limited. In March of 2020, the FDA issued an emergency use authorization for the agents to be administered to adolescents and adults hospitalized with COVID-19. One significant risk to the administration of chloroquine/hydroxychloroquine is QT prolongation. Currently, limited results of the use of these medications are available. Extensive information on chloroquine can be found in Chapter 25.

Systemic ribavirin is also being investigated for treatment and prevention of COVID-19. At the time this textbook went to press (July 2020), the safety and efficacy have not been established.

## Herpesvirus Infections

### Cytomegalovirus Infection and Retinitis

Cytomegalovirus (CMV) infection is common, and most people become infected by adulthood. Infection is usually asymptomatic in healthy, **immunocompetent** adults. Like other **herpesviruses**, CMV can cause a primary infection and then remain latent in body tissues, probably for life. This means the virus can be shed in secretions of an asymptomatic host and spread to others by contact with infected saliva, blood, urine, semen, breast milk, and cervical secretions. It also means the virus may lead to an opportunistic infection when the host becomes immunosuppressed. During pregnancy, CMV is transmitted to the fetus across the placenta and may cause infection in the brain, inner ears, eyes, liver, and bone marrow. Learning disabilities and mental retardation can result from congenital CMV infection. Children spread the virus to each other in saliva or urine, whereas adolescents and adults transmit the virus mainly through sexual contact.

*(Continued on page 436)*

**BOX 23.1** *Selected Viral Infections* (Continued)

Major populations at risk for development of active CMV infection are patients with cancer who receive immunosuppressant drugs and organ transplant recipients, who must receive immunosuppressant drugs to prevent their body's rejection of the transplanted organ. Patients with advanced HIV infection are also at risk, but the incidence has decreased with **active antiretroviral therapy**, or ART. Systemic CMV infection occurs mainly from reactivation of endogenous virus, although it may occur from an exogenous source. Active CMV infection may cause cellular necrosis and inflammation in various body tissues. Common manifestations of disease include pneumonitis, hepatitis, encephalitis, adrenal insufficiency, gastrointestinal inflammation, and gastric ulcerations.

In the eye, CMV infection produces retinitis, usually characterized by blurred vision and decreased visual acuity. Visual impairment is progressive and irreversible and, if untreated, may result in blindness. CMV retinitis may also indicate systemic CMV infection or may be entirely asymptomatic.

### Genital Herpes Infection

**Genital herpes** infection is caused by the herpes simplex virus (HSV) and produces recurrent, painful, blister-like lesions on skin and mucous membranes. HSV is usually transmitted from person to person by direct contact with open lesions or secretions, including genital secretions. Primary infection occurs at a site of viral entry, where the virus infects epithelial cells, produces progeny viruses, and eventually causes cell death. After primary infection, latent virus may become dormant within sensory nerve cells. In response to various stimuli (e.g., intense sunlight, emotional stress, febrile illness, menstruation), latent virus may become reactivated and lead to viral reproduction and shedding.

In the fetus, HSV may be transmitted from an infected birth canal, and neonatal herpes is a serious complication of maternal genital herpes. Neonatal herpes usually becomes evident within the first week of life and may be manifested by the typical clusters of blister-like lesions on skin or mucous membranes. Irritability, lethargy, jaundice, altered blood clotting, respiratory distress, seizures, or coma may also occur. The lesions may heal in 1 to 2 weeks, but neonatal herpes carries a high mortality rate. In immunosuppressed patients, HSV infection may result in severe, systemic disease.

### Herpes Zoster

Herpes zoster is caused by the varicella–zoster virus, which is highly contagious and present worldwide. Most children in the United States are infected by early school age. The virus produces chickenpox on first exposure and is spread from person to person by the respiratory route or by contact with secretions from skin lesions. Recovery from the primary infection leaves latent infection in nerve cells. Reactivation of the latent infection (usually later in life) causes herpes zoster (more commonly known as "shingles"), a localized cluster of painful, blister-like skin lesions. The skin lesions have the same appearance as those of chickenpox and genital herpes. Over several days, the vesicles become pustules and then rupture and heal. Because the virus remains in sensory nerve cells, pain can persist for months after the skin lesions heal. Most cases of herpes zoster infection occur among the elderly and the immunocompromised.

### Human Immunodeficiency Virus Infection

**Human immunodeficiency virus (HIV)** infection is caused by a **retrovirus** that infects the immune system. Two types of HIV virus have been identified: HIV-1 and HIV-2. Most infections in the United States are caused by HIV-1; HIV-2 infections occur mainly in Africa. HIV binds to receptors on the surface of CD4+ cells (especially T lymphocytes or helper T cells). HIV entry and replication eventually results in cell death. Because CD4+ cells play major roles in regulating immune function, their destruction results in serious impairment of the immune system.

The initial phase of HIV infection is characterized by influenza-like symptoms (e.g., fever, chills, muscle aches) that may last several weeks. During this time, the virus undergoes rapid replication. The next phase is characterized by a dramatic decline in the rate of viral replication, attributed to a partially effective immune response. During this phase, no visible manifestations of HIV infection may be present. However, replication of HIV continues and antibodies may be detected in the serum. During this period, the person is seropositive (HIV+) and infectious but asymptomatic. Eventually, the immune system is substantially damaged and the rate of viral reproduction accelerates. When **viral load** and immunodeficiency reach significant levels, the illness is termed acquired human immunodeficiency syndrome (AIDS) and serious opportunistic infections occur. With effective drug therapy, viral load decreases and the CD4+ cell count increases, so that HIV-infected people may live for many years without progression to AIDS.

HIV infection occurs in all age groups and can spread to a new host during any phase of infection. The virus is commonly spread by sexual intercourse, injection of intravenous drugs with contaminated needles, and mucous membrane contact with infected blood or body fluids and perinatally from mother to fetus. Although the virus is found in most body fluids, infection has primarily been associated with exposure to blood, semen, or vaginal secretions. The virus is not spread through casual contact. Health care workers may be infected by needlestick injuries. They should be aware that postexposure prophylaxis is available and may significantly reduce the risk of transmission.

### Human Papillomavirus (HPV) Infection

HPV infection, the most common sexually transmitted infection, is spread by contact with infected lesions. It affects both men and women and can cause genital warts and several types of cancer (e.g., cervical, vaginal, vulvar, anal, and penile). In women, 80% reportedly become infected within 5 years of becoming sexually active.

### Respiratory Syncytial Virus Infection

Respiratory syncytial virus (RSV) is a highly contagious virus that is present worldwide and infects most children by school age. Epidemics of RSV infection often occur in nurseries, day care centers, and pediatric hospital units during winter months. RSV infects and destroys respiratory epithelium in the bronchi, bronchioles, and alveoli. It is spread by respiratory droplets and secretions, direct contact with an infected person, and contact with fomites, including the hands of caregivers.

| BOX 23.1 | *Selected Viral Infections* (Continued) |
|---|---|

RSV is the most common cause of bronchiolitis and pneumonia in infants and causes severe illness in those younger than 6 months of age. These infants usually have wheezing, cough, respiratory distress, and fever. The infection is usually self-limited and resolves in 1 to 2 weeks. Antiviral therapy with ribavirin is used in some cases. The mortality rate from RSV infection is low in children who are generally healthy but increases substantially in those with congenital heart disease or immunosuppression. Recurrent infection occurs but is usually less severe than primary infection. In older children, RSV infection produces much milder disease but may be associated with acute exacerbations of asthma.

In adults, RSV infection causes colds and bronchitis, with symptoms of fever, cough, and nasal congestion. Infection occurs most often in those with household or other close contact with children, including pediatric health care workers. In older adults, RSV infection may cause pneumonia requiring hospitalization. In immunocompromised patients, RSV infection may cause severe and potentially fatal pneumonia.

### Viral Hepatitis

There are several types of viral **hepatitis**, and new hepatitis viruses are still being identified. Worldwide, viral hepatitis has increased in recent years. All hepatitis viruses have similar effects on the liver, although they differ in some other characteristics. Common types of viral hepatitis are described below. Vaccines are available to prevent hepatitis A and B (see Chap. 12).

Hepatitis A virus (HAV) is transmitted mainly by the fecal–oral route and close contact with an infected person; foodborne outbreaks also occur, usually from infected food handlers or contaminated produce in the United States. The virus survives for long periods in the environment (e.g., in water and soil) and on human hands and inanimate objects. It resists freezing, detergents, and acids but can be inactivated by chlorine and temperatures above 185°F.

The HAV reproduces only in liver and gastrointestinal cells, from which viral particles are released into blood and bile. The average incubation period is 25 to 30 days. The patient is infectious during the incubation period and for 7 to 10 days after symptoms develop. In infected adults, about 70% develop symptoms, including fever and jaundice, that may last as long as 2 months. Most recover without treatment and develop immunity against future HAV infections; 10% to 20% require hospitalization. In children, many are asymptomatic or develop flulike or nonspecific symptoms without jaundice. However, even children with few or no symptoms may shed virus in their stools and be a source of community infection for as long as 6 months. The availability of hepatitis A vaccine has greatly decreased the number of reported cases. The vaccine is recommended for children and adults at increased risk of contracting the disease (e.g., travelers to certain countries, men who have sex with men, drug abusers, recipients of clotting factor replacement) and for persons with chronic liver disease.

Hepatitis B virus (HBV) can be transmitted by contact with contaminated blood and other body fluids (e.g., perinatally, during sexual contact with an infected person, by sharing needles during IV drug use, and by undergoing acupuncture, hemodialysis, tattooing, or ear and body piercing). In addition, health care and public safety workers are at increased risk of developing HBV infection from injuries with contaminated equipment (e.g., contaminated needles) and from other exposures to infected body fluid. Any person exposed to infected body fluids should be evaluated for HBV infection; any person diagnosed with HBV infection should be evaluated for liver disease and for HIV infection. It is estimated that 70,000 Americans become infected with HBV every year and approximately 5000 of them will die of the complications caused by the infection. Many Americans have chronic HBV infection; asymptomatic chronic carriers of HBV may transmit the infection to others. Hepatitis B can lead to cirrhosis, liver cancer, liver failure, and death.

The HBV can live up to 3 days on various surfaces that appear clean. The incubation period is 30 to 180 days. Increased hepatitis B surface antigens and liver enzymes (ALT, AST) occur before symptoms of HBV infection develop. After symptoms develop, antibodies to the viral antigens are produced and the presence of antigens and viral DNA in the patient's blood indicate that the patient is infectious.

Hepatitis C virus (HCV) can be transmitted by contact with contaminated blood or other body fluids. Persons at high risk of exposure include health care and public safety workers; IV drug users; those with multiple sex partners; those undergoing hemodialysis, tattoos, or body piercings; and those who received blood transfusions before 1990, when screening blood for HCV was started. In addition, pregnant women may transmit the virus to their infants, and mothers with symptoms and high viral titers may transmit the virus to nursing infants.

The HCV incubation period is 14 to 80 days; infection is diagnosed by testing for viral DNA or antibodies. HCV infection affects people of all ages but is most often found among 20- to 39-year-olds. Infected persons can be asymptomatic for years, but most eventually develop chronic liver disease. In the United States, HCV infection is the leading cause of cirrhosis, liver cancer, and liver transplants. Effective drug therapy may cure HCV infection.

Other hepatitis viruses (e.g., D, G, and a "transfusion-transmissible" virus) have been identified; they, like HBV and HCV, are transmitted through contact with infected blood and body fluids.

The protein coat of the virus allows the immune system of the host to recognize the virus as a "foreign invader" and to produce antibodies against it. This system works well for most viruses but does not work for the influenza A virus, which can alter its protein covering so much and so often that the immune system does not recognize it as foreign to the body. Thus, last year's antibody cannot recognize and neutralize this year's virus.

Antibodies against infecting viruses can prevent the viruses from reaching the bloodstream or, if they are already in the bloodstream, prevent their invasion of host cells. After the virus has penetrated the cell, it is protected from antibody action, and the host depends on cell-mediated immunity (lymphocytes and macrophages) to eradicate the virus along with the cell harboring it.

## Clinical Manifestations

Viral infection may occur without signs and symptoms of illness. If illness does occur, the clinical course is usually short and self-limited. Recovery occurs as the virus is eliminated from the body. Some viruses (e.g., herpesvirus) can survive in host cells for many years and cause a chronic, latent infection that periodically becomes reactivated. Also, autoimmune diseases may be caused by viral alteration of host cells so that lymphocytes recognize the host's own tissues as being foreign.

Symptoms usually associated with acute viral infections include fever, headache, cough, malaise, muscle pain, nausea and vomiting, diarrhea, insomnia, and photophobia. White blood cell counts usually remain normal. Other signs and symptoms vary with the type of virus and body organs involved.

## Drug Therapy

Scientists have developed several vaccines (see Chap. 12) to prevent viral infections as well as numerous drugs to treat HIV and other viral infections. Most of these antiviral drugs inhibit viral reproduction but do not eliminate viruses from tissues. In general, available drugs are expensive, relatively toxic, and effective in a limited number of infections. Some may be useful in treating an established infection if given promptly and in chemoprophylaxis if given before or soon after exposure. Protection conferred by chemoprophylaxis is immediate but lasts only while the drug is being taken. The remainder of this chapter describes the subgroups of antiviral drugs. Table 23.1 summarizes the medications used to treat viral infections.

# DRUGS FOR HERPESVIRUS INFECTIONS

## DRUGS FOR HERPES SIMPLEX VIRUS AND VARICELLA–ZOSTER VIRUS

The herpesviruses include herpes simplex virus (HSV), varicella–zoster virus (VZV), and cytomegalovirus (CMV). There are two types of herpes viral infections: HSV-1 and HSV-2. HSV-1 causes fever blisters or cold sores on the lips, mouth, or face, and HSV-2 causes genital warts. **Acyclovir (Zovirax)**, the prototype antiviral agent used to combat the herpesviruses, is an oral, parenteral, and topical antiviral drug.

## Pharmacokinetics

After oral administration, the body absorbs 15% to 30% of the acyclovir dosage, reaching a peak of action in 1.5 to 2 hours. The drug is distributed to the tissues of the lower levels distributed

### TABLE 23.1

## Drugs Administered for the Treatment of Viral Infections

| Drug Class/Type | Prototype | Other Drugs in the Class/Related Drugs |
|---|---|---|
| **Drugs for herpesvirus infections** | | |
| Drugs for herpes simplex virus and varicella–zoster virus | Acyclovir (Zovirax) | Docosanol (Abreva)<br>Famciclovir<br>Penciclovir (Denavir)<br>Trifluridine<br>Valacyclovir (Valtrex) |
| Drugs for cytomegalovirus | Ganciclovir (Cytovene) | Cidofovir<br>Foscarnet (Foscavir)<br>Valganciclovir (Valcyte) |
| **Drugs for respiratory syncytial virus** | | |
| Antiviral agent | Ribavirin (Virazole) | |
| Monoclonal antibody | Palivizumab (Synagis) | |
| **Drugs for influenza** | | |
| Adamantanes | Amantadine hydrochloride (Gocovri, Osmolex ER) | Rimantadine |
| Endonuclease inhibitor | Baloxavir marboxil (Xofluza) | Peramivir (Rapivab)<br>Zanamivir (Relenza) |
| **Drugs for hepatitis B: nucleoside analogs** | | |
| | Lamivudine (Epivir, Epivir-HBV) | Adefovir dipivoxil (Hepsera)<br>Entecavir (Baraclude)<br>Ribavirin<br>Tenofovir alafenamide (Vemlidy)<br>Tenofovir disoproxil fumarate (Viread) |
| **Drugs for hepatitis C: polymerase inhibitors** | | |
| | Sofosbuvir (Solvaldi) | |

## TABLE 23.1

### Drugs Administered for the Treatment of Viral Infections (Continued)

| Drug Class/Type | Prototype | Other Drugs in the Class/Related Drugs |
|---|---|---|
| **Antiretroviral drugs** | | |
| Nucleoside/nucleotide reverse transcriptase inhibitors (NRTIs) | Zidovudine (Retrovir) | Abacavir sulfate (Ziagen) <br> Abacavir, lamivudine, and zidovudine (Trizivir) <br> Didanosine <br> Dolutegravir and lamivudine (Dovato) <br> Dolutegravir, abacavir, and lamivudine (Triumeq) <br> Elvitegravir, cobicistat, emtricitabine, and tenofovir disoproxil fumarate (Stribild) <br> Emtricitabine (Emtriva) <br> Emtricitabine and tenofovir (Truvada) <br> Emtricitabine, tenofovir, efavirenz (Atripla) <br> Lamivudine (Epivir, Epivir HBV) <br> Stavudine <br> Tenofovir disoproxil fumarate (Viread) <br> Zidovudine and lamivudine (Combivir) |
| Nonnucleoside/nonnucleotide reverse transcriptase inhibitors (NNRTIs) | Efavirenz (Sustiva) | Delavirdine mesylate <br> Etravirine (Intelence) <br> Nevirapine (Viramune) <br> Rilpivirine (Edurant) |
| Protease inhibitors (PIs) | Saquinavir mesylate (Invirase) | Atazanavir (Reyataz) <br> Darunavir (Prezista) <br> Fosamprenavir calcium (Lexiva) <br> Indinavir sulfate (Crixivan) <br> Lopinavir/ritonavir (Kaletra) <br> Nelfinavir mesylate (Viracept) <br> Ritonavir (Norvir) <br> Tipranavir (Aptivus) |
| Integrase strand transfer inhibitors (INSTIs) | Raltegravir (Isentress, Isentress HD) | Dolutegravir (Tivicay) |
| Fusion protein inhibitors | Enfuvirtide (Fuzeon) | |
| CCR5 antagonists | Maraviroc (Selzentry) | |
| P-450 Inhibitor | Cobicistat (Tybost) | |
| Integrase inhibitor, reverse transcriptase inhibitor, nucleoside, reverse transcriptase inhibitor, nucleotide | Ⓟ Bictegravir, emtricitabine, and tenofovir alafenamide (Biktarvy) | |

to the central nervous system (CNS). It is 9% to 33% protein bound and has a half-life of 2 to 3.5 hours. Acyclovir crosses the placenta and enters the breast milk. Excretion of unchanged drug occurs in the urine.

## Action

Following uptake by infected cells, acyclovir is converted to acyclovir monophosphate by the enzyme thymidine kinase. Acyclovir triphosphate inhibits DNA polymerase, thus interrupting viral DNA replication. This action reduces viral shedding and prevents formation of new lesions.

## Use

Immunocompromised patients take acyclovir for initial and recurrent cutaneous and mucosal HSV and VZV. Prescribers

also order the drug for the treatment of genital herpes (a herpesvirus that appears on the genitals); it decreases viral shedding as well as the duration of skin lesions and pain. Acyclovir does not eliminate inactive virus in the body and thus does not prevent recurrence of the disease unless oral drug therapy is continued. However, prolonged or repeated courses of drug therapy may result in the emergence of acyclovir-resistant viral strains, especially in immunocompromised patients. In patients with an altered immune response, authorities recommend the intravenous (IV) form for severe genital herpes, and nonimmunocompromised patients should also receive IV preparations. Acyclovir is effective against the herpes simplex virus. Parenteral acyclovir is used to treat viral encephalitis. It is administered orally for the treatment of HSV and VZV. Table 23.2 presents route and dosage information for acyclovir and other drugs used for HSV and VZV.

| TABLE 23.2 |
|---|
| **DRUGS AT A GLANCE: Drugs for Herpes Simplex Virus (HSV) and Varicella–Zoster Virus (VZV)** |

| Drug | Pregnancy Category | Routes and Dosage Ranges | |
|---|---|---|---|
| | | **Adults** | **Children** |
| **Acyclovir** (Zovirax; ✳ APO-Acyclovir, MYLAN-Acyclovir, TEVA-Acyclovir, Zovirax) | B | Genital herpes: 200 mg PO every 4 h, five times daily for 10 d for initial infection; 400 mg two times daily to prevent recurrence of chronic infection; 200 mg every 4 h five times daily for 5 d to treat recurrence<br>Herpes zoster: 800 mg PO every 4 h five times daily for 7–10 d<br>Chickenpox: 20 mg/kg PO (max dose 800 mg) four times daily for 5 d<br>Mucosal and cutaneous HSV infections in ICH: 5 mg/kg IV infused over 1 h, every 8 h for 7 d<br>VZV in ICH: 10 mg/kg IV infused over 1 h, every 8 h for 7 d<br>HSV encephalitis: 10 mg/kg IV infused over 1 h, every 8 h for 10 d<br>Topically to lesions every 3 h six times daily for 7 d | Younger than 12 y<br>10 or 20 mg/kg IV every 8 h for 7 or 10 d, depending on the condition being treated—chickenpox:<br>2 y and older and weight 40 kg or less, 20 mg/kg PO four times daily for 5 d<br>Weight above 40 kg, 800 mg PO four times daily for 5 d<br>12 y and older, topical, same as adults |
| Docosanol (Abreva) | C | Topically to lesions five times daily for up to 10 d | Older than 12 y: adult dosage |
| Famciclovir (✳ ACT-Famciclovir, APO-Famciclovir, Famvir, PMS Famciclovir, SANDOZ Famciclovir) | B | Herpes zoster: 500 mg PO every 8 h for 7 d<br>Genital herpes: 125 mg PO twice daily for 5 d | Safety and efficacy not established |
| Penciclovir (Denavir) | B | Topically every 2 h while awake for 4 d | Safety and efficacy not established |
| Trifluridine (✳ APO-Trifluridine, Viroptic) | C | Topically 1 drop in affected eye every 2 h: maximum dose 9 drops per day: when healing is complete reduce dose to 1 drop every 4 h for 7 d: maximum dose drops per day | ≥6 y: topically 1 drop in affected eye every 2 h: maximum dose 9 drops per day: when healing is complete reduce dose to 1 drop every 4 h for 7 d: maximum dose drops per day |
| Valacyclovir (Valtrex; ✳ APO-Valacyclovir, AURA-Valacyclovir, BIO-Valacyclovir, DOM-Valacyclovir, JAMP-Valacyclovir, MAR-Valacyclovir, SANDOZ-Valacyclovir, Valtrex) | B | Herpes labialis: 2 g PO twice daily for 1 d<br>Herpes zoster: 1 g PO every 8 h for 7 d<br>Recurrent genital herpes: PO 500 mg PO every 12 h daily for 5 d<br>Reduce dosage with renal impairment | Herpes labialis: adolescents, same as adults<br>Safety not established |

ICH, immunocompromised host.

## Use in Patients With Renal Impairment

There have been reports of renal failure with acyclovir use. It is necessary to reduce the dosage of acyclovir in patients with altered renal function according to the creatinine clearance (CrCl). In patients who are on hemodialysis, the half-life of acyclovir is approximately 5 hours.

## Use in Children

The half-life of acyclovir in neonates is 4 hours—longer than in adults. The treatment of HSV gingivostomatitis is an off-label use of acyclovir in infants and children.

## Adverse Effects

Acyclovir has minimal adverse effects. The most commonly reported adverse effects are malaise, headache, nausea, vomiting, and diarrhea. The parenteral form may lead to phlebitis at the injection site, hives, itching, rash, nausea, vomiting, elevated liver enzymes, and acute renal failure. The parenteral form may result in encephalopathy, a rare but potentially serious adverse effect. Other serious drug-related effects include thrombocytopenia purpura and hemolytic uremic syndrome.

## Contraindications

Contraindications to acyclovir include a known hypersensitivity to the drug, heart failure, renal disease, and lactation. Caution is necessary in patients who are receiving nephrotoxic agents.

## Nursing Implications

### Preventing Interactions

The most significant interactions with acyclovir include increased serum concentrations with probenecid, drowsiness with zidovudine, and renal insufficiency when combined with medications that cause renal toxicity. Hydantoins and valproic acid combined with acyclovir lead to decreased antiepileptic effects, placing patients at risk for seizure activity. The use of acyclovir and theophylline results in theophylline toxicity.

### Administering the Medication

With the topical preparation of acyclovir, it is important to wash the hands thoroughly prior to administration and apply with a gloved hand. It is crucial that the medication be prescribed and therapy started as soon as symptoms arise. With the oral medication, patients may take the drug without respect to food intake. With the parenteral form of acyclovir, it is necessary to infuse it over 1 hour to prevent renal damage. The nurse ensures that the patient is well hydrated with 2 to 3 L of fluid per 24 hours. Acyclovir is incompatible with blood products and protein-containing solutions. In patients who are obese, it is essential to calculate acyclovir dosages according to ideal body weight.

### Assessing for Therapeutic Effects

The nurse assesses for the healing of lesions, decreased pain, and itching. When administering acyclovir prophylactically for genital herpes, he or she assesses for fewer recurrences.

### Assessing for Adverse Effects

The nurse assesses for signs and symptoms of hypersensitivity to the acyclovir. With the topical drug, he or she assesses for burning, stinging, and pruritus. With the parenteral drug, the nurse assesses for phlebitis at the injection site. It is also necessary to assess for confusion, coma, seizures, and tremors. In addition, the nurse assesses the aspartate aminotransferase (AST) and alanine aminotransferase (ALT) for elevations, as well as blood urea nitrogen (BUN) and serum creatinine for increases.

### Patient Teaching

Box 23.2 identifies general patient teaching guidelines for the antiviral drugs.

## Other Drugs in the Class

Docosanol (Abreva) is an over-the-counter topical antiviral agent that works in the early stages of intracellular events of viral entry into the target cells. This action of the drug makes viral entry into the cell difficult, thus preventing viral replication. Uses include the treatment of HSV of the face and lips. The patient should notify his or her primary health care provider if symptoms do not resolve in 10 days.

Famciclovir is an oral antiviral agent administered for herpes zoster and recurrent genital herpes. It has greater

---

**BOX 23.2    Patient Teaching Guidelines for Antiviral Drugs**

- Prevention is better than treatment, partly because medications used to treat viral infections may cause serious adverse effects. Thus, whenever possible, it is important to use techniques to prevent viral infections, such as limiting exposure with those infected with a viral illness.
- Wash hands thoroughly for 20 seconds and do so frequently; this helps prevent most infections.
- Do not touch your face.
- Have immunizations against viral infections as indicated.
- With genital herpes, avoid sexual intercourse when visible lesions are present and always wash hands after touching any lesion.
- Understand that drugs may relieve symptoms but do not cure viral infections. For example, treatment of genital herpes does not prevent transmission to others, and treatment of cytomegalovirus (CMV) retinitis may not prevent disease progression.
- Ask a health care provider for information about managing adverse drug effects.
- If taking foscarnet or ganciclovir for CMV retinitis, have eye examinations approximately every 6 weeks.
- If taking ganciclovir, maintain regular appointments for the assessment of the complete blood count and renal function.
- Administer antiviral agents for recurrent genital herpes lesions as soon as signs and symptoms begin.
- Use gloves to apply topical antiviral ointment to lesions.

---

bioavailability than does acyclovir and is administered less frequently. A prodrug, famciclovir is metabolized to penciclovir, its active form, and is excreted mainly in the urine. Drug therapy should be started within 72 hours of the appearance of a rash or within 6 hours of the onset of genital herpes lesions. A CrCl less than 60 mL/min necessitates a dosage reduction. For patients receiving hemodialysis, dosage is calculated according to CrCl, with daily doses given after dialysis. Adverse effects of the medication include purpura, headache, nausea, vomiting, dizziness, paresthesias, and constipation. Patients on extended drug therapy should have periodic complete blood counts (CBCs) to identify blood dyscrasias.

Penciclovir (Denavir) is a topical drug used for the treatment of recurrent herpes labialis. The cold sore minimally absorbs the drug. The patient should apply the ointment every 2 hours for 4 days. If the lesion does not improve, it is important to notify the primary health care provider.

Trifluridine is an ophthalmic drug used to treat primary keratoconjunctivitis and recurring epithelial keratitis caused by type 1 or 2 HSV (see Chap. 59).

Valacyclovir (Valtrex) penetrates virus-infected cells, becomes activated by an enzyme, and inhibits viral DNA reproduction. Uses include the treatment of herpes simplex and herpes zoster infections. Metabolism occurs in the liver, and excretion takes place in the kidneys. In patients with renal impairment, the drug may accumulate, produce higher blood levels, have a longer half-life, and cause toxicity. Like famciclovir, valacyclovir has greater bioavailability than does acyclovir and is administered less frequently.

## NCLEX Success

1. A man with a fever, cough, and clear drainage from the nose presents to the clinic. A nurse practitioner diagnoses a viral infection. Which of the following describes the replication of the viral infection?

   A. The RNA of an infected person has invaded the man's mucous membranes.
   B. There are breaks in the cell membrane of the infected cells.
   C. Antibodies are defending against microbial cell invasion.
   D. The white blood cell count increases.

2. Why would patients with genital herpes receive acyclovir?

   A. It decreases viral shedding and pain related to outbreak.
   B. It eliminates future viral outbreaks.
   C. It prevents sterility in infected patients.
   D. It prevents the development of cytomegalovirus.

3. A woman is using topical acyclovir. Which of the following is the most important intervention to instruct the patient regarding medication administration?

   A. Administer the medication after meals to enhance absorption.
   B. Discontinue the medication when lesions are crusted over.
   C. Apply the medication to the lesions with a gloved hand.
   D. Increase oral fluids to enhance healing.

4. A man has an elevated uric acid level, and he receives a prescription for probenecid. He also has cold sores on his mouth due to exposure to the sun, which is being treated with acyclovir. What effect will occur with the administration of these medications?

   A. decreased serum acyclovir
   B. elevated aspartate aminotransferase and alanine aminotransferase
   C. increased serum uric acid
   D. increased serum acyclovir

5. A woman experiences recurrences of herpes simplex, with an outbreak on her lips. Which medication can she apply in the early stages of the viral illness?

   A. docosanol
   B. valganciclovir
   C. Neosporin
   D. tobramycin

### Clinical Application 23.1

- What is a cold sore? How does valacyclovir work to decrease Ms. Jackson's symptoms and ultimately heal the cold sore?
- What patient teaching does the nurse provide to Ms. Jackson?

## DRUGS FOR CYTOMEGALOVIRUS

CMV is a type of herpesvirus. The first agent developed for the treatment of CMV infection was **ganciclovir (Cytovene)**, the prototype. Prescribers use ganciclovir to treat CMV in immunocompromised patients, including those with AIDS and patients who have received transplants.

## Pharmacokinetics

With oral administration, the onset of action of ganciclovir is 2 to 4 hours, and with IV administration, the onset of action is 1 hour. The drug is distributed widely to all tissues, including the cerebrospinal fluid (CSF) and eye tissue. The half-life is 1.7 to 5.8 hours, and in renal impairment, the half-life is prolonged. It is excreted unchanged in the urine.

## Action

Like acyclovir, ganciclovir inhibits viral DNA synthesis. It is changed to a substrate that inhibits the binding of deoxyguanosine triphosphate to DNA polymerase.

## Use

The IV form of ganciclovir is for the treatment of CMV retinitis in immunocompromised patients. Also, this preparation is for the treatment or prevention of CMV in transplant recipients. Patients take oral ganciclovir for the prevention of CMV if they have advanced HIV infection or are at risk for disease development. In 2009, the Centers for Disease Control and Prevention (CDC) identified an unlabeled use of intravitreal ganciclovir plus systemic foscarnet for the treatment of VZV in patients with progressive outer retinal necrosis in patients with HIV. Table 23.3 summarizes route and dosage information for ganciclovir and related drugs.

### Use in Older Adults

Ganciclovir administration should proceed cautiously in older adults, who often have impaired organ function, have concomitant diseases, and use other drugs. Renal impairment is common in older adults, and risk of toxicity is greater because excretion of the drug occurs in the kidneys. Dose reduction, when indicated by decreased CrCl, may minimize these risks.

### Use in Patients With Renal Impairment

It is necessary to reduce the dosage of ganciclovir according to the CrCl. Hemodialysis patients should receive ganciclovir following dialysis. The IV dosage for dialysis patients is 1.25 mg/kg every 48 to 72 hours, with a maintenance dose of 0.625 mg/kg every 48 to 72 hours.

## TABLE 23.3

## DRUGS AT A GLANCE: Drugs for Cytomegalovirus (CMV)

| Drug | Pregnancy Category | Routes and Dosage Ranges | |
|---|---|---|---|
| | | **Adults** | **Children** |
| **Ganciclovir** (Cytovene; ❀ Cytovene) | C | CMV retinitis: induction therapy, 5 mg/kg/dose IV every 12 h for 14–21 d; maintenance therapy, 5 mg/kg/dose as a single daily dose for 7 d/wk or 6 mg/kg/d for 5 d/wk<br>Prevention of CMV disease in transplant patients: same as induction and maintenance therapy, but the induction course is 7–14 d | CMV CNS disease in HIV-exposed patients: 5 mg/kg/dose every 12 h plus foscarnet until symptoms improve followed by chronic suppression<br>CMV retinitis: same as adult dose (slow infusion)<br>Prevention of CMV in transplant patients: same as adult dose<br>Neonatal congenital CMV: 6 mg/kg/dose every 12 h for 6 wk; if HIV positive, a longer duration of therapy is considered |
| Cidofovir (❀ MAR-Cidofovir)<br>**Note:** Probenecid must be administered with each dose (25–40 mg/kg/dose in children) | C | Induction therapy, 5 mg/kg IV once weekly for 2 consecutive weeks; maintenance therapy, 5 mg/kg IV every 2 wk. Administer 1 L of normal saline IV before each infusion over 1–2 h and 1 L at the start of the infusion or immediately following over 1–3 h | Induction therapy, 5 mg/kg/dose IV once weekly for 2 consecutive weeks; maintenance therapy, 5 mg/kg/dose IV once every 2 wk until consecutive negative adenovirus sample. Hydrate with 20 mL/kg of normal saline for 1 h before induction therapy followed by 2 h of maintenance fluid |
| Foscarnet (Foscavir) | C | CMV retinitis: induction therapy, 60 mg/kg/dose IV every 8 h for 14–21 d or 90 mg/k IV every 12 h for 14–21 d; maintenance therapy, 90–120 mg every 12 h for 2 wk, followed by 120 mg/kg daily for ≥2 wk<br>Acyclovir-resistant HSV: 40 mg/kg/dose IV every 8–12 h for 14–21 d | CMV CNS disease: 60 mg/kg/dose IV every 8 h in combination with ganciclovir followed by 90–120 mg/kg/dose daily<br>CMV retinitis: 60 mg/kg/dose IV every 8 h for 14–21 d with or without ganciclovir followed by 90–120 mg/kg/dose daily<br>Acyclovir-resistant herpes simplex: 40–60 mg/kg/dose IV every 8 h until lesions heal<br>Chickenpox not responding to acyclovir: 40–60 mg/kg/dose IV every 8 h for 7–10 d |
| Valganciclovir (Valcyte; ❀ APO-AURA-Valganciclovir, TEVA-Valganciclovir, Valcyte) | C | CMV retinitis: 900 mg PO twice daily for 21 d, then 900 mg PO once daily<br>Prevention of CMV disease following kidney or heart transplant: 900 mg PO once daily beginning within 10 d of transplant; continue therapy until 100 d with heart or kidney transplant or 200 d for kidney transplant | 1–3 mo, 16 mg/kg/dose PO every 12 h<br>4 mo to 16 y, dose in mg = 7 × body surface × CrCl (begin within 10 d of transplant and continue until 100 d posttransplant); doses should be rounded to the nearest 25-mg increment; max dose 900 mg/d. |

## Adverse Effects

Adverse effects of ganciclovir include chills, fever, pruritus, anorexia, nausea, vomiting, anemia, leukopenia, neutropenia, thrombocytopenia, neuropathy, retinal detachment, hematuria, and sepsis. There may be increases in BUN and serum creatinine. Ganciclovir causes granulocytopenia and thrombocytopenia in 20% to 40% of recipients, often during the first 2 weeks of therapy. The U.S. Food and Drug Administration (FDA) has issued a **BLACK BOX WARNING ◆** for ganciclovir; granulocytopenia (neutropenia), anemia, and thrombocytopenia may occur. If severe bone marrow depression occurs, it is essential that the drug be discontinued; recovery usually occurs within a week of stopping the drug. A second **BLACK BOX WARNING ◆** advises female and male patients of childbearing age to maintain contraceptive precautions during ganciclovir therapy and for a minimum of 90 days after drug therapy.

## Contraindications

Patients should not receive ganciclovir if their neutrophil count is less than 500/mm³ or a platelet count below 25,000/mm³. A known hypersensitivity to ganciclovir or any of the antiviral agents is also a contraindication. Caution is warranted in renal impairment.

## Nursing Implications

### Preventing Interactions

Several drugs interact with ganciclovir. Imipenem combined with ganciclovir increases the risk of seizure activity.

Amphotericin B, antineoplastic agents, didanosine, dapsone, pentamidine, probenecid, trimethoprim–sulfamethoxazole, and zidovudine administered with ganciclovir increase the risk of bone marrow suppression. Cyclosporine and ganciclovir result in nephrotoxicity. Mycophenolate, probenecid, and tenofovir increase the serum concentration of ganciclovir–valganciclovir.

Some foods and herbs interact with ganciclovir (Box 23.3).

### Administering the Medication

Parenteral ganciclovir requires slow infusion, over at least 1 hour. Too rapid administration results in toxicity and excessive plasma levels. The medication is compatible with 5% dextrose and water, lactated Ringer's, and normal saline. Administration using intramuscular, subcutaneous, or IV push is contraindicated. Ganciclovir is a hazardous medication, and it is necessary to use appropriate precautions for handling and disposal. The nurse checks the manufacturer's guidelines and does not allow the powder or the reconstituted medication to touch the skin. The nurse does not administer the drug to patients with a platelet count less than 25,000/mm$^3$ or a neutrophil count less than 500/mm$^3$.

### Assessing for Therapeutic Effects

The nurse assesses the patient for improvement in vision and visual acuity related to retinitis. It is also important to assess for improvement in symptoms related to pneumonia, hepatitis, encephalitis, adrenal insufficiency, and gastrointestinal (GI) inflammation or ulcerations.

### Assessing for Adverse Effects

The nurse assesses BUN, creatinine, CrCl, CBC, and platelet count for impaired renal function and bone marrow depression. He or she assesses for signs and symptoms of hypersensitivity reactions. It is important to assess for neuropathic changes such as pain and diminished sensation.

### Patient Teaching

Box 23.2 identifies general patient teaching guidelines for the antiviral drugs.

## Other Drugs in the Class

Cidofovir is an IV drug indicated for treatment of CMS retinitis in patients with AIDS. After conversion to cidofovir diphosphate, it suppresses CMV replication by selective inhibition of viral DNA synthesis. Distribution in the CSF is limited. If the patient's serum creatinine increases by 0.3 to 0.4 mg/dL, it is necessary to reduce the dose to 3 mg/kg. If the creatinine is greater than 1.5 mg/dL, it is important to discontinue therapy. The FDA

has issued three **BLACK BOX WARNING** ◆ for cidofovir. The drug has possible carcinogenic and teratogenic adverse effects. It may also be nephrotoxic, and prior to administration, the patient should receive 1 L of normal saline and oral probenecid. In addition, it places the patient at risk for neutropenia.

Foscarnet (Foscavir) is an IV drug administered for CMV retinitis, acyclovir-resistant HSV, and other CMV infections related to diminished immune response. The infusion rate should not exceed 1 mg/kg/min. When given by central venous access, it is possible to administer 24 mg/mL undiluted, but when given through a peripheral vein, it is necessary to dilute the solution to 12 mg/mL. The nurse gives 750 to 1000 mL of normal saline or 5% dextrose and water to initiate diuresis. The patient should be well hydrated throughout the infusion of the medication. In addition to the warning related to potential renal impairment, the FDA has issued a **BLACK BOX WARNING** ◆ regarding seizures with use of foscarnet, which may occur related to impaired renal function, diminished serum calcium, and CNS conditions. It is important to use foscarnet cautiously in patients with renal disease and to assess for signs of renal impairment. Manifestations of renal impairment are most likely to occur during the second week of induction therapy but may appear any time during treatment. To minimize renal impairment, it helps to monitor renal function (e.g., at baseline; two or three times weekly during induction; at least every 1 or 2 weeks during maintenance therapy) and reduce the dosage accordingly. If the CrCl drops below 0.4 mL/min/kg, it is necessary to discontinue the drug.

Valganciclovir (Valcyte) is an oral drug administered for CMV retinitis and prevention of CMV infections following organ transplant. The medication inhibits viral reproduction after it is activated by a viral enzyme found in virus-infected cells. Valganciclovir has the same **BLACK BOX WARNING** ◆ as ganciclovir. Patients should take this drug with a high-fat diet to enhance absorption.

## NCLEX Success

6. **A man with human immunodeficiency virus is on hemodialysis for renal failure. Cytomegalovirus retinitis develops. Which of the following is most important when administering ganciclovir?**
   A. Administer the medication on an empty stomach.
   B. Assess the patient's vision following the medication administration.
   C. Administer ganciclovir after dialysis is completed.
   D. Assess the patient's sodium level following dialysis.

7. **A patient receives a prescription for valganciclovir for the prevention of cytomegalovirus infections following organ transplantation. Which of the following nursing interventions should be implemented?**
   A. Instruct the patient to take the medication following a meal high in fat.
   B. Instruct the patient to take the meal with large amounts of fluids.
   C. Instruct the patient to report abdominal pain.
   D. Instruct the patient to report diminished sense of hearing.

# DRUGS FOR RESPIRATORY SYNCYTIAL VIRUS

The prototype Ⓟ **ribavirin** (Virazole), a synthetic nucleoside antiviral drug, is one of the few antiviral drugs that is indicated for use in children. Its main use is for the treatment of respiratory syncytial virus (RSV) infections.

## Pharmacokinetics

Ribavirin, which is inhaled systemically, has a slow onset of action. It reaches its peak of action in 60 to 90 minutes. The medication is metabolized at the cellular level, with a 9.5-hour half-life. It is excreted in the feces and urine.

## Action and Use

Ribavirin inhibits the replication of RNA and DNA viruses to stop the influenza virus RNA polymerase activity. This action interferes with the elongation and initiation of RNA fragments, which stops protein synthesis. Inhaled ribavirin may be effective in infants and children with severe RSV infection of the lower respiratory tract. Table 23.4 presents route and dosage information for ribavirin.

## Adverse Effects

Adverse effects experienced by patients are fatigue, insomnia, headache, anemia, nausea, and anorexia. Less than 1% of the population experiences hypotension, cardiac arrest, conjunctivitis, bronchospasm, apnea, and decline in respiratory function. Health care workers caring for children treated with RSV may report headache, conjunctivitis, nausea, rash, dizziness, chest pain, bronchospasm, pharyngitis, and rhinitis. The FDA has issued a **BLACK BOX WARNING** ◆ for ribavirin; the drug causes significant teratogenic effects, according to animal studies. Pregnant women or those who plan to become pregnant should not care for children receiving inhalation therapy or be in the room when it is being administered.

## Contraindications

Contraindications to ribavirin include a known hypersensitivity to the drug or its components.

## Nursing Implications

### Preventing Interactions

There are no known drug or herb interactions with inhaled ribavirin. However, mixing the drug with other inhaled or aerosol medications is to be avoided.

### Administering the Medication

Administration in a well-ventilated room is necessary; there should be six air exchanges per hour. Patients who are mechanically ventilated require monitoring for malfunction or obstruction of the expiratory valve, which could result in high positive end-expiratory pressures. The nurse should know that when using a SPAG-2 unit for administration, it is important to discard solutions every 24 hours and when the liquid level is low.

### Assess for Therapeutic Effects

The nurse assesses respiratory status, including dyspnea, apnea, labored respirations, nasal flaring, contractions, shallow respirations, wheezing, rales, and rhonchi.

---

### TABLE 23.4

### DRUGS AT A GLANCE: Drugs for Respiratory Syncytial Virus (RSV) Infection

| Drug | Pregnancy Category | Routes and Dosage Ranges | |
|---|---|---|---|
| | | **Adults** | **Children** |
| Ⓟ **Ribavirin** (inhalation)* (Virazole) | X | Inhalation: 2 g over 2 h every 8 h Off-label use: RSV in hematopoietic cell or heart/lung transplant recipients | Inhalation, diluted to a concentration of 20 mg/mL for 12–18 h/d for 3–7 d |
| Ⓟ Palivizumab (Synagis) Monocolonal Antibody | Not for adult use | Not for adult use | Infants and children <24 months: IM 15 mg/kg once monthly throughout RSV season, first dose administered prior to commencement of RSV season; if hospitalized at the start of RSV season, palivizumab should be given 48–72 h before discharge or promptly after discharge The American Association of Pediatrics recommends a maximum of 5 doses per season; if hospitalization occurs for breakthrough RSV infection, monthly prophylaxis should be discontinued for the remainder of the season. |

*Ribavirin for the treatment of hepatitis is found in Table 23.6.

## Assess for Adverse Effects

The nurse assesses level of comfort; crying, grimacing, and anxiety could indicate pain. The level of activity may indicate increased fatigue. The nurse also assesses the airway for bronchospasm or alterations in pulmonary function, including cyanosis. In addition, he or she assesses vital signs for hypotension and changes in cardiac status. In infants, it is important to assess for sudden deterioration of respiratory function at the initiation of oral inhalation of ribavirin. If deterioration in respiratory function is noted, stop the treatment and notify the prescriber. If the oral inhalation ribavirin is reinstated, the infant should be continuously monitored and coadministration of bronchodilators may be prescribed.

# MONOCLONAL ANTIBODY FOR RESPIRATORY SYNCYTIAL VIRUS

Ⓟ **Palivizumab (Synagis)** is a monoclonal antibody approved for the treatment of RSV. It is only approved for use in infants and children less than 24 months of age.

## Pharmacokinetics

The bioavailability in infants and children less than 24 months of age without congenital heart disease is 70%. The half-life of the drug is 20 to 24.5 days, with a peak serum level in 3 to 5 days. Palivizumab concentrations are sufficient to inhibit RSV 2 days following administration. The excretion of palivizumab may increase in patients with chronic lung disease or in the presence of antipalivizumab antibodies.

## Action and Use

Palivizumab exhibits neutralizing and fusion-inhibiting activity against RSV, thus inhibiting its replication.

## Adverse Effects and Contraindications

The reported adverse effects are skin rash, fever, antibody development, angioedema, dyspnea, hypotonia, pruritus, respiratory failure, unresponsiveness, urticaria, hypersensitivity reaction, injection site reaction, and thrombocytopenia. Palivizumab is contraindicated in hypersensitivity reactions or hypersensitivity reaction to any humanized monoclonal antibodies.

## Nursing Implications

### Preventing Interactions

Palivizumab should not be combined with vitamins, minerals, or over-the-counter medications. The nurse should consult with the prescriber regarding specific drug interactions.

### Administering the Medication, Assessing for Therapeutic and Adverse Effects

Administer undiluted palivizumab deep into intramuscular tissues in the anterolateral aspect of the thigh. Never administer palivizumab in the gluteal muscle due to risk of damage to the sciatic nerve. Assess for injection reaction and hypersensitivity

reaction. The infant or child's lung sounds should be auscultated for clarity. In addition, assess pulmonary status for unlabored respirations and absence of retractions.

### Patient Teaching

Box 23.2 identifies general patient teaching guidelines for the antiviral drugs. In addition, the nurse instructs families about the risk of exposure with pregnancy and aspects of ribavirin administration.

> **! QSEN Alert: Evidence-Based Practice**
>
> Alansari, Toaimah, Almatar, El Tatawy, Davidson, and Qusad conducted a double-blind random study on 420 infants to determine if palivizumab would be helpful in young infants with acute RSV bronchiolitis. The infants in the study were ≤3 months of age who presented to the emergency department and were diagnosed with RSV bronchiolitis. The data showed that the palivizumab-treated infants were discharged in 29.5 hours, whereas the placebo group was discharged in 30.2 hours. For young infants with RSV, intravenous recombinant monoclonal anti-RSV antibody was not superior to normal saline for readmission and readiness for discharge.

---

**Clinical Application 23.2**

Ms. Jackson's 1-year-old child, James, is admitted to the pediatric medical division with a diagnosis of respiratory syncytial virus. Ms. Jackson is pregnant with twins.

- What precautions does the nurse need to take with Ms. Jackson and her child?
- What patient teaching does the nurse provide to Ms. Jackson and her family?
- What assessments does the nurse implement when caring for James?

---

 **NCLEX Success**

8. A 5-month-old infant is receiving ribavirin for respiratory syncytial virus. The nurse assesses the infant visually. Which of the following indicate that the infant's pulmonary status is impaired?

   A. shallow respirations
   B. nasal flaring
   C. respiratory rate of 36 breaths/min
   D. sleeping

9. When caring for an infant receiving ribavirin, the nurse notes the fluid level is low in the SPAG-2 unit. What action should the nurse take?

   A. Discard the remaining fluid and add more fluid.
   B. Add 10 mL of normal saline to the SPAG-2 unit.
   C. Discard the SPAG-2 unit.
   D. Add sterile water to the SPAG-2 unit.

# DRUGS FOR INFLUENZA

Two classes of drugs are used for the prophylaxis and treatment of influenza A. The first class is adamantanes, which includes **amantadine hydrochloride** (Gocovri, Osmolex ER). Amantadine is also discussed in Chapter 48 with regard to its use in the treatment of Parkinson's disease. The second class is the neuraminidase inhibitors, which includes **oseltamivir phosphate**.

## ADAMANTANES

Amantadine hydrochloride is a synthetic antiviral agent administered for the treatment of influenza A, an RNA virus. According to the Centers for Disease Control and Prevention (CDC), this drug is no longer recommended for the treatment or prophylaxis of influenza A; when used for this purpose, amantadine resistance has developed. This drug is not effective against influenza B. This chapter discusses **amantadine** because it may be used in the event of the reemergence of adamantane-susceptible strains.

## Pharmacokinetics

Amantadine is well absorbed, with an onset of action in 48 hours and a peak of action in 1 to 4 hours. It is distributed throughout the body fluids with the highest concentrations in the lung tissues. The medication is not metabolized, and 80% to 90% of the drug is eliminated unchanged in the urine.

## Action and Use

Amantadine blocks the uncoating of the virus, thus preventing penetration in the host. Its uses include prophylactic and symptomatic treatment of influenza A. Table 23.5 summarizes route and dosage information for the adamantanes and the neuraminidase inhibitors.

### Use in Older Adults

Dosage adjustment is warranted in older adults, according to the patient's renal function. It may be necessary to administer amantadine in two divided doses.

### Use in Patients With Renal Impairment

Dosage reduction is necessary in patients with impaired renal function according to the CrCl. Patients on hemodialysis should take amantadine 200 mg orally every 7 days.

## Adverse Effects

Use of amantadine is associated with several adverse effects. CNS effects may include depression as well as dizziness, light-headedness, nervousness with anxiety, and inability to concentrate. Cardiovascular adverse effects include orthostatic hypotension and peripheral edema. Other adverse effects are anorexia, constipation, nausea, diarrhea, dry nose, and bluish mottling of the skin on the legs and hands.

## Contraindications

Contraindications to amantadine include a known hypersensitivity to the medication.

# Nursing Implications

## Preventing Interactions

Anticholinergic agents administered during the course of amantadine therapy may enhance the anticholinergic effects such as urinary retention, dry mouth, narrow-angle glaucoma, and hypertension. Alcohol increases CNS depression.

## Administering the Medication

Patients should take the first dose of amantadine early in the morning and the second dose in the early evening, 12 hours later. They should take the drug with a full glass of water or with food to prevent disruptive sleep patterns. It is necessary to store the medication at room temperature in a tightly closed, light-protected container. High-risk patients who have not been vaccinated previously with the influenza A vaccine can receive amantadine with the vaccine.

## Assess for Therapeutic Effects

The nurse assesses for a decrease in flulike symptoms such as decreased fever, malaise, pain, cough, and rhinitis.

## Assess for Adverse Effects

The nurse assesses the patient's mental status regarding alertness and ability to cope. Also, it is necessary to assess for dizziness and light-headedness as well as for pedal edema and signs of orthostatic hypotension with position changes.

## Patient Teaching

Box 23.2 identifies general patient teaching guidelines for the antiviral drugs.

## Other Drugs in the Class

Rimantadine is an oral drug used to control outbreaks of influenza A. The drug can be used in combination with oseltamivir or zanamivir but is not recommended in combination with amantadine. It reaches a peak of action in 6 hours. Rimantadine is metabolized in the liver and is excreted unchanged in the urine. The serum half-life is 25.4 hours, which may be prolonged with liver or renal impairment.

## NEURAMINIDASE INHIBITORS

The neuroaminidase inhibitors are active against influenza A or B virus. The CDC recommends these antiviral medications be used for influenza; "on the basis of recent viral surveillance and resistance data, the greater than 99% of currently calculated influenza virus strains are sensitive to these medications." In this class, the prototype drug is **oseltamivir** (Tamiflu). The CDC recommends antiviral treatment of influenza or suspected influenza begin as soon as possible with baloxavir marboxil (Xofluza), oseltamivir, peramivir, and zanamivir. Baloxavir marboxil is an endonuclease inhibitor that will be discussed after the neuroaminidase inhibitors.

## Pharmacokinetics

Oseltamivir is well absorbed and distributed as oseltamivir carboxylate. The half-life of the drug is 1 to 3 hours. It is metabolized in the liver, and 90% is excreted in the urine with the remainder excreted in the feces.

**TABLE 23.5**

## DRUGS AT A GLANCE: Drugs for Influenza

| Drug | Pregnancy Category | Routes and Dosage Ranges | |
|---|---|---|---|
| | | **Adults** | **Children** |
| **Adamantanes** | | | |
| P **Amantadine hydrochloride** (Gocovri, Osmolex ER; ❋ PDP-Amantadine) | C | Influenza A prophylaxis: 200 mg PO daily or 100 mg PO twice daily for 10 d after exposure<br>Uncomplicated influenza: same as above; continue 24–48 h after symptoms subside | Not recommended for age <1 y<br>Influenza A prophylaxis: 1–9 y: 4.4–8.8 mg/kg/d PO in one or two divided doses not to exceed 150 mg/d<br>Uncomplicated influenza: same as above; continue 24–48 h after symptoms subside |
| Rimantadine | C | Influenza A: prophylaxis, 100 mg PO twice daily; treatment, 100 mg PO twice daily start within 48 h of symptoms for 5–7 d | 1–9 y, 5 mg/kg/d PO in divided doses (max dose: 150 mg/d)<br>10 y and older, same as adults |
| **Neuraminidase Inhibitors** | | | |
| P **Oseltamivir phosphate** (Tamiflu; ❋ NAT-Oseltamivir, Tamiflu) | C | Prophylaxis, 75 mg PO daily for 10 d begin within 2 d after exposure<br>Treatment, 75 mg PO twice daily for 5 d within 2 d of exposure | Birth to 1 y, consult manufacturer's recommendations<br>Infants <1 y, weight-based dosing; 3 mg/kg/dose twice daily for 5 d<br>1–12 y<br>Prophylaxis, ≤15 kg, 30 mg/d PO; 15–23 kg, 45 mg/d PO; 23–40 kg, 60 mg/d PO; >40 kg 75 mg/d; all for 10 d<br>Treatment, 30–75 mg PO twice daily for 5 d |
| Peramivir (Rapivab; ❋) | C | IV 600 mg in a single dose | No dosage available in children |
| Zanamivir (Relenza Diskhaler; ❋ Relenza Diskhaler) | C | Prophylaxis, 2 inhalations per day for 28 d<br>Treatment, 2 inhalations (10 mg total) every 12 h for 5 d (begin within 2 d of symptoms), first day 2 inhalations 2 h apart then every 12 h | Prophylaxis (5 y and older), same as adult<br>Treatment (7 y and older), same as adult |
| **Endonuclease Inhibitors** | | | |
| P Baloxavir marboxil (Xofluza) | Adverse effects were not observed in animal reproduction studies. | 40–<80 kg: 40 mg PO as a single dose within 48 h of influenza symptoms<br>>80 kg: 80 mg PO as a single dose within 48 h of influenza symptoms | Children >12 years of age, same as adult dosing |

## Action

Oseltamivir, in its active form oseltamivir carboxylate, inhibits the viral enzyme neuraminidase. This enzyme helps the newly formed virus to exit the host cell. By inhibiting this viral enzyme, oseltamivir carboxylate prevents new virus from infecting other cells.

## Use

Oseltamivir is an oral drug administered to adults and children 1 year or older who have contracted influenza A or B. The recipients of treatment must have been symptomatic for 2 days or less. Adults and children 1 year of age or older may also take it prophylactically. Table 23.5 gives route and dosage information for oseltamivir.

## Adverse Effects and Contraindications

The adverse effects of oseltamivir are nausea, vomiting, abdominal pain, diarrhea, conjunctivitis, and epistaxis. Contraindications include a known hypersensitivity to the medication. Women who are breast-feeding should not take oseltamivir.

## Nursing Implications

### Preventing Interactions

Probenecid increases the serum concentration of oseltamivir. It is necessary to assess for thrombocytopenia if these drugs are administered together. People should not take oseltamivir 48 hours before receiving the influenza virus vaccine or for 2 weeks after receiving the vaccine.

## Administering the Medication

According to the FDA, the manufacturer of the oral suspension of oseltamivir has changed the concentration from 12 to 6 mg/mL. The lower concentration allows for more accurate measurement because it does not become as frothy as the 12-mg concentration.

---

 **QSEN Alert: Patient-Centered Care**

People may take oseltamivir with food to improve tolerance and prevent GI upset. If necessary, adult capsules can be opened and the powder mixed in a sweetened liquid to make the drug more palatable (e.g., mixed with chocolate or strawberry syrup) to be administered to children.

---

## Assessing for Therapeutic Effects

The nurse assesses for a decrease in flulike symptoms such as fever, malaise, pain, cough, and rhinitis.

## Assessing for Adverse Effects

The nurse assesses the patient for GI upset, including nausea, vomiting, and diarrhea. It is also necessary to assess the nares for signs of bleeding and irritation as well as the conjunctiva for irritation, redness, and drainage.

## Patient Teaching

Box 23.2 identifies general patient teaching guidelines for the antiviral drugs.

## Other Drugs in the Class

Peramivir (Rapivab) is a parenteral antiviral agent that is given only to adults with influenza A or B. Geriatric patients with altered CrCl require a reduced dosage. Adverse effects are hypertension, insomnia, hyperglycemia, constipation, neutropenia, and increased AST and creatinine phosphokinase. During postmarketing of peramivir, users reported the following adverse effects: abnormal behavior, anaphylaxis, erythema, hallucinations, exfoliative dermatitis, skin rash, and Stevens-Johnson syndrome. When administering peramivir in the health care facility, the nurse must assess for wheezing, bronchospasm, and skin rash. It is also important to assess for neurologic abnormalities. In addition, it is necessary to obtain a baseline CBC and serum creatinine prior to the administration of the drug.

Zanamivir (Relenza) has a similar action to oseltamivir. Patients take the medication using a Diskhaler delivery system, which should be used cautiously in patients with chronic obstructive pulmonary disease and asthma because of the risk of bronchospasm. A rapid-acting inhaled bronchodilator should be available. It is important that the nurse instruct all patients about the use of the inhaler and report worsening respiratory symptoms or the occurrence of diarrhea, nausea, and vomiting. Zanamivir has an unlabeled use in H1N1 virus infection.

## ENDONUCLEASE INHIBITOR

Ⓟ **Baloxavir marboxil (Xofluza)** is an endonuclease inhibitor that blocks influenza. It is approved for the treatment of influenza A viruses, including H7N9 and H5N1. It is active against influenza viruses that are resistant to oseltamivir.

## Pharmacokinetics

Baloxavir is highly protein bound and metabolized completely, converted by UGT1A3 and CYP3A4 to an active metabolite. The medication's half-life is 79.1 hours. It reaches a peak in 4 hours. Eighty percent of the baloxavir is excreted in the feces with approximately 14% excreted in the urine.

## Action and Use

Baloxavir marboxil is converted to baloxavir. Baloxavir is an inhibitor of the endonuclease activity of the polymerase acidic protein. The endonuclease activity is responsible for influenza virus replication. Baloxavir has antiviral activity against both influenza A and B. It also has antiviral activity against virus strains that are currently resistant to other antiviral agents.

## Adverse Effects and Contraindications

Adverse effects reported with the administration of baloxavir marboxil include diarrhea that may include melena, erythema, facial swelling, skin rash, urticaria, delirium, and eyelid edema. The medication is contraindicated in patients with a known hypersensitivity to antiviral agents.

## Nursing Implications

### Administering the Medication

Baloxavir marboxil should be administered within 48 hours of the onset of influenza symptoms. Patients weighing 40 to less than 80 kg should be administered a 40-mg single dose. Patients weighing 80 kg or greater should be administered 80 mg orally. There are no dosage adjustments for renal or hepatic impairment.

### Assessing for Therapeutic and Adverse Effects

It is important to assess the patient for a decrease in influenza symptoms such as fever, cough, myalgia, and congestion. Assess the patient for diarrhea with blood, erythema, facial edema, and eyelid edema.

---

**NCLEX Success**

10. A 55-year-old woman takes oseltamivir for the treatment of influenza A. Which viral enzyme does it inhibit in the treatment of influenza?

   A. trypsin
   B. amylase
   C. lipase
   D. neuraminidase

11. A 25-year-old man with asthma develops influenza A. Which of the following medications is contraindicated for the treatment of influenza A in this case?

   A. acetaminophen
   B. pseudoephedrine
   C. oseltamivir
   D. zanamivir

# DRUGS FOR HEPATITIS B: NUCLEOSIDE ANALOGS

Drug therapy for hepatitis B virus (HBV) includes pegylated interferon and antiviral agents, particularly lamivudine. The goal of therapy is to reduce the risk of transmission to others and prevent long-term complications such as cirrhosis or hepatocellular carcinoma. The following section discusses the nucleoside analog ⬦ **lamivudine** (Epivir, Epivir-HBV) as the prototype antiviral agent for HBV.

## Pharmacokinetics

Lamivudine is rapidly absorbed in the GI tract, after which it is distributed with less than 36% of the drug bound by plasma protein. Approximately 4.2% of the drug is metabolized to a trans-sulfoxide metabolite. The half-life of the drug is 2 hours in children and 5 to 7 hours in adults. The drug is excreted unchanged in the urine.

## Action

Incorporation of a monophosphate form of lamivudine into the viral DNA of HBV polymerase results in the termination of the DNA chain. The drug also inhibits the transcription of the viral RNA chain in HBV. In addition, as a cytosine analog, lamivudine inhibits HIV reverse transcriptase of the viral RNA chain.

## Use

Prescribers order lamivudine for the treatment of chronic hepatitis B in patients who have evidence of hepatitis B viral replication and active inflammation of the liver. Patients with HIV may also take the drug when antiretroviral therapy with a multidrug regimen is necessary. An unlabeled use is for postexposure to HIV as part of a multidrug regimen. Table 23.6 gives route and dosage information for lamivudine and the other antiviral agents used for hepatitis.

### Use in Children

Pancreatitis is prevalent in children who take lamivudine. Close monitoring is necessary. If signs and symptoms of pancreatitis such as upper abdominal pain, back pain, and vomiting develop, it is essential to discontinue the drug.

### Use in Patients With Renal Impairment

The presence of renal impairment warrants a reduction in the lamivudine dosage according to the CrCl.

## Adverse Effects

A main adverse effect of lamivudine is pancreatitis. Other adverse effects include nausea, vomiting, diarrhea, abdominal pain, neutropenia, myalgia, neuropathy, and musculoskeletal pain. In addition, patients have reported headache; fatigue; insomnia; cough; sinusitis; and infections of the ear, nose, and throat. The FDA has issued a **BLACK BOX WARNING** ◆ for the nucleoside analogs stating that lactic acidosis and severe hepatomegaly with steatosis have been reported.

## Contraindications

Contraindications to lamivudine include a known hypersensitivity to the drug or any of the components of the drug.

## Nursing Implications

### Preventing Interactions

Several drugs interact with lamivudine. Trimethoprim–sulfamethoxazole increases the serum level of lamivudine. Ganciclovir–valganciclovir may enhance the adverse effects of lamivudine. Ribavirin increases the hepatotoxic effects of lamivudine. In addition, administration of lamivudine and zidovudine increases the serum level of zidovudine. Zalcitabine and lamivudine result in the inactivation of both drugs.

### Administering the Medication

Patients may take lamivudine with or without food.

### Assessing for Therapeutic Effects

The nurse assesses for decreased malaise, myalgia, loss of appetite, and abdominal pain. If the patient had jaundice, the nurse assesses for diminished yellowing of the skin and sclera. It is necessary to palpate the liver and lymph nodes for decreased size. Monitoring AST and ALT for decreasing serum levels is important. The administration of lamivudine decreases the effects of hepatitis, leading to an improvement in the serum liver enzyme levels.

### Assessing for Adverse Effects

The nurse assesses for abdominal pain, particularly in pediatric patients. Such pain may be indicative of pancreatitis. Also, the nurse assesses for GI effects such as nausea, vomiting, and diarrhea, as well as for headache, myalgia, and musculoskeletal pain. It is also necessary to assess for upper respiratory effects such as sinusitis and infections.

### Patient Teaching

Box 23.2 identifies general patient teaching guidelines for antiviral drugs. In addition, the nurse teaches the patient the signs of symptoms of lactic acidosis, including musculoskeletal pain.

## Other Drugs in the Class

Adefovir dipivoxil (Hepsera) is a purine nucleotide analog administered for chronic hepatitis B, with active viral replication producing elevation in AST/ALT. The drug requires cautious use in renal dysfunction. Experts do not recommend using adefovir for first-line therapy of chronic hepatitis B because of its weak antiviral activity, leading to viral resistance to the drug. (See discussion of tenofovir for use as a replacement drug.)

Entecavir (Baraclude), a potent antiviral agent, inhibits the HBV polymerase to reduce viral DNA levels. It is associated with a low rate of drug resistance and is preferred for patients with impaired kidney function. To aid in the absorption of the medication, administration on an empty stomach is necessary. The onset of action and the peak of action occur in ½ to 1 ½ hours. Excretion is in the urine.

Ribavirin is an oral antiviral drug administered in combination with peginterferon alfa-2a or peginterferon alfa-2b for chronic hepatitis B. People should take the drug on an empty

## TABLE 23.6

## DRUGS AT A GLANCE: Drugs for Hepatitis

| Drug | Pregnancy Category | Routes and Dosage Ranges | |
|------|---------------------|--------------------------|---|
| | | **Adults** | **Children** |
| **Nucleoside Analogs** | | | |
| **Lamivudine** (Epivir, Epivir-HBV; 3TC, APO-Lamivudine, Apo-Lamivudine HBV, Heptovir) | C | 100 mg PO daily | 2–17 y, 3 mg/kg PO daily up to max 100 mg daily |
| Adefovir dipivoxil (Hepsera; APO-Adefovir, Hepsera) | C | 10 mg PO daily | Younger than 12 y, safety and efficacy have not been established |
| Entecavir (Baraclude; ACCEL-Entecavir, APO-Entecavir, Auro Entecavir, JAMP-Entecavir, MINT-Entecavir, PMS-Entecavir) | C | PO 1 mg<br>CrCl 30–49 mL/min: decrease dose by 50%<br>CrCl 10–29 mL/min: decrease dose by 70% | PO 10–11 kg: 0.15 mg once daily<br>>11–14 kg: 0.2 mg once daily<br>>14–17 kg: 0.25 mg once daily<br>>17–20 kg: 0.3 mg once daily<br>>20–23 kg: 0.35 mg once daily<br>>26–30 kg: 0.4 mg once daily<br>>30 kg: 0.5 mg once daily |
| Ribavirin (Ibavyr) | X | <66 kg: 800 mg daily (400 mg in the AM and PM)<br>66–80 kg: 1000 mg daily (400 mg in AM and 600 mg in PM)<br>81–105 kg: 1200 mg daily (600 mg in AM and 600 mg in PM)<br>>105 kg: 1400 mg daily (600 mg in AM and 800 mg in PM) | <47 kg: 15 mg/kg/d in 2 divided doses<br>47–59 kg: 800 mg daily (400 mg in AM and PM)<br>60–73 kg: 1000 mg daily (400 mg in AM and 600 mg in PM)<br>>73 kg: 1200 mg daily (600 mg in AM and PM) |
| Tenofovir alafenamide (Vemlidy; Vemlidy) | Adverse effects not observed in animal reproduction studies* | PO 25 mg once daily | No dosage established |
| Tenofovir disoproxil fumarate (Viread; Viread) | B | 300 mg PO daily | Recommended only for ages 12 and older; see adult dosing |
| **Polymerase Inhibitors** | | | |
| Sofosbuvir (Solvaldi) | Sofosbuvir is not used as monotherapy; if used in combination with ribavirin it is contraindicated in pregnant females and males whose partner is pregnant. Use contraception when combined with ribavirin or peginterferon. | 400 mg PO with or without food | Oral pellets 1 or more spoonful of sprinkles on a nonacidic soft food |

stomach to aid in absorption and without antacids and nucleoside reverse transcriptase inhibitors (NRTIs). The FDA has issued a **BLACK BOX WARNING** ◆ for ribavirin, stating that it can produce hemolytic anemia, which could lead to myocardial infarction. Patients with unstable cardiovascular disease should not take the drug. Patients 3 years and older may take ribavirin (Copegus, Rebetol, Ribasphere, Virazole) with peginterferon alfa-2a or peginterferon alfa-2b (see Chap. 9) for the treatment of hepatitis C.

Adefovir (Hepsera) is used to treat chronic hepatitis B in patients with persistent elevation of the liver enzymes, AST and ALT. It is also administered for patients with lamivudine-resistant hepatitis B. In liver transplant patients treated with

adefovir, renal function must be closely monitored. Studies have shown that impaired renal function is a risk. Adefovir should not be administered with tenofovir.

Tenofovir disoproxil (Viread) is useful for the treatment of chronic hepatitis B in patients with compensated or decompensated liver disease. It is also used in combination with other antiretrovirals for HIV infection. Tenofovir disoproxil fumarate has primarily replaced adefovir, because tenofovir is more potent and effective without the combination of other medications. The approved dose is 10 mg daily. An increase in creatinine has been reported in 3% to 9% of patients. It is necessary to monitor patients who take tenofovir frequently for demineralization that may lead to pathologic fractures. The nurse teaches the patient to increase calcium intake with the use of dairy products.

Like tenofovir disoproxil, tenofovir alafenamide (Vemlidy) is also useful in the treatment of chronic hepatitis B in patient with compensated liver disease. It inhibits replication of HBV and inhibits HBV polymerase. There is no dosage adjustment with a creatinine clearance of greater than or equal to 50 mL/min with tenofovir. There is no dosage adjustment with a creatinine clearance of 15 mL/min with tenofovir alafenamide.

Telbivudine (Tyzeka) is an oral drug used for the treatment of hepatitis B. Its metabolite inhibits the hepatitis B DNA polymerase through competition with the natural nucleoside substrate. The DNA chain is then terminated, inhibiting the replication of hepatitis B. Telbivudine has a peak of action of 1 to 4 hours, with minimal protein binding. It is widely distributed in tissues and eliminated unchanged in the urine.

# DRUGS FOR HEPATITIS C: POLYMERASE INHIBITORS

Ⓟ **Sofosbuvir (Sovaldi)** is a polymerase inhibitor that treats patients infected with hepatitis C. Each patient diagnosed with hepatitis C should also be tested for hepatitis B virus prior to initiating sofosbuvir therapy. For patients coinfected with hepatitis B and hepatitis C, fulminant hepatitis or hepatic failure may develop or death may occur if hepatitis B is not treated.

## Pharmacokinetics

Sofosbuvir is 65% protein bound. During metabolism, the liver pharmacologically forms the drug to an active nucleoside analog triphosphate GS-461203. The dephosphorylation results in the formation of the nucleoside inactive metabolite GS-331007. Sofosbuvir's half-life elimination is 0.4 hours. It reaches a peak in ½ to 2 hours and is 80% excreted in the urine, with 14% excreted in the feces.

## Action and Use

Sofosbuvir is an antiviral agent used to treat hepatitis C. It inhibits hepatitis C virus NS5B RNA-dependent RNA polymerase, which is essential for viral replication. It acts as a chain terminator.

## Adverse Effects

Sofosbuvir is administered with ribavirin or peginterferon alfa. This section identifies the adverse effects reported with sofosbuvir combination therapy with ribavirin. The central nervous system adverse effects reported with sofosbuvir are fatigue, headache, insomnia, chills, and irritability. Pruritus and rash have been reported as dermatologic effects. Nausea, loss of appetite, and diarrhea are the gastrointestinal adverse effects. Six to twenty percent of patients developed anemia. Neutropenia is reported in less than one percent of patients. In postmarketing, patients have reported angioedema, bradycardia, and lactic acidosis. Sofosbuvir produces a rapid reduction in hepatitis C

viral load during direct-acting therapy for hepatitis C, and may lead to glucose metabolism with diabetes, resulting in potential hypoglycemia.

## Contraindications

There are no reported contraindications with sofosbuvir; however the contraindications noted with ribavirin or peginterferon alfa must be considered. Amiodarone administered with the sofosbuvir combination regimen can lead to fatal bradycardia with cardiac arrest.

## Nursing Implications

### Preventing Interactions

Amiodarone administered with the sofosbuvir combination regimen can lead to fatal bradycardia with cardiac arrest.

### Administering the Medication

Administer sofosbuvir with or without food. In pediatric patients the sofosbuvir pellets should be sprinkled in soft nonacidic foods such as pudding, mashed potatoes, or ice cream that are at or below room temperature.

### Assessing for Therapeutic Effects

Assess for decreased ALT and AST levels.

### Assessing for Adverse Effects

Assess for hypoglycemia in diabetic patients. Assess blood counts for anemia or neutropenia. Assess for signs and symptoms of fatigue. Assess for renal and hepatic adverse effects.

### Patient Teaching

See Box 23.2 for specific patient teaching guidelines for patients being administered antiviral agents. Diabetic patients must monitor blood sugar for hypoglycemia.

## NCLEX Success

12. A man is taking lamivudine. He states that he has severe upper abdominal pain. On assessment, he has guarding. What would the nurse suspect is wrong with the patient?

    A. hepatomegaly
    B. pancreatitis
    C. epiglottitis
    D. cardiomyopathy

13. A woman is taking lamivudine for chronic hepatitis B. She reports that her stools float and are clay colored. In addition, she complains of musculoskeletal pain. What would the nurse suspect has contributed to the development of these clinical manifestations?

    A. cirrhosis
    B. ascites
    C. lactic acidosis
    D. pulmonary edema

# DRUGS FOR HUMAN IMMUNODEFICIENCY VIRUS (ANTIRETROVIRAL DRUGS)

The cycle of HIV begins with the entry of the virus that finds and infuses. This is followed by reverse transcription, integration, replication, assembly, maturation, and budding. During entry, HIV binds to receptors on the surface of the CD4 cell. Health care providers use a variety of **antiretroviral drugs** to fight HIV, an infection of the immune system caused by a retrovirus. The broad classifications of these drugs are the nucleoside and nucleotide reverse transcriptase inhibitors (NRTIs), nonnucleoside reverse transcriptase inhibitors (NNRTIs), protease inhibitors (PIs), and the integrase strand transfer inhibitors (INSTIs). Other drug classifications used to treat HIV include the fusion protein inhibitors and CCR5 antagonists (Fig. 23.1). In general, newer drugs and drug combinations are more effective for viral suppression. The combination medications cause fewer serious adverse effects, and are more convenient for patients to take. The selection of an antiretroviral regimen is determined from the results of drug resistance testing.

The regimen usually consists of two NRTIs with an NNRTI or a PI. Antiretroviral therapy (ART) involves the use of several combinations of antiretroviral drugs in the treatment of HIV/AIDS. Authorities do not recommend using some of the older drugs for initial treatment but may suggest them when drug-resistant infections develop with the newer drugs. Patients often undergo genotypic or phenotypic testing for drug resistance to guide antiretroviral therapy.

When administering antiretroviral agents, it is important to distinguish whether the patient has taken antiretroviral agents in the past. Patients who have received antiretroviral agents are *treatment experienced*, whereas those who have not received them are *treatment naïve*.

The goal of ART is a reduction in morbidity and mortality. ART assists in improving patients' quality of life and suppressing conversion to AIDS. It is important to educate patients about the prevention of HIV transmission and mother-to-child transmission. The prevention of drug resistance is a goal that is accomplished by the administration of combination drug therapy. This allows the patient to take fewer medications allowing medication compliance.

The United States Department of Health and Human Services recommends one of the following regimens for early management of HIV:

- Dolutegravir plus tenofovir and either emtricitabine or lamivudine
- Bictegravir–tenofovir alafenamide–emtricitabine
- Ritonavir-boosted darunavir plus tenofovir and either emtricitabine or lamivudine

Combination ART is important to prevent opportunistic infections in patients with HIV-1 or HIV-2. Dolutegravir with tenofovir alafenamide–emtricitabine or bictegravir-emitricitabine–tenofovir alafenamide are the recommended combinations. Tenofovir disoproxil fumarate and emitricitabine (Truvada) combine an NRTI and NNRTI. This combination drug interferes with HIV viral RNA-dependent DNA polymerase, resulting in the inhibition of viral replication. Tenofovir alafenamide and emtricitabine (Descovy) also combines reverse transcriptase inhibitor nucleoside and reverse transcriptase inhibitor nucleotide. It interferes with HIV viral RNA-dependent DNA polymerase activity, thus inhibiting viral replication. Abacavir and lamivudine (Epzicom) is a third NRTI combination. Abacavir is a guanosine analogue that through phosphorylation becomes carbovir triphosphate to inhibit viral replication. Lamivudine is a cytosine analog that inhibits HIV reverse transcription, thus inhibiting RNA-dependent DNA polymerase of reverse transcriptase. Other regimens include INSTI raltegravir, elvitegravir/cobicistat, dolutegravir, PI of ritonavir-boosted lopinavir, or ritonavir-boosted darunavir. One of the newest combination medications for HIV is bictegravir, emtricitabine, and tenofovir alafenadmide (Biktarvy). This medication combines drugs from the following broad classifications: integrase inhibitor, reverse transcriptase inhibitor, nucleoside, reverse transcriptase inhibitor, and nucleotide. It will be described in detail later in the chapter.

It is important to be familiar with the action, adverse effects, and nursing implications of each medication. The nurse must also educate patients and caregivers about administration of the medications and drug–drug interactions. For questions regarding any of the drugs, the nurse should contact a pharmacist or infection control physician.

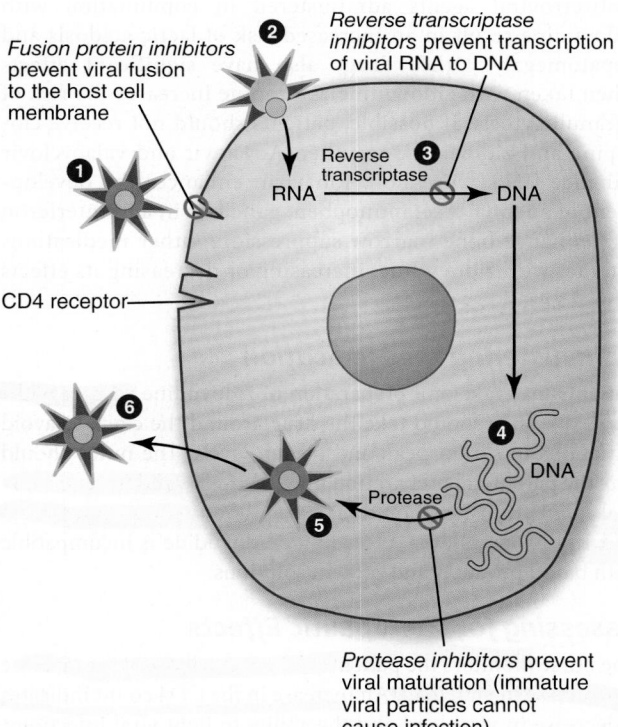

**FIGURE 23.1.** Human immunodeficiency virus (HIV) entry into cells and replication; actions of anti-HIV drugs. (1) The virus attaches to receptors (e.g., CD4 molecules) and coreceptors (CCR5 molecules) on the host cell membrane. (2) The virus becomes uncoated and releases its RNA into the host cell. (3) The enzyme reverse transcriptase converts RNA to DNA, which is necessary for viral replication. (4) The DNA codes for protein synthesis, which produces immature viral particles. (5) The enzyme protease assembles the immature viral particles into mature viruses. (6) Mature viruses are released from the host cell.

# NUCLEOSIDE REVERSE TRANSCRIPTASE INHIBITORS

The NRTIs are structurally similar to DNA components (adenosine, cytosine, guanosine, and thymidine) and thus easily enter human cells and viruses in human cells. For example, **zidovudine** (AZT, Retrovir), the prototype, is able to substitute for thymidine. The drugs are more active in slowing the progression of acute infection rather than in treating chronically infected cells. Thus, they do not cure HIV infection or prevent transmission of the virus through sexual contact or blood contamination.

## Pharmacokinetics

The oral preparation of zidovudine is quickly absorbed in the GI tract, reaching a peak of action in ½ to 1 ½ hours. The drug, which can cross the blood–brain barrier, is readily distributed to the CSF. It also crosses the placenta. Zidovudine is metabolized in the liver. It is 25% to 38% protein bound with a half-life of ½ to 3 hours. It is excreted in the urine; 72% to 74% is excreted as metabolites, with 14% to 18% excreted unchanged. (With the IV preparation, 45% to 60% is excreted as metabolites and 18% to 29% as unchanged drug.)

## Action

Like all NRTIs, zidovudine has the ability to incorporate into the DNA chains by viral reverse transcriptase. (HIV needs this enzyme to convert RNA to DNA and replicate.) Thus, the drug blocks the addition of further nucleotides and terminates viral replication.

## Use

Patients take zidovudine for the treatment of HIV infection—in combination with two or more other antiretroviral agents. Pregnant women who are infected with HIV take the drug as monotherapy to prevent the transmission of HIV to the fetus. Should the mother not receive antiviral therapy during her pregnancy, intravenous zidovudine is administered at the onset of labor. An unlabeled use is postexposure prophylaxis for HIV exposure with a multidrug regimen. Table 23.7 presents route and dosage information for zidovudine and other NRTIs.

### Use in Children

To prevent maternal–fetal HIV transmission in neonates, experts recommend that zidovudine be given as soon as possible after birth—6 to 12 hours after delivery. It is necessary to continue the dose until the neonate is 6 weeks of age. Infants born to mothers whose viral load (number of HIV RNA particles within the blood) is significantly below normal should receive zidovudine combined with nevirapine. If the infant develops a rash, there should be no dosage increase during the 14-day lead-in period.

### Use in Patients With Renal Impairment

For patients on hemodialysis or peritoneal dialysis and a CrCl less than 15 mL/min, the oral dose should be 100 mg every 6 to 8 hours or 300 mg daily. The IV dose should be 1 mg/kg every 6 to 8 hours.

## Adverse Effects

Patients administered zidovudine have reported headache and malaise. Other significant adverse effects include nausea, vomiting, and anorexia. The FDA has issued a **BLACK BOX WARNING** ◆ related to the adverse effects of granulocytopenia, aplastic or hemolytic anemia, pancytopenia with bone marrow hypoplasia, leukopenia, and lymphadenopathy with zidovudine. It is necessary to adjust the dosage in patients who develop anemia or neutropenia. Two other **BLACK BOX WARNING** ◆ for zidovudine relate to lactic acidosis and severe hepatomegaly with steatosis and symptomatic myopathy and myositis. The risk of liver disease increases in females, obesity, and pregnancy and with prolonged use. If clinical or laboratory signs of lactic acidosis or hepatotoxicity develop, it is essential that the drug be discontinued.

## Contraindications

Contraindications to zidovudine include a known hypersensitivity to the drug or history of lactic acidosis.

## Nursing Implications

### Preventing Interactions

Antiretroviral agents administered in combination with zidovudine result in an increased risk of lactic acidosis and hepatomegaly. Other drugs also have significant effects when taken with zidovudine. Clozapine increases the risk of agranulocytosis. If possible, patients should not receive clozapine and zidovudine together. Acyclovir and valacyclovir enhance CNS depression. Ribavirin enhances the development of anemia. Acetaminophen, ganciclovir, and interferon alfa enhance bone marrow suppression. Other medications interact with zidovudine, increasing or decreasing its effects (Box 23.4).

### Administering the Medication

Patients may take oral preparation of zidovudine with or without food. They should take the drug around the clock to avoid variations in serum peak and trough levels. The nurse should mix the parenteral preparation in 5% dextrose and water or normal saline. Infusion should take place over ½ hour in neonates and 1 hour in children and adults. Zidovudine is incompatible with blood products and protein solutions.

### Assessing for Therapeutic Effects

The nurse monitors the patient's CD4 and cell count for increase or decrease in viral load. An increase in the CD4 count indicates a decrease in viral load and the ability to fight viral infections. In addition, the nurse assesses the patient's clinical status for decrease in the development of opportunistic infections.

### Assessing for Adverse Effects

The nurse assesses for malaise, CNS depression, and GI symptoms such as nausea, vomiting, and diarrhea. He or she assesses for myalgia and hepatomegaly. The development of anemia usually occurs 2 to 4 weeks after the start of therapy. Neutropenia is most likely to occur in 6 to 8 weeks. It is important to obtain the patient's CBC as a baseline measure before therapy begins and

**TABLE 23.7**

**DRUGS AT A GLANCE: Antiretroviral Drugs: Nucleoside Reverse Transcriptase Inhibitors (NRTIs)**

| Drug | Pregnancy Category | Routes and Dosage Ranges | |
|---|---|---|---|
| | | **Adults** | **Children** |
| **Zidovudine** (Retrovir; ALTI-Zidovudine, APO-Zidovudine, AZT, Retrovir [AZT]) | C | 300 mg PO twice daily or 200 mg PO three times per day; 1 mg/kg/dose IV every 4 h<br>Prevention of maternal–fetal HIV transmission during labor and delivery (give when labor begins): 2 mg/kg IV as loading dose followed by a continuous IV infusion of 1 mg/kg/h until umbilical cord is clamped<br>Cesarean section: begin 3 h before surgery<br>Prevention of HIV following needlesticks: begin 2 h after exposure, 200 mg PO three times per day plus lamivudine 150 mg twice daily and a PI for high-risk exposure | Neonatal HIV: use in combination with other antiretroviral agents<br>Premature infants<br><35 wk gestational age, 2 mg/kg dose PO every 12 h or 1.5 mg/kg/dose IV every 12 h<br>Infants <30 wk, increase dose to every 8 h at 4 wk of age<br>Infants ≥30 wk, increase dose to every 8 h at 2 wk of age<br>Full-term infants, 2 mg/kg/dose PO every 6 h or 1.5 mg/kg/dose every 6 h<br>Prevention of maternal–fetal HIV transmission (zidovudine is used in neonates as monotherapy)<br>2 mg/kg/dose PO every 12 h or 1.5 mg/dose IV every 12 h; increase to every 8 h as follows:<br>Preterm infants<br><30 wk, increase dose to every 8 h at 4 wk of age<br>≥30 wk, increase above dose to every 8 h at 2 wk of age<br>Full-term infants<br>2 mg/kg PO every 6 h; alternate dosing<br><2.5 kg, 10 mg PO twice daily<br>>2.5 kg, 15 mg PO twice daily<br>1.5 mg/kg IV every 6 h<br>HIV:<br><6 wk, 2 mg/kg/dose PO every 6 h<br>6 wk to <12 y, 20 mg/m²/h IV continuous infusion<br>120 mg/m²/dose IV every 6 h<br>≥12 y, 1 mg/kg/dose IV intermittent infusion every 4 h around the clock |
| Abacavir sulfate (Ziagen; APO-ABaavir, MINT-Abacavir, Ziagen) | C | 300 mg PO twice daily or 600 mg daily<br>1 mg/kg/dose IV every 4 h<br>Hepatic impairment: 200 mg PO two times per day | 3 mo to 16 y, 8 mg/kg PO twice daily, not to exceed 300 mg/dose |
| Abacavir and lamivudine (Epzicom; APO-Abacavir,-Lamivudine, Kivexa, Mylan Abacavir/Lamivudine, Teva-Abacavir/Lamivudine) | C | Abacavir 600 mg and lamivudine 300 mg PO daily | Children and adolescents weighing ≥25 kg: same as adult |
| Abacavir, lamivudine, and zidovudine (Trizivir; APO Abacavir-Lamivud-Zidovud) | C | 1 tablet PO twice daily; not recommended for patients who weigh <40 kg | <40 kg: not recommended<br>≥40 kg: PO 1 tablet twice daily |

*(Continued on page 456)*

**TABLE 23.7**

## DRUGS AT A GLANCE: Antiretroviral Drugs: Nucleoside Reverse Transcriptase Inhibitors (NRTIs) [Continued]

| Drug | Pregnancy Category | Routes and Dosage Ranges | |
|------|--------------------|--------------------------|---|
| | | **Adults** | **Children** |
| Didanosine (✿ Videx EC) | B | Videx <br> <60 kg, 125 mg PO twice daily or 250 mg PO daily <br> ≥60 kg, 200 mg PO twice daily or 400 mg PO daily <br> Videx EC <br> 25 kg to <60 kg, 250 mg PO daily <br> ≥60 kg, 400 mg PO daily <br> When taken with tenofovir, <60 kg and CrCl ≥60 mL/min, 200 mg once daily; ≥60 kg and CrCl ≥60 mL/min: 250 mg once daily | Videx <br> 1 to <3 mo 50 mg/m², <br> ≥3–8 mo 100 mg/m² PO twice daily <br> >8 mo, 120 mg/m² PO twice daily (not to exceed adult dose) <br> Videx EC <br> ≥6 y <br> 20 to <25 kg, 200 mg PO once daily <br> 25 to <60 kg, 250 mg PO once daily <br> ≥60 kg, 400 mg PO once daily |
| Dolutegravir and lamivudine (Dovato; ✿ Dovato) Combination antiretroviral agent: Integrase inhibitor and reverse transcriptase inhibitor, nucleoside | The Health and Human Services perinatal HIV guidelines consider this fixed-dose combination a preferred regimen for pregnant females living with HIV. If females taking this fixed-dose combination drug become pregnant, they may continue if viral suppression is effective. | Dolutegravir 50 mg and lamivudine 300 mg PO with or without food 2 h before or 6 h after cation-containing antacids or laxatives, oral supplements with iron or calcium | Safety and efficacy not studied |
| Dolutegravir, abacavir, and lamivudine (Triumeq; ✿ Triumeq) Combination drug: integrase inhibitor and reverse transcriptase inhibitor | The Health and Human Services perinatal HIV guidelines consider this fixed dose combination a preferred regimen for pregnant females living with HIV. If females taking this fixed dose combination drug become pregnant, they may continue if viral suppression is effective. | Triumeq: Abacavir 600 mg, dolutegravir 50 mg, and lamivudine 300 mg <br> Administer with or without food. If the patient is on concomitant therapy with efavirenz, fosamprenavir/ritonavir, tipranavir/ritonavir, carbamazepine, or rifampin and additional daily single-component dolutegravir tablet should be administered 12 h after Triumeq. | Oral administration with or without food. Administer 2 h before or 6 h after cation-containing antacids or laxatives, sucralfate, oral supplements containing iron or calcium at the same time if administered with food. |
| Elvitegravir, cobicistat, emtricitabine, and tenofovir disoproxil fumarate (Stribild: ✿ Stribild) | The Health and Human Services perinatal HIV guidelines do not recommend this fixed dose combination for pregnant females living with HIV. If females taking this fixed dose combination drug become pregnant, alternative therapies should be considered. | Prior to initiation of therapy the patient should be tested for hepatitis B. Hepatic function must be monitored closely. <br> Combination medication of: <br> Elvitegravir: 150 mg <br> Cobicistat: 150 mg <br> Emitricitabine: 200 mg <br> Tenofovir disoproxil fumarate: 300 mg <br> One tablet PO daily | Children ≥ 12 years and weighing ≥35 kg one tablet PO once daily |
| Emtricitabine (Emtriva: ✿ Emtriva) | D | Capsules, 200 mg PO daily <br> Solution, 240 mg PO daily | 0–3 mo, 3 mg/kg/d PO <br> 3 mo to 17 y, >33 kg, 200 mg PO once daily <br> Solution, 6 mg/kg per PO per day |

**TABLE 23.7**

## DRUGS AT A GLANCE: Antiretroviral Drugs: Nucleoside Reverse Transcriptase Inhibitors (NRTIs) (Continued)

| Drug | Pregnancy Category | Routes and Dosage Ranges | |
|---|---|---|---|
| | | **Adults** | **Children** |
| Emtricitabine and tenofovir (Truvada; ❧ Truvada) | B | Emtricitabine 200 mg and tenofovir 300 mg, one tablet PO daily | Not intended for children |
| Emtricitabine, tenofovir, and efavirenz (Atripla: ❧ Atripla) | D | Emtricitabine 200 mg, tenofovir disoproxil 300 mg, and efavirenz 600 mg; 1 tablet PO daily | Not intended for children |
| Lamivudine (Epivir, Epivir-HBV; ❧ 3TC, APO-Lamivudine, APO-Lamivudine HBV, Heptovir) | C | 150 mg PO two times per day or 300 mg/d; PO as a single dose in combination with other antiretroviral agents | 1–3 mo, 4 mg/kg PO twice daily 3 mo to 16 y, 4 mg/kg PO two times per day; max dose 150 mg two times daily |
| Stavudine | C | <60 kg, 30 mg PO every 12 h ≥60 kg, 40 mg PO every 12 h | Birth to 13 d, 0.5 mg/kg PO every 12 h ≥14 d and <30 kg, 1 mg/kg PO every 12 h ≥30 kg, same as adults |
| Tenofovir disoproxil fumarate (Viread; ❧ APO-Tenofovir, Auro-Tenofir, JAMP-Tenofovir, MYLAN-Tenofovir Disoproxil, NAT-Tenofovir, PMS-Tenofovir, TEVA-Tenofovir, Viread) | B | 300 mg PO daily with meals | ≥12 y and ≥35 kg, same as adults |
| Zidovudine and lamivudine (Combivir; ❧ APO-Lamivudine-Zidovudine, Combivir, TEVA-Lamivudine/Zidovudine) | C | Zidovudine 300 mg and lamivudine 150 mg PO daily | Adolescents ≥30 kg, same as adults |

then every 2 weeks from then on. In addition, the nurse assesses the hemoglobin, hematocrit, and granulocyte count for hematologic toxicity. If the hemoglobin level is less than 7.5 g/dL or the reduction is greater than 25% of the baseline value, it may be necessary to interrupt therapy and administer transfusions. This is also the case if the granulocyte count is less than 750/mm³ or greater than 50% of the baseline measure.

### Patient Teaching

Box 23.5 identifies general patient teaching guidelines for antiretroviral drugs. Because lactic acidosis may develop, the nurse teaches the patient the signs and symptoms of this condition, including musculoskeletal pain.

## Other Drugs in the Class

Abacavir sulfate (Ziagen) inhibits the viral reverse transcriptase through competition with the natural DNA nucleoside and incorporation into viral DNA. It is contraindicated in moderate to severe hepatic impairment. Abacavir is administered in combination with other antiretroviral agents. The FDA has issued a **BLACK BOX WARNING** ◆ stating that patients taking abacavir may have serious and sometimes fatal hypersensitivity reactions. Patients who test positive for HLAB*5701 allele are at

---

**BOX 23.4** **Drug Interactions: Zidovudine**

**Drugs that Increase the Effect of Zidovudine**
- Divalproex, doxorubicin, fluconazole, flucytosine, indomethacin, methadone, pentamidine, probenecid, vincristine, valproic acid

  *Decrease the metabolism of zidovudine, thus increasing serum levels, leading to toxicity*

**Drugs that Decrease the Effect of Zidovudine**
- Protease inhibitors, rifamycin derivatives (excluding rifabutin)

  *Decrease serum concentration*

## BOX 23.5  *Patient Teaching Guidelines for Antiretroviral Drugs*

- Prevention is better than treatment, partly because medications used to treat viral infections may cause serious adverse effects. Thus, whenever possible, techniques to prevent viral infections should be used.
- Wash hands frequently and thoroughly; this helps prevent most infections.
- Have immunizations against viral infections as indicated.
- Always practice safe sex. Men should use a condom.
- In cases of intravenous drug use, use and promote the use of clean needles.
- Drugs may relieve symptoms but do not cure human immunodeficiency virus (HIV) infection, prevent transmission of the virus, or prevent other illnesses associated with advanced HIV infection.
- Effective treatment of HIV infection requires close adherence to drug therapy regimens involving several drugs and daily doses. Missing as few as one or two doses can decrease blood levels of antiretroviral drugs and result in increased HIV replication and development of drug-resistant viral strains.
- It is generally recommended that herbal products not be used with antiretroviral medications. St. John's wort may decrease blood levels of some anti-HIV medications and make them less effective; echinacea should be avoided because it may stimulate viral replication.
- Request information about adverse effects associated with the specific drugs you are taking and what you should do if they occur. Adverse effects vary among the drugs; some are potentially serious.
- Have regular blood tests, including viral load, CD4+ cell count, complete blood count, and others as indicated (e.g., tests of kidney and liver function).

- Keep your health care providers informed about all medications being taken; do not take any other drugs (including drugs of abuse, herbal preparations, vitamin/mineral supplements, nonprescription drugs) without consulting a health care provider. These preparations may make anti-HIV medications less effective or more toxic.
- Take the medications exactly as prescribed. Do not change doses or stop the medications without consulting a health care provider. If a dose is missed, do not double the next dose. The drugs must be taken consistently to suppress HIV infection and minimize adverse drug effects.
- These medications vary in their interactions with food and should be taken appropriately for optimal benefit. Unless otherwise instructed, take the drugs as follows:
  - Abacavir, Combivir, emtricitabine, famciclovir, fosamprenavir, Kaletra tablets, lamivudine, nevirapine, tenofovir, Trizivir, valacyclovir, and zidovudine with or without food. However, do not take abacavir or efavirenz with a high-fat meal.
  - Atripla, efavirenz, entecavir, or indinavir on an empty stomach or 1 hour before or 2 hours after a meal.
  - Atazanavir, darunavir, ganciclovir, Kaletra oral solution, nelfinavir, ritonavir, and tipranavir with food.
  - Saquinavir within 2 hours after a meal or with a full meal.
- To give nelfinavir to infants and young children, mix the oral powder can be mixed with a small amount of water, milk, or formula (if necessary). After it is mixed, give the entire amount to the child, who must take it all to obtain the full dose. Do not use acidic foods or juices (e.g., applesauce, orange juice, apple juice) because they produce a bitter taste.

greatest risk for hypersensitivity reactions. Patients may also be at risk for lactic acidosis.

Abacavir, lamivudine, and zidovudine (Trizivir) is used for HIV-1 treatment. The FDA has issued a **BLACK BOX WARNING ◆** stating that patients with the *HLA-B\*5701* allele are prone to a hypersensitivity reaction. The medications in this HIV drug work synergistically to inhibit reverse transcriptase by way of DNA chain termination after the incorporation of the nucleoside analogue and delay the emergence of mutations.

Didanosine is an oral antiretroviral that is administered 30 minutes before meals or 2 hours after meals. The drug blocks the HIV replication in T cells and monocytes to block viral DNA synthesis and replication. Patients should not combine it with alcohol due to the increased risk of pancreatitis. It is necessary to reduce the drug dosage in renal impairment.

Dolutegravir and lamivudine (Dovato) combines dolutegravir, an INSTI and lamivudine, a cytosine analog, to block the strand transfer step of retroviral DNA integration and inhibition of RNA and DNA polymerase activities of reverse transcriptase. The patient's CD4 count and viral DNA should be monitored closely.

Dolutegravir, abacavir, and lamivudine (Triumeq) has the same action as dolutegravir and lamivudine and also converts

cellular enzymes to the active metabolite, carbovir triphosphate, to inhibit the activity of reverse transcriptase through competition with the dGTP substrate and incorporating in the viral DNA.

Elvitegravir, cobicistat, emtricitabine, and tenofovir disoproxil fumarate (Stribild) combines an integrase inhibitor, reverse transcriptase inhibitor, nucleoside, and nucleotide reverse transcriptase inhibitor. The combination medication is administered orally with food. It is used to treat HIV-1 in adult and pediatric patients 12 years and older. It is contraindicated with alfuzoxin, carbamazepine, ergot derivatives, phenobarbital, phenytoin, rifampin, and sildenafil. The CD4, HIV RNA plasma levels, serum creatinine, serum phosphorous, and creatinine clearance should be monitored closely. The patient should be administered calcium and vitamin D supplements.

Emtricitabine (Emtriva) inhibits HIV-1 reverse transcriptase to inhibit HIV activity. Again, dosage reduction in renal impairment is necessary. Prior to beginning therapy, it is important to check liver function and assess it periodically throughout treatment. The nurse also assesses patients with depression for suicidal ideation. In addition, the nurse instructs patients to avoid driving or operating machinery until their response to the medication is known.

Emtricitabine and tenofovir (Truvada) is a reverse transcriptase inhibitor, nucleoside, and reverse transcriptase nucleotide. Emtricitabine is a cytosine analogue. Tenofovir is an analog of adenosine 5 monophosphate. This combination interferes with HIV viral RNA dependent DNA polymerase to inhibit viral replication.

Emtricitabine, tenofovir, and efavirenz (Atripla) adds the NNRTI of HIV-1 to block the RNA-dependent and DNA-dependent polymerase to assist in blocking HIV-1 replication.

Stavudine is an NRTI that is administered in combination with other antiretroviral medications. The World Health Organization recommends 30 mg every 12 hours in all adult and adolescent patients regardless of their weight. Geriatric patients require close monitoring for peripheral neuropathy. The dosage of stavudine should be reduced in patients with renal impairment.

## NCLEX Success

14. An infant is born to a mother infected with human immunodeficiency virus (HIV). When is it appropriate to administer zidovudine?

    A. following a positive HIV test
    B. within 6 to 12 hours after birth
    C. within the first 2 days of life
    D. only if the viral load is decreased

15. The mother of an infant infected with human immunodeficiency virus (HIV) has a low viral load and gives birth to a healthy baby boy. What is the most appropriate medical intervention?

    A. Administer the adult dose of stavudine to the infant.
    B. Administer zidovudine and nevirapine.
    C. Assess the infant's viral load.
    D. Perform HIV testing on delivery.

## NONNUCLEOSIDE REVERSE TRANSCRIPTASE INHIBITORS

The NNRTIs inhibit viral replication in infected cells by directly binding to reverse transcriptase and preventing its function. NRTIs and NNRTIs inhibit reverse transcriptase by different mechanisms, and therefore, they may have synergistic antiviral effects. The prototype NNRTI is ⓟ **efavirenz** (Sustiva).

## Pharmacokinetics

An oral drug, efavirenz is absorbed in the GI tract. Absorption is increased after consumption of a fatty meal. Its peak of action occurs in 3 to 5 hours. Efavirenz is approximately 99% protein bound, primarily to albumin. The drug is metabolized by the hepatic enzymes cytochrome P-450 (CYP) enzymes CYP3A4 and CYP2B6, which convert it to inactivated hydroxylated metabolites. The serum half-life is 52 to 76 hours after a single dose and 40 to 55 hours after multiple doses. It is eliminated as metabolites in the feces (16% to 61%) and the urine (14% to 34%).

## Action and Use

Efavirenz binds to reverse transcriptase to block RNA-dependent and DNA-dependent polymerase activities that includes HIV-1 replication. People take the medication in combination with other antiretroviral agents for HIV-1 infection. Table 23.8 presents route and dosage information for efavirenz and the other NNRTIs.

### Use in Patients With Hepatic Impairment

Patients with moderate to severe hepatic impairment should not take efavirenz.

## Adverse Effects

CNS adverse effects include dizziness, headache, insomnia, altered ability to concentrate, abnormal dreams, nervousness, and depression. Genitourinary adverse effects are renal calculus and hematuria. Patients may experience fever and fatigue, skin rash, erythema multiforme, Stevens-Johnson syndrome, and toxic epidermal necrolysis. In addition, patients may have increased levels of serum cholesterol, AST, and ALT.

## Contraindications

Contraindications to efavirenz include a known hypersensitivity to the medication and suicidal ideation. Because the drug may cause untoward fetal effects, particularly in the first trimester, women who are pregnant should not take it. Efavirenz is also contraindicated in breast-feeding women.

## Nursing Implications

### Preventing Interactions

Many medications and herbs interact with efavirenz, increasing or decreasing its effects (Boxes 23.6 and 23.7).

### Administering the Medication

Patients who experience CNS adverse effects, such as CNS depression, should take efavirenz at bedtime. They may take the medication on an empty stomach. After consuming a high-fat meal, patients should not take it for 2 hours. They should not discontinue efavirenz suddenly or without the consent of the prescriber.

### Assessing for Therapeutic Effects

The nurse assesses the CD4 count for increased ability to fight against viral infections.

### Assessing for Adverse Effects

The nurse assesses for skin rash and onset of Stevens-Johnson syndrome as well as for lack of concentration, increased nervousness, and impaired psychiatric effects. It is also necessary to assess for alterations in GI status such as nausea, vomiting, and diarrhea, as well as urinary output for bleeding and complaints of pain related to renal calculi. In addition, the nurse assesses the serum cholesterol, AST, and ALT values for possible increases.

### Patient Teaching

Box 23.5 identifies general patient teaching guidelines for antiretroviral drugs. The nurse should teach patients to use barrier

**TABLE 23.8**

**DRUGS AT A GLANCE: Antiretroviral Drugs: Nonnucleoside Reverse Transcriptase Inhibitors (NNRTIs)**

| Drug | Pregnancy Category | Routes and Dosage Ranges | |
|---|---|---|---|
| | | **Adults** | **Children** |
| P Efavirenz (Sustiva; Auro-Efavirenz, JAMP-Efavirenz, MYLAN-Efavirenz, Sustiva, TEVA-Efavirenz) | D | 600 mg PO daily<br>Dosage adjustments: with concomitant rifampin (if patient ≥50 kg), 800 mg PO daily; with concomitant voriconazole, efavirenz 300 mg PO daily and voriconazole 400 mg PO every 12 h | 3.5–5 kg: 100 mg daily<br>5–7.5 kg: 150 mg daily<br>7.5–15 kg: 200 mg daily<br>15 kg to <20 kg: 250 mg daily<br>20 kg to <25 mg: 300 mg daily<br>25 kg to <32.5 kg: 350 mg daily<br>32.5 kg to <40 kg: 400 mg daily<br>≥40 kg: 600 mg once daily |
| Delavirdine mesylate | C | 400 mg PO three times per day | ≥16 y: same as adult dose |
| Etravirine (Intelence; Intelence) | B | 200 mg PO twice daily after meals | Not recommended |
| Nevirapine (Viramune, Viramune XR; APO-Nevirapine XR, Auro-Nevirapine, JAMP-Nevirapine, MYLAN-Nevirapine) | B | Initial, 200 mg twice daily for 14 d; maintenance, 200 mg PO twice daily (immediate-release tablets) in combination with additional antiretroviral medications; 400 mg PO once daily (extended-release tablets) | Immediate-release tablets, 150 mg/m²/dose PO once daily for the first 14 d (max dose: 200 mg/d); increase dose to 150 mg/m²/dose PO twice daily if no rash or untoward effects (max 400 mg/d) |
| Rilpivirine (Edurant; Edurant) | B | PO 25 mg once daily | Children ≥12 y, refer to adult dosing |

contraceptives when taking efavirenz, not to drive or operate machinery until the effects of the medication are known, and to notify the prescriber in the event of pregnancy.

## Other Drugs in the Class

Delavirdine mesylate is an NNRTI that is indicated for combined use with other antiretroviral agents. The potential for life-threatening adverse effects has been noted when delavirdine is combined with CYP3A4 inducers. The drugs of greatest concern are dysrhythmic agents, clarithromycin, dapsone, rifabutin, benzodiazepines, calcium channel blockers, ergot derivatives, indinavir, saquinavir, quinidine, and warfarin. In patients who have an absence of hydrochloric acid in the gastric juices, it is necessary to administer the drug with an acidic beverage. Taking delavirdine requires mixing it with a minimum of

3 ounces of water. The solution should stand for a few minutes, and then the patient should drink the solution. After rinsing the glass, the patient should drink the rinse to obtain the entire dosage of the medication. Then he or she should rinse the mouth and swallow that solution.

Etravirine (Intelence) is an NNRTI that is used in combination with a minimum of two additional antiretroviral agents to treatment-experienced HIV patients. Patients should take it with food to aid absorption. Metabolism by CYP3A4, CYP2C9, and CYP2C19 occurs in the liver; this leads to reduced serum levels of other medications metabolized by the same substrates. For example, administration of etravirine with antifungal agents increases serum levels of etravirine and decreases antifungal activity.

Nevirapine (Viramune) is an NNRTI used in combination with other antiretroviral agents. Pregnant women with HIV may also take the drug in combination with zidovudine for the prevention of transmission of HIV to the fetus. It is essential that nevirapine not be given to children exposed to the drug

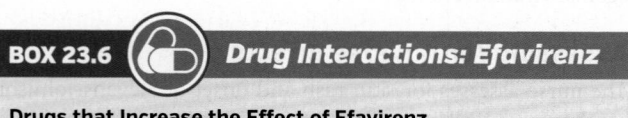

**BOX 23.6    *Drug Interactions: Efavirenz***

**Drugs that Increase the Effect of Efavirenz**
- Fluconazole, ritonavir
  *Increase serum levels*
- Alcohol
  *Increases central nervous system depression*

**Drugs that Decrease the Effects of Efavirenz**
- Rifampin, saquinavir
  *Decrease serum levels*

**BOX 23.7    *Herb and Dietary Interactions: Efavirenz***

- Fatty meal
  *Increases serum levels*
- St. John's wort
  *Decreases antiretroviral activity*

during prevention of transmission of HIV from the mother to the fetus. Patients may take the drug without regard to food intake. The **BLACK BOX WARNING ◆** issued by the FDA states that the most significant adverse effect of nevirapine is the abrupt onset of flulike symptoms, abdominal pain, fever with or without a rash, and jaundice. These adverse effects may progress to hepatic failure and encephalopathy.

Rilpivirine is useful in treatment-naïve patients whose viral load is less than 100,000 copies/mL and whose CD4 count is ≥200 cells/μL. It is administered alone or in combination with emtricitabine–tenofovir–disoproxil fumarate and rilpivirine–emtricitabine–tenofovir alafenamide. Caution is warranted in patients with long QT syndrome or torsade de pointes. It is important to avoid the use of rilpivirine in patients with reduced kidney function. During the administration of rilpivirine, it is necessary to monitor a patient's cholesterol levels because changes may occur (less than or equal to 48 weeks).

## NCLEX Success

16. A man infected with HIV is taking nevirapine (Viramune) and zidovudine (AZT). He develops a fever, malaise, and jaundice. He is at risk for which of the following conditions?

    A. hepatic failure
    B. heart failure
    C. pneumonia
    D. methicillin-resistant *Staphylococcus aureus*

17. An HIV-positive man who takes etravirine (Intelence) develops a fungal infection following a trip to the Caribbean. He is admitted to the hospital, where he receives intravenous amphotericin B for the fungal infection. What effect will etravirine have on amphotericin B?

    A. The antifungal activity will be diminished when combined with etravirine.
    B. The serum amphotericin B level will become toxic.
    C. The patient will require a stronger antifungal agent to prevent resistance.
    D. The two drugs are synergistic and will work together to fight the fungal infection.

## PROTEASE INHIBITORS

The PIs are antiretroviral drugs that exert their effects against HIV at a different phase of its life cycle than reverse transcriptase inhibitors. They inhibit the HIV enzyme protease, which is required to process viral protein precursors into mature particles capable of infecting other cells. Thus, they are active in both acutely and chronically infected cells. Compared with the NNRTIs and the integrase inhibitors, the PIs have a high genetic barrier to resistance. **Saquinavir mesylate** (Invirase) is the prototype PI. Note that other PIs have replaced saquinavir as the PI of choice because of increasing resistance and adverse effects. If saquinavir is administered, electrocardiogram (ECG)

monitoring for long QT syndrome is necessary. Reportedly, diminished resistance results with lopinavir/ritonavir (Kaletra), atazanavir/ritonavir, and darunavir/ritonavir.

The PIs are most commonly administered in combination with the nucleosides. In addition, ritonavir is a PI and cobicistat is a cytochrome P-450 inhibitor. Each of these medications is administered in combination with other antiretroviral agents to boost antiretroviral activity. These agents are described as boosting agents. Pharmacokinetic boosting improves the plasma trough concentrations and increases the drug's half-life and maximum concentration.

## Pharmacokinetics

Absorption of saquinavir mesylate is in the GI tract. However, absorption is enhanced when the drug is taken with a high-fat meal. It is 99% protein bound, and there is no distribution in the CSF. Saquinavir is metabolized by the liver enzyme CYP3A4 with extensive first-pass effect. The half-life is 13 hours. Saquinavir is excreted primarily in the feces (only 1% to 3% in the urine) within 5 days.

## Action

Saquinavir binds to the site of HIV-1 protease activity to prevent the cleavage of viral gag-pol polyproteins that are required for the maturation of the HIV virus. This action produces immature noninfectious viral particles.

## Use

The main purpose of using saquinavir is to reduce the viral load in HIV—in combination with other antiretroviral agents. Prescribers may also order it with colchicine for familial Mediterranean fever, gout prophylaxis, and gout flare-up and with phosphodiesterase-5 enzyme inhibitors for pulmonary hypertension or erectile dysfunction. Table 23.9 summarizes route and dosage information for saquinavir and the other PIs.

### Use in Older Adults

Administration in the elderly warrants caution because of the risk of organ dysfunction.

## Adverse Effects

Cardiovascular adverse effects include hypertension, hypotension, and chest pain. CNS adverse effects include back pain, fatigue, neuropathy, paresthesia, anxiety, depression, and suicidal ideation. Dermatologic adverse effects are pruritus, rash, and eczema. Hematologic adverse effects are thrombocytopenia, pancytopenia, and anemia. Elevations in creatinine kinase, AST and ALT, and bilirubin have occurred.

## Contraindications

Contraindications to saquinavir include a known hypersensitivity to the drug. Other conditions that preclude its use are congenital or acquired prolongation of the QT interval, atrioventricular block, hepatic impairment, refractory hypokalemia, or hypomagnesemia.

**TABLE 23.9**

## DRUGS AT A GLANCE: Antiretroviral Drugs: Protease Inhibitors (PIs)

| Drug | Pregnancy Category | Routes and Dosage Ranges | |
|---|---|---|---|
| | | **Adults** | **Children** |
| Ⓟ **Saquinavir mesylate** (Invirase; 🍁 Invirase) | B | 1000 mg PO twice daily with ritonavir 100 mg in combination with a full meal | 5 to <15 kg: 50 mg/kg/dose twice daily plus ritonavir 3 mg/kg/dose twice daily 15 to <40 kg: 50 mg/kg/dose twice daily plus ritonavir 2.5 mg/kg/dose twice daily ≥40 kg 1000 mg twice daily plus ritonavir 100 mg twice daily |
| Atazanavir (Reyataz; 🍁 MYLAN-Atazanavir, Reayataz, TEVA-Atazanavir) | B | Antiretroviral naïve, 300 mg PO once daily plus ritonavir 100 mg; patients who do not tolerate ritonavir: 400 mg PO once daily Antiretroviral experienced, 300 mg PO once daily plus ritonavir 100 mg Pregnant patients, 300 mg PO once daily plus ritonavir 100 mg once daily | 6–12 y Antiretroviral-naïve 15–24 kg, 150 mg PO once daily plus ritonavir 80 mg once daily 25–31 kg, 200 mg PO once daily plus ritonavir 100 mg PO once daily 32–38 kg, 250 mg once daily plus ritonavir 100 mg PO once daily ≥39 kg, 300 mg PO once daily plus 100 mg once daily Antiretroviral experienced 25–31 kg, 200 mg PO once daily plus ritonavir 100 mg PO once daily 32–38 kg, 250 mg PO once daily plus ritonavir 100 mg PO once daily ≥39 kg, 300 mg PO once daily plus 100 mg once daily |
| Darunavir (Prezista; 🍁 APO-Darunavir, Prezista) | C | Antiretroviral naïve, 800 mg PO once daily with ritonavir 100 mg Antiretroviral experienced, if genotypic testing is not possible, 600 mg PO with ritonavir 100 mg once daily | ≥6 y ≥20 to <30 kg, 375 mg PO twice daily with ritonavir 50 mg twice daily ≥30 to <40 mg, 450 mg PO twice daily with ritonavir 60 mg twice daily ≥40 kg, 600 mg PO twice daily with ritonavir 100 mg twice daily |
| Fosamprenavir calcium (Lexiva; 🍁 Telzir) | C | Unboosted regimen: 1400 mg PO twice daily Ritonavir-boosted regimen, 1400 mg PO plus ritonavir 100–200 mg once daily (not recommended in PI-experienced patients) *Or* 700 mg PO plus ritonavir 100 mg twice daily | Antiretroviral-naïve 2–5 y, 30 mg/kg/dose PO twice daily ≥6 y Unboosted regimen, 30 mg/kg/dose Ritonavir-boosted regimen, 18 mg/kg/dose plus 3 mg/kg/dose ritonavir PO twice daily (do not exceed adult dosage) |
| Indinavir sulfate (Crixivan) | C | Unboosted regimen, 800 mg PO every 8 h Boosted regimen, 800 mg PO twice daily with ritonavir 100–200 mg When combined with other antiretroviral agents, consult manufacturer's recommendations | Safety and efficacy not established |
| Lopinavir/ritonavir (Kaletra; 🍁 Kaletra) | C | Antiretroviral naïve or antiretroviral experienced, lopinavir 400 mg/ritonavir 100 mg PO twice daily Antiretroviral naïve or antiretroviral experienced with efavirenz, fosamprenavir, nelfinavir, nevirapine, lopinavir 500 mg/ritonavir 125 mg twice daily, or lopinavir 533 mg/ritonavir 133 mg solution PO twice daily Once-daily dosing, lopinavir 800 mg/ritonavir 200 mg PO once daily | 14 d to 6 mo, 16 mg/kg PO twice daily 6 mo to 18 y: <15 kg, 12 mg/kg PO twice daily 15–40 kg, 10 mg/kg PO twice daily >40 kg, lopinavir 400 mg/ritonavir 100 mg PO twice daily Combination therapy with efavirenz, fosamprenavir, nelfinavir, or nevirapine 6 mo to 18 y: <15 kg, 13 mg/kg PO twice daily 15–45 kg, 11 mg/kg PO twice daily >45 kg: same as adults |

| | **TABLE 23.9** | | |
| --- | --- | --- | --- |
| | **DRUGS AT A GLANCE: Antiretroviral Drugs: Protease Inhibitors (PIs)** (Continued) | | |

| Drug | Pregnancy Category | Routes and Dosage Ranges | |
| --- | --- | --- | --- |
| | | **Adults** | **Children** |
| Nelfinavir mesylate (Viracept; ✿ Viracept) | B | 750 mg PO three times per day or 1250 mg PO twice daily | 2–13 y: 45–55 mg/kg PO twice daily or 25–35 mg/kg PO three times daily not to exceed 2500 mg/d (mix oral powder in milk or water/do not mix with acidic juices) |
| Ritonavir (Norvir; ✿ Norvir) | B | 600 mg PO twice daily; increase dose as follows: 300 mg twice daily for 1 d, 400 mg twice daily for 2 d, and 500 mg twice daily for 1 d. Then increase by 100 mg twice daily every 2–3 d to recommended dosage of 600 mg PO twice daily | >1 mo: 350–400 mg/m² PO twice daily; initial dose 250 mg/m² PO twice daily; titrate upward every 2–3 d by 50 mg/m² PO twice daily |
| Tipranavir (Aptivus, ✿ Aptivus) | C | 500 mg PO twice daily (administer with ritonavir 200 mg PO twice daily) | ≥2 y: 14 mg/kg or 375 mg/m² PO twice daily; max 500 mg/dose (administer with ritonavir 6 mg/kg or 150 mg/m² twice daily) |

## Nursing Implications

### Preventing Interactions

Medications as well as herbs and foods interact with saquinavir, increasing or decreasing its effects (Boxes 23.8 and 23.9). The use of ergot alkaloids with PIs increases the risk of ergot toxicity.

### Administering the Medication

Patients should take saquinavir with ritonavir. To ensure maximum bioavailability, the nurse should instruct patients to take saquinavir within 2 hours of a meal or on a full stomach. Patients should have an ECG prior to the start of therapy and 3 to 4 days after therapy is begun. It is also necessary to measure serum potassium, magnesium, triglycerides, and cholesterol before the initiation of therapy.

### Assessing for Therapeutic Effects

The nurse assesses for an increase in T helper CD4 cells. The CD4 count is a measure of the ability to fight infections.

### Assessing for Adverse Effects

The nurse assesses for ECG-related changes, specifically QT prolongation. Also, he or she also assesses for signs and symptoms of peripheral neuropathy. In addition, the nurse assesses the mouth for signs of ulcerations related to increase gastric acid.

It is important to check laboratory results. The nurse assesses the CBC and bilirubin for anemia, thrombocytopenia, and pancytopenia; serum potassium and magnesium levels; and AST or ALT for elevation.

### Patient Teaching

Box 23.5 presents patient teaching guidelines for antiretroviral drugs.

## Other Drugs in the Class

Atazanavir (Reyataz) is a PI that is administered to treatment-naïve and treatment-experienced patients, often with ritonavir. It is necessary to take the drug with food. Monitoring of the patient's cholesterol level for increase of greater than 240 mg/dL is important. Contraindications to atazanavir include hypersensitivity to the drug—because of the risk of Stevens-Johnson syndrome.

Darunavir (Prezista) is very similar to atazanavir.

Fosamprenavir (Lexiva) is an oral PI administered with or without ritonavir. It is 63% absorbed and hydrolyzed to amprenavir by the stomach enzymes, reaching a peak of action in

| BOX 23.8 | Drug Interactions: Saquinavir |
| --- | --- |

**Drugs that Increase Effects of Saquinavir**
- Delavirdine, clarithromycin, indinavir, ketoconazole, ritonavir
  *Increase serum levels*

**Drugs that Decrease the Effects of Saquinavir**
- Carbamazepine, dexamethasone, phenobarbital, phenytoin, rifabutin, rifampin
  *Decrease serum levels*

| BOX 23.9 | Herb and Dietary Interactions: Saquinavir |
| --- | --- |

- St. John's wort
  *Decreases antiretroviral activity*
- Garlic
  *Decreases antiretroviral activity*
- Grapefruit juice (1 quart/d)
  *Increases plasma concentrations of saquinavir, leading to adverse effects*

2.5 hours. It is metabolized in the liver by CYP3A4 and eliminated in the urine and feces. Fosamprenavir has similar adverse effects as other drugs in the class.

Indinavir (Crixivan) is an oral PI administered with ritonavir. The medication binds to the site of HIV-1 protease activity to inhibit the functional proteins of infectious HIV, resulting in noninfectious viral particles. Patients should take it without food, and they should drink 48 ounces of fluids per day.

Lopinavir/ritonavir (Kaletra) is an oral PI administered in treatment-naïve and treatment-experienced patients. It is important to monitor patients who take lopinavir/ritonavir for significant adverse effects, including hypertriglyceridemia, myocardial infarction, and GI toxicity. Lopinavir, in this combination, may be part of a multidrug antiretroviral regimen. Patients should take it with food. Monitoring for signs and symptoms of pancreatitis, onset of diabetes, and triglyceride elevation is necessary. The nurse should instruct the patient about blood glucose testing and keeping regularly scheduled laboratory appointments to check amylase, triglycerides, inorganic phosphorus, thyroid function, and CBC.

Nelfinavir mesylate (Viracept) is an oral PI that patients should take with food to enhance absorption. It is distributed with 98% of the drug being protein bound. The nurse instructs the patient to take nelfinavir exactly as prescribed and not to alter the dose. The patient should report the onset of diarrhea. If necessary, the patient may mix the oral powder preparation of the drug with dietary supplements, regular or soy milk, or water but not with acidic liquids.

Ritonavir (Norvir) is an oral PI administered alone or in combination with other antiretroviral agents. Authorities do not recommend it as a primary PI. The medication is contraindicated with saquinavir in patients who have cardiac conduction insufficiency disorders. It is necessary to assess for GI distress, peripheral neuropathy, palpitations, syncope, tachycardia, and a prolonged QT interval.

Tipranavir (Aptivus) is a PI for treatment-experienced patients or patients with HIV-1 strains that are resistant to multiple PIs. Caution is warranted when administering it to patients receiving sulfonamides. It is necessary to monitor blood glucose to check for loss of glycemic control. The nurse instructs the patient to apply sunscreen because of possible photosensitivity reactions.

## CYTOCHROME P-450 INHIBITOR

Cobicistat (Tybost) is a boosting agent administered with atazanavir or darunavir or other retroviral agent. The purpose in combining cobicistat with antiretroviral agents is based on its action to increase exposure of CYP3A4 substrates in atazanavir or darunavir. This action increases the antiretroviral activity of these antiretroviral agents.

### NCLEX Success

18. Which of the following electrocardiographic changes warrant the discontinuation of saquinavir mesylate?
    A. prolongation of the QT interval
    B. inverted T wave
    C. elongated ST segment
    D. premature ventricular contraction

19. A 2-year-old child is started on nelfinavir mesylate. The nurse is instructing the mother on the proper administration of the medication. Which of the following is most appropriate to teach the mother?
    A. Squirt the medication in the mouth with a syringe.
    B. Tilt the head back and place the medicine in a nipple.
    C. Mix the medicine with water, milk, or formula.
    D. Mix the medicine in orange juice.

## INTEGRASE STRAND TRANSFER INHIBITORS

INSTIs block the action of integrase, a viral enzyme of HIV-1 essential for viral replication. The only member of this drug class approved by the FDA is Ⓟ **raltegravir** (Isentress, Insentress HD). This drug is comparable to efavirenz in terms of its ability to suppress HIV.

### Pharmacokinetics

Raltegravir is absorbed by the GI tract. The rate of absorption is doubled if the drug is taken with a high-fat meal. It is 83% protein bound. Raltegravir is metabolized by hepatic glucuronidation mediated by UGT1A1. The serum half-life is 9 hours. The drug is eliminated in the feces and urine.

### Action

Raltegravir blocks HIV-1 integrase to prevent the formation of the HIV-1 provirus to decrease the viral load and increase the active CD4 cells. Specifically, after HIV reverse transcriptase enters CD4 T cells, the enzyme transcribes viral RNA into DNA. As the integrase combines with viral DNA and other cellular cofactors, it forms the preintegration complex. The integrase removes the nucleotide from the 3' terminus to expose reactive hydroxyl groups. The preintegration complex enters the host cell nucleus, binding to host cell DNA. Integrase then nicks each strand of the host cell DNA, exposing 5' phosphate groups to enable covalent bonding of host and viral DNA. When the strand transfer is complete, the host cell enzymes repair the gaps between the viral and host DNA.

### Use

Raltegravir is a first-line antiviral agent that is administered with tenofovir and emtricitabine to treatment-experienced adults. These patients must have evidence of viral replication and HIV-1 strains resistant to multiple antiretroviral drugs. Table 23.10 supplies information about the route of administration and dosage for raltegravir.

### Adverse Effects and Contraindications

Few adverse effects occur with raltegravir. The most common include headache, dizziness, nausea, diarrhea, vomiting, abdominal pain, fever, and rhabdomyolysis. Sometimes serum glucose level, hepatic enzymes, and lipase level increase. However, in a double-blind study of treatment-naïve patients over 192 weeks

**TABLE 23.10**

**DRUGS AT A GLANCE: Antiretroviral Drugs: Integrase Strand Transfer Inhibitors (INSTIs), Fusion Protein Inhibitors, and CCR5 Antagonists**

| Drug | Pregnancy Category | Routes and Dosage Ranges | |
|------|-------------------|--------------------------|---|
| | | **Adults** | **Children** |
| **Integrase Strand Transfer Inhibitors (INSTIs)** | | | |
| ⓟ **Raltegravir** (Isentress, Isentress HD; 🍁 Isentress, Isentress HD) | C | 400 mg PO twice daily or 1200 mg PO once daily | 2 to <12 y 10 to <14 kg: 75 mg PO twice daily 14 to <20 kg: 100 mg PO twice daily 20 to <28 kg: 150 mg PO twice daily 28 to <40 kg: 200 mg PO twice daily ≥40 kg: 300 mg PO twice daily >12 y: see adults |
| Dolutegravir (Tivicay; 🍁 Tivicay) | Dolutegravir has a high level of transfer across the human placenta with increased risk of neural tube defects; may result in preterm delivery, stillbirth, low birth weight, and small for gestational age infants. | 10 mg, 25 mg, or 50 mg PO 2 h before or 6 h after cation antacids | Same as adults |
| **Fusion Protein Inhibitors** | | | |
| Enfuvirtide (Fuzeon; 🍁 Fuzeon) | B | 90 mg sub-Q twice daily | 6–16 y, 2 mg/kg sub-Q twice daily |
| **CCR5 Antagonists** | | | |
| Maraviroc (Selzentry; 🍁 Celsentri) | C | 300 mg PO twice daily | <16 y: safety and efficacy have not been established. >16 y, same as adults |
| **Cytochrome P-450 Inhibitor** | | | |
| Cobicistat (Tybost; 🍁 Tybost) | Not recommended in pregnancy | PO 150 mg with food and atazanavir or darunavir | No dosage approved |
| **Integrase inhibitor, Reverse Transcriptase inhibitor, Nucleoside, Reverse Transcriptase Inhibitor, Nucleotide** | | | |
| ⓟ **Bictegravir, emtricitabine, and tenofovir alafenamide (Biktarvy; 🍁 Biktarvy)** | The Health and Human Services perinatal HIV guidelines consider this fixed dose combination a preferred regimen for pregnant females living with HIV. If females taking this fixed dose combination drug become pregnant, they may continue if viral suppression is effective. | Bictegravir 50 mg/emtricitabine 200 mg/tenofovir alafenamide 25 mg PO once daily | Pediatric patients weighing >25 kg PO Bictegravir 50 mg/emtricitabine 200 mg/tenofovir alafenamide 25 mg once daily; in clinical trials the youngest patients were 6 years of age |

of follow-up, researchers found that patients showed excellent tolerance and lack of effect on lipids.

Contraindications include a known hypersensitivity to the medication. The drug is not suitable for treatment-naïve patients and breast-feeding women.

## Nursing Implications

### Preventing Interactions

Some medications interact with raltegravir, increasing or decreasing its effects (Box 23.10). St. John's wort decreases the effects of raltegravir.

**BOX 23.10    Drug Interactions: Raltegravir**

**Drugs that Increase the Effects of Raltegravir**
- Proton pump inhibitors
  *Increase the serum concentration*

**Drugs that Decrease the Effects of Raltegravir**
- Efavirenz, fosamprenavir, rifampin, tipranavir
  *Decrease the serum concentration*

### Administering the Medication

Patients may take raltegravir with or without meals.

### Assessing Therapeutic and Adverse Effects

The nurse assesses for an increase in T helper CD4 cells. The CD4 count measures the ability to fight against infections.

In addition, the nurse assesses for GI upset, headache, dizziness, fever, and rhabdomyolysis. It is necessary to monitor blood sugar, liver enzymes, and lipase levels for increases.

### Patient Teaching

Box 23.5 presents patient teaching guidelines for antiretroviral drugs.

## FUSION PROTEIN INHIBITORS

The drugs in this new class inhibit the HIV virus from binding to, fusing with, and entering the human cell. 🅟 **Enfuvirtide** (Fuzeon) is the only drug in this class. This drug is for use only by patients who have previously been treated with antiretroviral agents. Antiretroviral therapy–naïve patients should not use it.

## Pharmacokinetics

Following subcutaneous administration, enfuvirtide has a peak of action of 4 to 8 hours. The drug is 84% absorbed and distributed to the CSF in 2 to 18 hours. It is 92% protein bound. Enfuvirtide is metabolized by proteolytic hydrolysis in which it is catabolized into amino acids. The medication is not excreted; the amino acids are recycled.

## Action and Use

Enfuvirtide inhibits the fusion of the membrane of the HIV-1 virus with that of the cell, thus preventing HIV from entering the cell. It is used in combination with other antiretrovirals in treating HIV-1. Table 23.10 gives route of administration and dosage information for enfuvirtide.

## Adverse Effects and Contraindications

The most commonly reported adverse effects to enfuvirtide are fatigue, insomnia, nausea, and diarrhea. Injection site reactions such as rash, pain, discomfort, redness, hypersensitivity, rash, and nodule development may also occur. Researchers have reported bacterial pneumonia in 3% of the patients who used enfuvirtide. Less than 10% of the patients may have elevated serum creatine phosphokinase, myalgia, and limb pain.

## Contraindications

Contraindications to enfuvirtide include a hypersensitivity to the drug and lactation.

## Nursing Implications

### Preventing Interactions

PIs increase serum enfuvirtide levels.

### Administering the Medication

The nurse injects enfuvirtide subcutaneously into the upper arm, abdomen, or anterior thigh. Injection of the drug into blood vessels, navel, moles, scars, or other areas of skin change should never occur. Rotation of injection sites and assessment of the sites for reactions is necessary. It is important not to inject enfuvirtide into large nerves that are close to the skin near the buttocks, elbow, knee, or groin.

### Assessing for Therapeutic and Adverse Effects

The nurse assesses for an increase in T helper CD4 cells. The CD4 count measures the ability to fight against infections.

Also, the nurse assesses the injection site for signs of hypersensitivity such as rash, redness, nodules, or pain. He or she also assesses for diarrhea, nausea, or other signs of GI distress. In addition, it is necessary to assess the serum creatine phosphokinase for elevation along with myalgia or limb pain. Finally, the nurse assesses pulmonary status, looking for cough, fever, or bacterial pneumonia.

### Patient Teaching

The nurse instructs the patient or family about the proper technique for the administration of the enfuvirtide. Daily administration is necessary, and if a dose is missed, it is important to notify the primary care provider. Instruct the rotation of injection sites and assessment of site for changes. Box 23.5 provides general patient teaching guidelines for antiretroviral drugs.

## CCR5 ANTAGONISTS

Currently, there is only one member of this antiretroviral class, 🅟 **maraviroc** (Selzentry). It blocks the receptor site to which the HIV needs to interact to enter the cell.

## Pharmacokinetics

Maraviroc is absorbed in the GI tract. The drug has a slow onset of action, reaching a peak of action in ½ to 4 hours. Its half-life is 14 to 18 hours. Maraviroc is 76% protein bound. The drug is metabolized by the liver with the CYP3A enzyme to inactive metabolites. It is excreted in the urine (20%; 8% remains unchanged) and kidneys (76%; 25% remains unchanged).

## Action and Use

Maraviroc binds to the human chemokine receptor on the cell membrane. This action prevents the interaction of HIV-1 and CCR5 that is needed for HIV to enter the cell and replicate.

People with HIV take maraviroc in combination with other antiretroviral agents for detectable CCR5-tropic HIV-1 possessing evidence of viral replication. They may have HIV-1 strains that are resistant to many other antiretroviral drugs. Those with a CrCl less than 30 mL/min or with end-stage renal disease should not take maraviroc. Table 23.10 gives route of administration and dosage information for maraviroc.

## Adverse Effects

The most common adverse effects of maraviroc are fever; rash; upper respiratory infection with cough; vascular hypertension; and CNS depression with dizziness, anxiety, and depression. Other less significant adverse effects are lipodystrophy, pruritus, benign skin neoplasms, genital warts, elevated bilirubin, joint pain, conjunctivitis, and otitis media. The FDA has issued a **BLACK BOX WARNING** ◆ for maraviroc, stating that it may lead to drug-induced hepatotoxicity with allergic features following 1 month of treatment. Allergic reactions such as pruritic rash, fever, eosinophilia, fever, increased IgE, and symptoms of hepatitis that can be life threatening may precede this condition.

## Contraindications

Contraindications to maraviroc include severe renal impairment and use of medications that are potent CYP3A4 inhibitors.

## Nursing Implications

### Preventing Interactions

Several medications interact with maraviroc, increasing or decreasing its effects (Box 23.11). St. John's wort decreases the effects of the drug.

### Administering the Medication

Patients may take maraviroc before meals, with meals, or after meals. However, high-fat foods enhance absorption.

### Assessing for Therapeutic and Adverse Effects

The nurse assesses for an increase in T helper CD4 cells. The CD4 count measures the ability to fight against infections.

In addition, the nurse assesses the bilirubin, AST, and ALT levels for signs of hepatotoxicity. It is also necessary to assess the temperature for fever and monitor the IgE levels, which are indicative of the onset of hepatitis. The nurse assesses for rash or other skin changes such as the development of neoplasms. He or she assesses for cough and upper respiratory infection. Finally, the nurse assesses the ear canal for otitis media or complaints of ear pain.

### Patient Teaching

The nurse instructs the patient to use caution when changing positions due to possible drug-induced dizziness. He or she also tells the patient to report rash, yellow skin or eyes, muscle pain, or fatigue. In addition, the general patient teaching guidelines presented in Box 23.5 may be useful.

## COMBINATION MEDICATION FOR HIV-1: INTEGRASE INHIBITOR, REVERSE TRANSCRIPTASE INHIBITOR, NUCLEOSIDE, REVERSE TRANSCRIPTASE INHIBITOR, NUCLEOTIDE

ⓟ Bictegravir, emtricitabine, and tenofovir alafenamide (Biktarvy) is one of the newest antiretroviral agent for the treatment of HIV-1 in adult and pediatric patients. Approved for use in the United States in February 2018, it is a once-a-day treatment for HIV-1. This combination medication increases the immune response and assists in fighting infections. In 8 to 24 weeks the amount of HIV in the patient's system will be lowered or undetectable.

## Pharmacokinetics

Bictegravir is 99% protein bound; tenofovir alafenadmide is 80% protein bound; emtricitabine is only 4% protein bound. Bictegravir is metabolized by the CYP3A enzymes, and tenofovir alafenamide is converted intracellularly by hydrolysis. Bictegravir reaches a peak in 2 to 4 hours and has a 17.3-hour half-life. It is excreted in the feces and urine. Emtricitabine's half-life is 10.4 hours, with a peak in 1.5 to 2 hours. It is excreted in the feces and urine. Tenofovir alafenamide reaches a peak in 0.5 to 2 hours and has a half-life in 51 minutes. Tenofovir diphosphate's half-life is 150 to 180 hours. As with the other drugs, it is excreted in the feces and urine.

## Action and Use

Bictegravir inhibits HIV integrase and binds to the integrase site to block the transfer strand of DNA integration. Emtricitabine and tenofovir alafenamide are converted intracellularly to tenofovir and is phosphorylated by cellular kinases to tenofovir diphosphate. This action interferes with HIV and HIV viral RNA-dependent DNA polymerase activities to inhibit viral replication.

## Adverse Effects

Bictegravir, emtricitabine, and tenofovir alafenamide combination has the ability to increase the creatinine clearance, low density lipoprotein, amylase, as well as the ALT and AST. Diarrhea, nausea, abdominal pain, dyspepsia, flatulence, and vomiting are common gastrointestinal adverse effects.

## Contraindications

Bictegravir, emtricitabine, and tenofovir alafenamide combination is contraindicated with dofetilide and rifampin.

## Nursing Implications

### Preventing Interactions

Aminoglycoside, acyclovir, and valacyclovir increase serum concentrations of tenofovir. Adefovir diminishes the effect of tenofovir. Do not combine with medications that induce CYP3A4 action.

### Administering the Medication

Administer bictegravir, emtricitabine, and tenofovir alafenamide with or without food. Administer 2 hours before or 6 hours after aluminum or magnesium containing antacids. Administer with food with concomitant calcium- or iron-containing supplements or antacids.

### Assessing for Therapeutic and Adverse Effects

Assess CD4 count, HIV RNA plasma levels, serum creatinine, urine glucose, and serum phosphorous. Patients with chronic kidney disease are at risk for increased kidney damage.

Patients administered bictegravir, emtricitabine, and tenofovir alafenamide are at risk for bone loss and fracture; bone density should be monitored.

### Patient Teaching

In addition, the general patient teaching guidelines presented in Box 23.5 may be useful.

## NCLEX Success

20. **What is the action of raltegravir?**
    A. It blocks HIV integrase.
    B. It increases viral load.
    C. It diminishes cell membrane permeability.
    D. It increases white blood cell count.

21. **A patient has been admitted to the infectious disease division. The physician has ordered enfuvirtide 90 mg twice daily. What is the recommended route of administration of enfuvirtide?**
    A. intravenous
    B. oral
    C. intramuscular
    D. subcutaneous

22. **A physician prescribes maraviroc for a man with human immunodeficiency virus (HIV). The nurse should instruct the man to be alert for what adverse effect?**
    A. edema
    B. cardiac abnormality with chest pain
    C. yellowing of skin
    D. bronchospasm

## THE NURSING PROCESS

A concept map outlines the nursing process related to drug therapy considerations in this chapter. Additional nursing implications related to the disease process should also be considered in care decisions.

**Assessment**
- Assess for signs and symptoms of viral infections and resolution of signs and symptoms following the administration of antiviral medications.
- Assess renal and hepatic function.
- Assess viral hepatitis risk factors, exposure, and signs and symptoms of liver dysfunction.
- Assess baseline data to assist in monitoring response to drug therapy.
  - Vital signs, weight, and nutritional status
  - Signs and symptoms of disease and opportunistic infections associated with disease and immunosuppression
  - CBC; CD4+; lymphocyte count; plasma levels of viral RNA; and BUN, AST, ALT, AST, and creatinine

**Outcomes of Therapy**
The patient will
- Receive or take antiviral drugs as prescribed.
- Be safeguarded against new or recurrent infection.
- Act to prevent spread of viral infection to others and recurrence in self.
- Avoid preventable adverse drug effects and drug interactions.
- Receive emotional support and counseling to assist in coping with HIV infection or genital herpes.

**Nursing Interventions**
- Follow recommended policies and procedures for preventing spread of viral infections.
- Assist patients in learning ways to control spread and recurrence of viral infections.
- Assist patients to maintain immunizations against viral infections.
- For patients receiving systemic antiviral drugs, monitor serum creatinine and other tests of renal function, CBC, and fluid balance.
- For patients with HIV infection, help to schedule their drug therapy regimen as conveniently as possible (to promote adherence), monitor for changes in baseline data during each contact, prevent opportunistic infections (e.g., herpes infections) when possible, and manage adverse effects of drug therapy to promote quality of life.

**Evaluation**
- Observe for improvement in signs and symptoms of the viral infection for which a drug is given.
- Interview outpatients regarding their compliance with instructions for taking antiviral drugs.
- Interview and observe for use of infection control measures.
- Interview and observe for adverse drug effects.
- Observe the extent and severity of any symptoms in patients with HIV infection or viral hepatitis.

## KEY CONCEPTS

- Viral infections commonly occur in all age groups.
- Vaccinations, avoiding contact with people who have viral infections, and thorough hand hygiene are effective ways to prevent viral infections.
- Health care providers use a variety of antiviral drugs to fight viral infections.
- Because viruses are intracellular parasites, antiviral drugs are relatively toxic to human cells.
- Viral infections for which drug therapy is available include HSV, VZV, CMV, RSV, influenza, hepatitis B and C, and HIV infection.
- The FDA has issued two **BLACK BOX WARNING** ◆ for ganciclovir. The first states that granulocytopenia (neutropenia), anemia, and thrombocytopenia may occur. If severe bone marrow depression occurs, ganciclovir should be discontinued; recovery usually occurs within a week of stopping the drug. The second advises female and male patients of childbearing age to maintain contraceptive precautions during ganciclovir therapy and for a minimum of 90 days after drug therapy.
- The FDA has issued three **BLACK BOX WARNING** ◆ for cidofovir. The drug has possible carcinogenic and teratogenic adverse effects. It may also be nephrotoxic, and prior to administration, the patient should receive 1 L of normal saline and oral probenecid. In addition, it places the patient at risk for neutropenia.
- The FDA has issued a **BLACK BOX WARNING** ◆ for foscarnet. Seizures may occur related to impaired renal function, diminished serum calcium, and CNS conditions.
- Valganciclovir has the same **BLACK BOX WARNING** ◆ as ganciclovir.
- The FDA has issued two **BLACK BOX WARNING** ◆ for ribavirin. The first states that this drug causes significant teratogenic effects according to animal studies. Pregnant women or those who plan to become pregnant should not care for children receiving inhalation therapy or be in the room when it is being administered. Ribavirin is contraindicated in infants and children who have a known hypersensitivity to the drug or its components. The second states that the drug can produce hemolytic anemia, which could lead to myocardial infarction. Patients with unstable cardiovascular disease should not take the drug.
- Antiretroviral drugs are given in combination to increase effectiveness and decrease emergence of drug-resistant viruses. The antiretroviral drugs include the NRTIs, NNRTIs, PIs, the integrase strand transfer inhibitors, the fusion protein inhibitors, and the CCR5 antagonists.
- The FDA has issued a **BLACK BOX WARNING** ◆ for the nucleoside analogs, including lamivudine. There are reports of lactic acidosis and severe hepatomegaly with steatosis.
- The FDA has issued several **BLACK BOX WARNING** ◆ for zidovudine. One relates to the adverse effects of granulocytopenia, aplastic or hemolytic anemia, pancytopenia with bone marrow hypoplasia, leukopenia, and lymphadenopathy. Dosage adjustment is necessary in patients who develop anemia or neutropenia. Other warnings relate to lactic acidosis and severe hepatomegaly with steatosis and symptomatic myopathy and myositis.
- The FDA has issued a **BLACK BOX WARNING** ◆ for abacavir. Patients may have serious and sometimes fatal hypersensitivity reactions. Those who test positive for HLAB*5701 allele are at greatest risk for hypersensitivity reactions.
- A combination of abacavir, lamivudine, and zidovudine (Trizivir) is used for HIV-1 treatment. The FDA has issued a **BLACK BOX WARNING** ◆ that patients with the *HLA-B*5701* allele are prone to a hypersensitivity reaction.
- The FDA has issued a **BLACK BOX WARNING** ◆ for nevirapine. Its most significant adverse effect is the abrupt onset of flulike symptoms, abdominal pain, fever with or without a rash, and jaundice.
- The FDA has issued a **BLACK BOX WARNING** ◆ for maraviroc. Drug-induced hepatotoxicity with allergic features may occur following 1 month of treatment.

## CLINICAL REASONING CASE STUDY

### Meet the Patient

James Patterson, a 17-year-old man, is admitted to the hospital with severe pneumonia. He is diagnosed with *Pneumocystis jiroveci*. On further evaluation, he is tested for HIV. He tests positive, and he begins taking zidovudine, saquinavir, and ritonavir.

- What is the action of zidovudine?
- What is the action of saquinavir?
- What is the rationale for the administration of ritonavir with saquinavir and zidovudine?
- What testing should the patient have prior to beginning saquinavir and ritonavir therapy?
- What patient teaching does the nurse provide about HIV and antiretroviral therapy?

### Assessing Drug Information

- Zidovudine is an NRTI, which has components similar to those of DNA (adenosine, cytosine, guanosine, and thymidine). The drug easily enters human cells, as well as viruses, inhibiting reverse transcriptase, an enzyme required by retroviruses to convert RNA to DNA and allow replication. Zidovudine is active in slowing the progression of acute infection rather than treating chemically infected cells.
- Saquinavir is a PI that exerts effects against HIV by binding to the site of HIV-1 protease to prevent cleavage of viral gag-polyproteins required for the maturation of the HIV virus. This action produces immature noninfectious viral particles.
- Saquinavir is used with other antiretroviral agents to reduce viral load.
- Ritonavir increases the effect of other antiretroviral agents.

### Nursing Actions

- The nurse should tell Mr. Patterson about the importance of obtaining ECGs while taking saquinavir and ritonavir. ECGs are necessary prior to beginning therapy and 3 to 4 days after therapy is begun.
- Assess serum potassium, magnesium, triglycerides, and cholesterol before beginning therapy.
- The nurse provides the following instructions:
  - Take saquinavir within 2 hours of a meal or on a full stomach. The administration of a combination of antiretrovirals such as saquinavir and ritonavir ensures maximum bioavailability.
  - Take the oral preparation of zidovudine with or without food and around the clock to avoid variations in serum peak and trough levels.
  - When taking zidovudine, be aware of the signs and symptoms of lactic acidosis, which include musculoskeletal pain.
  - Prevent infection by using good hand hygiene.
  - Receive an annual influenza vaccine.
  - Practice safe sex by using a condom.
  - In case of intravenous drug use, utilize clean needles.
  - Maintain close adherence to the medications ordered.
  - Do not change doses or stop the medications without consulting a health care provider.
  - Take all antiretroviral medications consistently to suppress HIV infection and minimize adverse effects.
  - Do not take any other medications (including drugs of abuse, herbal preparations, vitamin/mineral supplements, nonprescription drugs) without informing your primary care provider.
  - Be aware of the interactions with food.
  - Do not take any herbal supplements. St. John's Wort may decrease blood levels of some anti-HIV medications and make them less effective.
  - Avoid echinacea because it may stimulate viral replication.
  - Have blood tests, including viral load, CD4+ cell count, CBC, and others as indicated.

---

*Visit* the Point® *at* **http://thePoint.lww.com/Frandsen12e** *for answers to NCLEX Success questions (in Appendix A), answers to Clinical Application Case Studies (in Appendix B), and more!*

## REFERENCES AND RESOURCES

Alansari, K., Toaimah, F. H., Almatrar, D. H., El Tatawy, L. A., Davidson, B. H., & Qusad, M. I. M. (2019). Monocolonal antibody treatment of RSV bronchiolitis in young infants: A randomized trial. *Pediatrics, 143*(3), 1–9. E20182308.

Centers for Disease Control and Prevention. (2020). Opening and mixing oseltamivir capsules with liquids if a child cannot swallow capsules. Retrieved from: https://www.cdc.gov/flu/highrisk/mixing-oseltamivir-qa.htm

Centers for Disease Control and Prevention. (2020). What you should know about flu antiviral drugs. Retrieved from: https://www.cdc.gov/flu/treatment/whatyoushould.htm

Fletcher, C. V. (2020). *Overview of antiretroviral agents used to treat HIV.* UpToDate. Lexi Comp, Inc.

Friel, T. J. (2020). *Epidemiology, clinical manifestations, and treatment of cytomegalovirus infection in immunocompetent adults.* UpToDate. Lexi Comp, Inc.

Gottlieb, G. S. (2020). *Treatment of HIV-2 infection.* UpToDate. Lexi Comp, Inc.

Hinkle, J. H., & Cheever, K. H. (2018). *Brunner & Suddarth's textbook of medical-surgical nursing* (14th ed.). Philadelphia, PA: Wolters Kluwer.

Klein, R. S. (2020). *Treatment of herpes simplex virus type 1 infection in immunocompetent patients.* UpToDate. Lexi Comp, Inc.

Lok, A. (2020). *Hepatitis B virus: Overview of management.* UpToDate. Lexi Comp, Inc.

McIntosh, K. (2020). *Coronaviruses.* UpToDate. Lexi Comp, Inc.

McIntosh, K. (2020). *Coronavirus disease 2019 (COVID-19).* UpToDate. Lexi Comp, Inc.

McIntosh, K. (2020). *Middle East respiratory syndrome coronavirus: Treatment and prevention.* UpToDate. Lexi Comp, Inc.

McIntosh, K. (2020). *Severe acute respiratory syndrome (SARS).* UpToDate. Lexi Comp, Inc.

Norris, T. L. (2019). *Porth's pathophysiology concepts of altered health states* (10th ed.). Philadelphia, PA: Wolters Kluwer.

Sax, P. E. (2020). *Acute and early HIV infection: Treatment.* UpToDate. Lexi Comp, Inc.

Sax, P. E. (2020). *Selecting antiretroviral regimens for the treatment-naïve HIV infected patient.* UpToDate. Lexi Comp, Inc.

UpToDate. (2020). *Drug information.* Lexi-Comp, Inc.

Zachary, K. C. (2020). *Pharmacology of antiviral drugs for influenza.* UpToDate. Lexi Comp, Inc.

# Drug Therapy for Fungal Infections

## LEARNING OBJECTIVES

*After studying this chapter, you should be able to:*

1. Describe the characteristics of fungi and fungal infections.
2. Discuss antibacterial drug therapy and immunosuppression as risk factors for development of fungal infections.
3. Identify the prototype and describe the action, use, adverse effects, contraindications, and nursing implications for polyenes.
4. Identify the prototype and describe the action, use, adverse effects, contraindications, and nursing implications for azoles.
5. Identify the prototype and describe the action, use, adverse effects, contraindications, and nursing implications for echinocandins.
6. Identify the prototype and describe the action, use, adverse effects, contraindications, and nursing implications for the pyrimidine analog.
7. Identify the prototype and describe the action, use, adverse effects, contraindications, and nursing implications for the miscellaneous antifungal agents.
8. Implement the nursing process when caring for patients undergoing drug therapy for fungal infections.

## CLINICAL APPLICATION CASE STUDY

Maria Angelo, age 21, is receiving antibiotic therapy for a strep throat. Following the completion of the course of antibiotics, she begins complaining of vaginal itching. She also notices a cheesy yellow vaginal discharge. Her primary care provider diagnoses *Candida albicans* vaginal infection and prescribes fluconazole (Diflucan) 150 mg PO, one dose.

## KEY TERMS

**Candidiasis:** infection either containing or caused by *Candida* fungi

**Dermatophytes:** fungal parasite that grows in or on the skin

**Fungi:** plantlike organisms that live as parasites on living tissue or as saprophytes on decaying organic matter

**Immunocompromised:** having an impaired or weakened immune system

**Molds:** fungi that are widely dispersed in the environment and either saprophytic or parasitic; multicellular organisms composed of colonies of tangled strands

**Mycoses:** disease induced by a fungus or resembling such a disease

**Yeasts:** unicellular fungi of the genus *Saccharomyces* or *Candida*

# INTRODUCTION

This chapter provides an introduction to the pharmacologic care of the patient diagnosed with a fungal infection. There are three broad classifications of antifungal agents prescribed in the treatment of fungal infections. The first group discussed is the polyenes, which are administered in the treatment of severe fungal infections. The second group discussed is the azoles, which are the most commonly prescribed antifungal medications. The azoles are administered orally, topically, and vaginally. The third group of antifungal agents is the echinocandins, which have fungicidal activity against *Candida*, including azole-resistant organisms, and fungistatic activity against *Aspergillus*. This chapter also discusses antifungal agents used in the treatment of dermatophytic infections.

## OVERVIEW OF FUNGAL INFECTIONS

### Etiology

**Fungi** are molds and yeasts that are widely dispersed in the environment and are either saprophytic (i.e., obtain food from dead organic matter) or parasitic (i.e., obtain nourishment from living organisms). **Molds** are multicellular organisms composed of colonies of tangled strands. They form a fuzzy coating on various surfaces (e.g., the mold that forms on spoiled food, the mildew that forms in damp environments). **Yeasts** are unicellular organisms. Some fungi, called **dermatophytes**, can grow only at the cooler temperatures of body surfaces. Other fungi, termed dimorphic, can grow as molds outside the body and as yeasts in the warm temperatures of the body. As molds, these fungi produce spores that can persist indefinitely in the environment and can be carried by the wind to distant locations. When these mold spores enter the body, most often by inhalation, they rapidly become yeasts that can invade body tissues. Dimorphic fungi include a number of human pathogens such as those that cause blastomycosis, histoplasmosis, and coccidioidomycosis.

Structurally, fungi are larger and more complex than bacteria. They have a thick, rigid cell wall, of which glucan is one of the components. Glucan is formed by the fungal enzyme, glucan synthase. Fungi also have a cell membrane composed mainly of ergosterol, a lipid that is similar to cholesterol in human cell membranes. Within the cell membrane, structures are mostly the same as those in human cells (e.g., a nucleus, mitochondria, Golgi apparatus, ribosomes attached to endoplasmic reticulum, a cytoskeleton with microtubules and filaments).

Fungal infections may be mild and superficial or life threatening and systemic. Fungi that are pathogenic in humans exist in soil, decaying plants, and other environmental habitats. Some are even part of the endogenous human flora. For example, *Candida albicans* organisms are part of the normal microbial flora of the skin, mouth, gastrointestinal (GI) tract, and vagina. Growth of *Candida* organisms is normally restrained by intact immune mechanisms and bacterial competition for nutrients. When these restraining forces are altered (e.g., by suppression of the immune system, antibacterial drug therapy), fungal overgrowth and opportunistic infection can occur, leading to the fungal infection called **candidiasis**. Dermatophytes cause superficial infections of the skin, hair, and nails. They obtain nourishment from keratin, a protein in skin, hair, and nails. Dermatophytic

infections include tinea pedis (athlete's foot) and tinea capitis (ringworm of the scalp) (see Chap. 61).

Systemic or invasive **mycoses** include the endemic mycoses that can cause disease (e.g., blastomycosis, coccidioidomycosis, histoplasmosis, sporotrichosis) in healthy hosts who are exposed to them in the environment and the opportunistic mycoses (e.g., aspergillosis, candidiasis, cryptococcosis) that cause serious infection, mainly in immunosuppressed hosts. The fungi that cause endemic mycoses exist as molds in the environment; they grow in soil and decaying organic matter. Infection is acquired by inhalation of airborne spores from contaminated soil. Histoplasmosis, coccidioidomycosis, and blastomycosis usually occur as pulmonary disease but may be systemic. These infections often mimic common bacterial infections, and their severity is determined both by the extent of the exposure to the organism and by the immune status of the host. The fungi that cause opportunistic mycoses may be part of the normal body flora (e.g., *Candida* species) or exist in the environment (*Aspergillus, Cryptococcus*). Infection occurs after inhalation or inoculation of the fungus into body tissues. Fungi may have characteristics that enhance their ability to cause disease. *Cryptococcus neoformans* organisms, for example, can become encapsulated, which allows them to evade the normal immune defense mechanism of phagocytosis. *Aspergillus* organisms produce protease, an enzyme that allows them to destroy structural proteins and penetrate body tissues.

Most fungal infections occur in healthy people but are more severe and invasive in **immunocompromised** hosts. Serious infections are increasing in incidence, largely because of human immunodeficiency virus (HIV) infections, the use of immunosuppressant drugs to treat patients with cancer or organ transplants, the use of indwelling intravenous (IV) catheters for prolonged drug therapy or parenteral nutrition, implantation of prosthetic devices, and widespread use of broad-spectrum antibacterial drugs.

## Pathophysiology and Clinical Manifestations

Pathophysiologic changes associated with fungal infections relate to the causal fungus and the tissue in which it has been colonized. Box 24.1 describes the characteristics of selected fungal infections and associated pathophysiologic changes. This box also identifies the clinical manifestations that result from fungal infection.

## Drug Therapy

Development of drugs that are effective against fungal cells without being excessively toxic to human cells has been limited because fungal cells are similar to human cells. Most of the available drugs target the fungal cell membrane and produce potentially serious toxicities and drug interactions. In general, antifungal drugs disrupt the structure and function of fungal cell components (Fig. 24.1).

Polyenes (e.g., amphotericin B), azoles (e.g., fluconazole), and the miscellaneous agent griseofulvin act on ergosterol to disrupt the fungal cell membrane. Amphotericin B (and nystatin) binds to ergosterol and forms holes in the membrane, causing leakage of fungal cell contents and lysis

| BOX 24.1 | *Selected Fungal Infections* |
|---|---|

Aspergillosis occurs in debilitated and immunocompromised people, including those with leukemia, lymphoma, or acquired immunodeficiency syndrome (AIDS), and those with neutropenia. Invasive aspergillosis is a serious illness characterized by inflammatory granulomatous lesions, which may develop in the bronchi, lungs, ear canal, skin, or mucous membranes of the eye, nose, or urethra. It may extend into blood vessels, which leads to infection of the brain, heart, kidneys, and other organs. It is associated with thrombosis, ischemic infarction of involved tissues, and progressive disease. It is often fatal.

Allergic bronchopulmonary aspergillosis, an allergic reaction to inhaled *Aspergillus* spores, may develop in people with asthma and cause bronchoconstriction, wheezing, dyspnea, cough, muscle aches, and fever. The condition is aggravated if the spores germinate and grow in the airways, thereby producing chronic exposure to the antigen and permanent fibrotic damage.

*Aspergillus* mold is widespread in the environment; spores are released into the air during soil excavations (e.g., for construction of buildings) or handling of decaying plant matter and are carried into most human environments. Spores have been found in water (e.g., hot water faucets, saunas, shower heads, swimming pools), public buildings and private homes (e.g., basements, bedding, humidifiers, ventilation ducts, potted plants, house dust), and foods (e.g., peppers and spices, pasta, peanuts, cashews, coffee beans). In hospitals, sources of infection include contaminated air from building renovations and new construction; hospital water, which may become aerosolized during activities such as patient showering; and cereals, powdered milk, tea, and soy sauce ingested by neutropenic patients. As *Aspergillus* molds grow, they produce toxins (e.g., aflatoxin, one of the strongest carcinogens known) that contaminate the food chain.

There are several species that cause invasive disease in humans, but *Aspergillus fumigatus* is the most common. *A. fumigatus* reproduces by releasing spores, which are small enough to reach the alveoli when inhaled. Most *Aspergillus* organisms enter the body through the respiratory system, and pulmonary aspergillosis is acquired by inhalation of the spores. Other potential entry sites include damaged skin (e.g., burn wounds, IV catheter insertion sites), operative wounds, the cornea, and the ear.

**Blastomycosis** occurs with inhalation of spores from a fungus that grows in soil and decaying organic matter. The organism is widespread in the United States. Sporadic cases most often occur in adult males who have extensive exposure to woods and streams with vocational or recreational activities. The infection may be asymptomatic or produce pulmonary symptoms resembling pneumonia, tuberculosis, or lung cancer. It may also be systemic and involve other organs, especially the skin and bone. Skin lesions (e.g., pustules, ulcerations, abscesses) may progress over a period of years and eventually involve large areas of the body. Bone invasion, with arthritis and bone destruction, occurs in 25% to 50% of patients.

Blastomycosis can occur in healthy people with sufficient exposure but is more severe and more likely to involve multiple organs and central nervous system (CNS) disease in immunocompromised patients.

**Candidiasis** occurs in patients with malignant lymphomas, diabetes mellitus, or AIDS and in patients receiving antibiotic, antineoplastic, corticosteroid, and immunosuppressant drug therapy. *Candida* organisms are found in soil, on inanimate objects, in hospital environments, and in food. In the human body, they are found on skin and in the GI and genitourinary tracts, including the urine of patients with indwelling bladder catheters. Historically, most infections arose from the normal endogenous organisms of the GI tract and were caused by *C. albicans*. In recent years, however, the incidence of infections caused by other candidal strains has greatly increased. Oral, intestinal, vaginal, and systemic candidiasis can occur. Early recognition and treatment of local infections may prevent systemic candidiasis.

- Oral candidiasis (thrush) produces painless white plaques on oral and pharyngeal mucosa. It often occurs in newborn infants who become infected during passage through an infected or colonized vagina. In older children and adults, thrush may occur as a complication of diabetes mellitus, as a result of poor oral hygiene, or after taking antibiotics or corticosteroids. It may also occur as an early manifestation of AIDS.
- GI candidiasis often occurs after broad-spectrum antibacterial therapy, which destroys a large part of the normal flora of the intestine. The main symptom is diarrhea.
- Vaginal candidiasis occurs in women who are pregnant, have diabetes mellitus, or take oral contraceptives or antibacterial drugs. The main symptom is a yellowish vaginal discharge. The infection may produce inflammation of the perineal area and spread to the buttocks and thighs.
- Skin candidiasis occurs in people with continuously moist skinfolds or moist surgical dressings. The organism also may cause diaper rash and perineal rashes. Skin lesions are red and macerated.
- Systemic or invasive candidiasis occurs when the organism gets into the bloodstream and is circulated throughout the body, with the brain, heart, kidneys, and eyes as the most common sites of infection. It occurs as a nosocomial infection in patients with serious illness or who are undergoing drug therapy that suppresses the immune system and may be fatal. Invasive infections may be present in any organ and may produce such disorders as urinary tract infection, endocarditis, and meningitis. It may be diagnosed by positive cultures of blood or tissue. Signs and symptoms depend on the severity of the infection and the organs affected and are indistinguishable from those occurring with bacterial infections.

The incidence of severe candidal infections has increased in recent years, in part because of increased numbers of neutropenic and immunodeficient patients. In addition, the frequent use of broad-spectrum antibiotics leads to extensive candidal colonization in debilitated patients, and the widespread use of medical devices (e.g., intravascular catheters, monitoring equipment, endotracheal tubes, urinary catheters) allows the organisms to reach sites that are normally sterile. People who use IV drugs also develop invasive candidiasis because the injections inoculate the fungi directly into the bloodstream.

**Coccidioidomycosis** is caused by an organism that grows as a mold in soil and decaying organic matter and is commonly found in the southwestern United States and Northern Mexico. Infection results from inhalation of spores that convert to yeasts in the warm environment of the body and often cause asymptomatic or mild respiratory infection. However, the organism may cause acute pulmonary infection

**BOX 24.1**    *Selected Fungal Infections* (Continued)

with fever, chest pain, cough, headache, and loss of appetite. Radiographs may show small nodules in the lung like those seen in tuberculosis. In some cases, chronic disease develops in which the organisms remain localized and cause large, organism-filled cavities in the lung. These cavities may become fibrotic and require surgical excision. In a few cases, severe, disseminated disease occurs, either soon after the primary infection or after years of chronic pulmonary disease. Disseminated coccidioidomycosis may produce acute or chronic meningitis or a generalized disease with lesions in many internal organs. Skin lesions appear as granulomas that may eventually heal or become ulcerations. Most patients with primary infection recover without treatment; patients with disseminated disease require long-term treatment.

Coccidioidomycosis may occur in healthy or immunocompromised people but is more severe and more likely to become systemic in immunocompromised patients. For example, patients with AIDS who live in endemic areas are highly susceptible to this infection. The severity of the disease also increases with intensity of exposure.

**Cryptococcosis** is caused by inhalation of spores of *C. neoformans*, an organism found worldwide, especially in bird droppings. The spores have also been found in fruits, vegetables, and dairy products.

When cryptococcosis occurs in healthy people, the primary infection is localized in the lungs, is asymptomatic or produces mild symptoms, and heals without treatment. However, pneumonia may occur and lead to spread of the organisms by the bloodstream. When cryptococcosis occurs in immunocompromised people, it is likely to be more severe and to become disseminated to the CNS, skin, and other organs. People with AIDS are highly susceptible, and cryptococcosis is a frequent opportunistic infection in this population. Infection most often affects the lungs and CNS. Cryptococcal pneumonia in patients with AIDS has a high mortality rate. Cryptococcal meningitis, the most common manifestation of disseminated disease, often produces abscesses in the brain. Clinical manifestations include headache, dizziness, and neck stiffness, and the condition is often mistaken for brain tumor. Later symptoms include coma, respiratory failure, and death if the meningitis is not treated effectively.

**Histoplasmosis** is a common infection that occurs worldwide, especially in the central and mideastern United States. The causative fungus is found in soil and organic debris around chicken houses, bird roosts, and caves inhabited by bats. Exposure to spores may result from activities such as demolishing or remodeling old buildings or cleaning chicken coops. Spores can be picked up by the wind and spread over large areas. Histoplasmosis develops when the spores are inhaled into the lungs, where they rapidly develop into the tissue-invasive yeast cells that reach the bloodstream and

become distributed throughout the body. In most cases, the organisms are destroyed or encapsulated by the host's immune system. The lung lesions heal by fibrosis and calcification and resemble the lesions of tuberculosis. Some people develop histoplasmosis years after the primary infection, probably from reactivation of a latent infection.

Clinical manifestations may vary widely. In people with a normal immune response, manifestations can be correlated with the extent of exposure. Most infections are asymptomatic or produce minimal symptoms for which treatment is not sought. When symptoms occur, they usually resemble an acute, influenza-like respiratory infection and improve within a few weeks. However, people exposed to large amounts of spores may have a high fever and severe pneumonia, which usually resolves with a low mortality rate. Some people, most often adult men with emphysema or other lung diseases, develop chronic pulmonary histoplasmosis with recurrent episodes of cough, fever, and weakness. In addition, histoplasmosis occasionally infects the liver, spleen, and other organs and is rapidly fatal if not treated effectively. The severe, disseminated form usually occurs in patients whose immune system is suppressed by diseases or drugs.

**Pneumocystosis** is caused by *Pneumocystis jiroveci*, an organism formerly considered a protozoan but now identified as a fungus. The organism is widespread in the environment, and most people are exposed at an early age. Infections are mild or asymptomatic in immunocompetent people. However, the organism can form cysts in the lungs, persist for long periods, and become activated in immunocompromised hosts. Activation produces an acute, life-threatening pneumonia (*Pneumocystis* pneumonia) characterized by cough, fever, dyspnea, and presence of the organism in sputum. Groups at risk include HIV-seropositive people, those receiving corticosteroids or antineoplastics and other immunosuppressive drugs, and caregivers of infected people.

**Sporotrichosis** occurs when contaminated soil or plant material is inoculated into the skin through small wounds (e.g., thorn pricks) on the fingers, hands, or arms. It is most likely to occur among people who handle sphagnum moss, roses, or baled hay. Thus, infection is a hazard for gardeners and greenhouse workers. It can occur in both healthy and immunocompromised people but is more severe and disseminated in immunocompromised hosts.

Initial lesions, which are usually small, painless bumps resembling insect bites, occur 1 week to 6 months after inoculation. The subcutaneous nodule develops into a necrotic ulcer, which heals slowly as new ulcers appear in adjacent areas. Local lymphatic channels and lymph nodes also develop abscesses, nodules, and ulcers that may persist for years if the disease is not treated effectively. In immunocompromised people, sporotrichosis may spread to various tissues, including the meninges.

of the cell. The azole drugs bind to an enzyme that is required for synthesis of ergosterol. This action causes production of a defective cell membrane, which also allows leakage of intracellular contents and destruction of the cell. Both types of drugs also affect cholesterol in human cell membranes, a characteristic considered mainly responsible for the drugs' adverse effects.

Echinocandins (e.g., caspofungin) disrupt fungal cell walls rather than fungal cell membranes. They inhibit glucan synthase, an enzyme required for synthesis of glucan. Glucan is a component of the fungal cell wall; its depletion leads to leakage of cellular contents and cell death. Because human cells do not contain cell walls, these drugs are less toxic than the polyene and azole antifungals.

**Figure 24.1.** Actions of antifungal drugs on fungal cells.

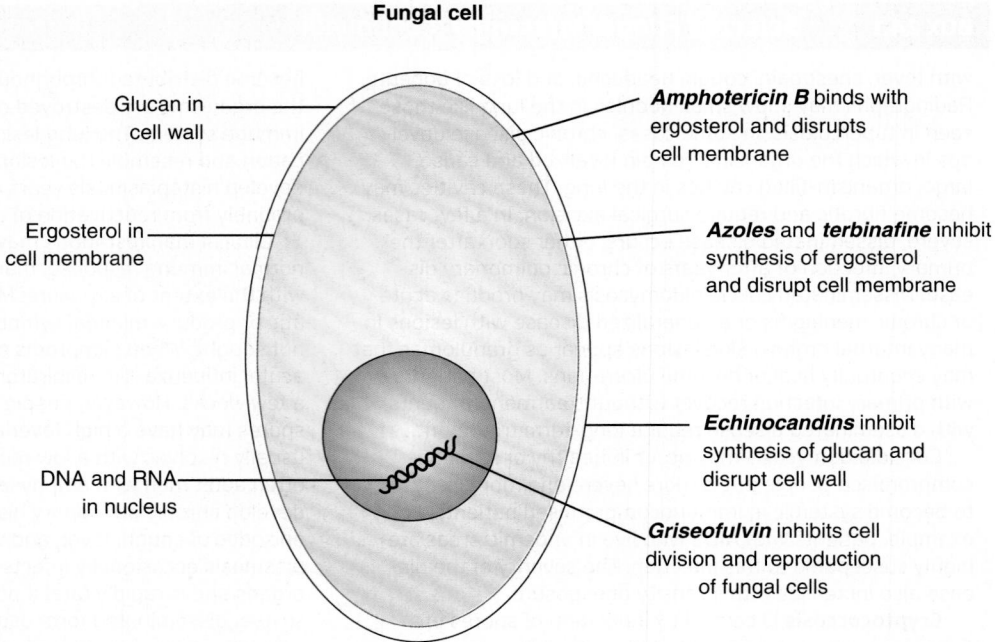

**Fungal cell**

Glucan in cell wall

**Amphotericin B** binds with ergosterol and disrupts cell membrane

Ergosterol in cell membrane

**Azoles** and **terbinafine** inhibit synthesis of ergosterol and disrupt cell membrane

**Echinocandins** inhibit synthesis of glucan and disrupt cell wall

DNA and RNA in nucleus

**Griseofulvin** inhibits cell division and reproduction of fungal cells

Drugs for superficial fungal infections of the skin and mucous membranes are often applied topically. Numerous preparations are available, many without a prescription. Drugs for systemic infections are given intravenously or orally. Patients with HIV infection or severe neutropenia due to treatment with cytotoxic cancer drugs require aggressive treatment of fungal infections, because they are at high risk for developing life-threatening systemic mycoses. Selected antifungal drugs are further described in the following sections.

Table 24.1 summarizes the medications used in the treatment of fungal infections.

## TABLE 24.1

### Drugs Administered for Fungal Infections (Antifungal Agents)

| Drug Class | Prototype | Other Drugs in the Class |
|---|---|---|
| Polyenes | Amphotericin B<br>• Deoxycholate formulation<br>• Lipid formulations (Abelcet, AmBisome) | Nystatin (Bio-Statin) |
| Azoles | Fluconazole (Diflucan) | Butoconazole (Femstat, Gynazole)*<br>Clotrimazole<br>Econazole (Ecoza)*<br>Itraconazole (Sporanox, Tolsura)<br>Ketoconazole (Extina, Nizoral)<br>Miconazole (Oravig)<br>Oxiconazole (Oxistat)*<br>Posaconazole (Noxafil)<br>Sulconazole (Exelderm)*<br>Terconazole (Terazol 3, Terazol 7)*<br>Tioconazole (Vagistat-1 [OTC])<br>Voriconazole (Vfend, Vfend IV)<br>Isavuconazole (Cresemba) |
| Echinocandins | Caspofungin (Cancidas) | Anidulafungin (Eraxis)<br>Micafungin (Mycamine) |
| Miscellaneous antifungal agents for superficial mycoses | Griseofulvin | Ciclopirox (Loprox, Penlac)*<br>Terbinafine (Lamisil)<br>Tolnaftate (Tinactin)* |
| Pyrimidine analog | Flucytosine (Ancobon) | |

*Topical antifungal agents.

## NCLEX Success

1. Which of the following patients is at greatest risk for developing a life-threatening system mycosis?
   A. a patient who develops a sexually transmitted disease and is being treated with doxycycline
   B. a patient with breast cancer being treated with the chemotherapeutic agent cyclophosphamide
   C. a patient who is taking warfarin for the prevention of a thromboembolism
   D. a patient with a strep throat who is being treated with cephalexin

2. A 32-year-old construction worker visits the occupational health clinic of the company where he is employed. The man has a high temperature, pain in the right middle and lower lobe of the lung, dyspnea, and malaise. During the admission interview, he states he has been working to restore homes in an urban area with 150-year-old houses. What does the nurse suspect is the cause of his symptoms?
   A. pneumocystosis
   B. sporotrichosis
   C. cryptococcosis
   D. histoplasmosis

## POLYENES

**Amphotericin B deoxycholate**, the prototype polyene, is active against most types of pathogenic fungi and is fungicidal or fungistatic, depending on the concentration in body fluids and the susceptibility of the causative fungus. Because of its toxicity, the drug is used only for serious fungal infections. It is usually given for 4 to 12 weeks. There are two additional formulations of amphotericin B. Amphotericin B lipid-based formulations include Abelcet and AmBisome.

## Pharmacokinetics

Amphotericin B must be given intravenously for systemic infections. After the infusion is complete, the drug is rapidly taken up by the liver and other organs. It is then slowly released back into the bloodstream. Despite its long-term use, little is known about its distribution and metabolic pathways. Drug concentrations in most body fluids are higher in the presence of inflammation; concentrations in cerebrospinal fluid (CSF) are low with or without inflammation. The drug has an initial serum half-life of 24 hours, which represents redistribution from the bloodstream to tissues. This is followed by a second elimination phase, with

a half-life of 15 days, which represents elimination from tissue storage sites. Most of the drug is thought to be metabolized in the tissues; some is excreted in the urine and can be detected for several weeks.

Lipid formulations (Abelcet, AmBisome) reach higher concentrations in diseased tissues than in normal tissues, so that larger doses can be given to increase therapeutic effects. At the same time, they cause less damage to normal tissues and decrease adverse effects. These products are much more expensive than the deoxycholate form. They are most likely to be used for patients with preexisting renal impairment or conditions in which other nephrotoxic drugs are routinely given (e.g., bone marrow transplant recipients) and when high doses are needed for difficult-to-treat infections. The lipid preparations differ in their characteristics and cannot be used interchangeably.

## Action

Amphotericin B binds to the sterols within the fungal cell membrane, resulting in a change in the membrane's permeability. This action destroys the fungal cells and prevents them from reproducing. Depending on the concentration of the medication, it has either a fungicidal or fungistatic effect.

## Use

Amphotericin B is reserved for patients with progressive and potentially fatal infections resulting from cryptococcosis, North American blastomycosis, systemic candidiasis, disseminated moniliasis, coccidioidomycosis, and histoplasmosis. It is also used for mucormycosis caused by the species of *Mucor*, *Rhizopus*, *Absidia*, *Conidiobolus*, and *Basidiobolus*; sporotrichosis; and aspergillosis. The drug is also given as an adjunctive agent in the treatment of American mucocutaneous leishmaniasis. A **BLACK BOX WARNING** ◆ issued by the U.S. Food and Drug Administration (FDA) states that amphotericin B should be reserved for progressive or potentially fatal infections. It is not recommended for use in noninvasive disease due to the risk of toxicity.

Abelcet is used in the treatment of aspergillosis. AmBisome is used in the treatment of cryptococcal meningitis in HIV-infected patients. Patients who are febrile and neutropenic are given AmBisome for presumed fungal infections. Also, AmBisome is administered in the treatment of *Aspergillus*, *Candida*, or *Cryptococcus* when conventional amphotericin is not tolerated.

Table 24.2 presents specific information about the use of polyenes, including dosages for adults and children.

### Use in Children

Children may take amphotericin B, but such use requires assessment of electrolytes due to magnesium wasting. Health care providers have used the drug successfully to treat children with serious fungal infections, without unusual or severe adverse effects.

### Use in Older Adults

Older adults, with the impaired renal and cardiovascular functions that usually accompany aging, are especially vulnerable to serious adverse effects. They require close monitoring to reduce the incidence and severity of nephrotoxicity, hypokalemia, and

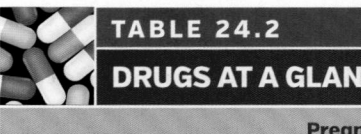

| TABLE 24.2 | | | | |
|---|---|---|---|---|
| **DRUGS AT A GLANCE: Polyenes** | | | | |
| **Drug** | **Pregnancy Category** | **Type of Infection Treated** | **Routes and Dosage Ranges** | |
| | | | **Adults** | **Children** |
| Ⓟ **Amphotericin B deoxycholate** (❈ Fungizone IV) | B | Serious, systemic fungal infections (e.g., candidiasis, histoplasmosis) Cutaneous candidiasis Oral candidiasis | Dosage is individualized according to the disease severity Initial IV dose: 0.25 mg/kg/d. Gradually increase dosage to 0.5–1 mg/kg/d, infused over 2–6 h Topical: Apply two to four times daily for 1–4 wk Oral suspension: 100 mg/mL, 1 mL swish and swallow four times per day | Same as for adults for IV, skin preparations, and oral suspension |
| Amphotericin B lipid complex (Abelcet; ❈ Abelcet) | B | Systemic infections in patients who do not tolerate Fungizone | IV 5 mg/kg/d | Same as adults |
| Liposomal amphotericin B (AmBisome; ❈ AmBisome) | B | Systemic infections in patients who do not tolerate Fungizone Empiric treatment of presumed fungal infections in febrile, neutropenic patients | IV 3–6 mg/kg/d | Same as adults |
| Nystatin (Bio-Statin; ❈ PMS-Nystatin, Nyaderm, TEVA-Nystatin) | C | Candidiasis of skin, mucous membrane, and intestinal tract | Oral or intestinal infection: PO tablets 1–2 (500,000–1,000,000 units) three times daily; oral suspension 4–6 mL (400,000–600,000 units) four times daily; oral troches 1–2 (200,000–400,000 units) four to five times daily Topically to skin lesions, two to three times daily Intravaginally, 1 vaginal tablet once daily for 14 d | Oral suspension, older than 1 y: same as adults; infants, 2 mL (200,000 units) four times daily Oral troches, same as adults for children old enough to suck on the lozenge until it dissolves |

other adverse drug reactions. Lipid formulations of amphotericin B are less nephrotoxic than the conventional deoxycholate formulation and may be preferred.

## Use in Patients With Renal Impairment

Amphotericin B deoxycholate is nephrotoxic. Renal impairment occurs in most patients (up to 80%) within the first 2 weeks of therapy but usually subsides with dosage reduction or drug discontinuation. Permanent impairment occurs in a few patients. Recommendations to decrease nephrotoxicity include hydrating patients with a liter of 0.9% sodium chloride solution intravenously and monitoring serum creatinine and blood urea nitrogen (BUN) at least weekly. If the patient's BUN exceeds 40 mg/dL or serum creatinine exceeds 3 mg/dL, the drug should be stopped, or dosage should be reduced until renal function recovers. Another strategy is to give a lipid formulation (e.g., Abelcet, AmBisome), which is less nephrotoxic. For patients who already have renal impairment or other risk factors for

development of renal impairment, a lipid formulation is indicated. Renal function should still be monitored frequently.

## Use in Patients With Hepatic Impairment

Although the main concern with amphotericin B is nephrotoxicity, monitoring of hepatic function during use is recommended.

## Use in Patients With Critical Illness

As previously stated, amphotericin B penetrates tissues well, except for the CSF, and only small amounts are excreted in the urine. With prolonged administration, the half-life increases from 1 to 15 days. Hemodialysis does not remove the drug. Lipid formulations may be preferred in critically ill patients because of less nephrotoxicity.

## Use in Patients Receiving Home Care

It is important that the home care nurse assess the patient's immune function with the administration of amphotericin B.

The patient's home should be kept meticulously clean and free of mold-producing substances such as potted plants, fresh flowers, and adhesive nonslip bathtub appliques. The bathroom should be cleaned daily with bleach, and air conditioning and air filtration systems should be kept clean.

## Adverse Effects

Adverse effects of amphotericin B are often severe, with the most serious being multiple organ failure, respiratory arrest, and cardiac arrest. Other adverse effects include the following:

- GI: nausea, vomiting, dyspepsia, bleeding (GI)
- Genitourinary: hypokalemia, azotemia, renal failure
- Hematologic: leukopenia, thrombocytopenia
- Electrolyte imbalances: hyperkalemia, hypomagnesemia, hyponatremia

## Contraindications

Patients with a known allergy to amphotericin B and impairment of renal function should not receive the drug. Women who are lactating should not take it except in life-threatening situations.

## Nursing Implications

### Preventing Interactions

Many medications interact with amphotericin B, increasing or decreasing its effect (Box 24.2). Researchers have not reported that any herbs interact with the drug.

### Administering the Drug

The pharmacy should reconstitute and prepare amphotericin B for IV administration. It is necessary to infuse the prepared solutions of amphotericin within 8 hours of reconstitution. The patient should receive a test dose to assess tolerance for the drug. Doubling maintenance doses and infusing them on alternate days is fine. Larger doses of the lipid preparations are

---

recommended to achieve therapeutic effects similar to those of the deoxycholate preparation. When possible, it is best to administer amphotericin B through a separate IV line. When injecting it into an existing IV line, flushing of the line with a 5% dextrose solution should occur before and after administration both with deoxycholate and lipid formulations. Do not use an in-line filter with the lipid formulations.

Specific instructions for administration of the various forms of amphotericin B are:

- IV form: give in 5% dextrose in water over 2 to 6 hours with the use of in-line filter. This drug should not be mixed with any other medications.
- Abelcet: give over 2 hours without the use of an in-line filter.
- Amphotericin cream or lotion: apply liberally to skin lesions and rub in gently.

Prior to beginning treatment, it is necessary to obtain a culture of the infection. However, treatment with amphotericin B should begin prior to return of the culture results. The nurse monitors injection sites for signs of phlebitis. He or she gives aspirin, antihistamines, and antiemetics, which are used to manage adverse effects, prior to the administration of amphotericin B. It is essential to assess the sodium balance throughout the administration. By maintaining the serum sodium level within normal range, the patient has decreased symptoms of drug discomfort. Small doses of corticosteroids assist in diminishing chills related to drug administration.

### Assessing for Therapeutic Effects

The nurse assesses for decrease in symptoms of the fungal infection. The administration of amphotericin B is consistent with the cure of infection. When the infection is controlled, the administration of amphotericin B continues with a maintenance dose for a period of time (Hinkle & Cheever, 2017).

### Assessing for Adverse Effects

The nurse assesses for severe chilling, headaches, malaise, nausea, vomiting, and generalized pain. (As previously stated, management of these symptoms requires aspirin, antihistamines, and antiemetics.) It is necessary to monitor the patient's electrolytes for hypokalemia and hyponatremia. When administering amphotericin topically, the nurse assesses for a hypersensitivity reaction at the site of the application. IV administration of amphotericin is irritating to the injection and requires assessment for phlebitis and thrombophlebitis.

### Patient Teaching

Box 24.3 identifies patient teaching guidelines for amphotericin B.

## Other Drugs in the Class

Nystatin has the same mechanism of action as amphotericin B. However, it is used only for topical therapy of oral, intestinal, and vaginal candidiasis because it is too toxic for systemic use. Although given orally for oral or intestinal infections, the drug is not absorbed systemically and is excreted in the feces. With oral use, adverse effects include nausea, vomiting, and diarrhea; with vaginal application, adverse effects include local irritation and burning.

---

**BOX 24.2 — Drug Interactions: Amphotericin B**

**Drugs That Increase the Effects of Amphotericin B**
- Antibiotics [*nephrotoxic*]
  *Increase the risk of nephrotoxicity*
- Antineoplastic agents
  *Increase renal toxicity, bronchospasm, and hypotension*
- Cardiac glycosides
  *Increase the risk of digitalis toxicity due to hypokalemia*
- Corticosteroid, corticotropin, skeletal muscle relaxants
  *Increase potassium depletion*

**Drugs That Decrease the Effects of Amphotericin B**
- Clotrimazole, fluconazole, ketoconazole
  *Increase resistance to fungal infection*
- Flucytosine
  *Increases flucytosine toxicity*

## BOX 24.3 *Patient Teaching Guidelines for Amphotericin B*

- Long-term use of amphotericin is necessary.
- You may not notice the effects of the medication for several weeks.
- Use good hygiene to prevent reinfection or spread of infection.
- You may experience side effects such as nausea and vomiting, so eat small, frequent meals.
- Be aware that topical administration of the medication may cause staining of clothes.
- Report skin irritations with the use of topical amphotericin.
- Report fever, chills, muscle aches, and headache.
- Report irritation at the injection site.

## NCLEX Success

3. A 53-year-old man has asthma. He is admitted to the emergency department with wheezing, dyspnea, muscle aches, and a high fever. He owns and operates a swimming pool business in which he sells above-ground swimming pools and hot tubs. His business has a showroom with functioning pools and hot tubs. What fungal infection do you suspect the patient is suffering from?

   A. blastomycosis
   B. histoplasmosis
   C. aspergillosis
   D. candidiasis

4. A patient was diagnosed with cryptococcal meningitis. Which of the following medications is administered to treat cryptococcal meningitis?

   A. amphotericin B
   B. Rocephin
   C. bleomycin
   D. mupirocin

5. When administering amphotericin B, what drug is administered to prevent the development of chilling, fever, malaise, and nausea?

   A. aminophylline
   B. ibuprofen
   C. penicillin G
   D. aspirin

## AZOLES

The azoles are the largest group of commonly used antifungal agents. Many are used topically, and some are available without a prescription for dermatologic (see Chap. 61) or vaginal use (e.g., butoconazole, clotrimazole, miconazole, terconazole, tioconazole). It is necessary to obtain a prescription to use azoles for other indications.

Systemic azoles include ketoconazole, fluconazole, itraconazole, posaconazole, and voriconazole. Although ketoconazole was the first azole developed, **fluconazole** (Diflucan) is considered to be the prototype medication of the class. Fluconazole and other drugs in the class have a broader spectrum of fungal activity, are distributed more effectively, and have fewer adverse effects and drug interactions.

### Pharmacokinetics

Fluconazole is administered orally or parenterally. The oral preparation has a slow onset of action with a peak of action in 1 to 2 hours and duration of action 2 to 4 days. The oral drug is well absorbed and reaches therapeutic levels in most body fluids and tissues, including the meninges. The IV preparation has a rapid onset of action, with a peak of action in 1 hour and the same duration of action 2 to 4 days. The azoles interact with cytochrome P450 (CYP) enzymes, which can potentially produce significant interactions with many other drugs (those in which there is a decrease in the metabolism and increase in the risk of toxicity with affected drugs).

Fluconazole is apparently a less potent inhibitor of CYP3A4 enzymes than ketoconazole and itraconazole. As a result, drug interactions with fluconazole are of lesser magnitude and usually occur only with dosages of 200 mg/day or more. However, fluconazole is a strong inhibitor of CYP2C9 enzymes. Fluconazole crosses the placenta and enters the breast milk. It is excreted in the urine.

### Action

Fluconazole binds to sterols in the fungal cell membrane. This action changes the membrane's permeability, producing a fungicidal or fungistatic effect depending on the drug concentration and the fungal organism.

### Use

Fluconazole and the other azoles discussed in this section are used systemically or both topically and systemically. Fluconazole is often the drug of choice for localized candidal infections (e.g., urinary tract infections, thrush) and is useful for systemic candidiasis. However, resistant strains of *Candida* organisms occur with extensive use of fluconazole. In vaginal candidiasis, a single oral dose of 150 mg is usually effective. Fluconazole is also used for long-term suppression of cryptococcal meningitis in patients with acquired immunodeficiency syndrome (AIDS), after initial use of amphotericin B. It is used prophylactically in the prevention of candidiasis in patients with bone marrow transplants.

Table 24.3 provides detailed information about the use of azoles, including dosages for adults and children.

### Use in Children

Fluconazole is commonly used in children with *Candida* infections. However, the maximum daily dosage should not exceed 600 mg/day.

### Use in Older Adults

Fluconazole is routinely administered to older patients with *Candida* infections. However, it is necessary to monitor the creatinine clearance and hepatic enzymes.

**TABLE 24.3**

# DRUGS AT A GLANCE: Azoles

| Drug | Pregnancy Category | Type of Infection Treated | Routes and Dosage Ranges | |
|---|---|---|---|---|
| | | | **Adults** | **Children** |
| **Fluconazole** (Diflucan; ✹ DOM-Fluconazole, Apo-Fluconazole, Diflucan) | C | Oropharyngeal, esophageal, vaginal, and systemic candidiasis Prevention of candidiasis after bone marrow transplantation Cryptococcal meningitis | Oropharyngeal candidiasis, PO, IV 200 mg first day and then 100 mg daily for 2 wk Esophageal candidiasis, PO, IV 200 mg first day and then 100 mg daily for at least 3 wk Vaginal candidiasis, PO 150 mg as a single dose Systemic candidiasis, PO, IV 400 mg first day and then 200 mg daily for at least 4 wk Prophylaxis, PO, IV 400 mg once daily Cryptococcal meningitis, PO, IV 400 mg first day and then 200–400 mg/d for 10–12 wk | Oropharyngeal candidiasis, PO, IV 6 mg/kg first day and then 3 mg/kg/d for at least 2 wk Esophageal candidiasis, PO, IV 6 mg/kg first day and then 3 mg/kg/d for at least 3 wk Systemic candidiasis, PO, IV 6–12 mg/kg/d Cryptococcal meningitis, PO, IV 12 mg/kg first day and then 6 mg/kg/d for 10–12 wk |
| Clotrimazole | C | Oropharyngeal candidiasis | Treatment, PO 10 mg dissolved slowly five times per day for 14 d Prophylaxis, PO 10 mg dissolved slowly three times daily for the duration of chemotherapy or until steroids are reduced to maintenance level | ≥3 y: 10 mg troche dissolved slowly five times per day |
| Itraconazole (Sporanox, Tolsura; ✹ Sporanox) | C | Systemic fungal infections, including aspergillosis and in neutropenic and immunocompromised hosts Onychomycosis Tinea infections | Systemic infection, PO 200 mg once or twice daily for 3 mo Blastomycosis, histoplasmosis, aspergillosis, IV 200 mg twice daily for 4 doses and then 200 mg/d Onychomycosis, fingernail, PO 200 mg twice daily for 1 wk, no drug for 3 wk, and then repeat dosage for 1 wk; toenail, PO 200 mg once daily for 12 consecutive wk Oral solution, 100–200 mg daily (10–20 mL), swish and swallow three times daily for 3–5 d Tinea infections, PO 100–200 mg daily for 1–4 wk | Safety and efficacy not established. 3- to 16-y-old patients have been treated with 100 mg daily for systemic infections and 6 mo- to 12-y-old patients have been treated with 5 mg/kg once daily for 2 wk without serious or unusual adverse effects |
| Isavuconazole (Cresemba) | C | Treatment of invasive aspergillosis and mucormycosis in adults | Aspergillosis, IV, PO 372 mg (isavuconazole 200 mg) every 8 h for 6 doses and then 372 mg (isavuconazole 200 mg)/d, starting 12–24 h after the last loading dose Mucormycosis, IV, PO 372 mg (isavuconazole 200 mg) every 8 h for 6 doses and then 372 mg (isavuconazole 200 mg)/d, starting 12–24 h after the last loading dose | Safety and efficacy not established |
| Ketoconazole (Extina, Nizoral; ✹ Apo-Ketoconazole, Teva-Ketoconazole) | C | Candidiasis, histoplasmosis, and coccidioidomycosis Cutaneous candidiasis Tinea infections | PO 200 mg once daily, increased to 400 mg once daily if necessary in severe infections Topically, once daily for 2–6 wk | 2 y and older: PO 3.3–6.6 mg/kg/d as a single dose |

**TABLE 24.3**

**DRUGS AT A GLANCE: Azoles** (Continued)

| Drug | Pregnancy Category | Type of Infection Treated | Routes and Dosage Ranges | |
|------|------|------|------|------|
| | | | **Adults** | **Children** |
| Posaconazole (Noxafil; ✳ Posanol) | C | Treatment of oropharyngeal candidiasis Prevention of invasive fungal infection | Prevention: PO 200 mg three times daily Oropharyngeal candidiasis PO 100 mg twice daily initially and then 200 mg once daily for 13 d | Adolescents ≥13 y: refer to adult dosing |
| Voriconazole (Vfend, Vfend IV; ✳ Apo-Voriconazole, Sandoz-Voriconazole, Teva-Voriconazole, Vfend) | D | Esophageal candidiasis Invasive aspergillosis Other serious fungal infections | Esophageal candidiasis, PO 200 mg every 12 h for weight of ≥40 kg; 100 mg every 12 h for weight <40 kg. Give at least 14 d or 7 d after symptoms resolve Aspergillosis and other serious infections, IV 6 mg/kg every 12 h for 2 doses (loading dose) and then 4 mg/kg every 12 h (maintenance dose) | Dosage not established except in off-label uses |

## Use With Renal Impairment

In patients with a creatinine clearance of 50 mL/minute or less, the patient should take 50% of the recommended dose. Patients receiving hemodialysis receive a full dose following each dialysis treatment.

## Use in Patients With Hepatic Impairment

The azoles may cause hepatotoxicity, ranging from mild elevations in alanine aminotransferase (ALT) and aspartate aminotransferase (AST) to clinical hepatitis, cholestasis, hepatic failure, and death. Fatal hepatic damage has occurred mainly in patients with serious underlying conditions, such as AIDS or malignancy, and with multiple concomitant medications. The drugs are relatively contraindicated in patients with increased liver enzymes, active liver disease, or a history of liver damage with other drugs. They should be used only if expected benefits outweigh risks of liver injury. It is necessary to check ALT, AST, and serum bilirubin before drug use, after several weeks of drug use, and every 1 to 2 months during long-term therapy. If ALT and AST increase to more than three times the normal range, the azole should be discontinued. Hepatotoxicity may be reversible if drug therapy is stopped.

## Use in Patients With Critical Illness

Fluconazole penetrates tissues well, including CSF. Although IV administration may be necessary in many critically ill patients, the drug is well absorbed when administered orally (or by nasogastric tube).

## Use in Patients Receiving Home Care

When administering the azoles in the home setting, it is important that the home care nurse instruct the patient and family on the management of the environment with the implementation of good hand hygiene, household cleanliness, removal of potted plants and fresh flowers, and the use of air conditioning and air filtration systems. The nurse should also tell the patient and family about measures to prevent the reinfection and spread of the fungal infection.

## Adverse Effects

Although fluconazole is usually well tolerated, it may cause nausea, vomiting, diarrhea, abdominal pain, headache, and skin rash. In addition, elevation of liver enzymes and hepatic necrosis have reportedly occurred, and alopecia often occurs in patients receiving prolonged, high-dose treatment.

In April 2016, the FDA released an alert because of a study conducted in Denmark. Researchers found that the administration of fluconazole 400 to 800 mg/day for the treatment of a yeast infection during pregnancy increased the woman's risk of miscarriage. A single dose of 150 mg was not linked to birth-related abnormalities.

## Contraindications

Fluconazole is contraindicated in patients who have experienced a hypersensitivity reaction to the azole medications. It is also contraindicated in pregnancy and lactation. It should be administered cautiously with renal or hepatic impairment.

## Nursing Implications

### Preventing Interactions

Azoles inhibit the metabolism of many drugs (by inhibiting CYP drug-metabolizing enzymes in the liver and small intestine, especially CYP3A4 enzymes), thus increasing the effects and possible toxicity of azoles. Many medications increase or decrease the effects of fluconazole (Box 24.4). Researchers have not identified any herbs that interact with fluconazole.

Although the main concern about azole drug interactions is increased toxicity of inhibited drugs, ketoconazole may be given with cyclosporine and tacrolimus to decrease dosages and costs of the immunosuppressant drugs. There may also be a reduced risk of fungal infections, which commonly occur in people with an impaired immune system.

---

**BOX 24.4** **Drug Interactions: Fluconazole**

**Drugs That Increase the Effects of Fluconazole**

- Benzodiazepines (alprazolam, midazolam, triazolam), calcium channel blockers (felodipine, nifedipine), cyclosporine, phenytoin, statins (atorvastatin, simvastatin), sulfonylureas, tacrolimus, theophylline, warfarin, vincristine, zidovudine
  *Increase serum levels and toxic effects of these drugs due to inhibition of cytochrome P450*

**Drugs That Decrease the Effects of Fluconazole**

- Cimetidine, rifampin
  *Decrease serum level of fluconazole*

---

**BOX 24.5** **Patient Teaching Guidelines for Fluconazole**

- Take the medication for the complete course to ensure adequate results.
- Implement hand hygiene and maintain environmental cleanliness.
- Have renal function tests as ordered.
- Have hepatic function tests as ordered.
- To avoid experiencing side effects such as nausea and vomiting, eat small, frequent meals.
- Report any skin eruption to the prescriber.
- Report any changes in stool or urine to the prescriber.
- Find out about adverse effects of the drug, and report any adverse effects to the prescriber.

---

The nurse should note that fluconazole is apparently a less potent inhibitor of CYP3A4 enzymes than ketoconazole and itraconazole. As a result, drug interactions with fluconazole are of lesser magnitude and usually occur only with dosages of 200 mg/day or more. However, fluconazole is a strong inhibitor of CYP2C9 enzymes, and concurrent administration of losartan, phenytoin, or warfarin results in greater risks of toxicity with the inhibited drugs.

### Administering the Medication

When administering IV fluconazole, it is necessary to follow the manufacturer's recommendations. Until the nurse prepares the medication for administration, he or she should not remove the overwrap of the package. The inner bag maintains the sterility of the medication. The nurse assesses the bag for minute leaks by squeezing it firmly. If any leaks are apparent, it is necessary to discard the medication. The nurse should never mix fluconazole with any other medications. Continuous infusion of fluconazole occurs at a maximum rate of 200 mg/hour. When administering the oral suspension, it is necessary to shake the elixir vigorously prior to pouring the dose. To decrease gastric upset, the nurse administers the medication with food.

### Assessing for Therapeutic Effects

When administering fluconazole, the nurse assesses the therapeutic effects of the medication. The patient who is treated for systemic mycoses should have a decrease in fever and malaise. There is also healing of skin and mucous membrane lesions. Treatment of intestinal candidiasis results in diminished diarrhea. The female patient who has experienced discomfort from vaginal candidiasis should have decreased burning and itching along with diminished vaginal discharge.

### Assessing for Adverse Effects

The nurse must assess the skin for signs of skin rash. The GI assessment should include assessing for nausea, vomiting, diarrhea, and abdominal pain. All of the azoles cause hepatotoxicity with an elevation of the AST and ALT levels. Thus, it is necessary to assess hepatic enzymes monthly during therapy. Assessment of renal function tests should occur weekly, with dosage reduction or discontinuation of the drug if renal toxicity results. All of the azoles (with the exception of isavuconazole) may cause prolongation of the QTc interval.

### Patient Teaching

Box 24.5 identifies patient teaching guidelines for fluconazole.

## Other Drugs in the Class

Ketoconazole (Extina, Nizoral) has largely been replaced by the newer drugs, but it may still be used for long-term therapy because it is less expensive than other azoles. It may also be used with cyclosporine and tacrolimus because it increases blood levels of these immunosuppressant drugs and allows smaller dosages in patients with organ transplants.

Itraconazole (Sporanox, Tolsura) is a broad-spectrum antifungal with activity against *Candida*, *Cryptococcus*, and *Aspergillus*. It can be given orally or intravenously. Drug absorption may be decreased in patients with achlorhydria and in those receiving a concurrent antacid, histamine $H_2$ antagonist, or proton pump inhibitor. Serum levels should be measured to ensure adequate absorption. Drug concentrations are higher in visceral organs than in serum; little drug appears in urine or CSF.

Usual doses may cause GI upset, and higher doses may cause hypokalemia, hypertension, edema, and heart failure. Itraconazole has many drug interactions. Drugs that increase the pH of gastric acid (e.g., antacids, histamine $H_2$ blockers, proton pump inhibitors) decrease absorption of itraconazole and should be given at least 2 hours after itraconazole. Drugs that induce drug-metabolizing enzymes (e.g., carbamazepine, phenytoin, rifampin) decrease serum levels of itraconazole. Itraconazole increases serum levels of cyclosporine, digoxin, oral sulfonylureas, and warfarin; it decreases serum levels of carbamazepine, phenytoin, and rifampin. The FDA has issued a **BLACK BOX WARNING ◆** about the risks of heart failure and drug interactions with itraconazole.

Posaconazole (Noxafil) is a second-generation azole with activity against *Candida*, *Cryptococcus*, and *Aspergillus*, and *Mucor*. It is available as an oral suspension; after administration, it reaches maximum concentration in the body in 3 to 5 hours and steady state in 7 to 10 days. Patients who take the suspension should receive a fatty meal to increase absorption. Acidic cola drinks or fruit juice also increase absorption. The drug is highly protein bound and eliminated mainly in feces. Patients with severe vomiting and diarrhea or renal impairment should be monitored for breakthrough fungal infections. If given with drugs metabolized by the CYP3A4 enzymes in the liver, posaconazole increases blood levels and risks of adverse effects with the other drugs.

Voriconazole (Vfend) is a second-generation azole with activity against species of *Candida*, *Cryptococcus*, and *Aspergillus*. It is well absorbed with oral administration and reaches peak serum levels in less than 2 hours. It is widely distributed in body tissues and metabolized in the liver by CYP2C9, CYP2C19, and CYP3A4. The metabolites are excreted renally. Transient visual disturbance is a common adverse effect, occurring in approximately 30% of recipients. Additional adverse effects such as torsades de pointes, cardiac arrest, and sudden death have been reported with voriconazole in critically ill individuals with comorbidities. Significant drug interactions include reduced voriconazole levels with enzyme inducers (e.g., rifampin, rifabutin, carbamazepine) and increased sirolimus levels with voriconazole administration, possibly to toxic levels. These drugs are contraindicated during voriconazole therapy, and concomitant administration of cyclosporine, tacrolimus, or warfarin requires vigilant monitoring. Dosage of voriconazole should be reduced with impaired liver function. The drug may exhibit interpatient variability, and voriconazole levels should be periodically monitored to ensure doses are within the range of 1 to 5 mcg/mL.

Isavuconazole (Cresemba), the newest of the azole antifungals, has a spectrum activity similar to that of the other azoles with respect to *Candida* species. It has slightly less activity against *Aspergillus* spp. compared to voriconazole but has similar *Mucorales* coverage compared to posaconazole. The drug is available in both IV and oral (PO) formulations; both are considered bioequivalent. Isavuconazole is considered to have fewer drug interactions compared to the other azole antifungals. Adverse reactions may include nausea, vomiting, diarrhea, headache, and abdominal pain. Unlike other azoles, the drug shortens the QTc interval. The clinical relevance of this is unknown.

> **(!) QSEN Alert: Evidence-Based Practice**
>
> Researchers conducted a retrospective study on pediatric patients with hemato-oncologic malignancy and neutropenia following the administration of chemotherapy [During et al., 2015]. These patients are at risk for the development of fungal infection. The administration of antifungal agents prophylactically is a common practice with these patients. It was found that fluconazole, itraconazole, and posaconazole are most commonly prescribed. The results of this study revealed that posaconazole had fewer adverse effects than did fluconazole and itraconazole. It is important that nurses observe patients for adverse effects related to nausea, vomiting, diarrhea, headache, fever, and erythema.

---

### Clinical Application 24.2

- Before Ms. Angelo takes fluconazole, what assessments should the nurse make?
- What is the action of fluconazole?
- Ms. Angelo returns to the primary care provider's office 2 weeks later. She has an active *Candida albicans* infection. The primary care provider prescribes fluconazole 200 mg PO for one dose and then 100 mg PO daily for 14 days. What adverse effects should the nurse tell the patient to watch for?

---

## NCLEX Success

6. A patient who is being treated for a seizure disorder with phenytoin receives a diagnosis of candidiasis. The prescriber orders fluconazole. What effect does fluconazole have on phenytoin?

   A. The dosage of phenytoin should be increased.
   B. The fluconazole will be ineffective with the phenytoin.
   C. The patient should be assessed for phenytoin toxicity.
   D. The fluconazole dosage will need to be increased.

7. A prescriber writes an order for fluconazole 250 mg IV per hour. Which of the following nursing interventions is most appropriate?

   A. Begin the IV infusion at 125 mg/hour and increase it to 250 mg/hour after 4 hours.
   B. Inform the prescriber that the maximum dose is 200 mg/hour IV.
   C. Administer the fluconazole at 250 mg/hour IV.
   D. Administer the fluconazole at 200 mg/hour IV.

8. A patient who is undergoing hemodialysis has received a diagnosis of a systemic *Candida* infection. Which of the following interventions should be implemented when administering fluconazole?

   A. Administer the full dose of fluconazole after dialysis.
   B. Administer the full dose of fluconazole before dialysis.
   C. Administer one half of the dose of fluconazole after dialysis.
   D. Administer one half of the dose of fluconazole before dialysis.

9. A patient is receiving a high dose of fluconazole intravenously. Which of the following laboratory values indicate the development of hepatic necrosis?

   A. creatinine clearance of 50 mL/minute
   B. blood urea nitrogen of 15 mg/dL
   C. aspartate aminotransferase of 10 U/L
   D. alanine aminotransferase of 200 U/L

10. A prescriber has ordered oral fluconazole. Which of the following patient teaching guidelines is important to implement?

    A. Administer the medication on an empty stomach.
    B. Administer the medication 2 hours following breakfast.
    C. Administer the medication with meals.
    D. Administer the medication with a full glass of water.

## ECHINOCANDINS

The echinocandins have fungal activity against *Candida*, including azole-resistant organisms, and fungistatic activity against *Aspergillus*. The prototype for this class of antifungals is **caspofungin** (Cancidas).

## Pharmacokinetics

Caspofungin is highly bound to plasma albumin. It is metabolized in the liver and by the plasma to inactive metabolites. (In older adults, the use of this drug requires reduced dosage if there is hepatic insufficiency.) It is excreted in the urine and feces. Its half-life is 9 to 11 hours.

## Action

Caspofungin inhibits the synthesis of the fungal cell wall, interfering with the reproduction and growth of susceptible fungi.

## Use

Caspofungin is used to treat invasive aspergillosis in patients who do not tolerate other antifungal drugs. It is also used to treat *Candida* infections related to intra-abdominal, pleural space, or esophageal abscesses or peritonitis. In addition, it is given to febrile neutropenic patients who possess a suspected fungal infection.

Table 24.4 provides information about the use of echinocandins, including dosages.

### Use in Children

Caspofungin is approved for use in children older than 3 months of age for the treatment of candidemia and invasive candidiasis. It is recommended that the dosage be established based on body surface area rather than weight. Both children and adults who are receiving rifampin or phenytoin with caspofungin require an increased dose. The combination of rifampin or phenytoin

with caspofungin leads to the inhibition of organic anion-transporting polypeptide-1 (OATP-1), producing caspofungin metabolism leading to its excretion.

### Use in Patients With Renal Impairment

No dosage adjustment is necessary when using in patients with renal impairment.

## Adverse Effects

Adverse effects of caspofungin include fever, headache, nausea, skin rash, vomiting, and phlebitis at the injection site.

## Contraindications

Caspofungin is contraindicated in patients who have experienced a hypersensitivity reaction to the medication. It should be not administered with mannitol.

## Nursing Implications

### Preventing Interactions

Certain medications interact with caspofungin, increasing or decreasing its effects (Box 24.6). Researchers have not reported that any herbs interact with caspofungin.

### Administering the Medication

It is essential to administer caspofungin intravenously, and the drug is incompatible with any other IV medication, including dextrose. The medication should be at room temperature prior

| TABLE 24.4 | | | | |
|---|---|---|---|---|
| **DRUGS AT A GLANCE: Echinocandins** | | | | |
| **Drug** | **Pregnancy Category** | **Type of Infection Treated** | **Routes and Dosage Ranges** | |
| | | | **Adults** | **Children** |
| Ⓟ **Caspofungin** (Cancidas; 🍁 Cancidas) | C | Invasive aspergillosis Candidiasis | IV infusion over 1 h, 70 mg initially and then 50 mg daily Hepatic impairment, 70 mg initially and then 35 mg daily | Safety and efficacy not established in children younger than 3 mo of age Infants and children 3 mo to 17 y are administered 70 mg/m$^2$/dose on the first day and 50 mg/m$^2$/dose daily. The dosage may be increased to 70 mg/m$^2$/dose daily |
| Anidulafungin (Eraxis; 🍁 Eraxis) | C | Treatment of candidemia, esophageal candidiasis, and other *Candida* infections | Candidemia, IV infusion 200 mg initially and then 100 mg daily Esophageal candidiasis, IV infusion 100 mg initially and then 50 mg daily | Dosage not established |
| Micafungin (Mycamine; 🍁 Mycamine) | C | Treatment of esophageal candidiasis Prevention of *Candida* infections in patients undergoing hematopoietic stem cell transplantation | Treatment: IV infusion 100–150 mg daily Prevention: IV infusion 50 mg daily | IV ≥4 mo of age ≤30 kg: 3 mg/kg once daily >30 kg: 2.5 mg/kg once daily |

to administration. It is necessary to reconstitute the 50- or 70-mg vials of caspofungin in 10.5 mL of normal saline or sterile water. The reconstituted medication yields 5 or 7 mg/mL, respectively. Reconstituted solutions are stable for 24 hours when stored at 25°C. Addition of the medication is to 250 mL of normal saline or half-normal saline follows. The nurse administers the medication slowly over 1 hour.

Prior to administering the first dose of caspofungin, the nurse assesses baseline liver and renal function along with electrolytes, complete blood count, and platelet count. During administration, the nurse assesses for hypersensitivity reactions and phlebitis at the infusion site. If it is administered concurrently with tacrolimus, it is necessary to assess serum blood levels.

### Assessing for Therapeutic Effects

The therapeutic effect of caspofungin is a decrease in the growth of fungi. The patient has decreased symptoms of malaise, fever, and GI symptoms.

### Assessing for Adverse Effects

When administering 50 mg daily of caspofungin, the nurse observes for nausea, vomiting, and phlebitis at the infusion site. When administering 50 to 70 mg, the nurse assesses for these adverse effects plus fever, headache, and abnormal laboratory reports (e.g., decreased white blood cells, hemoglobin and hematocrit, increased serum potassium, and liver aminotransferase enzymes). In addition, he or she assesses for a histamine reaction, including facial edema, wheezing, dyspnea, chest tightness, skin eruptions, and itching. Patients suffering from any cardiovascular disease warrant assessment for increasing weight and peripheral edema.

### Patient Teaching

Caspofungin is administered in the acute care setting. The patient should receive instruction about the histamine reaction to the medication and the necessity of reporting any cardiac symptoms.

## Other Drugs in the Class

Anidulafungin (Eraxis) is a semisynthetic antifungal medication that inhibits glucan synthase, an essential component in the fungal cell wall. It is used to treat esophageal candidiasis and other *Candida* infections. It produces similar adverse effects as caspofungin and warrants cautious use with hepatic impairment.

Micafungin (Mycamine), another echinocandin, is approved for use in adult and pediatric patients older than 4 years of age. Most frequently, the dose is 100 mg once daily.

# MISCELLANEOUS ANTIFUNGAL AGENTS FOR SUPERFICIAL MYCOSES

The miscellaneous antifungal agents are administered for dermatophyte infections of the scalp and nails. **Griseofulvin** is the prototype for this class.

## Pharmacokinetics

Griseofulvin is absorbed in the GI tract and metabolized in the liver. The serum half-life is 9 to 24 hours. The medication is excreted in the urine, feces, and perspiration.

## Action

Griseofulvin disrupts the metaphase of cell division by binding to keratin, making it resistant to fungal invasion.

## Use

Griseofulvin is used for the treatment of susceptible tinea infections of the skin, hair, and nails. Table 24.5 gives specific information about the use of miscellaneous antifungal agents, including dosages for adults and children.

### Use in Children

Safety has not been established in children 2 years of age and younger.

### Use in Patients With Hepatic Impairment

Patients with hepatic impairment should not take the drug.

**TABLE 24.5**

**DRUGS AT A GLANCE: Miscellaneous Antifungal Agents for Superficial Mycoses**

| Drug | Pregnancy Category | Type of Infection Treated | Routes and Dosage Ranges | |
|---|---|---|---|---|
| | | | **Adults** | **Children** |
| Griseofulvin (Gris-PEG) | C | Dermatophytosis (skin, hair, nails) | PO Microsize: 500–1000 mg/d in single or divided doses Ultramicrosize: 375 mg/d in single or divided doses. Up to 750 mg/d have been used to eradicate tinea unguium and tinea pedis | Children >2 y PO Microsize: 10–20 mg/kg/d in single or divided doses; tinea capitis, 20–25 mg/kg/d for 8–12 wk Ultramicrosize: 7.3 mg/kg/d in single dose or 2 divided doses. Maximum dosage is 750 mg/d |
| Terbinafine (Lamisil; ❋ Apo-Terbinafine, Lamisil, JAMP-Terbinafine) | | Tinea infections Onychomycosis of fingernails or toenails | Tinea infections, topically to skin, once or twice daily for at least 1 wk and no longer than 4 wk Onychomycosis, fingernail, PO 250 mg daily for 6 wk; toenail, PO 250 mg daily for 12 wk | |

## Adverse Effects

Adverse effects of griseofulvin include the following:

- Central nervous system (CNS): dizziness, fatigue, headache, insomnia, and mental confusion
- Dermatologic: erythema, photosensitivity, and urticaria
- GI: sometimes gastric upset with nausea and vomiting
- Other: hepatotoxicity and proteinuria

## Contraindications

Griseofulvin is contraindicated in patients with a known hypersensitivity reaction. It is also contraindicated with liver disease, porphyria, and pregnancy.

## Nursing Implications

### Preventing Interactions

Some medications interact with griseofulvin, increasing or decreasing its effect (Box 24.7). Substances that increase the effect of griseofulvin include alcohol and vitamin E.

### Administering the Medication

It is necessary to administer griseofulvin with meals to decrease gastric upset. Greater absorption occurs when the

drug is given with a high-fat meal. Storage in a tightly covered container at 15°C to 30°C is required. For treatment of tinea corporis, the duration of therapy is 2 to 4 weeks; for tinea capitis, it is 4 to 6 weeks but may be extended for 8 to 12 weeks; for tinea pedis, it is 4 to 8 weeks; and for tinea unguium, it is 4 to 6 months.

### Assessing for Therapeutic Effects

Tinea infections of skin (e.g., ringworm) improve in 3 to 8 weeks. Onychomycosis of toenails may require a year or more. The most effective therapeutic results are achieved when the patient has two to three consecutive negative cultures.

### Assessing for Adverse Effects

The nurse assesses for safety related to CNS depression. He or she also assesses for dermatologic reactions such as rash, photosensitivity, or urticaria. In addition, it is necessary to assess the urine for evidence of protein and check liver enzymes for signs and symptoms of hepatotoxicity. Finally, clinicians have reported hypersensitivity reactions in patients who are allergic to penicillin.

### Patient Teaching

Box 24.8 identifies patient teaching guidelines for griseofulvin.

**BOX 24.7** *Drug Interactions: Griseofulvin*

**Drugs That Increase the Effects of Griseofulvin**
- Estrogen
  *Possible breakthrough bleeding*

**Drugs That Decrease the Effects of Griseofulvin**
- Barbiturates and rifampin
  *Decrease griseofulvin drug action*

**BOX 24.8** *Patient Teaching Guidelines for Griseofulvin*

- Take the entire prescription to prevent reemergence of symptoms.
- Avoid exposure to sunlight or extreme artificial light.
- Know that oral contraceptive effects are diminished.

## Other Drugs in the Class

Terbinafine (Lamisil) is a broad-spectrum antifungal that inhibits an enzyme needed for synthesis of ergosterol, a structural component of fungal cell membranes. It has fungicidal activity against dermatophytes and has been used mainly for topical treatment of ringworm infections and oral treatment of onychomycosis. Therapeutic effects may not be evident until months after drug therapy is stopped, because of the time required for growth of healthy nail. The drug is metabolized to inactive metabolites and excreted in the urine.

Common adverse effects with oral terbinafine include headache, diarrhea, and abdominal discomfort, and with long-term use for onychomycosis, skin reactions and liver failure may also occur. Hepatotoxicity is uncommon but has occurred in people with and without preexisting liver disease and has led to liver transplant or death. Terbinafine is not recommended for patients with chronic or active liver disease, and serum ALT and AST should be checked before starting the drug. The FDA has issued a **BLACK BOX WARNING** ◆ for this drug regarding the risk of hepatotoxicity.

### NCLEX Success

13. When instructing a patient on the administration of griseofulvin, which of the following is most appropriate?
    A. Take the medication on an empty stomach.
    B. Take the medication while consuming a high-fat diet.
    C. Take the medication with a full glass of water.
    D. Take the medication 1 hour after a meal.

14. Which of the following patients should not receive griseofulvin?
    A. an 18-year-old woman who is taking oral contraceptives
    B. a 55-year-old man who is taking ibuprofen
    C. a 38-year-old man who is taking phenytoin
    D. a 35-year-old man who is allergic to penicillin

## PYRIMIDINE ANALOG

 **Flucytosine**, the prototype pyrimidine analog, is an antifungal agent used to treat cryptococcosis, candidiasis, and chromomycosis. This drug is similar in structure to cytosine. As the fungal agent attempts to use flucytosine in place of cytosine to construct DNA, fungal cell division is interrupted.

### ! QSEN Alert: Patient-Centered Care

Safety alerts for the administration of flucytosine include the following:
- The Institute for Safe Medication Practices (ISMP) states that flucytosine causes a significant risk of patient harm when used in error.
- Flucytosine is associated with hematologic, renal, and hepatic adverse effects. Assess complete blood count, blood urea nitrogen, creatinine, AST, and ALT.

## Pharmacokinetics

Flucytosine is absorbed by the GI tract and distributed to the CSF, aqueous humor, joints, peritoneal fluid, and bronchial secretions. It is 3% to 4% protein bound and metabolized by the liver. The serum half-life with normal renal function is 2 to 5 hours. In patients with anuria, the half-life ranges from 30 to 250 hours. In patients with end-stage renal disease, the serum half-life is 75 to 200 hours. Flucytosine is excreted in the urine, greater than 90% unchanged.

## Action

Flucytosine affects the cell membrane of the fungus to cause fungal death. The exact mechanism is unknown.

## Use

Flucytosine is used as an adjunctive agent with amphotericin B for the treatment of systemic fungal infections caused by *Candida* and *Cryptococcus*. Flucytosine is added to the therapy due to its anticandidal activity and ability to penetrate the CSF and brain tissue (Drew, 2017). It can be administered in combination with other antifungal agents for the treatment of chromomycosis and aspergillosis.

Table 24.6 presents specific information about the use of the pyrimidine analog flucytosine, including dosages for adults and children.

### Use in Children

Flucytosine should be used in combination with amphotericin B or another antifungal drug in children because of the development of resistance.

### TABLE 24.6

### DRUGS AT A GLANCE: Flucytosine

| Drug | Pregnancy Category | Type of Infection Treated | Routes and Dosage Ranges | |
|---|---|---|---|---|
| | | | **Adults** | **Children** |
| **Flucytosine** (Ancobon) | C | Serious infections caused by *Candida* and *Cryptococcus* | 50–150 mg/kg PO every 6 h | Neonates: 25–100 mg/kg/d PO in divided doses every 12–24 h<br>Infants and children: 50–150 mg/kg/d PO in divided doses every 6 h |

## Use in Older Adults

In the presence of renal insufficiency, the dosage of flucytosine should be reduced.

## Use in Patients With Renal Impairment

When administering flucytosine to patients with impaired renal function, a reduced dosage is used at the beginning. For patients with a creatinine clearance of 20 to 40 mL/minute, an individual dose is administered every 12 hours. For those with a creatinine clearance of 10 to 20 mL/minute, an individual dose is administered every 24 hours. For those with a creatinine clearance of less than 10 mL/minute, an individual dose is administered every 24 to 48 hours. The FDA has issued a **BLACK BOX WARNING ◆** indicating that flucytosine should be used with extreme caution in patients with renal impairment.

Patients receiving hemodialysis should be given 20 to 50 mg/kg following the dialysis treatment.

## Use in Patients With Hepatic Impairment

Hepatotoxicity and bone marrow toxicity appear to be related. Hepatic and hematologic function should be monitored closely, and the dose should be adjusted according to hepatic function and any signs and symptoms of hematologic toxicity (Cox, 2016).

## Adverse Effects

Adverse effects of flucytosine include the following:

- GI: nausea, vomiting, diarrhea, duodenal ulcer, and GI bleeding.
- Bone marrow depression: after 10 to 26 days of therapy. Bone marrow depression and hepatotoxicity are related to the administration of higher doses.
- Dermatologic: rash, photosensitivity, pruritus, and urticaria.

## Contraindications

Flucytosine is contraindicated in patients who have a known hypersensitivity to the medication or any component of the formulation. It is also contraindicated in pregnancy and lactation.

## Nursing Implication

### Preventing Interactions

Certain medications interact with flucytosine, increasing or decreasing its effect (Box 24.9). No documented interactions

---

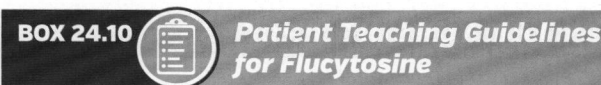

### BOX 24.10 · Patient Teaching Guidelines for Flucytosine

- Report any unusual bleeding such as bleeding of the gums or mouth.
- Take the entire course of treatment, which could be a minimum of 4 to 6 weeks.

---

between flucytosine and herbs exist. When the drug is given with food, the rate of absorption decreases.

### Administering the Medication

It is necessary to perform a culture and sensitivity before the initiation of therapy and at intervals throughout the course of treatment.

When treating endocarditis, it is necessary to give amphotericin B in combination with flucytosine. The oral dosage of amphotericin B is 25 to 37.5 mg/kg every 6 hours for at least 6 weeks after valve replacement. When treating meningoencephalitis caused by cryptococcal fungi, the oral dosage of amphotericin B is 25 mg/kg every 6 hours for 2 weeks. If the patient's clinical condition improves, the flucytosine and amphotericin B are discontinued, and the patient is started on fluconazole 400 mg/day. The administration of the medication with food decreases the rate but not the extent of drug absorption.

### Assessing for Therapeutic Effects

The patient has decreased symptoms of the fungal infection related to endocarditis and meningoencephalitis caused by *Candida* or *Cryptococcus*.

### Assessing for Adverse Effects

The nurse assesses for dermatologic reactions such as rash, photosensitivity, pruritus, and urticaria. He or she also assesses baseline hepatic and renal function prior to beginning therapy and at frequent intervals throughout therapy due to the adverse effect of hepatotoxicity and renal toxicity. It is necessary to check leukocyte and differential counts weekly as well as platelet counts to rule out bone marrow depression. In addition, the nurse assesses intake and output to determine any change in pattern or amount of urine output.

### Patient Teaching

Box 24.10 identifies patient teaching guidelines for flucytosine.

---

### BOX 24.9 · Drug Interactions: Flucytosine

**Drugs That Increase the Effects of Flucytosine**

- Amphotericin B

  *Increases serum levels of flucytosine*

**Drugs That Decrease the Effects of Flucytosine**

- *Saccharomyces boulardii* (probiotic; Florastor)

  *Flucytosine decreases the levels of Saccharomyces boulardii.*

---

### NCLEX Success

15. A patient with a fungal infection is taking flucytosine. Which of the following medications enhance the effectiveness of flucytosine in the treatment of the fungal infection?

    A. fluconazole
    B. fluorouracil
    C. vincristine
    D. amphotericin B

## THE NURSING PROCESS

A concept map outlines the nursing process related to drug therapy considerations in this chapter. Additional nursing implications related to the disease process should also be considered in care decisions.

**Assessment**

- Assess for superficial lesions of skin, hair, and nails, which are usually characterized by pain, burning, and itching. Some lesions are moist; others are dry and scaling.
- Assess warm, moist areas of the body; candidiasis occurs in such places. Skin lesions are likely to occur in perineal and intertriginous areas. They are usually moist, inflamed, pruritic areas with papules, vesicles, and pustules. Vaginal infection causes a cheesy vaginal discharge. Oral candidiasis has white patchy lesions on the buccal mucosa. Intestinal infection causes diarrhea. Systemic infection causes chills and fever, myalgia, arthralgia, and prostration.
- Assess for cough, fever, generalized malaise, and signs and symptoms of diminished pulmonary function. Blastomycosis, coccidioidomycosis, and histoplasmosis may be asymptomatic or mimic influenza, pneumonia, or tuberculosis, with cough, fever, malaise, and other pulmonary manifestations. Severe histoplasmosis may also cause fever, anemia, enlarged spleen and liver, leukopenia, and GI tract ulcers.
- Assess cognition and altered mental status. Cryptococcosis may involve the lungs, skin, and other body organs. In patients with AIDS or other immunosuppressant disorders, it often involves the CNS and produces mental status changes, headache, dizziness, and neck stiffness.
- Assess skin and lymph nodes. Sporotrichosis involves these areas. This infection usually produces small nodules that look like insect bites initially and ulcerations later. Nodules and ulcers also may develop in local lymphatic channels and nodes. The infection can spread to other parts of the body in immunocompromised patients.
- Assess for systemic mycoses producing severe symptoms that may be life-threatening. Confirmation involves recovery of organisms from specimens of body tissues or fluids.

**Outcomes of Therapy**

The patient will
- Take or receive systemic antifungal drugs as prescribed.
- Apply topical drugs accurately.
- Act to prevent recurrence of fungal infection.
- Avoid preventable adverse effects from systemic drugs.

**Nursing Interventions**

- Observe standard precautions while assessing or providing care to patients with skin lesions. Superficial infections (e.g., ringworm) are highly contagious and can be spread by sharing towels and hairbrushes. Systemic mycoses are not usually contagious.
- Decrease patient exposure to environmental fungi. For inpatients who are neutropenic or otherwise immunocompromised, do not allow soil-containing plants in the room and request regular cleaning and inspection of air-conditioning systems. For outpatients, assist to identify and avoid areas of potential exposure (e.g., soil contaminated by chicken, bird, or bat droppings; areas where buildings are being razed, constructed, or renovated). If exposure is unavoidable, instruct to spray areas with water to minimize airborne spores and to wear disposable clothing and a face mask. Patients working with landscaping are at risk for exposure to sporotrichosis; instruct to wear gloves and long sleeves. Implement measures for obese patients with skin candidiasis. Apply dry padding to intertriginous areas to help prevent irritation and candidal growth.
- Implement measures for patients with oropharyngeal ulcerations. Provide soothing oral hygiene, nonacidic fluids, and soft, bland foods.
- Implement measures for patients with systemic fungal infections. Monitor respiratory, cardiovascular, and neurologic status at least every 8 hours. Provide medications (e.g., analgesics, antihistamines, antipyretics, antiemetics) for patients receiving IV amphotericin B.

**Evaluation**

- Observe for relief of symptoms for which an antifungal drug was prescribed.
- Interview outpatients regarding their compliance with instructions for using antifungal drugs.
- Interview and observe for adverse drug effects with systemic antifungal agents.

## KEY CONCEPTS

- Serious fungal infections and infections with non*albicans Candida* strains are increasing.
- Patients whose immune systems are suppressed are at high risk for serious fungal infections.
- Fungal infections often require long-term drug therapy.
- Systemic antifungal drugs may cause serious adverse effects. For example, nephrotoxicity is associated with amphotericin B, and hepatotoxicity is associated with azole drugs.
- Liver function should be monitored with all systemic antifungal drugs, and both hepatic and renal function should be monitored with amphotericin B.

- A **BLACK BOX WARNING** ◆ states that amphotericin B be reserved for progressive or potentially fatal infections.
- A **BLACK BOX WARNING** ◆ points out the risks of heart failure and drug interactions associated with itraconazole.
- A **BLACK BOX WARNING** ◆ warns about the risk of hepatotoxicity with terfenadine.
- A **BLACK BOX WARNING** ◆ states that extreme caution be used when administering flucytosine to patients with renal impairment.

## CLINICAL REASONING CASE STUDY

**Meet the Patient**

Jacqueline Angelos is a 48-year-old woman who has developed cryptococcal meningoencephalitis. She is to receive flucytosine 25 mg/kg/dose with amphotericin B every 6 hours for 2 weeks. She has been taking ibuprofen (Motrin) 600 mg three times per day for the last 15 years. Her creatinine clearance (CrCl) is 10 to 20 mL/minute

- What is the action of flucytosine?
- Why is it administered with amphotericin B?
- How is the dosage of flucytosine affected due to the CrCl of 10 to 20 mL/minute?

**Assessing Drug Information**

- Flucytosine affects the cell membrane of the fungus causing fungal death. The exact mechanism of the drug is unknown.
- Amphotericin B is administered with flucytosine to enhance the effect of the flucytosine in the treatment of cryptococcal fungal infections.
- Ibuprofen is highly nephrotoxic when administered long term. Ms. Angelos has renal impairment so the flucytosine dosage must be reduced.
- Her creatinine clearance is 10 to 20 mL/minute and the maximum dose is 37.5 mg/kg every 24 hours.

**Nursing Actions**

- Administer flucytosine and amphotericin as prescribed.
- Assess neurological function.
- Assess CBC, AST, ALT, BUN, and creatinine.
- Assess for pain.
- Observe for any bleeding tendencies.

Visit the Point® at http://thePoint.lww.com/Frandsen12e for answers to NCLEX Success questions (in Appendix A), answers to Clinical Application Case Studies (in Appendix B), and more!

## REFERENCES AND RESOURCES

Cox, G. M. (2016). *Clinical management and monitoring during antifungal therapy of the HIV-infected patient with cryptococcal meningoencephalitis.* UpToDate. Lexi-Comp, Inc.

Drew, R. H. (2017). *Pharmacology of flucytosine (5-FC).* UpToDate. Lexi-Comp. Inc.

During, M., Eikemeier, M., Cabanillas Stanchi, K. M., Hartmann, U., Ebinger, M., Schwarze, C. P., et al. (2015). Antifungal prophylaxis with posaconazole versus fluconazole or itraconazole in pediatric patients with neutropenia. *European Journal of Clinical Microbiology Infectious Diseases, 34,* 1189–1200.

Hinkle, J. H., & Cheever, K. H. (2017). *Brunner & Suddarth's textbook of medical-surgical nursing* (14th ed.). Philadelphia, PA: Lippincott Williams & Wilkins.

Karch, A. (2017). *Focus on nursing pharmacology.* Philadelphia, PA: Lippincott Williams & Wilkins.

Kauffman, C. A. (2017). *Treatment of candidemia and invasive candidiasis.* UpToDate. Lexi-Comp, Inc.

Lewis, R. E. (2017). *Pharmacology of echinocandins.* UpToDate. Lexi-Comp, Inc.

Norris, T. L. (2019). *Porth's Pathophysiology: Concepts of altered health states* (10th ed.). Philadelphia, PA: Wolters Kluwer.

*Nursing 2020 drug handbook.* (2019). Philadelphia, PA: Lippincott Williams & Wilkins.

UpToDate. (2019). *Drug information.* Lexi-Comp, Inc.

# 25

# Drug Therapy for Parasitic Infections

## LEARNING OBJECTIVES

*After studying this chapter, you should be able to:*

1. Describe the etiology, pathophysiology, and clinical manifestations of parasitic infections.
2. Identify the prototype and describe the action, use, adverse effects, contraindications, and nursing implications for the amebicides.
3. Identify the prototype and describe the action, use, adverse effects, contraindications, and nursing implications for the antimalarial drugs.
4. Identify the prototype and describe the action, use, adverse effects, contraindications, and nursing implications for the anthelmintic drugs.
5. Identify the prototype and describe the action, use, adverse effects, contraindications, and nursing implications for the scabicides and pediculicides.
6. Implement the nursing process in the care of the patient being treated with antiparasitic agents.

## CLINICAL APPLICATION CASE STUDY

Lacy Michelson, a 35-year-old woman, is a missionary. She has just returned from a 2-year stay in a developing country. She comes to the clinic with severe diarrhea, fever, chills, headache, and myalgia. Ms. Michelson receives a diagnosis of giardiasis and malaria as well as a prescription for chloroquine 500 mg daily by mouth for 3 weeks and metronidazole 250 mg three times a day by mouth for 7 days.

## KEY TERMS

**Larvae:** developmental forms of a parasite

**Parasite:** organism that lives in or on the host and gains nutrition from the host

# INTRODUCTION

A **parasite** is a living organism that survives at the expense of another organism, called the host. Parasitic infestations are common human ailments worldwide. The effects of parasitic diseases on human hosts vary from minor to major and can be life threatening. Parasitic diseases discussed in this chapter are those caused by protozoa, helminths (worms), scabies, and pediculi (lice). There are currently no licensed vaccines to combat infection with any human parasite. Therefore, preventive measures, insecticide use, surveillance processes, and drug therapy are used to control parasitic infestations and any resulting diseases.

# OVERVIEW OF PARASITIC INFECTIONS

Protozoa can infect the digestive tract and other body tissues, and resulting infections include amebiasis, giardiasis, malaria, toxoplasmosis, and trichomoniasis. Helminths can also infect these sites, causing a number of infections. Scabies and pediculi affect the skin.

## Etiology and Pathophysiology

### Protozoal Infections
#### Amebiasis

Amebiasis is a common disease in Africa, Asia, and Latin America, but it can occur in any geographic region. In the United States, it is most likely to occur in residents of institutions for the mentally challenged, in men who have sex with men, and in travelers from countries with poor sanitation.

Amebiasis is caused by the pathogenic protozoan *Entamoeba histolytica*, which exists in two forms, cysts and trophozoites. Cysts are inactive; are resistant to drugs, heat, cold, and drying; and can survive outside the body for long periods. Transmission occurs by ingestion of food or water contaminated with human feces containing amebic cysts. After people ingest the cysts, some cysts remain intact to be expelled in feces and continue the chain of infection, and some open in the ileum to release amebae, which produce trophozoites. Trophozoites are active amebae that feed, multiply, move about, and produce clinical manifestations of amebiasis.

Trophozoites produce an enzyme that allows them to invade body tissues. They may form erosions and ulcerations in the intestinal wall with resultant diarrhea (this form of the disease is called intestinal amebiasis or amebic dysentery), or they may penetrate blood vessels and be carried to other organs, where they form abscesses. These abscesses are usually found in the liver (hepatic amebiasis) but also may occur in the lungs or brain.

#### Giardiasis

Giardiasis is a protozoal disease that may affect children more than adults. It occurs in areas with limited water treatment facilities and poor sanitary conditions and may cause community outbreaks of diarrhea. It also occurs in international travelers. Giardiasis is caused by *Giardia duodenalis* (also known as *Giardia lamblia*), a common intestinal parasite. The disease spreads by ingestion of food or water contaminated with human feces containing noninfective cysts with a hardy protective envelope or by contact with infected people or animals. Once in the small intestine, some protozoa escape from their envelopes and release trophozoites, which produce the infection seen 1 to 2 weeks after ingestion of the cysts. The resulting trophozoites and cysts then pass through the digestive system in the feces. Only the cysts are capable of surviving outside the host.

Person-to-person spread may occur in children in day care centers or in chlorinated water sources, such as pools, because *Giardia* cysts are resistant to chlorination. Transmission may also occur from ingestion of raw or undercooked food contaminated with cysts as well as by anal–oral sexual contact. The degree of infection ranges from asymptomatic to life threatening depending on the resistance of the host. Asymptomatic individuals are an important reservoir for spread of the infection.

### Clinical Application 25.1

- Ms. Michelson has received a diagnosis of a *Giardia* infection. What vitamin deficiency is she at risk for developing?
- What are the initial symptoms of giardiasis?

### Malaria

Malaria is a common cause of morbidity and mortality in many parts of the world, especially in tropical regions. In the United States, malaria is rare and affects travelers or immigrants from malarious areas.

Five species of protozoa of the genus *Plasmodium* (*P. falciparum, P. vivax, P. malariae, P. ovale,* and *P. knowlesi*) cause malaria in humans; the first two species pose the greatest threat. The bite of the female *Anopheles* mosquito, the malaria vector, spreads the parasites to people. *P. vivax, P. malariae,* and *P. ovale* cause recurrent malaria by forming reservoirs in the human host. In these types of malaria, signs and symptoms may occur months or years after the initial attack. *P. vivax* is the dominant malaria parasite in most countries outside of sub-Saharan Africa. *P. falciparum* is the most prevalent malaria parasite on the African continent but does not lead to formation of a reservoir. This type of malaria is responsible for most malaria-related deaths globally but may be cured and prevented from recurring. *P. knowlesi* normally affects animals, but this "monkey malaria" parasite can infect travelers to rainforests and fringe areas in Southeast Asia.

The plasmodia protozoa have a life cycle in which one stage of development occurs within the human body. When an uninfected *Anopheles* mosquito bites a person with malaria, it ingests blood that contains forms of the protozoan parasite. These forms produce sporozoites, which are transported to the mosquito's salivary glands. When the female mosquito bites the next person, the sporozoites are injected into that person's bloodstream. From the bloodstream, the organisms lodge in the liver and other tissues, where they reproduce and form merozoites. The liver cells containing the parasite eventually rupture and release the merozoites into the bloodstream, where they invade red blood cells. After a period of growth and reproduction, merozoites rupture red blood cells, invade other erythrocytes, and continue the cycle.

## Trichomoniasis

Trichomoniasis is a genitourinary infection caused by *Trichomonas vaginalis*, a single-cell protozoan. The disease is usually spread by men who have no signs and symptoms of infection who engage in sexual intercourse. Women are more likely than men to become infected.

## Helminthiasis

Helminthiasis, or infestation with parasitic worms, often occurs in many parts of the world. It affects about 1 billion people, making it one of the most common of all diseases. Although helminthiasis is quite frequent in topical areas, it is also found in other regions, including countries such as the United States and Canada. Box 25.1 describes the etiology and pathophysiology of some helminthic infections.

## Scabies and Pediculosis

Scabies and pediculosis are parasitic infestations of the skin. Scabies is caused by the "itch mite" (*Sarcoptes scabiei*), which burrows into the skin and lays eggs that hatch in 4 to 8 days. Pediculosis may be caused by one of three types of lice. *Pediculosis capitis* (head lice) is the most common type in the United States. It is diagnosed by finding louse eggs (nits) attached to hair shafts close to the scalp. *Pediculosis corporis* (body lice) is diagnosed by finding lice in clothing, especially in seams. *Pediculosis pubis* (pubic or crab lice) is diagnosed by the presence of nits in the pubic and genital areas. Although scabies and pediculosis are caused by different parasites, the conditions have two common characteristics:

- They are more likely to occur in areas of poverty, overcrowding, and poor sanitation. However, they may occur in people from any socioeconomic group, in any geographic area.
- They are highly communicable and transmitted by direct contact with an infected person or the person's personal effects (e.g., clothing, combs and hairbrushes, bed linens).

# Clinical Manifestations

Amebiasis may be asymptomatic. Affected people may have nausea, vomiting, diarrhea, abdominal cramping, and weakness. If the disease is severe, prolonged, and untreated, these people may experience symptoms from ulcerations of the colon or abscesses of the liver (hepatic amebiasis).

Giardiasis may be asymptomatic or produce diarrhea, abdominal cramping and distention, and flatulence. The clinical manifestations increase and decrease in intensity over months. If the infection is untreated, it may resolve spontaneously or progress to a chronic disease with anorexia, nausea, malaise, weight loss, and continued diarrhea with large, foul-smelling stools. Deficiencies of vitamin $B_{12}$, folate, and fat-soluble vitamins (see Chap. 35) may occur.

Malaria is an acute febrile illness that initially seems to resemble influenza in terms of its symptoms. In a nonimmune individual, symptoms appear a week or more (usually 10–15 days) after the infective mosquito bite. The first symptoms (fever, headache, chills, and vomiting) may be mild and difficult to identify as malaria. The characteristic paroxysms of chills, fever, and copious perspiration may not be present at the early stage of

---

**BOX 25.1** **Helminthic Infections**

**Hookworm infections** are caused by *Necator americanus*, a species found in the United States, and *Ancylostoma duodenale*, a species found in Europe, the Middle East, and North Africa. Hookworm is spread by ova-containing feces from infected people. Ova develop into larvae when deposited on the soil. Larvae burrow through the skin (e.g., if the person walks on the soil with bare feet), enter blood vessels, and migrate through the lungs to the pharynx, where they are swallowed. Larvae develop into adult hookworms in the small intestine and attach themselves to the intestinal mucosa.

**Pinworm infections** (enterobiasis), caused by *Enterobius vermicularis*, are the most common parasitic worm infections in the United States. They are highly communicable and often involve schoolchildren and household contacts. Infection occurs from contact with ova in food or water or on bed linens. The female pinworm migrates from the bowel to the perianal area to deposit eggs, especially at night. Touching or scratching the perianal area deposits ova on hands and any objects touched by the contaminated hands.

**Roundworm infections** (ascariasis), caused by *Ascaris lumbricoides*, are the most common parasitic worm infections in the world. They occur most often in tropical regions but may occur wherever sanitation is poor. The infection is transmitted by ingesting food or water contaminated with feces from infected people. Ova are swallowed and hatch into larvae in the intestine. The larvae penetrate blood vessels and migrate through the lungs before returning to the intestines, where they develop into adult worms.

**Tapeworms** attach themselves to the intestinal wall and may grow as long as several yards. Segments called *proglottids*, which contain tapeworm eggs, are expelled in feces. Tapeworms are transmitted by ingestion of contaminated, raw, or improperly cooked beef, pork, or fish. Beef and fish tapeworm infections are not usually considered serious illnesses. Pork tapeworm, which is uncommon in the United States, is more serious because it produces larvae that enter the bloodstream and migrate to other body tissues (i.e., muscles, liver, lungs, and brain).

**Threadworm infections** (strongyloidiasis), caused by *Strongyloides stercoralis*, are potentially serious infections. This worm burrows into the mucosa of the small intestine, where the female lays eggs. The eggs hatch into larvae that can penetrate all body tissues.

**Trichinosis**, a parasitic worm infection caused by *Trichinella spiralis*, occurs worldwide. It is caused by ingestion of inadequately cooked meat, especially pork. Encysted larvae are ingested in infected pork. In the intestine, the larvae excyst, mature, and produce eggs that hatch into new larvae. The larvae enter blood and lymphatic vessels and are transported throughout the body. They penetrate various body tissues (e.g., muscles and brain) and evoke inflammatory reactions. Eventually, the larvae are re-encysted or walled off in the tissues and may remain for 10 years or longer.

**Whipworm infections** (trichuriasis) are caused by *Trichuris trichiura*. Whipworms attach themselves to the wall of the colon.

disease. If not treated within 24 hours, *P. falciparum* malaria can progress to severe illness, often leading to death. During acute malarial attacks, the cycles occur every 36 to 72 hours. Clinical symptoms occur because of the large parasite burden. Children with severe malaria often develop severe anemia, respiratory distress in relation to metabolic acidosis, and/or cerebral malaria. In adults, multiorgan involvement is also frequent. In malaria-endemic areas, people may develop partial immunity, allowing asymptomatic infections to occur.

Trichomoniasis affects women and men differently. Women usually have vaginal burning, itching, and foul-smelling yellow–gray, frothy discharge. Men may be asymptomatic or have symptoms of urethritis.

Helminthiasis involves worm infestations; helminths are most often found in the gastrointestinal (GI) tract. However, several types penetrate body tissues or produce **larvae** (developmental forms of parasites) that migrate to the blood, lymph channels, lungs, liver, and other body tissues. Hookworm, roundworm, and threadworm larvae migrate through the lungs and may cause symptoms of pulmonary congestion. Hookworms may cause anemia by feeding on blood from the intestinal mucosa; fish tapeworms may cause megaloblastic or pernicious anemia by absorbing folic acid and vitamin $B_{12}$. Large masses of roundworms or tapeworms may cause intestinal obstruction. The major symptom usually associated with pinworms is intense itching in the perianal area (pruritus ani).

Scabies is characterized by burrows produced by the mite that create visible skin lesions, most often between the fingers, around the nails, and on the elbows and wrists. The lesions may also involve skin that is usually covered by clothing; the buttocks, belt line, penis, and skin around the nipples are likely places for mites to burrow.

Pediculosis leads to pruritus, which is usually the major symptom of the disease. This symptom results from an allergic reaction to parasite secretions. In addition to the intense discomfort associated with pruritus, scratching is likely to cause skin excoriation with secondary bacterial infection and formation of vesicles, pustules, and crusts.

## NCLEX Success

1. During the 2nd week of July, the emergency department of a local hospital treats 45 residents of one neighborhood for diarrhea. The neighborhood has a swimming pool, and in the past 10 days, 42 of the 45 affected people swam in the pool. What should the emergency department staff consider to be the cause of this outbreak of diarrhea?
   A. *Salmonella*
   B. *Clostridium difficile*
   C. *Pseudomonas*
   D. *Giardia*

2. A woman has received a diagnosis of *Trichomonas vaginalis*. What should the nurse teach the patient?
   A. Avoid yeast-containing foods.
   B. Wear a feminine pad to absorb the drainage.
   C. Use acetic acid douches.
   D. Avoid sexual intercourse.

## Drug Therapy

To combat parasitic diseases, health care professionals use antiparasitic drugs, including amebicides, antimalarials, other antiprotozoal agents, anthelmintics, scabicides, and pediculicides. Table 25.1 lists these drugs.

## AMEBICIDES

Amebicides, or drugs used to treat amebiasis, are classified according to their site of action. The prototype **Metronidazole** (Flagyl), a synthetic compound with amebicidal and trichomonacidal activity, is effective in both intestinal and extraintestinal amebiasis. Chloroquine is a tissue or extraintestinal amebicide because it acts in the bowel wall, liver, and other tissues. Chloroquine is

## TABLE 25.1

### Drugs Administered for Parasitic Infections

| Drug Class | Prototype | Other Drugs in the Class |
|---|---|---|
| Amebicide | Metronidazole (Flagyl) | Nitazoxanide (Alinia) Tinidazole (Tindamax) |
| Antibacterial | Tetracycline | Doxycycline |
| Antimalarial | Chloroquine phosphate | Quinine Artemether/lumefantrine (Coartem) Atovaquone/proguanil (Malarone) Chloroquine with primaquine Hydroxychloroquine (Plaquenil) Mefloquine Primaquine |
| Anthelmintic | Mebendazole (Emverm) | Ivermectin (Stromectol) |
| Scabicide/pediculicide | Permethrin (Elimite, Nix) | Lindane Malathion (Ovide) Spinosad (Natroba) |

discussed as an antimalarial agent because it is most commonly used for the prevention and treatment of malaria.

Tetracycline and doxycycline, which are antibacterial drugs (see Chap. 20), act against amebae in the intestinal lumen by altering the bacterial flora required for amebic viability. One of these drugs may be used with other amebicides in the treatment of all forms of amebiasis except asymptomatic intestinal amebiasis.

## Pharmacokinetics

Metronidazole is 80% absorbed by the GI tract, reaching a peak of action in 1 to 3 hours. The drug is widely distributed to the cerebrospinal fluid, bone, and cerebral and hepatic abscesses. Its half-life is 6 to 8 hours. Metronidazole is metabolized in the liver (30%–60%), with most excreted in the urine (77%) and some in the feces (14%). The drug readily crosses the placenta and enters the breast milk.

## Action and Use

Metronidazole diffuses across the cell membrane of anaerobic and aerobic microorganisms to cause cell death. The biochemical mechanism of action of the drug is unknown. Indications include intestinal amebiasis, amebic liver abscess, trichomoniasis, and bacterial vaginosis. The U.S. Food and Drug Administration (FDA) has not approved this drug or any other amebicide for the prophylaxis of amebiasis. The FDA has issued a **BLACK BOX WARNING ◆** for metronidazole and tinidazole, stating that these drugs should be used only for indicated conditions because they have produced carcinogenicity in rats. Table 25.2 gives route and dosage information for metronidazole and other amebicides.

## Adverse Effects and Contraindications

The adverse effects of metronidazole include headache, dizziness, ataxia, darkening of urine, diarrhea, nausea, vomiting, and an unpleasant metallic taste. Contraindications include a known hypersensitivity to the drug. Pregnancy is also a contraindication.

## Nursing Implications

### Preventing Interactions

Concomitant use of metronidazole with barbiturates increases the metabolism of the antiamebic drug, thus decreasing its therapeutic effect. Administration of metronidazole with anticoagulants (e.g., warfarin) increases bleeding tendencies due to decreased vitamin K metabolism. Ingesting alcoholic beverages or alcohol-containing medications while taking metronidazole may cause tachycardia, warmth or redness under the skin, a tingly feeling, and nausea and vomiting. Also, disulfiram and alcohol combined with metronidazole may lead to a disulfiram-like reaction, with tachycardia, nausea, flushing, and vomiting. No herbal interactions with metronidazole reportedly occur.

### Administering the Drug

Patients may take metronidazole with food to improve medication adsorption. It is important not to crush extended-release preparations. If the patient is unable to swallow regular metronidazole pills, it may be necessary to crush them.

### Assessing for Therapeutic Effects

The nurse assesses patients with intestinal amebiasis for decreased abdominal pain and diarrhea. It is necessary to assess stool

## TABLE 25.2

## DRUGS AT A GLANCE: Amebicides

| Drug | Pregnancy Category | Routes and Dosage Ranges | |
|---|---|---|---|
| | | **Adults** | **Children** |
| Ⓟ **Metronidazole** (Flagyl; ✳ Flagyl, PMS-Metronidazole) | B | Amebiasis: 750 mg PO for 5–10 d Giardiasis: 750 mg extended release PO daily for 7 d Trichomoniasis: 2 g PO in 1 d or 250 mg PO three times per day for 7 d | Amebiasis: 35–50 mg/kg/d PO in three divided doses for days |
| Nitazoxanide (Alinia) | B | *G. duodenalis* or *C. parvum*: 500 mg PO every 12 h for 3 d | 1–3 y: 100 mg PO every 12 h for 3 d (increase duration to 14 d in HIV exposed or patients infected with cryptosporidia) 4–11 y: 200 mg PO every 12 h for 3 d (increase duration to 14 d in HIV exposed or patients infected with cryptosporidia) ≥12 y: refer to adult dosing |
| Tinidazole (Tindamax) | C | Amebiasis: 2 g/d PO for 3 d Amebiasis, liver abscess: 2 g/d PO for 3–5 d Bacterial vaginosis: 2 g/d PO for 2 d or 1 g/d PO for 5 d Giardiasis: 2 g PO as single dose Trichomoniasis: 2 g PO as single dose | Intestinal amebiasis or amebiasis liver abscess (age > 3 y): 50 mg/kg/d PO for 3–5 d (max 2 g/d) |

*Assess stool*

specimens for amebic cysts and trophozoites periodically for 6 months. Also, the nurse checks the feces for increase in form that is indicative of diminished diarrhea stools and improved hydration.

It is important to assess women with trichomoniasis for decreased vaginal drainage and odor.

### Assessing for Adverse Effects

It is necessary to assess for headache; diminished muscular coordination; GI upset, including metallic taste; and hypersensitivity reactions such as rash and bronchospasm.

### Patient Teaching

Box 25.2 identifies patient teaching guidelines for antiparasitic drugs, including metronidazole.

## Other Drugs in the Class

Nitazoxanide (Alinia) is a less commonly used drug. In *Cryptosporidium parvum* infection, it inhibits the growth of sporozoites and oocysts. In *G. duodenalis* infection, it inhibits the growth of trophozoites. Nitazoxanide is administered with food for the treatment of diarrhea.

Tinidazole (Tindamax), a chemical relative of metronidazole, is approved for the treatment of amebiasis, giardiasis, bacterial vaginosis, and trichomoniasis. Cytochrome P4503A4

enzymes in the liver metabolize the drug, and caution is warranted with use in people with impaired liver function. The most common adverse effects are a bitter metallic taste and nausea.

## NCLEX Success

3. **A man with intestinal amebiasis has received a prescription for metronidazole. He later develops a cough and takes a prescription cough syrup. What adverse effect will he experience?**

   A. edema
   B. bronchospasm
   C. flushing
   D. bradycardia

4. **What assessment should the nurse implement when caring for a patient who is receiving metronidazole for intestinal amebiasis?**

   A. diminished diarrhea
   B. hypomagnesemia
   C. increased temperature
   D. hyperkalemia

---

**BOX 25.2**  *Patient Teaching Guidelines for Antiparasitic Drugs*

**General Considerations**

- Use measures to prevent parasitic infection or reinfection:
  - Support public health measures to maintain a clean environment (i.e., sanitary sewers, clean water, regulation of food-handling establishments and food-handling personnel).
  - When traveling to wilderness areas or to tropical or developing countries, check with the local health department about precautions needed to avoid parasitic infections.
  - Practice good hand hygiene and other personal hygienic practices.
  - When a family member or other close contact contracts a parasitic infection, be sure to complete prompt appropriate treatment and follow-up care.
  - Avoid ingesting raw fish and undercooked meat.
  - With vaginal infections, avoid sexual intercourse or use a condom.

**Self or Caregiver Administration**

- Use antiparasitic drugs as prescribed; their effectiveness depends on accurate use. Take the full course of the medication. For malaria prophylaxis, for example, take chloroquine at the same time each week, and set up a calendar with time and date of administration.
- Take atovaquone/proguanil, chloroquine and related drugs, oral metronidazole, and tinidazole with or after meals. Food increases absorption of atovaquone and decreases gastrointestinal irritation with the other drugs.
- Avoid alcoholic beverages while taking metronidazole or tinidazole and for 3 days after the drugs are stopped. Flushing, headache, nausea, sweating, and vomiting may occur if alcohol is ingested.
- Metronidazole has an unpleasant metallic taste. Taking this drug will make your urine dark in color. Do not be alarmed.

- Metronidazole is contraindicated in pregnancy. Let your health care provider/prescriber know if you think you could be pregnant before taking the medication.
- Have an ophthalmic examination at the start of chloroquine use and every 3 months during drug therapy. It is important to have complete blood count studies as ordered.
- Take or give most anthelmintics without regard to mealtimes or food ingestion. Mebendazole tablets should be chewed or crushed and mixed with food.
- Have a culture for ova and parasites 3 weeks after initial mebendazole use. Eat frequent small meals and maintain excellent hydration if diarrhea develops. Report fever and severe diarrhea.
- With a pinworm infection, adhere to the following instructions:
  - Disinfect the toilet facilities after use.
  - Launder bed linens, nightclothes, undergarments, and towels every day.
  - Family members should also be treated for pinworms due to the fact they are highly contagious.
  - Follow strict handwashing and excellent hygienic practices.
- Use pediculicides and scabicides as directed on the label or product insert. Instructions vary among preparations. Use gloves prior to applying permethrin cream rinse, cream, or lotion.
- With pediculosis and scabies, wash bed linens, towels, undergarments, and clothes daily.
- Inspect the head, genital area, and other parts of the body for lice and scabies to determine if they have been killed.
- With the administration of permethrin, report stinging, tingling, skin numbness, rash, itching, and rash to the prescriber.

# ANTIMALARIALS

Antimalarials act at different stages in the life cycle of plasmodial parasites. Some drugs such as **Chloroquine phosphate** are effective against erythrocytic forms and are therefore useful in preventing or treating acute attacks of malaria. Although these drugs do not prevent infection with the parasite, they do prevent clinical manifestations.

Widespread resistance in most malaria-endemic countries has led to decline in the use of chloroquine for treatment of malaria caused by *P. falciparum*, although it remains effective in most regions for disease caused by *P. vivax*. Other drugs such as primaquine act against exoerythrocytic or tissue forms of the parasite to prevent initial infection and recurrent attacks or to cure some types of malaria. Combination drug therapy, administered concomitantly or consecutively, is common with antimalarial drugs.

## Pharmacokinetics

Chloroquine is rapidly absorbed by the GI tract, and the drug is widely distributed and retained throughout the body tissues such as the central nervous system (CNS), eyes, cardiopulmonary system, liver, kidneys, and spleen. The peak of action is 1 to 2 hours with a serum half-life of 3 to 5 days. It is 55% protein bound and partially metabolized by the liver. Chloroquine is excreted by the kidneys. Small amounts of the drug are present in the urine for months following the discontinuation of drug therapy.

## Action and Use

Chloroquine inhibits DNA and RNA polymerase, thus interfering with the metabolism and hemoglobin used by parasites. The drug also inhibits prostaglandin effects while concentrating within the parasitic acid vesicles. It raises the internal pH to inhibit parasitic growth. Uses of chloroquine include the suppression and chemoprophylaxis of malaria. Health care providers also use it for the treatment of acute malaria caused by *P. malariae*, *P. ovale*, and *P. falciparum*, as well as for extraintestinal amebiasis. Table 25.3 gives route and dosage information for chloroquine and the other antimalarial drugs.

## TABLE 25.3

### DRUGS AT A GLANCE: Antimalarials

| Drug | Pregnancy Category | Routes and Dosage Ranges | |
|---|---|---|---|
| | | **Adults** | **Children** |
| **Chloroquine phosphate** (Aralen, Novo Chloroquine) | C | Prophylaxis: 500 mg/wk PO on the same day each week; start 1–2 wk prior to exposure; continue while in endemic area and for 4 wk after leaving the endemic area<br>Treatment: 1 g PO, followed by 500 mg 6, 24, and 48 h after first dose<br>Extraintestinal amebiasis: 1 g/d PO for 2 d followed by 500 mg/d for at least 2–3 wk | Prophylaxis: 8.3 mg/kg/wk PO on the same day each week (do not exceed 500 mg/dose); begin 1–2 wk prior to exposure; continue while in the endemic area and for 4 wk after leaving endemic area.<br>Treatment: 16.6 mg/kg PO (max 1000 mg), followed by 8.3 mg/kg (max 500 mg) 6, 24, and 48 h after first dose |
| Artemether/lumefantrine (Coartem) | C | 25–35 kg: 3 tablets PO at hour 0 and hour 8 the 1st day and then 3 tablets twice daily on day 2 and day 3 (total of 18 tablets per treatment course)<br>Patients ≥35 kg: 4 tablets at hour 0 and hour 8 the 1st day and then 4 tablets twice daily on day 2 and day 3 (total of 24 tablets per treatment course) | 5–15 kg: 1 tablet PO at hour 0 and hour 8 the 1st day and then 1 tablets twice daily on day 2 and day 3 (total of 6 tablets per treatment course)<br>15–25 kg: 2 tablets PO at hour 0 and hour 8 the 1st day and then 2 tablets twice daily on day 2 and day 3 (total of 12 tablets per treatment course)<br>25–35 kg: 3 tablets at hour 0 and hour 8 on the 1st day and then 3 tablets twice daily on day 2 and day 3 (total of 18 tablets per treatment course)<br>≥35 kg: 4 tablets PO at hour 0 and hour 8 the 1st day and then 4 tablets twice daily on day 2 and day 3 (total of 24 tablets per treatment course) |

**TABLE 25.3**

## DRUGS AT A GLANCE: Antimalarials (Continued)

| Drug | Pregnancy Category | Routes and Dosage Ranges | |
|---|---|---|---|
| | | **Adults** | **Children** |
| Atovaquone/ proguanil (Malarone; 🍁 Malarone) | C | Prophylaxis: 250 mg/100 mg PO once daily; start 1–2 d prior to entering malaria-endemic area and continue throughout the stay and for 7 d after returning<br>Acute treatment: 1 g/400 mg PO as a single dose, once daily for 3 consecutive days | Prophylaxis (begin 1–2 d prior to entering a malaria-endemic area; continue throughout the stay and for 7 d after returning; take as a single dose, once daily):<br>5–8 kg: 31.25/12.5 mg<br>9–10 kg: 46.8/18.75 mg<br>11–20 kg: 62.5/25 mg<br>21–30 kg: 125/50 mg<br>31–40 kg: 187.5/75 mg<br>>40 kg: 250/100 mg PO<br>Acute treatment:<br>5–8 kg: 125/50 mg<br>9–10 kg: 187.5/75 mg<br>11–20 kg: 250/100 mg<br>21–30 kg: 500/200 mg<br>31–40 kg: 750/300 mg<br>>40 kg: 1 g/400 mg PO as a single dose once daily for 3 consecutive days |
| Chloroquine with primaquine | Contraindicated in pregnant women | Prophylaxis: 1 tablet PO weekly for 2 wk before entering and 8 wk after leaving endemic area | Prophylaxis: same as adults for weight above 45 kg; 1/2 tablet for weight of 25–45 kg<br>For younger children, a suspension is prepared (e.g., 40 mg of chloroquine and 6 mg of primaquine in 5 mL); given weekly for 2 wk before entering and 8 wk after leaving malarious areas; dosages are 2.5 mL for weight of 5–7 kg; 5 mL for 8–11 kg; 7.5 mL for 12–15 kg; 10 mL for 16–20 kg; and 12.5 mL for 21–24 kg |
| Hydroxychloroquine (Plaquenil; 🍁 Plaquenil, Gen-Hydroxychloroquine) | | Prophylaxis: 400 mg once weekly for 2 wk before entering and 8 wk after leaving endemic area<br>Treatment of acute disease: 800 mg PO initially, then 400 mg 6 h later, and 400 mg/d for 2 d (total of four doses) | Prophylaxis: 5 mg/kg PO once weekly for 2 wk before entering and 8 wk after leaving endemic area<br>Treatment of acute disease: 13 mg/kg PO initially, then 6.5 mg/kg 6 h later, and 6.5 mg/kg/d PO for at 24 and 48 h (total of four doses) |
| Mefloquine | | Prophylaxis: 250 mg PO 1 wk before travel and then 250 mg weekly during travel and for 4 wk after leaving a endemic area<br>Treatment: 1250 mg (5 tablets) as a single dose | Prophylaxis: 1/4 tablet PO for 15–19 kg weight, 1/2 tablet for 20–30 kg, 3/4 tablet for 31–45 kg, and 1 tablet for above 45 kg, according to the schedule for adults |
| Primaquine (🍁 Primaquine) | Contraindicated | 15 mg once daily in combination with chloroquine for 14 d (maximum dose: 15 mg/d) | 0.39 mg/kg once daily for 14 d (maximum: 15 mg/d) |
| Quinine (🍁 Quinine) | | 650 mg PO every 8 h for 10–14 d | 25 mg/kg/d PO in divided doses every 8 h for 10–14 d |

## Adverse Effects

Adverse effects of chloroquine are usually mild because small doses are used for prophylaxis; administration of the larger doses required for treatment of acute attacks occurs only for short periods. CNS changes include visual disturbances with retinal damage and difficulty to focus. Cardiovascular adverse effects include electrocardiogram changes with prolonged QRS intervals and hypotension. Other significant adverse effects are nausea, vomiting, diarrhea, loss of appetite, skin rash, pruritus, and hair loss. Reportedly, ototoxicity and muscle weakness may also occur.

## Contraindications

Contraindications to chloroquine include a known hypersensitivity to 4-aminoquinoline compounds and the presence of retinal and visual field changes. Caution is necessary in porphyria, psoriasis, retinal disease, glucose-6-phosphate dehydrogenase (G6DP) deficiency, alcoholism, pregnancy, and lactation.

## Nursing Implications

### Preventing Interactions

Some medications interact with chloroquine, increasing or decreasing its effects (Box 25.3). When the drug is combined with alcohol, the risk of GI distress increases.

### Administering the Medication

For malaria prophylaxis, it is necessary to take chloroquine on the same day each week. The nurse may set up a calendar to assist with adherence. For malaria treatment, it is necessary to take the drug as prescribed (perhaps at the same time each day). It is appropriate to take chloroquine with food to reduce gastric distress. When administering chloroquine to children, it is essential to double-check the dosage because young people are especially sensitive to the 4-aminoquinoline compounds that the drug contains.

 *Concept Mastery Alert*

Teach patients taking chloroquine to avoid foods that acidify their urine, such as cranberries, prunes, plums, cheeses, meats, fish, eggs, and grains. These foods might interact with antimalarials and increase excretion, thus decreasing the effect of the drug.

### Assessing for Therapeutic and Adverse Effects

The nurse assesses for a decrease in signs and symptoms of malaria. Fever and chills usually subside in 24 to 48 hours. Blood smears for plasmodia are negative in 24 to 72 hours. Also, the nurse assesses for nausea, vomiting, diarrhea, pruritus, rash, headache, and visual changes.

### Patient Teaching

Box 25.2 identifies patient teaching guidelines for antiparasitic drugs, including chloroquine phosphate.

**BOX 25.3** *Drug Interactions: Chloroquine*

**Drugs That Increase the Effects of Chloroquine**
- Cimetidine
  *May increase the plasma concentration*

**Drugs That Decrease the Effects of Chloroquine**
- Magnesium trisilicate
  *May reduce bioavailability*
- Vitamin C
  *Increases urinary excretion*

## Other Drugs in the Class

Quinine was once the primary antimalarial drug, but synthetic agents that cause fewer adverse reactions have largely replaced it. However, this drug may still be useful in the treatment of chloroquine-resistant *P. falciparum* malaria. Also, it relaxes skeletal muscles and may be effective in the prevention and treatment of nocturnal leg cramps.

Artemisinin-based combination therapies (ACTs) are used for the treatment of uncomplicated malaria to prevent or delay development of drug resistance. The artemisinin component has the most rapid parasite clearance times of any antimalarial drug. The drugs appear to act by binding iron and breaking down peroxide bridges, resulting in the generation of free radicals that damage parasite proteins. Artemether/lumefantrine (Coartem), a combination product, is the only ACT recommended by the World Health Organization for the treatment of uncomplicated malaria in the United States.

People may take Coartem with a full meal for optimal absorption. It may be necessary (1) to crush the tablets and mix them in 5 to 10 mL of water and (2) to rinse the container and ingest the contents. If vomiting occurs, it is important to repeat the dosage in 2 hours. People with known QT prolongation should avoid taking Coartem. If people take this combination drug with grapefruit juice, the potential for QT prolongation is enhanced.

Chloroquine with primaquine is a mixture available in tablets containing chloroquine phosphate 500 mg (equivalent to 300 mg of chloroquine base) and primaquine phosphate 79 mg (equivalent to 45 mg of primaquine base). This combination is effective for prophylaxis of malaria and may be more acceptable to patients. It also may be more convenient for use in children because no pediatric formulation of primaquine is available.

 **QSEN Alert: Safety**

Before prescribing primaquine, health care providers should screen patients for G6DP deficiency. This genetic disorder, which occurs most often in males, causes hemolysis of red blood cells and can lead to hemolytic anemia.

Atovaquone–proguanil (Malarone) is a combination product with adult and pediatric formulations. Uses include the prevention and treatment of malaria, including chloroquine-resistant strains. The constituent drugs inhibit two different pathways in plasmodial reproduction. Atovaquone blocks the parasite mitochondrial electron transport chain, and proguanil inhibits the folate pathway and appears to act by a direct mechanism as well. This activity enhances atovaquone's mitochondrial membrane toxicity, and the combination maintains exceptional clinical efficacy for worldwide treatment and prevention, even if antifolate resistance is present. Adverse effects include vomiting, diarrhea, abdominal pain, headache, and pruritus.

Hydroxychloroquine (Plaquenil) is a derivative of chloroquine with essentially the same actions and uses with fewer adverse effects. Other uses of this drug include treatment of rheumatoid arthritis and lupus erythematosus.

Mefloquine is used to prevent *P. falciparum* malaria, including chloroquine-resistant strains, and to treat acute malaria caused by *P. falciparum* or *P. vivax*. The FDA has issued a **BLACK BOX WARNING** ◆ for mefloquine, warning that patients with major psychiatric disorders should not take the drug. Mefloquine can trigger neuropsychiatric adverse reactions that can persist after the drug has been discontinued. It should be administered with food and at least 8 oz of water, on the same day each week.

Primaquine is most commonly used to prevent recurrent attacks of malaria caused by *P. vivax* and *P. ovale*. Also, it may prevent the initial occurrence of malaria. When used to prevent initial occurrence of malaria (causal prophylaxis), people should take primaquine concurrently with a suppressive agent (e.g., chloroquine, hydroxychloroquine) after they have returned from a malarious area. Primaquine is not effective for treatment of acute attacks of malaria.

>  **QSEN Alert: Evidence-Based Practice**
>
> The World Health Organization (2015a,b) reviewed multiple studies that explored the safety of artemisinin-based combination therapies compared to quinine as first-line treatment of uncomplicated malaria in the first trimester of pregnancy. Findings indicated that the artemisinins are not associated with an increased risk of miscarriage, stillbirths, or major congenital malformations when compared to nonartemisinin regimens, and the rate of miscarriage was significantly less using artemisinin-based combination therapies than using quinine during the first trimester of pregnancy.

### NCLEX Success

5. A nurse who is scheduled to work at a hospital in Haiti in 2 weeks comes to the clinic for antimalarial medication. A health care provider should prescribe which of the following drugs prior to the nurse's trip?
   - A. primaquine
   - B. metronidazole
   - C. amitriptyline
   - D. clindamycin

6. Which of the following aspects of teaching is most important to provide to a patient who is taking chloroquine phosphate?
   - A. Take chloroquine with vitamin C.
   - B. Have frequent ophthalmologic examinations.
   - C. Administer antacids to reduce gastric distress.
   - D. Take chloroquine on an empty stomach.

### *Clinical Application 25.3*

- When providing patient teaching to Ms. Michelson regarding the chloroquine, what is most important that the nurse impart?

## ANTHELMINTICS

Health care providers use anthelmintics used for the treatment of helminthiasis. Most of these drugs act locally to kill or cause expulsion of parasitic worms from the intestines. Some of these medications act systemically against parasites that have penetrated various body tissues. The goal of anthelmintic therapy may be to eradicate the parasite completely or to decrease the magnitude of infestation ("worm burden"). **Mebendazole** (Emverm) is the prototype of this class of medications.

## Pharmacokinetics

Mebendazole is administered orally with a slow onset of action. The drug reaches peak of action in 2 to 4 hours. Approximately 2% to 10% is absorbed. It reaches its highest concentrations in the liver and muscle. Mebendazole is 95% protein bound and has an elimination half-life of 3 to 6 hours. The drug is metabolized extensively by the liver. It is excreted mostly in the feces and minimally in the urine.

## Action

Mebendazole blocks glucose uptake by susceptible helminths. The drug depletes glycogen stores that the worms need for survival and reproduction, resulting in their death.

## Use

Uses for mebendazole include the treatment of infections with *E. vermicularis* (pinworm), *T. trichiura* (whipworm), and *A. lumbricoides* (roundworm), as well as *A. duodenale* and *N. americanus* (hookworms). Unlabeled uses of this drug are infections with *Ancylostoma caninum* (eosinophilic enterocolitis), *Capillaria philippinensis* (capillariasis), *G. duodenalis* (giardiasis), *Mansonella perstans* (filariasis), and visceral larva migrans (toxocariasis). Table 25.4 presents route and dosage information for mebendazole and the other anthelmintics.

## Adverse Effects

Dizziness, drowsiness, headaches, seizures, transient abdominal pain, diarrhea, nausea, and vomiting may occur with mebendazole. Hematologic effects such as agranulocytosis, anemia, leukopenia, and neutropenia sometimes take place. The hepatic enzymes alanine aminotransferase (ALT) and aspartate aminotransferase (AST) may be increased. Genitourinary effects include casts in the urine, glomerulonephritis, and hematuria. Finally, hypersensitivity reactions have reportedly occurred.

## Contraindications

Contraindications to mebendazole include known hypersensitivity to the drug. It is also embryotoxic and teratogenic, particularly in the first trimester of pregnancy. Caution is necessary with lactation.

## Nursing Implications

### *Preventing Interactions*

Certain medications interact with mebendazole, increasing or decreasing its effects (Box 25.4). Serum levels of mebendazole may be increased with food.

### *Administering the Medication*

Administering mebendazole involves chewing and swallowing the tablets or crushing them and mixing them with food, whether solid or liquid. Taking the drug with food increases its serum levels.

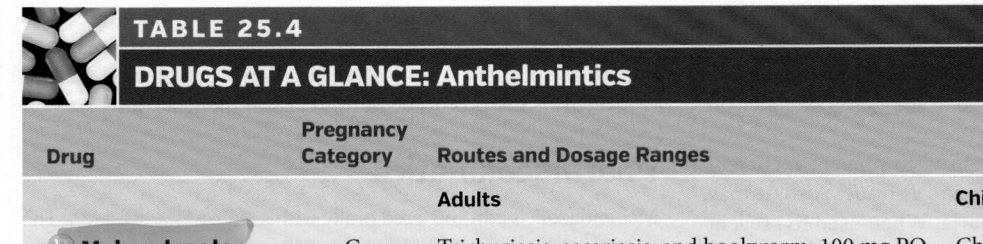

| Drug | Pregnancy Category | Routes and Dosage Ranges | |
|------|---------------------|--------------------------|---|
| | | **Adults** | **Children** |
| **Mebendazole** (Emverm; ✹ Vermox) | C | Trichuriasis, ascariasis, and hookworm: 100 mg PO morning and evening on 3 consecutive days<br>Enterobiasis: 1 tablet PO once; repeat treatment if not cured in 3 wk | Children 2 y of age and older, same as adults<br>Safety and efficacy have not been established younger than 2 y of age |
| Ivermectin (Stromectol) | C | Strongyloidiasis: PO 200 mcg/kg as a single dose | Children ≥15 kg: refer to adult dosing |

## Assessing for Adverse Effects

The nurse assesses for CNS depression, dizziness, and seizure activity. He or she also assesses for GI disorders, including nausea, vomiting, diarrhea, and alterations in fluid volume. In addition, it is important to assess the hepatic enzymes AST and ALT for elevations leading to hepatic failure. Finally, the nurse assesses for blood in the urine and glomerulonephritis. Assessing for rash and alterations in pulmonary status related to hypersensitivity to the medication is also necessary.

## Assessing for Therapeutic Effects

The nurse obtains a stool sample for culture for ova and parasites after 3 weeks of drug administration. A negative stool culture is the optimum outcome of drug therapy. There is a complete eradication of the parasite, and any "worm burden" is now nonexistent.

## Patient Teaching

Box 25.2 identifies patient teaching guidelines for antiparasitic drugs, including mebendazole.

## Other Drugs in the Class

Ivermectin (Stromectol), which is used for numerous parasitic infections, is most active against strongyloidiasis (caused by the roundworm *S. stercoralis*). Another use for this drug is in the oral treatment of resistant lice infestations. It has relatively few adverse effects but may cause some nausea and vomiting.

---

**BOX 25.4** *Drug Interactions: Mebendazole*

**Drugs That Increase the Effects of Mebendazole**

- Metronidazole
  *Enhances the toxic effect of mebendazole and the development of adverse effects*

**Drugs That Decrease the Effects of Mebendazole**

- Aminoquinolines (antimalarials), carbamazepine, phenytoin
  *Decrease the serum concentration*

---

**NCLEX Success**

7. A 4-year-old child receives a diagnosis of enterobiasis, an infection with *Enterobius vermicularis*. What is *E. vermicularis*?

   A. pinworm
   B. hookworm
   C. whipworm
   D. roundworm

8. A patient who has enterobiasis, which is caused by *Enterobius vermicularis*, is receiving treatment with mebendazole. Which of the following agents decreases the serum concentration of mebendazole?

   A. alcohol
   B. phenytoin
   C. ampicillin
   D. metronidazole

## SCABICIDES AND PEDICULICIDES

Topical and oral medications are administered for the treatment scabies as well as for head or pubic lice. **Permethrin** (Elimite, Nix), a pediculicide, is a first-line treatment and the prototype for the treatment of lice and scabies, caused by *P. capitis* and *S. scabiei*, respectively.

## Pharmacokinetics and Action

After topical administration of permethrin, 2% is absorbed through the skin and metabolized in the liver by ester hydrolysis to inactive metabolites. The drug is then excreted in the urine. It inhibits the influx of sodium ions through the nerve cell membrane channels of the parasites to delay the repolarization, resulting in the paralysis or death of the lice or scabies.

## Use

A single application of permethrin is useful in the treatment of infestation with *P. capitis* or *S. scabiei*. Prophylactic applications are effective during epidemics of lice. Table 25.5 presents route and dosage information for permethrin and related drugs.

| TABLE 25.5 |
|---|
| **DRUGS AT A GLANCE: Scabicides and Pediculicides** |

| Drug | Pregnancy Category | Routes and Dosage Ranges | |
|---|---|---|---|
| | | **Adults** | **Children** |
| ℗ **Permethrin** (Elimite, Nix; 🍁 Nix, Kwellada-P) | B | Head lice: apply large volume of cream, rinse to clean, damp hair to saturate hair and scalp; apply behind ears and at the base of the neck; leave on for 10 min before rinsing with water; repeat in 1 wk if lice and nits are present<br>Scabies: apply cream head to toe; leave on 8–14 h before washing off with water; reapply in 1 wk if mites appear. | Same as adults |
| Lindane | B | Head lice: rub lotion into affected area, leave in place for 12 h, then wash or shampoo (rub into the affected area for 4 min and rinse thoroughly)<br>Scabies: apply to the entire skin except the face, neck, and scalp; leave in place for 24 h; then remove by shower | Not recommend for use in children <50 kg due to safety concerns<br>>10 y: same as adults |
| Malathion (Ovide) | B | Head lice: apply to hair, rub in well to wet hair, then dry hair without covering or using a hair dryer; after 8–12 h, shampoo, rinse, and comb hair with a fine-toothed comb to remove dead lice and eggs; if necessary, repeat in 7–9 d | Contraindicated in neonates and infants<br>≥6 y: same as adults |
| Spinosad (Natroba) | B | Apply to dry scalp and rub in gently then apply to hair; leave on for 10 min and then rinse with warm water and shampoo; repeat in 7 d if the first treatment is ineffective | ≥6 mo: same as adults |

## Adverse Effects and Contraindications

The most common adverse effects of permethrin are pruritus, rash of the scalp, erythema, burning, tingling, numbness or pain of the scalp, and edema. Contraindications include a known hypersensitivity to chrysanthemums, pyrethroid, or pyrethrin, as well as age less than 2 months.

### Administering the Medication

 **QSEN Alert: Safety**

When administering permethrin for head lice, it is necessary to wear gloves and follow these directions:

- Wash the hair well and towel dry.
- Apply a large amount of cream rinse to saturate the hair and scalp as well as behind the ears and at the base of the neck.
- Leave the medication on for 10 minutes before rinsing it with water.

Administration should occur again in 1 week if lice and nits are present. The second time, the hair is dry and the drug stays on for 8 to 14 hours (e.g., overnight).

When administering permethrin for scabies, it is necessary to follow these directions:

- Apply the cream from head to toe.
- Leave it on for 8 to 14 hours, and then wash it off with water.

### Assessing for Therapeutic and Adverse Effects

The nurse assesses for lice or scabies. It is also necessary to assess the areas of application of permethrin for inflammation, pruritus,

erythema, and rash. The nurse asks the patient if there is any burning, stinging, tingling, scalp numbness or pain, or edema.

### Patient Teaching

Box 25.2 identifies patient teaching guidelines for antiparasitic drugs, including permethrin.

## Other Drugs in the Class

Lindane is a second-line drug for scabies and pediculosis. The FDA has issued a **BLACK BOX WARNING ◆** for lindane because neurologic toxicities, including seizures and death, have been reported even when it is taken as directed. The drug is also contraindicated in premature infants and individuals with known uncontrolled seizure disorders. Lindane is useful in people who cannot tolerate a safer, first-line drug for scabies; have hypersensitivity reactions to such a drug; or are resistant to treatment with such a drug. It is necessary to provide guidance about accurate use to individuals taking the drug.

Administration is topical, and absorption through intact skin is substantial. CNS toxicity has been reported with excessive use, especially in infants and children. The drug is available in a 1% concentration as a lotion and shampoo.

Malathion (Ovide) is a pediculicide used in the treatment of resistant head lice infestations, and pyrethrin preparations are available over the counter for treatment of pediculosis. These preparations require two applications approximately 10 days apart.

Spinosad (Natroba), a pediculicidal and ovicidal drug, is useful for the treatment of head lice. It causes insect paralysis and death due to excitation of the CNS of the parasite. Topical administration results in no absorption.

## NCLEX Success

9. A prescriber has ordered permethrin for an elderly patient who has received a diagnosis of scabies. What is the action of permethrin?
   A. It inhibits the influx of sodium through the nerve cell membranes to paralyze the parasite.
   B. It inhibits the influx of calcium through the nerve cell membranes to paralyze the parasite.
   C. It inhibits the influx of potassium through the nerve cell membranes to paralyze the parasite.
   D. It inhibits the influx of chloride through the nerve cell membranes to paralyze the parasite.

10. When applying spinosad to a dry scalp for treatment of head lice, how long should it be left on?
    A. 5 minutes
    B. 10 minutes
    C. 20 minutes
    D. 30 minutes

## THE NURSING PROCESS

A concept map outlines the nursing process related to drug therapy considerations in this chapter. Additional nursing implications related to the disease process should also be considered in care decisions.

**Assessment**
- Assess for exposure to parasites (e.g., overcrowded housing, institutional resident, history of parasites in environment, geographic location [travel to area of poor sanitation, an underdeveloped country, or a tropical region], and personal hygiene) and use of prophylactic measures, as appropriate.
- With vaginal trichomoniasis, assess in relation to sexual activity; sexual partners need simultaneous treatment to prevent reinfection.
- With pubic (crab) lice, assess sexual activity; lice transmission may occur with sexual or other close contact and contact with infested bed linens.
- Assess for signs and symptoms. These vary greatly, depending on the type and extent of parasitic infestation.

**Outcomes of Therapy**
The patient will
- Experience relief of symptoms for which antiparasitic drugs were taken.
- Self-administer drugs accurately.
- Avoid preventable adverse effects.
- Act to prevent recurrent infestation.
- Keep appointments for follow-up care.

**Nursing Interventions**
- Use environmental health measures to avoid exposure to or prevent transmission of parasitic diseases.
- Follow-up with examination and possibly treatment of household and other close contacts of people with helminthiasis, amebiasis, trichomoniasis, scabies, and pediculosis.
- Teach those traveling regarding measures to decrease exposure to mosquito bites (e.g., wear long-sleeved, dark clothing; use an effective insect repellent such as DEET; sleep in well-screened rooms or under mosquito netting).
- Use effective personal hygiene and other health measures to avoid exposure, prevent transmission of parasitic disease, or reinfection.
- Ensure follow-up measures, such as testing of stool specimens; vaginal examinations; anal swabs, smears, and cultures.
- With vaginal infections, avoid sexual intercourse, or have the male partner use a condom.

**Evaluation**
- Interview and observe for relief of symptoms.
- Interview outpatients regarding compliance with instructions for taking antiparasitic drugs and measures to prevent recurrence of infestation.
- Interview and observe for adverse drug effects.
- Interview and observe regarding food intake or changes in weight.

## KEY CONCEPTS

- Parasitic infestations injure host tissues.
- Amebiasis is caused by the pathogenic protozoan *E. histolytica*. It is transmitted by the fecal–oral route, such as by ingesting food or water contaminated with human feces containing amebic cysts.
- Helminthiasis is an infestation of parasitic worms and is most commonly found in the GI tract.
- Scabies and pediculosis are parasitic infestations of the skin.
- Scabies is caused by *S. scabiei*.
- Pediculosis is caused by three types of lice.
- Amebicides are effective against the protozoans that cause amebiasis.
- The U.S. Food and Drug Administration (FDA) has issued a **BLACK BOX WARNING ◆** for metronidazole and tinidazole, stating that the drug should only be used for conditions as indicated because it has produced carcinogenicity in rats.
- Travelers to malarious regions should generally receive chloroquine to prevent malaria and take precautions to avoid or minimize exposure to the causative mosquito.

- The FDA has issued a **BLACK BOX WARNING ◆** for mefloquine warning that patients with major psychiatric disorders should not take the drug. Mefloquine can trigger neuropsychiatric adverse reactions that can continue after mefloquine has been discontinued.
- Anthelmintics are used in the treatment of parasitic infections by hookworms, pinworms, roundworms, and whipworms.
- Scabies and pediculosis are treated with the topical agents.
- The FDA has issued a **BLACK BOX WARNING ◆** for lindane because neurologic toxicities, including seizures and death, have been reported even when it is taken as directed. The drug is also contraindicated in premature infants and individuals with known uncontrolled seizure disorders. Lindane is useful in people who cannot tolerate a safer, first-line drug for scabies; have hypersensitivity reactions to such a drug; or are resistance to treatment with such a drug. It is necessary to provide guidance about accurate use to individuals taking the drug.
- Personal and public health hygienic practices can prevent many parasitic infections and should be followed diligently.

## CLINICAL REASONING CASE STUDY

| | |
|---|---|
| **Meet the Patient** | Gabriela Cruz, a 17-year-old female high school student, has been taking ciprofloxacin for the past 10 days for the treatment of a "strep" throat. She visits the school nurse with the complaint of vaginal burning and itching along with a foul-smelling vaginal drainage. The school nurse, who is a family nurse practitioner, prescribes metronidazole (Flagyl) 500 mg every 6 to 8 hours for 7 days.<br><br>• What is the action of metronidazole?<br>• The nurse should provide what patient teaching to Ms. Cruz? |
| **Assessing Drug Information** | • Metronidazole is a synthetic compound that produces amebicidal and trichomonacidal activity, but the biochemical mechanism of action is unknown. The medication diffuses across the cell membrane of anaerobic and aerobic microorganisms and causes cell death.<br>• Prescribers order metronidazole for trichomoniasis and bacterial vaginosis as well as intestinal amebiasis and amebic liver abscess.<br>• Adverse effects include headache, dizziness, ataxia, darkening of urine, diarrhea, nausea, vomiting, and an unpleasant metallic taste. |
| **Nursing Actions** | • Explain to Ms. Cruz that the antibiotic she was taking changed the normal flora in her vagina and caused a yeast infection. If she is sexually active, she should be given a pregnancy test before starting metronidazole.<br>• In addition, be sure to give her the following instructions:<br>  • Understand that adverse effects of the medication.<br>  • Avoid sexual intercourse until after the course of the medication is completed—or use a condom.<br>  • Avoid alcoholic beverages or alcohol-containing medications while taking metronidazole or 3 days after completing the drug because the combination may cause tachycardia, flushing, a tingly feeling, nausea, and vomiting.<br>  • Do not stop using any medications without first talking to your provider. |

*Visit* thePoint *at* **http://thePoint.lww.com/Frandsen12e** *for answers to NCLEX Success questions (in Appendix A), answers to Clinical Application Case Studies (in Appendix B), and more!*

## REFERENCES AND RESOURCES

Guyton, A. C., & Hall, J. E. (2020). *Guyton & Hall textbook of medical physiology* (14th ed.). Philadelphia, PA: Elsevier.

Hinkle, J. H., & Cheever, K. H. (2018). *Brunner & Suddarth's textbook of medical-surgical nursing* (14th ed.). Philadelphia, PA: Lippincott Williams & Wilkins.

Karch, A. M., & Tucker, R. (2020). *Lippincott's pocket drug guide for nurses*. Philadelphia, PA: Lippincott Williams & Wilkins.

Leder, K., & Weller, P. F. (2020a). Treatment and prevention of cryptosporidiosis. In *UpToDate*. LexiComp, Inc.

Leder, K., & Weller, P. F. (2020b). Ascariasis. In *UpToDate*. LexiComp, Inc.

Porth, C. M. (2013). *Pathophysiology: Concepts of altered health status* (9th ed.). Philadelphia, PA: Lippincott Williams & Wilkins.

Pousibet-Puerto, J., Salas-Coronas, J., Sánchez-Crespo, A., et al. (2016). Impact of using artemisinin-based combination therapy (ACT) in the treatment of uncomplicated malaria from *Plasmodium falciparum* in a non-endemic zone. *Malaria Journal, 15*(339). doi:10.1186/s12936-016-1408-1

Savoia, D. (2016). New antimicrobial approaches: Reuse of old drugs. *Current Drug Targets, 17*(6), 731–738.

Tan, K. R., & Boundy, E. O. (2020). Prevention of malaria infection in travelers. In *UpToDate*. LexiComp, Inc.

Travassos, M., & Laufer, M. K. (2020). Antimalarial drugs: An overview. In *UpToDate*. LexiComp, Inc.

Weller, P. F. (2020). Anthelmintic therapies. In *UpToDate*. LexiComp, Inc.

Weller, P. F. (2016). Antiprotozoal therapies. In *UpToDate*. LexiComp, Inc.

World Health Organization. (2015a). *Guidelines for the treatment of malaria* (3rd ed.). Geneva: WHO. Retrieved October 22, 2016, from http://www.who.int/malaria/publications/atoz/9789241549127/en/

World Health Organization. (2015b). Recommendations on intermittent screening and treatment in pregnancy and the safety of ACTs in the first trimester. Geneva: WHO. Retrieved October 24, 2016, from http://www.who.int/malaria/publications/atoz/istp-and-act-in-pregnancy/en/

World Health Organization. (2016). Update on Artemisinin and ACT resistance. Geneva: WHO. Retrieved October 24, 2016, from http://www.who.int/malaria/publications/atoz/update-artemisinin-resistance-october2016/en/

# Drugs Affecting the Cardiovascular System

# 26

# Drug Therapy for Hypertension

## LEARNING OBJECTIVES

*After studying this chapter, you should be able to:*

1. Describe factors that regulate blood pressure.
2. Describe how hypertension is classified.
3. Discuss nonpharmacologic measures to control hypertension.
4. Identify the prototype and describe the action, use, contraindications, adverse effects, and nursing implications of the angiotensin-converting enzyme inhibitors.
5. Identify the prototype and describe the action, use, contraindications, adverse effects, and nursing implications of the angiotensin II receptor blockers.
6. Identify the prototype and describe the action, use, contraindications, adverse effects, and nursing implications of the calcium channel blockers.
7. Describe the rationale for using combination drugs in the management of hypertension.
8. Review the effects of alpha-adrenergic blockers, beta-adrenergic blockers, and diuretics in the management of hypertension.
9. Implement the nursing process when caring for patients with hypertension.

## CLINICAL APPLICATION CASE STUDY

Harold Caudill, a 55-year-old man, is married, has four children, and works as an automobile salesman. He has a history of primary hypertension. His medical history includes type 1 diabetes mellitus, with early signs of nephropathy. After having a myocardial infarction 2 years ago, he has been treated with metoprolol, a beta-adrenergic blocker. In addition, he has been taking the diuretic hydrochlorothiazide to treat the hypertension. His blood pressure today is 138/92 mm Hg, which is consistent with the readings on his last three visits. His physician has added captopril to his treatment regimen.

## KEY TERMS

**Angioedema:** sudden deep swelling or welts under skin, particularly around the eyes and lips

**Antiadrenergic:** decrease or block the effects of sympathetic nerve stimulation

**Autoregulation:** ability of body tissues to regulate their own blood flow

**Bradykinin:** peptide that causes vasodilation and lowers blood pressure

**Essential hypertension:** high blood pressure for which no cause can be found

**First-dose phenomenon:** orthostatic hypotension with palpitations, dizziness, and perhaps syncope 1 to 3 hours after the first dose of a drug or an increased dose

**Secondary hypertension:** high blood pressure from an identified cause, such as kidney disease

# INTRODUCTION

Antihypertensive drugs are used to treat hypertension, a common, chronic disorder estimated to affect more than 100 million adults and an unknown number of children and adolescents in the United States (Muntner et al., 2017). Hypertension increases risks of myocardial infarction (MI), heart failure, cerebral infarction and hemorrhage, and renal disease. To understand hypertension and antihypertensive drug therapy, it is necessary first to understand the physiologic mechanisms that normally control blood pressure, the characteristics of hypertension, and the characteristics of antihypertensive drugs.

# OVERVIEW OF HYPERTENSION

## Regulation of Blood Pressure

Arterial blood pressure reflects the force exerted on arterial walls by blood flow. Blood pressure normally remains constant because of homeostatic mechanisms that adjust blood flow to supply tissues with needed oxygen and nutrients. The two major determinants of arterial blood pressure are cardiac output (systolic pressure) and peripheral vascular resistance (diastolic pressure).

Cardiac output equals the product of the heart rate and stroke volume ($CO = HR \times SV$). Stroke volume is the amount of blood ejected with each heartbeat (~60–90 mL). Thus, cardiac output depends on stroke volume, which is dependent on the force of myocardial contraction, blood volume, and other factors. Peripheral vascular resistance is determined by local blood flow and the degree of constriction or dilation in arterioles and arteries (vascular tone).

## Autoregulation of Blood Flow

Autoregulation is the ability of body tissues to regulate their own blood flow. This is a critical homeostatic mechanism of major organs (e.g., heart, brain, kidneys) to preserve oxygenation and function. Local blood flow is regulated primarily by nutritional needs of the tissue, such as lack of oxygen or accumulation of products of cellular metabolism (e.g., carbon dioxide, lactic acid). Local tissues produce vasodilating and vasoconstricting substances to regulate local blood flow. Important tissue factors affecting vascular flow include histamine, bradykinin, serotonin, and prostaglandins.

Histamine is found mainly in mast cells surrounding blood vessels and is released when these tissues are injured. In some tissues, such as skeletal muscle, mast cell activity is mediated by the sympathetic nervous system (SNS), and histamine is released when SNS stimulation is blocked or withdrawn. In this case, vasodilation results from increased histamine release and the withdrawal of SNS vasoconstrictor activity. **Bradykinin** is released from a protein in body fluids. Kinins dilate arterioles, increase capillary permeability, and constrict venules; this increases blood flow to local tissues. Serotonin is released from aggregating platelets during the blood-clotting process. It causes vasoconstriction and plays a major role in control of bleeding. Prostaglandins are formed in response to tissue injury and include vasodilators (e.g., prostacyclin) and vasoconstrictors (e.g., thromboxane $A_2$).

An important component of regulating local blood flow is the production of several vasoactive substances by the endothelial cells that line blood vessels. Vasoconstricting substances, which increase vascular tone and blood pressure, include angiotensin II, endothelin 1, and thromboxane $A_2$. Vasodilating substances, which decrease vascular tone and blood pressure, include nitric oxide (NO) and prostacyclin. Excessive vasoconstrictors or deficient vasodilators may contribute to the development of atherosclerosis, hypertension, and other diseases. Injury to the endothelial lining of blood vessels by the sheer force of blood flow with hypertension or by rupture of atherosclerotic plaque leads to vasoconstriction, vasospasm, thrombus formation, and thickening of the blood vessel wall. All of these factors narrow the blood vessel lumen and increase peripheral vascular resistance.

Overall, regulation of blood pressure involves a complex, interacting, overlapping network of hormonal, neural, and vascular mechanisms, and any condition that affects heart rate, stroke volume, or peripheral vascular resistance affects arterial blood pressure. Many of these mechanisms are compensatory effects that attempt to restore balance when hypotension or hypertension occurs. Box 26.1 further describes these mechanisms.

---

**BOX 26.1**    *Mechanisms That Regulate Blood Pressure*

**Neural**

Neural regulation of blood pressure mainly involves the sympathetic nervous system (SNS). In the heart, SNS neurons control heart rate (chronotropy) and force of contraction (inotropy). In blood vessels, SNS neurons control muscle tone by maintaining a state of partial contraction, with additional constriction or dilation accomplished by altering this basal state. When hypotension and inadequate tissue perfusion occur, the SNS is activated and produces secretion of epinephrine and norepinephrine by the adrenal medulla; constriction of blood vessels in the skin, gastrointestinal tract, and kidneys; and stimulation of beta-adrenergic receptors in the heart, which increases heart rate and force of myocardial contraction. All of these mechanisms act to increase blood pressure, cardiac output, and tissue perfusion, especially of the brain and heart.

The SNS is activated by the vasomotor center in the brain, which constantly receives messages from baroreceptors and chemoreceptors located in the circulatory system. Adequate function of these receptors is essential for rapid and short-term regulation of blood pressure. The vasomotor center interprets the messages from these receptors and modifies cardiovascular functions to maintain adequate blood flow.

More specifically, baroreceptors detect changes in pressure or stretch. For example, when a person moves from a lying to a standing position, blood pressure falls and decreases stretch in the aorta and arteries. This elicits increased heart rate and vasoconstriction to restore adequate circulation. The increased heart rate occurs rapidly, and blood pressure is adjusted within 1 to 2 minutes. This quick response prevents orthostatic hypotension with dizziness and possible syncope. (Antihypertensive medications may blunt this response and cause orthostatic hypotension.)

Chemoreceptors, which are located in the aorta and carotid arteries, are in close contact with arterial blood and

---

*(Continued on page 510)*

**BOX 26.1** *Mechanisms That Regulate Blood Pressure* [Continued]

respond to changes in the oxygen, carbon dioxide, and hydrogen ion content of blood. Although their main function is to regulate ventilation, they also communicate with the vasomotor center and can induce vasoconstriction in response to lowered cardiac output.

Chemoreceptors are stimulated when blood pressure drops to a certain point because oxygen is decreased and carbon dioxide and hydrogen ions are increased in arterial blood.

The central nervous system [CNS] also regulates vasomotor tone and blood pressure. Inadequate blood flow to the brain results in ischemia of the vasomotor center. When this occurs, neurons in the vasomotor center stimulate widespread vasoconstriction in an attempt to raise blood pressure and restore blood flow. This reaction, the CNS ischemic response, is an emergency measure to preserve blood flow to vital brain centers. If blood flow is not restored within 3 to 10 minutes, the neurons of the vasomotor center are unable to function, the impulses that maintain vascular muscle tone stop, and blood pressure drops to a fatal level.

### Hormonal

The renin–angiotensin–aldosterone [RAA] system and vasopressin are important hormonal mechanisms in blood pressure regulation.

The RAA system is activated in response to hypotension and acts as a compensatory mechanism to restore adequate blood flow to body tissues. Renin is an enzyme that is synthesized, stored, and released from the kidneys in response to decreased blood pressure, SNS stimulation, or decreased sodium concentration in extracellular fluid. When released into the bloodstream, where its action lasts 30 to 60 minutes, renin converts angiotensinogen [a plasma protein] to angiotensin I. Angiotensin-converting enzyme [ACE] in the endothelium of pulmonary blood vessels then acts on angiotensin I to produce angiotensin II. Angiotensin II strongly constricts arterioles [and weakly constricts veins], increases peripheral resistance, and increases blood pressure by direct vasoconstriction, stimulation of the SNS, and stimulation of catecholamine release from the adrenal medulla. It also stimulates secretion of aldosterone from the adrenal cortex, which then causes the kidneys to retain sodium and water. Retention of sodium and water increases blood volume, cardiac output, and blood pressure.

Vasopressin, also called antidiuretic hormone or ADH, is a hormone secreted by the posterior pituitary gland that regulates reabsorption of water by the kidneys. It is released in response to decreased blood volume and decreased blood pressure. It causes retention of body fluids and vasoconstriction, both of which act to raise blood pressure.

### Vascular

The endothelial cells that line blood vessels synthesize and secrete several substances that play important roles in regulating cardiovascular functions, including blood pressure. These substances normally maintain a balance between vasoconstriction and vasodilation. When the endothelium is damaged [e.g., by trauma, hypertension, hypercholesterolemia, or atherosclerosis], the resulting imbalance promotes production of vasoconstricting substances and also causes blood vessels to lose their ability to relax in response to dilator substances. In addition, changes in structure of endothelial and vascular smooth muscle cells [vascular remodeling] further impair vascular functions.

Vasoconstrictors increase vascular tone [i.e., constrict or narrow blood vessels so that higher blood pressure is required to pump blood to body tissues]. Vasoconstricting substances produced by the endothelium include angiotensin II, endothelin 1, platelet-derived growth factor [PDGF], and thromboxane $A_2$. Endothelin 1 is the strongest endogenous vasoconstrictor known. Angiotensin II and thromboxane $A_2$ can also be produced by other types of cells, but endothelial cells can produce both. Thromboxane $A_2$, a product of arachidonic acid metabolism, also promotes platelet aggregation and thrombosis.

Vasodilators decrease vascular tone and blood pressure. Major vasodilating substances produced by the endothelium include NO and prostacyclin [prostaglandin I2].

Nitric oxide [NO] is a gas that can diffuse through cell membranes, trigger biochemical reactions, and then dissipate rapidly. It is formed by the action of the enzyme NO synthase on the amino acid L-arginine and continually released by normal endothelium. Its production is tightly regulated and depends on the amount of ionized calcium in the fluid portion of endothelial cells. Several substances [e.g., acetylcholine, bradykinin, catecholamines, substance P, and products of aggregating platelets such as adenosine diphosphate and serotonin] act on receptors in endothelial cell membranes to increase the cytosolic concentration of ionized calcium, activate NO synthase, and increase NO production. In addition, increased blood flow or blood pressure increases shear stress at the endothelial surface and stimulates production of NO.

Once produced, endothelium-derived NO produces vasodilation primarily by activating guanylyl cyclase in vascular smooth muscle cells and increasing intracellular cyclic 3′,5′-guanosine monophosphate as a second messenger. NO also inhibits platelet aggregation and production of platelet-derived vasoconstricting substances. Because NO is released into the vessel wall [to relax smooth muscle] and into the vessel lumen [to inactivate platelets], it is thought to have protective effects against vasoconstriction and thrombosis.

NO is also produced in leukocytes, fibroblasts, and vascular smooth muscle cells and may have pathologic effects when large amounts are produced. In these tissues, NO seems to have other functions, such as modifying nerve activity in the nervous system.

Prostacyclin is synthesized and released from endothelium in response to stimulation by several factors [e.g., bradykinin, interleukin-1, serotonin, thrombin, PDGF]. It produces vasodilation by activating adenylyl cyclase and increasing levels of cyclic adenosine monophosphate in smooth muscle cells. In addition, like NO, prostacyclin also inhibits platelet aggregation and production of platelet-derived vasoconstricting substances. The vasodilating effects of prostacyclin may occur independently or in conjunction with NO.

Overall, excessive vasoconstrictors or deficient vasodilators may contribute to the development of atherosclerosis, hypertension, and other diseases. Injury to the endothelial lining of blood vessels [e.g., by the sheer force of blood flow with hypertension or by rupture of atherosclerotic plaque] decreases vasodilators and leads to vasoconstriction, vasospasm, thrombus formation, and thickening of the blood vessel wall. All of these factors require the blood to flow through a narrowed lumen and increase blood pressure.

| BOX 26.1 | *Mechanisms That Regulate Blood Pressure* (Continued) |
|---|---|

**Vascular Remodeling**

Vascular remodeling is similar to the left ventricular remodeling that occurs in heart failure (see Chap. 30). It results from endothelial dysfunction and produces a thickening of the blood vessel wall and a narrowing of the blood vessel lumen. Thickening of the wall makes blood vessels less flexible and less able to respond to vasodilating substances. There are also changes in endothelial cell structure (i.e., the connections between endothelial cells become looser) that lead to increased permeability. The mechanisms of these vascular changes, which promote and aggravate hypertension, are described below.

As discussed in previous chapters, normal endothelium helps maintain a balance between vasoconstriction and vasodilation, procoagulation and anticoagulation, proinflammation and anti-inflammation, and progrowth and antigrowth. In the inflammatory process, normal endothelium acts as a physical barrier against the movement of leukocytes into the subendothelial space. Endothelial products such as NO may also inhibit leukocyte activity. However, inflammatory cytokines such as tumor necrosis factor alpha and interleukin-1

activate endothelial cells to produce adhesion molecules (which allow leukocytes to adhere to the endothelium), interleukin-8 (which attracts leukocytes to the endothelium and allows them to accumulate in subendothelial cells), and foam cells (lipid-filled monocyte/macrophages that form fatty streaks, the beginning lesions of atherosclerotic plaque). Although activation of endothelial cells may be a helpful component of the normal immune response, the resulting inflammation may contribute to disease development.

In terms of cell growth, normal endothelium limits the growth of vascular smooth muscle that underlies the endothelium and forms the vessel wall. Growth-inhibiting products of the endothelium include NO, which also inhibits platelet activation and production of growth-promoting substances. When the endothelium is damaged, endothelial cells become activated and also produce growth-promoting products. Other endothelial products (e.g., angiotensin II and endothelin 1) may also stimulate growth of vascular smooth muscle cells. Thus, damage or loss of endothelial cells stimulates growth of smooth muscle cells in the intimal layer of the blood vessel wall.

## Grades and Types of Hypertension

Normal or optimal blood pressure is the level at which minimal vascular damage occurs where blood flow remains sufficient for tissue oxygenation and waste removal. Hypertension is persistently high blood pressure that exceeds this level and results from abnormalities in regulatory mechanisms. It is usually defined as a systolic pressure above 130 mm Hg or a diastolic pressure above 80 mm Hg on multiple blood pressure measurements. The *Eighth Report of the Joint National Committee on Prevention, Detection, Evaluation, and Treatment of High Blood Pressure* (JNC 8), released in 2014, reviewed and updated the current evidence on the detection, evaluation, and treatment of high blood pressure (James et al., 2014). This commentary focused on key thresholds for initiation of pharmacologic treatment of hypertension, including blood pressure targets during treatment and recommendations for antihypertensive therapies. Based on this report and corresponding evidence, the American College of Cardiology (ACC) and American Heart Association (AHA) issued updated guidelines for the categories of hypertension in adults (in mm Hg) (Box 26.2) (Whelton et al., 2018).

| BOX 26.2 | *Classification of Hypertension (All Values in mm Hg)* |
|---|---|

- Normal = systolic less than 120 *and* diastolic less than 80
- Elevated = systolic 120–129 *and* diastolic less than 80
- Stage 1 hypertension = systolic 130–139 *or* diastolic 80–89
- Stage 2 hypertension = systolic greater than 140 *or* diastolic 90 or more

Source: James, P., Oparil, S., Carter, B., et al. (2014). 2014 evidence-based guideline for the management of high blood pressure in adults report from the panel members appointed to the Eighth Joint National Committee (JNC 8). *Journal of the American Medical Association, 311*(5), 507–520. doi:10.1001/jama.2013.284427

One of the significant changes to the classification of hypertension is the elimination of the prehypertension category and the addition of the elevated category. These recommendations have shifted focus from defining threshold levels of hypertension to defining treatment methods for patients with hypertension and establishing outcome measures for treatment effectiveness.

A systolic pressure of 140 mm Hg or greater, with a diastolic pressure of less than 80 mm Hg, is called isolated systolic hypertension and is more common in the elderly. Systolic–diastolic hypertension, which may also occur in older adults, involves elevations of both systolic and diastolic pressures. Both types increase cardiovascular morbidity and mortality, especially heart failure and stroke, and warrant treatment.

A hypertensive emergency or crisis is a systolic pressure of 180 mm Hg or more and/or a diastolic pressure of 120 mm Hg or more and possible target organ damage. (A hypertensive urgency is an episode of marked elevation in blood pressure without target organ damage. The goal of management is to lower blood pressure within 24 hours.)

## Etiology

Although it has frequently been indicated that the causes of primary hypertension, or **essential hypertension**, are not known, this is only partially true; genetic variations and inherited, behavioral, and environmental factors may increase blood pressure. These include obesity, high alcohol intake, insulin resistance, high salt intake in salt-sensitive people, aging, sedentary lifestyle, and stress. Furthermore, many of these factors are additive, such as obesity and alcohol intake. Primary hypertension makes up 90% to 95% of known cases. Appropriate therapy usually controls primary hypertension.

**Secondary hypertension** may result from renal, endocrine, or central nervous system (CNS) disorders and from drugs that stimulate the SNS or cause retention of sodium and water, producing adverse effects. Secondary hypertension can sometimes be cured by managing the underlying condition or cause. Hypertensive emergencies often result from such conditions as cerebral hemorrhage, dissecting aortic aneurysm, renal disease, pheochromocytoma, or eclampsia.

## Pathophysiology

Hypertension profoundly alters cardiovascular function by increasing the workload of the heart and causing thickening and sclerosis of arterial walls. The increased cardiac workload leads to myocardial hypertrophy as a compensatory mechanism, with eventual heart failure. As a result of endothelial dysfunction and arterial changes (vascular remodeling), the arterial lumen narrows, blood supply to tissues decreases, and the risk of thrombosis increases. In addition, necrotic areas may develop in arteries, and these may rupture with sustained high blood pressure. The areas of most serious damage are the heart, brain, kidneys, and eyes. These are often called target organs.

### Response to Hypotension

When hypotension (and decreased tissue perfusion) occurs, the SNS is stimulated, the hormones epinephrine and norepinephrine are secreted by the adrenal medulla, angiotensin II and aldosterone are formed, and the kidneys retain fluid. These compensatory mechanisms raise the blood pressure. Specific effects include the following:

- Constriction of arterioles, which increases peripheral vascular resistance
- Constriction of veins and increased venous tone
- Stimulation of cardiac beta-adrenergic receptors, which increases heart rate and force of myocardial contraction
- Activation of the renin–angiotensin–aldosterone mechanism

Chapter 29 contains an additional discussion of the effects and management of hypotension.

### Response to Hypertension

When arterial blood pressure is elevated, the following sequence of events occurs:

- Kidneys excrete more fluid (increase urine output).
- Fluid loss reduces both extracellular fluid volume and blood volume.
- Decreased blood volume reduces venous blood flow to the heart and therefore decreases cardiac output.
- Decreased cardiac output reduces arterial blood pressure.
- The vascular endothelium produces vasodilating substances (e.g., NO, prostacyclin), which reduce blood pressure.

## Clinical Manifestations

Initially, and perhaps for years, primary hypertension may produce no symptoms. If symptoms occur, they are usually vague and nonspecific. Hypertension may go undetected, or it may be incidentally discovered when blood pressure measurements are taken as part of a routine physical examination, screening test, or assessment of other disorders.

Symptoms associated with hypertension, if they occur, include severe headache, nausea, vomiting, visual disturbances, neurologic disturbances, disorientation, and decreased level of consciousness (drowsiness, stupor, coma). Hypertensive emergencies require immediate blood pressure reduction with parenteral antihypertensive drugs to limit damage to target organs. Eventually, symptoms reflect target organ damage associated with sustained elevations in blood pressure. Hypertension is often discovered after a person experiences angina pectoris, MI, heart failure, stroke, or renal disease.

## Therapy
### Goals of Treatment

After the diagnosis of hypertension is established, it is essential that a therapeutic regimen be designed and implemented. Based on guidelines published in 2018 (Whelton et al., 2018), treatment goals vary depending on the population being treated. In patients aged 60 years or older, without diabetes or chronic kidney disease, the treatment goal is a blood pressure of less than 150/90 mm Hg. In patients ages 30 to 59 years who are in general good health and patients 60 years or older with diabetes or chronic kidney disease, the goal of treatment is a blood pressure of less than 140/90 mm Hg. For patients 18 to 30 years of age, the panel recommends a treatment goal of blood pressure less than 140/90 mm Hg, but the evidence supporting the guidelines for this population is more limited.

Lowering blood pressure to any extent is considered beneficial in decreasing the incidence of coronary artery disease (CAD) and stroke. In most instances, it is better to lower blood pressure gradually and to avoid wide fluctuations in blood pressure. However, for patients who have difficulty achieving and maintaining blood pressure in the recommended ranges, referral to a hypertensive specialist is indicated.

### Nonpharmacologic Treatment

In their findings, the JNC 8 panel guidelines released recommendations for the management of hypertension (James et al., 2014). Initial interventions include lifestyle modifications (i.e., reduction of weight and sodium intake, regular physical activity, moderate alcohol intake, and no smoking) to achieve and maintain blood pressure below 120/80 mm Hg. Actual blood pressure trends and individual patient risk profiles determine if lifestyle changes with or without drug therapy are the initial treatment option.

#### Dietary Management

Recent management guidelines distinguish that key behavioral determinants of blood pressure are related to dietary consumption of calories and salt; there is a direct relationship between hypertension and body mass index (Whelton et al., 2018). According to this report, a diet low in sodium and fat along with an increased consumption of fruits, vegetables, and grains may decrease the systolic blood pressure by approximately 11 mm Hg. The Dietary Approaches to Stop Hypertension (DASH) study has demonstrated that people with elevated blood pressure or stage 1 hypertension can reduce their blood pressures by adhering to a diet abundant in fresh fruits and vegetables and low-fat dairy products even without restricting calorie or sodium intake. The effects of the DASH diet show blood pressure–lowering outcomes that parallel the degree of benefit from drug monotherapy and may include dietary sodium restriction. Effects are evident in people of all ethnicities, particularly

African Americans, and in those with significantly higher blood pressures.

Severe restrictions of sodium intake usually are not acceptable to people; however, moderate restrictions (4–6 g of salt a day) are beneficial and more easily implemented. Avoiding heavily salted foods (e.g., cured meats, sandwich meats, pretzels, potato chips) and not adding salt to food at the table can achieve this. Research and clinical observations indicate the following:

- Sodium restriction alone reduces blood pressure and is extremely effective when combined with lifestyle modifications.
- Sodium restriction potentiates the antihypertensive actions of diuretics and other antihypertensive drugs. Conversely, excessive sodium intake decreases the antihypertensive actions of all antihypertensive drugs. Patients with unrestricted salt intake who are taking thiazides may lose excessive potassium and become hypokalemic.
- Sodium restriction may decrease dosage requirements of antihypertensive drugs, thereby decreasing the incidence and severity of adverse effects.

### Lifestyle Management

Considerable evidence demonstrates that regular physical activity effectively reduces blood pressure. Research has demonstrated that both aerobic exercise and resistance training have a significant blood pressure lowering effect (Whelton et al., 2018). However, the direct benefits of exercise on blood pressure control are often difficult to isolate from those of the changes that often accompany exercise, such as improved diet, weight loss, decreased alcohol consumption, and decreased cigarette smoking. The 2017 AHA/ACC Lifestyle Management Guidelines note the importance of regular physical activity as part of a plan of care for adult men and women of all blood pressure levels, including those with hypertension. On average, aerobic physical activity decreases systolic blood pressure by 5 to 8 mm Hg for hypertensive patients. Data suggest that effective results can be expected with aerobic physical activity on interventions of, on average, at least 12 weeks' duration, three to four times per week, lasting on average 40 minutes per session. Besides aerobic activity, the JNC 8 recommendations also included achieving a weight loss goal of at least 10 lb if overweight, limiting alcohol consumption to two drinks or less per day for men and one drink or less per day for women, and ceasing smoking. In summary, it is estimated that each lifestyle change results in a 4 to 5 mm Hg decrease in systolic blood pressure and a 2- to 4–mm Hg decrease in diastolic blood pressure (Whelton et al., 2018).

### *Drug Management*

If lifestyle modifications alone do not produce the target blood pressure (or a systolic blood pressure ≥140 mm Hg or a diastolic blood pressure ≥90 mm Hg), it is important to initiate antihypertensive drug therapy and continue lifestyle modifications. Drugs used in the management of primary hypertension belong to several different groups, including ACE inhibitors; angiotensin II receptor blockers (ARBs), also called angiotensin II receptor antagonists; antiadrenergics; calcium channel blockers (CCBs); diuretics; and direct vasodilators. In general, these drugs act to decrease blood pressure by decreasing cardiac output or peripheral vascular resistance. Evidence indicates that management strategies need to account for race in drug selection for initial therapy.

For instance, recommendations for treatment of hypertension in individuals of African American descent, including those with diabetes, includes initial therapy with a CCB and/or thiazide-type diuretic. In non–African American populations, including those with diabetes, there is evidence to support initial drug therapy with an ACE inhibitor, ARB, CCB, and/or a thiazide-type diuretic. This chapter focuses on ACE inhibitors, ARBs, CCBs, and select adjuvant drugs (direct renin inhibitors, alpha$_1$-adrenergic blockers, alpha$_2$ agonists, beta-adrenergic blockers, alpha-/beta-adrenergic blockers, and diuretics); their sites of drug action are identified in Figure 26.1. Various other chapters in this book describe drugs discussed here—for example, chapters related to dysrhythmias (see Chap. 27), angina (see Chap. 28), heart failure (see Chap. 30), and fluid volume excess (see Chap. 34).

Table 26.1 outlines the antihypertensive drugs, and Table 26.2 lists antihypertensive–diuretic combination products. Product labeling and current recommendations are the basis for adult dosages. Product labeling and recent clinical research, along with the seminal recommendations from the National High Blood Pressure Education Program Working Group on High Blood Pressure in Children and Adolescents (2004) and Clinical Practice Guideline for Screening and Management of High Blood Pressure in Children and Adolescents (Flynn et al., 2017), are the basis for pediatric dosages.

Current guidelines (Whelton et al., 2018) suggest that thiazide diuretics (e.g., chlorthalidone, hydrochlorothiazide) be used as first-line therapy, either alone (monotherapy) or with an ACE inhibitor, ARB, or CCB. Monotherapy is reasonable if the patient has stage 1 hypertension and a BP goal less than 130/80 mm Hg. If the initial drug (and dose) does not produce the desired blood pressure within 1 month of initiating treatment, options for further management include increasing the dose, substituting another drug, or adding a second drug from a different group (James et al., 2014). If the patient has a systolic pressure greater than 140 mm Hg or a diastolic blood pressure greater than 90 mm Hg, initial drug therapy with a combination of two antihypertensives is recommended (Whelton et al., 2018). To minimize the impact of medication side effects, two or three medications may be combined at lower doses, rather than increasing doses of monotherapy, to achieve blood pressure treatment goals. If the response is still inadequate, addition of a third drug, including a diuretic if not previously prescribed, is recommended.

When current management is ineffective, it is necessary to reassess the patient's adherence to lifestyle modifications and drug therapy. In addition, it is also important to review other factors that may decrease the therapeutic response, such as the use of over-the-counter appetite suppressants, dietary or herbal supplements, or nasal decongestants, which raise blood pressure. Regardless of the medication selected, the primary determining factor in selecting the appropriate antihypertensive medication(s) and dose(s) is patient response to treatment, with attained blood pressure control being the ultimate outcome measure (Whelton et al., 2018).

Holistic management of hypertension should include consideration of age, ethnicity, and concomitant cardiovascular disorders when choosing an antihypertensive drug. Starting with a single drug, in the lowest available dose; changing to a drug from a different group, rather than increasing dosage of the first drug or adding a second drug, if the initial drug is ineffective or not well tolerated; and using long-acting drugs (i.e., a single

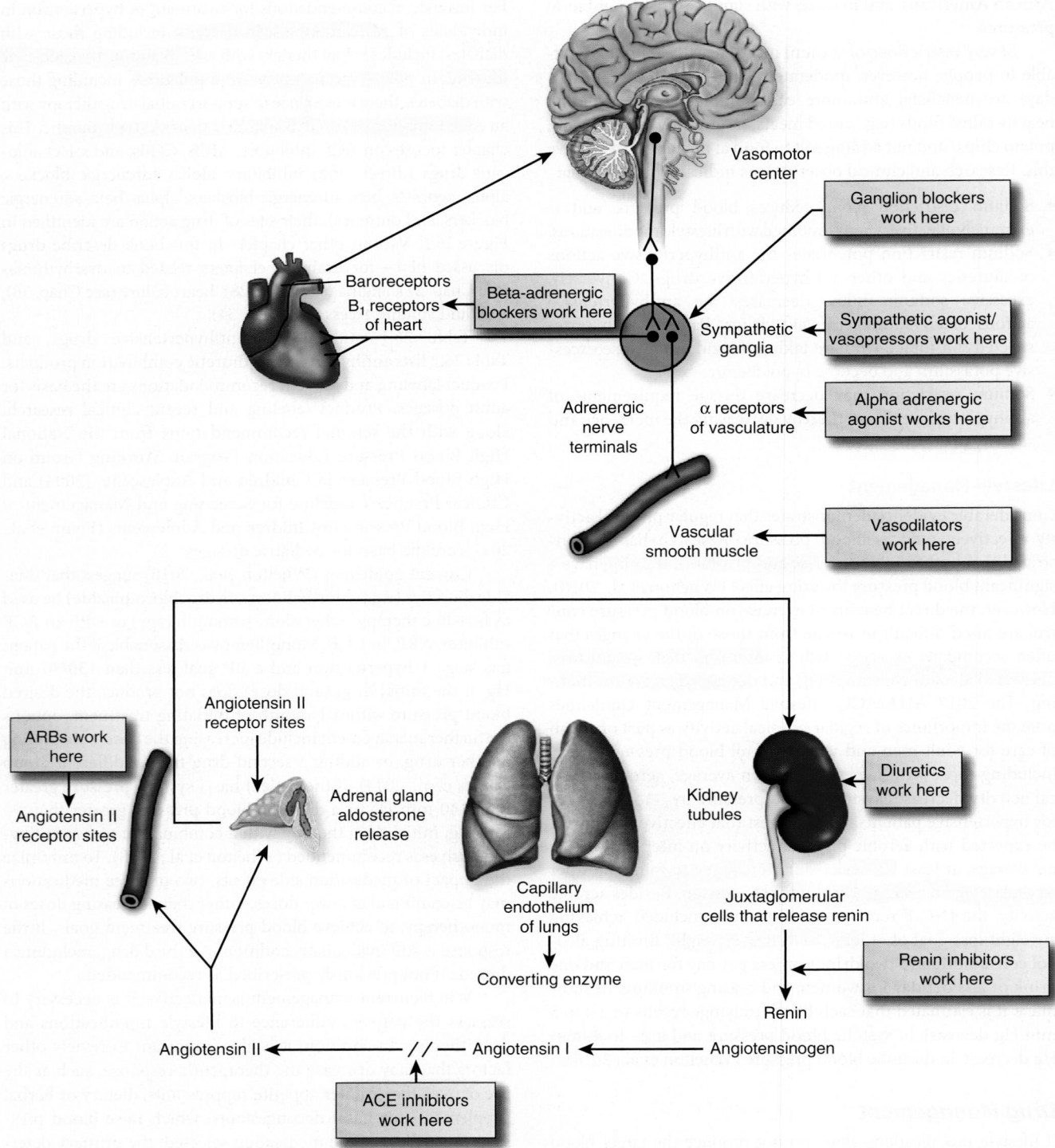

**Figure 26.1.** Sites of action of antihypertensive drugs. [Reprinted with permission from Karch, A. M. [2020]. *Focus on nursing pharmacology* [8th ed., Fig. 43.3, p. 734]. Philadelphia, PA: Wolters Kluwer.]

## TABLE 26.1

## Drugs Administered for the Treatment of Hypertension

| Drug Class | Prototype | Other Drugs in the Class |
|---|---|---|
| Angiotensin-converting enzyme (ACE) inhibitors | Captopril | Benazepril (Lotensin)<br>Enalapril (Vasotec)<br>Fosinopril (Monopril)<br>Lisinopril (Prinivil, Zestril)<br>Moexipril (Univasc)<br>Quinapril (Accupril)<br>Perindopril (Coversyl)<br>Ramipril (Altace)<br>Trandolapril (Mavik) |
| Angiotensin II receptor blockers (ARBs) | Losartan (Cozaar) | Azilsartan (Edarbi)<br>Candesartan (Atacand)<br>Eprosartan (Teveten)<br>Irbesartan (Avapro)<br>Olmesartan (Benicar)<br>Telmisartan (Micardis)<br>Valsartan (Diovan) |
| Calcium channel blockers | Amlodipine (Norvasc) | Diltiazem (sustained release) (Cardizem CD, Cartia XT)<br>Felodipine<br>Isradipine<br>Nicardipine<br>Nifedipine (Adalat CC, Procardia, Procardia XL)<br>Nisoldipine (Sular)<br>Verapamil (Calan, Calan SR, Tarka, Verelan) |
| **Adjuvant Medications** | | |
| *Direct renin inhibitors* | Aliskiren (Tekturna) | |
| **Antiadrenergics** | | |
| *Alpha₁-adrenergic blockers* | | Doxazosin (Cardura, Cardura XL)<br>Prazosin (Minipress)<br>Terazosin |
| *Alpha₂ agonists* | | Clonidine (Catapres)<br>Guanfacine<br>Methyldopa |
| *Beta-adrenergic blockers* | | Acebutolol<br>Atenolol (Tenormin)<br>Bisoprolol<br>Metoprolol (Lopressor)<br>Nadolol (Corgard)<br>Pindolol (Visken)<br>Propranolol (Inderal LA)<br>Timolol (Blocadren) |
| *Alpha-/beta-adrenergic blockers* | | Carvedilol (Coreg, Coreg CR)<br>Labetalol (Trandate, Normodyne) |
| **Diuretics** | | |
| *Thiazide* | Hydrochlorothiazide (Microzide) | Chlorothiazide (Diuril)<br>Chlorthalidone<br>Indapamide<br>Metolazone (Zaroxolyn) |
| *Loop* | Furosemide (Lasix) | Bumetanide (Bumex)<br>Torsemide (Demadex) |
| *Potassium sparing* | Spironolactone (Aldactone) | Amiloride (Midamor)<br>Triamterene (Dyrenium) |
| **Other vasodilators** | | Fenoldopam (Corlopam)<br>Hydralazine (Hydra-Zide, BiDil)<br>Minoxidil<br>Sodium nitroprusside (Nitropress) |

**TABLE 26.2**

## DRUGS AT A GLANCE: Oral Antihypertensive Combination Products*

| Trade Name | Components | | | | | | |
|---|---|---|---|---|---|---|---|
| | Angiotensin II Receptor Blocker | Angiotensin-Converting Enzyme Inhibitor | Beta-Adrenergic Blocker | Calcium Channel Blocker | Diuretic | Other | Dosage Ranges |
| Accuretic (🍁 Accuretic) | | Quinapril 10–20 mg | | | HCTZ 12.5–25 mg | | 1–2 tablets once daily |
| Aldactazide (🍁 Aldactazide 25 or 50, Teva-Spironolactone/HCTZ) | | | | | HCTZ 25–50 mg; spironolactone 25–50 mg | | 1–2 tablets once daily |
| Atacand HCT (🍁 APO-Candesartan HCTZ, Atacand, DOM-Candesartan) | Candesartan 16 or 32 mg | | | | HCTZ 12.5 or 25 mg | | 1 tablet daily |
| Avalide (🍁 Irbesartan-HCT, Avalide) | Irbesartan 150 mg | | | | HCTZ 12.5 mg | | 1 tablet daily |
| Azor | Olmesartan 20 or 40 mg | | | Amlodipine 5 or 10 mg | | | 1 tablet daily |
| Benicar HCT (🍁 Olmetec, ACT Olmesartan, RIVA-Olmesartan) | Olmesartan 20 or 40 mg | | | | HCTZ 12.5 or 25 mg | | 1–2 tablets daily |
| Corzide | | | Nadolol 40 or 80 mg | | Bendroflumethiazide 5 mg | | 1 tablet daily |
| Diovan HCT (🍁 Diovan HCT, Valsartan-HCT) | Valsartan 80, 160, or 320 mg | | | | HCTZ 12.5–25 mg | | 1 tablet daily |
| Dyazide | | | | | HCTZ 25 mg; triamterene 37.5 mg | | 1 tablet daily |
| Exforge | Valsartan 160 or 320 mg | | | Amlodipine 5 or 10 mg | | | 1–2 tablets once daily |
| Hyzaar (🍁 ACT Losartan/HCT, Hyzaar, ACT Losartan/HCT) | Losartan 100 mg | | | | HCTZ 12.5 mg | | 1 tablet daily |
| Lopressor HCT | | | Metoprolol 25, 50, or 100 mg | | HCTZ 12.5 or 25 mg | | 1–2 tablets daily |
| Lotrel | | Benazepril 10, 20, or mg | | Amlodipine 2.5 or 5 mg | | | 1 capsule daily |

**TABLE 26.2**

## DRUGS AT A GLANCE: Oral Antihypertensive Combination Products* (Continued)

| Trade Name | Angiotensin II Receptor Blocker | Angiotensin-Converting Enzyme Inhibitor | Beta-Adrenergic Blocker | Calcium Channel Blocker | Diuretic | Other | Dosage Ranges |
|---|---|---|---|---|---|---|---|
| Maxzide | | | | | HCTX 25–50 mg; triamterene 37.5–75 mg | | |
| Micardis HCT (Micardis Plus) | Telmisartan 40 or 80 mg | | | | HCTZ 12.5 or 25 mg | | 1–2 tablets daily |
| Tarka (Tarka) | | Trandolapril 1, 2, or 4 mg | | Verapamil 180 or 240 mg | | | 1 tablet daily |
| Tenoretic (Tenoretic) | | | Atenolol 50 or 100 mg | Chlorthalidone 25 mg | | | 1 tablet daily |
| Twynsta (Twynsta) | Telmisartan 40 or 80 mg | | | Amlodipine 5 or 10 mg | | | |
| Vaseretic (TEVA-Enalapril/HCTZ)  | | Enalapril 5 or 10 mg | | | HCTZ 12.5 or 25 mg | | 1–2 tablets daily |
| Zestoretic (APO-Lisinopril/HCTZ, Zestoretic) | | Lisinopril 10 or 20 mg | | | HCTZ 12.5 or 25 mg | | 1 tablet daily |
| Ziac (Ziac) | | Bisoprolol 2.5, 5, or 10 mg | | | HCTZ 6.25 mg | | 1 tablet daily |

*Note that one trade name product may be available in multiple formulations, with variable amounts of antihypertensive, diuretic, or both components. HCTZ, hydrochlorothiazide.

dose effective for 24 hours) are prudent considerations. Many patients require two or more drugs to achieve adequate blood pressure control. When this is the case, fixed-dose combinations or long-acting agents may be preferred, because they decrease the number of individual drugs and doses that are required and may increase compliance.

Variation exists in the response to drug therapy for hypertension in ethnic populations. Experts credit nearly 70% of the familial considerations related to blood pressure to shared genes rather than to shared environment. For most antihypertensive drugs, research studies comparing effects have indicated differences among different genetic or ethnic groups. For example, several studies indicate that beta-adrenergic blockers have greater effects in people of Asian heritage compared with those of Caucasian background. For hypertension, Asians in general need much smaller doses because they metabolize and excrete beta-adrenergic blockers slowly. Other populations known to metabolize beta-adrenergic blockers slowly include Arab and Egyptian Americans and possibly German Americans. In African Americans, thiazide diuretics and CCBs are effective and recommended as initial drug therapy. CCBs, alpha₁ receptor blockers, and the alpha-/beta-adrenergic blocker labetalol are reportedly equally effective in African Americans and Caucasians. ACE inhibitors, some ARBs (e.g., losartan and telmisartan), and beta-adrenergic blockers are less effective as monotherapy in African Americans. When beta-adrenergic blockers are used, they are usually one component of a multidrug regimen, and higher doses may be necessary. Overall, African Americans are more likely to have severe hypertension and require multiple drugs as a result of having low circulating renin, increased salt sensitivity, and a higher incidence of obesity.

### ! QSEN Alert: Evidence-Based Practice

Hypertension is a disease with wide-ranging implications for patient outcomes including short-term and long-term complications. The current guidelines represent significant changes in the assessment and diagnosis of hypertension as well as the latest in evidence-based practice standards for hypertension management (Whelton et al., 2018). These updated guidelines synthesize ongoing research and large-scale randomized controlled trials (RCTs), providing the best information available to guide health care teams in offering individualized treatment guidelines based on several factors, including age, race, and comorbidities. The updated guidelines reinforce management of hypertension as the ultimate goal, but the use of evidence-based data provides specific adjustments based on patient factors aimed at increasing the opportunities for patients to realize those treatment goals. This allows clinicians to treat the patient in a targeted manner versus merely treating the condition.

# ANGIOTENSIN-CONVERTING ENZYME INHIBITORS

Experts recommend  **captopril**, the prototype ACE inhibitor, and other drugs in this class as first-line agents for treating hypertension, particularly in patients with heart failure or asymptomatic left ventricular dysfunction. ACE inhibitors reduce proteinuria and slow progression of renal impairment in people with this disease. (However, they may cause or aggravate proteinuria and renal damage in people who do not have diabetes.) ACE inhibitors may be used alone or in combination with other antihypertensive agents, such as thiazide diuretics, CCBs, and beta-blockers, based on the patient's blood pressure.

## Pharmacokinetics

Captopril is well absorbed with oral administration (with absorption reduced by food), produces effects within 1 to 1½ hours, and has a prolonged serum half-life with impaired renal function. The drug is metabolized and excreted in the urine (half as unchanged drug) and is excreted in breast milk.

> ### ! QSEN Alert: Safety
>
> The metabolism of captopril is highly dependent on a patient's genetics and ethnicity. Current guidelines recommend that all nonblack individuals, including those with diabetes and chronic kidney disease, receive an ACE inhibitor as part of their drug therapy. ACE inhibitors are not recommended for treatment of hypertension in black patients unless they have chronic kidney disease.

## Action

ACE inhibitors such as captopril block the enzyme that normally converts angiotensin I to the potent vasoconstrictor angiotensin II. (ACE [also called kininase] is mainly located in the endothelial lining of blood vessels, which is the site of production of most angiotensin II. This same enzyme also metabolizes bradykinin, an endogenous substance with strong vasodilating properties.) By blocking production of angiotensin II, ACE inhibitors decrease vasoconstriction (thus having a vasodilating effect) and decrease aldosterone production (thus reducing retention of sodium and water). In addition to inhibiting formation of angiotensin II, these drugs also inhibit the breakdown of bradykinin, prolonging its vasodilating effects.

## Use

Health care providers use captopril to prevent or reverse the remodeling of heart muscle and blood vessel walls that impairs cardiovascular function and exacerbates cardiovascular disease processes. Widely used to treat heart failure and hypertension, the drug may also decrease morbidity and mortality in other cardiovascular disorders. Captopril may be effective as monotherapy in Caucasian patients with hypertension or in combination with a diuretic in African American hypertensive patients, but the 2017 Guideline for the Prevention, Detection, Evaluation, and Management of High Blood Pressure in Adults recommends thiazide diuretics or CCBs as preferred for monotherapy in the

absence of comorbidities (Whelton et al., 2018). Clinicians also recommend captopril and other ACE inhibitors for adults with hypertension and diabetes mellitus and kidney damage because they slow the progression of albuminuria. In addition, captopril improves post-MI survival when added to the standard therapy of aspirin, a beta-adrenergic blocker, and a thrombolytic.

Table 26.3 presents route and dosage information for captopril and other ACE inhibitors.

### Use in Children

Limited information is available on the safety and efficacy of captopril in children. Manufacturer information states that captopril should be used in children only when other measures to control blood pressure have not been successful.

### Use in Patients With Renal Impairment

Captopril and other ACE inhibitors are usually effective in patients with renal impairment, but responses may vary. Careful monitoring is required, especially during the first few weeks of therapy, to prevent irreversible renal failure. Manufacturer recommendations include a reduction in initial dosage and then slow titration over 1- to 2-week intervals to determine the minimum effective dose necessary to achieve desired blood pressure outcome. For some patients, it may not be possible to normalize blood pressure and maintain adequate renal perfusion.

### Use in Patients With Critical Illness

Health care providers may use captopril in patients who are critically ill. However, oral dosing may restrict use to patients who can tolerate oral medications. Urgent or emergent needs to reduce significant hypertension may require more effective management with drugs that can be administered intravenously or have a more rapid onset of action.

## Adverse Effects

Captopril is well tolerated and has a low incidence of serious adverse effects (e.g., neutropenia, agranulocytosis, proteinuria, glomerulonephritis, **angioedema** [sudden deep swelling or welts under skin, particularly around the eyes and lips]). However, a persistent cough develops in a significant number of patients, and this problem may lead to discontinuation of the drug. Also, acute hypotension may occur when captopril is started, especially in patients with fluid volume deficit. Starting with a low dose taken at bedtime or by stopping diuretics and reducing dosage of other antihypertensive drugs temporarily may prevent this reaction. Hyperkalemia may develop in patients with diabetes mellitus or renal impairment or who are taking nonsteroidal anti-inflammatory drugs (NSAIDs), potassium supplements, or potassium-sparing diuretics; these patients should be monitored for this condition.

## Contraindications

Contraindications to captopril and other ACE inhibitors include pregnancy, and it is important to discontinue them when pregnancy is detected. The U.S. Food and Drug Administration (FDA) has issued a **BLACK BOX WARNING ◆** for use of drugs that directly affect the renin–angiotensin system, such as ACE inhibitors, during pregnancy because their use can cause injury and even

| | | **TABLE 26.3** |
|---|---|---|
| | | **DRUGS AT A GLANCE: Angiotensin-Converting Enzyme Inhibitors** |

| Drug | Pregnancy Category | Routes and Dosage Ranges | |
|---|---|---|---|
| | | **Adults** | **Children 1–17 y of Age (Unless Otherwise Stated)** |
| **Captopril** (APO-Capto, PMS-Captopril, TEVA-Captopril) | D | 25 mg PO, 2–3 times daily initially, gradually increased to 50, 100, or 150 mg 2–3 times daily, if necessary; maximum dose 450 mg/d | 1.5 mg/kg/d PO in divided doses every 8 h; maximum dose 6 mg/kg/d Neonates, 0.03–0.15 mg/kg/d PO every 8–24 h; maximum dose 2 mg/kg/d |
| Benazepril | D | 10 mg PO once daily initially, increased to 40 mg daily if necessary, in 1 or 2 doses | 0.2 mg/kg PO once daily |
| Enalapril (Vasotec; ACT-Enalapril, APO-Enalapril) | D | 5 mg PO once daily, increased to 10–40 mg daily, in 1 or 2 doses, if necessary | 0.08 mg/kg PO; maximum dose 5 mg/d |
| Fosinopril (APO-Fosinopril, CO Fosinopril) | D | 10 mg PO once daily initially, increased to 40 mg daily if necessary in 1 or 2 doses | >50 kg, 5–10 mg PO once daily |
| Lisinopril (Zestril; APO-Lisinopril, DOM-Lisinopril) | D | 10 mg PO once daily, increased to 40 mg if necessary | ≥6 y, 0.07 mg/kg PO once daily; maximum dose 5 mg/d |
| Moexipril | D | Initial dose, 7.5 mg PO (3.75 mg for those who have renal impairment or are taking a diuretic). Maintenance dose, 7.5–30 mg daily, in 1 or 2 doses, adjusted according to blood pressure control | Safety and effectiveness in children have not been established |
| Quinapril (Accupril; Accupril, APO-Quinapril) | D | 10 mg PO once daily initially, increased to 20, 40, or 80 mg daily if necessary, in 1 or 2 doses; wait at least 2 wk between dose increments | 5–10 mg PO once daily; maximum dose 80 mg once daily |
| Perindopril (Coversyl, Auri-Perindopril) | D | 4 mg PO once daily initially; titrate to up to 16 mg/d based on patient response | Safety and effectiveness in children have not been established |
| Ramipril (ACT Ramipril, Altace) | D | 2.5 mg PO once daily, increased to 20 mg daily if necessary, in 1 or 2 doses | Safety and effectiveness in children have not been established |
| Trandolapril (Mavik, Odrik, SANDOZ Trandolapril) | D | Initial dose, 1 mg PO once daily (0.5 mg for those who have hepatic or renal impairment or are taking a diuretic; 2 mg for African Americans). Maintenance dose, PO 2–4 mg daily, in a single dose, adjusted according to blood pressure control | Safety and effectiveness in children have not been established |

death to a developing fetus. Additional contraindications to captopril include known hypersensitivity to the drug or occurrence of angioedema with previous treatment with an ACE inhibitor.

## Nursing Implications

### Preventing Interactions

Many medications interact with captopril, increasing or decreasing its effects (Box 26.3). Additionally, captopril may increase serum concentrations of digoxin and lithium and increase the risk of elevated serum levels and toxicity.

**! QSEN Alert: Safety**

Reportedly, taking captopril and other ACE inhibitors at the same time as potassium-containing salt substitutes (No Salt, Morton Salt Substitute, and others) or large amounts of high-potassium foods (bananas, oranges, and other fruit) increases the risk of hyperkalemia.

### Administering the Medication

People should take captopril 1 hour before or 2 hours after meals to enhance absorption. If they have difficulty swallowing, they

...PRIL

**BOX 26.3** *Drug Interactions: Captopril*

**Drugs That Increase the Effects of Captopril**

- Aliskiren
  *Increases the risk of hypotension, hyperkalemia, and renal impairment*
- Allopurinol
  *Increases the risk of severe hypersensitivity reactions, agranulocytosis, neutropenia, and serious infections*
- Amiloride, cyclosporine, potassium preparations, spironolactone, tizanidine, triamterene
  *Increase the risk of hyperkalemia*
- Leflunomide
  *Increases the risk of hepatic injury*

**Drugs That Decrease the Effects of Captopril**

- Iron
  *Decreases bioavailability*

may crush the tablets. It is necessary to assess blood pressure and pulse on an ongoing basis with initial dosage adjustment and intermittently during therapy.

### Assessing for Therapeutic Effects

The nurse monitors response to therapy, looking for a return of blood pressure to target limits without significant adverse effects.

### Assessing for Adverse Effects

The nurse observes acute hypotension when captopril is started, to make sure the patient does not have a fluid volume deficit that would worsen the likelihood of hypotension. He or she assesses for a persistent cough. Also, it is important to check serum potassium levels to ensure a decreased risk of hyperkalemia.

 **QSEN Alert: Safety**

It is important to instruct women of childbearing age to take measures to prevent pregnancy while taking captopril or other ACE inhibitors because the drugs are teratogenic.

### Patient Teaching

Box 26.4 contains additional patient education guidelines for patients taking antihypertensive drugs.

## Other Drugs in the Class

Because of their effectiveness in hypertension and beneficial effects on the heart, blood vessels, and kidneys, the ACE inhibitors are widely used with patients diagnosed with cardiovascular disorders. Drugs in this class also are used in the management of hypertension and heart failure because they decrease peripheral vascular resistance, cardiac workload, and ventricular remodeling. Adverse effects for the class are similar to those outlined with captopril. Specifically, there is an increased risk of cough, hyperkalemia, and angioedema, and the drugs pose a significant risk to a fetus if taken during pregnancy.

**Benazepril (Lotensin)** is indicated for the treatment of hypertension. Patients may take the drug alone or in combination with thiazide diuretics. Peak plasma concentrations occur within 30 minutes to 1 hour. Once-a-day dosing means that steady-state concentrations of the drug are reached after two or three doses.

**Enalapril (Vasotec)** is a prodrug used in the treatment of hypertension and heart failure (see Chap. 30). Prescribers may order the drug for use alone or in combination with antihypertensive agents, particularly thiazide diuretics.

**QSEN Alert: Safety**

Patients started on enalapril who are taking a diuretic occasionally may have symptomatic hypotension following the initial dose of enalapril. The nurse should advocate for the patient's safety and monitor adverse effects.

**Fosinopril (Monopril)** is indicated for the treatment of hypertension and heart failure. Patients may take the drug alone or in combination with thiazide diuretics. As with enalapril, symptomatic hypotension may occur following the initial dose if the patient has been taking a diuretic. A prodrug, fosinopril is absorbed very slowly after oral administration and is highly bound to protein. Time to peak concentration is about 3 hours.

**Lisinopril (Prinivil, Zestril)** is indicated for the treatment of hypertension and heart failure, and the drug is an adjunctive therapy in the management of MI. Prescribers may order it as monotherapy or in combination with thiazide diuretics. Peak serum concentrations of lisinopril occur within about 7 hours. The drug does not undergo metabolism and is excreted unchanged entirely in the urine.

**Moexipril (Univasc)**, which is administered orally and intravenously, is used in the treatment of hypertension. People may take the drug alone or in combination with thiazide diuretics. Peak serum concentrations occur within about 30 minutes. However, absorption is significantly delayed in the presence of food, and it is important to take the drug in a fasting state. In patients who are currently taking a diuretic, symptomatic hypotension may occasionally occur following the initial dose of moexipril. The nurse should advocate for the patient's safety.

**Perindopril (Coversyl)** is used alone or in combination with other therapies to treat mild to moderate essential hypertension. People should take it at least 1 hour prior to eating. Its peak effect occurs within 1 to 2 hours. Caution is necessary in patients older than 65 years of age; metabolism slows with age, and increased serum plasma levels of the mediation exacerbate fluid retention and hyponatremia.

**Quinapril (Accupril)** may be used as monotherapy or in combination with thiazide diuretics in the treatment of hypertension or heart failure. The blood pressure–lowering effect is greater in combination than that seen with either quinapril or the thiazide diuretic alone. Following oral administration, peak concentrations are reached within 1 hour; absorption is decreased with administration with a fatty meal. The drug is highly protein bound and is primarily excreted in the urine.

**Ramipril (Altace)** is used alone or in combination with other medications, including thiazide diuretics, in the treatment of hypertension. It is also used to reduce the risk of heart attack and stroke in at-risk patients as well as to improve survival in

**BOX 26.4** *Patient Teaching Guidelines for Antihypertensive Drugs*

**General Considerations**

- Hypertension is a major risk factor for heart attack, stroke, heart failure, and kidney failure. Although it rarely causes symptoms unless complications occur, it can be controlled by appropriate management. Consequently, you need to learn all you can about the disease process, the factors that cause or aggravate it, and its management. In few other conditions is your knowledge and understanding about your condition as important as with hypertension.

- For many people, lifestyle changes (i.e., a diet to avoid excessive salt and control weight and fat intake, regular exercise, and avoiding smoking) may be sufficient to control blood pressure. If drug therapy is prescribed, these measures should be continued without disruption.

- When drug therapy is needed, your prescriber will try to develop a regimen that works for you, including the drug (or drugs) that are best for you. There are numerous antihypertensive drugs, and many can be taken once a day, which makes their use more convenient and less disruptive of your usual activities of daily living. You may need several office visits to find the right drug or combination of drugs and the right dosage. Changes in drugs or dosages may also be needed later, especially if you develop other conditions or take other drugs that alter your response to the antihypertensive drugs.

- Antihypertensive drug therapy is usually long term, may require more than one drug, and may produce side effects. You need to know the brand and generic names of any prescribed drugs and how to take each drug for optimal benefit and minimal adverse effects.

- Antihypertensive drugs must be taken as prescribed for optimal benefits, even if you do not feel well when a medication is started or when dosage is increased. *No antihypertensive drug should be stopped abruptly. If problems develop, they should be discussed with the health care prescriber.* If treatment is stopped, blood pressure usually increases gradually as the medications are eliminated from the body. However, sometimes, blood pressure rapidly increases to pretreatment levels or even higher. With any of these situations, you are at risk of a heart attack or stroke. In addition, stopping one drug of a multidrug regimen may lead to increased adverse effects as well as decreased antihypertensive effectiveness. To avoid these problems, antihypertensive drugs should be tapered in dosage and discontinued gradually, as directed by your health care provider.

- Blood pressure measurements are the only way you can tell if your medication is working. Thus, you may want to monitor your blood pressure at home, especially when starting drug therapy, changing medications, or changing dosages. If so, a blood pressure machine may be purchased at a medical supply store. Follow instructions regarding use, take your blood pressure approximately the same time(s) each day (e.g., before morning and evening meals), and keep a record to show to your health care provider.

- People sometimes feel dizzy or faint while taking antihypertensive medications. This usually means your blood pressure drops momentarily and is most likely to occur when you start a medication, increase dosage, or stand up suddenly from a sitting or lying position. This can be prevented or decreased by moving to a standing position slowly, sleeping with the head of the bed elevated, wearing elastic stockings, exercising legs, avoiding prolonged standing, and avoiding hot baths. If episodes still occur, you should sit or lie down to avoid a fall and possible injury. You should discuss persistent dizziness with your prescriber; this may indicate a need for changing the timing or type of medication.

- It is very important to keep appointments for laboratory testing and follow-up care.

- As with all drugs, keep these medications in the original container, tightly closed, and out of reach of children.

**Self or Caregiver Administration**

- Take or give antihypertensive drugs at prescribed time intervals, about the same time each day. For example, take once-daily drugs as close to every 24 hours as you can manage; twice-a-day drugs should be taken every 12 hours. If ordered four times daily, take approximately every 6 hours. Taking doses too close together can increase dizziness, weakness, and other adverse effects. Taking doses too far apart may not control blood pressure adequately and may increase risks of heart attack or stroke.

- Take oral captopril on an empty stomach; food decreases drug absorption.

- If you are a sexually active woman, use birth control measures when taking angiotensin-converting enzyme (ACE) inhibitors.

- Take most other oral antihypertensive agents with or after food intake to decrease gastric irritation. Candesartan (Atacand), irbesartan (Avapro), losartan (Cozaar), telmisartan (Micardis), and valsartan (Diovan) may be taken with or without food.

- When taking losartan, take the following precautions:
  - Avoid potassium supplements and salt substitutes containing potassium, unless directed by prescriber.
  - Use birth control measures if you are a woman and you are sexually active.
  - Contact your health care provider immediately if you suspect that you are pregnant.
  - Discuss with your prescriber if you are considering breast-feeding.

- When taking aliskiren, use birth control measures if you are a woman and you are sexually active.

- When taking ACE inhibitors, angiotensin II receptor blockers (ARBs), and aliskiren, immediately report hypersensitivity reactions, especially lip or eyelid swelling, throat tightness, and difficulty breathing.

- Avoid taking aliskiren with a high-fat meal because this significantly decreases the amount of available drug.

- With prazosin, doxazosin, or terazosin, take the first dose and the first increased dose at bedtime to prevent dizziness and possible fainting.

- With the clonidine skin patch, apply to a hairless area on the upper arm or torso once every 7 days. Rotate sites.

patients with heart failure after a heart attack. After oral administration, peak concentration is reached in 1 hour.

Trandolapril (Mavik) is indicated for the treatment of hypertension alone or in combination with other antihypertensive agents such as hydrochlorothiazide. It is also used post-MI in patients who demonstrate left ventricular systolic dysfunction or in those who are symptomatic from heart failure immediately following an MI. The majority of drug is excreted in the stool, and the remainder is excreted in the urine. The extent of biliary excretion has not been determined.

## NCLEX Success

1. In administering a newly initiated order for captopril, an ACE inhibitor, discharge instructions should indicate that which of the following adverse effects is most common?
   A. tinnitus
   B. dry, nonproductive, persistent cough
   C. muscle weakness
   D. constipation

2. Which of the following is indicated for initial drug therapy in a patient newly diagnosed with uncomplicated hypertension (stage 1)? (Select all that apply.)
   A. calcium channel blocker
   B. potassium-sparing diuretic
   C. direct-acting vasodilator
   D. thiazide diuretic

3. A patient being treated with an ACE inhibitor could take which of the following drugs? (Select all that apply.)
   A. diuretics
   B. beta-adrenergic blockers
   C. angiotensin receptor blocker
   D. potassium

### Clinical Application 26.1

• Mr. Caudill states that he does not understand why he needs an additional medication considering his blood pressure is below 140 mm Hg systolic. How should the nurse respond?

## ANGIOTENSIN II RECEPTOR BLOCKERS

Scientists developed ARBs to block the strong blood pressure–raising effects of angiotensin II. ARBs are one of the recommended classes as first-line agents for controlling hypertension. These drugs resemble ACE inhibitors in their effects on blood pressure and hemodynamics and are as effective in the management of hypertension and possibly heart failure. However, they are less likely to cause hyperkalemia and angioedema than ACE

inhibitors, and the occurrence of a persistent cough is rare. The prototype ARB is **losartan** (Cozaar), the first ARB.

## Pharmacokinetics

Both losartan and its metabolite are highly bound to plasma albumin, and the drug's active metabolite is 40 times more potent than losartan and largely responsible for the duration of action. The drug undergoes extensive first-pass metabolism, has an onset of 6 hours, and reaches maximum concentrations 1 to 2 hours. Absorption is good. Metabolism is rapid; the cytochrome P450 liver enzymes process losartan to an active metabolite. Excretion is through the kidneys and the liver.

## Action

Instead of decreasing production of angiotensin II, like the ACE inhibitors, losartan blocks vasoconstricting and aldosterone-secreting effects of angiotensin II at various receptor sites and prevents angiotensin II from combining at various receptor sites. The drug also increases renal flow and enhances the excretion of chloride, calcium, magnesium, and phosphate.

Although multiple types of receptors have been identified, the angiotensin II receptors, type 1 (AT1) located in brain, renal, myocardial, vascular, and adrenal tissue, determine most of the effects of angiotensin II on cardiovascular and renal functions. ARBs block the AT1 receptors and decrease arterial blood pressure by decreasing systemic vascular resistance (see Fig. 26.1).

## Use

Prescribers primarily order losartan for use in the treatment of hypertension; the drug is effective in people with type 2 diabetes who have diabetic nephropathy. After drug therapy begins, maximal effects usually occur within 3 to 6 weeks. It is important to recognize that in African Americans, losartan and other ARBs may be ineffective when used alone. If losartan alone does not control blood pressure, a low dose of a diuretic may be added after 1 to 2 months. A combination product of losartan and hydrochlorothiazide is available.

Table 26.4 presents route and dosage information for losartan and other ARBs.

### Use in Older Adults

Losartan and other ARBs are metabolized by the liver and do not need dose reduction for adults with renal impairment. Use is not recommended in children or adults who have a glomerular filtration rate less than 30 mL/min/1.73 m².

### Use in Patients With Hepatic Impairment

Caution is warranted for use of all ARBs in biliary tract obstruction or hepatic impairment. Experts recommend a lower starting dose for losartan in affected patients because plasma concentrations of the drug and its active metabolite are increased and clearance is decreased approximately 50% with hepatic dysfunction.

### Use in Patients With Critical Illness

Health care providers may administer losartan to critically ill patients, but monitoring is necessary to ensure that the drug

## TABLE 26.4

## DRUGS AT A GLANCE: Angiotensin II Receptor Blockers

| Drug | Pregnancy Category | Routes and Dosage Ranges | |
|---|---|---|---|
| | | **Adults** | **Children 1–17 y of Age (Unless Otherwise Stated)** |
| **Losartan** (Cozaar; ACT Losartan, Cozaar) | C, first trimester; D, second and third trimesters | Initial dose, 50 mg PO once daily initially (25 mg for those who have hepatic impairment or are taking a diuretic). Maintenance dose, PO 35–100 mg daily, in 1 or 2 doses, adjusted according to blood pressure control | ≥6 y, 0.7 mg/kg PO once daily; maximum dose 50 mg daily |
| Azilsartan (Edarbi; Edarbi) | D | Initial dose 40 mg PO once daily, increase as needed up to 80 mg/d based on patient response | Safety and effectiveness in children have not been established |
| Candesartan (Atacand; ACH-Candesartan, Atacand) | D | 16 mg PO once daily initially, increased if necessary to a maximum of 32 mg daily, in 1 or 2 doses | 1 to <6 y, 0.05–0.4 mg/kg PO per day; 6 to <17 y of age <50 kg, 2–16 mg/d PO >50 kg, 4–32 mg/d PO |
| Eprosartan (Teveten) | D | 600 mg PO once daily; increase up to 800 mg/d in 1–2 doses | Safety and effectiveness in children have not been established |
| Irbesartan (Avapro; APO-Irbesartan, Avapro) | C, first trimester; D, second and third trimesters | 150 mg PO once daily initially, increased up to 300 mg, if necessary | 6–16 y: 75 mg PO once daily; maximum dose 150 mg |
| Olmesartan (Benicar; Olmetec, JAMP-Olmesartan) | C, first trimester; D, second and third trimesters | 20 mg PO once daily initially, increased to 40 mg after 2 wk | 6–16 y 20 to <35 kg, 10 mg PO once daily; maximum dose 20 mg/d >35 kg, 20 mg PO once daily; maximum dose 40 mg/d |
| Telmisartan (Micardis; APO-Telmisartan) | C, first trimester; D, second and third trimesters | 40 mg PO once daily initially, increased to maximum of 80 mg daily if necessary | Safety and effectiveness in children have not been established |
| Valsartan (Diovan; ACT Valsartan, Diovan, DOM-Valsartan) | D | 80 mg PO once daily initially, when used as monotherapy in patients who are not volume depleted; maintenance dose may be increased; however, adding a diuretic is more effective than increasing dose beyond 80 mg | 6–16 y, 1.3 mg/kg PO once daily initially up to 40 mg; increase to a maximum of up to 2.7 mg/kg (up to 160 mg) once daily |

produces the desired outcome without significant adverse effects. Also, it has significant drug–drug interactions and the potential to produce hyperkalemia, which could have potentially serious outcomes in the critically ill.

## Adverse Effects

Overall, losartan is generally well tolerated, with few side or adverse effects. Adverse effects include dizziness, muscle cramps or weakness, heartburn, diarrhea, and decreased sensitivity to touch. There are reports of angioedema, and it is important to evaluate this condition immediately.

## Contraindications

Contraindications to losartan include known hypersensitivity to the drug. Additionally, the FDA has issued a **BLACK BOX WARNING** ◆ regarding the use of losartan and

---

**BOX 26.5**   *Drug Interactions: Losartan*

**Drugs That Increase the Effects of Losartan**

- Alcohol, antihypertensive agents, and diuretics
  *Increase the risk of hypotension*
- Aliskiren
  *Increases the risk of hypotension, hyperkalemia, and renal impairment*
- Fluconazole
  *Increases the risk of hypotension through inhibited metabolism*

**Drugs That Decrease the Effects of Losartan**

- CYP2C9 inducers (e.g., rifampicin, secobarbital), CYP3A4 inducers (e.g., indinavir, clarithromycin) methylphenidate, nonsteroidal anti-inflammatory drugs, peginterferon alfa-2B, and yohimbine
  *Decrease serum levels*
- Indomethacin
  *Decreases antihypertensive effects*
- Phenobarbital and rifamycins
  *Increase metabolism and decrease antihypertensive effects*

CYP, cytochrome P450.

---

**BOX 26.6**   *Herb and Dietary Interactions: Losartan*

**Herbs and Foods That Increase the Effects of Losartan**

- Alfalfa
- Aloe
- American ginseng
- Bitter melon
- Black cohosh
- California poppy
- Celery
- Coleus
- Garlic
- Ginger
- Goldenseal
- Hawthorn
- Marshmallow
- Mistletoe
- Quinine
- Shepherd's purse
- St. John's wort

**Herbs and Foods That Decrease the Effects of Losartan**

- American ginseng
- Bayberry
- Blue cohosh
- Grapefruit juice
- Kola
- Licorice

---

other ARBs, which directly affect the renin–angiotensin system, because their use can cause injury and even death to a developing fetus. Therefore, pregnancy is a contraindication to use of losartan and other ARBs, and it is essential that the drugs be discontinued as soon as pregnancy is detected.

## Nursing Implications

### Preventing Interactions

Many medications and herbs interact with losartan, increasing or decreasing its effects (Boxes 26.5 and 26.6).

### Administering the Medication

People may take losartan without regard to meals.

### Assessing for Therapeutic Effects

The nurse monitors blood pressure to evaluate drug efficacy. Also, he or she observes for the presence of lifestyle modifications that will improve baseline blood pressure readings (e.g., weight loss, smoking cessation, restricted salt intake).

### Assessing for Adverse Effects

The nurse assesses kidney and liver function tests, as well as serum electrolyte levels, particularly potassium. Also, he or she observes for the presence of angioedema and other hypersensitivity reactions.

---

 **QSEN Alert: Safety**

It is important to instruct women of childbearing age to take measures to prevent pregnancy while taking losartan or other ARBs because the drugs are teratogenic.

---

### Patient Teaching

Box 26.4 contains patient education guidelines for the antihypertensive drugs.

## Other Drugs in the Class

Azilsartan (Edarbi) may be used as monotherapy or combined with other therapies for hypertension. Azilsartan is particularly potent in blocking the binding of angiotensin II to AT1 receptors, which enhances its ability to reduce blood pressure (Kurtz & Kajiya, 2012). It has a peak effect within 1 ½ to 3 hours of administration. Up to 10% of patients taking azilsartan experience gastrointestinal (GI) side effects, including diarrhea, and patients should be monitored for the adverse effects of angioedema, hyperkalemia, hypotension, and renal impairment. Although azilsartan is effective at lowering blood pressure in hypertensive patients, it is not preferred for monotherapy for the treatment of hypertension in patients with other cardiovascular disorders. Combination therapy may be necessary to achieve blood pressure goals.

Candesartan (Atacand) is used alone or in combination with other drugs to treat hypertension and heart failure. It is available in a fixed combination with hydrochlorothiazide (Avalide). The drug is highly protein bound, crosses the blood–brain barrier poorly, and is excreted in breast milk. After oral administration, the peak serum concentration is reached in about 3 to 4 hours.

Food with a high fat content does not affect the bioavailability of candesartan. A portion of the drug is excreted unchanged in the urine, with the remainder excreted in stool. The adverse effect profile is similar to losartan. Candesartan is slightly more effective in reducing blood pressure than losartan.

Eprosartan (Teveten) is used as monotherapy or in combination with other therapies to treat hypertension. It should be administered at least one hour before eating for maximum absorption, and peak action occurs within one to two hours. The drug is partially excreted through the kidney and should be used with caution in patients with renal impairment. Eprosartan has demonstrated positive effect on reducing blood pressure, but unlike many other drugs in this class, it has not demonstrated effectiveness at treating other cardiovascular disorders such as heart failure.

Irbesartan (Avapro) is used as monotherapy or in combination with other drugs to treat hypertension and is used to treat nephropathy in patients with type 2 diabetes. In patients with volume and salt depletions (e.g., those on hemodialysis), a lower initial dose is recommended. Like candesartan, irbesartan is a bit more effective in reducing blood pressure than losartan. The drug can be administered orally or intravenously. An oral preparation is available in a fixed combination with hydrochlorothiazide (Avapro HCT). Absorption of oral irbesartan is rapid, and peak concentrations occur within 30 minutes to 2 hours after dosing. Food does not affect the drug's bioavailability. Excretion of the drug and its metabolites occurs by both the renal and biliary routes.

Olmesartan (Benicar) is used alone or in combination with other drugs to treat hypertension. It is available in a fixed combination with hydrochlorothiazide (Benicar HCT) and with amlodipine (Azor). Absorption is good, and peak concentrations occur within 1 to 2 hours after dosing. Food does not affect the bioavailability of olmesartan. The drug is highly protein bound and crosses the blood–brain barrier poorly, but it is excreted in breast milk. The drug converts from olmesartan medoxomil to olmesartan during absorption; essentially, there is no further metabolism of olmesartan after conversion. Almost half of the absorbed drug is excreted in the urine. The remainder is excreted in the feces and via the bile. Hyperglycemia, dizziness, diarrhea, flulike symptoms, and a spruelike enteropathy are adverse effects. Concomitant use of olmesartan with aliskiren is contraindicated in patients with diabetes mellitus.

Telmisartan (Micardis) is used as monotherapy or in combination with other drugs to treat hypertension. It is available in a fixed combination with hydrochlorothiazide (Micardis HCT) and with amlodipine (Twynsta). It is also used in patients 55 years of age or older who are at high risk for developing major cardiovascular events for the risk reduction of death from cardiovascular causes, particularly MI or stroke, and who are unable to take ACE inhibitors. Administration of telmisartan is intravenous or oral. The drug is highly protein bound and is well absorbed, and peak concentrations occur within 30 minutes to 1 hour after dosing. Food slightly reduces bioavailability. Telmisartan is eliminated unchanged in feces via biliary excretion, and minute amounts are found in urine.

Valsartan (Diovan) is used as monotherapy or in combination with other drugs to treat hypertension. It is available in four fixed combinations: with hydrochlorothiazide (Diovan HCT), with amlodipine (Exforge), with amlodipine and hydrochlorothiazide (Exforge HCT), and with aliskiren (Valturna). The drug is available in oral (tablet and suspension) and intravenous forms. Following oral administration, peak plasma levels occur in 2 to 4 hours. With the tablet, food decreases the bioavailability and the peak plasma level. The suspension has a bioavailability about one and one half times the tablet. The drug is excreted primarily in the feces, with a small portion in the urine. Valsartan is excreted primarily as unchanged drug, with only one fifth of the dose recovered as metabolites.

## CALCIUM CHANNEL BLOCKERS

CCBs are first-line agents for controlling hypertension and may be used as monotherapy or in combination with other drugs. They may be especially useful for people with hypertension who also have angina pectoris, other cardiovascular disorders, or pulmonary disorders. Current guidelines recommend that CCBs be used alone or in combination with a thiazide diuretic to treat hypertension. These drugs are especially appropriate as the first-line treatment of hypertension for black patients. They may be used alone or in combination with thiazide-type diuretics. For the purposes of this discussion, amlodipine (Norvasc) serves as the prototype. Note that sustained-release forms of nifedipine, diltiazem, verapamil, and other long-acting drugs (e.g., amlodipine, felodipine) are recommended rather than the short-acting forms because they do not cause precipitous lowering of pressure.

In hypertension, CCBs mainly dilate peripheral arteries and decrease peripheral vascular resistance by relaxing vascular smooth muscle. As a group, the CCBs are well absorbed from the GI tract following oral administration and are highly bound to protein. The drugs are metabolized in the liver and excreted in the urine.

Most of the available CCBs have received FDA approval for use in hypertension. Nifedipine, a short-acting CCB, has been used to treat hypertensive emergencies or urgent hypertensive events.

Note that CCBs (e.g., verapamil) are used for several other cardiovascular disorders. Chapters 27 and 28, respectively, discuss the mechanism of action and use in the management of tachydysrhythmias and angina pectoris.

### Pharmacokinetics

Amlodipine is well absorbed with oral administration. Absorption is not reduced by the presence of food. Peak plasma concentration is achieved between 6 and 12 hours after oral administration. Significant initial reductions in blood pressure are achieved with 24 to 48 hours of the initial dose. Therapeutic plasma levels are reached in approximately 7 days with consistent daily dosing. The drug is metabolized in the liver and excreted in the urine.

### Action

Amlodipine inhibits the influx of calcium ions across cardiac and smooth muscle during depolarization, resulting in relaxation and vasodilation. This leads to lowered blood pressure.

### Use

Health care providers use amlodipine to treat hypertension alone or in combination with other antihypertensives. The drug can also be used to treat CAD, which is addressed in Chapter 28. Note that no dosage adjustment is necessary in patients with renal impairment.

Table 26.5 provides specific dosage information for amlodipine and other CCBs.

## Use in Children

Amlodipine has been shown to be effective in lowering blood pressure in children aged 6 to 17 years. Information on the effect of the drug on children younger than 6 years of age is limited. Small sample studies indicate that children younger than 6 years of age may have a weight-adjusted clearance of amlodipine greater than in older children, suggesting that larger-than-expected doses may be necessary in that age group to obtain the desired response.

## Use in Older Adults

Older patients have decreased clearance of the drug. Therefore, dosing should start with the lowest possible dose and be titrated as necessary.

## Use in Patients With Hepatic Impairment

Amlodipine is metabolized extensively by the liver. Consideration of the possibility of prolonged half-life and delayed clearance, resulting in drug accumulation, may be warranted. Reduced dosing is advised; titrate slowly if necessary.

### TABLE 26.5

### DRUGS AT A GLANCE: Calcium Channel Blockers

| Drug | Pregnancy Category | Routes and Dosage Ranges | |
|---|---|---|---|
| | | **Adults** | **Children 1–17 y of Age (Unless Otherwise Stated)** |
| **Amlodipine** (Norvasc; ACT AmLODIPine, DOM-AmLODIPine) | C | 5–10 mg PO once daily | <6 y, based on weight-based considerations and response |
| Diltiazem (sustained release) Cardizem CD, Cartia XT; ACT Diltiazem CD, APO-Diltiaz CD) | C | 60–120 mg PO twice daily | Safety and effectiveness have not been established |
| Felodipine (Plendil, SANDOZ Felodipine) | C | 5–10 mg PO once daily | Maximum 10 mg PO daily |
| Isradipine | C | 2.5–5 mg PO twice daily; may increase to up to 10 mg/d in two divided doses | Immediate release (PO), 0.25–0.2 mg/kg daily in 3–4 doses initially; maximum dose 0.8 mg/kg up to 20 mg daily Sustained release (PO), 0.15–0.2 mg/kg daily in two divided doses initially; maximum dose 0.8 mg/kg up to 20 mg daily |
| Nicardipine | C | Sustained release (PO), 30–60 mg daily up to 120 mg/d; twice daily IV infusion, 5–15 mg/h | 1–3 mcg/kg/min as IV infusion for rapid reduction of blood pressure |
| Nifedipine (Adalat CC, Procardia, Procardia XL; Adalat XL, DOM-NIFEdipine) | C | Sustained release (PO) only, 30–60 mg once daily, increased over 1–2 wk if necessary | Sustained release (PO), 0.25–0.5 mg/kg/d in 1–2 doses; maximum dose 3 mg/kg in 1–2 doses up to 120 mg |
| Nisoldipine (Sular) | C | 20 mg PO once daily initially, increased by 10 mg/wk or longer intervals to a maximum of 60 mg daily; average maintenance dose, 20–40 mg daily. Adults with liver impairment or >65 y, 10 mg PO once daily initially | Safety and effectiveness have not been established |
| Verapamil (Calan, Calan SR, Tarka, Verelan; APO-Verap, Isoptin SR) | C | Immediate release (PO), 40–120 mg 3 times daily Sustained release (PO), 180–240 mg once daily IV, see manufacturer's instructions | IV, see manufacturer's instructions |

## Adverse Effects

Amlodipine is generally well tolerated. Possible cardiovascular adverse effects occur most frequently and include peripheral edema of the hands, ankles, and feet and pulmonary edema, particularly in patients with heart failure. Other potential adverse effects include headache, drowsiness, fatigue, dizziness, flushing, palpitations, nausea, and abdominal pain.

## Contraindications

Contraindications include hypersensitivity to amlodipine or any of its components.

## Nursing Implications

### Preventing Interactions

Many medications interact with amlodipine, increasing or decreasing its effects (Box 26.7). Conivaptan, CYP3A4 strong inhibitors (e.g., ketoconazole), may increase plasma concentration levels. Avoid concurrent use. Cyclosporine may decrease the metabolism of CCBs. Monitor for hypotension.

Amlodipine also affects the action of several drugs. Simvastatin serum concentrations may increase when taken concurrently. Concurrent use should be avoided if possible and the simvastatin dose limited to 20 mg/day if patients must take the two drugs concurrently. Foods that affect the action of amlodipine include grapefruit juice (a CYP3A4 inhibitor), which may increase the serum level of the drug. St. John's wort (a CYP3A4 inducer) should be avoided because the herbal supplement may decrease the serum level of the drug.

### Administering the Medication

The drug can be given without regard for food.

### Assessing for Therapeutic Effects

The nurse monitors blood pressure to evaluate drug efficacy. Also, he or she observes for the presence of lifestyle modifications that will improve baseline blood pressure readings (e.g., losing weight, stopping smoking, restricting salt intake).

### Assessing for Adverse Effects

The nurse monitors blood pressure and assesses for chest pain frequently on initiation of drug therapy. In patients with severe CAD and/or heart failure, very close monitoring for chest pain, pulmonary edema, and peripheral edema is necessary.

### Patient Teaching

Box 26.4 contains patient education guidelines for the antihypertensive drugs, including amlodipine.

## Other Drugs in the Class

Diltiazem (Cardizem CD, Cartia XT) is administered for hypertension using the extended-release formulation. As a generic drug is available in once- and twice-daily dosing, it is important to verify that the appropriate extended-release formulation is administered. With diltiazem, the initial dosing for treatment of hypertension is 180 to 240 mg PO once daily (60–120 mg PO with twice-daily generic capsule). Diltiazem is also approved as a treatment to improve exercise tolerance for patients who experience angina by decreasing oxygen demand. Initial dose for management of exercise intolerance is 180 mg (extended release) PO once daily. It is necessary to monitor patients for dysrhythmias, atrioventricular heart block, bradycardia, heart failure, hypotension, headache, and dizziness.

Long-acting dihydropyridines are most commonly used to treat hypertension. If the nondihydropyridine CCBs (diltiazem, verapamil) are prescribed, the extended-release formulations are often used for hypertension; the two drugs can be given for control of angina and for rate control in patients with atrial fibrillation.

Nifedipine is available as Adalat CC, Procardia, and Procardia XL. The initial dose is 30 to 60 mg PO once daily with a maximum dose of 120 mg/day. Nifedipine should not be taken with grapefruit juice. Patients should be monitored for effects of excessive vasodilation, including hypotension, dizziness, and headache. Patient teaching must include that abrupt cessation of taking nifedipine could result in rebound tachycardia. Nifedipine immediate release should be used with caution in elderly patients. Patients taking nifedipine extended release should be monitored for sign and symptoms of GI obstruction.

> **⚠ QSEN Alert: Safety**
>
> Authorities no longer recommend puncturing a nifedipine capsule, because this practice is associated with an increased risk of adverse cardiovascular events precipitated by a rapid and severe decrease in blood pressure.

Verapamil (Calan, Calan SR, Tarka, Verelan) is another CCB used to treat hypertension. The initial dose is a 120- to 240-mg extended-release tablet PO once daily with reduced dosing for patients with hepatic or renal dysfunction and the elderly. It is important not to split or crush extended-release capsules or tablets and not to take the medication with grapefruit juice. The nurse should monitor patients for effects of excessive vasodilation, including hypotension, dizziness, and headache. Felodipine is also used to control hypertension. The initial dose is 5 mg PO once daily. Patients should take it with food and

---

**BOX 26.7** 💊 **Drug Interactions: Amlodipine**

**Drugs That Increase the Effects of Amlodipine**

- Adenosine
  *Increases bradycardia*
- Alfuzosin, amifostine, barbiturates, diazoxide, duloxetine, and antihypertensive agents
  *Increase hypotensive effects*
- Fluconazole and itraconazole
  *Inhibit metabolism of amlodipine and increase edema*

**Drugs That Decrease the Effects of Amlodipine**

- Rifampin, rifabutin, carbamazepine, and phenytoin
  *Decrease serum level of amlodipine*

should not crush or split the tablets. Patients require monitoring for headache, dizziness, chest pain, and palpitations. Felodipine is available only in extended-release form. Concurrent use with NSAIDs may decrease antihypertensive effects.

Isradipine is used alone or concomitantly with thiazide-type diuretics for treatment of hypertension in adults. As with other CCBs, isradipine is hepatically metabolized via cytochrome P450 isoenzyme CYP3A4, so numerous drug interactions can occur. Grapefruit juice (a CYP3A4 inhibitor) may increase the serum level of the drug, and St. John's wort (a CYP3A4 inducer) may decrease the serum level of the drug.

---

### Unfolding Patient Stories: Junetta Cooper • Part 2

Think back to Junetta Cooper from Chapter 1, a 75-year-old African American female with atherosclerotic heart disease and a 20-year history of hypertension controlled with hydrochlorothiazide. While hospitalized for a cardiac catheterization, her blood pressure is elevated and the health care team is considering the addition of amlodipine. Describe the ethnic variations in drug response that are associated with antihypertensive medications. How would the nurse explain why hydrochlorothiazide and amlodipine are selected for Junetta? What patient education should the nurse prepare if both medications are ordered for her?

Care for Junetta and other patients in a realistic virtual environment: *vSim for Nursing* (thepoint.lww.com/vSimPharm). Practice documenting these patients' care in DocuCare (thepoint.lww.com/DocuCareEHR).

---

Nicardipine is also used. The initial dose is 20 mg PO three times a day. The drug may be taken with or without food but should not be taken with a high-fat meal. It is necessary to monitor for hypotension, chest pain, palpitations, and tachycardia.

Nisoldipine (Sular) is a CCB that may be used to manage hypertension. The initial dose is 17 to 20 mg PO once daily. Patients should take the drug without food. The nurse should monitor for hypotension, chest pain, palpitations, and tachycardia.

---

### ! QSEN Alert: Safety

Abrupt discontinuation of CCBs may increase frequency and duration of chest pain.

---

## ADJUVANT MEDICATIONS USED TO TREAT HYPERTENSION

Prescribers may order other drugs for the treatment of hypertension. Table 26.6 presents route and dosage information for these drugs.

### Direct Renin Inhibitors

 **Aliskiren** (Tekturna), the only direct renin inhibitor, decreases plasma renin activity and inhibits the conversion of angiotensinogen to angiotensin I. The drug is used as monotherapy or in combination with other antihypertensive agents for the treatment of hypertension but should never be used in combination with an ACE inhibitor or an ARB. A fixed-dose combination with valsartan (Valturna) is available. Aliskiren is poorly absorbed, and steady-state blood levels are reached in about a week. Following oral administration, peak plasma levels are reached in 1 to 3 hours. If taken with a high-fat meal, bioavailability and peak levels are decreased by about 75%. The drug is excreted in the urine. Aliskiren is contraindicated in patients with chronic kidney disease because of the increased risk of renal impairment, hyperkalemia, and hypotension. Angioedema may occur.

---

### NCLEX Success

4. Which of the following drug classes are absolutely contraindicated for use in pregnant women? [Select all that apply.]
   A. ARBs
   B. calcium channel blockers
   C. direct renin inhibitors
   D. ACE inhibitors

5. Orthostatic hypotension is a potential outcome of hypertensive drugs that places the elderly at risk for injury from falls. Instructions given to the patient to decrease this effect include which of the following? [Select all that apply.]
   A. Take the dose at bedtime.
   B. Change position slowly when rising from bed or chair.
   C. Increase fluid intake by 500 mL/day.
   D. Decrease the dose until symptoms disappear.

6. Single-drug therapy with an ARB would be least effective in which of the following groups?
   A. people of Asian descent
   B. people of Caucasian descent
   C. people of Hispanic descent
   D. people of African descent

---

## Antiadrenergics

**Antiadrenergic** (sympatholytic) drugs inhibit activity of the SNS. When the SNS is stimulated, the nerve impulse travels from the brain and spinal cord to the ganglia. From the ganglia, the impulse travels along postganglionic fibers to effector organs (e.g., heart, blood vessels). Although SNS stimulation produces widespread effects in the body, the effects relevant to this discussion are the increases in heart rate, force of myocardial contraction, cardiac output, and blood pressure that occur. When the nerve impulse is inhibited or blocked at any location along its pathway, the result is decreased blood pressure.

Alpha$_1$-adrenergic receptor blockers (e.g., prazosin) dilate blood vessels and decrease peripheral vascular resistance. These drugs can be used alone or in multidrug regimens but are not routinely used as initial antihypertensive agents. One adverse effect, called the **first-dose phenomenon**, results in orthostatic

**TABLE 26.6**

## Adjunct Medications Used for the Treatment of Hypertension

| Drug | Pregnancy Category | Routes and Dosage Ranges | |
|---|---|---|---|
| | | **Adults** | **Children 1–17 y of Age (Unless Otherwise Stated)** |
| **Direct Renin Inhibitors** | | | |
| **Aliskiren** (Tekturna; ❋ Rasilez) | D | 150 mg PO once daily | Safety and effectiveness have not been established |
| **Antiadrenergics** *Alpha₁-Adrenergic Blockers* | | | |
| Doxazosin (Cardura, Cardura XL; ❋ APO-Doxazosin, DOM-Doxazosin) | C | 1 mg PO once daily initially, increased to 2 mg, then to 4, 8, and 16 mg daily if necessary | Safety and effectiveness have not been established |
| Prazosin (Minipress; ❋ APO-Prazo, Minipress) | C | 1 mg PO 2–3 times daily initially, increased if necessary to 20 mg in divided doses; average maintenance dose, 6–15 mg daily | Safety and effectiveness have not been established |
| Terazosin (❋ APO-Terazosin, PMS-Terazosin) | C | 1 mg PO at bedtime initially, may be increased gradually; usual maintenance dose, 1–5 mg once daily | Safety and effectiveness have not been established |
| *Alpha₂ Agonists* | | | |
| Clonidine (Catapres; ❋ APO-CloNIDine, MINT-CloNIDine) | C | 0.1 mg PO 2 times daily initially, gradually increased up to 2.4 mg daily, if necessary; average maintenance dose, 0.2–0.8 mg daily<br>Transdermal: 0.1 mg/24 h initially, patch applied once every 7 d and increase by 0.1 mg at 1- to 2-wk intervals; usual maintenance dose 0.1–0.3 mg/24 h patch applied once every 7 d | 5–25 mcg/kg/d PO, in divided doses, every 6 h; increase at 5- to 7-d intervals, if needed |
| Guanfacine (❋ Intuniv XR) | B | 1 mg PO daily at bedtime, increased to 2 mg after 3–4 wk and then to 3 mg if necessary | ≥12 y, 1 mg daily PO initially: maximum dose 2 mg daily |
| Methyldopa | B | 250 mg PO 2 or 3 times daily initially, increased gradually until blood pressure is controlled or a daily dose of 3 g is reached | 10 mg/kg/d PO in 2–4 divided doses initially, increased or decreased according to response; maximum dose 65 mg/kg/d or 3 g daily, whichever is less |
| *Beta-Adrenergic Blockers* | | | |
| Acebutolol (❋ APO-Acebutolol) | B | 400 mg PO once daily initially, increased to 800 mg daily if necessary | Safety and effectiveness have not been established. |
| Atenolol (Tenormin; ❋ APO-Atenol), BIO-Atenolol | D | 50 mg PO once daily initially, increased in 1–2 wk to 100 mg once daily, if necessary | 0.5–1 mg/kg/d PO in 1 or 2 doses; maximum dose 2 mg/kg up to 100 mg daily in 1 or 2 doses |
| Bisoprolol (❋ APO-Bisoprolol, RIVA-Bisoprolol) | C | 5 mg PO once daily, increased to a maximum of 20 mg daily if necessary | 10 mg PO in a fixed combination with hydrochlorothiazide 6.25 mg daily |
| Metoprolol (Lopressor; ❋ APO-Metoprolol, APO-Metoprolol SR) | C | 50 mg PO twice daily, gradually increased in weekly or longer intervals if necessary; maximum dose 400 mg daily | Immediate release (PO), 1–2 mg/kg/d in 2 doses; maximum dose 6 mg/kg/d not to exceed 200 mg/d<br>Sustained release (PO), 1 mg/kg once daily not to exceed 50 mg/d; maximum dose not to exceed 200 mg/d |

*(Continued on page 530)*

**TABLE 26.6**

## Adjunct Medications Used for the Treatment of Hypertension (Continued)

| Drug | Pregnancy Category | Routes and Dosage Ranges | |
|---|---|---|---|
| | | **Adults** | **Children 1–17 y of Age (Unless Otherwise Stated)** |
| Nadolol (Corgard) | C | 40 mg PO once daily initially, gradually increased if necessary; average dose, 80–320 mg daily | Safety and effectiveness have not been established |
| Pindolol (🍁 APO-Pindol, Visken) | B | 5 mg PO 2 or 3 times daily initially, increased by 10 mg/d at 3- to 4-wk intervals to a maximum of 60 mg daily | Safety and effectiveness have not been established |
| Propranolol (Inderal LA; 🍁 APO-Propranolol, Hemangiol) | C | 40 mg PO twice daily initially, gradually increased up to 640 mg daily | 1 mg/kg/d PO initially, gradually increased to a maximum of 10 mg/kg/d |
| Timolol | C | 10 mg PO twice daily initially, increased gradually if necessary; average daily dose, 20–40 mg; maximum daily dose, 60 mg | Safety and effectiveness have not been established |
| *Alpha–Beta-Adrenergic Blockers* | | | |
| Carvedilol (Coreg, Coreg CR) | C | 6.25 mg PO twice daily for 7–14 d, increase to 12.5 mg twice daily for 7–14 d, and then increase to a maximum dose of 25 mg twice daily if tolerated and needed | Not approved for children <18 y |
| Labetalol (🍁 Trandate, APO-Labetalol) | C | 100 mg PO twice daily, increased by 100 mg twice daily every 2–3 d if necessary; usual maintenance dose, 200–400 mg twice daily; severe hypertension may require 1200–2400 mg daily<br>IV injection, 20 mg slowly over 2 min, followed by 40–80 mg every 10 min until the desired blood pressure is achieved or 300 mg has been given<br>IV infusion, mix with IV fluids and infuse at a rate of 2 mg/min | 1–3 mg/kg PO daily initially twice daily; increase up to a maximum of 10–12 mg/kg or 1200 mg daily |
| **Diuretics** | | | |
| Hydrochlorothiazide (Microzide; 🍁 APO-Hydro, TEVA-Hydrochlorothiazide, Urozide) | B | Hypertension: 12.5–50 mg PO 1 or 2 times daily<br>Elderly: 12.5–25 PO mg/d | 2 mg/kg/d PO in 2 divided doses<br>Infants <6 mo, 2–3 mg/kg/d in 2 divided doses |
| Chlorothiazide (Diuril) | C | 500–2000 mg/d PO divided in 1–2 times doses<br>Elderly, 500 mg PO once daily or 1 g 3 times/wk<br>250–1000 mg IV once or twice daily; maximum dose 1000 mg | 22 mg/kg/d PO in 2 divided doses<br>Infants <6 mo, 20–40 mg/kg/d in 2 divided doses; maximum dose 375 mg/d<br>IV dosing not well established |
| Chlorthalidone (🍁 APO-Chlorthalidone) | C | 25–100 mg/d PO<br>Elderly, 12.5–25 mg/d PO or every other day | Not approved in children |
| Indapamide (🍁 APO-Indapamide, Lozide, MYLAN-Indapamide) | B | Hypertension: 1.25 mg PO in morning may increase to 5 mg/d | Dosage not established |

**TABLE 26.6**

## Adjunct Medications Used for the Treatment of Hypertension (Continued)

| Drug | Pregnancy Category | Routes and Dosage Ranges | |
|---|---|---|---|
| | | **Adults** | **Children 1–17 y of Age (Unless Otherwise Stated)** |
| Furosemide (Lasix; APO-Furosemide, Furosemide Special, MINT-Furosemide) | C | Hypertension: 20–40 mg PO twice daily, gradually increased if necessary<br>Hypertensive crisis: 40–80 mg IV injected over 1–2 min; with renal failure, much larger doses may be needed<br>PO, IV 5–20 mg once daily | 2 mg/kg PO 1 or 2 times daily initially, gradually increased by increments of 1–2 mg/kg per dose if necessary at intervals of 6–8 h; maximum daily dose 6 mg/kg 1 mg/kg IV initially; if diuretic response is not adequate, increase dosage by 1 mg/kg no sooner than 2 h after previous dose; maximum dose 6 mg/kg |
| Spironolactone (Aldactone, CaroSpir; Aldactone, TEVA-Spironolactone) | C; D in pregnancy-induced hypertension | 25–100 mg PO daily | Safety and effectiveness not established |
| Amiloride (Midamor) | B | 5–10 mg PO daily | Dosage not established |
| Triamterene (Dyrenium) | C | 100–300 mg PO daily in divided doses | 2–4 mg/kg/d PO in divided doses |
| **Other Vasodilators (Direct Acting)** | | | |
| Fenoldopam (Corlopam) | B | Infusion, IV, initial dose based on body weight and then flow rate titrated to achieve desired response; mix with 0.9% sodium chloride or 5% dextrose to a concentration of 40 mcg/mL (e.g., 40 mg of drug [4 mL of concentrate] in 1000 mL of IV fluid) | Infusion, IV, initial dose based on body weight (0.2 mcg/kg/min) and then flow rate titrated to achieve desired response; may increase dosage every 20–30 min by up to 0.3–0.5 mcg/kg/min; maximum dose 0.8 mcg/kg/min |
| Hydralazine (Hydra-zide, BiDil; APO-HydrALAZINE, Apresoline) | C | Chronic hypertension: 10 mg PO 4 times daily for 2–4 d, gradually increased up to 300 mg/d, if necessary<br>Hypertensive crisis: 10–20 mg IM, IV, increased to 40 mg if necessary; repeat dose as needed | Chronic hypertension: 0.75 mg/kg/d PO initially in 4 divided doses; gradually increase over 3–4 wk to a maximum dose of 7.5 mg/kg/d if necessary<br>Hypertensive crisis: 0.1–0.2 IM, IV mg/kg every 4–6 h as needed |
| Minoxidil (Loniten) | C | 5 mg PO once daily initially, increased gradually until blood pressure is controlled; average daily dose, 10–40 mg; maximum daily dose, 100 mg in single or divided doses | <12 y, 0.2 mg/kg/d PO initially as a single dose, increased gradually until blood pressure is controlled; average daily dose, 0.25–1.0 mg/kg; maximum dose 50 mg/d |
| Sodium nitroprusside (Nitropress; Nipride) | C | Infusion, IV, 0.5–10 mcg/kg/min; average dose, 3 mcg/kg/min; prepare solution by adding 50 mg of sodium nitroprusside to 250–1000 mL of 5% dextrose in water and cover promptly to protect from light | Same as adult |

Ortho

hypotension, with palpitations, dizziness, and perhaps syncope 1 to 3 hours after the first dose or an increased dose. To prevent this effect, first doses and first increased doses are taken at bedtime. Another effect, associated with long-term use or higher doses, leads to sodium and fluid retention and a need for concurrent diuretic therapy. Centrally acting sympatholytics (e.g., clonidine) stimulate presynaptic alpha$_2$ receptors in the brain and are classified as alpha$_2$ receptor agonists. Taking these drugs leads to the release of less norepinephrine and a reduction of sympathetic outflow from the vasomotor center. Stimulation of presynaptic alpha$_2$ receptors peripherally may also contribute to the decreased sympathetic activity. Reduced sympathetic activity leads to decreased cardiac output, heart rate, peripheral vascular resistance, and blood pressure. Chronic use of clonidine and related drugs may result in sodium and fluid retention, especially with higher doses.

Beta-adrenergic blockers are useful in the treatment of hypertension in patients with ischemic heart disease, especially in those (a) younger than 50 years of age with acute coronary syndrome or recent MI and (b) who have heart failure with reduced ejection fraction. Experts do not recommend beta-blockers as initial monotherapy unless they are specifically indicated; they are most effective when used in combination with ARBs (Mann et al., 2018, Sept 19). Most beta-adrenergic blockers have FDA approval for use in hypertension and are probably equally effective. However, the cardioselective drugs (see Chap. 28) are preferred for people with hypertension who also have asthma, peripheral vascular disease, or diabetes mellitus. Research studies demonstrate reduced morbidity and mortality with diuretics and beta-adrenergic blockers used in combination, especially after an MI.

Beta-adrenergic blockers (e.g., propranolol) decrease heart rate [chronotropy], force of myocardial contraction [inotropy], cardiac output, and renin release from the kidneys. The FDA has issued a **BLACK BOX WARNING ◆** for patients with CAD taking oral forms of atenolol, metoprolol, nadolol, propranolol, and timolol; abrupt withdrawal has resulted in exacerbation of angina, the incidence of ventricular dysrhythmias, and the occurrence of MIs. Beta-adrenergic blockers that normally undergo extensive first-pass hepatic metabolism (e.g., acebutolol, metoprolol, propranolol, timolol) may produce excessive blood levels in patients with cirrhosis because the blood containing the drug is shunted around the liver into the systemic circulation. It is necessary to start at a low dose and titrate the dosage carefully. Also, dosage reduction with bisoprolol and pindolol is important in patients with cirrhosis or other hepatic impairment.

Labetalol can be used as monotherapy for initial management of uncomplicated hypertension; however, thiazide diuretics are preferred by JNC 8. Administration is intravenous or oral. Occasionally following intravenous administration, orthostatic hypotension with loss of consciousness reportedly occurs; the hypotension can last for 3 hours or longer.

## Other Vasodilators (Direct Acting)

Vasodilator antihypertensive drugs directly relax smooth muscle in blood vessels, resulting in dilation and decreased peripheral vascular resistance. As they reduce afterload, they may be used in management of heart failure. The direct-acting vasodilators are effective in managing a hypertensive emergency.

Nitroprusside (Nitropress) is a potent vasodilator that acts on arterioles and venules. Given by continuous intravenous infusion, the drug has a rapid onset and short duration of action, and it requires continuous blood pressure monitoring. Intra-arterial blood pressure monitoring is the most effective during the infusion. Nitroprusside is metabolized to thiocyanate, and it is necessary to measure serum thiocyanate levels if the drug is given longer than 72 hours. If the serum thiocyanate level is more than 12 mg/dL, it is important to stop the infusion after 72 hours. The infusion should last no longer than 48 hours in patients with renal impairment. Hemodialysis reverses the symptoms of thiocyanate toxicity (e.g., nausea, vomiting, muscle twitching or spasm, seizures).

Hydralazine (Hydra-Zide, BiDil) and minoxidil act mainly on arterioles. These drugs have a limited effect on hypertension when used alone because the vasodilating action that lowers blood pressure also stimulates the SNS and triggers reflexive compensatory mechanisms (vasoconstriction, tachycardia, and increased cardiac output), which raise blood pressure. It is possible to prevent this effect during long-term therapy by also giving a drug that inhibits excessive sympathetic stimulation (e.g., propranolol, an adrenergic blocker). These drugs also cause sodium and water retention, which may be minimized by concomitant diuretic therapy. The FDA has issued a **BLACK BOX WARNING ◆** for minoxidil because the drug can exacerbate angina and precipitate pericardial effusion (which can progress to cardiac tamponade).

### *Clinical Application 26.2*

- Discuss the rationale for choosing captopril in Mr. Caudill's case.
- What should the nurse include in teaching Mr. Caudill to minimize adverse effects of the captopril and metoprolol?

## Diuretics

For mild to moderate hypertension, diuretics, particularly thiazide diuretics, are often first-line drugs. In cases of stage 1 hypertension, diuretics alone may lower blood pressure. When diuretic therapy begins, blood volume and cardiac output decrease. After long-term administration, cardiac output returns to normal, but there is a persistent decrease in peripheral vascular resistance. Authorities have attributed this to a persistent small reduction in extracellular water and plasma volume, decreased receptor sensitivity to vasopressor substances such as angiotensin, direct arteriolar vasodilation, and arteriolar vasodilation secondary to electrolyte depletion in the vessel wall. In hypertension that does not respond to a diuretic alone, the practitioner usually continues the diuretic and adds another antihypertensive drug or tries monotherapy with a different type of antihypertensive drug. Current hypertension management guidelines recommend initial drug therapy with two antihypertensive agents for patients with a blood pressure 20/10 mm Hg above goal, and diuretics are frequently part of this combination. Health care providers prefer diuretics for initial therapy in all people with hypertension but specifically older adults and African Americans. They should be included in any multidrug regimen for these and other populations.

Hydrochlorothiazide is most commonly used, although chlorthalidone reduces cardiovascular events. Diazoxide, usually in parenteral form, is indicated for short-term treatment of malignant hypertension. The selective aldosterone blocker, eplerenone, has demonstrated efficacy in African Americans.

Loop diuretics (e.g., furosemide) or potassium-sparing diuretics (e.g., spironolactone) may be useful in some circumstances. Loop diuretics are indicated in people with renal insufficiency. Potassium-sparing diuretics may precipitate hyperkalemia. Chapter 34 discusses diuretics.

## NCLEX Success

7. A patient with a history of hypertension comes to the emergency department with double vision and a blood pressure of 240/120 mm Hg. The physician on call orders sodium nitroprusside (Nitropress) by continuous infusion, with continual blood pressure monitoring. This drug's immediate action is to lower blood pressure by which of the following mechanisms?

   A. increasing peripheral vascular resistance
   B. increasing cardiac output
   C. dilating venous and arterial vessels
   D. decreasing heart rate

8. A patient in the intensive care unit has been receiving sodium nitroprusside for 2 days. The nurse needs to monitor for which of the following?

   A. thiocyanate toxicity
   B. hyperglycemia
   C. hyperkalemia
   D. metabolic alkalosis

## Unfolding Patient Stories: Mary Richards • Part 2

Think back to Chapter 3, where you met Mary Richards, an 82-year-old African American female who is hospitalized with symptoms of increased weakness and fatigue. She has a history of hypertension and chronic heart failure managed with furosemide, amlodipine, and digoxin. Upon admission, her current medications are discontinued; they will be replaced with hydrochlorothiazide, bisoprolol, and ramipril once she is stable. What are possible explanations for the medication changes? Why is it important for the nurse to understand the rationale for the adjustment? What nursing assessments verify the safe administration of the new medications and evaluate for potential side effects? What assessment findings would indicate to the nurse an improvement in heart failure and satisfactory medication response versus a need for additional or alternative medications?

Care for Mary and other patients in a realistic virtual environment: *vSim for Nursing* (thepoint.lww.com/vSimPharm). Practice documenting these patients' care in DocuCare (thepoint.lww.com/DocuCareEHR).

## THE NURSING PROCESS

A concept map outlining the nursing process related to drug therapy considerations in this chapter is found in the map below. Additional nursing implications related to the disease process should also be considered in care decisions.

**Assessment**
- Assess for conditions and risk factors that may lead to hypertension.
- Assess for the use of oral contraceptives, corticosteroids, appetite suppressants, nasal decongestants, and nonsteroidal anti-inflammatory agents, which may increase blood pressure.
- Assess for signs and symptoms of hypertension.
- Assess blood pressure accurately and repeatedly. As a rule, multiple measurements in which systolic pressure is greater than 140 mm Hg and/or diastolic pressure is greater than 90 mm Hg are necessary to establish a diagnosis of hypertension.

**Outcomes of Therapy**
The patient will
- Maintain drug regimen as ordered.
- Maintain blood pressure in the recommended range.
- Verbalize or demonstrate knowledge of prescribed drugs and recommended lifestyle changes.
- Recognize signs and symptoms that necessitate professional medical intervention.
- Keep follow-up appointments.

**Nursing Interventions**
- Implement measures that aid prevention, early detection, and management of hypertension.
- Support the patient with hypertension to adhere to prescribed therapy (see Box 26.4).
- Reinforce the patient's healthy lifestyle changes and supportive interpersonal relationships. Losing weight, stopping smoking, and other changes are most likely to be effective if attempted one at a time.
- Demonstrate and observe return demonstration of recommended techniques for measuring blood pressure. Proper technique is necessary to ensure that antihypertensive drugs and dosages are not changed on the basis of inaccurate blood pressures.

**Evaluation**
- Observe blood pressure measurement technique and for readings within goal or closer to normal ranges.
- Observe and interview regarding compliance with instructions about drug therapy and lifestyle changes.
- Observe and interview regarding adverse drug effects.

## KEY CONCEPTS

- Hypertension is defined in adults as a systolic pressure greater than 130 mm Hg or a diastolic pressure greater than 80 mm Hg on multiple blood pressure measurements.
- Key behavioral determinants of blood pressure are related to dietary consumption of calories and salt; the prevalence of hypertension rises proportionally to average body mass index and increased intake of salt.
- For patients with elevated blood pressure as well as those with stage 1 and 2 hypertension, current guidelines for hypertension management recommend nonpharmacologic interventions such as lifestyle modifications.
- For patients with stage 1 hypertension, monotherapy with antihypertensive medications is initially recommended.

- For patients with stage 2 hypertension, initial recommendations include combination therapy with two different classes of antihypertensives.
- First-line agents for hypertension management include thiazide diuretics, CCBs, and ACE inhibitors or ARBs.
- Thiazide diuretics reduce blood volume and decreases cardiac output. After long-term administration, cardiac output returns to normal, but there is a persistent decrease in peripheral vascular resistance, which reduces blood pressure.
- CCBs reduce blood pressure by dilating peripheral arteries and decreasing peripheral vascular resistance through relaxation of vascular smooth muscle.

- Long-acting dihydropyridines are most commonly used to treat hypertension. If the nondihydropyridine CCBs (diltiazem, verapamil) are prescribed, the extended-release formulations are often used for hypertension.
- Nifedipine, a short-acting CCB, has been used to treat hypertensive emergencies or urgencies. The capsule should not be punctured as this practice is associated with an increased risk of adverse cardiovascular events precipitated by a rapid and severe decrease in blood pressure.
- ACE inhibitors block the production of angiotensin II, which decreases vasoconstriction (thus having a vasodilating effect), and decrease aldosterone production (thus reducing retention of sodium and water).
- ARBs vasodilate and reduce blood pressure by blocking aldosterone-secreting effects of angiotensin II at various receptor sites and preventing angiotensin II from combining at various receptors sites.
- ACE inhibitors and ARBs are equally effective at controlling blood pressure but should not be used in combination with one another.

- The FDA has issued a **BLACK BOX WARNING** ◆ for ACE inhibitors and ARBs during pregnancy because their use can cause injury and even death to a developing fetus.
- Beta-adrenergic blockers are used to treat hypertension in patients with ischemic heart disease, especially in those with acute coronary syndrome, a recent MI, or heart failure with reduced ejection fraction.
- The FDA has issued a **BLACK BOX WARNING** ◆ for patients with CAD who are withdrawing from oral forms of atenolol, metoprolol, nadolol, propranolol, and timolol. Abrupt withdrawal has resulted in exacerbation of angina, the incidence of ventricular dysrhythmias, and the occurrence of MIs.
- African Americans are more likely to have severe hypertension and require multiple drugs as a result of having low circulating renin, increased salt sensitivity, and a higher incidence of obesity.
- In general, Asian Americans with hypertension require much smaller doses of beta-adrenergic blockers because they metabolize and excrete the drugs slowly.

## CLINICAL REASONING CASE STUDY

**Meet the Patient**

Mrs. Shea, a 54-year-old woman, is seen in her nurse practitioner's office, with a blood pressure of 180/98 and a heart rate of 136. She was diagnosed with hypertension 2 years ago and, until now, she has been controlling her blood pressure with captopril (Capoten) 50 mg orally twice daily. In taking her health history, the nurse learns that Mrs. Shea has recently started taking oral pseudoephedrine for sinus congestion. She tells the nurse, "I don't understand it; I have been taking my blood pressure medication regularly, as always. It has kept my blood pressure under control for 2 years. Why am I having these problems now?" What is the best response by the nurse to explain the relationship between the pseudoephedrine and Mrs. Shea's hypertension?

**Assessing Drug Information**

- Captopril (Capoten)
  - Captopril is an angiotensin-converting enzyme (ACE) inhibitor used as a first-line agent for treating hypertension. It is also used to treat heart failure and diabetic nephropathy.
  - ACE inhibitors such as captopril block the enzyme that normally converts angiotensin I to the potent vasoconstrictor angiotensin II decreasing vasoconstriction (thus having a vasodilating effect) and decreasing aldosterone production (thus reducing retention of sodium and water). In addition, ACE inhibitors also inhibit the breakdown of bradykinin, prolonging its vasodilating effects.
  - Adverse effects include a persistent cough (a major cause of discontinuation of the drug) and the risk of hyperkalemia in patients with diabetes mellitus or renal impairment or who are taking nonsteroidal anti-inflammatory drugs, potassium supplements, or potassium-sparing diuretics. Acute hypotension may occur when captopril is started, especially in patients with fluid volume deficit.
- Pseudoephedrine
  - Pseudoephedrine provides temporary symptomatic relief of nasal congestion due to common cold, upper respiratory allergies, and sinusitis.
  - Pseudoephedrine stimulates alpha receptors, causing vasoconstriction, which increases blood pressure. Pseudoephedrine also stimulates beta receptors, causing increased heart rate, which also increases the speed of conduction. All of these factors increase the heart rate and blood pressure.
  - Beta stimulation can induce adverse effects including cardiac dysrhythmias, increased myocardial oxygen requirement, hyperglycemia, hypokalemia, and hypophosphatemia.
  - The vasoconstriction produced could cause decreased renal perfusion and decreased urinary output and can also increase the risk of a cerebral hemorrhage related to hypertension.

**Nursing Actions**

- Instruct Mrs. Shea about the actions and adverse effects of pseudoephedrine and the importance of not taking over-the-counter medications before checking with her nurse practitioner to find a drug that will help to relieve her congestion while not adversely affecting her blood pressure.
- Verify that Mrs. Shea understands the drug therapy used to treat her hypertension and the nonpharmacologic measures to reduce blood pressure.
- See Box 26.4 for additional patient education guidelines.

*Visit* thePoint *at* **http://thePoint.lww.com/Frandsen12e**
*for answers to NCLEX Success questions (in Appendix A), answers
to Clinical Application Case Studies (in Appendix B), and more!*

## REFERENCES AND RESOURCES

Flynn, J. T., Kaelber, D. C., Baker-Smith, C. M., Blowey, D., Carroll, A. E., Daniels, S. R., et al. (2017). Clinical Practice Guideline for screening and management of high blood pressure in children and adolescents. *Pediatrics, 140*(3).

Gill, V., & Edelman, M. (2012). Pediatric hypertension: A cause for concern. *Nursing, 42*(3), 54–57.

Gupta-Malhotra, M., Banker, A., Shete, S., Hashmi, S. S., Tyson, J. E., Barratt, M. S., et al. (2015). Essential hypertension vs. secondary hypertension among children. *American Journal of Hypertension, 28*(1), 73–80. doi:10.1093/ajh/hpu083

Guyton, A. C., & Hall, J. E. (2011). *Textbook of medical physiology* (12th ed.). Philadelphia, PA: W. B. Saunders.

James, P., Oparil, S., Carter, B., Cushman, W., Dennison-Himmelfarb, C., Handler, J., et al. (2014). 2014 evidence-based guideline for the management of high blood pressure in adults report from the panel members appointed to the Eighth Joint National Committee (JNC 8). *Journal of the American Medical Association, 311*(5), 507–520. doi:10.1001/jama.2013.284427

Karch, A. M. (2018). *2019 Lippincott's pocket drug guide for nurses.* Philadelphia, PA: Lippincott Williams & Wilkins.

Kurtz, T., & Kajiya, T. (2012). Differential pharmacology and benefit/risk of azilsartan compared to other sartans. *Vascular Health Risk Management, 8*, 133–143.

Mann, J., Bakris, G., White, W., & Forman, J. (2018, Sept 19). Choice of drug therapy in primary (essential) hypertension. *Up To Date.* Retrieved from https://www.uptodate.com/contents/choice-of-drug-therapy-in-primary-essential-hypertension?search=hypertension%20treatment%20adult&source=search_result&selectedTitle=1~150&usage_type=default&display_rank=1

Muntner, P., Carey, R., Gidding, S., Jones, D., Taler, S., Wright, J., et al. (2017). Potential U.S. Population Impact of the 2017 American College of Cardiology/American Heart Association High Blood Pressure Guideline. *Journal of the American College of Cardiology,* doi:10.1016/j.jacc.2017.10.073

Norris, T. (2019). *Porth's pathophysiology: Concepts of altered health status* (10th ed.). Philadelphia, PA: Lippincott Williams & Wilkins.

Whelton, P. K., Carey, R. M., Aronow, W. S., Casey, D. E., Collins, K. J., Dennison Himmelfarb, C., et al. (2018). 2017 ACC/AHA/AAPA/ABC/ACPM/AGS/APhA/ASH/ASPC/NMA/PCNA guideline for the prevention, detection, evaluation, and management of high blood pressure in adults: A report of the American College of Cardiology/American Heart Association Task Force on Clinical Practice Guidelines. *Circulation, 138,* 484–e594. doi:10.1161/CIR.0000000000000596

# Drug Therapy for Dysrhythmias

## LEARNING OBJECTIVES

*After studying this chapter, you should be able to:*

1. Discuss the specific cardiac dysrhythmias in terms of their clinical significance, effect on normal cardiac electrophysiology, and alteration in cardiac function.
2. Describe the principles of therapy in the management of dysrhythmias, including measures that do not involve antidysrhythmic drugs.
3. Identify the prototype and describe the action, use, adverse effects, contraindications, and nursing implications for class I sodium channel blockers.
4. Recognize the prototype and outline the action, use, adverse effects, contraindications, and nursing implications for beta-adrenergic blockers.
5. Identify the prototype and explain the action, use, adverse effects, contraindications, and nursing implications for potassium channel blockers.
6. Identify the prototype and describe the action, use, adverse effects, contraindications, and nursing implications for calcium channel blockers.
7. Classify the drugs used in the management of emergency resuscitation.
8. Implement the nursing process when caring for patients who use selected antidysrhythmic drugs.

## CLINICAL APPLICATION CASE STUDY

Marjorie Johnson, a 62-year-old woman with a history of hypertension, goes to her primary health care provider complaining of fatigue and the sensation of her heart beating fast. Her primary care provider refers her to the emergency department, and she is admitted to the hospital with atrial fibrillation—a rate of 110 to 120 beats/minute.

## KEY TERMS

**Antidysrhythmic:** medication used for prevention and treatment of a cardiac dysrhythmia

**Automaticity:** ability of the heart to generate an electrical impulse

**Bradydysrhythmia:** dysrhythmia of less than 60 beats/minute

**Chronotropic:** influencing the rate of impulse formation

**Conductivity:** ability of the cardiac tissue to transmit electrical impulses

**Dysrhythmia:** abnormality in formation or conduction (or both) of electrical impulse in the heart affecting heart rate and/or rhythm

**Ectopic:** when an electrical impulse arises from an abnormal focus, anywhere other than the sinoatrial node

**Excitability:** ability of a cardiac muscle cell to respond to an electrical stimulus

**Paroxysmal supraventricular tachycardia:** episodic burst of a rapid heart rate that originates in a part of the heart above the ventricles

**Prodysrhythmic effect:** tendency of antidysrhythmic drugs to cause the development of new dysrhythmias

**Sinus rhythm:** electrical activity of the heart initiated by the sinoatrial node

**Tachydysrhythmia:** dysrhythmia of greater than 100 beats/minute

# INTRODUCTION

This chapter discusses the **antidysrhythmic** agents, the medications that are used for prevention and treatment of cardiac dysrhythmias. A **dysrhythmia** is an abnormality in heart rate or rhythm. It can become significant if it interferes with cardiac function, thereby altering the ability to adequately pump and causing inadequate perfusion of the body tissues.

# OVERVIEW OF DYSRHYTHMIAS

## Physiology

To aid in understanding antidysrhythmic drug therapy, it is necessary to review the physiology of the cardiac electrophysiologic conduction system. The heart is an electrical pump. The "electrical" activity resides primarily in the specialized myocardial tissues that can generate and conduct an electrical impulse. The mechanical or "pump" activity resides in contractile tissue. Normally, the synchronization of these activities results in effective cardiac contraction and distribution of blood throughout the body. Each heartbeat occurs at regular intervals and consists of four events: stimulation from an electrical impulse, transmission of the electrical impulse to adjacent conductive or contractile tissue, contraction of atria and then ventricles, and then relaxation of atria and then ventricles. Certain properties are inherent in myocardial cells that allow them to generate an electrical impulse. These properties are automaticity, excitability, and conductivity.

### Automaticity and Excitability

**Automaticity** is the heart's ability to generate an electrical impulse. Any part of the conduction system can spontaneously start an impulse, but the sinoatrial (SA) node normally has the fastest rate of automaticity and therefore the faster rate of spontaneous impulse formation.

Initiation of an electrical impulse depends predominately on the movement of sodium and calcium ions into a myocardial cell and movement of potassium ions out of the cell. Normally, the cell membrane becomes more permeable to sodium and opens certain channels to allow rapid movement of sodium into the cell. Calcium ions follow sodium ions into the cell at a slower rate and through different channels. As sodium and calcium ions move into cells, potassium ions move out of cells. The movement of the ions changes the membrane from its resting state of electrical neutrality to an activated state of electrical energy buildup. After the electrical energy is discharged (depolarization), muscle contraction occurs. The ease in which cardiac cells respond to this series of events is called cardiac **excitability**. The

greater the cardiac excitability, the more receptive the myocardial cells are to the conduction of the electrical impulse.

### Conductivity

**Conductivity** is the ability of cardiac tissue to transmit electrical impulses. The orderly, rhythmic transmission of impulses to all cells is needed for effective myocardial contraction. The cardiac conduction system is shown in Figure 27.1. Normally, electrical impulses originate in the SA node and are transmitted through internodal pathways to the atrioventricular (AV) node, where the impulse is delayed for a brief period. Then, the impulse travels through the bundle of His, bundle branches, Purkinje fibers, and throughout the ventricular muscle.

## Etiology

Cardiac dysrhythmias originate in any part of the conduction system or in atrial or ventricular muscle. They result from disturbances in electrical impulse formation (automaticity), conduction (conductivity), or both. The inherent characteristic of automaticity allows myocardial cells other than the SA node to depolarize and initiate the electrical impulse that culminates in contraction. This may occur when the SA node fails to initiate an impulse or does so at a slower rate than another conduction

**Figure 27.1.** The conducting system of the heart. Impulses originating in the sinoatrial [SA] node are transmitted through the atria, into the atrioventricular [AV] node to the bundle of His, and by way of Purkinje fibers through the ventricles. [Reprinted with permission from Hinkle, J. L., & Cheever, K. H. [2018]. *Brunner & Suddarth's textbook of medical-surgical nursing* [14th ed., Fig. 25-3, p. 676]. Philadelphia, PA: Wolters Kluwer Health | Lippincott Williams & Wilkins.]

focus in the heart. When the electrical impulse arises anywhere other than the SA node, the conduction focus is abnormal or ectopic. If the SA node fails to initiate an impulse, automaticity enables other myocardial cells to assume impulse generation. The impulse generation of alternate pacemaker sites with an SA node failure often results in **bradydysrhythmias**. If the ectopic focus depolarizes at a rate faster than the SA node, the ectopic focus becomes the dominant pacemaker. In many cases, an ectopic pacemaker overriding the SA node results in a **tachydysrhythmia**. Conditions such as hypoxia, ischemia, or hypokalemia may activate ectopic pacemakers. Ectopic foci indicate myocardial irritability, which can increase responsiveness to stimuli, leading to potentially serious impairment of cardiac function. Atrial fibrillation is the most common sustained dysrhythmia.

## Pathophysiology

Dysrhythmias may be clinically significant if they interfere with mechanical cardiac function and thus alter the heart's ability to pump sufficient blood to body tissues. Dysrhythmias affect the rate and rhythm of contraction, which can have a direct impact on cardiac output. The normal heart can maintain an adequate cardiac output with ventricular rates ranging from 40 to 150 beats/minute. The diseased heart, however, may not be able to maintain an adequate cardiac output with heart rates below 60 or above 120 beats/minute. These alterations in rates are referred to as dysrhythmias, which are usually categorized by rate, location, or patterns of conduction. Tachydysrhythmias are heart rates greater than 100 beats/minute. Bradydysrhythmias are those less than 60 beats/minute. Atropine, which is used to treat bradydysrhythmias, is discussed in Chapter 48, and digoxin, which is used to treat atrial fibrillation, is discussed in Chapter 30. Box 27.1 describes various types of dysrhythmias.

## Clinical Manifestations

Dysrhythmias may be asymptomatic or symptomatic. Mild or infrequent dysrhythmias may be perceived by the patient as palpitations or skipped heartbeats. More severe dysrhythmias may produce the following manifestations, which reflect decreased cardiac output and other hemodynamic changes:

- Hypotension, bradycardia or tachycardia, and irregular rhythm.
- Shortness of breath, dyspnea, and cough from impaired respiration.
- Syncope or mental confusion from reduced cerebral blood flow.
- Chest pain from decreased coronary artery blood flow. Angina pectoris or myocardial infarction may trigger a dysrhythmia or occur as result of a dysrhythmia.
- Oliguria from decreased renal blood flow.

## Nonpharmacologic Management

Management without the use of drugs may be preferable, at least initially, for several dysrhythmias. For example, sinus tachycardia usually results from such disorders as dehydration, fever, infection, or hypotension, and intervention and management should attempt to relieve the underlying cause. For **paroxysmal**

**supraventricular tachycardia** (episodic bursts of a rapid heart rate that originates in a part of the heart above the ventricles) with mild or moderate symptoms, Valsalva maneuver or other measures to increase vagal tone are preferred. For unstable patients with atrial tachycardia, immediate synchronized or unsynchronized cardioversion is the initial treatment for emergent rhythm management. For ventricular fibrillation, immediate defibrillation is the initial management of choice.

In addition to these strategies, use of other measures is increasing. The impetus for nonpharmacologic management developed mainly from studies demonstrating that antidysrhythmic drugs could worsen existing dysrhythmias, cause new dysrhythmias, and cause higher mortality rates in patients receiving the drugs than patients not receiving the drugs. Current technology allows clinicians to insert pacemakers and defibrillators (e.g., implantable cardioverter–defibrillators) to control bradydysrhythmias or tachydysrhythmias and to use radio waves (radiofrequency catheter ablation) or surgery to deactivate ectopic foci.

## Drug Therapy

All drugs used to combat dysrhythmias alter the electrical conduction system of the heart. The drugs used for the treatment of tachydysrhythmias are the focus of this chapter. They reduce automaticity, which is the spontaneous depolarization of myocardial cells, including ectopic pacemakers. They also slow conduction of electrical impulses through the heart and prolong the refractory period of myocardial cells so they are less likely to be prematurely activated by adjacent cells. Antidysrhythmic drug therapy is commonly indicated in the following conditions:

- Conversion of atrial fibrillation or atrial flutter to normal **sinus rhythm** (NSR).
- Maintaining NSR after electrical conversion from atrial fibrillation or atrial flutter.
- Suppression of a fast or irregular ventricular rate, which alters the cardiac output. Altered cardiac output leads to symptoms of decreased coronary, cerebral, and/or systemic circulation.
- Presence of dangerous dysrhythmias that may be fatal if not quickly terminated. For example, ventricular tachycardia may cause cardiac arrest.

The clinical use of antidysrhythmic drugs for tachydysrhythmias has changed over the years. Clinicians use drugs not just to suppress dysrhythmias but to prevent or relieve symptoms or prolong survival. Symptoms may manifest as chest pain, shortness of breath, anxiety, palpitations, or racing heart. This change resulted from study outcomes in which patients treated for some dysrhythmias had a higher mortality rate than patients who did not receive antidysrhythmic drug therapy. Researchers attributed the higher mortality rate to **prodysrhythmic effects**, which are those effects that worsen existing dysrhythmias or cause new dysrhythmias.

Many of the agents used to treat dysrhythmias do in fact produce prodysrhythmic effects. Thus, rational drug therapy for a cardiac dysrhythmia requires accurate identification of the dysrhythmia, understanding of the basic mechanisms causing the dysrhythmia, observation of the hemodynamic and electrocardiogram (ECG) effects of the dysrhythmia, knowledge of the pharmacologic actions of specific antidysrhythmic drugs, and

| BOX 27.1 | *Types of Dysrhythmias* |
|---|---|

Sinus bradycardia

Sinus tachycardia

Atrial flutter

*A lot P wave firing - but not conductive though*

Atrial fibrillation

Premature ventricular contraction

↑ PVC

Ventricular tachycardia

*Electricity coming from ventricles*

Ventricular fibrillation

*emergency*

BUFFALO  NEW YORK                                   PRIN

Asystole

*emergency*

the expectation that therapeutic effects will outweigh potential adverse effects. Even when these criteria are met, antidysrhythmic drug therapy is somewhat empiric.

Several different groups of drugs function as antidysrhythmics. They are classified according to their mechanisms of action and effects on the conduction system, even though they differ in other respects. Some drugs have characteristics of more than one group and may influence myocardial function beyond just conduction. **Chronotropic** medications affect heart rate. Inotropic medications affect the force of myocardial contractility. There are various types of antidysrhythmics: class I sodium channel blockers, class II beta-adrenergic blockers, class III potassium channel blockers, and class IV calcium channel blockers (Table 27.1).

## CLASS I SODIUM CHANNEL BLOCKERS

Class I drugs block cardiac sodium channels and slow conduction velocity, prolonging refractoriness and decreasing automaticity of sodium-dependent tissue. This results in a membrane-stabilizing effect and also decreases formation and conduction of electrical impulses. Within the category of class I drugs are subcategories, the class IA, class IB, and class IC medications.

## CLASS IA

The prototype class IA drug is **quinidine**. Quinidine is one of the most extensively researched class IA antidysrhythmic agents, but its use has declined as other drug classes are both more effective and safer. Table 27.2 presents dosages for quinidine and the other class IA sodium channel blockers.

## Pharmacokinetics

Quinidine is well absorbed after oral administration, with a usual onset of 1 to 3 hours. After intramuscular (IM) administration, onset occurs within 30 to 90 minutes, and after intravenous (IV) administration, the onset is rapid. Therapeutic serum levels (2–5 mcg/mL) are attained within 1 hour and persist for 6 to 8 hours. Note that measurements of levels vary with analytical

## TABLE 27.1

### Drugs Administered for the Treatment of Dysrhythmias

| Class of Antidysrhythmic Drug | Prototype | Other Drugs in the Class | Use |
|---|---|---|---|
| **Class I Sodium Channel Blockers** | | | |
| Class IA | Quinidine | Procainamide<br>Disopyramide (Norpace) | Maintenance of normal sinus rhythm after conversion of A-fib or atrial flutter; treatment of symptomatic PVCs, SVT, and VT; prevention of V-fib |
| Class IB | Lidocaine (Xylocaine) | | Treatment of symptomatic PVCs and VT; prevention of V-fib |
| Class IC | | Flecainide<br>Propafenone (Rythmol SR) | Treatment of life-threatening VT or V-fib and SVT unresponsive to other drugs; maintenance of sinus rhythm |
| **Class II Beta-Adrenergic Blockers** | | | |
| | Propranolol (Inderal LA) | Acebutolol<br>Esmolol<br>Sotalol (Betapace, Sorine, Sotylize) | Treatment of SVT |
| **Class III Potassium Channel Blockers** | | | |
| | Amiodarone (Nexterone, Pacerone) | Dofetilide (Tikosyn)<br>Dronedarone (Multaq)<br>Ibutilide (Corvert)<br>Sotalol (Betapace, Sorine, Sotylize) | Treatment of VT and V-fib; conversion of atrial flutter or A-fib to sinus rhythm; maintenance of sinus rhythm |
| **Class IV Calcium Channel Blockers** | | | |
| | Diltiazem (Cardizem, Cardizem CD, Cardizem LA, Tiazac) | Verapamil (Calan, Calan SR, Verelan, Verelan PM) | Treatment of SVT |
| **Unclassified** | | | |
| | | Adenosine (Adenocard)<br>Magnesium sulfate | Treatment of tachydysrhythmias; SVT<br>Treatment of torsades de pointes |

A-fib, atrial fibrillation; PVC, premature ventricular contraction; SVT, supraventricular tachycardia; V-fib, ventricular fibrillation; VT, ventricular tachycardia.

| TABLE 27.2 |
| :--- |
| **DRUGS AT A GLANCE: Class I Sodium Channel Blockers** |

| Drug | Pregnancy Category | Routes and Dosage Ranges | |
| :--- | :--- | :--- | :--- |
| | | **Adults** | **Children** |
| Class IA **Quinidine** (Apo-Quinidine, Quinate, Novo-Quinidin) | C | PO 200–400 mg every 6–8 h, or extended-action tablets, 300–600 mg every 8–12 h | PO 30 mg/kg/24 h in four equally divided doses every 6 h; IV (not recommended) 2–10 mg/kg/dose IV every 3–6 h |
| Procainamide (Apo-Procainamide, Procan SR) | C | PO maintenance dose of 50 mg/kg/d in divided doses every 6 h, 10–17 mg/kg at a rate of 25–50 mg/min (max dose 1 g) IV maintenance infusion 1–4 mg/min | PO 15–50 mg/kg/d in three to six divided doses every 3–6 h, maximum, 4 g/d IM 20–30 mg/kg/d divided every 4–6 h; maximum 4 g/d IV/IO loading dose 10–15 mg/kg over 30–60 min; maintenance dose of 20–80 mcg/kg/min continuous infusion; max 100 mg/d dose or 2 g/d; or 15 mg/kg given over 30–60 min, followed by maintenance infusion |
| Disopyramide (Norpace, Norpace CR; Rythmodan) | C | PO loading dose 200–300 mg (immediate release), maintenance dose 100–300 mg every 6 h depending on patient response | 12–18 y: PO 6–15 mg/kg/d in four equal divided doses 5–12 y: PO 10–15 mg/kg/d in four equal divided doses 1–4 y: PO 10–20 mg/kg/d in four equal divided doses <1 y: PO 10–30 mg/kg/d in four equal divided doses |
| Class IB **Lidocaine** (Xylocaine; Xylocaine, Xylocard) | B | IV (pulseless ventricular fibrillation or ventricular tachycardia) 1–1.5 mg/kg IV bolus; repeat 0.5–0.75 mg/kg every 5 to 10 min to max dose of 3 mg/kg IV infusion (with return of pulse) 1–4 mg/min (or 20–50 mcg/kg/min) | Safety and efficacy have not been established IV/IO loading dose 1 mg/kg bolus, followed by IV infusion of 20–50 mcg/kg/min with caution |
| Class IC Flecainide (Apo-Flecainide, Tambocor) | C | PO 50 mg every 12 h initially, increased by 50 mg every 12 h every 4 d until effective or reach maximum dose, 400 mg/d | Safety and efficacy in patients younger than 18 y have not been established |
| Propafenone (Rythmol SR; Apo-Propafenone, Rythmol) | C | PO 150 mg every 8 h initially, increase at 3–4 d intervals to 225 mg every 8 h, and then to 300 mg every 8 h; maximum dose of 900 mg/d PO (extended release) 225 mg every 12 h initially may increase at 5-d intervals; maximum 425 mg every 12 h | Safety and efficacy not established |

IO, intraosseous.

method used. Toxic symptoms are seen with serum levels greater than 8 mcg/mL. Quinidine is highly bound to serum albumin and has a half-life of about 6 to 7 hours. It is metabolized by the liver (about 80%) and excreted in the urine (about 20%) as well as the feces. In alkaline urine (i.e., pH > 7), renal excretion of quinidine decreases, and serum levels may rise.

## Action

Quinidine reduces automaticity and slows conduction throughout the cardiac system through direct and indirect anticholinergic effect on cardiac tissue, reducing myocardial contractility. In addition, it prolongs the refractory period of the myocardial cells.

## Use

Indications for quinidine include the treatment of (1) atrial dysrhythmias and (2) paroxysmal supraventricular tachycardia or chronic ventricular tachycardia without heart block. However, the drug is usually contraindicated in patients with severe, uncompensated heart failure or with heart block because it depresses myocardial contractility and conduction through the AV node. The U.S. Food and Drug Administration (FDA) has issued a **BLACK BOX WARNING ◆** for quinidine and other class 1A drugs (procainamide and disopyramide) because of their known prodysrhythmic properties; the drugs should be reserved for patients with life-threatening ventricular dysrhythmias. In clinical trials, the use of these drugs in individuals with non–life-threatening dysrhythmias has increased mortality, particularly in patients with structural heart disease.

### Use in Children

Pediatric patients take quinidine in the oral form. Although the IV route may be used, it is not recommended.

### Use in Older Adults

There are no recommendations for precautions regarding the use of quinidine in older adults. However, because of the likelihood that aging may result in renal and hepatic problems, precautions regarding the use of quinidine in older patients should be considered.

### Use in Patients With Renal Impairment

Reduced dosages of quinidine are necessary, with close monitoring. Caution is necessary, especially in patients with renal tubular acidosis.

### Use in Patients With Hepatic Impairment

Hepatic impairment increases the plasma half-life of several antidysrhythmic drugs, including quinidine, and patients with hepatic impairment usually receive a reduced dosage. Close monitoring is essential. In addition, caution is warranted, especially in patients with hepatic insufficiency.

### Use in Patients With Critical Illness

Critically ill patients often have multiple cardiovascular disorders as well as other conditions that increase the risk of acute, serious, and potentially life-threatening dysrhythmias. Patients may also have refractory dysrhythmias that require strong, potentially toxic antidysrhythmic drugs. Thus, antidysrhythmic drugs are often given intravenously in critical care settings for rapid reversal of a fast rhythm. After reversal, transitioning from IV drugs to oral ones is often necessary to prevent recurrence of the dysrhythmia. Frequently, potentials for renal and/or hepatic involvement are greater in patients who are critically ill. It is important to monitor responses to quinidine carefully, especially when beginning therapy.

### Use in Patients Receiving Home Care

Patients receiving chronic antidysrhythmic drug therapy are likely to have significant cardiovascular disease. At each visit to the home, the nurse assesses the patient's physical, mental, and functional status and evaluates pulse and blood pressure. In addition, he or she also instructs patients and caregivers to report symptoms (e.g., dizziness or fainting, chest pain) and avoid over-the-counter agents unless approved by a health care provider.

## Adverse Effects

Adverse effects of quinidine include central nervous system (CNS) changes, cardiac dysrhythmias, and gastrointestinal (GI) changes, as well as hematologic and hypersensitivity alterations. CNS changes include weakness, dizziness, headache, and fatigue. Cardiac dysrhythmias include conduction disturbances, including heart block and hypotension. GI effects include nausea, vomiting, diarrhea, and liver toxicity. Visual disturbances may also occur.

## Contraindications

Quinidine is contraindicated in patients with an allergy to the drug. It is also contraindicated in second- or third-degree heart block, prolonged QT syndrome, myasthenia gravis, pregnancy, lactation, and thrombocytopenic purpura.

## Nursing Implications

Prior to the start of any new therapy, it is necessary to assess for allergies, second- or third-degree heart block, prolonged QT syndrome, myasthenia gravis, pregnancy, lactation, and thrombocytopenic purpura. Physical assessment includes inspection of the skin for color and the presence of lesions, determination of orientation status, assessment of cranial nerves, determination of bilateral grip strength and reflexes, auscultation of pulse and blood pressure, interpretation of the ECG, checking for edema, and auscultation of bowel sounds. It is also necessary to evaluate hepatic and renal function as well as to perform a urinalysis and complete blood count. The findings of the physical assessment as well as results of the laboratory work and diagnostic tests help develop the nursing plan of care for the patient who is beginning sodium channel blocker therapy.

### Preventing Interactions

Preventing drug–drug and drug–food interactions requires knowledge of potential effects. Several medications interact with quinidine, increasing or decreasing its effect (Box 27.2). Use of quinidine with certain other drugs has specific results. Caution is warranted when using quinidine with concurrent antiarrhythmic medications. With succinylcholine, neuromuscular blocking effects may increase. With digoxin, increased digoxin level and toxicity result. With oral anticoagulants, anticoagulant effect increases, and bleeding may occur. Also, changes in dietary salt intake may alter the rate and extent of quinidine absorption. In addition, grapefruit juice, when given with quinidine, decreases the drug's metabolism and increases the risk of toxic drug effects. Ingesting large amounts of fruit juice or vitamin C may decrease urine pH, which increases the drug's clearance and results in decreased serum concentration.

### Administering the Medication

Two salt formulations of quinidine (gluconate and sulfate) are available. The oral preparations cannot be substituted on a milligram-per-milligram basis because of differences in the availability of the quinidine base. Oral preparations should be administered around the clock to maintain a constant serum level and with food or milk to minimize GI irritation. When administering quinidine in the IV form (gluconate), preparation includes diluting 800 mg in 50 mL of 5% dextrose. With an IV infusion, it is necessary to inject the quinidine slowly at a rate of 1 mL/minute. The nurse should note that if Y-site administration is needed, quinidine is not compatible with furosemide.

## BOX 27.2 — *Drug Interactions: Quinidine*

**Drugs That Increase the Effects of Quinidine**
- Cimetidine, amiodarone, verapamil, colchicine, conivaptan, darunavir, diltiazem, erythromycin
  *Increase the risk of possible quinidine toxicity*

**Drugs That Decrease the Effects of Quinidine**
- Sodium bicarbonate and sucralfate
  *Increase cardiac depressant effects*
- Phenobarbital, hydantoins, rifampin, and sucralfate
  *Decrease the serum levels of quinidine, leading to dysrhythmias*

### Assessing for Therapeutic Effects

The nurse assesses for improvement in symptoms and for return of an organized cardiac rhythm. Physical assessment includes inspection of the skin for adequate color and perfusion, clear mentation, and pulse and blood pressure within the patient's normal limits. It is also necessary to evaluate the adequacy of hepatic and renal function through laboratory testing.

### Assessing for Adverse Effects

The nurse monitors patients who are taking quinidine for adverse effects. Physical assessment of the body systems that are potentially affected by the action of quinidine provides this surveillance. Of particular concern are the CNS, cardiac, GI, and hematologic systems, as well as possible hypersensitivity. It is necessary to determine whether adverse effects, particularly diarrhea and other kinds of GI distress, the most frequently reported adverse problems, are manageable and are not complicating treatment.

### Patient Teaching

Quinidine, like any other drug, should be taken exactly as prescribed. Sustained-release tablets should not be chewed. If GI upset occurs, then the medication may be taken with food or milk. The nurse reinforces to the patient that frequent cardiac monitoring and blood tests are important for follow-up; these include regular checks of heart rhythm and blood counts. The additional patient teaching guidelines presented in Box 27.3 are important.

## Other Drugs in the Class

Procainamide and disopyramide (Norpace) have less prodysrhythmic properties than quinidine, but the FDA has issued a **BLACK BOX WARNING** ◆ for both drugs because of their known prodysrhythmic properties that can occur at normal plasma concentrations. As with quinidine, the drugs should be reserved for patients with life-threatening ventricular dysrhythmias because of the lack of evidence of improved survival with their use in patients without life-threatening dysrhythmias.

Procainamide produces drug-induced dysrhythmias, including prolongation of the QT interval, usually in relationship

## BOX 27.3 — *Patient Teaching Guidelines for Antidysrhythmic Drugs*

- A fast heartbeat normally occurs in response to exercise, fever, and other conditions so that more blood can be pumped and carried to body tissues. An irregular heartbeat occurs occasionally in most people. However, when your health care provider prescribes a long-term medication to slow or regularize your heartbeat, this means that you have a potentially serious condition. In addition, the medications can cause potentially serious adverse effects. So, it is extremely important that you take the medications exactly as prescribed. Taking extra doses is dangerous; skipping doses or waiting longer between doses may lead to loss of control of the heart problem.
- Report dizziness or fainting spells to your health care provider. This may mean the medication is decreasing your heart rate or blood pressure too much, which is more likely to occur when starting or increasing the dose of an antidysrhythmic drug. Drug dosages may need to be adjusted.
- Report any change in vision and complaints of nausea or vomiting, sun sensitivity, tremors, or loss of coordination to your health care provider. In addition, report unusual bleeding or bruising, fever, chills, intolerance to heat or cold, shortness of breath, difficulty breathing, cough, swelling of ankles or fingers, palpitation, or difficulty with vision.
- You may be given a drug classified as an antidysrhythmic or a drug from another group that has antidysrhythmic effects (e.g., a beta-adrenergic blocker such as propranolol, a calcium channel blocker such as diltiazem or verapamil). Follow the instructions for the specific drug ordered.
- Be sure you know the names (generic and brand) of the medication, why you are receiving it, and what effects you can expect (therapeutic and adverse).
- You will need continued medical supervision, along with periodic measurements of heart rate and blood pressure, blood tests, and electrocardiograms. Be sure to keep all health care appointments.
- Try to learn the triggers for your irregular heartbeats and avoid them when possible (e.g., excessive caffeinated beverages, strenuous or excessive exercise).
- Avoid over-the-counter cold and asthma remedies, appetite suppressants, and antisleep preparations, which are all stimulants that can cause or aggravate irregular heartbeats.
- Take or give medications at evenly spaced intervals to maintain adequate blood levels. Take your medications at the same time each day.
- Take amiodarone and quinidine with food to decrease gastrointestinal symptoms.
- Do not crush or chew sustained-release tablets or capsules.
- Do not drink grapefruit juice if you are taking quinidine because it decreases the metabolism of quinidine and increases the risk of toxic effects.
- Wear a medical alert tag if recommended stating the health condition you have or the medications you are taking.

to the plasma procainamide concentration. It also results in torsades de pointes and other polymorphic ventricular tachycardias. This and the frequency of adverse effects, including a lupus-like syndrome and the development of potentially severe bone marrow toxicity, limit the drug's use. In fact, the out-of-hospital administration of procainamide in cardiac arrest because of ventricular fibrillation or pulseless ventricular tachycardia has been associated with more pharmacologic management, more shocks, longer resuscitation times, and lower survival.

The use of disopyramide (Norpace) has decreased with the availability of newer drugs with less toxicity. In addition, disopyramide is a substrate of CYP3A4, part of the cytochrome P450; therefore, numerous clinically significant drug interactions are known to occur.

## CLASS IB

Class IB drugs shorten the repolarization phase. **Lidocaine** (Xylocaine), the prototype class IB drug, is used to treat serious ventricular dysrhythmias associated with acute myocardial infarction, cardiac catheterization, cardiac surgery, and digitalis-induced ventricular dysrhythmias. It decreases myocardial irritability (automaticity) in the ventricles by increasing the electrical stimulation threshold of ventricular myocardial cells. Lidocaine has little effect on atrial tissue and thus is not useful in treating atrial dysrhythmias. The drug differs from quinidine in that it must be given by injection, does not decrease AV conduction with usual therapeutic doses, and has a rapid onset and short duration of action. After IV administration of a bolus dose, therapeutic effects occur within 1 to 2 minutes and last approximately 10 to 20 minutes. This characteristic is advantageous in emergency management but limits the use of lidocaine to intensive care settings. Lidocaine is metabolized in the liver; thus, dosage must be reduced in patients with hepatic insufficiency or right-sided heart failure to avoid drug accumulation and toxicity. Serious adverse reactions with lidocaine are uncommon.

Therapeutic serum levels of lidocaine are 1.5 to 5 mcg/mL. Toxic serum levels are greater than 5 mcg/mL. Lidocaine is contraindicated in patients allergic to related local anesthetics (e.g., procaine). Anaphylactic reactions may occur in sensitized persons. Give lidocaine parenterally only as solutions labeled "for cardiac dysrhythmias," and do not use solutions containing epinephrine. Give an IV bolus over 2 minutes. Table 27.2 provides information about the dosages of lidocaine and related drugs.

---

### ⚠ QSEN Alert: Safety

Lidocaine solutions that contain epinephrine are for local anesthesia only. It is essential that epinephrine-containing lidocaine solutions never be given intravenously to patients with cardiac dysrhythmias because the epinephrine can cause or aggravate dysrhythmias. Rapid injection of lidocaine (within ~30 seconds) produces transient blood levels several times greater than therapeutic range limits. Therefore, there is an increased risk of toxicity without a concomitant increase in therapeutic effectiveness.

---

## CLASS IC

Class IC drugs have no effect on the repolarization phase but slow conduction velocity and the refractory period. Flecainide and propafenone (Rythmol SR) are oral agents that greatly

decrease conduction in the ventricles. These drugs may cause new dysrhythmias or aggravate preexisting dysrhythmias, sometimes causing sustained ventricular tachycardia or ventricular fibrillation. Thus, it is necessary to begin therapy in a hospital setting in patients with continuous ECG monitoring. The new or aggravated dysrhythmias are more likely to occur with high doses and rapid dose increases. Table 27.2 presents dosage information for these drugs.

Flecainide or propafenone may be used to suppress paroxysmal atrial flutter and fibrillation in patients with minimal or no heart disease. These class IC drugs are recommended for use in life-threatening ventricular dysrhythmias. The FDA has issued two **BLACK BOX WARNING ◆** for flecainide:

- Drug treatment increases the risk of nonfatal cardiac arrest and death in patients with recent myocardial infarction or chronic atrial fibrillation.
- It is necessary to monitor carefully for a risk of potentially fatal prodysrhythmic effects.

---

### NCLEX Success

1. A nurse is monitoring a patient who has been receiving quinidine in the critical care unit. The laboratory technician calls to report that the patient's serum quinidine level is 8 mcg/mL. The patient has also developed diarrhea. The priority action is to

   A. report the findings to the provider immediately
   B. administer the medication as ordered
   C. anticipate that the dosage of the medication will increase
   D. anticipate that the dosage of the medication will decrease

2. Ms. Ferguson, aged 58, is admitted to the coronary care unit for treatment of an acute anterior myocardial infarction. That evening, she experiences frequent episodes of ventricular tachycardia with hypotension. The provider tells the nurse to prepare an IV bolus dose of lidocaine. Why is lidocaine administered intravenously at this time—and not orally?

   A. Lidocaine absorption is too erratic when administered orally.
   B. Lidocaine is inactivated by hydrochloric acid.
   C. Most of an absorbed oral dose of lidocaine undergoes first-pass metabolism in the liver.
   D. The onset of action for oral lidocaine is greater than 8 hours.

---

## CLASS II BETA-ADRENERGIC BLOCKERS

Beta-adrenergic–blocking agents (see Chap. 26) exert antidysrhythmic effects by slowing the stimulation of beta receptors in the heart by the sympathetic nervous system, slowing SA and AV nodal conduction. Blockage of receptors in the SA node and ectopic pacemakers decreases automaticity, and blockage of receptors in the AV node increases the refractory period.

Beta-adrenergic blockers are effective for management of dysrhythmias resulting from excessive sympathetic activity. They are most often used to slow the ventricular rate of contraction in atrial flutter and atrial fibrillation.

Class II beta-adrenergic blockers are being used more extensively because of their effectiveness in reducing mortality in patients following myocardial infarction and heart failure. Reduced mortality may result from the ability of the drugs to prevent ventricular fibrillation. Emerging evidence suggests class II beta-adrenergic blockers reduce the development of atrial fibrillation in patients with heart failure. Propranolol (Inderal LA), the prototype class II drug, may be given orally for chronic therapy to prevent ventricular dysrhythmias, especially those precipitated by exercise. It may be administered intravenously for life-threatening dysrhythmias, including those that occur during anesthesia. Table 27.3 presents dosage information for propranolol and the other class II beta-adrenergic blockers.

## Pharmacokinetics

For the oral route, the onset of action of propranolol is 20 to 30 minutes, with a peak in 60 to 90 minutes and a duration of 6 to 12 hours. For the IV route, the onset of action is immediate, with a peak effect in 1 minute and a duration of more than 4 to 6 hours. The drug is metabolized in the liver, and its half-life is 3 to 5 hours (8–11 hours with the sustained release form of the medication). The drug is excreted in the urine.

## Action

Propranolol competitively blocks beta-adrenergic receptors in the heart and juxtaglomerular apparatus. This action causes a decrease in the influence of the sympathetic nervous system on these tissues and a decrease in the excitability of the heart, cardiac workload, and oxygen consumption. This then causes a release of renin and lowers the blood pressure. In addition, propranolol has a membrane-stabilizing effect that contributes to its antidysrhythmic action.

## Use

Propranolol is used in the treatment of cardiac dysrhythmias, especially supraventricular tachycardia. In addition, it has been found to be effective in the treatment of ventricular tachycardia. Other related cardiac indications for propranolol include hypertension, cardiomyopathy, and angina. The safety and efficacy of

### TABLE 27.3

### DRUGS AT A GLANCE: Class II Beta-Adrenergic Blockers

| Drug | Pregnancy Category | Routes and Dosage Ranges | |
|---|---|---|---|
| | | **Adults** | **Children** |
| **Propranolol** (Hemangeol, Inderal LA; ✸ Hemangiol, Inderal LA) *Beta₁ Beta₂* | C | PO 10–30 mg every 6–8 h; may increase to 40 mg every 6–8 h when rate controlled<br>IV 1–3 mg slow IVP with careful monitoring, not to exceed 1 mg/min; repeat every 2–5 min to a total of 5 mg or max dose of 0.1 mg/kg | PO 0.5–1.0 mg/kg/d in divided doses every 6–8 h to maximum daily dose of 16 mg/kg/d or 60 mg/d; IV 0.01–0.15 mg/kg slow IVP over 10 min; may give second dose in 6–8 h as needed to maximum age-dependent dose |
| Acebutolol (✸ Sectral) *Beta₁* | B | PO 200 mg every 12 h, increased gradually to 600–1200 mg/d in two divided doses | Safety and efficacy not established |
| Esmolol (✸ Brevibloc) *Beta₁* | C | IV loading dose 500 mcg/kg/min over 1 min, followed by a maintenance dose of 50 mcg/kg/min over 4 min. If no response in 5 min, repeat the same loading dose, and increase maintenance doses to 100 mcg/kg/min for 4 min, continue to increase by 50 mcg/kg/min up to 200 mcg/kg/min for 4 min. Once the desired response is attained, stop loading dose and increase infusion by no more than 25 mcg/kg/min. Average maintenance dose 50–200 mcg/kg/min. Infusion administered up to 24; up to 48 h may be well tolerated. Not to exceed 200 mcg/kg/min | IV loading dose 100–500 mcg/kg/min over 1 min, followed by a continuous IV infusion of 25–100 mcg/kg/min. Average maintenance dose 50–500 mcg/kg/min |
| Sotalol (Betapace, Sorine, Sotylize; ✸ Rylosol) *Beta₁ Beta₂* | B | PO 80 mg every 12 h initially, titrated to response; average dose, 240–320 mg daily | ≥2 y with normal renal function PO 30 mg/m² three times daily can titrate to a maximum of 60 mg/m² in hospital for at least 3 d<br>Infants and children <2 y: see manufacturer's instructions |

this drug have not been established in pediatric patients. There are no known precautions regarding administration of propranolol in older adults or in those with renal impairment.

### Use in Children

Propranolol is useful for the treatment of tachydysrhythmias in children. If the drug is administered orally, immediate-release formulations should be given. The dose should be individualized to the patient's response.

### Use in Patients With Hepatic Impairment

As previously stated, propranolol is metabolized in the liver. Therefore, it should be used cautiously with patients with hepatic impairment.

### Use in Patients With Critical Illness

Critically ill patients with cardiovascular disorders have an increased risk of acute, serious, and potentially life-threatening dysrhythmias. Thus, as with quinidine, it is important to monitor responses to propranolol carefully, especially when beginning therapy.

### Use in Patients Receiving Home Care

Patients receiving chronic antidysrhythmic drug therapy are likely to have significant cardiovascular disease. So, as with the administration of quinidine, the nurse assesses patients receiving beta-adrenergic agents both physically and mentally. It is important to assess for alterations in functional status and for changes in pulse and blood pressure.

## Adverse Effects

Some of the known adverse effects to propranolol include allergic reactions, specifically laryngospasm and CNS changes, including sleep disorders, agitation, fatigue, and dizziness. Specific cardiovascular effects are bradycardia, heart failure, cardiac dysrhythmias, SA or AV nodal block, peripheral vascular insufficiency, claudication, stroke, pulmonary edema, and hypotension. In addition, dermatologic, GI, genitourinary, musculoskeletal, and respiratory changes occur. Bronchospasm and laryngospasm are the most serious adverse respiratory effects, particularly in pediatric patients, who warrant careful monitoring.

## Contraindications

Contraindications to the use of propranolol include allergy to beta-adrenergic–blocking agents, sinus bradycardia, sick sinus syndrome, and second- or third-degree heart block. In addition, other contraindications may include cardiogenic shock, heart failure, bronchial asthma, bronchospasm, chronic obstructive pulmonary disease, pregnancy, and lactation.

## Nursing Implications

### Preventing Interactions

The nurse monitors for important drug–drug interactions when a patient is taking propranolol as well as interference with laboratory tests. Several medications interact with propranolol, increasing or decreasing its effect (Box 27.4). Also, concomitant use of propranolol and glycerin leads to prolonged hypoglycemic

---

**BOX 27.4** · **Drug Interactions: Propranolol**

**Drugs That Increase the Effects of Propranolol**
- Verapamil
  *Increases the risk of heart block effect*

**Drugs That Decrease the Effects of Propranolol**
- Indomethacin, ibuprofen, piroxicam, sulindac, and barbiturates
  *Decrease the effects of blocking the beta-adrenergic receptors in the heart; have less influence on the sympathetic nervous system, excitability of the heart, cardiac workload, and oxygen consumption*

---

effects. Additionally, propranolol interferes with glucose tolerance tests and insulin tolerance tests as well as with glaucoma screening tests.

### Administering the Medication

Routes of administration of propranolol (in adults) are oral as well as parenteral. Drug doses significantly differ for oral and parenteral forms; following oral administration, propranolol undergoes first-pass metabolism in the liver and only a portion of the drug reaches systemic circulation. Patients should take the oral form with meals. It is essential that the drug not be discontinued abruptly after long-term therapy; a hypersensitivity to catecholamines may have developed, exacerbating ventricular dysrhythmias. The FDA has issued a **BLACK BOX WARNING ◆** for propranolol and other beta-adrenergic blockers, stating that abrupt discontinuation of the drug can exacerbate cardiac ischemia, thus increasing the risk of angina pectoris and myocardial infarction. Gradual tapering over a 2-week period, with patient monitoring, is necessary.

### Assessing for Therapeutic Effects

After the nurse administers propranolol, he or she monitors the patient until it is determined that the dysrhythmia has resolved. If the patient has received the maximum amount of beta-adrenergic medication and the dysrhythmia persists, use of another pharmacologic agent may be necessary.

### Assessing for Adverse Effects

Allergic reaction, including laryngospasm, is one adverse effect. Cardiovascular effects include bradycardia, heart failure, cardiac dysrhythmias, SA or AV nodal block, peripheral vascular insufficiency, claudication, stroke, pulmonary edema, and hypotension. ECG changes to watch for include heart rates less than 60 beats/minute, abnormal heart rhythms, or heart blocks (first-, second-, or third-degree) and/or sinus exit blocks. Other adverse effects relate to the dermatologic, GI, genitourinary, and respiratory systems.

### Patient Teaching

The nurse instructs patients to take propranolol with meals. It is important that patients report night cough, swelling of the extremities, slow pulse, confusion, depression, rash, fever, or sore throat to the prescriber. Patients need to realize that they should not stop taking propranolol abruptly because this action can cause the dysrhythmia to worsen. In addition, the nurse should inform patients with diabetes mellitus that propranolol may mask the normal signs of hypoglycemia (e.g., cool, clammy skin; tachycardia); it is necessary to monitor blood or urine glucose carefully. Box 27.3 presents some patient teaching considerations for propranolol and other antidysrhythmics.

## Other Drugs in the Class

Acebutolol is a class II beta-adrenergic blocker used in the treatment of ventricular dysrhythmias and hypertension. The onset of beta-blockade action is 1 to 2 hours following oral administration. The drug's duration of action is 12 to 24 hours. Acebutolol undergoes extensive first-pass metabolism and is excreted in the feces and urine.

Esmolol is a short-acting class II beta-adrenergic blocker with $beta_1$ selectivity approved for the treatment of supraventricular tachycardia and atrial fibrillation/flutter. When given intravenously, the onset of beta-blockade is 2 to 10 minutes. The duration of hemodynamic effect of the drug is 10 to 30 minutes. Esmolol is metabolized and is excreted in the urine.

Sotalol (Betapace, Sorine, Sotylize), which is discussed in detail in the section on potassium channel blockers, has both beta-adrenergic–blocking and potassium channel–blocking activity. At lower doses, class II effects predominate. The drug is used to prevent or treat atrial fibrillation.

## CLASS III POTASSIUM CHANNEL BLOCKERS

Although all these drugs share a common mechanism of action, they are very different. The prototype potassium channel blocker amiodarone (Nexterone, Pacerone) has electrophysiologic characteristics of sodium channel blockers, beta-adrenergic blockers, and calcium channel blockers. Thus, it has vasodilating effects and decreases systemic vascular resistance, it prolongs conduction in all cardiac tissues and decreases heart rate, and it decreases contractility of the left ventricle. Multiple randomized control trials have demonstrated amiodarone is the most effective antiarrhythmic agent for preventing and maintaining atrial fibrillation (Al-Khatib et al., 2018). Amiodarone and lidocaine are the drugs of choice for emergent management of life-threatening ventricular dysrhythmias (Panchal et al., 2018). Table 27.4 presents dosage information for amiodarone and the other class III potassium channel blockers.

### TABLE 27.4

### DRUGS AT A GLANCE: Class III Potassium Channel Blockers

| Drug | Pregnancy Category | Routes and Dosage Ranges | |
|---|---|---|---|
| | | **Adults** | **Children** |
| **Amiodarone** (Nexterone, Pacerone; ❧ Cordarone) | D | IV loading dose 150 mg over 10 min (15 mg/min), then 360 mg over the next 6 h (1 mg/min), then 540 mg over the next 18 h (0.5 mg/min)<br>IV maintenance dose, 720 mg/24 h (0.5 mg/min)<br>PO loading dose 600–800 mg/d for 1–3 wk, with a gradual decrease to 100–200 mg/d for maintenance dose | IV, IO, loading dose, IV 5 mg/kg over 20–60 min; may repeat twice up to a maximum total dose of 15 mg/kg |
| Dofetilide (Tikosyn) | C | Creatinine clearance >60 mL/min, 500 mcg twice daily<br>Creatinine clearance 40–60 mL/min, 250 mcg twice daily<br>Creatinine clearance 20 to <40 mL/min, 125 mcg twice daily<br>Creatinine clearance <20 mL/min, use is contraindicated | Not recommended |
| Dronedarone (Multaq; ❧ Multaq) | X | PO 400 mg twice daily | Not recommended |
| Ibutilide (Corvert; ❧ Corvert) | C | Weight >60 kg: IV infusion 1 mg over 10 min<br>Weight <60 kg: IV infusion 0.01 mg/kg over 10 min<br>The dose can be repeated once, if normal sinus rhythm is not restored after 10 min | Not recommended |
| Sotalol (Betapace, Sorine, Sotylize; ❧ Rylosol) Class II and class III effects | B | PO 80 mg every 12 h initially, adjust gradually every 3 d; may require 240–320 mg daily. See manufacturer's recommendations for dosing in renal failure | ≥2 y with normal renal function PO 30 mg/m² three times daily can titrate to a maximum of 60 mg/m² in hospital for at least 3 d<br>Infants and children <2 y: see manufacturer's instructions |

IO, intraosseous.

## Pharmacokinetics

The oral form of amiodarone has an onset of 2 to 3 days, with a peak in 3 to 7 hours and a duration of 6 to 8 hours. However, the action may be delayed from 3 days up to 3 weeks. Onset of effect may be shorter in pediatric patients. The IV form has an immediate onset, with a peak in 20 minutes and a duration for as long as the infusion continues. Amiodarone is extensively metabolized in the liver and produces active metabolites. The drug and its metabolites accumulate in the liver, lungs, fat, skin, and other tissues. It has a half-life of 10 days. Because of the long serum half-life of amiodarone, loading doses are usually given. These loading doses reduce the time required for therapeutic effects. However, effects may persist for several weeks to months after the drug is discontinued.

## Action

Potassium channel blockers such as amiodarone prolong duration of the action potential, slow repolarization, and prolong the refractory period in both the atria and ventricles. To perform these actions, they block cardiac potassium channels.

## Use

Amiodarone is used for various types of life-threatening tachy-dysrhythmias, both ventricular and atrial dysrhythmias. The IV and oral forms of amiodarone differ in their electrophysiologic effects. The oral form is given to treat recurrent ventricular tachycardia or ventricular fibrillation and to maintain a NSR after conversion of atrial fibrillation and atrial flutter. The IV form is given mainly for acute suppression of refractory, hemodynamically destabilizing ventricular tachycardia and ventricular fibrillation. The major effect is slowing conduction through the AV node and prolonging the effective refractory period.

The FDA has issued a **BLACK BOX WARNING**  for amiodarone, recommending use only in patients with life-threatening dysrhythmias because of the risk of the development of potentially fatal pulmonary toxicity, hepatotoxicity, and worsening dysrhythmias. Low-dose amiodarone may be a pharmacologic choice for preventing recurrent atrial fibrillation after electrical or pharmacologic conversion. The low doses cause fewer adverse effects than the higher ones used for life-threatening ventricular dysrhythmias.

### Use in Children

Safety and efficacy have not been established in pediatric patients.

### Use in Patients With Hepatic Impairment

Amiodarone is hepatotoxic. Thus, it is necessary to evaluate the liver and monitor liver function tests closely in patients who take amiodarone.

### Use in Patients with Critical Illness

Amiodarone is used only for treatment of life-threatening recurrent ventricular dysrhythmias that do not respond to adequate doses of other antidysrhythmics or when patients do not respond to alternative agents. Yet because of the potential complications of use of the medication, authorities strongly recommend adjusting to the lowest possible IV dose to limit the side effects and switching to the oral form as soon as possible.

> **! QSEN Alert: Evidence-Based Practice**
>
> Over the past two decades, rapid response teams (RRTs) have been put in place with the goal of improving the identification and management of hospitalized patients who are worsening clinically. RRT remains a well-established patient safety strategy that is frequently used. Some form of RRT is present in most hospitals in the United States, although hospitalists are increasingly assuming RRT duties. Despite support from early research and anecdotal reports of the RRTs reducing overall patient death, the benefit has not been supported in multiple systematic reviews. At best, evidence indicates that RRTs slightly decrease unanticipated cardiac arrests but do not alter overall in-hospital mortality.

### Use in Patients Receiving Home Care

Because of the close monitoring needed even with changes in the drug dosage, careful patient assessment and evaluation are necessary. Continual monitoring of cardiac response to titrate the dosage is essential.

## Adverse Effects

Authorities consider most adverse effects of amiodarone to be dose dependent and reversible. However, maintenance dose selection is difficult because absorption and elimination are variable. With the use of amiodarone, CNS adverse effects, including malaise, fatigue, dizziness, tremors, and ataxia, are the most common. Other common adverse effects include bradycardia, cardiac dysrhythmias (which can be life-threatening), hypotension, and heart failure. GI conditions include nausea, vomiting, anorexia, and constipation.

Amiodarone is an iodine-rich drug that has been associated with thyroid dysfunction, with hypothyroidism occurring more frequently than hyperthyroidism. Respiratory adverse effects include serious, potentially fatal pulmonary toxicity (pulmonary fibrosis, pneumonitis, acute respiratory distress syndrome), which may begin with progressive dyspnea and cough with crackles, decreased breath sounds, and pleurisy. Liver function tests are abnormal. Hepatotoxicity may occur and can be life-threatening. Corneal microdeposits occur in almost all patients treated for more than 2 months and can lead to blurry vision. Photosensitivity is also an adverse effect and can result in solar dermatitis and blue-gray skin.

## Contraindications

Contraindications include hypersensitivity to amiodarone as well as sinus node dysfunction, heart block, cardiogenic shock, severe bradycardia, hypokalemia, lactation, and sensitivity to iodine. Caution is necessary when giving amiodarone to patients who are pregnant or have thyroid or liver dysfunction.

## Nursing Implications

> **! QSEN Alert: Safety**
>
> The names amrinone and amiodarone have given rise to confusion. Although the name amrinone has been changed to inamrinone, confusion may still occur. Caution is necessary.

## Preventing Interactions

When oral amiodarone is used long term, it increases the effects of numerous drugs, worsening existing dysrhythmias or producing new dysrhythmias. Drugs that interact with amiodarone include beta-adrenergic blockers, oral anticoagulants, digoxin, and phenytoin. The effects of interactions with amiodarone may not be apparent until about 7 weeks after the initiation of therapy.

## Administering the Medication

Careful patient assessment and evaluation with continual monitoring of cardiac response are necessary for titrating the dosage. Therapy should begin in the hospital with continual monitoring and emergency equipment on standby.

## Assessing for Therapeutic Effects

An effect of the medication is to increase the ventricular fibrillation threshold. The nurse assesses the patient's heart rate and the cardiac rhythm; the heart rate and rhythm should be regular, with a rate between 60 and 100 beats/minute.

## Assessing for Adverse Effects

If the nurse notes any change in heart rate greater than 100 beats/minute or less than 60 beats/minute or any change in the regularity of the rhythm, increased vigilance in assessing cardiac status is warranted. In addition, the nurse assesses for ectopy and calls its attention to the physician.

## Patient Teaching

Patients should understand that if drug dosages are changed in relation to response of dysrhythmias, they need to be hospitalized during the initiation of amiodarone therapy. Additionally, the nurse should stress the importance of keeping follow-up appointments, including chest x-ray, pulmonary function tests, liver function tests, and ophthalmic examinations. Box 27.3 presents patient teaching information for antidysrhythmic agents.

# Other Drugs in the Class

Dofetilide (Tikosyn) is indicated for the maintenance of NSR in symptomatic patients who are in atrial fibrillation for longer than 1 week. Adverse effects increase with decreasing creatinine clearance levels; thus, assessment of renal function is necessary and initial dosage is dependent on creatinine clearance levels. High dosages in patients with renal dysfunction result in accumulation of dofetilide and prodysrhythmia (torsades de pointes). The drug has an elimination half-life of approximately 10 hours, with the kidneys being the major route of elimination. It should initially be administered in a setting with personnel and equipment available for emergency use. The FDA has issued a **BLACK BOX WARNING** ◆ for dofetilide. It recommends that drug administration initially occur only in a facility that can provide calculations of creatinine clearance, continuous ECG monitoring, and cardiac resuscitation for a minimum of 3 days to minimize the risk of drug-induced dysrhythmia.

Dronedarone (Multaq) is ordered to reduce the risk of hospitalization for atrial fibrillation in patients with a history of persistent or paroxysmal atrial fibrillation. Structurally related to amiodarone, this related drug demonstrates electrophysiologic properties of all four antidysrhythmic classes (sodium channel blockers, potassium channel blockers, beta-adrenergic blockers, and calcium channel blockers). Thus, it inhibits sodium and potassium channels, which prolong the action potential and refractory period in myocardial tissue. The drug also decreases AV node conduction and sinus node function through inhibition of calcium channels and beta receptor blockade. Like amiodarone, the drug inhibits alpha 1 receptor–mediated increases in blood pressure, producing vasodilating effects and decreasing systemic vascular resistance.

The FDA has issued two **BLACK BOX WARNINGS** ◆ for dronedarone because it increases the risk of death, stroke, and heart failure. The drug is contraindicated in:

1. Patients with symptomatic heart failure (or New York Heart Association class IV heart failure) because the risk of death doubles in these patients who have had recent decompensation requiring hospitalization.
2. Patients in atrial fibrillation who will not or cannot be cardioverted into NSR. For those with permanent atrial fibrillation, dronedarone doubles the risk of death, stroke, and hospitalization for heart failure.

Ibutilide (Corvert) is indicated for the management of recent onset of atrial fibrillation or atrial flutter, in which the goal is conversion to NSR. The drug enhances the efficacy of cardioversion. It can convert atrial fibrillation to sinus rhythm more rapidly than procainamide or sotalol. Ibutilide is structurally similar to sotalol but lacks clinically significant beta-blocking activity. Studies have demonstrated that ibutilide has no significant advantage compared with amiodarone for the conversion of atrial fibrillation; however, severe hypotension does not occur with ibutilide. Ibutilide is widely distributed and has an elimination half-life of about 6 hours. Most of a dose is metabolized, and the metabolites are excreted in urine and feces. Adverse effects include supraventricular and ventricular dysrhythmias (particularly torsades de pointes) and hypotension. Patients with atrial fibrillation of more than 2 to 3 days' duration must be adequately anticoagulated, generally for at least 2 weeks prior to initiation of ibutilide. The FDA has issued a **BLACK BOX WARNING** ◆ recommending that ibutilide be initiated only in a setting of continue ECG monitoring with trained personnel and equipment available for emergency use.

Sotalol (Betapace, Sorine, Sotylize) is approved for prevention or management of ventricular tachycardia and fibrillation. It has also been used, usually in smaller doses, to prevent or treat atrial fibrillation. However, it is less effective than amiodarone in the prophylaxis of atrial fibrillation. As previously mentioned, the drug has both beta-adrenergic–blocking and potassium channel–blocking activities. Class II effects predominate at lower doses, and class III effects predominate at higher doses. Sotalol is well absorbed after oral administration, and peak serum levels are reached in 2 to 4 hours. It has an elimination half-life of approximately 12 hours, and 80% to 90% is excreted unchanged by the kidneys.

Contraindications to the use of sotalol include asthma, sinus bradycardia, heart block, prolonged QT syndrome, cardiogenic shock, heart failure, and previous hypersensitivity to sotalol. The dosage should be individualized, reduced with renal impairment, and increased slowly (e.g., every 2–3 days with normal renal function, at longer intervals with impaired renal function). Dysrhythmogenic effects are most likely to occur when therapy is started or when the dosage is increased. Heart failure may occur in patients with markedly depressed left ventricular systolic function. Most adverse effects are attributed to beta-adrenergic blocking activity. Like amiodarone, sotalol may be preferred over a class I agent because it is more effective in reducing recurrent ventricular tachycardia, ventricular fibrillation, and death. The FDA has issued a **BLACK BOX WARNING ◆** for sotalol. This recommends that the drug be initiated only in a facility that can provide cardiac resuscitation and continuous ECG monitoring in the event of life-threatening ventricular tachycardia.

### Clinical Application 27.1

Ms. Johnson begins an IV infusion of amiodarone as well as an anticoagulant. What is the therapeutic goal of the amiodarone infusion? What nursing actions would the nurse implement during the initiation of the infusion?

### NCLEX Success

3. The clinical use of class III agents rather than class I agents is preferred for patients with heart disease because the class III agents are associated with
   A. less ventricular fibrillation
   B. increased mortality
   C. more sustained effects
   D. milder adverse effects

4. Mr. Conley, who is 53 years of age, is about to be discharged from the hospital after treatment for recurrent ventricular fibrillation. To prevent breakthrough ventricular ectopy, his prescriber orders amiodarone, 1000 mg PO daily as a loading dose for 2 weeks. What patient teaching implications are important regarding this loading dose?
   A. Most of the drug is destroyed in the GI tract and thus a large dose needs to be given.
   B. Males require large dosages because of their faster metabolic rate.
   C. A history of ventricular dysrhythmia necessitates a higher dose.
   D. The drug has a long serum half-life.

### Clinical Application 27.2

• While Ms. Johnson is receiving the amiodarone infusion, her heart rate decreases to 52 beats/minute. The nurse continues to monitor the IV line and the ECG. What actions should the nurse take?

# CLASS IV CALCIUM CHANNEL BLOCKERS

**Diltiazem** (Cardizem, Cardizem CD, Cardizem LA, Tiazac), the prototype class IV drug, and verapamil are the only calcium channel blockers approved for management of dysrhythmias. Table 27.5 presents dosage information for these drugs. Additional discussion regarding calcium channel blockers is found in Chapters 26 and 28.

## Pharmacokinetics

When given intravenously, diltiazem acts within 15 minutes and lasts up to 6 hours. Diltiazem and verapamil are metabolized by the liver, and metabolites are primarily excreted by the kidneys.

## Action

Calcium channel blockers obstruct the movement of calcium into conductive and contractile myocardial cells by inhibiting the influx of calcium through its channels, causing a slower conduction through the SA and AV nodes. As antidysrhythmic agents, they act primarily against tachydysrhythmias at SA and AV nodes because the cardiac cells slow channels that depend on calcium influx are found mainly at these sites. Thus, they reduce automaticity of the SA and AV nodes, slow conduction, and prolong the refractory period in the AV node.

## Use

Diltiazem, as well as verapamil, is effective only in supraventricular tachycardias. The drug may be given intravenously to terminate acute paroxysmal supraventricular tachycardia, usually within 2 minutes, and in atrial fibrillation and atrial flutter. It is also effective in exercise-related tachycardias. One antidysrhythmic drug may not maintain an NSR, and the use of more than one agent is often necessary.

With diltiazem, the following usage information may be important:

• Safety and efficacy have not been established in pediatric patients.
• There are no recommendations regarding specific use in older adults.
• Impaired renal function is a contraindication.
• Impaired hepatic function is a contraindication.

### Use in Patients With Critical Illness

Cardiac function in the critically ill patient warrants carefully evaluation. Sick sinus syndrome, heart block (either second- or third-degree), severe hypertension, cardiogenic shock, and acute myocardial infarction with cardiogenic shock are all situations where use of diltiazem is contraindicated.

### Use in Patients Receiving Home Care

When patients are receiving home care and are taking diltiazem, it is necessary to perform a physical assessment, including pulse and blood pressure, with each visit. The home care nurse arranges for follow-up with a 12-lead ECG if alterations in cardiac rhythm occur (e.g., irregular rate or change in baseline heart rate).

| | Pregnancy | Routes and Dosage Ranges | |
|---|---|---|---|
| **Drug** | **Category** | **Adults** | **Children** |
| **Diltiazem** (Cardizem, Cardizem CD, Cardizem LA, Tiazac; ✹ Cardizem CD, Diltiazem-CD, Tiazac, Tiazac XC) | C | IV 0.25 mg/kg over 2 min. A second dose of 0.35 mg/kg IV over 2 min may be given in 15 min if no rhythm change, and an IV infusion of 5–15 mg/h may be given up to 24 h, if necessary | Safety and efficacy have not been established for use in the treatment of tachydysrhythmias |
| Verapamil (Calan, Calan SR, Verelan, Verelan PM; ✹ Apo-Verap, Verelan) | C | PO 240–480/daily in 3–4 divided doses IV loading dose 0.075–0.15 mg/kg over 2 min initially and then 10 mg 30 min later, if necessary IV maintenance dose 5 mg/h titrated to goal hear rate | 1–15 y: IV injection 0.1–0.3 mg/kg (usual range 2–5 mg for a single dose) over 2 min with continuous ECG monitoring; repeat in 30 min if necessary Verapamil is no longer included in PALS for management of tachydysrhythmias |

**TABLE 27.5**

**DRUGS AT A GLANCE: Class IV Calcium Channel Blockers**

PALS, pediatric advanced life support.

## Adverse Effects

Some of the most common adverse effects associated with diltiazem are CNS conditions, including dizziness, light-headedness, headache, and weakness. Cardiovascular adverse effects include peripheral edema, bradycardia, hypotension, and AV block. If asystole occurs, it is necessary to start cardiopulmonary resuscitation immediately. Dermatologic effect includes flushing. The GI effects most often noted are complaints of nausea and constipation.

## Contraindications

Contraindications to the use of diltiazem include allergy to diltiazem, impaired hepatic or renal function, sick sinus syndrome, heart block, severe hypertension, cardiogenic shock, acute myocardial infarction with cardiogenic shock, pulmonary congestion, and lactation. Diltiazem, as well as verapamil, is contraindicated in digoxin toxicity because it may worsen heart block. If diltiazem is used with propranolol or digoxin, it is necessary to exercise caution to avoid further impairment of myocardial contractility. Use of IV verapamil with IV propranolol should not take place; it may result in potentially fatal bradycardia and hypotension.

## Nursing Implications

### Preventing Interactions

Certain drugs increase the effects of diltiazem (Box 27.5). Also, diltiazem increases the serum levels and toxicity of cyclosporine. In addition, there is a decreased metabolism and increased risk of toxic effects if diltiazem is taken with grapefruit juice.

### Administering the Medication

Careful evaluation to determine the appropriate dosing of calcium channel blockers is warranted. Ensuring that the patient swallows the extended-release or the sustained-release preparations whole rather than cutting, crushing, or chewing is a must.

### Assessing for Therapeutic Effects

In determining the effects of the use of calcium channel blockers, the nurse monitors the cardiac rate and rhythm for a return to the patient's normal baseline.

### Assessing for Adverse Effects

When caring for patients who are receiving diltiazem, the nurse monitors carefully for changes in blood pressure and cardiac rhythm as well as output. (Checking the blood pressure is especially important if the patient is taking nitrates concurrently.) In addition, it is necessary to monitor the cardiac rhythm regularly during dosage stabilization and periodically during long-term therapy. The nurse should also observe for safety issues associated with the development of symptoms such as dizziness and light-headedness.

### Patient Teaching

It is important to instruct the patient to report any adverse effects. Box 27.3 outlines patient teaching guidelines.

---

**BOX 27.5** **Drug Interactions: Diltiazem**

**Drugs That Increase the Effects of Diltiazem**
- Amiodarone
  *Increases the risk of sinus arrest, decreased myocardial contractility, and hypotension*
- Atazanavir
  *Increases the risk of conduction disturbances and atrioventricular block*
- Beta-adrenergic blockers, flecainide
  *Cause additive reductions in heart rate, cardiac conduction, and contractility*

# UNCLASSIFIED ANTIDYSRHYTHMIC DRUGS

Adenosine (Adenocard), a naturally occurring component of all body cells, differs chemically from other antidysrhythmic drugs but acts like the calcium channel blockers. It depresses conduction at the AV node and is used to restore NSR in patients with paroxysmal supraventricular tachycardia; it is ineffective in other dysrhythmias. The drug has a very short duration of action (serum half-life of less than 10 seconds) and a high degree of effectiveness. It must be given by a rapid bolus injection, preferably through a central venous line. If given slowly, it is eliminated before it can reach cardiac tissues and exert its action.

Magnesium sulfate is another of the unclassified drugs that may be used intravenously in the management of polymorphic ventricular tachycardia (torsades de pointes). Recent American Heart Association (AHA) practice guidelines do not include routine use of magnesium during the management of cardiac arrest and life-threatening dysrhythmias beyond torsades de pointes. Magnesium assists with regulating the flow of sodium, potassium, and calcium across the cell membrane, which can prevent reinitiation of ventricular tachycardias. Its antidysrhythmic effects may derive from imbalances of magnesium, potassium, and calcium. Hypomagnesemia increases myocardial irritability and is a risk factor for both atrial and ventricular dysrhythmias. Thus, serum magnesium levels should be monitored in patients at risk and replacement therapy instituted when indicated. However, in some instances, magnesium sulfate seems to have antidysrhythmic effects even when serum magnesium levels are normal.

---

### Clinical Application 27.3

- Ms. Johnson's atrial fibrillation is converted to NSR pharmacologically. The physician prescribes amiodarone at 200 mg PO daily.
- Why is she taking amiodarone orally?
- What therapeutic level of amiodarone should be the goal for this patient?

---

# DRUG THERAPY IN EMERGENCY RESUSCITATION OF ADULTS

Drugs are essential for successful resuscitation in emergencies, but initial management of cardiac arrest must also include ensuring adequate ventilation, performing high-quality compressions, restoring circulating volume loss, and identifying the causal event. This section focuses on a brief overview of the best evidence related to the efficacy of drug therapy during resuscitation.

Strengthening systems of care for both out-of-hospital cardiac arrest and in-hospital cardiac arrest is also crucial for improved clinical outcomes. The AHA guidelines provide comprehensive algorithms for basic and advanced life support and post–cardiac arrest care and were comprehensively updated in 2015. Chapter 28 discusses the 2015 AHA recommendations for the evaluation and management of acute coronary syndromes.

## Oxygen

Oxygen is one of the most widely used therapeutic agents. The 2015 AHA guidelines strengthened its recommendation for the use of supplemental oxygen to achieve hyperoxia (an abnormally increased concentration of oxygen in tissues and organs) to produce the maximal feasible inspired oxygen during ongoing cardiopulmonary resuscitation or CPR. The use of supplemental oxygen to achieve adequate oxygenation in the early period following resuscitation should be reevaluated in light of the arterial blood gases and potential adverse effects of oxygen toxicity. Experts have cited a dose-dependent association between supernormal oxygen tension postresuscitation and risk of in-hospital death. Titration of oxygen to an oxygen saturation of at least 94% rather than continuing maximum oxygen delivery is emphasized.

## Epinephrine

Although no vasopressor medication has ever shown any long-term survival benefit in cardiac arrest, epinephrine is recommended for the treatment of asystole. The 2015 AHA guidelines recommend that epinephrine be administered as early as possible and in regular doses (1 mg IV every 3–5 minutes); data do not support improved survival with routine administration of high-dose epinephrine. In addition, because myocardial infarction is often the cause of ventricular fibrillation as the primary rhythm during cardiac arrest, some experts recommend a lower dose of epinephrine with ventricular fibrillation to minimize the vasoconstriction of the coronary arteries caused by epinephrine given at standard doses. Extreme vasoconstriction can produce lactic acidosis at the cellular level and result in metabolic acidosis.

## Atropine

The 2015 AHA guidelines no longer recommend the use of atropine for the treatment of asystole because data do not support the use of the drug. Research also does not support the use of atropine for pulseless electrical activity.

## Sodium Bicarbonate

Data do not indicate that sodium bicarbonate is generally effective during cardiac arrest, so the drug is not part of routine management. Experts still recommend the drug for use in patients with hyperkalemia and in those with tricyclic antidepressant overdose.

## Lidocaine

The 2015 AHA guidelines do not recommend the routine use of lidocaine after return of spontaneous circulation (ROSC). However, experts believe that it may be reasonable to continue lidocaine infusion in the immediate period after ventricular fibrillation or pulseless ventricular tachycardia if lidocaine was given intra-arrest and ROSC was achieved.

# Calcium Chloride

Calcium chloride is the first-line therapy for individuals who are hypercalcemic with sudden cardiac death. Calcium chloride is not recommended during cardiac resuscitation in the presence of ventricular fibrillation, in asystole or electromechanical dissociation, or with a risk of existing digitalis toxicity. Untreated hypomagnesemia may make hypocalcemia refractory to drug therapy, so abnormalities in magnesium and calcium should be corrected simultaneously.

## MAGNESIUM SULFATE

Magnesium sulfate is recommended during resuscitation only in patients with drug-induced QT prolongation and development of torsades de pointes.

## THE NURSING PROCESS

A concept map outlines the nursing process related to drug therapy considerations in this chapter. Additional nursing implications related to the disease process should also be considered in care decisions.

**Assessment**
- Assess the significance of symptoms in relation to the cardiac dysrhythmias.
- Identify conditions or risk factors that may precipitate the dysrhythmias.
- Observe for adverse drug effects used to manage the dysrhythmias.
- When ECG monitoring is available, assess for type and indications of the dysrhythmias.

**Outcomes of Therapy**
The patient will
- Receive or take antidysrhythmic drugs accurately.
- Avoid conditions that precipitate dysrhythmias, when feasible.
- Experience improved heart rate, circulation, and activity tolerance.
- Be monitored for therapeutic and adverse drug effects.
- Avoid preventable adverse drug effects.
- Have adverse drug effects promptly recognized and treated if they occur.
- Keep follow-up appointments for monitoring responses to treatment measures.

**Nursing Interventions**
- Use measures to detect, prevent, and/or minimize dysrhythmias.
- Manage underlying disease processes that contribute to dysrhythmia development. These include cardiovascular (e.g., acute myocardial infarction) and noncardiovascular (e.g., chronic lung disease) disorders.
- Prevent or treat other conditions that predispose to dysrhythmias (e.g., hypoxia, electrolyte imbalance, pain, acid–base imbalance, fluid alterations).
- Encourage the patient to recognize and avoid the negative effects of cigarette smoking, overeating, excessive coffee drinking, and other habits that may cause or aggravate dysrhythmias.
- Implement measures to minimize the incidence and severity of acute dysrhythmias and help the patient comply with drug therapy.
- Monitor heart rate and rhythm and blood pressure every 4 to 6 hours (or as often as clinical condition indicates or is the standard for the care environment where assessing the patient).
- During IV administration of antidysrhythmic drugs, maintain continuous cardiac monitoring and check blood pressure about every 1 to 5 minutes, depending on the onset of action of the drug.
- Check laboratory reports of serum electrolytes and serum drug levels when available. See Table 27.6 for commonly reported serum levels of antidysrhythmic agents. Report and treat abnormal values using established protocols and/or provider's orders.

**Evaluation**
- Interview and observe for symptom relief and stable vital signs and cardiac rhythm.
- Interview and observe for irregular rhythms, hypotension, and other adverse drug effects.
- Interview and observe for compliance with instructions for taking antidysrhythmic drugs and other aspects of care.

## TABLE 27.6

### Therapeutic Serum Drug Level Ranges of Some Common Antidysrhythmics

| Drug | Therapeutic Range |
| --- | --- |
| Quinidine | 2–6 mcg/mL |
| Procainamide | 4–8 mcg/mL |
| Disopyramide | 2–5 mcg/mL |
| Lidocaine | 1.5–5 mcg/mL |
| Flecainide | 0.2–1 mcg/mL |

*Na+ + Ca+ in   K+ out* (handwritten annotation)

## KEY CONCEPTS

- Atrial fibrillation is the most common dysrhythmia and is associated with increased morbidity and mortality.
- Initiation of an electrical impulse depends predominately on the movement of sodium and calcium ions into a myocardial cell and movement of potassium ions out of the cell.
- Quinidine, the prototype of class IA antidysrhythmics, reduces automaticity, slows conduction, and prolongs the refractory period. GI adverse effects, particularly diarrhea, limit compliance with dosing regimens.
- The FDA has issued a **BLACK BOX WARNING** ◆ for the class IA antidysrhythmics quinidine, procainamide, and disopyramide because of the prodysrhythmic properties of these drugs. These agents should be reserved for patients with life-threatening ventricular dysrhythmias. In clinical trials, the use of quinidine in non–life-threatening dysrhythmias has increased mortality, particularly in patients with structural heart disease.
- Lidocaine is the prototype of class IB antidysrhythmics used for treating serious ventricular dysrhythmias associated with acute myocardial infarction, cardiac catheterization, cardiac surgery, and digitalis-induced ventricular dysrhythmias.
- There are two **BLACK BOX WARNINGS** ◆ for flecainide, class IC antidysrhythmic.
- The drug increases the risk of nonfatal cardiac arrest and death in patients with recent myocardial infarction or chronic atrial fibrillation.
- In patients with cardiac dysrhythmias, it is necessary to monitor carefully for potentially fatal prodysrhythmic effects.
- As class II drugs, beta-adrenergic blockers are used because of their effectiveness in reducing mortality in postmyocardial infarction and heart failure patients.
- The FDA has issued a **BLACK BOX WARNING** ◆ for propranolol and other beta-adrenergic blockers; abrupt discontinuation of the drug can exacerbate cardiac ischemia, increasing the risk of angina pectoris and myocardial infarction.

- The class III antidysrhythmics, the potassium channel blockers, block potassium channels and prolong repolarization, which prolongs conduction in all cardiac tissues, decreases heart rate, and prevents dysrhythmic conduction. Amiodarone, the prototype class III antidysrhythmic, prolongs conduction in all cardiac tissues, decreases heart rate, and decreases contractility of the left ventricle The FDA has issued multiple **BLACK BOX WARNINGS** ◆ for amiodarone.
- The drug is recommended only for patients with life-threatening dysrhythmias because of the risk of the development of potentially fatal pulmonary toxicity and liver injury.
- Loading doses should be administered only in a hospital setting and with continuous ECG monitoring because of the slow onset of antiarrhythmic effect and the risk of life-threatening arrhythmias.
- The drug may pose life-threatening management problems in patients at risk for sudden death. Its use is only recommended in patients with life-threatening, recurrent ventricular dysrhythmias unresponsive to or intolerant of other antidysrhythmics or alternative drugs.
- The FDA has issued two **BLACK BOX WARNINGS** ◆ for dronedarone, another class III antidysrhythmic, because the drug increases the risk of death, stroke, and heart failure.
- It is contraindicated in patients with symptomatic heart failure (or New York Heart Association class IV heart failure); the risk of death doubles in these patients who have had recent decompensation requiring hospitalization.
- It is contraindicated in patients in atrial fibrillation who will not or cannot be cardioverted into NSR. For those with permanent atrial fibrillation, dronedarone doubles the risk of death, stroke, and hospitalization for heart failure.
- Class IV antidysrhythmics block the influx of calcium into the myocardial cells, which decreases contractility and slows heart rate. As class IV drugs, diltiazem and verapamil are the only calcium channel blockers approved for management of dysrhythmias.

## CLINICAL REASONING CASE STUDY

**Meet the Patient**

Cara Wright, a 62-year-old woman with a history of type 2 diabetes and hypertension, has been admitted to a telemetry unit with new-onset atrial fibrillation. She is placed on continuous cardiac monitoring and has a ventricular response rate of 124 beats/minute. Her blood pressure is 130/80 mm Hg. She complains of occasional shortness of breath and palpitations. The cardiologist explains to Mrs. Wright that treatment options depend on the results of a transesophageal echocardiogram. If no clot is found, she will receive ibutilide (Corvert) in the telemetry unit; if a clot is discovered, she will be started on the anticoagulant apixaban (Eliquis) for 3 weeks and then cardioverted. After the patient's husband arrives, she asks the nurse to tell her husband why she needs medication and to explain why apixaban might be prescribed instead of warfarin, which his mother used to take. How does the nurse best respond? Depending on the medication ordered, what additional patient teaching related to ibutilide or apixaban should the nurse provide?

**Assessing Drug Information**

- Ibutilide (Corvert)
  - Ibutilide (Corvert) is a class III antiarrhythmic agent used in patients with new-onset atrial fibrillation to try to convert the rhythm back to normal (sinus) rhythm and maintain that rhythm.
  - The drug is given intravenously while the patient is in the hospital so that the heart rhythm and rate can be monitored during and after administration.
  - The goal of drug therapy with ibutilide is to convert the heart rhythm back to normal.
- Apixaban (Eliquis)
  - Both warfarin (Coumadin) and apixaban (Eliquis) are anticoagulants used to treat or prevent blood clots, which reduces the risk of a stroke.
  - Warfarin works by blocking the body's ability to recycle vitamin K, which is necessary to form a blood clot. With less vitamin K in circulation, the body requires more time to form a clot. Frequent blood tests and dosage adjustments are required to maintain a therapeutic dose of warfarin. The drug is known to interact with other drugs and foods.
  - A newer drug, apixaban (Eliquis) can be given in a fixed dose and does not required monitoring with blood tests. The drug also causes fewer bleeding problems, including bleeding into the brain, when compared to warfarin.

**Nursing Actions**

- The nurse teaches Mrs. Wright and her husband that atrial fibrillation is an abnormal, fast electrical rhythm in the upper chambers of the heart. During atrial fibrillation, the upper chambers do not contract fully and blood flow can be impaired. When blood becomes stagnant to any degree, the mechanisms that form a clot are activated and clot can develop and can become dislodged and cause a stroke or heart attack. A transesophageal echocardiogram can detect a clot within the heart. If no clots are evident, the patient may receive ibutilide or undergo a cardioversion. If there is a clot, it is necessary to prescribe anticoagulants.
- If ibutilide is ordered, the nurse should have the proper emergency equipment available during administration of ibutilide and observe Mrs. Wright with continuous ECG monitoring for at least 4 hours following infusion or until the QT interval has returned to baseline. If symptomatic ventricular dysrhythmias, particularly polymorphic ventricular tachycardia (torsades de pointes), occur, the patient should undergo cardioversion.
- If anticoagulants are ordered, the nurse should instruct Mrs. Wright to take the drug as prescribed, use safety precautions to prevent injury, and report any signs of bleeding to her cardiologist. Additional teaching guidelines can be found in Chapter 9.

Visit thePoint® at **http://thePoint.lww.com/Frandsen12e** for answers to NCLEX Success questions (in Appendix A), answers to Clinical Application Case Studies (in Appendix B), and more!

## REFERENCES AND RESOURCES

Agency for Healthcare Research and Quality (AHRQ). (2019). *Patient safety primer: Rapid response systems.* Retrieved from https://psnet.ahrq.gov/primers/primer/4/rapid-response-systems

Al-Khatib, S. M., Stevenson, W. G., Ackerman, M. J., Bryant, W. J., Callans, D. J., Curtis, A. B., et al. (2018). 2017 AHA/ACC/HRS guideline for management of patients with ventricular arrhythmias and the prevention of sudden cardiac death: A report of the American College of Cardiology Foundation/American Heart Association Task Force on Clinical Practice Guidelines and the Heart Rhythm Society. *Circulation, 138*, e272–e391. doi:10.1161/CIR.0000000000000549

Callaway, C. W., Soar, J., Aibiki, M., Bottinger, B. W., Brooks, S. C., Deakin, C. D., et al. (2015). 2015 International consensus on cardiopulmonary resuscitation and emergency cardiovascular care science with treatment recommendations part 4: Advanced life support. *Circulation, 132*(16), S84–S145.

Damiani, E., Adrario, E., Girardis, M., Romano, R., Peilaia, P., Singer, M., et al. (2014). Arterial hyperoxia and mortality in critically ill patients: A systematic review and meta-analysis. *Critical Care, 18*(6), 711.

deSouza, I. S., Martindale, J. L., & Sinert, R. (2015). Antidysrhythmic drug therapy for the termination of stable, monomorphic ventricular tachycardia: A systematic review. *Emergency Medicine Journal, 32*(2), 161–167.

Hazinski, M. F., Nolan, J. P., & the International Liaison Committee on Resuscitation Editorial Board. (2015). Part 1: Executive summary: 2015 international consensus on cardiopulmonary resuscitation and emergency cardiovascular care science with treatment recommendations. *Circulation, 132*(16), S2–S39.

Karch, A. M. (2018). *2019 Lippincott's pocket drug guide for nurses.* Philadelphia, PA: Lippincott Williams & Wilkins.

Neumar, R. W., Shuster, M., Callaway, C. W., Gent, L.M., Atkins, D.L., Bhanji, F., et al. (2015). Part 1: Executive Summary: 2015 American Heart Association guidelines update for cardiopulmonary resuscitation and emergency cardiovascular care. *Circulation, 132*(18 Suppl 2), S315–S367. doi: 10.1161/CIR.0000000000000252.

Norris, T. (2019). *Porth's pathophysiology: Concepts of altered health status* (10th ed.). Philadelphia, PA: Lippincott Williams & Wilkins.

Panchal, A., Berg, L., Kudenchuk, P., Del Rios, M., Hirsch, K., Link, M., et al. (2018). 2018 American Heart Association focused update on advanced cardiovascular life support use of antiarrhythmic drugs during and immediately after cardiac arrest: An update to the American Heart Association guidelines for cardiopulmonary resuscitation and emergency cardiovascular care. *Circulation, 138*, e740–e749.

Sapp, J. L., Wells, G. A., Parkash, R., Stevenson, W. G., Blier, L., Sarrazin, J.-F., et al. (2016). Ventricular tachycardia ablation versus escalation of antiarrhythmic drugs. *The New England Journal of Medicine, 375*(2), 111–121.

UpToDate. (2019). *Drug information.* Lexi-Comp, Inc.

# Drug Therapy for Coronary Heart Disease

## LEARNING OBJECTIVES

*After studying this chapter, you should be able to:*

1. Relate the etiology and pathophysiology of coronary heart disease to its clinical manifestations.
2. Examine the nonpharmacologic measures beneficial in controlling or reversing risk factors for cardiovascular disease progression.
3. Identify the prototype and describe the action, use, contraindications, adverse effects, and nursing implications for the organic nitrates in the management of coronary heart disease.
4. Identify the prototype and outline the actions, use, adverse effects, contraindications, and nursing implications for the beta-adrenergic blockers in the management of coronary heart disease.
5. Identify the prototype and describe the actions, use, adverse effects, contraindications, and nursing implications for the calcium channel blockers in the management of coronary heart disease.
6. Evaluate evidence-based considerations in the use of adjuvant drugs administered in the management of patients with acute coronary syndromes.
7. Apply the nursing process in the care of patients with coronary heart disease.

## CLINICAL APPLICATION CASE STUDY

Richard Gerald, a 72-year-old man, has a history of hypertension and coronary artery disease. He stopped smoking and began a regular exercise program after having a non–ST-segment elevation myocardial infarction 2 months ago. He was discharged on nitroglycerin–in a sublingual form and as a transdermal patch (1 inch) every 4 hours while awake (off at night)–and on atenolol 50 mg orally daily.

## KEY TERMS

**Acute coronary syndromes:** umbrella term used to describe conditions brought on by sudden, reduced blood flow to the heart in situations where myocardial ischemia is suspected. These include unstable angina, non–ST-segment elevation myocardial infarction, and ST-segment elevation myocardial infarction.

**Afterload:** amount of vascular resistance that must be overcome to open the aortic valve on the left side of the heart (or pulmonic valve on the right) and eject the blood with systole

**Cardioselectivity:** ability of a beta-adrenergic blocker to selectively block beta$_1$ receptors

**Coronary artery vasospasm:** smooth muscle constriction of a coronary artery

**Coronary heart disease:** stable angina pectoris and acute coronary syndromes, which result from coronary artery disease or spasm

**Intima:** inner layer of an artery

**Media:** middle layer of a vessel

**Negative chronotropy:** causing slowing of the heart rate

**Preload:** passive stretch of the ventricles just prior to systole

## INTRODUCTION

The two broad categories of **coronary heart disease**, chronic coronary artery disease (CAD) and acute coronary syndromes, are on a continuum of disease progression. Stable angina is the classic initial manifestation of chronic CAD. As CAD worsens, the effects of ischemia may lead to **acute coronary syndromes**, an umbrella term used to describe the sequelae of unstable angina and myocardial infarction (MI) with or without elevation in the ST segment.

**Coronary artery vasospasm**, or smooth muscle constriction of a coronary artery, is another form of angina that can lead to MI, ventricular dysrhythmias, and sudden cardiac death. Termed variant angina (or Prinzmetal's or vasospastic angina), this form of angina is not due to an obstructive atherosclerotic lesion but results from the spasm of one or more coronary arteries that reduces blood flow to the myocardium. However, variant angina plays a key role in the development of atherosclerotic lesions.

This chapter introduces the pharmacologic care of the patient experiencing coronary heart disease. Nonpharmacologic treatment measures are also addressed. To understand clinical use of these drugs and nonpharmacologic treatment measures, it is necessary to understand the etiology, pathophysiology, and clinical manifestations of CAD.

## OVERVIEW OF CORONARY ARTERY DISEASE

### Etiology

CAD is the result of damage to the **intima**, or inner layer, of the coronary arteries, leading to a buildup of lipids and fibrous matter. A variety of irritants, including chemicals, drugs, or viruses, may cause additional injury. Box 28.1 outlines major risk factors associated with the development of CAD.

### Pathophysiology

In CAD, increased blood levels of low-density lipoprotein (LDL) irritate and damage the intima of the coronary artery. Once LDL has accumulated and damaged the protective layer of the vessel, fatty streaks form, with foam cells. These fatty streaks are yellow and flat and cause no significant coronary artery obstruction but are the earliest sign of arterial disease. The body responds by sending smooth muscle cells from the middle layer of the vessel, the **media**. This engulfs the fatty substance and the foam cells and produces a fibrous tissue, which stimulates calcium deposition. This cycle continues, and the fatty streak and foam cells eventually transform into a fibrous plaque along the intima, forming the fibrous cap, which is made up of smooth muscle cells, macrophages, foam cells, lymphocytes, collagen, and elastin. The

development of fixed atherosclerotic plaque narrows the lumen of the artery, which restricts the flow of oxygen-carrying blood. When oxygen supply is insufficient, especially during periods of high oxygen demand (e.g., with physical exertion), cardiac ischemia occurs and the patient may experience stable angina.

Over time, the plaque can harden or rupture, decreasing the diameter of the artery. Inflammation, a key determinant of the vulnerability of plaque, is related to an increase in the activity of macrophages at the site of the plaque; as macrophage activity increases, changes in the plaque core and cap make the plaque more vulnerable to rupture. With plaque rupture, the resulting injury to the endothelium causes platelets to aggregate at the site of injury, form a thrombus, and release chemical mediators that lead to vasoconstriction (e.g., thromboxane, serotonin, platelet-derived growth factor). The disrupted plaque and thrombi, together with the vasoconstriction, combine to further narrow the coronary artery and worsen ischemia. At this point, the intraluminal thrombi can occlude an artery outright or detach, move into the circulation, and eventually occlude smaller, distal branches of the artery causing thromboembolism and MI. Catecholamine release along with increased sympathetic tone as seen with tachycardia of any etiology, mental stress, or physical exertion can lead to further cardiac ischemia. Endothelial injury, with subsequent thrombus formation and vasoconstriction, may also result from therapeutic procedures (e.g., angioplasty, atherectomy). Figure 28.1 illustrates this process.

| BOX 28.1 | ***Risk Factors for the Development of Coronary Artery Disease*** |
|---|---|

- Smoking
- Abnormal cholesterol levels (high total cholesterol and low-density lipoprotein cholesterol and low high-density lipoprotein cholesterol (less than 40 mg/dL))
- High blood pressure (140/90 mm Hg or higher or taking blood pressure medication)
- Obesity (greater than 20% over ideal body weight; abdominal obesity)
- Diabetes mellitus or prediabetes
- High C-reactive protein (not attributed to other health conditions (1.0–2.9 mg/dL intermediate risk; greater than 3.0 mg/dL high risk))
- Physical conditioning (less than 30 minutes of moderate-intensity aerobic exercise less than three times weekly)
- Age (men ≥45 years; women ≥55 years)
- Ethnicity (higher risk of developing coronary artery disease in African Americans, American Indians, and Mexican Americans than Caucasians)
- History of preeclampsia in pregnancy
- Genetics (heart disease in father or brother less than 55 years; heart disease in mother or sister less than 65 years)

When blood flow is obstructed to all or a portion of a coronary artery, ischemia and ultimately death of the myocardium result. In myocardial cells, in areas of local ischemia, disruptions in intracellular sodium and calcium concentration homeostasis occur. A decreased efflux or increased influx of sodium may cause cellular sodium overload. What follows is an increased influx of calcium through sodium–calcium exchange. Failure to maintain the homeostasis of electrolytes leads to electrical instability and dysrhythmias, mechanical dysfunction from reduced contractility and increased diastolic tension, and mitochondrial dysfunction with a shift from aerobic to anaerobic metabolism.

## Clinical Manifestations

### Stable Angina

When intermittent myocardial oxygen demand surpasses oxygen supply to the heart muscle, the ischemia to the myocardium produces symptoms (Fig. 28.2). Stable angina (also called classic, typical, or exertional angina) is usually precipitated by situations that increase the workload of the heart, such as physical exertion, exposure to cold temperatures, and emotional upset. Recurrent episodes of stable angina usually have the same pattern of onset, duration, and intensity of symptoms.

Classic anginal pain is usually described as substernal chest pain of a constricting, squeezing, or suffocating nature. Pain may radiate to the jaw, neck, or shoulder; down the left or both arms; or to the back. The discomfort is sometimes mistaken for arthritis or for indigestion, because the pain may be associated with

**Figure 28.2.** Myocardial oxygen supply and demand. [Reprinted with permission from Norris, T. L. (2019). *Porth's pathophysiology: Concepts of altered health states* [10th ed., Fig. 27.4, p. 760]. Philadelphia, PA: Wolters Kluwer.]

nausea, vomiting, dizziness, diaphoresis, shortness of breath, or fear of impending doom. The discomfort is usually brief, typically lasting 5 minutes or less until the balance of oxygen supply and demand is restored. The traditional description of angina

**Figure 28.1.** Coronary heart disease, including two categories, stable angina and acute coronary syndromes, is a term used to describe clinical symptoms consistent with myocardial ischemia. Acute coronary syndromes encompass three clinical situations: unstable angina, ST-segment elevation myocardial infarction (STEMI), and non–ST-segment elevation MI (NSTEMI). A STEMI occurs with a complete occlusion of a coronary artery or major branch. To minimize myocardial damage, the artery must be opened quickly using thrombolytic therapy or PCI. [Reprinted with permission from Norris, T. L. (2019). *Porth's pathophysiology: Concepts of altered health states* [10th ed., Fig. 27.5, p. 765]. Philadelphia, PA: Wolters Kluwer.]

derives from studies in men. Women, who report pain other than in the chest, more commonly present with complaints of unusual fatigue, weakness, dizziness, and shortness of breath. The elderly and those with diabetes mellitus may have atypical symptoms or may present with silent myocardial ischemia. Note that patients with atypical presentations and those with silent ischemia are less likely to be diagnosed accurately and promptly, often placing them outside the therapeutic window of opportunity. They are less likely to receive appropriate treatment (i.e., thrombolytics and interventional therapies), resulting in poorer outcomes.

Variant angina occurs at rest or with minimal exertion, often at night and frequently at the same time each day. Individuals experience cycles of 3- to 6-month clusters of recurring attacks, followed by relatively symptom-free periods.

### Acute Coronary Syndromes

The symptoms of unstable angina (also called crescendo, rest, or preinfarction angina) are similar to those of stable angina. However, in unstable angina, the acute pain typically occurs at rest and usually lasts longer than 20 minutes. The intensity, timing, and characteristics of the pain show recent increases in severity and frequency, often develop with less exertion than previous episodes of angina, and may limit physical activity. Unstable angina differs from non–ST-elevation myocardial infarction (NSTEMI) in that the ischemia is not severe enough to cause sufficient myocardial damage to release detectable quantities of troponins. Because unstable angina often occurs hours or days before acute MI, early recognition and effective management are extremely important in preventing progression to infarction, heart failure, or sudden cardiac death.

In patients with acute coronary syndrome, early risk stratification is performed using a risk assessment system that predicts the risk of further cardiac episodes. Identifying patients at highest risk who may benefit from more aggressive therapeutic management is essential for improved outcomes. Factors that predict severe cardiac events include the presence and extent of ST-segment depression, elevated cardiac biomarkers, evidence of hemodynamic instability, and persistent chest pain despite appropriate medical therapy.

Patients who present without persistent ST-segment elevation may be experiencing an NSTEMI, formerly called a non–Q-wave MI. Their electrocardiogram (ECG) changes may show ST-segment depression or T-wave inversion, other changes, or no changes. An ST-segment elevation MI (STEMI), formerly called a Q-wave MI, is defined by persistent (greater than 20 minutes) ST elevation on ECG, which generally reflects an acute total coronary occlusion. Both NSTEMI and STEMI are characterized by a typical rise and/or fall in biomarkers of myocyte injury. Cardiac troponin I and troponin T are the preferred biomarkers of myocyte injury because they are more specific and sensitive than the traditional cardiac isoenzyme creatine kinase (CK)-MB.

## Nonpharmacologic Therapy

Nonpharmacologic management of CAD includes risk factor modification, patient education, and revascularization procedures. For patients at any stage of CAD development, irrespective of symptoms of myocardial ischemia, optimal management involves lifestyle changes and drugs to control or reverse risk

factors for disease progression. A growing body of evidence corroborates that risk factor management in patients with CAD improves survival, enhances quality of life, reduces recurrent events, and decreases the need for revascularization. Thus, efforts to assist patients in reducing blood pressure, weight, and serum cholesterol levels, when indicated, and developing an exercise program are necessary. For patients with diabetes mellitus, glucose and blood pressure control can reduce the microvascular changes associated with the condition.

In addition, people should avoid circumstances known to precipitate acute attacks, and those who smoke should stop. Smoking is harmful because of the following factors:

- Nicotine increases catecholamines, which, in turn, increase heart rate and blood pressure.
- Carboxyhemoglobin, formed from the inhalation of carbon monoxide in smoke, decreases delivery of blood and oxygen to the heart, decreases myocardial contractility, and increases the risks of life-threatening cardiac dysrhythmias (e.g., ventricular fibrillation) during ischemic episodes.
- Both nicotine and carbon monoxide increase platelet adhesiveness and aggregation, thereby promoting thrombosis.
- Smoking increases the risks of MI, sudden cardiac death, cerebrovascular disease (e.g., stroke), peripheral vascular disease (e.g., arterial insufficiency), and hypertension. It also reduces high-density lipoprotein (HDL) cholesterol.

Additional nonpharmacologic management strategies include surgical revascularization (e.g., coronary artery bypass graft) and interventional procedures that reduce blockages (e.g., primary percutaneous coronary intervention [PCI], intracoronary stent, laser therapy, rotational atherectomy).

Nonpharmacologic management improves patient outcomes. However, most patients still require antianginal and other cardiovascular medications to manage their disease.

## NCLEX Success

1. Mr. Smith, a 52-year-old man, is recovering from an acute non–ST-segment elevation myocardial infarction. His father died from an MI at age 44. He has smoked one pack of cigarettes a day for 30 years. Which of the following risk factors for heart disease does Mr. Smith have? (Select all that apply.)

   A. smoking
   B. genetics
   C. race
   D. age

2. A 63-year-old woman continues to complain of chest pain, although her cardiac catheterization showed no significant cardiac disease. She notes that the chest pain occurs at the same time each night and typically during the cold weather. What kind of angina is the patient likely experiencing?

   A. stable angina
   B. unstable angina
   C. variant angina
   D. acute coronary syndromes

# Drug Therapy

Upcoming sections discuss the drugs used to treat angina, myocardial ischemia, and infarction. Table 28.1 and the DRUGS AT A GLANCE tables list individual drugs used in the treatment of coronary heart disease, which include the organic nitrates, beta-adrenergic blockers, calcium channel blockers, and adjuvant drugs. These drugs relieve anginal pain by increasing blood supply to the myocardium as well as reducing the oxygen demand of the myocardium. In addition, this chapter includes a brief review of the current evidence related to the indications and effectiveness of additional drugs used in the management of acute MI.

# ORGANIC NITRATES

The most widely used nitrate is the prototype **nitroglycerin** (Nitro-Bid, Nitro-Dur). Available in multiple forms, it is indicated for the management and prevention of acute chest pain caused by myocardial ischemia.

## Pharmacokinetics

Nitroglycerin is 60% bound to protein, undergoes extensive first-pass metabolism in the liver, and has a half-life of 1 to 4 minutes. Excretion occurs in the urine. The onset of action, peak, and duration of action varies with the route of administration:

## TABLE 28.1

### Drugs Administered for the Treatment of Coronary Heart Disease

| Drug Class | Prototype | Other Drugs in the Class |
|---|---|---|
| Organic nitrates | Nitroglycerin (Nitro-Bid, others) | Isosorbide dinitrate (Isordil) Isosorbide mononitrate |
| Beta-adrenergic blockers | Atenolol (Tenormin) | Bisoprolol Carvedilol (Coreg) Esmolol (Brevibloc) Metoprolol (Lopressor, Toprol XL) Nadolol (Corgard) Propranolol (Inderal) |
| Calcium channel blockers | Nifedipine (Adalat, Procardia) | Amlodipine (Norvasc) Diltiazem (Cardizem) Felodipine Isradipine Nicardipine Verapamil (Calan, Verelan) |
| Adjunct medications | Ranolazine (Ranexa) | Dyslipidemic drugs Antihypertensive drugs Angiotensin-converting enzyme inhibitors Aspirin ADP receptor antagonists Glycoprotein IIb/IIIa receptor antagonists Morphine |

- Intravenous (IV) drip: onset, immediate; peak, immediate; duration of action, 3 to 5 minutes
- Sublingual (SL): onset, 1 to 3 minutes; peak, 4 to 8 minutes; duration of action, at least 25 minutes
- Translingual spray: onset, 1 to 3 minutes; peak, 4 to 10 minutes; duration of action, at least 25 minutes
- Oral (PO) tablets or capsules (sustained release): onset, about 60 minutes; peak, 2½ to 4 hours; duration of action, 4 to 8 hours
- Topical ointment: onset, 15 to 30 minutes; peak, 60 minutes; duration of action, 7 hours
- Topical transdermal disk: onset, about 30 minutes; peak, 120 minutes; duration of action, 10 to 12 hours

## Action

Organic nitrates are converted to nitric oxide, a potent vasodilator, which relaxes smooth muscle in blood vessel walls. The drugs relieve anginal pain by several mechanisms:

- Venous dilation, which reduces venous pressure and decreases venous return to the heart. This decreases blood volume and pressure within the heart (**preload**), which in turn decreases cardiac workload and oxygen demand. This is the main mechanism by which nitroglycerin relieves angina.
- Coronary artery dilation at higher doses, which can increase blood flow to ischemic areas of the myocardium.
- Arteriole dilation, which lowers peripheral vascular resistance (**afterload**). This results in lower systolic blood pressure and, consequently, reduced cardiac workload and balancing supply and demand in the heart.

## Use

For relief of sudden-onset angina, fast-acting preparations of nitroglycerin include SL tablets and transmucosal spray. Indications for these preparations include acute-onset chest pain and prophylaxis prior to activities known to provoke angina, such as walking, dancing, or mowing the lawn.

For management of recurrent, chronic angina, long-acting preparations include PO sustained-release tablets and transdermal ointment. With these longer-acting forms, intolerance to their hemodynamic effects may develop, and therefore, the drugs do not relieve chest pain.

> **! QSEN Alert: Safety**
>
> To avoid development of tolerance to nitroglycerin, it is essential to observe a 10- to 12-hour nitrate-free interval.

In clinical practice, patients taking nitrates are usually nitrate free during the night, while sleeping, to prevent nitrate tolerance. The oral form of the drug undergoes rapid metabolism in the liver, and relatively small portions ultimately reach the systemic circulation. Thus, the PO form does not relieve acute chest pain but may be useful prophylactically in chronic chest pain. Nitroglycerin ointment is indicated for prevention of chronic angina. This route is convenient to use when the patient can have nothing by mouth (NPO) before surgery and cannot take the usually PO dose.

Angina that is unresponsive to SL, PO, or transdermal preparations calls for IV nitroglycerin. Prescribers may typically order the IV form for management of pain associated with an MI. IV nitroglycerin is useful in the management of angina that is unresponsive to organic nitrates via other routes or to beta-adrenergic blockers. It also may be used to control blood pressure in perioperative or emergency situations and to reduce preload and afterload in severe heart failure. Table 28.2 presents route and dosage information for nitroglycerin and other nitrates.

 *Concept Mastery Alert*

> Nitroglycerin is given sublingually, transmucosally, or via IV, but is not given orally (i.e., it is not swallowed). Nitrates that are administered orally are isosorbide dinitrate and isosorbide mononitrate.

### Use in Children

IV nitroglycerin is the only form of nitroglycerin approved for use in children. It may be used to treat hypertension and heart failure. Caution and close monitoring are necessary.

### Use in Older Adults

Older adults may be more vulnerable to hypotension when taking nitroglycerin as a result of volume depletion, concurrent use of other medication, and loss of sympathetic tone.

 **QSEN Alert: Safety**

> Therefore, older adults may be at greater risk of falling than younger patients at the therapeutic doses of nitroglycerin because of the risk of hypotension.

### Use in Patients With Critical Illness

IV nitroglycerin is commonly used in the critical care setting. Angina related to MI may be a patient's principal issue in the intensive care unit (ICU). However, he or she may also have heart failure, hypertension, renal failure, and/or anemia and therefore could be receiving multiple drugs such as heparin, epoetin alfa, and dobutamine.

 **QSEN Alert: Safety**

> The nurse must always check IV compatibility when administering drugs by that route.

Close monitoring of vital signs, along with frequent titration of IV medications, is important in the critically ill.

## Adverse Effects

The majority of adverse effects of nitroglycerin are related to the hemodynamic changes responsible for preload reduction and vasodilation. The most common adverse effect is a severe headache, which is typically treated with acetaminophen. Other common adverse effects include dizziness, bradycardia, syncope, hypotension, and orthostatic hypotension.

## Contraindications

Contraindications to nitroglycerin include hypersensitivity reactions, severe anemia, hypotension, and hypovolemia.

**QSEN Alert: Safety**

> Men who take nitroglycerin or any other nitrate should not use phosphodiesterase enzyme type 5 inhibitors such as sildenafil (Viagra) and vardenafil (Levitra) for erectile dysfunction. The combined effect can produce profound, life-threatening hypotension.

Caution is necessary in the following situations:

- In the presence of head injury or cerebral hemorrhage because it may increase intracranial pressure.

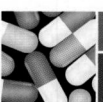

### TABLE 28.2

### DRUGS AT A GLANCE: Organic Nitrates

| Drug | Pregnancy Category | Routes and Dosage Ranges [Adults [Unless Indicated]] |
|---|---|---|
| Ⓟ **Nitroglycerin** (Nitro-Bid, Nitro-Dur, Nitrostat, Nitrolingual, Rectiv; ✳ Minitran, Nitro-Dur, Nitrostat) | C | Immediate-release tablets, 2.5–9 mg PO two or three times/day<br>Sustained-release tablets or capsules, 2.5 mg PO three or four times/day<br>Sublingual, 0.15–0.6 mg as needed for chest pain<br>Translingual spray, one or two metered doses (0.4 mg/dose) sprayed onto oral mucosa at onset of anginal pain, to a maximum of three doses in 15 min<br>Transmucosal tablet, 1 mg every 3–5 h while awake, placed between upper lip and gum or cheek and gum<br>Topical ointment, 1/2–2 inches every 4–8 h; do not rub in<br>Topical transdermal disk, applied once daily<br>IV, 5–10 mcg/min initially, increased in 10–20 mcg/min increments up to 100 mcg/min or more if necessary to relieve pain |
| Isosorbide dinitrate (Isordil, Dilatrate-SR; ✳ ISDN) | C | Sublingual, 5–10 mg as needed or every 2–4 h<br>Regular tablets, 5–80 mg PO two to three times/day<br>Sustained-release capsules, 40 mg PO one to two times daily, max 160 mg daily |
| Isosorbide mononitrate (✳ Imdur) | C | 5–20 mg PO twice daily, with first dose on arising and the second dose 7 h later<br>Extended-release tablets, 30–60 mg once daily PO in the morning, increased after several days; maximum dose 240 mg once daily |

*contra:*

- With the use of other antihypertensive agents such as beta-adrenergic blockers. It is essential to observe for extreme episodes of hypotension.
- With renal impairment.

## Nursing Implications

### Preventing Interactions

Many drugs interact with nitroglycerin, increasing or decreasing its effects (Box 28.2). Several herbs interact with nitroglycerin and cause profound hypotension or negate the effects of nitroglycerin (Box 28.3).

### Administering the Medication

It is important to take a patient's vital signs prior to administration of any form of nitroglycerin. The nurse should withhold the medication with hypotension (systolic blood pressure less than 90 or 30 mm Hg below the patient's normal blood pressure) as well as tachycardia with a heart rate greater than 100 beats/min.

Administration of SL nitroglycerin or translingual spray is essential as soon as chest pain develops. If a patient is hospitalized, it is necessary to call the patient's health care provider and obtain a 12-lead ECG at the onset of chest pain. The SL nitroglycerin container should stay in a dry, cool, dark environment, and replacement every 6 months is necessary. Exposure to light deactivates the nitroglycerin tablets. Once opened, the translingual spray has a shelf life of 2 to 3 years.

In acute coronary syndromes, after three SL doses, administered 5 minutes apart, patients outside of the hospital should seek medical attention. While hospitalized, IV dosing should be started and titrated to desired effect. Nitrate tolerance commonly develops within 24 hours in patients on a continuous infusion of nitroglycerin. Extended-release oral nitrate preparations are used post-MI if angina persists after revascularization.

Application of nitroglycerin ointment requires using the dose-measuring application papers supplied with ointment. It is necessary to do the following:

- Squeeze the ointment onto a measuring scale printed on paper; typically, this is 1 or 1/2 inch, depending on the practitioner's order.

**BOX 28.2** **Drug Interactions: Nitroglycerin**

**Drugs That Increase the Effects of Nitroglycerin**
- Adalat and other calcium channel blockers, alcohol, aripiprazole, benazepril and other angiotensin-converting enzyme inhibitors, codeine and other narcotics, diphenhydramine, tizanidine
  *Increase the risk of orthostatic hypotension*
- Sildenafil, tadalafil, vardenafil
  *Increase the risk of life-threatening hypotension*

*viagra*

**Drugs That Decrease the Effects of Nitroglycerin**
- Acetaminophen, chloral hydrate, dihydroergotamine, sulfonylureas, vasopressin
  *Decrease vasodilating effects*

**BOX 28.3** **Herb and Dietary Interactions: Nitroglycerin**

**Herbs and Foods That Increase the Effects of Nitroglycerin**
- *N*-Acetyl cysteine
- Arginine, folate, vitamin E
- Hawthorn

**Herbs and Foods That Decrease the Effects of Nitroglycerin**
- Vitamin C

- Use the paper to spread ointment onto a nonhairy area of skin (chest, abdomen, thighs; avoid distal extremities) in a thin, even layer, covering a 2- to 3-inch area.
- Do not allow the ointment to come in contact with the hand. Do not massage the ointment into the patient's skin because absorption will be increased and interfere with the sustained action.

People should take PO nitrates in the morning after a nitrate-free interval (typically during the night). They should take the tablets or capsules 1 to 2 hours before meals. It is important not to break, crush, or chew sustained-release preparations.

IV nitroglycerin preparations come in glass bottles, polyvinyl chloride (PVC)-free partial-additive bags, and di(2-ethylhexyl) phthalate (DEHP)-free, PVC-free plastic EXCEL containers. Nurses should use these only with special tubing provided by the manufacturer because PVC tubing absorbs up to 80% of the nitroglycerin. Inline IV filters that adsorb nitroglycerin should be avoided. In addition, nurses should ensure that IV nitroglycerin is administered via infusion pump and that patients are placed on cardiac monitors. Many hospitals require patients to be in ICUs or step-down units while the nitroglycerin drip is actively being titrated. As previously stated, it is essential to take vital signs frequently with IV administration and recheck them with each titration.

### Assessing for Therapeutic Effects

Therapeutic effects of some forms of nitroglycerin may include the relief of acute chest pain as well as a modest decrease in blood pressure. With oral preparations, a decreased frequency of chronic chest pain should occur. Overall, patients should report that they feel better, have no symptoms of cardiac ischemia (i.e., chest pain), and have a higher activity tolerance.

### Patient Teaching

Box 28.4 reviews general patient teaching guidelines regarding drugs for the management of coronary heart disease, including nitroglycerin.

## Other Drugs in the Class

Isosorbide dinitrate (Isordil) is useful for reducing the frequency and severity of acute anginal episodes, not for acute relief of anginal symptoms. When given sublingually, it acts in about 2 minutes, and its effects last for 2 to 3 hours. When higher doses are given orally, more drug escapes metabolism in the liver and produces systemic effects in approximately 30 minutes. Therapeutic effects last about 4 hours after PO administration. The effective PO dose is usually determined by increasing the dose until headache occurs, indicating the maximum tolerable dose. Sustained-release capsules also are available.

**BOX 28.4** *Patient Teaching Guidelines for Drugs Used for Coronary Heart Disease*

**General Considerations**

- Angina is chest pain that occurs because your heart is not getting enough blood and oxygen. The most common causes are hypertension and atherosclerosis of the coronary arteries. The chest pain usually lasts less than 5 minutes, and episodes can be managed for years without causing permanent heart damage. However, if the pain is severe or prolonged, a heart attack and heart damage may develop. Seek information about your heart condition to prevent or decrease episodes of angina and prevent a heart attack.

- Several types of drugs are used in coronary heart disease, and you may need a combination of drugs for the best effects. Most patients take one or more long-acting drugs to prevent anginal attacks and a fast, short-acting drug (usually nitroglycerin tablets that you dissolve under your tongue or a nitroglycerin solution that you spray into your mouth) to relieve acute attacks. Seek emergency care immediately if rest and three sublingual tablets or oral sprays 5 minutes apart do not relieve chest pain. The long-acting oral medications are not effective in relieving sudden anginal pain.

- As with any medications for serious or potentially serious conditions, it is extremely important to take antianginal medications as prescribed. Do not increase dosage or discontinue the drugs without specific instructions from your health care provider.

- With sublingual nitroglycerin tablets, keep them in the original container; carry them so that they are always within reach but not where they are exposed to body heat; and replace them approximately every 6 months because they become ineffective.

- It may be helpful to record the number and severity of anginal episodes, the number of nitroglycerin tablets required to relieve the attack, and the total number of tablets taken daily. Such a record can help your health care provider know when to change your medications or your dosages.

- Headache and dizziness may occur with nitrate antianginal drugs, especially sublingual nitroglycerin. These effects are usually temporary and dissipate with continued therapy. If dizziness occurs, avoid strenuous activity and stand up slowly for approximately an hour after taking the drugs. If headache is severe, you may take aspirin or acetaminophen with the nitrate drug. Do not reduce drug dosage or take the drug less often to avoid headache; loss of effectiveness may occur.

- Keep family members or support people informed about the location and use of medications for heart disease in case help is needed.

- Avoid over-the-counter decongestants, cold remedies, and diet pills, which stimulate the heart and constrict blood vessels and thus may cause angina.

- With nitrate drugs, avoid alcohol. Both the drugs and alcohol dilate blood vessels, and an excessive reduction in blood pressure (with dizziness and fainting) may occur with the combination.

- With a metabolic modulator, avoid concurrent intake of grapefruit juice; grapefruit juice increases serum drug levels.

- Several calcium channel blockers are available in both immediate-acting and long-acting (sustained-release) forms. The brand names often differ very little (e.g., Procardia is a brand name of immediate-release nifedipine; Procardia XL is a long-acting formulation). It is extremely important that the correct formulation is used consistently.

- Keep all appointments with your health care provider.

**Self- or Caregiver Administration**

- Take or give drugs for heart disease as instructed; specific instructions differ with the type of drug being taken.

- Take or give drugs for heart disease on a regular schedule, at evenly spaced intervals. This increases drug effectiveness in preventing acute attacks of angina. The only exception may be nitroglycerin transdermal paste, which you may be directed not to take at night.

- With nitroglycerin and other nitrate preparations:
  - Use according to instructions for the particular dosage form. The dosage forms were developed for specific routes of administration and are not interchangeable.
  - Take your blood pressure before administering the medication as possible, and anticipate that the drug can decrease blood pressure from original reading. For sublingual nitroglycerin tablets, place them under the tongue until they dissolve. Take at the first sign of an anginal attack, before severe pain develops. If chest pain is not relieved in 5 minutes, dissolve a second tablet under the tongue. If pain is not relieved within another 5 minutes, dissolve a third tablet. If pain continues or becomes more severe, notify your health care provider immediately or report to the nearest hospital emergency room. Sit down when you take the medications. This may help relieve pain and prevent dizziness from the drug.
  - Do not take medications for erectile dysfunction when taking nitroglycerin and other nitrate preparations.
  - For the translingual solution of nitroglycerin, spray onto or under the tongue; do not inhale the spray.
  - For transmucosal tablets of nitroglycerin, place them under the upper lip or between the cheek and gum and allow them to dissolve slowly over 3 to 5 hours. Do not chew or swallow the tablets.
  - For nitroglycerin ointment, use the special paper to measure the dose. Place the ointment on a nonhairy part of the upper body and apply with the applicator paper. Cover the area with plastic wrap or tape. Rotate application sites (because the ointment can irritate the skin) and wipe off the previous dose before applying a new dose. Wash hands after applying the ointment.
  - Use the measured paper for accurate dosage. Use the paper to apply the ointment because the drug is readily absorbed through the skin. Avoid skin contact except on the designated area of the body. Plastic wrap or tape aids absorption and prevents removal

**BOX 28.4** *Patient Teaching Guidelines for Drugs Used for Coronary Heart Disease*
(Continued)

of the drug. It also prevents soiling of clothes and linens.

- For nitroglycerin patches and ointment, apply at the same time each day to clean, dry, hairless areas on the upper body or arms. Note whether the directions require you to remove the patch or ointment at night. Rotate sites. Avoid applying below the knee or elbow or in areas of skin irritation or scar tissue. Correct application is necessary to promote effective and consistent drug absorption. The drug is not as well absorbed from distal portions of the extremities because of decreased blood flow. Rotation of sites decreases skin irritation. Also, dispose of used patches properly because there is enough residual nitroglycerin to be harmful, especially to children and pets.

- Take oral nitrates on an empty stomach with a glass of water. Oral isosorbide dinitrate is available in regular and sustained-release tablets; be sure each type is taken appropriately. Do not crush or chew sustained-release nitrate tablets.

- For sublingual isosorbide dinitrate tablets, place them under the tongue until they dissolve.

- If an oral nitrate and topical nitroglycerin are being used concurrently, stagger the times of administration. This minimizes dizziness from low blood pressure and headache, which are common adverse effects of nitrate drugs.

- Report all new dietary supplements to the prescriber because some herbs interact with nitroglycerin.

- With beta-adrenergic blockers:
  - Do not stop taking the drug abruptly because this can cause rebound tachycardia. If withdrawal of a beta-adrenergic blocker is planned by your prescriber, a gradual decrease in dose should occur, and you should limit physical activity to a minimum during this period.
  - Move slowly from a sitting to a standing position to avoid orthostatic hypotension.
  - Learn how to take your own pulse and blood pressure, report heart rate less than 55 beats/min to your health care provider, and withhold medication as instructed. Take your pulse and blood pressure more frequently when the medication is initiated and titrated up or down.
  - Be aware of possible adverse effects, including dizziness, wheezing, and low heart rate.
  - Take atenolol at the same time each day and avoid drinking large amounts of orange juice.
  - If you are a diabetic, especially if you are prone to low blood sugar levels, you may need to check your blood sugar levels more frequently and eat consistently because beta-adrenergic blockers mask symptoms of low blood sugar.

- With calcium channel blockers:
  - Increase water and fiber intake as tolerated to decrease constipation.
  - Elevate your feet during the day to avoid ankle swelling.
  - With sustained-release forms, which are usually taken once daily, do not take more often than prescribed and do not crush or chew.

Isosorbide mononitrate is the metabolite and active component of isosorbide dinitrate. It is well absorbed after PO administration and almost 100% bioavailable. Unlike other PO nitrates, this drug is not subject to first-pass hepatic metabolism. Onset of action occurs within 1 hour, peak effects occur between 1 and 4 hours, and the elimination half-life is approximately 5 hours. It is used only for prophylaxis of angina; it does not act rapidly enough to relieve acute attacks.

### Clinical Application 28.1

- Mr. Gerald returns to the clinic for follow-up. His blood pressure is 130/86 mm Hg, and his heart rate is 86 beats/min. He reports that he has been pain free since discharge. He is taking his atenolol as prescribed but reports that he is using the nitroglycerin patch four times a day around the clock because it is easier for his schedule. Given his vital signs, his provider increased the atenolol to 100 mg daily. Mr. Gerald asks the nurse why he needs to take atenolol at all, when he has no pain, and why the dose has been increased. How should the nurse respond? What patient teaching needs to be reinforced?

### NCLEX Success

3. The nurse removes a patient's transdermal nitroglycerin disk at bedtime as ordered to minimize nitrate tolerance. The patient awakens during the night and complains of anginal symptoms. The nurse's action is to do which of the following?

   A. notify the health care provider
   B. apply a new transdermal disk
   C. obtain further history of complaints
   D. administer a short-acting nitrate as ordered

4. The health care provider prescribes nitroglycerin 2% ointment, 1.5-inch dose every 4 hours. To accurately apply the ointment, the patient should be instructed to do which of the following?

   A. rub the ointment into the skin to enhance absorption
   B. leave previous ointment on for 4 hours after applying a new dose
   C. rotate application sites to decrease skin irritation
   D. place the ointment on a distal part of the lower body to increase absorption

5. Concurrent use of nitrates in any form or route of administration with phosphodiesterase enzyme inhibitors produces which of the following?
   A. enhanced erectile potential
   B. significant tachycardia
   C. severe hypotensive effects
   D. mild bronchodilation

6. A patient taking nitroglycerin for angina reports developing a headache after taking more than one tablet. The nurse should inform him of which of the following?
   A. Headache is a common side effect due to the vasodilating effects of the medication.
   B. A headache indicates that a person is allergic to the nitroglycerin.
   C. The experience of headache means that the levels of nitroglycerin are toxic.
   D. The experience of headache likely means that the tablets have passed their expiration date.

7. The nurse is educating a patient taking sublingual nitroglycerin 0.4 mg for anginal pain. Which of the following statements indicate that the patient understands the instructions? [Select all that apply.]
   A. "I should take one nitroglycerin tablet every 5 minutes for pain, up to a total of three tablets, as needed."
   B. "I should expect that the nitroglycerin will cause a stinging sensation when placed under my tongue."
   C. "I should store my nitroglycerin in the original dark bottle to protect the tablets from light."
   D. "I should replace my nitroglycerin tablets every month whether the bottle has been opened or not."
   E. "I should seek help for my anginal symptoms if I do not get relief with three sublingual tablets."

# BETA-ADRENERGIC BLOCKERS

Beta-adrenergic blockers have become the cornerstone of drug therapy regimens for people with angina, MI, hypertension, heart failure, and dysrhythmias. They inhibit the chronotropic, inotropic, and vasoconstrictor responses to the catecholamines epinephrine and norepinephrine by exerting effects on the three adrenergic receptors (beta₁, beta₂, and alpha). In the cardiac system, these drugs decrease cardiac workload by slowing heart rate, decreasing blood pressure, and reducing contractility. The drugs are as effective as the organic nitrates in reducing the frequency and severity of anginal symptoms during exercise. People taking the drugs do not develop tolerance during therapy as occurs with the organic nitrates. The 2013 ACCF/AHA Guidelines for the Management of Acute MI reported evidence from randomized controlled trials demonstrating that when beta-adrenergic blockers are started early in patients without signs of heart failure with acute MI (primarily STEMI), they reduce infarction size and early mortality. Also, with long-term use, these drugs lower the risk of death.

The ability of a drug in this class to selectively block beta₁ receptors, principally found in the myocardium, is known as **cardioselectivity**. Therefore, cardioselective beta-adrenergic blockers, such as atenolol, metoprolol, bisoprolol, and esmolol, offer the potential advantage of not interfering with bronchodilation or peripheral vasodilation. In addition to beta₁-blockade, noncardioselective beta-adrenergic blockers block beta₂ receptors found in smooth muscle in the lungs, blood vessels, and other organs. Examples of noncardioselective beta-adrenergic blockers include propranolol, labetalol, nadolol, carvedilol, and timolol. Labetalol and carvedilol block both beta- and alpha-receptors, thereby decreasing peripheral and coronary vascular resistance. During beta-adrenergic blocker therapy, the beta receptors undergo receptor up-regulation. This means that the number of receptors on the surface of target cells (the beta cells) becomes more sensitive to catecholamines.

Beta-adrenergic blockers are discussed elsewhere in the text in relation to heart failure (see Chap. 30), dysrhythmias (see Chap. 27), hypertension (see Chap. 26), and glaucoma (see Chap. 59). Propranolol (Inderal), the first beta-adrenergic blocker available, is discussed in detail in Chapter 27 and is particularly useful in preventing exercise-induced tachycardia, which can precipitate anginal attacks. This chapter discusses **atenolol** (Tenormin) and other beta-adrenergic blockers used to manage angina.

## Pharmacokinetics

With PO administration, atenolol undergoes limited first-pass metabolism in the liver. Absorption is rapid and consistent but incomplete. Approximately only 50% of an oral dose is absorbed from the gastrointestinal (GI) tract. The drug is modestly (6%–16%) bound to plasma, is distributed to the placenta, and is secreted in breast milk. It does not readily cross the blood–brain barrier. Peak blood levels occur between 2 and 4 hours after ingestion. With IV atenolol, onset of action is immediate, duration of action is dose dependent (half-life 6–7 hours), and peak blood levels are reached in 5 minutes. The drug is not metabolized and is excreted in the urine and feces.

## Action

Atenolol is a cardioselective beta-adrenergic blocker. The cardioselectivity is diminished at higher doses, where it inhibits beta₂ receptors in the bronchial and vascular musculature.

## Use

Atenolol is useful in the treatment of angina and hypertension as well as for the prophylaxis and treatment of MI. Health care providers use atenolol and other beta-adrenergic blockers in long-term management to decrease the frequency and severity of anginal attacks, decrease the need for sublingual nitroglycerin, and increase exercise tolerance. Evidence supports the use of a cardioselective beta-adrenergic blocker, such as atenolol, within the first 24 hours following an acute MI.

> **! QSEN Alert: Safety**
>
> It is important to note that nonselective beta-adrenergic blockers should not be used in patients with variant angina because they are ineffective and may increase the tendency to induce coronary artery vasospasm.

### TABLE 28.3

## DRUGS AT A GLANCE: Beta-Adrenergic Blockers

| Drug | Pregnancy Category | Routes and Dosage Ranges [Adults [Unless Indicated]] |
|---|---|---|
| **Atenolol** (Tenormin; ✽ Tenormin) | D | 50 mg PO once daily, initially, increased to 100 mg daily after 1 wk, if necessary |
| Bisoprolol (✽ Apo-Bisoprolol, Ava-Bisoprolol) | C | 5 mg PO once daily, initially, increased approximately every 3 d to 10 mg daily, then 20 mg once daily, if necessary |
| Carvedilol (Coreg, Coreg CR; ✽ Apo-Carvedilol, Auro-Carvedilol) | C | 3.125 mg PO twice a day with food, initially, increased every 2 wk as needed and tolerated to 6.25–25 mg PO twice a day; maximum recommended dose, ≤85 kg: 25 mg twice daily, >85 kg: 50 mg twice daily<br>Extended release, PO 10 mg once daily, initially, increased every 2 wk as needed and tolerated, max dose 80 mg/d |
| Metoprolol (Lopressor, Toprol XL, Kapspargo Sprinkle; ✽ Apo-Metoprolol) | C | 100–450 mg PO daily in two to three divided doses<br>Extended release, 100 mg PO daily in a single dose |
| Nadolol (Corgard) | C | 40–240 mg PO daily in a single dose |
| Propranolol (Inderal, Inderal LA, Hemangeol, InnoPran; ✽ Inderal LA, Hemangiol) | C | 80–3200 mg/d PO in divided doses two to four times/day<br>0.5–3 mg IV every 4 h until desired response is obtained<br>Extended release, 80 mg PO once daily, max dose 320 mg once daily |

Table 28.3 presents route and dosage information for atenolol and other beta-adrenergic blockers. The U.S. Food and Drug Administration (FDA) has issued a **BLACK BOX WARNING ◆** relating to the use of beta-adrenergic blockers in patients with CAD; abrupt withdrawal of oral forms may result in exacerbation of angina, increased incidence of ventricular dysrhythmias, MI, or death. Therefore, it is essential to slowly taper beta-adrenergic blockers before discontinuing them.

### Use in Older Adults

The prevalence of CAD increases with age and is the major cause of disability, morbidity, and mortality in older adults. The elderly have a higher incidence of multivessel coronary disease, decreased left ventricular function, and comorbid conditions. For this reason, beta-adrenergic blockers are one of the most frequently medications prescribed in older adults. Close monitoring of the patient's heart rate is essential because the incidence of sick sinus syndrome and chronotropic intolerance increases with age and predisposes these patients to bradycardia, syncope, and falls.

### Use in Patients With Renal Impairment

Atenolol is well tolerated in patients with renal impairment, but dosage reduction may be necessary. Study findings indicate beta-adrenergic blockers slow the deterioration of renal function in chronic kidney disease.

### Use in Patients With Critical Illness

Administration of atenolol in the critical care setting may occur to reduce cardiovascular mortality in the management of hemodynamically stable patients with definite or suspected acute MI. IV administration should occur in a controlled setting equipped to monitor heart rate, blood pressure, and ECG. Hypotension may also occur with use, so the patient should be closely monitored for symptoms of hypotension. Unlike nitroglycerin, IV beta-adrenergic blockers are rarely used in the ICU for control of angina.

## Adverse Effects

The major cardiac adverse reactions related to beta-adrenergic blockers such as atenolol include heart failure and substantial **negative chronotropy** (causing slowing of the heart rate). A small number of people with chronic heart failure may have an exacerbation of heart failure when they begin taking atenolol or other beta-adrenergic blockers. In these people, sympathetic drive is maintaining cardiac output. The beta-adrenergic blockers decrease this sympathetic drive and therefore cause a low cardiac output state and heart failure. The majority of patients with heart failure do benefit from beta-blockade, and symptoms of heart failure abate.

To manage the negative chronotropy, dosage adjustments may be necessary; the target heart rate should be 55 to 65 beats/min at rest. Use of beta-adrenergic blockers can lead to serious bradydysrhythmias and depression of the atrioventricular node. Noncardiac adverse effects include bronchospasm, especially in patients with chronic obstructive pulmonary disease (COPD) receiving high dosages because of beta$_2$ receptor blockade.

Note that many of the earlier signs of hypoglycemia are adrenergic warning symptoms (e.g., tremors, palpitation, tachycardia). Therefore, the use of beta-adrenergic blockers in patients with diabetes can mask the early warning symptoms of hypoglycemia.

## Contraindications

Contraindications to atenolol include known hypersensitivity to the drug, second- or third-degree heart block, and cardiogenic shock, as well as severe bradycardia, heart failure, or hypotension. Caution is warranted with milder bradycardia, heart failure, or hypotension, and asthma.

## Nursing Implications

### Preventing Interactions

Many medications interact with atenolol, increasing or decreasing its effects (Box 28.5). Additionally, some herbs decrease the effects of atenolol (Box 28.6).

## BOX 28.5 — *Drug Interactions: Atenolol*

**Drugs That Increase the Effects of Atenolol**

- Alcohol
  *Increases the risk of hypotension*
- Atazanavir, dolasetron, saquinavir
  *Increase the risk of heart block*
- Digoxin
  *Increases the risk of bradycardia*
- Diltiazem, verapamil
  *Increase the risk of bradycardia, heart block, and increased left ventricular end-diastolic pressure*
- Reserpine
  *Increases the risk of hypotension and significant bradycardia*
- Sildenafil, tadalafil, vardenafil
  *Increase the risk of life-threatening hypotension*

**Drugs That Decrease the Effects of Atenolol**

- Adrenergic drugs (e.g., epinephrine, isoproterenol)
  *Reverse bradycardia*
- Anticholinergic drugs (e.g., diphenhydramine, ipratropium)
  *Increase heart rate, offsetting slower heart rates of atenolol*
- Indomethacin
  *Decreases the hypotensive effects*

*[handwritten margin notes: "↑e effects", "viagra", "↓ effects"]*

### Administering the Medication

Prior to giving atenolol, the nurse should check the patient's vital signs. It is important to withhold atenolol and notify the prescriber for a resting heart rate of 60 beats/min and/or systolic blood pressure less than 90 mm Hg.

The nurse gives IV beta-adrenergic blockers over 2.5 minutes. Continuous telemetry is necessary for patients receiving an IV bolus or a continuous drip. The effectiveness of beta-adrenergic blockers in relation to relieving angina is dose dependent. It is necessary to titrate the dose of the beta-adrenergic blocker for a target heart rate of 50 to 60 beats/min with normal blood pressure. The nurse monitors the blood pressure every 5 minutes, while the drip is being titrated, and assesses for signs of bronchoconstriction at higher drug dosages where cardioselectivity may be lost.

### Assessing for Therapeutic Effects

The nurse evaluates for three main objectives in the patient with chronic angina. One, the patient's frequency and severity

## BOX 28.6 — *Herb and Dietary Interactions: Atenolol*

**Herbs and Foods That Decrease the Effects of Atenolol**

- Betel palm
- Calcium salts
- Orange juice

of angina are reduced. Two, the patient has improved exercise capacity. Three, there is a reduction or elimination in the use of sublingual nitroglycerin. Ideally, achievement of these goals results in fewer adverse effects.

### Assessing for Adverse Effects

The nurse closely monitors the patient's blood pressure and heart rate 2 to 4 hours after the first dose of atenolol. Signs of hypotension include dizziness and blurred vision; syncope is indicative of bradydysrhythmias. Increased shortness of breath and wheezing are adverse effects seen in patients with COPD who are taking noncardioselective beta-adrenergic blockers or high doses of cardioselective beta-adrenergic blockers. In patients with diabetes prone to hypoglycemia, more frequent assessment of serum glucose levels may be necessary.

### Patient Teaching

Box 28.4 includes patient teaching information regarding drugs for the management of coronary heart disease, including atenolol.

## Other Drugs in the Class

A variety of other beta-adrenergic blockers are used to treat stable angina.

Metoprolol (Lopressor, Toprol XL) is used alone or in combination with other medications to treat angina and hypertension. Like atenolol, metoprolol is cardioselective and improves survival after an MI. Extended-release tablets are used in the treatment of heart failure. The drug is lipid soluble and almost completely absorbed by the small intestine. Metoprolol has a short half-life, which allows for more rapid dose adjustments based on the patient's blood pressure and heart rate response. It is eliminated by hepatic metabolism and is excreted in the urine. It has a short plasma half-life. Adverse effects include bradycardia, hypotension, dizziness, fatigue, and impotence.

Bisoprolol (Zebeta) is used to manage hypertension (see Chap. 26) in patients with stable angina. The drug reduces the workload of the heart and decreases myocardial oxygen demand by decreasing heart rate and the force of myocardial contractions. It is generally well tolerated, and adverse effects are mild and transient; they include nausea, diarrhea, dizziness, fatigue, impotence, bradycardia, and hypotension. At higher doses, the cardioselective properties are diminished, and bisoprolol can cause shortness of breath and wheezing. The drug can mask the early warning symptoms of hypoglycemia, like most of the other beta-adrenergic blockers.

Propranolol (Inderal) is used to reduce the frequency and severity of acute attacks of angina. It is especially useful in preventing exercise-induced tachycardia, which can precipitate anginal attacks. Caution is warranted with hepatic impairment. Nonselective beta-adrenergic blockers such as propranolol can slow down the process of glycogenolysis. Therefore, the occurrence of hypoglycemia increases. Beta-adrenergic blockers also can mask the early symptoms of hypoglycemia such as palpitations and anxiety due to blocked catecholamines. Propranolol is well absorbed after oral administration. It is then metabolized extensively in the liver; a relatively small proportion of an oral dose (~30%) reaches the systemic circulation. For this reason, oral doses of propranolol are much higher than IV doses. Onset of action is 30 minutes after oral administration and 1 to 2 minutes after IV injection. It is important to instruct patients to take the drug at the same time each day, preferably with or immediately following meals, because food may enhance the bioavailability of propranolol. Erectile dysfunction and wheezing are common adverse effects. Also, patients should report shortness of breath, night cough, edema, slow pulse, confusion, depression, rash, fever, or sore throat. In addition, they should understand that propranolol should never be stopped abruptly. Cimetidine may increase beta-adrenergic blocking effects of propranolol by slowing its hepatic clearance and elimination.

Nadolol, which is also noncardioselective, has the same actions, uses, and adverse effects as propranolol, but it has a long half-life and can be given once daily. The drug is excreted by the kidneys, and it is necessary to reduce the dosage in patients with renal impairment.

### Clinical Application 28.2

- While reviewing his medication instructions with Mr. Gerald, the nurse learns that he has a history of erectile dysfunction and has some sildenafil, which was prescribed for him before his MI. What actions should the nurse take?

## CALCIUM CHANNEL BLOCKERS

Calcium channel blockers are used to treat an assortment of cardiovascular disorders, including stable angina pectoris and variant angina. Other indications include hypertension, hypertrophic cardiomyopathy, and supraventricular dysrhythmias. There are two main categories of calcium channel blockers: the dihydropyridines (nifedipine, amlodipine, nicardipine, nitrendipine) and the nondihydropyridines (verapamil and diltiazem). **Nifedipine** (Adalat, Procardia) is the prototype.

## Pharmacokinetics

Nifedipine is well absorbed after oral administration, with an onset of action of 20 minutes or less. It reaches peak plasma levels within 1 to 2 hours (6 hours or longer for sustained-release forms). Most of the drug is more than 90% protein bound. It undergoes extensive first-pass metabolism in the liver. Excretion occurs in the feces and urine.

## Action

Nifedipine inhibits the influx of calcium entering through slow channels, producing vasodilation of the peripheral blood vessels and coronary arteries. However, the drug has a minimal effect on the sinoatrial and atrioventricular nodes. Therefore, it does not affect the heart rate.

## Use

Nifedipine has been shown to be effective in the treatment for stable, variant, and unstable angina, mild-to-severe hypertension, and Raynaud's phenomenon. Table 28.4 contains route and dosage information for nifedipine and other calcium channel blockers.

### TABLE 28.4

### DRUGS AT A GLANCE: Calcium Channel Blockers

| Drugs | Pregnancy Category | Routes and Dosage Ranges (Adults [Unless Indicated]) |
|---|---|---|
| **Nifedipine** (Adalat CC, Procardia, Procardia XL; ✹ Adalat XL, Nifedipine ER) | C | Angina: immediate release, 10–30 mg PO three times daily; sustained release, 30–60 mg PO once daily, max 120 mg/d<br>Hypertension: sustained release only, 30–60 mg once daily, max 120 mg/d |
| Amlodipine (Norvasc; ✹ Norvasc) | C | 5–10 mg PO once daily |
| Diltiazem (Cardizem, Cardizem CD, Cartia XT, Matzim LA, Tiazac; ✹ ACT Diltiazem CD, Apo-Diltiaz SR, Tiazac, Tiazac XC) | C | Angina or hypertension (immediate release): 30 mg PO four times daily initially, titrate over 1–2 d, usual dose 120–320 mg/d PO in four divided doses<br>Hypertension (sustained release only): 180–240 mg PO once daily |
| Felodipine (✹ Plendil, Sandoz-Felodipine) | C | Hypertension: 5–10 mg PO once daily |
| Isradipine | C | Hypertension: 2.5–5 mg PO twice daily |
| Nicardipine | C | Angina: immediate release only, 20–40 mg PO three times daily<br>Hypertension: immediate release, same as for angina, above; sustained release, 30–60 mg PO twice daily |
| Verapamil (Calan, Calan SR, Verelan, Verelan PM; ✹ Covera-HS, Verapamil Hydrochloride Injection, Verelan, Isoptin SR) | C | Angina: 80–160 mg PO three times daily, max dose 480 mg/d<br>Dysrhythmias: 80–120 mg PO three to four times daily; injection, 5–10 mg IV over 2 min or longer, with continuous monitoring of electrocardiogram and blood pressure<br>Hypertension: 120–360 mg/d PO in three divided doses or 240 mg PO (sustained release) once daily |

### Use in Children

For primary hypertension, nifedipine and other long-acting calcium channel blockers are safe. They are especially useful in children who have asthma and cannot tolerate beta-adrenergic blockers.

### Use in Older Adults

Nifedipine and other calcium channel blockers are commonly used in older adults. This age group is more prone to orthostatic hypotension and is at high risk for falls while taking calcium channel blockers. Older adults may have higher plasma concentrations of nifedipine due to decreased hepatic metabolism of the drug, probably because of decreased hepatic blood flow.

### Use in Patients With Renal Impairment

With nifedipine, protein binding is decreased and the elimination half-life is prolonged with renal impairment; therefore, dosage adjustment may be necessary. In a few patients, reversible elevations in blood urea nitrogen and serum creatinine have occurred.

### Use in Patients With Hepatic Impairment

With nifedipine and other calcium channel blockers, impairment of liver function has profound effects on the pharmacokinetics and pharmacodynamics. Thus, use of these drugs requires caution. It is necessary to reduce dosages substantially and closely monitor patients for drug effects (including periodic measurements of liver enzymes). These recommendations stem from the following effects:

- An impaired liver produces fewer drug-binding plasma proteins such as albumin. This means that a greater proportion of a given dose is unbound and therefore active.
- In patients with cirrhosis, bioavailability of oral drugs is greatly increased and metabolism (of both oral and parenteral drugs) is greatly decreased. Both of these effects increase plasma levels of drug from a given dose (essentially an overdose). The effects result from shunting of blood around the liver so that drug molecules circulating in the bloodstream do not come in contact with drug-metabolizing enzymes and therefore are not metabolized.
- Although hepatotoxicity is uncommon, clinical symptoms of hepatitis, cholestasis, or jaundice and elevated liver enzymes (e.g., alkaline phosphatase, CK, lactate dehydrogenase [LDH], aspartate aminotransferase [AST], alanine aminotransferase [ALT]) have occurred, mainly with diltiazem, nifedipine, and verapamil. These changes resolve if the causative drug is stopped.

### Use in Patients Receiving Home Care

With patients taking nifedipine, the home health nurse should check patients' blood pressure and heart rate at each visit. Also, the nurse should note adverse effects of the drug and suggest measures to minimize fall risk.

## Adverse Effects

With nifedipine, cardiac adverse effects due to excessive vasodilation include hypotension, flushing, headache, dizziness, lower limb edema, and reflex tachycardia; these appear to be dose related. Noncardiac adverse effects include constipation, nausea, and gingival hyperplasia.

## Contraindications

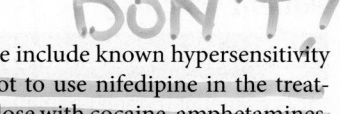

Contraindications to nifedipine include known hypersensitivity to the drug. It is important not to use nifedipine in the treatment of angina related to overdose with cocaine, amphetamines, or other alpha-adrenergic stimulants. This leads to unopposed stimulation of alpha-adrenergic receptors, causing vasoconstriction and severe, life-threatening hypertension.

## Nursing Implications

### Preventing Interactions

Many medications interact with nifedipine, increasing or decreasing its effect (Box 28.7). People should not take grapefruit juice with nifedipine because a twofold increase in the effects of the drug may occur. Nifedipine may interact with quinidine, decreasing plasma levels, and digoxin, increasing levels.

### Administering the Medication

People may take nifedipine with or without food. It is important not to crush or break sustained-release formulations. It is necessary to take the blood pressure prior to administering nifedipine and withhold the drug for a systolic blood pressure less than 90 mm Hg.

### Assessing for Therapeutic Effects

The nurse should note a reduction of angina episodes once the patient has started taking nifedipine. Ideally, in general, the systolic blood pressure should be less than 120 mm Hg.

### Assessing for Adverse Effects

The nurse should assess for excessive vasodilation. Symptoms include flushing, peripheral edema, and frequent headaches. Hypotension, dizziness, light-headedness, weakness, peripheral edema, headache, heart failure, pulmonary edema, nausea, and constipation may also occur.

**BOX 28.7    Drug Interactions: Nifedipine**

**Drugs That Increase the Effects of Nifedipine**

- Cisapride, dolasetron, pimozide
  *Increase risk of prolongation of QT interval, second- and third-degree heart block, and ventricular dysrhythmias*
- Itraconazole
  *Increases dose-related negative inotropic effect*
- Cimetidine
  *Increases peak plasma levels*
- Tizanidine
  *Increases the risk of hypotension*

**Drugs That Decrease the Effects of Nifedipine**

- Calcium-containing products
  *Saturate calcium channels*
- Carbamazepine, phenytoin, rifampin
  *Induce hepatic enzymes and increase the rate of metabolism*

## Patient Teaching

 **QSEN Alert: Safety**

It is essential to teach patients to not stop taking nifedipine abruptly. This may result in rebound tachycardia.

Box 28.4 outlines patient teaching guidelines regarding drugs for the management of coronary heart disease, including nifedipine.

## Other Drugs in the Class

The other calcium channel blockers vary in clinical indications for use; most are used for stable angina or hypertension, and only diltiazem and verapamil are used to manage supraventricular tachydysrhythmias. In patients with CAD, the drugs are effective as monotherapy but are commonly prescribed in combination with beta-adrenergic blockers. In addition, nimodipine is approved for use only in subarachnoid hemorrhage, in which it decreases spasm in cerebral blood vessels and limits the extent of brain damage.

In variant angina, calcium channel blockers reduce coronary artery vasospasm. In atrial fibrillation or flutter and other supraventricular tachydysrhythmias, diltiazem and verapamil slow the rate of ventricular response. In hypertension, the drugs lower blood pressure primarily by dilating peripheral arteries.

The dihydropyridines used to treat angina besides nifedipine include amlodipine and nicardipine. Amlodipine (Norvasc) is effective in patients with exertional angina, because the drug reduces afterload decreasing myocardial oxygen demand. It is also used for the treatment of coronary spasm in variant angina. The drug is well absorbed by the PO route. Amlodipine has a long elimination half-life (30–50 hours) and therefore can be given once daily. Common adverse effects include peripheral edema, fatigue, dizziness, nausea, palpitations, and headache.

Nicardipine (Cardene) is a dihydropyridine calcium channel blocker used for the treatment of chronic stable angina (exertional), hypertension, and Raynaud's phenomenon. The drug is available in oral and intravenous forms. The most common side effects are flushing, headaches, dizziness, and peripheral edema. The mechanism of action and clinical effects of nicardipine closely resemble those of nifedipine and the other dihydropyridines, amlodipine and felodipine, except that nicardipine is more selective for cerebral and coronary blood vessels.

Nondihydropyridines, such as diltiazem (Cardizem) and verapamil (Calan, Isoptin), block the slow calcium channels in the heart. They also decrease the heart rate by slowing conduction through the atrioventricular node and decrease sinoatrial node automaticity. Chapter 27 describes them well. Whereas nifedipine acts mainly on vascular smooth muscle to produce vasodilation, verapamil and diltiazem have greater effects on the cardiac conduction system. For this reason, these two drugs may also be used for supraventricular tachycardia. They are also effective in the treatment of angina, hypertension, and migraines. Diltiazem is a potent vasodilator of coronary and peripheral vessels, which decreases afterload and decreases workload on the heart. The drug has pharmacologic activity similar to verapamil, although diltiazem and verapamil differ chemically from the dihydropyridines and each other. Adverse effects include hypotension, bradycardia, dizziness, and flushing. Along with other calcium channel blockers, verapamil and diltiazem are known to induce gingival hyperplasia.

## ADJUVANT MEDICATIONS

### Ranolazine

The anti-ischemic metabolic modulator **ⓟ ranolazine** (Ranexa) is an approved first-line treatment for chronic angina. However, the drug does not relieve acute angina symptoms and has not shown a benefit in acute coronary syndromes. Conventional antianginal drugs significantly decrease one or more of the determinants of myocardial oxygen demand, such as heart rate, preload, afterload, or myocardial contractility, thus reducing myocardial ischemia. Ranolazine increases the energy production of the heart to preserve cardiac function without decreasing blood pressure or heart rate, but it does not relieve acute anginal attacks and does not have any benefit in treating acute coronary syndromes. Although its mechanism of action is not clearly understood, ranolazine works by preventing both calcium overload and the subsequent increase in diastolic tension. This is all related to inhibition of the late inward sodium channel. Because this sodium channel frequently fails to inactivate in a number of important myocardial disease states such as ischemia and hypertrophy, excess entry of sodium ions leads to activation of the sodium–calcium exchanger, thereby raising calcium concentration. Unlike the other classes of antianginal drugs, ranolazine decreases ischemia but does not possess negative inotropic or chronotropic effects. When compared to placebo in patients with CAD, ranolazine is associated with a decreased frequency of ventricular dysrhythmias, bradycardia, and new-onset atrial fibrillation.

Ranolazine should be reserved for use in two groups of patients: (1) in those who have not had an adequate response to beta-adrenergic blockers or (2) in combination with the blockers for relief of symptoms when initial treatment with the blockers has not been successful. Ranolazine has a dose-dependent ability to prolong the QT interval. Therefore, the drug is contraindicated in patients with preexisting QT-interval prolongation. It is also contraindicated in patients with hepatic disease and in patients taking other drugs that prolong the QT interval. Dose reduction of digoxin and simvastatin may be necessary with concurrent use because ranolazine affects the metabolic pathways of these drugs. Table 28.5 gives route and dosage information for ranolazine.

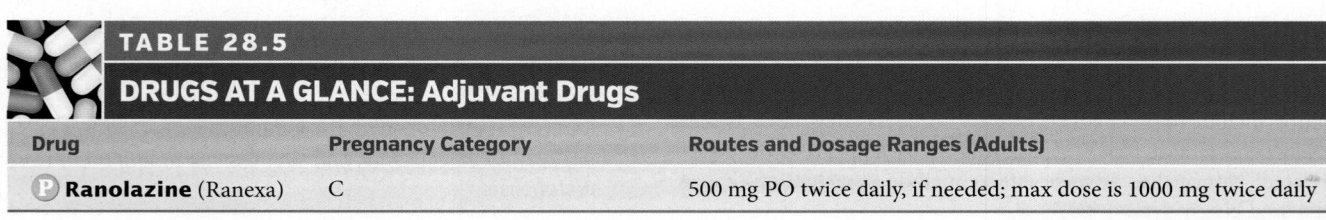

| | **TABLE 28.5** | |
| --- | --- | --- |
| | **DRUGS AT A GLANCE: Adjuvant Drugs** | |
| **Drug** | **Pregnancy Category** | **Routes and Dosage Ranges (Adults)** |
| ⓟ **Ranolazine** (Ranexa) | C | 500 mg PO twice daily, if needed; max dose is 1000 mg twice daily |

*Bad*

*good*

The routine use of oxygen in the setting of acute MIs has been common. However, evidence suggests that its use in acute MI patients with normal oxygen saturations [≥94% on pulse oximetry] results in no significant difference in mortality when compared to patients breathing room air. Researchers have demonstrated that giving supplemental oxygen to patients without hypoxia does not lead to improved outcomes and has the disadvantages of discomfort of use and additional cost. Abuzaid and colleagues, in a 2018 meta-analysis of seven studies [*n* = 7702], confirmed the lack of benefit of routine oxygen therapy in patients with acute MI with normal oxygen saturation levels.

In the 2015 AVOID study, Stub and associates randomly assigned 441 patients with a confirmed STEMI with normal oxygen saturations to either 8 L/min of oxygen or room air. Those who received oxygen had no improvement in infarction size in the acute phase and had a larger MI size at 6 months by cardiac magnetic resonance. These findings may result from the fact that hyperoxia has been shown to have a direct vasoconstrictive effect on the coronary arteries, which might occur with the administration of oxygen to patients with normal oxygen saturations. Oxygen should be administered with clinically significant hypoxemia [O₂ saturations less than 90%, dyspnea, or heart failure]. *only <90%*

## Dyslipidemic Drugs

Dyslipidemic drugs (i.e., atorvastatin, cholestyramine, niacin) are useful in the management of patients with major risk factors for atherosclerosis and vascular disorders such as CAD, stroke, and peripheral arterial insufficiency when lifestyle changes alone do not reduce blood lipids. These drugs have proven efficacy, and health care providers are increasingly using them to reduce morbidity and mortality from coronary heart disease and other atherosclerosis-related cardiovascular disorders. Prescribers order dyslipidemic drugs to decrease blood lipids, prevent or delay the development of atherosclerotic plaque, promote the regression of existing atherosclerotic plaque, and reduce morbidity and mortality from cardiovascular disease. Chapter 10 discusses the dyslipidemic drugs in detail.

## Antihypertensive Drugs

Antihypertensive drugs that decrease peripheral vascular resistance are useful in angina. Chapter 26 discusses antihypertensive drugs.

## Angiotensin-Converting Enzyme Inhibitors

Angiotensin-converting enzyme (ACE) inhibitors may be given to most patients routinely unless contraindicated, particularly in those with an anterior infarction, decreased left ventricular function, or heart failure. For those individuals who cannot tolerate an ACE inhibitor, an angiotensin receptor blocker can be given (see Chap. 26).

## Aspirin

Aspirin produces an antiplatelet effect by irreversibly acetylating the active site of cyclooxygenase-1 (COX-1), which at lower doses effectively suppress platelet aggregation without affecting important endothelial cell functions. A growing body of evidence supports the use of aspirin in both primary and secondary prevention of cardiovascular events. However, in primary prevention, benefits may be outweighed by the risk of major bleeding. In secondary prevention, aspirin has been shown to substantially reduce mortality when administered during an evolving MI and should be given, unless contraindicated, as soon as possible after the onset of symptoms. The loading dose is 162 to 325 mg of uncoated aspirin; chewing or crushing the tablet establishes a high blood level quickly. Evidence suggests that long-term use of lower doses as opposed to higher dosages does not significantly affect cardiovascular outcomes and causes less risk of bleeding. With NSTEMI and STEMI, enteric-coated aspirin should be avoided initially because the enteric coating delays and reduces drug absorption. Chapter 16 contains additional information regarding aspirin.

## Adenosine Diphosphate Receptor Antagonists

Clopidogrel and other adenosine diphosphate (ADP) receptor antagonists, prasugrel and ticagrelor, have antiplatelet effects similar to aspirin and inhibit the ADP (P2Y12) receptor on the surface of platelets. Clopidogrel has three shortcomings: delayed onset of action, irreversible inhibitory effects on platelets with no reversing agent or antidote, and significant individual variability in platelet response. Clopidogrel and ticagrelor are indicated for unstable angina and NSTEMI in patients who are to be treated medically or by planned primary PCI. Administering clopidogrel with aspirin (dual antiplatelet therapy) has been found superior to aspirin alone in decreasing the incidence of cardiovascular death and nonfatal MI—both acutely and for up to 9 to 11 months. Ticagrelor is used to reduce the rate of cardiovascular death, MI, and stroke in patients with a history of MI or acute coronary syndrome. The drug also decreases the rate of stent thrombosis in individuals requiring a stent for the treatment of acute coronary syndromes. Ticagrelor differs from clopidogrel and prasugrel in that receptor blockade is reversible. It is effective and relatively safe when compared to clopidogrel. The most recent data suggest that ticagrelor has broader applicability of use in individuals with acute coronary syndrome as compared to prasugrel. (However, prasugrel seems to be better tolerated.) In addition to aspirin, the ADP antagonists are usually continued for up to 12 months. Further information regarding the ADP receptor antagonists is found in Chapter 9.

## Glycoprotein IIb/IIIa Receptor Antagonists

The glycoprotein (GP) IIb/IIIa receptor antagonists eptifibatide and tirofiban inhibit platelet aggregation by preventing activation of GP IIb/IIIa receptors on the platelet surface and the subsequent binding of fibrinogen and von Willebrand factor to platelets. The drugs are used occasionally in combination with heparin or aspirin to prevent clotting before and during invasive heart procedures in patients with NSTEMI. Antiplatelet effects occur during intravenous drug infusion and diminish once the drug is stopped. Additional discussion regarding the GP IIb/IIIa receptors antagonists is found in Chapter 9.

## Morphine

Historically, morphine has been useful for relieving pain, reducing anxiety, and decreasing preload and remains a cornerstone in pain management in post-MI patients with unacceptable levels of pain (see Chapter 49). However, findings from the CRUSADE retrospective observational registry (57,039 patients with non–ST-elevation acute coronary syndrome) indicated that treating patients with morphine was associated with decreased survival. Although the exact cause of the negative outcome was not clear, recent studies (Kubica et al., 2015; Parodi et al., 2014) have suggested that morphine acts by interfering with the antiplatelet effect of the P2Y12 receptor blockers commonly given to this group of patients.

 **QSEN Alert: Evidence-Based Practice**

Interventions in acute MI are focused on the overall goal of prompt, complete, and sustained reperfusion of the myocardium. Interest in providing evidence-based decisions regarding management strategies that support that goal has given rise to concerns regarding morphine. One study found that the administration of morphine to patients following a NSTEMI increased the risk of death. Another study of patients following a STEMI indicated that morphine may interfere with platelet inhibition by disrupting the absorption of the antiplatelet drugs (P2Y12 inhibitors) and other medications. By impeding normal gastric activity, morphine may delay absorption and decrease peak plasma levels of orally administered drugs. Additional research is necessary to determine morphine's ongoing role in pain management following acute MI.

## Thrombolytic Drugs

The purpose of giving thrombolytic agents following a STEMI is to dissolve thrombi and reestablish blood flow as quickly as possible, prevent or limit tissue damage, and maximize functional improvement. These drugs stimulate conversion of plasminogen to plasmin, a proteolytic enzyme that breaks down fibrin, the framework of a thrombus. In coronary circulation, restoration of blood flow reduces morbidity and mortality by limiting MI size. Maximal benefit is achieved when thrombolytic drugs are administered within the first 2 to 3 hours, especially within the first hour. In addition, anticoagulant drugs, such as heparin and warfarin, as well as antiplatelet agents are given following thrombolytic therapy to decrease reformation of a thrombus. Thrombolytic treatment is not recommended as treatment for a NSTEMI.

Alternately, PCI (also called percutaneous transluminal coronary angioplasty) together with certain drugs may be used to reestablish blood flow with a STEMI. Adjunctive therapy with PCI includes antiplatelet and antithrombotic therapy to reduce thrombotic complications. Generally, aspirin, an ADP receptor antagonist, and a GP IIb/IIIa inhibitor are given. Intravenous fractionated heparin is also administered during the PCI to prevent acute coronary closure during the procedure. The goal in both approaches is to minimize total ischemic time and restore blood flow. Therapeutic effects include reversal of symptoms, stabilization of cardiac rhythm, decrease of the ST-segment elevation by 50%, and absence of bleeding complications. Chapter 9 discusses thrombolytic drugs in detail.

**NCLEX Success**

8. A 57-year-old man taking metoprolol presents to the cardiac clinic following a myocardial infarction. He reports that he continues to smoke. Smoking may contribute to what effect on beta-adrenergic blocking activity?
A. reduce the efficacy
B. potentiate an increase in intracranial pressure
C. precipitate ventricular fibrillation
D. increase the incidence of adverse effects

9. A 72-year-old woman with angina pectoris, who is being discontinued from beta-adrenergic blockers, asks the nurse, "Why can't I just stop taking the drug today if it's not working anyway?" The nurse instructs the patient that failure to taper the drug slowly may lead to which of the following?
A. worsening of her angina symptoms
B. significant bronchoconstriction
C. development of heart failure
D. drug fever

10. In caring for a patient with chronic angina who has been prescribed the new drug, ranolazine, the nurse is correct in counseling which of the following about this drug?
A. may be crushed if necessary
B. must not be taken with beta-adrenergic blockers
C. must not be taken with meals
D. should not be taken with grapefruit juice

11. Which of the following classes of medications protect the ischemic myocardium by blocking catecholamines and sympathetic nerve stimulation?
A. nitrates
B. beta-adrenergic blockers
C. adenosine diphosphate receptor antagonists
D. calcium channel blockers

12. Which of the following are expected outcomes for a patient on the 2nd day of hospitalization after revascularization following an ST-segment elevation myocardial infarction? (Select all that apply.)
A. The patient reports only minimal chest pain and diaphoresis with activity.
B. Electrocardiogram (ECG) monitors shows sinus tachycardia with only occasional premature ventricular contractions.
C. There is absence of bleeding complications.
D. 12-Lead ECG shows a decrease of the ST-segment elevations by 50% of the initial height.

## THE NURSING PROCESS

A concept map outlines the nursing process related to drug therapy considerations in this chapter. Additional nursing implications related to the disease process should also be considered in care decisions.

**Assessment**

- Assess the length of time and purpose for which patient is taking antianginal drugs (prophylaxis, treatment of acute attacks, or both). If the patient takes nitroglycerin, ask how often it is required, how many tablets are needed for relief of pain, how often the supply is replaced, and where the patient stores or carries the drug.
- Assess the frequency and duration of acute anginal attacks and whether either has increased recently. (An escalation could indicate worsening coronary atherosclerosis and increased risk of acute coronary syndromes.)
- Assess precipitating symptoms during an anginal event, such as chest pain or pressure (e.g., location, quality), shortness of breath, diaphoresis, nausea, and dizziness.
- Assess blood pressure and pulse, ECG reports, serum cholesterol, and cardiac enzymes.
- Assess whether previous invasive procedures were used to diagnose or treat CAD (e.g., cardiac catheterization, PCI, revascularization surgery).

**Outcomes of Therapy**

The patient will
- Receive or take drugs for coronary heart disease accurately.
- Experience relief of acute chest pain and other anginal symptoms.
- Have fewer episodes of acute chest pain and other anginal symptoms.
- Have increased activity tolerance.
- Identify and manage situations that precipitate anginal attacks.
- Be closely monitored for therapeutic and adverse effects, especially when drug therapy is initiated.
- Avoid preventable adverse effects.
- Verbalize essential information about the disease process, needed dietary and lifestyle changes to improve health status, and drug therapy.
- Identify available resources and support systems and demonstrate appropriate coping strategies.
- Recognize signs and symptoms that necessitate professional medical intervention.
- Keep appointments for follow-up care and monitoring.

**Nursing Interventions**

- Assist the patient to recognize and avoid precipitating factors (e.g., heavy meals, strenuous exercise) when possible.
- Support the patient while identifying resources, support systems, and effective coping strategies.
- Aid the patient during an acute event to manage symptoms of CAD:
  - Assume that any chest pain may be of cardiac origin.
  - Take a fast-acting nitroglycerin preparation (previously prescribed), up to three SL tablets or three sprays, each 5 minutes apart, as necessary.
  - If chest pain is not relieved with rest and nitroglycerin, assume that an MI has occurred until proven otherwise. In a health care setting, keep the patient at rest and notify the patient's prescriber immediately. Outside of a health care setting, call 911 for immediate assistance.
- Help the patient develop a more healthful lifestyle in terms of diet and weight control, adequate rest and sleep, regular exercise, and smoking cessation.
- Provide appropriate patient teaching related to drug therapy (see Box 28.4).

**Evaluation**

- Observe and interview for effective strategies used to relieve acute chest pain and frequency of symptoms.
- Identify CAD lifestyle factors that are being successfully modified or require modification (e.g., diet, weight, activity, smoking cessation).
- Observe effective coping strategies and appropriate use of support system and resources.
- Interview regarding success and adherence with drug therapy.
- Interview and observe for adverse drug effects.

## KEY CONCEPTS

- Angina results from deficit in myocardial oxygen supply (myocardial ischemia) in relation to myocardial oxygen demand, most often caused by atherosclerotic plaque in the coronary arteries.
- Cardiac troponin I and cardiac troponin T are the preferred biomarkers of myocyte injury because they are more specific and sensitive than the traditional cardiac isoenzyme CK-MB.
- The goals of antianginal drug therapy are to relieve acute anginal pain, reduce the number and severity of acute anginal attacks, improve exercise tolerance and quality of life, delay progression of CAD, prevent MI, and prevent sudden cardiac death.
- Because PO nitroglycerin is rapidly metabolized in the liver, relatively small proportions reach systemic circulation; transmucosal, transdermal, and IV preparations are more effective.
- Common drugs used for myocardial ischemia are the organic nitrates, the beta-adrenergic blockers, and the calcium channel blockers. Cardioselective beta-adrenergic blockers are more effective than nitrates or calcium channel blockers in decreasing the likelihood of silent ischemia, reducing infarction size, and improving mortality after STEMI.
- The FDA has issued a **BLACK BOX WARNING** ◆ concerning the use of beta-adrenergic blockers in patients with CAD; abrupt withdrawal of oral forms may lead to exacerbation of angina, increased incidence of ventricular dysrhythmias, MI, or death. Therefore, it is essential to slowly taper beta-adrenergic blockers before discontinuing them.
- Traditional antianginal drugs that act via hemodynamic mechanisms (e.g., beta-adrenergic blockers, calcium channel blockers, nitrates) can pose a problem in older adults because of the associated higher risk of drug interaction and greater incidence of adverse drug effects.
- Patients who take long-acting dosage forms of nitrates on a regular schedule develop tolerance to the vasodilating (antianginal) effects of the drugs. The use of a drug-free period, typically during sleep, reduces the development of this drug tolerance.

- Phosphodiesterase enzyme type 5 inhibitors for erectile dysfunction and nitrates both decrease blood pressure, and the combined effect can produce profound, life-threatening hypotension.
- Beta-adrenergic blockers can mask the early symptoms of hypoglycemia such as palpitations and anxiety due to blocked catecholamines. Patients may not recognize signs of hypoglycemia until confusion is present.
- In angina pectoris, calcium channel blockers improve blood supply to the myocardium by dilating coronary arteries and decrease the workload of the heart by dilating peripheral arteries; in variant angina, the drugs reduce coronary artery vasospasm.
- The metabolic modulator ranolazine increases the energy production of the heart to preserve cardiac function but does not relieve acute anginal attacks.
- Aspirin, antilipidemics, and antihypertensives are used in conjunction with antianginal drugs to prevent progression of myocardial ischemia to MI.
- Starting with relatively small doses of antianginal drugs and increasing them at appropriate intervals as necessary should achieve optimal benefit and minimal adverse effects.
- Aspirin has been shown to substantially reduce mortality when administered in an evolving MI and should be given, unless contraindicated, as soon as possible after the onset of symptoms.
- Oxygen should be administered with clinically significant hypoxemia ($O_2$ saturations less than 90%, dyspnea, or heart failure).
- The purpose of giving thrombolytic agents in STEMI is to dissolve thrombi to reestablish blood flow as quickly as possible, prevent or limit tissue damage, and maximize functional improvement.
- Desired therapeutic effects of early revascularization following a STEMI by thrombolytic agents or PCI include reversal of symptoms, stabilization of cardiac rhythm, decrease of the ST-segment elevations by 50% of the initial height, and absence of bleeding complications.

## CLINICAL REASONING CASE STUDY

**Meet the Patient**

Jonathan Trudeau, a 58-year-old accountant, is being evaluated at the cardiology clinic for angina. He is 5'9″ tall and weighs 220 pounds, with a waist measurement of 40 inches. He has a history of hypertension, for which he has been prescribed a thiazide diuretic. He admits that he has not been taking the medication lately. His blood pressure on this visit is 154/96 mm Hg. He smokes one pack of cigarettes per day. His LDL cholesterol level is 187 mg/dL. He has no history of diabetes, and his fasting glucose level is within normal limits. He states that he "works out at the gym" 3 days per week. He admits to episodes of midsternal chest pain accompanied by dyspnea and diaphoresis, which are associated with activity and usually relieved with rest. He states that these episodes have been increasing in frequency to once or twice weekly.

• Mr. Trudeau receives a prescription for SL nitroglycerin tablets to use as needed for chest pain and isosorbide mononitrate to take daily. He asks why he needs two prescriptions. How should the nurse respond?
• Mr. Trudeau continues to experience episodes of angina despite treatment with the nitrate. He receives a prescription for ranolazine (Ranexa). He asks whether he can stop taking the nitrate now. How should the nurse answer this question?
• The nurse is teaching Mr. Trudeau about nonpharmacologic management of his angina. What measures can he take to reduce his risk?

**Assessing Drug Information**

Sublingual nitroglycerin and isosorbide mononitrate are organic nitrates used to manage angina.
• Sublingual nitroglycerin is a rapid-acting nitrate taken at onset of acute anginal symptoms.
   • Mr. Trudeau should take three tablets, 5 minutes apart, and if chest pain persists, he should activate the emergency medical services (911).
   • For most nitroglycerin, the tablets should sting when placed under the tongue; potency may have been lost if the tablets do not produce this effect.
   • Adverse effects include hypotension, dizziness, and headache.
• Isosorbide mononitrate is a long-acting nitrate used to prevent further attacks of angina; it is not used to treat acute anginal symptoms.
• Ranolazine (Ranexa) blocks the influx of sodium into the cell during repolarization, reducing intracellular sodium concentrations. Decreased intracellular calcium reduces ventricular tension and myocardial oxygen consumption.
   • Designed to be used in combination with another antianginal agent for relief of chronic angina when initial treatment with another agent alone has not been successful.
   • Like isosorbide, the drug is not useful in the treatment of acute anginal attacks.
   • Exerts therapeutic effects without changing heart rate or blood pressure, but hypotension and bradycardia may be adverse effects.
   • Other adverse effects include prolonged QT interval on electrocardiogram (ECG), peripheral edema, dizziness, and headache.

**Nursing Actions**

• The nurse needs to instruct Mr. Trudeau on the following:
   • Carry nitroglycerin tablets in the original container and take for episodes of chest pain. Isosorbide and ranolazine will not help stop sudden chest pain.
   • Take care to sit or lie down prior to taking sublingual nitroglycerin, as a decrease in blood pressure or dizziness may occur.
   • Do not chew or break ranolazine tablets, avoid grapefruit juice, and do not double up on a missed dose.
   • Return to the clinic for regular ECG monitoring as directed, as ranolazine affects QT intervals and thus could precipitate dysrhythmias.
   • Resume taking the thiazide diuretic and have blood pressure monitored regularly.
   • Pursue nonpharmacologic measures to decrease cardiovascular risk.
       • Nutrition counseling can help with weight reduction.
       • Smoking cessation programs or aids can help with quitting smoking, which increases heart rate, blood pressure, and platelet adhesion while decreasing myocardial contractility and the amount of oxygen delivered to the myocardium.
       • A consistent exercise program should be maintained.

*Visit* thePoint° *at* **http://thePoint.lww.com/Frandsen12e** *for answers to NCLEX Success questions (in Appendix A), answers to Clinical Application Case Studies (in Appendix B), and more!*

## REFERENCES AND RESOURCES

Abuzaid, A., Fabrizio, C., Felpel, K., Al Ashry, H. S., Ranjan, P., Elbadawi, A., et al. (2018). Oxygen therapy in patients with acute myocardial infarction: A systematic review and meta-analysis. *American Journal of Medicine, 131*(6), 693.

Amsterdam, E. A., Wenger, N. K., Brindis, R. G., Casey, D. E. Jr, Ganiats, T. G., Holmes, D. R. Jr, et al. (2014). 2014 AHA/ACC Guideline for the management of patients with non–ST-elevation acute coronary syndromes: A report of the American College of Cardiology/American Heart Association Task Force on Practice Guidelines. *Journal of the American College of Cardiology, 64*(24), e139–e228.

DiPiro, J. T., Talbert, R. L., Yee, G. C., Wells, B. G., Posey, L. M., & Matzke, G. R. (2016). *Pharmacotherapy: A pathophysiologic approach* (10th ed.). New York, NY: McGraw-Hill Education.

Ettehad, D., Emdin, C.A., Kiran, A., Anderson, G., Callender, T., Emberson, J., et al. (2016). Blood pressure lowering for prevention of cardiovascular disease and death: A systematic review and meta-analysis. *The Lancet, 387*(10022), 957–967.

Guyton, A. C., & Hall, J. E. (2015). *Textbook of medical physiology* (13th ed.). Philadelphia, PA: Saunders.

Hazinski, M. F., Nolan, J. P., the International Liaison Committee on Resuscitation Editorial Board. (2015). Part 1: Executive summary: 2015 international consensus on cardiopulmonary resuscitation and emergency cardiovascular care science with treatment recommendations. *Circulation, 132*(16), S2–S39.

Hobl, E. L., Stimpfl, T., Ebner, J., Schoergenhofer, C., Derhaschnig, U., Sunder-Plassmann, R., et al. (2013). Morphine decreases clopidogrel concentrations and effects: A randomized, double-blind, placebo-controlled trial. *Journal of the American College of Cardiology, 63*(7), 630–635.

Kalra, B. S., & Roy, V. (2012). Efficacy of metabolic modulators in ischemic heart disease: An overview. *The Journal of Clinical Pharmacology, 52*(3), 292–305.

Karch, A. (2016). *Focus on nursing pharmacology*. Philadelphia, PA: Lippincott Williams & Wilkins.

Kubica, J., Adamski, P., Ostrowska, M., Sikora, J., Kubica, J. M., Sroka, W. D., et al. (2015). Morphine delays and attenuates ticagrelor exposure and action in patients with myocardial infarction: the randomized, double-blind, placebo-controlled IMPRESSION trial. *European Heart Journal, 37*(3), 245–252.

Mehta, L. S., Beckie, T. M., DeVon, H. A., Grines, C. L., Krumholz, H. M., Johnson, M. N., et al. (2016). Acute myocardial infarction in women: A scientific statement from the American Heart Association. *Circulation, 133*, 916–947.

Norris, T. L. (2019). *Porth's pathophysiology: Concepts of altered health states* (10th ed.). Philadelphia, PA: Wolters Kluwer.

O'Gara, P. T., Kushner, F. G., Ascheim, D. D., Casey, D. E. Jr, Chung, M. K., de Lemos, J. A., et al. (2013). 2013 ACCF/AHA guideline for the management of ST-elevation myocardial infarction: A report of the American College of Cardiology Foundation/American Heart Association Task Force on Practice Guidelines. *Journal of the American College of Cardiology, 61*(4), e78–e140.

Parodi, G., Bellandi, B., Xanthopoulou, I., Capranzano, P., Capodanno, D., Valenti, R., et al. (2014). Morphine is associated with a delayed activity of oral antiplatelet agents in patients with ST-elevation acute myocardial infarction undergoing primary percutaneous coronary intervention. *Circulation. Cardiovascular Interventions, 8*(1), pii: e001593.

Stub, D., Smith, K., Bernard, S., Nehme, Z., Stephenson, M., Bray, J. E., et al., AVOID Investigators (2015). Air versus oxygen in ST-segment-elevation myocardial infarction. *Circulation, 131*(24), 2143.

Thygesen, K., Alpert, J. S., Jaffe, A. S., Chaitman, B. R., Bax, J. J., Morrow, D. A., & White, H. D., Executive Group on behalf of the Joint European Society of Cardiology (ESC)/American College of Cardiology (ACC)/American Heart Association (AHA)/World Heart Federation (WHF) Task Force for the Universal Definition of Myocardial Infarction. (2018). Fourth universal definition of myocardial infarction. *Journal of the American College of Cardiology, 72*(18), 2231–2264. doi: 10.1016/j.jacc.2018.08.1038.

UpToDate. (2019). *Drug information*. Lexi-Comp, Inc.

Zipes, D. P., Libby, P., Bonow, R. O., Mann, D. L., & Tomaselli, G. F. (2018). *Braunwald's heart disease: A textbook of cardiovascular medicine* (11th ed.). New York, NY: Elsevier.

# Drug Therapy for Shock and Hypotension

## CLINICAL APPLICATION CASE STUDY

Karsen Sexton, a 78-year old man, lives alone. His daughter visits him twice a week. Today, she finds her father diaphoretic and disoriented, and she learns that he has had the flu for 3 days and has not been able to keep anything down. She calls 911, and Mr. Sexton is transported to the local medical center.

## KEY TERMS

**Chronotropic effect:** causing a change in heart rate

**Dromotropic effect:** causing a change in speed of electrical conduction in the heart

**Inotropic effect:** causing a change in myocardial contraction

**Normotensive:** having normal blood pressure

**Pressor:** effect that increases blood pressure

# INTRODUCTION

Blood pressure is important because the various organs adapt to keep blood flowing at certain pressures (autoregulation). Homeostatic mechanisms, including autonomic reflexes, capillary fluid shifts, and variations in neurohormones, normally maintain blood pressure. When hypotension (abnormally low blood pressure) occurs, shock develops if the homeostatic mechanisms are unable to raise blood pressure to the normal range.

Shock is a clinical condition initiated by compromised oxygen delivery, oxygen consumption, and/or oxygen utilization that leads to cellular and tissue hypoxia. This most commonly occurs when there is circulatory failure, producing hypotension (i.e., reduced tissue perfusion). Acute hypotension is a clinical indicator of shock; therefore, its management will be considered in relation to the underlying cause of shock. This chapter discusses the pharmacologic management of patients who experience shock.

# OVERVIEW OF ACUTE HYPOTENSION AND SHOCK

Shock is divided into four potential, although not necessarily exclusive, types based on the underlying cause: hypovolemic, cardiogenic, obstructive, and distributive. In each type, one or more circulatory mechanisms are compromised. Figure 29.1 illustrates how various factors are involved in the development

of shock. To understand the role of drug therapy in supporting restoration of balance to these mechanisms, the etiology, pathophysiology, and clinical manifestations of shock must be understood.

## Etiology

Identifying the etiology of shock is important because management varies among the four types. In hypovolemic, cardiogenic, and obstructive shock, low cardiac output and inadequate oxygen transport are characteristic. In distributive shock, the main deficit lies in peripheral circulation, with decreased systemic vascular resistance and altered oxygen extraction.

*Hypovolemic shock*, the most common type of shock, is caused by insufficient circulating volume from actual blood loss or relative loss from fluid shifts within the body. Hypovolemic shock may result from hemorrhage, trauma, burns, and medical conditions such as diabetic ketoacidosis or diabetes insipidus. In children, vomiting and diarrhea are the most typical causal conditions.

*Cardiogenic shock* occurs when the myocardium has lost its ability to contract efficiently and maintain an adequate cardiac output. Cardiogenic shock is seen with myocardial infarction, atrial and ventricular arrhythmias, and valve or ventricle septal rupture.

*Obstructive shock* may result when any kind of mass or fluid accumulation and/or blood clot outside of the heart interferes with the heart's ability to adequately pump a sufficient quantity of blood. Causes include pulmonary embolism, pulmonary hypertension, tension pneumothorax, constrictive pericarditis, and restrictive cardiomyopathy.

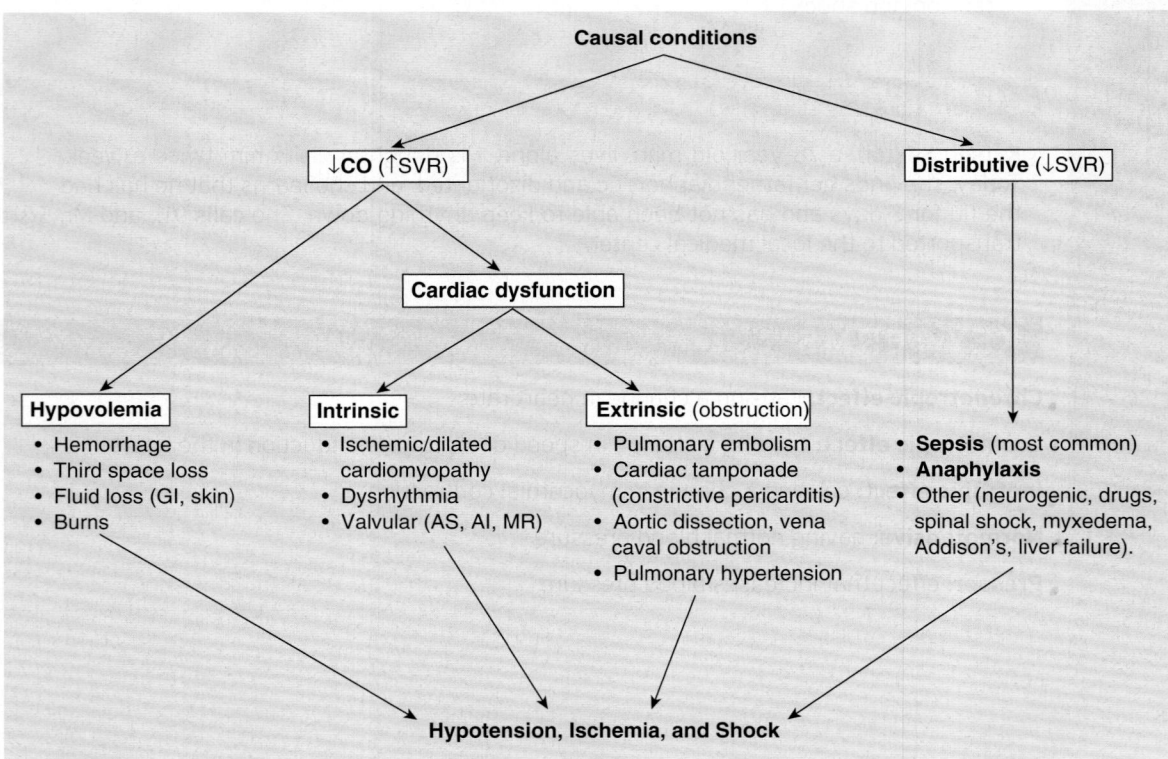

**Figure 29.1.** Impact of altered cardiac output and systemic vascular resistance on the development of hypotension, ischemia, and shock. AI, aortic insufficiency; AS, aortic stenosis; CO, cardiac output; GI, gastrointestinal; MR, mitral regurgitation; PE, pulmonary embolism; SVR, systemic vascular resistance. [Adapted with permission from Chowdhury, S. H., Cozma, A. I., & Chowdhury, J. H. (2017). *Essentials for the Canadian medical licensing exam* (2nd ed., Fig. 3.4). Philadelphia, PA: Wolters Kluwer.]

*Distributive* or *vasogenic shock* develops from impaired utilization of oxygen and thus production of energy by the cell. It is characterized by massive vasodilation, which results in a relative hypovolemia. Distributive shock can be further divided, depending on cause, into three subtypes.

- Anaphylactic shock, which is due to massive vasodilation caused by release of histamine in response to a severe allergic reaction.
- Neurogenic shock, which is a result of massive vasodilation of the peripheral blood vessels from high-level spinal cord injuries. In this injury, sudden loss of signals from the sympathetic nervous system causes loss of normal muscle tone in blood vessel walls, leading to decreased systemic vascular resistance and altered oxygen extraction.
- Septic shock, which is due to massive vasodilation caused by release of mediators of the inflammatory process in response to overwhelming infection. Almost any organism that gains access to the bloodstream can cause septic shock, but most often this kind of shock is associated with gram-negative and gram-positive bacteria and fungi.

## Pathophysiology

Shock is a physiologic continuum initiated by a precipitating event, such as an infection or an injury, which can progress through several stages if unchecked. Hypoxic injury results in an inadequate flow of nutrients and oxygen to the cell. If insufficient tissue perfusion continues, the cell relies on anaerobic metabolic pathways for energy production, cellular ATP stores are rapidly consumed, and difficulty regulating intracellular pH occurs. Inadequate supplies of ATP cause a loss of the normal ionic gradient on the cell membrane, and the sodium–potassium pump fails. This produces an efflux of potassium out of the cell and movement of sodium and calcium into the cell, causing intracellular edema. This may affect the conduction of electrical impulses within the cells and produce cardiac dysrhythmias. As calcium accumulates in the mitochondria, structural derangement of the organelles occurs, and this may signal the hallmark of irreversible cellular injury and eventual death. These pathophysiologic changes produce progressive clinical symptoms.

## Clinical Manifestations

Clinical symptoms vary with the stage and type of shock and the degree of impaired perfusion of vital organs (e.g., brain, heart, kidneys). Systemic arterial hypotension is usually present, but the magnitude of the hypotension may appear to be only moderate depending on the patient's baseline blood pressure. In **normotensive** adults, the systolic arterial pressure is less than 90 mm Hg, or the mean arterial pressure is less than 70 mm Hg, with associated tachycardia.

### *Stages of Shock*

The first two stages of shock are more responsive to treatment and are more likely to be reversible. End-stage shock is associated with irreversible end-organ damage and death.

*Compensated shock*, also known as preshock, is characterized by compensatory responses activated in an attempt to reverse the condition. An increase in heart rate and peripheral vasoconstriction may be sufficient to allow a person to appear asymptomatic and preserve a normal blood pressure. Decreases in oxygen supply cause a short-term transition to anaerobic metabolism, which is unable to sustain ATP production and cellular health for a prolonged period. Symptoms may include tachycardia, change in blood pressure, and potential elevated serum lactate levels (a marker of cellular hypoxia). Prompt recognition and treatment at this stage can completely halt any progression.

*Decompensated shock* occurs if the condition persists as compensatory mechanisms become overwhelmed, and signs and symptoms of organ dysfunction appear. When cardiac output or blood pressure is too low for prolonged periods, or when cytokine levels are elevated, endothelial damage occurs, and microvascular thrombosis further impairs capillary blood flow. The patient's symptoms reflect that the body is unable to maintain perfusion any longer. Hypotension, symptomatic tachycardia, dyspnea, restlessness, diaphoresis, metabolic acidosis, oliguria, and cool, clammy skin occur. These signs and symptoms of organ dysfunction typically correspond to significant pathophysiologic alterations. With rapid, appropriate treatment, this stage of shock can be reversed.

*Irreversible* or *end-stage shock* begins to take a permanent toll on the body's organs and tissues and leads to irreversible end-organ damage and multiple organ failure. Overall, organ failure is further accelerated by prior injury or disease. During this stage, the kidneys shut down, and anuria and acute renal failure develop. Lactic acidosis from anaerobic metabolism further depresses cardiac output and hypotension becomes severe and intractable to treatment. The end point of irreversible shock is death.

## TREATMENT OF HYPOTENSION AND SHOCK

In hypotension and shock, initial efforts involve identifying and treating the cause when possible. It may help to place the patient in a recumbent position; give blood transfusions, fluids, and electrolytes; and treat infections. If these measures are ineffective in raising the blood pressure enough to maintain perfusion to vital organs such as the brain, kidneys, and heart, adrenergic drugs may be used. The usual goal of drug therapy is to maintain tissue perfusion and a mean arterial pressure of at least 80 to 100 mm Hg.

 **QSEN Alert: Evidence-Based Practice**

Early rapid fluid replacement in hypovolemic shock can improve intravascular volume and delivery of oxygen to vital organs. However, too much fluid for too long can lead to tissue edema, which complicates an already leaking cellular microcirculation. Walley [2018] described the role that the endothelium and microvasculature play in subsequent organ dysfunction. With edema, the distance for diffusion of gases and metabolites increases, and the rise in tissue hydrostatic pressure further compresses the microcirculation; this results in impaired tissue perfusion. Optimal fluid resuscitation sufficient to improve microvascular function leads to improved microvascular flow, improved delivery of oxygen to the tissues, and enhanced organ function. Improved patient outcomes may occur when nurses assess for adverse signs of fluid resuscitation.

| TABLE 29.1 | | | |
|---|---|---|---|
| **Action of Adrenergic Receptors** | | | |
| **Adrenergic Receptor** | **Predominant Effect to Response Activation** | **Tissue or Organ Affected** | **Impact** |
| Beta₁ | Increased force of contraction | Heart | Positive **inotropic effect** |
| | Increased heart rate | Heart | Positive **chronotropic effect** |
| | Increased speed of electrical conduction | Heart | Positive or negative **dromotropic effect** |
| | Increased renin production | Kidneys | Increased blood pressure |
| Beta₂ | Bronchodilation | Lungs | |
| | Vasodilation | Blood vessels | Decreased blood pressure |
| | Glycogenolysis and gluconeogenesis | Liver | Hyperglycemia for energy |
| | Decreased insulin secretion | Pancreas | |
| Beta₃ | Lipolysis and increased release of free fatty acids into the blood | Adipose tissue | Generates energy |
| | Relaxation of smooth muscle | Uterus, urinary bladder, and gastrointestinal tract | |
| Alpha₁ | Vasoconstriction | Blood vessels | Pressor/vasopressor effect |
| Alpha₂ | Inhibition of release of norepinephrine into synapses of sympathetic nervous system | Surface membranes of target tissues and organs (presynaptic) | Antiadrenergic response in body |

# ADRENERGIC DRUGS

Three adrenergic receptors (beta₁, beta₂, and alpha) are targets of catecholamines, predominately epinephrine and norepinephrine. In order to understand the varying roles adrenergic agonists play in shock, it is necessary to recognize the inherent responses to activation of the adrenergic receptors (Table 29.1). The physiologic sequelae of shock depend on the type(s) of adrenergic receptor activated in response and the number of affected receptors in a particular part of the body.

The usefulness of adrenergic drugs stems mainly from the effects of these drugs on the heart, blood vessels, and bronchi. They are often used as emergency drugs in the treatment of acute cardiovascular and respiratory collapse. In addition, adrenergic drugs are useful in the treatment of allergic reactions. Patients who benefit from these drugs include those in need of restoration of blood pressure in reversing types of hypotensive states.

Adrenergic drugs produce effects similar to those produced by stimulation of the sympathetic nervous system and therefore have widespread effects on body tissues. Some adrenergic drugs, such as norepinephrine, epinephrine, and dopamine, are exogenous formulations of naturally occurring neurotransmitters and hormones. Other adrenergic medications, such as phenylephrine, pseudoephedrine, and isoproterenol, are synthetic chemical relatives of naturally occurring neurotransmitters and hormones. The adrenergic drugs in this chapter are discussed in relation to their use in hypotension and shock. In many cases, a combination of drugs is used, depending on the type of shock and the patient's response to treatment. In an emergency, the drugs may be used to maintain adequate perfusion of vital organs until sufficient fluid volume is replaced and adequate circulation is restored. Additional discussion regarding adrenergic receptors and other adrenergic

drugs that produce more localized therapeutic effects are discussed elsewhere (Chap. 31, Drug Therapy for Nasal Congestion and Cough; Chap. 33, Drug Therapy for Asthma, Airway Inflammation, and Bronchoconstriction; and Chap. 59, Drug Therapy for Disorders of the Eye).

Individual drugs are described in the following section, and indications for use and dosage ranges are listed in Table 29.2. **Norepinephrine** (Levophed) serves as the prototype adrenergic drug in the treatment of hypotension and shock.

> ### Concept Mastery Alert
>
> Agonists work by activating the receptor to which they bind. Beta₁ agonists mimic the action of epinephrine and norepinephrine to raise blood pressure to counteract shock or hypotension.

## Pharmacokinetics

Norepinephrine is administered via the intravenous (IV) route. Thus, it has an immediate onset of action with vasopressor duration of 1 to 2 minutes. The drug is metabolized via monoamine oxidase (MAO) and catechol O-methyltransferase, and it is excreted in the urine as inactive metabolites.

## Action

Norepinephrine is a pharmaceutical preparation of the naturally occurring catecholamine norepinephrine. It has predominant alpha-receptor agonist effects and results in potent peripheral arterial vasoconstriction. As a result, it increases blood pressure more than it increases heart rate, force of contraction, or cardiac output. The drug is useful in cardiogenic and septic shock, but reduced renal blood flow limits its prolonged use.

given central line

**TABLE 29.2**

## DRUGS AT A GLANCE: Drugs Used for Hypotension and Shock

| Generic/Trade Name | Pregnancy Category | Adults | Children |
|---|---|---|---|
|  **Norepinephrine** (Levophed; ✹ Levophed) | C | Hypotension and shock: IV infusion, 8–12 mcg/min initially, titrated to desired response; maintenance dose ranges from 2 to 4 mcg/min<br>Postcardiac arrest: IV infusion, 0.1–0.5 mcg/kg/min initially, titrated to desired response.<br>Sepsis and septic shock: IV infusion, 0.01–3 mcg/kg/min | Hypotension and shock: IV infusion, 0.05–0.1 mcg/kg/min; titrated to desired effect; maximum 2 mcg/kg/min |
| Dobutamine (✹ Dobutrex, Dobutamine Injection, USP) | B | Cardiac decompensation: IV 0.5–1 mcg/kg/min initially, maintenance dose 2–20 mcg/kg/min, increased to maximum of 40 mcg/kg/min if necessary | Cardiac decompensation: same as adult dosage |
| Dopamine | C | Hemodynamic support: IV 5–10 mcg/kg/min initially, maintenance 2–20 mcg/kg/min, gradually increasing to maximum 50 mcg/kg/min<br>Prepare by adding 200 mg of dopamine to 250 mL of IV fluid for a final concentration of 800 mcg/mL or to 500 mL IV fluid for a final concentration of 400 mcg/mL | Hemodynamic support: 2–20 mcg/kg/min, gradually increasing to maximum 50 mcg/kg/min |
| Epinephrine (Adrenalin, Auvi-Q, EpiPen; ✹ Adrenalin, Allerject, Anapen, EpiPen) | C | Anaphylaxis: IM (preferred), SubQ 0.2–0.5 mg using the 1 mg/mL solution; IV bolus 0.1 mg over 5–10 min using the 0.1 mg/mL solution, continuous infusion 2–15 mcg/min | IV infusion, 0.01 mcg/kg/min |
| Phenylephrine (Vazculep) | C | Hypotension and shock<br>IV bolus: 100–180 mcg/dose every 10–15 min as needed not to exceed 500 mcg<br>IV infusion: 100–180 mcg/min or alternatively 0.5 mcg/kg/min | Hypotension and shock<br>IV bolus: 5–20 mcg/kg/dose q10–15 min as needed<br>IV infusion: 0.1–0.5 mcg/kg/min<br>Titrate to effects |

## Use

Norepinephrine is used to treat severe hypotension and shock that persists after adequate fluid volume replacement. The drug is recommended as the first-choice vasopressor for the management of sepsis and septic shock.

> **! QSEN Alert: Evidence-Based Practice**
>
> A consensus committee of 68 international experts (Dellinger et al., 2013) updated guidelines related to the management of sepsis that stress initial fluid resuscitation to maintain a mean arterial pressure of 65 mm Hg or higher and the administration of vasopressors for hypotension that does not respond to fluids. The guidelines prefer the use of norepinephrine as a first-line drug for septic shock over dopamine. The committee's systematic review of randomized controlled trials and a meta-analysis found that norepinephrine was superior to dopamine in improving in-hospital and 28-day mortality and was associated with a lower risk of death and fewer dysrhythmias. If hypotension persists despite maximal doses of norepinephrine (or dopamine), second-line vasopressors are epinephrine, phenylephrine, and vasopressin. Early recognition and resuscitation measures to manage septic shock are critical to improved outcomes.

### Use in Children

Norepinephrine is used in children to treat refractory septic shock and persistent pulmonary hypertension. However, children are very sensitive to drug effects, including cardiac and central nervous system stimulation, and recommended doses usually should not be exceeded.

### Use in Older Adults

Norepinephrine must be used with caution in the geriatric patient population. However, because the drug has the capacity to reverse hypotension and shock, its benefit drug would outweigh any potential risk. However, because older adults often have chronic cardiovascular conditions (e.g., angina, dysrhythmias, heart failure, coronary artery disease, hypertension, peripheral vascular disease) that are aggravated by adrenergic drugs, careful monitoring by the nurse is required.

### Use in Patients With Renal Impairment

Norepinephrine warrants cautious use in patients with renal failure. Adrenergic drugs exert effects on the renal system that may cause problems for patients with renal impairment.

For example, the alpha$_1$ activity of norepinephrine causes constriction of renal arteries, thereby diminishing renal blood flow and urine production.

The renal system eliminates many adrenergic drugs, including norepinephrine, and their metabolites. In the presence of renal disease, these compounds may accumulate and cause increased adverse effects.

### Use in Patients With Critical Illness

Norepinephrine and other adrenergic drugs are important emergency drugs. Although they may save lives of critically ill patients, adrenergic drugs may result in adverse effects that require monitoring and intervention and may complicate the already complex care of the critically ill.

## Adverse Effects

Norepinephrine and other adrenergic drugs can cause significant adverse effects, including the following:

- Possible diminished renal perfusion and decreased urine output due to vasopressor action
- Possible decreased perfusion to the liver, with subsequent liver damage due to vasopressor action
- Possible irritable cardiac dysrhythmias due to beta$_1$ activity
- Possible increase in myocardial oxygen requirement due to beta$_1$ activity
- Hyperglycemia, hypokalemia, and hypophosphatemia due to beta$_1$ activity
- Severe hypertension and reflex bradycardia
- Limb ischemia due to profound vasoconstriction
- Extravasation at infusion site

### QSEN Alert: Safety

Note that the U.S. Food and Drug Administration (FDA) has issued a **BLACK BOX WARNING** ◆ regarding the potential risk of tissue damage with extravasation of norepinephrine. The drug should be infused into a large vein or central line if possible. The use of leg veins should be avoided in older adults and in those with occlusive disorders. If extravasation occurs, diluted phentolamine should be injected into the area with a small-gauge hypodermic needle as soon as possible to prevent sloughing and necrosis of the tissue.

*phentolamine antidote*

## Contraindications

Contraindications to using norepinephrine include cardiac dysrhythmias, angina pectoris, hypertension, hyperthyroidism, and cerebrovascular disease; stimulation of the sympathetic nervous system worsens these conditions. Narrow-angle glaucoma is a contraindication, because the drugs result in mydriasis, closure of the filtration angle of the eye, and increased intraocular pressure. Hypersensitivity to an adrenergic drug or any component is also a contraindication. For example, the norepinephrine preparation Levophed contains sulfites, to which some people may be allergic. However, the generic equivalent does not contain preservatives.

### NCLEX Success

1. When giving a drug with beta$_1$ agonist activity, the nurse knows that which of the following would provide therapeutic benefit? (Select all that apply.)
   A. vasoconstriction and elevation of the blood pressure
   B. relaxation of bronchial smooth muscle and bronchodilation
   C. elevated heart rate and improved force of myocardial contraction
   D. uterine contraction and induction of labor

2. The nurse teaches the patient with diabetes mellitus using adrenergic medications to anticipate which of the following?
   A. no change in blood glucose levels
   B. a decrease in blood glucose levels
   C. an increase in blood glucose levels
   D. more fluctuation in blood glucose levels

3. During administration of dopamine, a patient complains of pain at the infusion site. The nurse should recognize which of the following?
   A. Patient is hypersensitive to the drug, and infusion should be stopped.
   B. Infusion rate is too fast and should be slowed.
   C. Medication should be stopped, phentolamine should be infused, and the infusion site should be changed.
   D. Medication is probably not effective, and therefore, patient response should be assessed once all the medication is infused.

4. A patient in cardiogenic shock is started on dobutamine. The health care provider's order reads dobutamine 10 mcg/kg/min IV. What effect should the nurse expect after beginning drug therapy?
   A. enhanced cardiac contraction and contractility via stimulation of alpha$_1$, beta$_1$, and beta$_2$ receptors
   B. dilated blood vessels via stimulation of dopamine receptors
   C. increased cardiac output through stimulation of beta$_1$ receptors
   D. constricted blood vessels and increased cardiac output through stimulation of alpha$_1$ receptors

## Nursing Implications

### Preventing Interactions

Remember that norepinephrine reuptake is the major way that sympathetic nerve transmission is terminated. Drugs such as tricyclic antidepressants block norepinephrine reuptake, resulting in stimulation of alpha- and beta-adrenergic receptors. Concurrent use of MAO inhibitors and adrenergic drugs may lead to cardiac dysrhythmias, respiratory depression, and acute hypertensive crisis, with possible intracranial hemorrhage, convulsions, coma, and death. Therefore, MAO inhibitors must not be given with norepinephrine and other adrenergic drugs.

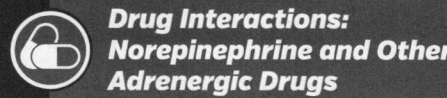

## BOX 29.1 — Drug Interactions: Norepinephrine and Other Adrenergic Drugs

**Drugs That Increase the Effects of Norepinephrine and Other Adrenergic Drugs**

- Anesthetics, general (e.g., propofol), cocaine
  *Increase the risk of ventricular irritability, serious cardiac dysrhythmias, or death*
- Anticholinergics (e.g., atropine)
  *Increase the risk of ventricular dysrhythmias*
- Antihistamines, tricyclic antidepressants (e.g., amitriptyline, imipramine), beta-adrenergic blocking agents (e.g., propranolol [Inderal]), doxapram [Dopram], methylphenidate [Ritalin]
  *Increase the pressor effect*
- Digoxin
  *Increases the risk of dysrhythmias*
- Ergot alkaloids
  *Increase blood pressure and ischemic response*
- Monoamine oxidase (MAO) inhibitors (e.g., isocarboxazid [Marplan]); xanthines (in caffeine-containing substances, such as coffee, tea, cola drinks, and theophylline)
  *Increase heart rate and blood pressure*

**Drugs That Decrease the Effects of Norepinephrine and Other Adrenergic Drugs**

- Anticholinesterases (e.g., neostigmine, pyridostigmine [Mestinon]) and other cholinergic drugs
  *Decrease the effects of norepinephrine*
- Antipsychotic drugs (e.g., haloperidol [Haldol]), chlorpromazine
  *Paradoxically decrease blood pressure*
- Phenothiazines, phentolamine
  *Inhibit or reverse the pressor effect*

Many other medications interact with norepinephrine, increasing or decreasing its effects (Box 29.1).

## Administering the Medication

Administration of norepinephrine should occur through a large vein or on an infusion pump, with titration as ordered to achieve the desired therapeutic response. Close nursing observation and monitoring during drug therapy is essential. Emergency and resuscitative equipment and other drugs should be immediately available to manage any adverse effects.

## Assessing for Therapeutic Effects

The nurse should observe signs of adequate tissue perfusion, including a mean arterial pressure of at least 65 mm Hg, heart rate less than 100 beats/min, unlabored breathing, and serum lactate levels and arterial blood gases within normal limits. In addition, urine output should be greater than 30 mL/h. There should be normal mentation; oxygen saturation by pulse oximetry greater than 90%; no dyspnea; and warm, dry skin with no signs of diminished perfusion. Laboratory values (blood urea nitrogen [BUN], creatinine, serum lactate level, aspartate aminotransferase [AST], alanine aminotransferase [ALT], and

lactate dehydrogenase [LDH]) should be within normal limits. In addition, with septic shock, patient should be afebrile with return of the white blood cell count to within normal limits.

## Assessing for Adverse Effects

The nurse should assess for signs of complications of vasopressor activity, including diminished renal perfusion, decreased urine output, decreased liver perfusion, and limb ischemia. The patient should be observed for cardiac dysrhythmias, signs of increased myocardial oxygen requirements, hyperglycemia, hypokalemia, and hypophosphatemia due to beta$_1$ activity. Ongoing assessment of blood pressure and heart rate is critical to avoid severe hypertension and reflex bradycardia. Monitoring the infusion site diligently for infiltration is essential.

### Clinical Application 29.1

Mr. Sexton's vital signs are temperature 97°F, pulse 122/min and regular, respirations 28/min, and blood pressure 76/52 mm Hg. His arterial blood gases are pH 7.12, O$_2$ 76 mm Hg, CO$_2$ 30 mm Hg, HCO$_3$ 20 mmol/L, and O$_2$ saturation 78%. He is in hypovolemic shock, and a physician in the emergency department administers a 1000-mL normal saline (NS) bolus and starts him on 35% oxygen by face mask.

Within 15 minutes of the start of the fluid bolus, Mr. Sexton is agitated and flushed and complains of palpitations. His vital signs have not improved, and he receives an additional fluid bolus. His blood pressure increases to 80/50 mm Hg, and his heart rate is 118 beats/min after receiving 2000 mL of NS. His physician then orders an additional 1000 mL of NS. A nurse gives him IV norepinephrine 8 mcg/min, titrated to a systolic blood pressure greater than 90 mm Hg after receiving the 3 L of IV fluids.

- What are the nursing implications for this patient's reaction to the fluid challenge?
- What assessment is needed relative to the therapeutic and adverse effects of norepinephrine?

## Patient Teaching

Patients who are recovering from critical illness will likely have different needs and may require additional services on discharge than they had prior to the shock experience. The nurse should facilitate opportunities to have the patient and family participate in the goal setting and plan of care for discharge as possible.

### ! QSEN Alert: Teamwork and Collaboration

Before discharge, the interprofessional team should assess the:

- Nature and complexity of posthospital care needs (e.g., patient safety, infection control)
- Impact of patient's illness on lifestyle of family or other caregiver and necessary interventions
- Readiness and availability of family or other caregiver to assist with care needs of patient at home during recovery
- Availability of community or other health care resources to assist with care
- Need for special equipment, supplies, or medication

---

**BOX 29.2** 📋 *Patient Teaching Guidelines for Hypotension and Shock*

---

### General Considerations

- Health care professionals use adrenergic drugs for short periods in the hospital setting to treat hypotension and shock. Although you will not be discharged on these drugs, patient teaching is aimed at supporting your recovery and preventing the condition from reoccurring.

- If you are receiving IV adrenergic drugs to stimulate your heart or raise your blood pressure, frequent cardiac monitoring and checks of flow rate, blood pressure, and urine output are necessary These measures increase the safety and benefits of drug therapy. Ask your nurse if you have concerns about your condition or questions about your drug regimen.

- Report adverse reactions such as fast pulse, palpitations, and chest pain so that drug dosage can be reevaluated and therapy changed if needed.

### Self-Administration

- Make sure you understand your medical condition and the reason for hospitalization and the measures to prevent reoccurrence. Specific considerations for types of shock are addressed below.

### For Hypovolemic Shock (Depending on What Caused the Volume Loss)

- Seek help for signs of shock (weak, rapid pulse; cool, clammy skin; faintness, postural dizziness, nausea) if you experience them again.

- Learn how to take your own pulse and blood pressure, and report heart rate greater than 100 beats/min to your health care provider. Take your pulse and blood pressure more frequently when you are not feeling well.

- If you have trouble keeping liquids down or have increased diarrhea, notify your health care provider.

- If you see blood in your urine or stool, or if you are coughing up blood, contact your health care provider.

- Stay hydrated when you are sick or exercising.

- Ask your nurse if you have concerns about your condition or questions about your drug regimen.

- Keep follow-up appointments.

### For Cardiogenic Shock

- Take care to prevent another heart attack because it is important in avoiding cardiogenic shock.

- Seek medical attention when you experience symptoms of a heart attack.

- Keep family members or support people informed about the location and use of antianginal medications in case help is needed.

- Avoid over-the-counter decongestants, cold remedies, and diet pills, which stimulate the heart and constrict blood vessels and thus may cause angina.

- Take all medications, particularly your heart medicine, as prescribed.

- Learn how to take your own pulse and blood pressure, report heart rate less than 55 beats/min to your health care provider, and withhold medication as instructed. Take your pulse and blood pressure more frequently when the medication is initiated and titrated up or down.

- Ask your nurse if you have concerns about your condition or questions about your drug regimen.

- Keep all laboratory and follow-up health care appointments.

### For Septic Shock

- Avoid coming into contact with people who are sick. Take care to prevent infection (get vaccinated, avoid spread of germs).

- If you are discharged on antibiotics, finish the full antibiotic treatment and seek medical attention if signs of infection reoccur.

- Ask your nurse if you have concerns about your condition or questions about your drug regimen.

- Keep all laboratory and health care appointments.

### For Anaphylactic Shock

- Learn to self-administer an injection of epinephrine if you have severe allergies. Always carry your injection kit with you. Seek immediate medical care after self-injection of epinephrine.

- Ask your nurse if you have concerns regarding your condition or how to self-administer epinephrine.

- If you have a food allergy, always ask about ingredients when eating food prepared by others. At a restaurant, tell your waiter or waitress about your food allergies.

- Wear a medical identification bracelet with the information about your allergy.

- If you have diabetes mellitus, monitor your glucose levels carefully because adrenergic medications may elevate them.

- Keep follow-up appointments.

---

Additional patient teaching guidelines for adrenergic drugs used to manage hypotension and shock, including norepinephrine, are outlined in Box 29.2.

## Other Drugs in the Class

Epinephrine (Adrenalin) is a naturally occurring catecholamine produced by the adrenal glands. Epinephrine is an agonist of alpha$_1$, beta$_1$, and beta$_2$ receptors. It can increase the mean arterial pressure by increasing the cardiac index and stroke volume, as well as systemic vascular resistance and heart rate. At low doses, epinephrine stimulates beta receptors, which increases cardiac output by increasing the rate and force of myocardial contractility. It also causes bronchodilation. Larger doses act on alpha receptors to increase blood pressure through vasoconstriction, although its effect of systemic vascular resistance is less than norepinephrine.

In hypotension and shock, epinephrine is administered intravenously. This route has an instant onset, a peak of 20 minutes, and a duration of 20 to 30 minutes. The drug produces an increase in blood pressure, a positive inotropic and positive chronotropic effect on the myocardium, hyperglycemia, bronchodilation, and vasoconstriction of arterioles in the skin, mucosa, and most viscera. Most epinephrine is rapidly metabolized in the liver to inactive metabolites, which are then excreted in the urine. The remaining epinephrine is deactivated by reuptake at synaptic receptor sites. Epinephrine decreases the splanchnic blood flow and may increase oxygen delivery and consumption. Administration may be associated with an increase in serum lactate levels.

## QSEN Alert: Safety

Ratio expressions of epinephrine concentrations are now prohibited on drug labels, and the metric system is now the expected method for expressing the strength of epinephrine. [A ratio expression of 1:1000 is equivalent in the metric system to 1 mg/mL, and 1:10,000 is equivalent to 0.1 mg/mL.]

Epinephrine is the adrenergic drug of choice for relief of anaphylactic shock, the most serious allergic reaction. People susceptible to severe allergic responses should carry a syringe of epinephrine at all times. EpiPen and EpiPen Jr are prefilled, auto-injection syringes for intramuscular self-administration of epinephrine in emergency situations (see Chap. 33). Epinephrine is also used as treatment of cardiac arrest (see Chap. 27). In addition, epinephrine is used as an additive to local anesthetics for vasoconstrictive effects, which include prolonging the action of the local anesthetic drug, preventing systemic absorption, and minimizing bleeding.

Dopamine, a naturally occurring precursor of norepinephrine and epinephrine, functions as a neurotransmitter. Its action is dose dependent and can stimulate alpha, beta, or dopaminergic receptors, depending on the dose being used. In addition, dopamine acts indirectly by releasing norepinephrine from sympathetic nerve endings and the adrenal glands. At low doses (1–5 mcg/kg/min), increased renal blood flow and urine output occur. At doses greater than 10 mcg/kg/min, stimulation of beta receptors takes place, and there is an increase in heart rate, myocardial contractility, and blood pressure. At the highest doses (20–50 mcg/kg/min), beta activity continues, but increasing alpha stimulation (vasoconstriction) may overcome its actions. Undesirable effects at higher doses are tachycardia and increased pulmonary shunting, as well as the potential for decreased splanchnic perfusion and increased pulmonary arterial wedge pressure. If dosages of dopamine exceeding 20 to 30 mcg/kg/min are needed, a more direct-acting vasopressor, such as epinephrine or norepinephrine may be more beneficial. Dopamine is useful in hypovolemic and cardiogenic shock. Adequate fluid therapy is necessary for maximal **pressor** (increased blood pressure) effect. Acidosis decreases the effectiveness of the drug.

Dobutamine is a sympathomimetic agent and beta$_1$-receptor agonist, although it has some beta$_2$-receptor and minimal alpha-receptor activity. It was developed to provide less vascular activity than dopamine. Dobutamine acts on beta$_1$ receptors in the heart to increase the force of myocardial contraction with a minimal increase in heart rate. In general, at usual doses, it is less likely to cause tachycardia, dysrhythmias, and significant increases in myocardial oxygen consumption than dopamine.

Dobutamine is most useful in cases of shock that require increased cardiac output without the need for blood pressure support. Caution is warranted when administering the drug in patients with moderate or severe hypotension (e.g., systolic blood pressure less than 80 mm Hg), because the peripheral vasodilation may cause a further fall in blood pressure.

However, it may increase blood pressure with large doses. In patients with an acute myocardial infarction, dobutamine may increase infarction size because of the potential for increases in myocardial oxygen consumption when oxygen supply is compromised. In addition, it may be useful for short-term management of patients experiencing cardiac decompensation who have not responded to medical therapy while awaiting heart transplant or mechanical circulatory support.

Dobutamine has a short plasma half-life and therefore requires administration by continuous IV infusion. A loading dose is not necessary because the drug has a rapid onset of action and reaches steady state within approximately 10 minutes after the infusion is begun. It is rapidly metabolized to inactive metabolites.

Phenylephrine (Vazculep) is a synthetic adrenergic drug that stimulates alpha-adrenergic receptors to produce vasoconstriction. As a result, it constricts arterioles and raises systolic and diastolic blood pressures. Phenylephrine resembles epinephrine but has fewer cardiac effects and a longer duration of action. Vasoconstriction decreases cardiac output and renal perfusion and increases peripheral vascular resistance and blood pressure. There is little cardiac stimulation because phenylephrine does not activate beta$_1$ receptors in the heart or beta$_2$ receptors in blood vessels. The drug is excreted primarily in the urine.

Phenylephrine may be given to increase blood pressure in hypotension and shock. Compared with norepinephrine, phenylephrine produces longer-lasting elevation of blood pressure (20–50 minutes with injection). When given systemically, phenylephrine produces a reflex bradycardia. This effect may be used therapeutically to relieve paroxysmal atrial tachycardia. However, other medications such as calcium channel blockers (see Chaps. 26 and 27) are more likely to be used for this purpose. As with norepinephrine, reduction of renal and mesenteric blood flow limits prolonged use. The FDA has issued a **BLACK BOX WARNING ◆** for parenteral use of Neo-Synephrine that alerts prescribers to be familiar with complete prescribing information before use.

## NCLEX Success

5. When the nurse responds to hypotension due to hypovolemic shock, which of the following should the nurse anticipate will be administered first?

   A. epinephrine
   B. dobutamine
   C. normal saline (IV)
   D. dopamine

6. A patient receiving norepinephrine for shock has an arterial line in place. The patient's blood pressure has been near 90/42 mm Hg for most of the morning. The blood pressure reading on the continuous monitor suddenly shows a blood pressure of 130/80 mm Hg. The nurse should do which of the following?

   A. decrease the rate of the norepinephrine
   B. call the health care provider
   C. stop the norepinephrine infusion
   D. confirm the blood pressure with a manual reading

7. **The preceptor asks the student nurse to describe the primary difference between distributive shock and hypovolemic shock. The best response is which of the following?**
   A. Hypovolemic shock results in decreased perfusion while distributive does not.
   B. Blood volume remains constant in distributive shock.
   C. Distributive shock is most commonly caused by trauma.
   D. Hypovolemic shock results in decreased vascular tone.

8. **Shock from anaphylaxis is a result of which type of shock?**
   A. hypovolemic
   B. distributive
   C. obstructive
   D. cardiogenic

*Clinical Application 29.2*

After 1 hour on the norepinephrine IV infusion, Mr. Sexton's blood pressure is 92/52 mm Hg. His urine output is 30 mL/h. His oxygen saturation is 92% on 40% face mask. He is able to answer questions when aroused and his skin is warm and dry. The patient's heart rate is 96 beats/min and regular. What are the appropriate actions by the nurse?

**THE NURSING PROCESS**

A concept map outlines the nursing process related to drug therapy considerations in this chapter. Additional nursing implications related to the disease process should also be considered in care decisions.

### Assessment

- Assess the patient's condition in relation to hypotension and shock.
- Check blood pressure; heart rate; urine output; skin temperature and color of extremities; level of consciousness; orientation to person, place, and time; and adequacy of respiration. In general, report blood pressure less than 90 mm Hg systolic, mean blood pressure greater than 65 mm Hg, heart rate greater than 100 beats/min, and urine output less than 30 mL/h.
- Assess electrocardiogram and cardiac status for alterations in rhythm or rate.
- Monitor and optimize hemodynamic status, noting and acting on indications of impaired cardiac function. Observe the trend in mixed venous oxygen saturation (SVO2), stroke index (SI), cardiac index (CI), pulmonary artery occlusive pressure (PAOP), and central venous pressure (CVP) values for effectiveness of treatments and indications for progress of patient toward goals.
- Monitor available laboratory reports for abnormal values. Decreased oxygen saturation levels indicate decreased oxygenation of tissues; abnormal arterial blood gases may indicate metabolic acidosis; an increased hematocrit may indicate hypovolemia; an increased eosinophil count may indicate anaphylaxis; the presence of bacteria in blood cultures may indicate sepsis; and increased serum creatinine and blood urea nitrogen may indicate impending renal failure.

### Outcomes of Therapy

The patient will
- Show improvement in tissue perfusion and relief of symptoms.
- Show improved hemodynamic status.
- Guard against recurrence of hypotension and shock, if possible.
- Assess for therapeutic and adverse effects of adrenergic drugs.
- Avoid preventable adverse effects of adrenergic drugs.

### Nursing Interventions

- Use measures to prevent or minimize hypotension and shock.
- Recognize impending shock so management can be initiated early.
- Recognize and manage the underlying cause of shock in a particular patient (e.g., replacing fluids; preventing further loss of blood or other body fluids).
- Monitor patients during shock and vasopressor drug therapy.
- Titrate adrenergic drug infusions to maintain blood pressure and tissue perfusion without causing hypertension.
- Check hemodynamic indices (including SVO2, SI, CI, PAOP, and CVP) every hour and blood pressure and pulse constantly or at least every 5 to 15 minutes during acute shock and titration of vasopressor drug therapy. Intra-arterial monitoring is more reliable than cuff blood pressure measurements in shock conditions.
- Monitor mental status, distal pulses, urine output, and skin temperature and color closely to assess tissue perfusion.
- If possible, administer all vasoactive medications via a central access line. Assess venipuncture sites frequently for signs of infiltration or extravasation. If peripheral sites are used, have phentolamine (Regitine), an alpha-adrenergic blocking agent that reverses vasoconstriction, readily available in any setting where IV adrenergic drugs are used. If infiltration occurs, instill phentolamine through the IV catheter prior to removal. If catheter has been removed, phentolamine may be administered subcutaneously, around the area of extravasation.
- Keep family members informed about patient status and management measures.
- When administering substances known to produce hypersensitivity reactions (penicillin and other antibiotics, allergy extracts, vaccines, local anesthetics), observe the recipient carefully for at least 30 minutes after administration. Have adrenergic and other emergency drugs and equipment readily available in case a reaction occurs.
- Place patient in a recumbent position to improve venous return and blood pressure.
- Provide patient teaching regarding drug therapy (see Box 29.2).

### Evaluation

- Observe for improved hemodynamic status, vital signs, color and temperature of skin, urine output, and mental responsiveness.

- Shock is a clinical condition of insufficient perfusion of cells and vital organs, causing tissue hypoxia.
- The overall goal in the treatment of hypotension and shock is to maximize oxygen delivery to the tissues by maintaining vascular volume and optimal hemoglobin levels.
- Blood pressure and heart rate should be monitored frequently during infusion of any drug used to manage shock.
- In hypotension and shock, drugs with alpha-adrenergic activity (e.g., norepinephrine, phenylephrine) are used to increase peripheral vascular resistance and raise blood pressure.
- The adrenergic catecholamines (e.g., dobutamine, dopamine, epinephrine, norepinephrine) are widely used in patients

with a low cardiac output that persists despite adequate fluid replacement and correction of electrolyte imbalance. Dobutamine is usually the cardiotonic agent of choice in critically ill patients.
- The FDA has issued a **BLACK BOX WARNING** ◆ regarding the potential risk of tissue damage with extravasation of norepinephrine. The drug should be infused into a large vein or central line if possible.
- The FDA has issued a **BLACK BOX WARNING** ◆ for parenteral use of phenylephrine that alerts prescribers to be familiar with complete prescribing information before use.

**CLINICAL REASONING CASE STUDY**

| | |
|---|---|
| **Meet the Patient** | Frank Lewis, a 77-year old man with diabetes and a history of hypertension, presents to the emergency department. He is pale and cool. His glucose is 274 mg/dL. His heart rate is 88 beats/min, blood pressure is 72/44 mm Hg, and oxygen saturation is 94% by pulse oximetry. He has a history of a ST-segment elevation myocardial infarction with resultant left ventricular heart failure. He is diagnosed with cardiogenic shock and is started on dopamine 10 mcg/kg/min intravenously.<br><br>• Administration of dopamine stimulates which adrenergic receptors? What is the action of the stimulus?<br>• What are the major adverse effects in the use of adrenergic agents?<br>• What assessment findings would indicate improvement in the patient's clinical condition? |
| **Assessing Drug Information** | • Vasopressors such as adrenergic agonists enhance coronary and cerebral blood flow with cardiogenic shock. Adrenergic drugs with both alpha- and beta-adrenergic effects, such as dopamine and dobutamine, are the drugs of choice to improve cardiac contractility, with dopamine the preferred agent in patients with hypotension.<br>• Dopamine stimulates adrenergic and dopaminergic receptors. Its hemodynamic effect depends on the dose. Lower doses primarily stimulate dopaminergic receptors that produce renal and mesenteric vasodilation. Higher doses produce cardiac stimulation and vasoconstriction.<br>• Adequate fluid therapy is necessary for the maximal pressor effect of dopamine. Acidosis decreases the effectiveness of dopamine. |
| **Nursing Actions** | • Observe Mr. Lewis for cardiac dysrhythmias, signs of increased myocardial oxygen requirements, hyperglycemia, hypokalemia, and hypophosphatemia due to beta$_1$ activity. Ongoing assessment of blood pressure and heart rate is critical to avoid severe hypertension and reflex bradycardia.<br>• Monitor the infusion site diligently for infiltration.<br>• With improvement in Mr. Lewis' condition, observe for signs of adequate tissue perfusion, including a mean arterial pressure of at least 65 mm Hg, heart rate less than 100 beats/min, unlabored breathing, and serum lactate levels and arterial blood gases within normal limits. Urine output should be greater than 30 mL/h. Assess for normal mentation, oxygen saturation by pulse oximetry greater than 90%, no dyspnea, and warm, dry skin with no signs of diminished perfusion. Laboratory values (BUN, creatinine, aminotransferases, LDH) should be within normal limits. |

Visit the Point® at **http://thePoint.lww.com/Frandsen12e** *for answers to NCLEX Success questions (in Appendix A), answers to Clinical Application Case Studies (in Appendix B), and more!*

## REFERENCES AND RESOURCES

Dellinger, R. P., Levy, M. M., Rhodes, A., Annane, D., Gerlach, H., Opal, S. M., et al.; Surviving Sepsis Campaign Guidelines Committee including the Pediatric Subgroup. (2013). Surviving sepsis campaign: International guidelines for management of severe sepsis and septic shock. *Critical Care Medicine, 41*(2), 580–630.

DiPiro, J. T., Talbert, R. L., Yee, G. C., Wells, B. G., Posey, L. M., & Matzke, G. R. (2016). *Pharmacotherapy: A pathophysiologic approach* (10th ed.). New York, NY: McGraw-Hill Education.

Griffiths, C. L., Vestal, M. L., & Hertel, K. A. (2018). Vasoactive agents in shock. *Nursing Critical Care, 13*(2), 6–13.

Kalkwarf, K. J., & Cotton, B. A. (2017). Resuscitation for hypovolemic shock. *The Surgical Clinics of North America, 97*(6), 1307–1321. doi:10.1016/j.suc.2017.07.011

Karch, A. M. (2018). *2019 Lippincott's pocket drug guide for nurses.* Philadelphia, PA: Lippincott Williams & Wilkins.

Norris, T. L. (2019). *Porth's pathophysiology: Concepts of altered health states* (10th ed.). Philadelphia, PA: Wolters Kluwer.

UpToDate. (2019). *Drug information.* Lexi-Comp, Inc.

Walley, K. R. (2018). Mitigating microvascular leak during fluid resuscitation of hemorrhagic shock. *Anesthesiology, 128,* 252–253.

# Drug Therapy for Heart Failure

*After studying this chapter, you should be able to:*

1. Recognize the clinical sequelae of heart failure characterized by left ventricular dysfunction.
2. Relate the pathophysiology of right-sided and left-sided heart failure to the clinical manifestations of each type of heart failure.
3. Identify the prototype and describe the action, use, adverse effects, contraindications, and nursing implications for the angiotensin receptor–neprilysin inhibitor combination.
4. Identify the prototype and describe the action, use, adverse effects, contraindications, and nursing implications for the sinoatrial node modulator.
5. Recognize the prototype and describe the action, use, adverse effects, contraindications, and nursing implications for the inotropes (cardiac glycosides).
6. Identify the prototype and describe the action, use, adverse effects, contraindications, and nursing implications for the phosphodiesterase inhibitors (cardiotonic–inotropic agents).
7. Identify the prototype and describe the action, use, adverse effects, contraindications, and nursing implications for the human B-type natriuretic peptides.
8. Identify the prototypes and describe the action, use, adverse effects, contraindications, and nursing implications for adjuvant drugs used in the treatment of heart failure.
9. Implement the nursing process in the care of patients undergoing drug therapy for heart failure with left ventricular dysfunction.

## CLINICAL APPLICATION CASE STUDY

Dr. Adams is a 59-year-old professor of history at a 4-year college. He tells the nurse practitioner at the campus health center that he has been experiencing increasing shortness of breath and fatigue for the past 2 months. Also, he says that his ankles seem to be swollen. The nurse practitioner asks Dr. Adams questions to ascertain his past medical history. He states that he has been taking enalapril maleate, 20 mg one time per day for hypertension for a number of years. He states he was diagnosed with atrial fibrillation 3 years ago and is taking amiodarone 200 mg one time per day. On examination, the nurse practitioner notes that Dr. Adams has pitting edema in his feet and ankles. The nurse practitioner advises Dr. Adams to make an appointment with his cardiologist immediately. The cardiologist diagnoses Dr. Adams with heart failure and prescribes digoxin (Lanoxin), 0.125 mg every morning, and spironolactone (Aldactone), 25 mg every morning, in addition to the enalapril maleate and amiodarone.

## KEY TERMS

**Catecholamines:** active amines (e.g., epinephrine, norepinephrine, dopamine) that have an effect on the cardiovascular system

**Chronotropic:** related to or impacting myocardial rate or heart rate/pulse

**Decompensation:** the inability of the heart to adequately circulate oxygenated blood to the body's vital organs

**Digitalis toxicity:** an accumulation of digitalis (digoxin) in the body that leads to nausea, vomiting, visual disturbances, atrial or ventricular tachydysrhythmias, ventricular fibrillation, sinoatrial block, and atrioventricular block

**Digitalization:** the administration of a loading dose of digoxin (Lanoxin) to achieve a therapeutic blood level of the medication more rapidly

**Ejection fraction:** the percentage of the total amount of blood in the left ventricle that is ejected with each heartbeat

**Endothelin:** a peptide that raises blood pressure, constricts blood vessels, and contributes to the onset of heart failure

**Inotropic:** related to or influencing the force of myocardial contractility

**Maintenance dose:** a dose administered on a routine basis to produce a therapeutic effect and control symptoms

**Phosphene:** intermittent enhanced brightness in a limited area of the visual field; appearance of halos or multiple images

**Renin:** an enzyme produced by the kidney that divides angiotensinogen to form angiotensin I, which is then changed to angiotensin II to produce vasoconstriction

**Therapeutic index:** the margin between effectiveness and toxicity in the blood level of a drug

**Ventricular remodeling:** dilation and hypertrophy of the ventricles in the initial phases of heart failure, causing the ventricle to assume a spherical shape

## INTRODUCTION

Despite significant advances in the management of cardiovascular disease, heart failure remains a leading cause of death in the United States and throughout the world. In the United States, heart failure is also a leading cause of repeated hospitalizations and accounts for over $30 billion in direct and indirect health care expenditures annually. This progressive complex clinical condition occurs when the heart cannot pump enough blood to meet the body tissue's needs for oxygen and nutrients. Heart failure can result from impaired relaxation and filling of either ventricle during diastole with or without preserved left ventricle ejection. Heart failure has a 50% mortality rate within 5 years of initial diagnosis, and patient outcomes depend on effective management and treatment. This chapter focuses on the management of patients with left ventricular systolic dysfunction, referred to simply as heart failure.

## OVERVIEW OF HEART FAILURE

It is important to understand the etiology, pathophysiology, and clinical manifestations of heart failure. This makes it easier to adequately understand the pharmacologic treatment of the problem.

### Etiology

Heart failure results from various conditions that prevent the contractile myocardial cells and the endothelial cells lining the heart and blood vessels from functioning properly. Hypertension, cardiomyopathy, and acute myocardial infarction can affect myocardial or endothelial cell function, leading to heart failure. Other leading causes of heart failure include cardiac dysrhythmias, heart valve disorders, volume overload, renal failure, and hypometabolic and hypermetabolic states.

Cardiac dysrhythmias are the result of abnormal electrical impulse conduction in the heart. The dysrhythmia impairs the pumping function of the heart by creating an abnormal rate and/or rhythm. When the rate or rhythm impairs the ability of the heart to adequately function and pump sufficient blood to meet the demands of homeostasis, heart failure results. Heart valve disorders disrupt the normal, unidirectional flow of blood through the heart and reduce cardiac output. Heart valve disorders from valve stenosis narrow or restrict blood flow resulting in increased myocardial workload and subsequent myocardial remodeling to compensate. Regurgitative heart valve disorders result in the backflow of blood in the heart and also increase myocardial workload to compensate for reduced cardiac output. Myocardial compensation for reduced cardiac output frequently results in the development of heart failure.

Endothelial dysfunction promotes processes that can lead to narrowing of the blood vessel lumen, such as the accumulation of atherosclerotic plaque, abnormal cell growth, inflammation, or platelet activation. The narrowing of the lumen can lead to blood clot formation and vasoconstriction.

Fluid volume overload impairs the pumping ability of the heart, contributing to the development of heart failure. Fluid volume overload can occur in patients with renal failure. Fluid volume overload can also be caused by the excessive administration of intravenous (IV) fluids or blood transfusions or therapy with certain medications such as corticosteroids, estrogens, and nonsteroidal anti-inflammatory drugs (NSAIDs), which all promote sodium and water retention.

Hyperthyroidism, a hypermetabolic disorder, and hypothyroidism, a hypometabolic disorder, are contributing factors in the development of heart failure. In hyperthyroidism, thyroid function is increased, which causes a rise in heart rate and myocardial contractility and ultimately cardiac output. The patient is prone to heart failure because of the demands of the increase in cardiac output. Mortality rates associated with heart failure are significantly increased in patients with hypothyroidism. In hypothyroidism, the systolic and diastolic functions of the heart are negatively impacted by the lack of adequate metabolic hormones. Additionally, hypo-

thyroidism contributes to the development of cardiac risk factors such as hyperlipidemia, endothelial dysfunction, and obesity.

## Pathophysiology

Heart failure is a condition that results in low cardiac output because the heart is unable to pump sufficient blood to meet the metabolic demands of the body. Normal compensatory mechanisms of the neurohormonal and renin–angiotensin–aldosterone systems (RAAS) work to overcome the systemic hypotension that accompanies the reduction in cardiac output. However, these compensation mechanisms worsen the fluid overload (preload) and increased afterload, which compound the inefficient contractility of the heart. The hypervolemia leads to activation of the natriuretic peptide (NP) system in an attempt to counterregulate the damaging effects of RAAS up-regulation. The pathophysiology of heart failure is shown in Figure 30.1 and explained in the following sections.

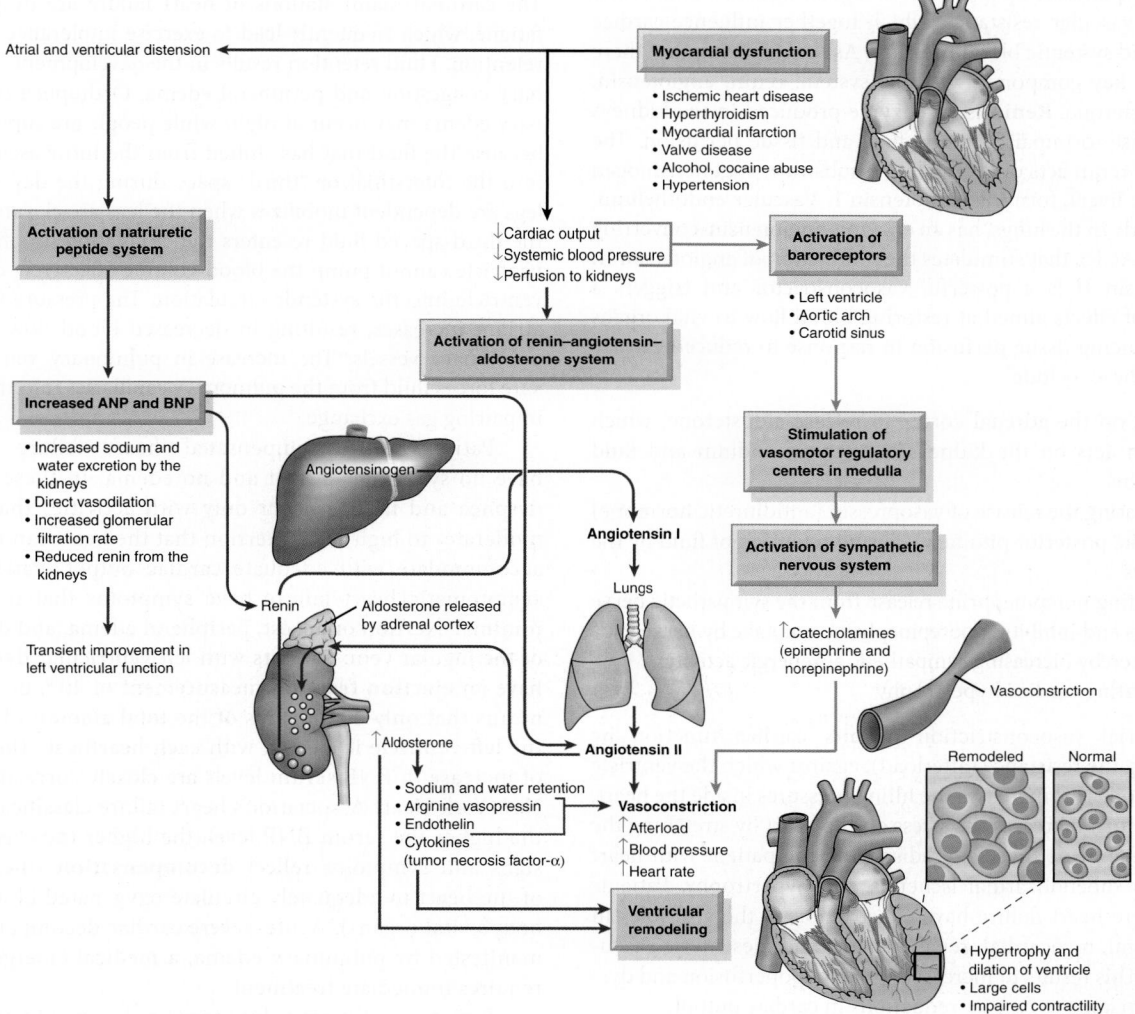

**Figure 30.1.** The pathophysiology of heart failure. A decrease in cardiac output activates multiple neurohormonal mechanisms that ultimately result in signs and symptoms of heart failure and are targeted with drug therapy. [Adapted from Hinkle, J. L., & Cheever, K. H. (2018). *Brunner & Suddarth's textbook of medical-surgical nursing* (14th ed.). Philadelphia, PA: Wolters Kluwer Health/Lippincott Williams & Wilkins.]

## Neurohormonal System

As a result of the hypoperfusion of the organs and tissues from the reduction in cardiac output, the neurohormonal system activates several feedback mechanisms. The baroreceptors in the aortic arch and carotid sinus that normally inhibit sympathetic nervous system activity are blunted in the patient who is experiencing heart failure. This results in high levels of circulating **catecholamines** (active amines, such as epinephrine, norepinephrine, and dopamine, that have a "flight or fight" effect on the cardiovascular system). The circulating catecholamines are inotropic and increase the force of myocardial contractility, as does the increased activity of the sympathetic nervous system. The increased sympathetic nervous system activity is **chronotropic**, increasing the patient's heart rate and constricting blood vessels. Levels of endothelin, a peptide secreted by the endothelial cells, are increased in heart failure. **Endothelin** is a potent vasoconstrictor and may exert additional direct toxic effects on the heart.

## Renin–Angiotensin–Aldosterone System

The RAAS plays an important role in regulating blood volume and systemic vascular resistance, which together influence cardiac output and systemic blood pressure. As the name implies, there are three key components to this system: renin, angiotensin, and aldosterone. **Renin** is an enzyme produced in the kidneys in response to impaired blood flow and tissue perfusion. The release of renin acts on a circulating substrate, angiotensinogen (from the liver), forming angiotensin I. Vascular endothelium, particularly in the lungs, has an enzyme, angiotensin-converting enzyme (ACE), that stimulates the production of angiotensin II. Angiotensin II is a powerful vasoconstrictor and triggers a cascade of effects aimed at restoring blood flow to vital organs and enhancing tissue perfusion in response to reduced cardiac output. These include

- Acting on the adrenal cortex to release aldosterone, which in turn acts on the kidneys to increase sodium and fluid retention
- Stimulating the release of vasopressin (antidiuretic hormone) from the posterior pituitary, causing retention of fluid by the kidneys
- Promoting norepinephrine release from the sympathetic nerve endings and inhibiting norepinephrine reuptake by nerve endings, thereby increasing sympathetic adrenergic activity
- Stimulating cardiac hypertrophy

Arterial vasoconstriction impairs cardiac function by increasing the resistance (afterload), against which the ventricle ejects blood. This increases the filling pressures inside the heart, which in turn increases the stress on the heart by stretching the walls of the heart muscle, predisposing the patient with heart failure to subendocardial ischemia and hypertrophy. Patients with severe heart failure have constriction of the arterioles in the cerebral, myocardial, renal, hepatic, and mesenteric vascular beds. This results in increased organ hypoperfusion and dysfunction related to further reductions in cardiac output.

## Natriuretic Peptide System

NPs are a family of related hormones that help maintain sodium and fluid balance. Two of the peptides, atrial or A-type NP (ANP) and brain or B-type NP (BNP; originally found in the brain), are most commonly associated with heart failure. ANP release is stimulated by atrial wall stress and stretch, and BNP release is stimulated by ventricular wall stress and stretch. ANP and BNP are not excreted by the same chamber of the heart, but they have very similar functions. Their release has several effects including increased sodium excretion by the kidneys, diuresis, direct vasodilation, increased glomerular filtration rate, and reduced renin from the kidneys. ANP and BNP are broken down by the neutral endopeptidase neprilysin, which also helps break down angiotensin II. However, despite elevated levels of NPs in heart failure from hypervolemia, they are ineffective at relieving excess volume. Circulating levels of ANP and BNP are increased in the presence of heart failure. BNP acts as a reliable biomarker of ventricular dilation and as such is useful to support clinical decision-making regarding the diagnosis of heart failure and to predict the severity of the disease.

# Clinical Manifestations

The cardinal manifestations of heart failure are dyspnea and fatigue, which frequently lead to exercise intolerance and fluid retention. Fluid retention results in the development of pulmonary congestion and peripheral edema. Orthopnea or pulmonary edema may occur at night while people are supine in bed because the fluid that has shifted from the intravascular space into the interstitial or "third" space during the day when the legs are dependent mobilizes when the legs are elevated. When the third-spaced fluid re-enters the circulation, the failing left ventricle cannot pump the blood volume effectively out of the ventricle into the systemic circulation. The pressure in the left atrium increases, resulting in decreased blood flow from the pulmonary vessels. The increase in pulmonary venous pressure forces fluid from the pulmonary capillaries into the alveoli, impairing gas exchange.

Patients with compensated heart failure typically have no symptoms at rest and no edema. In these patients, dyspnea and fatigue occur only with activities that require moderate- to high-level exertion that the heart can no longer accommodate with adequate cardiac output. Patients with symptomatic heart failure have symptoms that occur with minimal exertion or at rest, peripheral edema, and distention of the jugular vein. Patients with left ventricular dysfunction have an **ejection fraction** measurement of 40% or less. This means that only 40% or less of the total amount of blood in the left ventricle is ejected with each heartbeat. The amount of increase in BNP serum levels are closely correlated to the New York Heart Association's heart failure classification (i.e., the higher the serum BNP level, the higher the class). These signs and symptoms reflect **decompensation** (the inability of the heart to adequately circulate oxygenated blood to the body's vital organs). Acute, severe cardiac decompensation is manifested by pulmonary edema, a medical emergency that requires immediate treatment.

Symptoms of heart failure may be classified by the side of the heart that has failed first. Over time, left-sided heart failure will cause the right side to fail, producing symptoms associated with both sides of the heart. Clinical manifestations of left- and right-sided heart failure are illustrated in Figure 30.2.

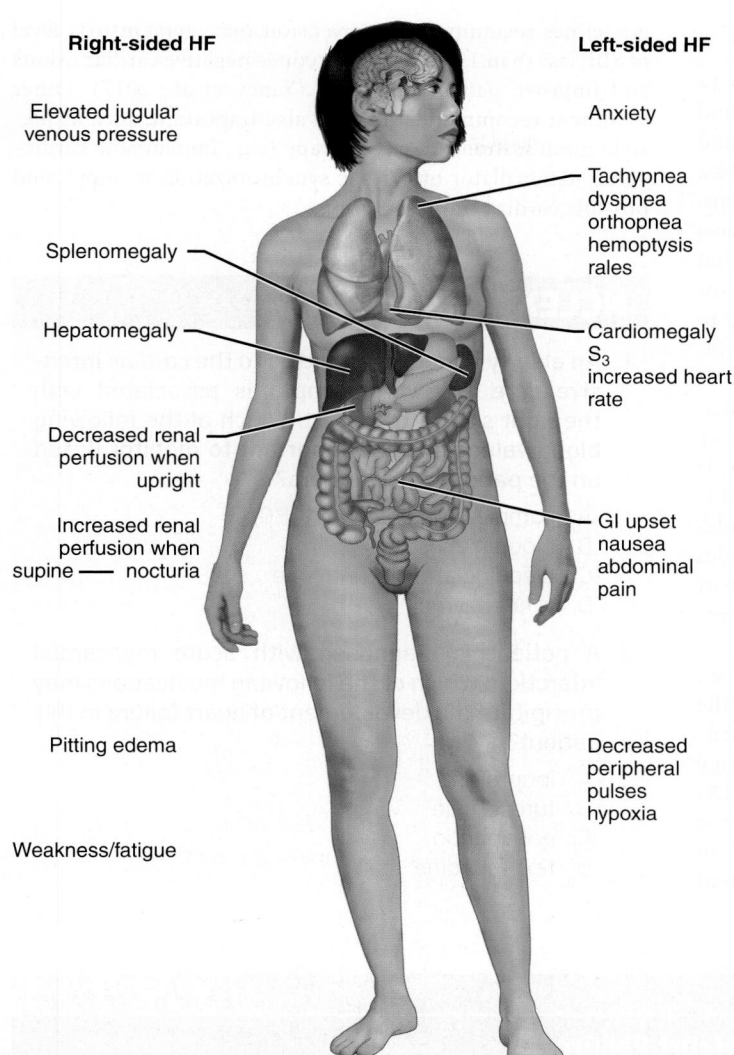

Right-sided HF

- Elevated jugular venous pressure
- Splenomegaly
- Hepatomegaly
- Decreased renal perfusion when upright
- Increased renal perfusion when supine — nocturia
- Pitting edema
- Weakness/fatigue

Left-sided HF

- Anxiety
- Tachypnea dyspnea orthopnea hemoptysis rales
- Cardiomegaly $S_3$ increased heart rate
- GI upset nausea abdominal pain
- Decreased peripheral pulses hypoxia

**Figure 30.2.** Classification of heart failure (HF) and its clinical manifestations. GI, gastrointestinal. (Reprinted with permission from Karch, A. M. (2020). *Focus on nursing pharmacology* (7th ed., Fig. 44.3). Philadelphia, PA: Wolters Kluwer.)

## Left-Sided Heart Failure

Left-sided heart failure results in a decrease in cardiac output related to an increase in left atrial and left ventricular end-diastolic pressures and congestion in the pulmonary circulation. The left side of the heart normally moves blood from the low-pressure pulmonary circulation to the higher-pressure arterial side of the systemic circulation. Increases in left-sided end-diastolic pressures impair left chamber filling resulting in increased pulmonary artery pressures and pulmonary congestion.

Left-sided heart failure is most commonly from a myocardial infarction or cardiomyopathy. Drugs may also cause or exacerbate heart failure by leading to direct myocardial toxicity; by producing negative inotropic, lusitropic (rate of myocardial relaxation), or chronotropic effects; by exacerbating hypertension; by delivering a high-sodium load; or by drug-to-drug interactions. For instance, traditional NSAIDs (i.e., ibuprofen, diclofenac, ketorolac, and indomethacin) act by nonselectively inhibiting both the cyclooxygenase (COX) isoenzymes (COX-1 and COX-2). Many of the adverse effects of NSAIDs are related to the inhibition of prostaglandin production through inhibition of COX-1. Prostaglandin inhibition has the potential to trigger heart failure by enhancing sodium and water retention, increasing systemic vascular resistance, and dampening the response to diuretics.

## Right-Sided Heart Failure

Right-sided heart failure results from an accumulation of blood in the systemic venous system. There are two pumps within the heart. The right-sided pump ejects unoxygenated blood from the systemic circulation into the pulmonary circulation. Failure of the right-sided pump results in an increase in the right atrial, right ventricular, end-diastolic, and systemic venous pressures. The increased pressures impair blood flow from systemic to pulmonary circulation, resulting in systemic fluid volume increases and peripheral edema.

The causes of right-sided heart failure are stenosis or regurgitation of the pulmonic or tricuspid valves, right-sided ventricular infarction, cardiomyopathy, or recurrent left-sided heart failure. In some cases, severe pneumonia, pulmonary embolus, or pulmonary hypertension can result in right-sided heart failure.

### Clinical Application 30.1

- Does Dr. Adams have symptoms of right- or left-sided heart failure? Why did his physician prescribe spironolactone?

## Drug Therapy

The goal of pharmacologic management in heart failure is to slow or reverse the progression of myocardial dysfunction and damage, improve patient symptoms, and reduce morbidity and mortality particularly related to repeated hospitalization risks. Drug therapy that manipulates neurohormonal mechanisms, the RAAS, and the NP system has demonstrated effectiveness in managing heart failure, thereby delaying disease progression and death. For example, ACE inhibitors, angiotensin II receptor blockers (ARB), and aldosterone receptor blockers are used to decrease arterial pressure, ventricular afterload, and blood volume and hence ventricular preload, and they also inhibit and reverse cardiac and vascular hypertrophy. First-line pharmacologic treatment for heart failure also includes diuretics to reduce blood volume and ventricular preload as well as beta-adrenergic blockers to reduce stimulation of the RAAS and myocardial oxygen demand. The introduction of a sinoatrial node modulator and an angiotensin receptor–neprilysin inhibitor provides additional pharmacologic alternatives in the treatment of heart failure. Medications used in the treatment of heart failure are listed in Table 30.1.

Guidelines for treatment of heart failure are based on signs and symptoms; the stages of heart failure indicate the severity of myocardial dysfunction. Drug therapy recommendations based on the 2013 American College of Cardiology Foundation (ACCF)/American Heart Association (AHA) Guidelines for the Management of Heart Failure and the subsequent 2017 update to the guidelines are outlined in Figure 30.3. The 2017 updated heart failure management guidelines recommend hypertension management to a level of SBP less than 130 mm Hg to reduce negative cardiac events and improve patient outcomes (Yancy et al., 2017). Other treatment recommendations are also important, such as lifestyle modifications, device therapy (e.g., implantable cardioverter–defibrillator or cardiac synchronization therapy), and possible cardiac transplantation.

### NCLEX Success

1. An elderly patient is admitted to the cardiac intensive care unit with symptoms associated with the right side of the heart. Which of the following blood values is most important to monitor based on the patient's risk factors?
   A. complete blood count (CBC)
   B. blood glucose
   C. bleeding and clotting time
   D. liver enzymes

2. A patient is diagnosed with acute myocardial infarction. Which of the following medications may precipitate the development of heart failure in this patient?
   A. ibuprofen
   B. furosemide
   C. gabapentin
   D. fexofenadine

### TABLE 30.1

### Drugs Administered for the Treatment of Heart Failure

| Drug Class | Prototype | Other Drugs in the Class |
| --- | --- | --- |
| Cardiac glycosides | Digoxin (Lanoxin) | |
| Phosphodiesterase inhibitors (cardiotonic–inotropic agents) | Milrinone | |
| Angiotensin receptor–neprilysin inhibitors | Sacubitril/valsartan (Entresto) | |
| Sinoatrial node modulators | Ivabradine (Corlanor) | |
| Angiotensin-converting enzyme inhibitors | Enalapril maleate (Epaned, Vasotec) | Captopril (Capoten)<br>Lisinopril (Prinivil, Zestril)<br>Quinapril hydrochloride (Accupril)<br>Ramipril (Altace) |
| Angiotensin II receptor blockers | Valsartan (Diovan) | See Chapter 26 |
| Beta-adrenergic blockers | Metoprolol succinate extended release (Toprol XL) | Bisoprolol<br>Carvedilol (Coreg) |
| Loop diuretics | Furosemide (Lasix) | Bumetanide (Bumex)<br>Ethacrynate sodium (Sodium Edecrin)<br>Ethacrynic acid (Edecrin)<br>Torsemide (Demadex) |
| Thiazide diuretics | Hydrochlorothiazide (Microzide) | Chlorothiazide sodium (Diuril)<br>Methyclothiazide (Enduron) |
| Aldosterone antagonists | Spironolactone (Aldactone) | Eplerenone (Inspra) |

**Figure 30.3.** Treatment options for various stages of HF. ACE, angiotensin-converting enzyme; ARBs, angiotensin receptor blockers; FDC, fixed-dose combination; HYD, hydralazine; ISDN, isosorbide dinitrate. Stage D (refractory symptoms requiring special interventions) is not shown. (Reprinted with permission from Whalen, K. (2018). *Lippincott illustrated reviews: Pharmacology* (7th ed., Fig. 18.11). Philadelphia, PA: Wolters Kluwer; modified from Yancy, C. W., et al. (2017). 2017 ACC/AHA/HFSA focused update of the 2013 ACCF/AHA guideline for the management of heart failure: A report of the American College of Cardiology/American Heart Association Task Force on Clinical Practice Guidelines and the Heart Failure Society of America. *Circulation, 136*, 1.)

# CARDIAC GLYCOSIDES

Cardiac glycosides exert positive inotropic effects on the contractility of the heart muscle. (**Inotropic** means related to, or influencing the force of, myocardial contractility.) **Digoxin** (Lanoxin), derived from the foxglove plant of the genus *Digitalis*, is the prototype drug of this class. Clinical trials support the use of digoxin in heart failure in patients with left ventricular dysfunction, especially in those with advanced disease, but it is no longer considered a first-line drug. Although digoxin improves symptoms and quality of life, there is no evidence to suggest that it improves survival; it is considered a second-line therapy. Other drugs (e.g., beta-adrenergic blockers, diuretics, and ACE inhibitors or ARB) have displayed mortality benefits in heart failure and should be maximized first before using digoxin.

## Pharmacokinetics

Digoxin is the only cardiac glycoside available in the United States. Both oral (tablet, elixir, capsules) and parenteral (IV, intramuscular [IM]) preparations are available. The elixir is absorbed more effectively than the tablet or capsule and is used primarily with infants and children. Digoxin dosages are summarized in Table 30.2.

When given orally, the onset of action occurs in 1 to 2 hours, with the peak effect of the medication occurring in 2 to 8 hours. Oral absorption is 50% to 80% complete, and the extent of absorption may be delayed by the presence of food but otherwise is unaffected. However, because digoxin is metabolized by sugar hydrolysis in the stomach and by colonic bacteria in the gut, only 10% of the dose of digoxin reaches systemic circulation after oral administration. When digoxin is given by the IV route, the onset of action occurs within 5 to 30 minutes and reaches a peak effect in 1 to 5 hours; complete absorption of the drug occurs with IV administration. It should be noted that metabolism is decreased in patients with decompensated heart failure. The drug is excreted by the kidneys as unchanged drug (50%–70%).

## Action

A patient with heart failure experiences decreased contractility of the heart, which impairs the heart's ability to pump blood adequately. Digoxin produces a cardiotonic (positive inotropic) effect that improves the contractility and pumping ability of the heart. Digoxin increases the force of myocardial contractility by inhibiting sodium, potassium, and adenosine triphosphatase (Na, K-ATPase), an enzyme in cardiac cell membranes that decreases the movement of sodium out of myocardial cells after contraction. As a result, calcium enters the cell in exchange for sodium, causing additional calcium to be released from intracellular binding sites and increasing myocardial contractility.

In a patient with an atrial fibrillation, which is a common comorbidity with heart failure, digoxin slows the rate of ventricular contraction (negative chronotropy) through several factors. First, digoxin has a direct depressant effect on cardiac contraction tissues, especially at the atrioventricular (AV) node. This action decreases the number of electrical impulses allowed to reach the ventricles from supraventricular sources.

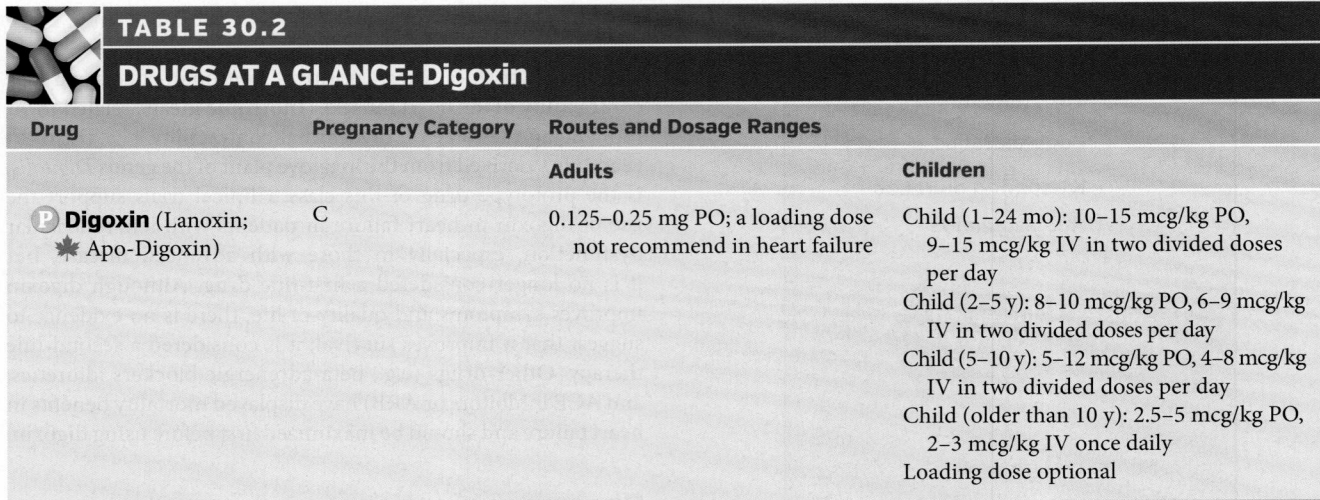

| Drug | Pregnancy Category | Routes and Dosage Ranges | |
|---|---|---|---|
| | | **Adults** | **Children** |
|  **Digoxin** (Lanoxin; ✷ Apo-Digoxin) | C | 0.125–0.25 mg PO; a loading dose not recommend in heart failure | Child (1–24 mo): 10–15 mcg/kg PO, 9–15 mcg/kg IV in two divided doses per day<br>Child (2–5 y): 8–10 mcg/kg PO, 6–9 mcg/kg IV in two divided doses per day<br>Child (5–10 y): 5–12 mcg/kg PO, 4–8 mcg/kg IV in two divided doses per day<br>Child (older than 10 y): 2.5–5 mcg/kg PO, 2–3 mcg/kg IV once daily<br>Loading dose optional |

Second, digoxin indirectly stimulates the vagus nerve. Third, increased efficiency of myocardial contraction and vagal stimulation decrease compensatory tachycardia that results from the sympathetic nervous system response to inadequate circulation.

## Use

The clinical indications for use of digoxin include the management of mild to moderate heart failure in adults and children. The drug is also used to control the ventricular response rate in adults with chronic atrial fibrillation.

### Use in Children

Digoxin is used in children with heart failure to enhance contractility. When used in children, digoxin therapy should be prescribed and supervised by a pediatric cardiologist when possible. The response to a given dose varies with age and size. The child's renal and hepatic function also affects the child's response to the medication, and the child should be carefully monitored for therapeutic response. There may be little difference between a therapeutic dose and a toxic dose. Very small amounts are often given to children. These factors increase the risk of dosage errors in children. In a hospital setting, institutional policies may require that each dose be verified with another nurse before it is administered. Liquid digoxin must be precisely measured in a syringe, and the dose should never be rounded. It is imperative that the dosage administered is accurate. Electrocardiographic monitoring is important when digoxin therapy is initiated.

As in adults, the dosage of digoxin in children is individualized and carefully titrated. Digoxin is primarily excreted by the kidneys, and the dosage should be reduced in the presence of renal impairment. In general, divided daily doses should be given to infants and children younger than 10 years of age, and adult dosages adjusted to weight should be given to children older than 10 years of age. Larger doses are usually needed to slow a too rapid ventricular rate in children with atrial fibrillation. Differences in bioavailability of different preparations (oral and parenteral) must be considered when switching from one preparation to another.

### ! QSEN Alert: Safety

How well neonates tolerate digoxin depends on their degree of maturity. Premature infants are especially sensitive to drug effects. The dosage must be reduced, and administration should be even more individualized and cautious than in more mature infants and children. Early signs of toxicity in newborns are undue slowing of the sinus rate, sinoatrial arrest, and prolongation of the P–R interval on electrocardiogram (ECG).

### Use in Older Adults

Digoxin is a frequent cause of adverse effects in older adults. Digoxin should not be used as first-line therapy for heart failure with adults greater than 65 years old. Reduced dosages are usually required because of decreased liver or kidney function, decreased lean body weight, and advanced cardiovascular disease. Impaired renal function leads to slower drug excretion and increased risk of accumulation.

### Use in Patients With Renal Impairment

Caution is necessary with the use of digoxin in patients with diminished renal function because renal impairment delays the drug's excretion, significantly increasing elimination half-life, drug accumulation, and adverse effects. Dosage must be reduced according to the creatinine clearance and severity of renal impairment; the nurse consults the prescriber's instructions for reduced dosages related to this value. Patients with advanced renal impairment can achieve therapeutic serum concentrations with a dosage of 0.125 mg three to five times per week.

In patients with reduced blood flow to the kidneys (e.g., as a result of fluid volume depletion or acute heart failure), digoxin may be reabsorbed in the renal tubules. As a result, less digoxin is excreted through the kidneys, and a **maintenance dose** (i.e., a dose administered on a routine basis to produce a therapeutic effect and control symptoms) may be even less than the dosage amount calculated according to creatinine clearance. It is necessary to reduce loading doses of digoxin as well.

Note that digoxin toxicity develops more often and lasts longer in patients with renal impairment. Patients with renal impairment who are receiving digoxin, even in small doses, must be monitored for adverse effects, and serum digoxin levels must be monitored periodically.

### Use in Patients With Hepatic Impairment

Hepatic function has little effect on digoxin clearance. Adjustments in the dosage amount are not required for patients with hepatic impairment.

### Use in Patients With Critical Illness

Critically ill patients often have multiple cardiovascular and other disorders that require drug therapy. Acute heart failure may be the patient's primary critical illness. However, that episode of heart failure may be precipitated by other illnesses and treatments that alter fluid balance, impair myocardial contractility, or increase the workload of the heart beyond its capacity to accommodate. As a part of digoxin treatment, carefully monitor renal function in the critically ill patient. Management of the critically ill patient is often symptomatic, with the choice of drug and dosage requiring careful titration and frequent monitoring of the patient's response. Cardiotonic, diuretic, and vasodilator drugs are often required. All of these medications should be used cautiously with careful monitoring in critically ill patients.

### Use in Patients Receiving Home Care

Oral digoxin is taken at home, and the home care nurse shares the responsibility for teaching patients and their caregivers how to use the drug effectively as well as how to recognize adverse responses that should be reported to the health care provider. Accurate dosing is vitally important because underuse may cause the recurrence of symptoms and overuse may cause toxicity. Either condition may be life threatening. The nurse instructs the patient and any caregivers that if symptoms of heart failure or digoxin toxicity develop, it is necessary to seek medical intervention immediately. The home care nurse also monitors the patient's response to the drug and changes in the patient's condition or drug therapy that increase the patient's risk for toxicity.

## Adverse Effects

Because of digoxin's narrow therapeutic index, the patient is at greater risk for developing digoxin toxicity. Digoxin's adverse effects can cause significant patient harm; the nurse must be extremely cautious with administration and monitoring. Factors that contribute to the development of digoxin toxicity are summarized in Box 30.1. Patients with hypokalemia can develop digoxin toxicity even when the serum digoxin level is not considered to be elevated.

Signs of toxicity include potentially life-threatening heart rhythm disturbances, ranging from slow to rapid ventricular rhythm. Premature ventricular contractions (PVCs) occur commonly with digoxin toxicity and are usually perceived as "skipped" heartbeats by patients. However, PVCs have many possible causes and therefore are not specific for digoxin toxicity. Other adverse effects include dizziness, nausea, vomiting, loss of appetite, abdominal discomfort, vision changes (yellow–green halos and problems with color perception), blurred vision, and mental changes. Box 30.2 identifies medications administered to treat digoxin toxicity.

## Contraindications

Digoxin is contraindicated in patients with severe myocarditis, second- or third-degree heart block, ventricular tachycardia, or ventricular fibrillation. Caution is necessary when administering the drug to patients with acute myocardial infarction, first-degree heart block, Stokes–Adams syndrome, or Wolff–Parkinson–White syndrome, because it may place these patients at risk for fatal dysrhythmias. Care is also warranted in patients with hypokalemia, hypomagnesemia, or hypercalcemia because of the increased risk of dysrhythmias. Renal impairment requires an alteration in dosage and cautious administration.

## Nursing Implications

### Preventing Interactions

Dosage must be reduced by approximately 50% with concurrent administration of amiodarone hydrochloride, quinidine, nifedipine, or verapamil. These drugs increase the serum digoxin level and increase the risk of toxicity if the dosage is not reduced. Many other medications and herbs interact with digoxin, increasing or decreasing its effect (Boxes 30.3 and 30.4).

### Administering the Medication

The administration of digoxin requires the nurse to thoroughly assess the patient's cardiac status. The nurse also obtains an accurate body mass assessment and assesses the patient for renal impairment to ensure that an accurate dosage of medication is administered. The nurse assesses the apical pulse at the point of maximal impulse for one full minute. If the rate is less than 60 beats/min in adults, 70 beats/min in older children, or 100 beats/min in younger children, the nurse does not give the drug and notifies the health care provider. The nurse also assesses the patient for a pulse deficit to monitor for therapeutic effect. The goal of therapy is to eliminate a pulse deficit in the patient with atrial fibrillation. In patients with atrial fibrillation, slowing

| **BOX 30.1** | *Factors That Contribute to Digoxin (Lanoxin) Toxicity* |
|---|---|
| • An accumulation of larger-than-necessary maintenance doses<br>• Rapid loading or digitalization, whether by one or more large doses or frequent administration of small doses<br>• Extremes in age (young and old)<br>• Electrolyte imbalance (hypokalemia, hypomagnesemia, hypercalcemia) | • Fluid imbalance (volume depletion or gastrointestinal losses)<br>• Hypoxia due to heart or lung disease (hypoxia increases myocardial sensitivity to digoxin)<br>• Hypothyroidism (slows metabolism of digoxin)<br>• Concurrent treatment with other drugs affecting the heart, such as quinidine, verapamil (Calan), or nifedipine (Procardia) |

| **BOX 30.2** | *Management of Digoxin (Lanoxin) Toxicity* |

- Digoxin is discontinued, not just reduced in dosage. (Most patients with mild or early toxicity recover completely within a few days after the drug is stopped.)

**In the Presence of Serious Cardiac Dysrhythmias:**

- Potassium chloride, a myocardial depressant that acts to decrease myocardial excitability, is administered if the potassium level is low. The dose and route depends on the severity of the toxicity, the serum potassium level, and the patient's response. Potassium is contraindicated in patients with renal failure and should be used with caution in the presence of cardiac conduction defects.
- Lidocaine is an antidysrhythmic local anesthetic agent used to decrease myocardial irritability.
- Atropine or isoproterenol is used to manage bradycardia or conduction defects.
- Other antidysrhythmic drugs may be used but are generally less effective in digoxin-induced dysrhythmias (as compared with dysrhythmias due to other causes).

- Digoxin immune fab (Digibind, DigiFab) is a digoxin-binding antidote derived from antidigoxin antibody fragments produced in sheep. It is recommended only for severe digitalis poisoning with life-threatening symptoms. Digoxin immune fab fragments combine with digoxin, pulling it out of the tissues and into the bloodstream. This causes serum digoxin levels to be high, but the drug is bound to the antibody and therefore inactive. Digoxin immune fab is given intravenously, as a bolus injection if the patient is in danger of immediate cardiac arrest, but preferably over 30 minutes. Dosage varies and is calculated according to the amount of digoxin ingested or the serum digoxin level based on the patient's weight. (The two commercial products vary in the amount of fragments they contain but each corresponds to binding of ~0.5 mg of digoxin per vial.) Dosing guidelines are provided by the manufacturer.

of the heart rate and elimination of the pulse deficit are clinical indicators that a therapeutic blood level has been achieved.

The patient should take digoxin with food or after meals to minimize gastric irritation and the side effects of anorexia, nausea, and vomiting. However, these symptoms probably arise from drug stimulation of chemoreceptors in the medulla rather than as a direct irritant effect of the drug on the gastrointestinal (GI) tract.

**Digitalization** is the administration of a loading dose (a dose larger than the regular prescribed daily dosage) of digoxin to reach the **therapeutic index** (the margin between effectiveness and toxicity in the blood level of the medication) that will produce therapeutic effects rapidly. The administration of digoxin for rapid digitalization is usually done for atrial tachydysrhythmias and is not recommended in heart failure.

If a loading dose is prescribed, the digitalizing dosage schedule requires the nurse to administer a total dose of 0.75 to 1.5 mg of digoxin in divided doses, 6 to 8 hours apart, over a 24-hour period. It is important to note that rapid digitalization places the patient at risk for developing digoxin toxicity. Thus, the nurse must be alert to signs and symptoms of toxicity, which include very slow or very rapid ventricular rhythm, nausea, vomiting, loss of appetite, abdominal distention, vision changes, blurred vision, and mental changes. During rapid digitalization, the patient is monitored continuously on a cardiac monitor.

When digoxin is administered for heart failure, drug therapy is accomplished by beginning with a maintenance dose of digoxin. The maintenance dose for digoxin in heart failure treatment is 0.125 to 0.25 mg once daily. If the patient is over 70 years old, has renal impairment, or has a lean body mass, the dose is lowered and may be administered every other day. The therapeutic effects with a maintenance dose occur within approximately 1 week. Although the therapeutic serum digoxin level is 0.8 to 2.0 ng/mL, the ideal therapeutic range for both men and women in heart failure may be 0.5 to 0.8 ng/mL. Higher serum levels are associated with an increased risk of adverse effects and toxicity without clear evidence of improved efficacy.

| **BOX 30.3** | *Drug Interactions: Digoxin* |

**Drugs That Increase the Effects of Digoxin**

- Adrenergic agents, such as epinephrine (Adrenaline), ephedrine sulfate, and isoproterenol hydrochloride (Isuprel)
  *Increase the risk of cardiac dysrhythmias*
- Antithyroid agents and conivaptan
  *Increase the serum concentration of digoxin*
- Calcium preparations
  *Increase absorption of oral digoxin by slowing transit time through the gastrointestinal tract*

**Drugs That Decrease the Effects of Digoxin**

- Antacids, cholestyramine, colestipol hydrochloride (Colestid), oral laxatives, and aminoglycosides (e.g., neomycin sulfate)
  *Decrease absorption of oral digoxin*
- Acarbose
  *Decreases the serum concentration of digoxin*

| **BOX 30.4** | *Herb and Dietary Interactions: Digoxin* |

**Herbs and Foods That Increase the Effects of Digoxin**

- Ginseng
- Hawthorn berries
- Licorice
- Milkweed

**Herbs and Foods That Decrease the Effects of Digoxin**

- Psyllium
- St. John's wort

The serum blood level is drawn prior to the administration of the digoxin dose. The blood sample is drawn at least 6 hours after the previous dose, because distribution of digoxin to the tissues requires about 6 hours. If the blood is drawn before 6 hours, the serum digoxin level may be elevated and not an accurate assessment of therapeutic levels.

When administering IV digoxin, the dose is administered by IV push slowly over at least 5 minutes. The oral and IV routes are not interchangeable because they vary in bioavailability. Note that IV administration of injectable digoxin is preferred over administering the drug intramuscularly, because the IM route can cause severe pain at the injection site. If the drug must be administered by the IM route, it should be injected deep into the muscle followed by massage.

Decreased absorption of digoxin can also result in digoxin toxicity or **digitalis toxicity** (an accumulation of digitalis in the body that leads to nausea, vomiting, visual disturbances, atrial or ventricular tachydysrhythmias, ventricular fibrillation, sinoatrial block, and AV block.) Factors that decrease the rate or extent of digoxin absorption include the presence of food in the GI tract, malabsorption syndromes, and the concurrent administration of antacids or cholestyramine. The administration of digoxin should take place at least 1 hour before the administration of an antacid. It is important to note that when digoxin is discontinued, it takes approximately 1 week for the drug to be eliminated from the body.

### Assessing for Therapeutic Effects

When administering digoxin and related medications in the treatment of heart failure, the nurse assesses the therapeutic effects of the medications. The pulmonary symptoms that develop with heart failure are a direct result of events initiated by inadequate cardiac output. The left side of the heart is unable to accommodate incoming blood flow from the lungs. The resulting back pressure in pulmonary veins and capillaries causes leakage of fluid from blood vessels into tissue spaces and alveoli. Fluid accumulation may result in severe respiratory difficulty and pulmonary edema, a life-threatening development. The improved strength of myocardial contraction resulting from cardiotonic–inotropic drugs reverses this potentially fatal chain of events. The nurse observes for signs and symptoms of pulmonary congestion, such as dyspnea, orthopnea, cyanosis, cough, hemoptysis, crackles, anxiety, and restlessness. The nurse also assesses the patient daily for edema. The absence of pitting edema, decreased size of ankles and abdominal girth, and decreased weight improves circulation and increases renal blood flow. The diminished fluid is indicative of an improved blood supply to the body tissues.

### Assessing for Adverse Effects

Digoxin's narrow therapeutic index predisposes a patient to adverse effects. Thus, it is important that the nurse assess the patient for signs and symptoms of digitalis toxicity, including bradycardia and cardiac dysrhythmias such as PVCs, paroxysmal atrial tachycardia with heart block, AV tachycardia, and AV block (also known as second- or third-degree heart block). These are the most severe adverse effects associated with digoxin therapy. They appear as abnormalities on ECGs and in pulse rate or rhythm. PVCs are among the most common digoxin-induced dysrhythmias. Excessive slowing of the heart rate is an extension of the drug's therapeutic action of slowing conduction through the AV node and possibly depressing the sinoatrial node as well. Electrocardiography is necessary for identification of nodal rhythms and heart block.

The GI assessment is crucial in determining the onset of digoxin toxicity. The nurse assesses the patient for anorexia, nausea, and vomiting, which are common with digoxin therapy because digoxin stimulates the vomiting center of the brain. The presence of these symptoms raises the suspicion for digitalis toxicity but is not specific because other conditions or medications (e.g., diuretics, potassium supplements) may also cause GI adverse effects. The nurse instructs the patient to report any of these symptoms immediately to the health care provider.

Other symptoms of digoxin toxicity include headache, dizziness, drowsiness, and confusion. These adverse effects are more commonly seen in older adults. Visual disturbances (such as blurred vision, photophobia, altered perception of color, and flickering dots) indicate acute toxicity and must be seen by a health care provider immediately.

### Patient Teaching

Box 30.5 identifies patient teaching guidelines for digoxin.

---

**Clinical Application 30.2**

- Dr. Adams' cardiologist has ordered digoxin to be administered. Why did the cardiologist prescribe digoxin?
- The cardiologist states to the nurse that he is going to begin with the maintenance dose and not use digitalization. What is meant by digitalization?
- In addition to digoxin, the cardiologist prescribed amiodarone, spironolactone, and enalapril maleate for Dr. Adams. How will digoxin, amiodarone, spironolactone, and enalapril maleate assist in decreasing Dr. Adams' symptoms?
- What are the potential interactions between these medications the nurse should be aware of?

---

**NCLEX Success**

3. A patient is taking digoxin for atrial fibrillation. Which of the following assessment findings would indicate that the digoxin should be held and the health care provider should be notified?
   A. respiratory rate of 20 breaths/min
   B. pulse rate of 80 beats/min
   C. respiratory rate of 12 breaths/min
   D. pulse rate of 52 beats/min

4. How does digoxin exert a negative chronotropic effect?
   A. Digoxin has a direct depressant effect on cardiac conduction tissue.
   B. Digoxin increases electrical impulses through the ventricles.
   C. Digoxin depresses the vagal nerve to increase contractility.
   D. Digoxin prevents calcium from entering the myocardial cell.

---

**BOX 30.5**    *Patient Teaching Guidelines for Digoxin (Lanoxin)*

- Digoxin may be used in the treatment of heart failure or atrial fibrillation.
  - In heart failure, digoxin strengthens the heartbeat to relieve symptoms such as ankle swelling, shortness of breath, and fatigue.
  - In atrial fibrillation, digoxin slows the heartbeat and decreases symptoms such as fatigue.
- Digoxin is administered long term because heart failure is a chronic condition.
- Digoxin is given daily at the same time to produce therapeutic blood levels.
- Overuse of digoxin will cause adverse effects.
- Use the same brand and type of digoxin all the time.
- Never miss a dose of digoxin. Take your prescribed dose at the same time every day, and keep a written record of the date and time of administration.
- If you forget to take your daily dose, and it is within 6 hours of the time you usually take the dose, take your daily dose.
- Do not take an extra dose.
- Do not take a double dose to make up for a missed dose.
- Count your pulse for a full minute prior to taking your daily dose of digoxin. If your pulse rate is less than 60 beats/min, hold the dose of digoxin, and notify your health care provider.

- Take digoxin with food or after a meal. Dairy products will delay absorption.
- If needed, the tablets can be crushed. Capsules should be swallowed whole.
- Digoxin elixir must be measured accurately. A few drops more could produce overdosage, with serious adverse effects; a few drops less could produce underdosage, with a loss or decrease of therapeutic effects.
- Do not take other prescription or nonprescription drugs without consulting a health care provider.
- Have periodic physical examinations, electrocardiograms, and blood tests as ordered. These tests are used to check digoxin and electrolyte (sodium, potassium, magnesium) levels, to monitor your body's response to the digoxin, and to determine needed dosage changes.
- Digoxin is one drug in the management regimen of several drugs for heart disease. Together, the drugs in the management regimen help maintain a balance in the cardiovascular system. Never change the regimen unless you are told to do so by your health care provider.
- Limit sodium intake and get an adequate intake of potassium if you are also taking a loop diuretic. Low potassium levels can contribute to causing adverse effects of digoxin.
  - Report adverse effects such as changes in heart rate or rhythm, nausea, vomiting, or visual changes to your health care provider immediately.

---

5. The home care nurse is visiting a patient who has a history of heart failure. The patient is taking digoxin 0.125 mg orally each day. During the assessment, the patient states he has been nauseated since the home care visit 3 days ago. The nurse suspects he has developed digoxin toxicity. Which of the following factors makes this patient more prone to the development of digoxin toxicity?

   A. creatinine level of 2.0 mg/dL
   B. potassium level of 4.0 mEq/L
   C. calcium level of 8.5 mg/100 mL
   D. magnesium level of 2.0 mg/100 mL

6. A patient being digitalized in the cardiac intensive care unit is noted to have frequent PVCs. What should the nurse suspect in this patient?

   A. myocardial infarction
   B. pulmonary embolism
   C. digitalis toxicity
   D. hyperkalemia

7. A patient is being treated for hypothyroidism. She is also taking digoxin for chronic heart failure. Which of the following factors places the patient at risk for digoxin toxicity?

   A. impaired renal function
   B. impaired liver function
   C. tachycardia
   D. decreased metabolic rate

# PHOSPHODIESTERASE INHIBITORS (CARDIOTONIC–INOTROPIC AGENTS)

**Milrinone** is the most commonly used phosphodiesterase inhibitor administered for short-term management of acute to severe heart failure in patients who do not respond to treatment with digoxin (Lanoxin), diuretics, and vasodilators.

## Pharmacokinetics

Milrinone is a potent inotropic agent that is given intravenously by bolus injection followed by continuous infusion. The flow rate of the drug is titrated to maintain adequate circulation. The IV administration of milrinone produces an immediate effect. The half-life of this medication is approximately 80 hours, which can lead to accumulation of the medication with prolonged infusions. Dosages for milrinone are given in Table 30.3.

## Action

Milrinone's therapeutic action is to increase the force of contraction of the ventricles, providing a positive inotropic effect and improving ejection fraction. It causes systemic and pulmonary vasodilation by exerting a direct relaxant effect on the vascular smooth muscle, decreasing both preload and afterload. The drug increases the levels of cyclic adenosine monophosphate (cAMP) in myocardial cells by inhibiting phosphodiesterase, the enzyme that normally metabolizes cAMP. The effects of this drug are additive to those of digoxin and vasodilators, increasing cardiac output in patients with

| Drug | Pregnancy Category | Routes and Dosage Ranges | |
|---|---|---|---|
| | | **Adults** | **Children** |
| Ⓟ **Milrinone** | C | General: Loading dose 50 mcg/kg IV bolus, given over 10 min<br>Maintenance infusion: 0.125–0.75 mcg/kg/min<br>Total dose not to exceed 1.13 mg/kg/d<br>Older adult: Total dose not to exceed 1.13 mg/kg/d<br>Renal impairment:<br>Creatinine clearance (mL/min)<br>5 mL/min infusion rate: 0.2 mcg/kg/min<br>10 mL/min infusion rate: 0.23 mcg/kg/min<br>20 mL/min infusion rate: 0.28 mcg/kg/min<br>30 mL/min infusion rate: 0.33 mcg/kg/min<br>40 mL/min infusion rate: 0.38 mcg/kg/min<br>50 mL/min infusion rate: 0.43 mcg/kg/min<br>Dilution: Dilute with 0.9% or 0.45% sodium chloride or<br>5% dextrose; administer the solution within 24 h | Limited data available, optimal dosing not established for children |

TABLE 30.3 / DRUGS AT A GLANCE: Phosphodiesterase Inhibitors (Cardiotonic–Inotropic Agents)

systolic heart failure. Because milrinone does not act through beta receptors such as dobutamine, concomitant use of beta-adrenergic blocking drugs does not diminish its effects.

## Use

Milrinone is indicated intermediate and long term as bridge therapy in heart failure. It is useful until a definitive decision is made regarding nonpharmacologic therapy (e.g., coronary revascularization, mechanical circulatory support, or heart transplantation) to optimize cardiac function and stabilize heart failure patients prior to definitive treatment. Milrinone may also be used as palliative therapy for symptom control in selected patients who are refractory to alternate therapy.

Milrinone (or dobutamine) should be considered for short-term IV administration (1) in patients with acute decompensated heart failure when cardiac output cannot be maintained with diuretics and vasodilators or (2) in patients who are in cardiogenic shock. Routine short-term use of milrinone or dobutamine is not recommended because the drugs are associated with increased mortality in patients with acute decompensated heart failure. Milrinone is not recommended for use in children. Because impairment of hepatic function has little effect on milrinone clearance, dosage adjustments are not required for patients with hepatic impairment.

### Use in Older Adults

Milrinone must be used cautiously in the elderly because the aging process results in decreased renal function. The administration of milrinone in older adults should not exceed 1.13 mg/kg/d.

### Use in Patients With Renal Impairment

The creatinine clearance level is used to determine the dosage administration for patients with renal impairment (see Table 30.3).

### Use in Patients With Critical Illness

Milrinone should be administered only in a cardiac intensive care unit. The patient's hemodynamic and clinical response to the medication is monitored carefully.

## Adverse Effects

The most serious adverse effect associated with the administration of milrinone is the development of potentially fatal ventricular dysrhythmias, which reportedly affect 12% of patients. Hypotension, supraventricular dysrhythmias, chest pain, angina, headache, thrombocytopenia, and hypokalemia may also occur.

## Contraindications

Milrinone, a pregnancy category C medication, should be administered cautiously in pregnant and lactating women. It is contraindicated in patients who are allergic to milrinone or bisulfites. It is also contraindicated in patients with severe aortic or pulmonic valvular disease.

## Nursing Implications

### Administering the Medication

Prior to administering milrinone, the nurse assesses the patient for allergy to milrinone or bisulfites. The nurse also obtains an accurate weight and assesses the patient for renal impairment to ensure that an accurate dosage of medication is administered. The patient's cardiac rhythm, blood pressure, and pulse are monitored continuously, and a baseline pulse and blood pressure are recorded. If a marked decline in blood pressure or pulse rate occurs, the rate of administration should be reduced. The nurse assesses for adventitious breath sounds prior to administration and periodically throughout the administration of the drug. A platelet count is drawn prior to administration and at least one time during drug therapy to rule out the adverse effect of thrombocytopenia. Serum electrolyte levels are monitored periodically throughout the administration of the drug. The nurse also monitors and records fluid intake and output.

Milrinone is not compatible with other medications and should not be mixed with any other medications during administration.

 **QSEN Alert: Safety**

Milrinone and furosemide [Lasix] should not be administered through the same IV line because a precipitate may form.

### Patient Teaching

Box 30.6 identifies patient teaching guidelines for milrinone.

### NCLEX Success

8. **Which of the following best describes the action of milrinone?**
   A. It relaxes the smooth muscles of the blood vessels to make the vessels wider.
   B. It provides an inotropic effect.
   C. It produces vasoconstriction to increase both preload and afterload.
   D. It decreases the levels of cyclic adenosine monophosphate [cAMP].

9. **During the administration of milrinone, the patient's blood pressure decreases from 170/96 to 96/60 mm Hg. What is the most appropriate nursing intervention?**
   A. Call the physician.
   B. Administer a vasoconstrictor.
   C. Reduce the infusion rate.
   D. Reassess the blood pressure.

## ANGIOTENSIN RECEPTOR– NEPRILYSIN INHIBITORS

The heart secretes cardiac NPs in response to changes in cardiac pressure. NPs have a wide range of effects to facilitate cardiac homeostasis related to pressures and volumes. Modulation of

**BOX 30.6**  *Patient Teaching Guidelines for Milrinone*

- While you are taking this medication, frequent monitoring of your blood pressure, pulse, and heart rhythm will be necessary.
- You may experience increased urination while you are taking this medication. Because bed rest must be maintained, please call for assistance with toileting.
- Report pain at the injection site to the nurse.
- Report any numbness or tingling, shortness of breath, or chest pain.

the natriuretic system through inhibition of the enzyme neprilysin, which degrades natriuretic (and other vasoactive) peptides, has demonstrated reduced risk of death and hospitalization when added to an ARB in people with chronic heart failure and a reduced ejection fraction. The prototype angiotensin receptor–neprilysin inhibitor (ARNI) **Sacubitril/valsartan** (Entresto) blocks the harmful effects of the RAAS and sustains the beneficial effects of the NPs while providing direct opposition to increases in angiotensin II. The drug simultaneously stimulates vasodilatation through the peptides degraded by neprilysin. ANRIs have demonstrated limited effectiveness in improving outcomes for patients with less severe heart failure, but are recommended when ejection fraction becomes significantly reduced (LVEF less than 40) (Solomon et al., 2012). The 2017 ACC/AHA/HFAS Focused Update of the Heart Failure Management Guidelines indicate ANRIs have a significant impact on improving mortality for patients with reduced ejection fraction heart failure (Yancy et al., 2017).

## Pharmacokinetics

Sacubitril, the prodrug, is strongly bound to protein and is converted to an active metabolite by esterases. Following oral administration, peak plasma sacubitril concentrations are reached in approximately 30 minutes. Sacubitril has a half-life of approximately 1½ hours, and the metabolite has a half-life of 11½ hours. The drug and its metabolite are excreted in the urine and feces. Following twice-daily dosing of the drug, steady-state levels of sacubitril and valsartan are reached in 3 days.

Valsartan selectively blocks the binding of angiotensin II to specific tissue receptors found in the vascular smooth muscle and adrenal glands. This, in turn, blocks the vasoconstrictive effect of the RAAS and the release of aldosterone, leading to a decrease in the patient's blood pressure. Chapter 26 contains additional information regarding the ARBs; all ARBs are approved singly or in combination with other medications for the treatment of hypertension. (Note that valsartan [Diovan], when used alone, is the only ARB to receive U.S. Food and Drug Administration [FDA] approval for the treatment of patients with moderate to severe heart failure and those unable to tolerate ACE inhibitors due to adverse effects, such as cough.) Valsartan produces direct antagonism of the angiotensin II receptors that produce more efficient blockade of the cardiovascular effects of angiotensin II and less adverse effects than ACE inhibitors. Patients with an allergy to ACE inhibitors may have cross-sensitivity reactions to valsartan and other ARBs.

## Action

Sacubitril is a neprilysin inhibitor, and valsartan is an ARB. The beneficial cardiovascular and renal effects in heart failure patients appear to result from the increased levels of NPs that are degraded by neprilysin. One method of increasing NP concentrations is to reduce their degradation, which is the action of sacubitril, while simultaneously inhibiting the effects of angiotensin II, which is the action of valsartan. Valsartan also inhibits angiotensin II–dependent aldosterone release.

## Use

Sacubitril/valsartan, when administered with other heart failure therapies (in place of an ACE inhibitor or other ARB therapy), has shown success in the management of chronic heart failure with a reduced ejection fraction. Dosages for sacubitril/valsartan are given in Table 30.4. Note that the safety and effectiveness of sacubitril/valsartan in children has not been established and that no changes in dosage are required in older adults.

### Use in Patients With Renal Impairment

In patients who have severe renal impairment, a dose reduction in sacubitril/valsartan is recommended. In patients who have compromised renal function, are elderly, or are volume-depleted (including those on diuretic therapy), concomitant use of NSAIDs may result in worsening of renal function, including possible acute renal failure. These effects are usually reversible.

### Use in Patients With Hepatic Impairment

In patients who have moderate hepatic impairment, a dose reduction in sacubitril/valsartan is recommended. The drug combination should not be used with severe hepatic impairment.

### Use in Patients With Critical Illness

Patients with heart failure and reduced ejection fraction often receive treatment in critical care units. Ongoing monitoring is necessary for prompt recognition of adverse effects, especially hypotension, hyperkalemia, and renal issues, which will further compromise the critically ill.

## Adverse Effects

The most common adverse effects of sacubitril/valsartan are hypotension, hyperkalemia, cough, dizziness, and renal impairment. Angioedema may also occur and African American patients are at greater risk. Angioedema associated with laryngeal edema may cause airway obstruction and be fatal.

> **! QSEN Alert: Safety**
>
> African Americans are at higher risk of developing angioedema with administration of sacubitril/valsartan.

## Contraindications

Sacubitril/valsartan is contraindicated with a hypersensitivity to any component, concomitant use with ACE inhibitors or with aliskiren in patients with diabetes, or a history of angioedema related to previous ACE inhibitor or ARB therapy. The FDA has issued a **BLACK BOX WARNING ◆** because the drug (valsartan component) can cause fetal harm when administered in pregnancy. The use of drugs that act on the RAAS during the second and third trimesters of pregnancy reduces fetal renal function and increases fetal and neonatal morbidity and death.

## Nursing Implications

### Preventing Interactions

Increases in serum lithium concentrations and lithium toxicity have been reported during concomitant administration of lithium with ARBs. Additional drug interactions that increase or decrease the effect of sacubitril/valsartan are found in Box 30.7. Patients should not take grapefruit juice (a CYP3A4 inhibitor) and St. John's wort (a CYP3A4 inducer) while taking the drug, because adverse effects may occur.

### Administering the Medication

Sacubitril/valsartan can be administered without regard to food. When switching from an ACE inhibitor to sacubitril/valsartan, there should be a "washout" period of 36 hours between administrations of the two drugs to reduce the risk of angioedema.

### Assessing for Therapeutic Effects

The nurse should assess for signs of improvement or stabilization of chronic heart failure. Patients with improved cardiac performance demonstrate increased activity tolerance and alertness, improved appetite, and decreased shortness of breath, cough, nocturia, and irregularity of heart rhythm or rate. Laboratory values (blood urea nitrogen, creatinine, potassium) are within acceptable limits. Patients report an improved quality of life and decreased hospitalizations.

### Assessing for Adverse Effects

The nurse should monitor vital signs and laboratory values and assess patient for the development of cough or dizziness.

| **TABLE 30.4** | | | |
|---|---|---|---|
| **DRUGS AT A GLANCE: Angiotensin Receptor–Neprilysin Inhibitors** | | | |
| Drug | Pregnancy Category | Routes and Dosage Ranges | |
| | | Adults | Children |
| ℗ **Sacubitril/valsartan** (Entresto; 🍁 Entresto) | None; approved in 2015 Valsartan: D | 49/51 mg PO twice daily initially and then double dose to 97/103 mg twice daily after 2–4 wk as tolerated. If a patient not currently taking an ACE inhibitor or ARB, an initial dose of 24/26 mg twice daily is recommended. | Not recommended for use in children |

**Drugs That Increase the Effects of Sacubitril/Valsartan**
- Angiotensin-converting enzyme inhibitors
  *Increase the risk of angioedema*
- Alcohol, antihypertensive agents, and diuretics
  *Increase the risk of hypotension*
- Aliskiren
  *Increases the risk of hypotension, hyperkalemia, and renal impairment*
- Eplerenone, drospirenone, and heparin
  *Increase the risk of hyperkalemia*

**Drugs That Decrease the Effects of Sacubitril/Valsartan**
- CYP2C9 inducers (e.g., rifampicin, secobarbital), CYP3A4 inducers (e.g., indinavir, clarithromycin), methylphenidate, nonsteroidal anti-inflammatory drugs, peginterferon alfa-2B, and yohimbine
  *Decrease serum levels*
- Indomethacin
  *Decreases antihypertensive effects*
- Phenobarbital and rifamycins
  *Increase metabolism and decrease antihypertensive effects*
- CYP, cytochrome P450.

*Patient Teaching*

Women of childbearing age should use effective birth control measures while taking sacubitril/valsartan, and they should notify their health care provider immediately if they become pregnant. Drugs that act directly on the RAAS can cause injury and death to the developing fetus. Box 30.8 identifies patient teaching guidelines for sacubitril/valsartan.

## SINOATRIAL NODE MODULATORS

Ⓟ **Ivabradine** (Corlanor), the only drug in its class, is an adjunctive therapy for moderate to severe heart failure when used with drugs with proven mortality benefits. Ivabradine reduces heart rate, which reduces myocardial demand and adverse outcomes for patients with reduced ejection fraction. Ivabradine is particularly beneficial in reducing hospitalizations for patients with severe heart failure and significantly reduced ejection fraction (Yancy et al., 2016). The FDA approved the drug in 2015 through the priority review program.

## Pharmacokinetics

Following oral administration, peak plasma ivabradine concentrations are attained in approximately 1 hour under fasting conditions (about 2 hours with food). The bioavailability of ivabradine is about 40%; the drug undergoes first-pass elimination in the liver and intestines. Metabolism is by CYP3A4-mediated oxidation. Ivabradine has an effective half-life of approximately 6 hours. The drug is excreted in the urine.

## Action

Ivabradine produces selective inhibition of the pacemaker ("funny" or f-channels) of the sinoatrial node, with resultant disruption of the current flow. This lengthens diastolic depolarization, resulting in a slower firing of the sinoatrial node and consequently a decrease in heart rate.

## Use

Ivabradine is useful for reducing the risk of hospitalization for worsening heart failure in patients with stable, symptomatic chronic heart failure with left ventricular ejection fraction 35% or less; in those who are in sinus rhythm with resting heart rate of 70 beats/min or more; and in those who are either on maximally tolerated doses of beta-adrenergic blockers or in those who have a contraindication to beta-adrenergic blockers. Dosages for ivabradine are given in Table 30.5. Dosage adjustments are based on resting heart rate. Note that no studies have focused on the use of ivabradine in children and that there are no indications that ivabradine dosages in older adults need to be different from those in younger adults.

**BOX 30.8** *Patient Teaching Guidelines for Sacubitril/Valsartan*

- While you are taking this medication, frequent monitoring of your blood pressure will be necessary.
- Do not start, stop, or change the dose of this drug without checking with your provider.
- Talk to your provider (1) if you are taking a salt substitute that contains potassium or a potassium supplement or (2) if you are taking a potassium supplement or a potassium-sparing diuretic.
- Avoid driving and performing other activities that require you to be alert until you see how this drug affects you.
- Get up slowly over a few minutes when sitting or lying down to decrease the chance of feeling dizzy or passing out; use caution and hold the handrail when climbing stairs.
- Have your blood pressure checked often.
- Have blood work checked as you have been told by your health care provider. Keep all appointments for laboratory work or provider visits.
- Make sure you drink adequate fluids particularly in hot weather or if you have too much sweating, vomiting or diarrhea. This could lead to low blood pressure.
- Seek medical attention if you have deep swelling or welts under your skin, particularly around your eyes and lips, because this may be a serious reaction called angioedema.
- Notify your provider if you are breast-feeding. You will need to talk about any risks to your baby.

| TABLE 30.5 | | | |
|---|---|---|---|
| **DRUGS AT A GLANCE: Sinoatrial Node Modulators** | | | |
| **Drug** | **Pregnancy Category** | **Routes and Dosage Ranges** | |
| | | **Adults** | **Children** |
| (P) **Ivabradine** (Corlanor; ✹ Corlanor) | None; approved in 2015 | 2.5–5 mg PO twice daily initially, and then after 2 wk, adjust dose to achieve a resting heart rate between 50 and 60 beats/min to maximum dose of 7.5 twice daily. | Not recommended for use in children |

## Use in Patients With Renal Impairment

Current data do not indicate the need for ivabradine dosage adjustments in patients with impaired renal function.

## Use in Patients With Hepatic Impairment

Current data do not indicate the need for ivabradine dosage adjustments in patients with mild to moderate hepatic dysfunction. No research has studied the effects of ivabradine in patients with severe impaired liver function, and these patients should not take the drug.

## Use in Patients With Critical Illness

Administration of ivabradine in the critical care setting may be necessary to reduce cardiovascular mortality in the management of patients who are experiencing worsening heart failure. These patients may also be receiving additional drugs that are metabolized by CYP3A4 or worsen heart failure. Ongoing, vigilant monitoring is warranted for prompt recognition of adverse effects, especially bradycardia, hypotension, and atrial fibrillation, which could further compromise the critically ill.

## Adverse Effects

The most common adverse reactions to ivabradine are bradycardia, hypotension, atrial fibrillation, and **phosphene** (intermittent enhanced brightness in a limited area of the visual field, halos, or multiple images).

## Contraindications

Ivabradine is contraindicated in acute decompensated heart failure, hypotension, a resting heart rate less than 60 beats/min, sinoatrial block or third-degree AV block, sick sinus syndrome, pacemaker dependence, severe hepatic impairment, and concurrent use with strong CYP3A4 inhibitors, macrolide antibiotics, HIV protease inhibitors, and nefazodone.

## Nursing Implications

### Preventing Interactions

Ivabradine is primarily metabolized by CYP3A4. Concomitant use of CYP3A4 inhibitors increases ivabradine plasma concentrations, and the use of CYP3A4 inducers decreases them. Increased plasma concentrations may exacerbate bradycardia and conduction disturbances. Additional drugs interact with ivabradine, increasing or decreasing its effect (Box 30.9). Also,

patients should not take grapefruit juice (a CYP3A4 inhibitor) or St. John's wort (a CYP3A4 inducer) while taking the drug because adverse effects may occur.

### Administering the Medication

Ivabradine should be taken with meals. Food delays absorption by approximately 1 hour and increases plasma exposure by 20% to 40%, extending the action of the drug in the body. As previously stated, patients should avoid drinking grapefruit juice.

### Assessing for Therapeutic Effects

Ivabradine causes a dose-dependent reduction in heart rate. The size of the effect is dependent on the baseline heart rate (greater heart rate reduction in patients with higher baseline heart rates). At recommended doses, the heart rate reduction is approximately 10 beats/min at rest and during exercise.

### Assessing for Adverse Effects

The nurse should regularly monitor cardiac rhythm, heart rate, and blood pressure. If atrial fibrillation, bradycardia, or hypotension occurs, discontinuation of ivabradine is warranted, and notification of the prescriber is necessary. The nurse should observe for patient reports of phosphenes.

### Patient Teaching

The nurse should advise patients to take the medication with meals and to avoid grapefruit juice and St. John's wort. Women of childbearing age should use effective birth control measures

**BOX 30.9** **Drug Interactions: Ivabradine**

**Drugs That Increase the Effects of Ivabradine**
- Moderate CYP3A4 inhibitors (diltiazem, verapamil)
  *Increase the risk of bradycardia*
- Azole antifungals, macrolide antibiotics, and protease inhibitors
  *Increase risk of adverse effects*

**Drugs That Decrease the Effects of Ivabradine**
- CYP3A4 inducers (rifampicin, barbiturates, phenytoin)
  *Decrease the effectiveness of ivabradine*

**BOX 30.10**     *Patient Teaching Guidelines for Ivabradine (Corlanor)*

- Check your blood pressure, pulse, and heart rhythm as you have been instructed. If your heart rate is less than 50 beats/min, do not take the next dose of medication, and call your provider. Keep all appointments for an electrocardiogram or other tests.
- Watch for changes in eyesight, including brightness with sudden changes in light. Be cautious while driving, including driving at night.

- Take your medication with food to maintain consistency in drug effect; avoid grapefruit and grapefruit juice.
- For women of childbearing age, use trustworthy birth control while taking this drug, and notify your prescriber if you become pregnant because this drug could harm the baby.

while taking ivabradine and should notify the health care provider immediately if they become pregnant. In animal studies, ivabradine caused miscarriage, heart and blood vessel problems, and infant death. Whether these effects occur in humans is not known. Also, it is not known if ivabradine passes into breast milk; mothers should not nurse while taking ivabradine. Box 30.10 identifies additional patient teaching guidelines for ivabradine.

# ADJUVANT MEDICATIONS USED TO TREAT HEART FAILURE

Adjuvant medications are administered for heart failure to support the treatment and resolution of symptoms. These adjuvant medications are summarized in Table 30.6.

## Angiotensin-Converting Enzyme Inhibitors

ACE inhibitors prolong morbidity and mortality in patients with heart failure with reduced ejection fractions and have served as the mainstay of heart failure management for over two decades. The prototype ACE inhibitor is 🄿 **enalapril maleate** (Epaned, Vasotec). Enalapril maleate blocks the conversion of angiotensin I to angiotensin II, which is a potent vasoconstrictor. By blocking the production of angiotensin II, enalapril maleate promotes vasodilation (decreasing blood pressure and left ventricular afterload) and decreases aldosterone secretion (increasing serum potassium levels and reducing sodium and water retention). The medication also increases prostaglandin synthesis to decrease blood pressure.

Enalapril maleate is used to treat hypertension, acute and chronic heart failure, and asymptomatic left ventricular dysfunction. The ACE inhibitors are the first choice of drugs used to treat chronic heart failure. All of the ACE inhibitors have similar effects, but enalapril, captopril (Capoten), lisinopril (Prinivil, Zestril), quinapril hydrochloride (Accupril), and ramipril (Altace) are approved for the treatment of heart failure. Additional information on these ACE inhibitors is found in Chapter 26.

The nurse assesses the patient's blood pressure and pulse prior to administration and periodically 4 to 6 hours after administration, because that is the peak of action. The nurse teaches the patient not to stop the medication without the primary health care provider's knowledge and how to recognize adverse effects that need to be reported immediately to the

health care provider. The nurse instructs women of childbearing age to use contraception while taking the medication because of the risk for fetal abnormalities or death.

### Clinical Application 30.3

Dr. Adams' wife brings her husband to the emergency department; she reports that since yesterday, he has not been eating, seems confused, and is not as active as usual. The results of a serum digoxin level and serum electrolyte panel reveal a digoxin level of 10 ng/mL and a calcium level of 12 mg/dL. His ECG shows that he is in Mobitz type II heart block with a heart rate of 42 beats/min. The patient is admitted to the intensive care unit, where he receives digoxin immune fab (Digibind) 9.5 mg intravenously over 30 minutes.
- What is digoxin immune fab (Digibind)? How does digoxin immune fab (Digibind) work?
- How is the development of digoxin toxicity related to the increase in serum calcium levels?

## Beta-Adrenergic Blocking Agents

Judicious use of beta-adrenergic blocking agents has been a cornerstone in the treatment of heart failure in light of increased evidence that supports their ability to decrease morbidity and mortality in patients with chronic heart failure. Beta-adrenergic blockers suppress the sympathetic nervous system and the resulting catecholamine excess that eventually damages myocardial cells, reduces myocardial beta receptors, and reduces cardiac output. As a result, over time, **ventricular remodeling** (dilation and hypertrophy of the ventricles) regresses, the heart returns toward a normal shape and function, and cardiac output increases. Although the prototype beta-adrenergic blocking agents is propranolol hydrochloride (Inderal), which is described in detail in Chapter 27, the prototype agent with heart failure is 🄿 **metoprolol succinate**.

Class II beta-adrenergic blockers are often administered in patients following myocardial infarction and heart failure because of their effectiveness in improving symptoms, reducing hospitalization, and improving survival. The ability to improve survival may result from the ability of the drug class to prevent ventricular fibrillation. With heart failure, the ACCF/AHA 2013 heart failure guidelines recommend the use of one of three

## TABLE 30.6

## DRUGS AT A GLANCE: Adjuvant Drugs for the Treatment of Heart Failure

| Drug | Pregnancy Category | Routes and Dosage Ranges | |
|---|---|---|---|
| | | **Adults** | **Children** |
| Ⓟ **Enalapril maleate** (Epaned, Vasotec; ✽ Taro-Enalapril, Teva-Enalapril, Vasotec) | C in first trimester D in second and third trimesters | 2.5–10 mg PO daily or BID in conjunction with diuretic and digitalis. Max dose 40 mg/d. Renal impairment: Use smaller initial dose and adjust upward to a maximum of 40 mg/d PO | 1 mo to 16 y: initial dose 0.1 mg/kg PO daily or two divided doses Maximum dose is 0.5 mg/kg/d |
| Ⓟ **Valsartan** (Diovan; ✽ Ran-Valsartan) | D | 20–40 mg PO twice daily initially; doubling dose as tolerated to a maximum dose of 320 mg/d | Not recommended for use in children with heart failure |
| Ⓟ **Metoprolol succinate** (Toprol XL; ✽ Lopressor SR, Metoprolol SR) | C | 12.5–25 mg once daily, to maximum dose of 200 mg | Limited data available, optimal dosing not established for children |
| Bisoprolol (✽ Mylan-Bisoprolol, Novo-Bisoprolol, PHL-Bisoprolol) | C | 1.25 mg PO once daily initially to maximum dose of 10 mg once daily | Not recommended for use in children |
| Carvedilol (Coreg, Coreg CR; ✽ Auro-Carvedilol, Dom-Carvedilol) | C | Coreg: 3.125 mg twice daily initially, doubling dose every 2 wk as tolerated; maximum dose based on weight and severity of HF; mild to moderate HF, <85 kg 25 mg twice daily, >85 kg 50 mg twice daily. Severe HF 25 mg twice daily Coreg CR (extended release): 10 mg once daily initially for 2 wk, doubling dose every 2 wk as tolerated; maximum dose 80 mg once daily | Limited data available, optimal dosing not established for children |
| Ⓟ **Furosemide** (Lasix; ✽ Lasix, Apo-Furosemide, Teva-Furosemide) | C | 20–80 mg PO daily; a second dose can be administered 6–8 h after the initial daily dose 20–40 mg IV push over 1–2 min; dose can be increased in increments of 20 mg in 2 h Renal impairment: Up to 4 mg/d has been tolerated IV bolus injection should not exceed 1 g/d given over 30 min | 0.5–2 mg/kg/dose PO every 6–24 h; max dose 6 mg/kg/d 0.5–2 mg/kg/dose IV or IM every 6–12 h; may increase dosage by 1 mg/kg in 2 h until desired effect is seen or reach max dose of 6 mg/kg/d |
| Ⓟ **Hydrochlorothiazide** (Microzide; ✽ Apo-Hydro, Urozide) | B | 25–100 mg PO daily until adequate fluid loss is attained and then 25–100 mg PO daily Total dose not to exceed 200 mg/d | Infants: 1–3 mg/kg/d PO in 1–2 doses; max dose 37.5 mg/d Children >2 y: 1–2 mg/kg/d PO in 1–2 doses; max dose 100 mg/d |
| Ⓟ **Spironolactone** (Aldactone; ✽ Aldactone, Teva-Spironolactone) | C | 12.5–25 mg once daily PO initially, to 50 mg/d maximum | Not approved for heart failure in children |

beta-adrenergic blocking agents: extended-release metoprolol succinate (Toprol XL), bisoprolol, and carvedilol (Coreg). These three drugs competitively block the beta-adrenergic receptors in the heart and juxtaglomerular apparatus to decrease the influence of the sympathetic nervous system on these tissues. The resultant diminished excitability of the heart reduces cardiac workload and oxygen consumption. In addition, these three drugs are beneficial in the management of stable, symptomatic heart failure. The drugs reduce the rate of hospitalizations and mortality in patients already receiving ACE inhibitors, diuretics, and/or digoxin.

Prior to the administration of metoprolol, bisoprolol, and carvedilol, the nurse determines if the patient has had any hypersensitivity reactions to beta-adrenergic blockers or conditions that contraindicate use of the medication. The patient should not take the herb betel palm, which blocks the reduction in heart rate produced by beta-adrenergic blocking agents, concurrently. The nurse assesses the patient's weight and cardiopulmonary status and for the presence of dizziness, drowsiness, syncope, or blurred vision. In addition, the nurse instructs the patient to report shortness of breath, night cough, edema, slow pulse, confusion, depression, rash, fever, or sore throat and explains that therapy with a beta-adrenergic blocker should never be stopped abruptly. The FDA has issued a **BLACK BOX WARNING ◆** for beta-adrenergic blocking agents for patients with coronary artery disease: rapid withdrawal of oral forms of these drugs may result in exacerbation of angina, increased incidence of ventricular dysrhythmias, and the occurrence of myocardial infarctions.

## Diuretics

The ability to manage the volume overload with diuretic drugs makes them a first-line drug category for symptom improvement in patients with heart failure. Diuretics are used to manage symptoms of fluid volume excess for mild, moderate, and severe heart failure and are often one of the first medications prescribed. Three drug classes of diuretics are used in heart failure: loop diuretics, thiazide diuretics, and aldosterone antagonists. A further discussion on diuretics is found in Chapter 34.

### Loop Diuretics

**Furosemide** (Lasix) is the prototype for the loop diuretics. Furosemide is administered to patients with moderate to severe heart failure to reduce edema. Loop diuretics cause profound diuresis and, unlike thiazide diuretics, are effective when the glomerular filtration rate is low. Furosemide is also used intravenously to manage symptoms and excess fluid volumes in acute decompensated heart failure. Furosemide is administered with food to prevent gastric upset. When a patient is being treated with furosemide, the nurse weighs the patient daily and reports any increase in weight of greater than 2 lb in 24 hours to the health care provider. It is necessary to assess fluid and electrolyte levels frequently to identify extracellular fluid overload or dehydration. The nurse withholds the medication in the event of fluid volume depletion and notifies the health care provider. The nurse assesses blood pressure, pulse, and respirations daily. Loop diuretics are potassium wasting; thus, a potassium-rich, low-sodium diet is recommended, and the nurse should instruct the patient on symptoms of hypokalemia such as weakness, fatigue, muscle cramps, and palpitations. Potassium supplements may also be necessary. In patients with diabetes mellitus, the nurse assesses blood glucose levels frequently because furosemide therapy may cause an increase in blood glucose levels.

### Thiazide Diuretics

The prototype drug for the thiazide diuretics is **hydrochlorothiazide** (Microzide). Hydrochlorothiazide (HCTZ) inhibits the reabsorption of sodium and chloride in the distal renal tubule, moderately increasing the excretion of sodium and water by the kidneys. It is administered primarily for hypertension but is sometimes beneficial in treating edema associated with early or mild heart failure. Decreasing the plasma volume increases cardiac output and decreases preload. In a clinical trial, chlorthalidone, a thiazide-like diuretic, reduced the incidence of new-onset heart failure with preserved ejection fraction compared to amlodipine, lisinopril, and doxazosin.

Prior to administering HCTZ, the nurse assesses the patient for allergy to thiazides and sulfonamides. The nurse also assesses the blood pressure and pulse before administering the medication and periodically following administration. HCTZ is also a potassium-wasting diuretic so a potassium-rich, low-sodium diet is recommended, and the nurse should instruct the patient on the symptoms of hypokalemia. In addition, potassium supplements may be necessary. The risk of toxicity and dysrhythmias in the presence of hypokalemia may be a concern, as with the loop diuretics. HCTZ is administered with food to prevent gastric upset. Throughout therapy, the nurse assesses the patient's lungs (for adventitious sounds), heart (for an $S_3$), and extremities (for peripheral edema), the patient's fluid and electrolyte status, and the patient's weight (daily). Any increase in weight of greater than 2 lb in 24 hours must be reported to the primary health care provider.

### Aldosterone Antagonists

Increased aldosterone is a major factor in the pathophysiology of heart failure. Increased aldosterone levels result in interstitial fibrosis, which may decrease systolic function and increase the risk of dysrhythmias.  **Spironolactone** (Aldactone), the prototype drug in this class, is an aldosterone antagonist that reduces aldosterone-induced retention of sodium and water and impaired vascular function by antagonizing the action of aldosterone at mineralocorticoid receptors. In patients with heart failure and inadequate renal function, spironolactone allows smaller doses of loop diuretics and potassium supplements to be administered as the drug reduces urinary potassium loss. Consequently, aldosterone antagonists are also referred to as potassium-sparing diuretics. Clinical trials have shown that the combination of spironolactone with other drugs improves cardiac function and reduces symptoms, hospitalizations, and mortality in patients with heart failure.

Spironolactone is used to decrease edema in patients with heart failure. A second drug in this class, eplerenone (Inspra), is approved for use in the management of heart failure after myocardial infarction to improve survival.

> **⚠ QSEN Alert: Evidence-Based Practice**
>
> Clinical trials have demonstrated mortality benefit with the addition of aldosterone antagonists to the treatment regimen of patients with heart failure and reduced ejection fraction. The 2013 ACCF/AHA guidelines report that these drugs are useful in heart failure because they inhibit sodium reabsorption and prevent other destructive aldosterone-mediated mechanisms in the heart. Spironolactone also produces nonspecific binding to various steroid receptors; thus, progestational and antiandrogenic adverse effects, including gynecomastia, menstrual irregularities, and impotence, can occur. However, because of the selectivity of eplerenone for the aldosterone receptor, these adverse effects seem to be less likely in patients who take eplerenone. Although

eplerenone is more selective, with the potential for fewer side effects, there is no evidence in clinical trials that its overall efficacy is superior to that of spironolactone and the cost of treatment may reduce overall use. The most severe side effect of spironolactone, hyperkalemia, also occurred with eplerenone; dosage reduction is recommended with rise in potassium level.

The nurse assesses the patient's blood pressure and pulse prior to administering an aldosterone antagonist. Prior to beginning therapy, it is necessary to obtain a baseline ECG and monitor electrolyte status and renal function. Because the risk of hyperkalemia increases in patients taking spironolactone and eplerenone, dose reduction or interruption of drug therapy may be necessary should hyperkalemia occur. The nurse instructs the patient to take salicylates only if prescribed by the health care provider, because salicylates can decrease the effects of aldosterone antagonists. The nurse also advises the patient to avoid using herb licorice, which blocks the effects of aldosterone antagonists. A patient taking eplerenone should avoid grapefruit juice because the combination leads to increased eplerenone levels.

## NCLEX Success

10. A patient is taking furosemide, 40 mg daily, to decrease extracellular fluid related to heart failure. During patient teaching, which of the following points is most important for the nurse to convey?
    A. Sodium intake should be increased due to fluid loss.
    B. Administration of the medication with food will decrease absorption.
    C. The skin should be protected from sun exposure using sunscreen.
    D. Foods that contain potassium should be encouraged to prevent hyperkalemia.

11. A 35-year-old woman has been prescribed enalapril maleate. What should the nurse teach the patient?
    A. Use effective contraception.
    B. Double the dose if one is missed.
    C. If dizziness occurs, it is not a concern.
    D. There is no change in dose with impaired renal function.

12. What is the purpose of administering an angiotensin II receptor blocker to a patient with heart failure?
    A. It will increase vasoconstriction to increase myocardial contractility.
    B. It will block the influx of calcium across the sinoatrial node.
    C. It will inhibit the enzyme that catalyzes cholesterol synthesis.
    D. It will block the renin–angiotensin II system to increase vasodilation.

13. A patient is diagnosed with heart failure. Which of the following nonpharmacological interventions will be a priority in decreasing edema?
    A. Administer a diuretic agent.
    B. Limit dietary sodium.
    C. Place the patient on bed rest.
    D. Increase dietary protein.

### Clinical Application 30.4

Dr. Adams is stable, and his cardiologist has discontinued the digoxin. Dr. Adams is preparing for discharge.
- What aspects of patient teaching are most important in the care of Dr. Adams?
- What dietary modifications are important in his care?

## THE NURSING PROCESS

A concept map outlines the nursing process related to drug therapy considerations in this chapter. Additional nursing implications related to the disease process should also be considered in care decisions.

**Assessment**

- Assess for current or potential heart failure.
  - Identify risk factors for heart failure.
    - Cardiovascular disorders: atherosclerosis, hypertension, coronary artery disease, myocardial infarction, cardiac dysrhythmias, cardiac valvular disease
    - Noncardiovascular disorders: severe infections, hyperthyroidism, pulmonary disease (e.g., cor pulmonale)
    - Other factors: fluid volume overload related to parenteral fluids or blood transfusions, increased age, third spacing
  - Interview and observe for signs and symptoms of chronic heart failure.
    - Mild heart failure: peripheral edema (feet and ankles), dyspnea on exertion, fatigue with ordinary activity
    - Moderate to severe heart failure: more extensive edema, dyspnea at rest, orthopnea, paroxysmal nocturnal dyspnea, cough related to congestion of the respiratory tract with venous blood, confusion from cerebral hypoxia, oliguria from decreased blood flow to the kidneys, anxiety
- Assess baseline vital signs, weight, edema, serum electrolytes (including potassium, magnesium, and calcium), and other laboratory values indicative of cardiovascular function.
- Assess for anticipated therapeutic effects (vital signs and heart rhythm within normal limits, adequate renal function, respiratory congestions and shortness of breath resolved, normal mentation, signs of adequate tissue perfusion, and reports of increased activity tolerance).
- Assess for adverse effects of disease and drug therapy.

**Outcomes of Therapy**

The patient will
- Take drug therapy safely and accurately.
- Experience improved breathing and less fatigue and edema.
- Verbalize understanding of disease process, recommended lifestyle changes, correct administration and rationale of drug therapy, and when and how to notify the provider.
- Be closely monitored for therapeutic and adverse effects, especially when other drugs are added to or removed from the management regimen.
- Maintain appointments with health care providers to monitor vital signs, serum electrolyte levels (especially potassium level), serum drug levels (such as digoxin), and renal function.

**Nursing Interventions**

- Implement measures to minimize and prevent heart failure and atrial dysrhythmias.
- Instruct the patient on lifestyle changes:
  - Balanced diet, avoidance of excessive saturated fat and salt, and weight control
  - Smoking cessation
  - Increased levels of regular exercise
  - Limited alcohol intake
- Implement measures to manage hypertension.
- Implement measures to reduce hypoxia.
- Avoid fluid overload, especially in elderly patients.
- Maintain management programs for heart failure, atrial dysrhythmias, and other cardiovascular or noncardiovascular disorders.
- Monitor vital signs, urine output, and serum potassium levels regularly, and compare with baseline values.
- Monitor ECGs when available and compare with baseline or previous ECGs.
- Implement appropriate teaching related to drug therapy.
- Administer oxygen, if needed, to relieve dyspnea, improve oxygen delivery, reduce the work of breathing, and decrease the constriction of pulmonary blood vessels.

**Evaluation**

- Interview and observe for relief of symptoms (weight loss, increased urine output, decreased peripheral edema, decreased or elimination of shortness of breath, improved activity tolerance, diminished heart rate, increased ability to perform self-care).
- Observe serum drug levels for normal or abnormal values.
- Interview regarding compliance with instructions for the administration of medications.
- Interview and observe for adverse drug effects.
- Observe for achievement of expected outcomes of drug therapy.

## KEY CONCEPTS

- Heart failure results from impaired myocardial contractility during systole (systolic dysfunction), impaired relaxation and filling of ventricles during diastole (diastolic dysfunction), or a combination of systolic and diastolic dysfunction.
- Myocardial dysfunction leads to compensation by the cardiovascular system, which ultimately worsens the myocardial dysfunction resulting in fluid volume overload and inadequate tissue perfusion.
- Cardinal manifestations of heart failure are dyspnea and fatigue, which lead to exercise intolerance and fluid retention, resulting in pulmonary congestion and peripheral edema.
- Pharmacologic management of heart failure is based on the classification or severity of the myocardial dysfunction and subsequent impact to ejection fraction and the patient signs and symptoms.
- First-line agents for mild to moderate heart failure include diuretics to reduce fluid volume, ACE inhibitors or ARBs to block compensation by the RAAS and lower blood pressure, and beta-adrenergic blockers to reduce heart rate and myocardial demand.
- Diuretics used in the management of heart failure include loop diuretics, thiazide diuretics, and aldosterone antagonists.
- The FDA has issued a **BLACK BOX WARNING ◆** for beta-adrenergic blocking agents for patients with coronary artery disease; withdrawing oral forms of the class may result in exacerbation of angina, increased incidence of ventricular dysrhythmias, and the occurrence of myocardial infarctions.
- Second-line pharmacologic management of heart failure includes digoxin (Lanoxin) which produces a cardiotonic or positive inotropic effect, improving myocardial contractility and pumping ability of the heart.
- Digitalis toxicity is one of the most commonly encountered drug-related reasons for hospitalization because digitalis has a narrow therapeutic index and the end point of effective therapy is often difficult to define and measure.
- The normal digoxin level is 0.8 to 2.0 ng/mL, although patients in heart failure may reduce the risk of adverse effects when the digoxin level is kept at the lower end of the range.
- Milrinone, a phosphodiesterase inhibitor, is administered for short-term management of acute decompensated heart failure in patients who do not respond to treatment with diuretics or vasodilators and who are in cardiogenic shock.
- Sacubitril, an ANRI, is administered as a combination drug with valsartan, an ARB, to inhibit cardiac NPs and block the RAAS to facilitate cardiac homeostasis through vasodilation and reduction of cardiac pressures. This medication has a significant positive impact on improving patient outcomes with moderate to severe heart failure.
- The FDA has issued a **BLACK BOX WARNING ◆** for the valsartan component of sacubitril/valsartan because valsartan acts on the RAAS during the second and third trimesters of pregnancy, reducing fetal renal function and increasing fetal and neonatal morbidity and death.
- Ivabradine, a sinoatrial node modulator, is an adjunct medication for the management of moderate to severe heart failure by reducing heart rate and myocardial demand which reduces adverse events and negative patient outcomes such as hospitalization.

## CLINICAL REASONING CASE STUDY

**Meet the Patient**

Karen Saxton, a 72-year-old woman, has been asymptomatic since being diagnosed with heart failure following a myocardial infarction 3 years ago. She presents to the emergency department complaining of shortness of breath, which has progressively worsened over the past 5 days. She woke last night not being able to catch her breath; her breathing improved when she sat on the edge of the bed for an hour. She reports that she sometimes needs to sleep on three pillows to breathe. Also, she has experienced episodes of shortness of breath during the past 2 months, especially on exertion. In addition, her feet have been swelling. making walking difficult. She says that she tires easily and has lost "all my pep—I can't do anything."

Pertinent findings include vital signs: temperature 99.2°F, blood pressure 106/52 mm Hg, pulse 142/min and irregular, and respirations 34/min and labored. Oxygen saturation on room air is 84%. Laboratory values are sodium 132 mEq/L, potassium 3.8 mEq/L, bicarbonate 20 mEq/L, blood urea nitrogen 18 mg/dL, and creatinine 1.0 mg/dL. Her left ventricular ejection fraction is 33%. A chest x-ray is consistent with pulmonary edema.

Mrs. Saxton was started on furosemide (Lasix), 20 mg PO once daily, spironolactone (Aldactone) 12.5 mg PO once daily, metoprolol succinate (Toprol XL) 25 mg PO once daily, and Enalapril (Vasotec) 12.5 mg twice daily.

• Discuss the rationale for prescribing these drugs.
• What assessment findings would demonstrate improvement in Mrs. Saxton's heart failure symptoms?
• What assessment finding would indicate adverse drug effects?

**Assessing Drug Information**

• The combined use of a loop diuretic, an aldosterone antagonist, a beta-adrenergic blocker, and an ACE inhibitor work to improve symptoms, slow, or reverse deterioration in myocardial function, and reduce mortality.
  • Furosemide (Lasix) is a potassium-wasting loop diuretic causes profound diuresis and unlike thiazide diuretics, is effective when the glomerular filtration rate is low.
  • Spironolactone (Aldactone), an aldosterone antagonist, reduces aldosterone-induced retention of sodium and water and impaired vascular function by antagonizing the action of aldosterone. In patients with heart failure and inadequate renal function, the addition of spironolactone allows smaller doses of loop diuretics and potassium supplements to be administered because the drug reduces urinary potassium loss.
  • Metoprolol succinate (Toprol XL), a beta-adrenergic blocker, competitively blocks the beta-adrenergic receptors in the heart and juxtaglomerular apparatus to decrease the influence of the sympathetic nervous system on these tissues reducing cardiac excitability, cardiac workload, and oxygen consumption.
  • Enalapril (Vasotec) blocks the production of angiotensin II, promotes vasodilation (decreasing blood pressure), decreases aldosterone secretion (increasing serum potassium levels and reducing sodium and water retention) and increases prostaglandin synthesis (decreasing blood pressure).

**Nursing Actions**

• Assess for improved myocardial function:
  • Systolic blood pressure > 90 mm Hg; heart rate below 100 beats/min and regular, respiratory rate of 20/min or less with no signs of labored breathing or complaints of shortness of breath; resolution of respiratory crackles on auscultation and chest x-ray congestion; signs of adequate tissue perfusion and clear mentation; and improvement or stabilization of reduced left ventricular ejection fraction.
  • Mrs. Saxton reports increased activity tolerance (decreased exertional dyspnea, orthopnea, and paroxysmal nocturnal dyspnea).
• Assess for adverse drug effects by assessing the patient's weight and cardiopulmonary status and for the presence of dizziness, drowsiness, syncope, or blurred vision.
• Assess for improvement of laboratory values: return of serum sodium level to normal limits and maintenance of serum potassium within normal limits.
• Assess for and instruct Mrs. Saxton to report shortness of breath, night cough, edema, slow pulse, confusion, depression, rash, fever, or sore throat.

---

*Visit* thePoint® *at* **http://thePoint.lww.com/Frandsen12e** *for answers to NCLEX Success questions (in Appendix A), answers to Clinical Application Case Studies (in Appendix B), and more!*

## REFERENCES AND RESOURCES

Borlaug, B. (2018). Treatment and prognosis of heart failure with mid-range ejection fraction. In D. Mancini (Ed.). *UpToDate*. Waltham, MA: UpToDate. Retrieved April 2, 2019.

DiPiro, J. T., Talbert, R. L., Yee, G. C., Wells, B. G., Posey, L. M., & Matzke, G. R. (2016). *Pharmacotherapy: A pathophysiologic approach* (10th ed.). New York, NY: McGraw-Hill Education.

Hinkle, J. L., & Cheever, K. H. (2018). *Brunner and Suddarth's: Textbook of medical-surgical nursing* (14th ed.). Philadelphia, PA: Lippincott Williams & Wilkins.

Inamdar, A. A., & Inamdar, A. C. (2016). Heart failure: Diagnosis, management and utilization. *Journal of Clinical Medicine, 5*(7), 62.

Jhund, P. S., & McMurray, J. V. (2016). The neprilysin pathway in heart failure: A review and guide on the use of sacubitril/valsartan. *Heart, 102*, 1342–1347.

Karch, A. M. (2018). *2019 Lippincott's nursing drug guide*. Philadelphia, PA: Lippincott Williams & Wilkins.

McMurray, J. J., Packer, M., Desai, A. S., Gong, J., Lefkowitz, M. P., Rizkala, A. R., et al. (2013). Dual angiotensin receptor and neprilysin inhibition as an alternative to angiotensin-converting enzyme inhibition in patients with chronic systolic heart failure: Rationale for and design of the Prospective comparison of ARNI with ACEI to Determine Impact on Global Mortality and morbidity in Heart Failure trial (PARADIGM-HF). *European Journal of Heart Failure, 15*(9), 1062.

Norris, T. L. (2019). *Porth's Pathophysiology: Concepts of altered health states* (10th ed.). Philadelphia, PA: Lippincott Williams & Wilkins.

Page, R. L., O'Bryant, C. L., Cheng, D., et al. (2016). Drugs that may cause or exacerbate heart failure: A scientific statement from the American Heart Association. *Circulation, 134*(9), e32–e69.

Post, T. W. (2019). *Use of beta blockers in heart failure with reduced ejection fraction*. Waltham, MA: UpToDate.

Solomon, S. D., Zile, M., Pieske, B., Voors, A., Shah, A., Kraigher-Krainer, E., et al. (2012). Prospective comparison of ARNI with ARB on management of heart failure with preserved ejection fraction. *Lancet, 380*(9851), 1387.

UpToDate. (2019). *Drug information.* Lexi-Comp, Inc.

Weeda, E. R., Nguyen, E., & White, C. M. (2016). Role of ivabradine in the treatment of patients with cardiovascular disease. *Annals of Pharmacotherapy, 50*(6), 475–485.

Yancy, C. W., Jessup, M., Bozkurt, B., Butler, J., Casey, D. E. Jr., Colvin, M. M., et al. (2017). 2017 ACC/AHA/HFSA Focused Update of the 2013 ACCF/AHA guideline for the management of heart failure: A report of the American College of Cardiology/American Heart Association Task Force on Clinical Practice Guidelines and the Heart Failure Society of America. *Circulation, 136*(6), e137–e161.

Yancy, C. W., Jessup, M., Bozkurt, B., Butler, J., Casey, D. E. Jr., Colvin, M. M., et al. (2016). 2016 ACC/AHA/HFSA focused update on new pharmacological therapy for heart failure: An update of the 2013 ACCF/AHA guideline for the management of heart failure. A report of the American College of Cardiology/American Heart Association Task Force on Clinical Practice Guidelines and the Heart Failure Society of America. *Circulation, 134*(13), e282–e293.

Yancy, C. W., Jessup, M., Bozkurt, B., Butler, J., Casey, D. E., Drazner, M. H., et al.; American College of Cardiology Foundation/American Heart Association Task Force on Practice Guidelines. (2013). 2013 ACCF/AHA guideline for the management of heart failure: A report of the American College of Cardiology Foundation/American Heart Association Task Force on practice guidelines. *Circulation, 128*(16), e240–e327.

# Drugs Affecting the Respiratory System

# Drug Therapy for Nasal Congestion and Cough

## LEARNING OBJECTIVES

*After studying this chapter, you should be able to:*

1. Describe characteristics of selected upper respiratory disorders and symptoms.
2. For the nasal decongestants, identify the prototype and describe the action, use, contraindications, adverse effects, and nursing implications.
3. For the antitussive agents, identify the prototype and describe the action, use, contraindications, adverse effects, and nursing implications.
4. For the expectorants, identify the prototype and describe the action, use, contraindications, adverse effects, and nursing implications.
5. For the mucolytics, identify the prototype and describe the action, use, contraindications, adverse effects, and nursing implications.
6. Recognize the concerns of using combination products to treat the common cold.
7. Implement the nursing process with patients receiving nasal decongestants, antitussives, expectorants, and mucolytic agents.

## CLINICAL APPLICATION CASE STUDY

Archie Hobbs is a 45-year-old welder at an industrial plant. The occupational nurse at the facility sees a high rate of colds. Mr. Hobbs comes to the health office complaining about his nasal congestion and cough.

## KEY TERMS

**Cough:** forceful expulsion of air from the lungs

**Rhinitis:** inflammation of nasal mucosa

**Rhinosinusitis:** inflammation of the nasal and paranasal sinus mucosa

**Sinusitis:** inflammation of the paranasal sinuses (air cells that connect with the nasal cavity and are lined by similar mucosa)

# INTRODUCTION

This chapter introduces the pharmacologic care of the patient who is receiving drugs used to treat upper respiratory disorders, such as the common cold and sinusitis, with symptoms such as nasal congestion, cough, and excessive secretions. A more extensive discussion of some of the many drugs used to treat these conditions appears in other chapters; their discussion here relates to their use in upper respiratory conditions.

## OVERVIEW OF NASAL CONGESTION AND OTHER RESPIRATORY SYMPTOMS

### Etiology and Pathophysiology

#### The Common Cold

The common cold, a viral infection of the upper respiratory tract, is the most common respiratory tract infection. Adults usually have 2 to 4 colds per year; schoolchildren may have as many as 10 colds annually. Many types of viruses, most often the rhinovirus, cause colds. Shedding of these viruses by infected people, mainly from nasal mucosa, can result in rapid spread to others.

The viruses can enter the body through mucous membranes. Cold viruses can survive for several hours on the skin and on hard surfaces, such as wood and plastic. There may also be airborne spread from sneezing and coughing, but this source is considered secondary. After the viruses gain entry, the incubation period is generally 5 days, the most contagious period is about 3 days after symptoms begin, and the cold usually lasts nearly 7 days. Because of the way cold viruses spread, frequent and thorough hand hygiene (by both infected and uninfected people) is the most important protective and preventive measure. The tendency for overmedication and inappropriate use of antibiotics for the common cold is widespread and poses significant risk of complications and drug resistance.

#### Rhinosinusitis

Some of the most common conditions that affect the upper respiratory system are inflammatory responses. **Sinusitis** is the inflammation of the mucous membranes lining the paranasal sinuses. **Rhinitis** is the inflammation and congestion of the nasal mucosa. Because sinusitis is almost always accompanied by inflammation of the contiguous nasal mucosa, the term **rhinosinusitis** is preferred. Sinusitis often results from a viral infection; allergic rhinitis occurs as a response to an allergen. Seasonal rhinitis, or hay fever, occurs in a specific season.

Ciliated mucous membranes help move fluid and microorganisms out of the sinuses and into the nasal cavity. (These membranes perform the same tasks in other parts of the respiratory tract.) This movement becomes impaired when sinus openings are blocked by nasal swelling, and the impairment is considered a major cause of sinus infections. Another contributing factor is decreased oxygen content in the sinuses, which contributes to the growth of microorganisms and impairs local defense mechanisms. In acute rhinosinusitis, the classic symptom triad is purulent nasal drainage, nasal obstruction, and facial pressure and/or pain. Figure 31.1 describes the pathophysiologic processes in rhinitis and rhinosinusitis.

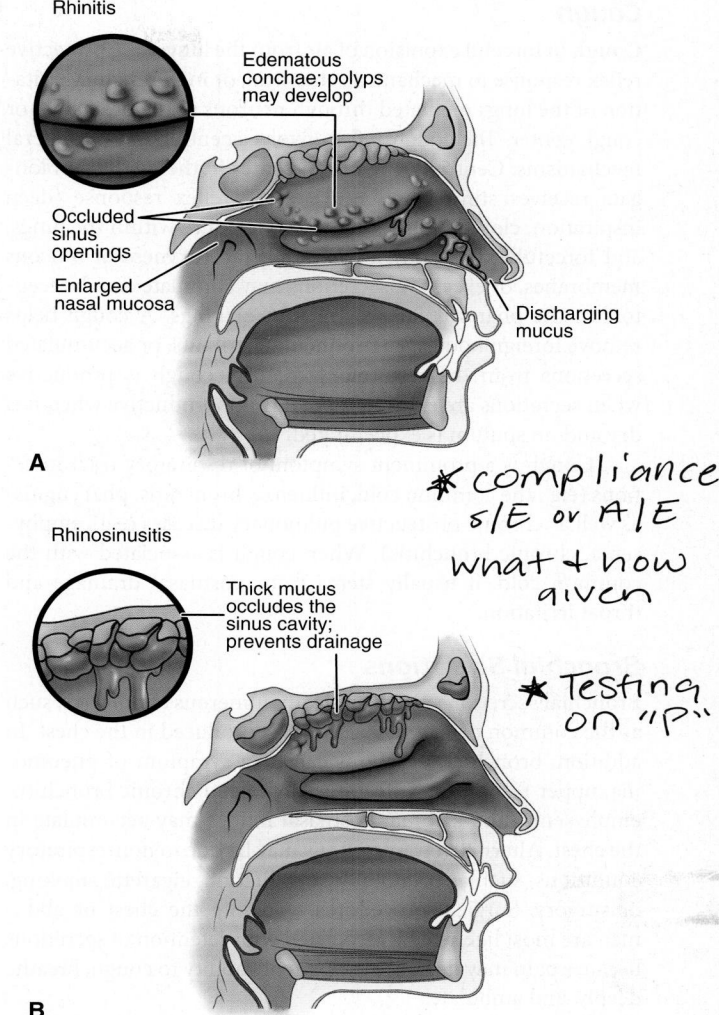

*(handwritten notes:)* ✱ compliance s/E or A/E what + how given
✱ Testing on "P"

**Figure 31.1.** Pathophysiologic processes in rhinitis and rhinosinusitis. Although pathophysiologic processes are similar in rhinitis and rhinosinusitis, they affect different structures. **A.** In rhinitis, the mucous membranes lining the nasal passages become inflamed, congested, and edematous. The swollen nasal conchae block the sinus openings, and the mucus is discharged from the nostrils. **B.** Rhinosinusitis is also marked by inflammation and congestion, with thickened mucous secretions filling the sinus cavities and occluding the openings. [Reprinted with permission from Hinkle, J. L., and Cheever, K. H. (2018). *Brunner & Suddarth's textbook of medical-surgical nursing* (14th ed., Fig. 22-1, p. 554). Philadelphia, PA: Wolters Kluwer.]

## Clinical Manifestations

### Nasal Congestion

Nasal congestion occurs when the nasal passages become blocked as membranes lining the nose become swollen due to inflamed blood vessels. The blood vessels in the nasal mucosa become dilated, and the mucous membranes become engorged with blood. Stimulation of the nasal membranes occurs at the same time, resulting in increased mucus secretion.

## Cough

**Cough** (a forceful expulsion of air from the lungs) is a protective reflex response to mechanical, chemical, or inflammatory irritation of the lungs mediated through neurons in the brainstem or cough center. The cough reflex involves central and peripheral mechanisms. Centrally, the cough center in the medulla oblongata receives stimuli and initiates the reflex response (deep inspiration, closed glottis, buildup of pressure within the lungs, and forceful exhalation). Peripherally, air, dryness of mucous membranes, or excessive secretions may stimulate cough receptors in the pharynx, larynx, trachea, or lungs. A cough helps remove foreign bodies, environmental irritants, or accumulated secretions from the respiratory tract. A cough is productive when secretions are expectorated; it is nonproductive when it is dry and no sputum is expectorated.

Cough is a prominent symptom of respiratory tract infections (e.g., the common cold, influenza, bronchitis, pharyngitis) as well as chronic obstructive pulmonary diseases (e.g., emphysema, chronic bronchitis). When cough is associated with the common cold, it usually stems from postnasal drainage and throat irritation.

### Bronchial Secretions

Bronchial secretions can result from numerous conditions, such as the common cold, where phlegm is produced in the chest. In addition, bronchial secretions can be a symptom of pneumonia, upper respiratory infections, acute and chronic bronchitis, emphysema, and asthma. Postnasal mucus may accumulate in the chest. Alternatively, secretions may be due to nonrespiratory conditions, such as immobility, debilitation, cigarette smoking, or surgery. Surgical procedures involving the chest or abdomen are most likely to be associated with retention of secretions because pain may decrease the patient's ability to cough, breathe deeply, and ambulate.

Excessive secretions may seriously impair respiration by obstructing airways and preventing airflow to and from alveoli, where gas exchange occurs. Secretions also may cause atelectasis (a condition in which part of the lung is airless and collapses) by blocking airflow, and they may cause or aggravate infections by supporting bacterial growth.

## Nonpharmacologic Measures

Given the anticipated progression and resolution of a virus, nonpharmacologic measures for symptom relief of a cold can be beneficial. Adequate fluid intake, humidification of the

environment, and sucking on hard candy or throat lozenges can help relieve mouth dryness and cough. Additional measures are described in the nursing process concept map.

> **! QSEN Alert: Evidence-Based Practice**
>
> A 2018 Cochrane systematic review of a sample of six studies in children with cough symptoms showed an initial benefit of administering honey on reducing cough frequency, cough severity, and impact of cough on sleep for both children over 1 year of age and for parents than no treatment and possibly to a greater extent than diphenhydramine. A dosage of 2.5 to 5 mL of liquid honey given before bedtime is suggested. The findings also suggest that the effects of honey may be comparable to dextromethorphan when given for 1 day. When honey is given up to 3 days, there was no advantage over salbutamol or placebo in decreasing cough severity and honey for a cough and probably had no advantage over salbutamol or placebo in the reduction of cough aggravation or severity. Overall, there was no strong evidence for or against using honey for the treatment of cough symptoms.

## Drug Therapy

Numerous drugs are available to treat nasal congestion and cough of respiratory disorders. Many are nonprescription drugs that can be obtained alone or in combination with products purchased as over-the-counter (OTC) medications. Available drugs include nasal decongestants, antitussives, expectorants, and mucolytics (Table 31.1). In addition, analgesic agents, such as acetaminophen or ibuprofen (for patients > 6 months of age), may provide symptomatic relief. For information on indications and considerations of administering drugs to reduce fever or pain, see Chapter 16.

## NASAL DECONGESTANTS

Indications for nasal decongestants are the relief of nasal obstruction and discharge. Adrenergic (sympathomimetic) drugs are most often used for this purpose (see Chap. 29). These agents relieve nasal congestion and swelling by constricting arterioles and reducing blood flow to the nasal mucosa. Oral and topical decongestants are available.  **Pseudoephedrine** (Sudafed) is the prototype. In the United States, the OTC sale of cold medicines containing pseudoephedrine is restricted due to the risk of their use in the illicit manufacturing of amphetamine drugs.

**TABLE 31.1**

### Drugs Administered for the Treatment of Nasal Congestion and Cough

| Drug Class | Prototype | Other Drugs in the Class |
|---|---|---|
| Nasal decongestants | Pseudoephedrine (Sudafed) | Oxymetazoline (Afrin) Phenylephrine (Vazculep) |
| Antitussives | Dextromethorphan (Delsym) | Benzonatate (Tessalon Perles) codeine Hydrocodone bitartrate (Hysingla, Zohydro ER) |
| Expectorants | Guaifenesin (glyceryl guaiacolate) (Mucinex, others) | |
| Mucolytics | Acetylcysteine (Acetadote, Cetylev) | |

### TABLE 31.2

### DRUGS AT A GLANCE: Nasal Decongestants

| Drug | Pregnancy Category | Routes and Dosage Ranges | |
| --- | --- | --- | --- |
| | | **Adults** | **Children** |
| (P) **Pseudoephedrine** (Sudafed) | C | Regular immediate-release tablets, PO 60 mg every 4–6 h<br>Extended-release tablets, PO 120 mg every 12 h or 240 mg every 24 h. Maximum, 240 mg in 24 h | *12 y and older*: same as adults for regular and extended-release tablets<br>*6–12 y*: PO 30 mg every 4–6 h. Maximum, 120 mg/24 h<br>*4 to <6 y*: PO 15 mg every 4–6 h. Maximum, 60 mg/24 h<br>*2–4 y*: PO 1 mg/kg/dose every 6 h. Maximum, 15 mg/dose<br>*Under 2 y*: Not recommended |
| Oxymetazoline (Afrin) 0.05% spray | C | Topically, 2–3 sprays in each nostril, every 10–12 h. Maximum, 2 doses/24 h | *6 y and older*: 2–3 sprays in each nostril, every 10–12 h not to exceed 3 days<br>*Under 6 y*: intranasal not recommended |
| Phenylephrine (Vazculep; ❋ Neo-Synephrine) | C | PO 10 mg every 4 h not to exceed 7 continuous days. Maximum, 60 mg/24 h<br>Intranasal, 2–3 sprays or drops of 0.25%, 0.5%, or 1% solution in each nostril no more often than every 4 h. Maximum, 6 doses/24 h. Not to exceed 3 continuous days | *12 y and older*: same as adults<br>*6 to <12 y*: PO 10 mg every 4 h. Maximum, 60 mg/24 h<br>Topically, 1–3 sprays or drops of 0.25% solution in each nostril no more often than every 4 h. Maximum, 6 doses/24 h. Not to exceed 3 continuous days<br>*2 to <6 y*: intranasal, 1 drop of 0.125% solution every 2–4 h. Maximum, 6 doses/24 h. Not to exceed 3 continuous days |

## Pharmacokinetics

The onset of action of oral pseudoephedrine is approximately 30 minutes and typically peaks in 1 to 2 hours. The drug has a half-life of 4 to 8 hours. Metabolism to an active metabolite occurs in the liver. Excretion is via the kidneys, and the extent of excretion is dependent on urine pH and flow rate.

## Action

Pseudoephedrine acts directly on adrenergic receptors and acts indirectly by releasing norepinephrine from its storage sites. The drug produces vasoconstriction, which shrinks nasal mucosa membranes, resulting in decreased nasal congestion. It may potentiate the drainage of sinus secretions. In addition, pseudoephedrine may increase irritability of the heart muscle, especially at high doses.

## Use

Uses of pseudoephedrine include the temporary relief of symptoms associated with nasal congestion due to the common cold, allergies, and sinuses. Health care providers may also use it to reduce local blood flow before nasal surgery and to aid in visualization of the nasal mucosa during diagnostic examinations.

Table 31.2 presents dosage information about various decongestants. It is not necessary to adjust dosages for pseudoephedrine in patients with hepatic impairment. Specific guidelines for adjustment in dosage in the presence of hepatic impairment are not available.

### Use in Children

Overall, pseudoephedrine appears to be effective in children older than 4 years of age, but research studies about the drug's safety and effectiveness in younger children are limited. The Food and Drug Administration (FDA) does not recommend OTC use of the drug in this age group due to the risk of serious and life-threatening adverse effects, including seizures, decreased level of consciousness, tachycardia, and death. The FDA also reports the drug's use with caution in children 2 years of age and older. One issue is that the low doses found in children's preparations may be insufficient to produce therapeutic effects. In addition, the risk of adverse effects and overdosing, particularly with liquid preparation, pose significant threats to safety. Extended-release tablets should not be administered to children younger than 12 years of age, and children should not be given drugs that are packaged for adults.

In children 4 years of age and older, pseudoephedrine and other OTC cough and cold products can be harmful if more than the recommended dose is used, they are given too often, or they contain more than one drug that is also inadvertently administered in a separate preparation.

 **QSEN Alert: Evidence-Based Practice**

Yin (2015) is exploring the efficacy of a comprehensive consumer-centered pediatric labeling and dosing strategy aimed at determining best practices in improving parental understanding and use of pediatric cough and cold medications. The research, which will conclude in 2018, is part of an ongoing 3-year funded project by the FDA's Safe Use Initiative. Each year, there are more than 20,000 US poison control center calls and 7000 pediatric emergency department visits related to therapeutic mistakes involving cough and cold medications. Parental confusion about the best use of these medications in young children is a contributing factor. Because the majority of cough and cold medications are OTC preparations, parents frequently do not seek guidance from health care providers prior to giving these drugs. Product container designs, carton labeling, and packaging are key factors in medication errors and occurrence of adverse events with cough and cold medications.

### Use in Older Adults

The increased risk of adverse effects from oral nasal decongestants (e.g., hypertension, cardiac dysrhythmias, nervousness, insomnia) is a major concern in older adults. Adverse effects from topical agents are less likely, but rebound nasal congestion and systemic effects may occur with overuse. Older patients with significant cardiovascular disease should avoid pseudoephedrine.

### Use in Patients With Renal Impairment

Because pseudoephedrine is excreted primarily via the kidneys, caution in patients with renal impairment is important. It may be necessary to reduce the dosage to avoid potential drug accumulation and drug toxicity.

### Use in Patients With Critical Illness

It is appropriate to use pseudoephedrine in patients with critical illness for relief of symptoms. However, caution is warranted with concomitant medications and comorbid disease, such as cardiovascular disorders, glaucoma, and diabetes. In addition, pseudoephedrine may produce central nervous system stimulation, so caution is also necessary in patients with seizure disorders.

### Use in Patients Receiving Home Care

People often take pseudoephedrine in the home. Household members may ask the home care nurse for advice about OTC remedies they are taking for conditions such as allergies, colds, coughs, and sinus headaches. Before recommending a particular product, the nurse needs to assess the intended recipient for conditions or other medications that contraindicate the product's use. For example, the nasal decongestant component may cause or aggravate a cardiovascular disorder (e.g., hypertension). The home care nurse also needs to evaluate other medications the patient is taking in terms of potential drug interactions with the cold remedy. In addition, the nurse must emphasize the need to read the label of any OTC medication for ingredients, precautions, contraindications, drug interactions, and administration instructions.

 **QSEN Alert: Safety**

The FDA encourages drug manufacturers to provide dosing instruments, such as syringes or cups, marked with the correct measurements for administration of liquid medications to children. These alternatives to household spoons for medication measurement contribute to accurate dosing in children.

## Adverse Effects

Some notable significant adverse reactions of pseudoephedrine include hypotension, dysrhythmia, impaired coordination, dizziness, excitability, headache, insomnia, restlessness, seizures, vertigo, dysuria, urinary retention, urinary difficulty, and thrombocytopenia. Some people may also experience blurred vision, tinnitus, chest tightness, dry nose, nasal congestion, and wheezing.

## Contraindications

Contraindications to pseudoephedrine use include severe hypertension or coronary artery disease because of the drug's cardiac-stimulating and vasoconstricting effects. Another contraindication is narrow-angle glaucoma. Caution is necessary with cardiac dysrhythmias, hyperthyroidism, diabetes mellitus, glaucoma, and prostatic hypertrophy. Patients who take tricyclic or monoamine oxidase inhibitor antidepressants should not receive pseudoephedrine.

## Nursing Implications

### Preventing Interactions

Many medications interact with pseudoephedrine, increasing its effect (Box 31.1). Caffeine can enhance the adverse effects of pseudoephedrine. The herb coleus may increase the effectiveness of the drug. Tannin-containing herbs such as green or black tea or witch hazel may decrease the absorption and effectiveness of the drug.

 **QSEN Alert: Evidence-Based Practice**

The Public Health Advisory issued by the FDA has recommended that OTC cough and cold products not be used to treat infants and children younger than 2 years of age. However, in an analysis of two large cohort studies, O'Donnell et al. (2015) found that caregivers continued to administer the drugs to these young children. Although a decrease in administration occurred in children younger than 1 year of age (from 25% to 7%) after the advisory, nearly 20% of children between ages 1 and 2 continued to receive OTC cough and cold products. It is important that the nurse emphasize the potential risk versus proven benefit to parents with young children. In patients of any age, in fact, the best available evidence should govern appropriate decisions regarding use of any medication.

### Administering the Medication

Patients may take the oral form of pseudoephedrine with or without food. It is important not to crush extended-release preparations.

**BOX 31.1**  **Drug Interactions: Pseudoephedrine**

**Drugs That Increase the Effects of Pseudoephedrine**

- Cocaine, digoxin, general anesthetics, monoamine oxidase (MAO) inhibitors, other adrenergic drugs, thyroid preparations, and xanthines
  *Increase the risk of cardiac dysrhythmias*
- Antihistamines, epinephrine, ergot alkaloids, MAO inhibitors, and methylphenidate
  *Increase the risk of hypertension due to vasoconstriction*

## Assessing for Therapeutic Effects

The nurse assesses for decreased nasal inflammation and congestion after administration of pseudoephedrine. Laboratory monitoring is not necessary.

## Assessing for Adverse Effects

The nurse must monitor for cardiac symptoms, particularly in patients with a cardiac history. If anaphylaxis, chest tightness, or throat swelling occurs, it is necessary to discontinue pseudoephedrine immediately.

## Patient Teaching

Box 31.2 outlines patient teaching guidelines for nasal decongestants such as pseudoephedrine.

## Other Drugs in the Class

Topical preparations (i.e., nasal solutions or sprays) are often preferred for short-term use. They are rapidly effective because they come into direct contact with nasal mucosa. Oxymetazoline (Afrin) is a commonly used nasal spray that acts directly on alpha receptors to produce vasoconstriction of the arterioles in nasal passages. If used longer than the recommended 3 days or in excessive amounts, however, rebound nasal congestion may occur. Topical decongestants are less likely to produce systemic effects than oral or parenteral products, but systemic adverse effects may occur; the nurse should watch for them. For patients with cardiovascular disease, topical nasal decongestants are usually preferred. Oral agents are usually contraindicated because of cardiovascular effects (e.g., increased force of myocardial contraction, increased heart rate, increased blood pressure).

*[handwritten annotations: "Addiction to topical spray!" "rebound congestion" "Mmm Read!" "nasal spray"]*

---

**BOX 31.2** — *Patient Teaching Guidelines for Nasal Decongestants, Antitussive Medications, Expectorants, and Mucolytics*

### General Considerations

- These drugs may relieve symptoms but do not cure the disorder causing the symptoms.
- An adequate fluid intake, humidification of the environment, and sucking on hard candy or throat lozenges can help relieve mouth dryness and cough.
- Over-the-counter (OTC) cold remedies should not be used longer than 1 week. Do not use nose drops or sprays more often or longer than recommended. Excessive or prolonged use may damage nasal mucosa and produce chronic nasal congestion.
- Do not increase dosage if symptoms are not relieved by recommended amounts.
- See a health care provider if symptoms persist longer than 1 week.
- Inform health care providers about any herbal supplements that are being taken.
- Read the labels of OTC allergy, cold, and sinus remedies for information about ingredients; many products contain more than the active ingredient. Understand dosages, conditions, or other medications with which the drugs should not be taken and adverse effects.
- Do not combine two drug preparations containing the same or similar active ingredients. For example, pseudoephedrine is the nasal decongestant component of most prescription and OTC sinus and multi-ingredient cold remedies. The recommended dose for immediate-release preparations is usually 30 to 60 mg of pseudoephedrine; doses in extended-release preparations are usually 120 mg. Taking more than one preparation containing pseudoephedrine (or phenylephrine, a similar drug) may increase dosage to toxic levels and cause irregular heartbeats and extreme nervousness.
- Note that many combination products contain acetaminophen or ibuprofen as pain relievers. If you are taking another form of one of these drugs (e.g., Tylenol or Advil), there is a risk of overdosage and adverse effects. Acetaminophen can cause liver damage; ibuprofen is a relative of aspirin that can cause gastrointestinal upset

and bleeding. Thus, you need to be sure your total daily dosage is not excessive (with Tylenol, above four doses of 1000 mg each; with ibuprofen, above 2400 mg).
- People with diabetes mellitus should read OTC labels for sugar content because many decongestants and cough medicines may contain sucrose, glucose, or corn syrup as a base.

### Self-Administration

- Take medications as prescribed or as directed on the labels of OTC preparations. Taking excessive amounts or taking recommended amounts too often can lead to serious adverse effects.
- Do not chew or crush long-acting tablets or capsules (e.g., those taken once or twice daily). Such actions can cause rapid drug absorption, high blood levels, and serious adverse effects, rather than the slow absorption and prolonged action intended with these products.
- For OTC drugs available in different dosage strengths, start with lower recommended doses rather than "maximum strength" formulations or the highest recommended doses. It is safer to see how the drugs affect you and then increase doses if necessary.
- With topical nasal decongestants:
  - Use only preparations labeled for intranasal use. For example, phenylephrine (Vazculep) is available in both nasal and eye formulations. The two types of solutions cannot be used interchangeably. In addition, phenylephrine preparations may contain 0.125%, 0.25%, 0.5%, or 1% of drug. Be sure the concentration is appropriate for the person to receive it (e.g., an infant, young child, older adult).
  - Blow the nose gently before instilling nasal solutions or sprays. This clears nasal passages and increases effectiveness of medications.
  - To instill nose drops, lie down or sit with the neck hyperextended and instill medication without touching the dropper to the nostrils (to avoid contamination of the dropper and medication). Rinse the medication dropper after each use.

**BOX 31.2** **Patient Teaching Guidelines for Nasal Decongestants, Antitussive Medications, Expectorants, and Mucolytics** (Continued)

- For nasal sprays, sit or stand, squeeze the container once to instill medication, and rinse the spray tip after each use. Most nasal sprays are designed to deliver one dose when used correctly.
- Report palpitations, dizziness, drowsiness, or rapid pulse. These effects may occur with nasal decongestants and cold remedies and may indicate excessive dosage.
- Take dextromethorphan as directed; increased intake can lead to increased central nervous system impairment. Take cough syrups undiluted and avoid eating and drinking for approximately 30 minutes.
- Part of the beneficial effect of cough syrups stems from soothing effects on the pharyngeal mucosa. Food or fluid removes the medication from the throat.

- If the cough has not improved after 7 days or if symptoms include high fever, skin rash, or persistent headache with cough, seek help from a health care provider.
- If you are taking acetylcysteine, understand that increasing fluid intake as directed helps loosen and mobilize secretions. In addition:
- The nebulization may initially cause an unpleasant odor, which soon resolves.
- If the mask leaves a sticky residue on the face, remove it with water.
- Clean the nebulizer equipment after use to minimize infections and prevent buildup of the drug on the equipment.

## NCLEX Success

1. In caring for a patient with nasal congestion, the nurse knows that adrenergic drugs are used as nasal decongestants to relieve symptoms by
   A. constricting arterioles and reducing blood flow to nasal mucosa
   B. stimulating air movement in the lungs
   C. stabilizing mast cells
   D. initiating the cough reflex

2. As the nurse caring for a patient with nasal congestion who is using the OTC decongestant oxymetazoline, the nurse counsels the patient that this medication should be used only for the time recommended on the package and no longer because excessive use may produce
   A. copious lower respiratory tract secretions
   B. ringing in the ears
   C. rebound nasal congestion
   D. a suppressed cough reflex

3. The FDA pediatric safety labeling changes, warning against the use of prescription opioid cough and cold medicines in children younger than 18 years, are based on available data and expert opinion that supports which of the following statements? (Select all that apply.)
   A. A cough should not be suppressed unless it is causing clinical consequences, such as consecutive nights of poor sleep and/or vomiting, rib fractures, or hypoxia.
   B. The safety labeling changes should protect children from unnecessary exposure to opioids.
   C. The risks for prescription opioid cough products typically outweigh the potential benefits in children of all ages.
   D. Addiction or abuse potential is a concern regarding the use of hydrocodone or codeine in children.

## ANTITUSSIVES

The goal of antitussive therapy is to suppress nonpurposeful coughing, not productive coughing. Locally acting agents (e.g., throat lozenges, cough drops) may suppress cough by increasing the flow of saliva and by containing demulcents or local anesthetics to decrease irritation of the pharyngeal mucosa. Flavored syrups are often used as vehicles for other drugs.

The nonnarcotic drug **dextromethorphan** (Delsym) is the antitussive prototype. It is the antitussive drug of choice in most circumstances and the antitussive ingredient in almost all OTC cough remedies (often designated by "DM" on the product label). (Note that some antitussives are narcotics [e.g., codeine, hydrocodone].)

## Pharmacokinetics

Following oral administration of dextromethorphan, absorption is rapid. Dextromethorphan undergoes first-pass metabolism in the liver, which results in conversion to an active metabolite, dextrorphan, by the cytochrome P450 enzyme CYP2D6. The rate of metabolism varies; about 10% of the Caucasian population has little or no CYP2D6 enzyme activity, leading to prolonged high drug levels. The duration of action is about 3 to 8 hours, with a peak cough-suppressing effect in 15 to 30 minutes. The half-life of the drug is 1 to 4 hours. Food decreases the rate and extent of absorption. The majority of drug and its metabolites are excreted in urine.

## Action

Antitussives suppress cough by depressing the cough center in the medulla oblongata or the cough receptors in the throat, trachea, or lungs, effectively elevating the threshold for coughing. Centrally acting antitussives include nonnarcotics and narcotics.

## Use

The major clinical indication for use of dextromethorphan is a dry, hacking, nonproductive cough that interferes with rest and sleep. It is not desirable to suppress a productive cough because

**TABLE 31.3**

## DRUGS AT A GLANCE: Antitussives

| Drug | Pregnancy Category | Routes and Dosage Ranges | |
|---|---|---|---|
| | | **Adults** | **Children** |
| Nonnarcotic | | | |
| ℗ **Dextromethorphan** (Delsym) | C | Liquid, lozenges, and syrup, 10–20 mg every 4 h or 20–30 mg every 6–8 h. Maximum, 120 mg/24 h Sustained-action liquid (Delsym), PO 60 mg every 12 h. Maximum 120 mg/24 h | *12 y and older*: Same as adults *6–12 y*: 5–10 mg every 4 h or 15 mg every 6–8 h. Maximum, 60 mg/24 h *2–6 y*: 2.5–7.5 mg every 4–8 h. Maximum, 30 mg/24 h Sustained-action liquid, 6–12 y: 30 mg every 12 h. *2–5 y*: 15 mg every 12 h |
| Benzonatate (Tessalon Perles) | C | PO 100–200 mg three times a day. Maximum, 600 mg/24 h | *10 y and older*: PO 100–200 mg three times a day. Maximum, 600 mg/24 h |
| Narcotic | | | |
| Codeine (✳ Codeine Contin, Teva-Codeine) | C (D during labor) | PO 10–20 mg every 4–6 h. Maximum, 120 mg/24 h | Not recommended for use in children <18 y |
| Hydrocodone bitartrate (Hysingla, Zohydro ER, ✳ pdp-Hydrocodone) | C (D during labor) | PO 1 (5 mg) tablet every 4–6 h up to 30 mg daily | Not recommended for use in children <18 y |

the secretions need to be removed. There is no information relating to the use of dextromethorphan in the elderly (compared with patients of other ages). Table 31.3 gives dosage information for various antitussives.

Recently, guidelines for treating diabetic neuropathy pain identified that moderate evidence existed for the use of dextromethorphan for this condition because it blocks pain receptors in the spinal cord. Chapter 41 discusses this use.

### Use in Children

Studies have not demonstrated that antitussives, particularly dextromethorphan, are effective in children and adolescents. The American Academy of Pediatrics and several other groups advise against the use of antitussives in young people. Adverse effects of dextromethorphan in children include behavioral disturbances and respiratory depression.

### Use in Patients Receiving Home Care

People often take dextromethorphan and other antitussives in the home care setting, and the nurse needs to assess the effectiveness of their use. The home care nurse also must emphasize the need to read the label of any OTC medication for ingredients, precautions, contraindications, drug interactions, and administration instructions. For children, it is necessary to use measuring devices specifically designed for the administration of medications.

## Adverse Effects

*proper measurement*

At normal doses, dextromethorphan is known to cause nausea, drowsiness, rash, and difficulty breathing. Doses exceeding recommendations can produce hallucinations and disassociation; dextromethorphan-containing OTC preparations have been used as recreational drugs.

## Contraindications

Contraindications to dextromethorphan and other antitussives include known hypersensitivity to the drugs. Caution is necessary in children with atopic syndrome caused by histamine release.

## Nursing Implications

### Preventing Interactions

Many medications interact with dextromethorphan, increasing its effect (Box 31.3). St. John's wort and tryptophan also interact with the antitussive to increase the risk of serotonin syndrome. No drugs appear to decrease the effect of dextromethorphan.

### Administering the Medication

It is necessary to administer dextromethorphan-containing cough syrups undiluted. The nurse instructs the patient to avoid eating and drinking for approximately 30 minutes. Some caution is warranted with lozenges, which should be dissolved in the mouth to decrease the risk of choking.

**BOX 31.3**  *Drug Interactions: Dextromethorphan*

**Drugs That Increase the Effects of Dextromethorphan**
- Monoamine oxidase inhibitors, serotonin reuptake inhibitors, tricyclic antidepressants, 5-HT1 receptor agonists, ergot alkaloids, lithium, and phenylpiperidine opioids
  *Increase the risk of serotonin syndrome*
- Alcohol
  *Increases central nervous system depression*

### Assessing for Therapeutic Effects

The nurse observes for decreased coughing.

### Assessing for Adverse Effects

The nurse observes for excessive suppression of the cough reflex (inability to cough effectively when secretions are present) or hallucinations with dosages that exceed recommendations.

### Patient Teaching

Box 31.2 outlines patient teaching guidelines for antitussives such as dextromethorphan.

## Other Drugs in the Class

Benzonatate (Tessalon Perles), another nonnarcotic antitussive agent, is a peripherally acting drug, unlike dextromethorphan. This antitussive drug acts by anesthetizing stretch receptors in the respiratory passages, thereby decreasing coughing. The nurse advises the patient to swallow the benzonatate capsules whole. Sucking or chewing them may cause numbness of the throat or mouth. Serious adverse effects include a choking feeling, chest pain or numbness, dizziness, confusion, and hallucinations.

Codeine and hydrocodone, which are both opioid narcotics, have antitussive effects in relatively small doses. Both are centrally acting drugs, like dextromethorphan. In the body, codeine is converted to morphine, and the potential for respiratory depression and death may occur. Other adverse reactions to the narcotic antitussives include nausea, vomiting, constipation, dizziness, drowsiness, pruritus, and drug dependence. Caution is necessary in people, especially children, who have asthma or other chronic breathing problems and who may be more susceptible to respiratory depression. Caution is also necessary in head injuries and increased intracranial pressure, acute abdominal disorders, seizure disorders, renal or hepatic impairment, and prostatic hypertrophy. A 2014 systematic review determined that there was no good evidence for or against the effectiveness of OTC medications (including guaifenesin, mucolytics, and combination medications) for acute cough. Additional information about these narcotics is found in Chapter 49.

### Clinical Application 31.1

- Mr. Hobbs works in an area with many other people. What should the nurse emphasize to help prevent the further spread of infection throughout the plant?

## EXPECTORANTS

Expectorants are agents given orally to liquefy respiratory secretions and allow for their easier removal. The drugs act by moistening the respiratory tract to make the mucus less tenacious. **Guaifenesin** (Mucinex, others) is the prototype expectorant. It is available alone and as an ingredient in many combination cough and cold remedies.

## Pharmacokinetics

Guaifenesin is well absorbed following oral administration. The onset of action is 4 to 6 hours, and the duration of action is unknown. The half-life is about 1 hour. Metabolism and excretion of guaifenesin and its metabolites occur in the urine.

## Action

Guaifenesin reduces the viscosity of tenacious secretions by irritating the gastric vagal receptors stimulating respiratory tract fluid. Thus, it increases the volume and decreases the viscosity of respiratory tract secretions.

## Use

Used with productive coughs, guaifenesin loosens mucus from the respiratory tract. The drug does not appear to cause unusual adverse effects or problems in older adults. There is no information identifying risk with the use of guaifenesin in older patients compared with younger ones. Table 31.4 presents dosage information for the expectorants.

It is important to note that with excessive respiratory tract secretions, mechanical measures (e.g., coughing, deep breathing, ambulation, chest physiotherapy, forcing fluids) are more likely to be effective than expectorant drug therapy. Research studies do not support the drug's overall effectiveness, and many authorities do not recommend its use.

### Use in Children

Guaifenesin does not appear to cause unusual problems in children. However, caution is necessary when the drug is used in children younger than 4 years of age. The extended-release tablets should not be used in children younger than 12 years of age.

### Use in Patients Receiving Home Care

People use guaifenesin in the home to help liquefy mucus that is making breathing difficult. The home care nurse must emphasize the need to increase fluid intake as recommended to help facilitate mobilization of secretions. Also, the nurse must stress

| Drug | Pregnancy Category | Routes and Dosage Ranges | |
|---|---|---|---|
| | | **Adults** | **Children** |
| **Guaifenesin** (glyceryl guaiacolate) (Mucinex, others) | C | PO 200–400 mg every 4 h. Maximum, 2400 mg/24 h | *12 y and older*: same as adults<br>*6 to <12 y*: PO 100–200 mg every 4 h. Maximum, 1200 mg/24 h<br>*4 to <6 y*: PO 50–100 mg every 4 h. Maximum, 600 mg/24 h<br>*2–4 y*: Limited data. 50–100 mg every 4 h. Maximum, 600 mg/24 h |

**TABLE 31.4**

**DRUGS AT A GLANCE: Expectorants**

the importance of reading the label of any OTC medication for ingredients, precautions, contraindications, drug interactions, and administration instructions. When giving medications to children, it is necessary to use only measuring devices specifically designed for the administration of medications to young patients.

## Adverse Effects

Adverse effects of guaifenesin include skin rash, headache, nausea, and vomiting.

## Contraindications

Hypersensitivity to guaifenesin is the major contraindication.

## Nursing Implications

### Administering the Medication

It is necessary to swallow sustained-release capsules or tablets of guaifenesin whole; patients should not break, crush, or chew them. Drinking plenty of water while taking the drug may help loosen mucus in the lungs. People can take it without regard to meals.

### Assessing for Therapeutic Effects

The nurse assesses for improvement in cold symptoms, specifically reduction of cough episodes and increased ability to mobilize secretions.

### Assessing for Adverse Effects

The nurse assesses for hypersensitivity to the drug and for signs of headache, nausea, and vomiting.

### Patient Teaching

Box 31.2 presents patient teaching guidelines for the expectorant guaifenesin.

> **⚠ QSEN Alert: Safety**
>
> It is important to note that guaifenesin liquefies mucus and increases the amount of mucus to be removed. Thus, suction equipment should be available (in the home, if necessary), and the patient and significant others require training in proper use.

> **Clinical Application 31.2**
>
> • Mr. Hobbs has been sick for more than 7 days. He feels that he is getting worse. When the nurse asks him what medication he is taking, he reports that he is using the oxymetazoline (Afrin) that was recommended the last time he was congested. What does the nurse tell him?

## MUCOLYTICS

Mucolytics are drugs that are used to liquefy mucus in the respiratory tract by attacking the protein bonds of the mucus. However, no well-designed studies have demonstrated their clinical efficacy. Administration is by inhalation; solutions may be nebulized into a facemask or mouthpiece or instilled directly into the respiratory tract through a tracheostomy. **Acetylcysteine** (Acetadote, Cetylev), the prototype, and sodium chloride solution are the only agents recommended for use as mucolytics.

## Pharmacokinetics

Acetylcysteine is rapidly absorbed following inhalation or instillation. The onset of action is 1 minute, the maximum peak effect occurs within 5 to 10 minutes, and the duration of action is 2 to 3 hours. Metabolism occurs in the liver, with drug excretion in the urine.

## Action

Acetylcysteine exerts its mucolytic action through its sulfhydryl group, which disrupts the disulfide bonds in the mucoproteins. This reduces the viscosity of mucous secretions.

> **▣ Concept Mastery Alert**
>
> Expectorants work by increasing production of respiratory secretions, which in turn appears to decrease the viscosity of the mucus. Mucolytics work by breaking down thick and tenacious mucus in the lower portions of the lungs.

## Use

Acetylcysteine is used as an adjunctive agent to liquefy viscous mucous secretions. Also, the oral drug is widely used as an antidote in the treatment of acetaminophen overdosage (see Table 2.1 and Chap. 16). Patients should receive an aerosolized bronchodilator 10 to 15 minutes before receiving acetylcysteine.

Table 31.5 presents dosage information for the mucolytics. No studies of acetylcysteine focus specifically on the use of the drug in older adults.

### Use in Children

Acetylcysteine does not appear to cause different adverse effects in children than in adults, although it has no proven benefit in children. No specific information compares the drug's use in children with use in other age groups. It should be noted that the development of more effective drugs has limited the use of acetylcysteine in the management of children with cystic fibrosis.

### Use in Patients With Critical Illness

Although people who are critically ill may receive acetylcysteine by inhalation, they more commonly receive it by mouth as an antidote to acetaminophen poisoning. Parameters for use in critically ill patients are consistent for use in other people.

### Use in Patients Receiving Home Care

People take acetylcysteine in the home in the treatment of certain lung conditions; the drug helps remove increased amounts of mucus that make breathing difficult. The home care nurse must emphasize the need to follow administration instructions, clean equipment on a scheduled basis, and increase fluid intake as recommended to help mobilize secretions. Because acetylcysteine liquefies mucus and increases the amount to be removed, suction equipment should be

liquids

**TABLE 31.5**

## DRUGS AT A GLANCE: Mucolytics

| Drug | Pregnancy Category | Routes and Dosage Ranges | |
|---|---|---|---|
| | | **Adults** | **Children** |
| Ⓟ **Acetylcysteine** (Acetadote, Parvolex) | B | Nebulization, 3–5 mL of a 20% solution or 6–10 mL of a 10% solution every 2–6 h<br>Instillation, 1–2 mL of a 10% or 20% solution every 1–4 h<br>Acetaminophen overdosage, PO 140 mg/kg initially, then 70 mg/kg every 4 h for 17 doses; dilute a 10% or 20% solution to a 5% solution with cola, fruit juice, or water | |

available. It is essential that the patient and significant others are trained in proper use.

## Adverse Effects

Adverse reactions with inhalation therapy using acetylcysteine include drowsiness, nausea, and vomiting. In some patients, the drug has the potential to cause airway inflammation and bronchospasm and inhibit ciliary function, which has limited its use.

## Contraindications

Contraindications include hypersensitivity to acetylcysteine.

## Nursing Implications

### Administering the Medication

It is necessary to give intermittent aerosol treatments. Typically, these are on arising, before meals, and at bedtime.

### Assessing for Therapeutic Effects

The nurse assesses the ability to mobilize secretions and the demonstration of improved respiratory function.

### Assessing for Adverse Effects

The nurse assesses for difficulty breathing, inability to expel secretions, bronchospasm, and chest tightness. Also, he or she observes for the additional adverse effects of nausea and vomiting.

### Patient Teaching

Box 31.2 outlines patient teaching guidelines for the mucolytic acetylcysteine.

## HERBAL REMEDIES AND OTHER PREPARATIONS

Herbal remedies and other preparations have been used as cold remedies. However, only herbal preparation and oral zinc preparations have demonstrated ability to reduce the duration and severity of cold symptoms in adults is (Box 31.4).

## COMBINATION PRODUCTS

Many combination products are available for treating symptoms of the common cold (Table 31.6). Many of the products contain an antihistamine, a nasal decongestant, and an

**BOX 31.4** *Herbal Remedies and Other Preparations Used as Cold Remedies*

**Echinacea** preparations differ in chemical composition depending on which of the nine species or parts of the plant (e.g., leaves, roots, whole plant) are used as well as the season of harvesting. Also, which constituents of the plants are pharmacologically active is unclear. Several well-designed randomized trials and a meta-analysis in adults have concluded that echinacea products are no better than placebo in effectively treating the common cold. In children, a randomized trial has found that the incidence of the development of a rash increased without demonstrated clinical efficacy.

**Vitamin C** is used to reduce the incidence and severity of colds and influenza. There is no clear consensus that vitamin C shortens the duration of colds and alleviates its symptoms in adults, although clinical trials with adults have been partially positive. For those adults regularly taking vitamin C, it appears that vitamin C plays a role in the defense

mechanisms of the respiratory system. A recent meta-analysis did not demonstrate the therapeutic benefit of vitamin C in reducing cold duration or severity of symptoms in children.

**Zinc sulfate** lozenges and syrup are marketed as cold remedies. Systematic reviews have demonstrated the efficacy of oral zinc preparations in reducing the duration and severity of cold symptoms in adults. A reduction of symptoms after 7 days was found in adults who started the oral zinc preparation within the first 24 hours of symptoms as compared to those who took a placebo. However, the efficacy of zinc in reducing the duration or severity of cold symptoms in children has not been established. More recently, nasal zinc gluconate preparations (Cold-Eeze, Zicam) have been developed, but the U.S. Food and Drug Administration has issued a public health advisory as multiple reports of long-standing or permanent loss of smell with nasal zinc outweighs any benefit.

## TABLE 31.6

## Representative Multi-ingredient Nonprescription Cold, Cough, and Sinus Remedies

| Trade Name | Ingredients | | | | |
| --- | --- | --- | --- | --- | --- |
| | **Antihistamine** | **Nasal Decongestant** | **Analgesic** | **Antitussive** | **Expectorant** |
| Advil Allergy & Congestion Relief | Chlorpheniramine 4 mg | Phenylephrine 10 mg | Ibuprofen 200 mg/tablet | | |
| Advil Cold and Sinus Tablets | | Pseudoephedrine 30 mg/tablet | Ibuprofen 200 mg/tablet | | |
| Comtrex Cold & Sinus Tablets | | Phenylephrine 5 mg/tablet | Acetaminophen 325 mg/tablet | Dextromethorphan 10 mg/tablet | |
| Contac Day and Night Cold & Flu Caplets | (Night only) Chlorpheniramine 2 mg/tablet | (Day and night) Phenylephrine 5 mg/tablet | (Day and night) Acetaminophen 500 mg/tablet | | |
| Coricidin D Cold & Flu | Chlorpheniramine 2 mg/tablet | Pseudoephedrine 30 mg/tablet | Acetaminophen 325 mg/tablet | | |
| Coricidin HBP Cold & Flu | Chlorpheniramine 2 mg/tablet | | Acetaminophen 325 mg/tablet | | |
| Motrin Sinus Headache Tablets | | Pseudoephedrine 30 mg/tablet | Ibuprofen 200 mg/tablet | | |
| Robitussin Severe Multi-Symptom Cough Cold & Flu | | Phenylephrine 10 mg/20 mL | Acetaminophen 650 mg/20 mL | Dextromethorphan 20 mg/20 mL | Guaifenesin 400 mg/20 mL |
| Sinutab Sinus Allergy Maximum Strength Caplets | Chlorpheniramine 2 mg/tablet | Pseudoephedrine 30 mg/tablet | Acetaminophen 500 mg/tablet | | |
| Theraflu Flu, Nighttime Severe Cold & Cough Hot Liquid Powder | Diphenhydramine 25 mg/packet | Phenylephrine 10 mg/packet | Acetaminophen 650 mg/packet | | |
| Vicks NyQuil Severe Cough, Cold & Flu LiquiCaps | Doxylamine 6.25 mg/caplet | | Acetaminophen 325 mg/caplet | Dextromethorphan 10 mg/caplet | |

analgesic. Some contain antitussives, expectorants, and other agents as well. Many cold remedies are OTC formulations. Commonly used ingredients include chlorpheniramine (antihistamine), pseudoephedrine (adrenergic nasal decongestant), acetaminophen (analgesic and antipyretic), dextromethorphan (antitussive), and guaifenesin (expectorant). Antihistamines are clearly useful in allergic conditions (e.g., allergic rhinitis; see Chap. 32), but their use to relieve cold symptoms is controversial. First-generation antihistamines (e.g., chlorpheniramine, diphenhydramine) have anticholinergic effects that may reduce sneezing, rhinorrhea, and cough. Also, their sedative effects may aid sleep. Many multi-ingredient cold remedies contain an antihistamine.

The use of OTC products containing pseudoephedrine to manufacture methamphetamine has increased at an alarming rate. Because of this trend, phenylephrine has largely replaced pseudoephedrine in many product formulations in the United States. The Combat Methamphetamine Epidemic Act of 2005 (see Table 1.1) applies to all cough and

cold products, including combination products that contain pseudoephedrine.

 **QSEN Alert: Safety**

By law, all phenylephrine-containing products, including liquids, gel caps, and pediatric formulas, are stored behind pharmacy counters to restrict purchase limits, control storage, and control sales.

Many products come in several formulations, with different ingredients, and are advertised for different purposes (e.g., allergy, sinus disorders, multisymptom cold, flu remedies). For example, allergy remedies contain an antihistamine; "nondrowsy" or "daytime" formulas contain a nasal decongestant but not an antihistamine; "PM" or "night" formulas contain a sedating antihistamine to promote sleep; pain, fever, and multisymptom formulas usually contain acetaminophen; and "maximum strength" preparations usually refer only to the amount of acetaminophen per dose, usually 1000 mg for adults. In addition, labels on OTC combination products list ingredients by generic name, without identifying the type of drug. This information can be confusing. As a result, consumers, including nurses and other health care providers, may not know what medications they are taking or whether some drugs increase or block the effects of other drugs. The FDA recommends that if parents and caregivers use cough and cold products in children older than 4 years of age, it is necessary to read labels carefully, use caution when administering multiple products, and use only measuring devices specifically designed for use with medications.

It is true that single-drug formulations allow flexibility and individualization of dosage, whereas combination products may contain unneeded ingredients and are more expensive. However, many people find combination products more convenient to use.

## Clinical Application 31.3

• Mr. Hobbs also complains of a productive cough. He has been taking chlorpheniramine to treat it. What advice should the nurse give to him with regard to the appropriate treatment of a productive cough?

## NCLEX Success

4. A common mucolytic used to liquefy mucus in the respiratory tract is
   A. acetylcysteine
   B. ipratropium
   C. dextromethorphan
   D. pseudoephedrine

5. Cold remedies listed as "nondrowsy" or labeled as "daytime" formulas do not contain
   A. a nasal decongestant
   B. a first-generation antihistamine
   C. a pain reliever
   D. any of the above

6. Which of the following herbal preparations appears to play a role in the defense mechanisms of the respiratory system in adults?
   A. echinacea
   B. vitamin C
   C. zinc gluconate
   D. valerian

A concept map outlines the nursing process related to drug therapy considerations in this chapter. Additional nursing implications related to the disease process should also be considered in care decisions.

**Assessment**
- Assess the patient's condition in relation to the presence of clinical signs and symptoms for which the drugs are used.
- Assess for the use of treatment measures, including over-the-counter medications, to relieve symptoms and duration of complaints.
- Assess for risk factors (smoking, crowds, contact with people with cold symptoms) that contributed to development of a cold.
- Review history of receiving influenza immunizations.
- Assess for conditions that increase risks of adverse effects or are contraindications to drug therapy.

**Outcomes of Therapy**
The patient will
- Experience relief of symptoms.
- Take drugs accurately and safely.
- Avoid overuse of decongestants.
- Avoid preventable adverse drug effects.
- Act to avoid recurrence of symptoms.

**Nursing Interventions**
- Encourage patients to use measures to prevent or minimize the incidence and severity of symptoms. Recommend to patients that they:
  - Avoid smoking cigarettes or breathing secondhand smoke, when possible. Cigarette smoke irritates respiratory tract mucosa, and this irritation causes cough, increased secretions, and decreased effectiveness of cilia in cleaning the respiratory tract.
  - Avoid or limit exposure to crowds, especially during winter when the incidence of colds and influenza is high.
  - Avoid contact with people who have colds or other respiratory infections. This is especially important for patients with chronic lung disease, because upper respiratory infections may precipitate acute attacks of asthma or bronchitis.
  - Maintain a fluid intake of 2000 to 3000 mL daily unless contraindicated by cardiovascular or renal disease.
  - Maintain nutrition, rest, activity, and other general health measures.
  - Practice good hand hygiene techniques.
  - Consider having an annual vaccination for influenza if they are young, elderly, work in high-risk areas, or have chronic respiratory, cardiovascular, or renal disorders.
- Provide appropriate teaching related to drug therapy (see Box 31.2).

**Evaluation**
- Interview and observe for relief of symptoms.
- Interview and observe for tachycardia, hypertension, drowsiness, and other adverse drug effects.
- Interview and observe for compliance with instructions about drug use and understanding about need for preventive measures.

## KEY CONCEPTS

- Frequent and thorough hand hygiene (by both infected and uninfected people) is the most important protective and preventive measure to prevent the spread of cold viruses.
- Inappropriate and widespread use of antibiotics for viral infections, such as the common cold, poses significant risk of complications and drug resistance.
- Retention of secretions commonly occurs with influenza, pneumonia, upper respiratory infections, acute and chronic bronchitis, emphysema, and acute attacks of asthma.
- Nonrespiratory conditions that predispose to secretion retention include immobility, debilitation, cigarette smoking, and postoperative status.

- An adequate fluid intake, humidification of the environment, and sucking on hard candy or throat lozenges can help relieve mouth dryness and cough.
- The goal of antitussive therapy is to suppress nonpurposeful coughing, not productive coughing.
- Rebound nasal swelling can occur with excessive or extended use of nasal sprays.
- First-generation antihistamines (e.g., chlorpheniramine, diphenhydramine) have anticholinergic effects that may reduce sneezing, rhinorrhea, and cough.

- There is limited or no support for the use of dietary or herbal supplements, such as echinacea, vitamin C, and zinc, to treat symptoms of the common cold.
- Several OTC cough and cold medicines for use in infants have been recalled voluntarily due to concerns about possible misuse that could result in overdoses.
- Parents and caregivers should be educated on the importance of safe storage of OTC cough and cold medicines to prevent unintentional ingestion by children.
- For children, it is necessary to use measuring devices specifically designed for the accurate administration of medications.

## CLINICAL REASONING CASE STUDY

**Meet the Patient**

Troy Farnsworth, a 76-year-old man with a history of coronary artery disease and hypertension, presents to the outpatient clinic where you work as a nurse. He is currently taking lisinopril 25 mg PO daily and hydrochlorothiazide 25 mg PO daily. His blood pressure is 140/86 mm Hg. He does not smoke. Mr. Farnsworth is complaining of symptoms of a cold that began 3 days ago and tells the nurse that he thinks he caught the virus from one of his grandchildren, who had been visiting the week before. To fight his cold, his wife has been giving him pseudoephedrine in the form of Sudafed, echinacea, and zinc in the form of Zicam. What should you tell him about measures for symptom relief, including the use of OTC nasal decongestants and cold remedies?

**Assessing Drug Information**

- Pseudoephedrine (Sudafed)
  - This nasal decongestant may increase irritability of the heart muscle, especially at high doses, because of the drug's stimulating and vasoconstricting effects on the heart.
  - People with hypertension, cardiac dysrhythmias, nervousness, and insomnia may have an increased risk of adverse effects from oral nasal decongestants.
  - Adverse effects from topical agents are less likely, but rebound nasal congestion and systemic effects may occur with overuse.
- Nasal zinc preparations (Cold-Eeze, Zicam)
  - The FDA has issued a public health advisory because of multiple reports of long-standing or permanent loss of smell with nasal zinc products.
  - A reduction of symptoms after 7 days was found in adults who started the oral zinc preparation within the first 24 hours of symptoms as compared to those who did not take them.
- Echinacea
  - Research in adults has concluded that echinacea products are no better than taking nothing in effectively treating the common cold.

**Nursing Actions**

- Instruct Mr. Farnsworth that people with high blood pressure have an increased risk of adverse effects from oral nasal decongestants and should not take them.
- Stress the importance of reading the labels on any OTC medications for ingredients, precautions, contraindications, drug interactions, and instructions for use before purchasing them.
- Instruct him to stop taking echinacea and the nasal zinc preparations.
- Instruct him to consider nonpharmacologic measures to relieve symptoms. He should:
  - Maintain a fluid intake of 2000 to 3000 mL daily and observe for the effect of the fluid intake on his blood pressure.
  - Maintain nutrition, rest, activity, and other general health measures.
  - Consider having an annual vaccination for influenza.
  - Avoid locations where he would be in contact with passive cigarette smoke.
- Underscore that he is contagious and should avoid unnecessary contact with others, particularly children and those with chronic health conditions.
- Emphasize that frequent and thorough hand hygiene by both he and his wife is the most important protective and preventive measure for a cold.
- Instruct Mr. Farnsworth to contact his health care provider if symptoms worsen or do not resolve within a week of developing cold symptoms, or if regular home blood pressure checks are higher than the values identified by his provider.

Visit thePoint* at **http://thePoint.lww.com/Frandsen12e** for answers to NCLEX Success questions (in Appendix A), answers to Clinical Application Case Studies (in Appendix B), and more!

## REFERENCES AND RESOURCES

FDA. Retrieved from http://www.fda.gov/ForConsumers/Consumer Updates/ucm048682.htm

Goodman, D. M. (2015). Cough and cold products—still in use despite the FDA advisory. *Journal of Pediatrics, 167*(1), 1–3.

Green, J. L., Wand, G. S., Reynolds, K. M., Banner, W., Bond, G. R., Kauffman, E., et al. (2017). Safety profile of cough and cold medication use in pediatrics. *Pediatrics, 139*(6), e20163070. doi: 10.1542/peds.2016-3070.

Guyton, A. C., & Hall, J. E. (2015). *Textbook of medical physiology* (13th ed.). Philadelphia, PA: Elsevier.

Hinkle, J. L., & Cheever, K. H. (2017). *Brunner & Suddarth's textbook of medical-surgical nursing* (14th ed.). Philadelphia, PA: Wolters Kluwer Health/Lippincott Williams & Wilkins.

Karch, A. M. (2019). *Lippincott's pocket drug guide for nurses.* Philadelphia, PA: Lippincott Williams & Wilkins.

MacGeorge, C., McElligott, J., Carter, E., Hinton, E., Basco, W., & Roberts, J. R. (2015). Parental perceptions of safety, efficacy and level of confusion regarding over the counter cough and cold medications. *Journal of Investigative Medicine, 63*(2), 421.

Norris, T. L. (2019). *Porth's pathophysiology: Concepts of altered health states* (10th ed.). Philadelphia, PA: Lippincott Williams & Wilkins.

Nursing 2019. (2019). *Drug handbook.* Philadelphia, PA: Wolters Kluwer Health/Lippincott Williams & Wilkins.

O'Donnell, K., Jonathan M., Mansbach, J. M., LoVecchio, F., Cheng, J., Piedra, P. A., et al. (2015). Use of cough and cold medications in severe bronchiolitis before and after a health advisory warning against their use. *Journal of Pediatrics, 167*(1), 196–198, e2.

Oduwole, O., Udoh, E. E., Oyo-Ita, A., & Meremikwu, M. M. (2018). Honey for acute cough in children. *Cochrane Database of Systematic Reviews*, (4), CD007094. doi: 10.1002/14651858.CD007094.pub5.

Patel, Z. M., & Hwang, P. H. (2019). *Uncomplicated acute sinusitis and rhinosinusitis in adults: Treatment. UpToDate.* LexiComp, Inc.

Sexton, D. J., & McClain, M. T. (2019). *The common cold in adults: Treatment and prevention. UpToDate.* LexiComp, Inc.

UpToDate. (2019). *Drug information.* Lexi-Comp, Inc.

Yin, S. (2015). Identifying best practices for the safe use of pediatric cough and cold medications. Retrieved from http://www.fda.gov/Drugs/DrugSafety/SafeUseInitiative/ucm516941.htm

# Drug Therapy to Decrease Histamine Effects and Allergic Response

## LEARNING OBJECTIVES

*After studying this chapter, you should be able to:*

1. Delineate the effects of histamines on selected body tissues.
2. Describe the types of hypersensitivity or allergic reactions.
3. Identify the effects of histamine that are blocked by histamine$_1$ (H$_1$) receptor antagonist drugs.
4. Discuss first-generation H$_1$ receptor antagonists in terms of prototype, indications and contraindications, major adverse effects, interactions, and administration.
5. Describe second-generation H$_1$ receptor antagonists in terms of prototype, indications and contraindications, major adverse effects, interactions, and administration.
6. Implement the nursing process in the care of patients receiving antihistamines.

## CLINICAL APPLICATION CASE STUDY

Gene Rudolph is a 72-year-old retired mail carrier. His medical history includes hypertension, benign prostatic hypertrophy, and coronary artery disease. He is visiting a medical clinic for a routine blood pressure check. He tells the nurse that he has been having symptoms of nasal congestion, sneezing, and watering of the eyes for the past several weeks and that the symptoms started after he began working in his garden.

## KEY TERMS

**Anaphylactic reactions:** severe, whole-body reaction after sensitization to an allergen causing a severe allergic response

**Anaphylactoid reactions:** anaphylaxis-like reaction to a substance without development of IgE antibody that may occur on first exposure to the causative agent

**Antihistamine:** drugs that antagonize the action of histamine, commonly the H$_1$ receptor antagonists

**Histamine:** first chemical mediator released in immune and inflammatory responses found mainly in mast cells surrounding blood vessels

**Hypersensitivity:** allergic reactions that are exaggerated responses by the immune system produce tissue injury and may cause serious disease

**Serum sickness:** type III hypersensitive response is an IgG- or IgM-mediated reaction characterized by formation of antigen–antibody complexes that induce an acute inflammatory reaction in the tissues

# INTRODUCTION

The drugs that antagonize the action of histamine are commonly called **antihistamines**. There are three main types of receptors for histamine, histamine$_1$ (H$_1$), histamine$_2$ (H$_2$), and histamine$_3$ (H$_3$) receptors. This chapter focuses on those drugs that specifically prevent or reduce most of the physiologic effects that histamine normally induces at H$_1$ receptor sites. (Prescribers use some H$_2$ receptor antagonists, such as cimetidine, to treat peptic ulcers.) To understand the use of antihistamines, it is necessary to understand histamine and its effects on body tissues, the characteristics of allergic reactions, and the selected conditions for which antihistamines are used.

## OVERVIEW OF HISTAMINE RELEASE AND THE ALLERGIC RESPONSE

### Etiology and Pathophysiology

#### Histamine and Its Receptors

**Histamine** is the first chemical mediator to be released in immune and inflammatory responses. It is synthesized and stored in most body tissues, with high concentrations in tissues exposed to environmental substances (e.g., the skin and mucosal surfaces of the eye, nose, lungs, and gastrointestinal [GI] tract). It is also found in the central nervous system (CNS). In these tissues, histamine is located mainly in secretory granules of mast cells (tissue cells surrounding capillaries) and basophils (circulating blood cells).

Histamine is discharged from mast cells and basophils in response to certain stimuli (e.g., allergic reactions, cellular injury, extreme cold). After it is released, it diffuses rapidly into other tissues, where it interacts with H$_1$ and H$_2$ receptors on target organs. H$_1$ receptors are located mainly on smooth muscle cells in blood vessels and the respiratory and GI tracts (Fig. 32.1). When histamine binds with these receptors and stimulates them, effects include the following:

- Contraction of smooth muscle in the bronchi and bronchioles (producing bronchoconstriction and respiratory distress).
- Stimulation of vagus nerve endings to produce reflex bronchoconstriction and cough.
- Increased permeability of veins and capillaries, which allows fluid to flow into subcutaneous tissues and form edema.
- Increased secretion of mucous glands. Mucosal edema and increased nasal mucus produce the nasal congestion characteristic of allergic rhinitis and the common cold.
- Stimulation of sensory peripheral nerve endings to cause pain and pruritus. Pruritus is especially prominent with allergic skin disorders.
- Dilation of capillaries in the skin, to cause flushing.

When H$_2$ receptors are stimulated, the main effects are increased secretion of gastric acid and pepsin, increased rate and force of myocardial contraction, and decreased immunologic and proinflammatory reactions (e.g., decreased release of histamine from basophils, decreased movement of neutrophils and basophils into areas of injury, inhibited T and B lymphocyte function). Stimulation of both H$_1$ and H$_2$ receptors causes peripheral vasodilation (with hypotension, headache, and skin flushing) and increases bronchial, intestinal, and salivary secretion of mucus.

**Figure 32.1.** Action of antihistamine drugs. Histamine$_1$ [H$_1$] receptor antagonists bind to H$_1$ receptors. This prevents histamine from binding to its receptors and acting on target tissues.

Unlike H$_1$ and H$_2$ receptors, H$_3$ receptors are primarily found in the brain and play a role in regulation of the release of histamine and other neurotransmitters from neurons. H$_3$ receptor agonists may be therapeutically useful in the treatment of various CNS, metabolic, and allergic disorders. Although several drugs affecting H$_3$ receptors are currently undergoing human trials, none is currently approved in the United States.

#### Hypersensitivity [Allergic] Reactions

In predisposed people, harmless environmental antigens that often do not cause a reaction sometimes may trigger an adaptive immune response, immunologic memory, and, on subsequent exposure to the environmental antigen, inflammation responses (see Chap. 16). **Hypersensitivity** involves allergic reactions—exaggerated responses by the immune system that produce tissue injury and may cause serious disease. The mechanisms that eliminate pathogens in adaptive immune responses are essentially identical to those of natural immunity. Allergic reactions may result from specific antibodies, sensitized T lymphocytes, or both, formed during exposure to an antigen. Treatments and interventions are covered in other chapters.

#### Types of Responses to Cell-Mediated Invasion

Hypersensitivity reactions are grouped into four types according to the mechanisms by which they are produced (Fig. 32.2). The substances that produce the effect for types I, II, and III hypersensitivity reactions are antibody molecules. The substances responsible for type IV reactions are antigen-specific T cells.

Type I (also called immediate hypersensitivity because it occurs within minutes of exposure to the antigen) is an immunoglobulin E (IgE)-induced response triggered by the interaction of antigen with antigen-specific IgE bound on mast cells, causing mast cell activation. Histamine and other mediators are released immediately, and cytokines, chemokines, and leukotrienes are synthesized after activation. Anaphylaxis is a type I

**Figure 32.2.** Types of hypersensitivity responses: **(A)** type I, atopic or anaphylactic; **(B)** type II, cytotoxic; **(C)** type III, immune complex; and **(D)** type IV, delayed. [Reprinted with permission from Timby, B. K., & Smith, N. E. (2018). *Introductory medical-surgical nursing* (12th ed., Fig. 34.1). Philadelphia, PA: Wolters Kluwer Health.]

response that may be mild (characterized mainly by urticaria, other dermatologic manifestations, or rhinitis) or severe and life-threatening (characterized by respiratory distress and cardiovascular collapse). It is uncommon and does not occur on first exposure to an antigen; it occurs with a second or later exposure, after antibody formation was induced by an earlier exposure. Severe anaphylaxis (sometimes called anaphylactic shock; see Chap. 29) is characterized by cardiovascular collapse from profound vasodilation and pooling of blood in the splanchnic system so that the patient has severe hypotension and functional hypovolemia. Respiratory distress often occurs from laryngeal edema and bronchoconstriction. Urticaria often occurs because the skin has many mast cells that release histamine. Anaphylaxis is a systemic reaction that usually involves the respiratory, cardiovascular, and dermatologic systems. Severe anaphylaxis may be fatal if not treated promptly and effectively. Antihistamines are helpful in treating urticaria and pruritus but are not effective in treating bronchoconstriction and hypotension. Epinephrine, rather than an antihistamine, is the drug of choice for treating severe anaphylaxis.

Type II responses are mediated by IgG or IgM, generating direct damage to the cell surface. These cytotoxic reactions include blood transfusion reactions, hemolytic disease of newborns, autoimmune hemolytic anemia, and some drug reactions. Hemolytic anemia (caused by destruction of erythrocytes) and

thrombocytopenia (caused by destruction of platelets), both type II hypersensitivity responses, are adverse effects of certain drugs (e.g., penicillin, methyldopa, heparin).

Type III is an IgG- or IgM-mediated reaction characterized by formation of antigen–antibody complexes that induce an acute inflammatory reaction in the tissues. **Serum sickness**, the prototype of these reactions, occurs when excess antigen combines with antibodies to form immune complexes. The complexes then diffuse into affected tissues, where they cause tissue damage by activating the complement system and initiating the immune response. If small amounts of immune complexes are deposited locally, the antigenic material can be phagocytized and digested by white blood cells and macrophages without tissue destruction. If large amounts are deposited locally or reach the bloodstream and become deposited in blood vessel walls, the lysosomal enzymes released during phagocytosis may cause permanent tissue destruction.

Type IV hypersensitivity (also called delayed hypersensitivity because of the lag time from exposure to antigen until the response is evident) is a cell-mediated response in which sensitized T lymphocytes react with an antigen to cause inflammation mediated by release of lymphokines, direct cytotoxicity, or both. The classic type IV hypersensitivity reaction is the tuberculin test, but similar reactions occur with contact dermatitis and some graft rejection.

## Clinical Manifestations

### Allergic Rhinitis

Allergic rhinitis is inflammation of nasal mucosa caused by a type I hypersensitivity reaction to inhaled allergens. It is a very common disorder characterized by nasal congestion, itching, sneezing, and watery drainage. Itching of the throat, eyes, and ears often occurs as well.

There are two types of allergic rhinitis. Seasonal disease (often called hay fever) produces acute symptoms in response to the protein components of airborne pollens from trees, grasses, and weeds, mainly in spring or fall. Perennial disease produces chronic symptoms in response to nonseasonal allergens such as dust mites, animal dander, and molds. Actually, mold spores can cause both seasonal and perennial allergies because they are present year round, with seasonal increases. Some people have both types, with chronic symptoms plus acute seasonal symptoms.

People with a personal or family history of other allergic disorders are likely to have allergic rhinitis. When mucous membranes in the nose become inflamed, nonallergenic irritants such as tobacco smoke, strong odors, air pollution, and climatic changes can worsen symptoms.

Allergic rhinitis is an immune response in which normal nasal breathing and filtering of air brings inhaled antigens into contact with mast cells and basophils in nasal mucosa, blood vessels, and submucosal tissues. With initial exposure, the inhaled antigens are processed by lymphocytes that produce IgE, an antigen-specific antibody that binds to mast cells. With later exposures, the IgE interacts with inhaled antigens and triggers the breakdown of the mast cell. This breakdown causes the release of histamine and other inflammatory mediators such as prostaglandins and leukotrienes (Fig. 32.3). These mediators, of which histamine may be the most important, dilate and engorge blood vessels to produce nasal congestion, stimulate secretion of mucus, and attract inflammatory cells (e.g., eosinophils, lymphocytes, monocytes, macrophages). In people with allergies, mast cells and basophils are increased in both number and reactivity. Thus, these cells may be capable of releasing large amounts of histamine and other mediators.

Allergic rhinitis that is not effectively treated may lead to chronic fatigue, impaired ability to perform usual activities of daily living, difficulty sleeping, sinus infections, postnasal drip, cough, and headache. In addition, this condition is a strong risk factor for asthma. Studies have demonstrated that although antihistamines relieve symptoms of allergic rhinitis, antihistamine are not successful or recommended for treatment of the common cold.

Chapters 17 and 31 describe the many drugs used to manage the condition besides antihistamines.

### Allergic Contact Dermatitis

Allergic contact dermatitis is a type IV hypersensitivity reaction resulting from direct contact with antigens to which a person

**Figure 32.3.** Allergic rhinitis: type I hypersensitivity reaction. **A.** The first exposure of mast cells in nasal mucosa to inhaled antigens (e.g., pollens from weeds, grasses, trees) leads to the formation of immunoglobulin E (IgE) antibody molecules. These molecules then bind to the surface membranes of mast cells. This process sensitizes mast cells to the effects of inhaled antigens (allergens). **B.** When sensitized mast cells are reexposed to inhaled pollens or other antigens, they release histamine and other chemical mediators, which then act on nasal mucosa to produce characteristic symptoms of allergic rhinitis.

has previously become sensitized (e.g., poison ivy or poison oak, cosmetics, hair dyes, metals, drugs applied topically to the skin). This reaction, which may be acute or chronic, usually occurs more than 24 hours after reexposure to an antigen and may last from days to weeks.

Affected areas of the skin are usually inflamed, warm, edematous, intensely pruritic, and tender to touch. Skin lesions are usually erythematous macules, papules, and vesicles (blisters) that may drain, develop crusts, and become infected. Lesion location may indicate the causative antigen.

### Allergic Food Reactions

Typically, food allergies are an immune response to the ingestion of a protein. Some food allergens such as shellfish, fish, corn, seeds, bananas, egg, milk, soy, peanut, and tree nuts have a higher inherent risk of triggering anaphylaxis than others. However, many other foods have been identified as allergens, including certain fruits and vegetables. Commonly, children allergic to milk, eggs, wheat, or soy outgrow their allergy. Exclusive breast-feeding has been found to be protective against the development of food allergies in early life but to increase the risk of food allergies as a person ages. There is no known preventive strategy to prevent food allergies except to delay introducing allergy-prone foods to infants until the GI tract has had time to mature. The timing for this varies from food to food and from infant to infant. The most common food allergy among adults is shellfish, often first presenting later in life.

### Allergic Drug Reactions

Virtually any drug may induce an immunologic response in susceptible people, and any body tissues may be affected. Allergic drug reactions are complex and diverse and may include any of the types of hypersensitivity described previously. A single drug may induce one or more of these states and multiple symptoms. There are no specific characteristics that identify drug-related reactions, although some reactions commonly attributed to drugs (e.g., skin rashes, drug fever, hematologic reactions, hepatic reactions) rarely occur with plant pollens and other naturally occurring antigens. Usually, however, the body responds to a drug as it does to other foreign materials (antigens). In addition, some coloring agents, preservatives, and other additives, rather than the drugs themselves, may cause reactions. The causal agent may be difficult to recognize in a person with atypical, resolving, or partially treated symptoms, as when skin signs such as urticaria are absent or masked by medications.

Allergic drug reactions should be considered when new signs and symptoms develop or when they differ from the usual manifestations of the illness being treated, especially if a reaction:

- Follows ingestion of a drug, especially one known to produce allergic reactions
- Is unpredictable and occurs in only a few patients when many patients receive the suspected drug
- Occurs approximately 7 to 10 days after initial exposure to the suspected drug (to allow antibody production)
- Follows a previous exposure to the same or similar drug (sensitizing exposure)
- Occurs minutes or hours after a second or subsequent exposure
- Occurs after small doses (reduces the likelihood that the reaction is due to dose-related drug toxicity)

- Occurs with other drugs that are chemically or immunologically similar to the suspected drug
- Produces signs and symptoms that differ from the usual pharmacologic actions of the suspected drug
- Produces signs and symptoms usually considered allergic in nature (e.g., anaphylaxis, urticaria, serum sickness)
- Produces similar signs and symptoms to previous allergic reactions to the same or a similar drug
- Increases eosinophils in blood or tissue
- Resolves within a few days of discontinuing the suspected drug

Virtually all drugs have been implicated in **anaphylactic reactions**. Penicillins and other antimicrobials, radiocontrast media, aspirin and other nonsteroidal anti-inflammatory drugs, and antineoplastics such as L-asparaginase and cisplatin are more common offenders. Less common causes include anesthetics (local and general), opioid analgesics, skeletal muscle relaxants used with general anesthetics, and vaccines. Approximately 10% of severe anaphylactic reactions are fatal. In many cases, it is unknown whether clinical manifestations are immunologic or nonimmunologic in origin.

Serum sickness is a delayed hypersensitivity reaction most often caused by drugs, such as antimicrobials. In addition, many drugs that produce anaphylaxis also produce serum sickness. With initial exposure to the antigen, symptoms usually develop within 7 to 10 days and include urticaria, lymphadenopathy, myalgia, arthralgia, and fever. The reaction usually resolves within a few days but may be severe or even fatal. With repeated exposure to the antigen, after prior sensitization of the host, accelerated serum sickness may develop within 2 to 4 days, with similar but often more severe signs and symptoms.

Systemic lupus erythematosus (SLE) is an autoimmune disorder that may be idiopathic from nondrug causes or induced by hydralazine, procainamide, isoniazid, and other drugs. Clinical manifestations vary greatly, depending on the location and severity of the inflammatory and immune processes, and may include skin lesions, fever, pneumonia, anemia, arthralgia, arthritis, nephritis, and others. Drug-induced lupus produces less renal and CNS involvement than idiopathic SLE.

Fever often occurs with allergic drug reactions. It may occur alone, with a skin rash and eosinophilia, or with other drug-induced allergic reactions such as serum sickness, SLE, vasculitis, and hepatitis. Dermatologic conditions (e.g., skin rash, urticaria, inflammation) commonly occur with allergic drug reactions and may be the first and most visible manifestations.

### Pseudoallergic Drug Reactions

Pseudoallergic drug reactions resemble immune responses (because histamine and other chemical mediators are released), but they do not produce antibodies or sensitized T lymphocytes. **Anaphylactoid reactions** are like anaphylaxis in terms of immediate occurrence, symptoms (rash or hives, difficulty breathing, swelling of body parts), and life-threatening severity. The main difference is that they are not antigen–antibody reactions and therefore may occur on first exposure to the causative agent. The drugs bind directly to mast cells, activate the cells, and cause the release of histamine and other vasoactive chemical mediators. Contrast media for radiologic diagnostic tests are often implicated.

# Drug Therapy

The $H_1$ receptor antagonist group contains several classes of antihistamines: alkylamines (e.g., chlorpheniramine), ethanolamines (e.g., clemastine), piperidines (e.g., cyproheptadine), piperazines (e.g., hydroxyzine pamoate), ethylenediamines (tripelennamine), phenothiazines (e.g., promethazine), and a miscellaneous group. Choosing an antihistamine is based on the desired effect, duration of action, adverse effects, and other characteristics of available drugs. For most people, a second-generation $H_1$ receptor antagonist is the first drug of choice. Metabolites of second-generation antihistamines (e.g., fexofenadine, desloratadine, and levocetirizine) are sometimes classed as third-generation antihistamines. These drugs were intended to have increased efficacy with fewer adverse drug reactions than second-generation drugs, although their ability to reduce side effects has not consistently been demonstrated. Table 32.1 lists the drugs given to block the effects of histamine. The $H_1$ receptor antagonists are categorized into first-, second-, and third-generation drugs. The second- and third-generation drugs are substantially more selective for peripheral histamine $H_1$ receptors, providing a better tolerability profile than first-generation agents. The following sections and the DRUGS AT A GLANCE tables describe selected $H_1$ receptor and $H_2$ receptor antagonists. (Chapter 33 discusses inhaled drugs used to decrease the histamine response.)

The receptor activity of drugs blocking the $H_2$ receptor blocking agents is not related to allergic responses but is used to prevent or treat peptic ulcer disease. Chapter 37 discusses these drugs, cimetidine (Tagamet), ranitidine (Zantac), famotidine (Pepcid), and nizatidine (Axid).

## FIRST-GENERATION $H_1$ RECEPTOR ANTAGONISTS

*H₂ is GI drugs*

The oldest $H_1$ receptor antagonists are relatively inexpensive and widely available. However, they have a limited role in the treatment of most patients because of their numerous adverse effects. They are effective in the relief of allergic symptoms but lack receptor selectivity. Their anticholinergic activity causes poor tolerability of some of these agents, especially compared with the second-

and third-generation $H_1$ receptor antagonists. Patient response and occurrence of adverse drug reactions vary greatly among classes and among drugs within classes. **Diphenhydramine**, the prototype first-generation antihistamine, has a high incidence of drowsiness and anticholinergic effects.

Drugs that block the $H_1$ receptors prevent or reduce most of the physiologic effects that histamine normally induces at $H_1$ receptor sites. Thus, they:

- Inhibit smooth muscle constriction in blood vessels and the respiratory and GI tracts
- Decrease capillary permeability
- Decrease salivation and tear formation

First-generation $H_1$ antagonists, chemically diverse antihistamines (also called nonselective or sedating agents), bind to both central and peripheral $H_1$ receptors and can cause CNS depression or stimulation. Many of these drugs are currently marketed with or without a prescription, both alone and in combination formulations such as sleep aids.

## Pharmacokinetics

Diphenhydramine is well absorbed after oral administration. Immediate-release oral forms act within 15 to 60 minutes and last 4 to 6 hours. Enteric-coated or sustained-release preparations last 8 to 12 hours. For most forms, administration is oral; for a few forms, administration is parenteral. Metabolism is primarily in the liver, and excretion of metabolites and small amounts of unchanged drug occurs in the urine within 24 hours.

## Action

Diphenhydramine and the other first-generation $H_1$ antagonists are structurally related to histamine and occupy the same receptor sites as histamine, which prevents histamine from acting on target tissues (see Fig. 32.1). Thus, the drugs are effective in inhibiting vascular permeability, edema formation, bronchoconstriction, and pruritus associated with histamine release. They do not prevent histamine release or reduce the amount released.

## TABLE 32.1

### Drugs Administered to Decrease Histamine Release and the Allergic Response*

| Drug Class | Prototype | Other Drugs in the Class |
|---|---|---|
| First-generation $H_1$ receptor antagonists | Diphenhydramine | Chlorpheniramine<br>Clemastine<br>Cyproheptadine<br>Dexchlorpheniramine (Polmon)<br>Hydroxyzine pamoate (Vistaril)<br>Promethazine |
| Second-generation $H_1$ receptor antagonists | Cetirizine (Zyrtec Allergy) | Azelastine (Astelin, Astepro)<br>Acrivastine and pseudoephedrine (Semprex-D)<br>Loratadine (Claritin)<br>Olopatadine (Patanase) |
| Third-generation $H_1$ receptor antagonists | Fexofenadine (Allegra) | Levocetirizine (Xyzal)<br>Desloratadine (Clarinex) |

*Table 33.1 lists inhaled drugs used to decrease the histamine response.

## Use

Indications for diphenhydramine include hypersensitivity reactions (allergic rhinitis, conjunctivitis, dermatitis), motion sickness, insomnia, and parkinsonism. Table 32.2 gives route and dosage information for some of the first-generation H₁ receptor antagonists.

### Use in Children

Young children may experience paradoxical excitement after receiving therapeutic dosages of diphenhydramine and other first-generation H₁ receptor antagonists. After overdose, hallucinations, convulsions, and death may occur. For safe use in children, close supervision and appropriate dosages are necessary.

Diphenhydramine is not recommended for use in newborn infants (premature or full term) or children with chickenpox or a flulike infection. When used in young children, doses should be small because of drug effects on the brain and nervous system.

b/c CNS ↑

### Use in Older Adults

Diphenhydramine and other first-generation H₁ receptor antagonists may cause confusion (with impaired thinking, judgment, and memory), dizziness, hypotension, sedation, syncope, unsteady gait, and paradoxical CNS stimulation in older adults. It is possible to misinterpret these effects, especially sedation, as senility or mental depression. Older men with prostatic hypertrophy may have difficulty voiding while taking these drugs. Some of these adverse reactions derive from anticholinergic effects of the drugs and are likely to be more severe if the patient is also taking other drugs with anticholinergic effects (e.g., tricyclic antidepressants, older antipsychotic drugs, some antiparkinson drugs). However, despite the increased risk of adverse effects, diphenhydramine is sometimes prescribed as a sleep aid for occasional use in older adults. As with many other drugs, smaller-than-usual dosages are indicated.

### Use in Patients With Renal Impairment

Little information is available about using first-generation H₁ receptor antagonists in patients with impaired renal function. In patients with severe renal impairment, it is necessary to give diphenhydramine at a dosing interval of 12 to 18 hours.

### Use in Patients With Hepatic Impairment

In patients with hepatic impairment, single doses of diphenhydramine are probably safe, but the effects of multiple doses have not been studied.

### Use in Patients With Critical Illness

The routine treatment of patients with critical illness does not often involve antihistamines. However, a patient who is having a blood transfusion or a diagnostic test may receive diphenhydramine, often by injection and usually as a single dose, to prevent allergic reactions.

### Use in Patients Receiving Home Care

People often take antihistamines in the home setting, especially for allergic rhinitis and other allergic disorders. Most people are familiar with the uses and side effects of antihistamines. The home care nurse is unlikely to be involved in antihistamine drug therapy unless visiting a patient for other care and purposes.

**QSEN Alert: Safety**

If diphenhydramine is being used, the home care nurse needs to assess for drowsiness and safety hazards in the environment (e.g., operating a car or other potentially hazardous machinery).

In most people, tolerance develops to the sedative effects within a few days if they are not taking other sedative-type drugs or alcoholic beverages. If a patient has an allergic disorder, the home care nurse may need to assist in identifying and alleviating environmental allergens (e.g., cigarette smoke, animal dander, dust mites).

*Concept Mastery Alert*

Because many patients self-manage allergy symptoms with OTC antihistamines, it is especially important to ask patients with glaucoma, peptic ulcer disease, and urinary retention and those who are pregnant about antihistamine use, as they may be contraindicated for these patients.

## Adverse Effects

Diphenhydramine and other first-generation H₁ receptor antagonists usually cause CNS depression (drowsiness, sedation) in therapeutic doses. Some studies have shown that cognitive and performance impairment occurs with the first-generation drugs even when the person does not feel drowsy or impaired. These drugs may cause CNS stimulation (anxiety, agitation) with excessive doses, especially in children. In addition, they have substantial anticholinergic effects (e.g., dry mouth, urinary retention, constipation, blurred vision).

H₂ is GI drugs

## Contraindications

Contraindications or caution is essential with diphenhydramine in pregnant women and in patients with hypersensitivity to the drugs, narrow-angle glaucoma, prostatic hypertrophy, stenosing peptic ulcer, and bladder neck obstruction.

## Nursing Implications

### Preventing Interactions

Several drugs interact with diphenhydramine, increasing its effects (Box 32.1). No drugs reportedly decrease the drug's effects, and no herbs appear to interact with it. Diphenhydramine may reduce the effectiveness of tamoxifen if used concomitantly.

**QSEN Alert: Safety**

It is important not to take diphenhydramine within 14 days of taking a monoamine oxidase inhibitor (isocarboxazid, phenelzine, or tranylcypromine) because of the risk of overstimulation of the sympathetic nervous system.

### Administering the Medication

People may take the oral form of diphenhydramine with or without food. Milk may help if stomach upset occurs.

### TABLE 32.2

## DRUGS AT A GLANCE: First-Generation H₁ Receptor Antagonists

| Drug | Pregnancy Category | Routes and Dosage Ranges | |
|------|-------------------|---------------------------|---|
| | | **Adults** | **Children** |
| Ⓟ **Diphenhydramine** (✽ Diphenhist, PMS-DiphenhydrAMINE) | B | Hypersensitivity reaction, motion sickness, parkinsonism: PO, 25–50 mg every 4–8 h; IV or deep IM injection 10–50 mg, increased if necessary to a max daily dose of 400 mg<br>Insomnia: PO 50 mg at bedtime<br>Cough (syrup): PO, 25 mg (10 mL) every 4 h, not to exceed 100 mg (40 mL) in 24 h | Weight >10 kg (22 lb), PO 12.5–25 mg every 6–8 h, 5 mg/kg/d, or 150 mg/m²/d; IV 5 mg/kg/d, or 150 mg/m²/d; max oral or parenteral dosage, 300 mg daily<br>Insomnia: ≥12 y, same as adults<br>Cough (syrup) PO 2–6 y, 6.25 mg (2.5 mL) every 4 h, not to exceed 25 mg (10 mL) in 24 h<br>6–12 y, PO 12.5 mg (5 mL) every 4 h, not to exceed 50 mg (20 mL) in 24 h |
| Chlorpheniramine (Aller-Chlor, Allergy-Time) | C | PO, 4 mg PO every 4–6 h; max dose, 24 mg in 24 h<br>Extended-release forms, PO 12 mg every 12 h; max dose, 24 mg in 24 h | 2–6 y, PO 1 mg every 4–6 h; max dose, 6 mg in 24 h<br>6–12 y, PO 2 mg every 4–6 h; max dose, 12 mg in 24 h<br>≥12 y, same as adults<br>Extended-release forms, ≥12 y, same as adults |
| Clemastine | B | Allergic rhinitis: PO 1.34 mg twice daily, increased up to a max of 8.04 mg daily, if necessary<br>Urticaria/angioedema: PO, 2.68 mg 1–3 times daily, increased up to a max of 8.04 mg daily, if necessary | Allergic rhinitis: 6–12 y (syrup only), PO 0.67 mg twice daily, increased up to a max of 4.02 mg daily, if necessary<br>≥12 y, same as adults<br>Urticaria/angioedema: PO 6 to <12 y (syrup only), PO 1.34 mg twice daily<br>≥12 y, same as adults |
| Cyproheptadine | B | PO, 4 mg every 8 h initially, increase if necessary; max dose 0.5 mg/kg/d | Calculate total daily dosage as 0.25 mg/kg or 8 mg/m²<br>2–6 y, 2 mg every 8–12 h; max dose, 12 mg/d<br>7 to <14 y, 4 mg PO every 8–12 h; max dose, 16 mg/d<br>≥14 y, same as adults |
| Dexchlorpheniramine (Polmon) | B | PO, Regular tablets and syrup, 2 mg every 4–6 h | 2–5 y, PO 0.5 mg every 4–6 h<br>6–11 y, PO 1 mg every 4–6 h<br>≥12 y, same as adults |
| Hydroxyzine Pamoate (Vistaril; ✽ Atarax, Novo-Hydroxyzin) | C | PO, 25 mg every 6–8 h<br>IM, 25–100 mg as needed | <6 y, PO 50 mg daily in divided dose<br>≥6 y, 50–100 PO mg daily in divided doses |
| Promethazine | C | PO, IM, rectally 25 mg, every 4–6 h as needed | ≥2 y, 0.5 mg/kg/dose (maximum dose 25 mg) every 12 h as needed |

**! QSEN Alert: Safety**

The nurse should give intramuscular antihistamines deeply into a large muscle mass to decrease tissue irritation; he or she injects intravenous (IV) antihistamines slowly, over a few minutes, because severe hypotension may result from rapid IV injection.

To prevent motion sickness, it is necessary to take the drug 30 to 60 minutes before travel.

### Assessing for Therapeutic Effects

The nurse observes for a verbal statement of therapeutic effect (relief of symptoms):

- For decreased nasal congestion when given for hypersensitivity
- For decreased dizziness and nausea when taken for motion sickness
- For drowsiness or sleep when given for insomnia

### Assessing for Adverse Effects

The nurse assesses for changes in level of consciousness; dryness of mouth, nose, and throat; blurred vision; urinary

retention; and constipation. He or she also assesses for gastric effects, such as anorexia, nausea, and vomiting. In addition, particularly in children, it is necessary to observe for paradoxical excitation (restlessness, insomnia, tremors, nervousness, palpitations).

### Patient Teaching

For children with allergies, family members should provide day care staff and school contacts with an emergency plan. Box 32.2 outlines patient teaching guidelines for diphenhydramine and other antihistamines.

## Other Drugs in the Class

Many of the first-generation $H_1$ receptor antagonists are available alone and in combination with adrenergic nasal decongestants, analgesics, and allergy, cold, and sinus remedies. Most are available as over-the-counter (OTC) drugs, without a prescription.

Chlorpheniramine causes slight to moderate drowsiness and may also have antidepressant properties. However, the chronic use of first-generation antihistamines, such as chlorpheniramine, should be avoided where possible because of sedation and interference with psychomotor performance. Dexchlorpheniramine (Polmon), which also produces minimal drowsiness, is used to treat runny nose, watery eyes, hives, itching, and other symptoms of allergies and the common cold. The drug has a similar adverse effects profile as diphenhydramine. Similar interaction patterns exist with other oral $H_1$ receptor antagonists and diphenhydramine (see Box 32.1).

Hydroxyzine pamoate (Vistaril) or promethazine may be given by injection for nausea and vomiting or to provide sedation but are not usually the first drugs of choice for these indications. The U.S. Food and Drug Administration (FDA) has issued a **BLACK BOX WARNING ◆** for promethazine because of the risk of severe chemical irritation and damage to tissues regardless of the route of administration. Patients younger than 2 years of age should not receive the drug; there is a potential for fatal respiratory depression. Although administration may be IV or intramuscular, the oral route should be used as soon as feasible. In addition, cholestatic jaundice has reportedly occurred with promethazine, and use of the drug warrants caution.

**BOX 32.2**      *Patient Teaching Guidelines for Antihistamines* (Continued)

dangerous drug interactions. Alcohol and other drugs that depress brain function may cause excessive sedation, respiratory depression, and death.

• Do not take more than one antihistamine at a time (e.g., two prescription drugs, two OTC drugs, or a combination of prescription and OTC drugs) because adverse effects are likely. If you do not know whether a particular medication is an antihistamine, consult a health care provider. For example, many OTC cold remedies and "nighttime" or "PM" allergy or sinus preparations contain an antihistamine. In addition, the active ingredient in OTC sleep aids is a sedating antihistamine, usually diphenhydramine.

• Avoid prolonged exposure to sunlight, and use sunscreens and protective clothing; some antihistamines may increase sensitivity to sunlight and risks of skin damage from sunburn.

• Report adverse effects, such as excessive drowsiness. The health care provider may be able to change drugs or dosages to decrease adverse effects.

• Store antihistamines out of reach of children to avoid accidental ingestion.

• If you experience an allergic reaction to a medication, obtain information about the drug thought responsible (including its various names), acceptable alternatives for future drug therapy, and potential sources of the drug. In addition, read the list of ingredients on labels of OTC drug preparations, inform all health care providers about the drug reaction before taking any newly prescribed drug, and wear a medical alert device that lists drugs to be avoided. Note that people may be allergic to additives (e.g., dyes, binders, others) rather than the active drug.

**Self-Administration**

• Take antihistamines only as prescribed or as instructed on packages of OTC preparations to increase beneficial effects and decrease adverse effects. If you miss a dose, do not take a double dose.

• Take most antihistamines with meals to decrease stomach upset. Take loratadine (Claritin) on an empty stomach for better absorption; cetirizine (Zyrtec Allergy) and desloratadine (Clarinex) may be taken with or without food. Do not take fexofenadine and related drugs with fruit juice.

• Do not chew or crush sustained-release tablets, and do not open sustained-release capsules. Such actions can cause rapid drug absorption, high blood levels, and serious adverse effects, rather than the slow absorption and prolonged action intended with these products.

---

In children, contraindications to promethazine include hepatic disease, Reye's syndrome, history of sleep apnea, or family history of sudden infant death syndrome.

## NCLEX Success

1. The nurse receives an order to administer diphenhydramine. This medication is recommended for use in which of the following?

    A. premature or full-term infants
    B. adults to prevent allergic reactions
    C. children with chickenpox
    D. children with a flulike infection

2. The nurse working in the emergency department anticipates an order of a severe allergic reaction with anaphylaxis, knowing that the drug of choice for severe allergic reactions with anaphylaxis is which of the following?   cookie (peanuts)

    A. diphenhydramine → then epinephrine prometh.
    B. cimetidine        signs of anaphylaxis
    C. epinephrine     limit H₁ reaction
    D. loratadine

3. Because of the action of antihistamines on target tissues, these drugs are effective in producing which of the following actions? (Select all that apply.)

    A. inhibiting vascular permeability
    B. reducing pruritus
    C. minimizing edema formation
    D. preventing histamine release

*Clinical Application 32.1*

• Mr. Rudolph tells the nurse that his wife has a prescription for diphenhydramine, which she takes intermittently at bedtime for insomnia. He says that he knows that diphenhydramine is used to treat allergies and asks if he can use it for his own symptoms. How should the nurse respond?

## SECOND-GENERATION H₁ RECEPTOR ANTAGONISTS

Unlike the first-generation H₁ receptor antagonists, the second-generation H₁ receptor antagonists do not readily enter the brain from the blood. **Cetirizine** (Zyrtec Allergy), the prototype, and other drugs in this class bind preferentially to peripheral rather than central H₁ receptors. This selectivity significantly reduces the occurrence of adverse drug reactions of the CNS, but drowsiness and CNS depression may occur. The second-generation H₁ receptor antagonists have supplanted the first-generation H₁ receptor antagonists in the symptomatic treatment of allergic rhinitis and in the relief of pruritus in urticaria. In addition, these drugs have a mild beneficial effect in chronic asthma. The drugs are used for treatment of atopic dermatitis or as adjunctive treatment of pruritus and other symptoms in anaphylaxis.

For most agents, onset of action is within 1 hour, and peak serum levels are achieved in 2 to 3 hours. The second-generation agents are also longer acting and require administration once or twice daily. The oral second-generation agents appear to be similarly efficacious to each other. Similar to the older first-generation antihistamines, this generation of agents has less effect on nasal congestion compared with glucocorticoid nasal sprays.

## Pharmacokinetics

Cetirizine is rapidly absorbed and reaches peak serum concentrations in 1 hour. The drug is 93% protein bound, and excretion of 50% of the unchanged drug occurs in urine and feces. The drug is present in breast milk.

## Action

Cetirizine competes with histamine for binding to histamine receptor sites on effector cells in the GI tract, blood vessels, and respiratory tract, preventing the activation of cells by histamine preventing allergy symptoms from occurring. Because the drug does not cross the blood–brain barrier, it does not cause the drowsiness associated with first-generation agents.

## Use

Health care providers use cetirizine for temporary relief of systems of respiratory allergies and urticaria (relief of pruritus). Table 32.3 presents route and dosage information for cetirizine and the other second-generation antihistamines.

 **QSEN Alert: Safety**

If an antihistamine is required during pregnancy, the lowest dose of chlorpheniramine, cetirizine, or loratadine is recommended. However, chlorpheniramine is not recommended during breast-feeding. If a mother takes a second-generation antihistamine while breast-feeding, the infant should be monitored for signs of irritability, jitteriness, or drowsiness.

### Use in Children

Prescription products may be used in children 6 months of age and older for symptoms associated with perennial allergic rhinitis and treatment of uncomplicated skin disorders associated with chronic idiopathic urticaria. OTC products for colds and other respiratory conditions are approved by the FDA in children ages 2 years and older and recommended with caution for use in children ≥2 years of age. Syrup formulations are available for use in younger children.

### Use in Older Adults

In general, second-generation antihistamines are much safer than first-generation agents for older adults because they are less likely to impair consciousness, thinking, or ability to perform activities of daily living (e.g., driving a car or operating various machines). However, the drugs should be used in caution with older adults as sedation has been reported and normal changes in renal function may increase adverse effects.

## TABLE 32.3

### DRUGS AT A GLANCE: Second-Generation H₁ Receptor Antagonists

| Drug | Pregnancy Category | Routes and Dosage Ranges | |
| --- | --- | --- | --- |
| | | **Adults** | **Children** |
| Ⓟ **Cetirizine** (Zyrtec Allergy) | B | PO, 5–10 mg once daily, to maximum dose of 10 mg daily<br>Renal or hepatic impairment: PO 5 mg once daily | 6–12 mo, PO 2.5 mg once daily (syrup available)<br>12 mo to 2 y, PO 0.5 mg once daily, to a maximum dose of 2.5 mg every 12 h, if needed<br>2–5 y, PO 2.5 mg (one-half tsp) once daily to a maximum dose of 2.5 mg every 12 h or 5 mg once daily, if needed<br>≥6 y, same as adults |
| Acrivastine and pseudoephedrine (Semprex-D) | B | PO, One capsule (acrivastine 8 mg/pseudoephedrine 60 mg) every 4–6 h, to maximum of 4 doses/24 h | ≥12, same as adults |
| Azelastine (Astelin, Astepro; 🍁 Astelin) | C | Nasal inhalation, (0.1% solution) two sprays per nostrils every 12 h | Nasal inhalation<br>≥6 mo to ≤5 y, (0.1% solution) one spray per nostrils every 12 h<br>6 to ≥12 y, (0.1%–0.15% solution) two sprays per nostrils every 12 h<br>12 y or older, same as adults |
| Loratadine (Alavert, Claritin) | B | 10 mg PO once daily<br>Renal or hepatic impairment: 10 mg PO every other day | 2–5 y, 5 mg PO daily (available in syrup)<br>≥6 y, same as adults |
| Olopatadine (Patanase) | C | Nasal inhalation, two sprays per nostrils every 12 h | Nasal inhalation, 6–11 y, one spray per nostrils every 12 h<br>≥12 y, same as adults |

### Use in Patients With Renal Impairment

The kidneys play a role in excretion of cetirizine. Therefore, use of the drug in people with renal impairment warrants caution, and authorities recommend a dosage adjustment. Although manufacturer labeling does not provide dosing adjustments with renal impairment, it is not uncommon to adjust dosing based on GFR in these people.

### Use in Patients Receiving Home Care

It is common for cetirizine to be administered in the home environment, particularly because the drug is available as an OTC preparation. As with first-generation antihistamines, the home care nurse may assess for the drug's effectiveness and provide patient teaching while visiting for other purposes. In general, patients likely tolerate the drug without serious adverse effects if renal function is not impaired.

## Adverse Effects

Adverse effects include drowsiness, headache, dizziness, nausea, vomiting, and fatigue.

## Contraindications

Contraindications include known sensitivity to cetirizine or any component of the formulation.

## Nursing Implications

### Preventing Interactions

Cetirizine does not appear to interact with many drugs, but concomitant use with drugs that also cause the potential for CNS depression may increase the risk of drowsiness and sedation. Theophylline is known to interact with the drug and slightly decreased the clearance of cetirizine. Potentially significant interactions may exist, requiring adjustment in dose or frequency, additional monitoring, or selection of an alternate drug.

### Administering the Medication

Administer usually once a day. Food has no effect on the overall absorption of cetirizine. However, food may increase the time it takes for peak levels of cetirizine to be reached in the blood. It is necessary to shake oral suspensions completely before administration.

### Assessing for Therapeutic Effects

The nurse assesses for relief of symptoms, including decreased nasal congestion with seasonal allergic rhinitis. In addition, he or she assesses for relief of pruritus in urticaria.

### Assessing for Adverse Effects

The nurse observes for headache, nausea, vomiting, and fatigue.

### Patient Teaching

Box 32.2 summarizes the patient teaching guidelines for antihistamines.

## Other Drugs in the Class

Other second-generation H₁ receptor antagonists have similar actions and adverse effect profiles. Acrivastine (Semprex-D) is formulated in combination with pseudoephedrine for symptom relief of seasonal allergic rhinitis. Some have sedative properties when taken at doses that exceed the recommended dose, including acrivastine, although cetirizine and intranasal azelastine may cause sedation at the recommended dose. Azelastine (Astelin, Astepro) and olopatadine (Patanase) are second-generation H₁ receptor antagonists that have been formulated as a nasal spray for topical use.

> ### QSEN Alert: Safety
>
> Olopatadine produces less sedation than azelastine, but patients should not perform activities that require alertness until they are sure they can engage in such activities safely.

Azelastine is available as an OTC preparation and may be used in children 5 years and older. Olopatadine is only available by prescription as a nasal spray and may be used in children 12 years of age and older. (However, olopatadine eye drops are available OTC.) Intranasal H₁ receptor antagonists are considered a first-line treatment for allergic rhinitis, although they are generally less effective than intranasal corticosteroids. Intranasal H₁ receptor antagonists are as effective as or superior to oral second-generation antihistamines for treating seasonal allergic rhinitis. Intranasal antihistamines have a clinically significant effect on nasal congestion. The nasal spray leaves an unpleasant taste; however, sniffing gently through the nose after each spray minimizes this taste. When applied to nasal mucosa, the drugs produce peak levels in 2 to 3 hours and last 12 to 24 hours. They are metabolized in the liver to an active metabolite and excreted mainly in feces.

Loratadine (Claritin) produces effects within 1 to 3 hours, which reach a maximum in 8 to 12 hours and last 24 hours or longer. The drug is metabolized in the liver, and its long duration of action is due, in part, to an active metabolite. The drug should be taken on an empty stomach.

## THIRD-GENERATION H₁ RECEPTOR ANTAGONISTS

Like the second-generation H₁ receptor antagonists, third-generation drugs do not readily enter the brain from the blood. Fexofenadine (the metabolite of terfenadine [no longer available]), desloratadine (the metabolite of loratadine), and levocetirizine (a purified isomer of cetirizine) are sometimes classified as third-generation agents. **Fexofenadine** (Allegra), the prototype, and other drugs in this class bind preferentially to peripheral rather than central H₁ receptors. This selectivity significantly reduces the occurrence of adverse drug reactions, such as drowsiness and sedation, while still providing effective relief of allergic conditions.

## Pharmacokinetics

Fexofenadine is rapidly absorbed and reaches peak serum concentrations in about 2.5 hours. It is 60% to 70% protein bound, and excretion of 95% of the unchanged drug occurs in bile and urine. Its effects last for 12 to 24 hours. The drug does not cross the blood–brain barrier, and whether the drug is excreted in breast milk is unknown.

**TABLE 32.4**

## DRUGS AT A GLANCE: Third-Generation H₁ Receptor Antagonists

| Drug | Pregnancy Category | Routes and Dosage Ranges | |
|------|-------------------|--------------------------|---|
| | | **Adults** | **Children** |
| **Fexofenadine** (Allegra Allergy; Allegra) | C | PO, 60 mg twice daily, to maximum of 120 mg/d<br>Renal impairment: 60 mg PO once daily<br>Once-daily formulations: 180 mg once daily (maximum 180 mg/d) | 6 mo to 2y, PO 15 mg twice daily<br>2–11 y, PO 30 mg twice daily, to maximum of 60 mg/d<br>≥12, same as adults, to maximum of 120 mg/d (available in syrup) |
| Desloratadine (Clarinex) | C | PO, 5 mg once daily | 6–11 mo, PO 1 mg once daily<br>12 mo to 5 y, 1.25 once daily<br>6–11 y, 2.5 mg once daily<br>≥12 y, same as adults |
| Levocetirizine (Xyzal) | B | PO, 5 mg once daily in evening | 6 mo to 5 y, PO 1.25 mg (one-half tsp) once daily in evening<br>6–11 y, PO 2.5 mg (one tsp) once daily in evening<br>≥12 y, same as adults |

## Action

Fexofenadine competes with histamine for binding to histamine receptor sites, preventing the activation of cells by histamine. Competition for the binding sites prevents activation of the H₁ receptors by histamine, thus preventing allergy symptoms from occurring. Because the drug does not cross the blood–brain barrier, it does not cause the drowsiness associated with first-generation agents.

## Use

Health care providers use fexofenadine for seasonal allergic rhinitis, other minor allergies, and urticaria (relief of pruritus). Table 32.4 presents route and dosage information for fexofenadine and the other third-generation antihistamines. A fexofenadine–pseudoephedrine combination (Allegra-D) is also available for cold and allergy relief, and it is important to review the package literature to ensure appropriate dosing.

### Use in Older Adults

As with second-generation antihistamines, fexofenadine and other third-generation drugs are much safer than the first-generation agents for older adults because they do not impair consciousness, thinking, or ability to perform activities of daily living (e.g., driving a car or operating various machines).

### Use in Patients With Renal Impairment

The kidneys play a role in excretion of fexofenadine. Therefore, use of the drug in people with renal impairment warrants caution, and authorities recommend a dosage adjustment.

### Use in Patients Receiving Home Care

It is common for fexofenadine to be administered in the home environment, particularly because the drug is available as an OTC preparation. As with first- and second-generation antihistamines, the home care nurse may assess for the drug's

effectiveness and provide patient teaching while visiting for other purposes. Patients likely tolerate the drug without serious adverse effects if renal function is not impaired.

## Adverse Effects

Adverse effects are usually minor and include headache, nausea, vomiting, dysmenorrhea, and fatigue.

## Contraindications

Contraindications include known sensitivity to fexofenadine.

## Nursing Implications

### Preventing Interactions

Several drugs may interact with fexofenadine, increasing or decreasing its effects (Box 32.3). Some herbs and foods also interact with this drug (Box 32.4).

**BOX 32.3** **Drug Interactions: Fexofenadine**

**Drugs That Increase the Effects of Fexofenadine**

- Alcohol, cannabinoids, dimethindene, doxylamine, dronabinol, droperidol, flunitrazepam, and oxycodone
  *Increase the potential for sedation*
- Azole antifungals (fluconazole, itraconazole, keto-conazole, miconazole) and macrolide antibacterials (azithromycin, clarithromycin, erythromycin)
  *Increase the plasma concentration*

**Drugs That Decrease the Effects of Fexofenadine**

- Antacids containing magnesium or aluminum
  *Decrease the absorption*
- Rifampin
  *Decreases the metabolism*

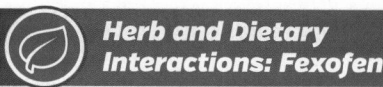
## Administering the Medication

Administration should occur with water only (fruit juice may decrease absorption). It is necessary to shake oral suspensions completely before administration. Oral disintegrating tablets should remain in the blister pack until use.

 **QSEN Alert: Safety**

Patients should take the tablets on an empty stomach. After placement on the tongue, the tablets dissolve in minutes, and swallowing, with or without water, may occur.

## Assessing for Therapeutic Effects

The nurse assesses for relief of symptoms, including decreased nasal congestion with seasonal allergic rhinitis. In addition, he or she assesses for relief of pruritus in urticaria.

## Assessing for Adverse Effects

The nurse observes for headache, nausea, vomiting, and fatigue. In women, it is also necessary to assess for dysmenorrhea.

## Patient Teaching

Box 32.2 summarizes the patient teaching guidelines for antihistamines.

# Other Drugs in the Class

Other third-generation $H_1$ receptor antagonists have similar actions and adverse effect profiles.

Levocetirizine (Xyzal) has an onset of action of 1 hour, and a single daily dose provides antihistamine activity for 28 hours. The drug can be used with children 6 years and older. It can be given with food, to decrease GI effects, or without food.

Desloratadine (Clarinex) is an active metabolite of loratadine. Desloratadine seems to offer no advantage over loratadine or other second-generation drugs. The drug may be used in children 6 months of age and older. It can be administered with food, to decrease GI effects, or without food.

 **QSEN Alert: Evidence-Based Practice**

National guidelines from the American Academy of Otolaryngology (Seidman et al., 2015) have revised the approach to the management of allergic rhinitis. The primary strategy to relieve the symptoms of allergic rhinitis is avoidance of the offending allergen. The group recommends allergy testing for patients with a clinical diagnosis of allergic rhinitis that does not respond to empiric treatment. If avoidance of allergens does not achieve symptom relief in patients with allergic rhinitis, indicated drugs may include the following:

- OTC second-generation antihistamines, such as loratadine, which should provide symptom relief in most situations for patients with primary complaints of sneezing and itching
- Prescription and other OTC drugs
  - Intranasal corticosteroids, such as fluticasone and flunisolide for adults and mometasone (see Chap. 33) for children, when symptoms are moderate to severe. If intranasal corticosteroids are not effective or the patient is not a candidate for corticosteroids:
  - Leukotriene receptor antagonists (see Chap. 33), which may be first-line therapy in patients with asthma concurrently
  - Intranasal OTC cromolyn
  - Intranasal antihistamines, such as OTC azelastine
- Ocular preparations, which may be considered for patients with allergic conjunctivitis if symptoms are not adequately controlled with oral antihistamines
- Prescription second-generation antihistamines, such as levocetirizine
- Oral decongestants to decrease nasal swelling and congestion

The use of evidence-based guidelines in the treatment of allergic rhinitis provides effective strategies for symptom relief. Appropriate drug therapy based on best practices maximizes symptom relief and reduces adverse effects. The nurse should educate patients regarding avoidance of the offending allergen and assess for effective symptom management.

**Clinical Application 32.2**

- Mr. Rudolph informs the nurse that he thinks he is allergic to the aspirin that he has been taking for his coronary artery disease because he becomes nauseated after taking his daily dose. What questions should the nurse ask Mr. Rudolph to help determine whether he has an allergy to aspirin?

# NCLEX Success

4. In explaining options for antihistamine medications to a patient, second-generation $H_1$ antagonists differ from first-generation $H_1$ antagonists in that they do which of the following?
   A. cause greater central nervous system sedation
   B. are available only by prescription
   C. are less expensive
   D. do not cross the blood–brain barrier

5. A patient has asked for an antihistamine to relieve symptoms of an upper respiratory infection. The nurse explains that studies have demonstrated that for treatment of the common cold, which of the following is true of antihistamines?
   A. are effective in relieving cold symptoms
   B. do not relieve symptoms and are not recommended
   C. should be compounded with other products to be effective
   D. relieve nonallergenic symptoms only

## THE NURSING PROCESS

A concept map outlines the nursing process related to drug therapy considerations in this chapter. Additional nursing implications related to the disease process should also be considered in care decisions.

**Assessment**

- Assess the patient's condition in relation to disorders for which antihistamines are used. For the patient with known allergies, try to determine the factors that precipitate or relieve allergic reactions and specific signs and symptoms experienced during a reaction.
- Assess every patient for a potential hypersensitivity reaction. For example, it is standard practice on first contact to ask a patient if he or she has any food, drug, or other allergies. The health care provider is likely to get more complete information by asking patients about allergic reactions to specific drugs (e.g., antibiotics such as penicillin, local anesthetics) rather than asking if they are allergic to or cannot take any drugs.
- If a drug allergy is identified, ask about specific signs and symptoms as well as any drugs currently being taken. With previous exposure and sensitization to the same or a similar drug, immediate allergic reactions may occur. With a new drug, antibody formation and allergic reactions usually require a week or longer. Most reactions appear within a month of starting a drug.
- When a suspected allergic reaction occurs (e.g., skin rash, fever, edema, dyspnea), interview the patient or consult medical records about the drug, dose, route, and time of administration. In addition, evaluate all the drugs a patient is taking as a potential cause of the reaction. This assessment may involve searching drug literature to see if the suspected drug is associated with allergic reactions and discussion with physicians and pharmacists.

**Outcomes of Therapy**

The patient will
- Experience relief of symptoms.
- Take antihistamines accurately.
- Avoid hazardous activities if sedation occurs from antihistamines.
- Avoid preventable adverse drug effects.
- Avoid taking sedative-type antihistamines with alcohol or other sedative drugs.

**Nursing Interventions**

- For patients with known allergies, assist in identifying and avoiding precipitating factors when possible. If it is a drug allergy, encourage the patient to carry a medical alert device that identifies the drug.
- Monitor the patient closely for excessive drowsiness during the first few days of therapy with antihistamines known to cause sedation.
- Encourage a fluid intake of 2000 to 3000 mL daily, if not contraindicated.
- When indicated, obtain an order and administer an antihistamine before situations known to elicit allergic reactions (e.g., blood transfusions, diagnostic tests that involve contrast media).
- For children with allergies, provide all family members, day care staff, and school personnel with an emergency plan.

**Evaluation**

- Observe for relief of symptoms.
- Interview and observe for correct drug usage.
- Interview and observe for excessive drowsiness.

---

## Unfolding Patient Stories: Yoa Li • Part 1

**Yoa Li** is a 26-year-old Asian male admitted to the hospital for an appendectomy. He is experiencing symptoms of allergic rhinitis. Recognizing he is NPO pending surgery, what are medication options to relieve nasal congestion and drainage that the nurse can recommend when informing the provider of his symptoms? (Yoa Li's story continues in Chapter 49.)

Care for Yoa and other patients in a realistic virtual environment: **vSim** *for Nursing* (thepoint.lww.com/vSimPharm). Practice documenting these patients' care in DocuCare (thepoint.lww.com/DocuCareEHR).

## KEY CONCEPTS

- Virtually any drug may induce an immunologic response in susceptible people, and any body tissue may be affected.
- Allergic rhinitis is inflammation of nasal mucosa caused by a type I hypersensitivity reaction to inhaled allergens.
- Anaphylaxis is a type I hypersensitivity reaction that is uncommon and does not occur on first exposure to an antigen; it occurs with a second or later exposure, after antibody formation was induced by an earlier exposure.
- Some food allergens such as shellfish, egg, milk, peanuts, and tree nuts have a higher inherent risk for triggering anaphylaxis than others.
- Patients with drug allergies should wear a medical alert bracelet identifying the drug.
- First-generation $H_1$ receptor antagonists may cause drowsiness and decreased mental alertness in both children and adults.

- First-generation $H_1$ receptor antagonists have substantial anticholinergic effects (e.g., cause dry mouth, urinary retention, constipation, blurred vision).
- The FDA has issued a **BLACK BOX WARNING ◆** regarding the risk of severe chemical irritation and damage to tissues with promethazine regardless of the route of administration. In addition, promethazine should not be used in patients younger than 2 years because of the potential for fatal respiratory depression.
- Second- and third-generation $H_1$ receptor antagonists cause less CNS depression because they are selective for peripheral $H_1$ receptors and do not cross the blood–brain barrier.
- For children with allergies, nurses should ensure that all family members as well as day care and school contacts have been provided with an emergency plan.

## CLINICAL REASONING CASE STUDY

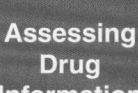

**Meet the Patient**

Amarjeet Kapoor, age 42, comes to the clinic with his wife with a red, itchy rash on both forearms. He has no shortness of breath, and his vital signs are temperature 980°F, pulse 92 beats/min, respiratory rate 22/min, blood pressure 130/82 mm Hg, and $O_2$ saturation on room air 94%. He says that the rash started this morning after he inadvertently ate mushrooms at a restaurant. After he developed a rash from mushrooms when he was a child, he has avoided mushrooms. The nurse practitioner orders diphenhydramine 50 mg now and 25 mg orally at bedtime for 2 days, as well as cetirizine 10 mg orally once daily until the rash disappears. The man has an appointment to return to the clinic in 3 days. What patient teaching information should the nurse provide?

**Assessing Drug Information**

- Diphenhydramine
  - The immediate-release form of a first-generation $H_1$ receptor antagonist acts in 15 to 60 minutes and lasts 4 to 6 hours.
  - Adverse effects may include excessive drowsiness or anxiety and agitation. Dry mouth, blurred vision, constipation, urinary retention, and tachycardia have been reported.
- Cetirizine (Zyrtec)
  - This drug is a second-generation $H_1$ receptor antagonist that binds preferentially to peripheral rather than central $H_1$ receptors. This selectivity significantly reduces the occurrence of adverse drug reactions, such as drowsiness and sedation, while still providing effective relief of allergic conditions.
  - It is an active metabolite of hydroxyzine that reaches maximal serum concentration in 1 hour and is about 93% protein bound. About half of a dose is metabolized in the liver; the other half is excreted unchanged in the urine.
  - It demonstrates a rapid onset of action and some mast cell-stabilizing activity.
  - Cetirizine and most of the second-generation medications have a longer duration of action than the first-generation medications.
  - The standard dose of 10 mg once daily is appropriate for adults and children aged 6 years and older (and may be increased to 10 mg twice daily in adults if needed).
  - Adverse effects include fatigue, dry mouth, and potential for drowsiness.

**Nursing Actions**

- Assess for allergies before any medications are administered.
- Assess for contraindications to antihistamines, such as pregnancy, narrow-angle glaucoma, prostatic hypertrophy, stenosing peptic ulcer, or bladder neck obstruction.
- Instruct Mr. Kapoor's wife to closely observe for excessive drowsiness during the first few days of treatment with antihistamines.
- Teach the patient to avoid alcoholic beverages and other central nervous system depressants while taking these medications.
- Caution Mr. Kapoor that he should not perform tasks that require mental alertness (drive or operate heavy equipment) while taking the drugs until he knows how it will affect him; they may cause drowsiness.
- Teach Mr. Kapoor to notify those who prepare his food about the mushroom allergy to avoid the reaction in the future.
- Reinforce the importance of not scratching the irritated areas; teach Mr. Kapoor alternatives to relieve this urge.

Visit thePoint® at **http://thePoint.lww.com/Frandsen12e** for answers to NCLEX Success questions (in Appendix A), answers to Clinical Application Case Studies (in Appendix B), and more!

## REFERENCES AND RESOURCES

deShazo, R. D., & Kemp, S. F. (2019). *Pharmacotherapy of allergic rhinitis.* UpToDate. Lexi-Comp, Inc.

Droessaert, V., Timmermans, M., Dekimpe, E., Seys, S., Ceuppens, J. J., Fokkens, W. J., et al. (2016). Real-life study showing better control of allergic rhinitis by immunotherapy than regular pharmacotherapy. *Rhinology, 54*(3), 214–220.

Guyton, A. C., & Hall, J. E. (2015). *Textbook of medical physiology* (13th ed.). Philadelphia, PA: Elsevier.

Hinkle, J. L., & Cheever, K. H. (2017). *Brunner & Suddarth's textbook of medical-surgical nursing* (14th ed.). Philadelphia, PA: Wolters Kluwer Health/Lippincott Williams & Wilkins.

Karch, A. M. (2019). *Lippincott's pocket drug guide for nurses.* Philadelphia, PA: Lippincott Williams & Wilkins.

National Guideline Clearinghouse. (2015). Guideline summary: Clinical practice guideline: Allergic rhinitis. National Guideline Clearinghouse. Retrieved from https://www.guideline.gov

Norris, T. L. (2019). *Porth's pathophysiology: Concepts of altered health states* (10th ed.). Philadelphia, PA: Wolters Kluwer.

Nursing2019. (2019). *Drug handbook.* Philadelphia, PA: Wolters Kluwer Health/Lippincott Williams & Wilkins.

Powell, R. J., Leech, S. C., Till, S., Huber, P. A., Nasser, S. M., & Clark, A. T. (2015). BSACI guideline for the management of chronic urticaria and angioedema. *Clinical and Experimental Allergy: Journal of the British Society for Allergy and Clinical Immunology, 45*(3), 547–565. doi:10.1111/cea.12494

Ridolo, E., Caminati, M., Martignago, I., Melli, V., Salvottini, C., Rossi, O., et al. (2016). Allergic rhinitis: Pharmacotherapy in pregnancy and old age. *Expert Review of Clinical Pharmacology, 9*(8), 1081–1089.

Seidman, M. D., Gurgel, R. K., Lin, S. Y., Swartz, S. R., Baroody, F. M., Bonner, J. R., et al. (2015). Clinical practice guideline: Allergic rhinitis. *Otolaryngology–Head and Neck Surgery, 152*(1), S1–S43.

UpToDate. (2019). *Drug information.* Lexi-Comp, Inc.

Wheatley, L. W., & Togias, A. (2015). Allergic rhinitis. *The New England Journal of Medicine, 372*(5), 456–463.

# Drug Therapy for Asthma, Airway Inflammation, and Bronchoconstriction

## CLINICAL APPLICATION CASE STUDY

Terry Lee, a 38-year-old man, presents to the emergency department in severe respiratory distress, with profound dyspnea, wheezing, and circumoral cyanosis. He received a diagnosis of asthma at age 10. Mr. Lee is admitted to the intensive care unit. His treatment regimen includes albuterol via inhalation every 20 minutes for four doses and intravenous corticosteroids every 6 hours.

## KEY TERMS

**Airway hyperresponsiveness:** exaggerated bronchoconstrictive response to stimuli

**Atopic sensitization:** predisposition toward developing certain allergic hypersensitivity reactions

**Bronchospasm (also called bronchoconstriction):** constriction of the air passages of the lung (as in asthma) by spasmodic contraction of the bronchial muscles

**Eosinophilic phenotype:** allergic response of individuals with severe asthma who have blood eosinophil counts of 150/μL or greater

**Leukotrienes:** strong chemical mediators of bronchoconstriction and inflammation, the major pathologic features of asthma

**Maintenance inhalant medications:** long-term control beta$_2$-agonists used to achieve and maintain prophylactic control of persistent asthma

**Mast cells:** cells releasing substances that produce bronchoconstriction and inflammation in response to causative stimuli

**Rescue inhalant medications:** quick-relief, short-acting beta$_2$-agonists used during periods of acute symptoms and exacerbations

**Status asthmaticus:** acute, severe asthma

**Triggers:** factors that initiate asthma symptoms

**Work-exacerbated asthma:** adverse respiratory outcome resulting from work-related conditions

## INTRODUCTION

This chapter describes drugs used to treat asthma and other respiratory disorders characterized by airway inflammation, bronchoconstriction, **airway hyperresponsiveness** (exaggerated bronchoconstrictive response to stimuli), and mucosal edema. These signs and symptoms characterize such features as asthma, chronic bronchitis, and emphysema, which are collectively considered the chronic lung diseases. Here, the emphasis is on asthma because of its widespread prevalence, especially in urban populations. To understand the use of drugs in the management of asthma, it is necessary to provide an overview of the condition and its prevalence, etiology, pathophysiology, and clinical manifestations.

## OVERVIEW OF ASTHMA

### Etiology

The causes of asthma are not known, but it appears to involve the relationship between host factors (predominantly genetic) and environmental exposures that occur at a critical time in immune system development. The strongest identifiable predisposing factor for asthma seems to be the genetic predisposition for the development of an immunoglobulin E (IgE)–mediated response (**atopic sensitization**) to common allergens. The condition may occur at any age but is especially common in children and older adults. Numerous stimuli may precipitate acute symptoms of asthma, and hyperresponsiveness to such stimuli may initiate both inflammation and bronchoconstriction. Viral infections of the respiratory tract are often the causative agents, especially in infants and young children, whose airways are small and easily obstructed. Asthma symptoms may persist for days or weeks after the viral infection resolves. Common environmental factors that cause asthma symptoms (**triggers**) vary from person to person and include outdoor allergens such as pollens and molds; indoor allergens, including dust mites, dander, and molds; and respiratory irritants, such as smoke from cigarettes and occupational environments. Children who are exposed to allergens and airway irritants such as tobacco smoke during infancy are at high risk for development of asthma. Authorities have suggested that strenuous physical activities; certain drugs; stress and emotion; and changes in season, weather, and temperature are asthma triggers.

**QSEN Alert: Evidence-Based Practice**

A review of literature by Sears (2015) explored predictors of remission or persistence of wheezing and asthma from early childhood to adulthood. Findings indicated that sensitization, especially to multiple allergens, increases the likelihood of development of classic childhood asthma. Persistence to adult asthma is strongly associated with allergic sensitization, greater severity and frequency of symptoms, abnormal lung function, and a greater degree of airway hyperresponsiveness, suggesting that early airway injury may contribute to lifelong disease. Remission is more likely in male subjects and those with less frequent and less severe symptoms, less atopic sensitization, a lesser degree of airway hyperresponsiveness, and no concomitant allergic disease. Treatment successfully controls symptoms, and exacerbations do not appear to change the natural progression of asthma. Drugs are useful while they are taken but are not effective in the long term.

Asthma is more prevalent in African Americans and Hispanics than in Caucasians. It results in death more often in African Americans. However, the differences are usually attributed to urban living and lesser access to health care rather than race or ethnicity.

Many people with asthma have sensitivities to certain drugs that can precipitate acute symptoms of asthma. In about 25% of patients with asthma, aspirin and other nonsteroidal anti-inflammatory drugs (NSAIDs) can precipitate an exacerbation. Research has also demonstrated an increased risk of asthma and its exacerbation with the use of acetaminophen.

Some patients are allergic to sulfites and may experience life-threatening asthma attacks if they ingest foods processed with these preservatives (e.g., beer, wine, dried fruit). Patients with severe asthma should be cautioned against ingesting food and drug products that contain sulfites or metabisulfites. The U.S. Food and Drug Administration (FDA) has banned the use of sulfites on foods meant to be served raw, such as salads in salad bars.

Gastroesophageal reflux disease (GERD), a common disorder characterized by heartburn and esophagitis, is also associated with asthma. Asthma that worsens at night may be associated with nighttime acid reflux. Although the precise mechanism of pulmonary symptoms of GERD in asthma is not known, experts suggest that microaspirations or a vagally mediated, reflex type of bronchoconstriction may be involved. Asthma, in turn, may also aggravate GERD, because antiasthma medications that dilate the airways also relax muscle tone in the gastroesophageal sphincter and may increase acid reflux. The results of randomized trials of acid suppression therapy suggest that gastroesophageal reflux is most likely not a contributor to asthma in patients without esophageal reflux symptoms.

**Work-exacerbated asthma** (WEA) (i.e., adverse respiratory outcomes resulting from repeated and prolonged work-related conditions) is also a major health problem. People with WEA often have symptoms while in the work environment, with improvement on days off and during vacations. Symptoms sometimes persist after termination of exposure. Different types of agents or conditions at work may exacerbate asthma. Cases of WEA with persistent work-related symptoms can have clinical characteristics (level of severity, medication needs) and adverse socioeconomic outcomes (unemployment, reduction in income) similar to those of cases of occupational asthma. Compared with adults with asthma unrelated to work, people with WEA report more days with symptoms, seek more medical care, and have a lower quality of life.

Management of WEA should focus on reducing work exposures and optimizing standard medical management, with a change in jobs only if these measures are not successful. Additional research is needed (1) to improve the understanding of the risk factors for WEA and its mechanisms and outcomes and (2) to inform and evaluate preventive interventions.

## Pathophysiology

### Asthma

Airway smooth muscle extends from the trachea through the bronchioles. The muscle wraps around the airways in a spiral pattern, and contraction causes a sphincter type of action that can completely occlude the airway lumen. **Bronchospasm (also called bronchoconstriction)** involves strong muscle contractions that narrow the airways. Airway inflammation, mucosal edema, and excessive mucus aggravate bronchoconstriction, and numerous stimuli described previously (in Etiology) may precipitate it. In some people, airway hyperresponsiveness occurs, and the bronchoconstrictive response is exaggerated.

In people with asthma, IgE plays a central role in the mechanism of immediate bronchoconstriction and the influx of inflammatory cells after exposure to an allergen. When lung tissues are exposed to causative stimuli, IgE molecules combine with **mast cells** and basophils, sensitizing them for a hypersensitivity reaction. This rapidly releases substances that mediate a reaction, leading to bronchoconstriction and airway inflammation. Mast cells, which are found throughout the body in connective tissues, are abundant in tissues surrounding capillaries in the lungs. When sensitized mast cells in the lungs or eosinophils in the blood are exposed to allergens or irritants, multiple cytokines and other chemical mediators (e.g., acetylcholine, cyclic guanosine monophosphate [GMP], histamine, interleukins [ILs], leukotrienes, prostaglandins, serotonin) important in allergic inflammation are synthesized and released. These chemicals act directly on target tissues of the airways, causing smooth muscle constriction, increased capillary permeability and fluid leakage, and changes in the mucus-secreting

properties of the airway epithelium. The influx of activated cells—including eosinophils and cytokine-producing T cells into the airway, eosinophil recruitment, mucus production, airway hyperresponsiveness, and remodeling features—contributes to the airway hyperresponsiveness that characterizes an asthma exacerbation.

Bronchoconstrictive substances are antagonized by cyclic adenosine monophosphate (cyclic AMP). Cyclic AMP is an intracellular substance that initiates various intracellular activities, depending on the type of cell. In lung cells, cyclic AMP inhibits release of bronchoconstrictive substances and thus indirectly promotes bronchodilation. In mild to moderate asthma, bronchoconstriction is usually recurrent and reversible, either spontaneously or with drug therapy.

In advanced or severe asthma, airway obstruction becomes less reversible and worsens because chronically inflamed airways undergo structural changes (e.g., fibrosis, enlarged smooth muscle cells, enlarged mucous glands), called "airway remodeling," that inhibit their function.

### Other Bronchoconstrictive Disorders

Other bronchoconstrictive disorders include such conditions as chronic bronchitis and emphysema. Although the pathophysiology of the diseases is different (Box 33.1), experts increasingly recognize that symptoms previously associated with one disorder may be reported in people with another condition. Importantly, people with mixed symptoms appear to have a poorer quality of life, higher mortality, and greater utilization of healthcare services.

## Clinical Manifestations

Asthma is an airway disorder characterized by airway inflammation, bronchoconstriction, and airway hyperresponsiveness to various stimuli. The airway hyperresponsiveness produces an exaggerated contractile response of the airways to stimuli. Resultant symptoms include intermittent dyspnea, wheezing, and cough, with variable expiratory airflow limitations. Wheezing is a high-pitched, whistling sound caused by turbulent airflow through an obstructed airway. Thus, any condition that produces significant airway occlusion can cause wheezing. However, a chronic cough may be the only symptom in some people with asthma. The presence of wheezing or coughing is not a dependable standard for evaluating the severity of an asthma attack.

Patients who use peak expiratory flow rate (PEFR) monitoring can assess the severity of airway constriction through trending of peak flow measurements. In general, a PEFR value 80% or greater of the patient's best PEFR (established when breathing is normal) is considered within a safe range; from 50% to 80% of the PEFR value is a moderate drop; and less than 50% of the patient's best PEFR value is considered a severe reduction in breathing function that requires urgent intervention.

 **QSEN Alert: Safety**

The nurse encourages patients to develop a written asthma action plan with their health care provider to identify the correct action for acute episodes of asthma should symptoms worsen or when the PEFR value is less than 50% of the best PEFR.

*prescriban*  *protocols to follow* — *divise tx plans*   (↓dose titbo)
effective ✓
— *multiple drugs used*

**654**   **Section 6 •** Drugs Affecting the Respiratory System

| **BOX 33.1** | *Other Bronchoconstrictive Disorders: Chronic Bronchitis and Emphysema* |
|---|---|

Chronic bronchitis and emphysema, commonly called chronic obstructive pulmonary disease (COPD), usually develop after long-standing exposure to airway irritants such as cigarette smoke. The conditions are also known as chronic obstructive lung disease (COLD), chronic obstructive airway disease (COAD), or chronic airflow limitation (CAL). In both conditions, bronchoconstriction and inflammation are more constant and less reversible than with asthma. Anatomic and physiologic changes occur over several years and lead to increasing dyspnea, activity intolerance, and reduced quality of life. Chronic bronchitis often leads to emphysema.

**Chronic Bronchitis**

Chronic bronchitis is defined in clinical terms as frequent cough with sputum production for 3 months per year, for two consecutive years. The hallmark of chronic bronchitis is an increase in the number and size of the goblet cells and mucous glands of the airway. This leads to increased mucus in the airways, a factor in narrowing of the airways and causing a cough with sputum. At the cellular level, inflammation infiltrates the airway walls leading to scarring and remodeling that thickens the walls; this further narrows the airways. As chronic bronchitis progresses, there is further thickening and scarring of the wall limitation of airflow.

**Emphysema**

Emphysema is an enlargement and destruction of the alveoli distal to the terminal bronchioles from long-term lung damage and inflammation. The changes to the alveolar walls decrease the surface area available for gas exchange. The elasticity of the lung also decreases leading to loss of supporting structures for the alveoli. Additionally, there is destruction of capillaries feeding the alveoli. The small airways that collapse early during expiration cause trapping of carbon dioxide and ultimate reduction of oxygen exchange at the alveoli.

Symptoms vary in incidence and severity from occasional episodes of mild respiratory distress, with normal functioning between exacerbations, to persistent, daily, or continual respiratory distress if not adequately controlled. Inflammation and damaged airway mucosa are chronically present, even when patients appear symptom free. Acute episodes of asthma may last minutes to hours.

Acute, severe asthma that does not respond to the usual use of bronchodilators and is characterized by severe respiratory distress is called **status asthmaticus**. This life-threatening condition requires emergency treatment due to the high probability of respiratory failure. Patients may show signs of acute breathlessness, chest tightness, agitation, confusion, or an inability to concentrate. In status asthmaticus, the lack of wheezing sound or coughing may indicate severe bronchoconstriction, impaired gas exchange in the lungs, and a worsening of the condition.

# Management

Management of asthma involves prevention of airway inflammation and avoidance of triggers for better symptom control. Because of asthma's significance as a world health problem, numerous agencies have published asthma guidelines related to the diagnosis, management, and education of asthma. Guidelines emphasize the importance of classifying asthma severity and the assessment of asthma control. Overall guidelines for adults and children with asthma (Box 33.2) center on symptom control and risk reduction. Although the focus of the discussion is on drug therapy, the nurse must consider the nonpharmacologic approaches in the management of the disease.

## Nonpharmacologic Approaches

Poor symptom control is a significant predictor of exacerbations of asthma. The nurse should identify any personal or environmental risk factors (e.g., cigarette smoke, mold, dander) that can be treated or modified. Efforts to modify risk factors to decrease the triggers of asthma (e.g., reducing work exposure, avoiding asthma triggers, decreasing stress) could minimize frequency or severity of asthma episodes.

In addition to avoidance of triggers, complementary and alternative medicine (CAM) treatments for asthma may be beneficial. These range from breathing exercises to herbal remedies. However, determining the safety and effectiveness of these therapies is problematic because of a lack of well-designed clinical trials. Overall, a review of asthma studies using a form of CAM therapies found insufficient evidence to support their use as effective asthma treatments; the use of these measures should not supersede or delay management of exacerbations.

## Drug Therapy

Bronchodilators and anti-inflammatory drugs are the pharmacologic cornerstones of asthma management. Bronchodilators used to prevent and treat bronchoconstriction include adrenergics, anticholinergics, and xanthines. Anti-inflammatory drugs, such as corticosteroids, leukotriene modifiers, mast cell stabilizers, and immunosuppressant monoclonal antibodies, are used to prevent and treat inflammation of the airways. Reducing inflammation also reduces bronchoconstriction by decreasing mucosal edema and mucous secretions that narrow airways and by decreasing airway hyperresponsiveness to various stimuli. Table 33.1 lists the drugs used for the treatment of asthma.

Overall, the severity of the disease process and a stepwise approach to the patient's response to therapy largely determine the choice of drug and route of administration. An aerosol, which is given by inhalation, acts directly on the airways. Therefore, people with mild asthma can usually take it in smaller doses, and it produces fewer adverse effects than oral or parenteral drugs. A selective, short-acting, inhaled beta$_2$-adrenergic agonist (e.g., albuterol) is the initial drug of choice for acute bronchospasm. Inflammation is a major component of asthma; thus, health care providers may give an inhaled corticosteroid early in the disease process, often adding a bronchodilator or mast cell stabilizer. In acute episodes of bronchoconstriction, prescribers often order that a corticosteroid be taken orally or intravenously for several days.

| BOX 33.2 | *Overall Guidelines for the Treatment of Asthma* |
| --- | --- |

## Goals of Therapy

- Minimal or no chronic symptoms day or night
- Minimal or no exacerbations or persistent airflow limitations
- Maintain normal activity levels; for children, no school/parent's work missed
- Minimal use of short-acting inhaled beta$_2$-agonist (less than one time per day, less than one canister per month)
- Minimal or no adverse effects from medications
- Minimize the risk of asthma-related deaths

## General Recommendations

- Establish and teach patients/parents/caregivers about quick-relief measures and long-term control measures. Assist to identify and control environmental factors that aggravate asthma. For acute attacks, gain control as quickly as possible (a short course of systemic corticosteroids may be needed); then step down to the least medication necessary to maintain control.
- Review the treatment regimen every 1 to 6 months. If control is adequate and goals are being met, a gradual stepwise reduction in medication may be possible. If control is inadequate, the treatment regimen may need to be changed. For example, frequent or increasing use of a short-acting beta$_2$-agonist (greater than two times a week with intermittent asthma; daily or increasing use with persistent asthma) may indicate the need to initiate or increase long-term control therapy. However, first reassess patients' medication techniques (e.g., correct use of inhalers), adherence, and environmental control measures.
- Maintain a good partnership between person with asthma and caregiver, and health care providers. Set mutually agreed to goals for individualized care, create written asthma action plan, and encourage self-management.

## Preferred Controller Relief (Adjusted Based on Individual Need and Response to Management)

- **Adults and children older than 5 years:** low-dose inhaled corticosteroid plus short-acting beta$_2$-agonist is preferred. Alternative options include leukotriene antagonist daily. A combination of inhaled steroids and long-acting beta$_2$-agonists leads to faster improvement than inhaled steroid use alone, increases lung function, improves quality of life, and reduces the risk of asthma-related hospitalization or death.
- **Children aged 5 years or younger:** administration of the daily low-dose inhaled corticosteroid by a nebulizer or metered-dose inhaler (MDI) with a holding chamber. Alternatives: a leukotriene modifier or intermittent inhaled corticosteroid.

## Rescuer Relief for Acute Exacerbations

- **Adults and children older than 5 years:** increase usual controller-double low-dose inhaled corticosteroid, short-acting, inhaled, beta$_2$-agonist started or increased, as needed.
- **Children aged 5 years or younger:** double low-dose inhaled corticosteroid short-acting beta$_2$-agonist by nebulizer or face mask and spacer or holding chamber.

### Low (L), Medium (M), and High (H) Doses of Inhaled Corticosteroids

| | Adults (mcg) | Children (6–11 y) (mcg) |
| --- | --- | --- |
| Beclomethasone (CFC) | L: 200–500<br>M: >500–1000<br>H: >1000 | L: 100–200<br>M: >200–400<br>H: >400 |
| Beclomethasone (HFA) | L: 100–200<br>M: 200–400<br>H: >400 | L: 50–100<br>M: >100–200<br>H: >200 |
| Budesonide (DPI) | L: 200–400<br>M: 400–800<br>H: >800 | L: 100–200<br>M: >200–400<br>H: >400 |
| Budesonide (nebules) | L: n/a<br>M: n/a<br>H: >n/a | L: 250–500<br>M: >500–1000<br>H: >1000 |
| Ciclesonide (HFA) | L: 80–160<br>M: >160–320<br>H: >320 | L: 80<br>M: >80–160<br>H: >160 |
| Fluticasone furoate (DPI) | L: 100<br>M: n/a<br>H: >200 | L: n/a<br>M: n/a<br>H: >n/a |
| Fluticasone propionate (DPI) | L: 100–250<br>M: >250–500<br>H: >500 | L: 100–200<br>M: 200–400<br>H: >400 |
| Fluticasone propionate (HFA) | L: 100–250<br>M: >250–500<br>H: >500 | L: 100–200<br>M: >200–500<br>H: >500 |
| Mometasone furoate | L: 110–220<br>M: >220–440<br>H: >440 | L: 110<br>M: >220–440<br>H: >440 |
| Triamcinolone acetonide | L: 400–1000<br>M: >1000–2000<br>H: >2000 | L: 400–800<br>M: >800–1200<br>H: >1200 |

CFC, chlorofluorocarbon propellant; DPI, dry powder inhaler; HFA, hydrofluoroalkane propellant; n/a, not applicable.

## TABLE 33.1

## Drugs Administered for the Treatment of Asthma

| Drug Class | Prototype | Other Drugs in the Class |
|---|---|---|
| Adrenergics | Albuterol (Proventil HFA, Ventolin HFA, ProAir RespiClick) | Epinephrine (Adrenalin)<br>Formoterol (Foradil)<br>Levalbuterol (Xopenex [MDI], Xopenex Concentrate, Xopenex HFA)<br>Metaproterenol (Alupent)<br>Salmeterol (Serevent)<br>Terbutaline |
| Anticholinergics | Ipratropium bromide (Atrovent) | Tiotropium (Spiriva) |
| Xanthines | Theophylline (Elixophyllin, Theo-24, Theochron) | |
| Corticosteroids | Beclomethasone (Qvar RediHaler Beconase AQ, QVAR) | Budesonide (Pulmicort Turbuhaler)<br>Ciclesonide<br>Flunisolide (Aerospan)<br>Fluticasone (Flonase)<br>Fluticasone aerosol (Flovent)<br>Fluticasone powder (Flovent Rota disk)<br>Mometasone (Asmanex Twisthaler, Nasonex)<br>Triamcinolone (Azmacort)<br>Hydrocortisone sodium phosphate and sodium succinate<br>Prednisone<br>Methylprednisolone sodium succinate |
| Leukotriene modifiers | Montelukast (Singulair) | Zafirlukast (Accolate)<br>Zileuton (Zyflo, Zyflo CR) |
| Immunosuppressant monoclonal antibodies | Omalizumab (Xolair) | Mepolizumab (Nucala)<br>Reslizumab (Cinqair)<br>Benralizumab (Fasenra) |
| Adjuvant medications | | |
| Mast cell stabilizer | | Cromolyn (NasalCrom) |

 **QSEN Alert: Evidence-Based Practice**

Evidence indicates that pregnant women with uncontrolled asthma experience problems in pregnancy [preeclampsia, preterm birth, low birth weight infants, increased risk of perinatal mortality]. Therefore, it is important to maintain optimal control of asthma in women prior to and during pregnancy. Well-controlled asthma during pregnancy creates little or no increased risk of adverse fetal or maternal complications [GINA, 2019].

The standard regimen for treatment of persistent moderate asthma is an inhaled corticosteroid on a regular schedule, two to four times daily, and a short-acting, inhaled beta$_2$-adrenergic agonist as needed for prevention or treatment of bronchoconstriction. For long-term asthma control, long-acting beta$_2$-agonists should be used in combination with inhaled corticosteroids and not as monotherapy. For more severe asthma, therapy may involve continuation of the inhaled corticosteroid with both a short-acting and a long-acting beta$_2$-agonist. The possible addition of a leukotriene modifier may also further control symptoms and reduce the need for corticosteroids and inhaled bronchodilators.

Management of status asthmaticus entails beta$_2$-agonists in high doses and as often as every 20 minutes for 1 to 2 hours (by metered-dose inhalers [MDIs] with spacer devices or by compressed-air nebulization). However, high doses of nebulized albuterol have been associated with tachycardia, hypokalemia, and hyperglycemia. After symptoms have subsided, dosage reduction usually may occur, with extended dosage intervals. People may take high doses of systemic corticosteroids for several days, intravenously or orally. If the patient is able to take an oral drug, there is no therapeutic advantage to intravenous (IV) administration.

 **QSEN Alert: Safety**

Because asthma can result in death in a matter of minutes, health care providers should counsel patients not to use dietary or herbal supplements in place of prescribed bronchodilating and anti-inflammatory medications. Delays in appropriate treatment can have serious, even fatal, consequences.

## ADRENERGICS

Specific effects of adrenergic medications depend mainly on the type of adrenergic receptor activated by the drug. Adrenergic receptors are those responses that are activated by adrenaline-like compounds. The drugs discussed in this chapter are more selective for specific adrenergic receptors or are primarily administered by inhalation to produce more localized therapeutic effects in the management of asthma and bronchoconstriction and thus have fewer systemic adverse effects.

Other adrenergic drugs affect multiple adrenergic receptors and have many clinical uses; other chapters discuss these drugs more extensively (see Chaps. 31 and 59).

Administering bronchodilators by inhalation (via nebulizer or MDI) is most effective and the treatment of first choice to relieve acute asthma. Two general types of inhaled beta$_2$-adrenergic agonists are used for asthma management: **rescue inhalant medications** (quick-relief, short-acting drugs) used during periods of acute symptoms and exacerbations and **maintenance inhalant medications** (long-term control drugs used to achieve and maintain prophylactic control of persistent asthma). Box 33.3 lists the rescue and maintenance medications used in asthma therapy. Ⓟ **Albuterol** (Proventil HFA, Ventolin HFA, ProAir RespiClick), the prototype adrenergic bronchodilator, is a rescue medication.

*safe in all age groups*

## Pharmacokinetics

Albuterol is rapidly absorbed following oral administration. With the oral drug, the onset of action is 15 to 30 minutes (extended release, 30 minutes), the peak is 2 to 3 hours, and the duration of action is 8 to 12 hours. With an MDI, the onset of action is 5 to 15 minutes, the peak activity is 1 to 1½ hours, and the duration of action is 3 to 6 hours. The drug quickly undergoes extensive metabolism in the liver. It enters breast milk.

## Action

Albuterol and other drugs in the class stimulate beta$_2$-adrenergic receptors in the smooth muscle of bronchi and bronchioles.

---

**BOX 33.3**  *Rescue and Maintenance Beta$_2$-Agonist Inhaled Medications*

**Short-Acting Rescue Medications**
- Albuterol
- Metaproterenol
- Levalbuterol
- Albuterol/ipratropium (combines a beta$_2$-agonist and an inhaled anticholinergic)

**Long-Acting Maintenance Medications**
- Formoterol
- Salmeterol
- Salmeterol/fluticasone (combines a beta$_2$-agonist bronchodilator and an inhaled steroid)
- Formoterol/budesonide (combines a beta$_2$-agonist bronchodilator and an inhaled steroid)
- Formoterol/mometasone (combines a beta$_2$-agonist bronchodilator and an inhaled steroid)

---

The receptors, in turn, stimulate the enzyme adenylyl cyclase to increase production of cyclic AMP. The increased cyclic AMP produces bronchodilation.

## Use

Health care providers use albuterol to treat or prevent bronchospasm in people with asthma and other reversible obstructive airway disease. They also use the drug to prevent exercise-induced bronchospasm. Table 33.2 gives route and dosage information for albuterol and other adrenergic bronchodilators. In general, children and adolescents may take antiasthmatic medications for the same indications as for adults.

### Use in Older Adults

Older adults often have chronic pulmonary disorders for which albuterol and other bronchodilators are used.

---

**❗ QSEN Alert: Safety**

The main risks with adrenergic bronchodilators, particularly in older adults, are excessive cardiac and central nervous system (CNS) stimulation.

---

As with other populations, administering the medications by inhalation and giving the lowest effective dose decrease adverse effects.

### Use in Patients With Critical Illness

People who are critically ill often use albuterol. Larger doses of bronchodilators (inhaled, systemic, or both) are usually required to relieve the symptoms of acute, severe bronchoconstriction, or status asthmaticus. Then, it is necessary to reduce doses to the smallest effective amounts to attain the most therapeutic effects and produce the fewest adverse effects.

### Use in Patients Receiving Home Care

Home administration of albuterol is common. Visits by a home care nurse should include assessment that the patient follows directions for administration; is not taking the drug more often than prescribed; is using the inhaler correctly; and is not manifesting signs of adverse effects, including excessive cardiac and CNS stimulation.

## Adverse Effects ♡ caution

Administration of albuterol by MDI is associated with fewer systemic effects than administration of higher dosages orally or by nebulizer. Muscle tremor is the most frequent adverse effect. Major adverse effects are excessive cardiac and CNS stimulation. Symptoms of cardiac stimulation include angina, tachycardia, and palpitations. Symptoms of CNS stimulation consist of agitation, anxiety, insomnia, seizures, and tremors. Other reported effects may include serious dysrhythmias and cardiac arrest.

## Contraindications

Contraindications to albuterol include known hypersensitivity to the drug, as well as cardiac tachydysrhythmias and severe

*Watch in cardiac patients*

## TABLE 33.2

## DRUGS AT A GLANCE: Adrenergic Bronchodilators

| Drug | Pregnancy Category | Routes and Dosage Ranges | |
|---|---|---|---|
| | | **Adults** | **Children** |
| Ⓟ **Albuterol** (Proventil HFA, Ventolin HFA, ProAir RespiClick; ✹ Airomir, Ventolin Discus, Ventolin HFA, Ventolin I.V. Infusion, Ventolin Nebules P.F.) | C | Inhalation* aerosol (90 mcg/actuation), 2 oral inhalations every 4–6 h; prevention of exercise-induced bronchospasm, 2 inhalations 5 min before exercise<br>Inhalation solution via nebulizer, 2.5 mg 3–4 times daily (in 2.5 mL sterile saline, over 5–15 min)<br>Regular tablets, 2–4 mg PO 3–4 times daily extended-release tablets, 4–8 mg PO every 12 h initially; increase if necessary to a max of 32 mg/d, in divided doses, every 12 h | Inhalation aerosol (90 mcg/actuation); ≥4 y, 4–8 puffs every 20 min for 3 doses then every 1–4 h; adolescents, 4–8 puffs every 20 min for up to 4 h and then every 1–4 h<br>Nebulizer solution, 12 y and older, same as adults; 2–12 y, 1.5 mg/kg (min dose 2.5 mg) every 20 min for 3 doses then 0.15–0.3 mg/kg to max of 10 mg every 1–4 h<br>Immediate-release tablets or syrup, 2–6 y 0.1–0.2 mg/kg/dose three times daily to max dose of 4 mg; 6–12 y, 2 mg 3–4 times daily; 12 y and older, same as adults; sustained-release tablets, ≥6 y, 0.3–0.6 mg/kg/d divided twice daily to max of 8 mg/d; 12 y and older, same as adults; 6–12 y, 4 mg PO every 12 h initially, increase if necessary to a max of 8 mg/dose twice daily |
| Epinephrine (Asthmanefrin Refill, S2; ✹ S2) | C | Nebulization, racemic (2.25% solution); OTC labeling hand-bulb nebulizer, add 0.5 mL to nebulizer, 1–3 inhalations; dose may be repeated after 3 h, if necessary, for 3 doses to max of 12 inhalations in 24 h | ≥4 y, inhalation, same as adults |
| Formoterol (Perforomist; ✹ Foradil, Oxeze Turbuhaler) | C | Nebulizer, 20 mcg/2 mL vial every 12 h | Perforomist not recommended in children |
| Levalbuterol (Xopenex [MDI], Xopenex Concentrate, Xopenex HFA) | C | Nebulizer, 0.63–1.25 mg 3 times daily, every 6–8 h to max of 2 inhalations every 4 h<br>MDI, 2 puffs every 4–6 h | ≤4 y, 0.31–1.25 mg every 4–6 h as needed<br>5–11 y, 0.31–0.63 mg every 8 h as needed<br>MDI ≤ 4 y and older, same as adults |
| Metaproterenol (✹ Orciprenaline) | C | PO, 20 mg 3–4 times/d | PO, <6 y 1.3–2.6 mg/kg/d divided every 6–8 h<br>6–9 y (or <27 kg), 10 mg/dose 3–4 times/d<br>>9 y (or ≥27 kg), same as adults |
| Salmeterol (Serevent Diskus; ✹ Serevent Diskhaler Disk, Serevent Diskus) | C | Inhalation powder, 1 inhalation (50 mcg) every 12 h | Inhalation powder: ≥4 y and older, same as adults |
| Terbutaline (✹ Bricanyl Turbohaler) | B | 2.5–5 mg PO every 6–8 h; max dose, 15 mg/d<br>0.25 mg sub-Q, repeated every 20 min to 3 h; hold with pulse >120 beats/min | <12 y, PO 0.05 mg/kg/dose 3 times/d to max of 0.15 mg/kg/dose 3–4 times/d or a total of 5 mg/24 h<br>12–15 y, 2.5 mg PO 3 times/d; max dose, 7.5 mg/d<br><12 y, sub-Q 0.005–0.01 mg/kg/dose to max of 0.4 mg/dose every 15–20 min for 3 doses; may repeat every 2–6 h as needed.<br>≥12 y, same as adults |

*Short-acting adrenergic bronchodilators are used mainly by inhalation, as needed, rather than on a regular schedule; MDI, metered-dose inhaler.

coronary artery disease. Caution is warranted in hypertension, hyperthyroidism, diabetes mellitus, and seizure disorders.

## Nursing Implications

### Preventing Interactions

Some drugs interact with albuterol. Beta-adrenergic blockers inhibit bronchodilation and can induce bronchospasm in patients with asthma who are taking albuterol. Thyroid hormones, theophylline, and some cold products can enhance the stimulatory adverse effects of the drug. Monoamine oxidase inhibitors should be avoided within 14 days of initiating treatment with albuterol to prevent hypertensive crisis. Caffeine-containing products, such as coffee, tea, or cola drinks, can also increase the adverse effects of cardiac and CNS stimulation.

### Administering the Medication

Self-administration of albuterol and the other beta$_2$-agonists is usually by MDI. Patients should use an albuterol inhaler before they use any other inhaler. This opens the airways and allows for better absorption of the other drug. The patient should wait 5 minutes or more between using different inhalers, such as one for a corticosteroid. Although most drug references still give a regular dosing schedule (e.g., every 4–6 hours) for beta$_2$-

agonists, asthma experts recommend that the drugs be used when needed (e.g., to treat acute dyspnea or prevent dyspnea during exercise). With overuse, they lose their bronchodilating effects because the beta$_2$-adrenergic receptors become unresponsive to stimulation. (However, this tolerance does not occur with the long-acting beta$_2$-agonists.)

### Assessing for Therapeutic Effects

The nurse observes for decreased dyspnea, wheezing, and respiratory secretions; relief of bronchospasm and wheezing; reduced rate and improved quality of respirations and pulmonary function; and reduced anxiety and restlessness.

### Assessing for Adverse Effects

The nurse observes for tachycardia, dysrhythmias, palpitations, restlessness, agitation, and insomnia. These signs and symptoms result from cardiac and CNS stimulation.

### Patient Teaching

In addition, the nurse helps patients recognize acute asthma attacks and have a plan to treat (or seek help for) exacerbations before respiratory distress becomes severe. Box 33.4 summarizes patient teaching guidelines for antiasthmatic drugs, including albuterol.

---

**BOX 33.4** · *Patient Teaching Guidelines for Antiasthmatic Drugs*

**General Considerations**

- The symptoms of asthma and other chronic lung diseases frequently overlap and are characterized by constant inflammation of the airways and periodic or persistent labored breathing from constriction or narrowing of the airways. Antiasthmatic drugs are often given in combination to combat these problems. Thus, it is extremely important to know the type and purpose of each drug.

- Except for the short-acting, inhaled bronchodilators (e.g., albuterol), antiasthmatic medications are used long term to control symptoms and prevent acute asthma attacks. This means they must be taken on a regular schedule and continued when symptom free.

- When an asthma attack (i.e., acute bronchospasm with shortness of breath, wheezing respirations, cough) occurs, a fast-acting, inhaled, short-acting bronchodilator (e.g., albuterol) is commonly used to relieve these symptoms. In addition, because most exacerbations are associated with added inflammation, inhaled corticosteroids are frequently increased.

- Try to prevent symptoms. For example, respiratory infections can precipitate difficulty in breathing. Avoiding infections (e.g., by good hand hygiene, avoiding people with infections, annual influenza vaccinations, and other measures) can prevent acute asthma attacks. If you are allergic to tobacco smoke, perfume, or flowers, try to avoid or minimize exposure. Other substances that irritate breathing passages may include aerosol hair spray, antiperspirants, cleaning products, and automobile exhaust.

A common cause of acute asthma attacks is not taking medications correctly. Some studies indicate that one third to two thirds of patients with asthma do not comply with instructions for using their medications. For instance, multiple studies have reported that less than one half of the patients use their inhaler correctly. Factors that contribute to nonadherence with drug therapy include long-term use, expense, and adverse effects. If you have difficulty taking medications as prescribed, discuss the situation with a health care provider. Cheaper medications or lower doses may be effective alternatives. Just stopping the medications may precipitate acute breathing problems.

- If unable to prevent symptoms, early recognition and treatment may help prevent severe distress and hospitalizations. A written asthma action plan can help with decision-making at the onset of acute exacerbation.

- Signs of impending difficulty include increased needs for bronchodilator inhalers, activity limitations, waking at night because of asthma symptoms, and variability in the PEFR, if you use a PEFR meter at home. The first treatment is to use a short-acting, inhaled bronchodilator. If this does not improve breathing, seek emergency care.

- Keep adequate supplies of medications on hand. Missing a few doses of long-term control or "preventive" medications may precipitate an acute asthma attack; not using an inhaled bronchodilator for early breathing difficulty may lead to more severe problems and the need for emergency treatment or hospitalization.

[Continued on page 660]

*Read!*

- Be sure you can use your metered-dose inhalers correctly. Drinking 2 to 3 quarts of fluids, as appropriate, daily helps thin secretions in the throat and lungs and makes them easier to remove.

- Avoid excessive intake of caffeine-containing fluids such as coffee, tea, and cola drinks. These beverages may increase bronchodilation but also may increase heart rate and cause palpitations, nervousness, and insomnia with bronchodilating drugs.

- Obtain an influenza vaccine annually and a pneumococcal vaccine at least once if you have chronic lung disease.

- Inform all health care providers about the medications you are taking and do not take over-the-counter drugs or herbal supplements without consulting a health care provider. Some drugs can decrease beneficial effects or increase adverse effects of antiasthmatic medications. For example, over-the-counter nasal decongestants, asthma remedies, cold remedies, and antisleep medications can increase the rapid heartbeat, palpitations, and nervousness often associated with bronchodilators. With herbal remedies, none are as effective as standard antiasthmatic medication, and they may cause serious or life-threatening adverse effects.

### Self-Administration

- Follow instructions carefully. Better breathing with minimal adverse effects depends on accurate use of prescribed medications. If help is needed with metered-dose inhalers, consult a health care provider.

- Use short-acting bronchodilator inhalers as needed, not on a regular schedule. If desired effects are not achieved or if symptoms worsen, inform your prescriber. Do not increase dosage or frequency of taking medication. Overuse increases adverse drug effects and decreases drug effectiveness.

- If taking formoterol or salmeterol, which are long-acting, inhaled bronchodilators, do not use more often than every 12 hours. If constricted breathing occurs, use a short-acting bronchodilator inhaler between doses of

a long-acting drug. Salmeterol does not relieve acute shortness of breath because it takes approximately 20 minutes to start acting and 1 to 4 hours to achieve maximal bronchodilating effects.

- If taking an oral or inhaled corticosteroid, take on a regular schedule, at approximately the same time each day. The purpose of these drugs is to relieve inflammation in the airways and prevent acute respiratory distress. They are not effective unless taken regularly.

- If taking oral theophylline, take fast-acting preparations before meals with a full glass of water, at regular intervals around the clock. If gastrointestinal upset occurs, take with food. Take long-acting preparations every 8 to 12 hours; do not chew or crush.

- Take zafirlukast 1 hour before or 2 hours after a meal; montelukast and immediate-release zileuton may be taken with or without food. Extended-release zileuton should be taken with food. Take montelukast in the evening or at bedtime. This schedule provides maximum beneficial effects during the night and early morning, when asthma symptoms often occur or worsen.

- Use inhalers correctly:
  1. Shake well immediately before each use.
  2. Remove the cap from the mouthpiece.
  3. Exhale to the end of a normal breath.
  4. With the inhaler in the upright position, place the mouthpiece just inside the mouth, and use the lips to form a tight seal or hold the mouthpiece approximately two finger widths from the open mouth.
  5. While pressing down on the inhaler, take a slow, deep breath for 3 to 5 seconds, hold the breath for approximately 10 seconds, and exhale slowly.
  6. Wait 3 to 5 minutes before taking a second inhalation of the drug.
  7. Rinse the mouth with water after each use.
  8. Rinse the mouthpiece and store the inhaler away from heat.
  9. If you have difficulty using an inhaler, ask your provider about a spacer device (a tube attached to the inhaler that makes it easier to use).

---

 **QSEN Alert: Safety**

It is essential to ensure that the patient has an adequate supply of albuterol for self-administration.

## Other Drugs in the Class

Epinephrine (Adrenalin) is an adrenergic that may be injected subcutaneously in an acute attack of bronchoconstriction, with therapeutic rescue effects in approximately 5 minutes and lasting for approximately 4 hours. However, an inhaled selective beta2-agonist is the drug of choice in this situation. Delivery by aerosol or nebulization of other selective beta2-agonists is effective, even to young children and to patients on mechanical ventilation, and there is seldom a need to give epinephrine or other nonselective adrenergic drugs by injection. Cardiac stimulation

is an adverse effect of bronchodilators, and in addition to beta2 receptor stimulation, epinephrine also stimulates beta1-adrenergic receptors in the heart to increase the rate and force of contraction.

Most prescription inhalers use hydrofluoroalkane (HFA) as a propellant.

Levalbuterol (Xopenex, Xopenex Concentrate, Xopenex [HFA]) is a short-acting beta2-adrenergic agonist used for prevention and treatment of bronchoconstriction. Formoterol (Foradil) and salmeterol (Serevent) are long-acting beta2-adrenergic agonists used only for prophylaxis of acute bronchoconstriction. They are not effective in acute attacks because they have a slower onset of action than the short-acting drugs (up to 20 minutes for salmeterol). Effects last 12 hours and the drugs should not be taken more frequently. If additional bronchodilating medication is needed, a short-acting agent (e.g., albuterol) should be used. The FDA has issued a BLACK BOX WARNING ◆ indicating that initiating salmeterol in people with significantly worsening or acutely deteriorating asthma may be life threatening.

Metaproterenol is a relatively selective, intermediate-acting beta$_2$-adrenergic agonist that may be given orally or by MDI. It is used to treat acute bronchospasm and to prevent exercise-induced asthma. In high doses, metaproterenol loses some of its selectivity and may cause cardiac and CNS stimulation.

Terbutaline is a relatively selective beta$_2$-adrenergic agonist and a long-acting bronchodilator. The drug is usually well tolerated, and when symptoms occur, they are minor and require little or no treatment. Common adverse effects include shakiness, drowsiness, and headaches. When given subcutaneously, terbutaline loses its selectivity and has little advantage over epinephrine. The drug is used to treat preterm labor, although it is not approved for this use, has not been shown to be effective, and causes some safety concerns. The nurse should be aware of the FDA's recommendation that oral and injectable terbutaline should not be used for prevention or treatment of preterm labor.

### Clinical Application 33.1

- Mr. Lee may experience adverse effects if albuterol is administered as ordered. For what signs and symptoms should the nurse be alert?
- Mr. Lee's wife is at his bedside. She expresses concern about his treatment with IV corticosteroids, stating that she has heard that many adverse effects are associated with these drugs. Discuss the rationale for the use of IV corticosteroids in this case.

## ANTICHOLINERGICS

The anticholinergic bronchodilators are most useful in the long-term management of asthma and other conditions producing bronchoconstriction, such as chronic bronchitis and emphysema. (For additional information about these drugs, see Chap. 48.) The two drugs in the class, the prototype ℗ **ipratropium** (Atrovent) and tiotropium, are ineffective in relieving acute bronchospasm by themselves, and they act synergistically with other adrenergic bronchodilators. Prescribers may order them for concomitant use. The drugs improve lung function about 10% to 15% over an inhaled beta$_2$-agonist alone.

### Pharmacokinetics

Ipratropium is rapidly absorbed via inhalation with an onset of action within 5 to 15 minutes, a peak effect in 1½ to 2 hours, and a duration of action of 2 to 5 hours. Absorption of the drug is negligible, with excretion in the kidneys and in the feces. Only about 15% of the drug reaches the lower airways.

### Action

Ipratropium is chemically related to atropine and blocks the muscarinic acetylcholine receptors in the smooth muscles of the bronchi in the lungs, inhibiting bronchoconstriction and mucus secretion.

### Use

Originally, ipratropium was formulated to be taken by inhalation for maintenance therapy of bronchoconstriction associated with asthma, chronic bronchitis, and emphysema. Improved pulmonary function usually occurs in a few minutes. Other uses include treatment of rhinorrhea associated with allergic rhinitis and the common cold. Table 33.3 presents route and dosage information for anticholinergics such as ipratropium.

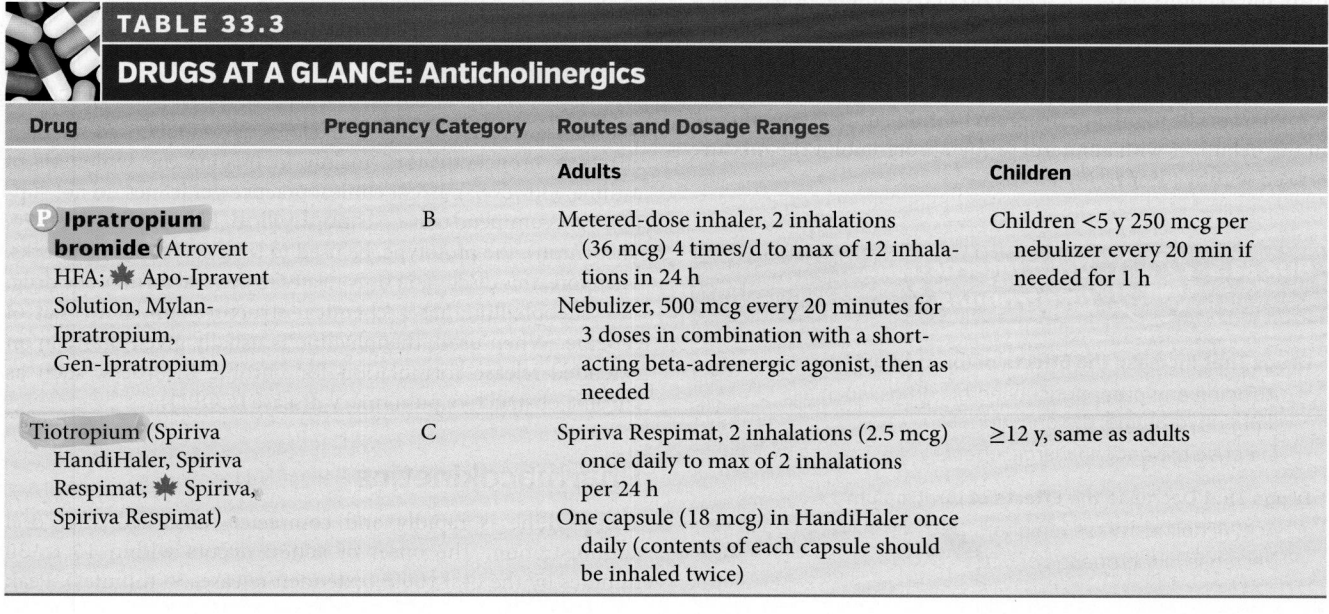

### TABLE 33.3

### DRUGS AT A GLANCE: Anticholinergics

| Drug | Pregnancy Category | Routes and Dosage Ranges | |
|---|---|---|---|
| | | **Adults** | **Children** |
| ℗ **Ipratropium bromide** (Atrovent HFA; ✳ Apo-Ipravent Solution, Mylan-Ipratropium, Gen-Ipratropium) | B | Metered-dose inhaler, 2 inhalations (36 mcg) 4 times/d to max of 12 inhalations in 24 h<br>Nebulizer, 500 mcg every 20 minutes for 3 doses in combination with a short-acting beta-adrenergic agonist, then as needed | Children <5 y 250 mcg per nebulizer every 20 min if needed for 1 h |
| Tiotropium (Spiriva HandiHaler, Spiriva Respimat; ✳ Spiriva, Spiriva Respimat) | C | Spiriva Respimat, 2 inhalations (2.5 mcg) once daily to max of 2 inhalations per 24 h<br>One capsule (18 mcg) in HandiHaler once daily (contents of each capsule should be inhaled twice) | ≥12 y, same as adults |

### Use in Patients With Critical Illness

Ipratropium can be used in the critical care setting, but it is ineffective in relieving acute bronchospasm. The drug may work synergistically with other adrenergic bronchodilators, and concomitant use may be effective. In patients who are critically ill, administering by nebulization may be necessary.

### Use in Patients Receiving Home Care

Ipratropium is used in the home setting. The drug poses minimal risk of adverse effects. A major role of the home care nurse is to assist patients in using the inhaled drug safely and effectively. Several studies have indicated that many people do not use MDIs and other inhalation devices correctly. If possible, the home care nurse needs to observe a patient using an inhalation device. If the nurse detects errors in technique, further education may be necessary. With inhaled medications, a spacer device may be useful, especially for children and older adults, because less muscle coordination is required to administer a dose. Adverse effects may be minimized, as well.

## Adverse Effects

Absorption of ipratropium is poor, and it produces few systemic effects. The most common adverse effects are cough, nervousness, nausea, gastrointestinal (GI) upset, headache, and dizziness.

## Contraindications

Ipratropium is contraindicated with known hypersensitivity to the drug or to atropine and related substances. Caution is recommended with use in patients with narrow-angle glaucoma, prostatic hypertrophy, and bladder neck obstruction because ipratropium can worsen these conditions.

## Nursing Implications

### Preventing Interactions

In general, ipratropium has been shown to have limited drug–drug interactions (Box 33.5) and no herbal interactions. When given as a nasal spray, no interactions reportedly occur.

### Administering the Medication

It is appropriate to mix ipratropium bromide inhalation solution in the nebulizer with albuterol or metaproterenol if the mixture is used within 1 hour.

---

**BOX 33.5** **Drug Interactions: Ipratropium**

**Drugs That Increase the Effects of Ipratropium**

- Atropine and other anticholinergic drugs, such as diphenhydramine, dimenhydrinate
  *Increase the anticholinergic effects*

**Drugs That Decrease the Effects of Ipratropium**

- Acetylcholinesterase inhibitors
  *Decrease in therapeutic effect*

---

### QSEN Alert: Safety

Administering anticholinergic drugs via the respiratory route instead of the systemic route results in less thickening of respiratory secretions and therefore a reduced incidence of mucus-plugged airways.

### Assessing for Therapeutic Effects

The nurse assesses for a reduced rate and improved quality of respirations and pulmonary function. The patient should report that breathing has improved and anxiety is reduced.

### Assessing for Adverse Effects

The nurse observes for the presence of a cough, nervousness, nausea, GI upset, headache, and dizziness.

### Patient Teaching

Box 33.4 summarizes patient teaching guidelines for antiasthmatic drugs such as ipratropium.

## Other Drugs in the Class

*[handwritten: at Hospital but Not gonna test on it]*

Tiotropium (Spiriva) is a long-acting, 24-hour, anticholinergic bronchodilator taken once daily by inhalation for maintenance therapy of bronchoconstriction associated with chronic bronchitis and emphysema. A muscarinic receptor antagonist, it is closely related to ipratropium but is not used for acute bronchospasm exacerbations. The drug has different pharmacokinetic and pharmacologic properties from ipratropium, and these differences may make it superior to ipratropium as an anticholinergic agent. A patient who is taking ipratropium should not take tiotropium. The primary adverse effect of tiotropium is dry mouth. Other effects include headache, dizziness, abdominal pain, constipation, diarrhea, flulike symptoms, and chest pain.

When taking tiotropium, the person places a capsule in a piercing chamber (HandiHaler) and then inhales the medication through the mouthpiece. It is necessary to repeat inhalations two to three times to ensure that the entire dose is received. When the drug is properly administered, the device makes a distinctive flutter or rattle.

## XANTHINES

The xanthines are a group of alkaloids commonly used for their effects as bronchodilators, mainly in treating the symptoms of asthma. However, current clinical practice guidelines do not support or recommend that **theophylline** (Elixophyllin, Theo-24, Theochron), the prototype, be used to treat acute asthma attacks. Therefore, this discussion only relates to the oral form of the drug.

Theophylline has a chemical structure similar to that of caffeine. When used, theophylline is usually given orally in an extended-release formulation for chronic disorders, such as chronic obstructive pulmonary disease (COPD).

## Pharmacokinetics

Theophylline is rapidly and completely absorbed after oral administration. The onset of action occurs within 15 to 30 minutes by the oral route (extended release, 30 minutes). Peak levels occur in 1 to 2 hours, and the duration of action is 4 to 6 hours (extended release, 12 hours). Metabolism in the liver is extensive. Excretion of metabolites and some unchanged drug involves the kidneys. The drug crosses the placenta, and it enters breast milk.

## Action

Theophylline works by relaxing bronchial smooth muscle, promoting bronchodilation. Additionally, the drug suppresses airway responsiveness to stimuli that trigger bronchospasm.

## Use

Theophylline was formerly used extensively in the prevention and treatment of bronchoconstriction associated with asthma, bronchitis, and emphysema. Now considered a second-line oral agent, a health care provider may add it to a regimen for severe disease that is inadequately controlled by first-line drugs. Most formulations contain anhydrous theophylline (100% theophylline) as the active ingredient, and sustained-action tablets (e.g., Theochron) are more commonly used than other formulations.

To determine theophylline dosage, prescribers should measure serum theophylline levels (therapeutic range is 5–15 mcg/mL; toxic levels are 20 mcg/mL or above). It is necessary to draw blood for serum levels 1 to 2 hours after patients have taken immediate-release dosage forms and about 4 hours after they have taken sustained-release forms. In addition, children and cigarette smokers usually need higher doses to maintain therapeutic blood levels because they metabolize theophylline rapidly, and patients with liver disease, congestive heart failure, COPD, or acute viral infections usually need smaller doses because these conditions impair theophylline metabolism. For obese patients, prescribers should calculate theophylline dosage on the basis of lean or ideal body weight because theophylline is not highly distributed in fatty tissue. Table 33.4 gives the route and dosage information for oral theophylline.

### Use in Children

Use of theophylline necessitates close monitoring because dosage needs and rates of metabolism vary widely. In children younger than 6 months of age, especially premature infants and neonates, drug elimination may be prolonged because of immature liver function. Experts do not recommend use of theophylline preparations in such young children, except for preterm infants with apnea.

Children 6 months to 16 years of age (approximately) metabolize theophylline more rapidly than younger or older patients. Thus, they may need higher doses than adults in proportion to size and weight. Authorities do not recommend long-acting dosage forms for use in children younger than 6 years of age. Children may become hyperactive and disruptive from the CNS-stimulating effects of theophylline. Tolerance to these effects usually develops with continued use of the drug.

### Use in Older Adults

It is important to monitor older patients who use theophylline carefully because effects of the drug are unpredictable. Typically, older adults require reduced doses.

### Use in Patients With Renal Impairment

Patients with renal impairment can take the usual doses of theophylline, but monitoring of serum drug levels is necessary.

### Use in Patients With Hepatic Impairment

Metabolism of theophylline takes place in the liver. This means that impaired liver function and decreased blood flow to the liver decrease metabolism; therefore, a dosage reduction is necessary.

### Use in Patients Receiving Home Care

With theophylline, the home care nurse needs to assess the patient and the environment for substances that may affect metabolism of theophylline and decrease therapeutic effects or increase adverse effects. The nurse assesses self-administration in the home. In addition, he or she assists with periodic office or clinic visits for blood tests and other follow-up care.

## Adverse Effects

The therapeutic range of theophylline is narrow, making it and other xanthines second-line asthma treatment. Signs and symptoms of theophylline overdose include anorexia, nausea, vomiting, agitation, nervousness, insomnia, tachycardia and other dysrhythmias, and tonic–clonic convulsions. Ventricular dysrhythmias or convulsions may be the first sign of toxicity. Serious adverse effects frequently occur

## TABLE 33.4

## DRUGS AT A GLANCE: Xanthines (Theophylline)

| Drug | Pregnancy Category | Routes and Dosage Ranges | |
|------|--------------------|---------------------------|---|
| | | Adults | Children |
| Ⓟ **Short-acting theophylline** (Elixophyllin, Theo-24, Theochron; Apo-theo LA, Theolair, Uniphyl) | C | 500 mg PO, initially, then 200–300 mg every 6–8 h | 7.5 mg/kg PO initially, then 5–6 mg/kg every 6–8 h |
| Long-acting theophylline (Theochron, others) | C | 150–300 mg PO every 8–12 h; max dose 13 mg/kg or 900 mg daily, whichever is less | 100–200 mg PO every 8–12 h; max dose 24 mg/kg/d |

at serum drug levels above 20 mg/mL. Overdoses with sustained-release preparations may cause a dramatic increase in serum drug concentrations much later (12 hours or longer) than the immediate-release preparations. Early treatment helps but does not prevent these delayed increases in serum drug levels. Theophylline also increases cardiac output, causes peripheral vasodilation, exerts a mild diuretic effect, and stimulates the CNS.

## Contraindications ~~Shy away~~

Contraindications to theophylline include acute gastritis and peptic ulcer disease. Caution is necessary in seizure disorders and cardiovascular disorders that could be aggravated by drug-induced cardiac stimulation.

## Nursing Implications

### Preventing Interactions

Because theophylline is metabolized by the cytochrome P450 (CYP) enzyme system, numerous drug–drug interactions using the same enzyme system exist (Box 33.6). Also, the rate of metabolism of theophylline is increased substantially in cigarette smokers (the half-life can be halved), although this metabolic increase may not be significant in those who smoke fewer than 10 cigarettes per day. In addition, caffeine reportedly produces additive cardiac and CNS stimulation. Finally, St. John's wort may decrease the effect of theophylline by increasing its metabolism.

*St. Johns wort - test question Pick it (doesn't work with others)*

### Administering the Medication

To help regulate theophylline dosage and avoid adverse effects, it is necessary to monitor serum drug levels. Patients should take immediate-release oral theophylline before meals with a full glass of water, at regular intervals around the clock. If GI upset occurs, they may take the drug with food to promote dissolution and absorption and decrease the associated nausea and vomiting. They should take sustained-release theophylline every 8 to 12 hours, with instructions not to chew or crush. Doing so causes immediate release of potentially toxic doses.

---

**BOX 33.6** 💊 **Drug Interactions: Theophylline**

**Drugs That Increase the Effects of Theophylline**

- Allopurinol, propranolol, quinolones [e.g., ciprofloxacin]
  *Decrease metabolism*
- Cimetidine, macrolides [e.g., erythromycin, clindamycin]
  *Decrease clearance and thereby increase plasma levels*

**Drugs That Decrease the Effects of Theophylline**

- Carbamazepine, phenytoin, rifampicin
  *Increase metabolism*
- Lithium
  *Increases excretion*
- Phenobarbital
  *Increases metabolism by way of enzyme induction*

---

### Assessing for Therapeutic Effects

The nurse observes for therapeutic serum levels of theophylline (5–15 mcg/mL). Chronic use of the drug results in improved arterial blood gas levels (normal values on room air: $PO_2$, 80–100 mm Hg; $PCO_2$, 35–45 mm Hg; pH, 7.35–7.45), improved exercise tolerance, and decreased incidence and severity of acute attacks of bronchospasm.

### Assessing for Adverse Effects

With theophylline, the nurse monitors the serum drug level and observes for tachycardia, dysrhythmias, palpitations, restlessness, agitation, insomnia, nausea, vomiting, and convulsions. Theophylline causes cardiac and CNS stimulation. Toxic serum concentrations (greater than 20 mcg/mL) lead to convulsions, which may occur without preceding symptoms of toxicity and may result in death. IV diazepam (Valium) may control seizures. In patients with seizures, treatment includes securing the airway, giving oxygen, injecting IV diazepam (0.1–0.3 mg/kg, up to 10 mg), monitoring vital signs, maintaining blood pressure, providing adequate hydration, and monitoring serum theophylline levels until they are between 15 and 20 mg/mL.

Theophylline also stimulates the chemoreceptor trigger zone in the medulla oblongata, causing nausea and vomiting. In patients without seizures, it may be necessary to induce vomiting, unless the level of consciousness is impaired. In these patients, precautions to prevent aspiration are necessary, especially in children. If overdose is identified within 1 hour of theophylline ingestion, gastric lavage may be helpful if health care providers are unable to induce vomiting or vomiting is contraindicated. Experts recommend administration of activated charcoal and a cathartic, especially for overdoses of sustained-release formulations—if the possible benefit exceeds the risk.

In addition, symptomatic treatment of dysrhythmias may be necessary.

### Patient Teaching

With theophylline, the nurse reinforces the importance of not exceeding the prescribed dose, not crushing long-acting formulations, reporting adverse effects, and keeping appointments for follow-up care. He or she also instructs patients who smoke to notify their prescriber if they stop smoking, because the dosage of theophylline may need to be reduced. Box 33.4 presents patient teaching guidelines for antiasthmatic drugs.

---

**NCLEX Success**

1. A woman begins using an albuterol inhaler and a beclomethasone inhaler for her asthma. She asks if it matters which inhaler she uses first. The best response by the nurse is which of the following?

   A. "You should use the albuterol inhaler first followed in 5 to 10 minutes by the beclomethasone inhaler."

   B. "You should use the beclomethasone inhaler first followed in 5 to 10 minutes by the albuterol inhaler."

   C. "The order in which you use the inhalers does not matter."

   D. "You should not use the inhalers one right after the other."

2. The nurse notes that a patient's serum theophylline level is 25 mcg/mL and that a scheduled dose of the medication is due. The nurse should do which of the following?

   A. Hold the scheduled dose, contact the health care provider, and assess the patient for signs of theophylline toxicity.
   B. Administer the dose as scheduled.
   C. Administer only half of the dose and repeat the theophylline level in 4 hours.
   D. Hold the dose until the next meal and administer at that time.

3. A 68-year-old man, well controlled on theophylline for 2 years, complains of insomnia, nervousness, nausea and vomiting, and tachycardia. He originally thought the nervousness was due to his recent smoking cessation. He had smoked one pack per day for 10 years. The nurse practitioner assesses the patient and tells him that he is likely experiencing theophylline toxicity. A serum theophylline level confirms the diagnosis. What is the best explanation for theophylline toxicity in this patient?

   A. Because of his age, the patient is likely having renal insufficiency.
   B. The patient is not taking the medication as prescribed.
   C. A concurrent medication is altering the metabolism of theophylline.
   D. The metabolism of theophylline has decreased with the recent smoking cessation.

## CORTICOSTEROIDS

Chapter 17 describes corticosteroids, which are often ordered for treatment of many inflammatory conditions. The ability of the corticosteroids to suppress airway inflammation produces beneficial effects, including decreased mucus secretion, decreased edema of airway mucosa, and repair of damaged epithelium, with subsequent reduction of airway reactivity. Corticosteroids are the most consistently effective long-term control medications for asthma. The inhaled drug **beclomethasone** (Qvar RediHaler) is the prototype corticosteroid in asthma. Current clinical practice guidelines and GINA recommend the addition of inhaled corticosteroids with administration of a short-acting (rescue) beta$_2$-adrenergic agonist.

### Pharmacokinetics

Beclomethasone is rapidly absorbed from the lower respiratory tract or nasal passages. The onset of action is rapid, and the drug peaks in 1 to 2 weeks. Therapeutic effects may not occur until 4 weeks after initial use. Metabolism occurs in the lungs, GI tract, and liver, and excretion predominately occurs in the feces. The drug crosses the placenta. Whether it enters breast milk is unknown.

## Action

Corticosteroids suppress the release of inflammatory mediators, block the generation of cytokines, and decrease the recruitment of airway eosinophils (Fig. 33.1). The drugs increase the number

**Figure 33.1.** Formation of leukotrienes and sites of action of leukotriene-modifying drugs and steroids. CysLT$_1$, cysteinyl leukotriene$_1$. [Reprinted with permission from Whalen, K. (2015). *Lippincott illustrated reviews: Pharmacology* (6th ed., Fig. 39.4). Philadelphia, PA: Wolters Kluwer.]

and sensitivity of beta$_2$-adrenergic receptors, which restores or increases the effectiveness of beta$_2$-adrenergic bronchodilators. The number of beta$_2$ receptors increases within approximately 4 hours, and improved responsiveness to beta$_2$-agonists occurs within approximately 2 hours.

## Use

Beclomethasone is effective in the prophylactic management of asthma. With inhalation, the drug controls asthma that requires corticosteroids as part of the treatment plan. In chronic asthma, patients usually take corticosteroids by inhalation, on a daily schedule. Often, they take them concomitantly with one or more bronchodilators and perhaps another anti-inflammatory drug such as a leukotriene modifier or a mast cell stabilizer. In some instances, the other drugs allow smaller doses of the corticosteroid. For acute flare-ups of symptoms during treatment of chronic asthma, a systemic corticosteroid may be needed temporarily to regain control. Intranasal administration helps relieve rhinitis that responds poorly to other treatment and minimizes the reoccurrence of nasal polyps after nasal surgery.

In early stages of progressive COPD, patients are unlikely to need corticosteroids. In later stages, however, they usually need periodic short-course therapy for episodes of respiratory distress and a scheduled inhaled corticosteroid for long-term control. When corticosteroids are needed for an acute exacerbation, administration is oral or parenteral.

Table 33.5 provides route and dosage information for beclomethasone and other corticosteroid antiasthmatic drugs.

## TABLE 33.5

## DRUGS AT A GLANCE: Corticosteroids

| Drug | Pregnancy Category | Routes and Dosage Ranges | |
|---|---|---|---|
| | | **Adults** | **Children** |
| Ⓟ **Beclomethasone** (Qvar RediHaler ✹ QVAR) | C | Oral inhalation, initial 40–80 mcg twice daily; max dose, 320 mcg twice daily; if on previous inhaled corticosteroids, 40–160 mcg twice daily; max dose 320 mcg twice daily | 5–11 y, oral inhalation, 40 mcg twice daily; max dose 80 mcg twice daily ≥12 y, 40–80 mcg twice daily; max dose 320 mcg twice daily |
| Ⓟ **Beclomethasone** (Beconase AQ, Qnasl, Qnasl Children; ✹ Apo-Beclomethasone, Mylan-Beclo AQ, Rivanase AQ) | C | Nasal inhalation, 2 sprays in each nostril twice daily (total dose 168–336 mcg/d) | ≥6 y, nasal inhalation, 2 sprays in each nostril twice daily (total dose 168–336 mcg/d) |
| Budesonide (Pulmicort, Pulmicort Flexhaler; ✹ Pulmicort Nebuamp, Pulmicort Turbuhaler) | B | Oral inhalation, 200–400 mcg twice daily | ≥6 y, oral inhalation 200 mcg twice daily |
| Ciclesonide (Alvesco ✹ Alvesco) | C | Oral inhalation, 80 mcg twice daily; max dose 160 mcg twice daily (if receiving bronchodilators alone); max dose 320 mcg twice daily (if receiving inhaled corticosteroids) | 2–11 y, oral inhalation, 40, 80, or 160 mcg once daily ≥12 y, same as adults |
| Flunisolide (Aerospan HFA) | C | Two inhalations twice daily; max dose eight inhalations daily | 6–11 y, oral inhalation: one inhalation twice daily; max dose four times daily |
| Fluticasone (Xhance; ✹ Flonase, Avamys) | C | 4 sprays in each nostril once daily (265 mcg/d) | ≥12 y, same as adults 4–11 y: 1 spray in each nostril once daily; may increase to 2 sprays in each nostril for desired effect |
| Fluticasone aerosol (Flovent Diskus, Arnuity Ellipta, Flovent HFA; ✹ Arnuity Ellipta, Flovent Diskus, Flovent HFA) | C | Aerosol, 88–220 mcg twice daily | Dosage not established |
| Fluticasone powder (Flovent Diskus) | C | Powder, 100–500 mcg twice daily | ≥12 y: same as adults 4–11 y, powder, 50–100 mcg twice daily |
| Mometasone (Asmanex HFA, Asmanex Twisthaler; ✹ Asmanex Twisthaler) | C | Aerosol, 100–200 mcg twice daily Inhalation powder (Twisthaler), 110–220 mcg twice daily | ≥12 y; same as adults 4–11 y, powder 110 mcg twice daily |

### TABLE 33.5

### DRUGS AT A GLANCE: Corticosteroids (Continued)

| Drug | Pregnancy Category | Routes and Dosage Ranges | |
|---|---|---|---|
| | | **Adults** | **Children** |
| Mometasone (Nasonex, Propel Mini; ❋ Apo-Mometasone, Mosaspray, Nasonex) | C | Nasal inhalation two sprays (50 mcg/spray) in each nostril once daily | ≥12 y, same as adults 2–11 y, 1 spray (50 mcg) in each nostril once daily |
| Prednisone (Deltasone, Prednisone Intensol, Rayos; ❋ Apo-Prednisone, JAA-Prednisone, Teva-Prednisone, Winpred) | C | Acute asthma: 40–60 mg/d PO for 3–10 d for a short burst | <12: 1–2 mg/kg/d PO for 3–10 d; maximum 60 mg daily ≥12 y, same as adults |
| Methylprednisolone sodium succinate (A-MethaPred, Depo-Medrol, ReadySharp Methylprednisolone, Solu-Medrol; ❋ Depo-Medrol, Medrol, Methylprednisolone acetate, Methylprednisolone sodium succinate, Solu-Medrol) | C | Oral 40–60 mg/d for a short burst; 7.5 mg to 60 mg/d for maintenance of asthma control<br>IV: 40–80 mg/d in divided doses once or twice daily<br>IM (acetate): 240 mg one-time dose in place of a short-course burst | <12 y: 1–2 mg/kg PO for 3–10 d; maximum dose: 60 mg daily<br>≥12 y, same as adults<br>IM (acetate): 7.5 mg/kg up to 240 mg as a one-time dose<br>IV: <12 y, 1–2 mg/kg/d; maximum of 60 mg/d<br>>12 y, same as adults |

## Use in Children

The effectiveness and safety of inhaled corticosteroids, including beclomethasone, in children older than 3 years of age are well established; few data are available on the use of inhaled drugs in those younger than 3 years. Major concerns about long-term use in children include decreased adrenal function, growth, and bone mass. Most corticosteroids are given by inhalation, and dosage, type of inhaler device, and characteristics of individual drugs influence the extent and severity of these systemic effects. Adrenal insufficiency is most likely to occur with systemic or high doses of inhaled corticosteroids. Although inhaled corticosteroids are the most effective anti-inflammatory medications available for asthma, high doses in children are still of concern, and monitoring of the effects is necessary. It is possible to reduce the risk by using (1) the lowest effective dose, (2) administration techniques that minimize swallowed drug, and (3) other antiasthmatic drugs to reduce corticosteroid dose. Research has not shown that nasal administration of beclomethasone affects growth. However, prolonged or high-dose use of nasal beclomethasone has the potential to influence growth.

## Use in Patients With Hepatic Impairment

Because elimination of beclomethasone and most corticosteroids is hepatic, dosage reductions may be appropriate.

## Use in Patients With Critical Illness

In critically ill patients, it may be necessary to replace inhaled or nasal beclomethasone with systemic corticosteroids in relatively high doses in patients whose respiratory distress is not relieved by multiple doses of inhaled beta₂-agonists. Administration of the systemic corticosteroid may be either IV or oral; IV administration offers no therapeutic advantage over oral administration. Relief of the symptoms of acute, severe bronchoconstriction or status asthmaticus usually requires larger doses of bronchodilators and corticosteroids (inhaled, systemic, or both). Then,

dose reduction to the smallest effective amounts for long-term control is necessary.

## Use in Patients Receiving Home Care

Administration of beclomethasone is common in the home setting. As with most inhaled medications, the nurse assesses the patient's ability to administer the medication as prescribed and his or her knowledge of what other medications and actions to use to treat exacerbations if symptoms occur. In addition, the nurse inspects the oral cavity to monitor for the presence of fungal infection (candidiasis).

## Adverse Effects

Common adverse effects of beclomethasone include headache, pharyngitis, cough, dry mouth, hoarseness, fungal infection (candidiasis), and nausea. It is possible to decrease local adverse effects of inhaled corticosteroids (oropharyngeal candidiasis, hoarseness) by reducing the dose, administering the drugs less often, rinsing the mouth and throat after use, or using a spacer device. These measures decrease the amount of drug deposited in the oral cavity.

## Contraindications

Contraindications to beclomethasone include an allergy to the drug. Recent nasal surgery, injury, or ulcers preclude use of the nasal preparation; the drug can interfere with healing and increase the risk of a nasal infection.

## Nursing Implications

### Preventing Interactions

Little, if any, of the beclomethasone is absorbed. Therefore, no clinically significant drug–drug or herbal interactions are known to occur.

### Administering the Medication

Patients should take inhaled or nasal beclomethasone on a regular schedule. After inhaling, they should rinse the mouth and throat to prevent fungal infection (candidiasis). The drug is not a rescue inhaler, and patients should not take it to resolve an acute asthma event. The recommended inhaled or nasal corticosteroid dose should be the lowest amount of drug required to control symptoms. *Can use spacer (clean it)*

### Assessing for Therapeutic Effects

The nurse assesses for reversal of asthma symptoms, including reduced airway inflammation, decreased mucus secretion, decreased edema of airway mucosa, and reduction of airway reactivity. With allergic rhinitis, the nurse assesses for the relief of rhinitis, including clearing of stuffy nose and postnasal drip.

### Assessing for Adverse Effects

With beclomethasone and other inhaled corticosteroids, the nurse observes for the presence of headache, hoarseness, cough, throat irritation, and fungal infection (candidiasis) of mouth and throat. Inhaled corticosteroids are unlikely to produce the serious adverse effects of long-term systemic therapy (see Chap. 17).

### Patient Teaching

*taper*

It is important to instruct patients that oral and nasal inhalations are not interchangeable.

>  **QSEN Alert: Safety**
>
> The nurse must remind patients that beclomethasone is not a fast-acting asthma treatment; the drug does not provide immediate relief from asthma-related breathing problems.

Box 33.4 outlines additional patient teaching guidelines.

## Other Drugs in the Class

Budesonide (Pulmicort, Pulmicort Flexhaler), ciclesonide, flunisolide (Aerospan), fluticasone (Flonase), and mometasone (Asmanex Twisthaler, Nasonex) are topical corticosteroids for inhalation. Topical administration minimizes systemic absorption and adverse effects; clinical effectiveness of inhaled drugs is due to direct local effects rather than systemic absorption. These preparations may substitute for or allow reduced dosage of systemic corticosteroids.

>  **QSEN Alert: Safety**
>
> In people with asthma who are taking an oral corticosteroid, it is necessary to reduce the oral dosage slowly (over weeks to months) when an inhaled corticosteroid is added.

The goal is to use the lowest oral dose necessary to control symptoms. Flunisolide and fluticasone also are available in nasal solutions for treatment of allergic rhinitis, which may play a role in bronchoconstriction. Because systemic absorption occurs in patients using inhaled corticosteroids (about 20% of a dose), high doses should be reserved for people who otherwise require oral corticosteroids.

Triamcinolone acetonide is not recommended for use in children younger than 2 years of age. Dose-related inhibition of growth has been reported in short and intermediate studies, but long-term studies have found few, if any, decreases in expected adult height. Inhaled corticosteroids have not been associated with significant decreases in bone mass, but more studies of high doses and of drug therapy in adolescents are needed.

Prednisone and methylprednisolone are given to patients who require systemic corticosteroids. Prednisone is given orally and is highlighted as a prototype drug in Chapter 17; methylprednisolone may be given intravenously to patients who are unable to take an oral medication.

## LEUKOTRIENE MODIFIERS

**Leukotrienes** are proinflammatory mediators produced by the immune system during trauma, infection, and inflammation. They can cause sustained constriction of bronchioles and immediate hypersensitivity reactions. They also increase mucus secretion and mucosal edema in the respiratory tract. Leukotrienes are formed by the lipoxygenase pathway of arachidonic acid metabolism (see Fig. 33.1) in response to cellular injury. Cysteinyl leukotrienes (cysLTs) are a family of inflammatory lipid mediators of various allergic and hypersensitivity reactions.

Leukotriene modifiers, or leukotriene receptor antagonists, are strong chemical mediators of bronchoconstriction and inflammation, the major pathologic features of asthma. These drugs are effective in a significant portion of patients with asthma. (However, clinical trials that compared leukotriene receptors to inhaled corticosteroids achieved treatment end points more consistently with inhaled corticosteroids.) The prototype leukotriene modifier is **montelukast** (Singulair). The drug antagonizes the cysteinyl leukotriene$_1$ receptor.

## Pharmacokinetics

Absorption from the GI tract is rapid. Extensive metabolism takes place in the liver via the CYP3A4, 2C8, and 2C9 enzyme systems, and the drug may interact with other medications metabolized by this system. Excretion of most metabolites occurs in the feces.

## Action

Montelukast prevents cysteinyl leukotrienes from binding to its receptors reducing the bronchoconstriction and ultimate inflammation caused by leukotrienes. The drug improves symptoms and pulmonary function tests, decreases nighttime symptoms, and decreases the use of beta$_2$-agonist drugs. The drug is not effective in relieving acute asthma attacks. However, patients may continue taking it concurrently with other drugs during acute episodes.

## Use

Health care providers use montelukast that is indicated for long-term treatment of asthma in adults and children. It is the only oral tablet approved for management of exercise-induced asthma. In addition, montelukast is the only leukotriene modifier approved for the management of allergic rhinitis or

## TABLE 33.6

## DRUGS AT A GLANCE: Leukotriene Modifiers

| Drug | Pregnancy Category | Routes and Dosage Ranges | |
|------|-------------------|--------------------------|---|
| | | **Adults** | **Children** |
| Ⓟ **Montelukast** (Singulair; 🍁 Singulair) | B | 10 mg PO once daily in the evening or at bedtime | ≥1–2 y, 4 mg (PO granules) once daily in the evening<br>≥2–6 y, 4 mg (PO granules or chewable tablet) once daily in the evening<br>≥6–14 y, 5 mg PO chewable tablet once daily in the evening<br>≥15 y, same as adults |
| Zafirlukast (Accolate; 🍁 Accolate) | B | 20 mg PO twice daily, 1 h before or 2 h after a meal | 5–11 y, 10 mg PO twice daily<br>≥12 y, same as adults |
| Zileuton (Zyflo, Zyflo CR) | C | Immediate release, 600 mg PO 4 times/d<br>Extended release, 1200 mg PO twice per day | ≥12 y, same as adults |

allergies, and it may result in relief of allergic conjunctivitis. The drug can be used with bronchodilators and corticosteroids and elicit a high degree of patient adherence and satisfaction. However, it is less effective than low doses of inhaled corticosteroids. Table 33.6 gives route and dosage information for montelukast and other leukotriene modifiers. Don't Forget

Note that the FDA has issued a **BLACK BOX WARNING ◆** for montelukast because neuropsychiatric events have been reported in adults, adolescents, and children who take the drug. These symptoms include agitation, aggressive behavior anxiousness, depression, disorientation, disturbance in attention, dream abnormalities, hallucinations, insomnia, irritability, memory impairment, restlessness, suicidal ideation, and tremor.

### Use in Children          age 12 ↓ ↑

Montelukast is approved for use in children 12 months of age and older. Film-coated tablets, chewable tablets, or granules are available.

### Use in Patients With Hepatic Impairment

Montelukast produces higher blood levels in patients with hepatic impairment, and drug elimination is slower in these patients. However, no dosage adjustment is necessary for patients with mild to moderate hepatic impairment.

### Use in Patients Receiving Home Care

Montelukast is self-administered at home for prevention of asthma symptoms. Prescribers often order the drug when inhaled corticosteroids and short-acting beta₂-agonists are unsuccessful in controlling asthma symptoms. The home health nurse assesses asthma severity and asthma control.

## Adverse Effects and Contraindications

Leukotriene modifiers seem relatively devoid of serious toxicity, and adverse effects are typically mild. The most common adverse effects reported are headache, nausea, vomiting, diarrhea, hyperkinesia, psychomotor hyperactivity, and infection.

Contraindications include known hypersensitivity to the drug.

## Nursing Implications

### Preventing Interactions

Montelukast is metabolized in the liver by the CYP enzyme system, and numerous drug–drug interactions exist, particularly in drugs that utilize the same enzyme system. Box 33.7 summarizes these interactions. St. John's wort may decrease the drug's effect by increasing metabolism of the drug.

### Administering the Medication

Oral administration of montelukast is effective. People can take it once or twice a day, in the evening or at bedtime. This schedule provides high drug concentrations during the night and early morning, when asthma symptoms tend to occur or worsen. Food does not significantly affect the drug's bioavailability; people may take it with or without food.

### Assessing for Therapeutic Effects

The nurse assesses for stability and improvement of asthma symptoms, relief of allergic rhinitis, or the absence of exercise-induced respiratory symptoms. If the patient's respiratory

**BOX 33.7**    **Drug Interactions: Montelukast**

**Drugs That Increase the Effects of Montelukast**
- Aspirin
  *Increases bleeding tendencies*

**Drugs That Decrease the Effects of Montelukast**
- Carbamazepine, erythromycin, phenobarbital, phenytoin, primidone, rifamycin antibiotics, theophylline
  *Decrease serum levels*

symptoms are not stable, it is necessary to determine the current frequency and severity of acute attacks as well as factors that precipitate or relieve acute attacks.

### Assessing for Adverse Effects

The nurse assesses for headache, nausea, diarrhea, signs of infection, and changes in behavior, including suicidal ideation.

### Patient Teaching

The nurse instructs the patient about recognizing signs and symptoms of infection and reporting them to his/her health care provider. Also, the nurse ensures that the patient understands appropriate use of the drug and realizes that the drug should not be used to manage acute asthma symptoms. Box 33.4 outlines additional patient teaching guidelines.

## Other Drugs in the Class

Zafirlukast (Accolate) was the first leukotriene modifier, but montelukast has overshadowed it. Like montelukast, zafirlukast antagonizes the cysteinyl leukotriene₁ receptor. Well absorbed with oral administration, metabolism of zafirlukast by the CYP enzyme system occurs in the liver, and the drug may interact with other drugs metabolized by the hepatic system. Excretion of most metabolites occurs in the feces. Blood levels of the drug are higher and elimination is slower in older adults than in younger adults. Zafirlukast is approved for use in children older than 5 years of age. The drug enters breast milk, and lactating women should not take it. People should take zafirlukast 1 hour before or 2 hours after a meal; food reduces the bioavailability by approximately 40%. Authorities recommend no dosage adjustments for zafirlukast in patients with renal impairment.

Zileuton (Zyflo, Zyflo CR), another leukotriene modifier, is a 5-lipoxygenase inhibitor that blocks the first step in leukotriene biosynthesis of the arachidonic acid cascade. Thus, the drug inhibits the formation of leukotrienes B4, C4, D4, and E4 and subsequently the formation of the cysLTs. The most common adverse effect is headache. The extended-release formulation should be taken with food; the immediate-release formulation can be given without regard to food. Zileuton is approved in the United States for use in children 12 years and older. Monitoring of serum alanine aminotransferase is recommended.

## IMMUNOSUPPRESSANT MONOCLONAL ANTIBODIES

Exposure to allergenic material in pollen, dander, and food can cause immune inflammation that leads to allergic asthma. With repeated stimulation of the allergen, IgE antibodies are produced. Monoclonal antibodies specifically bind to target cells or proteins in the hopes of stimulating the patient's immune system to attack those cells. Ⓟ **Omalizumab** (Xolair), a recombinant humanized IgE monoclonal antibody and the prototype, combines with free IgE-blocking receptors on the surfaces of mast cells and basophils so that there is less IgE available to combine with allergens. Omalizumab is the only available anti-IgE therapy approved as adjunctive therapy to inhaled corticosteroids, with the goal of reducing the prevalence of asthma exacerbations and hospitalizations. Chapter 13 further discusses the effects of altering the immune response to an allergen with monoclonal antibodies.

## Pharmacokinetics

Absorption is slow following subcutaneous injection. Metabolism occurs in the reticuloendothelial system and the endothelial cells in the liver. Half-life elimination is 26 days. Excretion is primarily through the liver, and intact IgG may be secreted in bile.

## Action

Omalizumab inhibits IgE binding to IgE receptors on mast cells and basophils. This limits the activation and release of mediators in the early and late phases of the allergic response.

## Use

Omalizumab is indicated as adjunctive therapy for moderate to severe persistent allergic asthma to a perennial aeroallergen that is not well controlled with a combination of a high-dose inhaled corticosteroid and a long-acting beta₂-agonist. Long-term treatment in patients with allergic asthma showed a decrease in asthma exacerbations and corticosteroid use. In addition, the drug is indicated for the treatment of chronic idiopathic urticaria.

Table 33.7 provides route and dosage information for omalizumab and other immunosuppressant monoclonal antibodies.

---

### TABLE 33.7

### DRUGS AT A GLANCE: Monoclonal Antibody

| | | | |
|---|---|---|---|
| Ⓟ **Omalizumab** (Xolair; 🍁 Xolair) | B | 150–375 mg every 2–4 weeks Sub-Q, based on body weight and level of total pretreatment serum IgE | ≥6–11 y, 75–375 mg every 2–4 weeks Sub-Q, based on body weight and level of total pretreatment serum IgE ≥12 y, same as adults |
| Mepolizumab (Nucala; 🍁 Nucala) | Not assigned 2015 | 100 mg Sub-Q once every 4 wk | ≥12 y, same as adults |
| Reslizumab (Cinqair; 🍁 Cinqair) | Not assigned 2016 | 3 mg/kg IV once every 4 wk | No data available on use in children |
| Benralizumab (Fasenra; 🍁 Fasenra) | Not assigned 2017 | 30 mg Sub-Q every 4 wk for the first 3 doses, then once every 8 wk | ≥12 y, same as adults |

### Use in Children

Omalizumab is approved for use in children older than 6 years of age.

### Use in Older Adults

Omalizumab is indicated in older adults.

### Use in Patients With Renal Impairment

The manufacturer's packaging provides no information regarding dosage adjustments in patients with renal impairment.

### Use in Patients With Hepatic Impairment

No dosage adjustments are recommended.

### Use in Patients With Critical Illness

Although omalizumab may be continued in patients with critical illness, the drug will not relieve symptoms of acute, severe bronchoconstriction or status asthmaticus, which usually requires larger doses of bronchodilators and corticosteroids (inhaled, systemic, or both).

### Use in Patients Receiving Home Care

Omalizumab is not self-administered at home because of the risk of anaphylaxis associated with the drug. People who receive home care may receive the drug in a healthcare setting and need to be assessed for signs of anaphylaxis. Because anaphylaxis may occur up to four days after the drug is administered, the patient and family need to be instructed to seek emergency medical treatment for signs of anaphylaxis, including trouble breathing or swallowing, swelling of throat and tongue, chest or throat tightness, cough, flushing, rash, or itching.

## Adverse Effects

The most common adverse effects of omalizumab include local reactions at the injection site, headache, nausea, and fatigue. Anaphylaxis presenting as bronchospasm, hypotension, syncope, urticaria, and/or angioedema of the throat or tongue has been reported following administration of the drug. Anaphylaxis has been reported with the first dose and has occurred more than 1 year after initial administration. Because of the risk of anaphylaxis, the FDA has issued a **BLACK BOX WARNING ◆** for omalizumab.

## Contraindications

Contraindications to omalizumab include a known allergy to the drug or a severe hypersensitivity reaction (anaphylaxis) with drug use.

## Nursing implications

### Preventing Interactions

No reported drug–drug interactions or herbal interactions occur that decrease or increase the effects of omalizumab.

### Administering the Medication

Administration of omalizumab must occur in the health care setting because of the risk of life-threatening anaphylaxis with administration. No more than 150 mg (contents of one vial) should be injected at one site. Doses of more than 150 mg should be given at two or more injection sites.

**!  QSEN Alert: Safety**

The nurse must take precautions with omalizumab to ensure correct product selection and dose–volume calculations. Pre-filled syringes and reconstituted lyophilized powder are available in different concentrations.

### Assessing for Therapeutic Effects

The nurse observes for a decrease in the number and severity of asthma exacerbations, better symptom control, and an improvement of airflow limitation. The patient should report a decreased need for rescue medications and oral corticosteroids, as well as an improved reported quality of life.

### Assessing for Adverse Effects

The nurse assesses for signs of anaphylaxis, local reactions at the injection sites, headache, nausea, and fatigue.

### Patient Teaching

The nurse instructs the patient and family to recognize the signs and symptoms of anaphylaxis and to report them to his or her health care provider. They should understand that the drug must be administered in a health care facility and that it may take several months before the patient begins to notice benefits from the drug. Management of local reactions at the site of injection involves the application of local cold compresses or the use of medications such as antihistamines or aspirin. Box 33.4 summarizes additional patient teaching guidelines for antiasthmatic drugs, including omalizumab.

### Other Drugs in the Class

Although omalizumab is the only monoclonal antibody that targets IgE, three other monoclonal antibodies target the production of eosinophils in the allergic response of individuals with severe asthma who have blood eosinophil counts of 150/μL or greater (**eosinophilic phenotype**). These include mepolizumab (Nucala) and reslizumab (Cinqair), and benralizumab (Fasenra), an anti-IL-5 receptor alpha antibody. IL-5 is a proeosinophilic cytokine that is a potent mediator of eosinophil hematopoiesis and contributes to eosinophilic inflammation in the airways. Mepolizumab and reslizumab are anti-IL-5 monoclonal antibodies, and benralizumab is a monoclonal antibody to IL-5. These drugs are considered add-on maintenance of treatment of severe asthma in adults and children ≥12 years of age with an eosinophilic phenotype. As with omalizumab, they are not indicated for the relief of acute bronchospasm or status asthmaticus. Table 33.7 contains route and dosage information for the other monoclonal antibodies.

## ADJUVANT MEDICATIONS USED TO TREAT ASTHMA

### Mast Cell Stabilizers  *= secretions bronchodilation*

Mast cell stabilizers are used as an alternative, but not preferred, medication for prophylaxis of acute asthma attacks in patients with mild, persistent asthma. They are not effective in acute bronchospasm or status asthmaticus and should not be used in these conditions. Use of one of these drugs may allow reduced dosage of bronchodilators and corticosteroids. Patients may take them prior to exercise or exposure to known allergens. Cromolyn (NasalCrom) stabilizes mast cells and prevents the release of bronchoconstrictive and inflammatory substances

*older drug - not rescue inhaler*
*see alot in pediatrics*

when mast cells are confronted with allergens and other stimuli. Administration of mast cell stabilizers is by inhalation. Cromolyn is available in a metered-dose aerosol and a solution for use with a power-operated nebulizer. A nasal solution is also marketed for prevention and treatment of allergic rhinitis. In patients with impaired renal or hepatic function, dosage reduction is necessary.

Serious toxicity is relatively absent with mast cell stabilizers. However, the propellants in the aerosols may aggravate coronary artery disease or dysrhythmias. With cromolyn, the nurse assesses for dysrhythmias, hypotension, chest pain, restlessness, dizziness, convulsions, CNS depression, anorexia, and nausea and vomiting. Sedation and coma may occur with overdosage.

## Combination Regimens

Combination regimens are commonly used, and one advantage is that smaller doses of each agent can usually be given. This may decrease adverse effects and allow dosages to be increased when exacerbation of symptoms occurs. Table 33.8 summarizes information about available combination inhalation products. Advair, which was developed to treat both inflammation and bronchoconstriction, is more effective than the individual components at the same doses and as effective as concurrent use of the same drugs at the same doses. In addition, the combination reduces the corticosteroid dose by 50% and is more effective than higher doses of fluticasone alone in reducing asthma exacerbations. The combination improves symptoms within 1 week. Additional combination products are likely to be marketed and may improve patient adherence to prescribed drug therapy.

### Clinical Application 33.2

- Mr. Lee's symptoms subside, and he is transferred to a medical unit. Mr. Lee tells the nurse that he hopes he does not have another asthma of this type again. What efforts does the nurse recommend to reduce the risk of future episodes?

### NCLEX  Success

4. When teaching a patient about the proper use of metered-dose inhalers, which of the following statements should be included?

   A. "Make sure that you puff out air repeatedly after you inhale the medication."
   B. "After you inhale the medication, hold the breath for approximately 10 seconds and exhale slowly."
   C. "After you inhale the medication once, repeat until you obtain relief."
   D. "Rinse out your mouth before using the inhaler to decrease the development of a mouth infection."

5. A man who is using a steroid inhaler complains of anorexia and discomfort when he eats. The nurse reports this to the care provider, and the patient receives a diagnosis of oropharyngeal candidiasis. It is possible to decrease this adverse effect by which of the following actions? (Select all that apply.)

   A. reducing the dose
   B. administering the drug more frequently
   C. rinsing the mouth after use
   D. using a spacer device

6. Montelukast is effective in relieving the inflammation and bronchoconstriction associated with acute asthmatic attacks through which principal action?

   A. stabilizing mast cells
   B. blocking leukotriene receptors
   C. binding to immunoglobulin E (IgE)
   D. decreasing prostaglandin synthesis

### TABLE 33.8
### DRUGS AT A GLANCE: Combination Regimens

| Drug | Pregnancy Category | Routes and Dosage Ranges | |
|---|---|---|---|
| | | **Adults** | **Children** |
| Fluticasone/salmeterol (Advair Diskus, Advair HFA, AirDuo RespiClick; ❈ Advair, Advair Diskus) | C | Advair Diskus: Oral inhalation, one inhalation, twice daily<br>Advair HFA: Oral inhalation, two inhalations, twice daily<br>AirDuo RespiClick: Oral inhalation, one inhalation, twice daily | ≥12 y, same as adults |
| Mometasone/formoterol (Dulera; ❈ Zenhale) | C | Oral inhalation, one inhalation, twice daily | ≥12 y, same as adults |
| Budesonide/formoterol (Symbicort; ❈ Symbicort) | C | Oral inhalation, two inhalations, twice daily | ≥12 y, same as adults |
| Ipratropium/albuterol (Combivent Respimat; ❈ Apo-Salvent-Ipravent Sterules, Combivent Respimat; Combivent UDV, ratio-Ipra Sal UDV, Teva-Combo Sterinebs) | C | Aerosol, two inhalations four times daily<br>Nebulizing solution, 1 vial four times daily, increased to six times daily if necessary | Dosage not established |

## THE NURSING PROCESS

A concept map outlines the nursing process related to drug therapy considerations in this chapter. Additional nursing implications related to the disease process should also be considered in care decisions.

### Assessment

- Assess for abnormal breathing patterns (e.g., rate below 12 or above 24 per minute, dyspnea, cough, orthopnea, wheezing, "noisy" respirations) because these may indicate respiratory distress. Severe respiratory distress is characterized by tachypnea, dyspnea, use of accessory muscles of respiration, and hypoxia.
- Assess for early signs of hypoxia, including mental confusion, restlessness, anxiety, and increased blood pressure and pulse rate. Late signs include cyanosis and decreased blood pressure and pulse rate. Hypoxemia is confirmed if arterial blood gas analysis shows decreased $PO_2$.
- In acute bronchospasm, assess for forceful expiration or wheezing, a characteristic feature of bronchospasm. The absence of wheezing in the presence of increased respiratory effort is an ominous sign.
- In chronic asthma, try to determine the frequency and severity of acute attacks; factors that precipitate or relieve acute attacks; antiasthmatic medications taken occasionally or regularly; allergies; and condition between acute attacks, such as restrictions in activities of daily living due to asthma.
- In chronic bronchitis or emphysema, assess for signs of respiratory distress, hypoxia, cough, amount and character of sputum, exercise tolerance (e.g., dyspnea on exertion, dyspnea at rest), medications, and nondrug treatment measures (e.g., breathing exercises, chest physiotherapy).

### Outcomes of Therapy

The patient will
- Self-administer bronchodilating and other drugs accurately.
- Experience relief of symptoms.
- Avoid preventable adverse drug effects.
- Avoid overusing bronchodilating drugs.
- Avoid exposure to stimuli or conditions that cause bronchospasm.

### Nursing Interventions

- Use measures to prevent or relieve bronchoconstriction when possible. A specific monitoring plan should be in place, whether peak expiratory flow rate (PEFR) or symptom monitoring. Some measures include coughing, deep breathing, percussion, and postural drainage to mobilize excessive respiratory tract secretions and preventing their retention.
- Help the patient identify and avoid exposure to conditions that precipitate bronchoconstriction.
- Assist patients with asthma to identify early signs of difficulty, including increased need for beta$_2$-adrenergic agonists, activity limitations, and waking at night with asthma symptoms.
- Monitor PEFR as an objective measure of airflow/airway obstruction and to help evaluate the patient's treatment regimen.
- Assist patients in obtaining meters and learning to measure PEFR.
- Assist patients and family in developing an action plan to manage acute attacks of bronchoconstriction, including when to seek emergency care.
- Encourage reduction of anxiety as it may aggravate bronchospasm. Stay with the patient and seek appropriate treatment during an acute asthma attack if feasible.
- Encourage smoking cessation as indicated and provide information, resources, and assistance in doing so.
- Provide appropriate patient teaching related to drug therapy (see Box 33.4).

### Evaluation

- Observe for relief of symptoms and improved arterial blood gas values.
- Interview and observe for correct drug administration, including use of inhalers.
- Interview and observe for tachydysrhythmias, nervousness, insomnia, and other adverse drug effects.
- Interview about and observe behaviors to avoid stimuli that cause bronchoconstriction and respiratory infections.

## Unfolding Patient Stories: Toua Xiong • Part 1

Toua Xiong has a 45-year history of smoking and is diagnosed with emphysema. The provider orders albuterol and ipratropium via metered-dose inhalers. What patient education would the nurse provide on the action and side effects of the medications? How would the nurse explain the use of an inhaler with a spacer and the sequence of medication delivery when the inhalers are ordered for the same time? (Toua Xiong's story continues in Chapter 60.)

Care for Toua and other patients in a realistic virtual environment: *vSim for Nursing* (thepoint.lww.com/vSim-Pharm). Practice documenting these patients' care in DocuCare (thepoint.lww.com/DocuCareEHR).

## KEY CONCEPTS

- Management of asthma involves prevention of airway inflammation and avoidance of triggers for better symptom control.
- Guidelines for asthma care highlight the importance of four essential components: assessment and monitoring, patient education, control of factors contributing to asthma severity, and pharmacologic treatment.
- It is important that a person with asthma to have a written asthma action plan based on the development of symptoms or decreased peak flow measurements.
- Maintenance $beta_2$-agonist inhaled medications are used to achieve and maintain control of persistent asthma, and rescue $beta_2$-agonist inhaled medications are used for quick-relief medications used during periods of acute symptoms and exacerbations.
- In an attack of acute, severe asthma, the lack of wheezing sound or coughing may indicate severe bronchoconstriction, impaired gas exchange in the lungs, and a worsening of the condition.
- Major groups of drugs used to treat asthma and other conditions causing bronchoconstriction include adrenergics, anticholinergics, xanthines, corticosteroids, leukotriene modifiers, and adjuvant medications (mast cell stabilizer and immunosuppressant monoclonal antibody).

- Because aerosol products act directly on the airways, drugs given by inhalation can usually be given in smaller doses and produce fewer adverse effects than oral or parenteral drugs.
- A selective, short-acting, inhaled $beta_2$-adrenergic agonist (e.g., albuterol) is the initial rescue drug of choice for acute bronchospasm; subcutaneous epinephrine may also be considered.
- The treatment of asthma exacerbations with theophylline is not supported or recommended by current clinical practice guidelines because of significant adverse effects.
- The FDA has issued a **BLACK BOX WARNING** ◆ that initiating salmeterol in people with significantly worsening or acutely deteriorating asthma may be life threatening.
- Cigarette smoking and drugs that stimulate drug-metabolizing enzymes in the liver (e.g., phenobarbital, phenytoin) increase the rate of metabolism and therefore dosage requirements of theophylline.
- Due to the risk of anaphylaxis with its use, the FDA has issued a **BLACK BOX WARNING** ◆ for omalizumab.
- Due to the risk of neuropsychiatric events, the FDA has issued a **BLACK BOX WARNING** ◆ for montelukast.

## CLINICAL REASONING CASE STUDY

**Meet the Patient**

Dion Carlson, an 8-year-old boy, arrives at the emergency department (ED) with severe asthma. This is the third time this month that his parents have brought him to the ED. Mrs. Carlson reports that they live in an old home that is full of mold and dust. In the ED, Dion receives inhaled albuterol two puffs every 20 minutes via multidose inhaler (MDI) for three treatments and inhaled beclomethasone 40 mcg via MDI and his symptoms resolve.

- What are the goals of therapy for Dion in the ED with an acute asthma exacerbation?
- What information should the nurse share about managing the potential triggers of the boy's asthma?

**Assessing Drug Information**

- Albuterol
  - As a beta$_2$ agonist, albuterol stimulates beta$_2$-adrenergic receptors in the smooth muscle of bronchi and bronchioles. The receptors, in turn, stimulate the enzyme adenyl cyclase to increase production of cyclic AMP. The increased cyclic AMP produces bronchodilation.
  - Albuterol is used as a rescue inhalant medication (quick-relief, short-acting drug) during periods of acute symptoms and exacerbations. It is used for the treatment or prevention of bronchospasm associated with reversible obstructive airway disease. The drug is also used in the prevention of exercise-induced bronchospasm.
  - Muscle tremor is the most frequent adverse effect. Major adverse effects are excessive cardiac and CNS stimulation. Symptoms of cardiac stimulation include angina, tachycardia, and palpitations. Symptoms of CNS stimulation consist of agitation, anxiety, insomnia, seizures, and tremors. Other reported effects may include serious dysrhythmias and cardiac arrest.
- Beclomethasone
  - Corticosteroids suppress the release of inflammatory mediators, block the generation of cytokines, and decrease the recruitment of airway eosinophils. The drugs increase the number and sensitivity of beta$_2$-adrenergic receptors, which restores or increases the effectiveness of beta$_2$-adrenergic bronchodilators. The number of beta$_2$ receptors increases within approximately 4 hours, and improved responsiveness to beta2-agonists occurs within approximately 2 hours.
  - Common adverse effects include headache, pharyngitis, cough, dry mouth, hoarseness, fungal infection (candidiasis), and nausea.

**Nursing Actions**

- Albuterol should be administered first to increase airway bronchodilation, allowing beclomethasone to reach the distal segments of the lungs.
- The nurse should frequently monitor Dion's response to therapy, oxygen status, and fluid requirements.
  - Rapidly reverse airflow obstruction by administration of inhaled bronchodilators and early institution of systemic glucocorticoids.
  - Correct hypoxemia (supplemental oxygen) and/or severe hypercapnia (correction of airflow obstruction with bronchoconstriction), if present.
  - Reduce likelihood of recurrence (third asthma exacerbation in the last month) by ensuring adequate baseline controller therapy and avoidance of triggers.
- Patient and family teaching considerations:
  - Successful treatment includes controlling and avoiding asthma triggers, such as dust and mold, which are likely contributing to the exacerbation of asthma. The nurse assesses the family's ability to improve the living condition in the home. Eliminating exposure to the triggers helps improve the successful management of the condition.
  - The parents should be able to verbalize how to use the maintenance inhalants and identify a plan for quick relief measures and long-term control measures of Dion's asthma symptoms.
  - In addition, the nurse emphasizes the importance of monitoring asthma symptoms and lung function.

---

*Visit* the Point® *at* **http://thePoint.lww.com/Frandsen12e** *for answers to NCLEX Success questions (in Appendix A), answers to Clinical Application Case Studies (in Appendix B), and more!*

## REFERENCES AND RESOURCES

Anise, A., & Hasnain-Wynia, R. (2016). Patient-centered outcomes research to improve asthma outcomes. *Journal of Allergy and Clinical Immunology, 138*(6), 1503–1510.

Banasiak, N. C. (2009). Childhood asthma practice guideline part three: Update of the 2007 National Guidelines for the Diagnosis and Treatment of Asthma. The National Asthma Education and Prevention Program. *Journal of Pediatric Health Care, 23*(1), 59–61.

Bateman, E. D., Reddel, H. K., van Zyl-Smit, R. N., & Agusti, A. (2015). The asthma-COPD overlap syndrome: Towards a revised taxonomy of chronic airways diseases? *Lancet Respiratory Medicine, 3,* 719–728.

DiPiro, J. T., Talbert, R. L., Yee, G. C., Wells, B. G., Posey, L. M., & Matzke, G. R. (2016). *Pharmacotherapy: A pathophysiologic approach* (10th ed.). New York: McGraw-Hill Education.

Fanta, C. H. (2016). *An overview of asthma management.* UpToDate. Lexicomp, Inc.

Global Initiative for Asthma (GINA). (2017). *Global strategy for asthma management and prevention.* Retrieved March 1, 2019, from http://www.ginasthma.org

Harber, P., Redlich, C. A., Henneberger, P., Lareau, S. C., & Sockrider, M. (2018). Work-exacerbated asthma. *American Journal of Respiratory and Critical Care Medicine, 197*(2), P1–P2.

Henneberger, P. K., Redlich, C. A., Callahan, D. B., Harber, P., Lemière, C., Martin, J., et al.; ATS Ad Hoc Committee on Work-Exacerbated Asthma. (2011). An official American Thoracic Society statement: Work-exacerbated asthma. *American Journal of Respiratory Critical Care Medicine, 184*(3),368–378.

Hess, D., & Dhand, R. (2019). *The use of inhaler devices in adults.* UpToDate. Lexi-Comp, Inc.

Hinkle, J. L., & Cheever, K. H. (2017). *Brunner & Suddarth's textbook of medical-surgical nursing* (14th ed.). Philadelphia, PA: Lippincott Williams & Wilkins.

Incorovaia, C., Mauro, M., Makri, E., Leo, G., & Ridolo, E. (2018). Two decades with omalizumab: What we still have to learn. *Biologics, 12,* 135–142. doi:10.2147/BTT.S180846

Karch A. M. (2018). *2019 Lippincott pocket drug guide for nurses.* Philadelphia, PA: Lippincott Williams & Wilkins.

Lippincott (2017). *Nursing 2019 drug handbook* (39th ed.). Philadelphia, PA: Lippincott Williams & Wilkins.

Norris, T. L. (2019). *Porth's Pathophysiology: Concepts of altered health states* (10th ed.). Philadelphia, PA: Wolters Kluwer.

Pavord, I. D., Beasley, R., Agusti, A., Anderson, G. P., Bel, E., Brusselle, G., et al. (2018). After asthma: Redefining airways diseases. *The Lancet Commissions, 391*(10118), 350–400. https://doi.org/10.1016/S0140-6736(17)30879-6

Reddel, H. K. (2019). The impact of the Global Initiative for Asthma (GINA): Compass, concepts, controversies and challenges. *Barcelona Respiratory Network Reviews, 5*(1), 4–18.

Reddel, H. K., FitzGerald, J. M., Bateman, E. D., Bacharier, L. B., Becker, A., Brusselle, G., et al. (2019). GINA 2019: A fundamental change in asthma management. *European Respiratory Journal, 53,* 1–7. doi:10.1183/13993003.01046-2019

Sears, M. R. (2015). Predicting asthma outcomes. *Journal of Allergy and Clinical Immunology, 136*(4), 829–836.

# Drugs Affecting the Renal and Digestive Systems

# Drug Therapy for Fluid Volume Excess

## LEARNING OBJECTIVES

*After studying this chapter, you should be able to:*

1. Recognize normal renal physiology and the conditions requiring diuretic administration.
2. Identify the loop diuretics in terms of their prototype, mechanism of action, indications for use, major adverse effects, and nursing implications.
3. Describe the thiazide diuretics in terms of their prototype, mechanism of action, indications for use, major adverse effects, and nursing implications.
4. Describe the potassium-sparing diuretics in terms of their prototype, mechanism of action, indications for use, major adverse effects, and nursing implications.
5. Discuss the rationale for using combination products containing a potassium-losing and a potassium-sparing diuretic.
6. Discuss the rationale for concomitant use of a loop diuretic and a thiazide or related diuretic.
7. Implement the nursing process in the care of patients receiving diuretics.

## CLINICAL APPLICATION CASE STUDY

Agnes Bass, a 68-year-old woman, presents to the emergency department in acute heart failure complaining of an inability to "catch my breath." Her initial vital signs are temperature 99°F, pulse 108 beats per minute, respirations 28 per minute, and blood pressure 172/90 mm Hg. Her $O_2$ saturation is 88% on room air. Mrs. Bass has a history of uncontrolled hypertension, and her husband reports that for the past 2 months, they did not have sufficient money to buy her medications.

## KEY TERMS

**Anasarca:** generalized massive edema

**Anuria:** no urine output

**Ascites:** accumulation of fluid in the abdominal cavity

**Ceiling threshold:** near-maximum response of a drug that is yielded by a certain dose

**Dependent edema:** localized edema occurring in the feet and ankles in people who are ambulatory

**Edema:** excessive accumulation of fluid in body tissues

## INTRODUCTION

Drugs used to treat fluid volume excess, thereby increasing urine formation and output, are referred to as diuretics. These drugs increase renal excretion of water, sodium, and other electrolytes. They are important therapeutic agents widely used in the management of both edematous (e.g., heart failure, renal and hepatic disease) and nonedematous (e.g., hypertension, ophthalmic surgery) conditions. Diuretics are also useful in preventing renal failure by their ability to sustain urine flow. To aid understanding of diuretic drug therapy, it is necessary to understand normal renal physiology.

## RENAL PHYSIOLOGY

The primary function of the kidneys is to regulate the volume, composition, and pH of body fluids. The kidneys receive approximately 25% of the cardiac output. From this large amount of blood flow, the normally functioning kidney is efficient in retaining substances needed by the body and eliminating those not needed.

### The Nephron

The nephron is the functional unit of the kidney; each kidney contains approximately 1 million nephrons. Each nephron is composed of a glomerulus and a tubule (Fig. 34.1). The glomerulus is a network of capillaries that receives blood from the renal artery. Bowman's capsule is a thin-walled structure that surrounds the glomerulus and then narrows and continues as the tubule. The tubule is a thin-walled structure of epithelial cells surrounded by peritubular capillaries. The tubule is divided into three main segments, the proximal tubule, loop of Henle, and distal tubule, which differ in structure and function. The tubules are often called convoluted tubules because of their many twists and turns. The convolutions provide a large surface area that brings the blood flowing through the peritubular capillaries

and the glomerular filtrate flowing through the tubular lumen into close proximity. Consequently, substances can be readily exchanged through the walls of the tubules.

The nephron functions by three processes: glomerular filtration, tubular reabsorption, and tubular secretion. These processes normally maintain the fluid volume, electrolyte concentration, and pH of body fluids within a relatively narrow range. They also remove waste products of cellular metabolism. A minimum daily urine output of approximately 400 mL is required to remove normal amounts of metabolic end products.

### Glomerular Filtration

Arterial blood enters the glomerulus by the afferent arteriole at the relatively high pressure of approximately 70 mm Hg. This pressure pushes water, electrolytes, and other solutes out of the capillaries into Bowman's capsule and then to the proximal tubule. This fluid, called glomerular filtrate, contains the same components as blood except for blood cells, fats, and proteins that are too large to be filtered.

The glomerular filtration rate (GFR) is about 180 L/d or 125 mL/min. Most of this fluid is reabsorbed as the glomerular filtrate travels through the tubules. The end product is about 2 L of urine daily. Because filtration is a nonselective process, the reabsorption and secretion processes determine the composition of the urine. After it is formed, urine flows into collecting tubules, which carry it to the renal pelvis and then through the ureters, bladder, and urethra for elimination from the body.

Blood that does not become part of the glomerular filtrate leaves the glomerulus through the efferent arteriole. The efferent arteriole branches into the peritubular capillaries that eventually empty into veins, which return the blood to systemic circulation.

### Tubular Reabsorption

In relation to renal function, the term reabsorption indicates movement of substances from the tubule (glomerular filtrate)

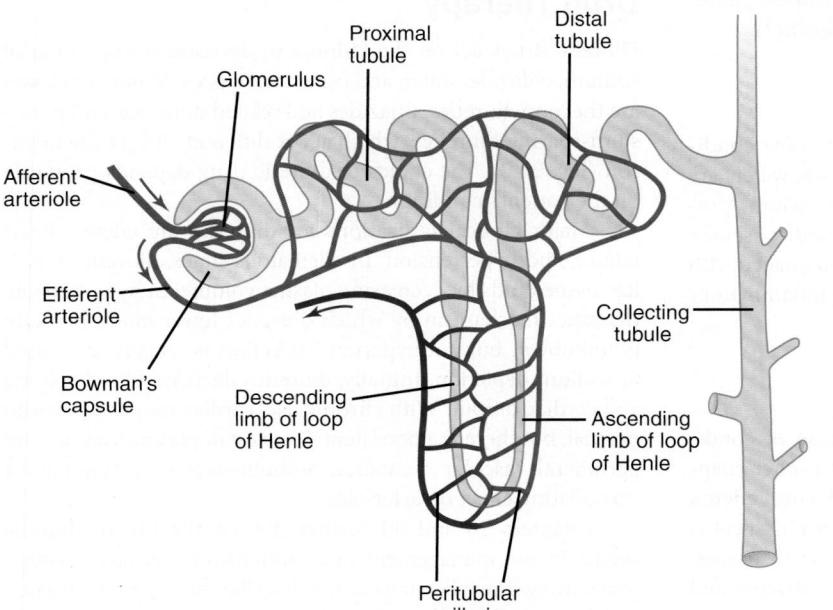

**Figure 34.1.** The nephron is the functional unit of the kidney.

to the blood in the peritubular capillaries. Most reabsorption occurs in the proximal tubule. Almost all glucose and amino acids are reabsorbed; about 80% of water, sodium, potassium, chloride, and most other substances is reabsorbed. As a result, about 20% of the glomerular filtrate enters the loop of Henle. In the descending limb of the loop of Henle, water is reabsorbed; in the ascending limb, sodium is reabsorbed. A large fraction of the total amount of sodium (up to 30%) filtered by the glomeruli is reabsorbed in the loop of Henle. Additional sodium is reabsorbed in the distal tubule, primarily by the exchange of sodium ions for potassium ions secreted by epithelial cells of tubular walls. Final reabsorption of water occurs in the distal tubule and small collecting tubules. The remaining water and solutes are now appropriately called urine.

Antidiuretic hormone from the posterior pituitary gland promotes reabsorption of water from the distal tubules and the collecting ducts of the kidneys. This conserves water needed by the body and produces more concentrated urine. Aldosterone, a hormone from the adrenal cortex, promotes sodium–potassium exchange mainly in the distal tubule and collecting ducts. Thus, aldosterone promotes sodium reabsorption and potassium loss.

## Tubular Secretion

The term *secretion*, in relation to renal function, indicates movement of substances from blood in the peritubular capillaries to glomerular filtrate flowing through the renal tubules. Secretion occurs in the proximal and distal tubules, across the epithelial cells that line the tubules. In the proximal tubule, uric acid, creatinine, hydrogen ions, and ammonia are secreted; in the distal tubule, potassium ions, hydrogen ions, and ammonia are secreted. Secretion of hydrogen ions is important in maintaining acid–base balance in body fluids.

## OVERVIEW OF CONDITIONS REQUIRING DIURETIC AGENTS

To adequately understand the pharmacologic treatment of fluid volume excess, it is important to understand the causes, pathophysiology, and clinical manifestations of renal disorders.

## Etiology

Many clinical conditions alter renal function. In some conditions, excessive amounts of substances (e.g., sodium, water) are retained; in others, needed substances (e.g., potassium, proteins) are eliminated. Causal conditions include cardiovascular, renal, hepatic, and other disorders, which may be managed with diuretic drugs. Burns and trauma or allergic and inflammatory reactions may also lead to fluid shifts or loss.

## Pathophysiology

Much of the pathophysiology related to the cause of conditions leading to the use of diuretics is discussed in other chapters. The pathophysiology of conditions producing **edema** formation (excessive accumulation of fluid in body tissues) is outlined below. Edema interferes with blood flow to tissues. Thus, it interferes with delivery of oxygen and nutrients and removal of metabolic waste products. If severe, edema may distort body features, impair movement, and interfere with activities of daily living.

Edema formation results from one or more of the following mechanisms that allow fluid to leave the bloodstream (intravascular compartment) and enter interstitial (third) spaces:

- Increased capillary permeability occurs as part of the response to tissue injury, including allergic and inflammatory reactions.
- Increased capillary hydrostatic pressure results from a sequence of events in which increased blood volume (from fluid overload or sodium and water retention) or obstruction of venous blood flow causes a high venous pressure and a high capillary pressure. This is the primary mechanism for edema formation in heart failure, pulmonary edema, and renal failure.
- Decreased plasma oncotic pressure may occur with decreased synthesis of plasma proteins (caused by liver disease or malnutrition) or increased loss of plasma proteins (caused by burn injuries or the nephrotic syndrome). Plasma proteins are important in keeping fluids within the bloodstream. When plasma proteins are lacking, fluid seeps through the capillaries and accumulates in tissues.

## Clinical Manifestations

Clinical manifestations reflect the alterations in fluid and electrolyte balance brought on by the inability of the kidneys to control the volume, composition, and pH of body fluids. Edema is a symptom of many disease processes and may occur in any part of the body. Specific manifestations of edema are determined by its location and extent. A common type of localized edema, known as **dependent edema**, occurs in the feet and ankles, especially with prolonged sitting or standing. A less common but more severe type of localized edema in the lungs is pulmonary edema, a life-threatening condition that occurs with circulatory overload (e.g., of intravenous [IV] fluids, blood transfusions) or acute heart failure. Generalized massive edema, or **anasarca**, interferes with the functions of many body organs and tissues.

## Drug Therapy

Diuretic drugs act on the kidneys to decrease reabsorption of sodium, chloride, water, and other substances. Major subclasses are the loop diuretics, thiazides and related diuretics, and potassium-sparing diuretics, which act at different sites in the nephron (Fig. 34.2). The choice of diuretic drug depends primarily on the patient's condition.

Major clinical indications for diuretics are edema, heart failure, and hypertension. In edematous states, diuretics mobilize tissue fluids by decreasing plasma volume. In hypertension, the exact mechanism by which diuretics lower blood pressure is unknown, but antihypertensive action is usually attributed to sodium depletion. Initially, diuretics decrease blood volume and cardiac output. With chronic use, cardiac output returns to normal, but there is a persistent decrease in plasma volume and peripheral vascular resistance. Sodium depletion may have a vasodilating effect on arterioles.

Chapters 26 and 30 further discuss the use of diuretic agents in the management of hypertension and heart failure, respectively. The following section describes the types of diuretics, and Table 34.1 lists individual drugs.

**Figure 34.2.** Diuretics act at different sites in the nephron to decrease reabsorption of sodium and water and to increase urine output. The main organ of the renal system is the kidney, which houses a tangled mass of nearly 1 million nephrons. The nephron is the structure known for its role in urine production. Different diuretic drugs work in different parts of the nephron: thiazide, thiazide-like, and potassium-sparing diuretics work in the distal convoluted tubule [1], loop diuretics in the ascending loop of Henle [2], and carbonic anhydrase inhibitors and osmotic diuretics in the proximal convoluted tubule [3]. Fluid and electrolyte alterations depend on where the specific diuretic works in the kidney. [Reprinted with permission from Aschenbrenner, D. S., & Venable, S. J. [2012]. *Drug therapy in nursing* [4th ed.]. Philadelphia, PA: Wolters Kluwer Health/Lippincott Williams & Wilkins.]

## TABLE 34.1

### Drugs Administered for the Treatment of Fluid Volume Excess

| Drug Class | Prototype | Other Drugs in the Class |
|---|---|---|
| **Loop diuretics** | Furosemide (Lasix) | Bumetanide (Bumex)<br>Ethacrynic acid (Edecrin)<br>Torsemide (Demadex) |
| **Thiazide-like diuretics** | Hydrochlorothiazide | Chlorothiazide (Diuril)<br>Chlorthalidone<br>Indapamide<br>Metolazone |
| **Potassium-sparing diuretics** | Spironolactone (Aldactone) | Amiloride (Midamor)<br>Eplerenone (Inspra)<br>Triamterene (Dyrenium) |
| **Osmotic diuretics** | Mannitol (Osmitrol) | |
| **Combination products** | | Aldactazide<br>Dyazide<br>Maxzide<br>Moduretic<br>(see Table 34.6 for details) |

# LOOP DIURETICS

Loop diuretics are the diuretics of choice when rapid effects are required (e.g., in pulmonary edema) and when renal function is impaired (creatinine clearance less than 30 mL/min). **Furosemide** (Lasix) is the most commonly used loop diuretic and serves as the prototype for the group. Dosage can be titrated upward as needed to produce greater diuretic effects. Overall, loop diuretics are the most effective and versatile diuretics available for clinical use and, unlike thiazide diuretics, are effective when the GFR is low.

## Pharmacokinetics

Furosemide is available in oral or IV forms. After oral administration, the diuretic effect of the drug occurs within 30 to 60 minutes, peaks in 1 to 2 hours, and lasts 6 to 8 hours. After IV administration, diuretic effects occur within 5 minutes, peak within 30 minutes, and last about 2 hours. Thus, furosemide produces extensive diuresis for short periods, after which the kidney tubules regain their ability to reabsorb sodium. Actually, the kidneys reabsorb more sodium than usual during this postdiuretic phase, so a high dietary intake of sodium can cause sodium retention and reduce or cancel the diuretic-induced sodium loss. Thus, dietary sodium restriction is required to achieve optimum therapeutic benefits. The drug is metabolized and excreted by the kidneys, and drug accumulation does not occur even with repeated doses.

## Action

Furosemide and other loop diuretics inhibit sodium and chloride reabsorption in the ascending limb of the loop of Henle, where reabsorption of most filtered sodium occurs. Thus, these potent drugs produce significant diuresis, their sodium-losing effect being up to 10 times greater than that of thiazide diuretics.

## Use

Furosemide is useful when given alone or in combination with other antihypertensive agents to treat hypertension. Uses include the management of acute pulmonary edema, heart failure, as well as hepatic and renal disease. It is feasible to titrate the dosage titrated upward as needed to produce greater diuretic effects. Table 34.2 presents route and dosage information for furosemide and the other loop diuretics.

### Use in Children

Furosemide is the loop diuretic used most often in children. Oral therapy is preferred when feasible, and authorities do not recommend doses greater than 6 mg/kg of body weight per day. For maintenance therapy, it is necessary to adjust the dose to the minimum effective level. In preterm infants, furosemide stimulates production of prostaglandin $E_2$ in the kidneys and may increase the incidence of patent ductus arteriosus and neonatal respiratory distress syndrome. In neonates, furosemide may be given with indomethacin to prevent nonsteroidal anti-inflammatory drug–induced nephrotoxicity (toxic or damaging effects to the kidney) during therapeutic closure of a patent ductus arteriosus. In both preterm and full-term infants, the half-life of furosemide is prolonged but becomes shorter as renal and hepatic functions develop.

### Use in Older Adults

In general, dose selection for the older adults requires caution, usually starting at the low end of the dosing range, reflecting the increased likelihood that older adults have decreased cardiac, renal, or hepatic function. Additionally, older adults often have concomitant disease or other drug therapy. It is necessary to monitor renal function because excessive diuresis, particularly in older adults, may cause dehydration, blood volume reduction with circulatory collapse, and the risk of vascular thrombosis and embolism.

### Use in Patients With Renal Impairment

Although furosemide and other loop diuretics are effective in patients with renal impairment, in those with chronic renal failure, the drugs have lower peak concentrations at their site of action, which decreases diuresis. Renal elimination is also prolonged. If renal dysfunction becomes more severe during treatment (e.g., oliguria, increases in blood urea nitrogen or creatinine), it may be necessary to discontinue the drug. High doses may produce fluid volume depletion and worsen renal function.

> **! QSEN Alert: Evidence-Based Practice**
>
> Polypharmacy for the treatment of chronic heart failure in adults is common. In 2018, the National Institute for Health and Clinical Excellence updated the clinical practice guideline, *Chronic Heart Failure in Adults: Diagnosis and management* [Clinical guideline no. 106], which continues to inform treatment decisions. The National Institute for Cardiovascular Outcomes Research has been compiling data through the National Heart Failure Audit to update the extent to which this guideline is used for care decisions in patients with chronic heart failure. One recommendation [no. 1.6.1] advocated that diuretics be routinely used for the relief of congestive symptoms and fluid retention in patients with heart failure. For the relief of these conditions, it is necessary to use diuretics routinely and adjust dosages according to the initiation of subsequent heart failure therapies. National findings from data collection since publication of the guidelines on the percentage of patients discharged with left ventricular systolic dysfunction found that 92% of patients were prescribed a loop diuretic on discharge.

### Use in Patients With Hepatic Impairment

Furosemide is often used to manage edema and **ascites** (accumulation of fluid in the abdominal cavity) in patients with hepatic impairment. Caution is warranted because diuretic-induced fluid and electrolyte imbalances may precipitate or worsen hepatic encephalopathy and coma. In patients with cirrhosis, diuretic therapy should begin in a hospital setting, with small doses and careful monitoring. To prevent hypokalemia and metabolic alkalosis, supplemental potassium or

**TABLE 34.2**

# DRUGS AT A GLANCE: Loop Diuretics

| Drug | Pregnancy Category | Routes and Dosage Ranges | |
|---|---|---|---|
| | | **Adults** | **Children** |
| P **Furosemide** (Lasix; ✸ APO-Furosemide, Furosemide Special, MINT-Furosemide) | C | Edema, heart failure: 20–80 mg PO, IM, IV as a single dose initially; if an adequate diuretic response is not obtained, dosage may be gradually increased by 20- to 40-mg increments at intervals of 6–8 h; for maintenance, dosage range and frequency of administration vary widely and must be individualized; max daily dose, 600 mg orally or 200 mg/dose IM and IV<br>Hypertension: 40 mg PO twice daily, gradually increased if necessary<br>Rapid mobilization of edema: 20–40 mg IV initially, injected slowly; dose may be repeated in 2 h<br>Acute pulmonary edema: initial dose is usually 40 mg IV over 1–2 min, which may be repeated in 60 min at a dose of 80 mg; max dose 200 mg<br>Acute renal failure: 40 mg IV initially, increased if necessary; max dose, 1–2 g/24 h<br>Hypertensive crisis: 40–80 mg IV injected over 1–2 min; with renal failure, much larger doses may be needed | Edema, heart failure: 2 mg/kg/dose PO initially; gradually increase by increments of 1–2 mg/kg per dose if necessary at intervals of 6–8 h; max daily dose, 6 mg/kg 1 mg/kg/dose IV initially; if diuretic response is not adequate, increase dosage by 1 mg/kg no sooner than 2 h after previous dose; maintenance dose at intervals of every 6–12 h; max dose, 6 mg/kg |
| Bumetanide (Bumex; ✸ Burinex) | C | Edema, heart failure: 0.5–2 mg PO per dose one to two times daily; may be repeated every 4–5 h to a max dose of 10 mg, if necessary; 0.5–1 mg IV, IM dose repeated in 2–3 h if necessary, may repeat in 2–3 h to a max daily dose of 10 mg; give IV injections over 1–2 min | Edema in infants and children: 0.015–0.1 mg/kg/dose PO, IM, IV every 6–24 h; max dose 10 mg daily |
| Ethacrynic acid (Edecrin; ✸ Edecrin, Sodium Edecrin) | B | Edema: 50–200 mg PO daily in one to two divided doses; max daily dose, 400 mg; rapid mobilization of edema: 50 mg IV or 0.5–1 mg/kg/dose injected slowly to a max of 100 mg/dose; repeat doses not routinely recommended | 1 mg/kg/dose once daily; increase at intervals of 2–3 d as indicated, to max of 3 mg/kg daily |
| Torsemide (Demadex) | B | Heart failure: 10–20 mg PO, IV daily; titrate by doubling the dose to a max of 200 mg daily<br>Hypertension: 5 mg PO daily up to 10 mg for appropriate response<br>Chronic renal failure: 20 mg daily PO, IV; titrate by doubling the dose to a max of 200 mg daily<br>Hepatic failure: 5–10 mg PO daily up to 40 mg for appropriate response | Safety and efficacy not established in children |

spironolactone may be necessary. Potassium imbalances may occur with diuretic therapy; Box 34.1 offers prevention and management strategies for potassium imbalances.

### Use in Patients With Critical Illness

Fast-acting, potent diuretics such as furosemide (and bumetanide) are the most likely diuretics to be used in critically ill patients (e.g., those with pulmonary edema). Although patients often receive IV bolus doses of the drugs, continuous IV infusions may be more effective and less likely to produce adverse effects in critically ill patients.

### Use in Patients Receiving Home Care

Furosemide is commonly used in the home setting. It is critical that the drug be administered safely and effectively and that

patient response is monitored. With each home visit, the nurse assesses nutritional status, blood pressure, weight, and use of over-the-counter medications that may aggravate edema or hypertension. In addition, the nurse may need to provide assistance in obtaining medications or blood for blood tests (e.g., serum potassium levels) and information as indicated.

A steady state of potassium within normal limits is necessary for cardiac function. Hypokalemia and hyperkalemia are cardiotoxic and should be prevented when possible.

## Adverse Effects

Adverse effects of furosemide include fluid and electrolyte imbalances (e.g., hyponatremia, hypokalemia, fluid volume deficit) and ototoxicity. It is usually possible to avoid ototoxicity, which is associated with high plasma drug levels (greater than

---

| BOX 34.1 | *Prevention and Management of Potassium Imbalances* |

**Hypokalemia (Serum Potassium Level < 3.5 mEq/L)**

Measures to prevent or manage hypokalemia include the following:

- Giving supplemental potassium, usually potassium chloride, in an average dosage range of 20 to 60 mEq daily. Sustained-release tablets are usually better tolerated than liquid preparations.
- Increasing food intake of potassium. The minimal daily requirement of potassium is unknown; usual recommendations are 40 to 50 mEq daily for the healthy adult. Potassium loss with diuretic drugs may be several times this amount. To provide 50 mEq of potassium daily, estimated amounts of certain foods include 1000 mL of orange juice, 1600 mL of apple or grape juice, 1200 mL of pineapple juice, 4 to 6 bananas, or 30 to 40 prunes.
  - Some of these foods are high in calories and may be contraindicated, at least in large amounts, for obese patients.

- Also, the amount of carbohydrate in these foods may be a concern for patients with diabetes mellitus.
- Restricting dietary sodium intake. This reduces potassium loss by decreasing the amount of sodium available for exchange with potassium in renal tubules.

**Hyperkalemia (Serum Potassium Level > 5 mEq/L)**

The following measures help prevent hyperkalemia:

- Avoiding use of potassium-sparing diuretics and potassium supplements in patients with renal impairment
- Avoiding excessive amounts of potassium chloride supplements
- Avoiding salt substitutes (half of which are commonly potassium chloride)
- Maintaining urine output, the major route for eliminating potassium from the body

---

50 mcg/mL), by dividing oral doses and by slow injection or continuous infusion of IV doses.

## Contraindications

Contraindications to furosemide include known sensitivity to the drug or anuria. Patients who are allergic to sulfonamides may also be allergic to furosemide. Pregnancy is another contraindication, unless the benefits to the mother outweigh the risks to the fetus.

## Nursing Implications

### Preventing Interactions

Several drugs and herbs may decrease or increase the effects of furosemide (Boxes 34.2 and 34.3, respectively). Additionally, furosemide may decrease the effects of insulin or oral antidiabetic drugs; blood glucose levels may rise.

### Administering the Medication

The nurse gives IV injections of furosemide over 1 to 2 minutes and administers high-dose furosemide continuous IV infusions

at a rate of 4 mg/min or less. This decreases or avoids high peak serum levels, which increases the risk of adverse effects, including ototoxicity. If using high doses of furosemide, a volume-controlled IV infusion at a rate of 4 mg or less per minute may be useful. For continuous infusion, it is necessary to mix furosemide with normal saline or lactated Ringer's solution because 5% dextrose in water, or D5W, may accelerate degradation of furosemide.

---

| BOX 34.2 | *Drug Interactions: Furosemide* |

**Drugs That Increase the Effects of Furosemide**
- Aminoglycosides, cephalosporins
  *Increase the risk of nephrotoxicity*
- Corticosteroids, digoxin
  *Increase the risk of hypokalemia*

**Drugs That Decrease the Effects of Furosemide**
- Ibuprofen
  *Inhibits prostaglandins*
- Phenytoin
  *Decreases absorption*

---

| BOX 34.3 | *Herb and Dietary Interactions: Furosemide, Hydrochlorothiazide, and Spironolactone* |

**Herbs and Foods That Increase the Effects of These Diuretics**
- Black cohosh
- California poppy
- Coleus
- Goldenseal
- Hawthorn
- Mistletoe
- Periwinkle
- Quinine
- Shepherd's purse

**Herbs and Foods That Decrease the Effects of These Diuretics**
- American ginseng
- Bayberry
- Blue cohosh
- Ginger
- Kola
- Licorice
- Foods

## Assessing for Therapeutic Effects

The nurse assesses for decreased or absent edema, increased urine output, and decreased blood pressure. In patients with heart failure or acute pulmonary edema, it is necessary to observe for decreased dyspnea, crackles, cyanosis, and cough.

## Assessing for Adverse Effects

Like any effective diuretic, furosemide may cause volume depletion and electrolyte imbalance, especially in patients receiving higher doses and a restricted salt intake. Hypokalemia may develop, especially with rapid diuresis, inadequate oral electrolyte intake, or when cirrhosis is present. Digitalis therapy may exaggerate metabolic effects of hypokalemia, particularly myocardial effects. The nurse should assess the patient for diminished hearing, a sign of ototoxicity. It is necessary to monitor serum electrolytes closely in children because of the frequent changes in kidney function and fluid distribution associated with growth and development.

## Patient Teaching

The reason for furosemide use should guide patient teaching. In most instances, it is necessary to initiate measures to limit sodium intake. Key considerations should include not adding salt to food during preparation or at the dinner table, reading food labels carefully to be aware of hidden sources of sodium, and avoiding processed or high-sodium foods. Loop diuretics are potassium wasting; thus, a potassium-rich, low-sodium diet is recommended. The nurse instructs the patient in the use of equipment needed to take routine blood pressure readings. The general teaching guidelines presented in Box 34.4 provide additional patient education information.

---

**BOX 34.4**  *Patient Teaching Guidelines for Diuretics*

### General Considerations

- Diuretics increase urine output and are commonly used to manage hypertension, heart failure, and edema (swelling) from heart, kidney, liver, and other disorders.
- While taking a diuretic drug, you need to maintain regular medical supervision so drug effects can be monitored and dosages adjusted when indicated.
- Reducing sodium intake in your diet helps diuretic drugs be more effective and allows smaller doses to be taken. Smaller doses are less likely to cause adverse effects. Thus, you need to avoid excessive table salt and obviously salty foods (e.g., ham, packaged sandwich meats, potato chips, dill pickles, most canned soups). These foods may aggravate edema or hypertension by causing sodium and water retention.
- Diuretics may cause blood potassium imbalances, and either too little or too much damages heart function. Periodic measurements of blood potassium and other substances are one of the major reasons for regular visits to a health care provider.
  - Too little potassium (hypokalemia) may result from the use of potassium-losing diuretics such as hydrochlorothiazide, furosemide (Lasix), and several others. To prevent or treat hypokalemia, your physician may prescribe a potassium chloride supplement or a combination of a potassium-losing and a potassium-saving diuretic (either separately or as a combined product such as Dyazide, Maxzide, or Aldactazide). He or she may also recommend increased dietary intake of potassium-containing foods (e.g., bananas, orange juice).
  - Too much potassium (hyperkalemia) can result from the use of potassium-saving diuretics, the overuse of potassium supplements, or the use of salt substitutes. Potassium-saving diuretics are not a major cause of hyperkalemia because they are usually given along with a potassium-losing diuretic. If potassium supplements are prescribed, they should be taken as directed. You should *not* use salt substitutes without consulting your primary health care provider because they contain potassium chloride instead of sodium chloride. Hyperkalemia is most likely to occur in people with decreased kidney function, which often occurs in older adults and people with diabetes.

- With diuretic therapy, you will have increased urination, which usually lasts only a few days or weeks if you do not have edema. If you do have edema (e.g., in your ankles), you can expect weight loss and decreased swelling as well as increased urination. It is a good idea to check and record your weight two to three times per week (at the same time of day with similar amount of clothing). Rapid changes in weight often indicate gain or loss of fluid.
- Some commonly used diuretics may increase blood sugar levels and cause or aggravate diabetes. If you have diabetes, you may need larger doses of your antidiabetic medications.
- Diuretics may cause sensitivity to sunlight. Thus, you need to avoid prolonged exposure to sunlight, use sunscreens, and wear protective clothing.
- Do not drink alcoholic beverages or take other medications without the approval of your health care provider.
- If you are taking a diuretic to lower your blood pressure, especially with other antihypertensive drugs, you may feel dizzy or faint when you stand up suddenly. This can be prevented or decreased by changing positions slowly. If dizziness is severe, notify your health care provider. Do not drive or operate dangerous machinery until the effects of the drug are known.

### Self or Caregiver Administration

- Take or give a diuretic early in the day, if ordered daily, to decrease nighttime trips to the bathroom. Fewer bathroom trips mean less interference with sleep and less risk of falls. Ask someone to help you to the bathroom if you are elderly, weak, dizzy, or unsteady in walking (or use a bedside commode).
- Take or give most diuretics with or after food to decrease stomach upset. Torsemide (Demadex) may be taken without regard to meals.
- If you are taking digoxin, a potassium-losing diuretic, and a potassium supplement, it is very important that you take these drugs as prescribed. This is a common combination of drugs for patients with heart failure, and the drugs work together to increase beneficial effects and avoid adverse effects. Stopping or changing the dose of one of these medications while continuing the others can lead to serious illness.

## Other Drugs in the Class

The pharmacologic characteristics of all loop diuretics are similar; use of another loop diuretic after a lack of response to one loop diuretic at adequate doses is not indicated. Instead, it is necessary to consider combining diuretics with different sites of action if aggressive diuresis is required.

Bumetanide (Bumex) may be used to produce diuresis in some patients who are allergic to or no longer respond to furosemide. It is more potent than furosemide by drug weight, and large doses can be given in small volumes. These drugs differ mainly in potency and produce similar effects at equivalent doses (e.g., furosemide 40 mg = bumetanide 1 mg). Bumetanide should be given by IV injection over 1 to 2 minutes.

Torsemide (Demadex) is indicated for the treatment of edema associated with heart failure, renal disease, or hepatic disease. It is also used for the treatment of hypertension alone or in combination with other antihypertensive agents. This drug is highly bioavailable after oral administration. Oral and IV doses are equivalent, and it is possible to switch patients from one route to the other without changing the dosage. To decrease or avoid high peak serum levels, which increase the risk of adverse effects, including ototoxicity, it is necessary to give torsemide intravenously over 2 minutes.

## THIAZIDE DIURETICS

Thiazide diuretics are synthetic drugs that are chemically related to the sulfonamides and differ mainly in their duration of action. **Hydrochlorothiazide**, the most commonly used drug in the class, is the prototype. It is not a strong diuretic and works efficiently only when urine flow is adequate. Thiazide diuretics are the drugs of choice for most patients who require diuretic therapy, especially for long-term management of heart failure and hypertension. All drugs in this group have similar effects.

## Pharmacokinetics

Hydrochlorothiazide is administered orally and is well absorbed, widely distributed in body fluids, and highly bound to plasma proteins. The drug accumulates only in the kidneys. Diuretic effects usually occur within 2 hours, peak at 4 to 6 hours, and last 6 to 24 hours. Antihypertensive effects usually last long enough to allow use of a single daily dose. Most of the drug is excreted unchanged by the kidneys within 3 to 6 hours.

## Action

Hydrochlorothiazide acts to decrease reabsorption of sodium, water, chloride, and bicarbonate in the distal convoluted tubule. Most sodium is reabsorbed before it reaches the distal convoluted tubule, and only a small amount is reabsorbed at this site.

## Use

Health care providers use hydrochlorothiazide to treat mild to moderate hypertension and the edema associated with heart failure and nephrotic syndrome. For most patients, this drug is effective. Table 34.3 presents route and dosage information for hydrochlorothiazide and the other thiazide diuretics.

### Use in Children

Children may take hydrochlorothiazide for hypertension, edema, bronchopulmonary dysplasia, hypercalciuria, and congenital nephrogenic diabetes insipidus. Chlorothiazide has more formulations, including a suspension, which may make thiazide preferable to hydrochlorothiazide in young patients. IV hydrochlorothiazide usually is not recommended. Thiazides do not commonly cause hyperglycemia, hyperuricemia, or hypercalcemia in children, as they do in adults.

### Use in Older Adults

Prescribers often order hydrochlorothiazide and other thiazide diuretics for the management of hypertension and heart failure, which are common in older adults. Older adults are especially sensitive to adverse drug effects, such as hypotension and electrolyte imbalance. The drug may aggravate renal or hepatic impairment. With rapid or excessive diuresis, myocardial infarction, renal impairment, or cerebral thrombosis may occur from fluid volume depletion and hypotension. The smallest effective dose is recommended. Adverse effects may exceed therapeutic benefits at doses greater than 25 mg.

### Use in Patients With Renal Impairment

Hydrochlorothiazide may be useful in managing edema due to renal disorders such as nephrotic syndrome and acute glomerulonephritis. However, its effectiveness decreases as the GFR decreases, and it becomes ineffective when the GFR is less than 30 mL/min. The drug may accumulate and increase adverse effects in patients with impaired renal function. Thus, it is necessary to perform renal function tests periodically.

### Use in Patients With Hepatic Impairment

Patients with severe hepatic impairment are at significant risk for thiazide-induced hypokalemic and hypochloremic alkalosis. Hepatic encephalopathy and death have occurred because of the electrolyte imbalances that accompany diuretic therapy. Blood ammonia levels may become increasingly elevated in people with previously elevated ammonia concentrations. Therapy with thiazide diuretics should be administered cautiously in patients with hepatic impairment and discontinued promptly if signs of impending hepatic coma (e.g., increased jaundice, tremors, confusion, and asterixis) appear.

### Use in Patients With Critical Illness

Hydrochlorothiazide is ineffective when immediate diuresis is required because of its slow onset of action. The loop diuretics are more likely to be administered in a critical care setting, because more potent diuretic agents may be necessary (see earlier discussion).

 **QSEN Alert: Safety**

It is important to note that hydrochlorothiazide should not be given the morning of surgery, because it may lead to volume depletion, causing the blood pressure to be labile and undergo frequent changes with general anesthesia.

| TABLE 34.3 | | | |
|---|---|---|---|
| **DRUGS AT A GLANCE: Thiazide-Like Diuretics** | | | |
| **Drug** | **Pregnancy Category** | **Routes and Dosage Ranges** | |
| | | **Adults** | **Children** |
|  **Hydrochlorothiazide** (✿ APO-Hydro, TEVA-Hydrochlorothiazide, Urozide) | B | Edema: 25–100 mg daily PO in one to two divided doses; max dose 200 mg/d<br>Hypertension: 12.5–50 mg PO 1 or 2 times daily<br>Elderly, 12.5–25 mg PO | <6 mo, 1–3 mg/kg/d in two divided doses; max 37.5 mg daily<br>>6 mo to <2 y, 1–2 mg/kg/d PO on one to two divided doses; max 37.5 mg daily<br>≥2–12 y 1–2 mg/kg/d PO on one to two divided doses; max 100 mg daily |
| Chlorothiazide (Diuril) | C | Hypertension: 500–2000 mg/d PO divided in 1–2 times doses<br>Heart failure: 250–500 mg PO once or twice daily; max 1000 mg/d<br>500–1000 mg IV once daily in combination with a loop diuretic | <6 mo, 10–30 mg/kg/d PO in two divided doses; max dose 375 mg daily<br>>6 mo, 10–20 mg/kg/d PO in one to two divided doses; max dose 375 mg daily in children <2 y or 1000 mg in children 2–12 y<br>5–10 mg/kg/d IV in two divided doses |
| Chlorthalidone (✿ APO-Chlorthalidone) | C | Edema: 50–100 mg PO daily; max 200 mg daily<br>Elderly, 12.5–25 mg/d PO (or every other day)<br>Heart failure: 12.5–25 mg PO once daily; max 100 mg daily | Hypertension: 0.3 mg/kg PO once daily up to 2 mg/kg/d; max 50 mg daily |
| Indapamide (✿ APO-Indapamide, Lozide, MYLAN-Indapamide) | B | Edema: 2.5–5 mg/d PO<br>Hypertension: 1.25 mg PO in morning; may increase to 5 mg/d | Dosage not established |
| Metolazone (✿ Zaroxolyn) | B | Edema: 5–20 mg PO, once daily<br>Hypertension: 2.5 mg once daily; max dose 20 mg daily | Edema, refractory: 0.2–0.4 mg/kg/d in doses every 12–24 h in combination with furosemide |

### Use in Patients Receiving Home Care

Diuretics are often taken in the home setting. The home care nurse may need to assist patients and caregivers in using the drugs safely and effectively, monitor patient responses, and provide information as indicated. With each home visit, the nurse assesses nutritional status, blood pressure, weight, and use of over-the-counter medications that may aggravate edema or hypertension.

## Adverse Effects

Adverse effects of hydrochlorothiazide include hypersensitivity reactions, hypotension, weakness, dizziness, diarrhea, constipation, electrolyte imbalances (e.g., hyponatremia, hypokalemia, hypochloremia), hyperglycemia, paresthesia, and erectile dysfunction.

## Contraindications

Contraindications to hydrochlorothiazide include known sensitivity to thiazides of sulfonamide-derived agents or renal decompensation or **anuria** (no urine output).

### ⚠ QSEN Alert: Safety

It is essential to use thiazide diuretics and related drugs cautiously in patients who are allergic to sulfonamide drugs because there is a known cross-sensitivity of some sulfonamide-allergic patients to a sulfonamide nonantibiotic.

Also, caution is necessary during pregnancy because the drug crosses the placenta and may have adverse effects on the fetus by compromising placental perfusion. It may cause an increased risk of congenital defects.

## Nursing Implications

### Preventing Interactions

Several drugs and herbs increase or decrease the effects of hydrochlorothiazide (Box 34.5; see Box 34.3). The thiazide diuretic can increase the effects of angiotensin-converting enzyme inhibitors, other hypertensive agents, allopurinol, calcitriol, and lithium.

**Drugs That Increase the Effects of Hydrochlorothiazide**

- Alcohol, barbiturates, monoamine oxidase inhibitors, opioids, phosphodiesterase 5 inhibitors, prostacyclin analogues
  *Increase hypotensive effects, possibly contributing to orthostasis*
- Beta-adrenergic blockers
  *Increase the risk of hyperglycemia, hyperlipidemia, and hyperuricemia*
- Carbamazepine
  *Increases the risk of hyponatremia*
- Chlorpropamide, corticosteroids, digoxin
  *Increase the risk of hypokalemia*

**Drugs That Decrease the Effects of Hydrochlorothiazide**

- Cholestyramine
  *May significantly decrease absorption*
- Methylphenidate, nonsteroidal anti-inflammatory drugs, yohimbine
  *Decrease hypotensive effects*

## Administering the Medication

Hydrochlorothiazide, like all thiazide diuretics, has a **ceiling threshold**, which means that a certain dose yields a near-maximum diuretic response. This dose, known as the ceiling dose, is dependent on the type of diuretic and the extent of a person's disease. As the maximum effect is reached, a subsequent increase in dose does not enhance efficacy. In addition, there is a direct correlation between the dosage increase and the possible onset of adverse effects. When the diuretic dose is less than at ceiling, fluid retention remains following diuresis.

## Assessing for Therapeutic Effects

The nurse assesses for the return of blood pressure to acceptable levels and improvement in the edema associated with heart failure and nephrotic syndrome.

## Assessing for Adverse Effects

Monitoring for transient or irreversible hearing impairment, tinnitus, or dizziness is important. Ototoxicity is more likely to occur with high serum drug levels (e.g., high doses or in patients with severe renal impairment) or when other ototoxic drugs (e.g., aminoglycoside antibiotics) are being taken concurrently.

## Patient Teaching

The nurse instructs the patient regarding the importance of taking the medication as prescribed, keeping follow-up appointments, and watching for signs and symptoms of adverse effects. Box 34.4 presents general patient teaching guidelines, which are a good reference.

## Other Drugs in the Class

Chlorothiazide is the only thiazide diuretic that can be given intravenously. Related diuretics are nonthiazides whose pharmacologic actions are essentially the same as those of the thiazides; they include chlorthalidone, indapamide, and metolazone. Chlorthalidone has a longer duration of action (48–72 hours), which is attributed to slower excretion.

Indapamide, a thiazide-related drug, is the first of a class of diuretics called the indolines. The drug is useful in the treatment of hypertension and can be given with other antihypertensive agents for an additive effect. People can take indapamide without regard to food. Its adverse effect profile is similar to that of hydrochlorothiazide.

Metolazone, another thiazide-related drug, is not generally recommended, but prescribers sometimes use it. Metolazone has some advantages over a thiazide because it is a stronger diuretic, causes less hypokalemia, and can produce diuresis in renal failure. In children, it is most often used with furosemide, in which case it is most effective when given 30 to 60 minutes before the furosemide dose.

---

### *Clinical Application 34.1*

After receiving oxygen at 2 L/min on nasal cannula, placement in a high Fowler's position, and administration of 40 mg of IV furosemide, Mrs. Bass's vital signs are temperature 99°F, pulse 102 beats per minute, respirations 26 per minute, blood pressure 172/90 mm Hg, and O₂ saturation 89%. Physical assessment findings include crackles on auscultation, productive cough, and bilateral 2+ peripheral edema to the knees. A cardiologist makes a diagnosis of biventricular heart failure.

- What is the rationale for the use of IV furosemide to treat the heart failure?
- What is the pathophysiology of fluid overload reflected in the assessment findings?

---

## NCLEX  Success

1. A patient receives intravenous (IV) furosemide 80 mg for symptoms of severe heart failure. The nurse recognizes that administering the drug slowly by IV push reduces the likelihood of which of the following adverse effects of drug therapy?

   A. hyponatremia
   B. hypokalemia
   C. fluid volume deficit
   D. ototoxicity

2. What assessment finding in a patient with heart failure receiving furosemide would indicate an improvement in fluid volume status?

   A. absence of crackles on auscultation of lungs
   B. complaints of proximal nocturnal dyspnea
   C. bounding radial pulse
   D. decrease in hematocrit

3. A man who is taking an oral hypoglycemic for management of his type 2 diabetes mellitus begins taking hydrochlorothiazide. The nurse should monitor for which of the following serum laboratory changes?

    A. hypocalcemia

    B. hypercalcemia

    C. hyperglycemia

    D. hypernatremia

## POTASSIUM-SPARING DIURETICS

Potassium-sparing diuretics act by competing for the aldosterone-sensitive Na+/K+ channel at the distal tubule of the nephron to decrease sodium and water reabsorption and potassium excretion. **Spironolactone** (Aldactone), the prototype drug in this class, is an aldosterone antagonist that reduces aldosterone-induced retention of sodium and water and impairs vascular function by antagonizing the action of aldosterone at mineralocorticoid receptors.

In patients with heart failure and inadequate renal function, the addition of spironolactone allows smaller doses of loop diuretics and potassium supplements to be administered as spironolactone reduces urinary potassium loss. Through this action, aldosterone antagonists are also referred to as potassium-sparing diuretics.

## Pharmacokinetics

Given orally, the effects of spironolactone are rather slow, requiring several days before full therapeutic effect is achieved; onset, peak, and duration occur between 24 and 48 hours. Absorption is best if the drug is administered with food. The half-life of the drug is 1.3 to 2 hours. Maximal effects may not occur for 6 weeks when the drug is used as an antihypertensive. It is excreted in the feces and urine.

## Action

Spironolactone competitively inhibits mineralocorticoid receptors and blocks the effects of aldosterone, a hormone secreted by the adrenal cortex, in the renal tubules. Spironolactone blocks the sodium-retaining effects of aldosterone, and aldosterone must be present for spironolactone to be effective. This effect promotes retention of sodium and water and excretion of potassium by stimulating the sodium–potassium exchange mechanism in the distal tubule. Independently, the drug is a weak diuretic because urine volume can only be slightly modified in the renal tubules; it can be combined with other diuretics to increase efficacy.

## Use

Primary uses of spironolactone include treatment of heart failure, ascites (in patients with liver disease), hypokalemia, and hypertension, as well as primary and secondary hyperaldosteronism. Also, prescribers often use spironolactone as adjunctive therapy in combination with other drugs to manage chronic heart failure. Clinical trials have shown that the addition of spironolactone improves cardiac function and reduces symptoms, hospitalizations, and mortality in patients with heart failure. Table 34.4 gives route and dosage information for spironolactone and other potassium-sparing diuretics.

### Use in Children

Spironolactone is used to treat hypertension in children. To decrease the delay in onset of effect of the drug, a loading dose of two to three times the daily amount may be administered initially. Also, it is possible to increase absorption of the drug by taking it with food.

In infants and children with isolated ventricular septal defects prior to closure, spironolactone may be added to furosemide for more aggressive diuretic therapy if needed to treat moderate heart failure. The drug is also used to diagnose primary hyperaldosteronism.

**TABLE 34.4**

### DRUGS AT A GLANCE: Potassium-Sparing Diuretics

| Drug | Pregnancy Category | Routes and Dosage Ranges | |
|------|-------------------|--------------------------|---|
| | | **Adults** | **Children** |
| **Spironolactone** (Aldactone; ❋ Aldactone, Teva-Spironolactone) | C | Edema: 25–200 PO mg daily in one to two divided doses<br>Heart failure: 12.5–25 mg PO in one to two divided doses once daily; max of 50 mg daily | Edema, hypertension: 1–17 y, 1 mg/kg/d divided every 12–24 h; max does 3.3 mg/kg/d, up to 100 mg daily |
| Amiloride (Midamor; ❋ Midamor) | B | Hypertension, heart failure: 5 mg PO once daily, may increase to 10 mg daily as necessary | Dosage not established |
| Eplerenone (Inspra; ❋ Inspra) | B | Hypertension: 50 mg PO once daily, with increase to 50 mg twice daily if response not adequate; may take 4 wk for full therapeutic response | Safety and effectiveness have not been established. |
| Triamterene (Dyrenium) | C | Edema: 100–300 mg PO daily in one to two divided doses; max to 300 mg daily | 1–2 mg/kg/d PO in two divided doses; max 3–4 mg/kg/d up to 300 mg daily |

### Use in Patients With Renal Impairment

Spironolactone accumulates in renal failure, and a reduction in dosage is warranted. Usually, practitioners do not use the drug in severe renal failure.

### Use in Patients With Hepatic Impairment

As mentioned earlier, there is an association between hepatic encephalopathy and the administration of diuretics, including some potassium-sparing diuretics. Although diuretics are used in the management of hepatic failure, they should be used cautiously and carefully monitored in patients with significant hepatic impairment because a rapid change in fluid and electrolyte balance may lead to hepatic coma. It is important to monitor susceptible patients carefully for signs and symptoms of hepatic encephalopathy such as tremors, confusion, increased jaundice, and coma. Because spironolactone is primarily metabolized in the liver, dosage reduction may be necessary in severe hepatic impairment.

### Use in Patients With Critical Illness

Diuretics other than spironolactone, which is administered orally, that can be administered intravenously are more likely to be used in critically ill patients to control the volume, composition, and pH of body fluids. Additionally, because critically ill patients can develop renal insufficiency, the risk of hyperkalemia with spironolactone is potentially harmful in most critically ill patients.

### Use in Patients Receiving Home Care

People may take spironolactone in the home care setting, and patients or family members may ask the home care nurse for advice about diuretic use or the clinical condition for which the drug is administered. The nurse should emphasize the need to read the labels of all over-the-counter medications as well as products, such as salt substitutes, for ingredients, adverse effects, and drug interactions that could complicate the patient's clinical condition. He or she should ensure that signs of hypotension and hyperkalemia and measures to manage these conditions are taught to the patient and the caregiver (see Box 34.4).

## Adverse Effects

Common adverse effects of spironolactone include dizziness, headache, abdominal cramping, and diarrhea. Because the drug also affects androgen receptors and other steroid receptors, it can cause deepening of the voice, gynecomastia, menstrual irregularities, and testicular atrophy. Its use has been known to cause an increased risk of gastric bleeding, although the mechanism is unknown. Because spironolactone may lead to a dose-related increase in serum potassium levels, assessment of serum potassium levels is important.

The U.S. Food and Drug Administration (FDA) has issued a **BLACK BOX WARNING** ◆ for spironolactone. Investigations have shown that the drug is tumorigenic with chronic toxicity in rats; unnecessary use should be avoided.

## Contraindications

Contraindications to spironolactone include known hypersensitivity to the drug. The presence of renal insufficiency is also a contraindication, as previously discussed, because use of spironolactone may cause hyperkalemia through the inhibition of aldosterone and the subsequent retention of potassium. Women should avoid taking spironolactone in the first trimester of pregnancy because antiandrogen effects have caused feminization of male fetuses in animal studies.

## Nursing Implications

### Preventing Interactions

Multiple drug and herbs interact with spironolactone, either increasing or decreasing its effects (Box 34.6; see Box 34.3). Also, spironolactone increases the half-life of digoxin, which could lead to digitalis toxicity. In addition, spironolactone may reduce renal clearance of lithium, producing a high risk of lithium toxicity.

### Administering the Medication

It is necessary to administer spironolactone at the same time each day, preferably during the morning, even if the patient feels well. As previously stated, taking the drug with food increases absorption, and this may decrease gastrointestinal irritation.

### Assessing for Therapeutic Effects

The nurse assesses for decrease or absence of edema, increased urine output, decreased blood pressure, or decreased ascites (in patients with liver disease). He or she measures and records weights to assist in determining the amount of mobilization of excess fluid. In patients with liver disease, it is necessary to assess abdominal girth to determine improvement in ascites.

### Assessing for Adverse Effects

The nurse observes for evidence of fluid and electrolyte imbalance, including hyperkalemia, hyponatremia, hypomagnesemia, and hypochloremic alkalosis. It is necessary to perform periodic laboratory tests to measure serum electrolytes at appropriate intervals, particularly in older adults and in people with significant renal or hepatic impairment.

**BOX 34.6**   **Drug Interactions: Spironolactone**

**Drugs That Increase the Effects of Spironolactone**
- Angiotensin-converting enzyme inhibitors, angiotensin II receptor blockers, potassium-containing drugs, tacrolimus
  *Increase the risk of hyperkalemia*
- Beta-adrenergic blockers
  *Increase the risk of hyperglycemia and hypertriglyceridemia*

**Drugs That Decrease the Effects of Spironolactone**
- Alcohol, antihypertensive drugs, in particular vasodilators and alpha-blockers
  *Increase the risk of hypotension and orthostasis*
- Salicylates
  *Interfere with the tubular secretion of active metabolite and decrease effectiveness*

### Patient Teaching

Routine blood pressure readings are necessary; the nurse instructs the patient in the use of equipment needed for these measurements. The nurse should instruct the patient that the drug may cause dizziness or drowsiness; the patient should curtail activities that require mental alertness (e.g., driving, operating machinery) until the effects of the drug are known. Use in pregnancy is appropriate only when the benefits to the mother outweigh the risks to the fetus. Box 34.4 contains additional patient teaching information.

## Other Drugs in the Class

Amiloride (Midamor) and triamterene (Dyrenium) act directly on the distal tubules but do not affect mineralocorticoid receptors. These drugs decrease the exchange of sodium for potassium and have similar diuretic activity. Amiloride enhances renal prostaglandin production, whereas triamterene decreases prostaglandin production. The drug is also effective in the treatment of lithium-induced nephrogenic diabetes insipidus. The choice of the specific potassium-sparing diuretic drug depends primarily on the patient's condition. Potassium-sparing diuretics are weak diuretics when used alone. Thus, they are usually given in combination with the so-called potassium-losing diuretics to increase diuretic activity and decrease potassium loss. The potassium-sparing diuretics are contraindicated in the presence of renal insufficiency because their use may cause hyperkalemia through the inhibition of aldosterone and subsequent retention of potassium. Hyperkalemia is the major adverse effect of these drugs.

Eplerenone (Inspra), like spironolactone, competitively inhibits mineralocorticoid receptors. The FDA has approved this drug for use in the management of heart failure after myocardial infarction—to improve survival. Because of the selectivity of eplerenone for aldosterone receptors, people tolerate it better than they do spironolactone; the incidence of endocrine adverse effects, including gynecomastia, menstrual irregularities, and impotence, is lower. Hyperkalemia, the most severe adverse effect of spironolactone, also occurs with eplerenone; dosage reduction is recommended with a rise in potassium level. Note that although eplerenone is more selective, with the potential for fewer adverse effects, there is no evidence in clinical trials that its overall efficacy is superior to that of spironolactone and the cost of treatment may reduce overall use.

**QSEN Alert: Safety**

It is essential that patients receiving potassium-sparing diuretics do not receive potassium supplements and do not eat foods high in potassium or use salt substitutes. [Salt substitutes contain mostly potassium chloride rather than sodium chloride.]

Box 34.1 presents strategies to manage hyperkalemia.

## ADJUVANT MEDICATIONS USED TO TREAT FLUID VOLUME EXCESS

### Osmotic Diuretics

Osmotic diuretics produce rapid diuresis by increasing the solute load (osmotic pressure) of the glomerular filtrate. The increased osmotic pressure causes water to be pulled from extravascular sites into the bloodstream, thereby increasing blood volume and decreasing reabsorption of water and electrolytes in the renal tubules. The drug is freely filterable at the glomerular level, but it is not reabsorbed by the renal tubules. **Mannitol** (Osmitrol), the prototype, is useful in managing oliguria or anuria, and it may prevent acute renal failure (ARF) during prolonged surgery, trauma, or infusion of cisplatin, an antineoplastic agent. Mannitol is effective even when renal circulation and GFR are reduced (e.g., in hypovolemic shock, trauma, dehydration). When administered early in ARF, the drug tends to clear cellular debris and prevent tubular cast formation. Other important clinical uses of hyperosmolar agents include reduction of intracranial pressure before or after neurosurgery, reduction of intraocular pressure before certain types of ophthalmic surgery (see Chap. 59), and urinary excretion of toxic substances.

The onset of diuretic action of mannitol is 1 to 3 hours, and reduction of intracranial pressure occurs in 15 to 30 minutes. Its half-life is approximately 1 to 1.6 hours. Excretion is primarily as unchanged drug in the urine.

Table 34.5 presents route and dosage information for mannitol.

| **TABLE 34.5** | | | |
|---|---|---|---|
| **DRUGS AT A GLANCE: Osmotic Diuretics** | | | |
| Drug | Pregnancy Category | Routes and Dosage Ranges | |
| | | **Adults** | **Children** |
| ⓟ **Mannitol** (Osmitrol; ✳ Osmitrol) | C | Cerebral edema: 0.25–1 g/kg IV as 15%–20% solution administered over at least 30 min, every 6–8 h as needed Intraocular pressure reduction: 1.5–2 g/kg IV administered over 30–60 min 1–1.5 h prior to surgery | Cerebral edema: 1 mo to 12 y: IV, 0.25–1.5 g/kg |

**TABLE 34.6**

## Combination Diuretic Products

| Drug Trade Name | Thiazide (Potassium-Losing) Diuretic | Potassium-Sparing Diuretic | Adult Dosage |
|---|---|---|---|
| Aldactazide 25 mg/25 mg (❀ Aldactazide 25) | HCTZ 25 mg | Spironolactone 25 mg | Hypertension, edema: 1–8 tablets PO daily |
| Aldactazide 50 mg/50 mg (❀ Aldactazide 50) | HCTZ 50 mg | Spironolactone 50 mg | Hypertension, edema: 1–4 tablets PO daily |
| Dyazide, Maxzide 25 mg/37.5 mg (❀ Apo-Trazide, Pro-Triazide, Teva-Triamterene HCTZ) | HCTZ 25 mg | Triamterene 37.5 mg | Hypertension, edema: 1–2 tablets/capsules PO once daily initially, then adjusted according to response |
| Maxzide 50 mg/75 mg (❀ Apo-Trazide, Pro-Triazide, Teva-Triamterene HCTZ) | HCTZ 50 mg | Triamterene 75 mg | Hypertension, edema: 1 tablet/ capsule PO daily |

HCTZ, hydrochlorothiazide.

### Clinical Application 34.2

- Mrs. Bass has improved, and her vital signs are temperature 98.6°F, pulse 84 beats per minute, respirations 18 per minute, blood pressure 132/80 mm Hg, and $O_2$ saturation 94% on room air. Her physician orders an extra dose of 20 mg of IV furosemide, to be given now. What administration guidelines should the nurse consider?

## Combination Products

Thiazide diuretics are available in numerous fixed-dose combinations with nondiuretic antihypertensive agents (see Chap. 26) and with potassium-sparing diuretics. Table 34.6 lists combination diuretic products. Fixed-dose combination products are not indicated for initial therapy of edema or hypertension because therapy should be titrated for the individual patient. However, if the fixed combination represents the dosage so determined, a major benefit of antihypertensive combinations is increased patient convenience and compliance. Additionally, a major purpose of diuretic combinations is prevention of potassium imbalances, typically by combining potassium-sparing and potassium-wasting diuretics.

To prevent or manage hypokalemia and to augment the diuretic effect, people may take a potassium-sparing diuretic concurrently with a potassium-losing diuretic. They may take the two drugs separately or in a fixed-dose combination product.

Alternatively, when an inadequate diuretic response occurs with one of the drugs, people sometimes take two potassium-losing diuretics concurrently. The combination of a loop and a thiazide diuretic has synergistic effects because the drugs act in different segments of the renal tubule. The synergistic effects probably result from the increased delivery of sodium to the distal tubule (where thiazides act) because a loop diuretic blocks sodium reabsorption in the loop of Henle. A commonly used combination is furosemide and hydrochlorothiazide (chlorothiazide can be given intravenously in patients who are unable to take an oral drug). Another combination is furosemide and metolazone. Generally, because a thiazide-loop diuretic combination can induce profound diuresis, with severe sodium, potassium, and volume depletion, only hospitalized patients who can be closely monitored should receive it. Ambulatory patients should take this combination in very low doses or only occasionally to avoid serious adverse events.

### NCLEX Success

4. Mrs. Conley, age 53, has had hypertension for 10 years and admits that she does not comply with her prescribed antihypertensive therapy. Recently, she has begun to experience shortness of breath and ankle swelling. A workup reveals the presence of chronic renal insufficiency. What classification of diuretic is the first drug of choice for the nurse practitioner to prescribe?
   A. thiazide
   B. loop
   C. osmotic
   D. potassium sparing

5. A nurse is instructing a patient on dietary considerations while taking spironolactone (Aldactone). Which of the following statements made by the patient indicates that teaching has been successful? **(Select all that apply.)**
   A. "I should not eat foods high in potassium while taking this medication."
   B. "I should use a salt substitute instead of regular salt."
   C. "I should call my nurse practitioner if I have any significant adverse effects from my medications."
   D. "I should not take large amounts of potassium chloride supplements."

6. A patient reports a drug allergy to sulfonamides. Which diuretic drug class should the nurse question if ordered for the patient?
   A. loop diuretics
   B. thiazides
   C. potassium-sparing diuretics
   D. osmotic diuretics

## THE NURSING PROCESS

A concept map outlines the nursing process related to drug therapy considerations in this chapter. Additional nursing implications related to the disease process should also be considered in care decisions.

**Assessment**

- Useful baseline data include serum electrolytes, creatinine, glucose, BUN, and uric acid, because diuretics may alter these values. Other data are blood pressure readings, weight, amount and appearance of urine output, and measurement of edematous areas such as ankles or abdomen.
- Observe for edema. Visible edema often occurs in the feet and legs of ambulatory patients. Rapid weight gain may indicate fluid retention.
  - With heart failure, numerous signs and symptoms result from edema of various organs and tissues. For example, congestion in the gastrointestinal tract may cause nausea and vomiting; liver congestion may cause abdominal pain and tenderness; and congestion in the lungs (pulmonary edema) causes rapid, labored breathing, hypoxemia, frothy sputum, and other manifestations of severe respiratory distress.
  - Cerebral edema may be manifested by confusion, headache, dizziness, convulsions, unconsciousness, bradycardia, or failure of the pupils to react to light.
  - Ascites, which occurs with hepatic cirrhosis, is an accumulation of fluid in the abdominal cavity. The abdomen appears much enlarged.
- With heart failure, fatigue and dyspnea, in addition to edema, are common symptoms.
- Hypertension (blood pressure greater than 140/90 mm Hg on several measurements) may be the only clinical manifestation present.

**Outcomes of Therapy**

The patient will
- Take or receive diuretic drugs as prescribed.
- Experience reduced edema and improved control of blood pressure.
- Reduce dietary intake of sodium and increase dietary intake of potassium.
- Avoid preventable adverse drug effects.
- Keep appointments for follow-up monitoring of blood pressure, edema, and serum electrolytes.

**Nursing Interventions**

- Promote measures to prevent or minimize conditions for which diuretic drugs are used.
  - With edema, helpful measures include the following:
    - Decreasing dietary sodium intake
    - Losing weight, if obese
    - Elevating legs when sitting
    - Avoiding prolonged standing or sitting
    - Wearing support hose or elastic stockings
    - Treating the condition causing edema
  - With heart failure and in older adults, it is necessary to administer IV fluids or blood transfusions carefully to avoid fluid overload and pulmonary edema. Fluid overload may occur with rapid administration or excessive amounts of IV fluids.
  - With hypertension, helpful measures include decreasing dietary sodium intake, exercising regularly, and losing weight, if obese.
  - With edematous patients, interventions to monitor fluid losses include weighing under standardized conditions, measuring urine output, and measuring edematous sites such as the ankles or the abdomen. After the patient reaches "dry weight," these measurements stabilize and can be done less often.
  - With patients who are taking digoxin, a potassium-losing diuretic, and a potassium supplement, help them understand that the drugs act together to increase therapeutic effectiveness and avoid adverse effects (e.g., hypokalemia, digoxin toxicity). Thus, stopping or changing dosage of one of these drugs can lead to serious illness.
- Provide patient teaching regarding drug therapy (see Box 34.3).

**Evaluation**

- Observe for reduced edema and body weight.
- Observe for reduced blood pressure.
- Observe for increased urine output.
- Monitor serum electrolytes for normal values.
- Interview regarding compliance with instructions for diet and drug therapy.
- Monitor compliance with follow-up appointments in outpatients.

### Clinical Application 34.3

● Mrs. Bass says that she enjoys snacks such as potato chips and pretzels. What response should the nurse make?

## KEY CONCEPTS

- Diuretic drugs act on the kidneys to decrease reabsorption of sodium, chloride, water, and other substances.
- A body weight change of 2.2 lb (1 kg) may indicate a gain or loss of 1000 mL of fluid.
- Excessive table salt and salty foods (e.g., ham, packaged sandwich meats, potato chips, dill pickles, most canned soups) may aggravate edema or hypertension.
- Thiazide diuretics are the drugs of choice for most patients who require diuretic therapy, especially for long-term management of heart failure and hypertension.
- High-dose furosemide continuous IV infusions should be given at a rate of 4 mg/min or less to decrease or avoid risks of adverse effects, including ototoxicity.

- There is a known cross-sensitivity of some sulfonamide-allergic patients to a sulfonamide nonantibiotic, such as the thiazides.
- Loop diuretics have a sodium-losing effect up to 10 times greater than that of thiazide diuretics.
- Patients with renal impairment should not take potassium-sparing diuretics because of the high risk of hyperkalemia.
- The U.S. FDA has issued a **BLACK BOX WARNING** ◆ for spironolactone, which has been shown to be tumorigenic with chronic toxicity in rats; unnecessary use should be avoided.
- When digoxin and diuretics are given concomitantly, the risk of digoxin toxicity is increased due to diuretic-induced hypokalemia.

## CLINICAL REASONING CASE STUDY

| | |
|---|---|
| **Meet the Patient** | Tonya Oliver, a 32-year-old executive, is diagnosed with hypertension and is starting hydrochlorothiazide. She is currently taking birth control pills and complains that she has peripheral edema in the evenings.<br>• What important information should be obtained from Mrs. Oliver before the discharging her from the clinic?<br>• What are important points to teach Mrs. Oliver about safe and effective drug usage?<br>• If on return to clinic, Mrs. Oliver's symptoms have not improved, what questions need answers? |
| **Assessing Drug Information** | • Hydrochlorothiazide acts to decrease reabsorption of sodium, water, chloride, and bicarbonate in the distal convoluted tubule. Most sodium is reabsorbed before it reaches the distal convoluted tubule and only a small amount is reabsorbed at this site.<br>• The drug is primarily used for the treatment of hypertension and edema due to heart failure, various forms of renal dysfunction (e.g., nephrotic syndrome, acute glomerulonephritis), corticosteroid and estrogen therapy.<br>• Adverse effects include dizziness; headache; weakness; tingling of hands, legs, or feet; erectile dysfunction; and respiratory distress. |
| **Nursing Actions** | • Assess drug allergies because there is a known cross-sensitivity between sulfonamides and sulfonamide nonantibiotics such as hydrochlorothiazide.<br>• Assess the consistency of Mrs. Oliver's birth control practices because it is necessary to use caution with hydrochlorothiazide during pregnancy.<br>　• The drug crosses the placenta and may have adverse effects on the fetus by compromising placental perfusion.<br>　• Mrs. Oliver should use alternate birth control if she does not take her birth control pills as directed.<br>　• It is essential that Mrs. Oliver be instructed to notify the nurse practitioner if she believes she is pregnant.<br>• Instruct Mrs. Oliver about the indications for use of hydrochlorothiazide, the major adverse effects, and symptoms that necessitate notification of the prescriber (e.g., respiratory distress, paresthesia).<br>• Emphasize that decreasing dietary sodium intake, exercising regularly, and losing weight (if overweight or obese).<br>• Tell Mrs. Oliver that women who take birth control pills are at risk for retention of sodium and water.<br>• Instruct Mrs. Oliver about keeping appointments for follow-up monitoring of blood pressure, edema, and serum electrolytes.<br>• Provide instruction about the process of measuring blood pressure and confirming return demonstration by Mrs. Oliver. Explain the importance of keeping a record of readings for analysis of therapeutic effect of treatment plan.<br>• If on return to the clinic, Mrs. Oliver's symptoms have not improved, consider whether:<br>　• The prescribed diuretic is being taken correctly.<br>　• The recommended diet is being followed.<br>　• There is worsening of the underlying condition that led to the edema.<br>　• Another disease or complication has developed. |

Visit **thePoint®** at **http://thePoint.lww.com/Frandsen12e** *for answers to NCLEX Success questions (in Appendix A), answers to Clinical Application Case Studies (in Appendix B), and more!*

## REFERENCES AND RESOURCES

Brater, D. C. (2016). *Mechanism of action of diuretics*. UpToDate, Lexicomp, Inc.

Dassanayaka, S., & Jones, S. P. (2015). Recent developments in heart failure. *Circulation Research, 117*(7), e58–e63.

DiPiro, J. T., Talbert, R. L., Yee, G. C., Wells, B. G., Posey, L. M., Fulton, D. R., et al. (2016). *Management of isolated ventricular septal defects in infants and children*. UpToDate, Lexicomp, Inc.

Hinkle, J. L., & Cheever, K. H. (2018). *Brunner and Suddarth's textbook of medical-surgical nursing* (14th ed.). Philadelphia, PA: Lippincott Williams & Wilkins.

Karch, A. M. (2019). *2019 Lippincott's pocket drug guide for nurses*. Philadelphia, PA: Lippincott Williams & Wilkins.

Matzke, G. R. (2016). *Pharmacotherapy: A pathophysiologic approach* (10th ed.). New York, NY: McGraw-Hill Education.

National Collaborating Centre for Acute and Chronic Conditions. (2018). *Chronic heart failure in adults: Diagnosis and management*. National Institute for Health and Clinical Excellence (NICE) (Clinical guideline no. 106). Retrieved January 24, 2020, from https://www.nice.org.uk/guidance/ng106

Norris, T. L. (2019). *Pathophysiology: Concepts of altered health status* (10th ed.). Philadelphia, PA: Lippincott Williams & Wilkins.

Yancy, C. W., Jessup, M., Bozkurt, B., Butler, J., Casey, D. E., Drazner, M. H., et al.; American College of Cardiology Foundation/American Heart Association Task Force on Practice Guidelines. (2013). 2013 ACCF/AHA guideline for the management of heart failure: A report of the American College of Cardiology Foundation/American Heart Association Task Force on practice guidelines. *Circulation, 128*(16), e240–e327.

# 35

# Nutritional Support Products, Vitamins, and Mineral Supplements

## LEARNING OBJECTIVES

*After studying this chapter, you should be able to:*

1. Discuss the need for vitamin and mineral supplements.
2. Describe the use of vitamins and minerals in specific groups of patients.
3. Identify fat-soluble vitamins used to treat deficiencies, including the nursing implications associated with their administration.
4. Identify water-soluble vitamins used to treat deficiencies, including the nursing implications associated with their administration.
5. Identify minerals used to treat deficiencies, including the nursing implications associated with their administration.
6. Discuss the chelating agents used to remove excess copper, iron, and lead from body tissues.
7. Recognize the benefit of nutritional supplements, including the nursing implications associated with their administration.
8. Apply nursing process skills to prevent, recognize, or treat nutritional imbalances, which may involve monitoring laboratory reports that indicate nutritional status.

## CLINICAL APPLICATION CASE STUDY

Jenny Martin, an 86-year-old woman, has lived alone for 10 years since her husband died. She sometimes must limit her food purchases to pay for her medicines and utilities. Thus, her nutritional status is poor. A neighbor, who has not seen Mrs. Martin for a couple of days, finds her lying on the kitchen floor, conscious but with slurred speech. Emergency medical personnel transport her to a hospital emergency department, where she is diagnosed with a left brain stroke with right hemiparesis, dysarthria, and dysphagia.

Mrs. Martin is unable to swallow foods safely, so the nurses insert a nasogastric tube. A dietician orders a high-calorie commercially prepared formula that contains carbohydrates, protein, fat, vitamins, and minerals.

## KEY TERMS

**Chelating agents:** drugs used to treat metal poisoning (e.g., from iron, lead, or mercury) that bind to the toxic metal, decrease binding of the metal within the body, and promote elimination of the metal

**Electrolytes:** electrically charged particles found in body fluids and cells (e.g., sodium or potassium ions)

**Enteral nutrition:** provision of fluid and nutrients to a functional gastrointestinal tract via a feeding tube in a patient who is unable to ingest enough fluid and food

**Fat-soluble vitamins:** vitamins that are accumulated and stored in the body when taken in excess

**Hyperkalemia:** greater than normal amount of potassium in the blood

**Hypokalemia:** less than normal amount of potassium in the blood

**Malabsorption:** impaired absorption of nutrients from the gastrointestinal tract

**Megaloblastic anemia:** anemia characterized by the presence in the blood of megaloblasts (large, abnormal blood cells) associated with vitamin $B_{12}$ deficiency

**Megavitamins:** large dose of vitamins in excess of the recommended dietary allowance

**Parenteral nutrition:** intravenous provision of fluid and nutrients to a patient who is unable to ingest enough fluid and food due to a nonfunctional gastrointestinal tract

**Water-soluble vitamins:** vitamins that are not stored in the body and are rapidly eliminated

# INTRODUCTION

Water, carbohydrates, proteins, fats, vitamins, and minerals are required to promote or maintain health, to prevent illness, and to promote recovery from illness or injury. Water is necessary for cellular metabolism and excretion of metabolic waste products; people need 2000 to 3000 mL daily. Carbohydrates and fats mainly provide energy for cellular metabolism. Energy is measured in kilocalories (kcal) per gram of food oxidized in the body. Carbohydrates and proteins supply 4 kcal/g, and fats supply 9 kcal/g. Proteins are structural and functional components of all body tissues; the recommended amount for adults is 50 to 60 g daily.

Vitamins are required for normal body metabolism, growth, and development. They are components of enzyme systems that release energy from ingested carbohydrates, proteins, and fats. They also are necessary for formation of genetic material, red blood cells, hormones, nerve cells, and bone and other tissues. Minerals and electrolytes are essential constituents of cell membranes, many essential enzymes, bone, teeth, and connective tissue. They function to maintain electrolyte and acid–base balance, maintain osmotic pressure, maintain nerve and muscle function, assist in transfer of compounds across cell membranes, and influence the growth process.

Patients' requirements for these nutrients vary widely, depending on age, sex, size, health or illness status, and other factors. This chapter discusses medications and products to improve nutritional status in patients with deficiency states and excess states of selected vitamins, minerals, and electrolytes.

# OVERVIEW OF ALTERED NUTRITIONAL STATES

## Etiology

Many patients may be unable to ingest, digest, absorb, or use sufficient nutrients to improve or maintain health. Debilitating illnesses often interfere with appetite and gastrointestinal (GI) function. Drugs often cause anorexia, nausea, vomiting, or diarrhea. The lack of certain vitamins and minerals may impair the function of body organs. Genetic disorders or traumatic injury may also affect nutritional status.

## Pathophysiology

Dietary intake must provide required amino acids, fatty acids, and lipids, as well as vitamins and minerals. Both deficient and excess amounts of these nutrients adversely influence health. Nutritional status directly affects enzyme function, immune response, and wound healing.

### Vitamins

Vitamins are organic compounds that help release energy from carbohydrates, fats, and proteins. They are necessary for the formation of genetic materials, red blood cells, hormones, and the nervous system, as well as for normal growth and development.

There are two types of vitamins: fat soluble and water soluble. **Fat-soluble vitamins**—vitamins A, D, E, and K—are stored in the body when taken in excess. They are absorbed from the intestine with dietary fat. Absorption requires the presence of bile salts and pancreatic lipase. (Note that vitamin D is discussed in Chapter 44 because of its major role in bone metabolism.) **Water-soluble vitamins**—B complex vitamins and vitamin C—are not stored in the body and are rapidly eliminated.

People can obtain vitamins from foods or supplements. Although experts believe foods to be the best source, studies indicate that most adults and children do not consume enough fruits, vegetables, cereal grains, dairy products, and other foods to consistently meet their vitamin requirements. In addition, some conditions increase requirements above the recommended amounts (e.g., pregnancy, lactation, and various illnesses). Historically, the major concern about vitamins concerned whether a person's intake was sufficient to promote health and prevent deficiency diseases. Hence, the Food and Nutrition Board of the National Academy of Sciences established recommendations for daily vitamin intake known as Dietary Reference Intakes (DRIs) (Box 35.1).

Vitamin deficiencies occur as a result of inadequate intake or disease processes that interfere with absorption or use of vitamins. Excess states occur with excessive intake of fat-soluble vitamins because these vitamins accumulate in the body. Excess states do not occur with dietary intake of water-soluble vitamins but may occur with vitamin supplements that exceed recommended amounts.

---

| **BOX 35.1** | *Dietary Reference Intakes* |
| --- | --- |

Dietary Reference Intakes (DRIs) are the recommended amounts of vitamins (see Table 35.1) and some minerals (see Table 35.2). The Food and Nutrition Board of the Institute of Medicine revised the current DRIs in 2006; the board intended them to replace the recommended dietary allowances (RDAs) used since 1989. DRIs consist of four subtypes of nutrient recommendations, as follows:

1. **Recommended dietary allowance (RDA)** is the amount estimated to meet the needs of approximately 98% of healthy children and adults in a specific age and gender group. The RDA is used to advise various groups about nutrient intake. It should be noted, however, that RDAs were established to prevent deficiencies and that they were extrapolated from studies of healthy adults. Thus, they may not be appropriate for all groups, such as young children and older adults.

2. **Estimated average requirement (EAR)** is the amount estimated to provide adequate intake in 50% of healthy persons in a specific group. The EAR is a median amount that takes into account the bioavailability of the nutrient and reduction of chronic disease. The EAR is used to determine the RDA.

3. **Adequate intake (AI)** is the amount thought to be sufficient when there is not enough reliable, scientific information to estimate an RDA. The AI is derived from data that show an average intake that appears to maintain health. Although an RDA is expected to meet the needs of all healthy people, an AI does not clearly

indicate the percentage of people whose needs will be met.

4. **Tolerable upper intake level (UL)** is the maximum intake considered unlikely to pose a health risk in almost all healthy people in a specified group. The UL is not intended to be a recommended level of intake.
   - **Vitamins.** The ULs for adults (ages 19–70 years and older) are D 100 mcg, E 1000 mg, $B_3$ (niacin) 35 mg, $B_6$ (pyridoxine) 100 mg, folate 1000 mcg, and C 2000 mg. With vitamin D, pyridoxine, and vitamin C, the UL refers to total intake from food, fortified food, and supplements. With niacin and folate, the UL applies to synthetic forms obtained from supplements, fortified food, or a combination of the two. With vitamin E, the UL applies to any form of supplemental alpha-tocopherol. *These ULs should not be exceeded.* There are inadequate data for establishing ULs for $B_1$ (thiamine), $B_2$ (riboflavin), $B_5$ (pantothenic acid), $B_{12}$ (cyanocobalamin), and biotin. As a result, consuming more than the recommended amounts of these vitamins should generally be avoided.
   - **Minerals.** ULs have been established for magnesium 350 mg, calcium 2.5 g, phosphorus 3 to 4 g, fluoride 10 mg, and selenium 400 mcg. *The UL should not be exceeded for any mineral–electrolyte because all minerals are toxic in overdose.* Except for magnesium, which is set for supplements only and excludes food and water sources, the stated UL amounts include those from both food and supplements.

---

Many authorities promote vitamin supplements as a means to improve health and prevent or treat illness. However, supplements can be harmful if overused. As a result, DRIs include tolerable upper intake levels (ULs) of some vitamins. Table 35.1 lists the function, recommended daily intake, food sources, and signs and symptoms of deficiency and excess of vitamins.

> **! QSEN Alert: Safety**
>
> No one should take more than the recommended ULs.

Although health care providers may order vitamin supplements, people mostly self-prescribe them. Because vitamins are essential nutrients, some people believe that large amounts (megadoses) promote health and provide other beneficial effects. However, excessive intake may cause harmful effects. People should never self-prescribe **megavitamins**, large doses of vitamins in excess of the recommended dietary allowance (RDA). Additional characteristics of vitamins include the following:

- Vitamins from supplements have the same physiologic effects as those obtained from foods.
- Synthetic vitamins have the same structure and function as do natural vitamins derived from plant and animal sources and are less expensive.
- Vitamin supplements do not require a prescription.
- Vitamin products vary widely in number, type, and amount of specific ingredients.

- Preparations should not contain more than the recommended amounts of vitamin A, vitamin D, and folic acid (a B complex vitamin).
- Multivitamin preparations often contain minerals as well. Large doses of all minerals are toxic.
- Vitamins are often marketed in combination products with each other (e.g., antioxidant vitamins) and with herbal products (e.g., B complex vitamins with ginseng). There is no reliable evidence to support the use of such products.

Some people believe that some vitamins (e.g., the vitamin A precursor beta-carotene, vitamin E, and vitamin C), with their antioxidant effects, prevent heart disease, cancer, and other illnesses. Antioxidants inactivate oxygen free radicals, which are potentially toxic substances formed during normal cell metabolism, and inhibit them from damaging body cells. However, the results of most research studies with antioxidant vitamin supplements have been disappointing and inconclusive. The consensus view is that dietary vitamins from several daily servings of grains, fruits, and vegetables and a daily multivitamin supplement are beneficial for most children and adults, but it is not possible to make recommendations about vitamin supplements to prevent various chronic illnesses on the basis of current evidence. Because parents' desires to promote health may lead them to give children unneeded supplements or to give them more than recommended amounts, it may be necessary to give parents information about the potential hazards of vitamin overdoses.

## TABLE 35.1

## Vitamins

| Vitamin/Function | Dietary Reference Intakes | Food Sources | Signs and Symptoms of Deficiency | Signs and Symptoms of Excess |
|---|---|---|---|---|
| **Fat-Soluble Vitamins** | | | | |
| **Vitamin A (retinol)** Required for normal vision, growth, bone development, skin, and mucous membranes | RDAs Females 14 y and older: 700 mcg Pregnancy, 19 y and older: 770 mcg 14–18 y: 750 mcg Lactation, 19 y and older: 1300 mcg Lactation, 14–18 y: 1200 mcg Males 14 y and older: 900 mcg Children 1–3 y: 300 mcg 4–8 y: 400 mcg 9–13 y: 600 mcg Infants (AIs) 1–6 mo, 400 mcg 7–12 mo, 500 mcg | Preformed vitamin A: meat, butter, fortified margarine, egg yolk, whole milk, cheese made from whole milk Carotenoids: turnip and collard greens, carrots, sweet potatoes, squash, apricots, peaches, cantaloupe | Night blindness; xerophthalmia, which may progress to corneal ulceration and blindness; changes in skin and mucous membranes that lead to skin lesions and infections; respiratory tract infections; urinary calculi | Anorexia; vomiting; irritability; skin changes (itching, desquamation, dermatitis); pain in muscles, bones, and joints; gingivitis; enlargement of spleen and liver; increased intracranial pressure; other neurologic signs Congenital abnormalities in newborns whose mothers took excessive vitamin A during pregnancy Acute toxicity, with increased intracranial pressure, bulging fontanelles, and vomiting, may occur in infants who are given vitamin A |
| **Vitamin D** (see Chap. 44) | | | | |
| **Vitamin E** (antioxidant) Essential in preventing destruction of certain fats, including the lipid portion of cell membranes | RDAs* Adults 15 mg; UL not >1000 mg Pregnancy ≤18 y: 15 mg; UL not >800 mg 19–50 y: 15 mg; UL not >1000 mg Lactation 19–50 y: 19 mg; UL not >1000 mg ≤18 y: 19 mg; UL not > 800 mg Children 1–3 y: 6 mg; UL not >200 mg 4–8 y: 7 mg; UL not >300 mg 9–13 y: 11 mg; UL not above 600 mg 14–18 y: 15 mg; UL not >800 mg Infants (AIs) 1–6 mo: 4 mg 7–12 mo: 5 mg | Cereals, green leafy vegetables, egg yolk, milk fat, butter, meat, vegetable oils | Deficiency is rare | Fatigue, headache, blurred vision, nausea, diarrhea |

*(Continued on page 700)*

**TABLE 35.1**

## Vitamins (Continued)

| Vitamin/Function | Dietary Reference Intakes | Food Sources | Signs and Symptoms of Deficiency | Signs and Symptoms of Excess |
|---|---|---|---|---|
| **Vitamin K**<br>Essential for normal blood clotting. It activates precursor proteins, found in the liver, into clotting factors II, VII, IX, and X | AIs<br>Males: 120 mcg/d<br>Females: 90 mcg/d (same dose in pregnancy and lactation)<br>RDAs<br>Children<br>1–3 y: 30 mcg<br>4–8 y: 55 mcg<br>9–13 y: 60 mcg<br>14–18 y: 75 mcg | Green leafy vegetables (spinach, kale, cabbage, lettuce), cauliflower, tomatoes, wheat bran, cheese, egg yolk, liver | Abnormal bleeding (petechiae, ecchymoses, epistaxis, hematemesis, melena, hematuria, hypovolemic shock) | Clinical manifestations rare; however, when vitamin K is given to someone who is receiving warfarin (Coumadin), the patient can be made "warfarin resistant" for 1 wk or more |
| **Water-Soluble Vitamins** | | | | |
| ***B Complex Vitamins***<br>**Vitamin B₁ (thiamine)**<br>A coenzyme in carbohydrate metabolism; essential for energy production | RDAs<br>Females<br>19 y and older: 1.1 mg<br>Pregnancy: 1.4 mg<br>Lactation: 1.4 mg<br>Males<br>19 y and older: 1.2 mg<br>Children<br>1–3 y: 0.5 mg<br>4–8 y: 0.6 mg<br>9–13 y: 0.9 mg<br>14–18 y: females, 1 mg; males, 1.2 mg<br>Infants (AIs)<br>0–6 mo: 0.2 mg<br>7–12 mo: 0.3 mg | Meat, poultry, fish, egg yolk, dried beans, whole-grain cereal products, peanuts | Mild deficiency: fatigue, anorexia; retarded growth; mental depression; irritability; apathy, lethargy<br>Severe deficiency (beriberi): peripheral neuritis; personality disturbances; heart failure; edema<br>Wernicke-Korsakoff syndrome in alcoholics | Not established |
| **Vitamin B₂ (riboflavin)**<br>A coenzyme in metabolism; necessary for growth; may function in production of corticosteroids and red blood cells and in gluconeogenesis | RDAs<br>19 y and older: 1.1 mg<br>Pregnancy: 1.4 mg<br>Lactation: 1.6 mg<br>Males<br>19 y and older: 1.3 mg<br>Children<br>1–3 y: 0.5 mg<br>4–8 y: 0.6 mg<br>9–13 y: 0.9 mg<br>14–18 y: females, 1 mg; males, 1.3 mg<br>Infants (AIs)<br>1–6 mo: 0.3 mg<br>7–12 mo: 0.4 mg | Milk, cheddar and cottage cheeses, meat, eggs, green leafy vegetables | Seborrheic dermatitis, glossitis, stomatitis, eye disorders (burning, itching, lacrimation, photophobia, vascularization of the cornea) | Not established |
| **Biotin**<br>Part of the vitamin B₂ complex; essential in fat and carbohydrate metabolism | AIs<br>Adults<br>30 mcg/d<br>Children<br>1–3 y: 8 mcg<br>4–8 y: 12 mcg<br>9–13 y: 20 mcg<br>14–18 y: 25 mcg<br>Infants<br>1–5 mo: 5 mcg<br>6–12 mo: 6 mcg | Meat, egg yolk, nuts, cereals, most vegetables | Anorexia, nausea; depression; muscle pain; dermatitis | Not established |

**TABLE 35.1**

## Vitamins (Continued)

| Vitamin/Function | Dietary Reference Intakes | Food Sources | Signs and Symptoms of Deficiency | Signs and Symptoms of Excess |
|---|---|---|---|---|
| **Vitamin B₃ (niacin)** Essential for glycolysis, fat synthesis, and tissue respiration. It functions as a coenzyme in many metabolic processes (after conversion to nicotinamide, the physiologically active form) | RDAs Females 19 y and older: 14 mg Pregnancy (all ages): 18 mg Lactation (all ages): 17 mg Males 19 y and older: 16 mg Children 1–3 y: 6 mg 4–8 y: 8 mg 9–13 y: 12 mg 14–18 y: females, 14 mg; males, 16 mg Infants (AIs) 0–5 mo: 2 mg 6–11 mo: 3 mg | Meat, poultry, fish, peanuts | Pellagra: erythematous skin lesions; GI problems (stomatitis, glossitis, enteritis, diarrhea); CNS problems (headache, dizziness, insomnia, depression, memory loss) Severe deficiency: delusions, hallucinations, impairment of peripheral motor and sensory nerves | Flushing, pruritus, hyperglycemia, increased liver enzymes, uricemia |
| **Vitamin B₅ (pantothenic acid)** Essential for metabolism of carbohydrate, fat, and protein (e.g., release of energy from carbohydrate; fatty acid metabolism; synthesis of cholesterol, steroid hormones, and phospholipids) | AIs Adults: 5 mg Females 14 y and older: 5 mg Pregnancy: 6 mg Lactation: 7 mg Males 14 y and older: 5 mg Children 1–3 y: 2 mg 4–8 y: 3 mg 9–13 y: 4 mg Infants 1–6 mo: 1.7 mg 7–12 mo: 1.8 mg | Eggs, liver, salmon, yeast, cauliflower, broccoli, lean beef, potatoes, tomatoes | No deficiency state established | Not established |
| **Vitamin B₆ (pyridoxine)** A coenzyme in metabolism of carbohydrate, protein, and fat; required for formation of tryptophan and conversion of tryptophan to niacin; helps release glycogen from the liver and muscle tissue; functions in metabolism of the central nervous system; helps maintain cellular immunity | RDAs Females 14–18 y: 1.2 mg 19–50 y: 1.3 mg 51 y and older: 1.5 mg Pregnancy: 1.9 mg Lactation: 2 mg Males 14–50 y: 1.3 mg 51 and older: 1.7 mg Children 1–3 y: 0.5 mg 4–8 y: 0.6 mg 9–13 y: 1 mg Infants (AIs) 1–6 mo: 0.1 mg 7–12 mo: 0.3 mg | Yeast, wheat germ, liver and other glandular meats, whole-grain cereals, potatoes, legumes | Skin and mucous membrane lesions (seborrheic dermatitis, intertrigo, stomatitis, glossitis), neurologic problems (seizures, peripheral neuritis, mental depression) | Not established |

*(Continued on page 702)*

**TABLE 35.1**

## Vitamins [Continued]

| Vitamin/Function | Dietary Reference Intakes | Food Sources | Signs and Symptoms of Deficiency | Signs and Symptoms of Excess |
|---|---|---|---|---|
| **Vitamin B$_{12}$ (cyanocobalamin)** Essential for normal metabolism of all body cells, normal red blood cells, normal nerve cells, growth, and metabolism of carbohydrate, protein, and fat | RDAs Females 14 y and older: 2.4 mcg Pregnancy: 2.6 mcg Lactation: 2.8 mcg Males 14 y and older: 2.4 mcg Children 1–3 y: 0.9 mcg 4–8 y: 1.2 mcg 9–13 y: 1.8 mcg Infants (AIs) 0–6 mo: 0.4 mcg 7–12 mo: 0.5 mcg | Meat, eggs, fish, cheese | Pernicious anemia: decreased numbers of RBCs; large, immature RBCs; fatigue; dyspnea Severe deficiency: leukopenia, infection, thrombocytopenia, cardiac dysrhythmias, heart failure Neurologic signs and symptoms: paresthesias in hands and feet, unsteady gait, depressed deep tendon reflexes, loss of memory, confusion, delusions, hallucinations, psychosis Nerve damage may be irreversible | Not established |
| **Folic acid (folate)** A B complex vitamin; essential for normal metabolism of all body cells, normal RBCs, and growth | RDAs Females 14 y and older: 400 mcg Pregnancy: 600 mcg Lactation: 500 mcg Males 14 y and older: 400 mcg Older adults (UL): 1000 mcg Children 1–3 y: 150 mcg 4–8 y: 200 mcg 9–13 y: 300 mcg Infants (AIs) 1–6 mo: 65 mcg 7–12 mo: 80 mcg | Liver, kidney beans, fresh green vegetables (spinach, broccoli, asparagus), fortified grain products (e.g., breads, cereals, rice) | Megaloblastic anemia that cannot be distinguished from the anemia produced by vitamin B$_{12}$ deficiency; impaired growth in children; glossitis; GI problems | Not established |
| **Vitamin C (ascorbic acid)** Essential for formation of skin, ligaments, cartilage, bone, and teeth; required for wound healing and tissue repair, metabolism of iron and folic acid, synthesis of fats and proteins, preservation of blood vessel integrity, and resistance to infection | RDAs Females 19 y and older: 75 mg Pregnancy: 19–50 y, 85 mg Lactation: 19–50 y, 120 mg Males 19 y and older: 90 mg Adult smokers: add additional 35 mg/d Children 1–3 y: 15 mg 4–8 y: 25 mg 9–13 y: 45 mg 14–18 y: male, 75 mg; female, 65 mg (pregnancy, 80 mg; lactation, 115 mg) Infants (AIs) 0–6 mo: 40 mg 7–12 mo: 50 mg | Fruits and vegetables, especially citrus fruits and juices | Mild deficiency: irritability, malaise, arthralgia, increased tendency to bleed Severe deficiency: scurvy and adverse effects on most body tissues (gingivitis; bleeding of gums, skin, joints, and other areas; disturbances of bone growth; anemia; and loosening of teeth); if not treated, coma and death may occur | Renal calculi |

ˈVitamin E activity is expressed in milligrams of alpha-tocopherol equivalents (alpha-TE).

AI, adequate intake; DRI, Dietary Reference Intake; GI, gastrointestinal; RBC, red blood cell; RDA, recommended dietary allowance; ULs, upper intake levels.

## Minerals

Minerals maintain acid–base balance and osmotic pressure. They make up part of enzymes, hormones, and vitamins. The body needs minerals for hemoglobin formation, muscle contraction, and skeletal development and maintenance. Minerals present in the body in large amounts (macrominerals) are sodium, potassium, chloride, calcium, magnesium, phosphorus, and sulfur. (Note: Calcium and phosphorus are discussed in Chapter 44 because they play major roles in bone metabolism.) Other minerals are required in small amounts (trace elements). Eight of these (chromium, cobalt, copper, fluoride, iodine, iron, selenium, and zinc) have relatively well-defined roles in human nutrition.

Minerals occur in the body and foods mainly in ionic form. When placed in solution, the components separate into **electrolytes**. Electrolytes are electrically charged particles found in body fluids and cells (e.g., sodium or potassium ions). At any given time, the body must maintain an equal number of positive and negative charges. Therefore, the ions are constantly combining and separating to maintain electrical neutrality or electrolyte balance.

Electrolytes also maintain the acid–base balance of body fluids. Acids are usually anions (e.g., bicarbonate, chloride, phosphate, or sulfate). Bases are usually cations (e.g., sodium, potassium, calcium, and magnesium). Mineral–electrolytes are obtained from foods or supplements. Although most minerals are supplied by a well-balanced diet, studies indicate that most adults and children do not ingest sufficient dietary calcium and that iron deficiency is common in some populations. In addition, some conditions increase requirements (e.g., pregnancy, lactation, and various illnesses), and some drug–drug interactions decrease absorption or use of minerals.

As with vitamins, goals for daily mineral intake have been established as DRIs. Thus far, DRIs and ULs have been established for calcium, fluoride, iron, magnesium, phosphorus, and selenium.

 **QSEN Alert: Safety**

People should not exceed the UL for any mineral–electrolyte.

Except for the stated amount for magnesium, which excludes food and water sources and considers supplements only, the ULs include those from both foods and supplements. Table 35.2 lists the function, recommended daily intake, and dietary sources of various minerals.

- Multivitamin–mineral combinations recommended for age and gender groups contain different amounts of some minerals (e.g., younger women need more iron than do postmenopausal women). It is necessary to consider this when choosing a product.
- Iron supplements other than those in multivitamin–mineral combinations are usually intended for temporary use in the presence of deficiency or a period of increased need (e.g., pregnancy). People should not take them otherwise because of risks of accumulation and toxicity.
- Most adolescent and adult females probably benefit from a calcium supplement to achieve the recommended amount (1000–1300 mg daily). It is important to consider the amounts consumed in dairy products and other foods and not exceed the UL of 2500 mg daily.

## Clinical Manifestations

Tables 35.1 and 35.2 list signs and symptoms associated with deficiency and excess of vitamins and minerals, respectively.

## Drug Therapy

Early recognition and treatment of vitamin disorders can prevent a mild deficiency or excess from becoming severe. For deficiency states, oral vitamin preparations are preferred when possible. Multiple deficiencies are common, and a multivitamin preparation used to treat them usually contains more than the recommended daily amount. Use for limited periods is best. When fat-soluble vitamins are given to correct a deficiency, there is a risk of producing excess states. When water-soluble vitamins are given, excesses are less likely but may occur with large doses. For excess states, the usual treatment is to stop administration of the vitamin preparation. There are no specific antidotes or antagonists.

It is important to titrate the amount of mineral supplement closely to the amount needed by the body as there is a risk of producing an excess state. Oral products are preferred for replacement because they are safer, less likely to produce toxicity, more convenient to administer, and less expensive than are parenteral preparations. The U.S. Food and Drug Administration (FDA) regulates the content of supplements for infants and children younger than 4 years of age; however, it does not regulate the content of preparations for older children.

### Children

Children need sufficient amounts of vitamins and minerals to support growth and normal body functioning. Dosages should not exceed recommended amounts. For infants (birth to 12 months), the only UL is for vitamin D. For other children, ULs vary according to age. A combined vitamin–mineral supplement every other day may be reasonable, especially for children who eat poorly.

There is a risk of overdose in children; this risk is more serious with the fat-soluble vitamins because they are stored long-term within the body. Also, all minerals and electrolytes are toxic in overdose. Because of manufacturers' marketing strategies, many supplements are available in flavors and shapes (e.g., animals, cartoon characters) designed to appeal to children.

 **QSEN Alert: Safety**

Because younger children may think of these supplements as candy and take more than recommended, it is essential that they be stored out of reach and dispensed by an adult.

### Older Adults

Vitamin requirements are the same for older adults as for younger adults, but deficiencies are common, especially with the fat-soluble vitamins A and D. It is important to assess every older adult regarding vitamin intake (from food and supplements) and use of drugs that interact with dietary nutrients. For most older adults, a daily multivitamin is probably desirable, even for those who seem healthy and able to eat a well-balanced diet. In addition, requirements may be increased during illnesses, especially those affecting GI function. Overdoses, especially of the fat-soluble vitamins A and D, may cause toxicity; it is necessary to avoid this.

### TABLE 35.2

## Minerals and Electrolytes

| Mineral/Function | Dietary Reference Intakes | Food Sources | Signs and Symptoms of Deficiency | Signs and Symptoms of Excess |
|---|---|---|---|---|
| **Macro Minerals** | | | | |
| **Sodium** Assists in regulating osmotic pressure, water balance, conduction of electrical impulses in nerves and muscles, and electrolyte and acid–base balance Influences permeability of cell membranes and assists in movement of substances across cell membranes Participates in many intracellular chemical reactions. Normal serum sodium = 135–145 mEq/L | Adults (AI) 19–50 y: 1.5 g 50–70 y: 1.3 g 71 y and over: 1.2 g Adults (UL): 2.3 g | Present in most foods; proteins contain large amounts; vegetables and cereals contain small to moderate amounts; fruits contain little or no sodium. Major source in the diet is table salt added to food in processing, cooking, or seasoning. One teaspoon contains 2.3 g of sodium. Water in some areas may contain significant amounts of sodium | Serum sodium <135 mEq/L; anorexia, nausea, and vomiting; ataxia; confusion; delirium; hypotension and tachycardia; muscle tremors; oliguria and increased blood urea nitrogen; seizures; weakness | Serum sodium >145 mEq/L, disorientation, dry skin and mucous membranes, fever, hyperactive reflexes, hypotension, muscle rigidity, tremors and spasms, irritability, cerebral hemorrhage, coma, oliguria, concentrated urine, increased blood urea nitrogen |
| **Potassium** Within cells, it helps maintain osmotic pressure, fluid, and electrolyte balance and acid–base balance. In extracellular fluid, it is required for conduction of nerve impulses and contraction of muscle. Helps transport glucose into cells and is required for glycogen formation and storage. Required for synthesis of muscle proteins. Normal serum potassium = 3.5–5 mEq/L | Adults (AI): 4.7 g Adults (UL): not established | Present in most foods, including meat, whole-grain breads or cereals, bananas, citrus fruits, tomatoes, and broccoli | Serum potassium <3.5 mEq/L; dysrhythmias and ECG changes; cardiac arrest; confusion; delirium; hyperglycemia; postural hypotension; muscle weakness; abdominal distension, constipation, paralytic ileus; polyuria; polydipsia, nocturia. Prolonged deficiency may increase blood urea nitrogen and serum creatinine | Serum potassium >5 mEq/L; muscle weakness; cardiotoxicity, with dysrhythmias or cardiac arrest. Cardiac effects are not usually severe until serum levels are 7 mEq/L or above |
| **Chloride** Helps maintain osmotic pressure and electrolyte, acid–base, and water balance. Forms hydrochloric acid in gastric mucosal cells. Normal serum chloride = 95–103 mEq/L | Adults (AI) 19–50 y: 2.3 g 50–70 y: 2 g 71 y and over: 1.8 g Adults (UL): 3.6 g | Most dietary chloride is ingested as sodium chloride, and foods high in sodium are also high in chloride | Serum chloride <95 mEq/L; arterial blood pH > 7.45; dehydration; hypotension; low respiratory rate and shallow respirations; paresthesias of face and extremities; muscle spasms and tetany, which cannot be distinguished from the tetany produced by hypocalcemia | Serum chloride >103 mEq/L; arterial blood pH < 7.35; increased rate and depth of respirations; lethargy, stupor, disorientation, and coma if acidosis is not treated |

## TABLE 35.2

## Minerals and Electrolytes (Continued)

| Mineral/Function | Dietary Reference Intakes | Food Sources | Signs and Symptoms of Deficiency | Signs and Symptoms of Excess |
|---|---|---|---|---|
| **Magnesium** Required for conduction of nerve impulses and contraction of muscle (especially important in function of cardiac and skeletal muscle). Serves as a component of many enzymes. Essential for metabolism of carbohydrate and protein. Normal serum magnesium = 1.5–2.5 mEq/L | Adults (RDA) Females 19–30 y: 310 mg 31 y and over: 320 mg Males 19–30 y: 400 mg 31 y and over: 420 mg Adults (UL): 350 mg/d from supplements only (does not include intake from food and water) | Present in many foods; diet that is adequate in other respects contains adequate magnesium. Good food sources include nuts, cereal grains, dark green vegetables, and seafood | Serum magnesium <1.5 mEq/L; ataxia; confusion; dizziness; irritability; muscle tremors, carpopedal spasm, nystagmus, and generalized spasticity; seizures; tachycardia, hypotension, premature atrial, and ventricular beats | Serum magnesium >2.5 mEq/L; skeletal muscle weakness; cardiac dysrhythmias, hypotension; respiratory insufficiency; coma |
| **Trace Elements** | | | | |
| **Chromium** Aids glucose use by increasing effectiveness of insulin and facilitating transport of glucose across cell membranes | Adults (AI) Females 19–50 y: 25 mcg 51 y and over: 20 mcg Males 19–50 y: 35 mcg 51 y and over: 30 mcg Adults (UL): undetermined | Brewer's yeast and whole wheat products | Impaired glucose tolerance (hyperglycemia, glucosuria); impaired growth and reproduction; decreased life span | Not established |
| **Cobalt** A component of vitamin $B_{12}$ that is required for normal function of all body cells and for maturation of red blood cells | ~1 mg in the form of vitamin $B_{12}$. There is no established RDA | Animal foods, including liver, muscle meats, and shellfish Fruits, vegetables, and cereals contain no cobalt as vitamin $B_{12}$ | Deficiency of vitamin $B_{12}$ produces pernicious anemia | Not established |
| **Copper** A component of many enzymes. Essential for correct functioning of the central nervous, cardiovascular, and skeletal systems. Important in formation of red blood cells, apparently by regulating storage and release of iron for hemoglobin | Adults (RDA): 900 mcg Adults (UL): 10,000 mcg | Many foods, including liver, shellfish, nuts, cereals, poultry, and dried fruits | Decreased serum levels; decreased iron absorption; anemia from impaired erythropoiesis; leukopenia. Death can occur. In infants, anemia, chronic malnutrition, and diarrhea or Menkes' syndrome (retarded growth and progressive mental deterioration) can occur. | Increased serum levels; Wilson's disease (a rare genetic disorder characterized by accumulation of copper in the brain, liver, and kidneys). Signs and symptoms vary according to affected organs |
| **Fluoride** A component of tooth enamel. Strengthens the bones. Adequate intake before ages 50–60 may decrease osteoporosis and fractures during later years. | Adults (AI) Females 19–70 y and over: 3 mg Pregnancy and lactation: 3 mg Males 19–70 y and over: 4 mg Children (AIs) 1–3 y: 0.7 mg 4–8 y: 1 mg | Beef, canned salmon, eggs. Very little in milk, cereal grains, fruits, and vegetables. Fluoride content of food depends on fluoride content of soil where they are grown. | Dental caries and possibly a greater incidence of osteoporosis | Mottling of teeth and osteosclerosis |

(Continued on page 706)

**TABLE 35.2**

## Minerals and Electrolytes (Continued)

| Mineral/Function | Dietary Reference Intakes | Food Sources | Signs and Symptoms of Deficiency | Signs and Symptoms of Excess |
|---|---|---|---|---|
| | 9–13 y: 2 mg<br>14–18 y: 3 mg<br>Infants (AIs)<br>   0–6 mo: 0.01 mg<br>7–12 mo: 0.5 mg<br>Adults (UL): 10 mg | | | |
| **Iodine**<br>Essential component of thyroid hormones | Adults (RDAs)<br>Females 14 y and over:<br>   150 mcg<br>Pregnancy: 220 mcg<br>Lactation: 290 mcg<br>Males 14 y and over:<br>   150 mcg<br>Children:<br>1–8 y: 90 mcg;<br>   9–13 y: 120 mcg<br>Infants<br>0–6 mo: 110 mcg<br>7–12 mo: 130 mcg | Iodized salt and seafood are the best sources. In vegetables, iodine content varies with the amount of iodine in soil where they are grown. In milk and eggs, content depends on the amount present in animal feed. | Thyroid gland enlargement; possible hypothyroidism | Iodism, with coryza, edema, fever, conjunctivitis, lymphadenopathy, stomatitis, vomiting |
| **Iron**<br>Essential component of hemoglobin, myoglobin, and several enzymes. Hemoglobin is required for transport and use of oxygen by body cells. Myoglobin aids oxygen transport and use by muscle cells. Enzymes are important for cellular metabolism. | Adults (RDAs)<br>Females<br>19–50 y: 18 mg<br>51 y and over: 8 mg<br>Pregnancy: 27 mg<br>Lactation:<br>14–18 y: 10 mg<br>19–50 y: 9 mg<br>Males: 8 mg<br>Children (RDAs)<br>1–3 y: 7 mg<br>4–8 y: 10 mg<br>9–13 y: 8 mg<br>14–18 y (girls): 15 mg<br>14–18 y (boys): 11 mg<br>Infants<br>0–6 mo: 0.27 mg<br>(AI) 7–12 mo: 11 mg<br>RDA<br>Adults (UL): 45 mg | Liver and other organ meats, lean meat, shellfish, dried beans and vegetables, egg yolks, dried fruits, molasses, whole-grain and enriched breads Milk and milk products contain essentially no iron | Iron deficiency anemia. With gradual development of anemia, minimal symptoms occur. With rapid development or severe anemia, dyspnea, fatigue, tachycardia, malaise, and drowsiness occur. | Acute iron intoxication: vomiting, diarrhea, melena, abdominal pain, shock, convulsions, and metabolic acidosis. Death may occur within 24 h if treatment is not prompt.<br>Chronic iron overload (hemochromatosis): cardiac dysrhythmias, heart failure, diabetes mellitus, bronze pigmentation of the skin, liver enlargement, arthropathy, and others |
| **Selenium**<br>Important for function of myocardium and probably other muscles | Adults (RDAs)<br>Females 19–70 y and<br>   over: 55 mcg<br>Pregnancy: 60 mcg<br>Lactation: 70 mcg<br>Males 19–70 y and over:<br>   55 mcg<br>Children (RDAs)<br>1–3 y: 20 mcg<br>4–8 y: 30 mcg<br>9–13 y: 40 mcg<br>14–18 y: 55 mcg<br>Infants (AIs)<br>0–6 mo: 15 mcg<br>7–12 mo: 20 mcg<br>Adult UL: 400 mcg | Fish, meat, bread, and cereals | Deficiency most likely with long-term IV therapy. Signs and symptoms include myocardial abnormalities and other muscle discomfort and weakness. | Highly toxic in excessive amounts. Signs and symptoms include fatigue, peripheral neuropathy, nausea, diarrhea, and alopecia. |

## TABLE 35.2

### Minerals and Electrolytes (Continued)

| Mineral/Function | Dietary Reference Intakes | Food Sources | Signs and Symptoms of Deficiency | Signs and Symptoms of Excess |
|---|---|---|---|---|
| **Zinc** A component of many enzymes that is essential for normal metabolism (e.g., carbonic anhydrase, lactic dehydrogenase, alkaline phosphatase). Necessary for normal cell growth, synthesis of nucleic acids (RNA and DNA), and synthesis of carbohydrates and proteins. May be essential for use of vitamin A | Adults (RDAs) Females 19–70 y and over: 8 mg Pregnancy: 14–18 y: 12 mg 19–50 y: 11 mg Lactation: 14–18 y: 13 mg 19–50 y: 12 mg Males 19–70 y and over: 11 mg Children 1–3 y: 3 mg 4–8 y: 5 mg 9–13 y: 8 mg 14–18 y (girls): 9 mg 14–18 y (boys): 11 mg Infants 0–6 mo (AI): 2 mg 7–12 mo (RDA): 3 mg Adult UL: 40 mg | Animal proteins such as meat, liver, eggs, and seafood. Wheat germ is also a good source. | Most evident in growing children and includes impaired growth, hypogonadism in boys, anorexia, and sensory impairment (loss of taste and smell). Also, if the patient has had surgery, wound healing may be delayed. | Unlikely with dietary intake but may develop with excessive ingestion or inhalation of zinc. Ingestion may cause nausea, vomiting, and diarrhea; inhalation may cause vomiting, headache, and fever. |

### Renal and Hepatic Impairment

Patients with acute renal failure who are unable to eat an adequate diet need a vitamin supplement to meet DRIs. Overall, a multivitamin with essential vitamins is recommended for daily use. Decreased renal function may promote mineral retention.

 **QSEN Alert: Patient-Centered Care**

It is important to monitor serum electrolyte levels closely and provide supplements only with great care.

Vitamin deficiencies commonly occur in patients with chronic liver disease because of poor intake and **malabsorption** (impaired absorption of nutrients from the GI tract). Hepatic failure results in depletion of hepatic stores of vitamin A and other vitamins.

### Critical Illness

Critically ill patients often have organ failure, which alters their ability to ingest and use essential nutrients. They may be undernourished with regard to vitamins and minerals.

The Nutrition Advisory Group of the American Medical Association has established guidelines for daily intake, and parenteral multivitamin formulations are available for adults and children. Close monitoring of serum electrolytes is necessary.

### Clinical Application 35.1

- Identify findings in the assessment of Mrs. Martin that would put her at risk for vitamin, mineral, and nutritional deficiency.

### NCLEX Success

1. Which one of the following findings in a nursing assessment of a newly admitted patient would be most likely to result in a vitamin deficiency?
   A. a history of liver disease
   B. use of self-prescribed megavitamins
   C. presence of a pressure ulcer
   D. frequent blood transfusions

2. A woman takes large amounts of vitamins, which she buys over the counter without a prescription. The nurse should teach the patient that excess consumption of which one of the following could result in a toxic overdose?
   A. folic acid
   B. vitamin A
   C. vitamin $B_1$
   D. vitamin C

## FAT-SOLUBLE VITAMINS

### VITAMIN A

The following discussion concerns vitamin A, or retinol.

## Pharmacokinetics and Use

After oral administration, vitamin A is absorbed from the GI tract along with dietary fat and is primarily stored in the liver. The body can store up to a year's supply of vitamin A in the liver. This vitamin, which is not soluble in the blood, is distributed by attaching to protein carriers in the blood. If a person consumes inadequate amounts of vitamin A, the body uses the vitamin stored in the liver. Vitamin A is metabolized in the liver and eliminated in the feces and urine.

The most important therapeutic use of vitamin A is for replacement in deficiency states. Table 35.3 gives route and dosage information.

## Adverse Effects and Contraindications

Signs and symptoms of vitamin A toxicity include hair loss, double vision, headaches, vomiting, bone abnormalities, and liver damage. If any signs or symptoms of vitamin A excess appear, it is necessary to stop intake of any known sources of vitamin A.

## TABLE 35.3

## DRUGS AT A GLANCE: Vitamins

| Drug | Pregnancy Category | Routes and Dosage Ranges | |
| --- | --- | --- | --- |
| | | **Adults** | **Children** |
| **Fat-Soluble Vitamins** | | | |
| Vitamin A (also called retinol) | A<br>X if dose is greater than RDA | Deficiency (severe): 500,000 international units PO or 100,000 international units IM daily for 3 d; then 50,000 international units PO or IM daily for 2 wk; then 10,000–20,000 international units PO daily for another 2 mo; follow with adequate dietary nutrition and retinol equivalent vitamin A supplements | Deficiency (severe):<br>1–8 y<br>17,500–35,000 international units IM daily for 10 d<br>Follow with oral therapeutic multivitamin containing additional vitamin A 5000–10,000 international units/d for 2 mo<br>Older than 8 y: see adult dose |
| Vitamin E | A (if within RDA) | Deficiency: 60–75 international units PO daily<br>Prevention of deficiency: 12–15 international units daily (vitamin E may be ordered in alpha-tocopherol equivalents or ATE; 1.40 international units = 1 ATE) | Deficiency: 1 international unit/kg/d PO of water-miscible vitamin E |
| Vitamin K or phytonadione (Mephyton; ❧ AquaMEPHYTON, Konakion, Mephyton) | C | Anti–coagulant-induced prothrombin deficiency: if major bleeding, 5–10 mg IV slowly; INR above 10 without bleeding, 2.5–5 mg oral; INR 4.5–10 without bleeding, 1–2.5 mg oral; INR below 4.5 without bleeding, no vitamin K<br>Hypoprothrombinemia due to other causes: 2.5–25 mg (rarely up to 50 mg) PO or subcutaneously or IM; repeat INR in 6–8 h; repeat dose if needed | Prevention of hemorrhagic disease: 0.5–1 mg IM within 1 h after birth<br>Treatment of hemorrhagic disease in newborns:<br>1–2 mg subcutaneously or IM daily |
| **Water-Soluble Vitamins** | | | |
| Vitamin B₁ (thiamine; ❧ Thiamiject) | A<br>If above RDA: C | Parenteral nutrition supplementation: 6 mg daily; may be increased to 25–50 mg daily with history of alcohol abuse<br>Deficiency (beriberi): 5–30 mg IM or IV three times daily if critically ill; then 5–30 mg/d in single or divided doses three times daily for 1 mo<br>Alcohol withdrawal syndrome: 100 mg IM or IV daily for several days, followed by 50–100 mg PO daily<br>Wernicke's encephalopathy: initially, 100 mg IV; then 50–100 mg IM or IV daily until patient is consuming a regular balanced diet | Deficiency (beriberi): 10–25 mg IM or IV once daily if critically ill; for noncritically ill children, 10–50 mg PO daily for 2 wk and then 5–10 mg PO daily for 1 mo |
| Vitamin B₂ (riboflavin) | A<br>If above RDA: C | Deficiency: 5–30 mg/d PO in divided doses | Deficiency: 3–10 mg/d PO in divided doses |

**TABLE 35.3**

## DRUGS AT A GLANCE: Vitamins (Continued)

| Drug | Pregnancy Category | Routes and Dosage Ranges | |
|---|---|---|---|
| | | **Adults** | **Children** |
| Vitamin B₃ (niacin, nicotinic acid; ❋ Niaspan, Niaspan FCT, Niodan) Nicotinamide (niacinamide) | C | Deficiency: up to 100 mg PO daily Pellagra: 50–100 mg oral 3–4 times daily; maximum 500 mg daily Hyperlipidemia: 100 mg oral three times daily; increase gradually as tolerated to 3 g daily in 2–3 divided doses; alternatively, extended-release tablets 500 mg once daily; increase by 500 mg at intervals of no sooner than 1 wk over 4–8 wk to maximum 2000 mg daily | Pellagra: 50–100 mg oral three times daily |
| Vitamin B₅ (calcium pantothenate) | A If above RDA: C | Deficiency: 4–7 mg PO daily | |
| Vitamin B₆ (pyridoxine) | A If above RDA: C | Deficiency: 100–200 PO daily or 10–20 mg IM or IV daily for several wk; then maintenance dose of 2–5 mg PO daily for several wk Prevention of vitamin B₆ deficiency during isoniazid therapy: 25–50 mg PO daily | Seizures related to vitamin B₆ deficiency (neonates and children): 10–100 mg IM or IV in a single dose |
| Vitamin B₁₂ (cyanocobalamin or hydroxocobalamin) (B₁₂ Compliance Injection; Physicians EZ Use B₁₂) ❋ Cobex; Cyano Vit B₁₂ | A If above RDA: C | Deficiency due to inadequate diet or causes other than pernicious anemia: as cyanocobalamin 1000–2000 mcg PO daily for 1–2 wk or 100 mcg deep subcutaneous or IM for 6–7 d; follow with same dose on alternate days for 7 doses; then every 3–4 d for 2–3 wk and monitor laboratory values; maintenance dose, 100 mcg oral daily or 100 mcg deep subcutaneous or IM daily; for subsequent prophylaxis, adequate nutrition and RDA of vitamin B₁₂ supplement PO Pernicious anemia: initially, cyanocobalamin 100 mcg deep subcutaneous or IM daily for 6–7 d; if response is observed, 100 mcg subcutaneously or IM every other day for seven doses; then, 100 mcg subcutaneously or IM every 3–4 d for 2–3 wk; then, 100 mcg subcutaneously or IM once monthly | Deficiency due to inadequate diet or causes other than pernicious anemia: as cyanocobalamin 0.2 mcg/kg deep subcutaneous or IM for 2 d; follow with 1000 mcg daily for 2–7 d; follow with 100 mcg weekly for 1 mo; for malabsorption, maintenance dose is 100 mcg deep subcutaneous or IM monthly; for subsequent prophylaxis, adequate nutrition and RDA of vitamin B₁₂ supplement PO Pernicious anemia: 30–50 mcg deep subcutaneous or IM daily for 2 or more wk to a total dose of 1000–5000 mcg; then maintenance dose of 100 mcg monthly |
| Intranasal cyanocobalamin (Nascobal) | C | Maintenance therapy for remission of pernicious anemia after parenteral vitamin B₁₂ therapy: intranasal cyanocobalamin 1 spray (500 mcg) in 1 nostril once weekly at least 1 h before or after hot liquids or foods | |
| Folic acid (FA-8; ❋ JAMP-Folic Acid) | A | Deficiency, megaloblastic anemia, hepatic disease, alcoholism: 0.4–1 mg PO, subcutaneously, IM, or IV daily; then maintenance dose of 0.4 mg/d Pregnancy/lactation maintenance dose: 0.8 mg/d | Deficiency, megaloblastic anemia, hepatic disease: 0.4–1 mg/d oral, subcutaneous, IM, or IV and then maintenance dose (infant 0.1 mg/d; children 1–3, 0.1–0.3 mg/d; children 4 and older and adolescents, use adult dose) |
| Vitamin C (ascorbic acid) (Acerola C 500; Asco-Tabs-1000; Ascocid; many other OTC brand names; ❋ Ascor L 500; Mega-C-Sodium) | A If above RDA: C | Deficiency, depending on severity: 100–300 mg oral daily or 300–1000 mg subcutaneous/IM/IV daily Burns: 1–2 g subcutaneous/IM/IV daily Wound healing: 300–500 mg subcutaneous/IM/IV daily for 7–10 d pre- and postoperatively | Deficiency, depending on severity: 100–300 mg PO daily |

Contraindications to vitamin A include a history of allergic reaction to the vitamin, hypervitaminosis A, and malabsorption syndrome (oral use only). Caution is warranted in pregnancy. Vitamin A toxicity during pregnancy can cause fetal defects (Dudek, 2018).

## Nursing Implications

### Preventing Interactions

Chronic use of mineral oil or bile acid sequestrants may cause vitamin A deficiency by preventing systemic absorption of vitamin A. Mineral oil combines with fat-soluble vitamins and prevents their absorption if both are taken at the same time. Bile salts increase the effects of vitamin A by increasing intestinal absorption of the vitamin. Large doses of vitamin A may increase the anticoagulant effects of warfarin. Antibiotics may cause diarrhea and subsequent malabsorption of vitamin A.

### Administering the Medication

People should take vitamin A preparations before meals, on an empty stomach. However, to prevent nausea, it may be necessary to take them after food or meals. (Intramuscular [IM] administration may be necessary.) Also, people should not take oral preparations of vitamin A at the same time as mineral oil; this laxative absorbs the vitamin and thus prevents its systemic absorption.

### Assessing for Therapeutic and Adverse Effects

The nurse observes for decreased signs and symptoms of deficiency, such as improved vision, especially in dim light or at night; less dryness in the eyes and conjunctiva (xerophthalmia); and improvement in skin lesions. Night blindness is usually better within a few days. Skin lesions may not disappear for several weeks.

In addition, the nurse observes for signs of hypervitaminosis A, such as anorexia, vomiting, irritability, headache, skin disorders, and pain in muscles, bones, and joints. Serum levels of vitamin A >1200 international unit/dL are toxic. Severity of manifestations depends largely on dose and duration of excess vitamin A intake. Very severe states produce additional clinical signs, including enlargement of the liver and spleen, altered liver function, increased intracranial pressure, and other neurologic manifestations.

### Patient Teaching

Box 35.2 identifies patient teaching guidelines for vitamins, including vitamin A.

## VITAMIN E

The following discussion concerns vitamin E, or alpha-tocopherol.

## Pharmacokinetics and Use

Vitamin E is absorbed from the GI tract if fat absorption is normal. It is primarily stored in adipose tissue. It is metabolized in the liver and eliminated primarily in bile.

The most important therapeutic use of vitamin E is for vitamin E replacement in the narrow, specific circumstances in which vitamin E deficiency occurs. Table 35.3 gives route and dosage information for vitamin E.

## Adverse Effects and Contraindications

Large amounts of vitamin E are relatively nontoxic but can interfere with vitamin K action (blood clotting) by decreasing platelet aggregation and producing a risk of bleeding. Excessive doses can also cause fatigue, headache, blurred vision, nausea, and diarrhea. If signs or symptoms of vitamin E excess appear, it is essential to stop the intake of any known source of vitamin E.

Contraindications to vitamin E include a history of allergic reaction to vitamin E or hypervitaminosis E. Patients with a history of bleeding disorders or thrombocytopenia should not take vitamin E.

## Nursing Implications

### Preventing Interactions

Mineral oil and cholestyramine decrease the absorption of vitamin E, which means that vitamin E should not be administered at the same time as these substances. Also, this vitamin may increase the anticoagulant effect of warfarin. Vitamin E may increase the absorption, hepatic storage, and use of vitamin A.

### Administering the Medication

People should take oral vitamin E preparations before meals on an empty stomach. However, to prevent nausea, people may also take them after food or meals.

### Assessing for Therapeutic and Adverse Effects

The nurse observes for decreased signs and symptoms of vitamin E deficiency. In addition, the nurse checks for signs of hypervitaminosis E, including bleeding, fatigue, headache, blurred vision, nausea, and diarrhea.

### Patient Teaching

Box 35.2 identifies patient teaching guidelines for vitamins, including vitamin E.

## VITAMIN K

The following discussion concerns vitamin K, or phytonadione.

## Pharmacokinetics and Use

After absorption, vitamin K is concentrated in the liver. Minimal amounts of the vitamin are stored. It crosses the placental barrier and enters breast milk. Onset of action after an oral dose is 6 to 12 hours and, after a subcutaneous dose, 1 to 2 hours. Metabolism occurs rapidly in the liver, and elimination is in the bile and urine.

Vitamin K has two important therapeutic uses: (1) to correct hypoprothrombinemia caused by inadequate levels of vitamin K and (2) to reverse the effects of warfarin (Coumadin) overdose. Table 35.3 gives route and dosage information for vitamin K.

**BOX 35.2** *Patient Teaching Guidelines for Vitamins*

## General Considerations

- Certain people may need vitamin supplements. Women who are pregnant as well as people who smoke, ingest large amounts of alcohol, have impaired immune systems, or are elderly may need to take oral vitamins.
- Avoid taking large doses of vitamins, which do not promote health, strength, or youth.
- Natural vitamins are advertised as being better than synthetic vitamins, but there is no evidence to support this claim. The two types are chemically identical, and the body uses them the same way. Natural vitamins are more expensive.
- Vitamins from supplements exert the same physiologic effects as those obtained from foods.
- Multivitamin preparations often contain minerals as well, usually in smaller amounts than those recommended for daily intake. Large doses of minerals are toxic.
- Supplementary vitamin preparations differ widely in amounts and types of vitamin content.
- When choosing a vitamin supplement, compare ingredients and costs. Store brands are usually effective and less expensive than name brands.

## Vitamin A

- Know about dietary sources of vitamin A. Retinol occurs in liver, milk, butter, cheese, cream, egg yolk, fortified milk, margarine, and ready-to-eat cereals. Beta-carotenes occur in spinach, collard greens, kale, mango, broccoli, carrots, peaches, pumpkin, red peppers, sweet potatoes, winter squash, watermelon, apricots, and cantaloupe.
- Understand that excessive amounts of vitamin A are stored in the body and often lead to toxic effects. High doses of vitamin A can result in headaches; diarrhea; nausea; loss of appetite; dry, itching skin; and elevated blood calcium.
- Do not take a supplementary vitamin product that contains more than recommended amounts of vitamin A because of possible adverse effects.
- If you are pregnant or could become pregnant, know that excessive doses of vitamin A during pregnancy may cause birth defects.

## Vitamin E

- Know about dietary sources of vitamin E. This vitamin occurs in vegetable oils, margarine, salad dressing, other foods made with vegetable oil, nuts, seeds, wheat germ, dark green vegetables, whole grains, and fortified cereals.
- Be familiar with the signs and symptoms of vitamin E overdose.
- Do not take a supplementary vitamin product that contains more than the recommended amounts of vitamin E.

## Vitamin K

- Know about dietary sources of vitamin K. This vitamin occurs in spinach, brussels sprouts, broccoli, cabbage, cauliflower, Swiss chard, lettuce, collard greens, carrots, green beans, asparagus, and eggs.
- Avoid excessive doses of vitamin K. Take this vitamin only as directed by a health care provider.
- Keep intake of vitamin K–containing foods constant. Avoid sudden increases or decreases in the amounts of these foods.
- If you are taking warfarin, report any use of vitamin K to your health care provider. During warfarin therapy, intake of vitamin K–containing foods should remain constant.

## Vitamin $B_1$, Vitamin $B_3$, and Vitamin $B_6$

- Know about dietary sources of vitamins $B_1$ (thiamine), $B_3$ (niacin), and $B_6$ (pyridoxine). Thiamine occurs in whole-grain and enriched breads and cereals, liver, nuts, wheat germ, pork, and dried peas and beans. Niacin occurs in all protein foods and whole-grain and enriched breads and cereals. Pyridoxine occurs in meats, fish, poultry, fruits, green leafy vegetables, whole grains, and dried peas and beans.
- Swallow extended-release products whole; do not break, crush, or chew them. Breaking the product delivers the entire dose at once and may cause adverse effects.
- Take oral niacin preparations, except for timed-release forms, with or after meals or at bedtime to decrease stomach irritation.
- After taking a dose of oral niacin, sit or lie down for approximately 30 minutes after taking a dose. Niacin causes blood vessels to dilate and may cause facial flushing, dizziness, and falls. Facial flushing can be decreased by taking aspirin 325 mg orally, 30 to 60 minutes before a dose of niacin (if aspirin is not contraindicated). Itching, tingling, and headache may occur. These effects usually subside with continued use of niacin.

## Vitamin $B_{12}$ and Folic Acid

- Know about dietary sources of vitamin $B_{12}$. This vitamin occurs in meat, fish, poultry, shellfish, milk, dairy products, eggs, and some fortified foods. Vitamin $B_{12}$ does not occur in plant sources. If you are a strict vegan who consumes no animal products, you are at risk for vitamin $B_{12}$ deficiency unless you take a supplementary source of the vitamin.
- Know about dietary sources of folic acid. This nutrient occurs in liver, okra, spinach, asparagus, dried peas and beans, seeds, and orange juice. Breads, cereals, and other grains are fortified with folic acid.
- Take prescribed vitamins as directed and for the appropriate time. If you have pernicious anemia, you must have vitamin $B_{12}$ injections for the remainder of your life. Any chronic vitamin $B_{12}$ deficiency requires lifelong treatment. If you are pregnant or breast-feeding, requirements may be greater; you usually may need additional vitamin supplements.
- Keep appointments for follow-up visits and obtain the necessary laboratory tests.

## Vitamin C

- Know about dietary sources of vitamin C. This vitamin occurs in citrus fruits and juices, red and green peppers, broccoli, cauliflower, Brussels sprouts, cantaloupe, kiwi fruit, mustard greens, strawberries, and tomatoes.
- Be aware that vitamin C improves the absorption of iron.
- Understand that vitamin C, which acidifies the urine, may alter the excretion of some drugs.

## Adverse Effects and Contraindications

No symptoms have been observed from excessive intake of vitamin K. Mild adverse effects of vitamin K intake may include facial flushing, alterations in taste, or redness and pain at the injection site. The FDA has issued a **BLACK BOX WARNING** ◆ stating that IV administration of vitamin K may result in an anaphylactic type of reaction with risks of shock, cardiorespiratory arrest, and death, even with drug dilution and slow administration.

Contraindications to vitamin K include a history of allergic reaction as well as a history of allergic reaction to benzyl alcohol or castor oil.

## Nursing Implications

### Preventing Interactions

Mineral oil as well as cholestyramine and other bile acid sequestrants inhibit the absorption of vitamin K if taken at the same time. Increased vitamin K levels decrease the anticoagulant effect of warfarin. It is necessary to avoid the use of vitamin K as a drug when a patient is receiving warfarin, and significant increases or decreases in dietary vitamin K may necessitate adjustment of the warfarin dose.

### Administering the Medication

The oral route for vitamin K administration is preferred when treating nonbleeding patients. The subcutaneous route demonstrates irregular absorption. The IV route is used if there is major bleeding. Both the IM route and the IV route are associated with severe hypersensitivity reactions. People may take the vitamin without regard to meals. They should avoid taking it at the same time as mineral oil or bile acid sequestrants.

It is necessary to protect all vitamin K preparations from light.

### Assessing for Therapeutic and Adverse Effects

The nurse observes for decreased signs and symptoms of vitamin K deficiency. This includes decreased bleeding and more nearly normal blood coagulation tests.

Oral vitamin K rarely produces adverse reactions. Following subcutaneous injection, the nurse observes the injection site for redness and pain. Use of the IM and IV routes requires close observation for anaphylactic reaction as evidenced by chills, fever, diaphoresis, dyspnea, hypotension, bronchospasm, respiratory arrest, cardiac arrest, shock, and death. The means for emergency resuscitation must be immediately available.

### Patient Teaching

Box 35.2 identifies patient teaching guidelines for vitamins, including vitamin K.

## WATER-SOLUBLE VITAMINS

### VITAMIN B COMPLEX: VITAMIN B$_1$, VITAMIN B$_3$, AND VITAMIN B$_6$

Most vitamin B complex deficiencies are multiple, rather than single, and treatment consists of administration of a multivitamin that contains several B complex vitamins. If a single deficiency seems predominant, that vitamin may be given alone or in addition to a multivitamin preparation. Three of the vitamin B complex vitamins are presented together in this section because they have much in common and are prototypical of the B complex vitamins as a whole: vitamin B$_1$ (thiamine), vitamin B$_3$ (niacin), and vitamin B$_6$ (pyridoxine). Vitamin B$_{12}$ (cyanocobalamin) and folic acid are discussed separately below because of their common use in the treatment of anemia.

## Pharmacokinetics and Use

Thiamine, niacin, and pyridoxine are absorbed from the GI tract. Thiamine is widely distributed and enters breast milk. Niacin crossed the placenta and enters breast milk. Pyridoxine is stored in the liver and crosses the placental barrier. Niacin and pyridoxine are metabolized in the liver. Thiamine, niacin, and pyridoxine are eliminated by the kidneys in the urine.

Table 35.3 gives route and dosage information for the B complex vitamins.

### Use in Patients With Renal or Hepatic Impairment

Both niacin and pyridoxine warrant caution in renal impairment. People with liver disease should not take niacin because it may increase liver enzymes and bilirubin and cause further liver damage. Long-acting dosage forms may be more hepatotoxic than the fast-acting forms.

## Adverse Effects and Contraindications

- Thiamine: history of an allergic reaction to the vitamin.
- Niacin: hepatic impairment, active peptic ulcer disease, arterial bleeding, and lactation. Caution is necessary with a history of jaundice, hepatobiliary disease, peptic ulcers, high alcohol consumption, renal impairment, unstable angina, gout glaucoma, and diabetes mellitus. Administration causes vasodilation, which may result in dizziness, hypotension, and injury from falls.
- Pyridoxine (IV form): cardiac disease. Caution is warranted with renal impairment.

## Nursing Implications

### Preventing Interactions

- Thiamine: no important drug interactions.
- Niacin: increases the risk of rhabdomyolysis from the statin antihyperlipidemics, increases the effectiveness of antihypertensives and vasoactive drugs, and increases the risk of bleeding from anticoagulants. Bile acid sequestrants decrease absorption.
- Pyridoxine: accelerates the peripheral conversion of levodopa into dopamine, thus decreasing the amount of levodopa that is available to cross into the central nervous system (CNS). Isoniazid decreases the effect of pyridoxine.

### Administering the Medication

- Thiamine: preferred route of administration is by mouth; people may take it without regard to food. It is necessary to swallow enteric-coated tablets whole, not chewed or crushed. The IM and IV routes are for severe deficiency states only.

- Niacin: people may take oral niacin, except for timed-release forms, with or after meals, which decreases anorexia, nausea, vomiting, diarrhea, and flatulence. They should swallow timed-release forms whole, not chewed or crushed. The nurse should instruct the patient to sit or lie down for about 30 minutes after administration because niacin causes vasodilation and possible dizziness and hypotension.
- Pyridoxine: the general route of administration is oral, and people should swallow sustained-release or enteric forms of pyridoxine whole, not chewed or crushed.

### Assessing for Therapeutic Effects

The nurse assesses for decreased signs and symptoms of deficiency. With B complex vitamins, it is necessary to observe for decreased or absent stomatitis, glossitis, seborrheic dermatitis, neurologic problems (neuritis, convulsions, mental deterioration, psychotic symptoms), cardiovascular problems (edema, heart failure), and eye problems (itching, burning, photophobia). Deficiencies of B complex vitamins commonly occur together and produce many similar manifestations.

### Assessing for Adverse Effects

Adverse reactions are generally unlikely to occur with B complex multivitamin preparations. They are most likely to develop with large IV doses and rapid administration. The nurse observes for the following:

- Niacin and thiamine (parenteral): hypotension and anaphylactic shock
- Niacin (oral): anorexia, nausea, vomiting, diarrhea, and postural hypotension

### Patient Teaching

Box 35.2 identifies patient teaching guidelines for vitamins, including vitamins $B_1$, $B_3$, and $B_6$.

## VITAMIN $B_{12}$ (CYANOCOBALAMIN) AND FOLIC ACID

The following discussion concerns vitamin $B_{12}$ (cyanocobalamin) and folic acid.

## Pharmacokinetics

- Vitamin $B_{12}$: requires intrinsic factor, produced by the stomach, for absorption. Normally, vitamin $B_{12}$ is widely distributed and stored principally in the liver (half-life in the liver is 400 days). Vitamin $B_{12}$ crosses the placenta and enters breast milk. It is converted into active coenzymes in the tissues and eliminated, very slowly, in the urine.
- Folic acid: absorbed from the proximal small intestine. Folic acid is distributed to all body tissues with high concentrations in the cerebrospinal fluid. The unused portion is stored in the liver. Folic acid crosses the placenta and enters breast milk. It is metabolized in the liver to active metabolites. Elimination is in the urine, at a more rapid rate than vitamin $B_{12}$.

## Use

Health care providers use vitamin $B_{12}$ to treat vitamin $B_{12}$ deficiency states, whether caused by dietary deficiency, malabsorption, or inadequate secretion of intrinsic factor. They use folic acid as a supplement during infancy, childhood, and pregnancy, as well as to treat folic acid deficiency caused by malabsorption (sprue) or alcoholism. Folate deficiency in alcoholism results from both poor dietary intake and interference with liver processing of folic acid. Deficiency states of both vitamin $B_{12}$ and folic acid present similarly as **megaloblastic anemia** (characterized by abnormally large, immature red blood cells). Proper diagnosis must establish which vitamin is deficient before treatment can begin. If megaloblastic anemia is severe, treatment usually involves both vitamin $B_{12}$ and folic acid.

In pernicious anemia (vitamin $B_{12}$ deficiency caused by absence of intrinsic factor), vitamin $B_{12}$ must be given by injection because oral forms are not absorbed from the GI tract. The injections must be continued for life. Vitamin $B_{12}$ is also given to prevent pernicious anemia in patients who are strict vegetarians, who have had a gastrectomy or bariatric surgery, or who have chronic small bowel disease. Although folic acid relieves hematologic disorders of pernicious anemia, giving folic acid alone allows continued neurologic deterioration. Thus, an accurate diagnosis is required.

Table 35.3 gives route and dosage information for vitamin $B_{12}$ and folic acid.

## Adverse Effects

- Vitamin $B_{12}$: rare. Hypokalemia sometimes results. There is a slight risk of anaphylactic shock and sudden death.
- Folic acid: uncommon. The most serious potential adverse effect is bronchospasm.

## Contraindications

- Vitamin $B_{12}$: history of a sensitivity to vitamin $B_{12}$, other cobalamins, or cobalt. Vitamin $B_{12}$ should be used with caution when treating folic acid deficiency.
- Folic acid: undiagnosed anemia because the vitamin may mask pernicious anemia. Other contraindication includes vitamin $B_{12}$ deficiency (the use of folic acid will improve the patient's megaloblastic anemia while doing nothing to reverse the neurologic problems associated with vitamin $B_{12}$ deficiency).

## Nursing Implications
### Preventing Interactions

- Vitamin $B_{12}$: effects decreased by omeprazole and metformin, which decrease absorption of vitamin $B_{12}$ from food.
- Folic acid: effects decreased by aspirin, chloramphenicol, nonsteroidal anti-inflammatory drugs, sulfa antibiotics, sulfonylureas, triamterene, and trimethoprim. Cholestyramine, oral contraceptives, and sulfasalazine decrease absorption of folic acid. Methotrexate and phenytoin act as antagonists to folic acid. Alcohol alters liver function and leads to poor hepatic storage of folic acid. Folic acid increases phenytoin metabolism, which decreases phenytoin levels.

## Administering the Medication

- Vitamin $B_{12}$: use of the oral form is most convenient, and administration with food increases absorption. Mixing the vitamin with fruit juice is fine, but it is important to consume the mixture quickly because ascorbic acid interferes with the stability of the vitamin. It is important to note that vitamin $B_{12}$ is not safe for IV administration.
- Folic acid: oral administration is preferable unless severe malabsorption is present, and people may take the vitamin without regard to food. Folic acid is also available in subcutaneous, IM, or IV forms. It is necessary to protect the parenteral forms from light and heat and store them at room temperature.

## Assessing for Therapeutic and Adverse Effects

With vitamin $B_{12}$ and folic acid, the nurse observes for increased appetite, strength, and feeling of well-being; increased reticulocyte counts; and increased number of normal red blood cells, hemoglobin, and hematocrit. Therapeutic effects may be rapid and dramatic.

## Patient Teaching

Box 35.2 presents patient teaching guidelines for vitamins, including vitamin $B_{12}$ and folic acid.

## VITAMIN C

The following section concerns vitamin C (ascorbic acid).

## Pharmacokinetics

Vitamin C is absorbed from the GI tract and is distributed generally. It crosses the placenta and enters breast milk. The vitamin is metabolized in the liver and eliminated by the kidneys.

## Use

The most important therapeutic use of vitamin C involves the prevention and treatment of scurvy. This vitamin is available alone for oral, IM, or IV administration. It is also an ingredient in most multivitamin preparations. There is no known benefit for taking large amounts of this vitamin, and the nurse should discourage its use.

Table 35.3 gives route and dosage information for vitamin C.

## Use in Patients With Renal Impairment

Patients with acute renal failure who are unable to eat an adequate diet need a vitamin supplement to meet DRIs. However, it is imperative to avoid large doses of vitamin C because of impaired urinary excretion. Also, oxalate (a product of vitamin C catabolism) may precipitate in renal tubules or form calcium oxalate stones, obstruct urine flow, and worsen renal function. In addition, dialysis removes vitamin C, and patients receiving dialysis require vitamin C replacement.

## Use in Critical Illness

Conditions that increase the need for vitamin C sometimes warrant larger doses of vitamin C. These conditions include extensive burns, delayed fracture or wound healing, delayed postoperative wound healing, or severe febrile or chronic disease states.

## Adverse Effects and Contraindications

Usual doses of vitamin C are well tolerated. The most common adverse effects of oral vitamin C (especially megadoses) are abdominal cramps, nausea, vomiting, and diarrhea.

Caution is warranted in patients who are prone to kidney stones, as well as in those with glucose-6-phosphate deficiency or sickle cell anemia.

## Nursing Implications
### Preventing Interactions

Vitamin C, which acidifies the urine, decreases the elimination of aspirin and other salicylates, which are eliminated more rapidly in alkaline urine.

### Administering the Medication

Vitamin C is available in various oral forms. Oral solutions may need mixing with food. Effervescent tablets may need dissolving in water immediately before use. Parenteral forms are also available.

### Assessing for Therapeutic and Adverse Effects

Vitamin C deficiency usually begins to resolve rapidly, with improvement seen after only a few days. The nurse assesses for decreased or absent malaise, irritability, and bleeding tendencies (easy bruising of skin, bleeding gums, nosebleeds, and so forth).

Adverse reactions are rare with usual doses and methods of administration.

### Patient Teaching

Box 35.2 presents patient teaching guidelines for vitamins, including vitamin C.

### Clinical Application 35.2

- Mrs. Martin's physician expresses concern about her nutritional status and decides to administer a vitamin supplement. Which vitamins might he or she order?
- The physician prescribes the anticoagulant warfarin (Coumadin) for Mrs. Martin to aid in preventing another stroke. If she receives an overdose of warfarin, why does the health care prescriber order vitamin K? If she is eventually able to eat solid food, what teaching does the nurse provide concerning vitamin K in her diet and warfarin?

## NCLEX Success

3. Which one of the following patients taking vitamin A supplements is of most concern to the nurse?

   A. a 21-year-old woman who is pregnant
   B. a 32-year-old man with poor night vision
   C. a 55-year-old man with hepatic cirrhosis
   D. a 79-year-old woman who is malnourished

4. The nurse administers vitamin K if a patient is bleeding from an overdose of which of the following?

   A. aspirin
   B. enoxaparin
   C. heparin
   D. warfarin

5. A nurse is planning to teach a patient about dietary sources of vitamin K. The nurse teaches that foods containing vitamin K include which of the following?

   A. spinach, brussels sprouts, and broccoli
   B. breads, cereals, and other grains
   C. citrus fruits and juices, as well as strawberries
   D. meat, fish, and poultry

6. The patient has pernicious anemia. Why does the nurse administer vitamin $B_{12}$ by the intramuscular route?

   A. The drug cannot be administered orally.
   B. The oral form has a bitter taste.
   C. The drug is not absorbed if taken orally.
   D. The oral form causes nausea and GI upset.

### ⚠ QSEN Alert: Evidence-Based Practice

The FDA-labeled indications for vitamin C are treatment of vitamin C deficiency or for use in conditions requiring increased vitamin C intake (such as burns or wound healing); as a dietary supplement; and for the prevention and treatment of scurvy. The FDA now also recognizes an off-label use for adults: treatment of severe sepsis or septic shock. Marik, Khangoora, Rivera, Hooper, and Catravas (2017) treated patients with severe sepsis or septic shock with standard treatments including broad-spectrum antibiotics, IV fluids, and vasopressors. Along with the standard treatments, they employed a regimen of vitamin C intravenous infusion 1.5 g every 6 hours, hydrocortisone IV push 50 mg every 6 hours, and thiamine intravenous infusion 200 mg every 12 hours. The researchers used the regimen of vitamin C and thiamine for 4 days and hydrocortisone for 7 days with a 3-day taper. Patients treated with the protocol were independent of vasopressors in a shorter time, had reduced mortality, and avoided new organ failure. Patients with sepsis have vitamin C and thiamine deficiencies. Experts believe vitamin C increases endogenous production of norepinephrine and vasopressin counteracting septic shock; it also improves microvascular function and has bacteriostatic activity. Hydrocortisone works synergistically with vitamin C to decrease production of inflammatory mediators, preserve microcirculatory function,

synthesize catecholamines, and increase vasopressor sensitivity. Thiamine reduces the risk of renal failure due to the high doses of vitamin C (Kuhn, Meissner, Mayes, & Bartels, 2018; Marik, 2017). Marik and Khangoora conclude early use of vitamin C, hydrocortisone, and thiamine may prove effective in preventing progressive organ dysfunction, including acute kidney injury, and reducing the mortality of patients with severe sepsis and septic shock (Marik et al., 2017, p. 1236). The three drugs in the protocol are also inexpensive and readily available.

# MINERALS

## IRON

Iron deficiency is usually the result not of normal elimination but of excessive menstruation or GI bleeding. The following discussion relates to the prototype drug ℗ **ferrous sulfate (Feosol)**. Ferrous sulfate is often the preparation of choice; it contains 20% elemental iron.

## Pharmacokinetics and Use

The fate of iron administered in drug form is the same as that of dietary iron. Only about 10% to 15% of ingested dietary iron is absorbed; although during pregnancy or iron deficiency, this percentage increases. Iron is stored in the small intestine (and in certain other cells) as ferritin as well as in the liver. When needed, iron is released into the bloodstream, bound to transferrin, and transported to the bone marrow for incorporation into hemoglobin. Iron crosses the placenta.

Iron is not metabolized; the iron in red blood cells is reused. Small amounts of iron are eliminated daily (about 0.5–1 mg) in urine, sweat, and sloughing of intestinal mucosal cells. Excess iron is excreted in feces, which turn dark green or black.

The most important therapeutic uses of ferrous sulfate are as a supplement during periods of increased iron use and as treatment for iron deficiency. Table 35.4 gives route and dosage information for ferrous sulfate and other iron preparations. Slow-release or enteric-coated iron products decrease absorption but may cause less gastric irritation.

## Adverse Effects and Contraindications

The most common adverse effects of ferrous sulfate and other oral iron preparations are GI discomfort, nausea, constipation, diarrhea, and black stools. Liquid forms of iron may temporarily stain the teeth. In iron overload, excess iron is deposited in the heart, liver, and endocrine glands resulting in organ damage and, if untreated, death.

Contraindications to ferrous sulfate include peptic ulceration, ulcerative colitis, regional enteritis, and repeated blood transfusions. Other contraindications are disorders that cause the accumulation of iron stores: hemosiderosis, primary hemochromatosis, and hemolytic anemia (unless iron deficiency anemia is also present).

**TABLE 35.4**

## DRUGS AT A GLANCE: Drugs Used in Mineral–Electrolyte and Acid–Base Imbalances

| Drug/Pregnancy Category | Indications for Use | Routes and Dosage Ranges | |
|---|---|---|---|
| | | **Adults** | **Children** |
| **Cation Exchange Resin** | | | |
| Sodium polystyrene sulfonate (Kayexalate; Kionex; ✹ Kayexalate) | Treatment of hyperkalemia | 15 g PO 1–4 times per day or 30–50 g rectal every 6 h | 1 g/kg/dose PO every 6 h or 1 g/kg/dose rectal every 2–6 h PO route more effective and preferred; in infants and small children, use lower dose by using practical exchange ratio of 1 mEqK$^+$/g resin as basis for calculation |
| **Chelating Agents (Metal Antagonists)** | | | |
| Deferasirox (Exjade; ✹ APO-Deferasirox; Exjade; Jadenu) | Chronic iron overload | Initially, 20 mg/kg PO daily on empty stomach 30 min before eating; adjust dose every 3–6 mo; should not exceed 40 mg/kg daily | Older than 2 y of age: same as adult; calculate dose to the nearest whole tablet size |
| Deferoxamine (Desferal; ✹ Desferal) | Acute iron intoxication Hemochromatosis due to blood transfusions Hemosiderosis due to hemolytic anemia | 1 g IV initially and then 500 mg IV every 4 h for two doses, then 500 mg every 4–12 h if needed; max dose 6 g/24 h; rate of IV infusion not to exceed 15 mg/kg/h IV route preferred | 15 mg/kg/h IV (maximum 80 mg/kg/d, not to exceed 6000 mg/24 h) IM route not preferred and rarely indicated |
| Penicillamine (Cuprimine; ✹ Cuprimine) NOTE: Penicillamine should always be administered with a supplement of pyridoxine 25–50 mg PO daily in both adults and children | Wilson's disease Rheumatoid arthritis Cystinuria | Wilson's disease: 750–1500 mg PO daily in divided doses (max dose 2000 mg PO daily; dose based on urinary copper excretion) Rheumatoid arthritis: 125–250 mg PO daily; may increase dose at 1–3-mo intervals up to 1–1.5 g PO daily Cystinuria: 1–4 g/d PO in four divided doses; initiate at 250 mg/d and gradually titrate up to reduce adverse effects; dose titrated based on urinary cystine excretion | Wilson's disease: 20 mg/kg/d PO in 2–3 divided doses (round off to the nearest 250 mg dose); dose adjusted based on urinary copper excretion Rheumatoid arthritis: initially 3 mg/kg/d PO (≤250 mg PO daily) for 3 mo; then, 6 mg/kg/d PO (≤500 mg PO daily) in two divided doses for 3 mo to a max of 10 mg/kg/d PO in 3–4 divided doses (max dose 1.5 g/d PO) |
| Succimer (Chemet) | Lead poisoning | See pediatric dosages | 10 mg/kg/dose or 350 mg/m$^2$/dose PO every 8 h for 5 d and then every 12 h for 14 d (max 500 mg/dose); treatment course may be repeated; 2-wk interval between courses recommended; capsule comes only in 100 mg; round the dose to nearest 100 mg; for young children who cannot swallow capsules, capsule contents can be sprinkled on soft food or given with a spoon |
| **Iron Preparations** | | | |
| Ferrous gluconate (Ferate) | Iron deficiency anemia | Doses in elemental iron (ferrous gluconate contains 12% elemental iron); 65–200 mg/d in 2–3 divided doses | 3–6 mg/kg/d in three divided doses; maximum daily dose 200 mg/d |

**TABLE 35.4**

## DRUGS AT A GLANCE: Drugs Used in Mineral–Electrolyte and Acid–Base Imbalances (Continued)

| Drug/Pregnancy Category | Indications for Use | Routes and Dosage Ranges | |
|---|---|---|---|
| | | **Adults** | **Children** |
| Ⓟ **Ferrous sulfate** (Fer-In-Sol; Fer-Iron; FeroSul; others; 🍁 PMS-Ferrous Sulfate) | Iron deficiency anemia | Doses in elemental iron (ferrous sulfate contains 20% elemental iron); ferrous sulfate doses given 65–200 mg/d in 2–3 divided doses or extended-release form once daily | 3–6 mg/kg/d in three divided doses; maximum daily dose 200 mg/d |
| Iron dextran injection (INFeD; 🍁 DexIron) | Iron deficiency anemia | Dosage is calculated for individual patients according to hemoglobin and weight (see manufacturer's literature); a 25-mg test dose is required before therapeutic doses are given | Same as adults; test dose 10–25 mg |
| **Magnesium Preparations** | | | |
| Magnesium oxide/B Magnesium hydroxide/A Magnesium sulfate/A | Hypomagnesemia Hypertension or seizures associated with toxemia of pregnancy | Hypomagnesemia: magnesium oxide 800 mg daily with food; magnesium sulfate 1 g IM every 6 h for four doses; magnesium sulfate 1–4 g IV well diluted, administer at rate of <1 g/h (do not exceed 12 g over 12 h) Constipation: magnesium hydroxide (milk of magnesia) 30–60 mL PO at bedtime Pre-eclampsia or eclampsia of pregnancy to prevent or control seizures: initially, magnesium sulfate 4 g in 5% dextrose or normal saline 250 mL infused IV along with magnesium sulfate 4–5 g deep IM into two suitable sites; then, 4–5 g deep IM every 4 h into alternate sites as needed; alternatively, magnesium sulfate 4–6 g in $D_5W$ or NS 250 mL infused IV as a loading dose; followed by 1–2 g IV hourly for at least 24 h; the total dose should not exceed 40 g in 24 h | Hypomagnesemia: magnesium oxide PO 10–20 mg/kg/dose up to four times per day; magnesium sulfate 25–50 mg/kg/dose IV every 6 h for 2–3 doses; maximum dose 2 g/dose; dilute in appropriate fluid prior to IV infusion; infuse IV solution slowly over 1–4 h |
| **Potassium Preparation** | | | |
| Ⓟ **Potassium chloride** (K-Tab; Klor-Con; 🍁 Apo-K; Micro-K; Slo-Pot 600) NOTE: Give potassium chloride by IV infusion only, *never* IM or IV push; rapid infusion may cause fatal hyperkalemia | Prevent or treat hypokalemia | Prevention of hypokalemia: potassium supplement 20–40 mEq PO daily in 1–2 divided doses; adjust dosage based on serum potassium levels Treatment of hypokalemia: potassium supplement 40–100 mEq PO daily in 2–4 divided doses; max dose of diluted potassium chloride IV is 40 mEq/L infused at 10 mEq/h—*do not* exceed 200 mEq daily; further doses based on serum potassium level and blood pH; give potassium replacement IV only with monitoring of ECG and serum potassium level | Prevention of hypokalemia: potassium supplement 1–2 mEq/kg/d in 1–2 divided doses Treatment of hypokalemia: potassium supplement 2–5 mEq/kg/d PO in divided doses (not to exceed 1–2 mEq/kg or 20 mEq whichever is less as single dose); by intermittent IV 0.5–1 mEq/kg/dose (max dose 40 mEq); infuse at rate <0.5 mEq/kg/h; if infusion exceeds 0.5 mEq/kg/h, continuous ECG monitoring and physician at bedside; frequently monitor serum potassium level |

*(Continued on page 718)*

**TABLE 35.4**

## DRUGS AT A GLANCE: Drugs Used in Mineral–Electrolyte and Acid–Base Imbalances (Continued)

| Drug/Pregnancy Category | Indications for Use | Routes and Dosage Ranges | |
|---|---|---|---|
| | | **Adults** | **Children** |
| **Sodium Preparation** | | | |
| Sodium chloride (NaCl or normal saline) injection | Hyponatremia | IV: Sodium fluid concentration is dependent on severity; use more concentrated solution (e.g., 3% NaCl) for more severe hyponatremia; increase serum sodium concentration by 4–6 mEq/L over 24 h | IV: use 0.9% isotonic solution or 0.3% hypertonic solution based on severity; acutely correct serum sodium by 5 mEq/L/dose increments using serum Na of 125 mEq/L as desired serum sodium; use serum correction rate of 2 mEq/L/h or less for first few hours; follow with rate of 0.5 mEq/L/h |
| **Zinc Preparation** | | | |
| Zinc sulfate (Orazinc; 🍁 Micro-Zn) | Prevent or treat zinc deficiency | Deficiency: zinc sulfate 110–220 mg (elemental zinc 25–50 mg) PO three times daily | Infants, children, and adolescents: elemental zinc 0.5–1 mg/kg/d once daily |
| **Multiple Mineral–Electrolyte Preparations** | | | |
| Oral solutions (Pedialyte) IV solutions (Normosol, Plasma-Lyte 148, Ringer's solution) | Prevent or treat fluid and electrolyte deficiencies | 2000–3000 mL/24 h IV, depending on individual fluid and electrolyte needs | Amount (PO, IV) individualized according to fluid and electrolyte needs based on estimated fluid loss, age, and weight (see manufacturer's literature) |

## Nursing Implications

### Preventing Interactions

In general, food decreases iron absorption. Examples include cereals, cheese, coffee, eggs, milk, tea, bran and whole-grain breads, and yogurt.

A few drugs increase iron absorption. Most notable is vitamin C, which increases iron absorption by acidifying gastric secretions. Vitamin C, taken at the same time as iron-containing foods or oral iron preparations, increases iron absorption. Taking ferrous sulfate with vitamin C–containing orange juice enhances iron absorption. Some oral iron preparations contain a small amount of vitamin C. Allopurinol may increase the concentration of iron in the liver.

Ferrous sulfate interferes with the absorption of the penicillamine, tetracycline, and fluoroquinolone antibiotics, possibly resulting in decreased antibiotic levels or effect. Ferrous sulfate also decreases the absorption of levodopa, methyldopa, and levothyroxine.

### Administering the Medication

People should take iron tablets or capsules before meals, with 8 oz of water or juice, if tolerated. They should not crush or chew sustained-release preparations. Oral iron preparations are better absorbed if taken on an empty stomach. However, because gastric irritation is a common adverse reaction, people more often take iron with or immediately after meals; this may decrease absorption. With liquid preparations, it is necessary to dilute them, take with a straw, and then rinse the mouth afterward to prevent temporary staining of teeth.

Certain interactions affect the timing of iron administration. Ferrous sulfate interferes with the absorption of the penicillamine, tetracycline, and fluoroquinolone antibiotics; therefore, it is necessary to take ferrous sulfate 2 to 4 hours before or after these antibiotics. Because some foods may affect iron absorption, people should take iron at least 2 hours before or after a caffeine-containing beverage or food.

### Assessing for Therapeutic and Adverse Effects

The nurse observes for increased vigor and feeling of well-being, improved appetite, less fatigue, and increased red blood cells, as well as hemoglobin, hematocrit, and reticulocyte count. Therapeutic effects are usually evident within a month unless other problems are also present (e.g., vitamin deficiency, achlorhydria, infection, or malabsorption).

The nurse assesses for GI upset, which may be related to dose. GI symptoms may decrease as therapy progresses. (Enteric-coated products reduce GI upset but also reduce the amount of iron absorbed.) It is also necessary to check for stool color depending on the iron preparation. Oral iron may turn stools black. Although this unabsorbed iron is harmless, it could mask melena.

*Patient Teaching*

Box 35.3 presents patient teaching guidelines for minerals and electrolytes, including iron.

### Clinical Application 35.3

Mrs. Martin appears to be anemic and requires iron supplementation.
- By what route is the iron ordered?
- How does the nurse determine if this iron therapy is successful?
- What adverse effects does the nurse observe for?

### NCLEX    Success

7. Teaching for a patient who is being started on an iron supplement should include information that the preparation

    A. may cause diarrhea
    B. may cause stools to be dark green or black
    C. should be taken with an antacid
    D. should not be taken with fruit juice

8. When assessing a patient for therapeutic effects of iron therapy, the nurse would check the result of which laboratory study?

    A. activated partial thromboplastin time
    B. international normalized ratio
    C. reticulocyte count
    D. white blood cell count

## Other Drugs Used to Treat Iron Deficiency

### Iron Dextran

Iron dextran (Dexferrum, INFeD) is a parenteral form of iron useful for treating iron deficiency anemia when oral supplements cannot be used. Indications for use include peptic ulcer or inflammatory bowel disease that may be aggravated by oral iron preparations, the patient's inability or unwillingness to take oral preparations, and a shortage of time for correcting the iron deficiency (e.g., late pregnancy, preoperative status, or excessive blood loss). The FDA has issued a **BLACK BOX WARNING ◆** for iron dextran regarding the risk of anaphylactic reactions and death. Because of this risk, administration should occur only when there is a clear indication. Contraindications include anemias not associated with iron deficiency and hypersensitivity to the drug. Caution is warranted in serious hepatic impairment, rheumatoid arthritis, or other inflammatory diseases as well as a significant history of allergies or asthma. The IV route is preferred to the IM route. It is necessary to give a small test dose before administering a therapeutic dose. The drug has a slow onset of action and peaks in 1 to 2 weeks. Dosage is calculated according to hemoglobin level and weight.

> **! QSEN Alert: Patient-Centered Care**
>
> Equipment and drugs for emergency resuscitation must always be available whenever iron dextran IV is administered. Anaphylactic reactions may occur.

### Iron Sucrose

Iron sucrose (Venofer) is a parenteral iron supplement given by IV infusion. This supplement is indicated for patients with

---

**BOX 35.3**    *Patient Teaching Guidelines for Minerals and Electrolytes*

**General Considerations**

- A well-balanced diet contains all the minerals needed for health in most people. Exceptions are iron and calcium, which are often needed as a dietary supplement in women and children. Note that herbal preparations of chamomile, feverfew, and St. John's wort may inhibit iron absorption. The safest action is to take mineral supplements only on a health care provider's advice, in the amounts and for length of time prescribed. All minerals are toxic when taken in excess.

- Keep all mineral or electrolyte substances out of reach of children to prevent accidental overdose. Acute iron intoxication is a common problem among young children and can be fatal. Supervise children about using fluoride supplements (e.g., remind them to spit out oral rinses and gels rather than swallow them).

- Keep appointments with health care providers for periodic blood tests and other follow-up procedures when mineral or electrolyte supplements are prescribed (e.g., potassium chloride). This helps prevent ingestion of excessive amounts.

- Minerals are often contained in multivitamin preparations, with percentages of the recommended dietary allowances supplied. These amounts differ in various preparations and should be included in estimations of daily intake.

**Iron**

- Know about dietary sources of iron. This mineral occurs in beef liver, red meats, fish, poultry, clams, tofu, oysters, lentils, dried peas and beans, fortified cereals, bread, and dried fruits.

- Avoid substituting one iron salt for another, because amounts of elemental iron may vary.

- Take iron preparations with or after meals, with approximately 240 mL of fluid, to prevent stomach upset. Do not take iron with coffee or other caffeine-containing beverages because caffeine decreases absorption. Take iron and caffeine preparations at least 2 hours apart.

- Do not crush or chew slow-release tablets or capsules.

- With liquid preparations, dilute with water, drink through a straw, and rinse the mouth afterward to avoid staining the teeth.
- Expect that stools will be dark green or black. Report constipation or change in color or consistency of stool to the health care provider.

**Potassium**

- Mix oral solutions or effervescent tablets with at least 120 mL of water or juice to improve the taste, dilute the drug, and decrease gastric irritation.
- Do not crush or chew slow-release preparations.
- Take after meals initially to decrease gastric irritation. If no nausea, vomiting, or other problems occur, the drug can be tried before meals because it is better absorbed from an empty stomach.

- *Do not stop taking the medication without notifying the health care provider who prescribed it, especially if you are also taking diuretics or digoxin.*
- Do not use salt substitutes except on the recommendation of a health care provider. Salt substitutes contain potassium chloride and may result in excessive intake.
- Serious problems may develop from either high or low levels of potassium in the blood. Know and recognize signs and symptoms of hypokalemia and hyperkalemia.
  - Signs and symptoms of hypokalemia: palpitations, confusion, dizziness, muscle weakness, abdominal distension, frequent voiding of large amounts of urine
  - Signs and symptoms of hyperkalemia: muscle weakness, palpitations, slow pulse, fatigue, shortness of breath

chronic kidney disease who are not on dialysis and for those who are peritoneal dialysis dependent or hemodialysis dependent. It may be given alone or concurrently with erythropoietin therapy. The major advantage of iron sucrose is a lesser risk of anaphylaxis than with iron dextran; however, hypersensitivity reactions, although rare, can be fatal. Test doses are not necessary. Common adverse effects include headache, heart failure, hypotension, nausea, leg cramps, and sepsis.

## POTASSIUM

The following discussion focuses on the prototype  **potassium chloride**, or KCl. The oral form of the drug has numerous trade names.

## Pharmacokinetics and Use

Potassium is absorbed from the GI tract. The potassium level is normally maintained by the kidneys.

Potassium chloride is usually the drug of choice for preventing or treating **hypokalemia** (less than normal amount of potassium in the blood) because deficiencies of potassium and chloride often occur together. Table 35.4 gives route and dosage information for this drug. Health care providers may order potassium chloride for patients who are receiving potassium-depleting diuretics (e.g., hydrochlorothiazide, furosemide), those who are receiving digoxin (hypokalemia increases the risk of digoxin toxicity), and those who are receiving IV fluids because of surgical procedures, GI disease, or other conditions. They may also use it to replace chloride in patients with hypochloremic metabolic acidosis.

## Adverse Effects and Contraindications

Adverse effects of oral potassium are nausea, vomiting, abdominal pain, and diarrhea. Adverse effects of IV potassium include postinfusion phlebitis at the IV site. Overdosage with oral or IV forms or rapid infusion of IV preparations produces **hyperkalemia** (greater than normal amount of potassium in the blood),

dysrhythmias, heart block, cardiac arrest, respiratory paralysis, and death. Hyperkalemia may occur with the following:

- Concurrent use of potassium chloride with angiotensin-converting enzyme inhibitors or potassium-sparing diuretics
- Salt substitutes that contain potassium instead of sodium if used with potassium supplements
- Penicillin G potassium (potassium salt of penicillin)

Contraindications to potassium supplementation include hyperkalemia, severe renal impairment, acute dehydration, heat cramps, and untreated Addison's disease. Caution is necessary in cardiac disease or renal impairment.

## Nursing Implications

### Administering the Medication

People should take oral preparations with or after meals; this decreases gastric irritation. They should not crush controlled-release or extended-release tablets. It is necessary to mix oral liquids, powders, and effervescent tablets in at least 120 mL of water, juice, or carbonated beverage to disguise the taste.

Intravenous (IV) potassium chloride is indicated when a patient cannot take an oral preparation or has severe hypokalemia. The nurse measures the serum potassium level and establishes that urine output is adequate before starting IV potassium therapy.

> **! QSEN Alert: Safety**
>
> It is essential to never give undiluted drug by the IV route or give it by the IV push route.

Well-diluted preparations prevent sudden hyperkalemia, cardiotoxic effects, and phlebitis at the venipuncture site. Careful administration is warranted.

### Patient Teaching

Box 35.3 identifies patient teaching guidelines for minerals and electrolytes, including potassium.

*Clinical Application 35.4*

- Serum electrolytes reveal that Mrs. Martin is hypokalemic. The health care provider orders potassium chloride per feeding tube. What steps does the nurse take to administer this medication, and what form of potassium chloride is preferable for administration per feeding tube? What adverse effects does the nurse assess for?
- Suppose Mrs. Martin is severely hypokalemic and the health care provider orders potassium chloride to be given intravenously. What nursing interventions ensure that the ordered potassium supplement is given correctly and safely? What adverse effects may occur if IV administration of this potassium preparation occurs too rapidly?

## NCLEX Success

9. Which one of the following mineral/electrolyte imbalances increases the chances of digoxin toxicity?

   A. hyperkalemia
   B. hypokalemia
   C. decreased serum iron levels
   D. elevated serum iron levels

10. A nurse should question the use of an oral potassium preparation with which one of the following drugs?

    A. ethacrynic acid
    B. furosemide
    C. hydrochlorothiazide
    D. spironolactone

11. The nurse should teach a patient to avoid large amounts of potassium-containing foods or a potassium supplement if the patient is taking which one of the following drugs for control of blood pressure?

    A. an angiotensin-converting enzyme inhibitor
    B. a beta-adrenergic blocker
    C. a calcium channel blocker
    D. a centrally acting alpha-agonist

## ADJUVANT MINERALS

Other medications may be necessary in a variety of conditions to support the treatment and resolution of symptoms. Table 35.4 contains information about some of the agents discussed in this section.

## Magnesium

Oral magnesium oxide or hydroxide may be useful for mild hypomagnesemia. Parenteral magnesium sulfate may be necessary for moderate to severe hypomagnesemia, convulsions associated with pregnancy, and prevention of hypomagnesemia in total parenteral nutrition. Therapeutic effects in these conditions are attributed to the preparations' depressant effects on the CNS as well as on smooth, skeletal, and cardiac muscles. (Discussion of the use of magnesium products as antacids and cathartics appears in Chapters 37 and 39, respectively.)

Oral magnesium salts may cause diarrhea. Contraindications to magnesium include impaired renal function or being comatose.

Oral preparations of magnesium oxide or hydroxide act in 3 to 6 hours, are minimally absorbed systemically, and are excreted in the urine. With parenteral magnesium sulfate, IM injections act in 1 hour and last 3 to 4 hours; IV administration produces immediate action that lasts 30 minutes.

## Zinc

Zinc sulfate and zinc gluconate are available over the counter in various forms and strengths. Zinc is also an ingredient in several vitamin–mineral combination products. Zinc preparations are given orally as a dietary supplement to prevent or treat zinc deficiency. They have a slow onset of action and a delayed peak. They are metabolized in the liver and excreted in feces. Adverse effects of zinc sulfate are dizziness, restlessness, nausea, vomiting, gastric ulcers, and diarrhea. The FDA recommends that intranasal zinc products not be used because of reports of loss of ability to smell (anosmia) following their use. Zinc-induced anosmia is characterized by rapid onset and stinging and burning.

## Multiple Mineral–Electrolyte Preparations

Oral electrolyte solutions (e.g., Pedialyte) contain several electrolytes and a small amount of dextrose. They are used to supply maintenance amounts of fluids and electrolytes when oral intake is restricted. They are especially useful in children for treatment of diarrhea and may prevent severe fluid and electrolyte depletion. The amount given must be carefully calculated, prescribed, and administered to avoid excessive intake. Oral solutions should not be used in severe circumstances in which IV fluid and electrolyte therapy is indicated, and they should not be mixed with other electrolyte-containing fluids, such as milk or fruit juices. In addition, they must be cautiously used in impaired renal function. There are numerous electrolyte solutions for IV use to maintain or replace electrolytes when the patient is unable to eat and drink.

## TREATMENT OF MINERAL EXCESS
## Penicillamine

Penicillamine (Cuprimine) is a **chelating agent**, which binds copper, lead, mercury, and zinc to form soluble complexes that are excreted in the urine. Its main use is the removal of excess copper in patients with Wilson's disease, a rare condition characterized by accumulation of copper in vital organs. Prophylactic use involves giving the agent to patients in whom this hereditary condition is likely to develop, before clinical manifestations occur. Other uses for penicillamine include cystinuria, a hereditary metabolic disorder characterized by large amounts of cystine in the urine and renal calculi; lead poisoning; and severe rheumatoid arthritis that does not respond to conventional treatment measures.

## Succimer

Succimer (Chemet) chelates lead to form water-soluble complexes that are excreted in the urine. Indications include the treatment of lead poisoning in children. After oral administration, peak blood levels are reached in 1 to 2 hours. The drug is metabolized in the liver and excreted in urine and feces, with a half-life of 2 days. The most common adverse effects are anorexia, nausea, vomiting, and diarrhea.

## Deferoxamine and Deferasirox

Acute iron overdosage requires treatment with these drugs as soon as possible, even if overdosage is only suspected and the amount taken is unknown. It is unnecessary to wait until the serum iron level is measured.

Deferoxamine (Desferal) is a parenteral drug used to remove excess iron from storage sites (e.g., ferritin, hemosiderin) in the body. It combines with iron to produce a water-soluble compound that can be excreted by the kidneys. IM, IV, and subcutaneous routes may be useful in certain circumstances. The urine becomes reddish brown from the iron content. A common adverse effect is pain or induration at the injection site. The most serious adverse effect is anaphylaxis.

Deferasirox (Exjade) is an iron-chelating agent used to treat chronic iron overload in children and adults who require frequent blood transfusions for severe, chronic anemia. This drug is absorbed with oral administration, with peak plasma levels in 1.5 to 4 hours. It is highly bound to serum albumin, metabolized in the liver, and excreted in bile and feces (with the iron, which binds to the drug). Oral administration should be at the same time each day, before a meal. Patients should not chew or swallow the tablets but dissolve them in water, orange juice, or apple juice. The most common adverse effects are skin rash, fever, headache, and GI problems (e.g., abdominal pain, vomiting, diarrhea, and constipation). The FDA has issued a **BLACK BOX WARNING** ◆ for deferasirox regarding the risk of hepatic and/or renal impairment and GI hemorrhage, all of which can be fatal. It is important to monitor liver and kidney function closely.

## Agents Used in the Treatment of Hyperkalemia

The first step in the treatment of hyperkalemia is to eliminate any exogenous sources of potassium. It is essential to treat acidosis, if present, because potassium leaves cells and enters the serum, causing acidosis. Health care providers use measures that antagonize the effects of potassium, cause potassium to leave the serum and reenter the cells, and remove potassium from the body. Serum potassium levels and electrocardiographic (ECG) changes are the primary determinants of the treatment regimen.

### Sodium Bicarbonate

Sodium bicarbonate is an agent used to control the acidosis associated with hyperkalemia. A dose of 50 mEq intravenously administered over 5 minutes causes rapid movement of potassium into cells. It may be necessary to give another dose if ECG changes persist. Experts do not recommend administration of sodium bicarbonate as the only therapy for acute management of hyperkalemia (Mount, 2019).

### Calcium Gluconate

Calcium gluconate is a mineral supplement. A 1000-mg dose (10 mL of a 10% solution) infused over 2 to 3 minutes with constant cardiac monitoring is given to decrease the cardiotoxic effects of hyperkalemia. It may be necessary to repeat the dose after 5 minutes if ECG changes persist or recur. Contraindications to calcium include digoxin use because hypercalcemia potentiates the cardiotoxic effects of digoxin. In patients with hyperkalemia due to digoxin toxicity, administration of digoxin-specific antibody fragments is the preferred therapy (Mount, 2019).

 *Concept Mastery Alert*

Digoxin toxicity is more likely in the presence of hypokalemia, hypomagnesemia, hypercalcemia, and myocardial ischemia.

### Glucose and Insulin

Intravenous glucose and insulin are a treatment for hyperkalemia. Infusion causes potassium to move into cells. Glucose, given with insulin, prevents hypoglycemia. A commonly used regimen is regular insulin 10 to 20 units in 10% dextrose 500 mL infused over 1 hour. Another regimen consists of a bolus of regular insulin 10 units followed immediately by 50 mL of 50% dextrose. To avoid hypoglycemia, experts recommend administration of IV fluids of 10% dextrose at 50 to 75 mL/hour (Mount, 2019). When glucose and insulin are used to lower serum potassium, blood glucose levels should be monitored every hour for 5 to 6 hours.

### Cation Exchange: Sodium Polystyrene Sulfonate

With less severe hyperkalemia, sodium polystyrene sulfonate (Kayexalate), a cation exchange resin, administered orally, removes potassium from the body in the stool. The resin is usually mixed with water and several daily doses may be required until serum potassium is normal.

 **QSEN Alert: Patient-Centered Care**

Although sorbitol has been given with sodium polystyrene sulfonate orally and as an enema for its laxative effect, recent studies showed an association between the combination and intestinal necrosis. The FDA no longer recommends that sodium polystyrene sulfonate be administered in sorbitol.

## NUTRITIONAL PRODUCTS

Various products are available to supplement or substitute for dietary intake. These may consist of vitamins, minerals, liquid enteral formulas, IV fluids and nutrition, and pancreatic enzymes.

Numerous liquid enteral formulas are available for oral or tube feedings, and many are nutritionally complete, except for water, when given in sufficient amounts (e.g., Ensure, Isocal, Sustacal, Resource). To meet fluid needs, it is necessary to give additional water. Most oral products come in a variety of flavors and contain 1 kcal/mL of formula. Additional products are available formulated for patients with special conditions (e.g., hepatic or renal failure, malabsorption syndromes) or needs (e.g., high protein, increased calories).

When the GI tract is functional but the patient cannot ingest sufficient food and fluid, the nurse can give high-protein, high-calorie foods (e.g., milkshakes) or nutritionally complete supplements (e.g., Ensure) with meals, between meals, and at bedtime. In patients with a feeding tube, **enteral nutrition** provides fluid and nutrients. When the GI tract is nonfunctional, the nurse often gives IV fluids or **parenteral nutrition**. Most of these solutions are nutritionally incomplete and are used short term to supply fluids, electrolytes, and a few calories; additional nutrition may be necessary.

## Use

For short-term use (e.g., 3–5 days), the goal is to provide adequate amounts of fluids and electrolytes and enough carbohydrates to minimize oxidation of body protein and fat for energy. The choice of specific solution depends on individual needs, but it should contain at least 5% dextrose. A frequently used solution is 5% dextrose in 0.45% sodium chloride, 2000 to 3000 mL per 24 hours (provides ~170 kcal/L, water, sodium, and chloride). Vitamins may be added. These solutions are nutritionally inadequate.

For long-term use (weeks to months), the goal is to provide all nutrients required for normal body functioning, including tissue repair. Basic solutions provide water, carbohydrates, proteins, vitamins, and minerals. Patients usually receive fat emulsions (e.g., Intralipid) that are usually given separately to provide additional calories and essential fatty acids (500 mL of 10% emulsion provides 550 kcal).

### Use in Children

For children with special needs in relation to nutrients, various enteral formulations are available. Some examples include Lofenalac for children with phenylketonuria; Nursoy and Soyalac, which contain soy protein, for children who are allergic to cow's milk; and Nutramigen and Pregestimil, which contain easily digested nutrients for children with malabsorption or other GI problems. However, parenteral nutrition may be necessary.

### Use in Patients With Renal Impairment

With enteral nutrition, Amin-Aid provides amino acids, carbohydrates, and a few electrolytes for patients with renal failure. With parenteral nutrition, several amino acid solutions are available for patients with renal failure (e.g., Aminosyn-RF). Nepro is a formulation for patients receiving dialysis. Suplena, which is lower in protein and some electrolytes than Nepro, is formulated for patients who are not receiving dialysis.

### Use in Patients With Hepatic Impairment

For enteral feedings (usually by GI tube) in patients with liver failure, Hepatic-Aid II is available. For parenteral feeding in patients with hepatic failure and hepatic encephalopathy, HepatAmine, a special formula of amino acids, may be useful.

Caution is warranted with the use of enteral and parenteral fat preparations in patients with hepatic impairment. Medium-chain triglycerides (e.g., MCT oil), which are used to provide calories in other malnourished patients, may lead to coma in patients with advanced cirrhosis. Patients who require parenteral nutrition may develop high serum triglyceride levels and pancreatitis if given usually amounts of IV fat emulsions.

## Adverse Effects

Adverse reactions, which are usually attributed to the hypertonicity of the preparations, include tachycardia, hypotension, dehydration, nausea, vomiting, diarrhea, and increased urine output. The risk of aspiration of formula is a consideration with tube feeding.

## Nursing Implications
### Administering the Medication

For oral supplemental feedings, it is necessary to chill liquids or pour them over ice and give them through a straw (unless contraindicated), from a closed container, between meals. This practice may improve formula taste and decrease formula odor. A straw directs the formula toward the back of the throat and decreases contact with taste buds. A closed container also decreases odor.

For tube feedings, the nurse adheres to guidelines for safe administration (positioning, placement of the tube, residual and aseptic management of formula and equipment). When medications are ordered, liquid preparations are preferable. Tablets or powders may stick in the tube lumen, which may mean the full dose of medication does not reach the stomach. Also, the obstruction of the tube is likely. It is important not to mix medications with tube feeding formula; this could interfere with drug absorption.

### Assessing for Therapeutic Effects

For patients receiving nutritional formulas, the nurse observes for weight gain and increased serum albumin. For infants and children receiving milk substitutes, the nurse observes for decreased diarrhea and weight gain. Therapeutic effects depend on the reason for use (i.e., prevention or treatment of undernutrition).

### Assessing for Adverse Effects

With commercial nutritional formulas (except Osmolite and Isocal), the nurse observes for tachycardia, hypotension, dehydration, nausea, vomiting, diarrhea, and increased urine output. These adverse reactions are usually attributed to the hypertonicity of the preparations. Beginning administration with small amounts of formula, given slowly, may prevent or minimize adverse effects.

## Patient Teaching

Box 35.4 presents patient teaching guidelines for nutritional products.

### Clinical Application 35.5

- Mrs. Martin has a percutaneous endoscopic gastrostomy tube. She is to receive a bolus tube feeding of 300 mL at 08:00, 12:00, 17:00, and 21:00 hours, with a flush of free water every 4 hours. What precautions does the nurse take to prevent aspiration of the tube feeding?
- Mrs. Martin receives several medications through the feeding tube. Explain what the nurse does if one of those medications cannot be crushed for administration through the tube. Describe the steps he or she takes to administer medications through the tube.

### NCLEX Success

12. The nurse has finished administering medication through a percutaneous endoscopic gastrostomy tube. Which one of the following steps should the nurse take next?
    A. Check the tube for proper placement.
    B. Lower the head of the bed to a comfortable position.
    C. Turn the pump on to continue the tube feeding.
    D. Flush the tube with water and record the amount.

13. The patient is to receive a bolus tube feeding and a medication per tube at 08:00. When should the medication be administered?
    A. prior to the feeding at 07:30
    B. mixed with the feeding at 08:00
    C. immediately after the feeding
    D. hold the medication

### BOX 35.4 — Patient Teaching Guidelines for Nutritional Products

- For oral supplements, take or give at the preferred time and temperature, when possible.
- For tube feedings:
  - Use or give with the patient in a sitting position, if possible, to decrease risks of aspirating formula into the lungs.
  - Be sure the tube is placed correctly before each tube feeding. Ask a health care provider how to check placement with your type of tube.
  - Be sure the solution is stored at room temperature. Cold formula may cause abdominal cramping.
  - Do not take or give more than 500 mL per feeding, including 60 to 90 mL of water for flushing the tube. This helps to avoid overfilling the stomach and possible vomiting.
  - Take or give slowly, over approximately 30 to 60 minutes. Rapid administration may cause nausea and vomiting.
  - With continuous feedings, change containers and tubing daily. With intermittent feedings, rinse all equipment after each use, and change at least every 24 hours. Most tube feeding formulas are milk based, and infection may occur if formulas become contaminated or equipment is not kept clean.
  - Ask a health care provider about the amount of free water. Most people receiving 1500 to 2000 mL of tube feeding daily need approximately 1000 mL or more of free water daily. However, patients' needs vary. Water can be mixed with the tube feeding for-

mula, given after the tube feeding, or given between bolus feedings. Be sure to include the amount of water used for flushing the tube in the total daily intake.

- For giving medications by tube:
  - Give liquid preparations when available.
  - When liquid preparations are not available, it may be necessary to crush some tablets and empty some capsules and mix them with 15 to 30 mL of water. Ask a health care provider which medications can safely be crushed or altered, because some (e.g., long-acting or enteric-coated) can be harmful if crushed.
  - Do not mix medications with the tube feeding formula because some medications may not be absorbed. If the absorption of a drug is affected by the tube feeding formula (e.g., phenytoin), discontinue the tube feeding for the recommended interval prior to drug administration; then, resume feeding at the recommended interval after drug administration.
  - Do not mix medications. Give each one separately.
  - Flush the tube with water before and after each medication to get the medication through the tube and to keep the tube open.
  - For more a more complete discussion of the care of patients with feeding tubes, administration of drugs through feeding tubes, and patient teaching guidelines for home use of feeding tubes, consult a textbook of nursing fundamentals or medical/surgical nursing.

## THE NURSING PROCESS

A concept map outlines the nursing process related to drug therapy considerations in this chapter. Additional nursing implications related to the disease process should also be considered in care decisions.

**Assessment**

- Assess dietary intake, nutritional deficiencies, and alcohol intake.
- Assess vitamin intake for deficiencies or megadoses.
- Assess body mass index (BMI).
- Assess deficiencies in B complex vitamins and vitamin C because these are more common.
- Assess for illness, anorexia, nausea, vomiting, and diarrhea.
- Assess for drug interactions and the influence on gains or losses of vitamins, minerals, or electrolytes (e.g., proton pump inhibitors decrease vitamin $B_{12}$).
- Assess minerals and electrolytes lost with gastric suction, polyuria, diarrhea, or diaphoresis.
- Assess complete blood count and electrolytes: sodium, potassium, chloride, carbon dioxide, and bicarbonate.

**Outcomes of Therapy**

The patient will
- Demonstrate improvement in nutritional status in relation to body needs.
- Maintain fluid and electrolyte balance as measured by appropriate intake and output and serum electrolyte values.
- Demonstrate appropriate intake of vitamins, minerals, and electrolytes.

**Nursing Interventions**

- Promote a well-balanced diet for all patients. Five daily servings of fruits and vegetables provide adequate vitamins unless the patient has increased requirements or conditions that interfere with absorption or use of vitamins. A diet that is adequate in protein and calories usually provides adequate minerals and electrolytes. Exceptions are calcium and iron, which are often needed as a dietary supplement in women and children.
- Provide relief for symptoms that are likely to interfere with nutrition, such as pain, nausea, vomiting, or diarrhea.
- Provide palatable supplements at appropriate times for patients who need increased protein–calorie intake and encourage patients to take them.
- Promote exercise and activity. For undernourished patients, this may increase appetite, improve digestion, and aid bowel elimination.
- Minimize the use of sedative-type drugs when appropriate. Although no one should be denied pain relief, strong analgesics and other sedatives may cause drowsiness, decreased desire or ability to eat and drink, constipation, and a feeling of fullness.
- Monitor weight, fluid intake, urine output, vital signs, blood glucose, serum electrolytes, and complete blood count for patients receiving parenteral nutrition. Obtain these values daily, weekly, or as institutional protocols dictate. Adjust monitoring based on patient status whether hospitalized or at home.
- Promote proper use of mineral supplements, which are recommended only for current or potential deficiencies and are toxic in excessive amounts.
- Follow institutional protocols in the care of patients with feeding tubes and in the administration of ordered tube feeding products, and medication administration. Use best practices in relation to assessing correct tube placement, maintaining patency of tubes, positioning of patients, prevention of aspiration, gravity or pump administration of feeding products, and administration of free water and flushes. Avoid the administration of crushed medications to prevent occlusion.

**Evaluation**

- Observe undernourished patients for quantity and quality of nutrient intake, weight gain, and improvement in laboratory tests of nutritional status (e.g., serum electrolytes, glucose, and proteins).
- Observe children for quantity and quality of food intake and appropriate increases in height and weight.
- Interview and observe for signs and symptoms of complications of enteral and parenteral nutrition.
- When specific vitamins/minerals/electrolytes are being administered, therapeutically observe for improvement in deficiency or excess states as evidenced by improvement in symptoms and absence of adverse effects.

## Unfolding Patient Stories: Jermaine Jones • Part 1

Jermaine Jones, a 34-year-old diagnosed with depression, is assessed by the nurse during a routine clinic visit. The nurse determines that he has lost 8 lb and consumes a beer in place of the evening meal when his wife is working late. What nursing interventions can be implemented to promote good nutrition? What nutritional supplements would the nurse consider for a poor nutritional intake? (Jermaine Jones's story continues in Chap. 55.)

Care for Jermaine and other patients in a realistic virtual environment: *vSim for Nursing* (thepoint.lww.com/vSimPharm). Practice documenting these patients' care in DocuCare (thepoint.lww.com/DocuCareEHR).

## KEY CONCEPTS

- Human nutrition to maintain health requires sufficient water, carbohydrates, proteins, fats, vitamins, and minerals.
- Patients with other health problems often have nutritional deficiencies, such as protein–calorie undernutrition and vitamin deficiencies.
- All patients require assessment for nutritional status. When problems are assessed, interventions to maintain or improve nutritional status are needed.
- Fat-soluble vitamins are A, D, E, and K; water-soluble vitamins are B complex and C.
- The best source of nutrients is foods. However, it may be necessary to use oral, enteral (via GI tubes), or parenteral (IV) feedings to meet a patient's nutritional needs.
- Techniques for safe administration of oral, enteral, and parenteral feedings must be consistently followed because complications and harm to patients may occur with all methods.

- Adverse effects may occur with large doses of vitamin and mineral supplements; people should not take more than the maximum recommended amounts.
- Although most adults and children probably benefit from a daily multivitamin, large doses of single vitamins do not prevent cancer or cardiovascular disease and should be avoided.
- The FDA has issued a **BLACK BOX WARNING** ◆ for vitamin K indicating that IV administration, even with drug dilution and slow administration, may result in an anaphylactic type of reaction with risks of shock, cardiorespiratory arrest, and death.
- The FDA has issued a **BLACK BOX WARNING** ◆ for iron dextran with regard to the risk of anaphylactic reactions and death.
- The FDA has issued a **BLACK BOX WARNING** ◆ for deferasirox; there is a risk of hepatic and/or renal impairment and GI hemorrhage, all of which may be fatal.

## CLINICAL REASONING CASE STUDY

**Meet the Patient**

Solomon Najjuma, a 65-year-old man, has had surgery for gastric cancer, and he has undergone a total gastrectomy. (Intrinsic factor is secreted by the parietal cells of the gastric mucosa and is necessary for the absorption of vitamin $B_{12}$.) Postoperatively Mr. Najjuma lacks the gastric mucosa and cannot secrete intrinsic factor, placing him at risk for vitamin $B_{12}$ deficiency (pernicious anemia).

- What are the signs and symptoms of pernicious anemia?
- What other body system is affected by a deficiency in vitamin $B_{12}$?
- The prescriber orders hydroxocobalamin 30 mcg intramuscularly once daily for 5 days, then hydroxocobalamin 100 mcg intramuscularly once monthly. Why is hydroxocobalamin ordered intramuscularly and not orally?
- For what length of time will he receive monthly injections of hydroxocobalamin?
- What patient teaching will be provided to Mr. Najjuma?
- What adverse effects should Mr. Najjuma be aware of?
- What laboratory tests are ordered to determine whether hydroxocobalamin is effective?

**Assessing Drug Information**

- Assess for the signs and symptoms of pernicious anemia (caused by vitamin $B_{12}$ deficiency): megaloblastic anemia (presence in the blood of large abnormal blood cells), a decreased number of red blood cells, fatigue, and dyspnea. The nervous system is also affected by vitamin B12 deficiency; symptoms include paresthesias of the hands and feet and an unsteady gait.
- Mr. Najjuma lacks gastric mucosa, which secretes intrinsic factor necessary to absorption of oral vitamin $B_{12}$. If he received hydroxocobalamin orally, he would not absorb it; he must receive it intramuscularly. He needs monthly injections for life.
- Adverse effects of hydroxocobalamin are rare. Serum potassium is monitored during the first 48 hours to detect hypokalemia. Redness, itching, or pain may occur at the injection site.
- The therapeutic effect will be evaluated with serum hemoglobin, hematocrit, red blood cell count, and reticulocyte count. Initial therapeutic effects can appear within 48 hours.

**Nursing Actions**

- Educate Mr. Najjuma about the action of hydroxocobalamin.
- Educate Mr. Najjuma about the proper administration of hydroxocobalamin.
- Educate Mr. Najjuma about the adverse effects of hydroxocobalamin.
- Educate Mr. Najjuma regarding follow-up care with his hematologist.

*Visit* thePoint® *at* **http://thePoint.lww.com/Frandsen12e** *for answers to NCLEX Success questions (in Appendix A), answers to Clinical Application Case Studies (in Appendix B), and more!*

## REFERENCES AND RESOURCES

Dudek, S. G. (2018). *Nutrition essentials for nursing practice* (8th ed.). Philadelphia, PA: Lippincott Williams & Wilkins.

Hinkle, J. H., & Cheever, K. H. (2018). *Brunner & Suddarth's textbook of medical-surgical nursing* (14th ed.). Philadelphia, PA: Wolters Kluwer Health/Lippincott Williams & Wilkins.

Hull, R. D., & Garcia, D. A. (2019). Management of warfarin-associated bleeding or supratherapeutic INR. *UpToDate.*

Kuhn, S., Meissner, K., Mayes, L. M., & Bartels, K. (2018). Vitamin C in sepsis. *Current Opinions in Anaesthesiology, 31*(1), 55–60.

Marik, P. E. (2017). Vitamin C for the treatment of sepsis: The scientific rationale. *Pharmacology & Therapeutics, 189*, 63–70.

Marik, P. E., Khangoora, V., Rivera, R., Hooper, M. H., & Catravas, J. (2017). Hydrocortisone, vitamin C, and thiamine for the treatment of severe sepsis and septic shock: A retrospective before-after study. *Chest, 151*(6), 1229–1238.

Mount, D. B. (2019). Treatment and prevention of hyperkalemia in adults. *UpToDate.*

Norris, T. L. (2019). *Porth's pathophysiology: Concepts of altered health states* (10th ed.). Philadelphia, PA: Wolters Kluwer.

*Nursing 2019 drug handbook.* (2019). Philadelphia, PA: Wolters Kluwer.

Pazirandeh, S., & Burns, D. L. (2019). Overview of vitamin K. *UpToDate.* Retrieved July 6, 2019.

Pazirandeh, S., Burns, D. L., & Griffin, I. J. (2019). Overview of dietary trace minerals. *UpToDate.*

Sexton, D. J., & McClain, M. T. (2019). The common cold in adults: Treatment and prevention. *UpToDate.*

Taylor, C., Lynn, P., & Bartlett, J. L. (2019). *Fundamentals of nursing: The art and science of person-centered nursing care* (9th ed.). Philadelphia, PA: Wolters Kluwer.

UpToDate. (2019). *Drug information.* Lexi-Comp, Inc.

# Drug Therapy for Weight Management

## LEARNING OBJECTIVES

*After studying this chapter, you should be able to:*

1. Identify the various factors associated with obesity.
2. Describe the clinical manifestations of obesity.
3. Identify the prototype and describe the action, use, adverse effects, contraindications, and nursing implications for the anorexiants.
4. Identify the prototype and describe the action, use, adverse effects, contraindications, and nursing implications for the lipase inhibitors.
5. Identify the prototype and describe the action, use, adverse effects, contraindications, and nursing implications for the miscellaneous drugs used for weight management.
6. Implement the nursing process in the care of patients who are overweight or obese.

## CLINICAL APPLICATION CASE STUDY

Halli Vargas is a 31-year-old woman who has had a weight problem all her life. She has been on any number of diets that have a "yo-yo" effect, with weight loss followed by weight gain. She stands 5 feet 5 inches tall and weighs 265 lb. Her nurse practitioner starts her on orlistat and prescribes a consultation with a dietitian.

## KEY TERMS

**Body mass index (BMI):** reflection of weight in relation to height; better indicator than weight alone for determining the fitness level of a person

**Central obesity:** concentration of fat in abdominal area resulting in an increase in waist size

**Obesity:** BMI of 30 or more $kg/m^2$

**Overweight:** BMI of 25 to 29.9 $kg/m^2$

# INTRODUCTION

Obesity, which affects 34% of the adult population in the United States, has reached epidemic proportions. It is associated with multiple chronic diseases, and its negative impact on morbidity, mortality, health care costs, and professional and personal quality of life has been well documented. Excess amounts of any of the dietary nutrients are converted to fat and stored in the body, resulting in extra weight and obesity. Although therapeutic lifestyle changes are the cornerstone of population-based interventions to manage obesity, they are often insufficient in achieving recommended treatment targets. Pharmacologic therapy may be necessary. However, once the agents are discontinued, people may regain weight. The importance of a safe and effective use of drugs coupled with therapeutic lifestyle changes has become critical. This chapter discusses obesity and weight management, specifically focusing on drugs to aid weight loss and maintain desired weight.

# OVERVIEW OF WEIGHT MANAGEMENT

A better indicator of weight problems than weight alone, **body mass index (BMI)** reflects weight in relation to height. **Overweight** is defined as a BMI of 25 to 29.9 kg/m². **Obesity** is defined as a BMI of 30 or more kg/m². The desirable range for BMI is 18.5 to 24.9 kg/m², with any values below 18.5 indicating underweight and any values of 25 or greater indicating excessive weight (Box 36.1). A large waist circumference (greater than 35 inches for women, greater than 40 inches for men) is another risk factor for overweight and obesity. Using these definitions, it is projected that 68% of adults in America are overweight and 34% are obese.

## Etiology

Carbohydrates, proteins, and fats are required for human nutrition. Either deficiencies or excesses impair health, cause illness, and interfere with recovery from illness or injury. Carbohydrates and fats serve primarily as sources of energy for cellular metabolism, and proteins are basic structural and functional components of all body cells and tissues. Energy is measured in kilocalories (kcal, commonly called calories) per gram of food oxidized in the body. Carbohydrates and proteins supply 4 kcal/g. Fats supply 9 kcal/g. Excessive amounts of any nutrient are converted to fat and stored in the body, resulting in excess weight and obesity.

The incidence of overweight and obesity has dramatically increased during the past 25 years. Obesity may occur in anyone but is more likely to occur in women, ethnic groups, and people of lower socioeconomic status. In general, more women than men are obese, whereas more men than women are overweight. African American women and Mexican American men and women have the highest rates of overweight and obesity in the United States. Women in lower socioeconomic classes are more likely to be obese than those in higher socioeconomic classes.

The etiology of excessive weight is thought to involve complex and often overlapping interactions among physiologic, genetic, environmental, psychosocial, and other factors.

---

**BOX 36.1** — *Calculation of Body Mass Index (BMI) and Height and Weight Indicators for Overweight and Obese*

**BMI**

BMI calculators are available online (http://www.nhlbisupport.com/bmi/) but can be calculated as weight in kilograms divided by height in meters, squared; or as weight in pounds divided by height in inches, squared, multiplied by a conversion factor of 704.5 (listed as 703 in some sources), as follows:

$$BMI = \frac{Weight\ (pounds)}{Height\ (inches)^2} \times 704.5$$

For example: A person who weighs 150 lb and is 5 feet 5 inches (65 inches) tall

$$BMI = \frac{150\ lb}{65\ in. \times 65\ in.} \times 704.5 = \frac{150}{4225} \times 704.5 = \frac{105675}{422.5} = 25$$

**Weight Compared With Height as an Indicator for Being Overweight or Obese**

| Height (ft/in.) | Weight (Pound) Indicating Overweight (BMI 25) | Weight (Pound) Indicating Obesity (BMI 30) |
|---|---|---|
| 5′2″ (62 in.) | 135 | 165 |
| 5′3″ | 140 | 170 |
| 5′4″ | 145 | 175 |
| 5′5″ | 150 | 180 |
| 5′6″ | 155 | 185 |
| 5′7″ | 160 | 190 |
| 5′8″ | 165 | 195 |
| 5′9″ | 170 | 200 |
| 5′10″ | 175 | 205 |
| 5′11″ | 180 | 210 |
| 6′0″ | 185 | 220 |
| 6′1″ | 190 | 225 |
| 6′2″ (74 in.) | 195 | 230 |

### Physiologic Factors

In general, increased weight is related to an energy imbalance in which energy intake (food/calorie consumption) exceeds energy expenditure. Total energy expenditure represents the energy expended at rest (i.e., the basal or resting metabolic rate), during physical activity, and during food consumption. When a person ingests food, about 10% of the energy content of that food is expended in the digestion, absorption, and metabolism of nutrients. Foods that contain carbohydrates and proteins stimulate energy expenditure; high-fat foods have little stimulatory effect. The energy required to metabolize and to use food reaches a maximum level about 1 hour after the food is ingested.

In addition, men tend to expend more energy than do women because they have proportionally more muscle mass. Energy expenditure usually decreases in older men and women of all ages because these groups have less muscle tissue and more adipose tissue. Muscle is more metabolically active (i.e., has higher energy needs and burns more calories) than is adipose tissue.

Excessive weight can result from eating more calories, exercising less, or a combination of the two factors. Consuming an extra 500 calories each day for a week results in 3500 excess calories or 1 lb of fat. Excess calories are converted to triglycerides and stored in fat cells. With continued intake of excessive calories, fat cells increase in both size and number.

 **QSEN Alert: Evidence-Based Practice**

Since the early 1960s, the National Health and Nutrition Examination Survey (NHANES) has used interviews and physical examinations to assess the health and nutrition of the American people. To obtain a representative picture of the U.S. population, NHANES has explored sedentary behaviors in all age groups. Yang and colleagues (2019) analyzed NHANES data from 2001 to 2016 regarding 51,896 individuals (children 5–11 years of age, adolescents 12–19 years of age, and adults 20 years of age and older) related to their sedentary behaviors. This study indicated the following:

- The estimated prevalence of watching television or videos for at least 2 hours per day remained high and stable.
- The estimated prevalence leisure-time computer use increased over the period for individuals in all age groups.
- Total sitting time increased in adolescents and adults.

Findings from the NHANES studies have suggested that levels of physical inactivity predispose patients to health risks, including obesity and cardiovascular disease. Therapeutic lifestyle changes to reduce sedentary behaviors could increase life expectancy in individuals in all age groups.

## Genetic Factors

Various studies indicate that a portion of weight variation within a given environment is genetic in origin. For example, identical twins raised in separate environments often have similar body types. However, most cases of human obesity result mainly from the combination of genetic susceptibility and environmental conditions. Although some people may be genetically predisposed to obesity, it may be possible to counteract a genetic predisposition by making healthy changes in diet, lifestyle, and environment.

## Environmental Factors

Environmental factors contributing to the greater number of overweight and obese people include increased food consumption and decreased physical activity. The ready availability and relatively low cost of a wide variety of foods, in addition to large portion sizes and high-calorie foods, promote overeating. In addition, many social gatherings are associated with eating or overeating.

In relation to physical activity, usual activities of daily living for many people, including work-related activities, require relatively little energy expenditure. In addition, few Americans are thought to exercise in the optimal frequency, intensity, or duration to maintain health and prevent excessive weight gain. For both adults and children, increased time watching television, playing video or computer games, and working on computers contribute to less physical activity and are thought to promote weight gain and obesity. In general, however, it is still unknown whether less physical activity leads to obesity or the physical effects of obesity lead to minimal physical activity.

## Psychosocial Factors

Psychosocial disorders may be either a cause or an effect of obesity. Although much is still unknown about the psychological aspects of obesity development, depression and/or abuse may play a role. Obese people often report symptoms of depression, and some people overeat and gain weight during depressive episodes. It may be that obesity and depression commonly occur together and reinforce each other. A depressed person is less likely to take the active measures in diet and exercise that are required to lose weight, even if obesity is a prominent factor in the development of depression.

## Other Factors

Diseases are rarely a major cause of the development of obesity. However, numerous disease processes may limit a person's ability to engage in calorie-burning physical activity. In addition, numerous prescription medications reportedly cause weight gain in some or most of the patients who take them (Box 36.2).

## Age Considerations
### Overweight and Obese Children

There has been a threefold increase in childhood obesity rates in the past 30 years; being overweight and obese is reaching epidemic proportions. It is estimated that nearly 17% of children and adolescents in the United States are overweight. Overweight is defined as a BMI above the 85th percentile for age and obesity as a BMI above the 95th percentile.

Childhood obesity is a major public health concern because obese children have or are at risk for developing hypertension, dyslipidemias, type 2 diabetes mellitus, and other disorders that may lead to reduced quality of life, major disability, and death at younger adult ages than nonobese children. Obesity, type 2 diabetes, and other health problems are mainly attributed to poor eating habits and too little exercise. In addition, the child who is obese after 6 years of age is highly likely to be obese as an adult and develop obesity-related health problems, especially if a parent is obese. Obesity in adults that began in childhood tends to be more severe.

Under pressure from parents and advocates to prevent obesity in youth, many school districts have banned soft drinks, candy, and junk foods from school vending machines and cafeterias. The American Beverage Association has agreed to a voluntary ban on the sale of all high-calorie drinks and all beverages in containers larger than 8, 10, and 12 oz in elementary, middle, and high schools, respectively. Several additional recent initiatives to combat childhood obesity have been implemented.

In children, treatment of obesity should focus on healthy eating and increasing physical activity. In general, children should not be put on "diets." For a child who is overweight, the recommended goal is to maintain weight or slow the rate of weight gain so that weight and BMI gradually decline as the child's height increases. If the child has already reached his or

| BOX 36.2 | *Effects of Selected Medications on Weight* |
| --- | --- |

## Antidepressants

Selective serotonin reuptake inhibitors, such as fluoxetine (Prozac, Sarafem) and related drugs, may promote weight loss with short-term use. However, with long-term use, they reportedly may cause as much weight gain as tricyclic antidepressants (TCAs) such as amitriptyline. TCAs have long been associated with excessive appetite and weight gain. Mirtazapine (Remeron) and phenelzine (Nardil) are also associated with weight gain. The effects of bupropion (Wellbutrin and Zyban) on weight are unclear from clinical trials. Gain was reported when bupropion was used as a smoking deterrent, but both gain and loss occurred when it was used as an antidepressant. However, anorexia and weight loss occurred at a higher percentage rate than did increased appetite and weight gain.

## Antidiabetic Drugs

Although little attention is paid to the topic in most literature about diabetic drugs, weight gain apparently occurs with insulin, sulfonylureas, and the glitazones (but not with metformin, acarbose, or miglitol). Almost all patients with type 2 diabetes eventually require insulin; those who are failing on oral agents generally gain a large amount of body fat when switched to insulin therapy. Although the mechanism of weight gain is unknown, it may be related to the chronic hyperinsulinism induced by long-acting insulins and the sulfonylureas (which increase insulin secretion). Less weight is gained when oral drugs are given during the day and an intermediate- or long-acting insulin is injected at bedtime. This strategy is thought to cause less daytime hyperinsulinemia than the more traditional insulin strategies.

For near-normal-weight patients with diabetes who require drug therapy, a sulfonylurea may be given. However, for obese patients, metformin is usually the initial drug of choice because it does not promote weight gain. Metformin may also be used to treat obese diabetic children, aged 10 to 16 years, who require drug therapy.

## Antiepileptic Drugs

Weight gain commonly occurs with the use of antiepileptic drugs (AEDs). This has been observed for many years with older drugs (e.g., phenytoin, valproic acid, carbamazepine) and with newer AEDs (e.g., gabapentin, lamotrigine, tiagabine). Mechanisms by which the drugs promote weight gain are unclear but may involve stimulation of appetite and/or a slowed metabolic rate. Consequences of weight gain may include increased risks of diabetes mellitus, hypertension, and other physical health problems as well as psychological distress over appearance, especially in children and adolescents.

## Antihistamines

Histamine$_1$ (H$_1$) antagonists (e.g., diphenhydramine, loratadine) reportedly increase appetite and cause weight gain.

## Antihypertensive Agents

The main antihypertensive drugs reported to cause weight gain are the beta-adrenergic blockers. The drugs can cause fatigue and decrease exercise tolerance and metabolic rate, all of which may contribute to weight gain. Other mechanisms may also be involved. As a result, some clinicians question the use of beta-adrenergic blockers in overweight or obese patients with uncomplicated hypertension. Alpha-blockers may also cause weight gain, but apparently at a low incidence. Angiotensin-converting enzyme (ACE) inhibitors and calcium channel blockers are not reported to promote weight gain.

## Antipsychotic Agents

Weight gain is often reported and extensively documented with antipsychotic drugs. Although the exact mechanism is unknown, weight gain has been associated with antihistaminic effects, anticholinergic effects, and blockade of serotonin receptors. In addition, dietary factors and activity levels may also play significant roles.

Clozapine and olanzapine reportedly cause significant weight gain in 40% or more of patients. Compared with clozapine and olanzapine, risperidone causes less weight gain, and quetiapine and ziprasidone cause the least weight gain. Weight gain may lead to noncompliance with drug therapy. In addition to weight gain, clozapine and olanzapine adversely affect glucose regulation and can aggravate preexisting diabetes or cause new-onset diabetes. The extent to which these effects are related to weight gain is unknown. For patients who are obese, diabetic, or at risk of developing diabetes, an antipsychotic drug that causes less weight gain would seem the better choice.

## Cholesterol-Lowering Agents

Weight gain has been reported with the statin group of drugs; mechanisms and extent are unknown.

## Corticosteroids

Systemic corticosteroids may cause increased appetite, weight gain, central obesity, and retention of sodium and fluid. Inhaled and intranasal corticosteroids have little effect on weight.

## Gastrointestinal Drugs

Increased appetite and weight gain have been reported with the proton pump inhibitors such as omeprazole and others. The mechanisms and extent are unknown.

## Hormonal Contraceptives

The weight gain associated with using hormonal contraceptives may be related more to retention of fluid and sodium than to increased body fat.

## Mood-Stabilizing Agent

Weight gain has been reported with long-term use of lithium, with approximately 20% of patients gaining 10 kg (22 lb) or more. This increased weight is attributed to fluid retention, consumption of high-calorie beverages as a result of increased thirst, or a decreased metabolic rate. Weight gain is a common reason for noncompliance with lithium therapy, and weight gain may be more common in women with lithium-induced hypothyroidism and in those who are already overweight.

her anticipated adult weight, maintenance of that weight and prevention of additional gain should be the long-term treatment goal. If the child already exceeds his or her optimal adult weight, the goal of treatment should be a slow weight loss of 10 to 12 lb per year until this weight is reached. As with adults, increased activity is necessary for successful weight loss or management in children. It is possible to implement these measures successfully mainly within a family unit, and family support to assist the child in weight control and a more healthful lifestyle is necessary. In addition, schools should teach children the basic principles of good nutrition and why eating a balanced diet is important to health.

## Overweight and Obese Older Adults

Although obesity is reported in older adults, the numbers are still significantly lower than the levels seen in the young adult population. It is speculated that socioeconomic factors may play a role in this age group when it comes to developing obesity.

Obesity does not appear to make a substantial difference to risks of death among older adults but is a major contributor to increased disability and reduced quality of life in later years. The development of type 2 diabetes mellitus remains a risk. Excess weight reduces the loss of bone mass, and overweight elderly people are less likely to suffer hip fractures, a major cause of morbidity and mortality; health risks of obesity are greater than any advantages.

# Pathophysiology

Obesity results from consistent ingestion of more calories than are used for energy, and it substantially increases risks of developing numerous health problems (Box 36.3). Most obesity-related disorders are attributed mainly to the multiple metabolic abnormalities associated with obesity. Abdominal fat out of proportion to total body fat (also called visceral or **central obesity**), which often occurs in men and postmenopausal women,

---

| BOX 36.3 | *Health Risks of Obesity* |
| --- | --- |

Obesity is associated with serious health risks. Several disease states and chronic health problems are more prevalent in obese patients, as well as increased mortality. Studies indicate that a high body mass index (BMI) is associated with an increased risk of death from all causes, among both men and women, and in all age groups. In addition, a higher death rate occurs in people who gain weight of 10 kg or more after 18 years of age. Some of the major health risks include the disorders listed below. In general, these conditions tend to worsen as the degree of obesity increases and improve with weight loss.

### Cancer

Obesity is associated with a higher prevalence of breast, colon, and endometrial cancers. With breast cancer, risks increase in postmenopausal women with increasing body weight. Women who gain more than 20 lb from age 18 to midlife have double the risk of breast cancer compared with women who maintain a stable weight during this period of their life. In addition, central obesity apparently increases the risk of breast cancer independent of overall obesity. In women with central obesity, this additional risk factor may be related to an excess of estrogen (from conversion of androstenedione to estradiol in peripheral fatty tissue) and a deficiency of sex hormone–binding globulin to combine with the estrogen.

Colon cancer seems to be more common in obese men and women. In addition, a high BMI may be a risk factor for a higher mortality rate with colon cancer. Endometrial cancer is clearly more common in obese women, with adult weight gain again increasing risk.

### Cardiovascular Disorders

Obesity is a major risk factor for cardiovascular disorders and increased mortality from cardiovascular disease. Studies have confirmed the relationship between obesity and increased risk of coronary heart disease (CHD) and stroke in both men and women. In addition, obesity during adolescence is associated with higher rates and greater severity of cardiovascular disease as adults.

Obesity increases risks by aggravating other risk factors such as hypertension, insulin resistance, low high-density lipoprotein [HDL] cholesterol, and hypertriglyceridemia. In addition, obesity seems to be an independent risk factor for cardiovascular disorders, and central obesity may be more important than BMI as a risk factor for death from cardiovascular disease. The increased mortality rate is seen even with modest excess body weight.

Hypertension, dyslipidemia, insulin resistance, and glucose intolerance are known cardiac risk factors that tend to cluster in obese people. Hypertension often occurs in obese people and is thought to play a major role in the increased incidence of cardiovascular disease and stroke observed in patients with obesity. Metabolic abnormalities that occur with obesity and type 2 diabetes mellitus (e.g., insulin resistance and the resultant hyperinsulinemia) aggravate hypertension and increase cardiovascular risks. The combination of obesity and hypertension is associated with cardiac changes (e.g., thickening of the ventricular wall, ischemia, and increased heart volume) that lead to heart failure more rapidly. Weight loss of as little as 4.5 kg (10 lb) can decrease blood pressure and cardiovascular risk in many people with obesity and hypertension.

### Diabetes Mellitus

Obesity is strongly associated with impaired glucose tolerance, insulin resistance, and diabetes mellitus. In addition, obesity during adolescence is associated with higher rates of diabetes as adults as well as more severe complications of diabetes at younger ages.

The cellular effects by which obesity causes insulin resistance are unknown. Proposed mechanisms include down-regulation of insulin receptors, abnormal postreceptor signals, and others. Whatever the mechanism, the impaired insulin response stimulates the pancreatic beta cells to increase insulin secretion, resulting in a relative excess of insulin called hyperinsulinemia, and causes impaired lipid metabolism (increased low-density lipoprotein [LDL] cholesterol and triglycerides and decreased HDL cholesterol). These metabolic changes increase hypertension and other

| **BOX 36.3** | *Health Risks of Obesity* [Continued] |

risk factors for cardiovascular disease. As with cardiovascular disease and diabetes in general, central obesity seems to increase the likelihood of serious disease. The abdominal fat of central obesity seems to be more insulin resistant than peripheral fat deposited over the buttocks and legs. Intentional weight loss significantly reduces mortality in obese people with diabetes.

### Dyslipidemias

Obesity strongly contributes to abnormal and undesirable changes in lipid metabolism (e.g., increased triglycerides and LDL cholesterol; decreased HDL cholesterol) that increase risks of cardiovascular disease and other health problems.

### Gallstones

Obesity apparently increases the risk of developing gallstones by altering production and metabolism of cholesterol and bile. The risk is higher in women, especially those who have had multiple pregnancies or who are taking oral contraceptives. However, rapid weight loss with very-low-calorie diets is also associated with gallstones.

### Metabolic Syndrome

Metabolic syndrome is a group of risk factors and chronic conditions that occur together and greatly increase the risks of diabetes mellitus, serious cardiovascular disease, and death. The syndrome is thought to be highly prevalent in the United States. Major characteristics include many of the health problems associated with obesity (e.g., dyslipidemias, hypertension, impaired glucose tolerance, insulin resistance, central obesity). More specifically, metabolic syndrome includes three or more of the following abnormalities:

- Central obesity (waist circumference over 40 inches for men and over 35 inches for women)
- Serum triglycerides of 150 mg/dL or more or taking medication for high triglycerides
- HDL cholesterol below 40 mg/dL in men and below 50 mg/dL in women or taking medication for low HDL cholesterol
- Blood pressure of 135/85 mm Hg or higher or taking medication for hypertension
- Serum glucose of 110 mg/dL or higher or taking medication for hyperglycemia

### Osteoarthritis

Obesity is associated with osteoarthritis (OA) of both weight-bearing joints, such as the hip and knee, and

non–weight-bearing joints. Extra weight can stress affected bones and joints, contract muscles that normally stabilize joints, and may alter the metabolism of cartilage, collagen, and bone. In general, obese people develop OA of the knees at an earlier age and are more likely than nonobese people to require knee replacement surgery.

The important role of obesity in OA is supported by the observation that weight loss delays onset and reduces symptoms and disability. Weight reduction may also decrease infection, wound complications, and blood loss if surgery is required. Despite the benefits of weight loss, however, persons with OA have difficulty losing weight because painful joints limit exercise and activity.

### Sleep Apnea

Sleep apnea commonly occurs in obese persons. A possible explanation is enlargement of soft tissue in the upper airways that leads to collapse of the upper airways with inspiration during sleep. The obstructed breathing leads to apnea with hypoxemia, hypercarbia, and a stress response. Sleep apnea is associated with increased risks of hypertension, possible right heart failure, and sudden death. Weight loss leads to improvement in sleep apnea.

### Miscellaneous Effects

Obesity is associated with numerous difficulties in addition to those described above. These may include the following:
- Nonalcoholic fatty liver disease, which is being increasingly recognized and which may lead to liver failure.
- Poor wound healing.
- Poor antibody response to hepatitis B vaccine.
- A negative perception of people who are obese that affects their education, socioeconomic, and employment status.
- High costs associated with treatment of the medical conditions caused or aggravated by obesity as well as the costs associated with weight loss efforts.
- In women, obesity is associated with menstrual irregularities, difficulty in becoming pregnant, and increased complications of pregnancy (e.g., gestational diabetes, higher rates of labor induction and cesarean section, and increased risk of neural tube and other congenital defects in offspring of obese women).
- In men, obesity is associated with infertility.
- In children and adolescents, obesity increases risk of bone fractures and muscle and joint pain. Knee pain is commonly reported, and changes in the knee joint make movement and exercise more difficult.

is considered a greater risk factor for disease and death than lower body obesity. In addition to the many health problems associated with obesity, obesity is increasingly being considered a chronic disease in its own right. Although it has been the focus of much research in recent years, no current theory adequately explains the disorder and its resistance to treatment.

## Clinical Manifestations

Common clinical manifestations that characterize overweight and obesity are increased body weight, excess body fat, and a BMI score of 25 kg/m² or greater. Other physical findings include

abnormal levels of lipids and lipoproteins, elevated serum levels of insulin, elevated blood pressure, and respiratory difficulties. These metabolic abnormalities place overweight and obese people at a significantly higher risk for hypertension, heart disease, diabetes, joint problems, and sleep apnea.

## Drug Therapy

The National Heart, Lung, and Blood Institute (NHLBI) of the National Institutes of Health and most other organizations generally recommend reserving drug therapy for people with a BMI of 30 or more kg/m² and health problems (e.g., hypertension,

*National Heart, Lung, and Blood Institute (NHLBI) Report: Clinical Guidelines on the Identification, Evaluation, and Treatment of Overweight and Obesity in Adults*

- Weight loss reduces health problems. People should decrease blood pressure if they are hypertensive; lower elevated levels of total cholesterol, low-density lipoprotein cholesterol, and triglycerides and raise low levels of high-density lipoprotein cholesterol if they are dyslipidemic; lower elevated blood glucose levels if they have type 2 diabetes.
- Body mass index is used to assess overweight and obesity and to estimate disease risks. Measure waist circumference initially and periodically to assess abdominal fat content. Weigh regularly to monitor body weight.
- The initial goal of weight loss therapy should be to reduce body weight by about 10% from baseline, at a rate of 1 to 2 lb per week for a period of 6 months. Steady weight loss over a longer period reduces fat stores in the body, limits the loss of vital protein tissues, and avoids the sharp decline in metabolic rate that accompanies rapid weight loss. After weight loss, weight maintenance should be the priority goal, because weight regain is a problem with all weight loss programs. In some cases, after a period of weight maintenance, additional losses may be desirable.
- Dietary recommendations include low-calorie diets for weight loss, mainly reducing caloric intake by 500 to 1000 calories daily. Reducing dietary fat can reduce calories. However, reducing dietary fat without reducing total caloric intake does not produce weight loss. Vitamin and mineral supplements that meet age-related requirements are usually recommended with weight loss programs that provide less than 1200 kcal for women or 1800 kcal for men.
- Physical activity recommendations should be part of any weight management program because physical activity contributes to weight loss, may decrease abdominal fat, increases cardiorespiratory fitness, and helps with weight maintenance. Initially, physical activity for 30 to 45 minutes, 3 to 5 days a week, is encouraged. On long term, adults should try to accumulate at least 30 minutes or more of moderate-intensity physical activity on most days of the week.

- In general, weight loss and weight maintenance programs should combine reduced-calorie diets, increased physical activity, and behavior therapy. After weight loss, weight loss maintenance with dietary therapy, physical activity, and behavior therapy should be continued indefinitely. Drug therapy can also be used. However, drug safety and efficacy beyond 1 to 2 years of total treatment have not been established.
- Behavioral modification can be helpful in a weight loss program. The goals are to help patients modify their eating, activity, and thinking habits that predispose to obesity. Techniques include identifying triggers that promote overeating and barriers that keep one from adopting a more healthful lifestyle. One strategy is keeping an accurate record of food/calorie intake and physical activity (most people tend to underestimate food intake and overestimate activity). In addition, stress management, stimulus control, and social support are helpful. Patients who eat more when stressed can learn to manage stress more healthfully. Counseling by a behavioral therapist may be needed. Stimulus control has to do with avoiding or minimizing circumstances that promote overeating (e.g., cooking calorie-dense foods; having high-calorie snacks and "junk food" readily available; eating high-fat, high-calorie foods at fast-food restaurants). Social support involves family, friends, coworkers, and fellow dieters who encourage weight loss efforts rather than sabotage them by urging one to eat high-calorie foods. In general, weight loss regimens that use several of these strategies are more effective.

Reprinted from NHLBI Obesity Education Initiative Expert Panel on the Identification, Evaluation, and Treatment of Obesity in Adults (US). (1998). *Clinical guidelines on the identification, evaluation, and treatment of overweight and obesity in adults: The evidence report.* Bethesda, MD: National Heart, Lung, and Blood Institute.

dyslipidemia, coronary heart disease [CHD], type 2 diabetes, sleep apnea) that are likely to improve with weight loss. A loss of 5% to 10% of body weight generally produces a decrease in blood pressure and improved serum lipid concentrations, increased insulin sensitivity, and reduced hyperglycemia, and it may also reduce any related mortality. Drug therapy for obesity should be part of a weight management program that also includes a sensible diet, physical activity, and behavioral modification, and it should be considered only after targeted lifestyle changes fail to achieve therapeutic target weight. A drug may produce adverse effects that can decrease overall benefit. The NHLBI clinical guidelines focus on the identification, evaluation, and treatment of obesity. These guidelines, outlined in Box 36.4, emphasize that drug therapy should be used to decrease medical risk and improve health rather than promote cosmetic weight loss.

Drug therapy for obesity has a problematic history, mainly because of a series of previous safety-related failures, serious adverse effects, and rapid weight regain when the drugs were stopped. The U.S. Food and Drug Administration (FDA) took some drugs (fenfluramine, dexfenfluramine, phenylpropanolamine, and sibutramine) and some components of many over-the-counter and herbal weight loss products (ephedra and ma huang) off the market because of their adverse effects. Currently, several drugs in various classes have received approval for short- and long-term use in weight management and treatment of obesity, including the noradrenergic sympathomimetic anorexiants (appetite suppressants), lipase inhibitors, and miscellaneous agents (e.g., serotinin-2C receptor agonists, glucagon-like peptide-1 [GLP-1] agonists, and bupropion–naltrexone). See Table 36.1 for a list of these agents.

# NORADRENERGIC SYMPATHOMIMETIC ANOREXIANTS

These adrenergic drugs (see Chap. 29) stimulate the release of norepinephrine and dopamine in the brain; this action in nerve terminals of the hypothalamic feeding center suppresses appetite. FDA approved for short-term use for weight loss, these agents include benzphetamine (Schedule III), diethylpropion (Schedule IV), phendimetrazine (Schedule III), and phentermine (Schedule IV). **P** **Phentermine**, the most frequently prescribed noradrenergic sympathomimetic anorexiant, is the prototype.

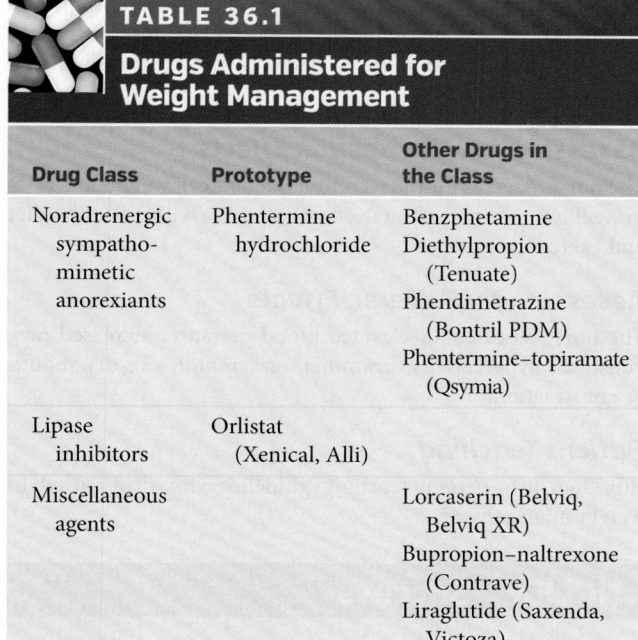

## TABLE 36.1

## Drugs Administered for Weight Management

| Drug Class | Prototype | Other Drugs in the Class |
|---|---|---|
| Noradrenergic sympatho-mimetic anorexiants | Phentermine hydrochloride | Benzphetamine Diethylpropion (Tenuate) Phendimetrazine (Bontril PDM) Phentermine–topiramate (Qsymia) |
| Lipase inhibitors | Orlistat (Xenical, Alli) | |
| Miscellaneous agents | | Lorcaserin (Belviq, Belviq XR) Bupropion–naltrexone (Contrave) Liraglutide (Saxenda, Victoza) |

## Pharmacokinetics

Phentermine is well absorbed orally, metabolized by the liver, and primarily excreted by the kidneys. Time to peak activity is 3 to 4.4 hours, and the half-life elimination is about 20 hours. Under acidic urinary conditions, the half-life is decreased.

## Action

Experts believe that phentermine inhibits the reuptake of both serotonin and norepinephrine. The drug causes appetite suppression, which is thought to result from direct stimulation of the satiety center in the hypothalamic and limbic region. As a sympathomimetic amine, the drug has pharmacologic activity similar to the amphetamines.

## Use

Phentermine is used to speed weight loss in people who are overweight. The drug is recommended only for short-term use (3 months or less). Combination with a healthy diet and exercise is important. Table 36.2 presents route and dosage information for phentermine and other noradrenergic sympathomimetic anorexiants.

Limited information is available about the use of phentermine in people with hepatic impairment.

### Use in Children

Phentermine may be useful in adolescents older than 16 years of age who are overweight or obese and may have complications of obesity. Phentermine should not be used in adolescents under 16 years of age; further research into the effectiveness and safety of antiobesity drugs in adolescents is needed.

### Use in Older Adults

It is important to use anorexiant drugs, including phentermine, very cautiously if at all in older adults. Older adults often have cardiovascular, renal, or hepatic impairments that increase the risk and seriousness of adverse drug effects.

### Use in Patients With Renal Impairment

Clearance of phentermine may be decreased in patients with renal impairment, resulting in an increased risk of toxicity.

## Adverse Effects

The most commonly reported adverse effects with phentermine are nervousness, palpitations, tachycardia, primary pulmonary

## TABLE 36.2

## DRUGS AT A GLANCE: Noradrenergic Sympathomimetic Anorexiants (in Adults Unless Specified)

| Drug | Pregnancy Category | Route and Dosage Ranges |
|---|---|---|
| Ⓟ **Phentermine hydrochloride** (Adipex-P) | X | Immediate release: 15–37.5 mg daily or divided twice daily Orally disintegrating tablet: 15–37.5 mg once daily in the morning Adolescents ≥16 y, same as adult dosage |
| Benzphetamine | X | Initial: 25 mg once daily; may titrate up to 25–50 mg 1–3 times daily. Maximum dose: 50 mg three times daily |
| Diethylpropion (Tenuate) | X | Immediate release: 25 mg three times daily before meals Controlled release: 75 mg every morning. |
| Phendimetrazine (Bontril PDM) | X | Immediate release: 17.5–35 mg 2 or 3 times daily, 1 h before meals. Maximum dose: 70 mg three times daily Sustained release: 105 mg daily in the morning |
| Phentermine–topiramate (Qsymia) | X | Initial: 3.75 mg phentermine/23 mg topiramate once daily in the morning for 14 d; then titrate; based on response: 7.5 mg phentermine/46 mg, topiramate daily for 12 wk, then 11.25 mg phentermine/69 mg topiramate daily for 14 d. Maximum dose: 15 mg phentermine/92 mg topiramate daily; reevaluate after 12 wk |

hypertension, hyperactivity, dry mouth, constipation, and systemic hypertension. Impotence, insomnia, and unpleasant taste may also occur. Tolerance to the drug may occur in as little as 4 to 6 weeks and is an indication for discontinuing the drug. Continued administration or use of large doses does not maintain appetite-suppressant effects. Instead, it increases the incidence of adverse effects.

 **QSEN Alert: Safety**

The nurse should emphasize to patients that phentermine may be habit forming and should be used only as prescribed. There may be an increased risk of drowsiness, so people who take phentermine should not drive a car or operate heavy machinery until they know how the drug affects them.

## Contraindications

Contraindications to phentermine use include moderate to severe hypertension, cardiovascular disease, hyperthyroidism, glaucoma, pregnancy, or breast-feeding and a history of drug abuse. Caution is warranted in anxiety or agitation because the drug may have central nervous system (CNS) stimulating effects. The drug is contraindicated within 14 days of treatment with a monoamine oxidase inhibitor.

## Nursing Implications

### Preventing Interactions

Several drugs interact with phentermine, increasing or decreasing its effect (Box 36.5). It is important to note that people with diabetes mellitus may require increased doses of insulin while taking phentermine because the drug produces effects similar to those caused by stimulating the sympathetic nervous system.

No herbal interactions have been identified.

### Administering the Medication

It is necessary to give sustained-release capsules before breakfast or at least 10 to 14 hours before bedtime and instruct patients to swallow the capsule whole and not chew, crush, or open them.

**BOX 36.5** **Drug Interactions: Phentermine**

**Drugs That Increase the Effects of Phentermine**
- Other tricyclic antidepressants, linezolid
  *Increase hypertensive effects*
- Other central nervous system stimulants, including alcohol
  *Have additive stimulant effects*
- Other sympathomimetic drugs (e.g., epinephrine)
  *Have additive hypertensive and other cardiovascular effects*

**Drugs That Decrease the Effects of Phentermine**
- Gastrointestinal acidifying agents, methenamine, multivitamins with minerals, urinary acidifying agents
  *May decrease serum concentration of phentermines*

Recipients should take immediate release multiple-dose preparations 30 minutes before meals, with the last dose of the day about 6 hours before going to bed to avoid the possibility of insomnia.

### Assessing for Therapeutic Effects

The nurse assesses for the recommended rate of weight loss (1–2 lb weekly), minimal adverse effects, and use with a healthy diet and exercise routine.

### Assessing for Adverse Effects

The nurse assesses for elevated blood pressure, increased nervousness, hyperactivity, insomnia, or symptoms of dry mouth or constipation.

### Patient Teaching

Box 36.6 lists patient teaching guidelines for drugs used in weight management.

**NCLEX Success**

1. Phentermine aids weight loss by doing which of the following?
   A. decreasing appetite
   B. increasing satiety and feelings of fullness
   C. increasing metabolism
   D. decreasing absorption of dietary fat

2. Mr. Johnson, a 42-year-old architect, is more than 40 lb overweight, and he has a 14-year history of type 1 diabetes mellitus. He is placed on phentermine and has been taking it for the last 8 weeks. His latest serum glycosylated ($A_{1c}$) hemoglobin levels have risen to 9% despite the fact that he has maintained a healthy diet and routine exercise program. Phentermine may cause an elevation of $A_{1c}$ levels by doing which of the following?
   A. producing stimulant effects to the sympathetic nervous system
   B. decreasing the level of fat-soluble vitamins
   C. decreasing metabolism to the pancreas
   D. increasing the absorption of dietary fat

## Other Drugs in the Class

The FDA has approved a phentermine–topiramate combination (Qsymia), a Schedule IV drug because of the phentermine, for long-term use in weight management. (Topiramate is an antiepileptic drug.) Both drugs affect appetite suppression and satiety enhancement through a combination of mechanisms. In clinical trials, researchers showed that phentermine–topiramate enhanced weight loss in the first year of use compared to a placebo. It is necessary to use this combination drug with caution in patients with CHD or hypertension or in pregnant women. Only certified retail or online pharmacies may fill prescriptions for this combination.

Other approved noradrenergic sympathomimetic drugs are benzphetamine, diethylpropion, and phendimetrazine. Their

**BOX 36.6** *Patient Teaching Guidelines for Weight Management and Drugs That Aid Weight Loss*

**General Considerations**

- Because of the extensive health problems associated with overweight and obesity, if your weight is within a normal range, you should try to prevent excessive weight gain by practicing a healthful lifestyle in terms of diet and exercise. You should try to:
  - Manage your weight by balancing calorie intake with physical activity
  - Increase your intake of fruits, vegetables, low-fat and fat-free dairy products, whole grains, and seafood
  - Limit your intake of sodium, saturated and trans fats, cholesterol, refined grains, and foods with added sugars
  - Spread your intake of daily fat, carbohydrate, and protein over three meals
- Further recommendations from the Dietary Guidelines for Americans 2015, published by the U.S. Department of Health and Human Services and the Department of Agriculture in December 2015 (updated every 5 years), are available online at http://www.healthierus.gov/dietaryguidelines.

**Self-Administration**

- Avoid caffeine.
- Take appetite suppressants in the morning to decrease appetite during the day and avoid interference with sleep at night.
- Do not crush or chew sustained-release products.
- With phentermine, monitor your blood pressure. As body weight decreases, blood pressure usually decreases.
- With orlistat (Xenical, Alli):
  - Take one capsule with each main meal or up to 1 hour after a meal, up to three capsules daily. If you miss a meal or eat a meal with no fat, you may omit a dose of orlistat.
  - Take a multivitamin containing fat-soluble vitamins (A, D, E, and K) daily, at least 2 hours before or after taking orlistat. Orlistat prevents absorption of fat-soluble vitamins from food or multivitamin preparations if taken at the same time.
  - Take the drug with a full glass of water.

mechanisms of action in reducing appetite appear to be secondary to CNS effects, including stimulation of the hypothalamus to release norepinephrine. Diethylpropion is also structurally similar to bupropion. Adverse effects include increases in heart rate, blood pressure, dry mouth, constipation, nervousness, and insomnia. The drugs may counteract the effects of blood pressure medications, so those with hypertension should be observed carefully. As with phentermine, these drugs are useful on a short-term adjunct in obese individuals when diet and exercise have not produced desired results.

## LIPASE INHIBITORS

Ⓟ **Orlistat** (Xenical, Alli), the only FDA-approved weight loss drug available without a prescription, is the prototype lipase inhibitor. A reversible inhibitor of gastric and pancreatic lipases, it slows absorption of dietary fats. Decreased fat absorption leads to decreased caloric intake, resulting in weight loss and improved serum cholesterol values (e.g., decreased total and low-density lipoprotein [LDL] cholesterol levels). The improvement in cholesterol levels is thought to be independent of weight loss effects.

## Pharmacokinetics

Orlistat is not absorbed systemically; it works in the gastrointestinal (GI) tract. Its half-life is 1 to 2 hours. Nearly the entire medication is excreted in feces, 83% as unchanged drug.

## Action

Orlistat binds to gastric and pancreatic lipases in the GI tract, and it can prevent the absorption of 30% of ingested fat. Triglycerides, cholesterol, and fat-soluble vitamins from fat-containing foods pass through the intestines unchanged and

are not absorbed. Increasing the dose does not increase the percentage.

## Use

Orlistat is intended for people who are clinically obese, not for those who want to lose a few pounds. It is still necessary to decrease consumption of high-fat foods because total caloric intake is a major determinant of weight, and adverse effects (e.g., diarrhea; fatty, malodorous stools) worsen with consumption of a large amount of fat.

The effects of long-term orlistat use are unknown. In addition to weight loss and reduced cholesterol levels, clinical trials found that orlistat results in reduced severity and improved management of other health problems associated with obesity, such as diabetes and hypertension. In general, studies have shown that the addition of orlistat therapy to diet and other lifestyle changes produces greater weight loss than addition of a placebo. In some patients with impaired glucose tolerance, weight loss with orlistat and lifestyle changes prevents or delays the occurrence of diabetes mellitus. After the medication is stopped, most patients regain weight.

Table 36.3 presents route and dosage information for orlistat.

### Use in Children

As previously discussed, encouraging weight control measures coupled with family involvement and support are vital to weight management in children. Methods that result in weight loss include leading a more active lifestyle, eating a low-fat diet with regular meals, avoiding high-calorie snacks, drinking water instead of calorie-containing beverages, and decreasing time spent watching television and playing computer games. Although experts do not generally recommend drug therapy for treatment of childhood obesity, the FDA has approved orlistat

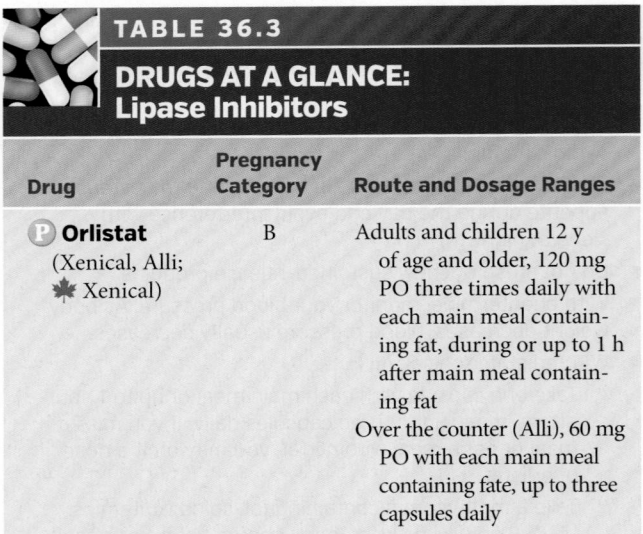

## TABLE 36.3

### DRUGS AT A GLANCE: Lipase Inhibitors

| Drug | Pregnancy Category | Route and Dosage Ranges |
|---|---|---|
| Orlistat (Xenical, Alli; Xenical) | B | Adults and children 12 y of age and older, 120 mg PO three times daily with each main meal containing fat, during or up to 1 h after main meal containing fat<br>Over the counter (Alli), 60 mg PO with each main meal containing fate, up to three capsules daily |

for use in children aged 12 and older and considers the drug to be safe and effective for weight reduction in overweight adolescents (see Table 36.3). In adolescents, who experience periods of growth spurts, BMI is a better indicator of weight loss because it accounts for weight related to growth.

### Use in Older Adults

Little information is available about the use of orlistat in people with renal or hepatic impairment. Manufacturer recommendations advise conservative use and lower dosages, because older adults often have decreased renal, cardiac, and hepatic function.

## Adverse Effects

The main adverse effects of orlistat are GI symptoms: abdominal pain, oily spotting, fecal urgency and incontinence, flatulence with discharge, fatty stools, and increased defecation. These effects occur in almost all users but usually subside after a few weeks of continued drug usage with moderation of fat intake.

In addition, the drug may cause pancreatitis or, rarely, liver dysfunction, including liver failure.

## Contraindications

Contraindications to orlistat include known allergy to the drug and chronic malabsorption syndrome or cholestasis.

## Nursing Implications

### Preventing Interactions

The body does not absorb orlistat, and no reported drug interactions affecting its action have occurred. However, orlistat may slightly reduce plasma concentrations of amiodarone. By partially inhibiting the absorption of dietary fat, the weight management drug may also decrease the plasma concentration of cyclosporine, which is highly lipid soluble; patients should take orlistat and cyclosporine 2 hours apart. Also, orlistat may decrease the serum concentration of levothyroxine; patients should take levothyroxine and orlistat at least 4 hours apart. In addition, concomitant use of orlistat may increase the lipid-lowering effects of pravastatin.

 **QSEN Alert: Safety**

Orlistat may reduce absorption of fat-soluble vitamins. This has implications for monitoring coagulation parameters if orlistat is use in conjunction with warfarin. The liver uses vitamin K to make blood-clotting proteins; therefore, a decrease in vitamin K increases the international normalized ratio and make it more difficult to manage warfarin therapy.

### Administering the Medication

It is necessary to take orlistat during or up to 1 hour after each main meal containing fat. (People may omit dose if a meal is missed or contains no fat.) Because the drug prevents absorption of the fat-soluble vitamins A, D, E, and K, people who take it should also take a multivitamin daily 2 hours before or after orlistat.

### Assessing for Therapeutic Effects

The nurse monitors weight loss and BMI. Most weight loss occurs in the first 6 months of therapy, but as patients continue to take orlistat, they can maintain the weight reduction. The metabolic improvements of weight loss are very beneficial for people with obesity-related health problems such as diabetes, dyslipidemia, hypertension, and metabolic syndrome.

### Assessing for Adverse Effects

The nurse assesses signs of common adverse GI effects (e.g., diarrhea, flatulence) and reduced concentrations of fat-soluble vitamins. To minimize GI effects, the nurse encourages patients to distribute fat calories over the three main meals and to avoid high-fat meals.

### Patient Teaching

Box 36.6 presents patient teaching guidelines for orlistat and other drugs used in weight management.

### NCLEX Success

3. Orlistat aids weight loss by doing which of the following?
   A. decreasing appetite
   B. increasing satiety and feelings of fullness
   C. increasing metabolism
   D. decreasing absorption of dietary fat

4. To decrease diarrhea with orlistat, it is important to instruct a patient to do which of the following?
   A. avoid large amounts of fatty foods
   B. drink eight glasses of water daily
   C. avoid caffeine-containing beverages
   D. increase physical activity

### Clinical Application 36.1

- In addition to proper administration of her medication, what strategies does the nurse review with Ms. Vargas to assist her in being successful with weight loss?
- Ms. Vargas says she needs to lose 140 lb and would like to accomplish this by her next birthday. How does the nurse respond?

## OTHER DRUGS USED FOR WEIGHT MANAGEMENT

Other drugs used for weight management, which have been approved for short-term use, include lorcaserin (Belviq, Belviq XR), bupropion–naltrexone (Contrave), and liraglutide (Saxenda, Victoza). Table 36.4 presents route and dosage information for these drugs. Amphetamines were once prescribed, but experts no longer recommend their use. These agents are controlled substances (Schedule II) with a high potential for abuse and dependence (see Chap. 57). Also, they can cause a life-threatening complication in patients who take antidepressants in the form of monoamine oxidase inhibitors (i.e., isocarboxazid, phenelzine).

Lorcaserin is believed to activate serotonin 5-hydroxy-tryptamine (5-HT) receptors, which stimulate select neurons in the hypothalamus. This leads to increased alpha-melanocor-tin–stimulating hormone release at melanocortin-4 receptors, resulting in satiety and decreased food intake. At recommended doses, lorcaserin has greater affinity for 5-HT receptors compared to other 5-HT receptor subtypes, the 5-HT receptor transporter, and 5-HT reuptake sites.

Bupropion is used for the prevention of weight gain during smoking cessation, as well as for the treatment of depression. It is a relatively weak inhibitor of the neuronal reuptake of dopamine and norepinephrine. Naltrexone is a pure opioid receptor antagonist used to treat alcohol and opioid dependence. Exactly how bupropion–naltrexone leads to weight loss is not fully understood. Effects may result from action on areas of the brain involved in the regulation of food intake, primarily the hypothalamus and the mesolimbic dopamine circuit. The combination is not commonly used as a first-line therapy for weight loss but may be beneficial for an individual who is obese and smokes and desires drug therapy for smoking cessation and obesity.

Liraglutide (Victoza, Saxenda) is a long-acting analog of endogenous GLP-1 that increases insulin secretion, decreases inappropriate glucagon secretion, increases B-cell growth/replication, and slows gastric emptying. The drug is prescribed for people with type 2 diabetes and is now used under the brand name Saxenda as a treatment for obese or overweight adults with at least one weight-related comorbid condition. It should not be used in those with a history of medullary thyroid cancer or pancreatitis.

## HERBAL AND DIETARY SUPPLEMENTS USED FOR WEIGHT MANAGEMENT

Many people use herbal or dietary supplements for weight loss, even though reliable evidence of safety and effectiveness is lacking. Some herbal products claim to decrease appetite and increase the rate at which the body burns calories. However, in most cases, there is no scientific evidence that they work at all. Research studies have not shown that bitter orange, chitosan, guar gum, green tea, or *Hoodia gordonii* is effective in producing weight loss. In addition, lack of evidence and safety concerns persist for chromium, ginseng, glucomannan, hydroxycitric acid, L-carnitine, psyllium, pyruvate supplements, St. John's wort, and conjugated linoleic acid.

Some supplements for weight loss contain cardiovascular and CNS stimulants that may cause serious, even life-threatening, adverse effects. For example, bitter orange exhibits a non–dose-related increase in heart rate and blood pressure with administration. In general, many consumers do not seem to appreciate the benefits of proven weight management techniques (e.g., appropriate diet and exercise) or the potential risks of taking unproven weight loss products. Box 36.7 contains more information about these herbal and dietary supplements.

**TABLE 36.4**

### DRUGS AT A GLANCE: Miscellaneous Weight Loss Agents (In Adults Unless Specified)

| Drug | Pregnancy Category | Route and Dosage Ranges |
|---|---|---|
| Lorcaserin (Belviq, Belviq XR) | X | Immediate release: 10 mg twice daily; reevaluate after 12 wk<br>Extended release: 20 mg once daily; reevaluate after 12 wk |
| Bupropion–naltrexone (Contrave) | X | Week 1: one tablet (8 mg naltrexone/90 mg bupropion) once daily<br>Week 2: one tablet twice daily<br>Week 3: two tablets in morning and one tablet in evening<br>Week 4: two tablets twice daily<br>Maximum daily dose: four tablets (32 mg naltrexone/360 mg bupropion); reevaluate after 12 wk |
| Liraglutide (Saxenda, Victoza; ✹ Victoza) | X | Initial: Victoza, 0.6 mg subcutaneously daily for 1 wk, increase by 0.6 mg to target of 1.8 mg once daily<br>Initial: Saxenda, 0.6 mg subcutaneously daily for 1 wk, increase by 0.6 mg to target of 3.0 mg once daily |

| BOX 36.7 | *Selected Herbal and Dietary Supplements Used in Weight Management* |
| --- | --- |

- Glucomannan expands on contact with body fluids. It is included in weight loss regimens because of its supposed ability to produce feelings of stomach fullness, thereby causing a person to eat less. It also has a laxative effect. There is little evidence to support its use as a weight loss aid. People with diabetes should not use products containing glucomannan; it may cause hypoglycemia alone and increases hypoglycemic effects of antidiabetic medications.
- Guarana, a major source of commercial caffeine, is a component of weight loss products as well as caffeine-containing soft drinks, "energy" drinks, body-building supplements, smoking-cessation products, vitamin supplements, candies, and chewing gums. Caffeine is the active ingredient; the amount varies among products, and it is not possible to determine the caffeine content of any particular product accurately. Advertisers promote guarana as a substance that decreases appetite and increases energy and mental alertness. Dysrhythmias contraindicate its use. It may aggravate gastroesophageal reflux disease and peptic ulcer disease.
- Adverse effects include diuresis, cardiovascular symptoms (premature ventricular contractions, tachycardia), central nervous system (CNS) symptoms (agitation, anxiety, insomnia, seizures, tremors), and GI symptoms (nausea, vomiting, diarrhea). Such effects are more likely to occur with higher doses or concomitant use of guarana and other sources of caffeine. Adverse drug–drug interactions include additive CNS and cardiovascular stimulation with beta-adrenergic agonists (e.g., epinephrine, albuterol

and related drugs, pseudoephedrine) and theophylline. In addition, concurrent use of cimetidine, fluoroquinolones, or oral contraceptives may increase or prolong serum caffeine levels and subsequent adverse effects.
- Guar gum is a dietary fiber included in weight loss products because it is presumed to be bulk forming and produces feelings of fullness. It may cause esophageal or intestinal obstruction if not taken with an adequate amount of water and may interfere with the absorption of other drugs if taken at the same time. In a meta-analysis of 20 clinical trials, the fiber was not effective in weight loss. Adverse effects include nausea, diarrhea, flatulence, and abdominal discomfort.
- Hydroxycitric acid (in Citrimax and other supplements) apparently suppresses appetite in animals, but there are no reliable studies that indicate its effectiveness in humans. One 12-week study did not show weight loss.
- In a meta-analysis of clinical trials comparing green tea preparations in overweight or obese adults, green tea did not significantly influence or help maintain weight loss.
- Laxative and diuretic herbs (e.g., aloe, rhubarb root, buckthorn, cascara, senna, parsley, juniper, dandelion leaves) are found in several commercial products. These products cause a significant loss of body fluids and electrolytes, not fat. Adverse effects may include low serum potassium levels, with subsequent cardiac dysrhythmias and other heart problems. In addition, long-term use of laxatives may lead to loss of normal bowel function and the necessity for continued use (i.e., laxative dependency).

### Clinical Application 36.2

- Ms. Vargas wants to know how orlistat will help her when nothing else in the past has been successful. How does the nurse respond?

### NCLEX Success

5. In counseling a patient about weight loss diets, the nurse knows that a recommended low-calorie or reduced-calorie diet does which of the following?

    A. provides about 500 to 800 kcal/d
    B. reduces daily intake to about 1800 kcal/d
    C. is required for weight loss
    D. focuses on high-fat, high-carbohydrate foods

6. Drug therapy for weight management may be prescribed for patients with which of the following?

    A. a body mass index (BMI) of 22 kg/m² and a desire to lose 10 lb
    B. a BMI of 24.5 kg/m² and physically fit
    C. a BMI of 30 kg/m² or more with weight-related health problems
    D. a BMI of 25 to 29 kg/m² and healthy

### Clinical Application 36.3

- Ms. Vargas' prescription is for orlistat three times a day. She takes the drug with breakfast, lunch, and dinner. She often has a meeting that runs through lunch, so she skips lunch but takes her pill on time. At her next clinic appointment, she discusses this with the nurse. How does the nurse respond?

# THE NURSING PROCESS

A concept map outlines the nursing process related to drug therapy considerations in this chapter. Additional nursing implications related to the disease process should also be considered in care decisions.

**Assessment**

- Assess usual drinking and eating patterns, including healthful (e.g., whole-grain breads and cereals, fruits, vegetables, low-fat dairy products) and unhealthful (e.g., sugar-containing beverages and desserts, fried foods, saturated fat, fast foods, high-calorie snack foods) intake. The best way is to ask the patient to keep a food diary for 2 or 3 days. If available, consult a nutritionist to assess a patient's diet and work with the patient to improve health and weight status.
- Assess any obviously overweight patient for health problems caused or aggravated by excessive weight (e.g., elevated blood pressure, other cardiovascular problems, diabetes mellitus, sleep apnea, osteoarthritis, and other musculoskeletal disorders).
- Calculate the BMI (see Box 36.1) and measure waist circumference.
- Check available reports of laboratory tests. Overweight patients may have abnormally high values for total and LDL cholesterol, triglycerides, and blood sugar and low values for HDL cholesterol. If no laboratory reports are available, ask patients if a health care provider has ever told them they have high cholesterol or blood sugar.
- List and review all prescription and nonprescription medications the patient is taking and ask about vitamins, herbals, and weight loss supplements.
- Assess motivation for weight loss and usual patterns of physical activity and exercise.

**Outcomes of Therapy**

The patient will
- Reduce the impact of excessive weight on chronic health problems.
- Modify lifestyle behaviors toward weight loss and weight maintenance at a more healthful level.
- Take weight loss drugs appropriately.
- Avoid unproven weight loss dietary supplements.

**Nursing Interventions**

- Support programs/efforts to help promote a healthful lifestyle and prevent obesity (e.g., in families and schools).
- Serve as a reliable source of information about weight loss and weight loss drugs and programs.
- For an obese patient who reports interest and motivation in losing weight, assist to formulate realistic goals. Losing 5% to 10% of body weight is a reasonable goal and can significantly reduce the medical problems associated with being overweight.
- Assist patients to identify factors that support weight loss efforts (e.g., family and friend encouragement) and factors that sabotage weight loss efforts (e.g., having high-calorie foods readily available, frequently eating at fast-food restaurants).
- Promote exercise and activity. For overweight and obese patients, exercise may decrease appetite and distract from eating behaviors as well as increase calorie expenditure.
- Refer patients to a dietitian or nutritionist as indicated.
- Be alert for the psychological consequences of obesity and refer patients for counseling if indicated.
- Instruct patient regarding symptoms of adverse drug effects and effective management of symptoms should they occur.
- Refer overweight and obese children to pediatric obesity specialists when possible.
- Provide appropriate teaching related to drug therapy (see Box 36.6).

**Evaluation**

- Evaluate the safe use of weight loss drugs and the patient's ability to manage any adverse effects.
- Observe overweight or obese patients for food intake, weight loss, decreased waist circumference, and appropriate use of exercise.
- Evaluate the patient's perception of level of success in managing weight loss.

## KEY CONCEPTS

- Being overweight and obese are major concerns because of their association with numerous health problems, including diabetes, hypertension, other cardiovascular disorders, and muscle and joint disorders.
- Ingesting 500 calories more per day than those used in exercise and physical activity leads to a weight gain of 1 lb in 1 week. Decreasing caloric intake or increasing caloric output of 500 cal/d for 1 week leads to a weight loss of 1 lb.
- Weight loss drugs are generally recommended only for people who are seriously overweight (BMI of 30 or more kg/m²) or who have a BMI greater than 27 kg/m² and health problems.

- Many people lose weight but regain it within a few months if they do not change their lifestyle habits and eat more healthfully and engage in more exercise.
- Noradrenergic sympathomimetic anorexiants are approved for short-term use for weight loss and include benzphetamine (Schedule III), diethylpropion (Schedule IV), phendimetrazine (Schedule III), and phentermine (Schedule IV).
- Orlistat prevents absorption of the fat-soluble vitamins, A, D, E, and K, so people taking the drug should also take a multivitamin containing these vitamins daily.

## CLINICAL REASONING CASE STUDY

**Meet the Patient**

Mrs. Cummings, a 41-year-old high school teacher, is a patient in the clinic at which a nurse works. She has requested assistance in losing weight. This woman is 5'7" tall and weighs 254 lb. She has had a lifelong battle with her weight, and nothing she has tried has been successful.

- How does the nurse calculate Mrs. Cummings' BMI?
- On the basis of Mrs. Cummings' BMI, does the nurse consider her clinically obese?
- The weight management provider orders phentermine 37.5 mg daily. What are some nursing interventions and patient teaching information will assist and support Mrs. Cummings to lose weight?

**Assessing Drug Information**

- Phentermine is a noradrenergic sympathomimetic anorexiant that causes appetite suppression, which is thought to result from direct stimulation of the satiety center in the hypothalamic and limbic region.
- The most commonly reported adverse effects with phentermine are nervousness, palpitations, tachycardia, primary pulmonary hypertension, hyperactivity, dry mouth, constipation, and systemic hypertension. Impotence, insomnia, and unpleasant taste may also occur.
- Contraindications to phentermine include pregnancy, breast feeding, moderate to severe hypertension, cardiovascular disease, hyperthyroidism, glaucoma, pregnancy, or a history of drug abuse.
- Teach the patient to avoid alcoholic beverages and other CNS depressants while taking phentermine.

**Nursing Actions**

- The nurse calculates BMI as (1) weight in kilograms (multiply weight in pounds by 0.45 [the metric conversion factor]) divided by height in meters (multiply height in inches by 0.025 [the metric conversion factor]) squared; or as weight in pounds divided by height in inches, squared, multiplied by a conversion factor of 704.5 (see Box 36.1), as follows:

$$\text{Option 2: BMI} = \frac{254 \text{ pounds}}{[67 \times 67 \text{ inches}]} \times 704.5 = \frac{254}{4489} \times 704.5 = 0.0566 \times 704.5 = 39.86$$

- Authorities consider that a person with a BMI of 30 kg/m² or more is clinically obese, so Mrs. Cummings' BMI is in the range of clinically obese.
- Nursing actions to support weight loss and weight maintenance should combine reduced-calorie diets, increased physical activity, and behavior therapy. The nurse helps Mrs. Cummings minimize circumstances that promote overeating (e.g., cooking calorie-dense foods; having high-calorie snacks and "junk food" readily available; and eating high-fat, high-calorie foods at fast-food restaurants). After weight loss, weight loss maintenance with dietary therapy, physical activity, and behavior therapy should continue indefinitely. Social support involves family, friends, coworkers, and fellow dieters who encourage weight loss efforts rather than sabotage them by urging the person who is trying to lose or maintain weight to eat high-calorie foods.
- Assess for allergies before administering any medications.
- Assess for contraindications to phentermine, such as pregnancy, moderate to severe hypertension, cardiovascular disease, hyperthyroidism, glaucoma, or a history of drug abuse. (If Mrs. Cummings becomes pregnant, she needs to stop the phentermine and notify her health care provider.)
- Teach Mrs. Cummings to avoid alcoholic beverages and other CNS depressants while taking phentermine.

Visit the Point® at **http://thePoint.lww.com/Frandsen12e** for answers to NCLEX Success questions (in Appendix A), answers to Clinical Application Case Studies (in Appendix B), and more!

## REFERENCES AND RESOURCES

American Heart Association. (2015). What is Metabolic Syndrome? Retrieved from https://www.heart.org/idc/groups/heart-public/@wcm/@hcm/documents/downloadable/ucm_300322.pdf

Centers for Disease Control and Prevention. (2015). Prevalence of Obesity Among Adults and Youth: United States, 2011–2014. Retrieved from https://www.cdc.gov/nchs/products/databriefs/db219.htm

Centers for Disease Control and Prevention. (2016). Overweight & Obesity. Retrieved from https://www.cdc.gov/obesity/data/childhood.html

Hinkle, J. H., & Cheever, K. H. (2018). *Brunner & Suddarth's textbook of medical-surgical nursing* (14th ed.). Philadelphia, PA: Wolters Kluwer.

Karch, A. M. (2014). *Lippincott's nursing drug guide*. Philadelphia, PA: Wolters Kluwer/Lippincott Williams & Wilkins.

Kim, G. W., Lin, J. E., Blomain, E. S., & Waldman, S. A. (2014). Antiobesity pharmacotherapy: New drugs and emerging targets. *Clinical Pharmacologic Therapy, 95*(1), 53–66.

Lippincott Williams & Wilkins. (2017). *Nursing 2017 drug handbook* (37th ed.). Philadelphia, PA: Lippincott Williams & Wilkins.

NHLBI Obesity Education Initiative Expert Panel on the Identification, Evaluation, and Treatment of Obesity in Adults (US). (1998). *Clinical guidelines on the identification, evaluation, and treatment of overweight and obesity in adults: The evidence report*. Bethesda, MD: National Heart, Lung, and Blood Institute.

National Institutes of Health. (2015). BMI Chart [Measurement instrument]. Retrieved from https://www.nhlbi.nih.gov/health/educational/lose_wt/BMI/bmi_tbl.htm

Perrault, L. (2016). *Obesity in adults: Drug therapy*. UpToDate. Lexi-Comp, Inc.

Perreault, L., & Apovian, C. (2019). *Obesity in adults: Overview of management*. UpToDate. Lexi-Comp, Inc.

UpToDate. (2019). *Drug information*. Lexi-Comp, Inc.

Yang, L., Cao, C., Kantor, E. D., et al. (2019). Trends in sedentary behavior among the US population, 2001–2016. *Journal of the American Medical Association, 321*(16), 1587–1597. doi:10.1001/jama.2019.3636

# Drug Therapy for Peptic Ulcer Disease and Hyperacidity

## LEARNING OBJECTIVES

*After studying this chapter, you should be able to:*

1. Describe the main elements of peptic ulcer disease and gastroesophageal reflux disease.
2. Discuss antacids in terms of the prototype, indications, and contraindications for use, routes of administration, and major adverse effects.
3. Describe histamine$_2$ receptor antagonists in terms of the prototype, indications, and contraindications for use, routes of administration, and major adverse effects.
4. Discuss proton pump inhibitors in terms of the prototype, indications, and contraindications for use, routes of administration, and major adverse effects.
5. Identify the adjuvant medications used to treat peptic ulcer and gastroesophageal reflux disease.
6. Implement the nursing process in the care of patients receiving antacids, proton pump inhibitors, and histamine$_2$ receptor antagonists.

## CLINICAL APPLICATION CASE STUDY

Stacy Carpenter, a 54-year-old woman, has chronic gastroesophageal reflux disease. She has been experiencing increasing gastric pain and is concerned that she is also developing a gastric ulcer. Presently, she takes omeprazole (Prilosec) 20 mg orally daily, as prescribed. In the past few weeks, she has begun taking three over-the-counter medications: famotidine (Pepcid) 10 mg twice a day as needed to control her heartburn, a combination antacid (Mylanta) 5 mL/dose, and bismuth (Pepto-Bismol) 10 mL. She has had no observable blood in her stools, which have not been discolored. She denies diarrhea or nausea. She does say that the gastric pain feels like someone is "sticking a knife" into her chest. The pain is relieved at times with a change in diet—to what she describes as "bland foods." She has quit drinking milk and limited her intake of other dairy foods because a friend told her these foods were "hard to digest."

## KEY TERMS

**Achlorhydria:** low or absent production of gastric acid in the stomach

**Cardia:** the part of the stomach that attaches to the esophagus

**Esophagitis:** inflammation of the esophagus

**Gastritis:** acute or chronic inflammation of the gastric mucosa

*Helicobacter pylori:* gram-negative bacterium found in the gastric mucosa of most patients with chronic gastritis

**Hydrogen, potassium adenosine triphosphatase:** enzyme system that catalyzes the production of gastric acid and acts as a gastric acid pump to move gastric acid from parietal cells in the mucosal lining of the stomach into the stomach lumen

**Pepsin:** proteolytic enzyme that helps digest protein foods

**Pyrosis:** heartburn

**Stress ulcers:** gastric mucosal lesions that develop in patients who are critically ill from trauma, shock, hemorrhage, sepsis, burns, acute respiratory distress syndrome, major surgical procedures, or other severe illnesses

# INTRODUCTION

Drugs to prevent or treat duodenal and peptic ulcers and acid reflux disorders consist of several groups of agents, most of which alter gastric acid and its effects on the mucosa of the upper gastrointestinal (GI) tract. To aid understanding of drug effects, this chapter presents an overview of both ulcer disease and gastroesophageal reflux disease (GERD) before providing details about specific drugs. Box 37.1 gives further descriptions of selected upper GI disorders.

# OVERVIEW OF PEPTIC ULCER DISEASE AND GASTROESOPHAGEAL REFLUX DISEASE

## Etiology and Pathophysiology

### Peptic Ulcer Disease

Peptic ulcer disease is characterized by ulcer formation in the esophagus, stomach, or duodenum areas of the GI mucosa that are exposed to gastric acid and pepsin. Gastric and duodenal ulcers are more common than esophageal ulcers. Infection with *Helicobacter pylori* and use of nonsteroidal anti-inflammatory drugs (NSAIDs) account for most cases of peptic ulcer disease. *H. pylori* is a gram-negative bacterium found in the gastric mucosa of most patients with chronic **gastritis** (inflammation of the gastric mucosa). This bacterium is spread mainly by the fecal–oral route. However, iatrogenic spread by contaminated endoscopes, biopsy forceps, and nasogastric tubes has also occurred. The frequency of people infected is related to race and ethnicity; about 60% of Hispanics, 54% of African Americans, and 20% to 29% of White Americans have detectable organisms. Up to 50% of the gastric ulcers and 80% of the duodenal ulcers are associated with this infection. The elimination of the organism significantly reduces the risk of ulcer recurrence and gastric cancer.

In addition, stress (e.g., major trauma, severe medical illness) can precipitate ulcer formation. Gastric ulcers are more likely to occur in older adults, especially in the sixth and seventh decades, and to be chronic in nature. Duodenal ulcers are strongly associated with *H. pylori* infection and NSAID ingestion, may occur at any age, occur about equally in men and women, are often manifested by abdominal pain, and are usually chronic in nature. They are also associated with cigarette smoking. Compared with nonsmokers, smokers are more likely to develop duodenal ulcers, their ulcers heal more slowly with treatment, and the ulcers recur more rapidly.

Peptic ulcers seem to result from an imbalance between cell-destructive and cell-protective effects (i.e., presence of increased destructive mechanisms or presence of decreased protective mechanisms). Cell-destructive effects include those of gastric acid (hydrochloric acid), pepsin, *H. pylori* infection, and NSAID ingestion. Gastric acid, a strong acid that can digest the stomach wall, is secreted by parietal cells in the mucosa of the stomach antrum, near the pylorus. The parietal cells contain receptors for acetylcholine, gastrin, and histamine, substances that stimulate gastric acid production. Acetylcholine is released by vagus nerve endings in response to stimuli, such as thinking about or ingesting food. Gastrin is a hormone released by cells in the stomach and duodenum in response to food ingestion and stretching of the stomach wall. It is secreted into the bloodstream and eventually circulated to the parietal cells. Histamine is released from cells in the gastric mucosa and diffuses into nearby parietal cells. The enzyme system **hydrogen, potassium adenosine triphosphatase** ($H^+$, $K^+$-ATPase) catalyzes the production of gastric acid and acts as a gastric acid (proton) pump to move gastric acid from parietal cells in the mucosal lining of the stomach into the stomach lumen.

**Pepsin**, a proteolytic enzyme, helps digest protein foods and also can digest the stomach wall. Pepsin is derived from a precursor called pepsinogen, which is secreted by chief cells in the gastric mucosa. Pepsinogen is converted to pepsin only in a highly acidic environment (i.e., when the pH of gastric juices is 3 or less).

After *H. pylori* moves into the body, the bacterium colonizes the mucus-secreting epithelial cells of the stomach mucosa and is thought to produce gastritis and ulceration by impairing mucosal function. Eradication of the microorganism accelerates ulcer healing and significantly decreases the rate of ulcer recurrence.

Cell-protective effects (e.g., secretion of mucus and bicarbonate, dilution of gastric acid by food and secretions, prevention of diffusion of hydrochloric acid from the stomach lumen back into the gastric mucosal lining, the presence of prostaglandin E, alkalinization of gastric secretions by pancreatic juices and bile, perhaps other mechanisms) normally prevent autodigestion of stomach and duodenal tissues and ulcer formation.

A gastric or duodenal ulcer may penetrate only the mucosal surface, or it may extend into the smooth muscle layers. When superficial lesions heal, no defects remain. When smooth muscle heals, however, scar tissue remains and the mucosa that regenerates to cover the scarred muscle tissue may be defective. These defects contribute to repeated episodes of ulceration.

**Selected Upper Gastrointestinal Disorders**

## Gastritis

Gastritis, a common disorder, is an acute or chronic inflammatory reaction of gastric mucosa. Patients with gastric or duodenal ulcers usually also have gastritis. Acute gastritis (also called gastropathy) usually results from irritation of the gastric mucosa by such substances as alcohol, aspirin or other nonsteroidal anti-inflammatory drugs (NSAIDs), and others. Chronic gastritis is usually caused by *Helicobacter pylori* (*H. pylori*) infection, and it persists unless the infection is treated effectively. *H. pylori* organisms may cause gastritis and ulceration by producing enzymes (e.g., urease, others) that break down mucosa; they also alter secretion of gastric acid.

## Nonsteroidal Anti-inflammatory Drug Gastropathy

NSAID gastropathy indicates damage to the gastroduodenal mucosa by aspirin and other NSAIDs. The damage may range from minor superficial erosions to ulceration and bleeding. NSAID gastropathy is one of the most common causes of gastric ulcers, and it may cause duodenal ulcers as well. Many people take NSAIDs daily for pain, arthritis, and other conditions. Chronic ingestion of NSAIDs causes local irritation of gastroduodenal mucosa, inhibits the synthesis of prostaglandins (which normally protect gastric mucosa by inhibiting acid secretion, stimulating secretion of bicarbonate and mucus, and maintaining mucosal blood flow), and increases the synthesis of leukotrienes and possibly other inflammatory substances that may contribute to mucosal injury.

## Stress Ulcers

Stress ulcers indicate gastric mucosal lesions that develop in patients who are critically ill from trauma, shock, hemorrhage, sepsis, burns, acute respiratory distress syndrome, major surgical procedures, or other severe illnesses. The lesions may be single or multiple ulcers or erosions. Stress ulcers are usually manifested by painless upper gastrointestinal (GI) bleeding. The frequency of occurrence has decreased, possibly because of improved management of sepsis, hypovolemia, and other disorders associated with critical illness and the prophylactic use of antiulcer drugs. However, there is concern about inappropriate use of stress ulcer prophylaxis.

Although the exact mechanisms of stress ulcer formation are unknown, several factors are thought to play a role, including mucosal ischemia, reflux of bile salts into the stomach, reduced GI tract motility, and systemic acidosis. Acidosis increases severity of lesions, and correction of acidosis decreases their formation. In addition, lesions do not form if the pH of gastric fluids is kept at about 3.5 or above, and lesions apparently form only when mucosal blood flow is diminished.

## Zollinger-Ellison Syndrome

Zollinger-Ellison syndrome is a rare condition characterized by excessive secretion of gastric acid and a high incidence of ulcers. It is caused by gastrin-secreting tumors in the pancreas, stomach, or duodenum. Approximately two thirds of the gastrinomas are malignant. Symptoms are those of peptic ulcer disease, and diagnosis is based on high levels of serum gastrin and gastric acid. Treatment may involve long-term use of a proton pump inhibitor to diminish gastric acid or surgical excision.

## *Gastroesophageal Reflux Disease*

GERD, the most common disorder of the esophagus, is a chronic digestive disease that occurs when stomach acid or, occasionally, bile refluxes into the esophagus. The backwash of acid irritates the lining of the esophagus. The main cause of GERD is thought to be an incompetent lower esophageal sphincter (LES). Normally, the LES is contracted or closed and prevents the reflux of gastric contents. It opens or relaxes on swallowing to allow passage of food or fluid and then contracts again. Several circumstances contribute to impaired contraction of the LES and the resulting reflux, including foods (e.g., fats, chocolate), fluids (e.g., alcohol, caffeinated beverages), medications (e.g., beta-adrenergics, calcium channel blockers, nitrates), gastric distention, cigarette smoking, and recumbent posture. GERD occurs in men, women, and children but is especially common during pregnancy and after 40 years of age.

The part of the stomach that connects to the esophagus is called the **cardia**. In healthy patients, the esophagus enters the stomach at an angle, forming a valve that prevents gastric contents from traveling back into the esophagus. In patients with GERD, pathophysiologic effects and symptoms result from failure of the cardia. Additionally, *H. pylori* infection is present in nearly half of all patients with GERD.

GERD is characterized by regurgitation of duodenal bile, enzymes, and stomach acid into the esophagus and exposure of esophageal mucosa to gastric acid and pepsin. The same amount of acid–pepsin exposure may lead to different amounts of mucosal damage, possibly related to individual variations in esophageal mucosal resistance.

## Clinical Manifestations

### *Peptic Ulcer Disease*

The clinical manifestations of a gastric ulcer are almost opposite to the clinical manifestations of duodenal ulcers; the main differences are the timing and severity of the pain. Gastric ulcers generally cause a dull aching pain, often right after eating. The intake of food does not relieve pain as is the case with a duodenal ulcer. The patient may experience bloating, indigestion, heartburn, or nausea. Gastric ulcers are often manifested by painless bleeding and take longer to heal than do duodenal ulcers. Duodenal ulcers cause heartburn, bloating, severe stomach pain, and a burning sensation at the back of the throat. The symptoms may be worse when the stomach is empty and may flare at night. Typically, the symptoms disappear and then return for a period of time.

### *Gastroesophageal Reflux Disease*

**Pyrosis** (heartburn), which increases with a recumbent position or bending over, is the main symptom of GERD. Effortless regurgitation of acidic fluid into the mouth, especially after a meal and at night, is often indicative. Important protective mechanisms for the esophagus, including gravity, swallowing, and saliva, are effective only when people are upright. At night during sleep in a recumbent position, the effect of gravity is negated, swallowing ceases, and the secretion of saliva is decreased. Consequently, reflux that occurs at night probably results in acid staying in the esophagus longer and causing greater damage. Many people experience both pyrosis and acid reflux from time to time. When they occur regularly, they may be signs of GERD. In addition, there may also be mild to severe **esophagitis** (inflammation of the esophagus) or esophageal ulceration. Pain on swallowing usually means erosive or ulcerative esophagitis.

## Drug Therapy

Drugs used in the treatment of acid–peptic disorders promote healing of lesions and prevent recurrence of lesions by decreasing cell-destructive effects or increasing cell-protective effects. Several types of drugs are used, alone and in various combinations. Figure 37.1 illustrates the sites of action for drugs used to treat GERD. Antacids neutralize gastric acid and decrease pepsin production, antimicrobials and bismuth can eliminate *H. pylori* infection, histamine$_2$ receptor antagonists (H$_2$RAs) and proton pump inhibitors (PPIs) decrease gastric acid secretion, sucralfate provides a barrier between mucosal erosions or ulcers

and gastric secretions, and misoprostol restores prostaglandin activity. The following sections describe the types of drugs and individual agents. Table 37.1 lists the drugs used for peptic ulcer disease and GERD.

Available drugs are safe and effective.

> **❗ QSEN Alert: Safety**
>
> Taking herbal supplements may delay drug treatment and have harmful consequences; therefore, it is important that nurses and other prescribers do not encourage the use of herbs for any acid–peptic disorder.

## ANTACIDS

People commonly take over-the-counter (OTC) antacids to offset the effects of GI acids. These drugs differ in their ability to neutralize gastric acid (50–80 mEq of acid is produced hourly), in onset of action, and in adverse effects. Commonly used antacids are mixtures of aluminum hydroxide and magnesium hydroxide, as well as other ingredients. The aluminum hydroxide–magnesium hydroxide–simethicone mixture  **Mylanta** is the prototype. (In this discussion, the trade name of the drug is used to refer to this antacid.)

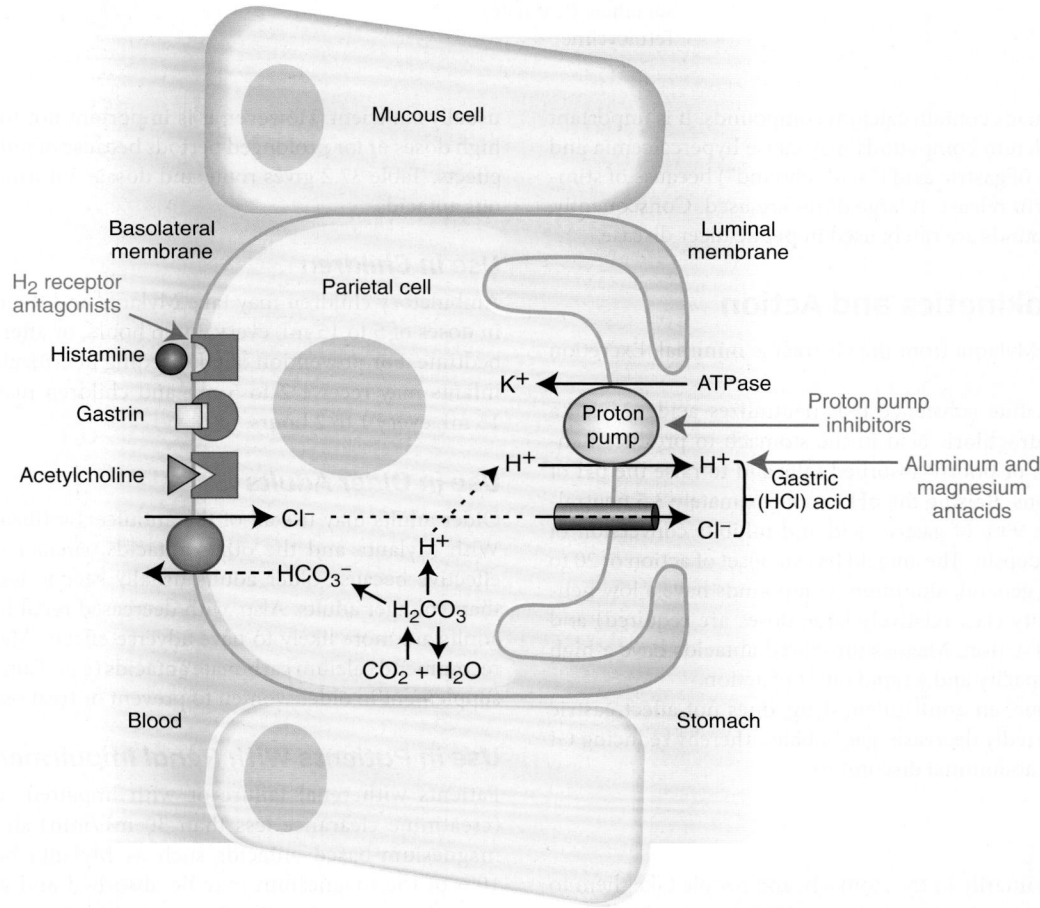

**Figure 37.1.** Sites of action of drugs for gastroesophageal reflux disease (see *red labels/arrows*). [Adapted with permission from Norris, T. L. (2019). *Porth's pathophysiology: Concepts of altered health states* (10th ed., Fig. 36.10, p. 1066). Philadelphia, PA: Wolters Kluwer.]

**TABLE 37.1**

## Drugs Administered for the Treatment of Peptic Ulcer Disease and Gastroesophageal Reflux Disease

| Drug Class | Prototype(s) | Other Drugs in the Class |
|---|---|---|
| Antacids | Mylanta<br>Mylanta Double Strength | Amphojel<br>Gelusil<br>Maalox suspension<br>Titralac, Tums |
| Histamine₂ receptor antagonists | Cimetidine (Tagamet) | Famotidine (Pepcid, Pepcid AC)<br>Famotidine 10 mg, calcium carbonate 800 mg, and magnesium hydroxide 165 mg (Pepcid Complete)<br>Nizatidine (Axid)<br>Ranitidine (Zantac) |
| Proton pump inhibitors | Omeprazole (Prilosec, Prilosec OTC) | Esomeprazole (Nexium, Nexium IV, Nexium delayed-release capsules, Esomep-EZS)<br>Dexlansoprazole (Dexilant)<br>Lansoprazole (Prevacid, Prevacid SoluTab)<br>Pantoprazole (Protonix, Protonix IV)<br>Rabeprazole (AcipHex, AcipHex Sprinkle) |
| Adjuvant medications | | Amoxicillin<br>Bismuth subsalicylate<br>Bismuth subcitrate potassium, metronidazole, and tetracycline (Pylera)<br>Clarithromycin<br>Metronidazole<br>Misoprostol (Cytotec)<br>Sucralfate (Carafate)<br>Tetracycline |

Some antacids contain calcium compounds. It is important to note that calcium compounds may cause hypercalcemia and hypersecretion of gastric acid ("acid rebound") because of stimulation of gastrin release, if large doses are used. Consequently, calcium compounds are rarely used in peptic ulcer disease.

## Pharmacokinetics and Action

Absorption of Mylanta from the GI tract is minimal. Excretion is in the urine.

As an alkaline substance that neutralizes acids, Mylanta reacts with hydrochloric acid in the stomach to produce neutral, less acidic, or poorly absorbed salts and to raise the pH of gastric secretions. Raising the pH to approximately 3.5 neutralizes more than 90% of gastric acid and inhibits conversion of pepsinogen to pepsin. The antacid has an onset of action of 20 to 60 minutes. In general, aluminum compounds have a low neutralizing capacity (i.e., relatively large doses are required) and a slow onset of action. Magnesium-based antacids have a high neutralizing capacity and a rapid onset of action.

Simethicone, an antiflatulent drug, does not affect gastric acidity. It reportedly decreases gas bubbles, thereby reducing GI distention and abdominal discomfort.

## Use

Antacids act primarily in the stomach, and people take them to prevent or treat peptic ulcer disease, GERD, esophagitis, heartburn, gastritis, GI bleeding, and stress ulcers. When pain relief is the goal of treatment, taking them on an as-needed basis is usually sufficient. However, it is important not to take them in high doses or for prolonged periods because of potential adverse effects. Table 37.2 gives route and dosage information for various antacids.

### Use in Children

Ambulatory children may take Mylanta and the other antacids in doses of 5 to 15 mL every 3 to 6 hours, or after meals, and at bedtime. For prevention of GI bleeding in critically ill children, infants may receive 2 to 5 mL and children may receive 5 to 15 mL every 1 to 2 hours.

### Use in Older Adults

Older adults may use all of the antiulcer, antiheartburn drugs. With Mylanta and the other antacids, smaller doses may be effective because older adults usually secrete less gastric acid than younger adults. Also, with decreased renal function, older adults are more likely to have adverse effects. Many physicians recommend calcium carbonate antacids (e.g., Tums) as a calcium supplement in older women to prevent or treat osteoporosis.

### Use in Patients With Renal Impairment

Patients with renal failure or with impaired renal function (creatinine clearance less than 30 mL/min) should not take magnesium-based antacids such as Mylanta because 5% to 10% of the magnesium may be absorbed and accumulate to cause hypermagnesemia. Patients with chronic renal failure and hyperphosphatemia may take aluminum-based antacids to decrease absorption of phosphates in food. (Aluminum binds with phosphate in the GI tract, preventing phosphate absorption and hyperphosphatemia that commonly occurs in renal failure.) However, aluminum may accumulate in patients with renal failure, leading to encephalopathy, erythropoietin-resistant anemia, and osteomalacia.

Antacids containing calcium carbonate are currently recommended for the purpose of controlling phosphate levels in patients with end-stage renal failure. Antacids with calcium carbonate can cause alkalosis and raise urine pH, and chronic use may cause renal stones and hypercalcemia.

### Use in Patients With Critical Illness

To prevent **stress ulcers** (gastric mucosal lesions that occur due to physiologic stress) in critically ill patients and to treat acute GI bleeding, nearly continuous neutralization of gastric acid is desirable. Dose and frequency of administration must be sufficient to neutralize the gastric acid: a continuous intragastric drip through a nasogastric tube is effective. For patients with a nasogastric tube in place, antacid dosage may be titrated by aspirating stomach contents, determining pH, and then basing the dose on the pH. (Most gastric acid is neutralized and most pepsin activity is eliminated at a pH above 3.5.)

### Use in Patients Receiving Home Care

People commonly take all of the antiulcer, antiheartburn drugs in the home setting, usually by self-administration. The home care nurse can assist patients by providing information about taking the drugs correctly and monitoring responses.

## Adverse Effects

Aluminum-containing antacids such as Mylanta can cause constipation. Hypophosphatemia and osteomalacia may develop in people who ingest large amounts of aluminum-based antacids over a long period because aluminum combines with phosphates in the GI tract and prevents phosphate absorption. Aluminum compounds are rarely used alone for acid–peptic disorders.

Mylanta also contains magnesium. Antacids with magnesium may cause diarrhea and hypermagnesemia. Older adults may experience neuromuscular effects.

## Contraindications

People with any signs of appendicitis or inflamed bowel (cramping, soreness, or pain in the lower abdomen) patients with renal failure should not take Mylanta.

## Nursing Implications

### Preventing Interactions

Because antacids are minimally absorbed, few drugs alter their effects. Anticholinergic drugs (e.g., atropine) increase effects by delaying gastric emptying and by decreasing acid secretion themselves. Cholinergic drugs (e.g., pyridostigmine [Mestinon]) decrease effects of antacids by increasing GI motility and rate of gastric emptying. No herbs are known to alter the effects of antacids.

However, antacids may prevent absorption of most drugs taken at the same time, including benzodiazepine antianxiety drugs, corticosteroids, digoxin, $H_2RAs$ (e.g., cimetidine), iron supplements, phenothiazine antipsychotic drugs, phenytoin, fluoroquinolone antibacterials, and tetracyclines. Antacids increase absorption of a few drugs including levodopa, quinidine, and valproic acid. To avoid or minimize these interactions, it is necessary to separate administration times by 1 to 2 hours.

### Administering the Medication

Typical prescribing practices with Mylanta and other antacids used to treat active ulcers are to take them 1 and 3 hours after meals and at bedtime for greater acid neutralization. This schedule is effective but inconvenient for many patients. More recently, lower doses taken less often have been found effective in healing duodenal or gastric ulcers, although less acid neutralization occurs.

Authorities once thought that liquid antacid preparations were more effective. Now, they consider tablets to be as effective as liquids.

> **! QSEN Alert: Safety**
>
> It is important to shake liquid antacid preparations well before measuring each dose, because these suspensions separate into layers with the medication consolidated at the bottom. Thorough mixing is necessary.

### Assessing for Therapeutic Effects

The nurse assesses for decreased epigastric pain in patients with gastric and duodenal ulcers or decreased heartburn in those with GERD. Antacids should relieve pain within a few minutes. Also, it is necessary to assess for decreased GI bleeding (e.g., absence of visible or occult blood in vomitus, gastric secretions, or feces). In addition, the nurse uses pH testing to evaluate the quantity, frequency, and duration of acid reflux episodes, as well as to check the pH of gastric contents. The minimum acceptable pH with antacid therapy is 3.5. Healing usually occurs within 4 to 8 weeks. Finally, the nurse assesses for radiologic or endoscopic reports of ulcer healing.

### Assessing for Adverse Effects

With antacids containing magnesium, such as Mylanta, the nurse assesses for diarrhea and hypermagnesemia. Combining such an antacid with one that contains aluminum or calcium may prevent this. Hypermagnesemia may occur in patients with impaired renal function. With the antacids containing calcium (Titralac, Tums), it is important to observe for constipation. (Combining this antacid with other antacids containing magnesium may prevent this effect.)

### Patient Teaching

Box 37.2 summarizes patient teaching information for antacids.

## HISTAMINE₂ RECEPTOR ANTAGONISTS

In addition to its other effects, histamine also causes strong stimulation of gastric acid secretion. Vagal stimulation causes release of histamine from cells in the gastric mucosa. The histamine then acts on receptors located on the parietal cells to increase production of hydrochloric acid. These receptors are

## TABLE 37.2

### DRUGS AT A GLANCE: Representative Antacid Products

| Drug | Pregnancy Category | Components | | | Route and Dosage Ranges (Adults) |
|------|-------------------|-----------|---|---|---------------------------------|
| | | **Magnesium Oxide or Hydroxide** | **Aluminum Hydroxide** | **Other** | |
| Mylanta | Not classified | 200 mg/tablet, 200 mg/5 mL | 200 mg/tablet, 200 mg/5 mL | Simethicone, 25 mg/ tablet, 20 mg/5 mL | 5–10 mL or 1–2 tablets PO every 2–4 h, between meals and at bedtime or as directed by physician |
| Mylanta Double Strength | Not classified | 400 mg/tablet, 400 mg/5 mL | 400 mg/tablet, 400 mg/5 mL | Simethicone, 30 mg/ tablet, 30 mg/5 mL | Same as Mylanta |
| Amphojel | Not classified | | 300 or 600 mg/tablet | | 600 mg PO five or six times daily |
| Gelusil | Not classified | 200 mg/tablet | 200 mg/tablet | Simethicone, 25 mg/tablet | 10 or more mL or two or more tablets PO after meals and at bedtime or as directed by physician to a max of 12 tablets or tsp/24 h |
| Maalox suspension | Not classified | 200 mg/5 mL | 225 mg/5 mL | | 30 mL PO four times daily, after directed by physician; max dose, 16 tsp/24 h |
| Titralac, Tums | Not classified | | | Calcium carbonate: 420 mg/tablet, 1 g/5 mL Glycine: 180 mg/tablet, 300 mg/5 mL | 1 tsp or 2 tablets PO after meals or as directed by physician to max of 19 tablets or 8 tsp/24 h |

called the $H_2$ receptors. Although traditional antihistamines or $H_1RAs$ prevent or reduce other effects of histamine, they do not block histamine effects on gastric acid production.

However, the $H_2RAs$ inhibit both basal secretion of gastric acid and the secretion stimulated by histamine, acetylcholine, and gastrin. **Cimetidine** (Tagamet HB) is the prototype of this class. An OTC preparation is available. Prescription forms are also obtainable.

## Pharmacokinetics

After oral administration, absorption is good. Cimetidine is distributed in almost all body tissues. Onset varies. After a single dose, peak blood level is reached in all routes in 1 to 1.5 hours, the half-life is 2 hours, and an effective concentration is maintained for about 6 hours. Onset of the drug after intravenous (IV) and intramuscular (IM) administration is rapid. Metabolism takes place in the liver. Excretion of the unchanged oral dose occurs unchanged in the urine within 24 hours; some excretion takes place in the bile, with elimination in the feces.

## Action

Cimetidine inhibits the action of histamine at the $H_2$ receptors of the stomach, decreasing the amount, acidity, and pepsin

content of gastric juices. A single dose can inhibit acid secretion for 6 to 12 hours, and a continuous IV infusion can inhibit secretion for prolonged periods.

Prescribers often advise taking antacids concurrently with $H_2RAs$ such as cimetidine to relieve pain. The pain relief usually occurs after 1 week. Patients should not take the antacid and the $H_2RA$ at the same time (except for Pepcid Complete) because the antacid reduces absorption of the $H_2RA$.

## Use

Indications for use of cimetidine include prevention and treatment of peptic ulcer disease, GERD, esophagitis, GI bleeding due to acute stress ulcers, and Zollinger-Ellison syndrome. With gastric or duodenal ulcers, healing occurs within 6 to 8 weeks; with esophagitis, healing occurs in about 12 weeks. The U.S. Food and Drug Administration (FDA) has approved the OTC preparations for the treatment of heartburn.

Table 37.3 gives route and dosage information for cimetidine and other $H_2RAs$.

### Use in Older Adults

With cimetidine, older adults are more likely to experience adverse effects, especially confusion, agitation, and disorientation.

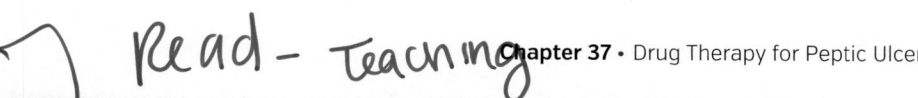

*Read - Teaching*

**BOX 37.2**    *Patient Teaching Guidelines: Drugs Used for Peptic Ulcer Disease and Gastroesophageal Reflux Disease*

**General Considerations**

- These drugs are commonly used to prevent and treat peptic ulcers and heartburn. Peptic ulcers usually form in the stomach or first part of the small bowel (duodenum), where tissues are exposed to stomach acid. Two common causes of peptic ulcer disease are stomach infection with a bacterium called *Helicobacter pylori* and taking nonsteroidal anti-inflammatory drugs (NSAIDs) such as ibuprofen and many others. Heartburn (also called gastroesophageal reflux disease) is caused by stomach acid splashing back onto the esophagus.

- Peptic ulcer disease and heartburn are chronic conditions that are usually managed on an outpatient basis. Complications such as bleeding require hospitalization. Overall, these conditions can range from mild to serious, and it is important to seek information about the disease process, ways to prevent or minimize symptoms, and drug therapy.

- With heartburn, try to minimize acid reflux by elevating the head of the bed; avoiding stomach distention by eating small meals; not lying down for 1 to 2 hours after eating; minimizing intake of fats, chocolate, citric juices, coffee, and alcohol; avoiding smoking (stimulates gastric acid production); and avoiding obesity, constipation, or other conditions that increase intra-abdominal pressure. In addition, take tablets and capsules with 8 oz of water and do not take medications at bedtime unless instructed to do so.

- Most medications for peptic ulcer disease and heartburn decrease stomach acid. An exception is the antibiotics used to treat ulcers caused by *H. pylori* infection. The strongest acid reducers are omeprazole (Prilosec), dexlansoprazole (Dexilant), esomeprazole (Nexium), lansoprazole (Prevacid), pantoprazole (Protonix), and rabeprazole (AcipHex). These are prescription drugs, except for omeprazole and lansoprazole, which is approved for nonprescription use. Histamine-blocking drugs such as cimetidine (Tagamet), famotidine (Pepcid), and others are available as both prescription and over-the-counter (OTC) preparations. OTC products are indicated for heartburn, and smaller doses are taken than for peptic ulcer disease. These drugs usually should not be taken longer than 2 weeks without the advice of a health care provider. (A 2-week treatment with Prilosec OTC can be repeated every 4 months if needed to control heartburn.) The concern is that OTC drugs may delay diagnosis and treatment of potentially serious illness. In addition, cimetidine can increase toxic effects of numerous drugs and should be avoided if you are taking other medications.

- Misoprostol (Cytotec) is given to prevent ulcers from NSAIDs, which are commonly used to relieve pain and inflammation with arthritis and other conditions. This drug should be taken only while taking a traditional NSAID such as ibuprofen. Do not take misoprostol if pregnant and do not become pregnant while taking the drug. If pregnancy occurs during misoprostol therapy, stop the drug and notify your prescriber immediately. Misoprostol can cause abdominal cramps and miscarriage. A related drug, celecoxib (Celebrex), is less likely to cause peptic ulcer disease.

- Numerous antacid preparations are available, but they are not equally safe in all people and should be selected carefully. For example, products that contain magnesium have a laxative effect and may cause diarrhea; those that contain aluminum or calcium may cause constipation (e.g., the antacids Titralac and Tums contain calcium). Some commonly used antacids (e.g., Maalox, Mylanta) are a mixture of magnesium and aluminum preparations, an attempt to avoid both constipation and diarrhea. People with kidney disease should not take products that contain magnesium because magnesium can accumulate in the body and cause serious adverse effects. Thus, it is important to read product labels and, if you have a chronic illness or take other medications, ask your physician or pharmacist to help you select an antacid and an appropriate dose.

- All $H_2$ receptor antagonists (e.g., cimetidine, famotidine) are available by prescription and OTC. When you obtain these drugs with a prescription, avoid concomitant use of OTC versions of the same or similar drugs.

**Self or Caregiver Administration**

- Take antiulcer drugs as directed. Underuse decreases therapeutic effectiveness; overuse increases adverse effects. For acute peptic ulcer disease or esophagitis, drugs are given in relatively high doses for 4 to 8 weeks to promote healing. For long-term maintenance therapy, dosage is reduced.

- With omeprazole, rabeprazole sodium, esomeprazole magnesium, and pantoprazole sodium, swallow the capsule whole; do not open, chew, or crush. With Prevacid, the capsule can be opened and the granules sprinkled on applesauce for patients who are unable to swallow capsules. Also, Prevacid granules are available in a packet for preparing a liquid suspension. Follow instructions for mixing the granules exactly. The granules should not be crushed or chewed.

- Take cimetidine with meals or at bedtime. Take famotidine, nizatidine, and ranitidine with or without food. Do not take an antacid for 1 hour before or after taking one of these drugs.

- Take sucralfate on an empty stomach at least 1 hour before meals and at bedtime. Also, do not take an antacid for 1 hour before or after taking sucralfate.

- Take misoprostol with food.

- For treatment of peptic ulcer disease, take antacids 1 and 3 hours after meals and at bedtime (4–7 doses daily), 1 to 2 hours before or after other medications. Antacids decrease absorption of many medications if taken at the same time. Also, chew chewable tablets thoroughly before swallowing and then drink a glass of water; allow effervescent tablets to dissolve completely and almost stop bubbling before drinking (this increases the surface area of drug available to neutralize gastric acid); and shake liquids well before measuring the dose. A high-fiber diet, adequate fluid intake (2000–3000 mL daily), and exercise may help prevent constipation if it occurs with Mylanta therapy.

- With Pepcid AC orally disintegrating tablets, open the blister package with dry hands immediately before use, place the tablet on the tongue, and allow the tablet to dissolve with saliva. Taking it with liquids is not necessary.

**TABLE 37.3**

## DRUGS AT A GLANCE: Histamine₂ Receptor Antagonists

| Drug | Pregnancy Category | Routes and Dosage Ranges | |
|---|---|---|---|
| | | **Adult** | **Children** |
| **ℙ Cimetidine** (Tagamet; ✹ Apo-Cimetidine, Novo-Cimetidine) | B | Duodenal or gastric ulcer: PO 800 mg once daily at bedtime or 300 mg four times daily or 400 mg twice daily<br>Maintenance: 400 mg PO at bedtime<br>IV injection, 300 mg diluted in 20 mL of 0.9% NaCl solution every 6–8 h<br>IV intermittent infusion: 300 mg diluted in 50 mL of dextrose or saline solution every 6 h<br>Impaired renal function (creatinine clearance <30 mL/min): 25 mg/h IV for prevention of GI bleeding; 300 mg PO or IV every 12 h, may increase to every 8 h if tolerated<br>300 mg IM every 6–8 h<br>GERD: 800 mg PO twice daily or 400 mg four times daily<br>Prevention of upper GI bleeding: 50 mg/h continuous IV infusion<br>Heartburn: 200 mg PO once or twice daily as needed<br>Impaired renal function: 300 mg PO or IV every 8–12 h | Not recommended for children younger than 12 y of age |
| Famotidine (Pepcid, Pepcid AC; ✹ Apo-famotidine; Pepcid, Pepcid AC) Famotidine 10 mg, calcium 800 mg, and magnesium hydroxide 165 mg (Pepcid Complete) | B | Duodenal or gastric ulcer: 40 mg PO or IV once daily at bedtime or 20 mg twice daily for 4–8 wk; maintenance, 20 mg PO or IV once daily at bedtime<br>Zollinger-Ellison syndrome: 20 mg PO every 6 h, increased if necessary<br>IV injection: 20 mg every 12 h, diluted to 5 or 10 mL with 5% dextrose or 0.9% sodium chloride<br>IV infusion: 20 mg every 12 h, diluted with 100 mL of 5% dextrose or 0.9% sodium chloride<br>Impaired renal function (creatinine clearance <50 mL/min): 20 mg PO or IV every 24–48 h<br>GERD: 20 mg PO twice daily for 6–12 wk<br>Heartburn (Pepcid Complete): 1–2 tablets PO chewed, daily as needed | GERD: <3 mo, 0.5 mg/kg/dose PO daily for 8 wk<br>3 mo ≤1 y: PO 0.5 mg/kg/dose twice daily, IV famotidine not adequately studied in patients <1 y with GERD<br>Peptic ulcer: 1–16 y, 0.5 mg/kg/d PO at bedtime or divided twice daily up to 40 mg/d<br>GERD with or without esophagitis: 1.0 mg/kg/d PO divided twice daily up to 40 mg twice daily |
| Nizatidine (Axid; ✹ Apo-Nizatidine, Novo-Nizatidine) | B | Duodenal or gastric ulcer: 300 mg PO once daily at bedtime or 150 mg PO twice daily; maintenance, 150 mg PO once daily at bedtime<br>GERD: 150 mg PO twice daily<br>Heartburn: 75 mg PO 30–60 min before meals<br>Impaired renal function (creatinine clearance [CrCl] 20–50 mL/min), 150 mg PO daily; CrCl <20 mL/min, 150 mg PO every 72 h | Dosing not established in children |
| Ranitidine (Zantac; ✹ ACT-Ranitidine, Dom-Ranitidine; Zantac) | B | Duodenal ulcer: 300 mg PO once daily at bedtime or 150 mg PO twice daily, maintenance 150 mg PO at bedtime<br>50 mg IM every 6–8 h<br>Injection, 50 mg IV diluted to 100 mL in 5% dextrose or 0.9% sodium chloride solution every 6–8 h<br>Intermittent infusion, 50 mg IV diluted in 100 mL of 5% dextrose or 0.9% sodium chloride solution<br>Gastric ulcer or GERD: 150 mg PO twice daily<br>Impaired renal function (CrCl < 50 mL/min): 150 mg PO every 24 h; 50 mg IV or IM every 18–24 h<br>Heartburn: 75 mg PO as needed<br>*H. pylori* infection: 400 mg PO twice daily for 4 wk in combination with clarithromycin | 1 mo to 16 y<br>Duodenal and gastric ulcers, 2–4 mg/kg PO twice daily to a max of 300 mg/d; maintenance, 2–4 mg/kg PO once daily to a max of 150 mg/d<br>GERD: 5–10 mg/kg/d PO, usually given as 2 divided doses |

GERD, gastroesophageal reflux disease, including erosive esophagitis; GI, gastrointestinal.

## Use in Patients With Renal Impairment

Use of cimetidine in patients with impaired renal function requires caution. It is necessary to reduce the dosage of cimetidine and other H$_2$RAs in the presence of impaired renal function because the drugs are eliminated through the kidneys. Cimetidine may cause mental confusion in patients with renal impairment. It also blocks secretion of creatinine in renal tubules, thereby decreasing creatinine clearance and increasing serum creatinine level. Any dosage increase, if necessary, should be cautious, with close monitoring of renal function.

 **QSEN Alert: Safety**

For patients on hemodialysis, cimetidine administration should occur at the end of dialysis.

## Use in Patients With Hepatic Impairment

The partial metabolism of cimetidine and other H$_2$RAs occurs in the liver, which means that drug levels are higher than anticipated in patients with impaired liver function. Cimetidine inhibits the hepatic metabolism of many other drugs; this is a major concern.

## Use in Patients With Critical Illness

H$_2$RAs are commonly used in critically ill patients to prevent stress-induced gastric ulceration. These are usually administered by intermittent IV infusion. Generally, information about the pharmacokinetics of these drugs in critically ill patients is limited. It appears that in patients who are critically ill, H$_2$RAs have a longer half-life and lower clearance rate than in people who are healthy.

## Use in Patients Receiving Home Care

People take cimetidine in the home care setting. The home care nurse can assist patients by providing information about taking the drug correctly and monitoring responses. It is necessary to assess for potential drug–drug interactions with cimetidine.

# Adverse Effects

Common adverse effects of cimetidine include diarrhea, dizziness, drowsiness, headache, confusion, and gynecomastia. They occur infrequently following the usual doses and standard duration of treatment. Adverse effects are more likely with prolonged use of high doses, with increasing age, and with impaired renal or hepatic function.

# Contraindications

Contraindications include known hypersensitivity to cimetidine. Caution is warranted in people with renal and hepatic impairment and in women who are lactating or pregnant.

# Nursing Implications

## Preventing Interactions

Antacids decrease absorption of cimetidine, so the drugs should not be given at the same time. No drugs are known to increase or decrease the effects of cimetidine. Additionally, no herbs increase or decrease the effects of cimetidine.

*↓ LOOK*

 **QSEN Alert: Safety**

However, cimetidine contributes to multiple-drug interactions. A known inhibitor of many isozymes of the cytochrome P450 (CYP450) drug-metabolizing system in the liver, it therefore interferes with the hepatic metabolism of other drugs. Consequently, the clearance of affected drugs from the body is slower; the increased serum levels mean that the drugs are more likely to cause adverse effects and toxicity unless dosage is reduced.

*D2D: true interaction check !*

Drugs that are affected by cimetidine include antidysrhythmics (lidocaine, propafenone, quinidine), the anticoagulant warfarin, anticonvulsants (carbamazepine, phenytoin), benzodiazepine antianxiety or hypnotic agents (alprazolam, diazepam, flurazepam, triazolam), beta-adrenergic blockers (labetalol, metoprolol, propranolol), the bronchodilator theophylline, calcium channel blocking agents (e.g., verapamil), tricyclic antidepressants (e.g., amitriptyline), and sulfonylurea antidiabetic drugs. In addition, cimetidine may increase serum levels (e.g., fluorouracil, procainamide and its active metabolite) and pharmacologic effects of other drugs (e.g., respiratory depression with opioid analgesics) by unidentified mechanisms. Cimetidine also may decrease effects of several drugs, including drugs that require an acidic environment for absorption (e.g., iron salts, indomethacin, fluconazole, tetracyclines) and miscellaneous drugs (e.g., digoxin, tocainide) by unknown mechanisms. The accumulation of the antihistamines, terfenadine and astemizole, may result in a prolongation of the QT interval and could lead to the development of ventricular dysrhythmias such as torsades de pointes. Cimetidine also may decrease the effects of drugs that require an acidic environment for absorption (e.g., iron salts, indomethacin, fluconazole, tetracyclines) and miscellaneous drugs (e.g., digoxin, tocainide) by unknown mechanisms.

## Administering the Medication

H$_2$RAs are available in a wide array of products, and it is essential to take precautions to ensure that the formulation, dosage strength, and method of administration are appropriate for the intended use.

Oral administration of a single oral dose occurs at bedtime, and administration of multiple oral doses of cimetidine occurs with meals and at bedtime.

 **QSEN Alert: Safety**

With the oral solution, it is important to measure the liquid with a marked measuring spoon or medicine cup, not with a tablespoon.

- IV administration requires dilution and administration over at least 2 minutes. For intermittent infusion, it is necessary to dilute and infuse over 15 to 20 minutes.

- IM administration does not require dilution. Injection is given deep into a large muscle group.

### Assessing for Therapeutic Effects

The nurse assesses for decreased epigastric pain with gastric and duodenal ulcers or decreased heartburn with GERD.

### Assessing for Adverse Effects

With H₂RAs, the nurse assesses for diarrhea or constipation, headache, dizziness, muscle aches, fatigue, skin rashes, mental confusion, delirium, coma, depression, and fever. Adverse effects are uncommon and usually mild with recommended doses. The nurse assesses for central nervous system effects, which have been associated with high doses in patients who are elderly or in those with impaired renal function. With long-term administration of cimetidine, other observed adverse effects include decreased sperm count and gynecomastia in men and galactorrhea in women.

### Patient Teaching

Box 37.2 summarizes patient teaching guidelines that apply to the H₂RAs.

## Other Drugs in the Class

Unlike cimetidine, ranitidine (Zantac), famotidine (Pepcid, Pepcid AC), and nizatidine (Axid AR) do not affect the cytochrome P450 drug-metabolizing system in the liver and therefore do not interfere with the metabolism of other drugs. Use of these other drugs may be preferable in patients who are critically ill because they often require numerous other drugs with which cimetidine may interact.

Ranitidine is more potent than cimetidine on a weight basis, and smaller doses can be given less frequently. Oral ranitidine reaches peak blood levels 1 to 3 hours after administration and is metabolized in the liver; approximately 30% is excreted unchanged in the urine. Parenteral ranitidine reaches peak blood levels in about 15 minutes; 65% to 80% is excreted unchanged in the urine. Famotidine and nizatidine pharmacokinetics are similar to cimetidine and ranitidine. Nizatidine is not available in a parenteral formulation. Compared with cimetidine, the other drugs cause similar effects except they are less likely to cause mental confusion and gynecomastia (antiandrogenic effects).

Ranitidine decreases absorption of diazepam if given at the same time and increases hypoglycemic effects of glipizide. Antacids probably decrease absorption of ranitidine. Nizatidine increases serum salicylate levels in people taking high doses of aspirin.

## PROTON PUMP INHIBITORS

PPIs are the most potent inhibitors of gastric acid secretion available. PPIs are similar to the H₂RAs in terms of effects but have a different mode of action. Compared with H₂RAs, PPIs suppress gastric acid more strongly, for a longer period. This effect provides faster symptom relief and faster healing in acid-related diseases. Rates of ulcer recurrence are similar. Because PPIs are more effective than H₂RAs, certainly in the short term, PPIs are more popular.  **Omeprazole** (Prilosec), the first drug in the class to be developed, is still widely used and serves as the prototype.

## Pharmacokinetics

Omeprazole is well absorbed after oral administration and highly bound to plasma proteins (about 95%). Metabolism occurs in the liver, and excretion takes place in the urine (about 75%) and bile or feces. The half-life of the drug is 1 to 1.5 hours. Acid-inhibiting effects occur within 2 hours and last 72 hours or longer. When the drug is discontinued, effects persist for 48 to 72 hours or longer, until the gastric parietal cells can synthesize additional H⁺, K⁺-ATPase.

## Action

Omeprazole binds irreversibly to the gastric proton pump (e.g., the enzyme H⁺, K⁺-ATPase) to prevent the "pumping" or release of gastric acid from parietal cells into the stomach lumen, thereby blocking the final step of acid production. Inhibition of the proton pump suppresses gastric acid secretion in response to all primary stimuli, histamine, gastrin, and acetylcholine. Thus, omeprazole and other drugs in the class inhibit both daytime (including meal-stimulated) and nocturnal (unstimulated) acid secretion.

## Use

Omeprazole and other PPIs are usually the drug class of choice for treatment of peptic ulcer disease, including duodenal and gastric ulcers; GERD with erosive esophagitis; and Zollinger-Ellison syndrome. With duodenal and gastric ulcers, healing may occur after 2 weeks compared to 4 weeks using H₂RAs. With GERD, PPIs usually eliminate symptoms within 1 to 2 weeks and heal esophagitis within 8 weeks. Lower doses can prevent recurrence of esophagitis, maintain symptom relief, and heal esophagitis. Higher doses or longer therapy may be needed for severe GERD.

In patients with *H. pylori*–associated ulcers, eradication of the bacterium with antimicrobial drugs is preferable to long-term maintenance therapy with antisecretory drugs. Therapy with a PPI and two antimicrobial drugs is the most effective regimen (see Medications Used to Treat *Helicobacter pylori*). Table 37.4 presents route and dosage information for omeprazole and other PPIs.

### Use in Children

Omeprazole and the other PPIs have gained widespread popularity in children and infants for the management of peptic ulcers and GERD as well as the eradication of *H. pylori*. These drugs are acid labile, and oral formulations consist of capsules that contain enteric-coated granules. A chewable form of omeprazole exists, and a pharmacist can prepare a liquid formulation.

### Use in Older Adults

Older adults tolerate PPIs well. PPIs are probably the drug of choice for treating symptomatic GERD because evidence suggests that patients 60 years of age and older require stronger antisecretory effects than younger adults. However, long-term use (greater than 1 year) is associated with increased risk of hip fractures in people older than 50 years of age; the risk of fractures increases the longer the medications are taken and is greater in people who take higher dosages of PPIs. The increased risk of fractures may be due to decreased calcium absorption due to **achlorhydria** (low or absent production of gastric acid in the stomach) from PPI therapy. It is important to consider appropriate dose and duration of therapy when treating GERD in older adults.

### Use in Patients With Hepatic Impairment

With omeprazole, bioavailability is increased because of decreased first-pass metabolism and plasma half-life is increased. Metabolism of PPIs occurs in the liver, and use of these drugs may cause transient elevations in liver function tests. However, dosage adjustments are not recommended.

### Use in Patients With Critical Illness

The PPIs are the strongest gastric acid suppressants used in patients who are critically ill. They usually tolerate the drugs well. IV administration, if necessary, is an option.

## Adverse Effects

Adverse effects are minimal with both short- and long-term use. Nausea, diarrhea, and headache are the most frequently reported adverse effects. Use of high-dose PPIs or long-term use of the drugs carries a possible increased risk of bone fractures. (As previously stated, this may increase in older patients.)

## Contraindications

Contraindications include known hypersensitivity to omeprazole.

## Nursing Implications

### Preventing Interactions

Drug interactions with the PPIs are relatively few. Omeprazole increases blood levels of some benzodiazepines (diazepam, flurazepam, triazolam), phenytoin, and warfarin, probably by inhibiting hepatic metabolism. Coadministration of clopidogrel with PPIs may reduce the cardioprotective effects of clopidogrel. Clarithromycin increases effects of omeprazole and may increase blood levels. No herbs have been reported to increase or decrease the effects of omeprazole.

### Administering the Medication

It is important that omeprazole be administered before food intake. Two 20-mg oral capsules or suspension packets are not equivalent to one 40-mg dose. The 20- and 40-mg dosages contain the same amount of sodium bicarbonate; substituting two 20-mg doses for one 40-mg dose results in the administration of too much sodium bicarbonate. The patient should swallow the tablets or capsules whole, without crushing or chewing, because the drug formulations are delayed-release and long-acting. Crushing or chewing destroys these effects.

### Assessing for Therapeutic Effects

The nurse assesses for decreased epigastric pain with gastric and duodenal ulcers and also assesses for decreased heartburn with GERDs.

### Assessing for Adverse Effects

The nurse observes for the presence of headache, diarrhea, abdominal pain, nausea, and vomiting.

### Patient Teaching

Box 37.2 lists general teaching guidelines that apply to PPIs.

## Other Drugs in the Class

The actions and pharmacokinetics of the other PPIs, including dexlansoprazole (Dexilant), esomeprazole (Nexium), lansoprazole (Prevacid), pantoprazole (Protonix), and rabeprazole (AcipHex), are similar to those of omeprazole. However, differences in their metabolism may lead to specific drug interactions. The PPIs are metabolized by the CYP450 system, with CPY2C19 having the predominant role in all PPIs but rabeprazole, which is metabolized primarily by CYP3A4.

Dexlansoprazole capsules should be swallowed whole and not chewed. However, the capsules may be opened and sprinkled on a tablespoon of applesauce if a person is not able to swallow

**TABLE 37.4**

## DRUGS AT A GLANCE: Proton Pump Inhibitors

| Drug | Pregnancy Category | Routes and Dosage Ranges | |
|---|---|---|---|
| | | **Adults** | **Children** |
| ℗ **Omeprazole** (Prilosec, Prilosec OTC; 🍁 Losec, Olex) | C | Gastric ulcer: 40 mg PO once daily for 4–8 wk<br>Duodenal ulcer: 20 mg PO once daily for 4–8 wk<br>GERD, with erosive esophagitis: 20 mg PO once daily<br>Zollinger-Ellison syndrome: 60 mg PO once daily<br>Heartburn: 20 mg PO for 14 d; may repeat treatment every 4 mo if needed<br>*H. pylori* infection: 40 mg PO daily for 14 d, then 20 mg daily for 14 d, with clarithromycin | 1–16 y<br>GERD:<br>5–10 kg, 5 mg<br>10–20 kg, 10 mg<br>≥20 kg, 20 mg PO |
| Dexlansoprazole (Dexilant; 🍁 Dexilant) | | GERD: 30 mg PO once daily for 4 wk | ≥12 y: 30 mg PO once daily for 4 wk |
| Esomeprazole (Nexium, Nexium IV, Nexium Delayed-Release Capsules, Esomep-EZS; 🍁 Nexium) | B | GERD: 20–40 mg PO once daily for 4–8 wk; maintenance, 20 mg PO once daily, 20–40 mg IV daily up to 10 d | 1 mo to <1 y, 0.5 mg/kg IV infused over 10–30 min<br>1–11 y, GERD, 30 mg PO once daily for up to 12 wk; >30 kg, 15 mg PO once daily for up to 12 wk<br>12–17 y, GERD, 10 mg PO once daily for up to 8 wk, <55 kg 10 mg IV; ≥55 kg 20 mg IV infused over 10–30 min<br>Healing erosive esophagitis: <20 kg 10 mg PO once daily for up to 8 wk; ≥20 kg 10 or 20 mg PO once daily for up to 8 wk |
| Lansoprazole (Prevacid, Prevacid SoluTab; 🍁 Prevacid, Prevacid FasTab) | B | Duodenal ulcer: 15 mg PO daily for healing and maintenance<br>Gastric ulcer: 30 mg PO once daily, up to 8 wk<br>Erosive esophagitis: 30 mg PO daily up to 8 wk; maintenance, 15 mg PO daily<br>*H. pylori* infection: 30 mg PO (with amoxicillin and clarithromycin) three times daily for 10–14 d<br>Hypersecretory conditions: 60–90 mg PO daily | 1–11 y, GERD: ≤30 kg, 30 mg PO once daily for up to 12 wk; >30 kg, 15 mg PO once daily for up to 12 wk<br>12–17 y<br>GERD: 30 mg PO once daily for up to 8 wk<br>Nonerosive GERD: 15 mg PO once daily for up to 8 wk<br>Healing erosive esophagitis: 15 mg PO once daily<br>Hypersecretory conditions: 60 mg PO once daily |
| Pantoprazole (Protonix, Protonix IV; 🍁 Panto IV, Pantoloc, Tecta) | B | GERD: 40 mg PO or IV once daily<br>Zollinger-Ellison syndrome: 40–80 mg PO or IV every 12 h | 5 y and more, GERD<br>>15 kg to <40 kg, 20 mg PO once daily for up to 8 wk<br>>40 kg, 40 mg PO once daily for up to 8 wk |
| Rabeprazole (AcipHex; AcipHex Sprinkle; 🍁 Pariet) | B | Duodenal ulcer: 20 mg PO once daily up to 4 wk<br>GERD: 20 mg PO once daily for healing and maintenance<br>Zollinger-Ellison syndrome: 60 mg PO once or twice daily | 12 y and more, GERD<br>20 mg PO once daily for up to 8 wk |

GERD, gastroesophageal reflux disease, including erosive esophagitis; GI, gastrointestinal; *H. pylori, Helicobacter pylori.*

the capsule. Capsules may also be opened and administered via a nasal gastric tube. Doses greater than 30 mg do not provide additional benefit during the maintenance phase. Note that two 30-mg orally disintegrating tablets are not interchangeable with one 60-mg delayed-release capsule.

Esomeprazole capsules can be opened, mixed with 50 mL of water, and swallowed or administered via nasogastric tube. Flush tube with water after administration. IV esomeprazole can be injected over no less than 3 minutes or infused over 10 to 30 minutes into a dedicated IV line. Flush the IV line with 5% dextrose or lactated Ringer's solution before and after esomeprazole administration.

Lansoprazole and rabeprazole should be used cautiously, and dosage should be reduced in patients with severe liver impairment. Those people with phenylketonuria should be advised that orally disintegrating tablets of lansoprazole may contain aspartame. Lansoprazole may cause drowsiness or dizziness. For patients who are unable to swallow capsules, they can have the lansoprazole (and esomeprazole) capsule opened and the granules mixed with applesauce or other acidic substances; this preserves the coating of the granules, allowing them to remain intact until they reach the small intestine. Chewing or crushing destroys the coating. For a liquid suspension, it is possible to mix the lansoprazole granules with 30 mL of water (use no other liquids), stir well, and swallow it immediately, without chewing the granules.

The nurse ensures that oral pantoprazole is taken with or without food as per the manufacturer's recommendations. The nurse may administer IV pantoprazole over 15 minutes, injecting the drug into a dedicated line or the Y-site of an IV infusion. Here are some specific directions regarding pantoprazole administration:

- Use the in-line filter provided; if injecting in a Y-site, place the filter below the Y-site closest to the patient.
- Flush the IV line with 5% dextrose, 0.9% NaCl, or lactated Ringer's solution before and after administration.

With regard to drug interactions, omeprazole and esomeprazole have the greatest potential. Esomeprazole appears to interfere with the metabolism of other drugs to a lesser degree than omeprazole. The metabolism of pantoprazole undergoes the same metabolism but is followed rapidly by sulfate conjugation. Because of this, pantoprazole has the lowest potential for drug interactions with other agents metabolized by the CYP450 system. Rabeprazole is metabolized by CYP2C19 but shows a strong affinity for CYP3A4 and is associated with very few known drug interactions. Although dexlansoprazole and lansoprazole are potent inhibitors of CYP2C19 and other CYP450 isoforms, these drugs are metabolized primarily by CYP3A4. Interactions with theophylline have been reported.

### Clinical Application 37.2

The patient education includes instructions for Ms. Carpenter about how to take her medication properly and measures to avoid gastric irritation.
- What content should the teaching plan include?
- What foods are included or excluded in her nutritional intake?

## ADJUVANT MEDICATIONS USED TO TREAT PEPTIC ULCER DISEASE AND GASTROESOPHAGEAL REFLUX DISEASE

Administration of adjuvant medications may support the treatment and resolution of symptoms of acid peptic disorders. Table 37.5 summarizes these adjuvant medications.

## Miscellaneous Medications

### Prostaglandin: Misoprostol

Naturally occurring prostaglandin E, which is produced in mucosal cells of the stomach and duodenum, inhibits gastric acid secretion and increases mucus and bicarbonate secretion, mucosal blood flow, and perhaps mucosal repair. It also inhibits the mucosal damage produced by gastric acid, aspirin, and NSAIDs. When synthesis of prostaglandin E is inhibited, erosion and ulceration of gastric mucosa may occur. This is the mechanism by which aspirin and other NSAIDs are thought to cause gastric and duodenal ulcers (see Chap. 16).

Misoprostol (Cytotec) (see Table 37.5) is a synthetic form of prostaglandin E approved for concurrent use with NSAIDs to protect gastric mucosa from NSAID-induced erosion and ulceration. It is indicated for patients at high risk for GI ulceration and bleeding, such as those taking high doses of NSAIDs for arthritis and older adults. The FDA has issued a **BLACK BOX WARNING ◆** to alert health care professionals that misoprostol is contraindicated in women of childbearing potential, unless effective contraceptive methods are being used, and during pregnancy, because it may induce abortion, premature birth, or birth defects. In fact, misoprostol is one of the drugs used for medical abortions in lieu of surgical evacuation.

The most common adverse effects are diarrhea (occurs in 10%–40% of recipients), which may be severe enough to lead to dosage reduction or stopping the drug, and abdominal cramping. Other adverse effects include nausea, vomiting, headache, uterine cramping, and vaginal bleeding. Older adults often take large doses of NSAIDs for arthritis and therefore are at risk for development of acute gastric ulcers and GI bleeding. Thus, they may be candidates for treatment with misoprostol. However, they may be unable to tolerate the misoprostol-induced diarrhea and abdominal discomfort. Dosage reduction to prevent severe diarrhea and abdominal cramping may be necessary.

### Sucralfate

Sucralfate (Carafate) is a preparation of sulfated sucrose and aluminum hydroxide that binds to normal and ulcerated mucosa. Prescribers use it to prevent and treat peptic ulcer disease. For ulcer treatment, it requires use for 4 to 8 weeks unless healing is confirmed by radiologic or endoscopic examination. When used long term to prevent ulcer recurrence, dosage reduction is necessary.

Sucralfate is effective even though it does not inhibit secretion of gastric acid or pepsin, and it has little neutralizing effect on gastric acid. Its mechanism of action is unclear, but it is thought to act locally on the gastric and duodenal mucosa. Possible mechanisms include binding to ulcer and forming a

**TABLE 37.5**

## DRUGS AT A GLANCE: Adjuvant Medications Used to Treat Peptic Ulcer Disease and Gastroesophageal Reflux Disease

| Drug | Pregnancy Category | Route and Dosage Ranges | |
|---|---|---|---|
| | | **Adults** | **Children** |
| Misoprostol (Cytotec) | X | 100–200 mg PO four times daily with meals and at bedtime | Safety and effectiveness not established |
| Sucralfate (Carafate; 🍁 Sucralfate-1, Sulcrate, Sulcrate Suspension Plus) | B | Active ulcer: 1 g PO four times daily before meals and at bedtime; maintenance, 1 g PO two times daily | Safety and effectiveness not established |
| Amoxicillin (Moxatag 🍁 Pro-Amox, Novamoxin) | B | 500 mg–1 g two to three times daily, Moxatag 775 mg ER | Dosing not established with *H. pylori* infection |
| Clarithromycin (🍁 ACCEL-Clarithromycin, ACT-Clarithromycin, APO-Clarithromycin, Biaxin) | C | 500 mg PO three times daily | Dosing not established with *H. pylori* infection |
| Metronidazole (🍁 Flagyl) | B | 250 mg PO four times daily | Dosing not established with *H. pylori* infection |
| Tetracycline (🍁 APO-Tetra, Nu-Tetra) | D | 500 mg PO four times daily | Dosing not established with *H. pylori* infection; tetracycline can discolor teeth in children 8 y of age or less |
| Bismuth subsalicylate | Not rated | 525 mg PO (2 tablets or 30 mL) four times daily | <3 y, consult physician<br>3–6 y, 1/3 tablet or 5 mL PO<br>6–9 y, 2/3 tablet or 10 mL PO<br>9–12 y, 1 tablet or 15 mL PO<br>Dosage may be repeated every 30–60 min, if needed, up to 8 doses in 24 h |

*H. pylori, Helicobacter pylori.*

protective barrier between the mucosa and gastric acid, pepsin, and bile salts; neutralizing pepsin; stimulating prostaglandin synthesis in the mucosa; and exerting healing effects through the aluminum component. Sucralfate is effective in healing duodenal ulcers and in maintenance therapy to prevent ulcer recurrence. In general, the rates of ulcer healing with sucralfate are similar to the rates with $H_2$RAs.

Adverse effects are low in incidence and severity because sucralfate is not absorbed systemically. Constipation and dry mouth are most often reported. Older adults tolerate sucralfate well. The main disadvantages of using sucralfate are that the tablet is large; it must be given at least twice daily; it requires an acid pH for activation and should not be given with an antacid, $H_2$RA, or PPI; and it may bind to other drugs and prevent their absorption. Sucralfate decreases absorption of ciprofloxacin and other fluoroquinolones, digoxin, phenytoin, warfarin, as well as the PPI lansoprazole. If a person takes both sucralfate and any of these drugs, to avoid or minimize this interaction, he or she should do the following:

- Take lansoprazole about 30 minutes before sucralfate.
- Take ciprofloxacin and other fluoroquinolones, digoxin, phenytoin, warfarin, or other drugs 2 hours before sucralfate, if it is possible.

In addition, antacids decrease the effects of sucralfate, and people should not take these within 30 minutes before or after administration of sucralfate.

## Medications Used to Treat *Helicobacter pylori*

### Combination Therapy With Antibiotics

Combination drug therapy that includes at least two antibiotics and an acid reducer (triple therapy), as well as occasionally bismuth subsalicylate, is recommended for patients with peptic ulcer disease who are known to be infected with *H. pylori*. If the selected antibiotics are not effective, the bacteria may become resistant to the action of some antibiotics. Combination regimens are the most effective way to help ensure that the bacteria do not acquire resistance to the selected antibiotics. A different combination of drug treatment may be required based on the treatment history. In situations where the first-line therapy is ineffective, rescue *H. pylori* therapy with esomeprazole, moxifloxacin, and amoxicillin has been effective and well tolerated. Data demonstrate that 14 days of treatment not only significantly improve the likelihood of eradication but also produce an increased rate of adverse events.

### QSEN Alert: Evidence-Based Practice

Over the past few decades, the effectiveness of standard triple therapy to eradicate *H. pylori* has declined as resistance in traditional regimens has increased. High-dose dual therapy with amoxicillin and a proton pump inhibitor for 14 days has been found to be an effective salvage regimen for treatment of *H. pylori* in patients who fail an initial attempt at eradication, particularly if resistance to metronidazole/clarithromycin or levofloxacin is suspected [Kwack, Lim, Lim, & Graham, 2016]. However, the role of amoxicillin as a first-line regimen remains unclear because findings are inconsistent in recent studies.

Over the past few years, an alternate approach to *H. pylori* treatment has demonstrated higher success rates by splitting up the antibiotics rather than taking them all at once. Sequential therapy may be more effective than standard triple therapy in light of the increasing frequency of resistant strains of *H. pylori*. Table 37.5 presents examples of drug combinations used to treat *H. pylori*. For convenience, some of the recommended drug combinations are packaged together (see Table 37.5).

Metronidazole (Flagyl), a nitroimidazole antibiotic, antiprotozoal medication, is sometimes included as part of a multidrug regimen (see Chap. 21).

### QSEN Alert: Safety

Consuming alcohol while using metronidazole has long been thought to have a disulfiram-like reaction with effects that can include flushing, tachycardia, diaphoresis, nausea, vomiting, or headache if alcohol ingestion occurs with use. It is important to tell patients that even a very small amount of alcohol can produce the reaction; the risk persists for up to 48 hours after completion of treatment.

Section IV of this book contains additional information about antibiotic therapy.

### Bismuth Subsalicylate

Prescribers use bismuth subsalicylate to coat ulcers, protecting them from stomach acid to treat *H. pylori*. Other uses include treatment of diarrhea and nausea. Commonly known as pink bismuth, it is the active ingredient in OTC medications such as Pepto-Bismol and Kaopectate. Bismuth subsalicylate is also used in combinations with other drugs to treat *H. pylori*. As salicylate, this drug can cause serious bleeding problems when used alone in patients with ulcers.

### QSEN Alert: Safety

People with an allergy to aspirin or other salicylates should not take bismuth subsalicylate.

People who are taking chewable tablets should chew them and then swallow them. If they are taking the liquid form of this medication, they should shake the bottle well and use a measuring device or cup. Adverse effects of bismuth subsalicylate include darkening of the stools or tongue, a harmless effect

that disappears once the drug is stopped, and ringing in the ears or hearing loss. If ear-related problems occur, it is necessary to discontinue the drug and have a prescriber evaluate the patient.

### QSEN Alert: Evidence-Based Practice

*H. pylori* infection is prevalent worldwide, but the elimination of this type of bacteria remains problematic. Jiang and Zhu [2018] investigated the addition of probiotics to the medication regimen. In a randomized controlled double-blinded study, these researchers investigated the effectiveness and safety of adding probiotics to the standard treatment for *H. pylori* infection. More than 200 subjects met the criteria of a positive breath test and confirmation through endoscopy of active gastritis or gastric ulcer. The control group was treated with a quadruple *H. pylori* eradication regimen of "colloidal bismuth pectin [0.2 g b.i.d.], lansoprazole [15 mg b.i.d.], amoxicillin [1.0 g b.i.d.], and clarithromycin [0.5 g b.i.d.] for 2 weeks, while the experimental group was treated with a quadruple *H. pylori* eradication regimen of colloidal bismuth pectin [0.2 g b.i.d.], lansoprazole [15 mg b.i.d.], amoxicillin [1.0 g b.i.d.], and clarithromycin [0.5 g b.i.d.], plus live combined bifidobacterium [2 capsules t.i.d.] for 2 weeks." The effectiveness rate of the control group was 84.7%, which was lower than that of the experimental group [84.7% vs. 94.6%, $p = .041$]. The total incidence of the adverse events in the control group was also statistically higher than in the experimental group [$p = .023$]. These findings confirmed that adding probiotics can improve the effectiveness and safety of standard *H. pylori* treatment.

## NCLEX Success

3. **Which fact regarding administration should the nurse include in patient teaching about the drug sucralfate?**
   A. Take sucralfate concurrently with an antacid.
   B. Take sucralfate after meals.
   C. Take sucralfate before meals.
   D. Take sucralfate 2 hours before meals.

4. **The nurse would question the use of misoprostol [Cytotec] in which population?**
   A. children under 5 years of age
   B. adults with concurrent use of antacid
   C. pregnant women at all stages of pregnancy
   D. older adults with concurrent use of cimetidine

5. **Adverse effects of cimetidine include which of the following? [Select all that apply.]**
   A. headache
   B. constipation
   C. gynecomastia
   D. diarrhea
   E. confusion

### Clinical Application 37.3

- What measures could Ms. Carpenter take to prevent or minimize GERD?
- What additional patient teaching regarding antacid therapy would the nurse provide Ms. Carpenter?

## THE NURSING PROCESS

A concept map outlines the nursing process related to drug therapy considerations in this chapter. Additional nursing implications related to the disease process should also be considered in care decisions.

**Assessment**
- Assess all patients for signs and symptoms of increased gastric acid secretion evidenced by heartburn, reflux, belching, abdominal pain, nausea, and any signs of hematemesis or blood in stools.
- Assess for history of aspirin, acetaminophen, ibuprofen, or other NSAID intake.
- Assess for times of pain occurrence (e.g., ask: does pain lessen after eating?, do certain foods exacerbate pain and discomfort?).
- Assess patients for smoking or alcohol intake.
- Assess patient for psychological stress.
- Assess patient for OTC "ulcer therapy."

**Outcomes of Therapy**
The patient will
- Take medications at specific times ordered.
- Decrease or eliminate smoking and alcohol intake.
- Remain upright after eating.
- Eat frequent small meals.
- Avoid foods high in fat and acidity.
- Maintain adequate levels of nutrition and fluids, rest and sleep, and exercise.
- Cope with anxiety and stress.
- Keep appointments for follow-up care.
- Prevent or recognize and promptly treat adverse drug effects.
- Avoid pregnancy.
- Maintain family and other emotional/social support systems.
- Receive optimal instructions and information about nutritional intake and avoidance of NSAIDs.

**Nursing Interventions**
- Instruct patients to verify times for medication therapy and the rationale for dosing intervals.
- Instruct patients about positioning after eating and while sleeping.
- Instruct patients about adverse effects of medications.
- Inform patients about additional diagnostic test results, changes in therapeutic regimen, and evidence of progress.
- Consult other health care team members (e.g., physician, dietitian, social worker) on the patient's behalf when indicated.
- Assist patients in learning strategies to manage day-to-day activities and stress relief measures.

**Evaluation**
- Interview and observe for accurate drug administration.
- Interview and observe for therapeutic and adverse drug effects with each patient contact.
- Interview regarding knowledge and attitude toward the drug therapy regimen, including follow-up care and symptoms to report to health care providers.
- Interview regarding a 24-hour dietary recall for diet compliance.
- Observe and assess outpatients regarding ability to comply with follow-up care.

**Unfolding Patient Stories: Suzanne Morris • Part 1**

 Suzanne Morris is 43 years old and diagnosed with peptic ulcer disease. She is prescribed triple combination therapy with amoxicillin, clarithromycin, and pantoprazole for *H. pylori*. What patient education would the nurse provide for each medication? (Suzanne Morris's story continues in Chap. 44.)

Care for Suzanne and other patients in a realistic virtual environment: *vSim for Nursing*. Practice documenting these patients' care in DocuCare (thepoint. lww.com/DocuCareEHR).

## KEY CONCEPTS

- The most common location for a peptic ulcer is in the duodenum followed by the stomach and esophagus.
- Experts have attributed peptic ulcers to an imbalance between cell-destructive and cell-protective effects.
- Cell-destructive effects include gastric acid (hydrochloric acid), pepsin, *H. pylori* infection, and ingestion of NSAIDs.
- Cell-protective effects include secretion of mucus and bicarbonate, dilution of hydrochloric acid by food and secretions, prevention of diffusion of hydrochloric acid from the stomach back into the gastric mucosal lining, the presence of prostaglandin E, and alkalinization of gastric secretions by pancreatic juices and bile.
- Antacids are alkaline substances that neutralize acids.
- Aluminum antacids have low neutralizing capacity and often cause constipation.
- Magnesium antacids have high neutralizing capacity and may cause diarrhea and hypermagnesemia.
- People with renal impairment should not take products that contain magnesium because magnesium can accumulate in the body and cause serious adverse effects.
- Calcium antacids have high neutralizing capacity and rapid onset. The drugs may cause rebound acidity and hypercalcemia and so are not used for the treatment of peptic ulcer disease or GERD.
- The treatment of choice for *H. pylori* infection is multiple-drug therapy to eradicate the infection and heal the ulcer.

- The $H_2RAs$ (e.g., cimetidine, famotidine, nizatidine, and ranitidine) inhibit secretion of gastric acid, decreasing the acidity of gastric juices. They are indicated for prevention and treatment of heartburn, peptic ulcer disease, GERD, esophagitis, GI bleeding due to stress ulcers, and hypersecretory syndromes such as Zollinger-Ellison syndrome.
- The PPIs (e.g., omeprazole, esomeprazole, lansoprazole, pantoprazole, rabeprazole) bind irreversibility to the gastric proton pump to prevent the release of gastric acid from parietal cells into the stomach lumen. They are considered drugs of choice for treatment of heartburn, gastric and duodenal ulcers, GERD, esophagitis, and hypersecretory syndromes such as Zollinger-Ellison syndrome.
- Misoprostol is a synthetic form of prostaglandin E approved for concurrent use with NSAIDs to protect the gastric mucosa from NSAID-induced erosion and ulceration.
- The FDA has issued a **BLACK BOX WARNING ◆** to alert health care professionals that misoprostol is contraindicated in women of childbearing potential, unless effective contraceptive methods are being used, and during pregnancy, because it may induce abortion, premature birth, or birth defects.
- Sucralfate forms a protective barrier over mucosal ulcerations, protecting them from exposure to gastric juices. It requires an acid pH to be effective.

**Meet the Patient**

Carla Sexton, a 54-year-old woman, is newly diagnosed with a duodenal ulcer associated with an *Helicobacter pylori* infection. She reports that she smokes a pack of cigarettes a day and consumes alcohol on occasion. Her physician places Ms. Sexton on omeprazole and Pylera, a combination drug that contains bismuth, metronidazole, and tetracycline. Ms. Sexton asks the nurse about the Pylera. When she is informed that it contains three drugs, she responds, "Wait a minute. I don't like to take a lot of medications. Isn't this treatment excessive?"

- What is the nurse's best response?
- What other patient teaching should be included in Ms. Sexton's plan of care?

**Assessing Drug Information**

- As part of a combination regimen, the drug combination is useful in treatment of infections due to *H. pylori*. In patients with *H. pylori*–associated ulcers, eradication of the bacterium with antimicrobial drugs is preferable to long-term maintenance therapy with antisecretory drugs.
  - Omeprazole irreversibly binds to the gastric proton pump to prevent the "pumping" or release of gastric acid from parietal cells into the stomach lumen in response to all primary stimuli, histamine, gastrin, and acetylcholine. This blocks the final step of acid production.
  - PPIs, including omeprazole, are the most potent inhibitors of gastric acid secretion available, and as such are typically the drug class of choice for treatment of peptic ulcer disease, including duodenal and gastric ulcers. With duodenal and gastric ulcers, healing may occur after 2 weeks compared to 4 weeks using H$_2$RAs.
  - Nausea, diarrhea, and headache are the most frequently reported adverse effects.
- Pylera (bismuth, metronidazole, and tetracycline) is used in combination with omeprazole for the treatment of patients with *H. pylori* infection.
  - Bismuth subsalicylate demonstrates both antisecretory and antimicrobial action as well as some anti-inflammatory action; the salicylate provides an antisecretory effect; and the bismuth exhibits antimicrobial action directly against bacterial and viral gastrointestinal pathogens. The protective coating protects ulcers from stomach acid.
  - Adverse effects of bismuth include anxiety, confusion, depression, headache, slurred speech, and tinnitus.
  - Metronidazole, a nitroimidazole antibiotic, reduces the risk of and complications from duodenal ulcers. In addition, *Clostridium difficile* infections associated with pseudomembranous colitis and *Mycoplasma*, *Chlamydia*, and *Rickettsia* infections are treated with the drug.
  - Adverse effects are numerous with metronidazole. Dermatological effects are skin rash, pruritus, and thrombophlebitis at the infusion site. Central nervous system effects include seizures, peripheral paresthesias, ataxia, confusion, dizziness, and headache. The most common GI effects are nausea, vomiting, diarrhea, and metallic taste. Consumption of alcohol when taking metronidazole will produce a disulfiram reaction. This reaction results in symptoms of flushing, headache, nausea, vomiting, and chest and abdominal pain.
  - Tetracycline, an antibiotic, penetrates microbial cells by passive diffusion and an active transport system. Intracellularly, it binds to the 30S ribosomes and possibly the 50S ribosomes and inhibits microbial protein synthesis.
  - Combined with other drugs, tetracycline may be effective in the eradication of *H. pylori*, thus reducing the risk of and complications from duodenal ulcers. It is also used to treat *Mycoplasma*, *Chlamydia*, and *Rickettsia*.
  - Adverse effects of tetracycline include hypersensitivity, superinfections, GI conditions such as flatulence, diarrhea, nausea, vomiting, and epigastric distress (commonly reported). Discoloration of the teeth and enamel hypoplasia may occur in children younger than 8 years of age.

**Nursing Actions**

- Assess for allergies before any medications are administered. People with an allergy to aspirin or other salicylates should not take bismuth subsalicylate.
- Instruct Ms. Sexton that combination drug therapy that includes at least two antibiotics and an acid reducer (triple therapy), as well as occasionally bismuth subsalicylate, is recommended for patients with peptic ulcer disease who are known to be infected with *H. pylori*.
- Instruct Ms. Sexton that drinking even a small amount of alcohol while taking Pylera may cause a disulfiram-like reaction; the risk persists for up to 48 hours after completion of treatment.
- The nurse should emphasize the importance of smoking cessation. With cigarette smoking, ulcers heal more slowly with treatment, and the ulcers recur more rapidly.
- Tell Ms. Sexton that she should seek medical attention if she develops sudden, sharp abdominal pain, has a rigid, hard abdomen that is tender to touch, vomits blood or passes dark, tarry black stools, or experiences fainting, excessive sweating, or confusion.

*Visit* thePoint® *at* **http://thePoint.lww.com/Frandsen12e** *for answers to NCLEX Success questions (in Appendix A), answers to Clinical Application Case Studies (in Appendix B), and more!*

## REFERENCES AND RESOURCES

Abadi, A. T. B., & Kusters, J. G. (2016). Management of *Helicobacter pylori* infections. *BMC Gastroenterology*, *16*(1), 94. doi:10.1186/s12876-016-0496-2

Alvi, S., Javeed, A., Akhtar, B., Sharif, A., & Akhtar, M. F. (2017). Probiotics for cure of Helicobacter pylori infection: A review. *International Journal of Food Properties*, *20*(1), 22115–22222.

American Gastroenterological Association (AGA) Institute. (2016). American Gastroenterological Association medical position statement on the management of gastroesophageal reflux disease. Researchers Identify Histologic Marker for GERD. Retrieved November 8, 2016, from www.gastro.org

Ansari, S., & Yamaoka, Y. (2018). Current understanding and management of *Helicobacter pylori* infection: An updated appraisal. *FIOOO Research*, 1–7.

Coyle, C., Crawford, G., Wilkinson, J., Thomas, S. J., & Bytzer, P. (2017). Randomized clinical trial: Addition of alginate-acid (Gaviscon Double Action) to proton pump inhibitor therapy in patients with breakthrough symptoms. *Alimentary Pharmacology & Therapeutics*, *45*, 1524–1533.

Diaconu, S., Predescu, A., Moldovean, A., Pop, C. S., & Fierbinteanu-Braticevid, C. (2017). Helicobacter pylori infection: Old and new. *Journal of Medicine and Life*, *118*(2), 112–117.

Gawron, A. J., French, D. D., Pandolfino, J. E., & Howden, C. W. (2014). Economic evaluation of gastroesophageal reflux disease medical management. *PharmacoEconomics*, *32*(8), 745–758.

Hussaini, S. Z. K., Hussaini, S. Z. H., Yasmeeen, R., Unnisa, B., et al. (2018). Comparison of efficacy and pharmacoeconomics of two *Helicobacter pylori* eradication regimens in peptic ulcer disease. *Perspectives in Clinical Research*, *9*(1), 4–8.

Jiang, L., & Zhu, W. (2018). Probiotics improved the effectiveness and safety of the quadruple *Helicobacter pylori* eradication therapy. *Biomedical Research*, *29*(10), 2053–2056.

Khoder, G., Al-Menhali, A., Yassir, F., & Karam, S. M. (2016). Potential role of probiotics in the management of gastric ulcer. *Experimental and Therapeutic Medicine*, *12*(1), 3–17.

Kwack, W., Lim, Y., Lim, C., & Graham, D. Y. (2016). High dose ilaprazole/amoxicillin as first-line regimen for helicobacter pylori infection in Korea. *Gastroenterology Research and Practice, 2016*:1648047. doi:10.1155/2016/1648047

Norris, T. L. (2019). *Pathophysiology: Concepts of altered health states* (10th ed.) Philadelphia, PA: Wolters Kluwer.

Phan, J., Benhammou, J. N., & Pisegna, J. R. (2015). Gastric hypersecretory states: Investigation and management. *Current Treatment Options in Gastroenterology*, *13*(4), 386–397.

Shinozaki, S., Osawa, H., Hayashi, Y., Sakamoto, H., et al. (2017). Vonoprazan 10 mg daily is effective for the treatment of patients with proton pump inhibitor-resistant gastroesophageal reflux disease. *Biomedical Reports*, *7*, 231–235.

Tooker, L. B., & Dexter, K. (2017). Zollinger-Ellison syndrome. Not your average peptic ulcer disease. *Clinician Reviews*, *27*(7), 32–34.

Wolfe, M. M. (2020). *Proton pump inhibitors: Overview of use and adverse effects in the treatment of acid related disorders.* UpToDate, Lexi-Comp, Inc.

UpToDate. (2019). *Drug information.* Lexi-Comp, Inc.

Yadlapati, R., Dukhout, L., Pandolfino, J. E., & Keswani, R. J. (2017). The quality of care for gastroesophageal reflux disease. *Digestive Diseases and Sciences*, *62*, 569–576.

# Drug Therapy for Nausea and Vomiting

*After studying this chapter, you should be able to:*

1. Identify patients at risk for developing nausea and vomiting.
2. Discuss the phenothiazines in terms of indications and contraindications for use, routes of administration, and major adverse effects.
3. Describe selected antihistamines used to control nausea and vomiting in terms of indications and contraindications for use, routes of administration, and major adverse effects.
4. Discuss the 5-hydroxytryptamine$_3$ receptor antagonists in terms of indications and contraindications for use, routes of administration, and major adverse effects.
5. Describe the substance P/neurokinin 1 antagonist aprepitant in terms of indications and contraindications for use, routes of administration, and major adverse effects.
6. Identify the prototype drug for each drug class.
7. Identify nonpharmacologic measures to reduce nausea and vomiting.
8. Implement the nursing process in the care of patients receiving drugs for the management of nausea and vomiting.

## CLINICAL APPLICATION CASE STUDY

Nellie Snyder is a 38-year-old woman with breast cancer who is receiving radiation and chemotherapy. She is experiencing significant nausea and vomiting.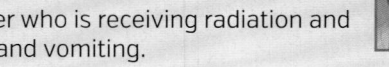

## KEY TERMS

**Anticipatory nausea and vomiting:** conditioned response prior to chemotherapy that is triggered by fears of recurrence of significant nausea and vomiting

**Cannabinoid:** derivative of marijuana

**Chemoreceptor trigger zone:** one of the central sites that relay stimuli to the vomiting center

**Emesis:** stomach contents produced with vomiting

**Emetogenic:** having the ability to cause vomiting

**Motion sickness:** action in which rapid changes in body motion stimulate receptors in the inner ear (vestibular branch of the auditory nerve, which is concerned with equilibrium) and nerve impulses are transmitted to the vomiting center

**Nausea:** an unpleasant sensation of abdominal discomfort accompanied by an urge to vomit

**Rescue antiemetic:** antiemetic use after a prophylactic antiemetic drug regimen was unsuccessful in preventing emesis

**Vomiting:** expulsion of stomach contents up through the esophagus and out of the mouth

**Vomiting center:** nucleus of cells in the medulla oblongata

## INTRODUCTION

Nausea and vomiting are common symptoms experienced by virtually everyone at some time. **Nausea**, an unpleasant sensation of abdominal discomfort accompanied by an urge to vomit, may occur without vomiting, and **vomiting**, the expulsion of stomach contents up through the esophagus and out of the mouth and occasionally nose, may occur without prior nausea, but the two symptoms often occur together. Antiemetic drugs are used to prevent or treat nausea and vomiting. They are usually contraindicated if their use may prevent or delay diagnosis or may mask signs and symptoms of drug toxicity.

## OVERVIEW OF NAUSEA AND VOMITING

### Etiology

Symptoms of nausea and vomiting may accompany almost any illness or stress situation. Causes of nausea and vomiting include the following:

- Gastrointestinal (GI) disorders, including infection or inflammation in the GI tract, liver, gallbladder, or pancreas; impaired GI motility and muscle tone (e.g., gastroparesis); and overeating or ingestion of foods or fluids that irritate the GI mucosa
- Cardiovascular, infectious, neurologic, or metabolic disorders
- Adverse effects of drug therapy; nausea and vomiting are the most common. Although the symptoms may occur with most drugs, they are especially associated with alcohol, aspirin, digoxin, anticancer drugs, antimicrobials, estrogen preparations, and opioid analgesics.
- Pain and other noxious stimuli, such as unpleasant sights and odors
- Emotional disturbances; physical or mental stress
- Radiation therapy
- Motion sickness
- Postoperative status, which may include pain, impaired GI motility, and receiving various medications
- Pregnancy
- Migraines

### Pathophysiology

Vomiting occurs when the **vomiting center** (a nucleus of cells in the medulla oblongata) is stimulated (Fig. 38.1). Five neurotransmitter receptors are significantly involved in the vomiting reflex; these include the muscarinic (M1), dopamine ($D_2$), histamine ($H_1$), 5-hydroxytryptamine$_3$ (5-HT$_3$), and substance P/neurokinin 1 (NK1) receptors. When stimulated, the vomiting center initiates efferent impulses that stimulate the salivary center; cause closure of the glottis, contraction of abdominal muscles and the diaphragm, relaxation of the gastroesophageal sphincter; and reverse peristalsis, which moves stomach contents toward the mouth for ejection.

Stimuli are then relayed to the vomiting center by afferent signals from the **chemoreceptor trigger zone** (CTZ), as well as the cerebral cortex, the sensory organs, and the vestibular apparatus. The CTZ, composed of neurons in the fourth ventricle, can be activated by a variety of stimuli, including the presence of emetic substances (e.g., toxins, chemotherapy, opioids, ipecac) in the blood and cerebrospinal fluid and stimuli from the pharynx and GI tract. In cancer chemotherapy, drugs that have the ability to cause vomiting are called **emetogenic**. They are thought to stimulate the release of serotonin from the enterochromaffin cells of the small intestine; this released serotonin then activates 5-HT$_3$ receptors located on vagal afferent nerves in the CTZ to initiate the vomiting reflex. Activation of the CTZ is also thought to play a role in the nausea and vomiting associated with pregnancy. **Anticipatory nausea and vomiting** triggered by memories and fear of nausea and vomiting is mediated by afferent signals from the higher centers of the cerebral cortex to the vomiting center. Noxious stimuli such as unpleasant odors or sights as well as pain are transmitted by afferent pathways from the sensory organs to the vomiting center. In **motion sickness**, rapid changes in body motion stimulate receptors in the inner ear (vestibular branch of the auditory nerve, which is concerned with equilibrium), and nerve impulses are transmitted to the vomiting center.

### Clinical Manifestations

As previously stated, nausea is an unpleasant abdominal sensation that is often, but not always, accompanied by vomiting. **Emesis** is the stomach contents produced with vomiting.

### Drug Therapy

Antiemetic drugs are indicated to prevent and treat nausea and vomiting associated with surgery, pain, motion sickness, cancer chemotherapy, radiation therapy, pregnancy, and other causes. Several classes of these drugs are available, which antagonize the neurotransmitter receptors that play a role in the physiology of nausea and vomiting by acting on the vomiting center, CTZ, cerebral cortex, vestibular apparatus, or a combination of these. The antiemetic drugs in this chapter are classified according to their primary action. However, some agents affect multiple receptors.

In general, the drugs are more effective in prophylaxis than treatment. Most antiemetic agents are available in oral, parenteral, and rectal dosage forms. Generally, oral forms are preferred for prophylactic use, and rectal or parenteral forms are preferred for therapeutic use. Prompt treatment of vomiting is more effective than in managing long-term vomiting.

Nurses should be aware that pregnant women should not take any medication without the guidance of their health care provider. Some antiemetics are dangerous during pregnancy and can cause damage to the fetus. However, when the nausea and vomiting associated with pregnancy are not controlled with lifestyle measures, some pharmacologic interventions may be appropriate. Interventions used depend on the severity of the disorder and are focused on improving the symptoms while minimizing risks to mother and fetus. See Chapter 6 for additional information on antiemetics used during pregnancy.

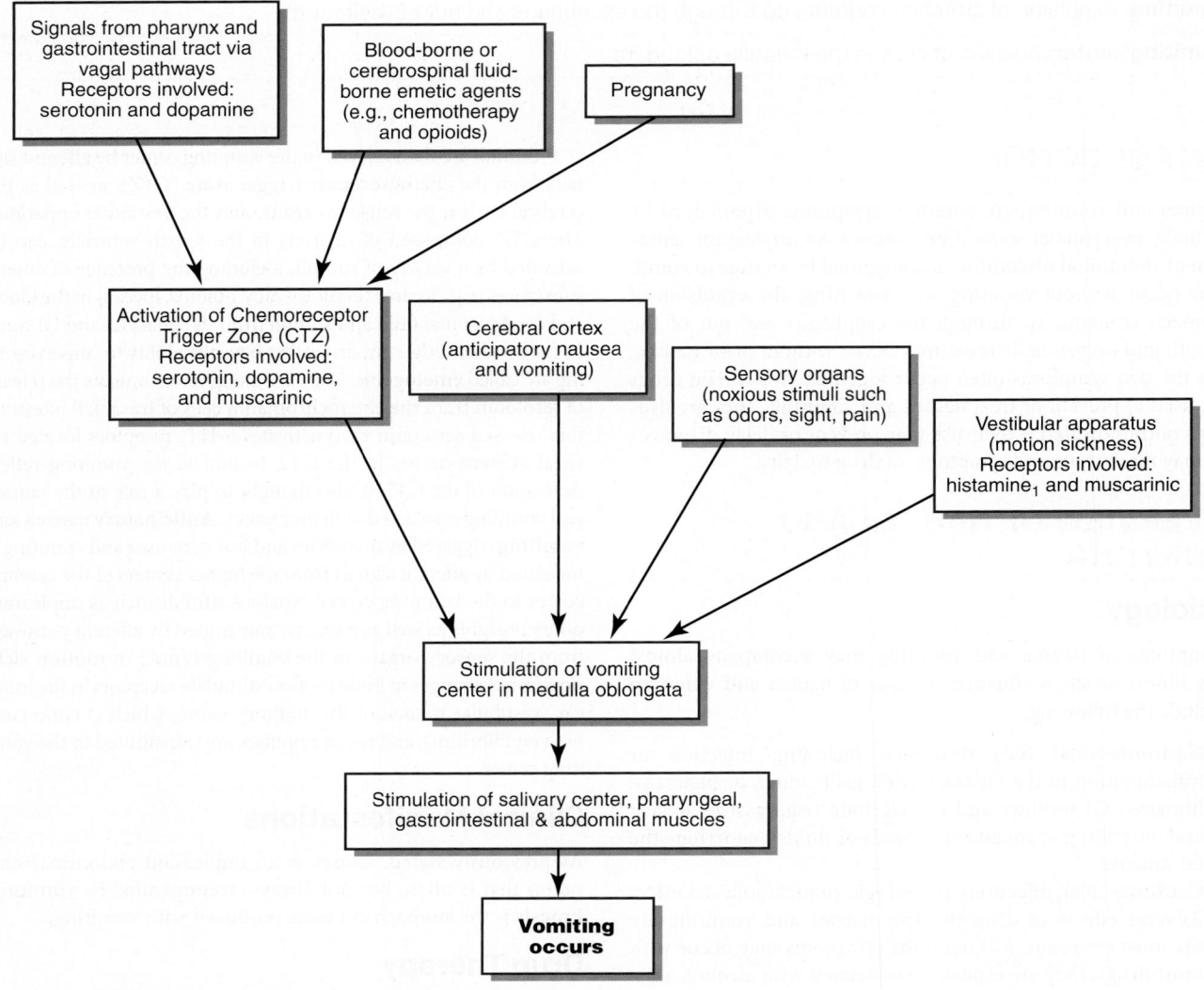

**Figure 38.1.** Pathophysiology of nausea and vomiting.

Table 38.1 and the following sections describe major antiemetic drugs.

## PHENOTHIAZINES

Phenothiazines are first-generation (typical) antipsychotic drugs that depress the central nervous system (CNS). They are the first group of drugs to exhibit extensive activity in the prevention of chemotherapy-induced emesis; they are also used to treat schizophrenia or psychosis (see Chap. 56). These drugs act primarily by antagonizing $D_2$-dopamine receptors in the area postrema of the midbrain, therefore decreasing the effect of dopamine in the brain. They also possess $M_1$-muscarinic and $H_1$-histamine blocking effects.

Dosage and route of administration depend primarily on the reason for use. Doses of phenothiazines are much smaller for antiemetic effects than for antipsychotic effects; not all phenothiazines are effective antiemetics. In this discussion, **promethazine** (Promethegan), with its antiemetic action, serves as the prototype.

**TABLE 38.1**

## Drugs Administered for the Treatment of Nausea and Vomiting

| Drug Class | Prototype | Other Drugs in the Class |
|---|---|---|
| Phenothiazines | Promethazine (Promethegan) | Chlorpromazine<br>Perphenazine<br>Prochlorperazine (Compro) |
| Antihistamines | Hydroxyzine (Vistaril) | Diphenhydramine<br>Dimenhydrinate<br>Doxylamine succinate with pyridoxine hydrochloride<br>   (Diclegis, Bonjesta)<br>Meclizine (Antivert, Dramamine Less Drowsy,<br>   Motion-Time) |
| 5-HT$_3$ (serotonin) receptor antagonists | Ondansetron (Zofran, Zuplenz) | Dolasetron<br>Granisetron (Sancuso, Sustol)<br>Palonosetron (Aloxi) |
| Substance P/neurokinin 1 receptor antagonists | Aprepitant (Emend) | Netupitant/palonosetron (Akynzeo)<br>Rolapitant (Varubi) |
| Miscellaneous agents | | Olanzapine (Zyprexa)<br>Dronabinol (Marinol, Syndros)<br>Nabilone (Cesamet)<br>Phosphorated carbohydrate solution (Emetrol)<br>Scopolamine (Transderm Scop) |

## Pharmacokinetics

Promethazine is rapidly absorbed following oral administration and undergoes extensive first-pass metabolism in the liver. Clinical effects are apparent within 20 minutes after oral, intramuscular, or rectal administration; the effects last 4 to 6 hours. Metabolism occurs in the liver, with excretion in the urine.

## Action

Promethazine and other phenothiazines have widespread effects on the body. The therapeutic effects in nausea and vomiting are attributed to their ability to block dopamine from receptor sites in the brain and CTZ.

## Use

Promethazine is used for the prevention and treatment of nausea and vomiting associated with surgery, anesthesia, migraines, chemotherapy, and motion sickness. Table 38.2 presents specific information about the use of promethazine and other phenothiazines in the treatment of nausea and vomiting, including dosages for adults and children.

### Use in Children

The U.S. Food and Drug Administration (FDA) has issued a **BLACK BOX WARNING** ◆ alerting nurses that promethazine is contraindicated in children younger than 2 years of age because of the risk of potentially fatal respiratory depression. In addition, promethazine should not be used in children with hepatic disease, Reye's syndrome, a history of sleep apnea, or a family history of sudden infant death syndrome. Newer agents, such as ondansetron and aprepitant, are recommended for management of postoperative nausea and vomiting in pediatric patients.

### Use in Older Adults

Older adults may have increased concerns with the adverse anticholinergic effects (e.g., dizziness, acute confusion, delirium, dry mouth, tachycardia, blurred vision, urinary retention, constipation).

### Use in Patients With Renal Impairment

A dose reduction may be necessary in patients with renal impairment to avoid the possibility of adverse effects, toxicity, or increased sensitivity to phenothiazines.

### Use in Patients With Hepatic Impairment

Phenothiazines are metabolized in the liver. Therefore, the presence of liver disease (e.g., cirrhosis, hepatitis) may slow metabolism and prolong drug elimination half-life, with resultant accumulation and increased risk of adverse effects. Thus, the drugs should be used cautiously in patients with hepatic impairment. Cholestatic jaundice may occur with promethazine.

## Adverse Effects

With promethazine, common side effects include blurred vision, urinary retention, dry mouth, photosensitivity, drowsiness, and confusion.

**TABLE 38.2**

**DRUGS AT A GLANCE: Phenothiazines**

| Drug | Pregnancy Category | Routes and Dosage Ranges | |
|---|---|---|---|
| | | **Adults** | **Children** |
| ⓟ **Promethazine** (Promethegan) | C | PO, IM, IV, rectal suppository 12.5–25 mg every 4–6 h (max dose PO, IM, rectal 50 mg; IV 25 mg) | >2 y: PO, IM, IV rectal suppository 0.25–1.0 mg/kg every 4–6 h (max dose 25 mg); use lowest dose possible to prevent respiratory depression |
| Chlorpromazine (❋ Teva-Chlorpromazine) | C | PO 10–25 mg every 4–6 h IM, IV 25–50 mg every 4–6 h IV (during surgery) 2 mg at 2-min intervals to not exceed 25 mg | >6 mo and ≤45.5 kg: PO, IM, IV 0.55 mg/kg/dose every 6–8 h as needed. Max for children <5 y or weighing <22.7 kg is 40 mg/d; max for children ≥5 y or weighing 22.7–45.5 kg is 75 mg/d >6 mo and >45.5 kg: PO 10–25 mg every 4–6 h as needed IM, IV 25 mg; if no hypotension, then 25–50 mg every 4–6 h as needed |
| Perphenazine (❋ PMS-Perphenazine) | C | PO 8–16 mg daily in divided doses Max daily dose 24 mg if necessary | >12 y: PO 8 mg daily in divided doses. Early dose reduction is desirable |
| Prochlorperazine (Compro; ❋ PMS-Prochlorperazine, Prochlorazine) | C | PO 10–25 mg 3 or 4 times daily (sustained-release capsule, 10 mg twice daily) IM 5–10 mg every 3–4 h to a maximum of 40 mg daily IV 2.5–10 mg every 3–4 h Rectal suppository 25 mg twice daily | >10 kg: PO 0.4 mg/kg/d, in 3 or 4 divided doses IM 0.2 mg/kg as a single dose Rectal suppository 0.4 mg/kg/d, in 3 or 4 divided doses |

## Contraindications

Contraindications to the use of promethazine include known hypersensitivity to the drug. Cautious use is necessary in people with glaucoma because the drug possesses antimuscarinic activity.

## Nursing Implications

### Preventing Interactions

Several medications interact with promethazine, increasing its effects (Box 38.1). Herbal interactions with promethazine have been reported with kava kava, St. John's wort, and valerian; an increased risk of CNS depression is a possibility. No herbs or foods that decrease the effects of promethazine have been identified.

### Administering the Medication

The FDA has issued a **BLACK BOX WARNING ◆** alerting nurses that promethazine is contraindicated for subcutaneous administration. The preferred parenteral route of administration is intramuscular, which reduces risk of surrounding muscle and tissue damage. However, the drug can cause pain at the injection site. The nurse avoids intravenous (IV) administration, if possible, because the drug can cause severe tissue injury.

### Assessing for Therapeutic Effects

The nurse observes for prevention or resolution of nausea and vomiting.

### Assessing for Adverse Effects

The nurse assesses for associated adverse anticholinergic effects (dry mouth, blurred vision, urinary retention, constipation, acute confusion, dizziness, tachycardia). It is necessary to be aware that hallucinations, convulsions, and sudden death may occur with excessive doses. The nurse also assesses tissue integrity with injection of the drug because the drug may cause severe tissue injury; burning and pain at the IV site justify immediate discontinuation of the drug.

**BOX 38.1    Drug Interactions: Promethazine**

**Drugs That Increase the Effects of Promethazine**

- Escitalopram, gabapentin, and zolpidem
  *Have additive respiratory depressant effects*
- Ethanol
  *Increases the risk of central nervous system depression and psychomotor impairment*
- Duloxetine
  *Increases the plasma concentration*

## BOX 38.2    *Patient Teaching Guidelines: Antiemetic Drugs*

**General Considerations**

- Try to identify the circumstances that cause or aggravate nausea and vomiting and avoid them when possible.
- Drugs are more effective in preventing nausea and vomiting than in stopping them. Thus, they should be taken before the causative event when possible.
- Do not eat, drink, or take oral medications during acute vomiting episodes, to avoid aggravating the stomach upset.
- Lying down may help nausea and vomiting to subside; activity tends to increase stomach upset.
- After your stomach has settled down, try to take enough fluids to prevent dehydration and potentially serious problems. Tea, broth, and gelatins are usually tolerated.
- Do not drive an automobile or operate dangerous machinery if drowsy from antiemetic drugs, to avoid injury.
- If you take antiemetic drugs regularly, do not drink alcohol or take other drugs without consulting a health care provider. Several drugs interact with antiemetic agents, to increase adverse effects.
- Dronabinol, which is derived from marijuana and recommended only for nausea and vomiting associated with cancer chemotherapy, can cause dizziness, drowsiness, mood changes, and other mind-altering effects. You

should avoid alcohol and other drugs that cause drowsiness. Also, do not drive or perform hazardous tasks requiring alertness, coordination, or physical dexterity, to decrease risks of injury.

**Self or Caregiver Administration**

- Take the drugs as prescribed. Do not increase dosage, take more often, or take when drowsy, dizzy, or unsteady on your feet. Several of the drugs cause sedation and other adverse effects, which are more severe if too much is taken.
- To prevent motion sickness, take medication 30 minutes before travel and then every 4 to 6 hours, if necessary, to avoid or minimize adverse effects.
- Take or give antiemetic drugs 30 to 60 minutes before a nausea-producing event, when possible. This includes cancer chemotherapy, radiation therapy, changing of painful dressings, or other treatments.
- Take dronabinol only when you can be supervised by a responsible adult because of its sedative and mind-altering effects.
- Aprepitant [Emend] reduces the effectiveness of oral contraceptives; therefore, use an alternative form of birth control during therapy and for 1 month after therapy.

### *Patient Teaching*

The nurse teaches patients taking promethazine to use the lowest effective dosage and not to take other drugs with respiratory depressant effects concurrently. Box 38.2 presents additional patient teaching guidelines.

## Other Drugs in the Class

Phenothiazines are effective antiemetic agents. However, because of their adverse effects (e.g., sedation, cognitive impairment, extrapyramidal reactions), they are mainly indicated if vomiting is severe and cannot be controlled by other measures or only when a few doses are needed. Prochlorperazine (Compro), which has a side effect profile similar to that of promethazine, is the most commonly used antiemetic in this class for the treatment of severe nausea and vomiting associated with anesthesia. Chlorpromazine is used less often than prochlorperazine for nausea and vomiting but is more commonly used in the treatment of psychosis and psychotic symptoms in other disorders (see Chap. 56). It is also used with intractable hiccups and treatment of nausea and vomiting associated with anesthesia. Perphenazine is used to manage severe nausea and vomiting. However, the FDA has issued a **BLACK BOX WARNING ◆** for perphenazine because elderly patients with dementia-related psychosis treated with perphenazine and other antipsychotic drugs have an increased risk of death. It is important to reduce the dose as soon as possible to minimize significant adverse effects, including bradycardia, cardiac arrest, hypotension, catatonic-like states, extrapyramidal symptoms, and a blue-gray discoloration of the skin.

## ANTIHISTAMINES

Antihistamines are used primarily to prevent histamine from exerting its widespread effects on body tissues (see Chap. 32). The antihistamines used as antiemetic agents are the "classic" antihistamines or $H_1$ receptor blocking agents (as differentiated from cimetidine and related drugs, which are $H_2$ receptor blocking agents). Not all antihistamines are effective as antiemetic agents. **Hydroxyzine** (Vistaril) is the prototype of the class.

## Pharmacokinetics

When administered orally, hydroxyzine is rapidly absorbed from the GI tract, with its effect noticeable within 30 minutes. The drug is metabolized in the liver, and the main metabolite is cetirizine. The half-life of hydroxyzine is, on average, 14 hours for adults, but it can be as short as 5 hours for small children and as long as 30 hours for elderly people. Hydroxyzine is excreted into the urine in the form of its metabolites.

## Action

Hydroxyzine and other antihistamines are thought to relieve nausea and vomiting by blocking the action of acetylcholine in the brain.

## Use

Hydroxyzine may be effective in treating nausea and vomiting and preventing and treating motion sickness. Hydroxyzine is also used as a sedative to treat anxiety. Additionally, the drug is given in combination with other medications during anesthesia. Table 38.3 presents dosage information for the antihistamines.

**TABLE 38.3**

## DRUGS AT A GLANCE: Antihistamines

| Drug | Pregnancy Category | Routes and Dosage Ranges | |
|---|---|---|---|
| | | **Adults** | **Children** |
| Ⓟ **Hydroxyzine** (Vistaril; ✹ NOVO-Hydroxyzine, Atarax, PMS-Hydroxyzine HCl) | D | PO IM 25–100 mg every 4–6 h as needed | IM 1.1 mg/kg in 4 divided doses (max 100 mg) |
| Dimenhydrinate (✹ Gravol) | B | PO 50–100 mg every 4–6 h as needed (max 400 mg in 24 h) IM 50 mg as needed IV 50 mg in 10 mL of sodium chloride injection, over 2 min (max 100 mg every 4 h) | 6–12 y: PO 25–50 mg every 4–6 h (max 150 mg in 24 h) IM 1.25 mg/kg four times daily (max 300 mg in 24 h) |
| Doxylamine succinate with pyridoxine hydrochloride (Diclegis, Bonjesta; ✹ Diclectin) | C | Nausea and vomiting of pregnancy: Doxylamine 10 mg/pyridoxine 10 mg/tablet (Diclegis): 2 tablets at bedtime on day 1 and 2; if symptoms continue, 1 tablet in morning and 2 tablets at bedtime on day 3; if symptoms continue, increase to 1 tablet in morning, 1 tablet in midafternoon, and 2 tablets at bedtime on day 4 (to max of doxylamine 40 mg/pyridoxine 40 mg [4 tablets] per day) Doxylamine 20 mg/pyridoxine 20 mg (Bonjesta): Initial: one tablet at bedtime on day 1; if symptoms persist on day 2, increase to 1 tablet in morning and 1 tablet at bedtime (maximum: doxylamine 40 mg/pyridoxine 40 mg [2 tablets] per day) | Not indicated for use in children |
| Meclizine (Antivert, Dramamine Less Drowsy, Motion-Time) | B | Motion sickness: PO 25–50 mg 1 h before travel Vertigo: PO 25–100 mg daily in divided doses | Motion sickness, >12 y: PO 25–50 mg/d divided into 2 or 3 doses |

## Use in Children

In children, the recommended dosage of hydroxyzine is based on age and weight.

## Use in Older Adults

According to the Beers Criteria (see Chap. 5), hydroxyzine is considered potentially inappropriate for use in older adults. Dosage reduction may be appropriate with older adults due to an increased sedative potential.

## Use in Patients With Renal Impairment

Because hydroxyzine is excreted in the urine, dosage adjustments and more intensive monitoring of adverse effects may be required in people with renal impairment.

## Use in Patients With Hepatic Impairment

Likewise, because hydroxyzine is metabolized in the liver, dosage adjustments and more intensive monitoring of adverse effects may be required in people with hepatic impairment.

## Use in Patients Receiving Home Care

Antiemetics are usually given orally or by rectal suppository in the home setting. The home care nurse may need to assess patients for possible causes of nausea and vomiting and assist patients and caregivers with appropriate use of the drugs and other interventions to prevent fluid and electrolyte depletion. Excessive sedation may occur with usual doses of antiemetics and is more likely with high doses. This may be minimized by avoiding high doses and assessing the patient's level of consciousness before each dose. Teaching safety precautions with sedating drugs may also be needed.

## Adverse Effects

With hydroxyzine, adverse anticholinergic effects include drowsiness, dizziness, confusion, dry mouth, thickened respiratory secretions, blurred vision, urinary retention, and tachycardia.

## Contraindications

Contraindications to hydroxyzine include known sensitivity to the drug.

## Nursing Implications

### Preventing Interactions

Many medications interact with hydroxyzine, increasing its effects (Box 38.3). Several medications that can cause CNS depression, such as sedatives, tranquilizers, muscle relaxants, and antidepressants, can have an increased sedative effect with the concomitant use of hydroxyzine. No herbs or foods appear to decrease or increase the effects of hydroxyzine.

### Administering the Medication

Oral administration of hydroxyzine is often unsuccessful with nausea and vomiting. It is important to give the medication intramuscularly deep into a large muscle, not subcutaneously. IV administration can result in a sterile abscess with damage to tissue.

### Assessing for Therapeutic Effects

The nurse assesses for the absence of nausea and vomiting.

### Assessing for Adverse Effects

The nurse assesses for the presence of anticholinergic effects, including blurred vision, urinary retention, constipation, thick secretions, and blurred vision. Patients with narrow-angle glaucoma, prostatic hyperplasia, and asthma are at greater risk for adverse effects.

### Patient Teaching

The nurse instructs patients to take medication as directed and to enhance safety precautions due to adverse effects. Adverse effects may impair thinking or reactions, so operating a motor vehicle should be avoided. Box 38.2 outlines additional patient teaching guidelines.

## Other Drugs in the Class

Diphenhydramine, dimenhydrinate, and meclizine (Antivert, Dramamine Less Drowsy, Motion-Time) are also used to prevent nausea, vomiting, dizziness, and vertigo associated with motion sickness. Meclizine is also given to manage vertigo associated with disease affecting the vestibular system. Dimenhydrinate is available over the counter, and meclizine is dispensed by prescription. The initial dose should be taken 1 hour prior to travel to reduce the risk of motion sickness. Thereafter, the dose may be repeated every 24 hours for the duration of the travel. For vestibular diseases, meclizine should be taken at the onset of symptoms. As with hydroxyzine, it is necessary to instruct patients taking dimenhydrate to use caution while driving,

operating machinery, or performing other hazardous activities due to the associated drowsiness. (The addition of theophylline to the formulation is designed to counteract drowsiness.) Dimenhydrinate typically takes a minimum of 4 hours to take full effect. Meclizine becomes effective in about 1 hour. This drug is less likely to cause drowsiness, but people taking the drug should use caution when participating in hazardous activities and avoid using alcohol.

In 2013, the FDA approved Diclegis, a combination of doxylamine succinate, an antihistamine, and pyridoxine, a form of vitamin B6, for the treatment of nausea and vomiting during pregnancy. Systematic reviews of clinical trials have shown that pyridoxine alone improves mild to moderate nausea in pregnancy but does not significantly reduce vomiting; however, the combination is effective.

Diclegis was the first medication specifically approved to treat nausea and vomiting during pregnancy after another combination of doxylamine and pyridoxine, Bendectin, was voluntarily withdrawn from the market in 1983 because of lawsuits alleging teratogenicity (there was no proven association between its use and birth defects). Currently, strong scientific evidence supports its safety and efficacy. In addition, numerous studies, including a meta-analysis of controlled studies on outcome of pregnancies in women taking the drug combination, have established the fetal safety of the combination.

 **QSEN Alert: Evidence-Based Practice**

In a randomized placebo-controlled trial in women with nausea and vomiting of pregnancy, Koren et al. (2015) found that a combination preparation of doxylamine succinate 10 mg and pyridoxine 10 mg administered in recommended doses was not associated with an increase in the rate of adverse events compared to a placebo. Data from patient diaries, clinical examination, and laboratory testing demonstrated that the combination preparation was safe and well tolerated by pregnant women.

**NCLEX Success**

1. The nurse knows that antiemetics are most effective when administered
   A. before an emetogenic event occurs
   B. during an episode of nausea but before vomiting has occurred
   C. after the patient has experienced nausea and vomiting
   D. any time; timing of administration has no impact on drug effectiveness

2. The nurse would question an order for which of the following antiemetics for treatment of motion sickness–induced nausea?
   A. prochlorperazine
   B. dimenhydrinate
   C. meclizine
   D. scopolamine

 **BOX 38.3 Drug Interactions: Hydroxyzine**

**Drugs That Increase the Effects of Hydroxyzine**
- Alcohol, gabapentin, levetiracetam, and lamotrigine
  *Increase the risk of respiratory depression*
- Seroquel
  *Increases the risk of severe extrapyramidal reactions*

# 5-HYDROXYTRYPTAMINE₃ (5-HT₃) OR SEROTONIN RECEPTOR ANTAGONISTS

The 5-HT$_3$ receptor antagonists approved for use in the United States are the cornerstones of therapy for the control of acute emesis caused by chemotherapy agents with moderate to high emetogenic potential. In addition, the class is usually considered drugs of first choice for postoperative nausea and vomiting. Ⓟ **Ondansetron** (Zofran, Zuplenz) is the prototype of the 5-HT$_3$ receptor antagonists.

## Pharmacokinetics

Oral ondansetron is well absorbed from the GI tract and undergoes some first-pass metabolism. The drug's half-life is 3 to 5.5 hours in most patients and 9 to 20 hours in patients with moderate or severe liver impairment. With the oral forms (disintegrating tablet or soluble film), action begins in 30 to 60 minutes and peaks in about 2 hours. With the IV form, onset and peak of drug action are immediate. The bioavailability is slightly increased by the presence of food but is unaffected by antacids.

## Action

Ondansetron and the other 5-HT$_3$ receptor antagonists antagonize serotonin receptors, preventing their activation by the effects of emetogenic drugs and toxins.

## Use

Ondansetron is used to prevent or treat moderate to severe nausea and vomiting associated with cancer chemotherapy, radiation therapy, and postoperative status. Table 38.4 presents dosage information for the 5-HT$_3$ receptor antagonists.

### Use in Children

The drug is indicated for use in children, although little information is available about its use in children younger than 6 months of age. The American Society of Clinical Oncology recommends the use of a 5-HT$_3$ receptor antagonist plus a corticosteroid before administering high-dose chemotherapy or chemotherapy with high to moderate emetic risk to pediatric oncology patients.

### Use in Older Adults

Dosage adjustment is not required in patients older than 65 years of age. Researchers have observed no overall differences in safety or effectiveness in older adults compared with younger patients.

### Use in Patients With Hepatic Impairment

The drug's half-life is significantly increased in patients with moderate to severe hepatic impairment. This increases the risk of adverse effects.

### Use in Patients Receiving Home Care

Oral administration of the drug may be given in the home setting. The home care nurse assesses for resolution of nausea and vomiting. Diarrhea is a common adverse effect; therefore, the nurse also needs to assist patients and caregivers with appropriate use of the drugs and other interventions to prevent fluid and electrolyte depletion.

## Adverse Effects

Adverse effects of ondansetron are usually mild to moderate. Common ones include diarrhea, headache, dizziness, constipation, fatigue, transient elevation of liver enzymes, and pain at the injection site.

## Contraindications

Contraindications to ondansetron include known hypersensitivity to the drug.

## Nursing Implications

### Preventing Interactions

Phenytoin, carbamazepine, rifampin, and other inducers of the cytochrome 450 (CYP) 3A4 enzymes increase the clearance of ondansetron and decrease serum concentrations. No dosage adjustment of ondansetron appears necessary for people taking these drugs based on available data. The use of ondansetron with apomorphine is contraindicated due to the potential of a significant drop of blood pressure or loss of consciousness with concurrent use. St. John's wort may decrease ondansetron levels.

### Administering the Medication

It is important to leave the disintegrating tablet in the blister pack until administration. Gentle removal is essential; it is necessary to peel back the blister backing and not push the tablet through the foil. The oral film dissolves rapidly on the tongue, without the need for water.

### Assessing for Therapeutic Effects

The nurse assesses for verbal reports of decreased nausea and the absence of vomiting.

### Assessing for Adverse Effects

Because headache and diarrhea are the most common adverse effects, the nurse gives special attention when assessing for these effects. It is also necessary to evaluate for stamina and balance. The nurse should note that the use of ondansetron may mask a progressive ileus and gastric distension following abdominal surgery or in patients with chemotherapy-induced nausea and vomiting.

### Patient Teaching

The drug may impair thinking or reactions, which means that it is necessary to advise patients to use caution with driving or other tasks requiring mental alertness. The nurse teaches patients with phenylketonuria that the oral disintegrating tablets contain phenylalanine. Box 38.2 presents other patient teaching guidelines.

## Other Drugs in the Class

The other 5-HT$_3$ receptor antagonist drugs may be less beneficial as rescue drugs in the treatment of chemotherapy-induced

## TABLE 38.4

## DRUGS AT A GLANCE: 5-Hydroxytryptamine₃ (5-HT₃ or Serotonin) Receptor Antagonists

| Drug | Pregnancy Category | Routes and Dosage Ranges | |
|---|---|---|---|
| | | **Adults** | **Children** |
| Ⓟ **Ondansetron** (Zofran, Zuplenz; 🍁 ACT Ondansetron, APO-Ondansetron, Zofran ODT) | B | Chemotherapy-induced nausea and vomiting (highly emetogenic chemotherapy): PO, 8 mg, given day chemotherapy is administered, IV 8 mg or 0.15 mg/kg given as a single dose on the day of chemotherapy; IV doses >16 mg not recommended by manufacturer due to the potential for prolongation of QT internal on electrocardiogram; given in regimen that includes dexamethasone and aprepitant or fosaprepitant<br>Chemotherapy-induced nausea and vomiting (moderately emetogenic chemotherapy): PO, 16 mg, given as 8 mg twice daily on day chemotherapy is administered, IV 8 mg or 0.15 mg/kg given as a single dose on day of chemotherapy; IV doses >16 mg not recommended due to the potential for prolongation of QT internal on electrocardiogram; given in regimen that includes dexamethasone and aprepitant or fosaprepitant<br>Prevention of radiation therapy-induced nausea and vomiting: PO 8 mg 1–2 h before irradiation then 8 mg every 8 h after first dose for 102 d after completion of radiation<br>Postoperative nausea and vomiting prevention: IV, IM 4 mg 1/2 h before end of anesthesia, IV 4 mg given over 2–5 min, PO 8 mg as an oral disintegrating tablet or soluble film ½–1 h before surgery; PO can be repeated in high-risk patients at discharge and on days 1 and 2 | Chemotherapy-induced nausea and vomiting:<br>>6 mo: IV 0.15 mg/kg for 3 doses, given ½ h before chemotherapy, repeat in 4 and 8 h. Infuse over 15 min<br>4–11 y: PO 4 mg given for 3 doses ½ h before chemotherapy, repeat in 8 and 16 h for 1–2 d after chemotherapy completed<br>≥12 y: PO 8 mg ½ h before chemotherapy, repeat<br>Postoperative nausea and vomiting, prevention<br>≥5 mo to 12 y:≤40 kg to IV 0.1 mg/kg, max 4 mg/dose<br>>40 kg: IV 4 mg<br>Given over 2–5 min; PO may be administered, if indicated |
| Dolasetron | C | Chemotherapy-induced nausea and vomiting: PO, 100 mg, given up to 1 h prior to chemotherapy<br>Postoperative nausea and vomiting: IV 12.5 mg 15 min before reversal of anesthesia, PO 100 mg within 2 h prior to surgery | Chemotherapy-induced nausea and vomiting (>2 y): PO 1.8 mg/kg (max 100 mg) given up to 1 h prior to chemotherapy<br>Postoperative nausea and vomiting (>2 y):<br>IV 0.35 mg/kg (max 12.5 mg) 15 min before the reversal of anesthesia or with nausea or vomiting<br>PO 1.2 mg/kg (max 100 mg) within 2 h prior to surgery |
| Granisetron (Sancuso, Sustol; 🍁 APO-Granisetron, NAT-Granisetron) | B | Chemotherapy-induced nausea and vomiting:<br>IV, 10 mcg/kg over 5 min, beginning ½ h prior to chemotherapy<br>PO, 2 mg, given up to 1 h prior to chemotherapy, or 1 mg given up to 1 h prior to chemotherapy and repeated in 12 h<br>PO, 2 mg, given up to 1 h prior to chemotherapy<br>Transdermal patch: apply one patch at least 24 h prior to chemotherapy for prophylaxis; remove patch 24 h after chemotherapy completion. Patch may be worn up to 7 d<br>Postoperative nausea and vomiting: IV 1 mg undiluted immediately before induction or reversal or after surgery | Chemotherapy-induced nausea and vomiting (2–16 y): IV 10 mcg/kg beginning ½ h prior to chemotherapy |
| Palonosetron (Aloxi; 🍁 Aloxi) | B | Prevention of chemotherapy-induced nausea and vomiting: IV 0.25 mg about 30 min prior to chemotherapy<br>Prevention of postoperative nausea and vomiting: IV 0.075 mg as a single dose immediately prior to induction of anesthesia | Prevention of chemotherapy-induced nausea and vomiting (≥1 mo): IV 20 mcg/kg (max 1.5 mg)<br>≥17 y: see adult dosage |

nausea and vomiting and more effective in the prevention of this condition. Granisetron (Sancuso, Sustol) may be given intravenously, orally, or subcutaneously. The oral route of dolasetron is approved for chemotherapy-related nausea and vomiting; the IV route is only used for prevention of postoperative nausea and vomiting. Palonosetron (Aloxi) is given only intravenously.

As with ondansetron, other 5-HT$_3$ receptor antagonists are associated with dose-dependent increases in electrocardiographic intervals, including PR, QRS duration, and QT interval. These drugs should be avoided in patients taking class I and class III antidysrhythmic agents because of concerns about the development of torsades de pointes, with prolongation of the QT interval.

### Clinical Application 38.1

- Ms. Snyder's oncologist orders ondansetron 32 mg IV to be administered 30 minutes prior to her chemotherapy and 8 to 16 mg PO every 8 hours as needed. She also receives metoclopramide 10 mg PO four times a day (30 minutes before meals and at bedtime). For what adverse effects of ondansetron does the nurse assess?

## SUBSTANCE P/NEUROKININ 1 ANTAGONISTS

Substance P is a peptide neurotransmitter in the neurokinin family. It plays a role in mediating acute chemotherapy-induced nausea and vomiting (along with serotonin) and is believed to be the primary mediator of delayed nausea and vomiting associated with chemotherapy. The oral drug **aprepitant** (Emend) and its parenteral version, fosaprepitant, are the prototype of the substance P/neurokinin 1 antagonists. Aprepitant and other substance P/neurokinin 1 antagonists are typically used in combination with a 5-HT$_3$ receptor and/or a glucocorticoid for patients receiving highly emetic chemotherapy.

## Pharmacokinetics

Aprepitant is orally absorbed, reaching peak levels 4 hours after administration. It is highly protein bound. The drug is metabolized in the liver and is excreted in urine and feces. Because aprepitant undergoes extensive hepatic metabolism by CYP450 enzyme systems, it has the potential for multiple drug interactions. After administration, the IV form, fosaprepitant, is rapidly converted in the body to aprepitant.

## Action

Aprepitant exerts its antiemetic effect by blocking the activity of substance P at NK1 receptors in the brain, inhibiting the signal to the brain that causes nausea. The drug has little or no effect on serotonin, dopamine, or corticosteroid receptors.

## Use

Prescribers often order aprepitant as part of combination therapy along with a 5-HT$_3$ receptor antagonist and corticosteroids

to treat both acute and delayed nausea and vomiting associated with chemotherapy. Other indications include prevention of postoperative nausea and vomiting. The FDA has stipulated that the IV prodrug of the oral formulation (fosaprepitant) should no longer be used to prevent nausea and vomiting associated with cancer chemotherapy in pediatric and adult patients because of the risk of abnormal heart rhythm.

Table 38.5 contains dosage information for aprepitant. No dosage adjustment is required in patients with renal disease, including those with end-stage renal disease receiving dialysis.

### Use in Children

Aprepitant appears to be well tolerated in children receiving the drug in combination with standard antiemetics for chemotherapy-induced nausea and vomiting. Additional evidence of efficacy is necessary in this population.

### Use in Patients With Hepatic Impairment

No adjustment is required in dosage for patients with mild to moderate hepatic impairment. However, no data are available regarding its use in people with severe hepatic impairment, and caution is warranted in cases of serious hepatic dysfunction.

### Use in Patients With Critical Illness

Aprepitant is used in patients with cancer who are receiving chemotherapy. The American Society of Clinical Oncology's antiemetic guidelines recommend the use of aprepitant in combination with a serotonin receptor antagonist and dexamethasone with chemotherapeutic drugs with high emetic risk. The drug is also recommended as part of a chemotherapy regimen in protocols including anthracycline, cyclophosphamide, and other chemotherapeutic agents known to cause moderate emetic risk.

## Adverse Effects

Aprepitant is well tolerated, with the most common adverse effects being fatigue, weakness, dizziness, abnormal heart rhythm, headache, and hiccups. Infusion site pain has been reported with IV administration.

## Contraindications

Contraindications to aprepitant include known hypersensitivity to the drug or use in combination with ranolazine, pimozide, or cisapride.

## Nursing Implications

### Preventing Interactions

Aprepitant is extensively metabolized by the CYP3A4 enzyme, which is particularly important in drug metabolism. Certain drugs may increase or decrease the effects of aprepitant and are affected by aprepitant's inhibitory effects (Box 38.4). It is essential to reduce oral doses of dexamethasone or methylprednisolone by 50% and the IV dose of methylprednisolone by 25% when coadministered with aprepitant because of CYP3A4 inhibition.

Aprepitant also produces significant interactions that alter the effectiveness of other medications. The drug reduces

## TABLE 38.5

# DRUGS AT A GLANCE: Substance P/Neurokinin 1 Receptor Antagonists

| Drug | Pregnancy Category | Routes and Dosage Ranges | |
|---|---|---|---|
| | | **Adults** | **Children** |
| ⓟ **Aprepitant** (Emend, Fosaprepitant dimeglumine, Cinvanti; 🍁 Emend, Emend Tri-Pack) | B | Prevention of nausea and vomiting associated with highly emetic and moderately emetic chemotherapy (administered as part of a four-drug treatment that also includes a 5-HT$_3$ receptor antagonist, olanzapine, and dexamethasone): Day 1: PO 125 mg 1 h before chemotherapy or IV 130 mg ½ h over 15 min before chemotherapy Days 2 and 3: PO 80 mg in the morning | ≥6 mo to <12 y (6–<30 kg) Day 1: PO suspension 3 mg/kg 1 h before chemotherapy and then 2 mg/kg on days 2 and 3. (regimen also includes a 5-HT$_3$ receptor antagonist, olanzapine, and dexamethasone, as indicated) ≥12 y: PO 125 mg prior to chemotherapy on day 1, followed by 80 mg once daily on days 2 and 3 (regimen also includes a 5-HT$_3$ antagonist, olanzapine, and dexamethasone, as indicated) |
| Netupitant/palonosetron (Akynzeo) | Unknown; approved in 2014 | Day 1: PO one capsule (netupitant 300 mg/palonosetron 0.5 mg) about 1 h before prior chemotherapy (regimen also includes dexamethasone) | Safety and efficacy in children not established |
| Rolapitant (Varubi) | Unknown; approved in 2015 | Day 1: PO one capsule about 1 h before prior chemotherapy (regimen also includes dexamethasone) Highly emetogenic: Day 1: PO 180 mg 1–2 h prior to chemotherapy (in combination with dexamethasone given on days 1, 2, 3, and 4 and a 5-HT$_3$ receptor antagonist) Moderately emetogenic: Day 1: PO 180 mg 1–2 h prior to chemotherapy (in combination with dexamethasone given on day 1 and a 5-HT$_3$ receptor antagonist and olanzapine, given as indicated) | Safety and efficacy in children not established |

the effectiveness of oral contraceptives for up to 28 days after administration; therefore, alternate contraceptive methods are recommended during treatment and for 1 month following administration of aprepitant.

## BOX 38.4   *Drug Interactions: Aprepitant*

### Drugs That Increase the Effects of Aprepitant

- CYP3A4 inhibitors, such as macrolide antibiotics, protease inhibitors, azole antifungal agents, nefazodone, cyclosporine, danazol, diltiazem, and verapamil
  *Alter metabolism, increasing serum levels*

### Drugs That Decrease the Effects of Aprepitant

- CYP3A4 inducers, such as carbamazepine, phenytoin, rifampin, phenobarbital, and nevirapine
  *Alter metabolism, decreasing serum levels*

### ❗ QSEN Alert: Safety

Aprepitant induces the metabolism of warfarin. It is necessary to monitor the international normalized ratio (INR) for 2 weeks after treatment is initiated, especially for the first 7 to 10 days, because a clinically significant drop in INR may occur.

Foods and herbs are also known to affect aprepitant concentrations. Grapefruit juice decreases the metabolism of aprepitant. Because this effect can last up to 24 hours, repeated juice consumption can result in a cumulative increase in the serum level of aprepitant. In contrast, St. John's wort is known to cause a decrease in serum levels.

## Administering the Medication

Patients should take aprepitant by mouth as directed with a full glass of water, with or without food. Typically, the first dose is taken 1 hour before chemotherapy and then daily in the morning for the next 2 days after the chemotherapy treatment. The recently approved IV form, fosaprepitant, a prodrug, in a dose of 150 mg, is bioequivalent to aprepitant, 125 mg, and it is appropriate to use these forms interchangeably.

### Assessing for Therapeutic Effects

The nurse assesses for the absence of nausea and vomiting after chemotherapy or during the postoperative period.

### Assessing for Adverse Effects

The nurse observes for the presence of adverse effects, such as fatigue, weakness, dizziness, headache, or hiccups. In addition, it is necessary to assess for a normal heart rhythm.

### Patient Teaching

The nurse instructs patients to take the medication as prescribed before the onset of nausea and vomiting. Alternate antiemetic medication (**rescue antiemetic**) may be necessary for who already have nausea and vomiting. Box 38.2 presents additional patient teaching guidelines.

## Other Drugs in the Class

Netupitant is available in an oral fixed combination tablet with palonosetron (Akynzeo). The combination of a selective 5-HT₃ receptor antagonist and a substance P/neurokinin 1 receptor antagonist is used for the prevention of acute and delayed nausea and vomiting associated with initial and repeat courses of cancer chemotherapy, including, but not limited to, highly emetogenic chemotherapy. Netupitant prevents nausea and vomiting during both the acute and delayed phases, and palonosetron prevents nausea and vomiting during the acute phase and after cancer chemotherapy.

Rolapitant (Varubi) has a longer plasma half-life (~7 days) than either aprepitant or fosaprepitant, but unlike these drugs, which are moderate inhibitors of CYP3A4, rolapitant does not inhibit this metabolic pathway. Therefore, no adjustment of dexamethasone is required. Rolapitant does inhibit the CYP2D6 enzyme, which is responsible for metabolizing certain drugs, such as thioridazine; the use of both drugs together is contraindicated. Adverse effects include headache, lack of energy and strength, dyspepsia, constipation, and erythema.

## MISCELLANEOUS ANTIEMETICS

Several miscellaneous agents are used individually or in multidrug regimens in the treatment of nausea and vomiting. Table 38.6 presents the dosage information for the miscellaneous agents.

### TABLE 38.6

### DRUGS AT A GLANCE: Miscellaneous Agents

| Drug | Pregnancy Category | Routes and Dosage Ranges | |
|---|---|---|---|
| | | **Adults** | **Children** |
| Olanzapine (Zyprexa; ✳ ACT Olanzapine OPT, TEVA-Olanzapine) | C | PO 10 mg on day 1 followed by 10 mg once daily, days 2–4 (in combination with dexamethasone and palonosetron on day 1 only) | Use in children not recommended for treatment of chemotherapy-induced nausea and vomiting |
| Dronabinol (Marinol, Syndros) | C | PO 5 mg/m² (square meter of body surface area) 1–3 h before chemotherapy and then every 2–4 h for a total of 4–6 doses daily. Dosage can be increased by 2.5 mg/m² increments to a maximal dose of 15 mg/m² if necessary | Same as adults for treatment of chemotherapy-induced nausea and vomiting |
| Nabilone (Cesamet; ✳ ACT-nabilone, Cesamet, PMS-nabilone) | C | PO initially, 1–2 mg twice daily; first dose 1–3 h before chemotherapy; may be administered 2–3 doses daily for course of chemotherapy continued to 48 h after the last dose | Limited data in select situations; first dose administered 1–3 h before chemotherapy <br> <18 kg: PO 0.5 mg twice daily <br> 19–30 kg: PO 1 mg twice daily <br> >30 kg: 1 mg 3 times daily |
| Phosphorated carbohydrate solution (Emetrol) | C | PO 15–30 mL repeated at 15-min intervals until vomiting ceases not to exceed 5 doses over 1 h | ≥2 y: PO 5–10 mL repeated at 15-min intervals until vomiting ceases not to exceed 5 doses over 1 h <br> ≥12 y: refer to adult dosing |
| Scopolamine (Transderm Scop; ✳ Buscopan, Transderm-V) | C | Motion sickness: PO, IM, subcutaneous, 0.6–1.0 mg as a single dose <br> Transdermal disc (1.5 mg scopolamine): placed behind the ear every 3 d if needed | Motion sickness: PO, subcutaneous, 0.006 mg as a single dose to max of 0.3 mg/dose; may be repeated every 6–8 h |

Although corticosteroids are used mainly as antiallergic, anti-inflammatory, and antistress agents (see Chap. 17), they have antiemetic effects as well. However, the mechanism by which the drugs exert antiemetic effects is unknown; they are thought to block prostaglandin activity in the cerebral cortex. Dexamethasone and methylprednisolone are commonly used in the management of chemotherapy-induced emesis and postoperative nausea and vomiting, either alone or in combination regimens with 5-HT$_3$ receptor antagonists and/or substance P/neurokinin 1 receptor antagonists. With short-term use, adverse effects associated with corticosteroids are mild (e.g., euphoria, insomnia, mild fluid retention).

Benzodiazepine antianxiety drugs (see Chap. 54) are not antiemetics, but they are often used in multidrug regimens to prevent nausea and vomiting associated with cancer chemotherapy. The drugs produce relaxation, relieve anxiety, and inhibit cerebral cortex input to the vomiting center. They are often prescribed for patients who experience anticipatory nausea and vomiting before administration of anticancer drugs. Lorazepam (Ativan) is commonly used for this purpose but is not recommended as a single-agent antiemetic.

Olanzapine (Zyprexa) is a second-generation (atypical) antipsychotic often used in the treatment of bipolar disorder and schizophrenia. Current practice guidelines by the American Society of Clinical Oncology (Hesketh, et al., 2017) recommend adding olanzapine to antiemetic prophylaxis to reduce the likelihood of nausea among adults who are treated with high emetic risk antineoplastic agents. In adults who did not receive olanzapine and who experience nausea or vomiting despite optimal prophylaxis, the drug should be considered in addition to continuing the standard antiemetic regimen. As antiemetic prophylaxis postoperatively in adults and children, the IV or oral formulations can be administered, as indicated.

Marijuana (*Cannabis*) is a schedule I drug, and over 33 U.S. states and the District of Columbia allow the use of medical marijuana with a prescription (or signed medical statement) for registered qualifying patients who would likely benefit from marijuana. Patients have used it to treat chemotherapy-induced nausea and vomiting. However, there remains insufficient evidence for a recommendation regarding its use in the most recent practice guidelines for management of chemotherapy- and radiation-induced nausea and vomiting (Hesketh, et al., 2017).

Dronabinol (Marinol, Syndros) and nabilone (Cesamet) are synthetic **cannabinoids** (derivatives of marijuana) that have demonstrated antiemetic activity and are FDA approved for the treatment of nausea and vomiting caused by chemotherapy. However, concern about their abuse potential and their rather unfavorable adverse effect profiles, especially in older adults, may limit their clinical utility. Both cannabinoids are approved in patients who have failed to respond adequately to conventional antiemetic treatments, and national clinical practice guidelines propose that this agent be considered as a rescue antiemetic for refractory nausea and vomiting. Onset of action occurs within 12 hours, with peak intensity within 24 hours and dissipation within 96 hours. Dronabinol is also an appetite stimulant approved for the treatment of anorexia in patients with AIDS. Synthetic cannabinoids have the same adverse effects as marijuana, including psychiatric symptoms (euphoria, tachycardia, abnormality in thinking, paranoia, drowsiness), and a high potential for abuse. Use caution when increasing the

dose of dronabinol and nabilone because there is an increased frequency of dose-related adverse reactions at higher dosages. In addition, the drugs may cause a withdrawal syndrome when abruptly discontinued. Withdrawal symptoms (e.g., insomnia, irritability, restlessness) are most likely to occur with high doses or prolonged use, and sleep disturbances may persist for several weeks.

---

**!  QSEN Alert: Safety**

Drugs with abuse potential are labeled in the Controlled Substance Act (see Chap. 1) on a schedule from I to V, from most to least risk of abuse, respectively. Marijuana is labeled schedule I as any cannabinoid found in the plant is automatically controlled in schedule I. Synthetic preparations nabilone and dronabinol, under the trade name Syndros, are schedule II drugs, and dronabinol, under the trade name Marinol, is a schedule III drug under federal narcotic laws. The difference in schedule classification of the trade name drugs of dronabinol may be the result of the date of approval, the research findings regarding abuse potential, and other factors. Assess individuals taking these drugs for adverse effects and withdrawal symptoms.

---

Phosphorated carbohydrate solution (Emetrol) is a hyperosmolar solution with phosphoric acid. This drug is thought to reduce smooth muscle contraction in the GI tract and is available as an over-the-counter medication in syrup form. Because this solution contains fructose, patients with diabetes mellitus should consult their health care provider before using it.

Scopolamine (Transderm Scop), an M1 muscarinic receptor antagonist, is a major anticholinergic drug (see Chap. 48) effective in relieving nausea and vomiting associated with motion sickness and radiation therapy. It is predominately used as a transdermal patch to prevent motion sickness.

---

**NCLEX  Success**

3. When administering 5-HT$_3$ receptor antagonists before cancer chemotherapy, the nurse should also be prepared to administer which of the following adjunctive medications?

   A. promethazine
   B. dexamethasone
   C. dronabinol
   D. hydroxyzine

4. A woman sends her partner to the store to purchase an over-the-counter product to resolve the vomiting she has experienced during a migraine. She has a history of diabetes mellitus and hypertension. She has an appointment with her health care provider in the morning. Which of the following drugs would be the best for the partner to purchase?

   A. promethazine
   B. phosphorated carbohydrate solution
   C. meclizine
   D. dimenhydrinate

5. A 30-year-old female has been ordered dronabinol. Which of the following statements are true for dronabinol? (Select all that apply.)

A. The drug is most effective when given every 2 hours.

B. It is approved for nausea and vomiting related to chemotherapy in people with cancer.

C. Adverse effects include drowsiness or euphoria.

D. Insufficient research is available to support its use as a treatment for nausea and vomiting.

E. It is approved as an appetite stimulant for anorexia in people with AIDS.

F. The drug is used as a first-line treatment in women with hyperemesis gravidarum associated with pregnancy.

---

### Clinical Application 38.2

- Ms. Snyder is concerned about the amount of medication she is receiving. She asks the nurse to withhold her antiemetics until she actually vomits. What is the best way to respond to Ms. Snyder?

---

## NONPHARMACOLOGIC MANAGEMENT

Nonpharmacologic techniques have become an acceptable adjunct to antiemetic drug therapy. The use of herbal supplements has also received support.

## Acupuncture and Acupressure

Practitioners use acupuncture and acupressure to stimulate the pericardium 6 site, which is generally thought to be effective in the management of chemotherapy-induced nausea and vomiting and motion sickness. Acupuncture is one of the most well studied of all the nonpharmacologic techniques, but interpretation of the results of randomized trials is hampered by a high risk of bias in most studies and a lack of standardization of treatment methods and comparison groups. Acupressure wristbands may also be useful in the treatment of nausea and vomiting associated with motion sickness.

## Herbal Supplements

The use of ginger in traditional Chinese and Indian medicine has a long history. Clinical trials indicate that the herb can effectively reduce nausea and vomiting associated with motion sickness, pregnancy, and surgery. Evidence of the herb's success against chemotherapy-induced nausea and vomiting is mixed. The herb's components are thought to interact with $5-HT_3$ receptors, which may account for the antiemetic activity.

---

### Clinical Application 38.3

- What nursing measures, in addition to the administration of antiemetic medication, should the nurse suggest to Ms. Snyder to reduce her nausea and vomiting?

## THE NURSING PROCESS

A concept map outlines the nursing process related to drug therapy considerations in this chapter. Additional nursing implications related to the disease process should also be considered in care decisions.

**Assessment**
- Identify risk factors for nausea and vomiting and frequency, duration, and precipitating causes.
- Interview for any measures, including antiemetic drugs, that successfully relieve nausea and vomiting.
- When possible, observe and measure the vomitus.

**Outcomes of Therapy**

The patient will
- Receive antiemetic drugs at appropriate times, by indicated routes.
- Take antiemetic drugs as prescribed for outpatient use.
- Obtain relief of nausea and vomiting.
- Eat and retain food and fluids.
- Report increased comfort.
- Maintain body weight.

**Nursing Interventions**
- Use measures to prevent or minimize nausea and vomiting.
- Assist patient to identify situations and avoid stimuli that cause or aggravate nausea and vomiting.
- Administer analgesics before painful diagnostic tests and dressing changes or other therapeutic measures, as pain may cause nausea and vomiting.
- Administer antiemetic drugs 30 to 60 minutes before a nausea-producing event, when possible (e.g., radiation therapy, cancer chemotherapy, travel).
- Adjust the timing of any oral drugs that cause gastric irritation, nausea, and vomiting by taking with or just after food if food does not alter the beneficial effects of drug.
- Assess the patient's condition and report to the health care provider reoccurring nausea and vomiting. In some instances, a drug (e.g., digoxin, an antibiotic) may need to be discontinued or reduced in dosage. In other instances (e.g., paralytic ileus, GI obstruction), preferred treatment is restriction of oral intake and nasogastric intubation.
- Suggest that a woman eat dry crackers before rising in the morning and ingest small, frequent protein meals to help prevent nausea and vomiting associated with pregnancy.
- Avoid administering oral intake of food, fluids, and drugs during acute episodes of nausea and vomiting. Oral intake may increase vomiting and risks of fluid and electrolyte imbalances.
- Give replacement fluids and electrolytes. Offer small amounts of food and fluids orally when tolerated and according to patient preference.
- Record vital signs, intake and output, and body weight at regular intervals if nausea or vomiting occurs frequently.
- Decrease environmental stimuli when possible (e.g., noise, odors). Allow the patient to lie quietly in bed when nauseated. Decreasing motion and activity may decrease stimulation of the vomiting center in the brain.
- Help the patient rinse his or her mouth after vomiting. Rinsing decreases the bad taste and corrosion of tooth enamel caused by gastric acid.
- Provide requested nonpharmacologic remedies when possible (e.g., a cool, wet washcloth to the face and neck).
- Provide appropriate education for any drug therapy (see Box 38.2).

**Evaluation**
- Observe and interview for decreased nausea and vomiting.
- Observe and interview regarding ability to maintain adequate intake of food and fluids and baseline weight.
- Observe and interview regarding appropriate use of antiemetic drugs.

- Antiemetic drugs are used to prevent or treat nausea and vomiting associated with surgery, pain, motion sickness, cancer chemotherapy, radiation therapy, pregnancy, and other causes.

- Antiemetic drugs are most effective when given before nausea and vomiting occurs.

- The vomiting center, CTZ, and GI tract contain benzodiazepine, cholinergic (muscarinic), dopamine, histamine, opiate, substance P/neurokinin, and serotonin receptors that are stimulated by emetogenic drugs and toxins. Antiemetic drugs produce their effects by blockade of one or more of these receptors.

- The antiemetic effect of phenothiazines such as prochlorperazine and promethazine is due to blockade of dopamine receptors in the brain and CTZ. They are used to treat nausea induced by drugs, radiation therapy, surgery, and other stimuli but are considered ineffective in motion sickness.

- The FDA has issued a **BLACK BOX WARNING** ◆ stating that promethazine is contraindicated in children younger than 2 years of age because of the risk of potentially fatal respiratory depression.

- A **BLACK BOX WARNING** ◆ alerts nurses that promethazine is contraindicated for subcutaneous administration. The preferred route of administration is intramuscular, which reduces the risk of surrounding muscle and tissue damage. The FDA has issued a **BLACK BOX WARNING** ◆ for perphenazine because elderly patients with dementia-related psychosis treated with perphenazine and other antipsychotic drugs are at an increased risk of death.

- Classic $H_1$-blocking antihistamine drugs such as dimenhydrinate are thought to produce an antiemetic effect due to their anticholinergic properties. Antihistamines are used to prevent and treat nausea and vomiting due to motion sickness.

- The antiemetic mechanism of action of corticosteroids such as dexamethasone and methylprednisolone is unknown. These drugs are commonly used alone or in combination with 5-HT$_3$ serotonin receptor antagonists and/or substance P/neurokinin 1 receptor antagonists in the management of chemotherapy-induced emesis and postoperative nausea and vomiting.

- 5-HT$_3$ serotonin receptor antagonists such as ondansetron, granisetron, dolasetron, and palonosetron antagonize serotonin receptors, preventing their activation by emetogenic drugs and toxins. They are used to prevent and treat moderate to severe nausea associated with cancer chemotherapy, radiation therapy, and postoperative conditions.

- Substance P, a peptide neurotransmitter in the neurokinin family, plays a role in acute and delayed chemotherapy-induced nausea and vomiting. Aprepitant antagonizes the neurokinin 1 receptor, preventing activation by emetogenic chemotherapeutic drugs.

- Benzodiazepines such as lorazepam produce relaxation, relieve anxiety, and inhibit cerebral cortex input to the vomiting center. They are prescribed for anticipatory nausea associated with cancer chemotherapy.

- Dronabinol and nabilone are cannabinoids used in the management of nausea and vomiting associated with chemotherapy unrelieved by other antiemetic drugs. Due to the drugs' potential for abuse, both are labeled Scheduled drugs under federal narcotic laws.

- Scopolamine is an anticholinergic drug effective in relieving nausea and vomiting associated with motion sickness and radiation therapy for cancer.

**CLINICAL REASONING CASE STUDY**

**Meet the Patient**

Lily Hayashi, a 27-year-old teacher, is in her 10th week of pregnancy and has had mild nausea and vomiting for the past month. She presents for her second prenatal visit and asks for something to treat her morning sickness. The nurse midwife discusses her options and tells her that she will place her on doxylamine succinate with pyridoxine hydrochloride (Diclegis) at her next visit if the nausea and vomiting worsen. Ms. Hayashi asks if this medication is safe for her baby. She also asks whether she should do something else if she continues to have nausea and vomiting. How should the nurse respond?

**Assessing Drug Information**

- The primary mechanism of diphenhydramine and other antihistamines for the treatment of nausea and vomiting of pregnancy is direct inhibition of histamine at the H1 receptor; the secondary mechanism is an indirect effect on the vestibular system by decreasing stimulation of the vomiting center. In addition, these agents, including diphenhydramine, inhibit the muscarinic receptor, which may mediate the emetic response. It is unclear how extra vitamin B$_6$ (pyridoxine) works as an antiemetic drug during pregnancy. The vitamin should not be taken in doses higher that prescribed.
- This drug may help treat pregnancy-associated nausea and vomiting not responsive to conservative management.
- Common adverse effects of antihistamines include sedation, dry mouth, blurred vision, lightheadedness, and constipation. Adverse effects of pyridoxine include drowsiness, headache, and paresthesia.

**Nursing Actions**

- Inform Ms. Hayashi that pregnant women should take antiemetic drugs only if the nausea and vomiting are severe enough to threaten maternal and fetal nutritional or metabolic status (hyperemesis gravidarum).
- Educate her about nonpharmacologic measures she can use. These may be beneficial so long as the vomiting does not become severe.
- Instruct Ms. Hayashi about eating habits that may ease her nausea:
  - Determine what foods she tolerates best and stick to those foods. Some women benefit by eliminating coffee, spicy, odorous, high-fat, acidic, and very sweet foods.
  - Snack before getting out of bed in the morning or during the night (e.g., crackers with peanut butter or cheese prior to bathroom trips).
  - Eat protein-dominant, salty, low-fat, bland, and/or dry foods (e.g., nuts, pretzels, toast, cereal, crackers) at meals.
  - Drink fluids at least 30 minutes before or after solid food to minimize the effect of a full stomach. Cold, clear, and carbonated or sour liquids (e.g., popsicles, lemonade, ginger ale) taken in small amounts are better tolerated; using a straw might help.
  - Peppermint tea or peppermint candies may reduce nausea after a meal.
- Suggest that she avoid environmental triggers that aggravate symptoms, such as:
  - Stuffy rooms, odors, heat, humidity, or noise.
  - Quickly changing position.
  - Not getting enough rest, particularly after eating.
  - Lying down soon after eating and lying on the left side (these actions may delay gastric emptying).
  - Hot solid foods, which have more odor than cold foods and require more preparation time.
  - Taking prenatal vitamins in the morning or on an empty stomach. (Taking prenatal vitamins before bed with a snack may be helpful).
- Tell her that scientific evidence has consistently shown that the drug combination of doxylamine succinate with pyridoxine hydrochloride is safe and effective and is a first-line treatment for nausea and vomiting during pregnancy.
- Should finances be a concern with the combination tablets, doxylamine is available in some over-the-counter sleeping pills (Unisom Sleep Tabs, Kirkland Signature Sleep Aid) as is pyridoxine (vitamin B$_6$). This may be a reasonable, less expensive option that Ms. Hayashi should discuss with her nurse midwife.
- Tell her to call the nurse midwife or seek emergency medical attention if nausea and vomiting worsen and she is not able to keep food or fluids down or develops dizziness, irritability or disorientation, somnolence, or less frequent urination.

Visit thePoint® at **http://thePoint.lww.com/Frandsen12e** for answers to NCLEX Success questions (in Appendix A), answers to Clinical Application Case Studies (in Appendix B), and more!

## REFERENCES AND RESOURCES

American College of Obstetricians and Gynecologists. (2015). ACOG Practice Bulletin #153. Clinical management guidelines for obstetrician-gynecologists: Nausea and vomiting of pregnancy. *Obstetrics and Gynecology, 126,* e12–e24.

Basch, E., Prestrud, A. A., Hesketh, P. J., Kris, M. G., Feyer, P. C., Somerfield, M. R., et al.; American Society of Clinical Oncology. (2011). Antiemetics: American Society of Clinical Oncology clinical practice guideline update. *Journal of Clinical Oncology, 29*(31), 4189–4198.

Bustos, M., Venkataramanan, R., & Caritis, S. (2017). Nausea and vomiting of pregnancy: What's new? *Autonomic Neuroscience: Basic and Clinical, 202,* 62–72. doi:10.1016/j.autneu.2016.05.002

DiPiro, J. T., Talbert, R. L., Yee, G. C., Wells, B. G., Posey, L. M., & Matzke, G. R. (2016). *Pharmacotherapy: A pathophysiologic approach* (10th ed.). New York, NY: McGraw-Hill Education.

Estoup, A. C., Moise-Campbell, C., Varma, M., & Stewart, D. G. (2016). The impact of marijuana legalization on adolescent use, consequences, and perceived risk. *Substance Use & Misuse, 51*(14), 1881–1887.

Fiaschi, L., Nelson-Piercy, C., Deb, S., King, R., & Tata, L. J. (2019). Clinical management of nausea and vomiting in pregnancy and hyperemesis gravidarum across primary and secondary care: A population-based study. *BJOG: An International Journal of Obstetrics & Gynaecology, 126,* 1201–1211. doi:10.1111/1471-0528.15662

Gan, T. J., & Habib, A. S. (2016). *Postoperative nausea and vomiting: A practical guide.* Cambridge, England: Cambridge University Press.

Grossman, S., & Porth, C. M. (2018). *Pathophysiology: Concepts of altered health status* (10th ed.). Philadelphia, PA: Lippincott Williams & Wilkins.

Hesketh, P. J. (2019). *Prevention and treatment of chemotherapy-induced nausea and vomiting in adults.* UpToDate. Lexi Comp, Inc.

Hesketh, P. J., Kris, M. G., Basch, E., Bohlke, K., Barbour, S. Y., Clark-Snow, R. A., et al. (2017). Antiemetics: American Society of Clinical Oncology Clinical Practice guideline update. *Journal of Clinical Oncology, 35*(28), 3240–3261.

Hinkle, J. H., & Cheever, K. H. (2017). *Brunner & Suddarth's textbook of medical-surgical nursing* (14th ed.). Philadelphia, PA: Lippincott Williams & Wilkins.

Karch, A. (2017). *Focus on nursing pharmacology.* Philadelphia, PA: Lippincott Williams & Wilkins.

Koren, G., Clark, S., Hankins, G. D., Caritis, S. N., Umans, J. G., Miodovnik, M., et al. (2015). Maternal safety of the delayed-release doxylamine and pyridoxine combination for nausea and vomiting of pregnancy: A randomized placebo controlled trial. *BMC Pregnancy and Childbirth, 15,* 59. doi:10.1186/s12884-015-0488-1

Koren, G., Clark, S., Hankins, G. D. V., Caritis, S. N., Umans, J. G., Miodovnik, M., et al. (2016). Demonstration of early efficacy results of the delayed-release combination of doxylamine-pyridoxine for the treatment of nausea and vomiting of pregnancy. *BMC Pregnancy and Childbirth, 16,* 371. doi:10.1186/s12884-016-1172-9

Longstreth, G. F., & Hesketh, P. J. (2019). *Characteristics of antiemetic drugs.* UpToDate, Lexi Comp, Inc.

Navari, R. M., & Aapro, M. (2016). Antiemetic prophylaxis for chemotherapy-induced nausea and vomiting. *New England Journal of Medicine, 374*(14), 1356–1367. doi:10.1056/NEJMra1515442

Smith, L. A., Azariah, F., Lavender, V. T., Stoner, N. S., & Bettiol, S. (2015). Cannabinoids for nausea and vomiting in adults with cancer receiving chemotherapy. *Cochrane Database of Systematic Reviews, 11,* CD009464.

UpToDate. (2019). *Drug information.* Lexi-Comp, Inc.

# Drug Therapy for Constipation and Elimination Problems

## LEARNING OBJECTIVES

*After studying this chapter, you should be able to:*

1. Discuss the etiology, physiology, and clinical manifestations for constipation and elimination problems.
2. Educate patients about nonpharmacologic measures to prevent or treat constipation.
3. Identify the prototype and describe the action, use, contraindications, adverse effects, and nursing implications of the laxatives.
4. Identify the prototype and describe the action, use, contraindications, adverse effects, and nursing implications of the cathartics.
5. Identify the prototype, indications, dosages, and routes for the miscellaneous agents used to treat constipation and other conditions.
6. Implement the nursing process in the care of patients with constipation.

## CLINICAL APPLICATION CASE STUDY

Doris Campbell, an 84-year-old woman, is complaining about being constipated. Her past health history includes arthritis, osteoporosis, hemorrhoids, and peptic ulcer disease. As a home care nurse, you frequently see patients who complain of constipation.

## KEY TERMS

**Constipation:** infrequent and painful expulsion of hard, dry stools

**Defecation:** bowel elimination that is normally stimulated by movements and reflexes in the gastrointestinal tract

**Fecal impaction:** mass of hard, dry stool in the rectum; caused by chronic constipation

**Flatulence:** expulsion of gas through the rectum

# INTRODUCTION

**Constipation** is a symptom, not a disease. It is the infrequent and painful expulsion of hard, dry stools. Generally, constipation is difficult to define clearly because normal frequency of stools varies as a symptom and differs from person to person. Drug therapy for constipation and elimination problems includes laxatives and cathartics, which are used to promote bowel elimination (defecation). The term *laxative* implies mild effects, with elimination of soft, formed stool. The term *cathartic* implies strong effects, with elimination of liquid or semiliquid stool. Although different effects may depend more on the dose than on the particular drug used, the names laxatives and cathartics are used in this chapter to specify the harshness of the level of response expected at normal doses of the drugs.

# OVERVIEW OF CONSTIPATION

## Etiology

Several factors can cause or contribute to constipation, although in most people, no single cause can be found. However, constipation occurs more frequently with age. Constipation may be associated with normal or slow bowel transit, defecatory dysfunction, or both. Several risk factors are associated with the development of constipation, including diet and lifestyle, particularly decreased levels of physical activity. Female sex, nonwhite status, advanced age, and low levels of education and income are related risk factors. In addition, certain drugs and disease process are associated with constipation.

## Physiology and Pathophysiology

**Defecation** is bowel elimination that is stimulated by movements and reflexes in the gastrointestinal (GI) tract. When the stomach and duodenum are distended with food or fluids, gastrocolic and duodenocolic reflexes cause propulsive movements in the colon, which move feces into the rectum and arouse the urge to defecate. When sensory nerve fibers in the rectum are stimulated by the fecal mass, the defecation reflex causes strong peristalsis, deep breathing, closure of the glottis, contraction of abdominal muscles, contraction of the rectum, relaxation of anal sphincters, and expulsion of the fecal mass.

The cerebral cortex normally controls the defecation reflex so that defecation can occur at acceptable times and places. Voluntary control inhibits the external anal sphincter to allow defecation or contracts the sphincter to prevent defecation. When the external sphincter remains contracted, the defecation reflex dissipates (defecatory dysfunction), and the urge to defecate usually does not recur until additional feces enter the rectum or several hours later. In people who often inhibit the defecation reflex or fail to respond to the urge to defecate, constipation develops as the reflex weakens.

## Clinical Manifestations

Constipation involves infrequent defecation. Because of variations in diet and other factors, there is no "normal" number of stools, but the traditional medical definition of functional constipation in adults includes three or fewer bowel movements per week. In adults, the use of a multisymptom criterion-based checklist (Rome III criteria for functional constipation) requires two or more of six symptoms during at least one fourth of the bowel movements. Along with fewer than three stools per week, symptoms include straining, a sensation of incomplete evacuation, a sensation of anorectal blockage, hard stools, and use of manual evacuation. Normal bowel elimination should produce a soft, formed stool without pain.

In children, the criteria that define constipation are slightly different. In those younger than 4 years of age, the Rome III criteria for functional constipation include two of the following symptoms: fewer than two stools per week, at least one episode of incontinence per week after the acquisition of toileting skills, stool retention, painful bowel movements, large mass of stool in rectum, and large-diameter stools that may obstruct the toilet. In those aged 4 and older, the criteria include two defecations in the toilet per week, stool retention, painful bowel movements, large mass of stool in rectum, large-diameter stools that may obstruct the toilet, and a history of retentive posturing or excessive volitional stool retention.

Physicians may measure the bowel transit time to find the cause of constipation or locate whether a specific part of the intestine is slowing down movement more than another. Because different people have different transit times, experts disagree on the usefulness of the test. Some providers do not recommend bowel transit time testing or do so only when lifestyle changes have not produced desired results.

## Lifestyle Changes

Nonpharmacologic treatment of people with constipation has included the use of fiber, fluid supplementation, prebiotics, probiotics, and behavioral therapy. There is some evidence that fiber supplements and adequate fluid intake improve the frequency and consistency of stools. Children with constipation should eat a balanced diet, containing juices that contain sorbitol, such as prune, pear, and apple juice (for infants) and whole grains, fruits, and vegetables (for children). Bowel transit time depends on what types of food eaten and the quantity of fluid ingested; research indicates that people who eat increased fruits, vegetables, and whole grains tend to have shorter transit times than do people who eat mostly sugars and starches. In addition, people should be advised to try to defecate after meals, thereby taking advantage of normal postprandial increases in colonic motility.

Behavioral interventions, such as biofeedback therapy, have been successful in improving symptoms of constipation.

**QSEN Alert: Teamwork and Collaboration**

Factors that improve the chance of successfully resolving constipation with biofeedback are the motivation of the patient and therapist; the intensity and frequency of the retraining program; and a team approach that includes a broad scope of participants, such as the patient and his or her significant others, behavioral psychologist, and dietitian. The role of significant others is especially important in children.

*Clinical Application 39.1*

- Given Mrs. Campbell's complaint of constipation, what does the nurse assess with regard to the patient's bowel pattern and risk of constipation?

## Drug Therapy

Laxatives and cathartics are given to prevent or treat constipation and are somewhat arbitrarily classified as:

- Laxatives: bulk-forming, lubricant or emollient, and surfactant agents (stool softeners)
- Cathartics: saline and stimulant agents
- Miscellaneous agents

Table 39.1 lists the specific drugs used for the treatment of constipation by class.

Clinically, the choice of a laxative or cathartic often depends on the reason for use and the patient's condition, as shown in Table 39.2. There are several indications for use:

- To relieve constipation in pregnant women, elderly patients whose abdominal and perineal muscles have become weak and atrophied, children with megacolon, and patients receiving drugs that decrease intestinal motility (e.g., opioid analgesics, drugs with anticholinergic effects)
- To prevent straining at stool in patients with coronary artery disease (e.g., post–myocardial infarction), hypertension, cerebrovascular disease, and hemorrhoids and other rectal conditions
- To empty the bowel in preparation for bowel surgery or diagnostic procedures (e.g., colonoscopy, barium enema)
- To accelerate elimination of potentially toxic substances from the GI tract (e.g., orally ingested drugs or toxic compounds)
- To prevent absorption of intestinal ammonia in patients with hepatic encephalopathy

- To obtain a stool specimen for parasitologic examination
- To accelerate excretion of parasites after anthelmintic drugs have been administered
- To reduce serum cholesterol levels (psyllium products)

In addition, safety, clinical response, cost, and convenience all influence the choice of the initial treatment selected.

## LAXATIVES

Bulk-forming laxatives are soluble fibers that are largely unabsorbed by the intestine. When water is added, these substances swell and become gellike. Bulk-forming laxatives are the most physiologic laxatives because their effect is similar to that of increased intake of dietary fiber. The bulk-forming laxative **psyllium** (Metamucil; others) is the prototype laxative.

## Pharmacokinetics

Psyllium usually acts within 12 to 24 hours, although it may take as long as 2 to 3 days to exert its full effects. Excretion is in the stool.

## Action

Psyllium is essentially unabsorbed by the body. It works by mechanical action to absorb excess water while stimulating normal bowel elimination. The drug adds bulk and size to the fecal mass that stimulates peristalsis and defecation. It also may act by pulling water into the intestinal lumen.

### TABLE 39.1

### Drugs Administered for the Treatment of Constipation

| Drug Class | Prototype(s) | Other Drugs in the Class |
|---|---|---|
| **Laxatives** | | |
| Bulk-forming | Psyllium preparations (Metamucil, Konsyl, Natural Fiber, Reguloid) | Methylcellulose (Citrucel, Soluble Fiber Therapy) <br> Polycarbophil (FiberCon, FiberGen, Fiber-Lax) |
| Lubricant laxative | | Mineral oil (GoodSense Mineral Oil, Fleet Oil, Fleet Mineral Oil Enema) |
| Stool softeners | | Docusate calcium (Surfak, Goldline DC, Sulfolax) <br> Docusate sodium (Colace, Docusil, Docuprene) |
| **Cathartics** | | |
| Stimulant | Bisacodyl (Dulcolax) | Castor oil <br> Glycerin (Glycerin, Pedia-Lax, Sani-Supp Pediatric) <br> Senna preparations (Ex-Lax Maximum Strength, Senokot) |
| Saline | | Magnesium citrate solution (Citroma, GoodSense Magnesium Citrate) <br> Magnesium hydroxide (Milk of Magnesia, Pedia-Lax, Phillips) <br> Polyethylene glycol (PEG) solution (GaviLAX, GlycoLax, HealthyLax, MiraLAX, PEGyLAX) <br> Polyethylene glycol–electrolyte solution (PEG-ES) (Colyte, GaviLyte-N, GoLYTELY, NuLYTELY, TriLyte) |
| Miscellaneous | | Lactulose (Constulose, Kristalose) <br> Lubiprostone (Amitiza) <br> Linaclotide (Linzess) <br> Plecanatide (Trulance) <br> Sorbitol <br> Prucalopride (*Motegrity*) <br> Tegaserod (Zelnorm) |

### TABLE 39.2

## Use of Laxatives and Cathartics for Specific Conditions

| Indication | Preferred Drug Regimen |
|---|---|
| For patients in whom straining is potentially harmful or painful such as those with coronary artery disease (e.g., post–myocardial infarction), hypertension, cerebrovascular disease, anal fissures, or hemorrhoids | Stool softeners (e.g., docusate sodium) are the agents of choice. |
| For occasional use to cleanse the bowel for endoscopic or radiologic examinations | Saline or stimulant cathartics are acceptable (e.g., magnesium citrate, polyethylene glycol–electrolyte solution, bisacodyl). These drugs should not be used more than once per week. Frequent use is likely to produce laxative abuse. |
| For long-term use of laxatives or cathartics in patients who are debilitated, older, or unable or unwilling to eat an adequate diet | Bulk-forming laxatives (e.g., Metamucil) usually are preferred. However, because obstruction may occur, these agents should not be given to patients with difficulty in swallowing or adhesions or strictures in the GI tract or to those who are unable or unwilling to drink adequate fluids. |
| To accelerate elimination of potentially toxic substances from the GI tract (e.g., orally ingested drugs or toxic compounds) | Sorbitol may be given with activated charcoal to remove toxic substances. |
| To prevent absorption of intestinal ammonia in patients with hepatic encephalopathy | Lactulose acidifies the stool and traps ammonia and eliminates it with other fecal material. |
| For fecal impaction | In adults, a rectal suppository (e.g., bisacodyl) or an enema (e.g., oil retention or Fleet Enema) is preferred. Oral laxatives are contraindicated when fecal impaction is present but may be given after the rectal mass is removed. In children, polyethylene glycol with or without electrolytes and mineral oil have been shown to be effective for initial disimpaction. After the impaction is relieved, measures should be taken to prevent recurrence. If dietary and other nonpharmacologic measures are ineffective or contraindicated, use of a bulk-forming agent daily or another laxative once or twice weekly may be necessary. |
| For adults with irritable bowel syndrome with constipation | If a trial of soluble fiber and polyethylene glycol is unsuccessful, lubiprostone, linaclotide, or plecanatide may be administered to adults. In women under 65 years of age, tegaserod may be considered. |

## Use

Uses of psyllium include treatment of occasional constipation or bowel irregularity. The drug may also help lower cholesterol when combined with a diet low in cholesterol and saturated fat. It may also be useful in the treatment of diarrhea. It should be noted that because psyllium, like most laxatives, is not absorbed or metabolized extensively, it can usually be used without difficulty in patients with hepatic impairment. Table 39.3 presents route and dosage information for the psyllium and other bulk-forming laxatives as well as surfactant and lubricant laxatives.

### Use in Children

Children should obtain adequate fiber from dietary intake. Although psyllium-containing products are available without a prescription, children should take them only under the supervision of a health care provider.

### Use in Older Adults

Psyllium is one of the many laxatives that is often used or overused in older adults. Nondrug measures to prevent constipation are much preferred to laxatives in such patients. If a laxative is required on a regular basis, a bulk-forming psyllium compound (e.g., Metamucil) is best because it is most physiologic in its action.

### Use in Patients With Critical Illness

Many patients with critical illness, including those with cancer, feel pain and require moderate to large amounts of opioid analgesics for pain control. The analgesics slow GI motility and cause constipation. The reduced mobility and altered bowel regimes that are often found in these patients increase the risk of constipation. Thus, they often need a bowel management program that includes routine administration of laxatives such as psyllium or another class of drug to relieve constipation.

### Use in Patients Receiving Home Care

Laxatives such as psyllium are commonly self-prescribed and self-administered in the home setting. When visiting patients for purposes other than providing care for patients who take laxatives, the home care nurse may become involved in their use. The functions of the home care nurse may include assessing usual patterns of bowel elimination, identifying patients at risk for constipation, promoting lifestyle interventions to prevent constipation, obtaining laxatives when indicated, and counseling about rational use of laxatives.

## Adverse Effects

Psyllium or any fiber product may result in severe **flatulence** (expulsion of gas through the rectum) and bloating. In addition,

## TABLE 39.3

## DRUGS AT A GLANCE: Laxatives

| Drug | Pregnancy Category | Routes and Dosage Ranges | |
|---|---|---|---|
| | | **Adults** | **Children** |
| **Bulk-Forming** | | | |
| Ⓟ **Psyllium preparations** (Metamucil, Konsyl, Natural Fiber, Reguloid; ✳ Metamucil) | B | PO 2.5–30 g daily in divided doses, stirred in at least 8 oz water or other liquid | 6–11 y: PO 1.25–15 g daily in divided doses in 8 oz water<br>12 y and older: PO same dosage as adults |
| Methylcellulose (Citrucel, Good Sense Fiber, Soluble Fiber Therapy) | Not classified | PO powder 2 g up to three times daily with water (8 oz or more)<br>PO caplets two up to six times daily | 6–11 y: PO 1 g in 8 oz water up to three times daily; 1 caplet up six times daily<br>12 y and older: PO same dosage as adults |
| Polycarbophil (FiberCon, Fiber-Lax) | C | PO 1250 mg 1–4 times daily or PRN with 8 oz of fluid; maximum dose 4 g/24 h | 6–12 y: PO 625 mg 1–4 times daily or PRN; maximum dose 2 g/24 h<br>12 y and older: PO same dosage as adults |
| **Stool Softeners** | | | |
| Docusate calcium (Surfak, Goldline DC; ✳ Apo-Docusate Calcium, PMS- Docusate Calcium) | C | PO 240 mg daily | 12 y and older: PO same dosage as adults |
| Docusate sodium (Colace, Docusil, ✳ Colace, Dosolax, Soflax, Taro-Docusate) | C | PO 50–360 mg once daily or in divided doses<br>Rectal 283 mg/5 mL in one enema 1–3 times daily | 2–6 y: products vary, consult labels<br>6–11 y: PO 100 mg daily<br>12 y and older: PO same dosage as adults |
| **Lubricants** | | | |
| Mineral oil (GoodSense Mineral Oil, Fleet Oil, Fleet Mineral Oil Enema) | B | PO 15–45 mL at bedtime or in divided doses, max 45 mL/d<br>Rectal enema, 118 mL as single dose | Older than 6 y: PO 5–15 mL at bedtime; rectal enema, 30–60 mL |

there have been reports of abdominal cramping and esophageal or bowel obstruction.

## Contraindications

Contraindications to the use of psyllium include the presence of undiagnosed abdominal pain. The danger is that the drugs may cause an inflamed organ (e.g., the appendix) to rupture and spill GI contents into the abdominal cavity with subsequent peritonitis, a life-threatening condition. Other contraindications are known allergy to the drug and intestinal obstruction and **fecal impaction**, a mass of hard, dry stool in the rectum.

> **⚠ QSEN Alert: Safety**
>
> People who have difficulty swallowing, including those with esophageal stricture or other narrowing or obstruction of the GI tract, should not take psyllium.

## Nursing Implications

### Preventing Interactions

With psyllium, no known drug or herbal interactions exist. However, the laxative may reduce or delay the absorption of certain medications, including carbamazepine, digoxin, lithium, tricyclic

antidepressants, and warfarin. People should take psyllium at least 1 hour before or 2 to 4 hours after taking other medications. There is also a potential risk of psyllium interfering with nutrient absorption, but clear evidence is not available.

### Administering the Medication

It is important to take the drug with at least 8 oz of water or another liquid. With the psyllium-containing preparation Metamucil, there have been reports of obstruction in the GI tract when the compound was taken with insufficient fluid. People should take capsules one at a time.

### Assessing for Therapeutic Effects

The nurse assesses for relief from constipation within 12 to 72 hours.

### Assessing for Adverse Effects

The nurse assesses for choking or trouble swallowing, severe stomach pain or cramping, nausea or vomiting, rectal bleeding, or constipation lasting longer than 7 days.

### Patient Teaching

Patients should take the medication as directed with a full glass of liquid, as soon as it is mixed. Maintaining adequate overall intake of fluids also helps improve bowel regularity.

**QSEN Alert: Safety**

Psyllium products may contain sugar, sodium, potassium, or artificial sweeteners. This may be of concern to patients who have diabetes, high blood pressure, renal disease, or phenylketonuria. It is important to teach patients to check the product label if they have these conditions.

Box 39.1 lists patient teaching guidelines for the laxatives and cathartics.

## Other Drugs in the Class

Other laxative products facilitate relief of constipation through different physiologic mechanisms. Surfactant and lubricant laxatives are briefly discussed in this section.

### Lubricant Laxative

Mineral oil is the only lubricant laxative used clinically. It lubricates the fecal mass and slows colonic absorption of water from

**BOX 39.1** **Patient Teaching Guidelines for Laxatives and Cathartics**

### General Considerations

- Diet, exercise, and fluid intake are important in maintaining normal bowel function and preventing or treating constipation.
- Eat foods high in dietary fiber daily. Fiber is the portion of plant food that is not digested. It is contained in fruits, vegetables, and whole-grain cereals and breads. Bran, the outer coating of cereal grains such as wheat or oats, is an excellent source of dietary fiber and is available in numerous cereal products.
- Drink at least 6 to 10 glasses (8 oz each) of fluid daily if not contraindicated.
- Exercise regularly. Walking and other activities aid movement of feces through the bowel.
- Establish a regular time and place for bowel elimination. The defecation urge is usually strongest after eating, and the defecation reflex is weakened or lost if repeatedly ignored.
- Laxative and cathartics use should be temporary and not regular, as a general rule. Regular use may prevent normal bowel function, cause adverse drug reactions, and delay treatment for conditions that cause constipation.
- *Never* take laxatives and cathartics when acute abdominal pain, nausea, or vomiting is present. Doing so may cause a ruptured appendix or other serious complication.
- After taking a strong laxative or cathartic, it takes 2 to 3 days of normal eating to produce enough feces in the bowel for a bowel movement. Frequent use of a strong laxative promotes loss of normal bowel function, loss of fluids and electrolytes that your body needs, and laxative dependence.
- If one is having chronic constipation and is unable or unwilling to eat enough fiber-containing foods in the diet, the next best action is regular use of a bulk-forming laxative (e.g., Metamucil) as a dietary supplement. These laxatives act the same way as increasing fiber in the diet and are usually best for long-term use. When taken daily, these can prevent constipation. However, these laxatives may take 2 to 3 days to work and are not effective in relieving acute constipation.
- Urine may be discolored if one takes a laxative containing senna (e.g., Senokot). The color change is not harmful.
- Some people use strong laxatives for weight control. This is an inappropriate use and a dangerous practice because it can lead to life-threatening fluid and electrolyte imbalances, including dehydration and cardiovascular problems.

### Self or Caregiver Administration
#### General Use

- Take all laxatives and cathartics as directed, and do not exceed recommended doses to avoid adverse effects.
- With bulk-forming laxatives, mix in 8 oz of fluid immediately before taking, and follow with additional fluid, if able. *Never* take the drug dry. Adequate fluid intake is essential with these drugs.
- With bisacodyl tablets, swallow whole (do not crush or chew), and do not take within 1 hour of an antacid or milk. This helps prevent stomach irritation, abdominal cramping, and possible vomiting.
- Take magnesium citrate or milk of magnesia on an empty stomach with 8 oz of fluid to increase effectiveness.
- Refrigerate magnesium citrate before taking to improve taste and retain effectiveness.
- Mix lactulose with fruit juice, water, or milk, if desired, to improve taste.
- Take lubiprostone (Amitiza) with food.
- Notify your health care provider if severe diarrhea develops while taking lubiprostone.

#### Use in Children

- Keep a diary or log to record bowel movements; the use of medication; and episodes of fecal incontinence, abdominal pain, and other symptoms.
- Plan, encourage, and observe a program of regular toilet sitting. A child should sit on the toilet shortly after a meal, for 5 to 10 minutes, two to three times per day. Toilet-sitting episodes should occur at the same time each day and be timed with a timer. (If a child's feet do not touch the floor sitting on a regular toilet seat, it is helpful to use a stool for foot support.)
- Structure a reward system tailored to the appropriate developmental period of the child. This system should provide rewards (stickers, reading a book, special toys used only during toilet sitting, handheld game) for effort (i.e., toilet sitting) rather than success (i.e., having a bowel movement in the toilet).
- Do not make negative comments about incontinence of stool. Do not scold or otherwise punish a child for soiling episodes or lack of success in having a bowel movement.
- Should aversion to using a school bathroom create constipation issues with school-age children, seek the aid of the school and teacher; the child may benefit from use of a private bathroom. It also may be helpful to have a change of clothing available in case a soiling episode occurs.

the fecal mass, but its exact mechanism of action is unknown. Effects usually occur in 6 to 8 hours. Oral mineral oil may cause several adverse effects and is not recommended for long-term use. Mineral oil is probably most useful as a retention enema to soften hard, dry feces and aid in their removal. Oral use of mineral oil may cause potentially serious adverse effects (decreased absorption of fat-soluble vitamins and some drugs; lipid pneumonia if aspirated into the lungs). Thus, mineral oil is not an oral laxative of choice in any condition, although occasional use in the alert patient is unlikely to be harmful. It should not be used regularly. With mineral oil, lipid pneumonia and decreased absorption of vitamins A, D, E, and K can occur.

 **QSEN Alert: Safety**

Lipid pneumonia can be prevented by not giving mineral oil to patients with dysphagia or impaired consciousness. Decreased absorption of fat-soluble vitamins can be prevented by not giving mineral oil with or shortly after meals or for longer than 2 weeks.

### Surfactant Laxatives (Stool Softeners)

Surfactant laxatives (e.g., docusate calcium or docusate sodium) decrease the surface tension of the fecal mass to allow water to penetrate into the stool. They also act as a detergent to facilitate admixing of fat and water in the stool. As a result, stools are softer and easier to expel. These agents have little, if any, laxative effect. Their main value is to prevent straining while expelling stool. They usually act within 1 to 3 days and should be taken daily.

**Clinical Application 39.2**

- Based on Mrs. Campbell's past health history, what is the most likely drug of choice to relieve her constipation?

**NCLEX Success**

1. Which of the following points should be included when teaching patients regarding measures to promote healthy bowel function? (Select all that apply.)
   A. increasing activity
   B. eating a low-residue diet
   C. maintaining adequate fluid intake
   D. establishing regular bowel habits

2. Which of the following oral medications is safe to use in a 60-year-old constipated patient with dysphagia?
   A. methylcellulose
   B. psyllium
   C. mineral oil
   D. docusate sodium

3. A laxative is contraindicated in a patient:
   A. with cancer taking daily narcotics for pain control
   B. complaining of abdominal pain and distention
   C. scheduled for a colonoscopy
   D. with limited mobility due to Parkinson's disease

## CATHARTICS

The stimulant cathartics are the strongest and most abused laxative products. Two types of cathartics exist: stimulant and saline. **Bisacodyl** (Dulcolax), a stimulant cathartic, is the prototype cathartic.

### Pharmacokinetics

Bisacodyl is very poorly absorbed in the small intestine following oral administration or in the large intestine following rectal administration. It has a half-life of 16 hours. The drug is metabolized in the liver. Bisacodyl is primarily excreted in the feces, and any systemically absorbed portion of the drug is excreted in the urine.

### Action

Bisacodyl and other stimulant cathartics act by irritating the GI mucosa and pulling water into the bowel lumen. As a result, feces move through the bowel too rapidly to allow colonic absorption of fecal water, so there is elimination of a watery stool.

### Use

Bisacodyl is prescribed for the relief of constipation and as part of bowel preparation before medical examinations and surgery. The drug is also used in the management of neurogenic bowel dysfunction. The use of bisacodyl is not restricted in patients with renal or hepatic impairment. Table 39.4 provides route and dosage information for bisacodyl as well as other stimulant and saline cathartics.

#### Use in Children

Stimulant laxatives are generally avoided in children younger than 6 years of age for occasional constipation, unless otherwise directed by a clinician. Bisacodyl can be used short term as rescue therapy or cautiously in children with difficult-to-treat constipation.

#### Use in Older Adults

There are no specific dosage recommendations for the use of bisacodyl in older adults. However, as with laxatives, cathartics are often used or overused in older adults. Measures such as maintaining adequate fluids, a high-fiber diet, and exercise are much preferred to cathartics.

#### Use in Patients With Critical Illness

In critically ill patients, an altered diet regimen, change in bowel habits, use of medications known to cause constipation, and decreased activity with bed rest increase the risk of constipation. Often, a bowel management program that includes routine laxative administration is necessary.

**TABLE 39.4**

## DRUGS AT A GLANCE: Cathartics

| Drug | Pregnancy Category | Routes and Dosage Ranges | |
|---|---|---|---|
| | | **Adults** | **Children** |
| **Stimulants** | | | |
| (P) **Bisacodyl** (Dulcolax, Correct; ✸ Apo-Bisacodyl, Bisacodyl-Odan) | B | PO 10–15 mg<br>Rectal suppository, 10 mg | 6 y and older: PO 5 mg; rectal suppository, 5 mg |
| Castor oil (GoodSense Castor Oil) | X | PO 15–60 mL as a single dose | 2–11 y: PO 5–15 mL as single dose<br>≥12 y: PO refer to adult dosing |
| Glycerin (Fleet Liquid Glycerin Supp, Pedia-Lax) | C | Rectal suppository, 1 adult suppository once daily as needed or directed | 2–6 y: rectal pediatric suppository once daily as directed |
| Senna preparations (Ex-Lax, Geri-kot, Senna-Tabs, Senokot) | C | Granules, PO 1 level tsp once or twice daily<br>Syrup, PO 10–15 mL once or twice daily<br>Tablets, PO 2 tablets once or twice daily<br>For geriatric, obstetric, or gynecologic patients, reduce all dosages by half | 2–6 y: PO syrup 2.5–3.75 mL at bedtime, not to exceed 3.75 mL twice daily<br>6–12 y: PO 5–7.5 mL at bedtime not to exceed 7.5 mL twice daily<br>≥12 y: 10–15 mL at bedtime not to exceed 15 mL twice daily<br>Tablets PO 2–6 y: PO ½ tablet (4.3 mg) at bedtime, not to exceed 1 tablet twice daily<br>6–12 y: PO 5–7.5 mL at bedtime, not to exceed 7.5 mL twice daily<br>≥12 y: 10–15 mL at bedtime, not to exceed 15 mL twice daily |
| **Saline** | | | |
| Magnesium citrate solution (Citroma, GoodSense Magnesium Citrate; ✸ Citro-Mag) | C | PO 195–300 mL given once or in divided doses | 2–6 y: PO 60–90 mL given once or in divided doses<br>6–11 y: PO 90–210 mL given once or in divided doses<br>12 y and older: PO same dosage as adults |
| Magnesium hydroxide (Milk of Magnesia, Pedia-Lax, Phillips Milk of Magnesia) | C | Tablet, chewable 311 mg/tablet: 8 tablets/d once daily at bedtime or in divided doses<br>Liquid: PO 2400–4800 once daily at bedtime or in divided doses | Liquid:<br>2–5 y: PO 400–1200 mg once daily at bedtime or in divided doses<br>6–11 y: PO 1200–2400 mg once daily at bedtime or in divided doses<br>12 y and older: PO same dosage as adults<br>Concentrated liquid:<br>2–5 y: PO 2.5–7.5 mL at bedtime<br>6–11 y: PO 7.5–15 mL at bedtime<br>12 y and older: PO same dosage as adults |
| Polyethylene glycol (PEG) solution (GaviLAX, GlycoLax, HealthyLax, MiraLAX, PEGyLAX; ✸ Lax-A-Day, Pegalax, Relaxa) | C | PO 17 g in 4–8 oz water or beverage or as ordered for bowel preparation before colonoscopy | Off-label: limited data available<br>Disimpaction: PO 1 to 1.5 g/kg/d by mouth for up to 6 days<br>Maintenance: PO 0.2 to 0.8 g/kg/d daily in 60 mL of noncarbonated beverage |
| Polyethylene glycol– electrolyte solution (PEG-ES) (Colyte, GaviLyte-N, GoLYTELY, NuLYTELY, TriLyte; ✸ Colyte, Klean-Prep, PegLyte) | C | For bowel cleansing before GI examination:<br>PO 240 mL every 10 min until 4 L is consumed or until rectal fluid clear | Disimpaction ≥ 6 mo: PO 25 mL/kg/h until rectal fluid clear to maximum of 1 L/h for 4 h per day for 2 d |

## Use in Patients Receiving Home Care

Bisacodyl is commonly self-prescribed and self-administered in the home setting. With all drugs used to treat constipation, it is important to identify patients at risk for developing constipation. The home care nurse assesses the usual patterns of bowel elimination, promotes lifestyle interventions to prevent constipation, and uses cathartics only as indicated.

## Adverse Effects

Common adverse effects of bisacodyl include abdominal pain and cramping, nausea, diarrhea, and weakness.

## Contraindications

Contraindications to bisacodyl include known allergy to the drug. Additionally, the presence of undiagnosed abdominal pain or intestinal obstruction or fecal impaction precludes its use.

## Nursing Implications

### Preventing Interactions

Medications interact with bisacodyl to decrease its effect (Box 39.2). Bisacodyl should not be taken within an hour after ingesting milk, because milk increases gastric pH and may reduce the resistance of the enteric coating of the tablet, resulting in earlier release of the drug.

### Administering the Medication

It is necessary to take bisacodyl on an empty stomach or at bedtime. Patients should swallow the drug whole.

 **QSEN Alert: Safety**

People should not use bisacodyl frequently or for longer than 1 week because it may produce serum electrolyte and acid–base imbalances (e.g., hypocalcemia, hypokalemia, metabolic acidosis, or alkalosis).

The nurse inserts bisacodyl rectal suppositories to the length of the index finger, next to the rectal mucosa.

### Assessing for Therapeutic Effects

Oral formulations produce laxative effects in 6 to 12 hours, and a single bedtime dose of bisacodyl usually produces a morning bowel movement. Rectal forms of bisacodyl typically produce a bowel movement within 15 minutes to 1 hour.

**BOX 39.2**  ***Drug Interactions: Bisacodyl***

**Drugs That Decrease the Effects of Bisacodyl**
- Anticholinergic drugs (e.g., atropine)
  *Slow intestinal motility, increasing constipation*
- H₂ receptor blockers (e.g., ranitidine)
  *Decrease stomach acid, resulting in premature tablet dissolution and gastric irritation*
- Proton pump inhibitors (e.g., omeprazole)
  *Decrease stomach acid, resulting in premature tablet dissolution and gastric irritation*

## Assessing for Adverse Effects

The nurse monitors for bowel elimination patterns and the presence of diarrhea. In addition, the nurse should monitor for the existence of abdominal pain and cramping, nausea, or weakness.

### Patient Teaching

With bisacodyl tablets, it is important to instruct the patient to swallow the tablets without chewing and not to take them within an hour after ingesting milk or gastric antacids or while receiving H₂ receptor blocker therapy. This prevents abdominal cramping and vomiting associated with premature tablet dissolution and gastric irritation.

Box 39.1 presents additional patient teaching guidelines for the laxatives and cathartics.

## Other Drugs in the Class

### Stimulant Cathartics

Besides bisacodyl, other stimulant cathartics are available. In addition to irritant, stimulant effects, glycerin exerts hyperosmotic effects in the colon. It usually acts within 30 minutes. Available in the form of rectal suppositories, glycerin is not given orally for laxative effects. Oral stimulant cathartics include castor oil and senna preparations.

### Saline Cathartics

Saline cathartics (e.g., magnesium citrate, milk of magnesia) are not well absorbed from the intestine. Consequently, the drugs increase osmotic pressure in the intestinal lumen and cause water to be retained. Distention of the bowel leads to increased peristalsis and decreased intestinal transit time for the fecal mass. The resultant stool is semifluid. These cathartics are used when rapid bowel evacuation is needed. With oral magnesium preparations, effects occur within ½ to 6 hours.

Saline cathartics are generally useful and safe for short-term treatment of constipation, cleansing the bowel before endoscopic examinations, and treating fecal impaction. However, they are not safe for frequent or prolonged usage or for certain patients because they may produce fluid and electrolyte imbalances. For example, patients with impaired renal function are at risk for hypermagnesemia with magnesium-containing laxatives because some of the magnesium is absorbed systemically. Patients with congestive heart failure are at risk for fluid retention and edema with sodium-containing cathartics. Saline cathartics containing phosphate, sodium, magnesium, or potassium salts are usually contraindicated or must be used cautiously in the presence of impaired renal function and in people who follow a sodium-restricted diet for hypertension. Ten percent or more of the magnesium in magnesium salts may be absorbed and cause hypermagnesemia, and potassium salts may cause hyperkalemia. Polyethylene glycol–electrolyte solution (PEG-ES) (e.g., NuLYTELY) is formulated for rapid and effective bowel cleansing without significant changes in water or electrolyte balance. The drug is a nonabsorbable oral solution that induces diarrhea within 30 to 60 minutes and rapidly evacuates the bowel, usually within 4 hours. It is a prescription drug used for bowel cleansing before GI examination (e.g., colonoscopy) and is contraindicated in patients with GI obstruction, gastric retention, colitis, or bowel perforation. Combination products, available by prescription, such as HalfLytely combine polyethylene glycol with a stimulant cathartic, bisacodyl, to evacuate the colon in preparation for a colonoscopy. Polyethylene glycol solution (MiraLAX) is an oral laxative that may be used to treat occasional constipation. Effects may require 2 to 4 days. It is an over-the-counter drug, and people should not take it for longer than 2 weeks. Refrigerating magnesium citrate and PEG-ES before giving increases palatability and retains potency.

4. **A nurse is caring for a patient preparing to undergo a colonoscopy. Which of the following drugs do health care providers commonly use to enhance bowel cleansing? (Select all that apply.)**

   A. polyethylene glycol–electrolyte solution
   B. bisacodyl
   C. psyllium
   D. docusate sodium

5. **Which of the following mechanism of action is shown by over-the-counter drug magnesium hydroxide (milk of magnesia)?**

   A. increased gastric secretions
   B. increased osmotic pressure in the intestinal lumen
   C. binding to diarrhea-causing bacteria for excretion
   D. decreased gastrointestinal motility

## MISCELLANEOUS AGENTS FOR CONSTIPATION

Several miscellaneous agents are used in the treatment of constipation. These drugs are discussed briefly below, and Table 39.5 gives dosage information.

Lactulose (Constulose, Kristalose) is a disaccharide that is not absorbed from the GI tract. It exerts laxative effects by pulling water into the intestinal lumen. It is used to treat constipation and hepatic encephalopathy. The latter condition usually results from alcoholic liver disease in which ammonia accumulates and causes stupor or coma. Metabolism of dietary protein and intestinal bacteria produces ammonia. Lactulose decreases production of ammonia in the intestine. The goal of treatment is usually to maintain two to three soft stools daily; effects usually occur within 24 to 48 hours. It is important to use the drug cautiously because it may produce electrolyte imbalances and dehydration.

 *Concept Mastery Alert*

Lactulose treats constipation by producing acid in the colon. It is catabolized by the bacterial flora in the colon into lactic acid and acetic acid. These acids lower the colonic pH; the reduced pH favors the formation of the nonabsorbable $NH_4^+$ from $NH_3$, trapping $NH_4^+$ in the colon and thus reducing plasma ammonia concentrations. In addition, the cathartic effects of a hyperosmolar load in the colon improve gastrointestinal transit, allowing less time for ammonia absorption.

Lubiprostone (Amitiza) is a chloride channel activator indicated for the treatment of chronic idiopathic constipation in adults, irritable bowel syndrome with constipation in women greater than 18 years of age, and opioid-induced constipation in adults. The drug acts locally in the apical membrane of the GI tract, producing increased intestinal fluid secretion and improved fecal transit. This mode of action is particularly beneficial in individuals with opioid-induced constipation as the effect bypasses the antisecretory effects of opiates, suppressing secretomotor neuron excitability.

The agent is more expensive compared to other treatment options for severe constipation, and its long-term safety has not been established. Lubiprostone is poorly absorbed into the circulation and exerts its effect locally, activating chloride channels in the GI tract to increase the secretion of chloride-rich fluids into the intestine. Increased intestinal fluid secretion stimulates intestinal motility, improving the passage of stool. It is metabolized by enzymes in the stomach and excreted in the urine and feces.

Adverse effects of lubiprostone include nausea, particularly in older adults, and severe diarrhea. Taking the drug with food may aid in decreasing nausea. Acute-onset dyspnea has been observed following the first and subsequent doses of lubiprostone that resolves within a few hours. Syncope and hypotension may also occur and generally resolve prior to the next dose or following discontinuation. Hypotension may require hospitalization, particularly in patients who are also taking drugs that produce a hypotensive effect. In addition, methadone may decrease the therapeutic effect of the agent.

Linaclotide (Linzess) and plecanatide (Trulance) are guanylate cyclase-C (GC-C) agonists that work to increase the secretion of chloride and water in the intestines by binding to GC-C on the surface of intestinal epithelium. This action softens stools and stimulates bowel movements. The drugs are used to treat adults with chronic idiopathic constipation and irritable bowel syndrome with constipation. The drugs should be given on an empty stomach at least 30 minutes before the first meal. Adverse effects include diarrhea and abdominal discomfort. The U.S. Food and Drug Administration (FDA) has issued a **BLACK BOX WARNING** ◆ for use of linaclotide and plecanatide in children. The drugs are contraindicated in children younger than 6 years of age. Death from dehydration was reported in nonclinical studies from administration of a single, adult oral dose of linaclotide. The drug should be avoided in children and adolescents 6 through 17 years of age.

Sorbitol is a monosaccharide that pulls water into the intestinal lumen and has laxative effects. It is often given with sodium polystyrene sulfonate (Kayexalate), a potassium-removing resin used to treat hyperkalemia, prevent constipation, and aid expulsion of the potassium–resin complex. It can also be given with activated charcoal to eliminate toxins in the body. Maternal use during pregnancy is not expected to result in fetal exposure to the drug.

Tegaserod (Zelnorm) is used as a short-term treatment of irritable bowel syndrome with constipation in women less than 65 years of age. Efficacy and safety have not been established in males. The drug is contraindicated with moderate to severe renal or liver disease and in women over the age of 65. The drug is also contraindicated in patients with a history of myocardial infarction, angina, stroke, or transient ischemic attack. Common adverse effects include headache and abdominal pain. The drug should be taken 30 minutes before meals as food decreases the drug's bioavailability and prolongs maximum effectiveness for 1 to 2 hours following a meal.

**TABLE 39.5**

## DRUGS AT A GLANCE: Miscellaneous Drugs Administered for the Treatment of Constipation

| Drug | Pregnancy Category | Routes and Dosage Ranges | |
|---|---|---|---|
| | | **Adults** | **Children** |
| Lactulose (Constulose, Enulose, Kristalose; ❧ Apo-Lactulose, Teva-Lactulose) | B | For constipation:<br>PO 10–20 g (15–30 mL) daily; maximum dose 60 mL daily<br>Portal systemic encephalopathy:<br>PO 20–30 g (30–45 mL) 3 or 4 times daily, adjusted to produce two or three soft stools daily<br>Rectally as retention enema, 300 mL with 700 mL water or normal saline, retained 30–60 min, every 4–6 h | Infants: PO 2.5–10 mL daily in divided doses<br>Older children: PO 40–90 mL daily in divided doses |
| Lubiprostone (Amitiza) | C | For chronic idiopathic constipation:<br>PO 24 mcg twice daily with food<br>For irritable bowel syndrome with constipation: females ≥18 y, 8 mcg twice daily<br>Opioid-induced constipation: PO 24 mcg twice daily | Safety and efficacy in children has not been established |
| Linaclotide (Linzess; ❧ Constella) | C | For chronic idiopathic constipation: PO 145 mcg once daily<br>For irritable bowel syndrome with constipation: PO 290 mcg once daily | ≤6 y: contraindicated<br>7–16 y: safety and efficacy not established |
| Plecanatide (Trulance) | Unknown; approved in 2017 | For chronic idiopathic constipation: PO 3 mg once daily | ≤6 y: contraindicated<br>7–16 y: safety and efficacy not established |
| Sorbitol | C | As hyperosmolar laxative, PO 30–150 mL (as 70% solution)<br>Rectal enema, 120 mL as 25%–30% solution | 2–11 y: PO 2 mg/kg (as 70% solution); rectal enema, 30–60 mL as 25%–30% solution<br>12 y and older: same as adult dose |
| Prucalopride (Motegrity; ❧ Resotran) | Unknown; approved in 2018 | For chronic idiopathic constipation: PO 2 mg once daily | Not approved for use in children |
| Tegaserod (Zelnorm) | B | For irritable bowel syndrome with constipation in women: PO 6 mg two times daily before meals | Not approved for use in children |

Prucalopride (*Motegrity*) is a serotonin 5-HT$_4$ receptor agonist used to treat chronic idiopathic constipation in adults. The drug enhances normal GI motility. Caution should be used with administration in people with renal impairment. Common adverse effects include headache, abdominal pain, nausea, and diarrhea. Diarrhea may be severe, particularly during the first week of treatment, and usually resolves within a few days. Dizziness has been reported, so patients should be instructed to avoid operating machinery and other tasks that require mental alertness. Suicide ideations have been reported, and patients should be monitored for worsening of depression or development of suicidal thoughts and behaviors.

### ⚠ QSEN Alert: Evidence-Based Practice

In a randomized, double-blind, controlled trial, Schoenfeld et al. (2018) explored the efficacy and safety of low-dose linaclotide for chronic irritable bowel syndrome with constipation in 1223 patients (mean age = 46 years, white = 71%, female = 77%). Inclusion criteria included less than three spontaneous bowel movements per week without the use of laxative, suppository, or enema during the preceding 24 hours and at least one of the following symptoms during 25% or more of bowel movements for at least 12 weeks within the preceding 6 months: straining, lumpy or hard stools, and a sensation of incomplete evacuation. Findings demonstrated that once-daily linaclotide (72 mcg) significantly improved symptoms in women and men in 12 weeks and the need to discontinue the drug due to diarrhea was low.

### *Clinical Application 39.3*

- Mrs. Campbell is concerned about not having a bowel movement. She takes a psyllium preparation at 8 AM. She does not have a result by noon, so she takes milk of magnesia. She has not had a stool by supper, so she takes a glycerin suppository. She has diarrhea throughout the night. What patient education is appropriate?

**THE NURSING PROCESS**

A concept map outlines the nursing process related to drug therapy considerations in this chapter. Additional nursing implications related to the disease process should also be considered in care decisions.

**Assessment**

- Assess patients for current or potential constipation.
- Signs and symptoms include the following:
  - Decreased number and frequency of stools (fewer than two to three stools per week, depending on age)
  - Passage of dry, hard stool
  - Abdominal distention and discomfort
  - Flatulence
  - Sensation of incomplete evacuation
  - History of retentive posturing or excessive volitional stool retention
  - Large mass of stool in rectum
- Presence of risk factors
  - Diet with minimal fiber (e.g., small amounts of fruits, vegetables, and whole-grain products)
  - Low fluid intake (e.g., less than 2000 mL daily)
  - Immobility or limited activity
  - Use of drugs that reduce intestinal function and motility (e.g., opioid analgesics, antacids containing aluminum or calcium, anticholinergics, calcium channel blockers, clozapine, diuretics, iron, phenothiazines, cholestyramine, colestipol, sucralfate, tricyclic antidepressants, vincristine)
  - Overuse of antidiarrheal agents, which may also cause constipation
  - Conditions that may reduce intestinal function and motility (e.g., depression, eating disorders such as anorexia nervosa, hypothyroidism, hypercalcemia, multiple sclerosis, Parkinson's disease, spinal lesions)
  - Hemorrhoids, anal fissures, or other conditions characterized by painful bowel elimination
  - Elderly or debilitated status

**Outcomes of Therapy**

The patient will
- Take drugs appropriately to promote normal bowel function and prevent constipation.
- Use nondrug measures to promote normal bowel function and prevent constipation.
- Regain normal patterns of bowel elimination.
- Avoid excessive losses of fluids and electrolytes from laxative use.
- Be protected from excessive fluid loss, hypotension, and other adverse drug effects, when possible.
- Be assisted to avoid constipation when at risk (e.g., has illness or injury that prevents activity and food and fluid intake; takes medications that decrease GI function).

**Nursing Interventions**

- Assist patients with constipation and caregivers to
  - Understand the importance of diet, exercise, and fluid intake in promoting normal bowel function and preventing constipation.
  - Increase activity and exercise.
  - Increase intake of dietary fiber (e.g., vegetables, fruits, cereal grains).
  - Drink at least 2000 mL of fluid daily, if not contraindicated.
  - Establish and maintain a routine for bowel elimination (e.g., going to the bathroom immediately after breakfast).
  - Recognize importance of and comply with drug therapy (see Box 39.1).
- Monitor patient responses.
  - Record number, amount, and type of bowel movements.
  - Record vital signs. Hypotension and weak pulse may indicate deficient fluid volume.

**Evaluation**

- Observe and interview for improved patterns of bowel elimination.
- Observe for use of nondrug measures to promote bowel function.
- Observe for appropriate use of laxatives.
- Observe and interview regarding adverse effects of laxatives.

## KEY CONCEPTS

- Constipation is the infrequent and painful expulsion of hard, dry stools.
- Lifestyle modifications such as fluid and fiber intake and exercise are preferred to medications in the treatment of constipation.
- Laxatives and cathartics are drugs to promote bowel elimination.
- Common reasons for abuse of laxatives and cathartics include eating disorders, desire for strict weight control, or the belief that a daily bowel movement is necessary for health.
- Laxatives and cathartics should not be used in the presence of undiagnosed abdominal pain or other signs of intestinal obstruction because of the risks of perforation and peritonitis.
- Bulk-forming laxatives add mass to the feces, stimulating peristalsis and defecation. They must be taken with water to avoid obstruction. Generally, bulk-forming drugs are the most desirable laxative for long-term use.
- Surfactant laxatives decrease the surface tension of the fecal mass to allow water and fat to penetrate into the stool, making it softer and easier to expel. They have little true laxative effect.
- Saline laxatives increase the osmotic pressure in the intestinal lumen, resulting in the retention of water, which distends the bowel and stimulates peristalsis. They produce a semifluid stool and may lead to fluid and electrolyte imbalances.
- Polyethylene glycol–electrolyte solution is a nonabsorbable oral solution that rapidly evacuates the bowel within 4 hours. It is useful for bowel cleansing before GI procedures.
- Stimulant cathartics are the strongest and most abused laxative products. They irritate the GI mucosa, pull water into the colon, and stimulate peristalsis. They produce a watery stool and may lead to fluid, electrolyte, and acid–base imbalances.
- Lubricant laxatives lubricate the fecal mass and slow colonic absorption of water from the fecal mass. These medications may interfere with the absorption of fat-soluble vitamins and, if aspirated, may result in a lipid aspiration pneumonia.
- Lactulose exerts an osmotic effect, pulling water into the colon and stimulating peristalsis. It is also useful in treating hepatic encephalopathy by decreasing the production of the waste product ammonia.
- Sorbitol is often given with sodium polystyrene sulfonate (Kayexalate) in the treatment of hyperkalemia to aid in the expulsion of the potassium–resin complex.
- Drug therapy for patients with irritable bowel syndrome with constipation includes lubiprostone (in women greater than 18 years of age), linaclotide, or plecanatide.
- Lubiprostone (Amitiza) aids in treating chronic idiopathic constipation by increasing intestinal fluid secretion, stimulating intestinal motility and defecation.
- Linaclotide should be given on an empty stomach at least 30 minutes before the first meal.
- The FDA has issued a **BLACK BOX WARNING ◆** for use of linaclotide in children. The drug is contraindicated in children younger than 6 years of age; death from dehydration has been reported in nonclinical studies from administration of a single, adult oral dose.

## CLINICAL REASONING CASE STUDY

**Meet the Patient**

Grace Park, a 6-year-old child, is seen in the pediatrician's office. Her mother reports that Grace has had occasional constipation since birth, which was well managed with increasing fiber in her diet. However, the constipation has become worse since her daughter started first grade. According to Mrs. Park, Grace has no more than two stools in the toilet each week but when she does, they are large-diameter stools that have obstructed the toilet on occasion. She has also become incontinent of stool at night. Grace complains of painful bowel movements, and she is reluctant to use the toilets at her elementary school to have a bowel movement. Physical examination reveals a markedly increased amount of stool in the colon. The pediatrician has prescribed polyethylene glycol (PEG) without electrolytes (MiraLAX) 1 g/kg/day by mouth for 6 days. The physician wants to see Grace on the sixth day and may consider a maintenance dose of PEG or other treatment options at that time.

- Grace weighs 44 lb. What is the daily dose in grams of PEG that should be administered?
- What patient teaching should the nurse provide to Grace and her mother?
- Mrs. Park asks the nurse how biofeedback can correct the constipation for Grace. What is the best response by the nurse?

**Assessing Drug Information**

- PEG is a mild oral cathartic that works by keeping more water in the stool so it is softer and easier to pass. The drug may take 24 hours or more to work.
- It is used for occasional constipation or for bowel preparation prior to bowel procedures (i.e., colonoscopy).
- It is well tolerated in children and adults but may cause loose, watery, or more frequent bowel movements. This may cause an increase in the soiling episodes Grace has experienced, especially during disimpaction; this should resolve. The most common side effects reported by patients include nausea, bloating, cramping, or gas.

**Nursing Actions**

- Grace weighs 44 lb or 20 kg (44/2.2). Tell Mrs. Park that her daughter should receive a daily dose of 20 g of laxative.
- Instruct Mrs. Park and Grace (as developmentally appropriate) as follows:
  - Provide a diet that is conducive to fecal regularity, including (1) increased intake of fruit and raw vegetables, bran, and whole-grain breads and cereals, as well as (2) adequate intake of fluids other than milk.
  - Keep a diary or log to record bowel movements; the use of medication; and episodes of fecal incontinence, abdominal pain, and other symptoms.
  - Plan, encourage, and observe a program of regular toilet-sitting. Grace should sit on the toilet shortly after a meal, for 5 to 10 minutes, two to three times per day. Toilet-sitting episodes should occur at the same time each day and be timed with a timer. (If her feet do not touch the floor sitting on a regular toilet seat, it is helpful to use a stool for foot support.)
  - Structure a reward system that is tailored to Grace; provide the reward (stickers, reading a book while sitting, or special toys used only during toilet-sitting) for effort (i.e., toilet-sitting) rather than success (i.e., having a bowel movement in the toilet). No one should make negative comments about incontinence of stool. Grace should not be scolded or otherwise punished for soiling episodes or lack of success in having a bowel movement.
  - To avoid reaccumulation of stool, ensure that a maintenance regimen of laxatives is started immediately after disimpaction based on the pediatrician's recommendations.
  - If Grace's aversion to using the school bathroom facilities persists and increases constipation, it may be helpful to seek the help of the school and teacher. Some children benefit from access to a private bathroom. Also, it may be helpful to have a change of clothing available in case a soiling episode occurs.

Visit thePoint® at **http://thePoint.lww.com/Frandsen12e** for answers to NCLEX Success questions (in Appendix A), answers to Clinical Application Case Studies (in Appendix B), and more!

## REFERENCES AND RESOURCES

Andy, U. U., Vaughan, C. P., Burgio, K. L., Alli, F. M., Goode, P. S., & Markland, A. D. (2016). Shared risk factors for constipation, fecal incontinence, and combined symptoms in older U.S. adults. *Journal of the American Geriatrics Society, 64*(11), e183–e188.

Carter, D., Bardan, E., & Dickman, R. (2018). Comparison of strategies and goals for treatment of chronic constipation among gastroenterologists and general practitioners. *Annals of Gastroenterology, 31*(1), 71–76. doi:10.20524/aog.2017.0214

Carter, D., Ron, Y., & Dickman, R. (2017). The Israeli Neurogastroenterology Association recommendations for the evaluation and treatment of chronic constipation. *Harefuah, 156*(11), 725–729.

DeMicco, M., Barrow, L., Hickey, B., Shailubhai, K., & Griffin, P. (2017). Randomized clinical trial: Efficacy and safety of plecanatide in the treatment of chronic idiopathic constipation. *Therapeutic Advances in Gastroenterology, 10*, 837–851.

DiPiro, J. T., Talbert, R. L., Yee, G. C., Wells, B. G., Posey, L. M., & Matzke, G. R. (2020). *Pharmacotherapy: A pathophysiologic approach* (11th ed., Kindle Edition). New York: McGraw-Hill Education.

Hinkle, J. H., & Cheever, K. H. (2018). *Brunner & Suddarth's textbook of medical-surgical nursing* (14th ed.). Philadelphia, PA: Wolters Kluwer.

Karch, A. M. (2019). *Focus on Nursing Pharmacology* (8th ed.). Philadelphia, PA: Wolters Kluwer.

Lacy, B. E., Mearin, F., Chang, L., Chey, W. D., Lembo, A. J., Simren, M., et al. (2016). Bowel disorders. *Gastroenterology, 150*, 1393–1407. e1395.

Lippincott Williams & Wilkins. (2019). *Nursing 2020 Drug Handbook* (40th ed.). Philadelphia, PA: Lippincott Williams & Wilkins.

Martinez de Andino, N. (2018). Current treatment paradigm and landscape for the management of chronic idiopathic constipation in adults: Focus on plecanatide. *Journal of the American Association of Nurse Practitioners, 30*, 412–420. doi:10.1097/JXX.0000000000000090

Norris, T. L. (2019). *Pathophysiology: Concepts of altered health status* (10th ed.). Philadelphia, PA: Wolters Kluwer.

Paquette, I. M., Varma, M., Ternent, C., Melton-Meaux, G., Rafferty, J. F., Feingold, D., et al. (2016). The American Society of Colon and Rectal Surgeons' Clinical Practice Guideline for the Evaluation and Management of Constipation. *Diseases of the Colon & Rectum, 59*(6), 479–492. doi:10.1097/DCR.0000000000000599

Philichi, L. (2018). Management of childhood functional constipation. *Journal of Pediatric Health Care, 32*(1), 103–111.

Schoenfeld, P., Lacy, B. E., Chey, W. D., Lembo, A. J., Kurtz, C. B., Reasner, D. S., et al. (2018). Low-dose linaclotide (72 μg) for chronic idiopathic constipation: A 12-week, randomized, double-blind, placebo-controlled trial. *American Journal of Gastroenterology, 113*(1), 105–114. doi: 10.1038/ajg.2017.230

Sood, M. R. (2020). Chronic functional constipation and fecal incontinence in infants and children: Treatment. In *UpToDate*. Lexi Comp, Inc.

Tabbers, M. M., DiLorenzo, C., Berger, M. Y., Faure, C., Langendam, M. W., Nurko, S., et al. (2014). Evaluation and treatment of functional constipation in infants and children: Evidence-based recommendations from ESPGHAN and NASPGHAN. *Journal of Pediatric Gastroenterology and Nutrition, 58*(2), 258–274.

UpToDate. (2019). *Drug information*. Lexi-Comp, Inc.

Wald, A. (2020). Management of chronic constipation in adults. In *UpToDate*. Lexi Comp, Inc.

Wald, A. (2020). Treatment of irritable bowel syndrome in adults. In *UpToDate*. Lexi Comp, Inc.

# Drug Therapy for Diarrhea

## LEARNING OBJECTIVES

*After studying this chapter, you should be able to:*

1. Identify the common causes of diarrhea.
2. Identify patients at risk for development of diarrhea.
3. Describe opioid-related antidiarrheal agents in terms of the prototype, indications and contraindications for use, routes of administration, and major adverse effects.
4. Identify adjuvant drugs used to manage diarrhea.
5. Apply the nursing process in the care of patients receiving drug therapy for diarrhea.

## CLINICAL APPLICATION CASE STUDY

Joseph Mendoza is a 47-year-old salesman who travels extensively as part of his job. He returned from a trip to Asia 2 days ago, and since his return, he has had abdominal cramping and bloating and an average of four watery bowel movements per day. Mr. Mendoza comes to the clinic seeking advice about how to manage his symptoms. He denies nausea and vomiting. His vital signs are temperature 99.4°F, pulse 82 beats/min, respirations 22 breaths/min, and blood pressure 124/72 mm Hg lying and 120/72 mm Hg standing.

## KEY TERMS

**Diarrhea:** increase in the liquidity of stool or frequency of defecation to more than 3 stools per day

**Inflammatory bowel disorders:** disorders in which inflamed mucous membranes secrete large amounts of fluids into the intestinal lumen, along with mucus, proteins, and blood; characterized by impaired absorption of water and electrolytes

**Irritable bowel syndrome:** functional disorder of intestinal motility with no evidence of inflammation or tissue changes

**Steatorrhea:** loose, fatty stool

**Traveler's diarrhea:** form of diarrhea caused by the enterotoxigenic strain of *Escherichia coli*, typically from fecal contamination of food or water

# INTRODUCTION

The focus of this chapter is the description of drugs used to relieve the symptoms of diarrhea, specifically the opioid-related agents. Topics of discussion include the general characteristics of these drugs, their mechanisms of action, indications for and contraindications to their use, and their nursing implications. The section on adjuvant medications briefly addresses specific drugs, including antibacterial agents, used to manage underlying disease processes that cause diarrhea.

# OVERVIEW OF DIARRHEA

## Pathophysiology

**Diarrhea**, an increase in the liquidity of stool or frequency of defecation to more than 3 stools per day, is a common condition experienced by virtually everyone. It is a symptom of numerous conditions and not a disease. Diarrhea is a manifestation of basic mechanisms that increase bowel motility, cause secretion or retention of fluids in the intestinal lumen (lactose intolerance or toxins such as cholera or laxatives and other drugs), or cause inflammation or irritation of the gastrointestinal (GI) tract (*Escherichia coli*, *Salmonella*, rotaviruses, *Giardia*). It is common for more than one of the mechanisms to be involved in the pathogenesis of a given situation. As a result, bowel contents are rapidly propelled toward the rectum, and absorption of fluids and electrolytes is limited.

## Clinical Manifestations

Diarrhea may be acute or chronic and mild or severe. Most episodes of acute diarrhea are defensive mechanisms by which the body tries to rid itself of irritants, toxins, and infectious agents. These episodes of frequent liquid or semiliquid stools are usually self-limiting and subside within 24 to 48 hours without serious consequences. If severe or prolonged, acute diarrhea may lead to serious fluid and electrolyte depletion, especially in young children and older adults. Chronic diarrhea may cause malnutrition and anemia and is often characterized by remissions and exacerbations.

Fever, vomiting, and bloody stools are associated with acute diarrhea, and the presence of these symptoms may help determine the cause. Fever is common and often linked with invasive pathogens. Vomiting is frequently found in illness caused by ingestion of bacterial toxins or viruses. Invasive and cytotoxin-releasing pathogens are known to cause bloody stools, and enterotoxigenic strain *E. coli* O157:H7 infection is suspected in the absence of fecal leukocytes. Bloody stools are not associated with viral agents and enterotoxins that release bacteria.

## Etiology

Some causes of diarrhea include the following:

- *Excessive use or abuse of laxatives*. Laxative abuse may accompany eating disorders such as anorexia nervosa or bulimia.
  - *Undigested, coarse, or highly spiced food in the GI tract*. The food acts as an irritant and attracts fluids in a defensive attempt to dilute the irritating agent. This may result from inadequate chewing of food or lack of digestive enzymes.

- *Lack of digestive enzymes*. Deficiency of pancreatic enzymes inhibits digestion and absorption of carbohydrates, proteins, and fats. Deficiency of lactase, which breaks down lactose to simple sugars (i.e., glucose and galactose) that can be absorbed by GI mucosa, inhibits digestion of milk and milk products. Lactase deficiency commonly occurs in people of African and Asian descent.
- *Intestinal infections with viruses, bacteria, or protozoa*. A common source of infection is ingested food or fluid contaminated by a variety of organisms.
  - *E. coli* O157:H7–related hemorrhagic colitis most commonly occurs with the ingestion of undercooked ground beef. A serious complication of *E. coli* O157:H7 colitis is hemolytic uremic syndrome (HUS), characterized by thrombocytopenia, microangiopathic hemolytic anemia, and renal failure. Children are especially susceptible to HUS, which is the leading cause of dialysis in pediatric patients. So-called **traveler's diarrhea** is usually caused by an enterotoxigenic strain of *E. coli* (ETEC). Fecal contamination of food or water is the most common source of ETEC-induced diarrhea.
  - Consumption of improperly prepared poultry may result in diarrhea due to infection with *Campylobacter jejuni*. In the United States, this is the most common bacterial organism identified in infectious diarrhea. In addition to diarrhea, vomiting, fever, and abdominal discomfort, *Campylobacter* bacteria produce neurotoxins, which may result in paralysis.
  - *Salmonella* infections may occur when contaminated poultry and other meats, eggs, and dairy products are ingested. Elderly patients are especially susceptible to *Salmonella*-associated colitis.
  - Several strains of *Shigella* may produce diarrhea. Infection most often results from direct person-to-person contact but may also occur via food or water contamination. Hand washing is especially important in preventing the spread of *Shigella* from person to person.
  - Other diarrhea-producing organisms associated with contamination of specific foods include *Vibrio vulnificus* and *Vibrio parahaemolyticus* contamination of raw shellfish and oysters (particularly in the Gulf Coast states), *Clostridium perfringens* contamination of inadequately heated or reheated meats, *Staphylococcus aureus* contamination of processed meats and custard-filled pastries, *Bacillus cereus* contamination of rice and bean sprouts, and *Listeria monocytogenes* contamination of hot dogs and luncheon meats. Newborns, pregnant women, and older and immunocompromised people are especially susceptible to *L. monocytogenes* infection.
  - Two of the most common viral organisms responsible for gastroenteritis and diarrhea are rotavirus or Norwalk-like virus (calicivirus). Vomiting is usually a prominent symptom accompanying virus-induced diarrhea.
- **Inflammatory bowel disorders**, such as gastroenteritis, diverticulitis, ulcerative colitis, and Crohn's disease. In these disorders, inflamed mucous membranes secrete large amounts of fluids into the intestinal lumen, along with mucus, proteins, and blood, and there is impaired absorption of water and electrolytes. In addition, when the ileum is diseased or a portion is surgically excised, large amounts of bile

salts reach the colon, where they act as cathartics and cause diarrhea. Bile salts are normally reabsorbed from the ileum.

- **Irritable bowel syndrome** (IBS) is a functional disorder of intestinal motility with no evidence of inflammation or tissue changes. It occurs more commonly in women than in men, affecting approximately 25 to 45 million adults in the United States. A change in bowel pattern (constipation, diarrhea, or a combination of both) accompanied by abdominal pain, bloating, and distention are the presenting symptoms. The etiology is unknown; however, activation of 5-HT$_3$ (serotonin) receptors, which affect the regulation of visceral pain, colonic motility, and GI secretions, is thought to be involved in the pathophysiology of IBS.

- *Drugs.* Many oral drugs irritate the GI tract and may cause diarrhea, including acarbose, antacids that contain magnesium, antibacterials, antineoplastic agents, colchicine, laxatives, metformin, metoclopramide, misoprostol, selective serotonin reuptake inhibitors, tacrine, and tacrolimus. Antibacterial drugs are commonly used offenders that also may cause diarrhea by altering the normal bacterial flora in the intestine.

  Antibiotic-associated colitis (also called pseudomembranous colitis) is a serious condition that results from oral or parenteral antibiotic therapy. By suppressing normal flora in the colon, antibiotics allow proliferation of other bacteria, especially gram-positive, anaerobic *Clostridioides difficile* organisms. These organisms produce a toxin that causes fever, abdominal pain, inflammatory lesions of the colon, and severe diarrhea with stools containing mucus, pus, and sometimes blood. Symptoms may develop within a few days or several weeks after the causative antibiotic is discontinued. Other enteric pathogens that may overgrow in the presence of antibiotic therapy and result in colitis include *Salmonella*, *C. perfringens* type A, *S. aureus*, and *Candida albicans*. Antibiotic-associated colitis is more often associated with ampicillin, cephalosporins, and clindamycin but may occur with any antibiotic or combination of antibiotics that alters intestinal microbial flora.

- *Intestinal neoplasms.* Tumors may increase intestinal motility by occupying space and stretching the intestinal wall. Diarrhea sometimes alternates with constipation in colon cancer.

- *Functional disorders.* Diarrhea may be a symptom of stress or anxiety in some patients. No organic disease process can be found in such circumstances.

- *Hyperthyroidism.* This condition increases bowel motility.

- *Surgical excision of portions of the intestine, especially the small intestine.* Such procedures decrease the absorptive area and increase fluidity of stools.

- *Human immunodeficiency virus (HIV) infection/acquired immunodeficiency syndrome (AIDS).* Diarrhea occurs in most patients with HIV infection, often as a chronic condition that contributes to malnutrition and weight loss. It may be caused by drug therapy, infection with a variety of microorganisms, or other factors.

## Nonpharmacologic Therapy

In most cases of acute, nonspecific diarrhea in adults, fluid losses are not severe, and patients need only simple replacement of fluids and electrolytes to replace those lost in the stool. Acceptable replacement fluids during the first 24 hours include clear liquids (e.g., flat ginger ale, decaffeinated cola drinks or tea, broth, gelatin)—2 to 3 L. Also, a diet consisting of bland foods (e.g., rice, soup, bread, salted crackers, cooked cereals, baked potatoes, eggs, applesauce) is best. People may resume their regular diet after 2 or 3 days.

## Drug Therapy

Antidiarrheal drugs include a variety of agents, most of which are discussed in other chapters. When used for treatment of diarrhea, health care providers may give the drugs to relieve the symptom or the underlying cause of the symptom. Overall, opiates and opiate derivatives (see Chap. 49) are the most effective agents for symptomatic treatment of diarrhea. Although morphine, codeine, and related drugs are effective in relieving diarrhea, they are rarely used for this purpose because of their adverse effects. The synthetic drugs diphenoxylate and loperamide have replaced these drugs. Uses include only treatment of diarrhea; they do not cause morphine-like adverse effects in recommended doses. Table 40.1 summarizes drugs used to manage diarrhea.

| **TABLE 40.1** | | |
| :--- | :--- | :--- |
| **Drug Therapy for Diarrhea** | | |
| **Drug Class** | **Prototype** | **Other Drugs in the Class** |
| Opiate-related antidiarrheals | Diphenoxylate with atropine sulfate (Lomotil) | Loperamide (Imodium A-D) Paregoric |
| Adjuvant antidiarrheal medications | | Alosetron (Lotronex) Bismuth subsalicylate (Pepto-Bismol) Cholestyramine (Questran) Colestipol (Colestid) Nitazoxanide (Alinia) Octreotide (Sandostatin) Pancreatin or pancrelipase (Viokase, Pancreaze, Creon) Polycarbophil preparations (FiberCon) Rifaximin (Xifaxan) |

# OPIATE-RELATED ANTIDIARRHEAL AGENTS

The oral opioid ⓟ **diphenoxylate with atropine** (Lomotil) is the prototype used to treat moderate to severe diarrhea. A Schedule V controlled substance, diphenoxylate requires a prescription.

## Pharmacokinetics

Diphenoxylate with atropine is well absorbed by the oral route with an onset of action of 45 to 60 minutes. The duration of action is 3 to 4 hours. The drug is metabolized in the liver to active metabolites and is excreted in bile and feces.

## Action

Diphenoxylate with atropine slows peristalsis by acting on the smooth muscles in the intestine.

## Use

Prescribers order diphenoxylate with atropine to treat diarrhea. Table 40.2 provides dosage information for diphenoxylate with atropine and other opiate-related drugs.

### Use in Children

Signs of atropine overdose may occur with usual doses with diphenoxylate, which contains atropine. Children younger than 2 years of age should not take the drug, and those from age 2 to less than 13 years should take the liquid preparation to enhance accuracy in dosage. If there is no improvement in symptoms in 48 hours, treatment with diphenoxylate with atropine is likely to be ineffective.

### Use in Older Adults

Diarrhea is less common than is constipation in older adults, but it may occur from laxative abuse and bowel-cleansing procedures before GI surgery or diagnostic tests. Fluid volume deficits may rapidly develop in older adults with diarrhea. General principles of fluid and electrolyte replacement, measures to decrease GI irritants, and drug therapy apply as for younger adults. Older people may safely take most antidiarrheal drugs, but cautious use is indicated to avoid inducing constipation.

### Use in Patients With Renal and/or Hepatic Impairment

Use of diphenoxylate with atropine warrants extreme caution in patients with severe hepatorenal disease because hepatic coma may be precipitated. Care is also necessary in patients with abnormal results of liver function tests.

### Use in Patients With Critical Illness

Use of diphenoxylate with atropine requires caution in critically ill patients because they may have renal or hepatic compromise. Episodes of acute diarrhea may be defensive mechanisms by which the body tries to rid itself of irritants, toxins, and infectious agents. Antibacterial drugs administered to the critically ill may cause diarrhea by altering the normal bacterial flora in the intestine. It is important to observe for fluid and electrolyte imbalance and assess the cause of diarrhea before treating the condition. Good hand washing techniques are particularly important in preventing the spread of organisms that can cause diarrhea.

## TABLE 40.2

## DRUGS AT A GLANCE: Opiate-Related Antidiarrheal Agents

| Drug | Pregnancy Category | Routes and Dosage Ranges | |
|---|---|---|---|
| | | **Adults** | **Children** |
| ⓟ **Diphenoxylate with atropine sulfate** (Lomotil; 🍁 Lomotil) | C | 5 mg (2 tablets or 10 mL of liquid) PO 3 or 4 times daily; max daily dose 20 mg | Liquid preparation (2.5-mg diphenoxylate and 0.025-mg atropine per 5 mL); contraindicated in children <2 y of age<br>2 y 1.5–3 mL PO four times daily<br>3 y 2–3 mL PO four times daily<br>4 y 2–4 mL PO four times daily<br>5 y 2.5–4.5 mL PO four times daily<br>6–8 y 2.5–5 mL PO four times daily<br>9–12 y 3.5–5 mL PO four times daily |
| Paregoric | C | 5–10 mL PO 1–4 times daily (max of 4 doses) until diarrhea is controlled | PO 0.25–0.5 mL/kg 1–4 times daily (maximum of 4 doses) until diarrhea is controlled |
| Loperamide (Imodium A-D; 🍁 Apo-Loperamide, Diarr-Eze) | C | 4 mg PO initially, then 2 mg after each loose stool to a maximal daily dose of 16 mg. For chronic diarrhea, dosage should be reduced to the lowest effective amount (average 4–8 mg daily) | Contraindicated in children <2 y of age<br>2–5 y, 13–20 kg: 1 mg three times daily<br>6–8 y, 20–30 kg: PO 2 mg twice daily<br>8–12 y, >30 kg: PO 2 mg three times daily |

### Use in Patients Receiving Home Care

People often take prescription drugs such as diphenoxylate with atropine and over-the-counter (OTC) antidiarrheal aids in the home setting. The role of the home care nurse may include advising patients and caregivers about appropriate use of the drugs, trying to identify the cause and severity of the diarrhea (i.e., risk of fluid and electrolyte deficit), and teaching strategies to manage current episodes and prevent future episodes.

## Adverse Effects

Adverse effects of diphenoxylate with atropine include tachycardia, dizziness, headache, flushing, nausea and vomiting, dry skin and mucous membranes, and urinary retention. Hypotension and respiratory depression have occurred, particularly with doses greater than ordered.

## Contraindications

Contraindications to the use of diphenoxylate with atropine include diarrhea caused by toxic materials, microorganisms that penetrate intestinal mucosa (e.g., pathogenic *E. coli*, *Salmonella*, *Shigella*), and antibiotic-associated colitis. In these circumstances, antidiarrheal drugs that slow peristalsis may aggravate and prolong diarrhea.

## Nursing Implications

### Preventing Interactions

Increased levels of diphenoxylate with atropine may result with the use of methotrimeprazine and pramlintide. Decreased drug levels may result from concurrent use of acetylcholinesterase inhibitors. Use of alcohol may increase central nervous system (CNS) depression. There are no known herbal interactions with diphenoxylate.

### Administering the Medication

Administration is oral.

> **QSEN Alert: Safety**
>
> With liquid diphenoxylate and atropine, it is necessary to use only the calibrated dropper furnished by the manufacturer for measuring doses accurately.

### Assessing for Therapeutic Effects

After drug administration, the nurse monitors the number and consistency of stools and fluid and electrolyte balance. Also, he or she assesses for the return of normal pattern of bowel movements and signs of normal fluid and electrolyte balance (adequate hydration, urine output, and skin turgor). In addition, it is important to assess for resumption of usual activities of daily living.

### Assessing for Adverse Effects

The nurse assesses for hypotension and respiratory depression due to the effects of diphenoxylate. He or she observes for signs of the effects of atropine, including tachycardia, thirst, flushing, urinary retention, and dry skin and mucous membranes.

### Patient Teaching

Once the diarrhea is under control, it is important that diphenoxylate with atropine be discontinued. The nurse ensures that patients who take this drug understand how to use it. Box 40.1 outlines patient teaching guidelines for antidiarrheal drugs.

**NCLEX Success**

1. An appropriate nursing measure when treating a 5-year-old child with a 1-day onset of mild diarrhea involves encouraging which of the following?
   - A. regular diet
   - B. intake of clear liquids
   - C. intake of milk products
   - D. no fluids for 24 hours

2. A hospitalized patient on antibiotic therapy begins to experience fever, abdominal pain, and diarrhea containing mucus, pus, and blood. The best nursing intervention in this situation is to do which of the following?
   - A. Continue the antibiotic because the patient has signs of a gastrointestinal infection.
   - B. Monitor the patient's vital signs and notify the provider if there is further deterioration.
   - C. Withhold the antibiotic and notify the provider of the patient's condition.
   - D. Encourage fluid intake because fever is a sign of dehydration.

## Other Drugs in the Class

The choice of antidiarrheal agent depends largely on the cause, severity, and duration of diarrhea. Loperamide (Imodium A-D) is a synthetic derivative of meperidine that decreases GI motility by its effect on intestinal muscles and is an unscheduled, nonprescription drug. Because loperamide does not penetrate the CNS well, it does not cause the CNS effects associated with opioid use and lacks potential for abuse. Although adverse effects are generally few and mild, loperamide can cause abdominal pain, constipation, drowsiness, fatigue, nausea, and vomiting. For nonprescription use, dosages for adults should not exceed 8 mg/day; with supervision by a health care provider, maximum daily dosage is 16 mg/day. In general, it is necessary to discontinue loperamide after 48 hours if clinical improvement has not occurred. The Food and Drug Administration (FDA) has issued a **BLACK BOX WARNING ◆** because torsades de pointes, cardiac arrest, and death have been reported in people using higher than recommended dosages of loperamide. With loperamide, the nurse monitors patients with hepatic impairment for signs of CNS toxicity. The drug normally undergoes extensive first-pass metabolism, which may be lessened by liver disease. As a result, a larger portion of a dose reaches the systemic circulation and may cause adverse effects. Treatment of overdose may involve naloxone, gastric lavage, and administration of activated charcoal. A dosage adjustment may be necessary.

## BOX 40.1   *Patient Teaching Guidelines for Antidiarrheals*

**General Considerations**

- Taking a medication to stop diarrhea is not always needed or desirable because diarrhea may mean the body is trying to rid itself of irritants or bacteria. Treatment is indicated if diarrhea is severe, is prolonged, or occurs in young children or older adults, who are highly susceptible to excessive losses of body fluids and electrolytes.
- Try to drink 2 to 3 quarts of fluid daily. This helps prevent dehydration from fluid loss in stools. Water, clear broths, and noncarbonated, caffeine-free beverages are recommended because they are unlikely to cause further diarrhea.
- Avoid highly spiced or "laxative" foods, such as fresh fruits and vegetables, until diarrhea is controlled.
- Frequent and thorough hand washing and careful food storage and preparation can help prevent diarrhea.
- Consult a health care provider if diarrhea is accompanied by severe abdominal pain or fever or lasts longer than 3 days or if stools contain blood or mucus. These signs and symptoms may indicate more serious disorders for which other treatment measures are needed.
- Stop antidiarrheal drugs when diarrhea is controlled to avoid adverse effects such as constipation.
- Bismuth subsalicylate [Pepto-Bismol] and loperamide [Imodium A-D] are available over the counter; diphenoxylate [Lomotil] is a prescription drug.
- Diphenoxylate and loperamide may cause dizziness or drowsiness and should be used with caution if driving or performing other tasks requiring alertness, coordination, or physical dexterity. In addition, alcohol and other drugs that cause drowsiness should be avoided.
- Pepto-Bismol may temporarily discolor bowel movements a grayish-black.
- Keep antidiarrheal drugs out of reach of children.

**Self or Caregiver Administration**

- Do not administer Pepto-Bismol to children due to the risk of Reye's syndrome.

- Take or give antidiarrheal drugs only as prescribed or directed on nonprescription drug labels.
- Do not exceed maximal daily doses of diphenoxylate [Lomotil], loperamide, or paregoric.
- With liquid diphenoxylate, use only the calibrated dropper furnished by the manufacturer for accurate measurement of dosages.
- Use caution driving or operating heavy machinery with diphenoxylate and atropine, which may cause drowsiness or dizziness, until the effects of the medication are known.
- Diphenoxylate can cause dry mouth, so sucking on hard candy or chewing gum may alleviate the problem.
- With Pepto-Bismol liquid, shake the bottle well before measuring the dose; with tablets, chew them well or allow them to dissolve in the mouth.
- Add at least 30 mL of water to each dose of paregoric to help the drug dose reach the stomach. The mixture appears milky.
- Take cholestyramine or colestipol with at least 4 oz of water. These drugs should never be taken without fluids because they may block the gastrointestinal tract. Also, do not take within 4 hours of other drugs because they may combine with and inactivate other drugs.
- Take rifaximin with or without food for 3 days. Notify your health care prescriber if your condition worsens or does not improve after 1 to 2 days.
- Use caution driving or operating machinery if experiencing dizziness while using rifaximin.
- With Alinia, if you have diabetes, be aware that the oral suspension contains 1.48 g of sucrose per 5 mL.
- With Lotronex, if you become constipated, notice blood in your bowel movements, or experience a new worse or different pain in your stomach or abdomen, *stop* taking the drug and notify your health care prescriber.

---

Paregoric is a schedule III drug alone and a schedule V in the small amounts combined with other drugs; it contains 0.4 mg/mL of morphine. The main effects of paregoric are to increase the muscular tone of the intestine, to inhibit normal peristalsis, and to suppress coughing. Practitioners use it as an antidiarrheal and as an antitussive. In recommended doses over the short term, paregoric does not produce euphoria, analgesia, or dependence.

### ! QSEN Alert: Safety

Confusing paregoric [camphorated tincture of opium] with the much more potent drug opium tincture is a common and potentially fatal drug error. Opium tincture is much more concentrated than is paregoric and contains 10 mg/mL of morphine. Labels on opium tincture packaging should identify it as a poison, giving the strength of morphine as 10 mg/mL and containing the statement, "Warning! Do not use opium tincture in place of paregoric."

### *Clinical Application 40.1*

- What factors does the nurse practitioner include in assessment of Mr. Mendoza?
- What recommendations for management of the diarrhea does the nurse practitioner most likely make?

## ADJUVANT MEDICATIONS USED TO TREAT DIARRHEA

Specific drug therapy for diarrhea depends on the cause of the symptoms and may include the use of hormones, bulk-forming products, enzymatic replacement therapy, bile salt–binding drugs, antibacterial agents, and 5-HT₃ serotonin receptor antagonists. Table 40.3 presents route and dosage information for these drugs.

**TABLE 40.3**

## DRUGS AT A GLANCE: Adjuvant Antidiarrheal Medications

| Drug | Pregnancy Category | Routes and Dosage Ranges | |
|------|--------------------|--------------------------|--|
| | | **Adults** | **Children** |
| Alosetron (Lotronex) | B | 0.5 mg PO twice a day; may increase to 1 mg after 4 wk if needed | Not recommended |
| Bismuth subsalicylate (Pepto-Bismol) | C | 2 tablets or 30 mL PO every 30–60 min, if needed, up to 8 doses in 24 h | Under 3 y, consult pediatrician<br>3–6 y, 1/3 tablet or 5 mL PO every 30–60 min as needed<br>6–9 y, 2/3 tablet or 10 mL PO every 30–60 min as needed<br>9–12 y, 1 tablet or 15 mL PO every 30–60 min as needed |
| Cholestyramine (Questran; ✻ Novo-Cholamine)<br>Binds and inactivates bile salts in the intestine (see Chap. 10) | C | 16–32 g/d in 120–180 mL of water PO, in 2–4 divided doses before or during meals and at bedtime | Safety and effectiveness not established |
| Colestipol (Colestid; ✻ Colestid)<br>Binds and inactivates bile salts in the intestine (see Chap. 10) | C | 15–30 g/d in 120–180 mL of water PO, in 2–4 divided doses before or during meals and at bedtime | Safety and effectiveness not established |
| Nitazoxanide (Alinia)<br>Inhibits growth of certain protozoa | B | 500 mg (tablet or suspension) PO every 12 h for 3 d | 12–47 mo, 5 mL (100 mg) PO every 12 h for 3 d<br>4–11 y, 10 mL (200 mg) PO every 12 h for 3 d<br>≥12 y, see adult dose |
| Octreotide (Sandostatin; ✻ Ocphyl, Sandostatin)<br>Decreases secretions and motility in GI tract (see Chap. 24) | B | 100–150 mcg every 8 h SC, 50–100 mcg every 8 h IV divided over 2–4 doses; start at 200–300 mcg/d divided over 2–4 doses for 2 wk and then individualize dose to response | 1–10 mcg/kg every 12 h SC, IV |
| Pancreatin or pancrelipase (Viokase, Pancreaze, Creon; ✻ Cotazym, Pancrex V, Photozyme)<br>Replaces pancreatic enzymes | C | 1–3 tablets or capsules PO or 1–2 packets of powder with meals and snacks | 1–3 tablets or capsules PO or 1–2 packets of powder with each meal |
| Polycarbophil preparations (FiberCon, Care One Fiber; ✻ Equalactin)<br>Absorbs water and toxins and decreases fluidity of stools (see Chap. 39) | C | 1 g PO, 1–4 times daily; do not exceed 4 g in 24 h; for severe diarrhea, repeat dose every 30 min but do not exceed max dose | Under 6 y, products vary, so consult labels; for severe diarrhea, repeat dose every 30 min but do not exceed max dose<br>6–12 y, 500 mg PO 1–4 times daily; do not exceed 2 g in 24 h |
| Rifaximin (Xifaxan; ✻ Zaxine)<br>Affects *E. coli* in the GI tract | C | 550 mg PO 3 times a day for 14 d | ≥12 y, see adult dosing |

AIDS, acquired immunodeficiency syndrome; GI, gastrointestinal; HIV, human immunodeficiency virus.

## Bismuth Salts

Bismuth salts have antibacterial and antiviral activity. Bismuth subsalicylate (Pepto-Bismol), a commonly used OTC drug, also has antisecretory and possibly anti-inflammatory effects because of its salicylate component.

 **QSEN Alert: Safety**

People with an allergy to aspirin and aspirin products should not take bismuth subsalicylate as the drug is a salicylate.

This salt causes a temporary and harmless darkening of the tongue or stool.

## Octreotide

Octreotide acetate (Sandostatin) is a synthetic form of somatostatin, a hormone produced in the anterior pituitary gland and in the pancreas. The drug may be effective in diarrhea because it decreases GI secretion and motility. Uses include diarrhea associated with carcinoid syndrome, intestinal tumors, HIV/AIDS, and diarrhea that does not respond to other antidiarrheal drugs. Commonly reported adverse effects are diarrhea, headache, cardiac dysrhythmias, and injection site pain.

## Polycarbophil

Polycarbophil (e.g., FiberCon) and psyllium are most often used as bulk-forming laxatives. They are occasionally used in diarrhea to adsorb toxins and water, decreasing the fluidity of stools. Polycarbophil is the only adsorbent drug evaluated to be effective by the FDA OTC review panel. Polycarbophil absorbs large amounts of water and produces stools of gelatin-like consistency. It may cause abdominal discomfort and bloating and may reduce the absorption of coadministered medications.

## Enzymatic Replacement

In diarrhea caused by enzyme deficiency, pancreatic enzymes are given rather than antidiarrheal drugs. Practitioners recommend pancreatin or pancrelipase (Viokase, Pancreaze, Cotazym) when a deficiency of pancreatic enzymes results in malabsorption of nutrients and **steatorrhea**, which is a loose fatty stool.

## Bile-Binding Drugs

Cholestyramine (Questran) and colestipol (Colestid) are useful in treating diarrhea due to bile salt accumulation in conditions such as Crohn's disease or surgical excision of the ileum.

## Antibacterial Drugs

Practitioners recommend antibacterial drugs for bacterial enteritis when diarrhea lasts longer than 48 hours, when the patient passes six or more loose stools in 24 hours, when diarrhea is associated with fever, or when blood or pus is present in the stools. In bacterial gastroenteritis or diarrhea, the choice of antibacterial drug depends on the causative microorganism and susceptibility tests. Antibacterial drugs are effective in preventing traveler's diarrhea, but authorities usually do not recommend them because their use may promote the emergence of drug-resistant microorganisms. Although effective in reducing diarrhea due to *Salmonella* and *E. coli* intestinal infections, antibiotics may induce a prolonged carrier state during which the infection can be transmitted to other people.

Rifaximin (Xifaxan) is a structural analog of the antimycobacterial drug rifampin. This nonsystemic antibiotic remains in the gut and is not absorbed into the bloodstream. Researchers developed it specifically to treat traveler's diarrhea due to noninvasive strains of *E. coli* in patients older than 12 years of age. Use for diarrhea in the presence of fever or bloody stools or due to pathogens other than *E. coli* is not warranted. As with the use of other broad-spectrum antibiotics, superinfections may occur, requiring termination of the rifaximin. Adverse effects of rifaximin may include flatulence, headache, stomach pain, urgent bowel movements, nausea, constipation, fever, vomiting, and dizziness.

### ! QSEN Alert: Evidence-Based Practice

The American College of Gastroenterology (ACG) guideline provides recommendations for the diagnosis, management, and prevention of acute diarrheal infections in adults in US-based and travel settings. The ACG (Riddle, DuPont, & Connor, 2016) provided the treatment recommendations based on systematic review of the related literature.

Recommendations regarding treatment of US-based acute diarrheal infections include the use of balanced electrolyte rehydration, probiotics or prebiotics, and administration of bismuth subsalicylates to control the frequency of stools. The group did not recommend the use of antibiotics for community-acquired diarrhea because the infection is typically viral in nature, and its duration is not shortened by the use of antibiotics. Further, there is not sufficient evidence that empiric antimicrobial treatment for routine acute diarrheal infection should be used except in cases where the likelihood of a bacterial basis is sufficient to justify the potential adverse effects of antibiotic administration.

The guidelines reinforced that prevention strategies for acute diarrheal illness in travel settings include the use of bismuth for travelers who can adhere to the frequent dosing requirements and do not have contraindications to use. In addition, administration of antibiotic prophylaxis has demonstrated moderate to good effectiveness and may be considered in high-risk groups for short-term use. However, the use of probiotics and prebiotics for prevention of traveler's diarrhea is not consistently strong and is currently not recommended.

Nitazoxanide (Alinia) is an antiprotozoal agent used specifically for treating diarrhea resulting from infection with *Giardia lamblia* or *Cryptosporidium parvum* (see Chap. 25). Caution is necessary when administering nitazoxanide concurrently with highly plasma protein–bound medications such as warfarin, because the active metabolite of nitazoxanide is highly plasma protein bound, and such concurrent use may result in competitive drug interactions.

### Selective 5-HT₃ Receptor Antagonist

Alosetron (Lotronex) is a selective $5\text{-}HT_3$ receptor antagonist indicated for treating women with chronic severe diarrhea-predominant IBS that has not responded to conventional therapy. Clinical studies have not demonstrated safety and efficacy of alosetron in men. Alosetron is rapidly absorbed orally with a bioavailability of 50% to 60%. It is moderately plasma protein bound (82%). Extensively metabolized by the cytochrome 450 enzyme system (CYP2C9, CYP3A4, and CYP1A2), its multiple metabolites produced are excreted primarily in the urine. Caution is essential with concurrent administration with CYP1A2 and CYP3A4 inhibitors. Contraindications include concurrent administration with fluvoxamine and severe hepatic impairment is also a contraindication. Reduced dosages to prevent drug accumulation and toxicity may be necessary in some women older than 65 years of age.

An FDA-issued **BLACK BOX WARNING** ◆ alerts nurses to the serious GI adverse effects of alosetron. Severe constipation, with possible obstruction, perforation, and hemorrhage, is the most common problem. Ischemic colitis (reduced blood flow to the intestinal tract resulting in tissue damage) has also occurred. These serious conditions have resulted in hospitalizations, blood loss necessitating transfusion, surgery, and death in severe cases. It is important not to give alosetron to patients with a history of GI disorders, including chronic or severe constipation or sequelae of constipation, intestinal obstruction, stricture, toxic megacolon, GI perforation and/or adhesions, ischemic colitis, impaired intestinal circulation, thrombophlebitis or hypercoagulable state, Crohn's disease or ulcerative colitis, and diverticulitis.

To ensure safe and appropriate use of alosetron, the drug manufacturer has established a prescribing program, and only qualified health care providers enrolled in the program can prescribe this medication. Pharmacists must provide patients with a medication guide developed by the manufacturer at the time the medication is dispensed that includes the risks of taking alosetron and the situations under which the drug should be immediately discontinued. Each patient must sign a patient–physician agreement indicating that he or she (1) understands the risks of taking alosetron and agrees to take the medication; (2) will discontinue taking alosetron if constipation occurs; (3) will immediately notify the physician if constipation or signs of ischemic colitis occur; and (4) will stop taking alosetron and contact the physician after 4 weeks of therapy with alosetron if the symptoms of IBS are not controlled.

## NCLEX Success

3. **A woman with diarrhea begins to complain of eye pain after administration of diphenoxylate with atropine. The nurse should do which of the following?**

   A. Offer an over-the-counter analgesic such as acetaminophen.
   B. Discontinue the diphenoxylate with atropine and notify the provider.
   C. Tell the patient that this is a common side effect and will soon pass.
   D. Apply a cool compress to the eyes for relief of the discomfort.

4. **A man tells the nurse that he has bought the over-the-counter drug bismuth subsalicylate for the next episode of diarrhea. The nurse should assess for what allergy that would contraindicate use of bismuth subsalicylate?**

   A. penicillin
   B. acetaminophen
   C. aspirin
   D. sulfa

## Clinical Application 40.2

- Mr. Mendoza's culture report identifies an enterotoxigenic strain of *E. coli* (ETEC). What is the most likely drug of choice for him?

## THE NURSING PROCESS

A concept map outlines the nursing process related to drug therapy considerations in this chapter. Additional nursing implications related to the disease process should also be considered in care decisions.

**Assessment**

- Try to determine the duration of diarrhea; number of stools per day; amount, consistency, color, odor, and presence of abnormal components (e.g., undigested food, blood, pus, mucus) in each stool; precipitating factors; accompanying signs and symptoms (i.e., nausea, vomiting, fever, abdominal pain, or cramping); and measures used to relieve diarrhea. When possible, look at stool specimens for possible clues to causation. Blood may indicate inflammation, infection, or neoplastic disease; pus or mucus may indicate inflammation or infection. Infections caused by *Shigella* organisms produce blood-tinged mucus. Infections caused by *Salmonella* or *E. coli* usually produce green, liquid or semiliquid stools. Inflammatory bowel disorders often produce nonbloody mucus.
- Try to determine the cause of the diarrhea. This includes questioning about such causes as chronic inflammatory diseases of the bowel, food intake, possible exposure to contaminated food, living or traveling in areas of poor sanitation, and use of laxatives or other drugs that may cause diarrhea. When available, check laboratory reports on stool specimens (e.g., culture reports).
- With severe or prolonged diarrhea, especially in young children and older adults, assess for dehydration, hypokalemia, and other fluid and electrolyte disorders.

**Outcomes of Therapy**

The patient will
- Take antidiarrheal drugs appropriately.
- Obtain relief from acute diarrhea (reduced number of liquid stools, reduced abdominal discomfort).
- Maintain fluid and electrolyte balance.
- Maintain adequate nutritional intake.
- Avoid adverse effects of antidiarrheal medications.
- Reestablish normal bowel patterns after an episode of acute diarrhea.
- Have fewer liquid stools with chronic diarrhea.

**Nursing Interventions**

- Provide instruction about the use of measures to prevent diarrhea.
- Prepare and store food properly and avoid improperly stored foods and those prepared under unsanitary conditions. Dairy products, cream pies, and other foods may cause diarrhea (food poisoning) if not refrigerated.
- Wash hands before handling any foods, after handling raw poultry or meat, and always before eating.
- Chew food well.
- Do not overuse laxatives (i.e., amount per dose or frequency of use). Many OTC products contain senna or other strong stimulant laxatives.
- Provide education about drug therapy (see Box 40.1).
- Provide supportive care, which is necessary regardless of whether antidiarrheal drugs are used.
- Replace fluids and electrolytes (2–3 quarts daily). Fluids such as weak tea; water; bouillon; clear soup; noncarbonated, caffeine-free beverages; and gelatin are usually tolerated and helpful. If the patient cannot tolerate adequate amounts of oral liquids or if diarrhea is severe or prolonged, intravenous fluids may be needed (i.e., solutions containing dextrose, sodium chloride, and potassium chloride).
- Avoid foods and fluids that may further irritate GI mucosa (e.g., highly spiced foods; "laxative" foods, such as raw fruits and vegetables).
- Increase frequency and length of rest periods, and decrease activity. Exercise and activity stimulate peristalsis.
- If perianal irritation occurs because of frequent liquid stools, cleanse the area with mild soap and water after each bowel movement, then apply an emollient, such as white petrolatum (Vaseline).

**Evaluation**

- Observe and interview for decreased number of liquid or loose stools.
- Observe for signs of adequate food and fluid intake (e.g., good skin turgor and urine output, stable weight).
- Observe for appropriate use of antidiarrheal drugs.
- Observe and interview for return of prediarrheal patterns of bowel elimination.
- Interview regarding knowledge and use of measures to prevent or minimize diarrhea.

## KEY CONCEPTS

- Diarrhea is the frequent expulsion of liquid or semiliquid stools resulting from increased bowel motility, increased secretion or retention of fluids in the intestinal lumen, or inflammation/irritation of the GI tract.
- Overall, opiates and opiate derivatives are the most effective nonspecific therapy for symptomatic treatment of diarrhea.
- Use of antidiarrheal medications to treat diarrhea if it is caused by toxin-producing substances or poisoning is inappropriate.
- Specific drug therapy for diarrhea is directed at the cause of the symptoms and may include enzymatic replacement therapy, bile salt–binding drugs, antibacterial agents, and 5-HT$_3$ receptor antagonists.
- Octreotide, a synthetic form of somatostatin, decreases GI secretion and motility. Uses include diarrhea associated with carcinoid syndrome, intestinal tumors, HIV/AIDS, and diarrhea that does not respond to other antidiarrheal drugs.
- Bismuth subsalicylate has antisecretory, antimicrobial, and possibly anti-inflammatory effects. Uses include control of traveler's diarrhea and relief of abdominal cramping.
- The FDA has issued a **BLACK BOX WARNING ◆** because torsades de pointes, cardiac arrest, and death have been reported in people using higher than recommended dosages of loperamide.
- Polycarbophil treats diarrhea by adsorbing toxins and water, decreasing the fluidity of stools.
- In bacterial gastroenteritis or diarrhea, the choice of antibacterial drug depends on the causative organism and susceptibility tests.
- Because of the risk of severe GI adverse effects, use of alosetron is subject to a mandated prescribing program; the FDA has issued a **BLACK BOX WARNING ◆** for alosetron alerting nurses to the serious GI adverse effects of alosetron. Severe constipation, with possible obstruction, perforation, and hemorrhage, is the most common problem. Ischemic colitis (reduced blood flow to the intestinal tract resulting in tissue damage) has also occurred. These serious conditions have resulted in hospitalizations, blood loss necessitating transfusion, surgery, and death in severe cases. Only qualified health care providers enrolled in the program can prescribe this medication. Pharmacists are required to distribute educational materials when dispensing alosetron. Patients must sign a patient–physician agreement before taking this medication.

## CLINICAL REASONING CASE STUDY

### Meet the Patient

Yasmine Hassan, a mother of a 5-year-old child, calls the health department because her son's stools have been semiliquid for the past 24 hours. She has asked the nurse who has been contacted to recommend an over-the-counter antidiarrheal drug. The nurse asks Mrs. Hassan to bring her son, Adam, to the clinic for evaluation by the nurse practitioner. At the visit, stool cultures are obtained and are negative. The nurse practitioner recommends loperamide (Imodium A-D) 1 mg three times daily.

- What drug information regarding loperamide is important in children?
- What nursing interventions and patient teaching should be implemented by the nurse?

### Assessing Drug Information

- Loperamide decreases GI motility by its effect on intestinal muscles and decreases the frequency of diarrhea. Although loperamide is a synthetic derivative of meperidine, the drug does not penetrate the CNS well, so it does not cause the CNS effects associated with opioid use and lacks potential for abuse.
- Uses include control of acute nonspecific diarrhea in patients aged 2 years or older, mild traveler's diarrhea, irritable bowel syndrome, chronic diarrhea due to bowel resection, and chronic diarrhea secondary to inflammatory bowel disease.
- Although adverse effects are generally few and mild, loperamide can cause abdominal pain, constipation, drowsiness, fatigue, nausea, and vomiting.

### Nursing Actions

- A liquid preparation of loperamide is available. To measure doses accurately, calibrated devices (plastic medicine cups, oral syringes, oral droppers, or cylindrical dosing spoons) rather than using household utensils should be used. Teach parents to use these.
- Educate Mrs. Hassan about encouraging adequate fluids. Clear liquids, such as Pedialyte or popsicles, and bland foods are appropriate in the diet of a young child to replace fluid and electrolytes lost in the stool during diarrhea.
- Suggest that a diet consisting of bland foods (e.g., rice, soup, bread, salted crackers, cooked cereals, baked potatoes, eggs, applesauce) may be well-tolerated.
- Educate Mrs. Hassan about the course of diarrhea. Tell her that the diarrheal episodes are usually self-limiting and subside within 24 to 48 hours without serious consequences. If diarrhea lasts longer than 2 days, symptoms worsen, blood appears in the stool, or abdominal swelling or bulging develops, loperamide should be discontinued and she should call the clinic. The drug is for short-term use only.
- Follow-up with Mrs. Hassan the following day to see if the diarrhea is improving and the child is tolerating liquids to maintain adequate hydration.

Visit thePoint® at **http://thePoint.lww.com/Frandsen12e** *for answers to NCLEX Success questions (in Appendix A), answers to Clinical Application Case Studies (in Appendix B), and more!*

## REFERENCES AND RESOURCES

Centers for Disease Control and Prevention. (2016). *Travelers' diarrhea.* Retrieved December 30, 2019, from https://wwwnc.cdc.gov/travel/page/travelers-diarrhea

DiPiro, J. T., Talbert, R. L., Yee, G. C., Wells, B. G., Posey, L. M., & Matzke, G. R. (2020). *Pharmacotherapy: A pathophysiologic approach* (11th ed., Kindle Edition). New York: McGraw-Hill Education.

Fabel, P. H., & Shealy, K. M. (2017). Diarrhea, constipation, and irritable bowel syndrome. In J. T. DiPiro, R. L. Talbert, G. C. Yee, G. R. Matzke, B. G. Wells, & L. M. Posey (Eds.), *Pharmacotherapy: A pathophysiologic approach* (10th ed., pp. 511–526). New York: McGraw-Hill Education.

Heywood, A. E., & Zwar, N. (2018). Improving access and provision of pre-travel healthcare for travelers visiting friends and relatives: A review of the evidence. *Journal of Travel Medicine, 25*(1). doi: 10.1093/jtm/tay010

Hinkle, J. L., & Cheever, K. H. (2018). *Brunner & Suddarth's textbook of medical-surgical nursing* (14th ed.). Philadelphia: Wolters Kluwer.

Karch, A. M. (2019). *Focus on Nursing Pharmacology* (8th ed.) Philadelphia: Lippincott Williams & Wilkins.

LaRocque, P., & Harris, J. B. (2019). Approach to the adult with acute diarrhea in resource-rich settings. In *UpToDate*. Lexi-Comp, Inc.

Norris, T. L. (2019). *Pathophysiology: Concepts of altered health status* (10th ed.). Philadelphia: Wolters Kluwer.

Riddle, M. S., DuPont, H. L., & Connor, B. A. (2016). ACG Clinical Guideline: Diagnosis, treatment, and prevention of acute diarrheal infections in adults. *American Journal of Gastroenterology, 111*(5), 602–622.

UpToDate. (2019). *Drug information.* Lexi-Comp, Inc.

# Drugs Affecting the Endocrine System

# Drug Therapy for Diabetes Mellitus

*After studying this chapter, you should be able to:*

1. Differentiate between type 1 and type 2 diabetes mellitus.
2. Understand the major effects of endogenous insulin on body tissues.
3. Identify the clinical manifestations of type 1 and type 2 diabetes mellitus.
4. Identify the prototype and describe the action, use, adverse effects, contraindications, and nursing implications for the insulins.
5. Discuss characteristics of the various types of insulins and insulin analogs.
6. Identify the various prototypes, and describe the actions, uses, adverse effects, contraindications, and nursing implications for the oral antidiabetic drugs.
7. Identify the different prototypes and describe the actions, uses, adverse effects, contraindications, and nursing implications for the sulfonylureas, alpha-glucosidase inhibitors, amylin analogs, biguanide, thiazolidinediones, meglitinides, dipeptidyl peptidase 4 (DPP-4) inhibitors, amylin analogs, incretin mimetics, and sodium glucose cotransporter 2 inhibitors.
8. Apply the pharmacokinetics, pharmacodynamics, and pharmacotherapeutics of the angiotensin-converting enzyme inhibitors, angiotensin II receptor blockers, and the statins in the care of the diabetic patient.
9. Implement the nursing process in the care of patients receiving medications for the treatment of diabetes mellitus.
   - Explain the benefits of maintaining glycemic control in preventing complications of diabetes.
   - Assist patients or caregivers in learning how to manage diabetes care, including administration of medication agents used to manage diabetes.
   - Assess and monitor patients' adherence to prescribed management strategies.

## CLINICAL APPLICATION CASE STUDY

Alfred Smith, a 56-year-old librarian, visits his physician because he has been feeling more tired and weak than usual for the past 2 months. On questioning, the physician learns that Mr. Smith often gets up in the middle of the night to urinate and drink a glass of water. He also has numbness and tingling in his hands and feet, as well as blurred vision, which affects his job. Laboratory results show an impaired fasting glucose of 160 mg/dL and urinalysis of 4+ glucose. His lipid panel also shows total cholesterol of 240 mg/dL, high-density lipoprotein cholesterol of 22 mg/dL, and triglycerides of 400 mg/dL. Mr. Smith receives a diagnosis of type 2 diabetes, and his physician places him on metformin (Glucophage XR) 500 mg by mouth once daily. He also receives information about a diet and exercise routine to help control his diabetes.

# KEY TERMS

**Blood glucose level:** blood sugar level in the body

**Blood glucose meter:** device that measures how much glucose is in the blood

**Diabetes mellitus:** chronic disease characterized by disordered metabolism of carbohydrates, fats, and protein, and hyperglycemia, due to a deficiency in the amount on action of insulin; the three main forms of diabetes are type 1, type 2, and gestational diabetes.

**Glucagon:** pancreatic hormone that raises blood glucose levels by stimulating the liver to convert glycogen into glucose; it opposes insulin.

**Gluconeogenesis:** formation of glucose from noncarbohydrate sources such as fats and amino acids

**Glucose:** sugar in the blood; major stimulus of insulin secretion

**Impaired fasting glucose:** fasting blood glucose level between 100 and 125 mg/dL; also referred to as prediabetes

**Insulin:** protein hormone secreted by beta cells in the pancreas; facilitates glucose utilization by cells. Absence of insulin results in diabetes mellitus.

**Insulin pump:** wearable delivery system for continuous subcutaneous insulin infusion; the insulin dosage is programmed into the pump, and the appropriate amount of insulin is injected through a needle into the adipose tissue.

**Ketoacidosis:** metabolic acidosis due to accumulation of ketone bodies formed by the breakdown of fatty acids and amino acids for energy in the absence of insulin

**Lancet:** sharp instrument used to prick the finger for a blood test

## INTRODUCTION

**Diabetes mellitus** is characterized as a disease of insulin availability that eventually results in high blood glucose concentrations. Treatment of diabetes mellitus includes drugs to maintain **blood glucose levels** within the normal range and prevent complications. Insulin and oral antidiabetic agents are two of the several types of medications used to lower blood **glucose** in diabetes mellitus. New drug therapies include amylin analogs, incretin mimetics, and dipeptidyl peptidase 4 (DPP-4) inhibitors. It is important that nurses understand the characteristic of diabetes mellitus and the clinical use of insulin, oral hypoglycemic medications, and the newer drugs. They also need to be familiar with the effects of dietary herbal supplements on blood glucose levels.

## OVERVIEW OF DIABETES

Metabolic problems occur early in people with diabetes mellitus and are related to changes in the metabolism of carbohydrate, fat, and protein. A major clinical manifestation of disordered metabolism is hyperglycemia, or fasting blood glucose levels exceeding 126 mg/dL. A person with a fasting blood glucose level between 100 and 125 mg/dL is said to have **impaired fasting glucose** (IFG), or prediabetes. Fasting plasma glucose, a 75-g glucose tolerance test, and hemoglobin A1C are used to test for prediabetes and type 2 diabetes. Plasma blood glucose is used to diagnose the acute onset of type 1 diabetes in individuals with symptoms of hyperglycemia.

Vascular problems include atherosclerosis throughout the body. Macrovascular (moderate and large vessels) clinical manifestations include hypertension, myocardial infarction, stroke, and peripheral vascular disease. Changes in small blood vessels (microvasculature) especially affect the retina and kidney, resulting in retinopathy and chronic kidney disease.

## Etiology

The two major classifications of diabetes mellitus are type 1 and type 2. Although both are characterized by hyperglycemia, they differ in onset, course, pathology, and treatment. Other types of diabetes may be induced by disease processes such as slowly progressing autoimmune disorders, certain drugs, and pregnancy (see Chap. 6).

### Type 1 Diabetes

Type 1 diabetes, a common chronic disorder of childhood, results from an autoimmune disorder that destroys pancreatic beta cells. Although it may occur at any age, it usually appears after 4 years of age and peaks in incidence at 10 to 12 years for girls and 12 to 14 years for boys. A subtype of type 1 diabetes, latent autoimmune diabetes of the adult, begins in adulthood. Symptoms of traditional type 1 diabetes usually develop when 10% to 20% of functioning beta cells remain, but they may occur at any time if acute illness or stress increases the body's demand for **insulin** (a protein hormone secreted by the beta cells) beyond the capacity of the remaining beta cells to secrete insulin. Eventually, destruction of all beta cells occurs, resulting in no insulin production.

Type 1 diabetes usually has a sudden onset; produces severe symptoms; is difficult to control; produces a high incidence of complications, such as diabetic **ketoacidosis** (DKA) and renal failure; and requires administration of exogenous insulin. About 10% of people with diabetes have type 1 disease.

## Type 2 Diabetes

Type 2 diabetes is characterized by hyperglycemia and insulin resistance. The hyperglycemia results from increased production of glucose by the liver and decreased uptake of glucose in liver, muscle, and fat cells. Insulin resistance means that higher-than-usual concentrations of insulin are required. Thus, insulin is present but unable to work effectively (i.e., inhibits hepatic production of glucose and causes glucose to move from the bloodstream into liver, muscle, and fat cells). Most insulin resistance is attributed to impaired insulin action at the cellular level, possibly related to postreceptor, intracellular mechanisms.

Historically, the onset of type 2 diabetes occurred after 40 years of age. More recently, however, type 2 diabetes is increasing in prevalence among children and adolescents. Compared with type 1, it usually has a gradual (insidious) onset, produces less severe symptoms initially, is easier to control, causes less DKA and renal failure but more myocardial infarctions and strokes, and does not necessarily require exogenous insulin because endogenous insulin is still produced. About 90% of people with diabetes have type 2 disease; 20% to 30% of them require exogenous insulin at some point in their lives.

Type 2 is a heterogeneous disease, and etiology probably involves multiple factors such as a genetic predisposition and environmental factors. Obesity is a major cause. With obesity and chronic ingestion of excess calories, along with a sedentary lifestyle, more insulin is required. The increased need leads to prolonged stimulation and eventual "fatigue" of pancreatic beta cells. As a result, the cells become less responsive to elevated blood glucose levels and less able to produce enough insulin to meet metabolic needs. Thus, insulin is secreted but is inadequate or ineffective, especially when insulin demand is increased by obesity, pregnancy, aging, or other factors.

A risk factor for the development of type 2 diabetes is the presence of metabolic syndrome. This syndrome is characterized by a group of risk factors, including abdominal obesity (excessive fat tissue in and around the abdomen), hypertriglyceridemia, low high-density lipoprotein (HDL) cholesterol, hypertension, and/or IFG. People with metabolic syndrome have an increased risk of coronary heart disease and other diseases related to plaque buildup in artery walls (e.g., stroke and peripheral vascular disease) and type 2 diabetes. Metabolic syndrome has become increasingly common in the United States. Estimates indicate that more than 50 million Americans have it.

The Centers for Disease Control (CDC) in 2017 reported the prevalence of diagnosed and undiagnosed diabetes is 30.3 million people of all ages. This is 9.4% of the US population. Approximately 7.2 million individuals were not aware of having diabetes. In the United States, African Americans, Hispanics, Native Americans, Native Alaskans, and some Asian Americans and Pacific Islanders are at high risk for type 2 diabetes. Prevalence rates are about 9% in Asian Americans, 13.8% in non-Hispanic blacks, 12.7% in non-Hispanic whites, 12.1% in Hispanics, and 15.1% in Native Americans and Alaskans.

The Native American population aged 15 to 19 has the highest prevalence of type 2 diabetes in youth of that age. The Pima Indian adolescents have prevalence of 51 per 1000 and the Navajo adolescents of 1.45 per 1000. The non-Hispanic Black adolescents are 1.06 per 1000 individuals. Hispanic youth are 0.79 per 1000. The CDC reports that 132,000 children and adolescents under the age of 18 years are diagnosed with diabetes mellitus. Of these, approximately 5% are diagnosed with type 1.

# Pathophysiology

## Endogenous Insulin

Beta cells in the pancreas secrete insulin. The average adult pancreas secretes 40 to 60 units of insulin daily. This includes a basal amount of 1 to 2 units/hour and additional amounts (4–6 units/hour) after meals or when the blood glucose level exceeds 100 mg/dL. In a fasting state, serum insulin levels are low, and the body uses stored glucose and amino acids for energy needs of tissues that require glucose. After a meal, serum insulin levels increase and peak in a few minutes and then decrease to baseline levels in 2 to 3 hours.

Amylin, a pancreatic hormone secreted with insulin, delays gastric emptying, increases satiety, and suppresses **glucagon** (hormone that raises blood glucose levels by stimulating the liver to convert glycogen into glucose) secretion, thus complementing the effects of insulin on blood glucose. A synthetic form of amylin, pramlintide, has been developed to assist with glucose control in patients with diabetes (see later discussion).

Insulin is secreted into the portal circulation and transported to the liver, where about half is used or degraded. The other half reaches the systemic circulation, where it circulates mainly in an unbound form and is transported to body cells.

At the cellular level (Fig. 41.1), insulin binds with and activates receptors on the cell membranes of about 80% of body cells. Liver,

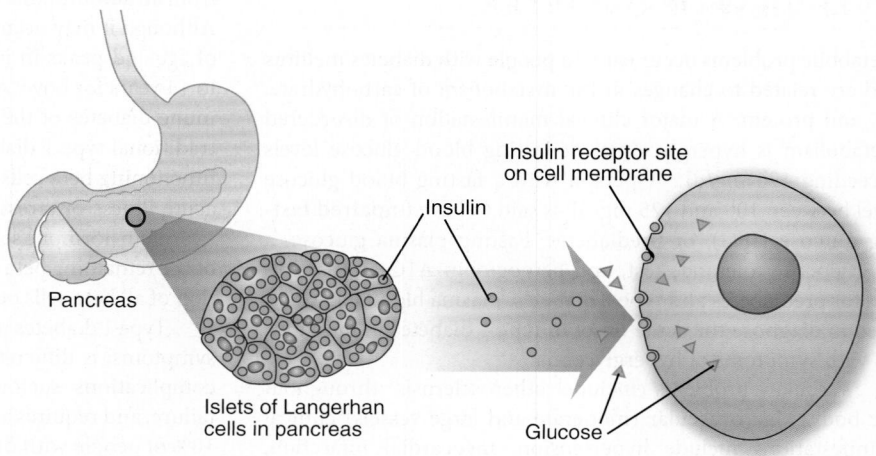

**Figure 41.1.** Normal glucose metabolism. After insulin binds with receptors on the cell membrane, glucose can move into the cell, promoting cellular metabolism and energy production.

Pancreas

Islets of Langerhan cells in pancreas

Insulin

Insulin receptor site on cell membrane

Glucose

muscle, and fat cells have many insulin receptors and are primary tissues for insulin action. After insulin–receptor binding occurs, cell membranes become highly permeable to glucose and allow rapid entry of glucose into the cells. The cell membranes also become more permeable to amino acids, fatty acids, and electrolytes such as potassium, magnesium, and phosphate ions. Cellular metabolism is altered by the movement of these substances into the cells, by activation of some enzymes and inactivation of others, by movement of proteins between intracellular compartments, by changes in the amounts of proteins produced, and perhaps by other mechanisms. Overall, the changes in cellular metabolism stimulate anabolic effects (e.g., utilization and storage of glucose, amino acids, and fatty acids) and inhibit catabolic processes (e.g., breakdown of glycogen, fat, and protein). After binding to insulin and entering the cell, receptors may be degraded or recycled back to the cell surface.

Insulin is cleared from circulating blood in 10 to 15 minutes because of rapid binding to peripheral tissues or metabolic breakdown. The insulin that does not combine with receptors is metabolized in the liver, kidneys, plasma, and muscles. In the kidneys, insulin is filtered by the glomeruli and reabsorbed by the tubules, which also degrade it. Severe renal impairment slows the clearance of insulin from the blood.

Insulin plays a major role in metabolism of carbohydrate, fat, and protein (Box 41.1). Food particles are broken down into molecules of glucose, lipids, and amino acids, respectively. The molecules enter the cells and are converted to energy for cellular activities. The energy can be used immediately or converted to storage forms for later use. When carrying out its metabolic functions, the overall effect of insulin is to lower blood glucose levels, primarily by the following mechanisms:

- In the liver, insulin acts to decrease breakdown of glycogen (glycogenolysis), form new glucose from fatty acids and amino acids (**gluconeogenesis**), and form ketone bodies (ketogenesis). At the same time, it acts to increase synthesis and storage of glycogen and fatty acids.

- In adipose tissue, insulin acts to decrease breakdown of fat (lipolysis) and to increase production of glycerol and fatty acids.
- In muscle tissue, insulin acts to decrease protein breakdown and amino acid output and to increase amino acid uptake, protein synthesis, and glycogen synthesis.

## Regulation of Insulin Secretion

Insulin decreases blood sugar and regulates the amount of glucose available for cellular metabolism and energy needs, during both fasting and feeding. Insulin secretion involves coordination of various nutrients, hormones, the autonomic nervous system, and other factors.

Glucose is the major stimulus of insulin secretion; others include amino acids, fatty acids, ketone bodies (which are acidotic substances in themselves), and stimulation of beta$_2$-adrenergic receptors or vagal nerves. Oral glucose is more effective than intravenous (IV) glucose because glucose or food in the digestive tract stimulates vagal activity and induces the release of gastrointestinal (GI) hormones called incretins. Incretin hormones stimulate the release of insulin when glucose levels are normal or elevated. In addition, incretin hormones reduce glucagon production and delay gastric emptying. Two incretin hormones have been identified: glucose-dependent insulinotropic peptide and glucagon-like peptide-1 (GLP-1). GLP-1 also appears to improve insulin sensitivity and may increase the formation of new beta cells in the pancreas. The therapeutic uses of incretin hormones have recently been investigated, and this has led to the development of new drugs to treat diabetes mellitus.

Several hormones raise blood glucose levels and stimulate insulin secretion, including cortisol, glucagon, growth hormone, epinephrine, estrogen, and progesterone. Excessive, prolonged, endogenous secretion or administration of pharmacologic preparations of these hormones can exhaust the ability of pancreatic beta cells to produce insulin and thereby cause or aggravate diabetes mellitus.

---

| **BOX 41.1** | *Effects of Insulin on Metabolism* |
| --- | --- |

### Carbohydrate Metabolism

- Insulin increases glucose transport into the liver, skeletal muscle, adipose tissue, the heart, and some smooth muscle organs (such as the uterus); it must be present for muscle and fat tissues to use glucose for energy.
- Insulin regulates glucose metabolism to produce energy for cellular functions. If excess glucose is present after this need is met, it is converted to glycogen and stored for future energy needs or converted to fat and stored. The excess glucose transported to liver cells is converted to fat only after glycogen stores are saturated. When insulin is absent or blood glucose levels are low, these stored forms of glucose can be reconverted. The liver is especially important in restoring blood sugar levels by breaking down glycogen or by forming new glucose.

### Fat Metabolism

- Insulin promotes transport of glucose into fat cells, where it is broken down. One of the breakdown products is alpha-glycerophosphate, which combines with fatty acids to form triglycerides. This is the mechanism by which insulin promotes fat storage.

- When insulin is lacking, fat is released into the bloodstream as free fatty acids. Blood concentrations of triglycerides, cholesterol, and phospholipids are also increased. The high blood lipid concentration probably accounts for the atherosclerosis that tends to develop early and progress more rapidly in people with diabetes mellitus. Also, when more fatty acids are released than the body can use as fuel, some fatty acids are converted into ketones. Excessive amounts of ketones produce acidosis and coma.

### Protein Metabolism

- Insulin increases the total amount of body protein by increasing transport of amino acids into cells and synthesis of protein within the cells. The basic mechanism of these effects is unknown.
- Insulin potentiates the effects of growth hormone.
- Lack of insulin causes protein breakdown into amino acids, which are released into the bloodstream and transported to the liver for energy or gluconeogenesis. The lost proteins are not replaced by synthesis of new proteins, and protein wasting causes abnormal functioning of many body organs, severe weakness, and weight loss.

Factors that inhibit insulin secretion include stimulation of pancreatic alpha$_2$-adrenergic receptors and stress conditions such as hypoxia, hypothermia, surgery, or severe burns.

## Clinical Manifestations

Most signs and symptoms stem from a lack of effective insulin and the subsequent metabolic abnormalities. The incidence and severity depend on the amount of effective insulin, and conditions such as infection, rapid growth, pregnancy, or other factors may increase demand for insulin. Most early symptoms result from disordered carbohydrate metabolism, which causes excess glucose to accumulate in the blood (hyperglycemia). Hyperglycemia produces glucosuria, which, in turn, produces polydipsia, polyuria, dehydration, and polyphagia.

Glucosuria usually appears when the blood glucose level is approximately twice the normal value and the kidneys receive more glucose than can be reabsorbed. However, renal threshold varies, and the amount of glucose lost in the urine does not accurately reflect blood glucose. In children, glucose tends to appear in urine at much lower or even normal blood glucose

levels. In older people, the kidneys may be less able to excrete excess glucose from the blood. As a result, blood glucose levels may be high with little or no glucose in the urine.

When large amounts of glucose are present, water is pulled into the renal tubule. This results in a greatly increased urine output (polyuria). The excessive loss of fluid in urine leads to increased thirst (polydipsia) and, if fluid intake is inadequate, to dehydration. Dehydration also occurs because high blood glucose levels increase osmotic pressure in the bloodstream and fluid is pulled out of the cells in the body's attempt to regain homeostasis. Polyphagia (increased appetite) occurs because the body cannot use ingested foods. People with uncontrolled diabetes lose weight because of abnormal metabolism.

Complications of diabetes mellitus are common and potentially disabling or life threatening. Diabetes is a leading cause of myocardial infarction, stroke, blindness, leg amputation, and kidney failure. These complications result from hyperglycemia and other metabolic abnormalities that accompany a lack of effective insulin. The metabolic abnormalities associated with hyperglycemia can cause early, acute complications, such as DKA or hyperosmolar hyperglycemic nonketotic coma (HHNC; Box 41.2).

---

**BOX 41.2**    *Acute Complications of Diabetes Mellitus*

### Diabetic Ketoacidosis

This life-threatening complication occurs with severe insulin deficiency. In the absence of insulin, glucose cannot be used by body cells for energy, and fat is mobilized from adipose tissue to furnish a fuel source. The mobilized fat circulates in the bloodstream, from which it is extracted by the liver and broken down into glycerol and fatty acids. The fatty acids are further changed in the liver to ketones (e.g., acetoacetic acid, acetone), which then enter the bloodstream and are circulated to body cells for metabolic conversion to energy, carbon dioxide, and water.

The ketones are produced more rapidly than body cells can use them, and their accumulation produces acidemia (a drop in blood pH and an increase in blood hydrogen ions). The body attempts to buffer the acidic hydrogen ions by exchanging them for intracellular potassium ions. Hydrogen ions enter body cells, and potassium ions leave the cells to be excreted in the urine. Another attempt to remove excess acid involves the lungs. Deep, labored respirations, called *Kussmaul's respirations*, eliminate more carbon dioxide and prevent formation of carbonic acid. A third attempt to regain homeostasis involves the kidneys, which excrete some of the ketones, thereby producing acetone in the urine.

Two major causes of diabetic ketoacidosis (DKA) are omission of insulin and illnesses such as infection, trauma, myocardial infarction, or stroke. DKA worsens as the compensatory mechanisms fail. Clinical signs and symptoms become progressively more severe. Early ones include blurred vision, anorexia, nausea and vomiting, thirst, and polyuria. Later ones include drowsiness, which progresses to stupor and coma; Kussmaul's respirations; dehydration and other signs of fluid and electrolyte imbalances; and decreased blood pressure, increased pulse, and other signs of shock.

Insulin therapy is a major part of any treatment for DKA. Patients with DKA have a deficiency in the total amount of insulin in the body and a resistance to the action of the insulin that is available, probably due to acidosis, hyperosmolality, infection, and other factors. To be effective, insulin therapy must be individualized according to frequent measurements

of blood glucose. Low doses, given by continuous intravenous (IV) infusion, are preferred in most circumstances so that the brain has time to equilibrate and account for fluid shifts.

Additional measures include identification and treatment of conditions that precipitate DKA, administration of IV fluids to correct hyperosmolality and dehydration, administration of potassium supplements to restore and maintain normal serum potassium levels, and administration of sodium bicarbonate to correct metabolic acidosis. Infection is one of the most common causes of DKA. If no obvious source of infection is identified, cultures of blood, urine, and throat swabs are recommended. When infection is identified, antimicrobial drug therapy may be indicated.

### Hyperosmolar Hyperglycemic Nonketotic Coma

Hyperosmolar hyperglycemic nonketotic coma (HHNC) is another type of diabetic coma that is potentially life threatening. It is relatively rare and carries a high mortality rate. The term *hyperosmolar* refers to an excessive amount of glucose, electrolytes, and other solutes in the blood in relation to the amount of water.

Like DKA, HHNC is characterized by hyperglycemia, which leads to osmotic diuresis and resultant thirst, polyuria, dehydration, and electrolyte losses, as well as neurologic signs ranging from drowsiness to stupor to coma. Additional clinical problems may include hypovolemic shock, thrombosis, renal problems, or stroke. In contrast with DKA, hyperosmolar coma occurs in people with previously unknown or mild diabetes, usually after an illness; occurs in hyperglycemic conditions other than diabetes (e.g., severe burns, corticosteroid drug therapy); and does not cause ketosis.

Treatment of HHNC is similar to that of DKA in that insulin, IV fluids, and potassium supplements are major components. Regular insulin is given by continuous IV infusion, and dosage is individualized according to frequent measurements of blood glucose levels. IV fluids are given to correct the profound dehydration and hyperosmolality, and potassium is given IV to replace the large amounts lost in urine during a hyperglycemic state.

Eventually, metabolic abnormalities lead to damage in blood vessels and other body tissues. For example, atherosclerosis develops earlier, progresses more rapidly, and becomes more severe in people with diabetes. Microvascular changes lead to nephropathy, retinopathy, and peripheral neuropathy. Other complications include musculoskeletal disorders, increased numbers and severity of infections, and complications of pregnancy.

The American Diabetes Association (2018) recommends that patients aim to achieve normal or near normal glycemic index with an A1C goal of less than 7%. The range of less than 6.5% is considered normal, and greater than 8% is appropriate for patients with severe hypoglycemia or patients with diminished life expectancy, comorbid conditions, or advanced age.

The ADA also recommends that an adult diabetic patient's hemoglobin A1C is tested each year to determine if the treatment goals are met. For a patient not meeting the goals of therapy, the hemoglobin A1C should be tested quarterly.

---

**⚠ QSEN Alert: Evidence-Based Practice**

Aljack, Abdalla, Idris, and Ismail (2019) investigated the effect of serum vitamin D level in patients with type 2 diabetes mellitus and its association with the development of diabetic nephropathy and cardiovascular disease. In the study, type 2 diabetic patients who were deficient in serum vitamin D also exhibited an increase in the C-reactive protein. The authors concluded that type 2 diabetes and deficiency in serum vitamin D placed them at increased risk of cardiovascular disease and peripheral neuropathy. Monitor serum vitamin D levels in patients with type 2 diabetes and provide supplementation as indicated by the primary care provider.

---

## Drug Therapy

Medications used in the treatment of diabetes mellitus depend on the type of diabetes and degree of glycemic control. Health care providers use many medications to control diabetes (Table 41.1). Insulin is the prototype drug for treatment of type 1 diabetes. Several different classes of other drugs are also available for the treatment of type 2 diabetes (Fig. 41.2). Patients with diabetes may be using herbal supplements, and nurses should be aware that some of these substances affect blood glucose levels (Box 41.3).

---

**_Clinical Application 41.1_**

- What additional condition does Mr. Smith have?
- What are the complications related to this diagnosis?

---

**NCLEX  Success**

1. A patient presents with a blood pressure of 162/88 mm Hg, heart rate of 100 bpm, triglycerides of 378 mg/dL, and HDL of 25 mg/dL. Which of the following are characteristics of metabolic syndrome? (Select all that apply.)
   A. blood pressure of 162/88 mm Hg
   B. heart rate of 100 bpm
   C. triglycerides of 378 mg/dL
   D. HDL of 25 mg/dL

2. A patient who has just arrived at the emergency department may be suffering from diabetic ketoacidosis. Which of the following would confirm the diagnosis?
   A. elevated serum potassium
   B. increased respiratory rate
   C. increased pH
   D. elevated blood glucose level

---

## INSULINS

Insulin in its various forms is the only effective drug treatment for type 1 diabetes, where pancreatic beta cells are unable to secrete endogenous insulin and metabolism is severely impaired. **Regular insulin** (HumuLIN R U-500, HumuLIN R U-500 KwikPen) is the prototype. Over-the-counter (OTC) preparations include HumuLIN R, NovoLIN R, and NovoLIN R ReliON. Insulin is also necessary in patients with type 2 diabetes who cannot control their disease with diet, weight control, and oral agents. Any person with diabetes may need insulin during times of stress, such as illness, infection, or surgery. Other uses of insulin include control of diabetes induced by chronic pancreatitis, surgical excision of pancreatic tissue, hormones and other drugs, and pregnancy (gestational diabetes). In patients who do not have diabetes, health care providers use insulin to prevent or treat hyperglycemia induced by IV parenteral nutrition and to treat hyperkalemia. In hyperkalemia, an IV infusion of insulin and dextrose solution causes potassium to move from the blood into the cells; it does not eliminate potassium from the body.

All insulin in the United States is human insulin. Pork and bovine insulins, which were more antigenic, are no longer manufactured in the United States. The name human insulin means that the synthetic product is identical to endogenous insulin (i.e., has the same number and sequence of amino acids).

### Types of Insulin

Insulins differ in onset and duration of action. They are usually categorized as short, intermediate, or long acting. The synthesis of insulin analogs involves altering the type or sequence of amino acids in insulin molecules.

Rapid-acting insulins have a rapid onset (15 minutes or less) and a short duration of action (4–8 hours). Rapid-acting products include insulin lispro (HumaLOG, Admelog, HumaLOG KwikPen), insulin aspart (NovoLOG, Fiasp, NovoLOG FlexPen), and insulin glulisine (Apidra, Apidra SoloStar). Lispro, the first insulin analog to be marketed, is identical to human insulin except for the reversal of two amino acids (lysine and Proline). It is absorbed more rapidly and has a shorter half-life after subcutaneous injection than regular (short-acting) human insulin. As a result, it is similar to physiologic insulin secretion after a meal, more effective at decreasing postprandial hyperglycemia, and less likely to cause hypoglycemia before the next meal. Injection just before a meal produces hypoglycemic effects similar to those of an injection of conventional regular insulin given 30 minutes before a meal. Aspart has an even more rapid onset and shorter duration of action. Glulisine has the shortest onset of action (5–10 minutes).

## TABLE 41.1

## Drugs Administered for the Treatment of Diabetes Mellitus

| Drug Class | Prototype | Other Drugs in the Class |
|---|---|---|
| Insulins | Insulin (HumuLIN R U-500, HumuLIN R U-500 KwikPen, *over-the-counter* HumuLIN R, NovoLIN R, NovoLIN R ReliON) | Rapid-acting insulins or analogs:<br>Insulin lispro (HumuLIN N KwikPen, HumuLIN N, NovoLin N ReliOn, Novolin N)<br>Insulin aspart (NovoLOG, Fiasp, NovoLOG FlexPen)<br>Insulin glulisine (Apidra, Apidra SoloStar).<br>Intermediate-acting insulin:<br>Isophane insulin suspension (NPH Humulin N, Novolin N)<br>Long-acting insulins:<br>Insulin glargine (Lantus)<br>Insulin detemir (Levemir) |
| Sulfonylureas | Glyburide (Glynase) | Glimepiride (Amaryl)<br>Glipizide (Glucotrol, Glucotrol XL, GlipiZIDE)<br>Chlorpropamide<br>Tolazamide<br>Tolbutamide |
| Biguanide | Metformin (Fortamet, Glucophage, Glucophage XR, Glumetza, Riomet, Metformin ER) | |
| Alpha-glucosidase inhibitors | Acarbose (Precose) | Miglitol (Glyset) |
| Thiazolidinediones | Rosiglitazone (Avandia) | Pioglitazone (Actos) |
| Meglitinides | Repaglinide (Prandin) | Nateglinide (Starlix) |
| Dipeptidyl peptidase 4 (DPP-4) inhibitor | Sitagliptin (Januvia) | Alogliptin (Nesina)<br>Linagliptin (Tradjenta)<br>Saxagliptin (Onglyza) |
| Glucagon-like peptide-1 receptor agonist (incretin mimetics) | Exenatide (Bydureon, Byetta) | Albiglutide (Tanzeum)<br>Dulaglutide (Trulicity)<br>Liraglutide (Saxenda, Victoza)<br>Lixisenatide (Adlyxin, Adlyxin Starter Kit) |
| Amylin analogs | Pramlintide (SymlinPen 120, SymlinPen 60) | |
| Angiotensin-converting enzyme inhibitors | Enalapril maleate (Vasotec) | Benazepril hydrochloride (Lotensin)<br>Captopril (Capoten)<br>Fosinopril (Monopril)<br>Lisinopril (Prinivil, Zestril)<br>Moexipril hydrochloride (Univasc)<br>Perindopril erbumine (Aceon, Coversyl)<br>Quinapril hydrochloride (Accupril)<br>Ramipril (Altace)<br>Trandolapril (Mavik, Gopten) |
| Angiotensin II receptor antagonists | Losartan (Cozaar) | Azilsartan medoxomil (Edarbi)<br>Candesartan cilexetil (Atacand)<br>Eprosartan mesylate (Teveten)<br>Irbesartan (Avapro)<br>Olmesartan medoxomil (Benicar) |
| Thiazide-like diuretics | Hydrochlorothiazide (HCTZ) | Hydrochlorothiazide (Hydrodiuril) |
| Antiplatelet | Acetylsalicylic acid (Aspirin) | Acetylsalicylic acid/Methocarbamol (Robaxisal) |
| HMG-CoA reductase inhibitors | Simvastatin (Zocor) | Atorvastatin calcium (Lipitor)<br>Fluvastatin (Lescol, Lescol SL)<br>Lovastatin (Altoprev, Mevacor)<br>Pitavastatin calcium (Livalo)<br>Pravastatin (Pravachol)<br>Rosuvastatin (Crestor) |

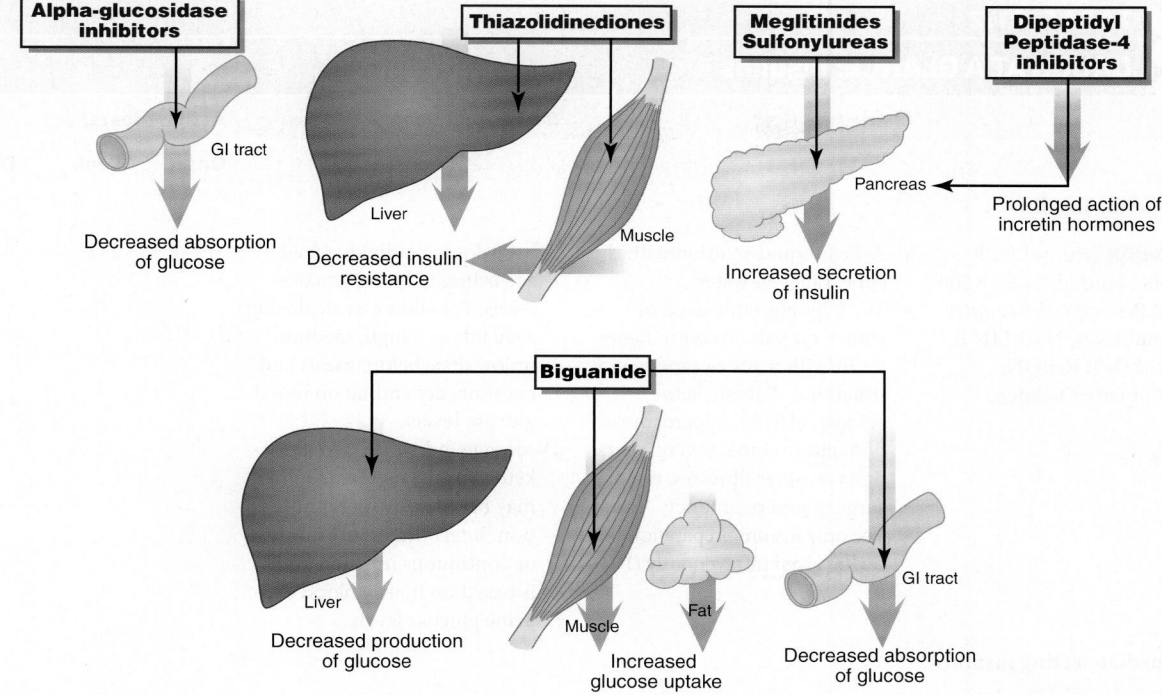

**Figure 41.2.** Actions of oral antidiabetic drugs. The drugs lower blood sugar by decreasing absorption or production of glucose, by increasing secretion of insulin, or by increasing the effectiveness of available insulin (decreasing insulin resistance).

Afrezza is an inhaled regular insulin analog. The U.S. Food and Drug Administration has issued a **BLACK BOX WARNING ◆** for this insulin, stating that patients with diabetes and chronic lung disease who take it are at risk for acute bronchospasm. Acute bronchospasm has been reported in patients with asthma and chronic obstructive pulmonary disease, and Afrezza is contraindicated in these patients who need insulin. The Institute for Safe Medication Practices also lists Afrezza as a drug with heightened risk for significant patient harm. Before ordering Afrezza, prescribers should collect a detailed medical history, perform a physical examination, and evaluate the patient's spirometry. The insulin requirements can vary with the use of Afrezza; thus, careful blood glucose monitoring is necessary. Afrezza is administered at the beginning of every meal. The cartridges should be stored at room temperature.

Intermediate-acting insulin preparations such as isophane (NPH) suspension possess zinc insulin crystals that have been modified by protamine in a neural buffer. The addition of zinc assists in slowing the absorption and thus prolongs the duration of action.

Long-acting insulin preparations include insulin glargine and insulin detemir. Health care providers use them to provide a basal amount of insulin through 24 hours, similar to normal, endogenous insulin secretion.

Several mixtures of an intermediate- and a short-acting insulin are available and in common use. U-100, the main insulin concentration in the United States, contains 100 units of insulin per milliliter of solution. Accurate measurement requires an orange-tipped syringe designed for use only with U-100 insulin.

After subcutaneous injection, insulin is absorbed most rapidly from the abdomen, followed by the upper arm, thigh, and buttocks. Absorption is delayed or decreased by injection into subcutaneous tissue with lipodystrophy or other lesions, by circulatory problems such as edema or hypotension, by insulin-binding antibodies (which develop after 2 or 3 months of insulin administration), and by injecting cold (i.e., refrigerated) insulin. Absorption may also be increased when administered in an extremity before the patient engages in a sport that requires use of the specific extremity (i.e., swimming, tennis, or jogging).

Table 41.2 gives information about insulins, including routes and dosages.

---

**BOX 41.3** 🌿 ***Herb and Dietary Interactions: Antidiabetic Drugs***

**Herbs That Increase the Risk of Hypoglycemia When Used With Antidiabetic Drugs**

- Alfalfa
- Aloe
- Bilberry
- Bitter melon
- Burdock
- Celery
- Coriander
- Damiana
- Dandelion root
- Fenugreek
- Garcinia
- Garlic
- Ginseng
- Gymnema
- Juniper
- Marshmallow
- Stinging nettle

## TABLE 41.2

## DRUGS AT A GLANCE: Insulins

| Drug | Characteristics* | Routes and Dosage Ranges† | Action (Hours) | | |
|---|---|---|---|---|---|
| | | | Onset | Peak | Duration |
| **Short-acting insulin** | | | | | |
| **Insulin** (HumuLIN R U-500, HumuLIN R U-500 KwikPen, *over-the-counter* HumuLIN R, NovoLIN R, NovoLIN R ReliON; ✹ Entuzity Kwikpen) | • A clear liquid solution with the appearance of water<br>• The hypoglycemic drug of choice for patients with diabetes in/with acute or emergency situations, diabetic keto-acidosis (DKA), hyperosmolar nonketotic coma, severe infections or other illnesses, major surgery, and pregnancy<br>• The only insulin preparation that can be given intravenously (IV) | Sub-Q, dosage individualized according to blood glucose levels. For sliding-scale dosing available as a high, medium, or low dose before meals and bedtime, depending on blood glucose levels<br>IV, dosage individualized. For ketoacidosis, regular insulin may be given by direct injection, intermittent infusion, or continuous infusion and is based on hourly blood and urine glucose levels | 1/2–1 | 2–3 | 5–7 |
| **Intermediate-acting insulins** | | | | | |
| Isophane insulin suspension (HumuLIN N KwikPen, HumuLIN N, NovoLin N ReliOn, Novolin N) | • Commonly used for long-term administration<br>• Modified by addition of prot-amine (a protein) and zinc<br>• A suspension with a cloudy appearance when correctly mixed in the drug vial<br>• Given *only* sub-Q<br>• Hypoglycemic reactions are more likely to occur during mid to late afternoon<br>• Not recommended for use in acute situations | Sub-Q, dosage individualized. Initially, 7–26 units may be given once or twice daily | 1–1½ | 8–12 | 18–24 |
| **Insulin mixtures** | | | | | |
| NPH 70%, regular 30% (Humulin 70/30, Novolin 70/30; ✹ Humulin 70/30, Novolin ge 30/70, Novoline ge 40/60, Novolin ge 50/50)<br>NPH 50%, regular 50% (Humulin 50/50) | • Controls postprandial hyperglycemia<br>• Not recommended for DKA or hyperosmolar hyperglycemic reaction | | | | |
| **Insulin analogs** | | | | | |
| Insulin lispro (HumaLOG, Admelog, HumaLOG KwikPen; ✹ HumaLOG, HumaLOG KwikPen) | • A synthetic insulin of recom-binant DNA origin, created by reversing two amino acids<br>• Has a faster onset and a shorter duration of action than human regular insulin<br>• Intended for use with a longer-acting insulin | Sub-Q, dosage individualized, 15 min before meals. May also be given in external insulin pumps | 1/4 | 1–1½ | 6–8 |
| Insulin aspart (NovoLOG, Fiasp, NovoLOG FlexPen; ✹ NovoRapid) | Similar to lispro | Sub-Q, dosage individualized | 1/4 | 1–3 | 3–5 |

## TABLE 41.2

## DRUGS AT A GLANCE: Insulins (Continued)

| Drug | Characteristics* | Routes and Dosage Ranges† | Action (Hours) | | |
|---|---|---|---|---|---|
| | | | **Onset** | **Peak** | **Duration** |
| Insulin glargine (Solostar; 🍁 SoloStar). | • Long-acting<br>• Provides basal amount of insulin<br>• Must *not* be diluted or mixed with any other insulin or solutions | Sub-Q, dosage individualized, once daily at bedtime | 1.1 | None | 24 |
| Insulin glulisine (Apidra; 🍁 Apidra SoloStar; Apidra) | • Clear, colorless solution<br>• More rapid onset of action and shorter duration of action than regular human insulin<br>• Should be used in regimens that include a longer-acting insulin or basal insulin analog<br>• May be mixed with NPH insulin for injection only. Draw up Apidra first and then NPH insulin. Do NOT mix Apidra with other insulins in sub-Q infusion pumps | Sub-Q by injection or continuous infusion pump, dosage individualized<br>When used as a mealtime insulin, give up to 15 min before or within 20 min of beginning the meal | 1/12–1/6 (5–10 min) | 1 | 4 |
| Insulin detemir (Levemir, Levemir FlexTouch; 🍁 Levemir) | • Long-acting<br>• Provides basal amount of insulin<br>• Must not be diluted or mixed with other insulins | Sub-Q once or twice daily, dosage individualized | 1 | None | 6–23 |
| **Analog mixtures** | | | | | |
| Insulin lispro protamine (HumaLOG Mix, HumaLOG Mix 50/50, HumaLOG Mix 50/50 KwikPen, HumaLOG Mix 75/25, HumaLOG Mix 75/25 KwikPen; 🍁 Humalog Mix 25, Humalog Mix 50)<br>Insulin lispro 25% (Humalog Mix 75/25) | • Same onset, peak, and duration as individual components | Sub-Q, dosage individualized | | | |
| Insulin, recombinant (Afrezza) | | Initial dose: insulin-naive patients, 4 units at each meal<br>Patients previously on sub-Q mealtime (prandial) insulin:<br>≤4 units injected dose per meal: 4 units inhalation dose per meal<br>5–8 units injected dose per meal: 8 units inhalation per meal<br>9–12 units injected dose per meal: 12 units inhalation dose per meal<br>13–16 units injected dose per meal: 16 units inhalation per meal<br>17–20 units injected dose per meal: 20 units inhalation dose per meal | 12–15 min | | 160–180 min |

*All insulins are in U.S. Food and Drug Administration Pregnancy Category B.
†When mixing insulins, always draw up the clear insulin first, and then add the cloudy insulin.

## Choice of Insulin

When insulin therapy is indicated, the physician may choose from several preparations that vary in composition, onset, duration of action, and other characteristics. Some factors to be considered include the following:

- Regular insulin (insulin injection) has a rapid onset of action and can be given intravenously. Therefore, it is the insulin of choice during acute situations, such as DKA, severe infection or other illness, and surgical procedures.
- Isophane insulin (NPH) is often used for long-term insulin therapy. For many patients, a combination of NPH and short-acting insulin provides more consistent control of blood glucose levels. Although several regimens are used, a common one is a mixture of regular and NPH insulins administered before the morning and evening meals. A commercial mixture is more convenient and probably more accurate than a mixture prepared by a patient or caregiver, if the proportions of insulins are appropriate for the patient.
- Insulin lispro, aspart, or glulisine may be used instead of regular subcutaneous insulin in most situations, but safe use requires both health care providers and patients to be aware of differences. All rapid-acting insulins are approved for use in external **insulin pumps** that administer a continuous subcutaneous infusion.
- Insulin glargine or insulin detemir may be used to provide a basal amount of insulin over 24 hours, with a short-acting or rapid-acting insulin at meal times. Short-acting insulin, such as regular, will act in 15 to 30 minutes, whereas rapid-acting insulin begins to act immediately upon administration.

## Pharmacokinetics

Regular insulin is rapidly absorbed after IV, intramuscular (IM), and subcutaneous administration. Afrezza is the newest rapid-acting insulin on the market. It is inhaled and rapidly absorbed. All of these forms of regular insulin are considered to be of short duration with a slow action. It is primarily metabolized in the liver, and a small amount is metabolized in the kidneys. Less than 2% of the drug is excreted in the urine.

## Action

Insulin and its analogs (structurally similar chemicals) replace endogenous insulin, and this exogenous insulin has the same effects as the pancreatic hormone. The insulins lower blood glucose levels by increasing glucose uptake by body cells, especially skeletal muscle and fat cells, and by decreasing glucose production in the liver.

## Use

Insulin is used to lower blood glucose, and the dosage must be individualized according to blood glucose levels. **Blood glucose meters** are devices that measure how much glucose is in the blood. A specially coated test strip containing a fresh sample of blood (obtained by pricking the skin, usually the finger or forearm, with a **lancet**) is inserted in the meter, which then measures the amount of glucose in the blood. The goal is to administer enough insulin to alleviate symptoms of hyperglycemia and to

reestablish metabolic balance without causing hypoglycemia (Box 41.4). An initial dose of 0.4 to 1 units/kg/d may be started and then adjusted to maintain blood glucose levels (tested before meals and at bedtime) of 80 to 130 mg/dL in adults. For children and adolescents, insulin is used to maintain glucose levels (tested before meals and at bedtime) of 90 to 150 mg/dL. However, many factors influence blood glucose response to exogenous insulin and therefore influence insulin requirements.

- Factors that increase insulin requirements include weight gain, increased caloric intake, pregnancy, decreased activity, acute infections, hyperadrenocorticism (Cushing's disease), primary hyperparathyroidism, acromegaly, hypokalemia, and drugs such as corticosteroids, epinephrine, levothyroxine, and thiazide diuretics. Patients who are obese may require 2 units/kg/d because of resistance to insulin in peripheral tissues.
- Factors that decrease insulin requirements include weight reduction; decreased caloric intake; increased physical activity; development of renal insufficiency; stopping administration of corticosteroids, epinephrine, levothyroxine, and diuretics; hypothyroidism; hypopituitarism; recovery from hyperthyroidism; recovery from acute infections; and the "honeymoon period," which may occur with type 1 diabetes.
- People who need less than 0.5 units/kg/d may produce some endogenous insulin, or their tissues may be more responsive to insulin because of exercise and good physical conditioning.
- In acute situations, dosage of regular insulin needs frequent adjustments based on measurements of blood glucose. When insulin is given intravenously in a continuous infusion, 20% to 30% binds to the IV fluid container and the infusion tubing.
- Dosage of insulin for long-term therapy is determined by blood glucose levels at various times of the day and is adjusted when indicated (e.g., because of illness or changes in physical activity). Titrating insulin dosage may be difficult and time consuming; it requires cooperation and collaboration between patients and health care providers.
- Insulin has been used successfully with all currently available types of oral agents (alpha-glucosidase inhibitors, biguanide, thiazolidinediones, meglitinides, and sulfonylureas).

### Use in Children

Effective management of type 1 diabetes requires a consistent schedule of meals, snacks, blood glucose monitoring, insulin injections and dose adjustments, and exercise. Insulin is the only drug indicated for use as replacement therapy because affected children cannot produce insulin. Three decades of research support the effectiveness and safety of children with type 1 diabetes receiving either multiple daily injections of insulin or continuous subcutaneous administration through an insulin pump. Rotation of injection sites is important in infants and young children because of the relatively small areas for injection at each anatomic site and to prevent lipodystrophy. Young children usually adjust to injections and blood glucose monitoring better when the parents express less anxiety about these vital procedures. Parents of infants and young children should be taught to monitor blood glucose more frequently than children ages 3 and older. Infants are at the highest risk of severe hyperglycemia, which can be difficult to detect due to the infant's inability to communicate the symptoms. In addition, the clinical signs are less specific than those experienced by an older child. Infants

| BOX 41.4 | *Hypoglycemia: Characteristics and Management* |
|---|---|

Hypoglycemia may occur with insulin, meglitinides, oral sulfonylureas, amylin analogs (pramlintide [Symlin]), and incretin mimetics (exenatide [Byetta]). When hypoglycemia is suspected, the blood glucose level should be measured if possible, although signs and symptoms and the plasma glucose level at which they occur vary from person to person. Hypoglycemia is blood glucose below 60 to 70 mg/dL and is especially dangerous at approximately 40 mg/dL or below. Central nervous system effects may lead to accidental injury or permanent brain damage; cardiovascular effects may lead to cardiac dysrhythmias or myocardial infarction. Causes of hypoglycemia include:

- Intensive insulin therapy (i.e., continuous subcutaneous [sub-Q] infusion or three or more injections daily)
- Omitting or delaying meals
- An excessive or incorrect dose of insulin or an oral agent that causes hypoglycemia
- Altered sensitivity to insulin
- Decreased clearance of insulin or an oral agent (e.g., with renal insufficiency)
- Decreased glucose intake
- Decreased production of glucose in the liver
- Giving an insulin injection via the intramuscular (IM) rather than the sub-Q route
- Drug interactions that decrease blood glucose levels
- Increased physical exertion
- Ethanol ingestion

### Hormones That Raise Blood Sugar

Normally, when hypoglycemia occurs, several hormones (glucagon, epinephrine, growth hormone, and cortisol) work to restore and maintain blood glucose levels. Glucagon and epinephrine, the dominant counterregulatory hormones, act rapidly because they are activated as soon as blood glucose levels start declining. Growth hormone and cortisol act more slowly, about 2 hours after hypoglycemia occurs.

People with diabetes who develop hypoglycemia may have impaired secretion of these hormones, especially those patients with type 1 diabetes. Decreased secretion of glucagon is often evident in patients who have had diabetes for 5 years or longer. Decreased secretion of epinephrine also occurs in people who have been treated with insulin for several years. Decreased epinephrine decreases tachycardia, a common sign of hypoglycemia, and may delay recognition and treatment.

### The Conscious Patient

Treatment of hypoglycemic reactions consists of immediate administration of a rapidly absorbed carbohydrate. For the conscious patient who is able to swallow, the carbohydrate is given orally. Foods and fluids that provide approximately 15 g of carbohydrate include:

- Liquids or fruit juices.
- Teaspoons of sugar.
- Commercial glucose products (e.g., Glutose, B-D Glucose). These products must be swallowed to be effective.
- Symptoms usually subside within 15 to 20 minutes. If they do not subside, the patient should take another 10 to 15 g of oral carbohydrate.
- *If acarbose or miglitol has been taken with insulin or a sulfonylurea and a hypoglycemic reaction occurs, glucose (oral or intravenous [IV]) or glucagon must be given for treatment.* Sucrose (table sugar) and other oral carbohydrates do not relieve hypoglycemia because the presence of acarbose or miglitol prevents their digestion and absorption from the gastrointestinal tract.

### The Unconscious Patient

Carbohydrate cannot be given orally. Therefore, the choices are parenteral glucose or glucagon.

- In the health care facility, administer 25% to 50% dextrose solution.
- In home or elsewhere, give sub-Q or IM glucagon 0.5 to 1 mg if available, and there is someone to inject it.
- Glucagon is a pancreatic hormone that increases blood sugar by converting liver glycogen to glucose. It is effective only when liver glycogen is present. Some patients cannot respond to glucagon because glycogen stores are depleted by conditions such as starvation, adrenal insufficiency, or chronic hypoglycemia. The hyperglycemic effect of glucagon occurs more slowly than that of IV glucose and is of relatively brief duration. If the patient does not respond to one or two doses of glucagon within 20 minutes, IV glucose is indicated.

### Avoid Overtreatment

Caution is necessary in the treatment of hypoglycemia. Although the main goal of treatment is to relieve hypoglycemia and restore the brain's supply of glucose, a secondary goal is to avoid overtreatment and excessive hyperglycemia.

---

may present with poor feeding, lethargy, hypotonia, or jitteriness (Levitsky & Misra, 2019).

A healthful, varied diet, rich in whole grains, fruits, and vegetables and limited in simple sugars, is recommended. According to the American Diabetes Association, medical nutrition therapy should be tailored to a person's specific health issues and personal preferences to help maintain optimum health by controlling blood glucose levels, blood pressure, cholesterol, and other risk factors.

It is essential to synchronize food intake with insulin injections, and this coordination usually involves three meals and three snacks, all at regularly scheduled times. Such a schedule is difficult to maintain in children, but it is extremely important in promoting normal growth and development. A major factor in optimal treatment is a supportive family in which at least one member is thoroughly educated about the disease and its

management. Less-than-optimal treatment can lead to stunted growth, delayed puberty, and early development of complications such as retinopathy, nephropathy, or neuropathy.

Physical activity and exercise are recommended and encouraged for all children with type 1 diabetes. The goal is 60 minutes of moderate- to vigorous-intensity aerobic activity daily. The child and family members should be educated about checking blood glucose levels before, during, and after exercise. A pre-exercise glucose of 90 to 250 mg/dL is optimal, and the child should have access to carbohydrate snacks in the event the blood sugar decreases during exercise. The effects of a hypoglycemia after exercise and overnight should be taught to the child and caregivers. Strategies to reduce the postexercise hypoglycemia include reducing mealtime dosing preceding the exercise, increasing carbohydrate intake preceding exercise, eating bedtime snacks, using continuous glucose monitoring, and/or reducing basal insulin doses.

Infections and other illnesses may cause wide fluctuations in blood glucose levels and interfere with metabolic control. For example, viral infections cause hypoglycemia; others, especially chronic infections, may cause hyperglycemia and insulin resistance and may precipitate ketoacidosis. As a result, insulin requirements may vary widely during illness episodes and should be based on blood glucose and urine ketone levels. Hypoglycemia often develops in young children, partly because of anorexia and smaller glycogen reserves.

During illness, children are highly susceptible to dehydration, and an adequate fluid intake is very important. Many clinicians recommend sugar-containing liquids (e.g., regular sodas, clear juices, and regular gelatin desserts) if blood glucose values are lower than 250 mg/dL. When blood glucose values are above 250 mg/dL, children should receive diet soda, unsweetened tea, and other fluids without sugar.

Administration of insulin for infants and toddlers who weigh less than 10 kg or require less than 5 units of insulin per day can be difficult because small doses are difficult to measure in a U-100 syringe. Use of diluted insulin allows more accurate administration. The most common dilution strength is U-10 (10 units/mL), and a diluent is available from insulin manufacturers for this purpose. It is necessary to clearly label vials of diluted insulin and discard them after 1 month.

Avoiding hypoglycemia is a major goal in infants and young children because of potentially damaging effects on growth and development. There may be a delay in recognition of hypoglycemia because signs and symptoms are vague and children may be unable to communicate them to parents or caregivers. Most pediatric endocrinologists recommend maintaining blood glucose levels between 100 and 200 mg/dL to prevent hypoglycemia. It is important never to skip the bedtime snack and blood glucose measurement.

Signs and symptoms of hypoglycemia in older children are similar to those in adults (e.g., hunger, sweating, and tachycardia). In young children, hypoglycemia may be manifested by changes in behavior, including severe hunger, irritability, and lethargy. In addition, mental functioning may be impaired in all age groups, even with mild hypoglycemia. Any time, hypoglycemia is suspected; it is essential that blood glucose be tested.

Adolescents may resist adhering to their prescribed treatment regimens, and effective management may be especially difficult during this developmental period. Adolescents and young adults may delay, omit, or decrease dosage of insulin to fit in socially (e.g., by eating more, "sleeping in," drinking alcohol) or to control their weight. Omitting or decreasing insulin dosage may lead to repeated episodes of ketoacidosis. Also, adolescent females may develop eating disorders.

Health care professionals are increasingly identifying type 2 diabetes in children. This trend is attributed mainly to obesity and inadequate exercise because most children with type 2 disease are seriously overweight and have poor eating habits. In addition, most are members of high-risk racial and ethnic groups and have relatives with diabetes. Management involves exercise; weight loss; a more healthful diet; and, in some cases, drug therapy, including insulin. It is also important to attend to treating comorbid conditions such as hypertension and hyperlipidemia.

## Use in Older Adults

It is estimated that at least 20% of people older than 65 years of age have diabetes. General precautions for safe and effective use of oral hypoglycemic drugs apply to older adults, including close monitoring of blood glucose levels; however, control of cardiovascular risk factors may play a greater role in reducing morbidity and mortality in this population. In addition, older adults may have impaired vision, poor manual dexterity, or other problems that decrease their ability to perform needed tasks (e.g., self-administration of insulin, monitoring blood glucose levels, managing diet, and exercise).

## Use in Patients With Renal Impairment

Frequent monitoring of blood glucose levels and dosage adjustments may be necessary. It is difficult to predict dosage needs because, on the one hand, less insulin is degraded by the kidneys (normally about 25%), and this may lead to higher blood levels of insulin if dosage is not reduced. On the other hand, muscles and possibly other tissues are less sensitive to insulin, and this insulin resistance may result in an increased blood glucose level if dosage is not increased. Overall, vigilance is required to prevent dangerous hypoglycemia, especially in patients whose renal function is unstable or worsening.

## Use in Patients With Hepatic Impairment

Higher blood levels of insulin may occur in patients with hepatic impairment because less insulin may be degraded. Careful monitoring of blood glucose levels and insulin dosage reductions may be needed to prevent hypoglycemia.

## Use in Patients With Critical Illness

Critically ill patients, with and without diabetes mellitus, often experience hyperglycemia associated with insulin resistance. Hyperglycemia may complicate the progress of critically ill patients, resulting in increased complications such as postoperative infections, poor recovery, and increased mortality. Tight glycemic control is a key factor in preventing complications and improving mortality in the patient in an intensive care unit.

Insulin is more likely to be used in critical illness than any of the oral agents. Reasons include the greater ability to titrate dosage needs in patients who are often debilitated and unstable, with varying degrees of cardiovascular, liver, and kidney impairment. One important consideration with IV insulin therapy is that 30% or more of a dose may adsorb into containers of IV fluid or infusion sets. In addition, many critically ill patients are unable to take oral drugs. Surgery may require use of insulin. Box 41.5 provides information about perioperative insulin therapy.

Some critically ill patients are also at risk for serious hypoglycemia, especially if they are debilitated, sedated, or unable to recognize and communicate symptoms. Vigilant monitoring is essential for any patient who has diabetes and a critical illness.

## Use in Patients Receiving Home Care

Most insulins are taken at home, and the home care nurse shares the responsibility for teaching patients how to use the drug effectively and how to recognize medication responses that should be reported to the health care provider. Accurate dosing is extremely important so that blood glucose levels can be maintained at a normal level. Hyperglycemia and hypoglycemia are both unwanted effects of poor glycemic control. The nurse instructs the patient and any caregivers that if symptoms of hypoglycemia develop, it is essential to take corrective steps immediately. The home care nurse also monitors the patient's response to insulin and changes

## BOX 41.5 *Perioperative Insulin Therapy*

Patients with diabetes who undergo major surgery have increased risks of both surgical and diabetic complications. Risks associated with surgery and anesthesia are greater if diabetes is not well controlled and complications of diabetes (e.g., hypertension, diabetic kidney disease, vascular damage) are already evident. Hyperglycemia and poor metabolic control are associated with increased susceptibility to infection, poor wound healing, and fluid and electrolyte imbalances. Risks of diabetic complications are increased because the stress of surgery increases insulin requirements and may precipitate diabetic ketoacidosis. Metabolic responses to stress include increased secretion of catecholamines, cortisol, glucagon, and growth hormone, all of which increase blood glucose levels. In addition to hyperglycemia, protein breakdown, lipolysis, ketogenesis, and insulin resistance occur. The risk of hypoglycemia is also increased.

The goals of treatment are to avoid hypoglycemia, severe hyperglycemia, ketoacidosis, and fluid and electrolyte imbalances. Maintenance of blood glucose levels between 80 and 180 mg/dL during the perioperative period is desirable. Because surgery is a stressful event that increases blood glucose levels and the body's need for insulin, insulin therapy is usually required. A 25% reduction of the insulin dose in the evening before surgery is likely to achieve perioperative blood glucose in the target range with decreased risk for hypoglycemia. Oral hypoglycemic agents such as metformin are withheld the day of the surgery. If NPH is used, give half of the NPH dose or 60% to 80% of a long-acting analog or pump basal insulin. Blood glucose is monitored every 4 to 6 hours while the patient is NPO, and prescribers should dose with short-acting insulin as needed.

The goal of insulin therapy is to avoid ketosis from inadequate insulin and hypoglycemia from excessive insulin. Specific actions depend largely on the severity of diabetes and the type of surgical procedure. Diabetes should be well controlled before any type of surgery. Minor procedures usually require little change in the usual treatment program; major operations usually require a different medication regimen.

---

in the patient's condition or drug therapy that increases the patient's risk for hypoglycemic episodes.

When a patient is receiving a combination of insulins for management of diabetes, the nurse assists the patient in understanding that the different types of insulins have different onsets and therapeutic ranges. As a result, the medications work together to be more effective and maintain a more stable glycemic control. Changing medications or dosages can upset the balance and lead to hyperglycemia or hypoglycemia. If the patient is unable to take the medications for any reason, it is essential to notify the health care provider.

### Contraindications

The only clear-cut contraindication to the use of insulin is hypoglycemia, because of the risk of brain damage (see Box 41.4).

## Nursing Implications

### Preventing Interactions

Patients who take insulin may have other diseases that require therapeutic drugs. Certain medications can interfere with insulin, increasing or decreasing the effects, thus causing hypoglycemia or hyperglycemia (Box 41.6). Some herbs increase the risk of hypoglycemia (see Box 41.3).

### Administering the Medication

Oral administration of insulins is not effective because the proteins are destroyed by proteolytic enzymes in the GI tract. Sub-Q administration is preferred, and for regular insulin, the IV route may be appropriate.

>  **QSEN Alert: Safety**
>
> Before administering insulin, patient safety requires that two nurses always check the dosage.

### Timing

Patients with type 1 diabetes administer rapid-acting or short-acting insulin prior to meals. Patients with type 2 diabetes may

## BOX 41.6 *Drug Interactions: Insulin*

**Drugs That Increase the Effects of Insulin**
- Angiotensin-converting enzyme inhibitors (e.g., captopril)
  *Increase the risk of hypoglycemia*
- Alcohol
  *May promote increased hypoglycemia; inhibits gluconeogenesis (in people with or without diabetes)*
- Antidiabetic drugs, oral
  *May alter blood glucose levels; increasingly being used with insulin in the treatment of type 2 diabetes (The risks of hypoglycemia are greater with the combination.)*
- Antimicrobials (sulfonamides, tetracyclines)
  *Increase the risk of hypoglycemia*
- Beta-adrenergic blocking agents (e.g., propranolol)
  *Increase hypoglycemia by inhibiting the effects of catecholamines on gluconeogenesis and glycogenolysis (effects that normally raise blood glucose levels in response to hypoglycemia); may also mask signs and symptoms of hypoglycemia (e.g., tachycardia, tremors) that normally occur with a hypoglycemia-induced activation of the sympathetic nervous system*

**Drugs That Decrease the Effects of Insulin**
- Adrenergics (e.g., albuterol, epinephrine)
  *Increase insulin requirements*
- Anabolic corticosteroids (e.g., prednisone)
  *Increase insulin requirements*
- Estrogens and oral contraceptives
  *Increase insulin requirements*
- Glucagon
  *Raises blood glucose by converting liver glycogen to glucose*
- Levothyroxine
  *Increases insulin requirements due to hyperglycemia*
- Phenytoin
  *Raises blood sugar by inhibiting insulin secretion*
- Thiazide diuretics (e.g., hydrochlorothiazide)
  *Increase risk of hyperglycemia due to change in glucose control*

take at least two insulin injections daily, with one half to two thirds of the total daily dose in the morning before breakfast and the remaining one half or one third before the evening meal or at bedtime. With regular insulin before meals, it is very important that the medication be injected 30 to 45 minutes before meals so that the insulin is available when blood sugar increases after meals. With insulin lispro, aspart, or glulisine before meals, it is important to inject the medication about 15 minutes before eating. Insulin glargine or detemir is most commonly given at bedtime. However, it may be administered in the morning or in split doses as needed.

For the patient who uses an external insulin pump, it is important for the patient to understand the pharmacokinetics of the insulin used in the pump. The health care provider overseeing the patient's insulin pump sets the basal insulin settings that provide the continuous insulin needed throughout the day. However, the patient needs to have an understanding of how much and when to administer the insulin for meals. Figure 41.3 presents information concerning the insulin pump.

### Selection of Subcutaneous Sites for Injections and Pumps

Several factors affect insulin absorption from injection sites, including the site location, environmental temperature, and exercise or massage. Studies indicate that insulin is absorbed fastest from the abdomen, followed by the deltoid, thigh, and hip.

Because of these differences, many clinicians recommend rotating injection sites within areas. This technique decreases rotations between areas and promotes more consistent blood glucose levels. With regard to temperature, insulin is absorbed more rapidly in warmer sites and environments. In relation to exercise, people who exercise should avoid injecting insulin into subcutaneous tissue near the muscles to be used. The increased blood flow that accompanies exercise promotes rapid absorption and may lead to hypoglycemia.

For the patient with an insulin pump, the most commonly recommended sites are the abdomen and lower back so that absorption rates remain consistent (see Fig. 41.3). It is extremely important that the patient rotate sites and avoid placing a site into scar tissue, which also affects insulin absorption.

### Timing of Food Intake

Patients receiving insulin need food at the peak action time of the insulin and at bedtime. They usually take the food as a between-meal and a bedtime snack. These snacks help prevent hypoglycemic reactions between meals and at night. When hypoglycemia occurs during sleep, there may be a delay in recognition and treatment, which may allow the reaction to become more severe.

### *Assessing for Therapeutic Effects*

Patients with type 1 diabetes self-monitor their blood glucose by testing 6 to 10 times daily. Patients with type 2 diabetes and using basal insulin may test their blood glucose up to four times a day. In patients with type 2 diabetes not using insulin, routine glucose

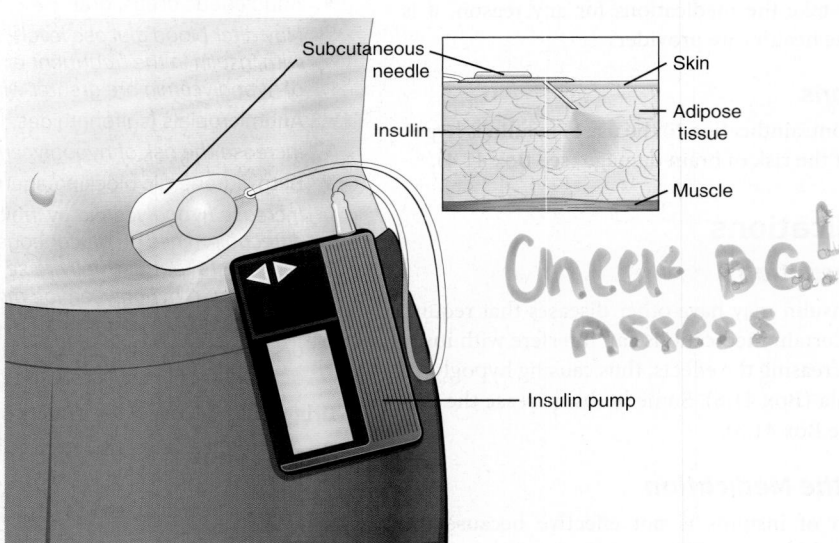

**Figure 41.3.** Continuous subcutaneous (sub-Q) insulin infusion pump. The insulin dosage is programmed into the pump's computer, and the appropriate amount of insulin is injected into the adipose tissue through a needle inserted into the sub-Q area. Insulin pumps are being increasingly used, especially by adolescents and young adults who want flexibility in diet and exercise. These devices allow continuous subcutaneous administration of regular insulin, insulin aspart, or insulin glulisine. A basal amount of insulin is injected (e.g., 1 unit/hour or a calculated fraction of the dose used previously) continuously, with bolus injections before meals. This method of insulin administration maintains more normal blood glucose levels and avoids wide fluctuations. Candidates for insulin pumps include patients with diabetes that is poorly controlled with other methods and those who are able and willing to care for the devices properly. The MiniMed Paradigm Real-Time System (Medtronic), the world's first integrated insulin pump and continuous glucose monitoring system, is now available in the United States. The Guardian RT System is an insulin pump and displays glucose readings every 5 minutes. It sounds an alarm when glucose levels reach high or low glucose limits preset by the clinical professional. The study completed on the RT System demonstrated that patients using the RT continuous glucose monitoring technology had better control of their blood glucose than did patients using fingersticks only.

## TABLE 41.3

### Estimated Average Glucose (eAG)

| A1C (%) | eAG (mg/dL) |
|---|---|
| 5 | 97 |
| 5.5 | 111 |
| 6 | 126 |
| 6.5 | 140 |
| 7 | 154 |
| 7.5 | 169 |
| 8 | 183 |
| 8.5 | 197 |
| 9 | 212 |
| 9.5 | 226 |
| 10 | 240 |
| 10.5 | 255 |
| 11 | 269 |
| 11.5 | 283 |
| 12 | 298 |

Reprinted with permission from Gebel, E. (2011). Back to Basics: Blood Glucose. Retrieved January 6, 2020, from http://www.diabetesforecast.org/2011/apr/back-to-basics-blood-glucose.html

monitoring has limited clinical benefit. The more often the patient can check blood glucose levels, the greater possibility of tighter glucose control. The goal of the patient taking insulin is to maintain blood glucose levels within normal range. Health care providers also look at the glycosylated hemoglobin (hemoglobin A1C) levels to assess the effectiveness of treatment. Because glucose stays attached to hemoglobin for the life of the red blood cell, which is about 120 days, the hemoglobin A1C level reflects the average blood glucose level over the past 3 months. The normal hemoglobin A1C level is less than 7% (Table 41.3).

### Assessing for Adverse Effects

Assessing for signs and symptoms of hypoglycemia is essential (see Box 41.4). It is necessary to assess for tachycardia, palpitations, nervousness, weakness, confusion, hunger, and sweating. A decrease in blood glucose activates the sympathetic nervous system to produce a stress response. The nurse also assesses for such central nervous system effects as mental confusion, incoherent speech, visual changes, convulsions, and coma. In addition, he or she assesses the skin and subcutaneous fat for dimpling, atrophy, or hypertrophy of the injection sites. These effects are indicative of lipodystrophy that prevents proper absorption of insulin.

### ! QSEN Alert: Patient-Centered Care

Patients who work outdoors in hot weather and have insulin pumps are at risk for not receiving the insulin because of its inactivation with increased temperatures.

### Patient Teaching

It is important to teach the patient and family about all aspects of diabetes care (Box 41.7). It is also essential to teach them about the insulins and their administration (Box 41.8).

### Clinical Application 41.2

Mr. Smith comes back 6 months later after an increase in glyburide of up to 20 mg daily because of poor glycemic control and failure to adhere to a diet and exercise regimen. His physician orders 6 units of Humulin 70/30 once daily in the morning.
- At what time does the nurse tell Mr. Smith to expect hypoglycemia to occur?
- What teaching does the nurse provide to Mr. Smith about preparing and injecting the insulin?

### NCLEX Success

3. A patient is taking NPH insulin once daily in the morning. What is the most likely time for a hypoglycemic reaction?
   - A. 1 to 3 hours after administration
   - B. 4 to 12 hours after administration
   - C. 12 to 18 hours after administration
   - D. 18 to 24 hours after administration

4. A patient with newly diagnosed type 1 diabetes is beginning daily insulin injections. The nurse is preparing to teach the patient about insulin injections. What should the nurse include in the teaching plan?
   - A. Understand that ketones in the urine indicate the need for a decrease in the number of units of insulin.
   - B. Administer the insulin at the same time every day regardless of meals.
   - C. Rotate the insulin injection sites.
   - D. Increase the insulin dosage just prior to exercise.

5. When teaching a patient who has recently received a diagnosis of diabetes how to self-administer short-acting and intermediate-acting insulin subcutaneously, which of the following instructions is correct?
   - A. Understand that the order of drawing up the two insulins into the syringe does not matter.
   - B. Draw the short-acting insulin into the syringe first, followed by the intermediate-acting insulin.
   - C. Draw the intermediate-acting insulin into the syringe first, followed by the short-acting insulin.
   - D. Give yourself two injections because mixing these insulins together is unsafe.

6. **Which of the following insulins cannot be administered in a continuous subcutaneous insulin infusion pump?**
   A. insulin lispro
   B. insulin aspart
   C. insulin glulisine
   D. insulin glargine

7. **A nurse is caring for a patient who is "nothing by mouth" (NPO) before surgery scheduled at 10:00 AM. He routinely receives 30 units of Humulin 70/30 every morning at 7:00 AM. What is the appropriate nursing action in this situation?**
   A. Administer 30 units of Humulin 70/30 subcutaneously.
   B. Hold the insulin because the patient is NPO.
   C. Give the patient a light breakfast and administer the insulin as ordered.
   D. Contact the physician for a presurgery insulin order.

---

**BOX 41.7**  *Patient Teaching Guidelines for Antidiabetic Drugs (General)*

- Wear or carry diabetic identification (e.g., a MedicAlert necklace or bracelet) at all times, to aid treatment if needed.
- Learn as much as you can about diabetes and its management. Few other diseases require as much adaptation in activities of daily living, and you must be well informed to control the disease, minimize complications, and achieve an optimal quality of life. Although much information is available from health care providers (physicians, nurses, nurse diabetes educators, nutritionists), an additional major resource is the:

  American Diabetes Association
  1660 Duke St.
  Alexandria, VA 22314
  1-800-ADA-DISC
  http://www.diabetes.org

- In general, a consistent schedule of diet, exercise, and medication produces the best control of blood sugar levels and the least risk of complications.
- Diet, weight control, and exercise are extremely important in managing diabetes. Maintaining normal weight and avoiding excessive caloric intake decrease the need for medication and decrease the workload of the pancreas. Exercise helps body tissues use insulin better, which means that glucose moves out of the bloodstream and into muscles and other body tissues. This promotes more normal blood glucose levels and decreases long-term complications of diabetes.
- Take antidiabetic medication as prescribed. If unable to take a medication, notify a health care provider. To control blood sugar most effectively, medications are balanced with diet and exercise. If you take insulin, you need to know what type(s) you are taking, how to obtain more, and how to store it. Unopened vials of insulin should be refrigerated. An opened vial may be stored at room temperature for 28 days. DO NOT freeze insulin. Regular and isophane (NPH) insulins and mixtures (e.g., Humulin) are available

over the counter; lispro (Humalog), aspart (NovoLog), glargine (Lantus), glulisine (Apidra), and detemir (Levemir) require a prescription. Keep several days' supply of insulin and syringes on hand to allow for weather or other conditions that might prevent replacement of insulin or other supplies when needed. If you take Byetta, you should store it in the original package in the refrigerator and discard unused portion after 30 days. Alert your health care provider if you experience acute abdominal discomfort while taking Byetta. If you take Symlin, opened vials can be kept in the refrigerator or at room temperature for up to 28 days.

- You need to know the signs and symptoms of high blood sugar (hyperglycemia): increased blood glucose and excessive thirst, hunger, and urine output. Persistent hyperglycemia may indicate a need to change some aspect of the treatment program, such as diet or medication.
- You need to know the symptoms of low blood sugar (hypoglycemia): sweating, nervousness, hunger, weakness, tremors, and mental confusion. Hypoglycemia may indicate too much medication or exercise or too little food. Treatment is a rapidly absorbed source of sugar, which usually reverses symptoms within 10 to 20 minutes. If you are alert and able to swallow, take 4 oz of fruit juice; 4 to 6 oz of a sugar-containing soft drink; a piece of fruit or 1/3 cup of raisins; two to three glucose tablets (5 g each); a tube of glucose gel; 1 cup of skim milk, tea, or coffee with two teaspoons of sugar; or eight Life Savers candies. Avoid taking so much sugar that hyperglycemia occurs.
- If you take acarbose (Precose) or miglitol (Glyset) along with insulin, glimepiride (Amaryl), glipizide (Glucotrol), or glyburide (DiaBeta, Glynase) and a hypoglycemic reaction occurs, you must take some form of glucose (or glucagon) for treatment. Sucrose (table sugar) and other oral carbohydrates do not relieve hypoglycemia because the presence of acarbose or miglitol prevents their digestion and absorption from the gastrointestinal (GI) tract.
- You need to have a family member or another person who is able to recognize and manage hypoglycemia in

case you are unable to obtain or swallow a source of glucose. If you take insulin, glucagon should be available in the home, and a caregiver should know how to give it.

- The best way to prevent, delay, or decrease the severity of diabetes complications is to maintain blood sugar at a normal or near-normal level. Other measures include regular visits to health care providers, preferably a team of specialists in diabetes care; regular vision and glaucoma testing; and special foot care. In addition, if you have hypertension or elevated lipid levels, treatment can help prevent heart attacks and strokes.

- Take only drugs prescribed by a physician who knows you have diabetes. Avoid other prescriptions and over-the-counter drugs unless these are discussed with the physician treating the diabetes because adverse reactions and interactions may occur. For example, nasal decongestants [alone or in cold remedies] and asthma medications may cause tachycardia and nervousness, which may be interpreted as hypoglycemia. In addition, liquid cold remedies and cough syrups may contain sugar and raise blood glucose levels.

- If you wish to take any kind of herbal or dietary supplement, you should discuss this with the health care provider who is managing your diabetes. There has been little study of these preparations in relation to diabetes; many can increase or decrease blood sugar and alter diabetes control. If you start a supplement, you need to check your blood sugar frequently to see how it affects your blood glucose level.

- Test blood regularly for glucose. A schedule individualized to your needs is best. Testing should be done more often when medication dosages are changed or when you are ill. Current blood glucose technology allows the selection of the fingertip or other location such as the forearm to obtain the blood sample. Glucose concentrations measured at different sites may vary. The fingertips are the most accurate site and should be the preferred test site if hypoglycemia is suspected.

- Reduce insulin dosage or eat extra food if you expect to exercise more than usual. Specific recommendations should be individualized and worked out with health care providers in relation to the type of exercise.

- Ask for written instructions about managing "sick days," and call your physician if unsure about what you need to do. Although each person needs individualized instructions, some general guidelines include the following:
  - Continue your antidiabetic medications unless instructed otherwise. Additional insulin also may be needed, especially if ketosis develops. Ketones [acetone] in the urine indicate insulin deficiency or insulin resistance.
  - Check blood glucose levels before meals and at least four times daily; test urine for ketones when the blood glucose level exceeds 250 mg/dL or with each urination. If unable to test urine, have someone else do it.
  - Rest, keep warm, do not exercise, and keep someone with you if possible.
  - If unable to eat solid food, take easily digested liquids or semiliquid foods. About 15 g of carbohydrate every 1 to 2 hours is usually enough and can be provided by half cup of apple juice, applesauce, cola, cranberry juice, eggnog, cream of wheat cereal, custard, vanilla ice cream, regular gelatin, or frozen yogurt.
  - Drink 2 to 3 quarts of fluids daily, especially if you have a fever. Water, tea, broths, clear soups, diet soda, or carbohydrate-containing fluids are acceptable.
  - Record the amount of fluid intake as well as the number of times you urinate, vomit, or have loose stools.
  - Seek medical attention if a premeal blood glucose level is more than 250 mg/dL, if urine acetone is present, if you have fever above 100°F, if you have several episodes of vomiting or diarrhea, or if you have difficulty in breathing, chest pain, severe abdominal pain, or severe dehydration.
  - Understand that an illness is a stress response and can increase or decrease your blood glucose. The body will have increased secretions of glucagon, epinephrine, growth hormone, cortisol, and hormones that raise blood glucose levels, and this will require an increase in medication to lower blood sugar. If you are unable to eat, hypoglycemia will result. Illnesses that lower blood sugar include viral infections, nausea, and vomiting. These conditions can result in dehydration and changes in fluids and electrolytes, leading to diabetic ketoacidosis.

## SULFONYLUREAS

The sulfonylureas are the oldest and largest group of oral agents used in patients living with type 2 diabetes. However, they are not commonly prescribed due to the increased risk of hypoglycemia. The sulfonylureas stimulate insulin secretion in patients who still have some beta cell production in the pancreas. Second-generation sulfonylureas have largely replaced first-generation sulfonylureas (e.g., chlorpropamide, tolazamide, tolbutamide). **Glyburide** (Glynase) is the prototype sulfonylurea. It is chemically related to sulfonamide antibacterial drugs.

### Pharmacokinetics

After oral administration, glyburide is well absorbed and more than 90% bound to plasma proteins. The drug is metabolized to inactive metabolites in the liver. These products are excreted

mainly by the kidneys; however, any whole drug is excreted about equally in urine and bile.

### Action

Glyburide lowers blood glucose mainly by increasing secretion of insulin. It may also increase peripheral use of glucose, decrease production of glucose in the liver, increase the number of insulin receptors, and alter postreceptor actions to increase tissue responsiveness to insulin. Because the drug stimulates pancreatic beta cells to produce more insulin, it is effective only when functioning pancreatic beta cells are present.

### Use

Health care professionals use glyburide in combination with diet to lower blood sugar in patients with type 2 diabetes mellitus. It

## BOX 41.8 — *Patient Teaching Guidelines for Insulin*

- Use correct techniques for injecting insulin:
- Follow instructions for times of administration as nearly as possible. Different types of insulin have different onsets, peaks, and durations of action. Accurate timing (e.g., in relation to meals) can increase beneficial effects and decrease risks of hypoglycemic reactions.
- Wash hands; wash injection site, if needed.
- Draw up insulin in a good light, being very careful to draw up the correct dose. If you have trouble seeing the syringe markers, get a magnifier or ask someone else to draw up the insulin. Prefilled syringes or cartridges for pen devices are also available.
- Instructions may vary about cleaning the top of the insulin vial and the injection site with an alcohol swab and about pulling back on the plunger after injection to see if any blood enters the syringe. These techniques have been commonly used, but many diabetes experts do not believe they are necessary.

- Inject straight into the fat layer under the skin, at a 90-degree angle. If very thin, pinch up a skinfold and inject at a 45-degree angle.
- Rotate injection sites. Your health care provider may suggest a rotation plan. Many people rotate between the abdomen and the thighs. Insulin is absorbed fastest from the abdomen. Do not inject insulin within 2 inches of the "belly button" or into any skin lesions.
- If it is necessary to mix two insulin preparations, ask for specific instructions about the technique, and then follow it consistently. There is a risk of inaccurate dosage of both insulins unless measured very carefully. Commercial mixtures are also available for some combinations.
- Change insulin dosage only if instructed to do so and the circumstances are specified.
- Carry sugar, candy, or a commercial glucose preparation for immediate use if a hypoglycemic reaction occurs.

---

is usually necessary to start with a low dosage and increase it gradually until the fasting blood glucose level is 110 mg/dL or less. The lowest dose that achieves normal fasting and postprandial blood sugar levels is recommended (Table 41.4).

### Use in Older Adults

Older adults tend to be more sensitive to glyburide. In addition, older adults may have other disease states and may take other drugs that complicate management of diabetes. In addition,

---

## TABLE 41.4

### DRUGS AT A GLANCE: Sulfonylureas

| Drug | Pregnancy Category | Routes and Dosage Ranges | |
|---|---|---|---|
| | | **Adults** | **Children** |
| Ⓟ **Glyburide** (Glynase; ✿ APO-GlyBURIDE, DiaBeta, DOM-GlyBURIDE, SANDOZ-GlyBURIDE, TEVA-GlyBURIDE) | C | Initial dose, 2.5–5 mg PO with breakfast<br>Maintenance dose, 1.25–20 mg/d PO given as single or divided doses; increase in increments of no more than 2.5 mg at weekly intervals based on patient's blood glucose<br>Older adult initial: 1.25 mg/d PO | Not recommended |
| Chlorpropamide (✿ APO-ChlorproPAMIDE) | C | PO 250 mg daily; may be increased or decreased by 50–125 mg at 3–5-d intervals; titrate after 5–7 d<br>Maintenance: 100–250 mg daily<br>Severe diabetes: 500 mg daily avoid doses >750 mg daily | Not recommended |
| Glimepiride (Amaryl; ✿ Amaryl, Apo-Glimepiride; Novo-Glimepiride, PMS-Glimepiride, ratio-Glimepiride, Sandoz-Glimepiride) | C | Initial dose, 1–2 mg PO once daily, with breakfast or first main meal; max starting dose, 2 mg or less<br>Maintenance dose, 1–4 mg once daily; after a dose of 2 mg is reached, increase dose in increments of 2 mg or less at 1- to 2-wk intervals, based on blood glucose levels; max recommended dose, 8 mg once daily<br>When administered with insulin, administer glimepiride 8 mg PO once daily with insulin at the breakfast or the first main meal of the day | Safety and efficacy not established |
| Glipizide (GlipiZIDE XL Glucotrol; ✿ Glucotrol XL) | C | Initial dose, 5 mg PO daily in a single dose, 30 min before breakfast; max dose, 40 mg daily<br>In elderly, may start with 2.5 mg daily<br>Extended-release, once daily with breakfast | Safety and efficacy not established |

**TABLE 41.4**

**DRUGS AT A GLANCE: Sulfonylureas** (Continued)

| Drug | Pregnancy Category | Routes and Dosage Ranges | |
|---|---|---|---|
| | | **Adults** | **Children** |
| Tolazamide | C | PO 100–250 mg/d; 500 mg in 2 divided doses | Safety and efficacy not established |
| Tolbutamide | C | PO 1–2 g/d as a single dose in the morning or in divided doses throughout the day; maintenance dose, 0.25 mg to 3 g/d<br>Geriatric:<br>Initial dose: 250 mg one to three times per day | Safety and efficacy not established |

hypoglycemia is a concern. Drugs with a short duration of action and inactive metabolites are considered safer, especially in elderly people with impaired liver or kidney function. Therapy usually begins with a low dose, which is then increased or decreased according to blood glucose levels and clinical response.

### Use in Patients With Renal Impairment

The kidneys are mainly responsible for excretion of metabolites, and renal impairment may lead to accumulation and hypoglycemia. Therefore, use of glyburide requires caution, with close monitoring of renal function, in patients with mild to moderate renal impairment. Use in severe renal impairment is contraindicated. Renal insufficiency may increase risks of adverse effects with oral hypoglycemic drugs, thereby increasing dosage requirements.

### Use in Patients With Hepatic Impairment

Caution is warranted with use of glyburide, and monitoring of liver function is necessary. Metabolism of glyburide takes place in the liver, and hepatic impairment may result in higher serum drug levels and inadequate release of hepatic glucose in response to hypoglycemia. Glyburide may cause hypoglycemia in patients with liver disease.

## Adverse Effects

The main adverse effect is hypoglycemia.

## Contraindications

Contraindications include hypersensitivity to sulfa-based medications as well as sensitivity to glyburide itself. Other contraindications include severe renal or hepatic impairment. Caution is necessary with pregnancy, lactation, pituitary, or thyroid disorders.

## Nursing Implications

In the event of high stress such as infections, surgery, or trauma, a change to insulin therapy may be warranted. In the event of severe hypoglycemia, it is necessary to administer IV glucose.

### Preventing Interactions

Drugs may interact with glyburide, increasing or decreasing its effects (Box 41.9). Some herbs may increase its effects (see

Box 41.3). It is extremely important that the patient inform the health care provider of all newly prescribed medications so that the patient and caregivers can be prepared to monitor for side effects related to other drugs.

**BOX 41.9** **Drug Interactions: Glyburide**

**Drugs That Increase the Effects of Glyburide**
- Acarbose, miglitol, metformin, pioglitazone, and rosiglitazone
  *Increase risk of hypoglycemia*
- Alcohol (acute ingestion)
  *Causes hypoglycemia*
- Cimetidine
  *May inhibit metabolism of sulfonylureas, thereby increasing and prolonging hypoglycemic effect*
- Insulin
  *May cause hypoglycemia*

**Drugs That Decrease the Effects of Glyburide**
- Alcohol (acute ingestion)
  *Accelerates metabolism of sulfonylureas, shortening their half-lives; may produce a flushing response*
- Beta-adrenergic blocking agents
  *Decrease hypoglycemic effects, possibly by decreasing release of insulin in the pancreas*
- Corticosteroids, diuretics, epinephrine, estrogens, and oral contraceptives
  *Have hyperglycemic effects*
- Glucagon
  *Raises blood glucose levels*
- Nicotinic acid (large doses)
  *Has hyperglycemic effect*
- Phenytoin
  *Inhibits insulin secretion and has hyperglycemic effects*
- Rifampin
  *Increases the rate of metabolism of sulfonylureas by inducing liver metabolizing enzymes*
- Thyroid preparations
  *Antagonize hypoglycemic effects of oral antidiabetic drugs*

### Administering the Medication

Patients should take glyburide before breakfast in the morning or in divided doses before meals if the patient experiences gastric distress.

### Patient Teaching

Box 41.7 presents general patient teaching guidelines for the antidiabetic drugs. Box 41.10 presents patient teaching guidelines for the oral antidiabetic drugs, including glyburide.

## Other Drugs in the Class

Other drugs in this class include glimepiride and glipizide, which resemble glyburide in terms of therapeutic and adverse effects. Tolazamide and tolbutamide are older oral hypoglycemic medications that have been replaced by glyburide, glimepiride, and glipizide.

Glimepiride (Amaryl) stimulates the release of insulin from functioning beta cells in the pancreas and improves binding between insulin and the insulin receptors. People may take this sulfonylurea in combination with metformin or insulin for better control of glucose with diet and exercise. A reduced dosage is necessary in elderly patients as well as in patients who are malnourished or have renal or hepatic impairment. Use of glimepiride entails avoidance of alcohol.

Glipizide (Glucotrol, Glucotrol XL, GlipiZIDE XL) also stimulates the release of insulin from functioning beta cells in the pancreas and improves binding between insulin and the insulin receptors; in addition, it may increase the number of insulin receptors. People should take the drug 30 minutes before breakfast to provide the greatest reduction in blood glucose. When beginning therapy with elderly patients, it is necessary to start with 2.5 mg/day orally, monitor them for 24 hours, and then increase the dose after several days as needed. Glipizide is associated with an increased risk of cardiovascular mortality and hematologic adverse effects such as leukopenia, thrombocytopenia, and anemia. As with the previous second-generation sulfonylureas, dosage reduction is warranted with impaired liver function.

Tolazamide and tolbutamide are both administered as adjuncts to diet in managing mild to moderate type 2 diabetes mellitus. Patients who have glucose-6-phosphate dehydrogenase deficiency are at increased risk for sulfonylurea-induced hemolytic anemia. Each drug stimulates the release of insulin from pancreatic beta cells and reduces glucose output from the liver.

## BIGUANIDE

The only drug available in this class is the prototype **metformin** (Fortamet, Glucophage, Glucophage XR, Glumetza, Riomet). Experts prefer to call it an antihyperglycemic rather than a hypoglycemic because it does not cause hypoglycemia, even in large doses, when used alone.

## Pharmacokinetics

Absorption of metformin occurs in the small intestine, and it circulates without binding to plasma proteins. The drug has a serum half-life of 1.3 to 4.5 hours. It is not metabolized in the liver and is excreted unchanged in the urine.

---

**BOX 41.10**  *Patient Teaching Guidelines for Oral or Injectable Antidiabetic Drugs*

- Take oral drugs as directed. Recommendations usually include the following:
  - Take glipizide or glyburide (DiaBeta) approximately 30 minutes before meals; take glimepiride with breakfast or the first main meal. Take Glucotrol XL with breakfast.
  - Take acarbose or miglitol (Glyset) with the first bite of each main meal. The drugs need to be in the gastrointestinal tract with food because they act by decreasing absorption of sugar in the food. Starting with a small dose and increasing it gradually helps to prevent bloating, "gas pains," and diarrhea.
  - Take metformin (Glucophage) with meals to decrease stomach upset.
    - Take Glucophage XR with the evening meal.
    - If a diagnostic test is ordered requiring a contrast media with iodine, stop metformin 48 hours before the test, and do not begin taking it again until 48 hours after the test.
  - Take repaglinide (Prandin) or nateglinide (Starlix) about 15 to 30 minutes before meals (two, three, or four times daily). Doses may vary from 0.5 to 4.0 mg, depending on fasting blood glucose levels. Dosage

changes should be at least 1 week apart. If you skip a meal, you should skip that dose of repaglinide or nateglinide; if you eat an extra meal, you should take an extra dose.
  - Take pioglitazone (Actos), rosiglitazone (Avandia), and sitagliptin (Januvia) without regard to meals. If you take rosiglitazone or pioglitazone, report shortness of breath, chest pain, swelling, and fatigue.
- If you take glimepiride, glipizide, glyburide, repaglinide, or nateglinide alone or in combination with other antidiabetic drugs, be prepared to handle hypoglycemic reactions (as with insulin; see Box 41.7). Acarbose, miglitol, metformin, pioglitazone, and rosiglitazone do not cause hypoglycemia when taken alone. Do not skip meals and snacks. This increases the risk of hypoglycemic reactions.
- If you exercise vigorously, you may need to decrease your dose of antidiabetic drug or eat more. Ask for specific instructions related to the type and frequency of the exercise. Follow the recommended diet and exercise program as ordered by the health care provider.
- Do not stop taking your diabetic medications without consulting your health care provider.

*concious pt: feed/inject 15 grams*
*unconscious pt: IV/IM glucagon  D25 D50*

# Action

Metformin reduces the production of glucose by the liver. It also decreases the intestinal absorption of glucose to increase insulin sensitivity. This action increases the uptake of glucose, thus enhancing its utilization to produce energy.

# Use

People may take metformin alone or in combination with insulin or other oral agents. Prescribers widely order it as the initial drug in newly diagnosed type 2 diabetes, mainly because it does not cause the weight gain associated with most other oral agents. Authorities consider metformin to be weight neutral and ideal for overweight people with type 2 diabetes, who have been known to lose weight on this medication, further improving insulin sensitivity. Table 41.5 presents dosage information about metformin.

## Use in Children

The most common dosage administered to provide a clinical response in children with type 2 diabetes is 1500 to 2000 mg/day. The starting dose should be lower, with gradual increases every 1 to 2 weeks. The gradual increase in dose will decrease the gastrointestinal symptoms that occur with metformin administration.

## Use in Older Adults

Dosage titration to the maximum amount recommended for younger adults is not appropriate for older adults. Contraindications to use of metformin in older adults often include cardiovascular disorders that increase risks of fluid retention and congestive heart failure. A **BLACK BOX WARNING ◆** for metformin states that patients 80 years of age or older should not take the drug because of the risk of lactic acidosis.

## Use in Patients With Renal Impairment

With metformin, periodic tests of renal function are necessary for determining dosages. Assessment of renal function should occur before starting the drug and at least annually during long-term therapy. It is essential to discontinue the metformin if renal impairment occurs or if serum lactate increases. As with other oral hypoglycemic drugs, patients taking this drug should continue their diet, exercise, and blood glucose testing regimens.

Parenteral radiographic contrast media containing iodine (e.g., Cholografin, Hypaque) may cause renal failure and have been associated with lactic acidosis in patients receiving metformin. It is important to discontinue metformin at least 48 hours before diagnostic tests are performed with these materials and resume the drug at least 48 hours after the tests are done and tests indicate that renal function is normal.

## Use in Patients With Hepatic Impairment

Metformin is not recommended for use in patients with clinical or laboratory evidence of hepatic impairment because risks of lactic acidosis may be increased.

# Adverse Effects

The primary adverse effect of metformin is lactic acidosis. Other adverse effects include hypersensitivity reactions, dizziness, nausea, vomiting, abdominal discomfort or cramping, malabsorption of amino acids, and diarrhea.

# Contraindications

Contraindications to metformin include diabetes complicated by fever, severe infections, severe trauma, major surgery, acidosis, or pregnancy (insulin is indicated in these conditions). Patients with serious hepatic or renal impairment, cardiac or respiratory insufficiency, hypoxia, or a history of lactic acidosis should not take the drug because these conditions may increase production of lactate and the risk of potentially fatal lactic acidosis (see note above about **BLACK BOX WARNING ◆**).

# Nursing Implications

## Preventing Interactions

Some drugs increase the effects of metformin (Box 41.11). Use with sulfonylureas, furosemide, cationic drugs such as digoxin, and vancomycin increases the risk of hypoglycemia. Box 41.3 lists herbs that interact with metformin.

## TABLE 41.5

## DRUGS AT A GLANCE: Metformin (Biguanide)

| Drug | Pregnancy Category | Routes and Dosage Ranges | |
|---|---|---|---|
| | | **Adults** | **Children** |
| **Metformin** (Fortamet, Glucophage, Glucophage XR, Glumetza, Riomet, Metformin ER; 🍁 ACT MetFORMIN, APO-MetFORMIN ER, Glumetza, Glycon, JAMP-MetFORMIN) | B | 500 mg bid or 850 mg once daily PO; max dosage: 2550 mg/d in divided doses<br>Fortamet: 500–1000 mg once daily; dosage may be increased by 500 mg at 1–2 wk; maximum daily dose, 2000 mg/d<br>Glucophage XR: 500 mg once daily; increase by 500 mg weekly; maximum daily dose, 2000 mg/d<br>Glumetza: 1000 mg once daily; increase by 500 mg weekly; maximum daily dose, 2000 mg/d | 10 y, 500 mg bid PO with meals; max dosage, 2000 mg/d in divided doses<br>17 y and older, see adult dose |

**BOX 41.11** **Drug Interactions: Metformin**

**Drugs That Decrease the Effects of Metformin**
- Corticosteroids (systemic and inhaled)
  *Result in hyperglycemia*
- Luteinizing hormone, somatotropin, and thiazide diuretics
  *Increase risk of hyperglycemia*

**Drugs That Increase the Effects of Metformin**
- Alcohol
  *Increases risk of hypoglycemia and lactic acidosis*
- Cephalexin, cimetidine, dalfampridine, and glycopyrrolate
  *Interferes with metabolism and increases blood levels*
- Corticosteroids (oral and inhaled)
  *May suppress the hypothalamic–pituitary–adrenal axis, leading to adrenal crisis, leading to hypoglycemia*
- Furosemide
  *Increases blood levels*
- Pegvisomant
  *Increases risk of hypoglycemia*
- Sulfonylurea hypoglycemic agents
  *Increases risk of hypoglycemia*

### Administering the Medication

The nurse should ensure that renal function is assessed before starting metformin and at least annually during long-term therapy. Patients should take metformin with meals. They should swallow the extended-release formulation whole and take it with the evening meal. They should discontinue the drug immediately if they are diagnosed with a myocardial infarction.

### Assessing for Therapeutic Effects

The nurse assesses fasting, preprandial, and postprandial blood glucose for normal or near-normal levels. Also, the nurse assesses for improvement in hemoglobin A1C levels.

### Assessing for Adverse Effects

The nurse assesses the skin for eczema, pruritus, erythema, and urticaria. All of these symptoms are indicative of a hypersensitivity reaction. It is also necessary to assess the GI response to the medication. In addition, the nurse assesses for abdominal pain, nausea, vomiting, and diarrhea. It is essential to check the liver function to determine the onset of lactic acidosis. Blood lactate levels are above 5 mmol/L, and blood pH is below 7.35. Symptoms and signs of lactic acidosis may include drowsiness, malaise, respiratory distress, bradycardia, and hypotension.

### Patient Teaching

Box 41.7 presents general patient teaching guidelines for the antidiabetic drugs. Box 41.10 presents patient teaching guidelines for the oral antidiabetic drugs.

## ALPHA-GLUCOSIDASE INHIBITORS

Alpha-glucosidase inhibitors inhibit alpha-glucosidase enzymes (e.g., sucrase, maltase, amylase) in the GI tract, thereby delaying digestion of complex carbohydrates into glucose and other simple sugars. **Acarbose** (Precose), the prototype alpha-glucosidase inhibitor, is known best for improving glycosylated hemoglobin levels. The drug is obtained through the fermentation process of microorganisms. Because acarbose does not enhance insulin, it works best when given with a sulfonylurea to control blood glucose levels.

## Pharmacokinetics

Acarbose has a rapid onset of action and peaks in 1 hour. The drug is metabolized by the digestive enzymes and intestinal bacteria in the GI tract. It is minimally distributed and excreted in the urine and feces.

## Action and Use

Acarbose works to delay the digestion of carbohydrates to diminish the increase in blood glucose after meals.

It may be necessary to combine acarbose with insulin or an oral agent, usually a sulfonylurea. Low initial doses and gradual increases decrease GI upset (e.g., bloating, diarrhea) and promote patient adherence. Patients taking acarbose should continue their diet, exercise, and blood glucose testing routines. Acarbose does not alter insulin secretion or cause hypoglycemia. Table 41.6 presents dosage information for acarbose and other alpha-glucosidase inhibitors.

### Use in Older Adults

Some older adults have other complex diseases such as congestive heart failure, for which they may take digoxin. Acarbose can decrease digoxin levels, and patients who take both drugs need close monitoring. In addition, aging adults may have fat loss, resulting in weight reduction. In adults who weigh less than 60 kg, it is necessary to decrease the maximum dosage.

### Use in Patients With Renal Impairment

Alpha-glucosidase inhibitors, which are excreted by the kidneys, accumulate in patients with renal impairment. However, dosage reduction is not helpful because the drugs act locally, within the GI tract.

## Adverse Effects

There are no serious adverse effects of acarbose. However, acarbose can cause gastric upset because the drug is metabolized in the GI tract. It also has the potential to produce leukopenia, thrombocytopenia, and anemia.

## Contraindications

Contraindications to acarbose include hypersensitivity, DKA, hepatic cirrhosis, inflammatory or malabsorptive intestinal disorders, and severe renal impairment.

## Nursing Implications

### Preventing Interactions

As mentioned previously, acarbose can decrease digoxin levels, and thus, patients taking digoxin require close monitoring.

**TABLE 41.6**

**DRUGS AT A GLANCE: Alpha-Glucosidase Inhibitors**

| Drug | Pregnancy Category | Routes and Dosage Ranges | |
|---|---|---|---|
| | | **Adults** | **Children** |
| Ⓟ **Acarbose** (Precose; ✿ Glucobay) | B | Monotherapy: initially 25 mg PO three times per day with first bite of each meal; may start with 25 mg/d and gradually increase if gastrointestinal (GI) side effects are a problem<br>Patients weighing 60 kg or less, max dosage 50–100 mg three times per day PO<br>Patients weighing more than 60 kg, max dosage 100 mg three times per day PO | Not recommended for use in children |
| Miglitol (Glyset) | B | Monotherapy: initial dose 25 mg PO three times per day at the first bite of each meal; may start at 25 mg PO daily if severe GI effects are seen<br>Maintenance: 100 mg PO three times per day | Safety and efficacy not established |

Certain drugs may decrease the effects of acarbose (Box 41.12). The herbs that interact with acarbose are the same as those that may affect other antidiabetic agents (see Box 41.3).

### Administering the Medication

People should take acarbose at the beginning of each meal so that it is present in the GI tract with food and able to delay digestion of carbohydrates.

### Assessing for Therapeutic and Adverse Effects

After acarbose administration, the increase in blood glucose levels after a meal is smaller. The nurse assesses the patient's response to the medication—diminished blood glucose levels without signs and symptoms of hypoglycemia.

The nurse also assesses for GI effects such as diarrhea, abdominal pain, and flatulence. He or she should assess the complete blood (cell) count for leukopenia, thrombocytopenia, and anemia.

### Patient Teaching

Box 41.7 presents general patient teaching guidelines for the antidiabetic drugs. Box 41.10 presents patient teaching guidelines for the oral antidiabetic drugs.

**BOX 41.12** 🔵 *Drug Interactions: Acarbose*

**Drugs That Decrease the Effects of Acarbose**
- Corticosteroids (systemic and inhaled)
  *Result in hyperglycemia*
- Luteinizing hormone, somatotropin, and thiazide diuretics
  *Increase risk of hyperglycemia*

**Drugs That Increase the Effects of Acarbose**
- Corticosteroids (inhaled)
  *May suppress the hypothalamic–pituitary–adrenal axis, leading to adrenal crisis, leading to hypoglycemia*
- Pegvisomant
  *Increased risk of hypoglycemia*

### Other Drugs in the Class

Miglitol (Glyset) has the same action, use, adverse effects, and contraindications as acarbose.

## THIAZOLIDINEDIONES

Thiazolidinediones are sometimes called "glitazones" and are also referred to as insulin sensitizers. These drugs decrease insulin resistance, a major factor in the pathophysiology of type 2 diabetes. Ⓟ **Rosiglitazone maleate** (Avandia) is the prototype for the thiazolidinediones.

### Pharmacokinetics

Rosiglitazone has a delayed onset of action and takes up to 12 weeks to reach its maximum effects. It is 99.8% protein bound primarily by albumin. The medication is metabolized in the liver by cytochrome P450 (CYP) 2C8, and a minor portion is metabolized by CYP2C9. The serum half-life is 3 to 4 hours. The peak plasma level is reached in 1 hour, with delayed absorption when taken with food. Sixty-four percent of the medication is excreted in the urine and 23% in the feces.

### Action

Rosiglitazone stimulates receptors on muscle, fat, and liver cells, thus increasing or restoring the effectiveness of circulating insulin. This change results in increased uptake of glucose by peripheral tissues and decreased production of glucose by the liver. In addition, this drug decreases insulin resistance, a major factor in the pathophysiology of type 2 diabetes.

### Use

Patients may take rosiglitazone as monotherapy with diet and exercise or in combination with insulin, metformin, a sulfonylurea, an amylin analog (pramlintide), or glucagon-like peptide-1 receptor agonist (exenatide). Table 41.7 presents dosage information for rosiglitazone.

**TABLE 41.7**

**DRUGS AT A GLANCE: Thiazolidinediones**

| Drug | Pregnancy Category | Routes and Dosage Ranges | |
|---|---|---|---|
| | | **Adults** | **Children** |
| **Rosiglitazone** (Avandia; ❦ Avandia) | C | 4 mg as a single oral dose or divided into two doses; if adequate response not seen in 8–12 wk, may be increased to 8 mg PO daily | Not recommended |
| Pioglitazone (Actos; ❦ ACCEL Pioglitazone, ACH-Pioglitazone, ACT Pioglitazone, JAMP-Pioglitazone) | C | PO 15–30 mg once daily; max dosage 45 mg<br>Combination therapy with sulfonylurea or metformin: 15–30 mg daily PO added to the established dose of the other agent; if hypoglycemia occurs, reduce the dose of the other agent<br>Combination therapy with insulin: decrease insulin does by 10%–25%; individualize based on glycemic response | Safety and efficacy not established |

### Use in Patients With Hepatic Impairment

Rosiglitazone has been associated with hepatotoxicity and requires monitoring of liver enzymes. Liver function tests (e.g., serum aminotransferase enzymes) should be checked before starting therapy and periodically thereafter. After initiation of thiazolidinedione therapy, it is important to measure liver enzymes every 2 months for 1 year and then periodically.

## Adverse Effects

GI adverse effects of thiazolidinedione include liver injury and diarrhea. The most common respiratory adverse effects are sinusitis, upper respiratory infection, rhinitis, and dyspnea. Congestive heart failure and myocardial infarction are the most severe adverse effects.

## Contraindications

Contraindications to rosiglitazone use include active liver disease or a serum alanine aminotransferase value more than 2.5 times the upper limit of normal, as well as hypersensitivity to the drug.

Caution is necessary when patients are at risk for congestive heart failure. Authorities do not recommend rosiglitazone for patients who have symptomatic congestive heart failure. Rosiglitazone increases plasma volume and may cause fluid retention. In one study, heart failure developed in 4.5% of rosiglitazone users within 10 months and in 12.4% of users within 36 months. In people who did not take a thiazolidinedione, 2.6% developed heart failure within 10 months and 8.4% within 36 months. The FDA has issued a **BLACK BOX WARNING** ◆ alerting health care professionals about the risk of congestive heart failure in patients using pioglitazone and rosiglitazone. Assess the patient for excessive weight gain, dyspnea, and edema. A meta-analysis of several studies and clinical trials have raised concerns about increased risk of myocardial ischemic events, including angina, myocardial infarction (heart attack), and heart-related deaths, with rosiglitazone. It is not recommended for patients with symptomatic heart failure.

## Nursing Implications

### Preventing Interactions

Rosiglitazone serum levels may increase if the antidiabetic drug is taken with gemfibrozil, so it is essential to monitor the patient closely and make dosage adjustments if necessary. Box 41.3 lists the herbs that interact with rosiglitazone.

### Administering the Medication

It is important to take rosiglitazone with meals. A patient may take a missed dose at the next meal. (However, if the patient skips a dose for an entire day, he or she should not take a double dose.)

### Assessing for Therapeutic Effects

The nurse assesses fasting, preprandial, and postprandial blood glucose for normal or near-normal levels. Also, the nurse assesses for improvement in hemoglobin A1C levels.

### Assessing for Adverse Effects

The nurse assesses the patient's cardiopulmonary status by auscultating the lungs for crackles or gurgles and auscultating the heart for an audible $S_3$ that indicates heart failure. Also, it is necessary to assess for signs of hepatic insufficiency and check liver enzymes. In addition, it is essential to assess for upper respiratory congestion.

### Patient Teaching

The nurse teaches patients to report any signs or symptoms of congestive heart failure (e.g., dyspnea, fatigue, peripheral edema) to appropriate health care personnel. Box 41.7 presents general patient teaching guidelines for the antidiabetic drugs. Box 41.10 presents patient teaching guidelines for the oral antidiabetic drugs.

## Other Drugs in the Class

Pioglitazone (Actos) acts by resensitizing the tissues to insulin. This drug stimulates the insulin receptor sites, lowering blood glucose levels to improve the action of insulin. As with rosiglitazone, it has a risk of heart failure in patients. People may take pioglitazone without regard to meals. They may take a missed dose at the next scheduled time. In 2016, the FDA issued a safety announcement regarding pioglitazone. This drug may be linked to an increased risk of bladder cancer. Patients treated with pioglitazone and diagnosed with bladder cancer should be changed to a different medication to treat type 2 diabetes.

# MEGLITINIDES

Meglitinides are nonsulfonylureas that lower blood sugar by stimulating pancreatic secretion of insulin. 🄳**Repaglinide** (Prandin) is the prototype meglitinide drug. The ability of repaglinide to work effectively depends on the existence of functioning beta cells left in the pancreas. Administration in combination with metformin or insulin results in a greater reduction in a patient's hemoglobin A1C than when either medication is administered alone.

## Pharmacokinetics

Absorption of repaglinide from the GI tract is good, and peak plasma level occurs within 1 hour. The drug has a plasma half-life of 1 to 1.5 hours and is highly bound (greater than 98%) to plasma proteins. Metabolism occurs in the liver. Excretion of metabolites is in urine and feces. Metabolism and removal of repaglinide from the bloodstream occurs within 3 to 4 hours after a dose. This decreases the workload of pancreatic beta cells (i.e., decreases duration of beta-cell stimulation), allows serum insulin levels to return to normal before the next meal, and decreases risks of hypoglycemic episodes.

## Action

Repaglinide works by closing potassium channels in pancreatic beta cells, which causes calcium channels to open and release insulin. The ability to lower blood glucose is dependent on the amount of functioning beta cells in the pancreas.

## Use

Repaglinide can be used as monotherapy with diet and exercise or in combination with metformin or thiazolidinediones.

Dosage is flexible, depending on food intake, but patients should eat within a few minutes after taking a dose to avoid hypoglycemia. Table 41.8 presents dosage information for the meglitinides, including repaglinide.

### Use in Patients With Renal Impairment

Assessment of renal function should occur before initiation of treatment with repaglinide and periodically during therapy. The drug requires a decrease in initial dosage in patients with renal disease as well as for those with moderate to severe renal dysfunction. It is necessary to make incremental dosage changes cautiously in patients with renal impairment or renal failure requiring hemodialysis.

### Use in Patients With Hepatic Impairment

Cautious use of repaglinide is warranted in patients with moderate to severe hepatic impairment. It is necessary to make incremental dosage changes very slowly, because serum drug levels are higher for a long period.

## Adverse Effects

Hypoglycemia is the most common adverse effect of repaglinide. Other adverse effects are upper respiratory congestion and gastric upset.

## Contraindications

Repaglinide is contraindicated in patients with hypersensitivity. It is also contraindicated in patients with type 1 diabetes or patients with DKA.

## Nursing Implications

### Preventing Interactions

The risk of severe hypoglycemia is associated with the use of repaglinide with gemfibrozil and itraconazole. Therefore, such drug combinations should be avoided (Box 41.13).

### Administering the Medication

Patients should take repaglinide just before or up to 30 minutes before meals. If a meal is skipped, the drug dose should be skipped; if a meal is added, a drug dose should be added.

| | | TABLE 41.8 | | |
|---|---|---|---|---|
| | | **DRUGS AT A GLANCE: Meglitinides** | | |
| **Drug** | **Pregnancy Category** | **Routes and Dosage Ranges** | | |
| | | **Adults** | | **Children** |
| 🄳**Repaglinide** (Prandin; ✳ ACT Repaglinide, APO-Repaglinide, Auro-Repaglinide) | C | 0.5–4 mg PO taken three or four times a day 15–30 min before meals; max dosage 16 mg/d PO; wait 1 wk before making dose adjustment<br>Severe renal impairment: starting dose 0.5 mg PO | | Not recommended |
| Nateglinide (Starlix) | C | 120 mg PO three times daily, 1–30 min before meals; omit dose if skipped a meal<br>60 mg PO three times per day may be tried if patient is near HbA1C goal | | Safety and efficacy not established |

## BOX 41.13   *Drug Interactions: Repaglinide*

### Drugs That Increase the Effects of Repaglinide

- Cimetidine, erythromycin, ketoconazole, and miconazole

  *Increase serum concentrations of repaglinide, leading to hypoglycemia*

- Corticosteroids (oral or inhaled)

  *May suppress the hypothalamic–pituitary–adrenal axis, leading to adrenal crisis, leading to hypoglycemia*

- Nonsteroidal anti-inflammatory drugs and other agents that are highly bound to plasma proteins

  *May displace drug from binding sites, increasing blood levels*

- Pegvisomant

  *Increases the risk of hypoglycemia*

- Sulfonamides

  *May inhibit hepatic metabolism, increasing blood levels*

### Drugs That Decrease the Effects of Repaglinide

- Adrenergics, corticosteroids, estrogens, niacin, oral contraceptives, and thiazide diuretics

  *Increase the risk of hyperglycemia*

- Corticosteroids (systemic and inhaled)

  *Diminish the effect of acarbose, resulting in hyperglycemia*

- Luteinizing hormone, somatotropin, and thiazide diuretics

  *Increase the risk of hyperglycemia*

- Carbamazepine and rifampin

  *Induce drug-metabolizing enzymes in the liver, which leads to faster inactivation*

### Assessing for Adverse and Therapeutic Effects

The nurse assesses fasting, preprandial, and postprandial blood glucose for normal or near-normal levels. It is also important to assess for improvement in hemoglobin A1C levels.

The nurse assesses for dizziness, weakness, and hunger. In addition, he or she assesses for gastric upset and respiratory congestion.

### Patient Teaching

When instructing patients who have been prescribed meglitinides, it is necessary to inform them that if they skip a meal, then they should also skip the dose. If they add a meal, then they need to take a dose before the meal. Box 41.7 presents general patient teaching guidelines for the antidiabetic drugs. Box 41.10 presents patient teaching guidelines for the oral antidiabetic drugs, including repaglinide. The nurse teaches patients taking repaglinide to know and recognize the signs and symptoms of hypoglycemia and how to treat the condition immediately.

## Other Drugs in the Class

Nateglinide (Starlix) is a nonsulfonylurea, known as a meglitinide analog, that blocks the ATP-dependent potassium channels to depolarize the membrane and facilitate calcium to reenter the calcium channels. The increase in intracellular calcium then stimulates the release of insulin from pancreatic beta cells. The drug is rapidly absorbed, reaching a peak of action in 1 hour. It is 98% protein bound to albumin and metabolized in liver by hydroxylation. The drug then undergoes glucuronide conjugation by CYP2C9 and CYP3A4. When combined with metformin or insulin, Rapaglinide is more effective than Nateglinide in lowering hemoglobin A1C.

## NCLEX   Success

8. The nurse is assessing a patient who has just begun taking glyburide. Which of the following is a therapeutic outcome for this patient? (Select all that apply.)

   A. a glycosylated hemoglobin (hemoglobin A1C) of 10%
   B. a decrease in polyuria
   C. a decrease in polyphagia
   D. a fasting blood glucose of 108 mg/dL

9. A patient with type 2 diabetes calls the nurse to report the following symptoms: blood glucose of 378 mg/dL, excessive urination, and feelings of becoming drowsier. To determine a possible diagnosis, which of the following questions is most important?

   A. "Has there been any change in diet?"
   B. "Has there been any fever?"
   C. "Have there been any ketones in the urine?"
   D. "Have you increased the amount of fluid intake?"

10. A patient with type 2 diabetes is scheduled to have a cardiac catheterization in 1 week, and the nurse makes a preprocedure phone call. The nurse instructs the patient to stop taking which medication 2 days before the procedure?

    A. sitagliptin
    B. insulin
    C. glyburide
    D. metformin

11. A man with type 2 diabetes mellitus has a blood glucose of more than 500 mg/dL. He is complaining of excessive urination, extreme thirst, and weakness, and he also notes recent weight loss. The nurse would expect to find which diagnosis in his chart?

    A. hypoglycemia
    B. diabetic ketoacidosis
    C. hyperglycemic hyperosmolar nonketotic syndrome
    D. hypothyroidism

12. The nurse is monitoring a patient newly diagnosed with type 2 diabetes mellitus taking repaglinide for complications. Which of the following, if exhibited by the patient, would indicate hypoglycemia and require immediate treatment?

    A. polyuria
    B. diaphoresis
    C. decreased heart rate
    D. hypertension

# DIPEPTIDYL PEPTIDASE 4 INHIBITORS

GLP-1 has been known for some time to have a hypoglycemic action via its ability to stimulate insulin secretion. Recent advances have overcome the problems associated with short half-life and inactivation of the incretin hormone. The DPP-4 enzyme inhibitor Ⓟ **sitagliptin** (Januvia) is a new medication that solves these problems.

## Pharmacokinetics

Sitagliptin is rapidly absorbed and distributed with 3% protein bound. The drug is metabolized minimally by CYP3A4 and CYP2C8, resulting in a 12-hour circulating half-life for GLP-1. The peak of action is 1 to 4 hours. Eighty-seven percent of the medication is excreted in the urine with 79% unchanged. Approximately 13% is excreted in the feces.

## Action

Sitagliptin minimizes the rate of inactivation of the incretin hormones to increase hormone levels and prolong their activity. Incretin hormones stimulate insulin release in response to a meal to normalize glucose levels. This action increases and lengthens the release of insulin and decreases hepatic glucose production to promote glycemic control.

## Use

Patients with type 2 diabetes mellitus take sitagliptin in addition to following an exercise and diet regimen. They may also take it in combination with metformin and/or thiazolidinediones. Table 41.9 presents dosage information for sitagliptin and other DPP-4 enzyme inhibitors.

### Use in Patients With Renal Impairment

Caution is warranted in renal insufficiency because sitagliptin is excreted by the kidneys. Patients with an elevated creatinine clearance require decreased dosages initially. Dosage adjustments are also necessary in the earlier stages of chronic kidney diseases.

## Adverse Effects

Common adverse effects of sitagliptin are upper respiratory tract infection, stuffy or runny nose, sore throat, and headache.

## Contraindications

Contraindications to sitagliptin use include type 1 diabetes mellitus, insulin use, or the common production of ketones in the urine. Another contraindication is end-stage renal disease. Strict avoidance of other medications known to cause hypoglycemia, such as sulfonylureas, is warranted.

The FDA has identified a risk of heart failure associated with DPP-4 inhibitors. This risk is more pronounced in patients with kidney and heart disease.

## Nursing Implications

### Administering the Medication

Patients should take sitagliptin once daily with or without food. If they forget to take a dose, they should take it as soon as possible. However, if a dose is skipped, patients should take only one dose per day.

### Assessing for Therapeutic and Adverse Effects

The nurse assesses fasting, preprandial, and postprandial blood glucose for normal or near-normal levels. It is also important to

## TABLE 41.9

### DRUGS AT A GLANCE: Dipeptidyl Peptidase 4 (DPP-4) Inhibitors

| Drug | Pregnancy Category | Routes and Dosage Ranges | |
|------|--------------------|--------------------------|---|
| | | **Adults** | **Children** |
| Ⓟ **Sitagliptin** (Januvia; 🍁 Januvia) | B | 100 mg/d PO as monotherapy or combined with metformin, pioglitazone, rosiglitazone, or other oral drugs<br>Renal impairment: creatinine clearance of 30–50 mL/min, 50 mg/d PO; creatinine clearance <30 mL/min, 25 mg/d PO | Not recommended |
| Alogliptin (Nesina; 🍁 Nesina) | Adverse events were not observed in animal reproduction studies | 25 mg PO once daily | Not recommended |
| Linagliptin (Tradjenta; 🍁 Tradjenta) | B | 5 mg PO once daily | Safety and efficacy not established |
| Saxagliptin (Onglyza; 🍁 Onglyza) | B | 2.5–5 mg PO daily<br>Limit dose to 2.5 mg when used with a strong CYP3A4/5 inhibitor or with renal impairment | Safety and efficacy not established |

**BOX 41.14** *Patient Teaching Guidelines for the Newer Antidiabetic Drugs*

- Use correct technique for injecting amylin analogs and incretin mimetics:
  - Inject pramlintide (Symlin) subcutaneously into the abdomen or thighs before meals. Do not mix in same syringe with insulin. Insulin dosages may be reduced by 50% when taking pramlintide.
  - Inject exenatide (Byetta) subcutaneously into the abdomen, thigh, or upper arm within 60 minutes before morning and evening meal.
  - Rotate the injection site of pramlintide and do not give in the same site where insulin is administered.

assess for improvement in hemoglobin A1C levels. In addition, the nurse assesses the patient for signs and symptoms of upper respiratory infection.

> **! QSEN: Safety**
>
> In 2015, the FDA issued a warning that the DPP-4 inhibitors may cause joint pain that can be severe or cause disability. Patients should be instructed not to stop the medication and consult with the prescriber.

### Patient Teaching

Box 41.7 presents general patient teaching guidelines for the antidiabetic drugs. Box 41.14 gives some patient teaching guidelines for the newer antidiabetic drugs, including sitagliptin.

## Other Drugs in the Class

Alogliptin (Nesina), linagliptin (Tradjenta), and saxagliptin (Onglyza) inhibit DPP-4 to prolong the incretin levels. The incretin hormones and glucose-dependent insulinotropic polypeptide regulate the glucose homeostasis. The synthesis of insulin increases, allowing the release of insulin from beta cells. In addition, glucagon secretion from the alpha cells decreases. This decrease also reduces production of hepatic glucose. It is important to note that alogliptin and saxagliptin have the potential to increase the risk of heart failure when administered to patients with heart or kidney disease.

**NCLEX Success**

13. A patient with type 2 diabetes begins taking sitagliptin for the management of blood glucose levels. Which statement by the patient indicates an understanding of this medication?
    A. "I will take two doses in the morning if my blood sugar is high."
    B. "By taking this medication, I am able to eat more."
    C. "Now that I am taking this medication, I don't have to exercise anymore."
    D. "I will take this medicine once a day."

14. The nurse caring for a patient with diabetes mellitus has lipodystrophy of the abdomen. What should the nurse assess?
    A. Does the patient administer the injection at a 45-degree angle?
    B. Does the patient aspirate for blood prior to giving the injection?
    C. Does the patient pinch the skin appropriately?
    D. Does the patient rotate sites for giving each injection?

15. Based on the action of pramlintide, which of the following is a primary nursing intervention?
    A. Administer glucagon during the peak of action.
    B. Assess blood sugar at 2.4 hours after medication administration.
    C. Assess respiratory status for the onset of an upper respiratory infection.
    D. Provide a meal immediately after the administration of the subcutaneous injection.

## AMYLIN ANALOGS

Some people with type 1 or type 2 diabetes cannot achieve optimal glucose control with insulin therapy alone. **Pramlintide acetate** (SymlinPen 120, SymlinPen 60) is a newer drug used as an adjunctive treatment with mealtime insulin that is important in the regulation of glucose control during the postprandial period. A synthetic analog of amylin, pramlintide is a peptide hormone secreted with insulin by the beta cells of the pancreas.

## Pharmacokinetics

Pramlintide has a rapid onset of action, reaching its peak in 20 minutes, with a 3-hour duration of action. Sixty percent of the drug is protein bound. It is metabolized primarily in the renal system and excreted in the urine.

## Action

Pramlintide slows gastric emptying, which helps regulate the postprandial rise in blood glucose. The drug also suppresses postprandial glucagon secretion, thus helping maintain better blood glucose control. It also increases the sense of satiety, possibly reducing food intake and promoting weight loss.

## Use

Taken immediately before meals, pramlintide mimics the body's natural processes. Oral hypoglycemic drugs and insulin dosages are usually up to 50% lower as well, depending on the patient's response to the drug. Patients with type 2 disease may combine pramlintide and insulin therapy with metformin or sulfonylureas. Table 41.10 gives dosage information for pramlintide.

## Adverse Effects

Nausea, another frequent adverse effect of pramlintide, tends to decrease with time. Careful titration of the dosage to the

| | Pregnancy Category | Routes and Dosage Ranges | |
|---|---|---|---|
| **TABLE 41.10** | | | |
| **DRUGS AT A GLANCE: Amylin Analog (Pramlintide)** | | | |
| **Drug** | **Pregnancy Category** | **Routes and Dosage Ranges** | |
| | | **Adults** | **Children** |
| **Pramlintide** (Symlin, Symlin Pen; ❈ SymlinPen 60, SymlinPen 120) | C | Type 2 diabetes: initially 60 mcg sub-Q injection immediately prior to major meals. Dose can be increased to 120 mcg if needed<br>Type 1 diabetes: initially 15 mcg sub-Q injection immediately prior to major meals; titrate 15-mcg increments to maintenance dose of 30 or 60 mcg as tolerated | Not recommended |

therapeutic level may reduce it. A **◆ BLACK BOX WARNING ◆** alerts nurses to the danger of severe insulin-induced hypoglycemia with pramlintide therapy, especially in type 1 diabetes.

## Contraindications

The only contraindications to pramlintide are hypersensitivity and gastroparesis.

## Nursing Implications

### Preventing Interactions

Some drugs may increase the effects of pramlintide (Box 41.15). Pramlintide also can cause increased effects of gastric emptying if combined with anticholinergic drugs or drugs that slow gastric absorption of nutrients. It is essential to avoid pramlintide with such drugs.

### Administering the Medication

Subcutaneous injection of pramlintide before meals is necessary. The patient should not use pramlintide if a meal is skipped or if a dose is forgotten. It is necessary to inject pramlintide into a site (thigh or abdomen) that is at least 2 inches away from the insulin site injection. Opened vials of pramlintide may be stored in a refrigerator or at room temperature for up to 28 days.

It is essential not to mix pramlintide in the same injection with mealtime insulin. Patients with type 2 diabetes should take oral hypoglycemic drugs at least 1 hour before or 2 hours after injecting pramlintide.

### Assessing for Therapeutic and Adverse Effects

The nurse assesses fasting, preprandial, and postprandial blood glucose for normal or near-normal levels. It is also important to assess for improvement in the hemoglobin A1C levels.

**BOX 41.15**    *Drug Interactions: Pramlintide*

**Drugs That Increase the Effects of Pramlintide**
- Anticholinergics
  *May further slow gastrointestinal motility and intestinal absorption of drug*
- Alpha-glucosidase inhibitors
  *Increase risk of hypoglycemia*

In addition, the nurse teaches the signs and symptoms of hypoglycemia, as well as its treatment. This is the only serious adverse effect.

### Patient Teaching

Box 41.7 presents general patient teaching guidelines for the antidiabetic drugs. Box 41.14 gives some patient teaching guidelines for the newer antidiabetic drugs, including pramlintide.

## GLUCAGON-LIKE PEPTIDE-1 RECEPTOR AGONISTS (INCRETIN MIMETICS)

Before starting a patient with type 2 diabetes on insulin, the provider should consider a new option for treatment of diabetes. The glucagon-like peptide-1 receptor agonist is also known as the incretin mimetic **exenatide** (Bydureon, Byetta 10 MCG Pen, Byetta 5 MCG PEN), a synthetic GLP-1 analog; it is possible to improve glycemic control in patients with type 2 diabetes who are already taking an oral hypoglycemic medication but having difficulty in achieving glycemic control.

## Pharmacokinetics

Exenatide has a rapid onset, and the peak effect occurs in 2 hours. The drug is metabolized minimally and has proteolytic degradation following glomerular filtration. It remains in the body for 8 to 10 hours, which means that dosages must be 6 hours apart. It has a 2.4-hour half-life and is excreted in the urine. Exenatide also crosses the placenta; thus, this drug must be used cautiously in patients who are pregnant.

## Action

Exenatide acts as a natural helper hormone by stimulating the pancreas to secrete the right amount of insulin based on the food that was just eaten. This helps reduce the problem of high blood glucose after meals. The drug also halts gluconeogenesis by the liver, keeping it from making too much glucose after a meal. Exenatide slows gastric emptying, which serves to reduce the sudden rise of blood glucose after a meal, and it also quickly stimulates a feeling of satiety when eating. This fosters a sense of fullness, which causes the patient to eat less and potentially lose weight.

## Use

When oral medications, diet, and exercise together have not assisted in reaching the target hemoglobin A1C goal, prescribers may now order exenatide. The FDA has approved its use with oral medications such as sulfonylureas, metformin, and/or thiazolidinediones. Major advantages of exenatide over insulin are increased satiety and weight loss. Exenatide is also now being used as monotherapy in combination with diet and exercise for newly diagnosed adults with type 2 diabetes. Table 41.11 provides route and dosage information for exenatide and other incretin mimetics.

## Adverse Effects

Major adverse effects of exenatide are hypoglycemia, GI distress, and nausea. Many patients experience nausea at first, and health care providers should encourage them to continue the medication if at all possible because the nausea usually subsides and becomes a feeling of fullness. A rare but serious side effect is the development of acute pancreatitis.

## Contraindications

Contraindications to exenatide include a known hypersensitivity to the drug. Patients with liver disease or elevated liver enzymes should not receive it with HMG-CoA reductase inhibitors. Lactation is also a contraindication.

The FDA has issued a **BLACK BOX WARNING ◆** for exenatide; C-cell thyroid cancer has developed in studies of animals who were given the drug. Patients should routinely be monitored for thyroid nodules, and the drug is contraindicated in patients with a family history of endocrine neoplasia syndrome type 2.

### TABLE 41.11

### DRUGS AT A GLANCE: Glucagon-Like Peptide-1 Receptor Agonist (Incretin Mimetics)

| Drug | Pregnancy Category | Routes and Dosage Ranges | |
|---|---|---|---|
| | | Adults | Children |
| ℗ **Exenatide** (Bydureon, Bydureon BCise, Byetta 10 MCG Pen, Byetta 5; ❋ Bydureon, Byetta 10 MCG PEN, Byetta 5 MCG PEN) | C | 5 mcg by subcutaneous injection within 60 min before morning and evening meals or two main meals of day ~6 h apart; may be increased to 10 mcg twice a day after 1 mo of therapy if needed | Not recommended for use in children |
| Albiglutide | C | 30 mg by subcutaneous injection once weekly; may increase to 50 mg once weekly if inadequate glycemic response. Titration to 50 mg once weekly occurred at week 12 in a monotherapy trial and after a minimum of 4 wk in combination therapy trials | Not recommended for use in children |
| Dulaglutide (Trulicity; ❋ Trulicity) | C | 0.75 mg by subcutaneous injection once weekly; may increase to 1.5 mg once weekly if adequate glycemic response; maximum 1.5 mg once weekly | Not recommended for use in children |
| Liraglutide (Saxenda, Victoza; ❋ Saxenda, Victoza) | C | Initially 0.6 mg sub-Q once daily for 1 wk; then increase dose to 1.2–1.8 mg once daily to achieve glycemic control | >10 years old and Adolescents: 0.6 mg subcutaneous once daily for at least 1 wk; may increase by 0.6 mg/d increments at weekly intervals to achieve glycemic control. Maximum daily dose: 1.8 mg/d |
| Lixisenatide (Adlyxin, Adlyxin Starter Pack; ❋ Adlyxin) | Lixisenatide is not recommended for use in pregnancy | 10 mcg subcutaneous once daily for 14 d; on day 15, increase to 20 mcg one daily; maintenance dose: 20 mcg once daily | Not recommended for use in children |
| Semaglutide (Ozempic; ❋ Ozempic) | Semaglutide produced adverse fetal effects in animals. It should be stopped at least 2 mo before a planned pregnancy in both men and women. It should not be administered with pregnancy or lactation | 0.25 mg subcutaneous once weekly for 4 wk then increase to 0.5 mg once weekly for at least 4 wk. Maximum dose is 1 mg once weekly. Missed doses should be administered as soon as possible within 5 d. If >5 d has lapsed, skip the missed dose, and resume the next scheduled day | Not recommended for use in children |

## Nursing Implications

### Preventing Interactions

Like pramlintide, exenatide may reduce the absorption of concurrently administered oral medications due to slow gastric emptying (see Box 41.15).

### Administering the Medication

Patients administer exenatide subcutaneously twice a day within 60 minutes of the morning and evening meal (at least 6 or more hours apart). No dosage adjustment is necessary based on blood glucose levels or the amount of food a patient is able to consume. If patients forget a dose, they should not inject exenatide after a meal. Injection sites include the subcutaneous tissue of the upper arm or leg and the abdomen areas.

It is essential that exenatide be stored at all times in the original packaging in a refrigerator at 36°F to 46°F, protected from light, kept dry, and discarded once opened after 30 days.

### Assessing for Therapeutic Effects

The nurse assesses fasting, preprandial, and postprandial blood glucose for normal or near-normal levels. It is also important to assess for improvement in hemoglobin A1C levels.

### Assessing for Adverse Effects

It is important that patients and their caregivers recognize the signs and symptoms of hypoglycemia, a possible adverse effect of exenatide, and be prepared to treat hypoglycemia with fast-acting sugar or glucagon. If patients are unable to eat or plan to skip a meal, they should not take the drug. Patients taking exenatide should report any unusual abdominal discomfort to their health care providers because acute pancreatitis is a possible adverse effect of the medication.

### Patient Teaching

Box 41.7 presents general patient teaching guidelines for the antidiabetic drugs. Box 41.14 gives some patient teaching guidelines for the newer antidiabetic drugs.

### Other Drugs in the Class

Albiglutide (Tanzeum) and dulaglutide (Trulicity) are injected subcutaneously. They are agonists of human GLP-1 receptor to enhance glucose-dependent insulin secretion and slow gastric emptying. As with exenatide, all drugs in the class possess a

**BLACK BOX WARNING ◆**; C-cell thyroid cancer has developed in studies of animals who were given the drug. Routine monitoring for thyroid nodules is warranted, and a family history of endocrine neoplasia syndrome type 2 is a contraindication. Dulaglutide has an increased risk for the development of pancreatitis. Instruct the patient to notify the prescriber of persistent severe abdominal pain. Lixisenatide was approved by the FDA in 2016. It is for stand-alone therapy or in combination with insulin or other oral agents. It is contraindicated in patients who have an increased serum or urinary ketone level. Semaglutide should be discontinued at least 2 months prior to a planned pregnancy. Adverse events with congenital malformations were noted in animal reproduction studies.

## SODIUM GLUCOSE COTRANSPORTER 2 (SGLT2) INHIBITORS

In 2013, the FDA approved the first SGLT2 inhibitor. The prototype of this class is **canagliflozin** (Invokana). The drug inhibits renal SGLT2, thus blocking reabsorption of glucose in the kidney. In addition, it promotes the excretion of excess glucose in the urine. All the SGLT2 inhibitors provide renal protection by decreasing the protein loss and reducing the damage caused by hyperfiltration.

### Pharmacokinetics

Canagliflozin is 99% bound to albumin. The peak of action is 1 to 2 hours. For a 100-mg dose, the half-life of the drug is 10.6 hours, and for a 300-mg dose, it is 13.1 hours. The drug is metabolized by glucuronidation. The elimination of the drug is 30% in the urine and 52% in the feces.

### Action

The proximal renal tubule is the site where the majority of filtered glucose is reabsorbed, and in this tubule, canagliflozin inhibits SGLT2. This action provides the patient with type 2 diabetes greater excretion of glucose by the kidney.

### Use

Prescribers order canagliflozin in combination with other antidiabetic agents to promote improvement in glycemic control in patients with type 2 diabetes. Table 41.12 gives route and dosage information for canagliflozin and other SGLT2 inhibitors.

### TABLE 41.12

### DRUGS AT A GLANCE: Sodium Glucose Cotransporter 2 (SGLT2) Inhibitors

| Drug | Pregnancy Category | Routes and Dosage Ranges | |
|---|---|---|---|
| | | Adults | Children |
| Canagliflozin (Invokana; ☘ Invokana) | C | PO 100 mg once daily prior to the first meal of the day; may increase to 300 mg once daily to patients with eGFR >60 mL/m² | Not recommended for use in children |
| Dapagliflozin (Farxiga; ☘ Farxiga) | C | PO 5 mg once daily; may increase to 10 mg daily | Not recommended for use in children |
| Empagliflozin (Jardiance; ☘ Jardiance) | C | PO 10 mg once daily; may increase to 25 mg once daily | Not recommended for use in children |

### Use in Patients With Hepatic Impairment

Patients with severe hepatic impairment should not take canagliflozin.

### Use in Patients With Renal Impairment

In patients with an estimated glomerular filtration rate of 45 to 59 mL/min, the dosage of canagliflozin should not exceed 100 mg daily. It is not recommended that patients with an estimated glomerular filtration rate less than 45 mL/min take canagliflozin.

## Adverse Effects

The loss of body fluids leads to dehydration, hypotension, syncope, and dehydration. The metabolic adverse effects include increased low-density lipoprotein, hyperphosphatemia, hyperkalemia, hypermagnesemia, and increased creatinine. Because of increases in urine glucose, patients are prone to genital mycotic infections. Approximately 12% of women develop vulvovaginal candidiasis. Four percent of men develop inflammation of the glans penis; this includes balanitis/balanoposthitis, balanitis candida, and fungal genital infection. The administration of potassium-sparing diuretics with SGLT2 inhibitors causes hyperkalemia.

In addition, in June 2016, the FDA identified the risk of acute kidney injury with canagliflozin. Health Canada found evidence of a link between bone-related adverse effects, including demineralization of the bone and risk of bone fractures. In May 2017, an FDA alert was issued. Canagliflozin causes an increased risk of leg and foot amputations.

## Contraindications

Severe renal impairment and hypersensitivity reactions contraindicate the administration of canagliflozin.

## Nursing Implications

### Preventing Interactions

SGLT2 inhibitors combined with angiotensin-converting enzyme (ACE) inhibitors, angiotensin II receptor blockers (ARBs), and loop diuretics that have hypotensive effects will lead to symptoms of syncope, hypotension, and hyperkalemia. In addition, hyperkalemia will result with potassium-sparing diuretics. St. John's wort will decrease the serum concentration of the SGLT2 inhibitors, leading to hyperglycemia. Certain drugs may interact with canagliflozin (Box 41.16).

### Administering the Drug

Prior to administering SGLT2 inhibitors, patients should be well hydrated. The initial dose should be low. Patients should take the drugs with the first meal of the day. Box 41.17 gives patient teaching guidelines for canagliflozin and the other SGLT2 inhibitors.

### Assessing for Therapeutic Effects

The nurse assesses fasting, preprandial, and postprandial blood glucose for normal or near-normal levels. It is also important to assess for improvement in hemoglobin A1C levels.

### Assessing for Adverse Effects

It is imperative to assess the patient's hydration level and blood pressure for signs and symptoms of syncope and hypotension. The nurse should assess the potassium level and alert the prescriber of hyperkalemia. In the event of hyperkalemia, it is important to check the patient's cardiac rhythm for dysrhythmia.

## Other Drugs in the Class

Following the development of canagliflozin, dapagliflozin (Farxiga) and empagliflozin (Jardiance) became available. These two drugs have the same action, use, adverse effects, and contraindications as canagliflozin.

## COMBINATION DRUG THERAPY FOR TYPE 2 DIABETES

Combination drug therapy is an increasing trend in type 2 diabetes that is not controlled by diet, exercise, and single-drug therapy. Useful combinations include drugs with different mechanisms of action, and several rational combinations are currently available. Most studies have involved combinations of two drugs; some three-drug combinations are also being used. All combination therapy should be monitored with periodic measurements of fasting plasma glucose and glycosylated hemoglobin levels. If adequate glycemic control is not achieved, oral drugs may need to be discontinued and insulin therapy started. A list of some two-drug combinations are as follows:

- **Insulin plus a sulfonylurea.** Advantages include lower fasting blood glucose levels, decreased glycosylated hemoglobin levels, increased secretion of endogenous insulin, smaller daily doses of insulin, and no significant change in body

---

**BOX 41.16** **Drug Interactions: Canagliflozin**

**Drugs That Increase the Effects of Canagliflozin**
- Alpha-lipoic acid, androgens, insulin, or antidiabetic agents (oral or subcutaneous, monoamine oxidase inhibitors, pegvisomant, quinolone antibiotics, salicylates, selective serotonin reuptake inhibitors)
  *Increase hypoglycemic effects*

**Drugs That Decrease the Effects of Canagliflozin**
- Carbamazepine, efavirenz, fosphenytoin, phenobarbital, phenytoin, primidone, and ritonavir
  *Decreases the serum concentration of canagliflozin*

---

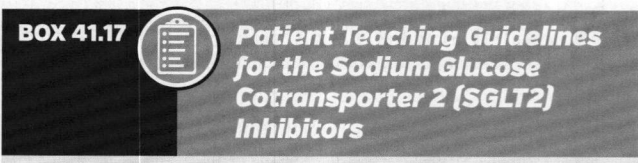

**BOX 41.17** **Patient Teaching Guidelines for the Sodium Glucose Cotransporter 2 (SGLT2) Inhibitors**

- Administer without regard to food with the first meal of the day.
- For patients with stable glycemic control, hemoglobin A1C should be monitored every 6 months.
- Maintain adequate hydration of 2000 to 3000 mL/day.
- Instruct on hypotension and syncope.
- Do not consume salt substitutes.

weight. The role of insulin analogs in combination therapy is not clear. One regimen, called BIDS, uses bedtime insulin, usually NPH, with a daytime sulfonylurea, usually glyburide.

- **Insulin plus a glitazone.** Thiazolidinediones increase the effectiveness of insulin, whether endogenous or exogenous.
- **Sulfonylurea plus acarbose or miglitol.** This combination is approved by the U.S. Food and Drug Administration (FDA) for patients who do not achieve adequate glycemic control with one of the drugs alone.
- **Sulfonylurea plus metformin.** Glimepiride is approved by the FDA for this combination.
- **Sulfonylurea plus a thiazolidinedione.** The sulfonylurea increases insulin, and the thiazolidinedione increases insulin effectiveness.
- **Metformin plus a meglitinide.** If one of the drugs alone does not produce adequate glycemic control, the other one may be added. Dosage of each drug should be titrated to the minimal dose required to achieve the desired effects.
- **Metformin plus a thiazolidinedione.** If metformin alone does not produce adequate glycemic control, a thiazolidinedione may be added. Pioglitazone is approved by the FDA for this combination.
- **Metformin or thiazolidinedione plus sitagliptin.** Sitagliptin may be added as adjunctive therapy with metformin or a thiazolidinedione to achieve desired glycemic control.
- **Metformin or sulfonylurea plus exenatide.** Exenatide may be added as adjunctive therapy with metformin or a sulfonylurea to achieve desired glycemic control.
- **Mealtime insulin plus metformin, thiazolidinedione, and/or sulfonylurea plus pramlintide.** Pramlintide may be

given with mealtime insulin in people with type 2 diabetes to achieve better postprandial glucose control.

- **Dapagliflozin and saxagliptin (Qtern) was approved by the FDA in February 2017.** This drug combination is an adjunct to diet and exercise to improve glycemic control in patient with type 2 diabetes. It is designed to treat increase glucose levels for patients not controlled on dapagliflozin alone or currently taking dapagliflozin and saxagliptin.

## ADJUVANT MEDICATIONS USED TO TREAT DIABETES

For most patients, the goals of treatment are to maintain blood glucose at normal or near-normal levels; promote normal metabolism of carbohydrate, fat, and protein; prevent acute and long-term complications; and prevent hypoglycemic episodes. There is strong evidence that strict control of blood sugar delays the onset and slows progression of complications of diabetes. In addition to glycemic control, other measures can be used to help prevent complications of diabetes. Table 41.13 summarizes these adjuvant medications.

### Angiotensin-Converting Enzyme Inhibitors

The prototype ACE inhibitor is ⓟ **enalapril maleate** (Vasotec). Enalapril maleate blocks the conversion of angiotensin I to angiotensin II, thereby decreasing blood pressure. Enalapril maleate has protective effects on the kidneys in both type 1 and type 2 diabetes and in both normotensive and hypertensive people. Although ACE inhibitors are also used in the treatment of

---

**TABLE 41.13**

### DRUGS AT A GLANCE: Adjuvant Drugs for the Treatment of Diabetes Mellitus

| Drug | Pregnancy Category | Routes and Dosage Ranges | |
|---|---|---|---|
| | | **Adults** | **Children** |
| ⓟ **Enalapril maleate** (Epaned, Vasotec; 🍁 ACT Epaned, APO Epaned, JAMP Epaned, NOVO Vasotec) | D | 2.5 mg PO daily or twice daily; maintenance daily dosage is 2.5–20 mg daily<br>Renal impairment: use smaller initial dose, and adjust upward to a max of 40 mg/d PO | 1 mo to 16 y: initial dose 0.08 mg/kg PO once daily<br>Maximum dose: 5 mg |
| ⓟ **Losartan** (Cozaar; 🍁 ACT Losartan, AG-Losartan, SANDOZ Losartan, TEVA Losartan) | D | 50 mg PO once daily; can be increased to 100 mg once daily based on blood pressure response<br>Diabetic nephropathy: 50 mg PO once daily; can be increased to 100 mg once daily based on blood pressure response | ≥6 y to ≤16 y: 0.7 mg/kg once daily<br>Maximum initial dose: 50 mg/d |
| ⓟ **Hydrochlorothiazide** (🍁 APO Hydro, BIO Hydrochlorothiazide) | B | 25 mg/d in morning. May not need more than 50 mg with other ACES and ARBS | 2–12 y: 1–2 mg/kg/d (0.5–1 mg/lb) orally daily as a single dose or in 2 divided doses<br>Maximum dose: 100 mg/d |
| ⓟ **Acetylsalicylic acid (ASA)** (Aspirin; 🍁 Novasen; Asaphen) | D | 75–162 mg/d | Not recommended |
| ⓟ **Simvastatin** (Zocor; Zocor, FloLipid; 🍁 ACT Simvastatin, AG Simvastatin, Auro Simvastatin) | X | 20–40 mg PO once daily in the evening<br>Renal impairment: starting dose 5 mg/d PO and increase slowly | 10–17 y: 10 mg/d PO in evening |

hypertension, their ability to delay nephropathy seems to be independent of antihypertensive effects. Additional measures to preserve renal function include effective treatment of hypertension, limited intake of dietary protein, prompt treatment of urinary tract infections, and avoidance of nephrotoxic drugs when possible. Serum potassium levels and creatinine levels should be monitored.

## Angiotensin II Receptor Blockers

**Ⓟ Losartan** (Cozaar) is the prototype ARB. In renal studies of patients with diabetes and nephropathy, losartan reduced the incidence of end-stage renal disease in 28% of the patients. ARBs do not prevent nephropathy but reduce the rate of progression. Serum potassium levels and creatinine levels should be monitored.

## Thiazide-Like Diuretics

**Ⓟ Hydrochlorothiazide** (HCTZ) is the prototype thiazide-like diuretics. Thiazide-like diuretics have been shown to reduce cardiovascular events in diabetes. Serum potassium levels and creatinine levels should be monitored.

## Antiplatelet Agent

Aspirin therapy is considered a primary prevention strategy in patients with diabetes who are at increased cardiovascular risk.

## HMG-CoA Reductase Inhibitors

The prototype HMG-CoA reductase inhibitor is **Ⓟ simvastatin** (Zocor). Simvastatin inhibits HMG-CoA reductase, the enzyme that catalyzes the first step in cholesterol synthesis, which ultimately reduces serum cholesterol. Current research suggests that a number of treatment strategies may be beneficial in reducing the cardiovascular disease risk associated with type 2 diabetes mellitus. Some clinicians are recommending the routine use of statins such as simvastatin to reduce the risk of occlusive arterial disease in all patients with diabetes, regardless of cholesterol level.

### Clinical Application 41.3

In addition to the addition of insulin to Mr. Smith's medication regimen, the physician also prescribes enalapril maleate (Vasotec) and simvastatin (Zocor) for Mr. Smith.
- What is the purpose of adding these medications for Mr. Smith, and how will they assist him in his treatment of diabetes mellitus?

### NCLEX Success

16. A patient who is newly diagnosed with diabetes mellitus demonstrates extreme anxiety. The most appropriate intervention to decrease the patient's anxiety would be to do which of the following?
    A. convey empathy, trust, and respect toward the patient
    B. administer an antianxiety medication
    C. ensure that the patient knows the correct medical terminology to understand what is going on
    D. ignore the signs and symptoms of anxiety so they will disappear more quickly

17. The nurse is educating a patient about proper foot care. Which instruction does the nurse include in the teaching plan?
    A. Always use a pumice stone on callused areas of the feet.
    B. Use a heavy moisturizing cream on the feet at all times.
    C. Wash feet in cold water only.
    D. Always have a podiatrist cut toenails.

18. A patient with DKA is admitted to the hospital. Which of the following does the nurse expect to see?
    A. increased pH and increased heart rate
    B. increased respiratory rate and decrease in urine output
    C. elevated potassium and increase in blood pressure
    D. elevated blood glucose and decreased plasma bicarbonate

19. A 58-year-old woman with type 2 diabetes mellitus takes glyburide (DiaBeta) 5 mg by mouth daily, and this drug controls her diabetes well. However, recently, her fasting blood glucose has measured between 200 and 220 mg/dL. Which of the following medications may have been added to the patient's regimen?
    A. atenolol
    B. prednisone
    C. enalapril maleate
    D. levothyroxine sodium

20. A nurse administers 10 units of lispro to a patient with type 1 diabetes, based on the number of carbohydrates the patient will consume at breakfast. At 9:30, the patient tells the nurse he feels shaky and is sweating and states "I think my blood sugar is low." What is the nurse's next action?
    A. Test the patient's blood glucose.
    B. Call the prescriber for orders.
    C. Review the blood sugar trends.
    D. Prepare to administer glucagon.

### Clinical Application 41.4

The goal of care for Mr. Smith is to increase his ability to achieve good glycemic control and prevent complications related to diabetes mellitus.
- In addition to his primary physician, what other types of health care providers should be involved in his care to allow him to achieve this goal?
- What additional teaching could the nurse provide to Mr. Smith to help prevent physical and emotional complications?

# THE NURSING PROCESS

A concept map outlines the nursing process related to drug therapy considerations in this chapter. Additional nursing implications related to the disease process should also be considered in care decisions.

**Assessment**

- Assess the patient's history, including age at onset of diabetes, prescribed control measures and their effectiveness, the ease or difficulty of adhering to the prescribed treatment, occurrence of complications such as ketoacidosis, and whether other disease processes have interfered with diabetes control.
- Assess the patient's:
  - **Diet**. Ask about the prescribed nutritional plan and use of herbal or dietary.
  - **Activity**. Ask the patient to describe usual activities of daily living, and exercise.
  - **Medication**. Assess the type or insulin or anti-diabetic agent. Assess hypoglycemic reactions due to the medication administered.
  - **Monitoring methods**. Testing the blood for glucose and the urine for ketones (e.g., when blood sugar is elevated, when ill and unable to eat) are the two main methods of self-monitoring glycemic control.
  - **Skin and mucous membranes**. Inspect for signs of infection and other lesions. Women with diabetes are susceptible to monilial vaginitis and infections under the breasts. Check the sites of insulin injection for atrophy (dimpling or indentation), hypertrophy (nodules or lumps), and fibrosis (hardened areas). Inspect the feet for calluses, ulcers, and signs of infection. Check pedal pulses, color, and temperature in both feet to evaluate arterial blood flow.
  - **Eyes**. Ask about difficulties with vision and if eyes are examined regularly. Cardiovascular system. Assess blood pressure and ask about chest pain and pain in the legs with exercise (intermittent claudication).
  - **Genitourinary system**. Assess for signs of urinary tract infection, polyuria, and impotence in men.
  - **Blood glucose levels**. Assess blood sugar reports for abnormal levels. Two or more fasting blood glucose levels greater than 126 mg/dL or two random levels greater than 200 mg/dL are diagnostic of diabetes. Decreased blood sugar levels are especially dangerous at 40 mg/dL or below.
  - **Glycosylated hemoglobin level**. Assess the glycosylated hemoglobin (also called glycated hemoglobin and HbA1c) level when available.

**Outcomes of Therapy**

The patient will
- Learn self-care activities.
- Manage drug therapy to prevent or minimize hypoglycemia and other adverse effects.
- Develop a consistent pattern of diet and exercise.
- Use available resources to learn about the disease process and how to manage it.
- Take diabetes medications accurately.
- Self-monitor blood glucose and urine ketones appropriately.
- Keep appointments for follow-up and monitoring procedures by a health care provider.

**Nursing Interventions**

- Instruct the patient and family about diet, exercise, and the use of insulin or antidiabetic agents.
- Self-monitoring of blood glucose levels allows the patients to see the effects of diet, exercise, and hypoglycemic medications on blood glucose levels and may promote compliance.
- Test urine for ketones when the patient is sick, when blood glucose levels are greater than 200 mg/dL, and when episodes of nocturnal hypoglycemia are suspected. Instruct patients and family to test urine when indicated.
- Promote early recognition and treatment of problems by observing for signs and symptoms of urinary tract infection, peripheral vascular disease, vision changes, ketoacidosis, hypoglycemia, and others.
- Discuss the importance of regular visits to health care facilities for blood sugar measurements, weights, blood pressure measurements, and eye examinations.
- Perform and teach correct foot care. Also, teach the patient to report any lesions on the feet to the physician.
- Provide appropriate patient teaching for any drug therapy and combination drug therapy for patients with type 2 diabetes mellitus (Boxes 41.7, 41.10, 41.14, and 41.17).

**Evaluation**

- Check blood sugar reports regularly for normal or abnormal values.
- Check glycosylated hemoglobin reports when available.
- Interview and observe for therapeutic and adverse responses to diabetic drugs.
- Interview and observe for compliance with prescribed treatment.
- Interview patients and family members about the frequency and length of hospitalizations for diabetes mellitus.

## KEY CONCEPTS

- A person with a fasting blood glucose level between 100 and 125 mg/dL is said to have IFG or prediabetes.
- The two major classifications of diabetes mellitus are type 1 and type 2.
- Insulin plays a role in the metabolism of carbohydrates, fats, and proteins.
- Insulin decreases blood sugar and regulates the amount of glucose available for cellular metabolism and energy needs, during fasting and with the intake of food.
- Various forms of insulin are effective for the treatment of type 1 diabetes and in some patients with type 2 diabetes.
- The dosage of insulin must be individualized according to the blood glucose levels.
- The goal of insulin administration is to alleviate the symptoms of hyperglycemia and reestablish metabolic balance without hypoglycemia.
- The goal of the patient taking insulin is to maintain blood glucose levels within normal range. The normal hemoglobin A1C level is under 7%.
- The FDA has issued a **BLACK BOX WARNING** ◆ for the inhaled insulin Afrezza, because individuals with diabetes and chronic lung disease who take it are at risk for acute bronchospasm.
- Self-monitoring of blood glucose is an important tool for achieving glycemic control. It is necessary to individualize the frequency of self-monitoring of blood glucose based on type of diabetes, glucose goals, and other factors.
- The second-generation sulfonylureas are administered for type 2 diabetes to stimulate the release of insulin from the functioning beta cells.
- Alpha-glucosidase inhibitors inhibit alpha-glucosidase in the GI tract to delay digestion of complex carbohydrates in glucose and other simple sugars.
- Metformin is a biguanide that reduces blood sugar without causing hypoglycemia.
- The FDA has issued a **BLACK BOX WARNING** ◆ for metformin. There is a risk of lactic acidosis, and patients 80 years of age or older should not take this drug. Also, people should not take it with alcohol.
- Thiazolidinediones stimulate the receptors on muscle, fat, and liver cells to increase and restore the effectiveness of circulating insulin.
- The FDA has issued a **BLACK BOX WARNING** ◆ alerting health care professionals about the risk of congestive heart failure in patients using pioglitazone and rosiglitazone.
- A **BLACK BOX WARNING** ◆ alerts nurses to the danger of severe insulin-induced hypoglycemia with pramlintide therapy, especially in type 1 diabetes.
- The FDA has issued a **BLACK BOX WARNING** ◆ for incretin mimetics; C-cell thyroid cancer has developed in animals in studies. Patients should routinely be monitored for thyroid nodules. These drugs are contraindicated in patients with a family history of endocrine neoplasia syndrome type 2.
- Exercise is perhaps the best therapy for the prevention of both type 2 diabetes and the metabolic syndrome. Exercise acts as an extremely strong hypoglycemic agent.
- Diabetes self-management education involves a continuum of services ranging from the teaching of survival skills to comprehensive self-management education programs to intensive management.
- Assessment of educational needs is necessary at time of diagnosis and whenever there is poor clinical control or a major change in therapy.

## CLINICAL REASONING CASE STUDY

**Meet the Patient**

Maria Ortiz, a 20-year-old woman, received a diagnosis of type 1 diabetes mellitus last year. She has been having difficulty obtaining tight glycemic control. In the spring, her prescriber ordered a continuous Humalog insulin infusion by insulin pump. Her glycemic control has improved. She is seeing the nurse practitioner at the university she attends. She informs the nurse practitioner that she will be starting a new job as a lifeguard when she returns home.

- Why is only regular or short-acting insulin used in the insulin pump?
- What is the onset of action, peak of action, and duration of action for Humalog insulin?
- What patient education should the nurse practitioner provide for Ms. Ortiz?
- What other members of the health care team would the nurse practitioner include in the teaching plan?

**Assessing Drug Information**

- Only regular or short-acting insulin is used in an insulin pump because it most closely mimics insulin secreted by the human body. Also, because insulin is continuously given by the pump, it needs to a have a quick onset and peak.
- The onset of action for Humalog insulin is 15 minutes, and it peaks in 1 to 1.5 hours. This form of insulin possesses a 6- to 8-hour duration of action.
- Ms. Ortiz should check her blood glucose often so that the health care provider responsible for monitoring and adjusting the insulin pump can make the necessary changes.
- Given the fact Ms. Ortiz will be working outside in what may be high temperatures, she may want to have a small amount of insulin in the pump at all times and change the setting more often. In extreme temperatures, the effect of insulin weakens. She should protect the pump and insulin from direct sunlight. It helps to place it in a pocket or in an insulin pump pouch, where it is protected from extreme temperatures and sunlight.

**Nursing Actions**

- Refer Ms. Ortiz to a nutritionist, exercise scientist, diabetic educator, and a support group. The nutritionist will help in terms of counting carbohydrates to determine the number of units of insulin that are needed. The exercise scientist will help determine how exercise will influence her blood glucose levels. The diabetes educator will assist in educating her about site placement, rotation, and care. The diabetes support group will consist of patients and family members who share their stories to promote compliance with diet, the medication regime, and an exercise program.
- Instruct Ms. Ortiz about the use of her insulin pump and protecting the insulin from heat and direct sunlight.
- Assess Ms. Ortiz's blood glucose level based on her diet, exercise, and insulin.

Visit the Point® at **http://thePoint.lww.com/Frandsen12e** *for answers to NCLEX Success questions (in Appendix A), answers to Clinical Application Case Studies (in Appendix B), and more!*

## REFERENCES AND RESOURCES

Aljack, H. A., Abdalla, M. K., Idris, O. F., & Ismail, A. M. (2019). Vitamin D deficiency increases risk of nephropathy and cardiovascular diseases in Type 2 diabetes mellitus patients. *Journal of Research in Medical Sciences, 24*(47), 1–7. doi:10.4103/jrms.JRMS_303_18

American Diabetes Association. (2018). Glycemic targets: Standards of medical care in diabetes. *Diabetes Care, 41,* S55.

American Diabetes Association. (2019). Standards of medical care in diabetes. *Journal of Clinical and Applied Research and Education, 42*(1), S1–S187.

Centers for Disease Control. (2017). *National diabetes statistic report, 2017 estimates of diabetes and its burden in the United States.* Retrieved August 8, 2019, from https://www.cdc.gov/diabetes/pdfs/data/statistics/national-diabetes-statistics-report.pdf

Hinkle, J. L., & Cheever, K. H. (2018). *Brunner & Suddarth's textbook of medical-surgical nursing* (14th ed.). Philadelphia, PA: Wolters Kluwer.

Karch, A. M. (2019). *2019 Lippincott's nursing drug guide.* Philadelphia, PA: Lippincott Williams & Wilkins.

Laffel, L., & Svoren, B. (2019). Epidemiology, presentation, and diagnosis of type 2 diabetes mellitus in children and adolescents. UpToDate. Lexi-Comp Inc.

Levitsky, L., & Misra, M. (2019). Management of type 1 diabetes mellitus in children and adolescents. UpToDate. Lexi-Comp Inc.

Lippincott. (2019). *Nursing 2019 Drug handbook.* Philadelphia, PA: Wolters Kluwer.

McCulloch, D. K. (2019a). Overview of medical care in adults with diabetes mellitus. UpToDate. Lexi-Comp Inc.

McCulloch, D. K. (2019b). Sulfonylureas and meglitinides in the treatment of diabetes mellitus. UpToDate. Lexi-Comp Inc.

Norris, T. L. (2019). *Porth's Pathophysiology: Concepts of altered health states* (10th ed.). Philadelphia, PA: Wolters Kluwer.

UpToDate. (2019). *Drug Information.* Lexi-Comp, Inc.

U.S. Food and Drug Administration. (2015). FDA drug safety communication: FDA warns that DPP-4 inhibitors for type 2 diabetes may cause severe joint pain. Retrieved August 8, 2019, from https://www.fda.gov/drugs/drug-safety-and-availability/fda-drug-safety-communication-fda-warns-dpp-4-inhibitors-type-2-diabetes-may-cause-severe-joint-pain

U.S. Food and Drug Administration. (2016a). FDA approves Adlyxin to treat type 2 diabetes. Retrieved August 9, 2019, from https://www.fda.gov/news-events/press-announcements/fda-approves-adlyxin-treat-type-2-diabetes

U.S. Food and Drug Administration. (2016b). Updated FDA review concludes that use of type 2 diabetes medicine pioglitazone may be linked to an increased risk of bladder cancer. Retrieved August 8, 2019, from https://www.fda.gov/media/101952/download

# Drug Therapy for Hyperthyroidism and Hypothyroidism

## LEARNING OBJECTIVES

*After studying this chapter, you should be able to:*

1. Understand the physiologic effects of thyroid hormone.
2. Describe the etiology, pathophysiology, and clinical manifestations of hyperthyroidism.
3. Describe the etiology, pathophysiology, and clinical manifestations of hypothyroidism.
4. Identify the prototype and describe the action, use, adverse effects, contraindications, and nursing implications of the drugs administered for the treatment of hyperthyroidism.
5. Identify the prototype and describe the action, use, adverse effects, contraindications, and nursing implications of the drugs administered for the treatment of hypothyroidism.
6. Implement the nursing process in the care of the patient receiving medications for the treatment of hyperthyroidism or hypothyroidism.

## CLINICAL APPLICATION CASE STUDY

Brenda Zalewski, a 45-year-old woman, had a goiter as a child and a thyroidectomy at age 12. She has been taking a synthetic thyroid preparation since that time. Ms. Zalewski takes a maintenance dose of levothyroxine [Synthroid] 0.1 mg orally daily. She is 5 feet 8 inches tall and weighs 215 lbs.

## KEY TERMS

**Cretinism:** congenital hypothyroidism that occurs when a child is born with a poorly functioning or absent thyroid gland

**Euthyroid:** normal thyroid gland functioning

**Goiter:** visible enlargement of the thyroid gland

**Graves' disease:** antibody-mediated autoimmune disease resulting in hyperthyroidism; the most common cause of hyperthyroidism

**Hyperthyroidism:** excessive secretion of thyroid hormone; usually involves an enlarged thyroid gland that has an increased number of cells and an increased rate of secretion

**Hypothyroidism:** diminished secretion of thyroid hormone; occurs when disease or destruction of thyroid gland tissue causes inadequate production of thyroid hormones

**Myxedema:** hypothyroidism that occurs after early childhood, more often in women than in men

**Myxedema coma:** severe, life-threatening hypothyroidism

**Thyroid storm:** rare but severe complication characterized by extreme symptoms of hyperthyroidism; most likely to occur in patients with hyperthyroidism that has been inadequately treated, especially when stressful situations occur; also known as thyrotoxic crisis

**Thyroiditis:** common cause of primary hypothyroidism; an autoimmune disorder characterized by inflammation of the thyroid gland

# INTRODUCTION

This chapter introduces the pharmacologic care of the patient experiencing increased or decreased function of the thyroid gland. To fully appreciate the management of hyperthyroidism and hypothyroidism, the two types of thyroid disorders requiring drug therapy, it is necessary to understand the normal physiology, etiology, clinical manifestations, and pathophysiology of the thyroid gland.

# OVERVIEW OF THE THYROID GLAND

## Physiology

Normal serum levels of thyroid hormones and a **euthyroid** physiologic state (normal thyroid function) require a functioning thyroid gland and feedback mechanism. The thyroid gland produces three hormones: thyroxine, triiodothyronine, and calcitonin. Thyroxine (also called $T_4$) contains four atoms of iodine, and triiodothyronine (also called $T_3$) contains three atoms of iodine. Chapter 44 discusses calcitonin functions in calcium metabolism.

Production of $T_3$ and $T_4$ depends on the presence of iodine and tyrosine in the thyroid gland. In a series of chemical reactions, iodine atoms become attached to tyrosine, an amino acid derived from dietary protein, to form the thyroid hormones $T_3$ and $T_4$. After they are formed, the hormones are stored within the chemically inactive thyroglobulin molecule. Tyrosine forms the basic structure of thyroglobulin. Thyroid hormones are released into the circulation when the thyroid gland is stimulated by thyroid-stimulating hormone (TSH or thyrotropin) from the anterior pituitary gland (Fig. 42.1) through a negative feedback mechanism. The hormones become largely bound to plasma proteins, with only the small unbound ones remaining biologically active. $T_3$, the most active thyroid hormone, mediates the cellular actions of the other thyroid hormone. $T_3$ is more potent than $T_4$ and has a more rapid onset but a shorter duration of action. $T_3$ binds to two receptors that regulate the expression of many genes. The bound thyroid hormones are released to tissue cells very slowly. In tissue cells, the hormones combine with intracellular proteins so they are again stored. They are released slowly within the cell and used over a period of days or weeks. When they are used by the cells, the thyroid hormones release iodine atoms. Most of the iodine is reabsorbed and used to produce new thyroid hormones; the remainder is excreted in the urine.

Thyroid hormones have profound effects on many major physiologic processes, such as metabolism, growth, and development. By controlling the rate of cellular metabolism, these hormones influence the functioning of virtually every cell in the body. The heart, skeletal muscle, liver, and kidneys are especially responsive to the stimulating effects of the hormones. The brain, spleen, and gonads are less responsive. Normal levels of thyroid hormones are essential for normal growth and development. Experts consider them especially critical for fetal and neonatal brain and skeletal development and maturation, and a deficiency in thyroid hormones is not compatible with human health.

Thyroid hormones also influence linear growth; brain function, including intelligence and memory; neural development; dentition; and bone development. These hormones are thought to act mainly by controlling intracellular protein synthesis. Some specific physiologic effects include:

- Increased rate of cellular metabolism and oxygen consumption with a resultant increase in heat production
- Increased heart rate, force of contraction, systemic vascular resistance, and cardiac output (increased cardiac workload)
- Increased carbohydrate metabolism
- Increased fat metabolism, including increased lipolytic effects of other hormones and metabolism of cholesterol to bile acids
- Inhibition of pituitary secretion of TSH

## Etiology and Pathophysiology

### Hyperthyroidism

**Hyperthyroidism** is characterized by excessive synthesis and secretion of thyroid hormone(s) by the thyroid and usually involves an enlarged thyroid gland that has an increased number of cells. Endogenous hyperthyroidism most commonly results from Graves' disease or nodular thyroid goiter. Other causes include thyroiditis, overtreatment with thyroid drugs, functioning thyroid carcinoma, and pituitary adenoma that secretes excessive amounts of TSH.

**Graves' disease** is an autoimmune disorder in which thyrotropin receptor antibodies stimulate the TSH receptors, increasing thyroid hormone production and release. In nodular thyroid goiter, growth of established nodules and new nodule formation trigger the hyperthyroidism. Graves' disease is the most common cause of hyperthyroidism in the United States; however, the prevalence of toxic nodular goiter increases in older adults and in regions with dietary iodine deficiency. The hyperplastic thyroid gland may secrete 5 to 15 times the normal amount of thyroid hormone. As a result, body metabolism is greatly increased. Specific physiologic effects vary (see Clinical Manifestations), depending on the amount of circulating thyroid hormone, and they usually increase in incidence and severity over time if hyperthyroidism is not treated.

Subclinical hyperthyroidism is defined as a reduced TSH (less than 0.1 microunit/L) and normal $T_3$ and $T_4$ levels. The most common cause is excess thyroid hormone therapy.

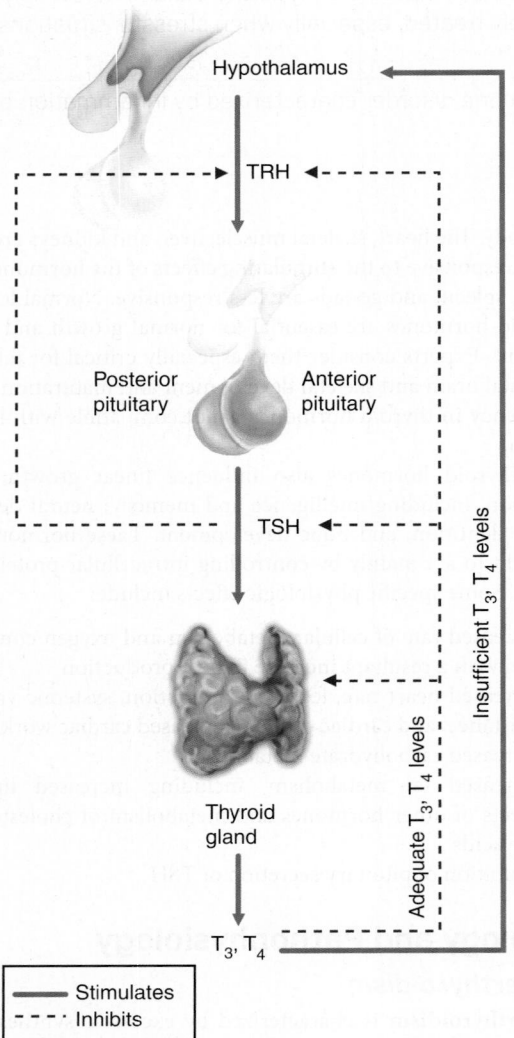

Hypothalamus

TRH

Posterior pituitary     Anterior pituitary

TSH

Thyroid gland

$T_3$, $T_4$

Adequate $T_3$, $T_4$ levels

Insufficient $T_3$, $T_4$ levels

—— Stimulates
- - - - Inhibits

**Figure 42.1.** Thyroid-releasing hormone (TRH) from the hypothalamus stimulates the anterior pituitary to release thyroid-stimulating hormone (TSH). It also inhibits the hypothalamus from releasing TRH. TSH stimulates the thyroid gland to release $T_3$ and $T_4$. It also inhibits the hypothalamus from releasing TRH and the anterior pituitary from releasing more TSH. The release of $T_3$ and $T_4$ from the thyroid gland inhibits TRH release from the hypothalamus, TSH release from the pituitary, and further $T_3$ and $T_4$ release from the thyroid gland. Falling $T_3$ and $T_4$ levels stimulate the hypothalamus to release TRH, and the process repeatedly continues to maintain effective hormone levels. ACTH, adrenocorticotropic hormone; CRH, corticotropin-releasing hormone; FSH, follicle-stimulating hormone; GH, growth hormone; GHRH, growth hormone–releasing hormone; GnRH, gonadotropin-releasing hormone; LH, luteinizing hormone; PIF, prolactin-inhibiting factor; PRL, prolactin; PRF, prolactin-releasing factor; SRIF, somatotropin release–inhibiting factor.

Subclinical hyperthyroidism is a risk factor for osteoporosis in postmenopausal women who do not take estrogen replacement therapy, because it leads to reduced bone mineral density. It also greatly increases the risk of atrial fibrillation in patients older than 60 years of age.

## Hypothyroidism

**Hypothyroidism** is characterized by diminished secretion of thyroid hormone. Primary hypothyroidism occurs when disease or destruction of thyroid gland tissue causes inadequate production of thyroid hormones. Common causes of primary hypothyroidism include chronic (Hashimoto's) **thyroiditis**, an autoimmune disorder characterized by inflammation of the thyroid gland, and treatment of hyperthyroidism with antithyroid drugs, radiation therapy, or surgery. Other causes include previous radiation to the thyroid area of the neck and treatment with amiodarone, lithium, or iodine preparations. Secondary hypothyroidism occurs when there is decreased TSH from the anterior pituitary gland or decreased thyrotropin-releasing hormone (TRH) secreted from the hypothalamus, which disrupts the negative feedback mechanism.

# Clinical Manifestations

Several signs and symptoms of altered thyroid function are characteristic. Table 42.1 lists the specific effects of hyperthyroidism and hypothyroidism.

## Hyperthyroidism

**Thyroid storm** or thyrotoxic crisis is a rare but severe complication characterized by extreme symptoms of hyperthyroidism, such as severe tachycardia, fever, dehydration, heart failure, and coma. It is most likely to occur in patients with inadequately treated hyperthyroidism, especially when stressful situations occur (e.g., trauma, infection, surgery, emotional upset).

It should be noted that iodine is present in foods (especially seafood and kelp) and in radiographic contrast dyes. Reports of iodine-induced hyperthyroidism have been reported after ingestion of dietary sources of iodine.

## Hypothyroidism

Hypothyroidism is the result from a congenital or acquired defect that results in thyroid hormone deficiency. Congenital hypothyroidism, or **cretinism**, occurs when a child is born with a poorly functioning or absent thyroid gland. Now uncommon in the United States, cretinism once occurred because of a lack of iodine in the mother's diet; however, salt with iodine supplements has virtually eliminated frank iodine deficiency. Symptoms are rarely present at birth but develop gradually during infancy and early childhood, and they include poor growth and development, lethargy and inactivity, feeding problems, slow pulse, subnormal temperature, and constipation. If cretinism is untreated until the child is several months old, irreversible mental retardation is likely to result.

Hypothyroidism occurring after early childhood, or **myxedema**, may be caused when inflammatory diseases of the thyroid or another acquired defect destroys parts of the gland. The condition occurs much more often in women than in men. Myxedema may be classed subclinical or clinical. Subclinical hypothyroidism, the most common thyroid disorder, involves a mildly elevated serum TSH and normal serum thyroxine levels. It is usually asymptomatic. If the thyroid gland cannot secrete enough hormones despite excessive release of TSH, hypothyroidism occurs, and a **goiter** (visible enlargement of the thyroid gland) may occur from the overstimulation. Clinical hypothyroidism produces variable signs and symptoms, depending on the amount of circulating thyroid hormone. Initially, manifestations (see Table 42.1) are mild and vague. They usually increase

**TABLE 42.1**

## Thyroid Disorders and Their Effects on Body Systems

| Hypothyroidism | Hyperthyroidism |
|---|---|
| **Cardiovascular Effects** | |
| Increased capillary fragility | |
| Decreased cardiac output | Increased cardiac output |
| Decreased blood pressure | Increased systolic blood pressure<br>Decreased diastolic blood pressure |
| Decreased heart rate | Tachycardia |
| Cardiac enlargement | Cardiac dysrhythmias |
| Heart failure | Heart failure |
| Anemia | |
| More rapid development of atherosclerosis and its complications (e.g., coronary artery and peripheral vascular disease) | |
| | Increased blood volume |
| **Central Nervous System Effects** | |
| Apathy and lethargy | Nervousness |
| Emotional dullness | Emotional instability |
| Slow speech, perhaps slurring and hoarseness as well | Restlessness |
| Hypoactive reflexes | Hyperactive reflexes |
| Forgetfulness and mental sluggishness | Anxiety |
| Excessive drowsiness and sleeping | Insomnia |
| **Metabolic Effects** | |
| Intolerance of cold | Intolerance of heat |
| Subnormal temperature | Low-grade fever |
| Increased serum cholesterol | |
| Weight gain | Weight loss despite increased appetite |
| **Gastrointestinal Effects** | |
| Decreased appetite | Increased appetite |
| Constipation | Abdominal cramps<br>Diarrhea<br>Nausea and vomiting |
| **Muscular Effects** | |
| Weakness | Weakness |
| Fatigue | Fatigue |
| Vague aches and pains | Muscle atrophy<br>Tremors |
| **Integumentary Effects** | |
| Dry, coarse, and thickened skin | Moist, warm, flushed skin due to vasodilation and increased sweating |
| Puffy appearance of the face and eyelids | Localized edema around the eyeballs, which produces characteristic eye changes, including exophthalmos |
| Dry and thinned hair<br>Thick and hard nails | Hair and nails soft |

## TABLE 42.1

### Thyroid Disorders and Their Effects on Body Systems (Continued)

| Hypothyroidism | Hyperthyroidism |
| --- | --- |
| **Reproductive Effects** | |
| Prolonged menstrual periods<br>Infertility or sterility<br>Decreased libido | Amenorrhea or oligomenorrhea |
| **Miscellaneous Effects** | |
| Increased susceptibility to infection | Increased susceptibility to infection |
| Increased sensitivity to narcotics, barbiturates, and anesthetics due to slowed metabolism of these drugs | |
| | Dyspnea<br>Hoarse, rapid speech<br>Polyuria<br>Excessive perspiration |

in incidence and severity over time as the thyroid gland gradually atrophies and functioning glandular tissue is replaced by nonfunctioning fibrous connective tissue.

**Myxedema coma** is a severe, life-threatening hypothyroidism characterized by coma, hypothermia, cardiovascular collapse, hypoventilation, and severe metabolic disorders such as hyponatremia, hypoglycemia, and lactic acidosis. Predisposing factors include exposure to cold, infection, trauma, respiratory disease, and administration of central nervous system (CNS) depressants (e.g., anesthetics, analgesics, sedatives).

### ! QSEN Alert: Safety

A person with severe hypothyroidism cannot metabolize and excrete the CNS depressants. It is necessary to assess the patient for signs of adverse drug effects.

### NCLEX Success

1. A 62-year-old woman has a reduced thyroid-stimulating hormone level of 0.07 microunit/L and a normal $T_3$ and $T_4$. Which of the following symptoms is she at risk for developing?
   A. sinus bradycardia
   B. premature ventricular contractions
   C. atrial fibrillation
   D. prolong QT interval

2. An infant has diminished growth and development with a very slow pulse and below-normal temperature. Based on the symptoms, what disorder is suspected?
   A. cretinism
   B. Cushing's disease
   C. Addison's disease
   D. thyroid storm

3. A patient has been treated for ventricular dysrhythmias with amiodarone. What is the patient at risk for developing?
   A. Graves' disease
   B. thyroiditis
   C. thyroid storm
   D. cretinism

## Drug Therapy

The goal of treatment is to restore the euthyroid state and normal metabolism. In hyperthyroidism, the goals are to reduce thyroid hormone production to relieve symptoms, return serum TSH and thyroid hormone levels to normal, and avoid complete destruction of the thyroid gland. Antithyroid drugs act by decreasing the production or release of thyroid hormones. The thioamide drugs inhibit the synthesis of thyroid hormones. Iodine preparations inhibit the release of thyroid hormones and cause them to be stored within the thyroid gland. Radioactive iodine emits rays that destroy the thyroid gland tissue.

In hypothyroidism, the goal of thyroid replacement therapy is to administer a dosage in sufficient amounts to compensate for the thyroid deficit to resolve symptoms and restore serum TSH and thyroid hormone to normal. TSH is the most reliable marker of adequacy of replacement therapy, and a serum value within the reference range is often considered the therapeutic target. Table 42.2 summarizes the drugs administered for thyroid disease.

## ANTITHYROID DRUGS

### Propylthiouracil and Related Drugs

 **Propylthiouracil** is the prototype of the thioamide antithyroid drugs. The U.S. Food and Drug Administration (FDA) approved it for the treatment of hyperthyroidism more than 60 years ago.

## TABLE 42.2

### Drugs Administered for the Treatment of Hyperthyroidism and Hypothyroidism

| Drug Class | Prototype | Other Drugs in the Class |
|---|---|---|
| Antithyroid drug | Propylthiouracil | Methimazole (Tapazole)<br>Strong iodine solution (Lugol solution)<br>Saturated solution of potassium iodide (SSKI; ThyroShield)<br>Sodium iodide $^{131}$I (Hicon) |
| Beta-adrenergic–blocking agent | Propranolol hydrochloride (Inderal) | |
| Thyroid drug | Levothyroxine (Synthroid, Levoxyl) | |

## Pharmacokinetics

Propylthiouracil is well absorbed with oral administration, and peak plasma levels occur within 30 minutes. The drug's plasma half-life is 1 to 2 hours. However, its duration of action depends on the half-life within the thyroid gland rather than the plasma half-life. Because this time is relatively short, the drug must be given every 8 hours. It is metabolized in the liver and excreted in urine.

## Action

Propylthiouracil acts by inhibiting production of thyroid hormones and peripheral conversion of $T_4$ to the more active $T_3$. The drug does not interfere with release of thyroid hormones previously produced and stored. Thus, therapeutic effects do not occur for several days or weeks until the stored hormones have been used.

## Use

Health care providers may use propylthiouracil alone to treat hyperthyroidism, as part of the preoperative preparation for thyroidectomy, before or after radioactive iodine therapy, and in the treatment of thyroid storm. Treatment of hyperthyroidism changes the rate of body metabolism, including the rate of metabolism of many drugs. In the hyperthyroid state, drug metabolism may be very rapid, and higher doses of most drugs may be necessary to achieve therapeutic results. When the patient becomes euthyroid, the rate of drug metabolism decreases. Consequently, it is necessary to evaluate and likely reduce doses of all medications to avoid severe adverse effects. Table 42.3 contains the standard route and dosage information for propylthiouracil and other antithyroid drugs.

### Use in Children

Due to severe liver toxicity, propylthiouracil is not recommended for children (UpToDate, 2019). The FDA no longer approves propylthiouracil for pediatric patients. Use is limited to patients who have developed minor toxic reactions to methimazole and who are not candidates for surgery or radioactive iodine treatment. Administration to pediatric patients should be for a limited duration and a short course of therapy. Aspartate aminotransferase (AST) and alanine aminotransferase (ALT) levels should be monitored. If the levels rise two to three times the upper normal limits and do not lower within a week, then therapy should be discontinued.

### Use in Older Adults

Propylthiouracil (or methimazole) may be useful. However, radioactive iodine is often preferable because it is associated with fewer adverse effects than other antithyroid drugs or surgery. It is necessary that patients be monitored closely for hypothyroidism, which usually develops within 1 year after receiving treatment for hyperthyroidism.

### Use in Patients With Hepatic Impairment

The FDA has issued a **BLACK BOX WARNING**  for propylthiouracil stating that severe liver injury resulting in death or acute liver failure may occur within 6 months of treatment. Routine liver function testing to assess for liver failure is important.

## Adverse Effects

Administration of propylthiouracil may have several adverse effects, including the following:

- Signs and symptoms of hypothyroidism: bradycardia, heart failure, anemia, coronary artery disease, peripheral vascular disease, slow speech and body movements, emotional and mental dullness, excessive sleeping, increased weight, constipation, and skin changes
- Hematologic effects: leukopenia, agranulocytosis (puts patient at risk for sepsis, rare but severe, earliest symptoms likely to be sore throat and fever), and hypoprothrombinemia
- Dermatologic effects: rash, pruritus, and alopecia
- CNS effects: headache, dizziness, loss of taste, drowsiness, and paresthesias
- Gastrointestinal (GI) effects: nausea, vomiting, abdominal discomfort, gastric irritation, and cholestatic hepatitis
- Other reported effects: lymphadenopathy, edema, joint pain, and drug fever

## Contraindications

The only contraindication to propylthiouracil is a known hypersensitivity reaction to the medication.

### ! QSEN Alert: Evidence-Based Practice

Wall, Weaver, Litt, and Rae (2017) conducted a case report and review of literature to provide evidence of the clinical symptoms, diagnosis, prevention, and management of propylthiouracil-associated vasculitis in the intensive care setting. The

| | TABLE 42.3 | | | |
|---|---|---|---|---|
| | **DRUGS AT A GLANCE: Drugs for Hyperthyroidism (Antithyroid Drugs)** | | | |
| **Drug** | **Pregnancy Category** | **Routes and Dosage Ranges** | | |
| | | **Adults** | **Children** | |
| Ⓟ **Propylthiouracil** (✱ Propyl-Thyracil) | D | 300–400 mg/d PO in divided doses every 8 h, until the patient is euthyroid; then 100–150 mg/d in three divided doses, for maintenance | Dosing is no longer FDA approved for pediatric patients | |
| Methimazole (Tapazole; ✱ Tapazole, APO-Methimazole, DOM-Methimazole, Mar-Methimazole, PHL-Methimazole) | D | 15–60 mg/d PO initially, in divided doses every 8 h until the patient is euthyroid; maintenance, 5–15 mg/d PO in two or three doses | 0.4 mg/kg/d PO initially, in three divided doses every 8 h; maintenance dose, one half initial dose | |
| Potassium iodide and iodine (Lugol solution) | D | Thyroidectomy preparation: 5–7 drops PO three times per day for 10 d before surgery<br>Thyrotoxic crisis: 4–8 drops every 6–8 h; initial dose ≥1 h following the initial dose of either propylthiouracil or methimazole | Thyroidectomy preparation: 3–5 drops PO three times per day for 10 d before surgery<br>Thyrotoxic crisis: 4–8 drops every 6 h; initial dose 2 h following the initial dose of either propylthiouracil or methimazole | |
| Potassium iodide saturated solution of potassium iodide (iOSAT, ThyroSafe, ThyroShield, Pima, SSKI) | D | Thyroidectomy preparation: 50–100 mg PO three times per day for 10 d before surgery | Thyroidectomy preparation: 150–350 mg PO three times per day for 10 d before surgery | |
| Sodium iodide I$^{131}$ (Iodotope, i3odine Max, Hicon) | D | Dosage (PO, IV) as calculated by a radiologist trained in nuclear medicine | Dosage (PO, IV) as calculated by a radiologist trained in nuclear medicine | |

case reports described the onset of rashes in patients taking propylthiouracil. Of the 128 cases of propylthiouracil-associated vasculitis, the majority were women who presented with a rash, fever, and arthralgia. The patients were treated with steroids. Eight of the patients progressed to end-stage renal disease, two required intubation, and five died of multiple organ failure that was related to the vasculitis. The result of the analysis is screening with myeloperoxidase–antinuclear cytoplasmic antibodies. Patients who screen positive should be evaluated for skin manifestations, and aggressive wound care should be implemented.

## Nursing Implications

### Preventing Interactions

Propylthiouracil may increase the effect of anticoagulants, which may put patients at risk for bleeding. Also, use with amiodarone, potassium iodide, and sodium iodide reverses thyroid hormone efficacy. Lithium acts synergistically with propylthiouracil to produce hypothyroidism.

### Administering the Drug

Patients should take propylthiouracil around the clock in evenly divided doses. If they choose to take one dose of the medication without food, they should take all doses without food. (The same is true if they take it with food.)

### Assessing for Therapeutic Effects

The nurse assesses for a slower pulse rate, slow speech, normal level of activity without the signs of hyperactivity, decreased nervousness and tremors, increased sleep patterns, and weight gain. The therapeutic effects should be apparent in 1 to 2 weeks, but a euthyroid state may not occur for 6 to 8 weeks.

### Assessing for Adverse Effects

The nurse assesses the patient's heart rate and peripheral pulses for increases, the lung sounds for crackles, and the heart sounds for an audible $S_3$; these are all indicative of heart failure. It is also necessary to assess for slow speech and emotional status (dullness). In addition, the nurse checks for increased periods of rest, increased weight, constipation, and skin changes. Finally, he or she assesses for CNS depression and gastric irritation, as well as for fever or sore throat, the first signs of agranulocytosis. It is important to assess the white blood count for leukopenia.

### Patient Teaching

All patients should receive instructions about the signs and symptoms of acute liver failure and seek immediate medical treatment should those symptoms occur. Box 42.1 identifies additional patient teaching guidelines for propylthiouracil.

**BOX 42.1** *Patient Teaching Guidelines for Propylthiouracil*

- To decrease the production of thyroid hormone by an overactive thyroid gland, it is necessary to take antithyroid drugs for 1 year or longer to return thyroid hormone levels to normal.
- Have periodic tests of thyroid function. Dosage adjustments may be necessary.
- Have periodic tests of liver function tests during the first 6 months of treatment.
- Ask the prescriber if it is necessary to avoid or restrict amounts of seafood or iodized salt. It may be necessary to reduce or omit these sources of iodide during antithyroid drug therapy.
- Take this drug at regular intervals around the clock, usually every 8 hours.
- Report fever, sore throat, unusual bleeding or bruising, headache, skin rash, yellowing of the skin, or vomiting to

the prescriber. If these adverse effects occur, he or she may reduce the drug dosage or have you stop taking the drug.
- Consult a health care provider before taking over-the-counter drugs. Some drugs contain iodide, which can increase the likelihood of goiter and the risk of adverse effects from excessive doses of iodide. For example, some cough syrups, asthma medications, and multivitamins may contain iodide.
- Take your pulse daily and report rates above 100 and below 60 beats/min to the prescriber.
- Check your weight two to three times per week, and if it increases suddenly, call your health care provider.
- Consult a health care provider if signs or symptoms of a rash occur.

## Other Drugs in the Class

Methimazole (Tapazole) is similar to propylthiouracil in terms of action, use, and adverse effects. It is also well absorbed with oral administration and rapidly reaches peak plasma levels.

 **QSEN Alert: Safety**

Because of the risk of fetal abnormalities associated with methimazole, women of childbearing age should have a pregnancy test before beginning the drug. Pregnant women should avoid methimazole during the first trimester; it is safe to use in the second and third trimesters.

Strong iodine solution (Lugol solution) and saturated solution of potassium iodide (SSKI) are iodine preparations sometimes used in short-term treatment of hyperthyroidism. These drugs inhibit release of thyroid hormones, causing them to accumulate in the thyroid gland. Lugol solution is usually used to treat thyrotoxic crisis and to decrease the size and vascularity of the thyroid gland before thyroidectomy. SSKI is more often used as an expectorant but may be given as preparation for thyroidectomy. Iodine preparations should not be followed by propylthiouracil, methimazole, or radioactive iodine because the latter drugs cause release of stored thyroid hormone and may precipitate acute hyperthyroidism.

Sodium iodide $^{131}$I (Hicon) is a radioactive isotope of iodine. The thyroid gland cannot differentiate between regular iodide and radioactive iodide, so it picks up the radioactive iodide from the circulating blood. As a result, small amounts of radioactive iodide can be used as a diagnostic test of thyroid function, and larger doses are used therapeutically to treat hyperthyroidism. Therapeutic doses act by emitting beta and gamma rays, which destroy thyroid tissue and thereby decrease production of thyroid hormones. The drug is also used to treat thyroid cancer. It is safe, effective, inexpensive, and convenient. One disadvantage is hypothyroidism, which usually develops within a few months and requires lifelong thyroid hormone replacement therapy. Another disadvantage is the delay in therapeutic benefits. Results

may not be apparent for 3 months or longer, during which time it is necessary to bring severe hyperthyroidism under control with one of the thioamide antithyroid drugs. Note that after radioactive iodine therapy, patients should not expectorate or cough freely because their saliva will be radioactive for 24 hours.

## ADJUVANT MEDICATION USED TO TREAT HYPERTHYROIDISM

The drug Ⓟ **propranolol** (Inderal) is a beta-adrenergic–blocking agent that is recommended in all patients with symptomatic hyperthyroidism. It is particularly useful in older adults who have resting heart rates greater than 90 beats/min or have a history of cardiovascular conditions, such as dysrhythmias, angina pectoris, and hypertension. When given to patients with hyperthyroidism, propranolol blocks beta-adrenergic receptors in various organs and thereby controls symptoms of hyperthyroidism resulting from excessive stimulation of the sympathetic nervous system. These symptoms include tachycardia, palpitations, excessive sweating, tremors, and nervousness. Propranolol is useful for controlling symptoms during the delayed response to thioamide drugs and radioactive iodine, before thyroidectomy, and in treating thyrotoxic crisis. When patients become euthyroid and definitive treatment has controlled hyperthyroid symptoms, it is necessary to taper propranolol and discontinue it. Table 42.4 gives route and dosage information for propranolol.

## NCLEX Success

4. A patient with a diagnosis of hyperthyroidism has a blood pressure of 170/98 mm Hg. Which of the following medications might a physician prescribe to treat hypertension?

   A. propylthiouracil
   B. propranolol
   C. furosemide
   D. hydrochlorothiazide with triamterene

| TABLE 42.4 | | | |
|---|---|---|---|
| **DRUGS AT A GLANCE: Adjuvant Drugs for the Treatment of Hyperthyroidism (Propranolol)** | | | |
| **Drug** | **Pregnancy Category** | **Routes and Dosage Ranges** | |
| | | **Adults** | **Children** |
| ⓟ **Propranolol hydrochloride** (Inderal, Inderal LA, Innopran XL; ✳ Inderal, Inderal LA, Hemangeol, InnoPran XL) | C | Thyrotoxicosis: 10–40 mg/d PO every 6–8 h | Thyrotoxicosis: same as adults |

**5. How does propranolol control symptoms of hyperthyroidism?**

A. Propranolol blocks the alpha-adrenergic receptor sites.

B. Propranolol stimulates the thyroid gland to decrease thyroid production.

C. Propranolol impedes the beta-adrenergic receptors in various organs.

D. Propranolol lowers blood pressure to decrease metabolism.

**6. A woman taking propylthiouracil develops a sore throat and fever. What does the nurse suspect is wrong with this woman?**

A. She has developed a goiter.

B. She has an elevated liver function.

C. She has developed a hypersensitivity reaction.

D. She has agranulocytosis.

# THYROID DRUGS

ⓟ **Levothyroxine** (Synthroid, Levoxyl), a synthetic preparation of thyroxine, serves as the prototype thyroid drug and is considered the standard of care for long-term treatment of hypothyroidism. This potent form of $T_4$ contains a uniform amount of hormone and can be administered orally and parenterally.

## Pharmacokinetics

Absorption of levothyroxine varies after oral administration from 48% to 79%. Taking the drug on an empty stomach increases absorption. In malabsorption syndromes, this results in excessive loss of the drug in the feces. Most (99%) of the circulating drug is bound to serum proteins, including thyroid-binding globulin as well as thyroid-binding prealbumin and albumin. Levothyroxine has a long half-life, about 6 to 7 days in a euthyroid state, but it is prolonged to 9 to 10 days in hypothyroidism and shortened to 3 to 4 days in hyperthyroidism. The drug is metabolized in the liver and excreted in the urine.

## Action

Levothyroxine increases the metabolic rate in the body's tissues, increasing oxygen consumption, respiratory rate, and heart rate. It also increases the metabolism of fats, carbohydrates, and proteins and enhances the growth process.

## Use

Health care providers use levothyroxine as replacement therapy for people with hypothyroidism. Other uses include the following:

• Treatment and prevention of euthyroid goiters in patients with pituitary suppression of TSH
• Management of thyroid cancer
• Prevention of goitrogenesis, hypothyroidism, and thyrotoxicosis during pregnancy (in combination with antithyroid medications)
• Treatment of myxedema coma

Table 42.5 provides route and dosage information for levothyroxine. It is important to note that the FDA has issued a **BLACK BOX WARNING ◆** cautioning prescribers not to order thyroid hormones, either alone or with other therapeutic agents, for the treatment of obesity or for weight loss. Significant and serious complications may develop in euthyroid people who take thyroid hormones.

### Use in Children

Replacement therapy is necessary because thyroid hormone is essential for normal growth and development. As in adults, levothyroxine is the drug of choice in children, and dosage needs may change with growth. After thyroid drugs are started, determination of the maintenance dosage requires periodic radioimmunoassay of serum thyroxine levels and periodic radiographs to follow bone development. To monitor drug effects on growth in children, it is important to record height and weight and compare them with growth charts at regular intervals. Close monitoring for adverse drug effects is necessary.

### Use in Older Adults

Thyroid hormone replacement with levothyroxine increases the workload of the heart and may cause serious adverse effects in older adults, especially those with cardiovascular disease. In such patients, cautious treatment is necessary because of a high risk of adverse effects on the cardiovascular system. Thus, use of smaller initial dosages and smaller drug increments at longer intervals than younger adults is essential. It is important to have periodic measurements of serum TSH levels to monitor drug therapy and to adjust doses when indicated. Also, regular monitoring of blood pressure and pulse is essential. In general, levothyroxine should not be given if the resting heart rate is more than 100 beats/min.

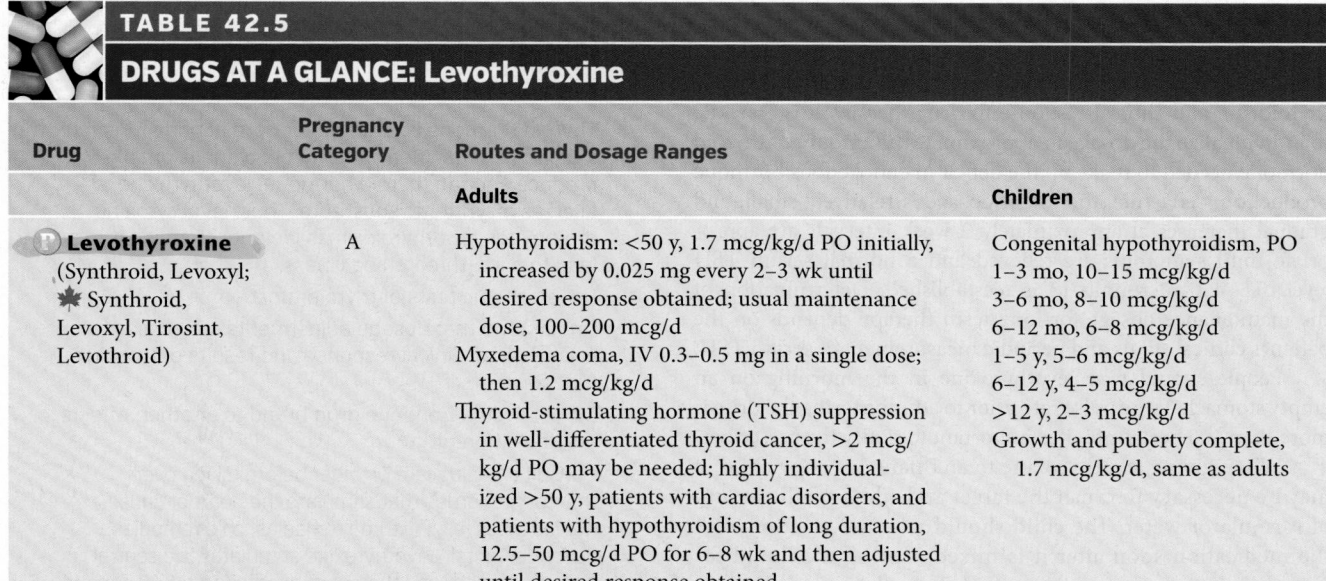

| TABLE 42.5 — DRUGS AT A GLANCE: Levothyroxine | | | |
|---|---|---|---|
| **Drug** | **Pregnancy Category** | **Routes and Dosage Ranges** | |
| | | **Adults** | **Children** |
|  **Levothyroxine** (Synthroid, Levoxyl; ❋ Synthroid, Levoxyl, Tirosint, Levothroid) | A | Hypothyroidism: <50 y, 1.7 mcg/kg/d PO initially, increased by 0.025 mg every 2–3 wk until desired response obtained; usual maintenance dose, 100–200 mcg/d<br>Myxedema coma, IV 0.3–0.5 mg in a single dose; then 1.2 mcg/kg/d<br>Thyroid-stimulating hormone (TSH) suppression in well-differentiated thyroid cancer, >2 mcg/kg/d PO may be needed; highly individualized >50 y, patients with cardiac disorders, and patients with hypothyroidism of long duration, 12.5–50 mcg/d PO for 6–8 wk and then adjusted until desired response obtained | Congenital hypothyroidism, PO<br>1–3 mo, 10–15 mcg/kg/d<br>3–6 mo, 8–10 mcg/kg/d<br>6–12 mo, 6–8 mcg/kg/d<br>1–5 y, 5–6 mcg/kg/d<br>6–12 y, 4–5 mcg/kg/d<br>>12 y, 2–3 mcg/kg/d<br>Growth and puberty complete, 1.7 mcg/kg/d, same as adults |

## Use in Patients With Hepatic Impairment

> **❗ QSEN Alert: Safety**
>
> Hepatic metabolism of levothyroxine in patients with hypothyroidism is slow, so drug metabolism may be delayed. Many drugs given to these patients have a prolonged effect. It is therefore important to assess drug reactions in patients with hepatic impairment.

## Use in Patients With Critical Illness

Management of patients in thyroid storm or thyrotoxic crisis is common in the critical care unit. Increased rate of cellular metabolism and oxygen consumption occurs with a resultant increase in heat production. The hypermetabolic state increases the metabolism of medications, so increased or more frequent dosing may be necessary.

## Adverse Effects

Adverse effects of levothyroxine include signs and symptoms of hyperthyroidism. Other more serious adverse effects are tachycardia, cardiac dysrhythmias, angina pectoris, myocardial infarction, and heart failure. Nervousness, hyperactivity, insomnia, diarrhea, abdominal cramps, nausea, vomiting, weight loss, fever, and an intolerance to heat have also been reported.

Most adverse reactions stem from excessive doses, and signs and symptoms produced are the same as those occurring with hyperthyroidism. Excessive thyroid hormones make the heart work very hard and fast in attempting to meet tissue demands for oxygenated blood and nutrients. Symptoms of myocardial ischemia occur when the increased cardiac workload is prolonged. Cardiovascular problems are more likely to occur in patients who are elderly or who already have heart disease.

## Contraindications

Contraindications to levothyroxine include a known hypersensitivity to active or extraneous constituents of the drug, thyrotoxicosis,

and acute myocardial infarction related to hypothyroidism. Caution is warranted in Addison's disease. Affected patients require corticosteroids prior to administration of levothyroxine. Thyroid hormones increase tissue metabolism and tissue demands for adrenocortical hormones. If adrenal insufficiency is not treated first, administration of thyroid hormone may cause acute adrenocortical insufficiency, a life-threatening condition. Also, caution is necessary during lactation and with coronary artery disease or angina.

## Nursing Implications

### Preventing Interactions

Many medications interact with levothyroxine, increasing and decreasing its effects (Box 42.2).

> **BOX 42.2** **Drug Interactions: Levothyroxine**
>
> **Drugs That Increase the Effects of Levothyroxine**
> - Activating antidepressants (bupropion, venlafaxine), adrenergic asthmatic agents (albuterol, epinephrine), nasal decongestants
>   *Increase the effects of thyroid hormones*
>
> **Drugs That Decrease the Effects of Levothyroxine**
> - Antacids, cholestyramine, iron, sucralfate
>   *Decrease the absorption of levothyroxine*
> - Antihypertensives, propranolol
>   *Decrease cardiac-stimulating effects*
> - Estrogens, oral contraceptives
>   *Increase thyroxine-binding globulin, thereby increasing the amount of bound, inactive levothyroxine in patients with hypothyroidism*
> - Phenytoin, rifampin
>   *Induce enzymes, leading to more rapid metabolism*

## Administering the Medication

Several factors affect the dosage of levothyroxine: the choice of drug, age and general condition, severity and duration of hypothyroidism, and clinical response to drug therapy. It is essential to individualize the dosage to approximate the amount of thyroid hormone needed to make up the deficit in endogenous hormone production. As a rule, the initial dosage is relatively small, and gradual increases at approximately 2-week intervals are appropriate until symptoms are relieved and a normal serum TSH level (0.5–4.2 microunits/L) is reestablished. Determination of the maintenance dosage for long-term therapy depends on the patient's clinical status and periodic measurement of serum TSH.

People should take levothyroxine in the morning on an empty stomach. If the pulse rate prior to administering the drug is more than 100 beats/min, it is important to notify the prescriber.

When giving levothyroxine to an infant or young child, it may be necessary to crush the tablet and add a small amount of formula or water. The child should take the solution with the medication soon after it is mixed; storing the liquid for long periods is a practice to avoid. It is also appropriate to sprinkle the crushed tablet on a small amount of food and then administer it.

## Assessing for Therapeutic Effects

In hypothyroidism, thyroid replacement therapy is lifelong. Medical supervision is necessary frequently during early treatment and at least annually after the patient's condition has stabilized, and maintenance dosage has been determined. The brand of medication should be consistent; patients should not change brands. The nurse assesses for the following conditions:

- Increasing energy and diminished sleep
- Level of alertness and interest in the environment and surroundings
- Increased pulse rate and blood pressure
- Bowel regularity and decreased symptoms of constipation
- Reversal of coarseness of the skin and hair
- Laboratory values (should decrease as the thyroid hormone is replaced): serum cholesterol, creatinine phosphokinase, lactate dehydrogenase, and aspartate aminotransferase

In patients with cretinism, the nurse records the patient's height periodically to determine an increased in linear growth.

In patients with myxedema, the nurse assesses for decreased edema and loss of weight.

## Assessing for Adverse Effects

The nurse assesses for tachycardia and any cardiac dysrhythmias. Excessive thyroid hormones make the heart work very hard and fast in an attempt to meet the tissue demands for oxygenated blood and nutrients. It is necessary to assess for chest pain, edema, and signs of heart failure. Symptoms of myocardial infarction occur when the myocardium does not have an adequate supply of oxygenated blood. Symptoms of heart failure occur when the increased cardiac workload is prolonged.

**BOX 42.3** | *Patient Teaching Guidelines for Levothyroxine*

- Thyroid hormone is required for normal body functioning and for life. When your thyroid gland is unable to produce enough thyroid hormone, levothyroxine is used as a synthetic substitute. Thus, levothyroxine therapy for hypothyroidism is lifelong; stopping it may lead to a life-threatening illness.
- Have periodic tests of thyroid function.
- Understand that dosage adjustments may occur according to clinical response and results of thyroid function tests.
- Do not switch from one drug brand to another; effects may be different.
- Consult a health care provider before taking over-the-counter drugs that stimulate the heart or cause nervousness (e.g., asthma remedies, cold remedies, decongestants). Levothyroxine stimulates the central nervous system and the heart; excessive stimulation may occur if it is taken with other stimulating drugs. In addition, you should probably limit your intake of caffeine-containing beverages to two to three servings daily.
- Take the drug every morning, on an empty stomach, for best absorption. Also, do not take the drug with an antacid (e.g., Tums, Maalox), an iron preparation, or sucralfate (Carafate). These drugs decrease absorption of levothyroxine. If it is necessary to take one of these drugs, take levothyroxine 2 hours before or 4 to 6 hours after the other drug.
- Take the drug at about the same time each day for more consistent blood levels and more normal body metabolism.
- Report chest pain, heart palpitations, nervousness, or insomnia to the prescriber. These adverse effects result from excessive stimulation and may indicate that drug dosage or intake of other stimulants needs to be reduced.

## Patient Teaching

Box 42.3 provides patient teaching guidelines for levothyroxine.

### Clinical Application 42.1

While Ms. Zalewski is in the hospital, the nurse is administering her medications. Hospital routine is to administer all once-daily medications at 9:00 AM. When reviewing the medication administration orders, the nurse notes that Ms. Zalewski is to receive levothyroxine (Synthroid) at 9:00 AM. Patients usually receive their breakfast trays between 8:00 and 8:30 AM.

- What action should the nurse take with regard to the administration of levothyroxine?

## NCLEX Success

7. A patient asks the nurse when the daily dose of levothyroxine should be taken. Which of the following instructions is most appropriate to teach the patient?

   A. Take it before breakfast on an empty stomach.
   B. Take it with meals every 8 hours in divided doses.
   C. Take it every night at bedtime with a snack.
   D. Take it every day at the same without regard to meals.

8. What should the nurse assess prior to the administration of levothyroxine?

   A. blood glucose
   B. heart rate
   C. lung sounds
   D. urine output

9. The home care nurse is visiting with a patient who has a diagnosis of hypothyroidism. The patient is being treated with levothyroxine. The assessment of the patient reveals the following findings: an audible S3, crackles in the lower lobes, edema of the lower extremities, and a heart rate of 120 beats/min. What does the nurse suspect the patient has developed?

   A. myocardial infarction
   B. thrombophlebitis
   C. pulmonary embolism
   D. heart failure

10. A 21-year-old woman is taking levothyroxine for hypothyroidism. She has recently become sexually active and would like to take an oral contraceptive. Which of the following aspects of patient teaching is most accurate?

    A. A low-dose oral contraceptive agent is permissible with levothyroxine.
    B. Oral contraceptive agents increase the amount of thyroid hormone.
    C. For protection from pregnancy, it is necessary to use an oral contraceptive and an alternative form of birth control.
    D. Oral contraceptive agents result in diminished levothyroxine levels due to inactivation.

11. A patient diagnosed with a thyroid condition is preparing for a laboratory draw. The nurse is reviewing the laboratory orders. Which laboratory data are necessary for this patient?

    A. complete blood count (CBC)
    B. comprehensive metabolic panel (CMP)
    C. cluster of differentiation 4 (CD4)
    D. thyroid-stimulating hormone (TSH)

## Clinical Application 42.2

Ms. Zalewski has been discharged from the hospital and is being seen by the home care nurse. During the visit, the nurse reviews all of Ms. Zalewski's medications. Ms. Zalewski states she is taking aluminum hydroxide gel (Amphojel) every morning when she arises to prevent gastric distress after breakfast.

- How will the administration of Amphojel affect her levothyroxine?
- What patient teaching should the home care nurse provide to Ms. Zalewski?

# THE NURSING PROCESS

A concept map outlines the nursing process related to drug therapy considerations in this chapter. Additional nursing implications related to the disease process should also be considered in care decisions.

**Assessment**

- Assess for signs and symptoms of thyroid disorders (see Table 42.1). During the course of treatment with thyroid or antithyroid drugs, the patient should be monitored for indicators of hypothyroidism, euthyroidism, and hyperthyroidism, which can indicate therapeutic and adverse drug effects.
- Check laboratory reports for serum TSH (normal = 0.5–4.2 microunits/mL) when available. An elevated serum TSH is the first indication of primary hypothyroidism and commonly occurs in middle-aged women, even in the absence of other signs and symptoms. Serum TSH is used to monitor response to drugs that alter thyroid function.

**Outcomes of Therapy**

The patient will
- Achieve normal blood levels of thyroid hormone.
- Receive or take drugs accurately.
- Experience relief of symptoms of hypothyroidism or hyperthyroidism.
- Be assisted to cope with symptoms until therapy becomes effective.
- Avoid preventable adverse drug effects.
- Maintain the therapeutic and avoid the adverse effects of drug therapy.

**Nursing Interventions**

- Use nondrug measures to control symptoms, increase effectiveness of drug therapy, and decrease adverse reactions. Some areas for intervention include the following:
  - Patients with hypothyroidism are very intolerant of cold, due to their slow metabolism rate. Chilling and shivering should be prevented because of added strain on the heart. Provide blankets and warm clothes as needed. Patients with hyperthyroidism are very intolerant of heat and perspire excessively, due to their rapid metabolism rate. Provide cooling baths and lightweight clothing as needed.
  - Hypothyroid patients are often overweight because of a slow metabolism rate. Thus, a low-calorie, weight-reduction diet may be indicated. In addition, an increased intake of high-fiber foods is usually needed to prevent constipation as a result of decreased GI secretions and motility. Hyperthyroid patients are often underweight because of a rapid metabolism rate. They often need extra calories and nutrients to prevent tissue breakdown. With hypothyroidism, patients need an adequate intake of low-calorie fluids to prevent constipation. With hyperthyroidism, patients need large amounts of fluids (3000–4000 mL/d) unless contraindicated by cardiac or renal disease. With hypothyroidism, encourage activity to maintain cardiovascular, respiratory, GI, and musculoskeletal function. With hyperthyroidism, encourage rest and quiet, nonstrenuous activity. Because patients differ in what they find restful, this must be determined with each patient.
  - Hypothyroid patients are likely to have edema and dry skin. When edema is present, inspect pressure points, turn often, and avoid trauma when possible. Edema increases risks of skin breakdown and decubitus ulcer formation. Also, increased capillary fragility increases the likelihood of bruising from seemingly minor trauma. When skin is dry, use soap sparingly and lotions and other lubricants freely.
  - Hyperthyroid patients may have exophthalmos. In mild cases, use measures to protect the eye. For example, dark glasses, local lubricants, and patching of the eyes at night may be needed. If the eyelids cannot close, they are sometimes taped shut to avoid corneal abrasion. In severe exophthalmos, corticosteroids and diuretics are usually given.

**Evaluation**

- Interview and observe for compliance with instructions for taking medications.
- Observe for relief of symptoms.
- Check laboratory reports for normal blood levels of TSH or thyroid hormones.
- Interview and observe for adverse drug effects.
- Check appointment records for compliance with follow-up procedures.

## KEY CONCEPTS

- Propylthiouracil is the prototype thioamide antithyroid drug and is used alone to treat hyperthyroidism, as part of the preoperative preparation for thyroidectomy, before or after radioactive iodine therapy, and in the treatment of thyroid storm.

- The FDA no longer approves propylthiouracil for pediatric patients. Use is limited to patients who have developed minor toxic reactions to methimazole and who are not candidates for surgery or radioactive iodine treatment.

- The nurse helps ensure that patients who take antithyroid drugs are monitored closely for hypothyroidism, which may typically develop within a year after receiving treatment for hyperthyroidism.

- The FDA has issued **BLACK BOX WARNING ◆** for propylthiouracil. Severe liver injury resulting in death or acute liver failure may occur within 6 months of treatment. All patients should receive instruction about the signs and symptoms of acute liver failure. Routine liver function testing is necessary to assess for liver failure.

- Levothyroxine (Synthroid, Levoxyl), a synthetic preparation of $T_4$, is the drug of choice for long-term treatment of hypothyroidism.

- Thyroid replacement therapy in the patient with hypothyroidism is lifelong; no clear-cut guidelines exist regarding the duration of antithyroid drug therapy because exacerbations and remissions can occur. Replacement therapy usually continues until the patient is euthyroid for 6 to 12 months.

- For congenital hypothyroidism (cretinism), drug therapy should begin within 6 weeks of birth and continued for life, or mental retardation may result.

- People with hypothyroidism are especially likely to experience respiratory depression and myxedema coma with opioid analgesics and other sedating drugs.

- The FDA has issued a **BLACK BOX WARNING ◆** regarding the use of thyroid hormones for the treatment of obesity or for weight loss, either alone or with other therapeutic agents. Significant and serious complications may develop in euthyroid people who take thyroid hormones.

## CLINICAL REASONING CASE STUDY

| | |
|---|---|
| **Meet the Patient** | Rose Conley, a 72-year-old woman, is diagnosed with Graves' disease. She is tachycardic and extremely nervous. Her endocrinologist orders radioactive iodine.<br><br>• Why is radioactive iodine ordered in a patient with Graves' disease?<br>• What is the action of radioactive iodine?<br>• What condition is the patient at risk for in 1 year?<br>• What patient teaching should the nurse implement with Mrs. Conley? |
| **Assessing Drug Information** | • Radioactive iodine therapy is the treatment of choice for almost all patients with Graves' disease because it destroys thyroid tissue and thereby decreases production of thyroid hormones. Peak results take 6 to 12 weeks (several treatments may be necessary); however, a single dose controls hyperthyroidism in most patients. For hyperthyroidism, radioactive iodine is often preferred because it is associated with fewer adverse effects than other antithyroid drugs or surgery.<br>• Sodium iodide $^{131}I$ (Hicon) is a radioactive isotope of iodine. The thyroid gland cannot differentiate between regular iodide and radioactive iodide, so it picks up the radioactive iodide from the circulating blood. Small amounts of radioactive iodide can also be used as a diagnostic test of thyroid function.<br>• The drug is administered orally or parenterally, and the dosage is determined by a radiologist trained in nuclear medicine.<br>• The patient should be monitored closely for hypothyroidism, which usually develops within 1 year of receiving treatment for hyperthyroidism. |
| **Nursing Actions** | • After radioactive iodine therapy, tell Mrs. Conley not to expectorate or cough freely because saliva will be radioactive for 24 hours.<br>• Assess orthostatic blood pressure and monitor electrocardiographic readings, noting the heart rate and rhythm as well as the presence of dysrhythmias.<br>• Investigate reports of chest pain.<br>• Observe signs of severe thirst, dry mucous membranes, poor capillary refill, weak or thready pulse, and decreased urine output.<br>• Observe behavior indicative of level of anxiety.<br>• Encourage Mrs. Conley to initiate necessary lifestyle changes (e.g., planned rest periods, adequate nutrition, limited caffeine) and participate in the treatment regimen.<br>• Stress the need for keeping laboratory appointments for repeated measurement of serum $T_4$ levels.<br>• Emphasize the importance of continued medical follow-up.<br>• Teach Mrs. Conley and her significant others to watch for signs of hypothyroidism (see Table 42.1). |

Visit thePoint® at **http://thePoint.lww.com/Frandsen12e** for answers to NCLEX Success questions (in Appendix A), answers to Clinical Application Case Studies (in Appendix B), and more!

## REFERENCES AND RESOURCES

Hinkle, J. H., & Cheever, K. H. (2018). *Brunner & Suddarth's textbook of medical-surgical nursing* (14th ed.). Philadelphia, PA: Lippincott Williams & Wilkins.

Norris, T. L. (2019). *Porth's pathophysiology concepts of altered health states* (10th ed.). Philadelphia, PA: Wolters Kluwer.

UpToDate. (2019). *Drug Information*. Lexi-Comp, Inc.

Wall, A. E., Weaver, S. M., Litt, J., & Rae, L. (2017). Propylthiouracil-associated leukocytoclastic necrotizing cutaneous vasculitis: A case report and review of literature. *Journal of Burn Care & Research, 38*(3), e678–e685. doi:10.1097/BCR.0000000000000464

# Drug Therapy for Pituitary and Hypothalamic Dysfunction

## LEARNING OBJECTIVES

*After studying this chapter, you should be able to:*

1. Describe the functions of the anterior and posterior pituitary hormones as well as the hypothalamic hormones.
2. Identify the pathophysiology and clinical manifestations of central precocious puberty, acromegaly, growth deficiency in children, and diabetes insipidus.
3. Identify the prototype and describe the action, use, adverse effects, contraindications, and nursing implications of the anterior pituitary hormone used to treat growth hormone deficiency in children.
4. Identify the prototype and describe the action, use, adverse effects, contraindications, and nursing implications of the posterior pituitary hormone used to treat diabetes insipidus.
5. Identify the prototype and describe the action, use, adverse effects, contraindications, and nursing implications of the hypothalamic hormone drugs used to treat precocious puberty.
6. Identify the prototype and describe the action, use, adverse effects, contraindications, and nursing implications of the hypothalamic hormone drugs used to treat acromegaly.
7. Implement the nursing process in the care of the patient receiving specific pituitary and hypothalamic hormones.

## CLINICAL APPLICATION CASE STUDY

Jose Rojas is a 24-year-old man who has suffered a head injury while riding his motorcycle without a helmet. He has been admitted for observation, with multiple abrasions and a blow to the head. He begins to produce massive amounts of clear, pale-yellow urine. The health care provider diagnoses diabetes insipidus and orders desmopressin 0.2 mL intranasally in two divided doses.

## KEY TERMS

**Acromegaly:** a chronic disease, resulting from excessive secretion of growth hormone (GH); characterized by an abnormal pattern of bone and connective tissue growth associated with an increased incidence of diabetes mellitus and hypertension

**Antidiuretic hormone:** functions to regulate water balance; also known as vasopressin. This hormone is secreted when body fluids become concentrated and when blood volume is low

**Corticotropin:** anterior pituitary hormone obtained from animal pituitary glands; also referred to as adrenocorticotropic hormone. This hormone may be used as a diagnostic test to differentiate primary adrenal insufficiency from secondary adrenal insufficiency caused by inadequate pituitary secretion of corticotropin

**Corticotropin-releasing hormone or factor:** causes release of corticotropin in response to stress and threatening stimuli; most often secreted during sleep

**Dwarfism:** a condition marked by severely decreased linear growth and frequently severely delayed mental, emotional, dental, and sexual growth; some forms can be attributed to lack of growth hormone

**Gonadotropin-releasing hormone:** causes release of follicle-stimulating hormone and luteinizing hormone

**Growth hormone:** stimulates the growth of body tissues; regulates cell division and protein synthesis required for normal growth and promotes an increase in cell size and number, including growth of muscle cells and lengthening of bone

**Inhibiting hormone:** hormones produced in the hypothalamus that control the release of other hormones by inhibition of their release. The main inhibiting hormone in the hypothalamus uses somatostatin in communication with the anterior pituitary to inhibit somatropin

**Releasing hormone:** hormones produced by the hypothalamus to accelerate secretion of a major hormone of the pituitary gland
- Hypothalamus uses growth hormone–releasing hormone to communicate with the pituitary to release somatotropin
- Hypothalamus uses corticotropin-releasing hormone to communicate with the pituitary to release corticotropin
- Hypothalamus uses thyrotropin-releasing hormone to communicate with the pituitary to release thyrotropin
- Hypothalamus uses gonadotropin to communicate with the pituitary to release more gonadotropin

**Thyroid-stimulating hormone (thyrotropin):** regulates secretion of thyroid hormones

# INTRODUCTION

This chapter introduces the pharmacologic care of the patient experiencing increased or decreased function of the hormones secreted by the hypothalamus and pituitary gland. It focuses on drug therapy for chronic precocious puberty, acromegaly, growth hormone (GH) deficiency in children, and diabetes insipidus.

The hypothalamus of the brain and the pituitary gland interact to control most metabolic functions of the body and to maintain homeostasis (Fig. 43.1). They are anatomically connected by a funnel-shaped hypophyseal stalk. The hypothalamus controls secretions of the pituitary gland. The pituitary gland, in turn, regulates secretions or functions of other body tissues called target tissues. The pituitary gland is actually two glands, each with different structures and functions. The anterior pituitary is composed of different types of glandular cells that synthesize and secrete different hormones. The posterior pituitary is anatomically an extension of the hypothalamus and is composed mainly of nerve fibers. Although it does not manufacture any hormones itself, it stores and releases hormones synthesized in the hypothalamus. Hormones are chemical messengers with specific regulatory effect on the cells that control various bodily functions.

## OVERVIEW OF PITUITARY AND HYPOTHALAMIC DYSFUNCTION

### Physiology

#### Anterior Pituitary Hormones

The anterior pituitary gland produces seven hormones. Two of these, GH and prolactin, act directly on their target tissues; the other five act indirectly by stimulating target tissues to produce other hormones.

**Corticotropin,** also called adrenocorticotropic hormone (ACTH), stimulates the adrenal cortex to produce corticosteroids (see Chap. 17). The hypothalamus and plasma levels of cortisol, the major corticosteroid, control secretion of corticotropin. A negative feedback mechanism inhibits the release of cortisol when plasma levels are adequate for body needs. After corticotropin administration, there is a greater release of cortisol by way of negative feedback. Thus, the therapeutic effects are greater with corticotropin than with glucocorticoids, leading to a decrease in ACTH and changing the structure of the pituitary.

**Growth hormone** (GH, also called somatotropin) stimulates growth of body tissues. It regulates cell division and protein synthesis required for normal growth and promotes an increase in cell size and number, including growth of muscle cells and lengthening of bone. These effects occur mainly via altered metabolism of carbohydrate, protein, and fat by direct and indirect effects. Authorities often consider GH an insulin antagonist because it suppresses the abilities of insulin to stimulate uptake of glucose in peripheral tissues and enhance glucose synthesis in the liver. Paradoxically, administration of GH produces hyperinsulinemia by stimulating insulin secretion. In addition, GH stimulates protein anabolism in many tissues. The hormone also enhances fat utilization by stimulating triglyceride breakdown and oxidation in fat-storing cells.

Levels of GH rise rapidly during adolescence, peak in the 20s, and then start to decline. In children, deficient GH produces some forms of **dwarfism**, a condition marked by severely decreased linear growth and, frequently, severely delayed mental, emotional, dental, and sexual growth. If untreated, excessive GH in preadolescents produces gigantism, resulting in heights of 8 or 9 feet.

In adults, deficient GH (less than expected for age) can cause increased fat, reduced skeletal and heart muscle mass, reduced strength, reduced ability to exercise, and worsened cholesterol

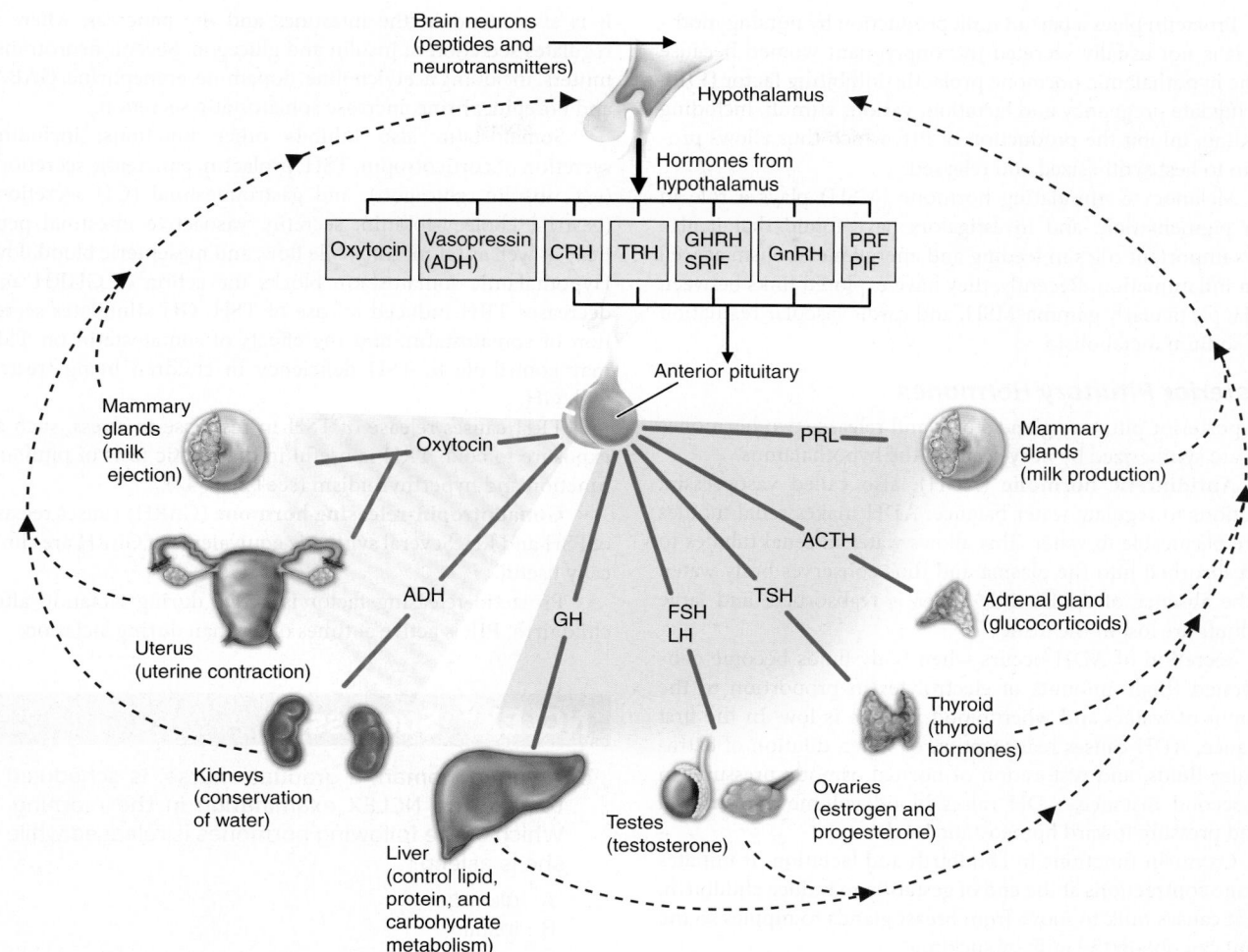

**Figure 43.1.** Hypothalamic and pituitary hormones and their target organs. The hypothalamus produces hormones that act on the anterior pituitary or are stored in the posterior pituitary. The anterior pituitary produces hormones that act on various body tissues and stimulate production of other hormones. ACTH, adrenocorticotropic hormone; ADH, antidiuretic hormone; CRH, corticotropin-releasing hormone or factor; FSH, follicle-stimulating hormone; GH, growth hormone; GnRH, gonadotropin-releasing hormone; LH, luteinizing hormone; PIF, prolactin-inhibiting factor; T₃, triiodothyronine; T₄, thyroxine; TRH, thyrotropin-releasing hormone; TSH, thyroid-stimulating hormone.

levels (i.e., increased low-density lipoprotein cholesterol and decreased high-density lipoprotein cholesterol), which increases the risk of cardiovascular disease. Excessive GH in adults produces **acromegaly**, a chronic disease characterized by an abnormal pattern of bone and connective tissue growth associated with an increased incidence of diabetes mellitus and hypertension.

**Thyroid-stimulating hormone** (TSH; also called thyrotropin) regulates secretion of thyroid hormones. Thyrotropin secretion is controlled by a negative feedback mechanism in proportion to metabolic needs. Thus, increased thyroid hormones in body fluids inhibit secretion of thyrotropin by the anterior pituitary and of thyrotropin-releasing hormone (TRH) by the hypothalamus.

Follicle-stimulating hormone (FSH), one of the gonadotropins, stimulates functions of sex glands. In people of both sexes, the anterior pituitary produces FSH, beginning at puberty. It acts on the ovaries in a cyclical fashion during the reproductive years, stimulating growth of ovarian follicles. These follicles then produce estrogen, which prepares the endometrium

for implantation of a fertilized ovum. FSH acts on the testes to stimulate the production and growth of sperm (spermatogenesis), but it does not stimulate secretion of male sex hormones.

Luteinizing hormone (LH; also called interstitial cell–stimulating hormone), another gonadotropin, stimulates hormone production by the gonads of both sexes. In women, LH is important in the maturation and rupture of the ovarian follicle (ovulation). After ovulation, LH acts on the cells of the collapsed follicular sac to produce the corpus luteum, which then produces progesterone during the last half of the menstrual cycle. When blood progesterone levels rise, a negative feedback effect acts on hypothalamic and anterior pituitary secretion of gonadotropins. Decreased pituitary secretion of LH causes the corpus luteum to die and stop producing progesterone. Lack of progesterone causes slough and discharge of the endometrial lining as menstrual flow. (Of course, if the ovum has been fertilized and attached to the endometrium, menstruation does not occur.) In men, LH stimulates the Leydig cells in the spaces between the seminiferous tubules to secrete androgens, mainly testosterone.

Prolactin plays a part in milk production by nursing mothers. It is not usually secreted in nonpregnant women because of the hypothalamic hormone prolactin-inhibiting factor (PIF). During late pregnancy and lactation, various stimuli, including suckling, inhibit the production of PIF, which thus allows prolactin to best synthesized and released.

Melanocyte-stimulating hormone (MSH) plays a role in skin pigmentation, and investigators have found that it also plays important roles in feeding and energy metabolism as well as in inflammation. Recently, they have explored links between MSH, particularly gamma-MSH, and cardiovascular regulation and sodium metabolism.

### Posterior Pituitary Hormones

The posterior pituitary gland stores and releases two hormones that are synthesized by nerve cells in the hypothalamus.

**Antidiuretic hormone** (ADH), also called vasopressin, functions to regulate water balance. ADH makes renal tubules more permeable to water. This allows water in renal tubules to be reabsorbed into the plasma and thus conserves body water. In the absence of ADH, little water is reabsorbed, and large amounts are lost in the urine.

Secretion of ADH occurs when body fluids become concentrated (high amounts of electrolytes in proportion to the amount of water) and when blood volume is low. In the first instance, ADH causes reabsorption of water, dilution of extracellular fluids, and restoration of normal osmotic pressure. In the second instance, ADH raises blood volume and arterial blood pressure toward homeostatic levels.

Oxytocin functions in childbirth and lactation. It initiates uterine contractions at the end of gestation to induce childbirth, and it causes milk to move from breast glands to nipples so the infant can obtain the milk by suckling.

### Hypothalamic Hormones

The hypothalamus produces **releasing hormones** and **inhibiting hormones**. Their primary purpose is to control the release of other hormones produced by the anterior pituitary gland, either by stimulating or by inhibiting their release.

**Corticotropin-releasing hormone or factor** (CRH or CRF) causes release of corticotropin in response to stress and threatening stimuli. Secretion of CRH most often occurs during sleep; it is under the influence of several neurotransmitters. Acetylcholine and serotonin stimulate its secretion, and gamma-aminobutyric acid (GABA) and norepinephrine inhibit its secretion. ADH increases the ability of CRH to stimulate corticotropin secretion, and somatostatin and elevated levels of glucocorticoids decrease or prevent this ability. Health care providers use CRH in the diagnosis of Cushing's disease, a disorder characterized by excess cortisol.

Growth hormone–releasing hormone (GHRH) causes release of GH in response to low blood levels of GH. The neurotransmitters dopamine, norepinephrine, epinephrine, GABA, acetylcholine, and serotonin stimulate the secretion of hypothalamic GHRH. Somatostatin blocks the stimulatory effect of GHRH on secretion of GH. Uses of GHRH include testing pituitary function and stimulating growth in children with GHRH deficiency.

As previously mentioned, somatostatin (growth-inhibiting hormone) inhibits release of GH and is distributed throughout the brain and spinal cord, where it functions as a neurotransmitter.

It is also found in the intestines and the pancreas, where it regulates secretion of insulin and glucagon. Several neurotransmitters, including acetylcholine, dopamine, epinephrine, GABA, and norepinephrine, increase somatostatin secretion.

Somatostatin also inhibits other functions, including secretion of corticotropin, TSH, prolactin, pancreatic secretions (e.g., insulin, glucagon), and gastrointestinal (GI) secretions (gastrin, cholecystokinin, secretin, vasoactive intestinal peptide) as well as GI motility, bile flow, and mesenteric blood flow. Hypothalamic somatostatin blocks the action of GHRH and decreases TRH-induced release of TSH. GH stimulates secretion of somatostatin, and the effects of somatostatin on TSH may contribute to TSH deficiency in children being treated with GH.

TRH causes release of TSH in response to stress, such as exposure to cold. TRH is useful in diagnostic tests of pituitary function and hyperthyroidism (see Chap. 42).

**Gonadotropin-releasing hormone** (GnRH) causes release of FSH and LH. Several synthetic equivalents of GnRH are clinically useful.

Prolactin-releasing factor is active during lactation after childbirth. PIF is active at times other than during lactation.

## Pathophysiology and Clinical Manifestations

### Precocious Puberty

Children diagnosed with precocious puberty develop secondary sexual characteristics prior to the age of 9 (boys) and 7½ to 8 (girls). The Lawson Wilkins Pediatric Endocrine Society recommends that African American girls who develop breast and/or pubic hair prior to age 6 and Caucasian girls who develop these characteristics prior to the age of 7 be evaluated for precocious puberty. The three types of precocious puberty involve different pathologic processes.

The first type, central precocious puberty, is also known as gonadotropin-dependent precocious puberty. The cause of this disorder is early maturation of the hypothalamic–pituitary–gonadal axis. Breast enlargement and pubic hair development occur in girls, and testicular enlargement and pubic hair development occur in boys. Other signs of this disorder include accelerated linear bone growth, increased bone age, and pubertal levels of some gonadal hormones (FSH and LH in girls; testosterone in boys). Idiopathic central precocious puberty is often due to the presence of genetic variants that are associated with early puberty. The most common lesion that results in central precocious puberty is hamartomas. These are benign tumors of the tuber cinereum. Central nervous system (CNS) irradiation rarely results in the development of central precocious puberty, but it can result in GH deficiency.

The second type, peripheral precocity, also known as gonadotropin-independent precocious puberty, is a result of excess secretion of the estrogen and androgen sex hormones from the gonads or adrenal glands. In girls, pituitary tumors are rare but do cause this type of precocious puberty. Exposure to estrogen creams used by menopausal care providers of girls may also lead to precocious puberty. A follicular cyst of the ovaries is the most common cause of peripheral precocity. Ovarian tumors may also cause peripheral precocity. In boys, Leydig cell tumors may be the cause. These tumors, which result in an asymmetric enlargement of the testes, are benign; surgical removal is appropriate.

The third type, benign or nonprogressive pubertal variants previously called incomplete precocious puberty, is isolated breast development in girls or hormone-mediated characteristics (e.g., acne or axillary or pubic hair) in boys. It is necessary to confirm the diagnosis using radiographic examination of the bone age—determining when the epiphyseal maturation is marginally advanced.

## Acromegaly

Acromegaly results from persistent hypersecretion of GH due to the presence of a somatotroph adenoma of the anterior pituitary or a hypothalamic tumor that releases GHRH. The hypersecretion of GH then results in the liver secretion of insulin-like growth factor 1 (IGF-1). This activity produces the clinical manifestations of acromegaly. The diagnosis of acromegaly should be ruled out in patients who present with typical clinical features of GH excess. The onset of these clinical manifestations is slow, as is its progression. Patients may complain of headaches with visual changes. Women have menstrual abnormalities, hot flashes, and vaginal atrophy from decreased estrogen levels. Men have erectile dysfunction, diminished libido, and decreased testicular size. Other signs and symptoms are thickening of the skin, linear bone growth, and enlargement of the liver, lungs, kidney, thyroid, and heart. High serum levels of GH and IGF-1 result in impaired glucose tolerance, hyperinsulinism, and insulin resistance.

## Growth Hormone Deficiency in Children

The definition of growth deficiency in children is growth below the third percentile of the established normal values. There are several causes of GH deficiency. Mutation of a transcription factor (POUF1; also known as PIT-1) leads to variable recessive peptide hormone deficiencies that may be associated with anterior pituitary hypoplasia. Also, mutation of a transcription factor (PROP1), which causes a failure to activate POUF1/PIT-1 gene expression, results in pituitary hypoplasia and/or familial multiple pituitary hormone deficiency. In addition, mutations in the anterior pituitary cells are sources of GH deficiency.

Idiopathic short stature is present when a child's stature falls below two standard deviations of the mean for age. The child has no endocrine, metabolic, or other condition to account for the GH deficiency.

## Diabetes Insipidus

Diabetes insipidus is a condition that results from a dysfunction in the posterior pituitary lobe. Excretion of large quantities of dilute urine results due to a deficiency in the production of ADH. With the absence of ADH, the kidneys filter the water but do not reabsorb it. When this occurs, the circulating fluid volume decreases, producing increased thirst and large amounts of urine production.

Diabetes insipidus may be idiopathic, hereditary, or acquired. Causes include lesions in the posterior pituitary, hypothalamus, or infundibular stem that interfere with ADH synthesis, transport, and release. These lesions in the CNS can be the result of a tumor, aneurysm, or thrombus. Other causes are the removal of the pituitary gland, immunologic disorders, or infections.

Characteristic features include polyuria, with excretion of dilute urine ranging from 4 L to as much as 30 L; extreme polydipsia, with the consumption of copious amounts of water or other fluids; and hypernatremia, with increased serum osmolality. The dehydration produces dizziness, weakness, and weight loss. Children present with enuresis, irritability, diminished sleep, and decreased weight gain along with diminished linear growth. If diabetes insipidus goes untreated, it may produce circulatory collapse and CNS depression or damage in both adults and children.

### Clinical Application 43.1

- How has Mr. Rojas' head injury contributed to the development of diabetes insipidus?
- Why is he producing large amounts of dilute urine?

### NCLEX Success

4. A nurse is educating grandparents about child safety. Which of the following prevents precocious puberty?
   A. keeping acetaminophen out of a child's reach
   B. keeping estrogen cream out of a child's reach
   C. keeping nitroglycerin paste out of a child's reach
   D. keeping hydrocortisone out of a child's reach

5. Two weeks ago, a 4-year-old girl fell from a backyard swing and hit her head. Her mother states her potty-trained daughter has been wetting the bed for the past 3 nights. What do you suspect the bedwetting is related to?

A. regression in development due to changes in the home
B. drinking juices prior to bedtime
C. a urinary tract infection
D. possible diabetes insipidus

6. A man has received a diagnosis of acromegaly. Which of the following symptoms can cause alterations in the man's psychosocial integrity?

A. increased libido
B. tachycardia
C. increased linear growth
D. erectile dysfunction

## Drug Therapy

Although pituitary and hypothalamic hormones have few therapeutic uses, they have important functions when used in certain circumstances. Hypothalamic hormones are synthesized into drug formulations that are administered to treat endometriosis, metastatic breast cancer, advanced prostate cancer, uterine fibroid tumors, vasoactive intestinal tumors, and diarrhea, as well as central precocious puberty. Manufacturers have

**TABLE 43.1**

### Drugs Administered for the Treatment of Hypothalamic Hormonal Changes

| Drug Class | Prototypes | Other Drugs in the Class |
|---|---|---|
| Hypothalamic hormones | Leuprolide acetate (Lupron) Octreotide acetate (Sandostatin, Sandostatin LAR Depot) | Goserelin (Zoladex) Histrelin (Vantas, Supprelin LA) Lanreotide (Somatuline Depot) Nafarelin (Synarel) Pasireotide (Signifor, Signifor LAR) Triptorelin (Trelstar Mixject) |

synthesized more drug formulations. Tables 43.1 and 43.2 list the exogenous hormones used in the treatment of hormonal dysfunction.

## ANTERIOR PITUITARY HORMONE DRUGS FOR GROWTH DEFICIENCY IN CHILDREN

The prototype anterior pituitary hormone is GH. Administered therapeutically, GH is not natural but rather synthesized from bacteria using recombinant DNA technology. **Somatropin**

**TABLE 43.2**

### Drugs Administered for the Treatment of Pituitary Hormonal Changes

| Hormone | Hormonal Action |
|---|---|
| **Anterior Pituitary Hormones** | |
| Corticotropin (Acthrel, HP Acthar Gel) | Stimulates the synthesis of hormones by the adrenal cortex |
| Cosyntropin (Cortrosyn) | Stimulates the adrenal cortex to synthesize and secrete adrenocortical hormones |
| Follitropin alfa/beta (Follistim AQ, Gonal-F, Gonal-F RFF Redi-Ject) | Stimulates ovulation |
| Human chorionic gonadotropin (Pregnyl) | Induces ovulation |
| Menotropins (Menopur) | Induces ovulation |
| Pegvisomant (Somavert) | GH receptor antagonist |
| Recombinant chorionic gonadotropin alpha (Ovidrel) | Induces ovulation |
| Somatropin (Genotropin, Humatrope, Norditropin, Nutropin, Serostim) | Stimulates skeletal, linear, muscle, and organ growth |
| Thyrotropin alfa (Thyrogen) | Stimulates the secretion of thyroglobulin |
| Urofollitropin (Bravelle) | Stimulates ovulation |
| **Posterior Pituitary Hormones** | |
| Desmopressin (DDAVP, Stimate) | Increases the permeability of renal tubular epithelium to cAMP leading to concentrated urine |
| Vasopressin (Vasostrict) | Increases cAMP |
| Oxytocin (Pitocin) | Increases uterine contractility |

(Genotropin, Humatrope; others) is therapeutically equivalent to endogenous GH produced by the anterior pituitary gland.

## Pharmacokinetics

Somatropin is well absorbed. Most of the drug is metabolized in the liver and kidneys. A small amount is excreted unchanged by the kidneys.

## Action

Somatropin has the same sequence of amino acids as endogenous GH; it stimulates skeletal, linear, muscle, and organ growth. Stimulation of cartilage growth at the epiphyseal plate promotes linear growth. Lean body mass and bone mass increase, and fat mass decreases. Stimulation of erythropoietin results in an increase of red blood cells. The drug increases protein synthesis and hepatic glucose output. Absorption of nutrients from the GI tract improves.

## Use

The main clinical use of somatropin is for children whose growth is impaired by a deficiency of endogenous GH. The drug is ineffective when impaired growth results from other causes or after puberty, when epiphyses of the long bones have closed. Also, it is useful in the treatment of growth failure associated with chronic kidney disease as well as short stature associated with Turner's syndrome, being born small for gestational age, Prader-Willi syndrome, idiopathic short stature, certain genetic mutations, and Noonan's syndrome. In addition, somatropin is useful in adults with GH deficiency. Table 43.3 gives route and dosage information for somatropin and other anterior pituitary hormone drugs.

### TABLE 43.3

### DRUGS AT A GLANCE: Anterior Pituitary Hormone Drugs

| Drug | Pregnancy Category | Routes and Dosage Ranges | |
|---|---|---|---|
| | | Adults | Children |
| **Somatropin** (Genotropin, Humatrope, Norditropin, Nutropin, Serostim; ❋ Omnitrope, Genotropin GoQuick, Genotropin MiniQuick, Humatrope, Norditropin, NordiFlex, Norditropin Simplex, Nutropin AQ NuSpin, Nutropin AQ pen, Saizen, Serostim) | C | Humatrope, adjust dose based on individual requirements ≤0.006 mg/kg and gradually increase to maximum of 0.0125 mg/kg subcutaneously daily<br>Norditropin, begin at 0.004 mg/kg subcutaneously daily and increase to maximum of 0.016 mg/kg daily after 6 wk | 0.18–0.3 mg/kg/wk subcutaneously divided equally and given six times weekly or once daily |
| Corticotropin (Acthar; ❋ ACTH 40) | C | Diagnostic use, up to 80 units IM, subcutaneous as a single injection HP Acthar Gel, 40–80 units IM, subcutaneous every 24–72 h 80–120 units IM daily for 2–3 wk | Infants and children <2 y: 75 units/m²/dose twice daily IM for 2 wk; followed by a gradual taper over a 2-wk period |
| Cosyntropin (Cortrosyn; ❋ Cortrosyn, Synacthen Depot) | C | 0.25 mg IM, IV (equivalent to 25 units ACTH) | Older than 2 y, same as adult dose<br>Younger than 2 y, 0.125 mg IM, IV |
| Human chorionic gonadotropin (hCG) (Novarel, Pregnyl; ❋ Pregnyl) | X | Ovulation induction: IM: 5000–10,000 units 1 d following last dose of menotropin<br>Cryptorchidism and male hypogonadism: 500–4000 units IM 2–3 times per week for several weeks | Preadolescent boys, cryptorchidism and hypogonadism: see adult dose |
| Recombinant chorionic gonadotropin alpha (Ovidrel; ❋ Ovidrel) | X | 250 mcg subcutaneous in 1 dose, 1 d after treatment with menotropins | |
| Follitropin alfa/beta (Gonal-t, Gonal-F RFF Redi-Ject; ❋ Gonal-F, Gonal-F Pen) | X | 75 IU subcutaneous of FSH to maximum daily dose of 300 units<br>Prefilled pen, 300–900 IU IV of FSH as individualized dosage | |

(*Continued on page 872*)

| TABLE 43.3 | | | |
|---|---|---|---|
| **DRUGS AT A GLANCE: Anterior Pituitary Hormone Drugs** (Continued) | | | |

| Drug | Pregnancy Category | Routes and Dosage Ranges | |
|---|---|---|---|
| | | **Adults** | **Children** |
| Menotropins (Menopur; ❋ Menopur) | X | Initially 225 units subcutaneously; can be increased to maximum daily dose of 450 units for a maximum of 20 d to be followed by hCG to induce ovulation | |
| Pegvisomant (Somavert; ❋ Somavert) | C | Load, 40 mg subcutaneous Maintenance, 10 mg daily subcutaneous, titrate by 5 mg increments or decrements every 4–6 wk according to IGF-1 levels to maximum of 30 mg/d | |
| Thyrotropin alfa (Thyrogen; ❋ Thyrogen) | C | 0.9 mg IM every 24 h for 2 doses or every 72 h for 3 doses | Younger than 16 y, dosage not established |
| Urofollitropin | X | 150 IU subcutaneous of FSH daily for the first 5 d Adjust dose every 2 d as needed to maximum daily dose of 450 units | |

## Use in Children

When constituting somatotropin for infants, it is important to reconstitute the medication in sterile water. Risk of malignancy is increased in children with short stature who receive the drug. It is contraindicated in children with Prader-Willi syndrome suffering from severe obesity because of the risk of respiratory failure.

## Use in Older Adults

Reduced dosages may be necessary to minimize adverse effects. Patients who are 65 years of age or older may be more sensitive to the action of GH. Clinicians should avoid using GH in the elderly except as hormone replacement following pituitary gland removal. Treatment should begin at the low end of the dosage range.

## Use in Patients With Renal or Hepatic Impairment

Although chronic renal impairment or severe hepatic disease decreases renal or hepatic metabolism, respectively, there are no recommended dosing changes in patients with renal or hepatic dysfunction. Patients on dialysis should take somatropin before bedtime or 3 to 4 hours after the procedure. Children receiving the drug for chronic renal insufficiency should take it until renal transplantation.

## Use in Patients With Critical Illness

It is important not to initiate somatropin in patients with acute critical illness because of complications following open heart or abdominal surgery, trauma, or acute respiratory failure. Increased mortality may occur.

## Adverse Effects

Adverse effects are not common and are fewer in children than in adults. Mild edema, headache, localized muscle pain, weakness, and hyperglycemia may occur. Patients with diabetes are more likely to develop hyperglycemia; they require close monitoring, and diabetic medications may require adjustment. Antibodies to the drug may develop, but this does not interfere with its growth-stimulating effects. Otitis media may occur in children. Hypersensitivity reactions are possible.

Patients with chronic renal failure, Turner's syndrome, and Prader-Willi syndrome are at increased risk for intracranial hypertension; symptoms include headache, papilledema, visual changes, nausea, and vomiting. When intracranial hypertension occurs, it is important to stop treatment, but it is appropriate to start the drugs again after symptoms resolve.

A special set of warnings accompanies the use of somatropin in treating short stature in patients with Prader-Willi syndrome. Fatalities have been reported following the use of somatropin in these patients. Risk factors associated with these fatalities are severe obesity, sleep apnea, respiratory impairment, respiratory infection, and male sex. It is essential to discontinue use of somatropin if any signs of upper airway obstruction occur or if snoring develops or increases.

## Contraindications

Contraindications to somatropin include closed epiphyses, pre-proliferative or severe nonproliferative diabetic retinopathy, active malignancy, acute critical illness (as described previously), or active underlying intracranial lesions. Patients with Prader-Willi syndrome who have severe obesity or severe respiratory impairment should not take the drug.

Caution is necessary in hypothyroidism, GH deficiency caused by intracranial lesions, and diabetes.

## Nursing Implications

### Preventing Interactions

Long-term use of corticotropin or corticosteroids inhibits the growth response to somatropin. Patients require monitoring to determine this lack of effect. Somatropin decreases insulin sensitivity, resulting in hyperglycemia. Patients most at risk for increased insulin sensitivity are those with obesity, Turner's syndrome, or a family history of diabetes mellitus. Antihyperglycemic drugs may require dosage adjustments.

### Administering the Medication

Administration may be subcutaneous or intramuscular (IM). The subcutaneous route is preferred; here are guidelines for its use:

- To prepare the solution, inject the supplied diluent into the vial containing the drug by aiming the stream of liquid against the glass wall of the vial.
- Swirl the vial gently. Do not shake it.
- After reconstitution, make sure the solution is clear. Do not inject a cloudy solution.
- Rotate injection sites.
- Store the reconstituted drug in the refrigerator; use within the time period recommended by the manufacturer.
- If the patient develops sensitivity to the diluent, reconstitute the drug with sterile water for injection. When administering the drug to infants, use only sterile water as the diluent. With sterile water, administer only one dose per vial and use the reconstituted drug within 24 hours; discard any unused portion.
- There is a preservative-free form of somatropin. Not all forms are approved for IM injection.
- Administer the correct dosage daily.

For patients on hemodialysis, give the drug before bedtime or 3 to 4 hours after dialysis. For long-term cycling peritoneal dialysis, give the drug in the morning after completion of dialysis. For long-term ambulatory dialysis, give the drug in the evening at the time of the overnight exchange.

>  **QSEN Alert: Safety**
>
> When administering somatropin, it is essential that after one nurse calculates the dosage, another nurse rechecks the calculation.

### Assessing for Therapeutic Effects

The nurse observes for increased skeletal growth and development. Appropriate increases in height and weight should occur. It is necessary to measure the child's height frequently. The child should take somatropin until a satisfactory height has been achieved, epiphyseal closure occurs, or until no further stimulation of growth occurs. Periodic tests of growth curve and bone age are also important.

### Assessing for Adverse Effects

It is important to have periodic tests of serum glucose levels and thyroid function as well as frequent eye examinations. Monitoring of serum and urine calcium should occur. Hypercalciuria may develop within 2 to 3 months after the start of therapy. Assess the patient for flank pain and colic. Patients who fail to respond to somatropin should receive testing for GH antibodies. Children who have GH deficiency may develop slipped capital femoral epiphyses more frequently, and those

with scoliosis may see a progression of the condition. The nurse assesses the patient for severe hip or knee pain or the development of a limp.

The nurse carefully assesses patients with malignancies or GH deficiency secondary to an intracranial lesion to ensure that enlargement or recurrence of the lesion is not occurring. Reportedly, there is an increased risk of a second neoplasm in adults who had cancer as children and who have been treated with somatropin. It is necessary to monitor patients with Prader-Willi syndrome carefully for signs of respiratory infection.

### Patient Teaching

Box 43.1 presents patient teaching information for somatropin.

## Other Anterior Pituitary Hormone Drugs

Corticotropin (HP Acthar Gel), which is obtained from animal pituitary glands, is mainly of historical interest. Corticotropin (ACTH) is effective in treating infantile seizures in patients 2 months to 2 years of age. For therapeutic purposes, adrenal corticosteroids have replaced it. It may be used occasionally as a diagnostic test to differentiate primary adrenal insufficiency (Addison's disease, which is associated with atrophy of the adrenal gland) from secondary adrenal insufficiency caused by inadequate pituitary secretion of corticotropin. However, cosyntropin (Cortrosyn), a synthetic formulation, is more commonly used to test for suspected adrenal insufficiency (see Chap. 45).

>  **QSEN Alert: Patient-Centered Care**
>
> Acute relapses of multiple sclerosis with new or worsening neurologic symptoms that persist for greater than 24 hours and are not attributable to heat overexertion or infection can be treated with repository corticotropin injection. This treatment is particularly beneficial in patients who are allergic to corticosteroid therapy. The exact mechanism of action of the drug is unknown, but it has been attributed to its ability to stimulate the adrenal corticosteroids, leading to an indirect modulation of multiple inflammatory processes.

Human chorionic gonadotropin (hCG) produces physiologic effects similar to those of naturally occurring LH. In males, it is used to evaluate the ability of Leydig cells to produce testosterone, to treat hypogonadism caused by pituitary deficiency, and to treat cryptorchidism (undescended testicle) in preadolescent boys. In females, recombinant hCG choriogonadotropin alpha (Ovidrel) is used in combination with menotropins to induce ovulation in the treatment of infertility. Excessive doses or prolonged administration can lead to sexual precocity, edema, and breast enlargement caused by oversecretion of testosterone and estrogen (see Chap. 6).

Menotropins (Menopur) are available in a gonadotropin preparation obtained from the urine of postmenopausal women that contains both FSH and LH. The drug is usually combined with hCG to induce ovulation in the treatment of infertility caused by lack of pituitary gonadotropins (see Chap. 6).

Pegvisomant (Somavert) is a GH receptor antagonist used in the treatment of acromegaly in adults who are unable to tolerate or are resistant to other management strategies. The drug selectively binds to GH receptors, blocking the binding of endogenous GH. In general, it is necessary to individualize the dosage according to response. Dosage reduction of hypoglycemic agents may be required because the drug may increase glucose tolerance. Increased dosages of pegvisomant may be necessary when administered with narcotics. Caution is warranted in the elderly and in renal or hepatic disease. At the initiation of therapy, baseline liver function tests should be assessed. Liver function should be assessed monthly for the first 6 months, quarterly for the next 6 months, and biannually the following year.

Thyrotropin alfa (Thyrogen) is a synthetic formulation of TSH used as a diagnostic adjunct for serum thyroglobulin testing in people with well-differentiated thyroid cancer who have previously undergone a thyroidectomy. The test may or may not involve radioiodine imaging. Because there is a risk of missing the diagnosis of thyroid cancer. Thyroid hormone withdrawal thyroglobulin testing radioactive imaging is the standard test for evaluating the presence, extent, and location of thyroid cancer. Thyrotropin alfa requires caution in patients with coronary artery disease and with a large amount of residual thyroid tissue; the drug produces a temporary rise of thyroid hormone concentration in the blood.

Urofollitropin and follitropin alfa/beta (Gonal-F) are drug preparations of FSH. The purpose of these drugs is to stimulate ovarian function in the treatment of infertility, and women may take them sequentially with hCG. Urofollitropin, which is extracted from the urine of postmenopausal women, acts directly on the ovaries to stimulate follicular ovulation. Follitropin alfa and follitropin beta are recombinant products that appear to be well tolerated and have similar efficacy. A new liquid formulation of follitropin alfa/beta (Gonal-F RFF Rediject) is available in a prefilled and ready-to-use multidose FSH injection (see Chap. 6).

## NCLEX Success

7. A boy with type 1 diabetes mellitus receives a prescription for somatropin. How will this medication affect the boy's insulin needs?

   A. His insulin needs will decrease.
   B. He will need a sulfonylurea added to his insulin.
   C. His insulin needs will remain the same.
   D. His insulin needs will increase.

8. A girl is taking somatropin. Her mother asks the nurse when her daughter will no longer need the medication. Which of the following is the nurse's best response?

   A. It will be stopped if she develops obesity.
   B. It will be stopped when she has stopped growing.
   C. It will be stopped when she no longer wants to take the medication.
   D. It will be stopped if she has a test showing that the epiphysis of the bone is open.

# POSTERIOR PITUITARY HORMONE DRUGS FOR DIABETES INSIPIDUS

**Desmopressin acetate** (DDAVP, Stimate) is the prototype posterior pituitary hormone medication. It is a synthetic analogue of ADH. It reduces urine volume and serum osmolality in patients with diabetes insipidus. It increases the reabsorption of water by the kidney.

## Pharmacokinetics

For the intranasal form, the onset of action is 15 to 30 minutes and the peak of action of 60 to 90 minutes. For the intravenous (IV) form, the onset of action is 30 minutes and peak of action is 1.5 to 2 hours. For the oral form, the onset of action is 60 minutes and the peak of action is 60 to 90 minutes. For the subcutaneous form, the onset of action, peak of action, and duration of action are unknown. For all forms, the duration of action is approximately 6 to 14 hours. The half-life of the intranasal, IV and subcutaneous, and oral preparations is approximately 3.5, 3, and 2 to 3 hours, respectively. Elimination of all forms of the medication takes place in the urine.

## Action

Desmopressin increases cyclic adenosine monophosphate (cAMP) in the cells of the renal tubule to increase the water permeability, decreasing urine volume and increasing its osmolality. The drug increases the plasma level of von Willebrand factor, clotting factor VIII, and tissue plasminogen activator (a protein involved in the breakdown of blood clots) to shorten the activated partial thromboplastin and bleeding times.

## Use

The main clinical use for desmopressin is for the treatment of neurogenic diabetes insipidus. However, synthetic hormones are useful for other purposes. Table 43.4 contains route and dosage information for desmopressin and other posterior pituitary hormones.

### Use in Patients With Renal Impairment

A creatinine clearance less than 50 mL/minutes contraindicates the use of desmopressin.

## Adverse Effects and Contraindications

Adverse effects of desmopressin reportedly occur in less than 5% of cases. The most common effects are erythema, swelling, and burning of the parenteral injection site. Other adverse effects include drowsiness, headache, dizziness, lethargy,

**TABLE 43.4**

**DRUGS AT A GLANCE: Posterior Pituitary Hormone Drugs**

| Drug | Pregnancy Category | Routes and Dosage Ranges | |
|---|---|---|---|
| | | **Adults** | **Children** |
| **Desmopressin** (DDAVP, Stimate;  DDAVP, Apo-Desmopressin) | C | Diabetes insipidus: intranasally 0.1–0.4 mL/d, in 1–3 doses, or, give 0.5–1 mL, IV or subcutaneously daily in two divided doses. For PO administration to adults and children over 4 y of age: Initially, 0.05 mg, orally twice daily Hemophilia A, von Willebrand's disease: IV 0.3 mcg/kg in 50 mL sterile saline, infused over 15–30 min (if used preoperatively give 30 min prior to procedure) | Diabetes insipidus: 3 mo to 12 y, 0.05–0.3 mL/d in 1–2 doses intranasally Hemophilia A, von Willebrand's disease: Weight more than 10 kg, same as adult dosage Weight 10 kg or less, 0.3 mcg/kg IV in 10 mL of sterile saline |
| Vasopressin (Vasostrict) | C | 0.25–0.5 mL (5–10 units) IM, subcutaneously, intranasally on cotton pledgets 2–3 times daily | 0.125–0.5 mL (2.5–10 units) IM, subcutaneously, intranasally on cotton pledgets 3–4 times daily |
| Oxytocin (Pitocin; Oxytocic Agent) | C | Induction of labor: initially, 10 units in 1000 mL of $D_5W$, lactated Ringer's, or normal saline infused IV at 0.5–2 mU/min titrated every 30–60 min until 9–10 mU/min or normal contraction pattern has been achieved Postpartum hemorrhage: 10–40 units in 1000 mL of $D_5W$, lactated Ringer's, or normal saline, IV, infused at rate to control bleeding, not to exceed 40 mU/min | |

shortness of breath, gastric irritation with heartburn, abdominal cramping, vulval pain, nasal congestion, and nasal irritation. The U.S. Food and Drug Administration (FDA) has issued a **BLACK BOX WARNING ◆** stating that severe hyponatremia may develop as a result of the medication, leading to seizures and death. Another **BLACK BOX WARNING ◆** stipulates that changes in fluid volume status may result in cardiac arrest in patients with known cardiovascular disease.

Contraindications include hypersensitivity to the drug or any component of its formulation.

## Nursing Implications

### Preventing Interactions

Several medications interact with desmopressin, increasing or decreasing its effects (Box 43.2).

**BOX 43.2   Drug Interactions: Desmopressin**

**Drugs That Increase the Effects of Desmopressin**
- Carbamazepine and chlorpropamide
  *Increase the risk of antidiuretic effects*
- Selective serotonin reuptake inhibitors and tricyclic antidepressants
  *Increase the risk of hyponatremia*

**Drugs That Decrease the Effects of Desmopressin**
- Alcohol
  *Decreases the diuretic effect*

### Administering the Medication

Guidelines for administration are as follows:

- Use the IM, IV, and subcutaneous preparations for central diabetes insipidus. Withdraw the dosage from the ampule and administer it using a small gauge needle and syringe (e.g., an insulin syringe).
- For hemophilia A, von Willebrand's disease (type 1), and prevention of surgical bleeding in patients with uremia, dilute in normal saline solution and infuse over 15 to 30 minutes.
- For intranasal administration, ensure that nasal passages are intact, clean, and free of obstruction before giving intranasally. The nasal spray pump delivers only doses of 10 mcg DDAVP. If doses other than these are necessary, use the nasal tube delivery system as directed below.
- Insert the top of the dropper into the tube in a downward position. Then squeeze the dropper until the solution reaches the desired calibrated dose and disconnect the dropper.
- Hold the tube 3/4 inch from the end and insert one end into the nostril until the fingertips reach the nostril. Place the opposite end into the patient's mouth while the patient holds his or her breath.
- Have the patient tilt the head back and blow into the tube, and into the nostril, with a strong, short puff. (In children, the nurse or an adult needs to blow into the tube.)

### Assessing for Therapeutic Effects

The desired therapeutic effects are decreased urine output, increased urine specific gravity, decreased signs of dehydration, and decreased thirst. It is important to assess the serum electrolytes, particularly the sodium and potassium levels. The sodium level should be 135 to 145 mEq/L. The nurse assesses serum osmolality; it should be in the normal range of 285 to 295 mOsm/kg H$_2$O. It is necessary to interview the patient to determine if he or she is thirsty. The nurse assesses skin turgor, mucous membranes, and production of tears for signs of rehydration. In patients with von Willebrand's disease, it is important to determine the factor VIII coagulant effect; the normal factor VIII is 55% to 145%.

### Assessing for Adverse Effects

The nurse assesses for hyponatremia, which can lead to diminished mental status and seizures. Serum osmolality may be less than 285 mOsm/kg H$_2$O. It is also necessary to assess fluid volume status for signs of dehydration, as well as urine output and urine specific gravity. Also, the nurse assesses the parenteral injection site for rash or erythema.

### Patient Teaching

Box 43.3 presents patient teaching information for desmopressin.

## Other Posterior Pituitary Hormone Drugs

Vasopressin (Vasostrict) once received approval from the FDA for the treatment of central diabetes insipidus, although it has since been discontinued. However, the Vasostrict formulation is used to increase blood pressure in patients experiencing septic or postcardiotomy syndrome. Patients with postcardiotomy syndrome have a febrile illness with inflammation of the pleura or pericardium. This condition can also occur following a myocardial infarction with the placement of a pacemaker. Therapeutically, vasopressin replaces ADH; the drug increases tubular reabsorption of water. It stimulates the arginine vasopressin, oxytocin, and purinergic receptors. The stimulation of these receptors yields an increase in systemic vascular resistance and mean arterial blood pressure to decrease the heart rate. In addition, the stimulation of the receptors causes an increase in cAMP, which in turn increases water permeability, decreasing urine output.

---

**BOX 43.3**  **Patient Teaching Guidelines for Desmopressin**

- Report drowsiness, headache, dizziness, lethargy, shortness of breath, gastric irritation with heartburn, abdominal cramping, vulval pain, nasal congestion, and nasal irritation to the health care provider.
- When using the DDAVP nasal spray pump, insert the top of the dropper into the tube in a downward position. Squeeze the dropper until the solution reaches the desired calibrated dose and disconnect the dropper. Then hold the tube 3/4 inch from the end and insert it into the nostril until the fingertips reach the nostril. Place the opposite end of the tube in the mouth while holding your breath. Tilt the head back and blow into the tube with a strong, short puff into the nostril.
- When administering subcutaneously, rotate injection sites.

---

Oxytocin (Pitocin) is a synthetic drug that exerts the same physiologic effects as the posterior pituitary hormone. Thus, it promotes uterine contractility and is used clinically to induce labor and in the postpartum period to control bleeding. It is essential that oxytocin be used only when clearly indicated and when the patient can be supervised by well-trained personnel, as in a hospital (see Chap. 6).

- What are the signs and symptoms of diabetes insipidus?
- What is the action of desmopressin?
- What is the therapeutic effect of desmopressin?
- How does the nurse administer desmopressin intranasally using a rhinal tube?

---

**NCLEX Success**

9. The nurse is administering intranasal desmopressin to a child. What does he or she need to do differently from administering this drug to an adult?

    A. The nurse should question the order, because intranasal desmopressin is contraindicated in children.

    B. The nurse should encourage the mother to administer the medication in the hospital.

    C. The nurse needs to blow in the tube to administer the medication.

    D. The nurse should use parenteral administration in the child.

10. A patient has just received desmopressin. Which electrolyte is most important to assess?

    A. sodium
    B. chloride
    C. potassium
    D. calcium

---

# HYPOTHALAMIC HORMONE DRUGS

## DRUGS FOR CENTRAL PRECOCIOUS PUBERTY

Ⓟ **Leuprolide acetate** (Eligard, Lupron) is equivalent to GnRH. The drug is more potent than the natural hormone.

## Pharmacokinetics

Leuprolide has a transient onset of action. The drug is 43% to 49% protein bound. It is metabolized to pentapeptide in the hypothalamus and anterior pituitary and is excreted in the urine.

## Action

An LH-releasing hormone agonist, leuprolide acts as a potent inhibitor of gonadotropin secretion, thus suppressing production of ovarian and testicular steroids. This action decreases LH and FSH to decrease testosterone in males and estrogen in females. (Testosterone levels are below levels required for reproduction.)

## Use

Leuprolide is useful for the treatment of central precocious puberty in children. Experts recommended that the drug be administered to girls until age 11 and boys until age 12. Other uses include treatment of advanced prostate cancer, and endometriosis and uterine fibroids. Table 43.5 gives route and dosage information for the hypothalamic hormones.

## Adverse Effects and Contraindications

The most common adverse effect of leuprolide is pain at the injection site. Less than 2% of the people who receive the drug have reported vasodilation, labile emotions, rash, acne, and allergic reaction.

Contraindications include known hypersensitivity to the medication's formulation, GnRH, or GnRH antagonists.

### TABLE 43.5

### DRUGS AT A GLANCE: Hypothalamic Hormones

| Drug | Pregnancy Category | Routes and Dosage Ranges | |
|---|---|---|---|
| | | **Adults** | **Children** |
| Ⓟ **Leuprolide acetate** (Eligard, Lupron Depot; 🍁 Eligard, Lupron, Lupron Depot) | X | Advanced prostate cancer: 1 mg subcutaneously daily<br>Endometriosis: 3.75 mg IM depot injection once monthly for up to 6 mo or 11.25 mg IM every 3 mo for up to 6 mo<br>Uterine fibroids: 3.75 mg IM depot injection once monthly for up to 3 consecutive mo or 11.25 mg IM depot injection for 1 dose | Central precocious puberty: 50 mcg/kg/d subcutaneously (may be titrated up to 10 mcg/kg/d) Depot-Ped, IM 5 kg or less, 7.5 mg 25–37.5 kg, 11.25 mg More than 37.5 kg, 15 mg every mo |
| Ⓟ **Octreotide acetate** (Sandostatin; 🍁 Sandostatin LAR) | B | Acromegaly: 50–100 mcg subcutaneous or IV 3 times daily; long-acting, give 20 mg, IM (intragluteally), at 4-wk intervals for 3 mo | Dosage not established |
| Goserelin (Zoladex; 🍁 Zoladex, Zoladex LA) | X<br>Pregnancy category D: with the treatment of breast cancer | Implant into upper abdominal wall, 3.6 mg subcutaneously every 28 d or 10.8 mg SC every 3 mo | |
| Histrelin (Vantas, Supprelin LA) | X | Implant, 1 subcutaneously every 12 mo | Central precocious puberty: Supprelin LA, implant subcutaneously every 12 mo |
| Lanreotide (Somatuline Depot; 🍁 Somatuline Autogel) | C | Subcutaneous: initial dose 90 mg once every 4 wk for 3 mo; after initial 90 d of therapy, adjust dose based on clinical response | ≥16 y: refer to adult dosing |
| Nafarelin (Synarel; 🍁 Synarel) | X | 1 spray (200 mcg) in one nostril in the morning and 1 spray in the other nostril in the evening (400 mcg/d), starting between the 2nd and 4th day of the menstrual cycle<br>If regular menstruation persists after 2 mo, may increase dose to 2 sprays in the morning and evening; total duration of therapy not to exceed 6 mo | Central precocious puberty: 2 sprays (400 mcg) in each nostril morning and evening (1600 mcg/d), until resumption of puberty is desired |
| Pasireotide (Signifor LAR; 🍁 Signifor LAR) | C | Initial 40 mg IM once every 28 d for patients who have not normalized IGF-1 levels after 3 mo; increase to a maximum dose of 60 mg | Dosage not established |
| Triptorelin (Trelstar Mixject; 🍁 Trelstar, Decapeptyl) | X | Advanced prostate carcinoma: 3.75 mg once every 4 wk, 11.25 mg once every 12 wk, or 22.5 mg once every 24 wk IM<br>Controlled ovarian hyperstimulation for assisted reproductive technologies: 0.1 mg subcutaneously once daily initiated on day 2 or 3 or days 21–23 of menstrual cycle | |

# Nursing Implications

## Preventing Interactions

Leuprolide may decrease the therapeutic effect of antidiabetic drugs, resulting in hyperglycemia.

## Administering the Medication

Administration of Lupron Depot should occur as a single injection. The depot suspension is stable for 24 hours after reconstitution. It is important to rotate the injection sites and not to use areas of the body that are compressed or rubbed.

## Assessing for Therapeutic Effects

The nurse assesses for a decrease in mature sexual characteristics. Gonadotropins (testosterone in males; estrogen in females) should decrease to prepubertal levels. These effects occur within 2 to 4 weeks after therapy has begun.

## Assessing for Adverse Effects

The nurse assesses for pain at the injection sites. It is also necessary to assess for signs of a hypersensitivity reaction to the medication such as a rash or erythema.

## Patient Teaching

Box 43.4 presents patient teaching information for leuprolide.

# Other Hypothalamic Hormone Drugs

Goserelin (Zoladex), histrelin (Vantas), nafarelin (Synarel), and triptorelin (Trelstar Mixject) are equivalent to GnRH. After initial stimulation of LH and FSH secretion, chronic administration of therapeutic doses inhibits gonadotropin secretion. This action results in decreased production of testosterone and estrogen, which is reversible when administration is stopped. In children with central precocious puberty, gonadotropins decline to prepubertal levels. As with leuprolide, these effects occur within 2 to 4 weeks of beginning drug treatment.

Oral administration of these GnRH equivalents is ineffective, because enzymes in the GI tract destroy the medication. Administration of most of these drugs is by injection; they are available in depot preparations that nurses can give once a month (or less often). Adverse effects are basically those of testosterone or estrogen deficiency. The drugs may also cause or aggravate depression.

---

**BOX 43.4**    *Patient Teaching Guidelines for Leuprolide*

- Administer the medication subcutaneously or intramuscularly.
- Use a calendar to mark the dates of future injections.
- Report any pain, burning, itching, or tingling of the injection site to the health care provider.
- A sexually active female prescribed leuprolide should use a nonhormonal form of birth control.

---

# DRUGS FOR ACROMEGALY

**Octreotide acetate** (Sandostatin, Sandostatin LAR Depot) has pharmacologic actions similar to the anterior pituitary hormone somatostatin. Scientists first synthesized this somatostatin analogue in 1979.

## Pharmacokinetics

Octreotide is rapidly and completely absorbed when given IV and subcutaneously with a rapid onset and a peak in 30 minutes. It is released slowly in the microsphere of the muscle; therefore, when given intramuscularly, the onset and duration is unknown, but the peak occurs in 1 to 2 weeks. Its half-life is 1.5 hours. Octreotide is metabolized in the liver and excreted by the kidneys.

## Action

Octreotide mimics the natural hormone somatostatin by inhibiting serotonin release. The drug also inhibits gastrin, vasoactive intestinal peptide, insulin, glucagon, secretin, motilin, and pancreatic polypeptide. In acromegaly, it suppresses GH and IGF-1. In fact, octreotide inhibits GH, glucagon, and insulin more than endogenous somatostatin. The drug also suppresses LH response to GnRH and the secretion of TSH.

## Use

Prescribers order octreotide for patients with acromegaly to reduce levels of GH. In addition, they use it to (1) treat secretory diarrhea and GI bleeding and (2) inhibit tumor GH and solid tumors. Table 43.5 presents route and dosage information for this drug.

### Use in Older Adults

In older adults, the elimination half-life of octreotide is 46% greater, and the drug's clearance is 26% less. Thus, it is necessary to reduce the dosage of the medication to the lower recommended range.

### Use in Patients With Renal and Hepatic Impairment

For patients on renal dialysis, it is essential to reduce the dosage of the drug by 50%. For those with cirrhosis of the liver, the initial dosage should be 10 mg intramuscularly over 4 weeks. It is necessary to titrate the dosage weekly based on the patient's response.

## Adverse Effects

Octreotide may cause CNS effects such as headache, dizziness, light-headedness, and fatigue. Cardiac effects such as bradycardia and heart failure may also occur. Other effects include hyperglycemia, pruritus, abdominal pain, loose stools, nausea, and cholelithiasis. Reportedly, approximately 20% of patients report back pain, myalgia, upper respiratory infections, and shortness of breath.

## Contraindications

Contraindications to octreotide include a known hypersensitivity to the drug or any component of the formulation. It is important to use the drug cautiously in patients with pancreatitis, gallbladder or bile disorders, cardiac abnormalities, diabetes, or nutritional disorders; the medication may cause or exacerbate these conditions.

## Nursing Implications

### Preventing Interactions

The combination of octreotide with alfuzosin, artemether, chloroquine, ciprofloxacin, dronedarone, indacaterol, levofloxacin, lumefantrine, pimozide, propafenone, quetiapine, quinine, tetrabenazine, thioridazine, toremifene, vandetanib, vemurafenib, and ziprasidone results in a prolonged QTc with an increased risk of ventricular dysrhythmia and cardiac arrest. The combination of octreotide and codeine increases the metabolism of codeine, and the combination of cyclosporine and octreotide decreases the serum concentration of cyclosporine. The administration of octreotide with food may alter the absorption of dietary fats. Many herbs increase the effects of octreotide (Box 43.5).

### Administering the Medication

Administration is by injection. It is important to administer the medication between meals to prevent fat malabsorption. Storage of the ampules requires refrigeration. For IV administration, dilute in 50 to 200 mL 5% dextrose in water or normal saline and infuse over 15 to 30 minutes. It may be given by IV push over 3 minutes.

With a depot injection, administration should occur immediately after the medication is mixed. The nurse administers the depot injections intramuscularly, deep in the intragluteal site—never in the deltoid. With an IM or subcutaneous injection, he or she rotates the sites of administration.

It is necessary to withdraw the drug for 4 weeks once per year.

### Assessing for Therapeutic Effects

The nurse assesses for diminished bone growth. He or she must interview the patient to determine if headaches and visual changes have subsided. Also, it is necessary to assess women for a decrease in hot flashes and regulation of the menstrual cycle.

### Assessing for Adverse Effects

The nurse assesses for alertness (e.g., Is there any fatigue?). It is necessary to interview the patient and ask about headache or light-headedness. The nurse checks the blood glucose for glucose tolerance. Approximately 2% to 27% of the patients develop hyperglycemia. Also, the nurse assesses the heart rate for bradycardia and an audible $S_3$, indicating the onset of heart failure. In addition, he or she assesses for abdominal pain, nausea, or pain between the shoulder blades, indicating the onset of cholelithiasis. Finally, it is important to check for musculoskeletal pain, fever, cough, and congestion, including the respiratory rate and effort that indicates the onset of shortness of breath.

### Other Drugs in the Class

Lanreotide (Somatuline Depot) is administered subcutaneously for the treatment of acromegaly and gastroenteropancreatic neuroendocrine tumor. It is important to assess for GI symptoms. It was reported that 20% of patients experience gallbladder-related symptoms and cholelithiasis.

Pasireotide (Signifor, Signifor LAR) is administered deep intramuscularly for acromegaly and Cushing's disease. The nurse assesses for elevation of aspartate aminotransferase and alanine aminotransferase as well as for bradycardia and QT prolongation. Hazardous drug handling protocols must be in place to administer this medication. Doing the receipt of the drug, unpacking the drug, and storing it, gloves must be worn.

### Patient Teaching

Box 43.6 presents patient teaching information for octreotide.

---

**BOX 43.5** 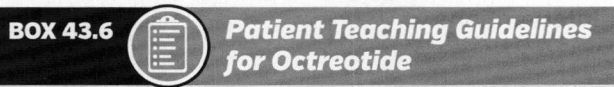 **Herb and Dietary Interactions: Octreotide**

**Herbs and Foods That Increase the Effects of Octreotide**
- Alfalfa
- Aloe
- Bilberry
- Bitter melon
- Burdock
- Celery
- Damiana
- Fenugreek
- Garcinia
- Garlic
- Ginger
- Ginseng
- Gymnema
- Marshmallow
- Stinging nettle

---

**BOX 43.6** **Patient Teaching Guidelines for Octreotide**

- Administer the medication subcutaneously or intramuscularly.
- Contact the health care provider to determine the time for withdrawal of the medication. It should be withdrawn for 4 weeks one time per year.
- Have follow-up diagnostic tests and keep the schedule of those tests.
- Monitor blood glucose.
- Notify the health care provider if abdominal pain or pain between the shoulder blades develops.
- Have follow-up gallbladder ultrasounds to detect cholelithiasis.

## NCLEX Success

11. A 30-year-old woman is receiving treatment for acromegaly. Her health care provider has prescribed octreotide for subcutaneous administration three times per day. What is the most important information to teach the patient?

    A. to rotate the sites of the injections and use the sites infrequently
    B. to administer all injections in the dorsogluteal muscle
    C. to administer the injections with food
    D. to take an antacid if you experience gastric upset

12. A man with acromegaly is planning a mission trip to Haiti to assist with rebuilding houses damaged in a recent earthquake. He is taking chloroquine to prevent malaria and octreotide for acromegaly. What is he at risk for developing?

    A. diarrhea
    B. ventricular dysrhythmia
    C. hepatotoxicity
    D. urinary retention

## THE NURSING PROCESS

A concept map outlines the nursing process related to drug therapy considerations in this chapter. Additional nursing implications related to the disease process should also be considered in care decisions.

**Assessment**

- Assess for disorders for which hypothalamic and pituitary hormones are given.
- Assess for the following:
  - For children with impaired growth, assess height and weight (actual and compared with growth charts) and diagnostic radiographic reports of bone age.
  - For patients with diabetes insipidus, assess baseline blood pressure, weight, ratio of fluid intake to urine output, urine specific gravity, and laboratory reports of serum electrolytes.

**Outcomes of Therapy**

The patient will
- Experience relief of symptoms without serious adverse effects.
- Take or receive the drug accurately.
- Adhere to procedures for monitoring and follow-up.

**Nursing Interventions**

- For children receiving GH, help the family set reasonable goals for increased height and weight and comply with accurate drug administration and follow-up procedures (e.g., periodic radiographs to determine bone growth and progress toward epiphyseal closure; recording height and weight at least weekly).
- For patients with diabetes insipidus, help them develop a daily routine to monitor their response to drug therapy (e.g., weigh themselves; monitor fluid intake and urine output for approximately equal amounts; check urine specific gravity [should be at least 1.015] and replace fluids accordingly).

**Evaluation**

- Interview and observe for adherence to instructions for taking the drug(s).
- Observe for relief of symptoms for which pituitary hormones were prescribed.
- Observe for effective coping with the underlying condition and the effects of treatment.

## KEY CONCEPTS

- The pituitary gland and the hypothalamus interact to control most metabolic functions of the body and to maintain homeostasis.
- Hormones are chemical messengers with specific regulatory effect on the cells that control various bodily functions.
- The hypothalamus produces a releasing hormone to accelerate the secretion of a given hormone or an inhibiting hormone that decreases hormone secretion that corresponds to each of the major hormones of the anterior pituitary gland.
- The anterior pituitary gland produces seven hormones. Two of these, GH and prolactin, act directly on their target tissues; the other five act indirectly by stimulating target tissues to produce other hormones.
- The posterior pituitary gland stores and releases two hormones that are synthesized by nerve cells in the hypothalamus.
- Children diagnosed with precocious puberty develop secondary sexual characteristics prior to the age of 9 in boys and 7½ to 8 in girls.
- Acromegaly is caused by persistent hypersecretion of GH due to the presence of a somatotroph adenoma of the anterior pituitary or a hypothalamic tumor that releases GHRH.
- The diagnosis of growth deficiency in children is established when the child's growth is below the third percentile for growth patterns of the established norm referenced charts. There are several causes of GH deficiency.

- Leuprolide is an LH-releasing hormone agonist that acts as a potent inhibitor of gonadotropin secretion to suppress ovarian and testicular steroid production.
- Diabetes insipidus is a condition that results from a dysfunction in the posterior pituitary lobe. An affected patient excretes large quantities of dilute urine due to a deficiency in the production of ADH (vasopressin).
- Octreotide acetate has pharmacologic actions similar to the anterior pituitary hormone somatostatin. Its many uses include acromegaly.
- GH administered therapeutically is not natural GH but rather GH synthesized from bacteria by recombinant DNA technology. Somatropin is therapeutically equivalent to endogenous GH produced by the anterior pituitary gland.
- The posterior pituitary hormone medications are desmopressin acetate and vasopressin. They are synthetic equivalents of ADH. Oxytocin is a synthetic drug that exerts the same physiologic effects as the posterior pituitary hormone.
- The FDA has issued a **BLACK BOX WARNING** ◆ stating that patients taking desmopressin can develop hyponatremia, leading to seizures and death.
- Another **BLACK BOX WARNING** ◆ states that changes in fluid volume status associated with the administration of desmopressin can lead to cardiac arrest in patients with known cardiovascular disease.

## CLINICAL REASONING CASE STUDY

**Meet the Patient**

A pediatrician diagnoses a 1-year-old girl with growth hormone deficiency. To treat the condition, the primary care provider prescribes somatropin 0.06 mg/kg intramuscularly three times per week. The girl weighs 22 lbs.

- How much somatropin should the child receive?
- What is the action of somatropin?
- What should the nurse teach the mother about the medication?

**Assessing Drug Information**

- Calculate the child's weight in kilograms.

$$\frac{22}{2.2} = 10 \text{ kg}$$

- Calculate the dosage of somatropin to be administered three times per week.

$$10 \text{ kg} \times 0.06 \text{ mg/kg} = 0.6 \text{ mg}$$

Thus, the child should receive 0.6 mg (intramuscularly) three times per week.

- Somatropin, which has the same sequence of amino acids as endogenous growth hormone, stimulates skeletal, linear, muscle, and organ growth. Stimulation of cartilage growth at the epiphyseal plate promotes linear growth. Lean body mass and bone mass increase, and fat mass decreases. Also, stimulation of erythropoietin increases red blood cells. In addition, the drug increases protein synthesis and hepatic glucose output, and improves absorption of nutrients from the gastrointestinal tract.

**Nursing Actions**

- Explain the importance of follow-up visits and diagnostic tests.
- Explain the expected rate of linear growth and the importance of measuring the height at intervals. Report any lack of progress to the health care practitioner.
- Explain the increased risk of slipped capital epiphyses. Report any new-onset limping or hip or knee pain.
- Instruct the family how to monitor glucose level as ordered by the health care practitioner.
- Instruct the mother about how to administer the drug.
- Observe the mother administering the drug.

*Visit* thePoint® *at* **http://thePoint.lww.com/Frandsen12e** *for answers to NCLEX Success questions (in Appendix A), answers to Clinical Application Case Studies (in Appendix B), and more!*

## REFERENCES AND RESOURCES

Glaze, D. G. (2020). Management and prognosis of infantile spasms. In *UpToDate*. Lexi-Comp, Inc.

Harrington, J., & Palmert, M. R. (2020). Definition, etiology, and evaluation of precocious puberty. In *UpToDate*. Lexi-Comp, Inc.

Hinkle, J. H., & Cheever, K. H. (2018). *Brunner & Suddarth's textbook of medical-surgical nursing* (14th ed.). Philadelphia, PA: Wolters Kluwer.

Kutz, C. F., & Dix, A. L. Repository corticotropin injection in multiple sclerosis: an update. *Neurodegenerative Disease Management, 8*(4), 217–225.

Liddle, R. A. (2016). Physiology of somatostatin and its analogues. In *UpToDate*. Lexi-Comp, Inc.

Melmed, S., & Katzneson, L. (2020). Diagnosis of acromegaly. In *UpToDate*. Lexi-Comp, Inc.

Norris, T. L. (2019). *Porth's pathophysiology concepts of altered health states* (10th ed.). Philadelphia, PA: Wolters Kluwer.

*Nursing 2020 drug handbook*. (2020). Philadelphia, PA: Wolters Kluwer.

UpToDate. (2020). *Drug information*. Lexi-Comp, Inc.

# Drug Therapy to Regulate Calcium and Bone Metabolism

## LEARNING OBJECTIVES

*After studying this chapter, you should be able to:*

1. Examine the roles of parathyroid hormone, calcitonin, and vitamin D in regulating calcium metabolism.

2. Evaluate the use of calcium and vitamin D supplements, as well as calcitonin, in the treatment of osteoporosis.

3. Identify the prototype and describe the action, use, adverse effects, contraindications, and nursing implications of the bisphosphonates used in the treatment of osteoporosis.

4. Outline appropriate management strategies of hypercalcemia as a medical emergency.

5. Implement the nursing process in the care of the patient receiving drug therapy to regulate calcium and bone metabolism.

## CLINICAL APPLICATION CASE STUDY

Carolyn Taylor, a 68-year-old retired teacher, has chronic venous insufficiency and osteoporosis. She has suffered two fractures from falls in recent years. Mrs. Taylor has been menopausal for 16 years and has not been on estrogen replacement therapy due to her vascular disease. Her health care provider prescribes alendronate once weekly.

## KEY TERMS

**Bisphosphonates:** class of drugs that binds to bone and inhibits calcium resorption from bone

**Calcitonin:** hormone from the thyroid gland whose secretion is controlled by the concentration of ionized calcium in the blood flowing through the thyroid gland lowers serum calcium in the presence of hypercalcemia

**Hypercalcemia:** abnormally high blood calcium level (greater than 10.5 mg/dL)

**Hyperparathyroidism:** excessive production of parathyroid hormone (PTH)

**Hypocalcemia:** abnormally low blood calcium level (less than 8.5 mg/dL)

**Hypoparathyroidism:** insufficient production of PTH

**Osteoporosis:** decreased bone density and weak, fragile bones that often lead to fractures, pain, and disability

**Paget's disease:** inflammatory skeletal disease that affects older people

**Parathyroid hormone (PTH):** hormone secreted by the parathyroid gland secretion is stimulated by low serum calcium levels and inhibited by normal or high levels

**Tetany:** neuromuscular irritability characterized by numbness and tingling of the lips, fingers, and toes, twitching of facial muscle, spasms of skeletal muscle, carpopedal spasm, laryngospasm, and convulsions

**Vitamin D (calciferol):** fat-soluble vitamin that includes both ergocalciferol (obtained from foods) and cholecalciferol (formed by exposure of skin to sunlight) functions as a hormone and plays an important role in calcium and bone metabolism

# INTRODUCTION

Three hormones regulate calcium and bone metabolism—parathyroid hormone (PTH), calcitonin, and vitamin D—and act to maintain normal serum levels of calcium. When serum calcium levels are decreased, hormonal mechanisms raise them; when they are elevated, hormonal mechanisms lower them (Fig. 44.1). Overall, the hormones alter absorption of dietary calcium from the gastrointestinal (GI) tract, movement of

calcium from bone to serum, and excretion of calcium through the kidneys.

Disorders of calcium and bone metabolism include hypocalcemia, hypercalcemia, osteoporosis, Paget's disease, and bone breakdown associated with breast cancer and multiple myeloma. Drugs used to treat these disorders mainly alter serum calcium levels or strengthen bone. This chapter describes the characteristics of the hormones, calcium, phosphorus, and some associated disorders.

**Figure 44.1.** Hormonal regulation of serum calcium levels. When serum calcium levels are low (hypocalcemia), there is increased secretion of parathyroid hormone (PTH) and increased activation of vitamin D. These mechanisms lead to decreased loss of calcium in the urine, increased absorption of calcium from the intestine, and increased resorption of calcium from bone. These mechanisms work together to raise calcium levels to normal. When serum calcium levels are high (hypercalcemia), there is decreased secretion of PTH and increased secretion of calcitonin. These mechanisms lead to increased loss of calcium from the intestine and decreased resorption of calcium from bone. These mechanisms lower serum calcium levels to normal.

# OVERVIEW OF CALCIUM AND BONE METABOLISM

## Etiology and Pathophysiology

**Hypocalcemia**, a low serum calcium level, stimulates **parathyroid hormone (PTH)** secretion, and **hypercalcemia**, a high serum calcium level, inhibits it (a negative feedback system). Because phosphate is closely related to calcium in body functions, PTH also regulates phosphate metabolism. In general, when serum calcium levels increase, serum phosphate levels decrease, and vice versa. Thus, an inverse relationship exists between calcium and phosphate.

When the serum calcium level falls below the normal range, PTH raises the level by acting on bone, intestines, and kidneys. In bone, breakdown is increased, so that calcium moves from bone into the serum. In the intestines, there is increased absorption of calcium ingested in food (PTH activates vitamin D, which increases intestinal absorption). In the kidneys, there is increased reabsorption of calcium in the renal tubules and less

urinary excretion. The opposite effects occur with phosphate (PTH decreases serum phosphate and increases urinary phosphate excretion).

Calcium and phosphorus are discussed together because they are closely related physiologically. These mineral nutrients occur in many of the same foods, from which they are absorbed together. Calcium and phosphorus both play critical roles in cellular structure and function and, as calcium phosphate, in formation and maintenance of bones and teeth. Box 44.1 summarizes their characteristics and functions.

Disorders of parathyroid function are related to **hypoparathyroidism** (insufficient production of PTH) or **hyperparathyroidism** (excessive production of PTH). Most often, the cause of hypoparathyroidism is removal of or damage to the parathyroid glands during neck surgery. Most often, the cause of hyperparathyroidism is a tumor or hyperplasia of a parathyroid gland. It also may result from ectopic secretion of PTH by malignant tumors (carcinomas of the lung, pancreas, kidney, ovary, prostate gland, or bladder). Clinical manifestations and treatment of hypoparathyroidism are the

---

**BOX 44.1**    *Characteristics and Functions of Calcium and Phosphorus*

### Calcium

Calcium is the most abundant cation in the body. Approximately 99% is located in the bones and teeth; the rest is in the extracellular fluid and soft tissues. Approximately half of serum calcium is bound, mostly to serum proteins, and is physiologically inactive. The other half is ionized and physiologically active. Ionized calcium can leave the vascular compartment and enter cells, where it participates in intracellular functions. An adequate amount of free (ionized) calcium is required for normal function of all body cells.

Of the calcium obtained from the diet, only 30% to 50% is absorbed from the small intestine; the rest is lost in feces. Absorption is increased in the presence of vitamin D, lactose, moderate amounts of fat, and high protein intake; increased acidity of gastric secretions; and a physiologic need. Absorption is inhibited by vitamin D deficiency; a high-fat diet; the presence of oxalic acid (from beet greens, chard), which combines with calcium to form insoluble calcium oxalate in the intestine; alkalinity of intestinal secretions, which leads to formation of insoluble calcium phosphate; diarrhea or other conditions of rapid intestinal motility, which do not allow sufficient time for absorption; and immobilization.

Calcium is lost from the body in feces, urine, and sweat. Even when there is deficient intake, approximately 150 mg is lost daily through the intestines (in mucosal and biliary secretions and sloughed intestinal cells). In lactating women, relatively large amounts are lost in breast milk.

### Functions

- Calcium participates in many metabolic processes, including the regulation of:
  - Cell membrane permeability and function
  - Nerve cell excitability and transmission of impulses (e.g., it is required for release of neurotransmitters at synapses)
  - Contraction of cardiac, skeletal, and smooth muscles
  - Conduction of electrical impulses in the heart

- Blood coagulation and platelet adhesion processes
- Hormone secretion
- Enzyme activity
- Catecholamine release from the adrenal medulla
- Release of chemical mediators (e.g., histamine from mast cells)
- Calcium is required for building and maintaining bones and teeth. Bone calcium is composed mainly of calcium phosphate and calcium carbonate. In addition to these bound forms, a small amount of calcium is available for exchange with serum. This acts as a reserve supply of calcium. Calcium is constantly shifting between bone and serum as bone is formed and broken down. When serum calcium levels become low, calcium moves into serum.

### Requirements and Sources

The calcium requirement of normal adults is approximately 1000 mg daily. Increased daily amounts are needed by growing children (1300 mg), pregnant or lactating women (1200 mg), and postmenopausal women (1200 mg to prevent osteoporosis).

The best sources of calcium are milk and milk products. Three 8-oz glasses of milk daily contain approximately the amount needed by healthy adults. Calcium in milk is readily used by the body because milk also contains lactose and vitamin D, both of which are involved in calcium absorption. Other sources of calcium include vegetables (e.g., broccoli, spinach, kale, mustard greens) and seafood (e.g., clams, oysters).

### Phosphorus

Phosphorus is one of the most important elements in normal body function. Most phosphorus is combined with calcium in bones and teeth as calcium phosphate (~80%). The remainder is distributed in every body cell and in extracellular fluid. It is combined with carbohydrates, lipids, proteins, and various other compounds.

*(Continued on page 886)*

Phosphorus is obtained from the diet, and approximately 70% of dietary phosphorus is absorbed from the GI tract. The most efficient absorption occurs when calcium and phosphorus are ingested in approximately equal amounts. Because this equal ratio is present in milk, milk is probably the best source of phosphorus. In general, factors that increase or decrease calcium absorption act the same way on phosphorus absorption. Vitamin D enhances, but is not essential for, phosphorus absorption. Large amounts of calcium or aluminum in the GI tract may combine with phosphate to form insoluble compounds and thereby decrease absorption of phosphorus.

Phosphorus is lost from the body primarily in urine. In people with acute or chronic renal failure, phosphorus intake is restricted because excretion is impaired.

### Functions

Phosphorus, most of which is located intracellularly as the phosphate ion, performs many metabolic functions:

- It is an essential component of deoxyribonucleic acid, ribonucleic acid, and other nucleic acids in body cells. Thus, it is required for cell reproduction and body growth.
- It combines with fatty acids to form phospholipids, which are components of all cell membranes in the body. This

reaction also prevents buildup of excessive amounts of free fatty acids.

- It forms a phosphate buffer system, which helps to maintain acid–base balance. When excess hydrogen ions are present in kidney tubules, phosphate combines with them and allows their excretion in urine. At the same time, bicarbonate is retained by the kidneys and contributes to alkalinity of body fluids. Although there are other buffering systems in the body, failure of the phosphate system leads to metabolic acidosis (retained hydrogen ions or acid and lost bicarbonate ions or base).
- It is necessary for cellular use of glucose and production of energy.
- It is necessary for proper function of several B vitamins (i.e., the vitamins function as coenzymes in various chemical reactions only when combined with phosphate).

### Requirements and Sources

Daily requirements for phosphorus are approximately 700 mg for normal adults and 1250 mg for growing children and pregnant or lactating women. Phosphorus is widely available in foods. Good sources are milk and other dairy products, meat, poultry, fish, eggs, and nuts. There is little risk of phosphorus deficiency with an adequate intake of calcium and protein.

same as those of hypocalcemia. Clinical manifestations and treatment of hyperparathyroidism are the same as those of hypercalcemia.

**Calcitonin** is a hormone from the thyroid gland whose secretion is controlled by the concentration of ionized calcium in the blood flowing through the thyroid gland. When the serum level of ionized calcium increases, secretion of calcitonin increases. The function of calcitonin is to lower serum calcium in the presence of hypercalcemia, which it does by decreasing movement of calcium from bone to serum and increasing urinary excretion of calcium. The action of calcitonin is rapid but of short duration. Thus, this hormone has little effect on long-term calcium metabolism.

**Vitamin D (calciferol)** is a fat-soluble vitamin that includes both ergocalciferol (obtained from foods) and cholecalciferol (formed by exposure of the skin to sunlight). It functions as a hormone and plays an important role in calcium and bone metabolism. The main action of vitamin D is to raise serum calcium levels by increasing intestinal absorption of calcium and mobilizing calcium from bone. It also promotes bone formation by providing adequate serum concentrations of minerals. Vitamin D is not physiologically active in the body. It must be converted to an intermediate metabolite in the liver and then to an active metabolite (1,25-dihydroxyvitamin D or calcitriol) in the kidneys. PTH and adequate hepatic and renal function are required to produce the active metabolite.

Deficiency of vitamin D causes inadequate absorption of calcium and phosphorus. This, in turn, leads to low levels of serum calcium and stimulation of PTH secretion. In children, this sequence of events produces inadequate mineralization of bone (rickets), a rare condition in the United States. In adults, vitamin D deficiency causes osteomalacia, a condition characterized by decreased bone density and strength.

Bone is a mineralized connective tissue that functions as structural support and a reservoir for calcium, phosphorus,

magnesium, sodium, and carbonate. The role of bone in maintaining serum calcium levels takes precedence over its structural function (bone may be weakened or destroyed as calcium leaves bone and enters serum). Bone tissue is constantly being formed and broken down in a process called remodeling. Bone tissue removal is referred to as resorption. During childhood, adolescence, and early adulthood, formation usually exceeds breakdown (resorption) as the person attains adult height and peak bone mass. After approximately 35 years of age, resorption is greater than formation. **Osteoporosis** occurs when bone strength (bone density and bone quality) is impaired, leading to increased porousness and vulnerability to fracture. Hormonal deficiencies, some diseases, and some medications (e.g., glucocorticoids) can also increase resorption, resulting in loss of bone mass and osteoporosis. Table 44.1 presents an overview of the prevention and treatment of osteoporosis.

## Clinical Manifestations

The calcium disorders are hypocalcemia and hypercalcemia, either of which can be life threatening. Hypocalcemic emergencies, for example, may result in **tetany** (neuromuscular irritability). The bone disorders discussed in this chapter are those characterized by increased resorption of calcium and loss of bone mass. These disorders weaken the bone, possibly leading to osteoporosis, with fractures, pain, and disability. Box 44.2 describes the selected calcium and bone disorders.

## Drug Therapy

Health care providers use a variety of drugs to regulate calcium and bone metabolism:

- Treatment of hypocalcemia and prevention and treatment of osteoporosis: calcium and vitamin D supplements

## TABLE 44.1

## Prevention and Treatment of Osteoporosis

| Prevention/Treatment | Rationale |
|---|---|
| Adequate dietary intake of calcium at all ages<br>Calcium supplementation if needed | Promotes normal bone development and maintenance<br>Promotes peak bone mass<br>Allows for more bone loss before osteoporosis develops |
| Adequate dietary intake of vitamin D<br>Vitamin D supplementation if at risk (older adults and patients on chronic corticosteroid therapy) | Ensures adequate stores of vitamin D to maintain normal serum and bony calcium |
| Lifestyle changes<br>Adequate exercise<br>Smoking cessation | Vigorous, weight-bearing exercise promotes and maintains strong bone<br>Smoking decreases the amount of active estrogen that accelerates bone loss |
| Use of bisphosphonates (e.g., alendronate) | Used for prevention and treatment<br>Reduces bone resorption and increases bone mass and strength |
| Preventive measures for patients on chronic corticosteroid therapy (prednisone >7.5 mg daily)<br>Calcium and vitamin D supplements<br>Lifestyle changes<br>Use of bisphosphonates<br>Use of low doses of corticosteroids or nonsystemic route, if possible | Corticosteroids decrease calcium absorption, increasing risk of osteoporosis. Lower doses or nonsystemic routes decrease corticosteroid effect on calcium absorption |
| Preventive measures for patients taking phenytoin<br>Calcium and vitamin D supplements<br>Drug treatment if bone density is low | Phenytoin increases hepatic metabolism of vitamin D |
| Treatment in women (if actual bone loss is present)<br>Calcium/vitamin D supplements<br>Alendronate 10 mg daily or 70 mg weekly<br>OR<br>Risedronate 5 mg daily or 35 mg weekly or 150 mg monthly<br>Dose reduction if on corticosteroids | Bisphosphonates decrease the rate of bone breakdown, slow the rate of bone loss, increase bone mineral density, reduce the risk of vertebral fractures, and slow the progression of vertebral deformities and loss of height |
| Treatment in men<br>Calcium/vitamin D supplements<br>Use of bisphosphonates<br>Testosterone supplements<br>Dose reduction if on corticosteroids | Low testosterone levels may contribute to osteoporosis in men |

- Treatment of hypercalcemia: bisphosphonates, calcitonin, corticosteroids, 0.9% sodium chloride intravenous (IV) infusion, and other agents
- Treatment of osteoporosis: bisphosphonates, calcitonin, estrogens, and antiestrogens

### Clinical Application 44.1

- Mrs. Taylor, who has osteoporosis, should take preventive measures in addition to taking her prescribed medication. One important measure is to increase the intake of foods that contain high levels of calcium. What dietary recommendations should the nurse make?

### ! QSEN Alert: Evidence-Based Practice

In study results published in 2018, Bajger reviewed 12 studies comparing patients' preferences and satisfaction using oral bisphosphonates compared with denosumab. Patients take oral bisphosphonates usually daily or weekly. Denosumab is administered subcutaneously every 6 months. Four major themes emerged. First, as to the attributes of the medications, patients favored medication regimens that were effective and convenient. The most likely reasons for stopping therapy were adverse effects and inconvenience. Second, comparing oral bisphosphonates with denosumab, patients preferred the convenience of twice-yearly injections of denosumab rather than daily or weekly bisphosphonates. Patients found the gastrointestinal adverse effects of oral bisphosphonates more intolerable than the skin infections and flulike symptoms associated with denosumab. Third, more patients adhered to the denosumab treatment regimen, preferring the more convenient administration schedule and less concern about adverse effects. Finally, what are the implications for practice? Patient satisfaction is an important factor in adherence to the treatment regimen. Patients who reported dissatisfaction with the treatment regimen were more likely to discontinue taking the medication. Practitioners must listen to patients' concerns and tailor drug regimens to fit individual needs and preferences.

### Hypocalcemia

Hypocalcemia is an abnormally low blood calcium level (i.e., less than 8.5 mg/dL). Causes may include inadequate intake of calcium and vitamin D, numerous disorders (e.g., diarrhea or malabsorption syndromes that cause inadequate absorption of calcium and vitamin D, hypoparathyroidism, renal failure, severe hypomagnesemia, hypermagnesemia, acute pancreatitis, rhabdomyolysis, tumor lysis syndrome, vitamin D deficiency), and several drugs (e.g., cisplatin, cytosine arabinoside, foscarnet, ketoconazole, pentamidine, agents used to treat hypercalcemia). Calcium deficits caused by inadequate dietary intake affect bone tissue rather than serum calcium levels. Two mechanisms result in hypocalcemia associated with renal failure. First, inability to excrete phosphate in urine leads to accumulation of phosphate in the blood (hyperphosphatemia). Because phosphate levels are inversely related to calcium levels, hyperphosphatemia induces hypocalcemia. Second, when kidney function is impaired, vitamin D conversion to its active metabolite is impaired. This results in decreased intestinal absorption of calcium.

Clinical manifestations are characterized by increased neuromuscular irritability, which may progress to tetany. Tetany is characterized by numbness and tingling of the lips, fingers, and toes; twitching of facial muscles; spasms of skeletal muscle; carpopedal spasm; laryngospasm; and convulsions. In young children, hypocalcemia may be manifested by convulsions rather than tetany and erroneously diagnosed as epilepsy. This may be a serious error because anticonvulsant drugs used for epilepsy may further decrease serum calcium levels. Severe hypocalcemia may cause lethargy or confusion.

### Hypercalcemia

Hypercalcemia is an abnormally high blood calcium level (i.e., greater than 10.5 mg/dL). It may be caused by hyperparathyroidism, hyperthyroidism, malignant neoplasms, vitamin D or vitamin A intoxication, aluminum intoxication, prolonged immobilization, adrenocortical insufficiency, and ingestion of thiazide diuretics, estrogens, and lithium. Cancer is a common cause, especially carcinomas (of the breast, lung, head and neck, or kidney) and multiple myeloma. Cancer stimulates bone breakdown, which increases serum calcium levels. Increased urine output leads to fluid volume deficit. This leads, in turn, to increased reabsorption of calcium in renal tubules and decreased renal excretion of calcium. Decreased renal excretion potentiates hypercalcemia. Patients at risk for hypercalcemia should be monitored for early signs and symptoms, so treatment can be started before severe hypercalcemia develops.

Clinical manifestations are caused by the decreased ability of nerves to respond to stimuli and the decreased ability of

muscles to contract and relax. Hypercalcemia has a depressant effect on nerve and muscle function. GI problems with hypercalcemia include anorexia, nausea, vomiting, constipation, and abdominal pain. Central nervous system problems include apathy, depression, poor memory, headache, and drowsiness. Severe hypercalcemia may produce lethargy, syncope, disorientation, hallucinations, coma, and death. Other signs and symptoms include weakness and decreased tone in skeletal and smooth muscle, dysphagia, polyuria, polyphagia, and cardiac dysrhythmias. In addition, calcium may be deposited in various tissues, such as the conjunctiva, cornea, and kidneys. Calcium deposits in the kidneys (renal calculi) may lead to irreversible damage and impairment of function.

### Osteoporosis

Osteoporosis is characterized by decreased bone density (osteopenia) and weak, fragile bones that often lead to fractures, pain, and disability. Although any bones may be affected, common fracture sites are the vertebrae of the lower dorsal and lumbar spines, wrists, and hips. Risk factors include female sex, advanced age, small stature, lean body mass, White or Asian race, positive family history, low calcium intake, menopause, sedentary lifestyle, nulliparity, smoking, excessive ingestion of alcohol or caffeine, high protein intake, high phosphate intake, hyperthyroidism, and chronic use of certain medications (e.g., corticosteroids, phenytoin). Postmenopausal women are at high risk because of estrogen deficiency, age-related bone loss, and a low peak bone mass. Osteoporosis occurs in men but less often than in women. Both men and women who take high doses of corticosteroids are at high risk because the drugs demineralize bone. In addition, renal transplant recipients can acquire osteoporosis from corticosteroid therapy, decreased renal function, increased PTH secretion, and cyclosporine immunosuppressant therapy.

Osteopenia or early osteoporosis may be present and undetected unless radiography or a bone density measurement is done. If detected, treatment is needed to slow bone loss. If undetected or untreated, clinical manifestations of osteoporosis include shortened stature (a measurable loss of height), back pain, spinal deformity, or a fracture. Fractures often occur with common bending or lifting movements or falling.

### Paget's Disease

Paget's disease is an inflammatory skeletal disease that affects older people. Its etiology is unknown. It is characterized by a high rate of bone turnover and results in bone deformity and pain. It is treated with nonnarcotic analgesics and drugs that decrease bone resorption (e.g., bisphosphonates, calcitonin).

## CALCIUM PREPARATIONS

Calcium is available in many different forms. These preparations differ mainly in the amounts of calcium they contain and their routes of administration. It is important to note that even if people have normal serum levels of calcium, their diets may not contain enough calcium; they may need calcium supplements. Experts believe that the diets of most people of all ages, but especially of young women and older adults, are deficient in calcium.

## Pharmacokinetics and Action

Absorption of calcium occurs in the small intestine, where approximately one third of the amount consumed is actually absorbed. PTH and vitamin D increase the absorption of calcium. Excretion primarily occurs in the feces, with the remainder excreted by the kidneys. PTH decreases renal excretion of calcium.

Oral and IV calcium preparations replace lost calcium and help maintain normal calcium levels.

# Use

Oral calcium (e.g., calcium carbonate or calcium citrate) provides supplemental calcium when diet alone is insufficient to meet body requirements. Also, it is useful for treatment of chronic, nonemergent hypocalcemia, regardless of the cause. In addition, it provides relief from symptoms of acid indigestion and heartburn. Finally, it can decrease bone loss and fractures, especially in women. Calcium citrate is reportedly better absorbed than calcium carbonate.

IV calcium is essential for the treatment of acute, severe hypocalcemia, which is a medical emergency. It may be necessary to give repeated doses, to give a continuous infusion, or to use oral supplements to avoid symptoms of hypocalcemia and maintain normal serum calcium levels (measured every 4–6 hours). In calcium blocker overdose, calcium gluconate is given by IV infusion to help reverse the vasodilation and decreased myocardial contractility caused by the calcium channel blocker.

Table 44.2 gives route and dosage information for several calcium supplements.

## TABLE 44.2

## DRUGS AT A GLANCE: Calcium and Vitamin D Preparations

| Drug | Pregnancy Category | Routes and Dosage Ranges | |
|---|---|---|---|
| | | **Adults** | **Children** |
| **Oral Calcium Products** | | | |
| Calcium acetate (PhosLo; ❋ PhosLo) 25% calcium | C | 1334 mg PO with each meal; increase gradually to 2001–2668 mg with each meal | Limited data available<br>Individualize dose; initial dose 667–1000 mg with each meal; titrate to response |
| Calcium carbonate precipitated (Os-Cal, Tums; ❋ Apo-Cal, Os-Cal, Tums) 40% calcium | C | 500–4000 mg daily in 1–3 divided doses | 2–4 y: 750 mg twice daily<br>5–18 y: 750 mg three times daily |
| Calcium citrate (Cal-Citrate; ❋ Osteocit) 21% calcium | Not rated | 19–50 y: 1000 mg daily<br>Females 51 y and older: 1200 mg daily<br>Males 51–70 y: 1000 mg daily | 1–6 mo: 200 mg/d<br>7–12 mo: 260 mg/d<br>1–3 y: 700 mg/d<br>4–8 y: 1000 mg/d<br>9–18 y: 1300 mg/d |
| Calcium gluconate 9% calcium; (❋ Calcium Sandoz) | C | 19–50 y: 1000 mg/d<br>Females 51 y and older: 1200 mg/d<br>Males 51–70 y: 1000 mg/d | Same as above for calcium citrate |
| **Parenteral Calcium Products** | | | |
| Calcium chloride 10 mL of 10% solution contains 273 mg (13.6 mEq) of calcium; ❋ (Calciject) | C | Hypocalcemia: 200–1000 mg IV every 1–3 d | Hypocalcemia: 2.7–5 mg/kg/dose IV every 4–6 h |
| Calcium gluconate 10 mL of 10% solution contains 93 mg (4.65 mEq) of calcium; calcium gluconate preferred over calcium chloride | C | Hypocalcemia (IV)<br>Mild: 1000–2000 mg over 2 h<br>Moderate to severe: 4000 mg over 4 h<br>Severe (with seizures): 1000–2000 mg over 10 min; repeat until symptoms resolve | Hypocalcemia (infants, children, adolescents), 200–500 mg/kg/d IV as continuous infusion or in four divided doses; maximum dose infants/children, 1000 mg/dose; adolescents 2000–3000 mg/dose<br>Symptomatic (with seizures): 100–200 mg/kg/dose over 5–10 min; repeat after 6 h or follow with continuous infusion of 200–800 mg/kg/d |
| **Vitamin D Preparations** | | | |
| Calcitriol (Rocaltrol; ❋ Rocaltrol) | C | 0.25 mcg PO daily initially; then adjusted according to serum calcium levels (usual daily maintenance dose 0.5–1 mcg) | 1–5 y: 0.25–0.75 mcg PO daily<br>6 y or older: refer to adult dose |
| Cholecalciferol (vitamin D3) (Delta-D; D-Vi-Sol; ❋ D-Tabs; EURO-D) | C | DRI (19–70 y): 600 IU PO daily | DRI<br>Birth to 12 mo: AI, 400 PO IU/d<br>1–18 y: RDA, 600 PO IU/d |

*(Continued on page 890)*

**TABLE 44.2**

## DRUGS AT A GLANCE: Calcium and Vitamin D Preparations (Continued)

| Drug | Pregnancy Category | Routes and Dosage Ranges | |
|---|---|---|---|
| | | **Adults** | **Children** |
| Ergocalciferol (vitamin D2) (Calciferol, Drisdol; ✹ D-Forte, SANDOZ D-Forte) | C | 19–70 y: 600 IU/d PO | Same as cholecalciferol |
| Paricalcitol (Zemplar; ✹ Zemplar) | C | Secondary hyperparathyroidism associated with chronic renal failure: 0.04–0.1 mcg/kg IV every other day initially; increase by 2–4 mcg at 2- to 4-wk intervals if necessary; reduce dosage or stop therapy if hypercalcemia occurs | Secondary hyperparathyroidism associated with chronic renal failure 5 y and older: same as adults (small studies only) |

AI, adequate intake; DRI, dietary reference intake; RDA, recommended dietary allowance.

### Use in Older Adults

Hypocalcemia is uncommon in older adults because calcium moves from bone to blood to maintain normal serum levels. However, calcium deficiency commonly occurs because of long-term dietary deficiencies of calcium and impaired absorption of calcium from the intestine. As previously stated, osteoporosis is a concern in some women. Although osteoporosis develops in older men, it occurs less often, at a later age, and to a lesser extent than in older women. Both men and women who take corticosteroids are at risk for osteoporosis. The risk is higher with systemic corticosteroids but may also occur with oral or inhaled drugs, especially at higher doses.

### Use in Patients With Renal Impairment

Patients with renal impairment or failure often have disturbances in calcium and bone metabolism. Calcium acetate may be used to prevent or treat hyperphosphatemia. The calcium reduces blood levels of phosphate by reducing its absorption from foods. It binds with dietary phosphate to produce calcium phosphate, which is insoluble and excreted in feces.

## Adverse Effects

Hypercalcemia produces adverse effects in several body systems. GI effects include anorexia, nausea, vomiting, abdominal pain, and constipation. Central nervous system effects are apathy, poor memory, depression, drowsiness, and disorientation. Cardiac effects include dysrhythmias, and an electrocardiogram (ECG) shows a prolonged QT interval and an inverted T wave. Weakness and decreased tone in skeletal and smooth muscles, dysphagia, polyuria, and polydipsia may also occur.

## Contraindications

Contraindications to calcium preparations include cancer with bone metastases, as well as ventricular fibrillation, hypercalcemia, hypophosphatemia, and renal calculi.

## Nursing Implications

### Preventing Interactions

Several medications and foods interact with calcium supplements, increasing or decreasing their effects (Boxes 44.3 and 44.4).

Also, it is important to note that oral calcium preparations interfere with the absorption of numerous drugs, including atenolol and fluoroquinolones, when the calcium is taken at the same time. In the case of oral tetracyclines, the calcium combines with the antibiotic, preventing its absorption.

In addition, calcium preparations and digoxin have similar effects on the myocardium. Therefore, if a patient taking digoxin receives calcium, the risks of digoxin toxicity and cardiac dysrhythmias increase. It is essential to use this combination very cautiously. Use of calcium with phenytoin decreases absorption of both drugs. IV calcium antagonizes the effects of verapamil.

**BOX 44.3** **Drug Interactions: Calcium Preparations**

**Drugs That Increase the Effects of Calcium**
- Thiazide diuretics
  *Reduce calcium losses in the urine*
- Vitamin D
  *Increases absorption of calcium*

**Drugs That Decrease the Effects of Calcium**
- Calcitonin
  *Interferes with absorption of calcium*
- Corticosteroids (prednisone and others)
  *Lower calcium levels by various mechanisms*
- Phosphates
  *Lower calcium levels by various mechanisms*

## Administering the Medication

Calcium is available in many different forms; the nurse ensures that the form being given is the correct one. The nurse also makes sure to:

- Administer oral preparations with or after meals to increase absorption. If used as an antacid, administer after a meal.
- Administer oral preparations separately from atenolol and fluoroquinolones and more than 2 to 3 hours before or after giving oral tetracycline.
- Dilute IV preparations in a compatible fluid and administer slowly as a continuous infusion or in divided doses; check pulse and blood pressure closely; monitor the ECG if possible. IV solutions may cause dysrhythmias and hypotension if administered too rapidly.
  - Carefully observe the IV site during administration because IV calcium is irritating to tissues.
  - Do not administer parenteral forms intramuscularly.

## Assessing for Therapeutic Effects

The nurse observes for relief of symptoms of neuromuscular irritability and tetany, such as decreased muscle spasms, decreased paresthesias, absence of Chvostek's sign, and absence of Trousseau's sign. He or she also assesses laboratory results for return of serum calcium levels to the normal range of 8.5 to 10.5 mg/dL.

Once the hypocalcemia is stabilized, the aim of treatment is management of the underlying cause or prevention of recurrence. If diarrhea or malabsorption is the cause, treatment of the underlying condition decreases loss of calcium from the body and increases absorption. It is also necessary to measure serum magnesium levels; treatment of hypomagnesemia is essential before treatment of hypocalcemia can be effective.

## Assessing for Adverse Effects

The nurse assesses for increased thirst, inability to eat, and increased urination, as well as for constipation and abdominal pain. It is necessary to assess for diminished memory, disorientation, and drowsiness. The nurse checks the ECG for a prolonged QT interval and inverted T wave that results from hypercalcemia.

## Patient Teaching

Box 44.5 presents patient teaching guidelines for calcium preparations.

**Clinical Application 44.2**

- What instructions should the nurse give Mrs. Taylor about taking oral calcium supplements?

## NCLEX Success

1. The nurse must administer a tetracycline antibiotic to a patient who takes an oral calcium supplement with each meal. When should the nurse administer the tetracycline?

   A. 2 hours before meals
   B. 30 minutes before meals
   C. with meals
   D. 1 hour after meals

2. The nurse is administering a continuous IV infusion of calcium properly diluted in a compatible IV fluid. Which one of the following would it be most important for the nurse to monitor?

   A. cardiac rhythm
   B. urine output
   C. hearing changes
   D. musculoskeletal pain

# VITAMIN D

Vitamin D is a fat-soluble vitamin used in chronic hypocalcemia if calcium supplements alone cannot maintain serum calcium levels within a normal range. It is also used to prevent deficiency states and treat hypoparathyroidism and osteoporosis. Although authorities agree that dietary intake is better than supplements, some suggest a vitamin D supplement for people who ingest less than the recommended amount. The recommended dietary allowance, or RDA, for vitamin D is 15 mcg/day 1 to 70 years of age and 20 mcg/day for adults 71 years and older to prevent and treat osteoporosis. Adequate intake for infants 0 to 12 months is 10 mcg/day.

## Pharmacokinetics and Action

As a drug, vitamin D is absorbed from the GI tract. It is stored in the liver, skin, and other tissues for months. It is metabolized into its active form in the liver and kidneys. Half of an oral dose is eliminated in the bile.

Vitamin D increases calcium and phosphorus absorption from the GI tract. It also promotes movement of calcium and phosphorus from the bones to maintain normal serum calcium levels. In the kidneys, vitamin D decreases elimination of calcium and phosphorus.

## Use

Vitamin D is useful for the treatment of rickets, other vitamin D deficiency diseases, and hypoparathyroidism. It is important to take vitamin D supplements cautiously and not overuse them; excessive amounts can cause serious problems, including hypercalcemia. Table 44.2 gives route and dosage information for some vitamin D preparations.

Vitamin D is also useful if a calcium preparation alone cannot maintain serum calcium levels within a normal range. When vitamin D is given to treat hypocalcemia, frequent measurements of serum calcium levels determine dosage. Usually, people take higher doses initially, and lower doses are appropriate for maintenance therapy. Calcium salts and vitamin D are available over the counter in many combined preparations promoted as dietary supplements (Table 44.3). These mixtures are not indicated for maintenance therapy in chronic hypocalcemia.

### Use in Children

Authorities recommend vitamin D supplementation for infants who are partially or completely breast-fed because breast milk contains only small quantities of vitamin D.

### Use in Patients With Renal Impairment

Renal disease interferes with metabolism of vitamin D precursors to the active form of vitamin D in the kidneys. If vitamin D therapy is necessary for the treatment of osteomalacia associated with renal impairment, calcitriol (Rocaltrol) is preferable. Calcitriol is the active form of vitamin D and thus undergoes no metabolism.

| **TABLE 44.3** | | |
| --- | --- | --- |
| **Selected Calcium/Vitamin D Combination Products\*** | | |
| **Drug** | **Calcium (mg of Elemental Calcium)/ Tablet or Capsule** | **Vitamin D International Units/Tablet** |
| Caltrate 600 + D3 | 600 | 800 |
| Citracal Maximum | 315 | 250 |
| Citracal + D Slow Release | 600 | 500 |
| Citracal Calcium Gummies | 250 | 500 |
| Os-Cal Calcium + D3 | 500 | 200 |
| Os-Cal Extra + D3 | 500 | 600 |
| Os-Cal Chewable | 500 | 600 |

\*In general, the upper intake level for vitamin D is 100 mcg/d.

## Adverse Effects

The principal adverse effects of excessive vitamin D use are hypervitaminosis D and hypercalcemia. This is most likely to occur with chronic ingestion of high doses daily. In children, accidental ingestion may lead to acute toxicity. Of particular significance with vitamin D excess are kidney stones, irreversible kidney damage, and muscle and bone weakness. Box 44.2 discusses symptoms of hypercalcemia, such as tetany.

## Contraindications

Contraindications to vitamin D include hypercalcemia and vitamin D toxicity. It is necessary to withhold all preparations containing vitamin D.

## Nursing Implications

### Preventing Interactions

Several medications interact with vitamin D, increasing or decreasing its effects (Box 44.6).

**BOX 44.6    Drug Interactions: Vitamin D**

**Drugs That Increase the Effects of Vitamin D**
- Thiazide diuretics
  *Inhibit renal excretion*

**Drugs That Decrease the Effects of Vitamin D**
- Cholestyramine resin
  *Decreases the intestinal absorption of vitamin D*
- Mineral oil
  *Prevents the absorption of vitamin D*
- Phenytoin
  *Accelerates vitamin D metabolism in the liver*

## Administering the Medication

People may take vitamin D without regard to food. It is important not to take both the vitamin and magnesium-containing antacids or mineral oil.

## Assessing for Therapeutic Effects

The nurse observes for a decrease in symptoms of hypocalcemia and symptoms of rickets or osteomalacia. It is necessary to check that the following laboratory results are normal: serum calcium level, blood urea nitrogen and serum creatinine, and serum phosphate. Improved bone health, as documented by radiograph, should be evident.

## Assessing for Adverse Effects

It is important to monitor serum calcium. If hypercalcemia occurs, the nurse must stop the drug and notify the health care provider. It is necessary to observe for signs and symptoms of vitamin D excess, including headache, somnolence, weakness, irritability, hypertension, cardiac dysrhythmias, kidney stones, polydipsia, polyuria, and bone and muscle pain.

## Patient Teaching

Box 44.7 presents patient teaching guidelines for vitamin D.

### Clinical Application 44.3

- Mrs. Taylor has developed end-stage renal disease and receives hemodialysis three times per week. She requires a vitamin D supplement. Why would she receive the active form of vitamin D, calcitriol (Rocaltrol)?

### BOX 44.7 Patient Teaching Guidelines for Vitamin D

- Take vitamin D supplements only if recommended by your primary health care provider.
- Avoid unapproved over-the-counter drugs and magnesium-containing antacids.
- Immediately report early symptoms of vitamin D intoxication: weakness, nausea, vomiting, dry mouth, constipation, muscle or bone pain, and metallic taste.
- Be aware that certain drugs interact with vitamin D such as thiazide diuretics, phenytoin, cholestyramine resin, and mineral oil and increase or decrease the effects of the vitamin.
- Learn about good dietary sources of vitamin D. Food sources of vitamin D include cod-liver oil, oysters, mackerel, most fish, egg yolks, fortified milk, some ready-to-eat cereals, and margarine.
- Understand that a source of vitamin D besides diet is sunlight on the skin. Adequate sun exposure allows the body to produce enough vitamin D to meet daily requirements. Factors that limit vitamin D production through sun exposure include lack of exposure, geographic location, season, use of sunblock, and darker skin pigmentation.

# BISPHOSPHONATES

**Bisphosphonates** are drugs that bind to bone and inhibit calcium resorption from bone. Although indications vary, the drugs are used mainly in the treatment of hypercalcemia and osteoporosis. **Alendronate** (Fosamax) is the prototype bisphosphonate.

## Pharmacokinetics and Action

Alendronate is poorly absorbed from the intestinal tract. It is not metabolized. The drug bound to bone is slowly released into the bloodstream. Most of the drug that is not bound to bone is excreted in the urine.

Alendronate suppresses osteoclast activity on newly formed resorption surfaces, which reduces bone turnover. This means that bone formation exceeds resorption at remodeling sites, leading to progressive gains in bone mass.

## Use

Although the main use of alendronate is to prevent and treat osteoporosis in postmenopausal women, it is also used to treat osteoporosis in men. Other uses include the treatment of **Paget's disease**, an inflammatory bone disease that affects older people, and glucocorticoid-induced osteoporosis in both sexes. Table 44.4 gives route and dosage information for alendronate and other bisphosphonates.

### Use in Children

Alendronate is beginning to be used for disorders characterized by bone fragility and poor bone calcification such as osteogenesis imperfecta and osteopenia associated with cystic fibrosis. Another use is with osteopenia in nonambulatory patients (e.g., cerebral palsy or muscular dystrophy); patients who are unable to remain upright following administration may not be able to use the drug. Limited data exists for pediatric use. See Table 44.4.

### Use in Patients With Renal Impairment

Experts do not recommend using alendronate in severe renal impairment (creatinine clearance [CrCl] <35 mL/min).

## Adverse Effects

Adverse effects of alendronate are usually minor if the doses taken for prevention or treatment of osteoporosis are used and the drug is taken as directed. Patients who do not follow the dosing instructions are at greater risk for esophagitis, dysphagia, and esophageal ulcers/erosions. Other effects include headache, musculoskeletal pain (sometimes severe), and decreased serum calcium. More severe effects may occur with the higher doses taken for Paget's disease.

Rare adverse effects include atypical femur fracture and osteonecrosis of the jaw. Patients on long-term therapy are at greater risk for femur fracture. Greater risk of osteonecrosis of the jaw occurs with higher drug potency, higher cumulative dose, and parenteral route of administration. Experts recommend a drug holiday of 2 to 3 years for women with low risk for fracture after 3 to 5 years of bisphosphonate therapy (Aggarwal & Masuda, 2018).

## Contraindications

Contraindications to alendronate include hypersensitivity to the drug, abnormalities of the esophagus that delay esophageal

### TABLE 44.4

## DRUGS AT A GLANCE: Bisphosphonates

| Drug | Pregnancy Category | Routes and Dosage Ranges | |
|---|---|---|---|
| | | **Adults** | **Children** |
| Ⓟ **Alendronate** (Fosamax; ※ ACH-Alendronate, ACT Alendronate, etc.; multiple brand names) | C | Osteoporosis: Women (postmenopausal) Prevention: 5 mg once daily PO or 35 mg PO once weekly Treatment: 10 mg once daily PO or 70 mg PO once weekly Men: Same as women Glucocorticoid-induced disease: 10 mg PO once daily or 70 mg PO weekly Paget's disease: 40 mg PO daily for 6 mo; repeat if necessary CrCl ≥ 35 mL/min: No dosage adjustment CrCl < 35 mL/min: Use not recommended | Osteogenesis imperfecta: Children 2 y or older and adolescents 30 kg or less, 5 mg PO once daily; 30 to <40 kg, 5 or 10 mg PO once daily; 40 kg or greater, 10 mg PO once daily Osteopenia associated with cystic fibrosis: Children 5 y or older and adolescents 25 kg or less, 5 mg PO once daily; >25 kg, 10 mg PO once daily Osteopenia/osteoporosis, rheumatology patients: Children 4 y or older and adolescents 20 kg or less, 5 mg PO once daily; >20–30 kg, 5 or 10 mg PO once daily; >30 kg, 10 mg PO once daily |
| Ibandronate (Boniva) | C | Osteoporosis (postmenopausal women): Prevention: 150 mg PO every month Treatment: 150 mg PO every month or 3 mg IV every 3 mo | No use established |
| Pamidronate (Aredia; ※ PMS-Pamidronate; Pamidronate Disodium Omega) | D | Hypercalcemia of malignancy: 60–90 mg IV as a single dose over 2–24 h Breast cancer: 90 mg IV over 2 h every 3–4 wk Multiple myeloma: 90 mg IV over 4 h once monthly Paget's disease: 30 mg IV over 4 h once daily for 3 consecutive days | Hypercalcemia: Initial treatment 0.5–1 mg/kg IV (maximum dose 90 mg); repeat if needed at interval of 24 h or more Osteogenesis imperfecta: Infants/children <2 y: First cycle 0.25 mg/kg IV day one and then 0.5 mg/kg/dose IV days two and three; subsequent cycles 0.5 mg/kg/dose once daily for 3 d; repeat cycles every 2 mo for total 9 mg/kg yearly Children 2–3 y: First cycle 0.38 mg/kg IV day 1 and then 0.75 mg/kg/dose IV days two and three; subsequent cycles 0.75 mg/kg/dose once daily for 3 d; repeat cycles every 3 mo for total 9 mg/kg yearly Children >3 y and adolescents: First cycle 0.5 mg/kg IV day one and then 1 mg/kg/dose days two and three; subsequent cycles 1 mg/kg/dose once daily for 3 d; repeat cycles every 4 mo for total 9 mg/kg yearly |
| Risedronate (Actonel; ※ Actonel, Actonel DR) | C | Osteoporosis (postmenopausal women) Prevention/treatment: 5 mg PO once daily or 35 mg PO once weekly or 150 mg PO once monthly. If glucocorticoid induced, 5 mg PO once daily Paget's disease: 30 mg PO (immediate release) once daily for 2 mo | No use established |
| Zoledronic acid (Reclast, Zometa; ※ Aclasta, TARO-Zoledronic Acid) | D | Osteoporosis: 5 mg IV once per year Hypercalcemia of malignancy: 4 mg IV; max given as a single dose | No use established |

CrCl, creatinine clearance.

emptying, and inability to stand or sit upright for at least 30 minutes. People with hypocalcemia require correction of the low serum calcium levels before beginning therapy with alendronate.

Caution is warranted with active upper GI conditions.

## Nursing Implications

### Preventing Interactions

Several medications interact with alendronate, increasing or decreasing its effects (Box 44.8). Any food interferes with absorption of alendronate.

### Administering the Medication

The nurse ensures proper administration of alendronate. It is always necessary to take the drug with a full glass of water, not juice or coffee, at least 30 minutes before breakfast and before taking other drugs. The person must remain upright (either with head elevated 90 degrees if in bed, sitting upright in a chair, or standing) for at least 30 minutes after administration. These interventions promote absorption and decrease esophageal and gastric irritation.

### Assessing for Therapeutic and Adverse Effects

The nurse observes for improved bone density and absence of fractures. Early osteopenia and osteoporosis are asymptomatic. Measurement of bone density is the only way to quantify bone loss.

It is also necessary to observe for GI adverse effects, including abdominal distention, acid regurgitation, dysphagia, esophagitis, and flatulence.

### Patient Teaching

Box 44.9 gives patient teaching guidelines for alendronate.

## Other Drugs in the Class

Other bisphosphonates include ibandronate (Boniva), pamidronate (Aredia), risedronate (Actonel), and zoledronic acid (Reclast, Zometa). Ibandronate, risedronate, and zoledronic acid (Reclast), like alendronate, are used to prevent and treat osteoporosis. Both ibandronate and risedronate are available in oral preparations to be taken once monthly. Zoledronic acid, as Reclast, is administered IV once a year. Pamidronate is not approved by the U.S. Food and Drug Administration (FDA) for osteoporosis but may be useful for various bone-related conditions such as Paget's disease and bone lesions.

---

**BOX 44.8  Drug Interactions: Alendronate**

**Drugs That Increase the Effects of Alendronate**
- Aspirin and nonsteroidal anti-inflammatory drugs
  *Increase the risk of gastrointestinal effects when combined with alendronate*

**Drugs That Decrease the Effects of Alendronate**
- Antacids and calcium supplements
  *Interfere with alendronate absorption if they are taken within 2 hours of the drug*

---

**BOX 44.9  Patient Teaching Guidelines for Alendronate**

- Take tablets on waking only with 6 to 8 oz of water or more at least 30 minutes before eating or drinking anything else, including food, beverages, or other drugs. Waiting longer than 30 minutes improves absorption.
- Do not lie down for at least 30 minutes after taking alendronate to reduce the risk of esophageal irritation and aid movement of the drug to the stomach.
- Report adverse effects to the health care provider immediately, especially esophageal pain, irritation, or burning; heartburn; dyspepsia, nausea, or vomiting; or difficulty swallowing.

---

Common adverse effects of bisphosphonates include nausea and vomiting. Serious adverse effects may include anemia, jaw osteonecrosis, neutropenia, infections, and renal damage.

**Clinical Application 44.4**

- The nurse is giving instructions to Mrs. Taylor on the proper administration method for taking alendronate. What important instructions must the nurse include?

**NCLEX Success**

3. A man has a serum calcium level of 6.8 mg/dL. The health care provider orders a vitamin D supplement. Which one of the following laboratory values for serum calcium indicates that the vitamin D is effective?
   A. 5.5 mg/dL
   B. 6.8 mg/dL
   C. 7.5 mg/dL
   D. 8.5 mg/dL

4. The nurse is caring for a patient who takes alendronate. Which adverse effects should the nurse observe for?
   A. numbness and tingling of the extremities
   B. irregular pulse rate and angina
   C. acid reflux and difficulty swallowing
   D. rash and skin lesions

5. The health care provider has prescribed alendronate for the patient. Which one of the following should the nurse include in discharge teaching?
   A. "Take alendronate first thing in the morning with orange juice."
   B. "Take alendronate at bedtime with a glass of milk."
   C. "Take alendronate first thing in the morning with water."
   D. "Take alendronate on a full stomach after breakfast."

# OTHER MEDICATIONS USED TO TREAT BONE DISORDERS AND HYPERCALCEMIA

Other drugs are used to treat bone disorders and hypercalcemia. Table 44.5 presents route and dosage information for these drugs.

Calcitonin (Miacalcin) is used in the treatment of hypercalcemia, Paget's disease, and postmenopausal osteoporosis. In hypercalcemia, calcitonin lowers serum calcium levels by inhibiting bone resorption. Calcitonin is most likely to be effective in hypercalcemia caused by hyperparathyroidism, prolonged immobilization, or certain malignant neoplasms. In acute hypercalcemia, health care providers may use calcitonin along with other measures to lower serum calcium rapidly. A single injection of calcitonin decreases serum calcium levels in approximately 2 hours, and its effects last approximately 6 to 8 hours. In Paget's disease, calcitonin slows the rate of bone turnover, improves bone lesions on radiologic examination, and relieves bone pain. In osteoporosis, calcitonin prevents further bone loss in the presence of adequate calcium and vitamin D.

Denosumab (Prolia, Xgeva) is an antiresorptive drug. Prolia is used to treat osteoporosis in postmenopausal women at high risk of fracture. Xgeva is used to prevent skeletal-related events in bone metastases from solid tumors. Denosumab decreases bone resorption and increases bone mass and strength. The drug is administered subcutaneously at 6-month intervals. Adverse effects include fatigue, weakness, back pain, extremity pain, hypocalcemia, hypophosphatemia, nausea, diarrhea, peripheral edema, hypertension, headache, skin rash, and dermatitis.

Glucocorticoids (e.g., prednisone, hydrocortisone) are useful in the treatment of hypercalcemia due to malignancies or vitamin D intoxication. These drugs lower serum calcium levels by inhibiting cytokine release, by direct cytolytic effects on some tumor cells, by inhibiting calcium absorption from the intestine, and by increasing calcium excretion in the urine. The serum calcium level decreases in approximately 5 to 10 days, and after it stabilizes, gradual dosage reduction to the minimum needed to control symptoms of hypercalcemia is necessary. High dosage or prolonged administration leads to serious adverse effects.

Phosphate salts (Neutra-Phos) inhibit intestinal absorption of calcium and increase deposition of calcium in bone. (Neutra-Phos is an oral combination of sodium phosphate and

## TABLE 44.5

### DRUGS AT A GLANCE: Drugs Used to Treat Other Bone Disorders and Hypercalcemia

| Drug | Pregnancy Category | Routes and Dosage Ranges | |
|---|---|---|---|
| | | **Adults** | **Children** |
| Calcitonin (Miacalcin; 🍁 Calcimar) | C | Hypercalcemia: 4 units/kg subcutaneously or IM every 12 h; can be increased after 1–2 d to 8 units/kg every 12 h; max dose 8 units/kg every 6 h<br>Paget's disease: 100 units/d subcutaneously or IM<br>Postmenopausal osteoporosis: nasal spray, 200 units daily (1 spray in 1 nostril daily); subcutaneously or IM, 100 units daily | Osteogenesis imperfecta:<br>Infants >6 mo, children, and adolescents: 2 units/kg/dose subcutaneously or IM three times/wk |
| Denosumab (Prolia, Xgeva; 🍁 Prolia, Xgeva) | D | Osteoporosis, bone loss in the breast, and prostate cancer treatment (Prolia): 60 mg subcutaneously every 6 mo<br>Prevention of skeletal-related events with solid tumor bone metastases (Xgeva): 120 mg subcutaneously every 4 wk | Treatment of giant cell tumor of the bone (Xgeva):<br>Skeletally mature adolescents weighing 45 kg or more, 120 mg subcutaneously once every 4 wk (during the 1st mo, give additional 120 mg on days 8 and 15) |
| Potassium phosphate; sodium phosphate | C | Hypercalcemia: elemental phosphorus 250–500 mg PO four times per day | Hypercalcemia: 4 y of age or older, elemental phosphorus 250 mg PO four times per day |
| Prednisone (Deltasone, Prednisone; 🍁 APO-PredniSONE; TEVA-PredniSONE) | C/D | Hypercalcemia: prednisone, 20–40 mg PO daily | Consult pediatric literature |
| Raloxifene (Evista; 🍁 ACT Raloxifene, APO-Raloxifene, Evista) | X | Postmenopausal osteoporosis: prevention/treatment, 60 mg PO once daily | No use established |
| Teriparatide (Forteo; 🍁 Forteo) | C | Postmenopausal osteoporosis, osteoporosis in men, Glucocorticoid-induced osteoporosis: 20 mcg subcutaneous daily for up to 2 y (first dose, sitting, or lying down) | No use established |

potassium phosphate.) Oral salts are effective in the treatment of hypercalcemia due to any cause. A potential adverse effect of phosphates is calcification of soft tissues due to deposition of calcium phosphate, which can lead to severe impairment of function in the kidneys and other organs. It is important to give phosphates only when hypercalcemia is accompanied by hypophosphatemia (serum phosphate <3 mg/dL) and renal function is normal to minimize the risk of soft tissue calcification. Frequent monitoring of serum calcium, phosphate, and creatinine levels is necessary, and the dose reduction should occur if serum phosphate exceeds 4.5 mg/dL or the product of serum calcium and phosphate exceeds 60 mg/dL.

Raloxifene (Evista) is a selective estrogen receptor modulator that is used to prevent or treat postmenopausal osteoporosis. It acts like estrogen in some body tissues and prevents the action of estrogen in other body tissues. It has estrogenic effects in bone tissue, thereby decreasing bone breakdown and increasing bone mass density. It has antiestrogen effects in breast and uterine tissue. Raloxifene increases the risk of deep vein thrombosis or pulmonary emboli; the risk of death due to stroke may be increased in women with coronary heart disease or in women at risk for coronary events.

Teriparatide (Forteo) is a recombinant DNA version of PTH that is approved for the treatment of osteoporosis in women. This drug increases bone formation by increasing the number of bone-building cells (osteoblasts). It also increases serum levels of calcium and the active form of vitamin D. In clinical trials, teriparatide increased vertebral bone mineral density and decreased vertebral fractures. Experts recommend the drug for use in patients with severe osteoporosis or those who have not responded adequately to other treatments. Patients with an increased risk of osteosarcoma, such as those with Paget's disease, prior radiation, unexplained elevation of alkaline phosphatase, and open epiphyses, should avoid using teriparatide. Adverse effects include nausea, headache, back pain, dizziness, syncope, and leg cramps. It is necessary to administer the drug with the patient sitting or lying down to prevent orthostatic hypotension.

Teriparatide is rapidly and well absorbed after subcutaneous injection. Bioavailability is 95%, and peak serum levels occur in 30 minutes. The drug is metabolized and excreted through the liver, kidneys, and bone. It is not expected to accumulate in bone or other tissues, to interact significantly with other drugs, or to require dosage adjustment with renal or hepatic impairment.

## Emergency Treatment of Hypercalcemia

Acute hypercalcemia (severe symptoms or a serum calcium level greater than 14 mg/dL) is a medical emergency, and rehydration is a priority. It is essential to administer an IV saline solution (0.9% sodium chloride) at an initial rate of 200 to 300 mL/h and then adjust it to maintain a urine output of 100 to 150 mL/h. Authorities no longer recommend the routine use of loop diuretics, such as furosemide, in the absence of heart failure or renal insufficiency. Because sodium, potassium, and water are also lost in the urine, replacement with IV fluids is necessary.

In addition, symptomatic patients should receive calcitonin subcutaneously. Long-term control of hypercalcemia requires addition of a bisphosphonate; zoledronic acid and pamidronate are preferred agents. These two bisphosphonates are given intravenously and reach their maximum effect in 2 to 4 days (Shane & Berenson, 2019).

## THE NURSING PROCESS

A concept map outlines the nursing process related to drug therapy considerations in this chapter. Additional nursing implications related to the disease process should also be considered in care decisions.

**Assessment**

- Assess for risk factors and manifestations of hypocalcemia and calcium deficiency:
- Assess dietary intake of dairy products, other calcium-containing foods, and vitamin D.
- Assess serum calcium. The normal total serum calcium level is approximately 8.5 to 10.5 mg/dL (SI units 2.2–2.6 mmol/L). Approximately half of the total serum calcium (4–5 mg/dL) should be free ionized calcium, the physiologically active form. To interpret serum calcium levels accurately, serum albumin levels and acid–base status must be considered. Low serum albumin decreases the total serum level of calcium by decreasing the amount of calcium that is bound to protein; however, the ionized concentration is unaffected by serum albumin levels. Metabolic and respiratory alkalosis increase the binding of calcium to serum proteins, thereby maintaining normal serum calcium but decreasing the ionized values. Conversely, metabolic and respiratory acidosis decrease binding and therefore increase the concentration of ionized calcium.
- Assess Chvostek's and Trousseau's signs.
- Assess for conditions in which hypercalcemia is likely to occur: cancer, prolonged immobilization, or vitamin D overdose.
- Assess ECG changes indicative of hypercalcemia, which include a shortened QT interval and an inverted T wave.
- Assess for risk factors and manifestations of osteoporosis, especially in postmenopausal women and in men and women on chronic corticosteroid therapy.
- If Paget's disease is suspected, assess for an elevated serum alkaline phosphatase level and abnormal bone scan reports.

**Outcomes of Therapy**

The patient will
- Achieve and maintain normal serum levels of calcium.
- Increase dietary intake of calcium-containing foods to prevent or treat osteoporosis.
- Use calcium or vitamin D supplements in recommended amounts.
- Adhere to instructions for safe drug use and follow-up treatment of hypocalcemia, hypercalcemia, or osteoporosis.
- Be monitored closely for therapeutic and adverse effects of drugs used to treat hypercalcemia.

**Nursing Interventions**

- Assist all patients in meeting the recommended daily requirements of calcium and vitamin D. Instruct the patient that the best dietary source is milk and other dairy products, including yogurt.
- Recommend that adults drink at least two 8 oz glasses of milk daily (unless contraindicated by the patient's condition). This supplies half of the daily recommended amount of calcium.
- Instruct parents that children need approximately four glasses of milk or an equivalent amount of calcium in milk and other foods to support normal growth and development.
- Teach pregnant and lactating women to consume four glasses of milk or the equivalent to meet increased needs, in addition to prescribed vitamin and mineral supplements.
- Instruct postmenopausal women who take estrogens to consume at least 1000 mg of calcium daily. Those who do not take estrogen need at least 1500 mg.
- Instruct patients on calorie restrictions to consume low-calorie sources such as skim milk and low-fat yogurt.
- Educate patients about additional sources of vitamin D. Sun exposure is also needed to supply adequate amounts of vitamin D.
- Instruct patients who have an inadequate intake of calcium to take a calcium supplement to prevent osteoporosis.
- Instruct patients with hypercalcemia to drink 3000 to 4000 mL of fluid daily to prevent renal calculi.

**Evaluation**

- Check laboratory reports of serum calcium levels for normal values.
- Interview and observe for relief of symptoms of hypocalcemia, hypercalcemia, or osteoporosis.
- Interview and observe intake of calcium-containing foods.
- Question about normal calcium requirements and how to meet them.
- Interview and observe for accurate drug usage and adherence to follow-up procedures.
- Interview and observe for therapeutic and adverse drug effects.

## Unfolding Patient Stories: Suzanne Morris • Part 2

Think back to Suzanne Morris, the 43-year-old female from Chapter 37 who is treated for peptic ulcer disease (PUD) with amoxicillin, clarithromycin, and pantoprazole. During the clinic visit, she expresses concern about a family history of osteoporosis. What patient education should the nurse provide on factors that can influence the development of osteoporosis? If Suzanne's diet is insufficient, what oral supplements would the nurse consider for osteoporosis prevention? What are the nursing implications when administering oral supplements for osteoporosis prevention with her current medications for PUD?

Care for Suzanne and other patients in a realistic virtual environment: **vSim** *for Nursing* (thepoint.lww.com/vSimPharm). Practice documenting these patients' care in DocuCare (thepoint.lww.com/DocuCareEHR).

## KEY CONCEPTS

- Hypoparathyroidism is most often caused by removal of or damage to the parathyroid glands during neck surgery.
- Hyperparathyroidism is most often caused by a tumor or hyperplasia of a parathyroid gland.
- Deficiency of vitamin D causes inadequate absorption of calcium and phosphorus.
- In general, intake of calcium should not exceed 2500 mg from all sources. The upper intake level for vitamin D is 1000 mg/day (4000 IU/day).
- Calcium deficiency commonly occurs in the elderly because of long-term dietary deficiencies of calcium and vitamin D, impaired absorption of calcium from the intestine, lack of exposure to sunlight, and impaired liver or kidney metabolism of vitamin D to its active form.
- Postmenopausal women are at high risk for osteoporosis.
- Both men and women who take corticosteroids are at risk for osteoporosis.

## CLINICAL REASONING CASE STUDY

**Meet the Patient**

Ralph Lansing is an 80-year-old man with bruising from the top of his left hip extending to the ankle. He sees his health care provider. Mr. Lansing's alkaline phosphatase level is extremely elevated at 220 units/L. He receives a diagnosis of Paget's disease.

- What is the action of alendronate?
- What are the adverse effects of alendronate?
- As a result of increased age, Mr. Lansing has a CrCl of 40 mL/min. Will this require an adjustment in the dosage of alendronate?
- What patient teaching should the nurse provide?

**Assessing Drug Information**

- Alendronate suppresses osteoclast activity on newly formed resorption surfaces, which reduces bone turnover. This means that bone formation exceeds resorption at remodeling sites, leading to progressive gains in bone mass.
- Adverse effects of alendronate are usually minor if the doses taken for prevention or treatment of osteoporosis are used and the drug is taken as directed. Patients who do not follow the dosing instructions are at greater risk for esophagitis, dysphagia, and esophageal ulcers/erosions. Other effects include headache, musculoskeletal pain (sometimes severe), and decreased serum calcium. More severe effects may occur with the doses taken for Paget's disease, which are higher than those taken for osteoporosis.
- Rare adverse effects of alendronate include atypical femur fracture and osteonecrosis of the jaw. Patients on long-term therapy are at greater risk for femur fracture.

**Nursing Actions**

- Understand that no dosage adjustment is needed with a CrCl *of at least* 35 mL/min. Mr. Lansing's CrCl is 40 mL/min. A CrCl less than 35 mL/min contraindicates the use of alendronate.
- Ensure proper administration of alendronate. Instruct Mr. Lansing to always take the drug on waking with 6 to 8 oz of water (not juice or coffee) at least 30 minutes before breakfast and before taking other drugs. He should remain upright (either with head elevated 90 degrees if in bed, sitting upright in a chair, or standing) for at least 30 minutes after administration. This reduces the risk of esophageal irritation and aids movement of the drug to the stomach. (Waiting longer than 30 minutes improves absorption.)
- Instruct Mr. Lansing to report adverse effects to his health care provider immediately, especially esophageal pain, irritation, or burning; heartburn; dyspepsia; nausea and vomiting; and difficulty swallowing.

Visit thePoint® at **http://thePoint.lww.com/Frandsen12e** for answers to NCLEX Success questions (in Appendix A), answers to Clinical Application Case Studies (in Appendix B), and more!

## REFERENCES AND RESOURCES

Aggarwal, L., & Masuda, C. (2018). Osteoporosis: A quick update. *The Journal of Family Practice, 67*(2), 59–65.

Bajger, B. (2018). Osteoporosis treatment preferences and satisfaction in postmenopausal women: Denosumab compared with oral bisphosphonates. *Australian Journal of Advanced Nursing, 35*(3), 39–49.

Hinkle, J. L., & Cheever, K. H. (2018). *Brunner & Suddarth's textbook of medical-surgical nursing* (14th ed.). Philadelphia, PA: Wolters Kluwer Health/Lippincott Williams & Wilkins.

*Nursing 2019 Drug handbook.* Philadelphia, PA: Wolters Kluwer.

Shane, E., & Berenson, J. R. (2019). *Treatment of hypercalcemia.* UptoDate. Retrieved July 5, 2019.

UpToDate. (2019). *Drug information.* Lexi-Comp, Inc.

# Drug Therapy for Adrenal Cortex Disorders

## LEARNING OBJECTIVES

*After studying this chapter, you should be able to:*

1. Associate the etiology and pathophysiology of Addison's disease with its major manifestations.
2. Associate the etiology and pathophysiology of Cushing's disease with its major manifestations.
3. Explain how corticotropin [ACTH] is used in the diagnosis of adrenocortical insufficiency.
4. Explain how cosyntropin [Cortrosyn] is used in the diagnosis of adrenocortical insufficiency.
5. Identify the prototypes and describe the action, use, adverse effects, contraindications, and nursing implications for the drugs used in the treatment of Addison's disease.
6. Identify the prototypes and describe the action, use, adverse effects, contraindications, and nursing implications for the drugs used in the treatment of Cushing's disease.
7. Implement the nursing process in the care of the patient with Addison's disease or Cushing's disease.

## CLINICAL APPLICATION CASE STUDY

Rosa James is a 68-year-old woman who is being seen by her nurse practitioner with symptoms of muscle weakness and fatigue. She states that she has felt depressed. Physical assessment reveals dark pigmentation of the mucous membranes and skin on the knuckles, knees, and elbows. She appears dehydrated with poor skin turgor. Her blood pressure is 84/50 mm Hg. Blood chemistry reveals sodium level of 132 mEq/L and a potassium level of 5.5 mEq/L. Mrs. James is admitted to the hospital with suspected Addison's disease, and an endocrine consult is ordered.

## KEY TERMS

**Acute adrenal crisis (or addisonian crisis):** acute adrenocortical insufficiency

**Adrenocortical excess:** increase in adrenocortical function

**Adrenocortical insufficiency:** decrease in adrenocortical function

# INTRODUCTION

This chapter introduces the pharmacologic care of the patient with adrenocortical insufficiency and the patient with adrenocortical excess. The adrenal glands are attached to the upper portion of each kidney. The adrenal cortex of each adrenal gland secretes steroid hormones. The hypothalamic–pituitary–adrenal (HPA) axis regulates hormone secretion. The hypothalamus secretes corticotropin-releasing hormone (CRH), which in turn stimulates the pituitary gland to secrete adrenocorticotropic hormone (ACTH) (Fig. 45.1). The ACTH then stimulates the adrenal cortex to secrete glucocorticoid hormone (cortisol). As the levels of adrenal or steroid hormones increase, the levels of CRH and ACTH decrease through a negative feedback mechanism. For discussion of corticosteroids, see Chapter 17, and for discussion about the types of hormones secreted by the hypothalamus, including CRH, see Chapter 43.

# OVERVIEW OF ADDISON'S DISEASE

## Etiology and Pathophysiology

There are two forms of **adrenocortical insufficiency**. Primary adrenal insufficiency, or Addison's disease, occurs when adrenal cortical hormones are deficient. ACTH levels are elevated because the feedback mechanism is not working. Secondary adrenal insufficiency occurs when there is a disorder in the HPA system.

Primary adrenal insufficiency most commonly results from an autoimmune disorder that has destroyed the layers of the adrenal cortex. Other causes of adrenal cortex destruction include metastatic carcinoma, fungal infections such as

histoplasmosis, cytomegalovirus, amyloid disease, and hemochromatosis. Hemorrhage of the adrenal cortex related to anticoagulant therapy, coronary artery bypass graft surgery, giving birth, or trauma also leads to primary adrenal insufficiency.

Secondary adrenal cortical insufficiency results from hypopituitarism or surgical removal of pituitary gland. The abrupt withdrawal of oral glucocorticoids also causes secondary adrenal insufficiency. Patients who have endogenous steroid production from a nonendocrine tumor have adrenocortical insufficiency.

Primary adrenocortical insufficiency is associated with the destruction of the adrenal cortex. The resulting deficiency in the mineralocorticoids causes an increase in the loss of urinary sodium, chloride, and water. The patient becomes hyponatremic, and the cardiac output decreases. This progression of the disease is known as **acute adrenal (or addisonian) crisis**. The loss of sodium leads to retention of potassium, resulting in symptoms of hyperkalemia.

**Clinical Application 45.1**

- Mrs. James is hyponatremic. When assessing her cardiac status, what findings would the nurse expect?
- On the 2nd day of Mrs. James' hospital admission, her sodium level is 125 mEq/L. What condition does the nurse suspect?

## Clinical Manifestations

Clinical manifestations of adrenocortical insufficiency are evident when approximately 90% of the adrenal cortex has been destroyed. These signs and symptoms reflect loss of sodium, water, and chloride.

**Figure 45.1.** The adrenal glands are located on the top of each kidney. Adrenocorticotropic hormone is secreted by the pituitary gland.

Findings include decreased cardiac output, dehydration, weakness, and fatigue. Excessive sodium loss results in cardiovascular collapse and shock. Other symptoms include lethargy, weakness, fever, anorexia, nausea, vomiting, and weight loss. Hyperkalemia and hypoglycemia are present. (Any patient with unexplained severe hypoglycemia requires assessment for adrenal insufficiency.) Hyperpigmentation of the gums and mucous membranes is also present; they may be bluish black. Women have diminished axillary and pubic hair, but men have few effects from the lack of androgens due to the production of hormones by the testes.

Acute adrenal crisis, or addisonian crisis, is a life-threatening condition that occurs when Addison's disease is the underlying problem and the patient is exposed to minor illness or increased stress. Nausea, vomiting, hypotension, muscle weakness, and vascular collapse are present. There may be a craving for salt.

### QSEN: Evidence-Based Practice

In this study by Iwasaku, Shinzawa, Tanaka, Kimachi, and Kawakami (2017), the researchers sought to determine the characteristics of adrenal crisis. The research goal was to determine if comorbidities and glucocorticoid therapy increased the risk of adrenal crisis. In this retrospective study, 7.4 million patient charts were reviewed. The study identified 504 patients with adrenal crisis. Twenty-three of the patients had primary adrenal insufficiency. One hundred and thirty-six patients had central adrenal insufficiency. The remaining adrenal crisis patients, accounting for 68.5%, had comorbidities such as cancer, autoimmune diseases, and renal failure. The study found that predisposing factors for adrenal crisis were complicated if the patient had adrenal insufficiency, were older, and presented with comorbid conditions.

### NCLEX Success

1. A man is admitted to the emergency department. He is hypotensive with nausea, vomiting, and muscle weakness. He has been taking enoxaparin 40 mg subcutaneously daily for the past 2 weeks. It is suspected that he has developed which of the following disorders?

    A. hyperglycemia related to diabetes insipidus
    B. sepsis related to his heart surgery
    C. hemorrhage of the adrenal cortex
    D. hyponatremia and cardiovascular collapse

2. A woman visits the clinic. She states that she has been satisfying her recent cravings for salt by eating large quantities of potato chips and other salty foods. She has been under a great deal of stress, and last week she received treatment for pneumonia. What do these symptoms suggest?

    A. heart failure
    B. acute adrenal crisis
    C. hypernatremia
    D. thyrotoxicosis

### Diagnosis

Patients commonly present to their primary health care provider with vague symptoms of adrenocortical insufficiency. However, as the adrenocortical insufficiency progresses, acute hypotension results and acute adrenal crisis may develop. Making the diagnosis of adrenocortical insufficiency involves laboratory work. This includes early morning serum cortisol and plasma ACTH levels. A serum cortisol level less than 3 mcg/dL, or 80 nmol/L, is indicative of adrenocortical insufficiency. (The normal morning level of serum cortisol is greater—10–20 mcg/dL, or 275–555 nmol/L.) An ACTH level greater than 22.0 nmol/L is indicative of (primary) adrenocortical insufficiency. (The normal morning level of ACTH is less than 18 nmol/L.)

Confirming the diagnosis of adrenocortical insufficiency requires a short plasma corticotropin stimulation test. The examiner administers corticotropin in the morning, and a subnormal blood cortisol level in the morning and afternoon confirms the diagnosis. A higher cortisol level in the morning is a sign that a person does not have adrenal insufficiency. In a patient with adrenal insufficiency, the response to the corticotropin, or ACTH, is the same both morning and afternoon.

Another test that confirms the diagnosis of adrenocortical insufficiency is the standard high-dose test. It is a three-step process:

1. Measurement of baseline serum cortisol
2. Intravenous (IV) administration of 250 mcg of ACTH 30 minutes later
3. Measurement of serum cortisol 30 to 60 minutes later

An increase of *at least* 18 to 20 mcg/dL is considered normal. No increase in serum cortisol indicates the presence of adrenocortical insufficiency.

Diagnosis of secondary adrenocortical insufficiency in its early stages requires the low-dose test. It is also used for the diagnosis of chronic partial pituitary ACTH deficiency. This test involves the administration of 1 mcg of cosyntropin (Cortrosyn) as an IV bolus. Normally, an increase in cortisol occurs in 20 minutes. In patients with adrenocortical insufficiency, there is no increase in the serum cortisol level.

## OVERVIEW OF CUSHING'S DISEASE

### Etiology and Pathophysiology

The cause of Cushing's disease is **adrenocortical excess**. In the majority of patients, the increased adrenocortical function results from excessive corticotropin, leading to hyperplasia of the adrenal cortex. In a smaller percentage of patients, it is the result of a cortisol-secreting adrenal tumor, whether from too much corticotropin (ACTH) or a primary tumor of the adrenal gland. A malignant tumor of the adrenal gland can produce many corticosteroids, whereas the benign adrenal tumor only produces one corticosteroid that is secreted by the adrenal gland. Other, much less common causes are hyperplasia of the adrenal gland or ectopic production of ACTH by malignancies such as bronchogenic carcinoma. Long-term treatment with pharmacologic glucocorticoids leads to iatrogenic Cushing's syndrome.

### Clinical Manifestations

Patients with Cushing's disease often present with classic signs and symptoms. These include obesity, with a heavy trunk and thin extremities, a fatty "buffalo hump" at the neck and supraclavicular region, and a moon-faced appearance. The skin becomes fragile and tears easily, and broad purple striae and bruises may develop. Wound healing may be impaired. The hair is thin. Women have virilization with the appearance of masculine traits such as increased facial hair, breast atrophy, enlarged clitoris, disrupted menses, and voice deepening. Libido is diminished or absent in men and women. Depression, weakness, and lassitude may also occur.

The excessive secretion of corticotropin leads to osteoporosis and fractures, which are caused by the increase in calcium reabsorption from the bone. Blood glucose levels are also increased, and glucose intolerance may occur as a result of increased hepatic gluconeogenesis and resistance to insulin. Peptic ulcers may develop because of increased secretion of gastric acid and pepsin.

### ! QSEN Alert: Evidence-Based Practice

Researchers from the Endocrine Society updated current clinical practice guidelines regarding the treatment of Cushing's syndrome [Nieman et al., 2015] using the related best available evidence from systematic reviews and individual studies. Two recommendations highlight the effects of severe hypercortisolism and the importance of nursing assessment following surgery to treat Cushing's syndrome. One, severe hypercortisolism impairs immunity and predisposes patients to severe, systemic infection, including sepsis due to bacterial, fungal, and opportunistic pathogens. Two, hypercortisolism alters coagulation factors for up to 1 year after surgical intervention and carries an increased risk of venous thrombosis, especially in the 4 weeks after surgery. Nurses participating in the care of patients with Cushing's disease should be aware of the risks and assess and educate patients the risk of infection, thrombosis, and bleeding.

## Diagnosis

The diagnosis of Cushing's disease requires an overnight dexamethasone suppression test. The patient takes dexamethasone, a synthetic glucocorticoid, 1 mg orally at 11 PM. He or she then has a serum cortisol level drawn at 8 AM. A cortisol level of less than 5 mcg/dL indicates that the HPA axis is functioning normally. Cortisol levels are higher in patients with adrenal or ectopic tumors.

### NCLEX Success

3. A women receives a diagnosis of Cushing's disease. She has an excess of which of the following hormones?

    A. luteinizing hormone
    B. glucose
    C. insulin
    D. corticotropin

4. A man has a low level of adrenocorticotropic hormone and a high level of cortisol. What disease does he have?

    A. Cushing's disease
    B. Addison's disease
    C. adrenal cortex hemorrhage
    D. myocardial infarction

# DRUGS USED TO TREAT ADDISON'S DISEASE

The goal of treatment for Addison's disease is to replace the adrenocorticoids to correct adrenal insufficiency. It is important to replace both the mineralocorticoid and adrenocorticoid. Lifetime hormone replacement is necessary. Table 45.1 summarizes the adrenocorticoid and mineralocorticoids administered for the treatment of adrenocortical insufficiency.

## ADRENOCORTICOIDS/ MINERALOCORTICOIDS

The prototype  **hydrocortisone** (Solu-Cortef), a combination of a mineralocorticoid and adrenocorticoid, is useful in acute and chronic adrenal insufficiency.

## Pharmacokinetics and Action

The oral preparation of hydrocortisone has a 1- to 2-hour onset of action, a peak of action in 1 to 2 hours, and a duration of action of 1 to 1.5 days. The parenteral preparation of the drug has an immediate onset of action, an unknown peak of action, and a duration of action of 1 to 1.5 days. Metabolism occurs in the liver. Excretion is in the kidneys.

## Action

Hydrocortisone enters the cells and binds to the receptors in the cytoplasm to decrease inflammation; it suppresses the migration of polymorphonuclear lymphocytes and decreases capillary permeability. The mineralocorticoid in the drug increases the retention of sodium.

## Use

Health care providers used hydrocortisone to replace adrenocorticoids and mineralocorticoids in patients with Addison's disease. The drug is also useful in congenital adrenal hyperplasia. Table 45.2 gives route and dosage information for adrenocorticoids and mineralocorticoids.

### Use in Children

It is necessary to individualize the dose depending on the severity of the adrenal insufficiency and the response to the medication. The drug may affect growth velocity, and it is important to

### TABLE 45.1

#### Drugs Administered for Addison's Disease

| Drug Class | Prototypes | Other Drugs in the Class |
| --- | --- | --- |
| Adrenocorticoid/ mineralocorticoids | Hydrocortisone (Cortef, Solu-Cortef) | None |
| Mineralocorticoids | Fludrocortisone | None |

| | | | |
|---|---|---|---|
| **TABLE 45.2** | | | |
| **DRUGS AT A GLANCE: Adrenocorticoids/Mineralocorticoids and Mineralocorticoids** | | | |
| **Drug** | **Pregnancy Category** | **Routes and Dosage Ranges** | |
| | | **Adults** | **Children** |
| Ⓟ **Hydrocortisone** (Cortef, Solu-Cortef; ✹ Cortef, Solu-Cortef) | C | 100–500 mg IV and every 2, 4, or 6 h based on condition and response  15–25 mg PO initially and individualized to patient response | Infants, 2–3 mg/kg IV (preferred) IM, PO initially; maximum dose: 100 mg/dose; then 1–5 mg/kg/dose every 6 h individualized to patient response  <5 y, 25–50 mg once followed by 25–50 mg/d in divided doses every 6 h for 24 h then individualized to patient response  ≥5 y, 50–100 mg once followed by 50 mg/d in divided doses every 6 h for 24 h then individualized to patient response  Adolescents, 100 mg once followed by 100 mg/d in divided doses every 6 h for 24 h then individualized to patient response |
| Ⓟ **Fludrocortisone** (Florinef) | C | 0.1 mg PO daily initially with ranges of 0.1 mg three times weekly to 0.2 mg daily | 0.05–0.2 mg daily |

carefully assess growth and development with infants and children. Also, the nurse assesses neonate's respiratory status closely after the administration of parenteral hydrocortisone. Some preparations contain benzyl alcohol, which may cause gasping syndrome in neonates.

### Use in Older Adults

Elderly people should receive the lowest possible dosage because of the increased risk of adverse effects with systemic corticosteroids.

## Adverse Effects

Hydrocortisone has significant adverse effects, including the following:

- Cardiac effects: fluctuations in blood pressure, shock, dysrhythmias, myocardial infarction, embolism, circulatory collapse, heart failure, and cardiac arrest
- Central nervous system (CNS) effects: vertigo, headache, and depression
- Dermatologic effects: fragile skin that tears easily, petechiae, ecchymoses
- Gastrointestinal (GI) effects: peptic or esophageal ulcers, pancreatitis, increased appetite, and weight gain
- Hematologic effects: sodium and fluid retention
- Metabolic effects: hyperglycemia and Cushing's syndrome
- Musculoskeletal effects: osteoporosis and spontaneous fractures (long-term administration)
- Reproductive (female) effects: amenorrhea and irregular menses
- Other effects: immunosuppression, muscle weakness, impaired wound healing, and anaphylaxis

## Contraindications

Contraindications to hydrocortisone include a known hypersensitivity to the drug or any component of the formulation as well as a serious infection. The U.S. Food and Drug Administration (FDA) has issued a **BLACK BOX WARNING ◆** stating that patients who are being treated with hydrocortisone should not receive live virus vaccines.

## Nursing Implications

### Preventing Interactions

Several medications interact with hydrocortisone, increasing or decreasing its effects (Box 45.1). Echinacea may increase the effects of hydrocortisone, whereas St. John's wort may decrease the drug's effects. Hydrocortisone has numerous other interactions. Combination of hydrocortisone with certain drugs may result in the following effects:

- Salicylates: increased serum salicylate levels
- Acetylcholinesterase drugs: diminished therapeutic effect

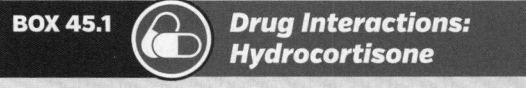

**BOX 45.1** **Drug Interactions: Hydrocortisone**

**Drugs That Increase the Effects of Hydrocortisone**
- Estrogen, hormonal contraceptives, ketoconazole, troleandomycin
  *Increase steroid blood levels*

**Drugs That Decrease the Effects of Hydrocortisone**
- Cholestyramine, phenobarbital, phenytoin, rifampin
  *Decrease steroid blood levels*

- Anticoagulants: increased bleeding; it is necessary to monitor the prothrombin time and the international normalized ratio closely
- Food: interference with calcium absorption
- Alcohol: increased risk of gastric mucosal irritation and development of gastric ulcers

### Administering the Medication

People should take the oral preparation with food to decrease gastric irritation.

 **QSEN Alert: Safety**

Administration of hydrocortisone should take place every morning before 9 AM. This minimizes HPA suppression.

It is necessary to dilute hydrocortisone sodium succinate to 50 mg/mL and administer the drug as an IV bolus over 30 seconds or over 10 minutes for doses ≥500 mg. For intermittent IV infusion, dilution to 1 mg/mL and administration over 20 to 30 minutes is appropriate.

### Assessing for Therapeutic Effects

The nurse assesses the patient's blood pressure, pulse, and respirations for improved cardiac function. He or she also assesses the sodium level and fluid volume status for return to normal range with retention of sodium and water. It is important to assess for increased strength and energy as well as for improved mood and ability to cope with stress.

### Assessing for Adverse Effects

The nurse assesses for hypertension, heart failure, or alterations in cardiac output. It is important to assess for normal menses and diminished virilization in women. Also, the nurse checks the patient's ability to fight infection (e.g., normal white blood cell count). In addition, he or she assesses the serum blood sugar to rule out hypoglycemia or hyperglycemia.

### Patient Teaching

Box 45.2 presents patient teaching guidelines for hydrocortisone.

#### Clinical Application 45.2

- Mrs. James' endocrinologist orders hydrocortisone 200 mg intravenously every 4 hours. How does the nurse dilute the drug and over what period does he or she administer it?
- One hour following the administration of the medication, the endocrinologist orders blood glucose testing. What is the rationale for blood glucose testing?
- What is the action of hydrocortisone?

## MINERALOCORTICOIDS

If a patient with Addison's disease requires additional mineralocorticoid supplementation, then ⬤ **fludrocortisone**, a synthetic steroid, is useful. A patient usually takes it in

 **BOX 45.2** *Patient Teaching Guidelines for Hydrocortisone*

- Take the oral preparation of hydrocortisone every day at 9:00 AM.
- Space other doses of hydrocortisone evenly throughout the day.
- Do not stop the medication abruptly or without notifying the prescriber.
- Inform the health care provider of increased stress. The dosage of the medication may need to be increased.
- Increase calcium intake if hydrocortisone is administered for a prolonged period.
- Administer antacids between doses of hydrocortisone to prevent gastric irritation.
- Monitor blood sugar daily.
- Wear a medic alert bracelet.
- Report swelling, weight gain, muscle weakness, tarry stools, moon face, fever, infection, inability of wounds to heal, and fatigue.

combination with a glucocorticoid. It is important to note that fludrocortisone has also proved effective for the treatment of orthostatic hypotension in older adults.

## Pharmacokinetics and Action

Fludrocortisone is absorbed rapidly and completely and is 42% protein bound. The drug reaches a peak serum level in approximately 1.7 hours, and it has a 3.5-hour serum half-life. Metabolism occurs in the liver. The site of excretion is unknown.

Fludrocortisone has strong mineralocorticoid action. This drug produces sodium retention and potassium excretion to increase blood pressure.

## Use

Health care providers use fludrocortisone for partial replacement of mineralocorticoids in the treatment of primary and secondary adrenocortical insufficiency resulting from Addison's disease.

### Use in Children

In young children who have taken high doses of fludrocortisone for long periods, the drug may cause hypercorticism or suppression of the HPA axis. This suppression can lead to adrenal crisis.

### Use in Older Adults

Use of fludrocortisone warrants caution in older adults because they are at risk for adverse effects of the drug. It is essential that the lowest possible dose is used for the shortest possible period.

### Use in Patients With Hepatic Impairment

Patients with hepatic impairment or cirrhosis who take fludrocortisone for long periods require close monitoring for fluid retention.

# Adverse Effects and Contraindications

The endocrine and metabolic effects of fludrocortisone are HPA axis suppression, growth suppression, hyperglycemia, and hypokalemia alkalosis. The most commonly reported cardiopulmonary adverse effects include heart failure, edema, and hypertension. Other adverse effects include peptic ulcer, acne, bruising, rash, cataracts, muscle weakness, and diaphoresis.

Contraindications include known hypersensitivity to the medication or any component of its formulation as well as a systemic fungal infection.

# Nursing Implications

### Preventing Interactions

Many medications interact with fludrocortisone, increasing or decreasing its effects (Box 45.3). Amphotericin B, indacaterol, loop diuretics, and thiazide diuretics in combination with fludrocortisone enhance the hypokalemic effect of fludrocortisone. Warfarin in combination with fludrocortisone enhances the anticoagulant effect, placing the patient at risk for hemorrhage.

### Administering the Medication

People should take fludrocortisone concomitantly with a glucocorticoid to enhance effectiveness and produce a more normal adrenal response. It is necessary to store the drug in an airtight, light-protected container at a temperature of 59°F to 86°F.

### Assessing for Therapeutic Effects

The nurse assesses sodium levels for increased values and potassium levels for decreased values. It is also important to assess intake, output, and blood pressure. The nurse monitors the patient's weight and assesses fluid volume status. If the weight increases by 5 lbs in 1 week, it is necessary to notify the prescriber.

### Assessing for Adverse Effects

In children, it is essential to assess growth patterns. In all patients, the nurse assesses the patient's fluid and electrolyte status for hypokalemia and alkalosis. He or she assesses for

**BOX 45.3** **Drug Interactions: Fludrocortisone**

**Drugs That Decrease the Effects of Fludrocortisone**
- Acetylcholinesterase inhibitors, neuromuscular agents
  *Increase muscle weakness*
- Aminoglutethimide
  *Increases metabolism of fludrocortisone*
- Antacids
  *Decrease bioavailability of fludrocortisone*
- Barbiturates, primidone
  *Decrease serum concentration of fludrocortisone*

**Drugs That Increase the Effects of Fludrocortisone**
- Antifungal agents, calcium channel blockers, macrolide antibiotics
  *Decrease the metabolism of corticosteroids*
- Aprepitant, estrogens, fosaprepitant, mifepristone, mitotane, telaprevir
  *Increase serum concentration of fludrocortisone*

**BOX 45.4** **Patient Teaching Guidelines for Fludrocortisone**

- Eat foods high in potassium such as bananas, potatoes, and orange juice.
- Consume foods high in calcium and vitamins A and D such as dairy products.
- Take supplements containing vitamins B6 and C, folate, zinc, and phosphorous.
- Decrease sodium in the diet and limit salt intake.
- Report muscle weakness, numbness, fatigue, depression, increased urination, changes in heart rhythm, epigastric pain, and tarry stools.
- Monitor weight and report an increase of 5 lbs to the primary health care provider.
- See an ophthalmologist every 6 months to determine if cataracts have formed.
- Have periodic laboratory tests as ordered by the prescriber.
- Report swelling of feet, hands, and shortness of breath to the primary health care provider.
- Report any infections or injuries to the primary health care provider.
- Wear medical alert identification.

pedal edema, hypertension, crackles in the lungs, and an audible $S_3$ that is indicative of heart failure. It is important to assess the GI system for burning, epigastric pain, and bleeding, which are signs of peptic ulcer disease. The nurse assesses the skin for bruising and rash. He or she also assesses for muscle weakness.

### Patient Teaching

Box 45.4 contains patient teaching guidelines for fludrocortisone.

## NCLEX Success

5. A patient is taking fludrocortisone acetate for adrenal insufficiency. Which of the following symptoms indicates that the patient is hypokalemic?
   A. tetany
   B. irregular pulse rate
   C. decreased pulse rate
   D. muscle weakness

6. The administration of fludrocortisone is necessary in which of the following conditions?
   A. hypoglycemia
   B. hypernatremia
   C. hypercalcemia
   D. hyperphosphatemia

7. A woman receives a prescription of hydrocortisone for adrenal insufficiency. It is necessary to report which of the following conditions to the primary health care provider?
   A. fever
   B. headache
   C. insomnia
   D. neuropathic pain

# DRUGS USED TO TREAT CUSHING'S DISEASE

The treatment of Cushing's disease depends on the cause of the medical condition. The most common treatment of hypercortisolism is transsphenoidal surgery. Drug therapy is indicated in several situations: when surgery is contraindicated, in preparation for surgery, in occult ectopic ACTH syndrome, with a recurrence of hypercortisolism following surgery, and with treatment using radiation therapy to the pituitary.

# GLUCOCORTICOID RECEPTOR ANTAGONISTS

Glucocorticoid receptor antagonists are administered when surgery to treat corticotroph tumors is delayed or contraindicated. The two medications used to normalize the 24-hour urinary cortisol are cabergoline and pasireotide. Cabergoline is an ergot derivative. Its off-label use is to normalize urinary free cortisol levels in the treatment of Cushing's syndrome. Pasireotide is a somatostatin analog to maximize the reduction of urinary free cortisol. The maximum reduction of cortisol is usually noted in approximately 2 months.

Cabergoline is a long-acting dopamine receptor agonist. It has a high affinity for $D_2$ receptors in the anterior pituitary. It inhibits lactation and hyperprolactinemia. Cabergoline is administered orally with food. Cabergoline is extensively distributed to the pituitary gland. It is 40% to 42% protein bound, with a half-life of 63 to 69 hours. Metabolism of the drug takes place in the liver by hydrolysis. The peak of action is 2 to 3 hours, with 60% excretion in the feces and approximately 20% in the urine. Patients with impaired liver function will see an increase in cabergoline levels. Hot flashes, edema, and orthostatic hypotension are the most commonly reported adverse effects. Patients who have a history of cardiac valvular disease should not be administered cabergoline. It is also contraindicated in patients with a known ergot hypersensitivity.

Pasireotide (Signifor, Signifor LAR) is administered subcutaneously for Cushing's disease. The initial dose is 0.6 or 0.9 mg subcutaneously twice daily. The recommended maintenance dose is 0.3 to 0.9 mg twice daily. Signifor LAR is administered 10 mg once every 28 days. The maximum dose is 40 mg. Pasireotide binds to somatostatin receptor with high affinity for $sst_1$, $sst_2$, $sst_3$, and $sst_5$. It inhibits ACTH secretion and causes decreased cortisol secretion. Patients with severe hepatic impairment should avoid this medication. If symptoms of hepatic impairment develop, the medication should be discontinued. Gloves should be worn when unpacking, administering, or disposing of pasireotide. Assess the patient for peripheral edema, hyperglycemia, diarrhea, and prolonged partial thromboplastin time. Assess the serum alanine aminotransferase and serum aspartate aminotransferase; if there is an elevation of ALT and AST, the medication dosage should be reduced or discontinued. In addition, assess the blood glucose for elevation.

# 11-DEOXYCORTISOL INHIBITORS

In Cushing's disease, the goal of drug therapy is to inhibit one or more enzymes contained in cortisol synthesis. The antifungal drug (see Chap. 24) **ketoconazole** has the ability to inhibit these enzymes. It also prevents the conversion of

## TABLE 45.3

### Drugs Administered for Cushing's Disease

| Drug Class | Prototype | Other Drugs in the Class |
|---|---|---|
| Glucocorticoid receptor antagonists | N/A | Ergot derivative: Cabergoline<br>Somatostatin analog: Pasireotide (Signifor, Signifor LAR) |
| 11-Deoxycortisol inhibitors | Ketoconazole | Metyrapone (Metopirone) Etomidate (Amidate) |
| Antineoplastics | Mitotane (Lysodren) | None |

11-deoxycortisol to cortisol. Table 45.3 identifies the drugs administered for the treatment of Cushing's disease.

## Pharmacokinetics and Action

Ketoconazole is absorbed rapidly in the GI tract. The drug is protein bound. It is metabolized in the liver and excreted by the kidneys.

Ketoconazole acts by inhibiting the first step in cortisol biosynthesis and the conversion of deoxycortisol to cortisol.

## Use

Health care providers use ketoconazole to control cortisol secretion in Cushing's disease. Table 45.4 presents route and dosage information for the drugs used in Cushing's disease.

## Adverse Effects and Contraindications

The most commonly reported adverse effects associated with ketoconazole include pruritus, headache, sedation, nausea, vomiting, and abdominal pain. Gynecomastia, impotence, and decreased libido may occur and are related to the decrease in testosterone production. The FDA has issued a **BLACK BOX WARNING ◆** stating that ketoconazole can cause hepatotoxicity. Therefore, caution is warranted in patients with hepatic impairment.

Contraindications include a known hypersensitivity to the medication.

## Nursing Implications

### Preventing Interactions

Some medications interact with ketoconazole, decreasing its effects (Box 45.5). Ketoconazole combined with echinacea puts the patient at risk for hepatotoxicity. In addition, a **BLACK BOX WARNING ◆** alerts that ketoconazole increases the plasma concentration of methadone, pimozide, cisapride, disopyramide, dronedarone, and ranolazine, and it may prolong QT intervals on an electrocardiogram. Coadministration increases the risk of life-threatening ventricular dysrhythmias, such as torsades de pointes.

### Administering the Medication

People should take ketoconazole with water, coffee, tea, or fruit juice. The presence of stomach acid enhances absorption.

## TABLE 45.4

## DRUGS AT A GLANCE: Glucocorticoid Receptor Antagonists, 11-Deoxycortisol Inhibitors, and Antineoplastics

| Drug | Pregnancy Category | Routes and Dosage Ranges | |
|---|---|---|---|
| | | **Adults** | **Children** |
| **Glucocorticoid Receptor Antagonists** | | | |
| Cabergoline | Discontinue use during pregnancy | 0.5 mg PO daily | Not administered to children |
| Pasireotide (Signifor, Signifor LAR) | Alternative agents should be used during pregnancy | 0.6 or 0.9 mg subcutaneous two times per day. Signifor LAR: Initial: 10 mg once every 28 d; may increase dose to a maximum of 40 mg once every 28 d | Not administered to children |
| **11-Deoxycortisol Inhibitors** | | | |
| **Ketoconazole** (✳ Apo-Ketoconazole, Teva-Ketoconazole) | C | 200–400 mg PO 2–3 times per day | Not administered to children |
| Metyrapone (Metopirone) | C | 250 mg PO four times daily (max dose 6000 mg). Diagnostic test for hypothalamic–pituitary adrenocorticotropic hormone (ACTH) function: single dose, 30 mg/kg (max 3 g) at midnight; multiple dose, 750 mg/kg every 4 h for 6 doses | Diagnostic test for ACTH function: single dose, 30 mg/kg (min 250 mg; max 750 mg) at midnight; multiple dose, 15 mg/kg every 4 h for 6 doses |
| Etomidate (Amidate) | | 0.04–0.05 mg/kg IV per hour titrated to serum cortisol level | Same as adults |
| **Antineoplastics** | | | |
| **Mitotane** (Lysodren; ✳ Lysodren) | | Adrenocortical carcinoma: 2–6 g/d in 3–4 divided doses and then increase incrementally to 9–10 g/d in 3–4 divided doses; max tolerated range is 2–16 g/d, usually 9–10 g/d; max studied dose is 18–19 g/d. Cushing's syndrome: 500 mg PO three times per day; max dose 4000–8000 mg in three divided doses per day | Safety and efficacy not established |

## Assessing for Therapeutic Effects and Adverse Effects

The nurse assesses for a decrease in blood pressure. He or she checks the blood glucose for normal levels. It is also important to assess for increased muscle strength and cardiopulmonary status without edema or crackles in the lower lobes and audible $S_3$.

Assessing for adverse effects is also necessary. The nurse assesses for skin irritation and pruritus; nausea, vomiting, and headache; and diminished libido, gynecomastia, and impotence.

### BOX 45.5 Drug Interactions: Ketoconazole

**Drugs That Decrease the Effects of Ketoconazole**
- Antacids, anticholinergics
  *Decrease absorption, thus decreasing serum levels*
- Isoniazid, rifampin
  *Increase metabolism*

## Patient Teaching

Box 45.6 presents patient teaching guidelines for ketoconazole.

### BOX 45.6 Patient Teaching Guidelines for Ketoconazole

- Take the medication with water, coffee, tea, or fruit juice. Acidic drinks enhance absorption.
- Take the drug with food to prevent gastrointestinal upset.
- Do not take antacids.
- Maintain serum liver enzyme laboratory tests as ordered by the prescriber.
- Report clay-colored stools, extreme thirst, and yellowing of skin or eyes. These signs and symptoms indicate elevated liver enzymes.

**QSEN Alert: Patient-Centered Care**

Stomach acid increases the absorption of some medications, like ketoconazole. Coffee, tea, and fruit juice increase the acidity in the stomach, enhancing the absorption of these medications.

## Other Drugs in the Class

Metyrapone and etomidate are also administered for their inhibition of 11-deoxycortisol. Metyrapone (Metopirone) blocks the final step in cortisol biosynthesis and increases adrenal androgen production. The drug also decreases cortisol production. It is administered as an adjunctive agent to prevent further release of ACTH in patients with mild Cushing's disease or following radiation therapy of the pituitary gland.

Etomidate (Amidate) also blocks the production of cortisol. Normally administered to produce sedation, it is a local anesthetic and is discussed in Chapter 50. Prescribers order it for patients with ectopic secretion of ACTH (Cushing's disease).

 **QSEN Alert: Safety**

Studies have not demonstrated sedation with etomidate at recommended doses for Cushing's disease. However, patients should be managed in an intensive care unit with sedation scoring every 2 hours for the first 24 hours, then every 12 hours, to assess for sedation.

Etomidate lowers serum cortisol to normal in approximately 10 hours. Cortisol levels should be measured every 4 to 6 hours.

## ANTINEOPLASTICS

Health care providers use the antineoplastic drug **mitotane** (Lysodren) for the treatment of adrenocortical carcinoma. The drug may also be useful for therapy of Cushing's disease caused by such carcinoma.

## Pharmacokinetics and Action

Mitotane is absorbed rapidly, with approximately 40% of the drug absorbed in the GI tract. The onset of action is 2 to 4 weeks. The half-life of mitotane is 18 to 159 days. The drug is metabolized in the liver and deposited in the adipose tissues. It is eliminated in the urine and feces.

Mitotane is an adrenolytic agent that causes the adrenal cortex to atrophy. The drug affects the mitochondrial adrenal cortical cells, resulting in decreased production of cortisol. It also alters the peripheral metabolism of steroids.

## Use

Mitotane is used for the treatment of an inoperable adrenocortical carcinoma. Its unlabeled use is for treatment of Cushing's syndrome. Table 45.4 gives route and dosing information for mitotane.

## Adverse Effects and Contraindications

The CNS effects of mitotane include depression, lethargy, and dizziness. GI effects are anorexia, nausea, vomiting, and diarrhea. Neuromuscular effects include weakness and muscle tremors.

Contraindications include known hypersensitivity to the drug.

## Nursing Implications

### Preventing Interactions

Mitotane increases the metabolism of phenytoin, phenobarbital, and warfarin. The antineoplastic drug decreases the effect of potassium-sparing diuretics. Alcohol increases the CNS depression associated with mitotane.

### Administering the Medication

The FDA has issued a  **BLACK BOX WARNING** ◆ stating that it is necessary to withhold mitotane in the event the patient develops shock or with trauma, because the primary action of the drug is adrenal suppression and adrenal crisis can occur. The onset of shock or trauma should lead to a temporary discontinuation of mitotane followed by the administration of steroids.

 **QSEN Alert: Safety**

The Institute for Safe Medication Practices considers mitotane to be a drug that has a heightened risk of causing significant patient harm when used in error.

### Assessing for Therapeutic Effects

The nurse assesses for a decrease in blood pressure. It is necessary to check the blood glucose for normal levels. The nurse also assesses for increased muscle strength and cardiopulmonary status without edema or crackles in the lower lobes and audible $S_3$.

### Assessing for Adverse Effects

The nurse assesses for CNS depression. Such depression may place the patient at risk for injury. It is also important to assess the gait for safety with walking. The nurse assesses for decreased weight related to anorexia or fluid and electrolyte balance related to nausea and vomiting, as well as for muscle weakness and tremors.

### Patient Teaching

Box 45.7 presents patient teaching guidelines for mitotane.

## NCLEX Success

8. A woman has received a diagnosis of Cushing's disease and is taking ketoconazole. Which of the following conditions affects the treatment plan?

    A. hypertension with administration of hydrochlorothiazide
    B. type 2 diabetes with the administration of metformin
    C. migraine headaches with the administration of ergotamine
    D. heart failure with the administration of digoxin

9. A man is receiving mitotane for an inoperable adrenocortical carcinoma. He is admitted to the emergency department following an automobile accident. He is diaphoretic and unresponsive. He has a blood pressure of 80/30 mm Hg. What medication should the nurse anticipate administering?

    A. a steroid
    B. an anticoagulant
    C. a beta-adrenergic blocker
    D. a sulfonylurea

10. A patient is taking ketoconazole for the treatment of Cushing's disease. When providing patient teaching, which of the following is most important?

    A. Take antibiotics at the first sign of a sore throat.
    B. Have prothrombin times drawn monthly.
    C. Salt cravings mean that it is fine to increase salt intake.
    D. Take the medication with juice or an acidic beverage.

## THE NURSING PROCESS

A concept map outlines the nursing process related to drug therapy considerations in this chapter. Additional nursing implications related to the disease process should also be considered in care decisions.

**Assessment**

- For the patient with Addison's disease, the major focus of the assessment should be on the severity of symptoms and the effectiveness of drug therapy for the treatment of the disease. Assess for dehydration, hypovolemia, hypoglycemia, hyperkalemia, weight loss, hyperpigmentation of gums and mucous membranes, and depression.
- For the patient with Cushing's disease, the major focus of the assessment should be on the severity of symptoms, body image, and drug therapy of the treatment of the disease. Assess for glucose intolerance, fragile skin tissues, truncal obesity, peripheral edema, osteoporosis, moon face, buffalo hump, irritability, and decreased wound healing.

**Outcomes of Therapy**

The patient will
- Take the drug correctly.
- Practice measures to decrease the need for corticosteroids and minimize adverse effects.
- Be monitored regularly for adverse drug effects.
- Keep appointments for follow-up care.
- Be assisted to cope with body image changes.
- Verbalize or demonstrate essential drug information.

**Nursing Interventions**

- For the patient taking long-term, systemic mineralocorticoid/glucocorticoid therapy, use supplementary drugs as ordered and nondrug measures to decrease dosage and adverse effects of corticosteroid drugs. Specific measures include the following:
- Help set reasonable goals of drug therapy. For example, partial relief of symptoms may be better than complete relief if the latter requires larger doses or longer periods of treatment with systemic drugs.
- Dietary changes may be beneficial. Salt restriction may help prevent hypernatremia, fluid retention, and edema. Foods high in potassium may help prevent hypokalemia. A diet high in protein, calcium, and vitamin D may help prevent osteoporosis. Increased intake of vitamin C may help decrease bleeding in the skin and soft tissues.
- Avoid exposing the patient to potential sources of infection by washing hands frequently, using aseptic technique when changing dressings, keeping health care personnel and visitors with colds or other infections away from the patient, and following other appropriate measures.
- Handle tissues very gently during any procedures (e.g., bathing, assisting out of bed, venipunctures).

**Evaluation**

- Interview and observe for relief of symptoms for which mineralocorticoids, adrenocorticoids, cortisol, 11-deoxycortisol inhibitors, and antineoplastic agents have been prescribed.
- Interview and observe for accurate drug administration.
- Interview and observe for use of nondrug measures indicated for the condition being treated.
- Interview and observe for adverse drug effects on a regular basis.
- Interview regarding drug knowledge and effects to be reported to health care providers.

## KEY CONCEPTS

- In adrenocortical insufficiency, the deficiency in mineralocorticoids causes a loss of urinary sodium, chloride, and water, leading to decreased cardiac output.
- Primary adrenocortical insufficiency is known as Addison's disease. This chronic metabolic disorder requires lifetime hormone replacement.
- Clinical manifestations of Addison's disease include lethargy, weakness, fever, anorexia, nausea, vomiting, and weight loss. Excessive sodium loss results in cardiovascular collapse and shock. Hyperkalemia and hypoglycemia are present.
- Secondary adrenocortical insufficiency is a disorder of the HPA system.
- In Cushing's disease, adrenocortical excess resulting from excessive corticotropin leads to hyperplasia of the adrenal cortex.
- Clinical manifestations of Cushing's disease include a buffalo hump, heavy trunk, thin extremities, fragile skin, impaired wound healing, and bruising. A woman has masculine traits.

- The goal of treatment for Addison's disease is to replace the adrenocorticoids to correct adrenal insufficiency. It is important to replace both the mineralocorticoid and adrenocorticoid.
- Health care providers give hydrocortisone systemically for acute and chronic adrenal insufficiency.
- A **BLACK BOX WARNING ◆** stipulates that patients who are being treated with hydrocortisone should not receive live virus vaccines.
- Patients who have a mineralocorticoid deficiency may take fludrocortisone. They usually combine it with a glucocorticoid for Addison's disease.
- Ketoconazole is an antifungal drug (see Chap. 24) that is administered for the treatment of Cushing's disease.

- The FDA has issued a **BLACK BOX WARNING ◆** stating that ketoconazole can cause hepatotoxicity. Caution is necessary in hepatic impairment.
- A **BLACK BOX WARNING ◆** alerts nurses that ketoconazole increases the plasma concentration of methadone, pimozide, cisapride, disopyramide, dronedarone, and ranolazine, and it may prolong QT intervals, increasing the risk of life-threatening ventricular dysrhythmias.
- Mitotane is an antineoplastic drug that is administered for the treatment of adrenocortical carcinoma.
- The FDA has issued a **BLACK BOX WARNING ◆** stating that it is necessary to withhold mitotane in the event the patient develops shock or with trauma. The primary action of mitotane is adrenal suppression.

## CLINICAL REASONING CASE STUDY

**Meet the Patient**

Richard Chan, a 50-year-old man, is admitted to the hospital with a fractured hip. While hospitalized, he receives a diagnosis of hyperplasia of the adrenal gland (Cushing's disease) after an overnight dexamethasone suppression test revealed that there is no suppression of cortisol. The endocrinologist prescribes ketoconazole 300 mg orally twice daily.

- What is the cause of adrenal gland hyperplasia?
- Mr. Chan asks if the Cushing's disease contributed to the fracture. What is the best response by the nurse?
- What blood test should be monitored during the administration of ketoconazole?

**Assessing Drug Information**

- Ketoconazole acts by inhibiting the first step in cortisol biosynthesis and the conversion of deoxycortisol to cortisol.
- The most commonly reported adverse effects associated with ketoconazole include pruritus, headache, sedation, nausea, vomiting, and abdominal pain. Gynecomastia, impotence, and decreased libido may occur and are related to the decrease in testosterone production.
- Because of the risk of hepatotoxicity with ketoconazole, it is necessary to measure liver enzymes routinely.

**Nursing Actions**

- Explain to Mr. Chan that the excessive secretion of corticotropin with Cushing's disease results in osteoporosis and fractures; this likely contributed to the fracture.
- Instruct him to take ketoconazole with water, coffee, tea, or fruit juice because the presence of stomach acid enhances absorption. Additional patient teaching guidelines are found in Box 45.6.
- Assess for the therapeutic effects of ketoconazole, including decreasing blood pressure and normalizing blood glucose levels. It is also important to assess for increased muscle strength and cardiopulmonary status without edema or crackles in the lower lobes and the absence of an audible $S_3$ heart sound.

---

*Visit* **thePoint** *at* **http://thePoint.lww.com/Frandsen12e** *for answers to NCLEX Success questions (in Appendix A), answers to Clinical Application Case Studies (in Appendix B), and more!*

## REFERENCES AND RESOURCES

Hinkle, J. L., & Cheever, K. H. (2018). *Brunner & Suddarth's textbook of medical-surgical nursing* (14th ed.). Philadelphia: Wolters Kluwer.

Hunt, D. (2012). Is it Addison's disease or Cushing's syndrome? Two patient scenarios provide hints to help you differentiate these endocrine disorders. *American Nurse, 7*(1), 8–11.

Iwasaku, M., Shinzawa, M., Tanaka, S., Kimachi, K., & Kawakami, K. (2017). Clinical characteristics of adrenal crisis in adult population with and without predisposing chronic adrenal insufficiency; a retrospective cohort study. *BMC Endocrine Disorders, 14*(58), 1–10. doi:10.1186/s12802-017-0208-0

Nieman, L. K. (2020a). Clinical manifestations of adrenal insufficiency in adults. In *UpToDate.* Lexi-Comp, Inc.

Nieman, L. K. (2020b). Medical therapy of hypercortisolism (Cushing's syndrome). In *UpToDate.* Lexi-Comp, Inc.

Nieman, L. K. (2020c). Overview of the treatment of Cushing's syndrome. In *UpToDate.* Lexi-Comp, Inc.

Nieman, L. K. (2020d). Treatment of adrenal insufficiency in adults. In *UpToDate.* Lexi-Comp, Inc.

Nieman, L. K., Biller, B. M. K., Findling, J. W., Murad, M. H., Newell-Price, J., Savage, M. O., et al. (2015). Treatment of Cushing's syndrome: An Endocrine Society clinical practice guideline. *Journal of Clinical Endocrinology and Metabolism, 100*(8), 2807–2831.

Norris, T. L. (2019). *Porth's pathophysiology: Concepts of altered health status* (10th ed.). Philadelphia: Wolters Kluwer.

UpToDate. (2019). *Drug information.* Lexi-Comp, Inc.

# Drugs Affecting the Autonomic and Central Nervous System

# Physiology of the Autonomic and Central Nervous Systems and Indications for the Use of Drug Therapy

## LEARNING OBJECTIVES

*After studying this chapter, you should be able to:*

1. Identify the physiologic effects of the sympathetic nervous system.
2. Differentiate the subtypes and functions of sympathetic nervous system receptors.
3. Identify the physiologic effects of the parasympathetic nervous system.
4. Differentiate the subtypes and functions of parasympathetic nervous system receptors.
5. Describe signal transduction and the intracellular events that occur when receptors of the autonomic nervous system are stimulated.
6. Recognize the terminology and general characteristics of drugs affecting the autonomic nervous system.

## CLINICAL APPLICATION CASE STUDY

Jennifer Johnson is a 35-year-old woman who runs 5 miles daily before work. One morning while running, she encounters a bear on the jogging trail. She begins to hyperventilate and can feel her heart racing. She also begins to sweat profusely, and her pupils begin to dilate. The bear runs into the woods when a car approaches.

## KEY TERMS

**Affinity:** rate of binding of ligands that demonstrates a tendency or strength of the effect

**Agonist:** a ligand that can bind to a receptor, alter the function of the receptor, and trigger a physiologic response for that receptor

**Antagonist:** a ligand that binds to a receptor but fails to activate the physiologic response for that receptor

**Downregulation:** a process by which a cell decreases the quantity of a cellular component in response to an external variable; also called desensitization

**First messenger:** extracellular ligand that binds to a cell surface receptor and initiates intracellular activity

**Ligands:** substances, such as neurotransmitters, medications, and hormones, that bind to receptors in the autonomic nervous system

**Second messenger:** molecule inside the cell that is the link between events occurring outside the cell and resulting events that will occur inside the cell

**Signal transduction:** cascade of intracellular events that occur when receptors located on target tissues are stimulated by a ligand

**Upregulation:** a process by which a cell increases the quantity of a cellular component in response to an external variable; also called hypersensitization

## INTRODUCTION

The nervous system has two main divisions: the central nervous system (CNS) and the peripheral nervous system (PNS) (Fig. 46.1). The CNS includes the brain and spinal cord. It receives and processes incoming sensory information and responds by sending out signals that initiate or modify body processes. The PNS includes all the neurons and ganglia found outside the CNS. Afferent neurons carry sensory input from the periphery to the CNS and modify motor output through the action of reflex arcs. Efferent neurons carry motor signals from the CNS to the peripheral areas of the body. Ganglia are nerve cell clusters that house the cell bodies of the afferent nerves.

The efferent portion of the PNS has two subdivisions: the somatic nervous system and the autonomic nervous system (ANS). The somatic nervous system innervates skeletal muscles and controls voluntary movement. The ANS, without conscious thought or effort, controls involuntary activities in smooth muscle, in secretory glands, and in the visceral organs of the body such as the heart.

## STRUCTURE AND FUNCTION OF THE AUTONOMIC NERVOUS SYSTEM

Structural centers in the CNS, including the hypothalamus, brainstem, and spinal cord, regulate the ANS. There are two parts of the ANS: the sympathetic nervous system (SNS) and the parasympathetic nervous system. The functions of the ANS can be broadly described as activities designed to maintain a constant internal environment (homeostasis), to respond to stress or emergencies, and to repair body tissues.

Nerve impulses are generated and transmitted to body tissues in the SNS and the parasympathetic nervous system, as

**Figure 46.1.** Divisions of the human nervous system. The nervous system can be divided anatomically into the central (brain and spinal cord) nervous system (CNS) and the peripheral (sensory organs and nerves) nervous system (PNS). The nervous system can be functionally divided into the somatic nervous system and the autonomic nervous system (ANS). The somatic nervous system leads to contraction of muscle fibers through efferent (motor) neurons. The autonomic nervous system controls the heart, glands, and hollow organs and is essential in maintaining homeostasis. (Reprinted with permission from Plowman, S. A., & Smith, D. L. (2017). *Exercise physiology for health, fitness, and performance* (5th ed.). Philadelphia, PA: Wolters Kluwer.)

they are in the CNS. Preganglionic nerve impulses travel from the CNS along the presynaptic nerves to ganglia. Ganglia are bundles of nerve tissue composed of the terminal end of the presynaptic neuron and clusters of postsynaptic neuron cell bodies. A neurotransmitter is released from the terminal end of the presynaptic neuron, allowing the nervous impulse to bridge the synapse between the presynaptic and postsynaptic nerves. The postganglionic impulses travel from the ganglia to target or effector tissues of the heart, blood vessels, glands, other visceral organs, and smooth muscle. A neurotransmitter is released from the terminal end of the postsynaptic neuron, allowing the impulse to reach the effector tissue, stimulate a receptor, and bring about a response (Fig. 46.2).

The primary neurotransmitters of the ANS are acetylcholine and norepinephrine. Acetylcholine is synthesized from acetyl-coenzyme A and choline. It is released at preganglionic fibers of both the SNS and parasympathetic nervous system and at postganglionic fibers of the parasympathetic nervous system. Acetylcholine is also released from postganglionic sympathetic neurons that innervate the sweat glands and from motor neurons of the somatic nervous system that innervate the skeletal muscles. The nerve fibers that secrete acetylcholine are called cholinergic fibers. Acetylcholine acts on receptors in body organs and tissues to cause parasympathetic effects.

Norepinephrine is synthesized from the amino acid tyrosine by a series of enzymatic conversions that also produce dopamine and epinephrine (i.e., tyrosine → dopamine → norepinephrine → epinephrine). Except in the adrenal medulla, where most of the norepinephrine is converted to epinephrine, the chemical reaction stops with norepinephrine. This neurotransmitter is released at most postganglionic fibers of the SNS. Norepinephrine-secreting nerve fibers are called adrenergic fibers. Norepinephrine acts on receptors in body organs and tissues to cause sympathetic effects.

Neurotransmitters, such as acetylcholine and norepinephrine, as well as medications and hormones that can bind to receptors in the ANS, are collectively called **ligands**. The rate of binding is called **affinity**, and this rate typifies a tendency or strength of the effect. A ligand that can bind to a receptor, alter the function of the receptor, and trigger a physiologic response is called an **agonist** for that receptor. Ligands that bind to a receptor but fail to activate the physiologic response are receptor **antagonists**. When receptors located on target tissues are stimulated by a ligand, a cascade of intracellular events known as **signal transduction** is initiated.

The extracellular ligand that binds to the receptor to initiate the intracellular activity is the **first messenger**. In most cases, this ligand–receptor interaction activates a cell membrane–bound G protein and an effector enzyme, which then activate a

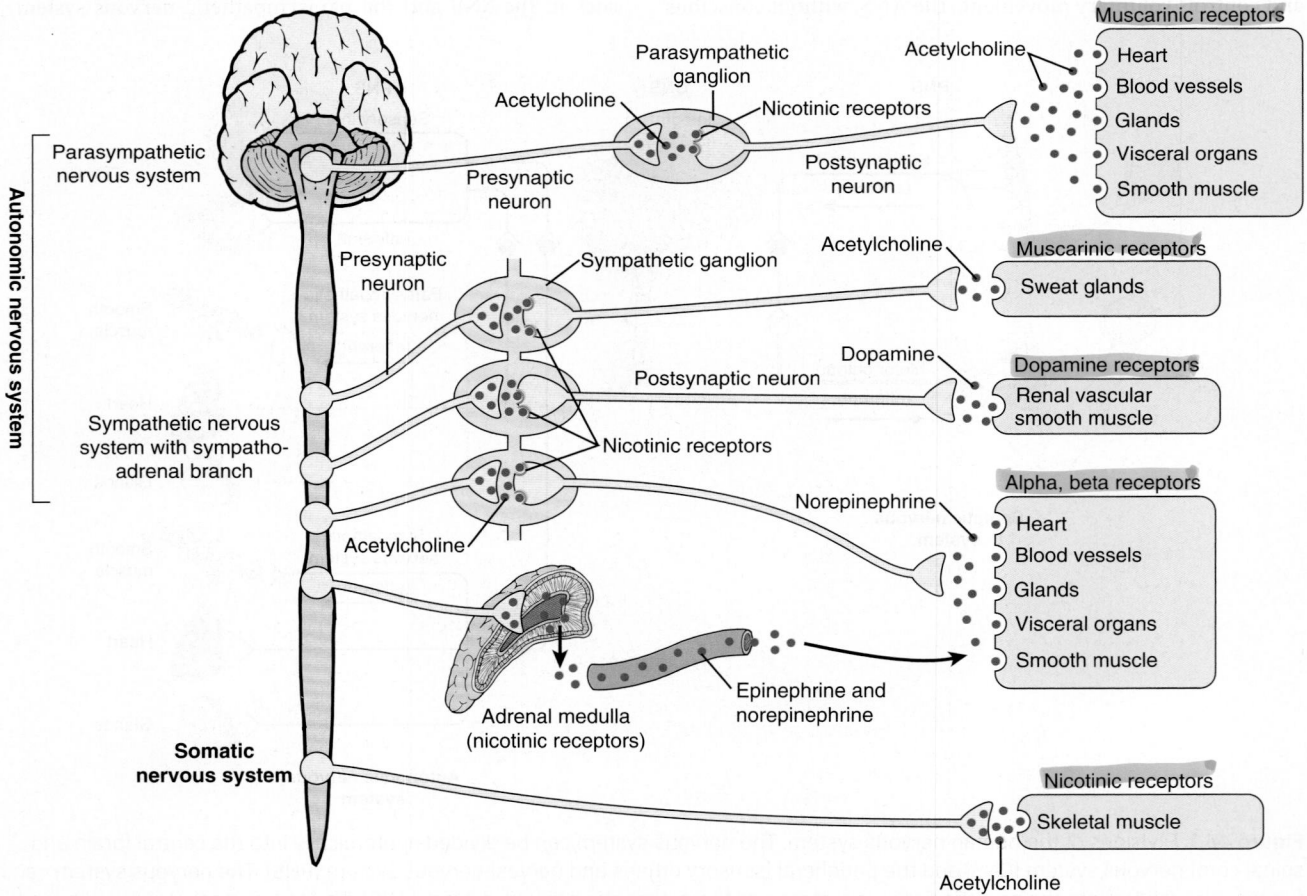

**Figure 46.2.** Organization of the autonomic and somatic nervous systems. [Reprinted with permission from Brophy, K., Scarlett-Ferguson, H., Webber, K. S., Abrams, A. C., Pennington, S. S., & Lammon, C. B. [2011]. *Clinical drug therapy for Canadian practice* [2nd ed.]. Philadelphia, PA: Wolters Kluwer Health | Lippincott Williams & Wilkins.]

molecule inside the cell called a **second messenger**. This messenger is the link between events that are occurring outside the cell (i.e., receptor activation by the ligand) and resulting events that will occur inside the cell, such as opening ion channels, stimulating other enzymes, and increasing intracellular calcium levels. These intracellular events ultimately produce the physiologic responses to neurotransmitter and hormone release or drug administration. Figure 46.3 illustrates the intracellular events of signal transduction that occur when an adrenergic beta-receptor is stimulated by epinephrine.

Involuntary muscles in organs and tissues in the body are innervated by both divisions of the ANS. However, most organs are predominantly controlled by one system. For example, in the gastrointestinal tract, the parasympathetic nervous system predominates, and stimulation of the parasympathetic nervous system regulates the routine activities of digestion and elimination.

The two divisions of the ANS are usually antagonistic in their actions on a particular organ. When the sympathetic system excites a particular organ, the parasympathetic system often inhibits it and vice versa. Stimulation of the ANS causes excitatory effects in some organs but inhibitory effects in others. For example, sympathetic stimulation of the heart causes an increased rate and force of myocardial contraction, and parasympathetic stimulation decreases rate and force of contraction, thereby resting the heart. In the gastrointestinal tract, stimulation of the parasympathetic nervous system promotes digestion, and sympathetic stimulation decreases blood flow and impairs digestion. Exceptions to this antagonistic action include sweating and regulation of arteriolar blood vessel diameter, which is controlled by the SNS.

## Sympathetic Nervous System

The SNS is stimulated by physical or emotional stress, such as strenuous exercise or work, pain, hemorrhage, intense emotions, and temperature extremes. The reaction produced by the SNS is essentially a whole-body response and includes:

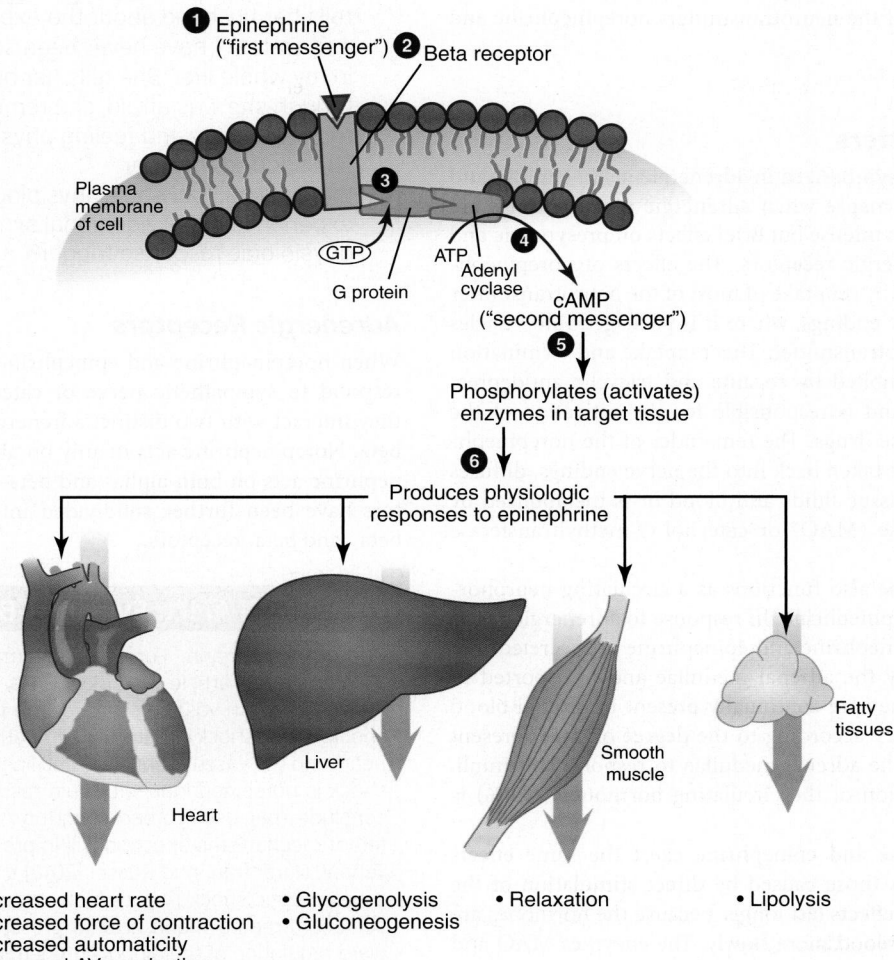

**Figure 46.3.** Signal transduction mechanism for an adrenergic beta-receptor. Epinephrine [1], the "first messenger," interacts with a beta-receptor [2]. This hormone–receptor complex activates a G protein, which reacts with a guanosine triphosphate [GTP] [3]. The activated G protein then activates the enzyme adenyl cyclase, which [4] catalyzes the conversion of adenosine triphosphate [ATP] to cyclic adenosine monophosphate [cAMP], the "second messenger" [5]. cAMP activates enzymes, which bring about the biologic responses to epinephrine [6]. AV, atrioventricular. [Reprinted with permission from Brophy, K., Scarlett-Ferguson, H., Webber, K. S., Abrams, A. C., Pennington, S. S., & Lammon, C. B. [2011]. *Clinical drug therapy for Canadian practice* [2nd ed.]. Philadelphia, PA: Wolters Kluwer Health | Lippincott Williams & Wilkins.]

SNS ! Fight or Flight

- Increased arterial blood pressure and cardiac output
- Increased blood flow to the brain, heart, and skeletal muscles; decreased blood flow to the viscera, skin, and other organs not needed for "fight or flight" (whether real or imaginary)
- Increased rate of cellular metabolism, with increased oxygen consumption and carbon dioxide production
- Increased breakdown of muscle glycogen for energy
- Increased blood glucose
- Increased mental activity and ability to think clearly
- Increased muscle strength
- Increased rate of blood coagulation
- Increased rate and depth of respiration
- Pupil dilation to aid vision
- Increased sweating (Note that acetylcholine is the neurotransmitter for this sympathetic response—not the normal postganglionic neurotransmitter, which is norepinephrine.)

These responses are protective mechanisms designed to help the person cope with the stress or escape from it. The intensity and duration of the sympathetic response depend on the existing amounts of the neurotransmitters norepinephrine and epinephrine.

## Neurotransmitters

Norepinephrine is synthesized in adrenergic nerve endings and released into the synapse when adrenergic nerve endings are stimulated. It exerts intense but brief effects on presynaptic and postsynaptic adrenergic receptors. The effects of norepinephrine are terminated by reuptake of most of the neurotransmitter back into the nerve endings, where it is packaged into vesicles for reuse as a neurotransmitter. This reuptake and termination process can be inhibited by cocaine and tricyclic antidepressant medications and is responsible for the activation of the SNS seen with these drugs. The remainder of the norepinephrine, which was not taken back into the nerve endings, diffuses into surrounding tissue fluids and blood or is metabolized by monoamine oxidase (MAO) or catechol-O-methyltransferase (COMT).

Norepinephrine also functions as a circulating neurohormone, along with epinephrine. In response to adrenergic nerve stimulation, norepinephrine and epinephrine are secreted into the bloodstream by the adrenal medullae and transported to all body tissues. They are continually present in arterial blood in amounts that vary according to the degree of stress present and the ability of the adrenal medullae to respond to stimuli. The larger proportion of the circulating hormones (~80%) is epinephrine.

Norepinephrine and epinephrine exert the same effects on target tissues as those caused by direct stimulation of the SNS. However, the effects last longer because the hormones are removed from the blood more slowly. The enzymes MAO and COMT metabolize these hormones, mainly in the liver. Box 46.1 outlines the strength and type of response to activation of alpha- and beta-receptors.

Dopamine is also an adrenergic neurotransmitter and a catecholamine. In the brain, dopamine is essential for normal function. In peripheral tissues, its main effects are on the heart and blood vessels of the renal system and viscera, where it produces vasodilation.

---

**BOX 46.1** **Response to Activation of Alpha- and Beta-Receptors**

Activation of alpha₁ and beta₁ receptors causes stimulatory responses:
- When activating alpha₁ receptors, norepinephrine causes a greater response than does epinephrine.
- When activating beta₁ receptors, epinephrine and norepinephrine cause equal responses.

Activation of alpha₂, beta₂, and beta₃ receptors causes inhibitory responses:
- When activating alpha₂ receptors, epinephrine causes a greater or equal response than does norepinephrine.
- When activating beta₂ receptors, epinephrine causes a significantly greater response than does norepinephrine.

---

### Clinical Application 46.1

- When Mrs. Johnson returns home, she tells her husband about the experience and states "I have never been so scared in my whole life." She tells her husband that even though she was afraid, she remembers being able to think clearly and feeling physically stronger after she spotted the bear.
- Explain Mrs. Johnson's physiologic response to the experience. What additional symptoms does this physiologic response trigger?

## Adrenergic Receptors

When norepinephrine and epinephrine act on body cells that respond to sympathetic nerve or catecholamine stimulation, they interact with two distinct adrenergic receptors, alpha and beta. Norepinephrine acts mainly on alpha-receptors, and epinephrine acts on both alpha- and beta-receptors. These receptors have been further subdivided into alpha₁, alpha₂, beta₁, beta₂, and beta₃ receptors.

---

**! QSEN Alert: Evidence-Based Practice**

Chawla, Ostermann, Forni, and Tidmarsh (2019) published a commentary article in *Critical Care*, promoting the use of broad-spectrum vasopressors for the management of septic shock. Septic shock impairs the sympathetic modulation of the heart and the vasculature. The first-line vasopressor for septic shock is norepinephrine with fluid resuscitation. The authors conclude that using broad-spectrum vasopressors with different mechanisms of action will improve outcomes of shock. Teboul, Durantrau, and Russel (2018) suggest that patients in severe septic shock require high doses of norepinephrine to achieve targeted mean arterial pressure, due to the downward regulation of the *alpha₁* adrenergic receptors. High-dose norepinephrine can injure the myocardial cells, so the use of vasopressin can be administered as adjunctive medication to reduce the dosage of norepinephrine. Vasopressin will elevate blood pressure and restore vascular tone. Other vasopressors that can also improve outcomes are selepressin or terlipressin. The oral vasopressin midodrine has had positive outcomes in the recovery phase of septic shock and has shortened the patient's stay in the intensive care unit.

When dopamine acts on body cells that respond to adrenergic stimulation, it can activate $alpha_1$ and $beta_1$ receptors as well as dopaminergic receptors. Only dopamine can activate dopaminergic receptors. Dopamine receptors are located in the brain, in blood vessels of the kidneys and other viscera, and probably in presynaptic sympathetic nerve terminals. Activation (agonism) of these receptors may result in stimulation or inhibition of cellular function. Like alpha- and beta-receptors, dopamine receptors are divided into several subtypes ($D_1$–$D_5$), and specific effects depend on which subtype of receptor is activated. Additional discussion about the adrenergic receptors is found in Table 29.1, which describes the locations of adrenergic receptors in the body and the response that occurs when each receptor is stimulated.

The intracellular events resulting from signal transduction after stimulation of adrenergic receptors are thought to include the following mechanisms:

- *Alpha$_1$ receptors*: Activation of $alpha_1$ receptors in smooth muscle cells is thought to open ion channels, allow calcium ions to move into the cell, and produce muscle contraction (e.g., vasoconstriction, gastrointestinal and bladder sphincter contraction).
- *Alpha$_2$ receptors*: In the brain, some of the norepinephrine released into the synaptic cleft between neurons returns to the nerve endings from which it was released and stimulates presynaptic $alpha_2$ receptors. This negative feedback prevents calcium-mediated release of norepinephrine from storage vesicles into the synapse, resulting in decreased sympathetic outflow and an antiadrenergic effect. In addition, $alpha_2$ receptors cause a decrease in cyclic adenosine monophosphate (cAMP), resulting in smooth muscle contraction.
- *Beta$_1$, beta$_2$, and beta$_3$ receptors*: Activation of these receptors stimulates activity of adenyl cyclase (an enzyme in cell membranes), which increases intracellular cAMP activity. cAMP serves as a second messenger and can initiate several different intracellular actions, such as cardiac contraction, smooth muscle relaxation, and glycogenolysis. An enzyme called phosphodiesterase rapidly degrades cAMP to 5′-adenosine monophosphate. Drugs such as theophylline inhibit phosphodiesterase and increase cAMP concentrations, resulting in bronchodilation (see Chap. 33).
- *Dopaminergic receptors $D_1$ and $D_5$*: Activation of these receptors is thought to stimulate the production of cAMP, as does activation of $beta_1$ and $beta_2$ receptors.
- *Dopaminergic receptors $D_2$, $D_3$, and $D_4$*: Activation of this receptor is thought to inhibit formation of cAMP and to alter calcium and potassium ion currents. $D_3$ and $D_4$ receptors are grouped with $D_2$ receptors, but the effects of their activation have not been clearly delineated.

The number of receptors and the binding activity of receptors to target organs and tissues are dynamic and may be altered. These phenomena are most clearly understood with beta-receptors. For example, when chronically exposed to high concentrations of substances that stimulate their function, the beta-receptors decrease in number and become less efficient in stimulating adenyl cyclase. The resulting decrease in beta-adrenergic responsiveness is called desensitization or **downregulation** of receptors. Conversely, when chronically exposed to substances that block their function, the receptors may increase in number and become more efficient in stimulating adenyl cyclase. The resulting increase in beta-adrenergic responsiveness, called hypersensitization or **upregulation**, may lead to an exaggerated response when the blocking substance is withdrawn.

## NCLEX Success

1. Activation of the sympathetic nervous system will result in which of the following? [Select all that apply.]
   A. increased rate and depth of respiration
   B. pupil dilation to aid vision
   C. increased blood pressure and heart rate
   D. increased urine output

2. Which of the following statements is correct regarding the sympathetic and the parasympathetic nervous systems?
   A. Acetylcholine activates muscarinic receptors.
   B. Activation of the sympathetic nervous system causes a decrease in blood pressure.
   C. Acetylcholine activates adrenergic receptors.
   D. Norepinephrine activates cholinergic receptors.

3. The sympathetic nervous system is also called the
   A. fight-or-flight system
   B. eat-drink-and-rest system
   C. autonomic nervous system
   D. somatic nervous system

4. A drug that has the same effects on the human body as stimulation of the sympathetic nervous system is called which of the following? [Select all that apply.]
   A. sympathomimetic agent
   B. adrenergic drug
   C. beta-adrenergic agonist drug
   D. alpha-adrenergic blocking agent

5. When the body is exposed to high concentrations of substances that stimulate their function, the resulting decrease in beta-adrenergic responsiveness is called which of the following? [Select all that apply.]
   A. desensitization
   B. downregulation
   C. fight or flight
   D. norepinephrine reuptake

## Parasympathetic Nervous System

Experts often describe processes stimulated by the parasympathetic nervous system as "rest and digest" because of their resting, reparative, or vegetative functions. They include digestion, excretion, cardiac deceleration, anabolism, and near vision.

PNS "Rest & digest"

Approximately 75% of all parasympathetic nerve fibers are in the vagus nerves. These nerves supply the thoracic and abdominal organs; their branches go to the heart, lungs, esophagus, stomach, small intestine, proximal half of colon, the liver, gallbladder, pancreas, and upper portions of the ureters. Other parasympathetic fibers supply pupillary sphincters and circular muscles of the eye; lacrimal, nasal, submaxillary, and parotid glands; descending colon and rectum; lower portions of the ureters and bladder; and genitalia.

Specific body responses to parasympathetic stimulation include:

- Dilation of blood vessels in the skin
- Decreased heart rate, possibly bradycardia
- Increased secretion of digestive enzymes and motility of the gastrointestinal tract
- Constriction of smooth muscle of bronchi
- Increased secretions from glands in the lungs, stomach, intestines, and skin (sweat glands)
- Constricted pupils (from contraction of the circular muscle of the iris) and accommodation to near vision (from contraction of the ciliary muscle of the eye)
- Contraction of smooth muscle in the urinary bladder
- Contraction of skeletal muscle
- Release of nitrous oxide from the endothelium of blood vessels, resulting in decreased platelet aggregation, decreased inflammation, relaxation of vascular smooth muscle, and dilation of blood vessels

## Neurotransmitters

Parasympathetic responses are regulated by acetylcholine, a neurotransmitter in the brain, ANS, and neuromuscular junctions. Acetylcholine is formed in cholinergic nerve endings from choline and acetyl-coenzyme A, in a chemical reaction catalyzed by choline acetyltransferase. After its release from the nerve ending, the effect of acetylcholine on receptors of the parasympathetic nervous system is brief and measured in milliseconds. The action of acetylcholine on receptors is terminated because of rapid metabolism by acetylcholinesterase, an enzyme present in the nerve ending and on the surface of the receptor organ. Acetylcholinesterase splits the active acetylcholine into inactive acetate and choline. The choline is taken up again by the presynaptic nerve terminal and reused to form more acetylcholine. Acetylcholine exerts excitatory effects at nerve synapses and neuromuscular junctions and inhibitory effects at some peripheral sites such as the heart.

## Cholinergic Receptors

When acetylcholine acts on body cells that respond to parasympathetic nerve stimulation, it interacts with two types of *cholinergic* receptors: *nicotinic* and *muscarinic*. Nicotinic receptors are located in motor nerves and skeletal muscles. When they are activated by acetylcholine, the cell membrane depolarizes and produces muscle contraction. Muscarinic receptors are located in most internal organs, including the cardiovascular, respiratory, gastrointestinal, and genitourinary systems. When muscarinic receptors are activated by acetylcholine, the affected cells may be excited or inhibited in their functions.

Nicotinic and muscarinic receptors have been further subdivided; two types of nicotinic and five types of muscarinic receptors have been identified. Although the subtypes of cholinergic receptors have not been as well characterized as those of the adrenergic receptors, the intracellular events resulting from signal transduction after receptor stimulation are thought to include the following mechanisms:

- *Muscarinic$_1$ receptors:* Muscarinic$_1$ receptors are expressed primarily in the CNS, autonomic ganglia, and the gastric and salivary glands. Activation of these receptors results in a series of processes during which phospholipids in the cell membrane and inside the cell are broken down. One of the products of phospholipid metabolism is inositol phosphate. Inositol phosphate acts as a second messenger to increase the intracellular concentration of calcium. Calcium also acts as a second messenger and functions to activate several intracellular enzymes, initiate contraction of smooth muscle cells, increase secretions of exocrine glands, increase cognitive function, and decrease dopamine release.
- *Muscarinic$_2$ receptors:* Receptor activation results in inhibition of adenyl cyclase in the heart, smooth muscle, and brain. As a result, less cAMP is formed to act as a second messenger and stimulate intracellular activity. Receptor stimulation also results in activation of potassium channels in cell membranes of the heart. The overall consequences of M$_2$ activation are inhibition of cardiac function, increased contraction of smooth muscle, and inhibition of neuronal transmission.
- *Muscarinic$_3$ receptors:* Muscarinic$_3$ receptors are expressed primarily in the CNS, smooth muscle, glands, and heart. Activation apparently causes the same cascade of intracellular processes as with activation of the M$_1$ receptors, resulting in decreased dopamine release, increased smooth muscle contraction, and increased glandular secretion. In addition, nitrous oxide is generated from vascular endothelial cells, resulting in dilation of vessels.
- *Muscarinic$_4$ receptors:* Activation of these receptors in the CNS results in a molecular response similar to M$_2$ receptor activation. Muscarinic$_4$ activation results in inhibition of acetylcholine release in the striatum, a subcortical portion of the forebrain. These receptors have a regulatory effect on dopaminergic neurotransmission, and activation facilitates dopamine release. Alterations in M$_4$ receptors may contribute to disorders such as Parkinson's disease.
- *Muscarinic$_5$ receptors:* Receptor activation results in a molecular response similar to M$_1$ receptor activation. The receptor has been identified in CNS tissues (especially the substantia nigra); its activation results in dilation of cerebral arteries and arterioles and facilitation of dopamine release. In addition, stimulation of M$_5$ receptors decreases cAMP levels.

**! QSEN Alert: Safety**

Muscarinic$_5$ activation also plays a role in augmentation of drug-seeking behavior and reward.

Although five muscarinic receptor subtypes have been identified, currently available drug therapies do not selectively differentiate among the various receptor subtypes:

- *Nicotinic$_n$ receptors:* These receptors are located on autonomic ganglia and the adrenal medulla. Activation results in enhanced transmission of nerve impulses at all parasympathetic and sympathetic ganglia and release of epinephrine from the adrenal medullae.

- *Nicotinic$_m$ receptors*: These are located at neuromuscular junctions in skeletal muscle. Their activation causes muscle contraction.
- *Nicotinic$_{CNS}$ receptors*: These receptors are located on presynaptic nerve fibers in the brain and spinal cord. Their activation promotes the release of acetylcholine in the cerebral cortex.

Nicotinic receptors are composed of five different protein subunits. The protein subunits that make up a nicotinic$_n$ receptor vary from those that make up a nicotinic$_m$ receptor, thus allowing the development of medications that are more selective in their actions.

---

### ! QSEN Alert: Safety

Neuromuscular-blocking medications such as pancuronium, which act selectively at nicotinic$_m$ receptors, can paralyze skeletal muscles in patients when limiting movement is therapeutic (such as in the ventilated patient or during surgery), without adversely affecting the other functions of the ANS.

## CHARACTERISTICS OF AUTONOMIC DRUGS

Many drugs are used clinically because of their ability to stimulate or block activity of the SNS or parasympathetic nervous system. Drugs that stimulate an activity act like endogenous neurotransmitter substances; drugs that block an activity prevent the actions of both endogenous substances and stimulating drugs. Specific drugs that either stimulate or block the SNS are well described in the cardiac section of this text. Chapters 47 and 48 discuss the influence of drugs on the PNS.

Because ANS receptors are widespread throughout the body, drugs that act on the ANS usually affect the entire body rather than certain organs and tissues. Drug effects depend on which branch of the ANS is involved and whether it is stimulated or inhibited by drug therapy. Thus, knowledge of the physiology of the ANS is required if drug effects are to be understood and predicted. In addition, it is becoming increasingly important to understand receptor activity and the consequences of stimulation or inhibition. More drugs are being developed to stimulate or inhibit particular subtypes of receptors. This is part of the continuing effort to design drugs that act more selectively on particular body tissues and decrease adverse effects on other body tissues. For example, drugs such as terbutaline (see Chap. 33) have been developed to stimulate beta$_2$ receptors in the respiratory tract and produce bronchodilation (a desired effect) with decreased stimulation of beta$_1$ receptors in the heart (an adverse effect).

The terminology used to describe autonomic drugs is often confusing because different terms are used to refer to the same phenomenon. Thus, sympathomimetic, adrenergic, and alpha- and beta-adrenergic agonists are used to describe a drug that has the same effects on the human body as stimulation of the SNS. Parasympathomimetic, cholinomimetic, and cholinergic are used to describe a drug that has the same effects on the body as stimulation of the parasympathetic nervous system. There are also drugs that oppose or block stimulation of these systems. Sympatholytic, antiadrenergic, and alpha- and beta-adrenergic blocking drugs inhibit sympathetic stimulation. Parasympatholytic, anticholinergic, and cholinergic blocking drugs inhibit parasympathetic stimulation. This text uses the terms adrenergic, antiadrenergic, cholinergic, and anticholinergic when describing medications.

*Same effect*

*Block oppose effect*

6. During a teaching session for a patient who is receiving a respiratory inhaler that stimulates beta$_2$ receptors in the respiratory tract, the patient asks why he needs to take the inhaler. The best response by the nurse is that the effect of a beta$_2$ receptor is

   A. prevention of bronchospasm
   B. reduction of sputum production
   C. maintenance of respiratory rate
   D. suppression of cough

7. Functions stimulated by the parasympathetic nervous system include which of the following? (Select all that apply.)

   A. digestion
   B. excretion
   C. catabolism
   D. anabolism *build up*

8. A drug that has the same effects on the body as stimulation of the parasympathetic nervous system is described as

   A. cholinergic
   B. sympatholytic
   C. antiadrenergic
   D. parasympatholytic *NO*

9. Activation of the parasympathetic system will result in which of the following? (Select all that apply.)

   A. dilation of blood vessels in the skin
   B. decreased heart rate
   C. increased motility of the gastrointestinal tract
   D. constriction of smooth muscle of bronchi

## THE NURSING PROCESS

A concept map outlines the nursing process related to drug therapy considerations in this chapter. Additional nursing implications related to the disease process should also be considered in care decisions.

**Assessment**
- Assess for potential contraindications to the use of adrenergic medications: angina, hypertension, and tachydysrhythmias.
- Throughout treatment, monitor vital signs, level of consciousness, and gas exchange.
- Assess for the therapeutic effects of adrenergic drug therapy.
- Assess for the adverse effects of adrenergic drug therapy.
- Assess for patient's understanding about drug therapy and use of over-the-counter medications.

**Outcomes of Therapy**
The patient will
- Receive or take drugs that affect the sympathetic and parasympathetic nervous systems accurately.
- Recognize that many of these drugs should not be stopped abruptly.
- Have fewer episodes of symptoms.
- Be closely monitored for therapeutic and adverse effects, especially when drug therapy is started.
- Avoid preventable adverse effects.
- Verbalize essential information about the drug therapy.
- Demonstrate appropriate coping strategies.
- Recognize signs and symptoms that necessitate professional medical intervention.
- Keep appointments for follow-up care and monitoring.

**Nursing Interventions**
- Use appropriate measures to prevent symptoms.
- Provide appropriate patient teaching related to drug therapy.

**Evaluation**
- Observe and interview for relief of symptoms.
- Observe effective coping strategies and appropriate use of support system and resources.
- Interview regarding success and adherence with drug therapy.
- Interview and observe for adverse drug effects.

## KEY CONCEPTS

- The ANS controls involuntary activities in smooth muscle, secretory glands, and the visceral organs of the body such as the heart.
- The ANS functions to maintain homeostasis, to respond to stress, and to repair body tissues.
- The ANS is composed of the sympathetic and parasympathetic nervous systems; these two divisions are usually antagonistic in their actions on a particular organ. Exceptions to this antagonism are sweating and regulation of arteriolar diameter, which are controlled by the sympathetic nervous system.
- Release of neurotransmitters allows nerve impulses in the ANS to bridge synapses and travel from presynaptic to postsynaptic nerves, eventually stimulating receptors located on effector organs.

- Stimulation of receptors in the SNS produces adrenergic effects. Blockade of receptors produces antiadrenergic effects.
- Stimulation of receptors in the parasympathetic nervous system produces cholinergic effects. Blockade of receptors produces anticholinergic effects.
- Drugs that activate ANS receptors stimulate the ANS; these medications function like endogenous neurotransmitters.
- Drugs that block the activity of ANS receptors prevent the actions of both endogenous neurotransmitters and ANS agonists.
- Adrenergic receptors include alpha- and beta-receptors as well as dopamine receptors; there are several subtypes.
- Cholinergic receptors include muscarinic and nicotinic receptors; there are several subtypes.
- The number of receptors in the ANS is dynamic and can be upregulated or downregulated as needed.

## CLINICAL REASONING CASE STUDY

| | |
|---|---|
| **Meet the Patient** | Michele Washington, a 65-year-old woman with a history of asthma, presents to the emergency department (ED) with significant wheezing on auscultation. Her vital signs are temperature 99°F orally, pulse 112 beats/min, respiratory rate 32 per minute, and blood pressure 146/88 mm Hg. She is having moderate difficulty breathing. She has been using an albuterol inhaler but has not been able to afford to purchase the inhaler for the last month. She is provided an albuterol inhaler in the ED, which is effective in causing bronchodilation. A nursing student asks the nurse taking care of Ms. Washington why Ms. Washington did not receive a drug such as epinephrine.<br>• What would be the best response by the nurse?<br>• What signs and symptoms may indicate worsening of the patient's condition? |
| **Assessing Drug Information** | • Epinephrine is effective in producing bronchodilation and can be administered nasally, subcutaneously, or intravenously. Because epinephrine affects both beta$_1$ and beta$_2$ adrenergic receptors, untoward adverse effects could result from beta$_1$ stimulation, particularly because her pulse and blood pressure are already elevated.<br>• Albuterol is a beta$_2$-selective drug that is equally effective in causing bronchodilation with a much lower risk of adverse cardiovascular effects. |
| **Nursing Actions** | • Observe Ms. Washington for signs of worsening respiratory status (e.g., rate below 12 or above 24 per minute, dyspnea, cough, orthopnea, wheezing, "noisy" respirations).<br>  • Severe respiratory distress is characterized by tachypnea, dyspnea, use of accessory muscles of respiration, and hypoxia.<br>  • Early signs of hypoxia include mental confusion, restlessness, anxiety, and increased blood pressure and pulse rate. Late signs include cyanosis and decreased blood pressure and pulse rate. Hypoxemia is confirmed if arterial blood gas analysis shows decreased PO$_2$.<br>  • Assess for improvement in Ms. Washington's pulmonary function. General assessment factors include rate and character of respiration, skin color, arterial blood gas analysis, and pulmonary function tests. Assess for the return of stable vital signs.<br>  • Once acute event has resolved, try to determine the frequency and severity of acute attacks; factors that precipitate or relieve acute attacks; allergies; and condition between acute attacks, such as restrictions in activities of daily living due to asthma.<br>  • Consult to social services to determine what options are available for financial assistance in obtaining the prescribed inhaler and other essentials. |

*Visit* thePoint® *at* **http://thePoint.lww.com/Frandsen12e** *for answers to NCLEX Success questions (in Appendix A), answers to Clinical Application Case Studies (in Appendix B), and more!*

## REFERENCES AND RESOURCES

Chawla, L. S., Ostermann, M., Forni, L., & Tidmarsh, G. F. (2019). Broad spectrum vasopressors: A new approach to the initial managements of septic shock. *Critical Care, 23*(124), 1–3. doi:10.1186/s13054-019-2420-y

Manaker, S. (2019). Use of vasopressors and inotropes. *UpToDate.* Lexi-Comp, Inc.

Norris, T. L. (2019). *Porth's pathophysiology: Concepts of altered health states* (10th ed.). Philadelphia, PA: Wolters Kluwer Health/Lippincott Williams & Wilkins.

Nursing 2019. (2019). *Drug handbook.* Philadelphia, PA: Wolters Kluwer Health/Lippincott Williams & Wilkins.

Teboul, J. L., Duranteau, J., & Russel, J. A. (2018). Intensive care medicine in 2050: vasopressors in sepsis. *Intensive Care Medicine, 44,* 1130–1132. doi:10.1007/s00134-017-4909-7

UpToDate. (2019). *Drug information.* Lexi-Comp, Inc.

# Drug Therapy for Myasthenia Gravis, Alzheimer's Disease, and Other Conditions Treated with Cholinergic Agents

## LEARNING OBJECTIVES

*After studying this chapter, you should be able to:*

1. Understand the pathophysiology and major manifestations of myasthenia gravis.
2. Identify the prototype and describe the action, use, adverse effects, contraindications, and nursing implications for acetylcholinesterase inhibitors used in myasthenia gravis.
3. Understand the pathophysiology and major manifestations of Alzheimer's disease.
4. Identify the prototype and describe the action, use, adverse effects, contraindications, and nursing implications for reversible cholinesterase inhibitors used in Alzheimer's disease.
5. Understand the etiology, pathophysiology, and clinical manifestations of urinary retention.
6. Identify the prototype and describe the action, use, adverse effects, contraindications, and nursing implications for cholinergic agonist drugs.
7. Describe the pharmacologic care of the patient with toxicity of acetylcholinesterase agents.
8. Be able to implement the nursing process in the care of patients undergoing drug therapy for myasthenia gravis, Alzheimer's disease, and urinary retention.

## CLINICAL APPLICATION CASE STUDY

Mary Collins, a 35-year-old woman, is admitted to the emergency department with shortness of breath, difficulty swallowing, and a drooping eyelid on the left side. The physician on duty suspects that she is suffering from myasthenia gravis and orders atropine 0.6 mg in the intravenous (IV) form followed by neostigmine 1.5 mg IV.

## KEY TERMS

**Acetylcholine:** neurotransmitter in the cholinergic system located in many areas of the brain, with high concentrations in the motor cortex and basal ganglia (also a neurotransmitter in the autonomic nervous system and at peripheral neuromuscular junctions); exerts excitatory effects at synapses and at the nerve–muscle junction and inhibitory effects at some peripheral sites, such as organs supplied by the vagus nerve

**Acetylcholinesterase:** enzyme that acts on the neurotransmitter acetylcholine, breaking it into choline and an acetate group; found mainly at neuromuscular junctions, its activity serves to terminate synaptic transmission

**Alzheimer's disease:** most common type of dementia; characterized by a significant loss of neurons in addition to shrinkage of large cortical neurons, with plaques and neurofibrillary tangles ᵛ **Anticholinesterase inhibitor drugs:** drugs that inhibit the destruction of acetylcholinesterase to facilitate impulse transmissions across the myoneural junction, mimicking the cholinergic effect on the skeletal muscle

ᶠ **Cholinergic drugs:** agents that stimulate the parasympathetic nervous system in the same manner as acetylcholine

ᵗ **Myasthenia gravis:** chronic autoimmune neuromuscular disease characterized by varying degrees of weakness of the skeletal (voluntary) muscles of the body

## INTRODUCTION

The neuromuscular conditions myasthenia gravis and Alzheimer's disease are characterized by disruptions in neurologic and auto-immune processes. This chapter discusses the acetylcholinesterase inhibitor medications used for the treatment of myasthenia gravis as well as the medications used to improve memory related to Alzheimer's disease. It also covers selected drugs used to treat atony of the gastrointestinal (GI) and urinary smooth muscle, which may result in paralytic ileus and urinary retention.

## OVERVIEW OF MYASTHENIA GRAVIS

**Myasthenia gravis** is a chronic autoimmune neuromuscular disease characterized by varying degrees of painless weakness of the skeletal (voluntary) muscles of the body. The hallmark of the disorder is muscle weakness that increases during periods of activity and improves after periods of rest. The name myasthenia gravis, which is Latin and Greek in origin, literally means "grave muscle weakness." With the therapies, currently available, however, most cases of myasthenia gravis are not as "grave" as the name implies. In fact, most people who have myasthenia gravis have a normal life expectancy.

Myasthenia gravis occurs in all ethnic groups and both genders. It most commonly affects young adult women (younger than 40 years of age) and older men (older than 60 years of age).

### Etiology

Myasthenia gravis results from a defect in the transmission of nerve impulses to muscles. Normally, when impulses travel down the nerve, the nerve endings release a neurotransmitter called **acetylcholine**. Acetylcholine travels from the neuromuscular junction and binds to acetylcholine receptors, which are activated and generate a muscle contraction.

### Pathophysiology

Myasthenia gravis occurs when normal communication between the nerve and muscle is interrupted at the neuromuscular junction—the place where nerve cells connect with the muscles they control. Antibodies produced by the body's own immune system block, alter, or destroy the receptors for acetylcholine at the neuromuscular junction, which prevents muscle contraction from occurring. Because the immune system, which normally protects the body from foreign organisms, mistakenly attacks itself, myasthenia gravis is known as an autoimmune disease.

### Clinical Manifestations

Although myasthenia gravis may affect any voluntary muscle, muscles that control eye and eyelid movement, facial expression,

and swallowing are most frequently affected. The onset of the disorder may be sudden, and symptoms often are not immediately recognized as myasthenia gravis. In most cases, the first noticeable symptom is weakness of the eye muscles. In others, difficulty in swallowing and slurred speech may be the first signs. The degree of muscle weakness involved in myasthenia gravis varies greatly among people, ranging from a localized form limited to eye muscles (ocular myasthenia) to a severe or generalized form in which many muscles—sometimes including those that control breathing—are affected.

Symptoms, which vary in type and severity, may include a drooping of one or both eyelids (ptosis), blurred or double vision (diplopia) due to weakness of the muscles that control eye movements, unstable or waddling gait, a change in facial expression, difficulty in chewing and swallowing, shortness of breath, impaired speech (dysarthria), and weakness in the arms, hands, fingers, legs, and neck.

### Diagnosis

In the past, bedside edrophonium tests were used to diagnose myasthenia gravis. In many cases, false-positive results were obtained. Currently, laboratory tests for autoantibodies and repetitive nerve stimulation studies are used for diagnosis. Single-fiber electromyography is definitive (Bird 2019a).

### Myasthenia Crisis

Myasthenia crisis is characterized by respiratory insufficiency, worsening of tongue and swallowing muscle weakness, and in rare cases, respiratory failure. It can be precipitated by infection, surgery, pregnancy, or a spontaneous response of myasthenia gravis. Current management and treatment include plasma exchange, intravenous immune globulin (IVIG), high-dose glucocorticoids, and monitoring and assessment of respiratory muscle strength (Bird 2019b).

### Drug Therapy

**Cholinergic drugs** stimulate the parasympathetic nervous system in the same manner as acetylcholine. These drugs act directly to stimulate the cholinergic receptors. Figure 47.1 shows the mechanism of action by interacting with the postsynaptic cholinergic receptor. The **acetylcholinesterase inhibitor drugs** are cholinergic drugs that inhibit the enzyme **acetylcholinesterase**, thereby slowing acetylcholine metabolism at autonomic nerve synapses. The acetylcholinesterase inhibitor drugs are also known as indirect-acting cholinergics. Other cholinergic drugs act directly to stimulate cholinergic receptors (Fig. 47.2).

Acetylcholinesterase inhibitor drugs are classified as either reversible or irreversible inhibitors of acetylcholinesterase. The reversible inhibitors exhibit a moderate duration of action and

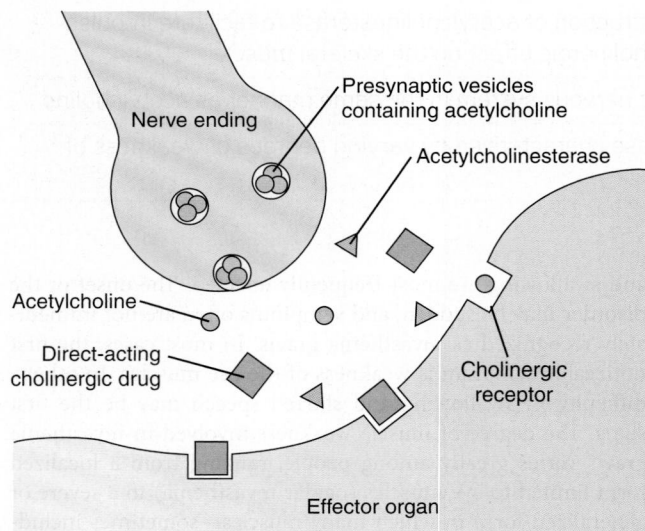

**Figure 47.1.** Mechanism of drug action. Direct-acting cholinergic drugs interact with postsynaptic cholinergic receptors on target effector organs, activating the organ in a similar fashion as the neurotransmitter acetylcholine.

have several therapeutic uses—in myasthenia gravis and, as described later in this chapter, in Alzheimer's disease. Table 47.1 lists medications used to treat myasthenia gravis (Bird 2019c).

## ACETYLCHOLINESTERASE INHIBITORS (INDIRECT-ACTING CHOLINERGICS)

The initial therapy for mild to moderate myasthenia gravis is an oral acetylcholinesterase inhibitor. **ⓟ Neostigmine** (Bloxiverz) is the prototype drug of the class, although pyridostigmine is more commonly prescribed. (Pyridostigmine is discussed in the Other Drugs in the Class section. Health care providers use neostigmine for the long-term treatment of myasthenia gravis and as an antidote for tubocurarine and other nondepolarizing skeletal muscle relaxants used in surgery.

## Pharmacokinetics

In the United States, neostigmine is available for IV use only. In Canada, the drug is available in oral and parenteral formulations. When administered intravenously, its onset of action is 10 to 30 minutes, it peaks in 20 to 30 minutes, and its half-life is 24 to 113 minutes. When administered intramuscularly, the duration of action is 2.5 to 4 hours, and the half-life is 51 to 90 minutes. Neostigmine is 15% to 25% protein bound to albumin. The drug is metabolized in the liver and excreted 50% unchanged in the urine. The remainder is excreted as metabolites.

## Action

Neostigmine decreases the inactivation of acetylcholine in the synapse by the enzyme acetylcholinesterase. Thus, acetylcholine accumulates in the synapse and enhances the activation of postsynaptic muscarinic as well as nicotinic receptors (see Fig. 47.2). In addition to the cholinergic drug effects described above, the added effect of indirect-acting cholinergic drugs on nicotinic receptors in skeletal muscles results in improved skeletal muscle tone and strength.

In a patient with myasthenia gravis, specific effects of neostigmine include decreasing the heart rate, increasing the tone of GI smooth muscle, and stimulating the salivary glands to increase secretions. In addition, this drug increases tone and contractility of smooth muscle (detrusor) in the urinary bladder and relaxes the sphincter and bronchial smooth muscles (see Fig. 47.2).

## Use

The major use of neostigmine is in the diagnosis and treatment of myasthenia gravis. In addition, prescribers order it to reverse the action of nondepolarizing neuromuscular blocking agents, such as tubocurarine, which is used in surgery. Neostigmine does not reverse the neuromuscular blockade produced by depolarizing neuromuscular blocking agents such as succinylcholine.

**Figure 47.2.** Mechanism of action of acetylcholinesterase inhibitor drugs is by way of indirect action on the cholinergic receptors. This prevents the enzymatic breakdown of the neurotransmitter acetylcholine. The acetylcholine remains in the synapse and continues to interact with cholinergic receptors on target effector organs, producing a cholinergic response.

| TABLE 47.1 |
| --- |

## Drugs Administered for the Treatment of Myasthenia Gravis, Alzheimer's Disease, and Urinary Retention

| Drug Class | Prototype | Other Drugs in the Class |
| --- | --- | --- |
| Acetylcholinesterase inhibitors | Neostigmine (Prostigmin, Bloxiverz) | Physostigmine<br>Pyridostigmine (Mestinon, Regonol) |
| Cholinesterase inhibitors | Donepezil (Aricept) | Galantamine (Razadyne, Razadyne ER)<br>Rivastigmine (Exelon, Exelon Patch) |
| NMDA receptor antagonist | Memantine (Namenda, Namenda XR) | |
| Cholinesterase–NMDA receptor antagonist | Donepezil–memantine (Namzaric) | |
| Cholinergic agonist | Bethanechol (Urecholine) | |

Table 47.2 presents dosage information for neostigmine and related drugs.

### Use in Older Adults

Older adults are more likely to experience adverse drug effects because of age-related physiologic changes and superimposed pathologic conditions.

### Use in Patients With Renal Impairment

Neostigmine undergoes tubular excretion in the kidneys. Therefore, renal impairment may result in accumulation and increased adverse effects, especially with chronic use. It is necessary to monitor patients with renal impairment and urinary obstruction carefully and give the drug at the lowest possible loading dose.

### Use in Patients With Hepatic Impairment

Neostigmine undergoes metabolism in the liver, and hepatic disease may interfere with this, resulting in increased adverse effects. However, no dosage adjustments are necessary in patients with hepatic impairment.

### Use in Patients With Critical Illness

Neostigmine has specific uses in critical illness. These include reversal of skeletal muscle paralysis caused by nondepolarizing muscle relaxants, improvement of muscle strength, and use as an antidote to anticholinergic poisoning. In this last case, drugs such as atropine or tricyclic antidepressants are also required.

### Use in Patients Receiving Home Care

In the United States, use of neostigmine in the home is not common because the oral form has been discontinued, although in Canada, oral administration for the treatment of long-term conditions such as myasthenia gravis may occur. Self-administration of neostigmine may be a problem for the patient, who may have diplopia or diminished muscle strength. Strict adherence to timely medication administration promotes optimal blood levels of drugs and optimal symptom control. In the event the patient develops muscle weakness, it is essential that the primary care provider be notified immediately. For information about treatment of myasthenia gravis in the home using pyridostigmine, see Other Drugs in the Class.

> ### Clinical Application 47.1
>
> Following the administration of neostigmine, Ms. Collins is able to swallow and breathe more effectively.
> - Why is neostigmine administered?
> - What is the action of neostigmine?
> - Why has Ms. Collins' breathing improved, and why is she now able to swallow?

## Adverse Effects

### Specific Effects

Neostigmine has several adverse effects. Cardiovascular adverse effects of neostigmine are cardiac dysrhythmias, diminished cardiac output, hypotension, syncope, and cardiac arrest. Development of respiratory depression indicates cholinergic crisis. Other respiratory adverse effects include increased pharyngeal and tracheobronchial secretions, laryngospasm, bronchospasm, bronchiolar constriction, shortness of breath, and respiratory paralysis. Caution is necessary when the drug is used in patients with asthma. (IV atropine sulfate is the specific antidote for cholinergic agents.) Conditions such as excessive salivation, nausea, emesis, frequent urination, or diarrhea require a reduction in dosage.

### Toxicity of Neostigmine and Other Acetylcholinesterase Inhibitors

Cholinergic crisis is a drug-induced overstimulation of the parasympathetic nervous system, requiring discontinuation of any anticholinesterase drug that the patient has been receiving. Atropine sulfate should be readily available whenever cholinergic drugs are given. It is important to note that atropine reverses only the muscarinic effects of cholinergic drugs, primarily in the heart, smooth muscle, and glands. Atropine does not interact with nicotinic receptors and therefore cannot reverse the nicotinic effects of skeletal muscle weakness due to overdose of indirect anticholinergic drugs.

Atropine sulfate is also administered for the management of mushroom poisoning. Muscarine, an alkaloid that is found

*Record Symptoms*

### TABLE 47.2

## DRUGS AT A GLANCE: Acetylcholinesterase Inhibitors

| Drug | Pregnancy Category | Routes and Dosage Ranges | |
|------|--------------------|--------------------------|---|
| | | **Adults** | **Children** |
| **P Neostigmine** (Bloxiverz; ✳ Prostigmin) | C | Diagnosis of myasthenia gravis: 0.022 mg/kg IM<br>Treatment of myasthenia gravis: Dosage individualized to patient needs. PO 15–375 mg/d in 3 or 4 divided doses. SC, IV, or IM 0.5–2.5 mg based on patient response<br>Prevention/treatment of postoperative distention and urinary retention:<br>Prevention: 0.25 mg as soon as possible postoperatively; repeat every 4–6 h for 2–3 d. Treatment: 0.5–1 mg IM or SC, repeat every 3 h for 5 doses<br>Antidote for nondepolarizing neuromuscular blockers: Give atropine sulfate 0.6–1.2 mg IV several minutes before slow IV injection of neostigmine 0.5–2.5 mg. Repeat as needed; total dose not to exceed 5 mg<br>Bloxiverz IV: Adults: 0.03 mg/kg for neuromuscular blockers with a short half-life (e.g., rocuronium); 0.07 mg/kg for neuromuscular blockers with a longer half-life (e.g., vecuronium, pancuronium); the dose may be repeated for a total dose of 0.07 mg/kg or 5 mg (choose the lowest dose); administer atropine IV (0.6–1.2) several minutes in a separate syringe prior to neostigmine. Inject slowly directly into vein or into tubing of running IV, each 0.5 mg over 1 min. | Diagnosis of myasthenia gravis: 0.04 mg/kg IM<br>Treatment of myasthenia gravis: PO 0.3–0.6 mg/kg every 3–4 h SC, IV, IM 0.01–0.04 mg/kg/dose every 2–3 h as needed<br>Prevention/treatment of postoperative distention and urinary retention: safety and efficacy not established<br>Antidote for nondepolarizing neuromuscular blockers for infants, children, adolescents IV; see adult dosing. |
| Physostigmine | C | Initially, IM, IV 0.5–2 mg. Give IV slowly, no faster than 1 mg/min to avoid adverse effects of bradycardia, respiratory distress, and seizures. May repeat every 10–30 min until response occurs. | Infants, children, and adolescents: IM and IV<br>Initial: 0.02 mg/kg; maximum: 0.5 mg per dose; may repeat every 5–10 min until response occurs (maximum total dose, 2 mg) |
| Pyridostigmine (Mestinon, Regonol; ✳ Mestinon, Mestinon-SR) | C | Initially, PO 60–1500 mg/d; usually 600 mg/d divided into 5–6 doses. Individualize dose to control symptoms. IM, IV slowly: 1/30th the oral dose | Neonates of mothers with myasthenia gravis who have difficulty with sucking/breathing/swallowing: 0.05–0.15 mg/kg IM. Change to syrup as soon as possible.<br>Children: 7 mg/kg (200 mg/m²)/d in 5–6 divided doses |

*mushroom*

in small quantities in the *Amanita muscaria* mushroom, is the source of the name for the muscarinic receptors in the parasympathetic nervous system; muscarine can stimulate these receptors. Some mushrooms found in North America, such as *Clitocybe* and *Inocybe* mushrooms, however, contain much larger quantities of muscarine. Accidental or intentional ingestion of these mushrooms results in cholinergic crisis and is potentially fatal.

## Contraindications

Contraindications to neostigmine include known hypersensitivity. Patients with lung disease, such as bronchial asthma, or heart disease, such as sick sinus syndrome, should not take the drug. In addition, it is necessary to use caution in patients with peritonitis as well as benign prostatic hypertrophy and other urinary retention problems.

## Nursing Implications

### Preventing Interactions

Several drugs interact with neostigmine (Box 47.1), increasing or decreasing its effects.

**BOX 47.1** *Drug Interactions: Neostigmine*

**Drugs That Increase the Effects of Neostigmine**
- Aminoglycoside antibiotics (e.g., gentamicin)
  *Increase neuromuscular blocking*

**Drugs That Decrease the Effects of Neostigmine**
- Atropine
  *Decreases the effects of neostigmine by unknown mechanism*
- Corticosteroids
  *May result in muscular depression*

## Administering the Medication

It is important to administer IV neostigmine slowly and have atropine available as an antidote in the event of a cholinergic crisis or hypersensitivity to neostigmine.

### Clinical Application 47.2

Thirty minutes after the administration of neostigmine, Ms. Collins develops copious salivary secretions and respiratory depression.
- What do these symptoms indicate?
- What medication will be administered?

**! QSEN Alert: Patient-Centered Care**

When administering neostigmine to older patients, it is essential to observe for signs of cholinergic reactions, particularly when the drug is given intravenously. Treatment for myasthenic crisis includes administration of additional acetylcholinesterase inhibitors, glucocorticoids, immunoglobulin, and measures to maintain respirations until the medications are effective in improving muscle strength (Bird, 2019).

## Assessing for Therapeutic Effects

The nurse assesses the patient's response to the medication. When neostigmine is given to patients with myasthenia gravis, it is necessary to observe for increased muscle strength; decreased difficulty with chewing, swallowing, and speech; and decreased or absent ptosis of eyelids.

## Assessing for Adverse Effects

The nurse assesses for increased central nervous system (CNS) effects such as convulsions, dizziness, and drowsiness. He or she assesses for increased secretions, bronchospasm, laryngospasm, and respiratory failure. It is necessary to assess for nausea and vomiting, which are common GI effects. In addition, the nurse observes neonates of mothers with myasthenia gravis who have received neostigmine for difficulty breathing, swallowing, or sucking.

**! QSEN Alert: Safety**

It is important to avoid the following drugs in patients with myasthenia gravis. They may exacerbate the symptoms of the disease.
- Fluoroquinolones
- Aminoglycosides
- Neuromuscular blocking agents
- Lidocaine and procaine
- Penicillamine
- Beta-blockers
- Anticonvulsants
- Statins
- Glucocorticoids
- Live attenuated vaccines

### Patient Teaching

Box 47.2 identifies patient teaching guidelines for neostigmine.

## Other Drugs in the Class

Physostigmine is the only acetylcholinesterase inhibitor. It is a carbamate that prolongs both central and peripheral effects of acetylcholine. It is capable of crossing the blood–brain barrier.

**BOX 47.2** *Patient Teaching Guidelines for Acetylcholinesterase Inhibitors: Neostigmine*

- Wear a medical alert identification device if you are taking long-term cholinergic drug therapy for myasthenia gravis.
- Record symptoms of myasthenia gravis and effects of drug therapy, especially when drug therapy is initiated and medication doses are being titrated. The amount of medication required to control symptoms of myasthenia gravis varies greatly, and the physician needs this information to adjust the dosage correctly.
- Do not overexert yourself if you have myasthenia gravis. Rest between activities. Although the dose of medication may be increased during periods of increased activity, it is desirable to space activities to obtain optimal benefit from the drug, at the lowest possible dose, with the fewest adverse effects.
- Report increased muscle weakness, difficulty breathing, or recurrent of myasthenic symptoms to your physician. These are signs of drug underdosage (myasthenic crisis) and indicate a need to increase or change drug therapy.
- Report adverse reactions, including abdominal cramps, diarrhea, excessive oral secretions, difficulty in breathing, and muscle weakness. These are signs of drug overdosage (cholinergic crisis) and require immediate discontinuation of drugs and treatment by a physician. Respiratory failure can result if this condition is not recognized and treated properly. Atropine may be administered for overdose of cholinergic drugs.

Unlike other drugs in this group, physostigmine is not a quaternary amine and does not carry a positive charge; therefore, it is more lipid soluble. It is sometimes used as an antidote for overdose of anticholinergic drugs, including atropine, antihistamines, tricyclic antidepressants, and phenothiazine antipsychotics. However, its potential for causing serious adverse effects limits its usefulness. It should be administered intravenously no faster than 0.5 mg/minute to prevent bradycardia, seizures, and respiratory depression.

Pyridostigmine (Mestinon, Regonol) is similar to neostigmine in terms of action, use, and adverse effects. It inhibits the destruction of acetylcholine to enable the transmission of impulses across the neuromuscular junction. Pyridostigmine is the drug of choice in the treatment of myasthenia gravis. The initial immediate-release oral dose is 60 to 1500 mg/day; usually 600 mg/day, divided into five to six doses. The availability of a sustained-release form, which is effective for 6 to 12 hours, is an added advantage. The sustained-release dose is 180 to 540 mg twice daily, with 6 hours between doses. When this form is taken at bedtime, the patient does not have to take other medications during the night and does not awaken too weak to swallow. In some cases, it may be necessary for immediate-release and sustained-release to be used concurrently.

Pyridostigmine's adverse effects of abdominal cramping, diarrhea, increased salivation and bronchial secretions, nausea, sweating, and bradycardia can be controlled with the administration of glycopyrrolate, propantheline, and hyoscyamine. The diarrhea can be controlled by loperamide or diphenoxylate.

## NCLEX Success

1. A patient has received neostigmine intravenously. Which of the following is a serious adverse effect of neostigmine?

    A. bronchospasm
    B. headache
    C. nausea
    D. sweating

2. What is the therapeutic effect for the administration of pyridostigmine extended-release at bedtime?

    A. increases urinary frequency
    B. allows for increased swallowing
    C. decreases heart rate
    D. prevents hallucinations

3. A woman presents with muscle weakness. The physician orders neostigmine to confirm a diagnosis of myasthenia gravis. What drug should the nurse have available when the neostigmine is administered?

    A. pralidoxime
    B. diphenhydramine
    C. atropine
    D. travoprost

# IMMUNOSUPPRESSIVE THERAPY FOR MYASTHENIA GRAVIS

Patients who do not achieve control of symptoms on pyridostigmine may require immunosuppressive therapy to treat underlying immune dysregulation. Prescribers may use glucocorticoids initially and later add a nonsteroidal immunosuppressive agent such as azathioprine or mycophenolate. These drugs reduce the long-term use of glucocorticoids (Bird, 2019b).

## Azathioprine

Prescribers use azathioprine on an off-label basis for the treatment of myasthenia gravis. The drug blocks the purine pathway and inhibits RNA, DNA, and protein synthesis. Azathioprine is well absorbed orally and is 30% protein bound. The metabolism of the drug is by 6-mercaptopurine via glutathione S-transferase reduction. The initial dose administered is 50 mg orally per day, with the dose increased every 1 to 2 weeks to a target of 2.5 to 3 mg/kg/day. The drug may be administered as monotherapy or in combination with pyridostigmine and/or glucocorticoids. The dose increase in the medication should be 25 mg/day with a gradual increase to 25 to 50 mg/day every 2 weeks up to 150 mg/day if flulike symptoms develop. Adverse effects include malaise, hepatotoxicity, increased risk of infection, and myalgia.

## Mycophenolate

Mycophenolate (CellCept), another drug used on an off-label basis for myasthenia gravis, may be appropriate for patients who remain significantly asymptomatic on pyridostigmine. Mycophenolate inhibits inosine monophosphate dehydrogenase, which then inhibits de novo guanosine nucleotide synthesis. The drug exhibits a cytotoxic effect on T and B lymphocytes, which are dependent on these pathways for proliferation. Mycophenolate is rapidly and extensively absorbed. It must be administered on an empty stomach. The initial therapy is 500 mg orally twice daily, with an increase to a maintenance dose of 1 to 1.5 g.

The U.S. Food and Drug Administration (FDA) has issued a **BLACK BOX WARNING ◆** for mycophenolate. It states that women of childbearing age must be instructed about the increased risk of congenital malformations and first trimester pregnancy loss. Prior to beginning therapy, a negative pregnancy test is required. Two types of birth control are recommended.

# OVERVIEW OF ALZHEIMER'S DISEASE

## Etiology

**Alzheimer's disease** is the most common form of dementia, a general term for memory loss and other intellectual abilities serious enough to interfere with daily life. Alzheimer's disease accounts for 60% to 80% of dementia cases. As many as 5% of people with the disease have early-onset Alzheimer's disease (also known as younger onset), which often develops when a person is in their 40s or 50s. About 10% of people 65 years of age and older have Alzheimer's dementia, and two thirds of these are women.

## Pathophysiology

Patients who suffer from Alzheimer's disease have a deficiency in cholinergic function in the cortex and basal forebrain. This deficiency leads to diminished cognitive function. Significant loss of neurons also occurs, in addition to shrinkage of large cortical neurons. The neuropathologic hallmarks of Alzheimer's disease are neuritic plaques and neurofibrillary tangles, although these lesions are not unique to Alzheimer's disease and can be found in other neurodegenerative disorders and in clinically normal people as well. The number and distribution of the plaques and tangles appear to contribute to the development of dementia.

Classic neuritic plaques are spherical structures consisting of a central core of fibrous protein known as amyloid that is surrounded by degenerating or dystrophic nerve endings (neurites). Two other types of amyloid-related plaques are recognized in the brains of patients with Alzheimer's disease: diffuse plaques, which contain poorly defined amyloid but no well-circumscribed amyloid core, and "burnt-out" plaques, which consist of an isolated dense amyloid core.

Neurofibrillary tangles, found in the cytoplasm of abnormal neurons, consist of fibrous proteins that are wound around each other. These tangles are resistant to breakdown and persist in brain tissue.

## Clinical Manifestations

The most common early symptom of Alzheimer's disease is difficulty remembering newly learned information because the neurologic changes typically begin in the part of the brain that affects learning. As Alzheimer's disease advances through the brain, it leads to increasingly severe symptoms, including disorientation and mood and behavior changes; deepening confusion about events, time, and place; unfounded suspicions about family, friends, and professional caregivers; more serious memory loss and behavior changes; and difficulty speaking, swallowing, and walking.

## Drug Therapy

The goal of drug therapy for Alzheimer's disease is to slow the loss of memory and cognition, thus preserving the independence of the individual person for as long as possible. Studies have shown that vitamin E, estrogen, and anti-inflammatory agents lower the risk of Alzheimer's disease. Practice guidelines developed by the Alzheimer's Association (2018) recommend early diagnosis and treatment of Alzheimer's disease with cholinesterase inhibitors for all patients with mild to moderate symptoms. Although these drugs do not cure the disease, they do delay the onset of the disease somewhat and bring about a slight improvement in cognition and function. Improvement in cognitive function is seen in approximately 12 weeks with continuous therapy. The reversible cholinesterase inhibitors are also known as indirect-acting cholinergic drugs that improve memory by elevating acetylcholine in the cerebral cortex of the brain. Tacrine (available as Cognex) was the first U.S. FDA-approved drug for use in the treatment of Alzheimer's disease. Now, it is no longer marketed in the United States, and other related drugs have taken its place.

**QSEN Alert: Evidence-Based Practice**

Hamina et al. (2017) conducted a study on patients with and without a diagnosis of Alzheimer's disease to determine the use of analgesics, nonsteroidal anti-inflammatory drugs (NSAIDs), and opioids. The report indicated that 34.9% of patients with Alzheimer's disease used analgesics in place of NSAIDs or opioids. The patients most commonly used acetaminophen.

## CHOLINESTERASE INHIBITORS: REVERSIBLE INDIRECT-ACTING CHOLINERGICS

This class of drugs for the treatment of Alzheimer's disease or dementia interferes with enzyme that allows for the production of acetylcholinesterase to increase acetylcholine and improve memory.

**Donepezil** (Aricept) is the prototype drug in this class. Treatment of Alzheimer's disease is the primary use for this centrally acting reversible cholinesterase inhibitor. This drug interferes with enzyme that allows for the production of acetylcholinesterase, thus increasing acetylcholine and improving memory. Table 47.1 lists the cholinesterase inhibitors used in the management of Alzheimer's disease.

## Pharmacokinetics

Absorption of donepezil after oral administration is good, and it is unaffected by food. The drug is highly bound (96%) to plasma proteins. The peak of action occurs in 3 to 8 hours. Metabolism takes place in the liver, producing several metabolites, some of which are pharmacologically active. Excretion of these metabolites and some unchanged drug occurs mainly in urine.

## Action

Donepezil increases acetylcholine in the brain by inhibiting its metabolism, leading to elevated acetylcholine levels in the cortex. This slows the neuronal degradation that occurs in Alzheimer's disease.

## Use

As previously stated, health care providers use donepezil to treat mild, moderate, or severe Alzheimer's disease. Long-term studies have shown that the drug delays the progression of the disease for up to 55 weeks. Other uses include enhancing memory in other neurologic conditions such as multiple sclerosis, treating myasthenia gravis, or treating overdoses of atropine and centrally acting anticholinergic drugs (e.g., those used for parkinsonism). Table 47.3 presents dosage information for donepezil and related drugs.

### Use in Older Adults

Older adults are more likely to experience adverse drug effects because of age-related physiologic changes and superimposed pathologic conditions.

## TABLE 47.3

# DRUGS AT A GLANCE: Drugs Used for the Treatment of Alzheimer's Disease

| Drug | Pregnancy Category | Routes and Dosage Ranges | |
|---|---|---|---|
| | | **Adults** | **Children** |
| **Cholinesterase Inhibitors** | | | |
| Ⓟ **Donepezil** (Aricept; ❉ Aricept, Aricept RDT | C | 5 mg PO daily at bedtime for 4–6 wk, then increase to 10 mg daily if needed | Dosage not established |
| Galantamine (Razadyne, Razadyne ER; ❉ Auro-Galantamine ER, Mylan-Galantamine ER, Reminyl ER) | C | 8 mg PO daily initially, with food; increase to 16 mg/d after 4 wk if needed. May continue to increase every 4 wk up to max dose of 24 mg/d | Dosage not established |
| Rivastigmine (Exelon, ❉ Exelon, | C | 1.5 mg PO twice daily with food initially. May titrate to higher doses at 1.5 mg intervals every 2 wk to a maximum dose of 6 mg twice daily TDS initially 4.6 mg/24 h patch. Increase to 9.5 mg/24 h patch after 4 wk. Max dose 13.3 mg/24 h patch | Dosage not established |
| **NMDA Receptor Antagonist** | | | |
| Ⓟ **Memantine** (Namenda, Namenda Titration Pack, Namenda XR, Namenda XR Titration Pack; ❉ Ebixa) | B | 5 mg PO daily, increase dose by 5 mg/wk to a target dose of 20 mg daily; doses >5 mg should be given twice/d. Severe renal impairment: 5 mg PO 2 times/d | Dosage not established |
| **Acetylcholinesterase–NMDA Receptor Antagonist** | | | |
| Donepezil–memantine (Namzaric) | Adverse effects have been observed in some animal reproduction studies. | Recommended starting dose is 7 mg/10 mg daily, with a maximum dose of 28/10 mg daily; administer in evening without regard to meals | Dosage not established |

TDS, transdermal delivery system.

## *Use in Patients With Hepatic Impairment*

Liver disease may impair the hepatic metabolism of donepezil, resulting in increased adverse effects. It is important to monitor a patient's liver function and clinical response to the medication carefully.

## *Use in Patients With Critical Illness*

Donepezil has several specific uses in critical illness, which include reducing cognitive dysfunction. Commonly, critically ill patients may have delirium, a form of acute cognitive dysfunction that manifests as a fluctuating change in mental status, with inattention and altered level of consciousness. As many as 80% of mechanically ventilated patients are in the intensive care unit; this makes donepezil an important management drug.

## *Use in Patients Receiving Home Care*

Patients with Alzheimer's disease may have problems with remembering to take medications and may easily underdose or overdose themselves. It is important for the home care nurse to work with responsible family members in such cases to ensure accurate drug administration.

## Adverse Effects

The most common adverse effects of donepezil are headache, dizziness, depression, vertigo, and insomnia. Possible drug-related GI conditions include nausea, vomiting, diarrhea, abdominal muscle cramps, anorexia, and GI bleeding. The most serious adverse effects are breathing problems (e.g., asthma, chronic obstructive pulmonary disease), fainting, and heart disease (e.g., sick sinus syndrome, other heart conduction disorders). Dyspnea has been reported and is more common in patients who have previous lung disease. In addition, fatigue and anorexia may occur. Other adverse effects include seizures and trouble urinating.

## Contraindications

Contraindications to donepezil include known hypersensitivity to the drug. Patients with lung disease or heart disease such as sick sinus syndrome should not take this medication.

## BOX 47.3 — Drug Interactions: Donepezil

**Drugs That Increase the Effects of Donepezil**
- Theophylline
  *Increases the risk of toxicity*
- Cholinesterase inhibitors
  *Increase the risk of toxicity*

**Drugs That Decrease the Effects of Donepezil**
- Anticholinergics
  *Decrease the efficacy*
- Nonsteroidal anti-inflammatory drugs
  *Increase the risk of gastrointestinal bleeding*

## Nursing Implications

### Preventing Interactions

Many medications interact with donepezil, increasing or decreasing its effects (Box 47.3).

### Administering the Medication

Before administering donepezil, the nurse assesses the patient for allergy, orientation, and contraindications. Administration should occur at bedtime each day. If the patient is taking an oral disintegrating tablet, the nurse ensures that the medication is dissolved on the tongue.

### QSEN Alert: Safety

The brand names for donepezil (Aricept) and rabeprazole (AcipHex) are a source of confusion. It is essential to use caution when administering either of these drugs.

### Assessing for Therapeutic Effects

The nurse assesses for improved memory and reduction of dementia. This involves assessing daily for memory changes, forgetfulness, and mood.

### Assessing for Adverse Effects

The nurse assesses for signs and symptoms of GI upset such as nausea, diarrhea, insomnia, and vomiting. If GI bleeding is suspected, it is important to obtain an order for laboratory tests such as complete blood count and bleeding time.

### Patient Teaching

Box 47.4 identifies patient teaching guidelines for donepezil.

## Other Drugs in the Class

Galantamine hydrobromide (Razadyne, Razadyne ER) is similar to donepezil in its action. Indications include mild to moderate dementia and vascular dementia (unlabeled use). Contraindications include severe hepatic or renal impairment. The most common adverse effects are insomnia, tremor, dizziness, somnolence, headache, bradycardia, and syncope. Patients

## BOX 47.4 — Patient Teaching Guidelines for Cholinesterase Inhibitors: Donepezil

- Take this drug exactly as prescribed, at bedtime.
- Place orally disintegrating tablet on your tongue; allow it to dissolve and then drink water.
- Know that this drug does not cure the disease but is thought to slow down the degeneration associated with the disease.
- Continue taking this drug if no change in symptoms is noted.
- Arrange for regular blood tests and follow-up visits while adjusting to this drug.
- Note that the following side effects may occur: nausea, vomiting (eat frequent small meals), insomnia, fatigue, and confusion (use caution if driving or performing tasks that require alertness).
- Report severe nausea, vomiting, changes in stool or urine color, diarrhea, changes in neurologic functioning, and yellowing of the eyes or skin to your health care provider.

and families should receive instructions about reporting any changes in mental status. To decrease gastric upset, it is necessary to take the medication with food.

Rivastigmine (Exelon, Exelon Patch) is a long-acting central cholinesterase inhibitor approved for the treatment of mild to moderate dementia due to Alzheimer's disease as well as Parkinson's disease. Like other drugs in this class, rivastigmine is not a cure for Alzheimer's disease but does slow the progression of symptoms. Oral rivastigmine lasts 12 hours, making twice-a-day dosing possible. Rivastigmine transdermal is applied as a patch once a day. The site of the transdermal application should be rotated. The site used should not be used again for a period of 14 days. Before a new patch is applied, the old patch should be removed and the area cleaned. The patch should be applied to dry, clean skin. Metabolism occurs in the liver, and excretion takes place in the feces. The side effect profile of rivastigmine is similar to that of donepezil. To minimize certain adverse effects (e.g., nausea, vomiting, loss of appetite), it is typically necessary to increase dosages slowly until the therapeutic dosage is reached. Patients may take the drug with food to decrease GI distress.

## NCLEX Success

4. A nurse is teaching family members how to administer donepezil for Alzheimer's disease. The instructions should include which of the following?
   A. Take the medication with food.
   B. Take the medication on an empty stomach.
   C. Take the medication at bedtime.
   D. Take the medication at the start of each day.

5. A 74-year-old man has Alzheimer's disease. She has been prescribed rivastigmine. Which of the following instructions is most appropriate?
   A. Change patch every 48 hours.
   B. Apply the rivastigmine transdermal patch to the same site.
   C. Apply the rivastigmine transdermal patch to a clean, dry area.
   D. Administer oral rivastigmine with transdermal patch until a blood level is attained.

6. A woman diagnosed with Alzheimer's disease has used donepezil for 4 years. Her daughter notices her memory is worsening. Which of the following medications might be more successful for enhancing her memory?
   A. tacrine
   B. rivastigmine
   C. memantine
   D. galantamine

# N-METHYL-D-ASPARTATE RECEPTOR ANTAGONIST

Ⓟ **Memantine [Namenda]**, the prototype *N*-methyl-D-aspartate (NMDA) receptor antagonist, was approved for use in 2003. The drug is administered to patients with moderate to severe Alzheimer's disease. Its neuroprotective action is different from that of the cholinesterase inhibitors.

## Pharmacokinetics

Memantine is well absorbed orally, with 100% absorption in the GI tract. It is easily distributed and easily transported across the blood–brain barrier. The drug is 45% protein bound. Its peak of action occurs in 3 to 7 hours with the immediate-release formulation and in 9 to 12 hours with the extended-release formulation. It is partially metabolized by the liver, independent of the cytochrome P450 enzyme system. The terminal elimination half-life is 60 to 80 hours.

## Action

Glutamate is an excitatory amino acid in the CNS and is known to contribute to origin and development of Alzheimer's disease. In Alzheimer's patients, overstimulation of the glutamate receptors occurs, leading to cell death. NMDA is a glutamate receptor in which memantine induces an antagonistic effect. When the NMDA receptors are overstimulated, magnesium is prevented from reentering and blocking the channel from closing. Thus, an influx of calcium results, and neuronal cell death subsequently occurs. Memantine has the ability to bind to the magnesium site to block the excitatory function by slowing intracellular calcium accumulation. This action prevents nerve damage but does not have an effect on glutamate.

## Use

Memantine is used to slow the progression of moderate to severe Alzheimer's disease.

## Contraindications

Contraindications include any hypersensitivity reaction to memantine. Also, patients with renal failure should not take the drug.

## Nursing Implications

### Preventing Interactions

Memantine interacts with carbonic anhydrase and alkalinizing agents, resulting in increased serum concentration of memantine. Also, trimethoprim may lead to memantine toxicity.

### Administering the Medication

Memantine should be administered without regard to meals. The extended-release capsule should be swallowed whole; it should not be chewed. The capsule can be opened and sprinkled on applesauce, which must be consumed immediately. The liquid formulation should be squirted in the corner of the patient's mouth and should not be mixed with any other liquid.

### Assessing for Therapeutic Effects

The nurse assesses for improved memory and reduction in dementia. He or she should also assess for changes in memory and mood.

### Assessing for Adverse Effects

The nurse should assess the patient for changes in blood pressure. Hypertension occurs in 4% of patients who take memantine, and hypotension may result with the extended-release formulation. He or she should assess for CNS adverse effects such as dizziness, confusion, anxiety, fatigue, and hallucinations. In addition, he or she should assess for diarrhea, constipation, vomiting, abdominal pain, urinary incontinence, back pain, and cough. Finally, he or she should assess for signs and symptoms of a hypersensitivity reaction.

### Patient Teaching

Instruct the patient's caregiver about the administration of memantine. Because of the CNS effects, the patient should be protected from falls related to dizziness. In the event the patient develops GI symptoms, urinary incontinence, back pain, or cough, the prescriber should be notified. In addition, the caregiver should be instructed about hypersensitivity reactions, including skin rash, dyspnea, or bronchospasm.

# CHOLINESTERASE INHIBITOR– N-METHYL-D-ASPARTATE RECEPTOR ANTAGONIST

Donepezil and memantine are available as a combination of a cholinesterase inhibitor and an NMDA—as Namzaric. For the actions of this combination drug, see previous discussions. Donepezil–memantine is administered to patients with moderate to severe dementia. This oral agent is for patients who are stabilized on 10 mg donepezil once daily but are not taking memantine. Initial dose of memantine extended-release of 7 mg combined with donepezil 10 mg once daily. The dosage can be increased weekly with a maintenance dose of memantine extended-release of 28 mg and donepezil 10 mg daily.

The nurse must assess for cardiovascular adverse effects. The donepezil may cause bradycardia and heart block. Patients should be protected from falls; there is a risk of syncopal episodes. Diarrhea, nausea, and vomiting may develop and commonly resolve in 1 to 3 weeks. As with other medications administered for Alzheimer's disease, it is important to monitor the patient's mental status and ability to perform activities of daily living.

# OVERVIEW OF URINARY RETENTION

## Etiology and Pathophysiology

Urinary retention may be due to several factors. The most common cause is a lack of nerve innervation; this condition is also known as neurogenic bladder. Other causes include diabetes, prostate enlargement, pregnancy, neurologic disorders such as multiple sclerosis or Parkinson's disease, as well as surgery with general anesthesia. Surgery with general anesthesia that involves perineal or anal regions results in a reflex spasm of the sphincters (Hinkle & Cheever, 2018). There may be a reduction of bladder muscle innervation in the postoperative period.

The two most common neurogenic bladder disorders are the failure to store urine, known as the spastic bladder, or the failure to empty urine from the bladder, known as the flaccid bladder. The spastic bladder results from neurologic lesions above the level of the sacral micturition reflexes. The flaccid bladder results from lesions at the sacral micturition reflex.

## Clinical Manifestations and Drug Therapy

A neurogenic bladder results in urinary retention or leakage. The patient may describe a sensation of bladder fullness or incomplete bladder emptying. The pharmacologic treatment of urinary retention is administration of a cholinergic agonist (see Table 47.1).

# CHOLINERGIC AGONIST

Ⓟ **Bethanechol** (Urecholine) is the prototype cholinergic agonist.

## Pharmacokinetics

Bethanechol is well absorbed in the GI tract. The onset of action is 30 minutes, and the medication reaches its peak in 60 to 90 minutes. The duration of action is 1 to 6 hours. The site of metabolism and elimination is not known. The drug does not cross the blood–brain barrier but does cross the placenta, and it enters breast milk.

## Action

Bethanechol is a sympathomimetic agent that acts at the cholinergic receptors in the urinary and GI tracts to increase muscle tone. The increased tone of the detrusor muscle in the urinary bladder allows for bladder emptying.

## Use

Bethanechol is administered during the acute postoperative and postpartum periods for the treatment of nonobstructed urinary retention and neurogenic atony of the bladder muscle. Table 47.4 gives dosage information for this drug.

## Adverse Effects

Cardiovascular adverse effects to bethanechol include transient heart block, orthostatic hypotension with large doses, and cardiac arrest. Reported GI adverse effects are abdominal discomfort, increased salivation, nausea, vomiting, and fecal incontinence. Genitourinary effects include urinary urgency. Other adverse effects are flushing, sweating, malaise, and dyspnea.

## Contraindications

Contraindications to bethanechol include known hypersensitivity to the drug or other cholinergic agent as well as hyperthyroidism, peptic ulcer disease, intestinal obstruction, asthma, bradycardia, coronary artery disease, epilepsy, and parkinsonism. Patients should not take bethanechol in the postoperative phase of bladder neck or GI surgery.

## Nursing Implications

### Preventing Interactions

Several drugs, including cholinergic agents, atropine, procainamide, epinephrine, and ganglionic blockers, increase the effects of bethanechol. This causes a significant drop in blood pressure.

| **TABLE 47.4** | | | |
|---|---|---|---|
| **DRUGS AT A GLANCE: Cholinergic Agonist Used for the Treatment of Urinary Retention** | | | |
| **Drug** | **Pregnancy Category** | **Routes and Dosage Ranges** | |
| | | **Adults** | **Children** |
| Ⓟ **Bethanechol** (Urecholine; 🍁 Duvoid, PHL-Bethanechol, PMS Bethanechol) | C | 10–50 mg PO 3–4 times/d; initial dose of 5–10 mg with gradual increases hourly until desired effect is seen; or until 50 mg is given | Safety and efficacy not established |

## Administering the Medication

Administration of bethanechol should occur 1 hour before meals or 2 hours after meals to prevent nausea and vomiting. Therapy should begin using the lowest possible dosage, which is then increased as tolerated.

## Assessing for Therapeutic Effects

The nurse assesses the patient's ability to void 1 hour following the administration of the medication. He or she interviews the patient regarding the relief of symptoms of bladder fullness.

## Assessing for Adverse Effects

The nurse assesses the patient's blood pressure lying, sitting, and standing. It is also necessary to assess an electrocardiogram for signs of heart block or impending cardiac arrest. In addition, the nurse assesses for cholinergic crisis with sweating and flushing. Finally, he or she assesses for GI effects such as abdominal pain, nausea, and vomiting.

## Patient Teaching

Box 47.5 identifies patient teaching guidelines for bethanechol.

### NCLEX Success

7. The nurse should be prepared to administer which of the following drugs as an antidote to cholinergic drug overdose?
   A. epinephrine
   B. diphenhydramine
   C. atropine
   D. propranolol

8. The nurse who is working in the genitourinary surgical division of the health center has an order to administer bethanechol to a patient. Which of the following statements by the patient would require the nurse to hold the medication and notify the prescriber?
   A. "I was diagnosed with hyperthyroidism this year."
   B. "I have not eaten any breakfast."
   C. "I have not urinated for 6 hours."
   D. "My mother was allergic to bethanechol."

9. The nurse has administered bethanechol to a patient who has not voided in 8 hours. What is the priority assessment following the administration of bethanechol?
   A. Assess the patient's blood pressure in 2 hours.
   B. Assess the cardiac status every 15 minutes.
   C. Assess the patient's urinary output in 1 hour.
   D. Assess the patient's fluid intake for 24 hours.

10. A 40-year-old patient is taking bethanechol for urinary retention. The physician increases the dosage from 30 to 40 mg. For which of the following adverse effects should the nurse assess?
    A. pulmonary edema
    B. bronchospasm
    C. orthostatic hypotension
    D. pulse deficit

**BOX 47.5**   **Patient Teaching Guidelines for Bethanechol**

- Take the medication on an empty stomach.
- Take the medication only as prescribed.
- Report difficulty urinating to your health care provider.
- Report diarrhea, headache, belching, substernal pressure, or pain to your health care provider.

## IRREVERSIBLE ANTICHOLINESTERASE TOXICITY

Most irreversible anticholinesterase agents are highly lipid soluble and can enter the body by a variety of routes, including the eye, skin, respiratory system, and GI tract. Because they readily cross the blood–brain barrier, their effects are seen peripherally as well as centrally.

Some of the agents used by terrorists are irreversible anticholinesterases. In 1995, a terrorist group released sarin gas on a number of subway trains in Tokyo, Japan. Sarin is a toxic nerve gas that produces a cholinergic crisis characterized by excessive cholinergic (muscarinic) stimulation and neuromuscular blockade. This cholinergic crisis occurs because the irreversible anticholinesterase poison binds to the enzyme anticholinesterase and inactivates it. Consequently, acetylcholine remains in cholinergic synapses and causes excessive stimulation of muscarinic and nicotinic receptors. Other nerve gases that produce these effects include tabun and soman. In addition, the organophosphate insecticides malathion and parathion have the same cholinergic effects.

Emergency treatment includes decontamination procedures such as removing contaminated clothing, flushing the poison from skin and eyes, and using activated charcoal and lavage to remove ingested poison from the GI tract. Pharmacologic treatment includes administering atropine to counteract the muscarinic effects of the poison (e.g., salivation, urination, defecation, bronchial secretions, laryngospasm, bronchospasm). Atropine acts by blocking the acetylcholine at the parasympathetic sites of the smooth muscle, salivary glands, and the CNS to dry secretions and increase cardiac output. The severity of the poisoning dictates the dosage of atropine. The U.S. Department of Defense uses atropine in the form of AtroPen for the initial treatment of muscarinic symptoms.

In addition, a second drug is necessary to relieve the neuromuscular blockade produced by nicotinic effects of the poison. This drug, pralidoxime (Protopam), a cholinesterase reactivator, is a specific antidote for overdose with irreversible anticholinesterase agents. (Other indications for pralidoxime include control of overdose by anticholinesterase drugs used to treat myasthenia gravis.) It treats toxicity by causing the anticholinesterase poison to release the enzyme acetylcholinesterase. The reactivated acetylcholinesterase can then degrade excess acetylcholine at the cholinergic synapses, including the neuromuscular junction. It is important to note that pralidoxime cannot cross the blood–brain barrier; thus, it is effective only in the peripheral areas of the body. It is essential that pralidoxime is given as soon after the poisoning as possible. If too much time passes, the bond between the irreversible anticholinesterase agent and acetylcholinesterase becomes stronger, and pralidoxime is unable to release the enzyme from the poison.

Because pralidoxime is excreted in the urine, dosage reduction is necessary in the presence of renal impairment. During the administration of the medication, continuous monitoring of the patient is essential due to the risk of tachycardia and cardiac arrest. The peak onset of action is 5 to 15 minutes. The half-life is 74 to 77 minutes. Excretion of unchanged drug occurs in the urine.

Treatment of anticholinesterase overdose may also require diazepam or lorazepam to control seizures. The mechanism of action of diazepam is not understood, but the drug is thought to act in the limbic system. It potentiates gamma-aminobutyric acid, an inhibitory neurotransmitter. Close monitoring of the patient's electrocardiogram during drug administration is necessary. Mechanical ventilation may be necessary to treat respiratory paralysis.

Table 47.5 summarizes the miscellaneous medications used for the treatment of irreversible anticholinesterase toxicity.

## TABLE 47.5

### DRUGS AT A GLANCE: Miscellaneous Drugs Used for Treatment of Irreversible Anticholinesterase Toxicity

| Drug | Pregnancy Category | Routes and Dosage Ranges | |
| --- | --- | --- | --- |
| | | **Adults** | **Children** |
| Atropine sulfate (AtroPen) | C | Neuromuscular blockade reversal: IV 15–30 mcg/kg administered with neostigmine or 7–10 mcg/kg administered with edrophonium<br>Muscarine-containing mushroom poisoning: IV 1–2 mg; titrate and repeat as needed<br>Organophosphate or carbamate insecticide or nerve agent poisoning: AtroPen: Mild symptoms: IM 2 mg at initial exposure<br>If severe symptoms develop after first dose, rapidly give two additional doses within 10 min; do not exceed three doses. | Mushroom poisoning (muscarine): IV 0.02 mg/kg/dose; minimum dose 0.1 mg; titrate and repeat as needed.<br>AtroPen: IM < 7 kg: 0.25 mg/dose (yellow pen)<br>6.8–18 kg: 0.5 mg/dose (blue pen)<br>18–41 kg: 1 mg/dose (dark red pen)<br>>41 kg: 2 mg/dose (green pen)<br>Administer the weight-based dose as soon as exposure is known or suspected: 2 additional doses should be repeated in rapid succession 10 min after the first dose; do not administer more than 3 doses. |
| Pralidoxime (Protopam) | C | Use in conjunction with atropine<br>1–2 g IV or IM; repeat in 1–2 h if muscle weakness has not been relieved, then at 10–12 h intervals if cholinergic signs recur.<br>Organophosphate poisoning: loading dose 1000–2000 mg IV, repeat bolus of 1000–2000 mg after 1 h and repeat 10–12 h thereafter.<br>Mild symptoms: 600 mg IM, repeat every 15 min (maximum dose 1800 mg).<br>Severe symptoms: 600 mg; repeat twice in rapid succession to deliver a total of 1800 mg.<br>Persistent symptoms: repeat entire series beginning 1 h after last injection. | Use in conjunction with atropine<br>20–50 mg/kg/dose; repeat in 1–2 h if muscle weakness is not improved, then 10–12 h intervals if cholinergic signs recur<br>Organophosphate poisoning (<16 y): 20–50 mg/kg IV (max dose 2000 mg/dose); repeat after 1 h and every 10–12 h if muscle weakness persists.<br>Mild symptoms: 15 mg/kg repeat every 15 min for persistent symptoms (max dose: 45 mg/kg; may administer in rapid succession)<br>Severe symptoms: 15 mg/kg; repeat twice in rapid succession 45 mg/kg total dose<br>Persistent symptoms: may repeat entire series (45 mg/kg) beginning 1 h after last dose |
| Diazepam (Valium; Diastat AcuDial, Diastat Pediatric, Diazepam Intensol) (✳ Apo-Diazepam, BIO-Diazepam, Diazemuls, Diastat, Valium) | D | 5–10 mg IV slowly; may repeat in 10–15 min; max dose: 30 mg | Infants, children, adolescents; IV 0.15–0.2 mg/kg max dose: 10 mg; may repeat once |

## THE NURSING PROCESS

A concept map outlines the nursing process related to drug therapy considerations in this chapter. Additional nursing implications related to the disease process should also be considered in care decisions.

**Assessment**

- Myasthenia gravis
  - Assess for muscle weakness in mild to moderate disease: ptosis (drooping) of the upper eyelid and diplopia (double vision) caused by weakness of the eye muscles.
  - In severe disease, assess for difficulty in chewing, swallowing, and speaking; accumulation of oral secretions, which the patient may be unable to expectorate or swallow; decreased skeletal muscle activity, including impaired chest expansion; and eventual respiratory failure.
- Alzheimer's disease
  - Assess for abilities and limitations in relation to memory, cognitive functioning, and self-care activities.
  - Assess for preexisting conditions that may be aggravated by a cholinergic drug.
- Urinary retention
  - Assess for bladder distention.
  - Assess for time and amount of previous urination and fluid intake.

**Outcomes of Therapy**

The patient will
- Verbalize or demonstrate correct drug administration
- Improve in self-care abilities
- Regain usual patterns of urinary and bowel elimination
- Maintain effective oxygenation of tissues
- Report adverse drug effects
- For patients with myasthenia gravis, at least one family member will verbalize or demonstrate correct drug administration, symptoms of too much or too little drug, and emergency care procedures.
- For patients with dementia, a caregiver will verbalize or demonstrate correct drug administration and knowledge of adverse effects to be reported to a health care provider.

**Nursing Interventions**

- Use measures to prevent or decrease the need for cholinergic drugs. Ambulation, adequate fluid intake, and judicious use of opioid analgesics or other sedative-type drugs help prevent postoperative urinary retention.
- In myasthenia gravis:
  - Schedule activities to avoid excessive fatigue and to allow adequate rest periods. This may be beneficial, because muscle weakness is aggravated by exercise and improved by rest.
  - Recommend that one or more family members be trained in cardiopulmonary resuscitation.
- In Alzheimer's disease, assist and teach caregivers to
  - Maintain a quiet, stable environment and daily routines to decrease confusion (e.g., verbal or written reminders, simple directions, adequate lighting, calendars, personal objects within view and reach).
  - Avoid altering dosage or stopping the drug without consulting the prescribing physician.
  - Be sure that the patient keeps appointments for supervision and blood tests.
- With long-term drug use, assist patients and families to establish a schedule of drug administration that best meets the patient's needs.
- Do not give cholinergic drugs for bladder atony and urinary retention or for paralytic ileus in the presence of an obstruction.

**Evaluation**

- Observe and interview about the adequacy of urinary elimination.
- Observe abilities and limitations in self-care.
- Question the patient and at least one family member of the patient with myasthenia gravis about correct drug usage, symptoms of underdosage and overdosage, and emergency care procedures.
- Question caregivers of patients with dementia about the patient's level of functioning and response to medication.

## KEY CONCEPTS

- Cholinergic drugs stimulate the parasympathetic nervous system in the same manner as acetylcholine.
- The acetylcholinesterase inhibitor drugs are cholinergic drugs, also known as indirect-acting cholinergics, which inhibit the enzyme acetylcholinesterase, thereby slowing acetylcholine metabolism at autonomic nerve synapses.
- Acetylcholinesterase inhibitor drugs are classified as either reversible or irreversible inhibitors of acetylcholinesterase.
- Neostigmine (Bloxiverz) is the prototype acetylcholinesterase inhibitor drug.
- Cholinergic crisis is a drug-induced overstimulation of the parasympathetic nervous system, requiring discontinuation of any anticholinesterase drug.
- Atropine sulfate should be readily available whenever cholinergic drugs are given.
- Pyridostigmine is the drug of choice in the treatment of myasthenia gravis.
- Patients suffering from Alzheimer's disease have a deficiency in cholinergic function in the cortex and basal forebrain. This deficiency leads to diminished cognitive function. Patients also have a significant loss of neurons, in addition to shrinkage of large cortical neurons.

- Donepezil (Aricept) is the prototype centrally acting reversible cholinesterase inhibitor. The primary use for this drug is treatment of Alzheimer's disease.
- Memantine (Namenda) is an NMDA receptor antagonist that was approved for use in 2003. It is administered to patients with moderate to severe Alzheimer's disease.
- Donepezil, a cholinesterase, and memantine, an NMDA receptor antagonist, are components of Namzaric, a combination drug administered for moderate to severe Alzheimer's disease.
- Bethanechol (Urecholine) is the prototype cholinergic agonist used to increase the contraction of the detrusor muscle to relieve urinary retention.
- Atropine reverses muscarinic effects resulting from overdose of cholinergic drugs but does not reverse the nicotinic effects of skeletal muscle weakness or paralysis resulting from overdose of indirect cholinergic drugs.
- Pralidoxime, a cholinesterase reactivator, is the specific treatment for neuromuscular blockade caused by overdose with irreversible cholinergic drugs.

## CLINICAL REASONING CASE STUDY

**Meet the Patient**

Leola Patke has been living alone but recently moved in with her son and daughter-in-law after being diagnosed with Alzheimer's disease. She has been taking donepezil (Aricept) for moderate Alzheimer's disease. In the past few weeks, her family states that she has become increasingly more forgetful and has had episodes where she roams the house at night. She also has increased anxiety. The geriatrician has prescribed memantine (Namenda) 5 mg orally once daily in addition to her donepezil.

- What is the action of donepezil?
- What is the rationale for prescribing memantine in addition to donepezil?
- Mrs. Patke's son and his wife note improvement in her ability to perform activities of daily living and her memory. What medication could Mrs. Patke be administered in place of donepezil and memantine?
- What patient teaching does the nurse provide to the family?

**Assessing Drug Information**

- Donepezil increases acetylcholine in the brain by inhibiting its metabolism, leading to elevated acetylcholine levels in the cortex. This slows the neuronal degradation that occurs in Alzheimer's disease.
- Memantine is used to slow the progression of moderate to severe Alzheimer's disease.
- In Alzheimer's patients, there is an overstimulation of the glutamate receptors leading to cell death. *N*-methyl-D-aspartate (NMDA) is a glutamate receptor in which memantine induces an antagonistic effect. An overstimulation of NMDA receptors prevent magnesium from reentering and blocking the channel from closing, resulting in an influx of calcium. This action results in neuronal cell death. Memantine has the ability to bind to the magnesium site to block the excitatory function by slowing intracellular calcium accumulation. This action prevents nerve damage but does not have an effect on glutamate.
- Donepezil–memantine is a combination drug that is administered to patients with moderate to severe dementia.

**Nursing Actions**

- Instruct the patient and family that donepezil should be taken at bedtime. The orally disintegrating tablets should be placed on the tongue and allowed to dissolve; this should be followed by drinking water.
- Continue taking the donepezil if no change in symptoms is noted.
- Note that the following side effects may occur: nausea, vomiting (eat frequent small meals), insomnia, fatigue, and confusion (protect Mrs. Patke from injury).
- Report severe nausea, vomiting, changes in stool or urine color, diarrhea, changes in neurologic functioning, and yellowing of the eyes or skin to your health care provider.
- Instruct the patient and family to administer memantine without regard to meals. The extended-release formulation should be swallowed whole. It should not be chewed. The capsule can be opened and sprinkled on applesauce, which must be consumed immediately. The liquid formulation should be squirted in the corner of the patient's mouth. It should not be mixed with any other liquid.

*Visit* thePoint® *at* **http://thePoint.lww.com/Frandsen12e** *for answers to NCLEX Success questions (in Appendix A), answers to Clinical Application Case Studies (in Appendix B), and more!*

## REFERENCES AND RESOURCES

Alzheimer's Association. (2018). *2018 Alzheimer's disease facts and figures.* Retrieved February 7, 2019, from www.alz.org

Alzheimer's Association. (2019). *What is Alzheimer's disease?* Retrieved February 12, 2019, from www.alz.org

Lippincott. (2020). *Nursing 2020 drug handbook.* Philadelphia, PA: Lippincott, Williams, and Wilkins.

Bird, S. J. (2019a). Diagnosis of myasthenia gravis. In *UpToDate.* Lexi Comp, Inc.

Bird, S. J. (2019b). Myasthenic crisis. In *UpToDate.* Lexi Comp, Inc.

Bird, S. (2019c). Overview of the treatment of Myasthenia gravis. In *UpToDate.* Lexi Comp, Inc.

Hamina, A., Taipale, H., Tanskanen, A., Tolppanen, A. M., Tihonen, J., & Hartikainen, S. (2017). Differences in analgesic use in community-dwelling persons with and without Alzheimer's disease. *European Journal of Pain, 21,* 658–667. doi:10.1002/ejp.969

Hinkle, J. H., & Cheever, K. H. (2018). *Brunner & Suddarth's textbook of medical-surgical nursing* (14th ed.). Philadelphia, PA: Lippincott Williams & Wilkins.

Karch, A. M. (2019). *2019 Lippincott Pocket Drug guide for nurses.* Philadelphia, PA: Lippincott Williams & Wilkins.

Norris, T. (2019). *Porth's pathophysiology concepts of altered health states* (10th ed.). Philadelphia, PA: Lippincott Williams & Wilkins.

Press, D., & Alexander, M. (2018). Treatment of dementia. *UptoDate.* Lexi Comp, Inc.

UpToDate. (2019). *Drug information.* Lexi-Comp, Inc.

Wright, C. (2017). Treatment and prevention of vascular dementia. In *UpToDate.* Lexi Comp, Inc.

# Drug Therapy for Parkinson's Disease, Urinary Spasticity, and Disorders Requiring Anticholinergic Drug Therapy

## LEARNING OBJECTIVES

*After studying this chapter, you should be able to:*

1. Describe the major characteristics and manifestations of Parkinson's disease.
2. Understand the pathophysiology of Parkinson's disease.
3. Describe the types of commonly used antiparkinson drugs.
4. Identify the prototype and describe the action, use, adverse effects, contraindications, and nursing implications for the dopamine receptor agonists.
5. Identify the prototype and describe the action, use, adverse effects, contraindications, and nursing implications for the catechol-*O*-methyltransferase (COMT) inhibitors.
6. Identify the prototype and describe the action, use, adverse effects, contraindications, and nursing implications for a COMT inhibitor and decarboxylase inhibitor/dopamine precursor.
7. Implement the nursing process in the care of patients undergoing drug therapy for Parkinson's disease.
8. Describe the general characteristics of anticholinergic drugs.
9. Identify the prototype and describe the action, use, adverse effects, contraindications, and nursing implications for belladonna alkaloids and derivatives.
10. Identify the prototype and describe the action, use, adverse effects, contraindications, and nursing implications for centrally acting anticholinergic drugs.
11. Identify the prototype and describe the action, use, adverse effects, contraindications, and nursing implications for anticholinergic medications used for gastrointestinal and urinary disorders.
12. Implement the nursing process in the administration of anticholinergic agents.

## CLINICAL APPLICATION CASE STUDY

Lee Stokes is a 61-year-old man who visits his primary health care provider. He is experiencing pill-rolling movement of the right hand and fingers; slow, stooped movement; a shuffling gait with the absence of arm movement; and excessive salivation. His physician diagnosed Mr. Stokes with Parkinson's disease and started him on levodopa–carbidopa (Sinemet) 25-mg carbidopa–100-mg levodopa four times a day and benztropine mesylate at bedtime.

# KEY TERMS

**Akinesia:** rigid limbs

**Anticholinergic drug:** drug that inhibits the actions of acetylcholine in the brain

**Antimuscarinic drug:** drug that interacts with muscarinic cholinergic receptors in the brain, secretory glands, heart, and smooth muscle to produce an anticholinergic response

**Basal ganglia:** area in the midbrain that controls smooth voluntary movement

**Bradykinesia:** inability to move

**Catechol-O-methyltransferase inhibitor:** medication that inhibits the metabolism of levodopa in the periphery

**Cycloplegia:** paralysis in the ciliary muscle of the eye

**Dopamine receptor agonist:** drug that corrects the neurotransmitter imbalance by increasing levels of dopamine

**Extrapyramidal reactions:** movement disorders such as tardive dyskinesia (inability to initiate movement), akathisia (inability to remain motionless), dystonia, and drug-induced parkinsonism that may occur with use of antiparkinsonism and antipsychotic drugs

**Hypertensive crisis:** severe increase in blood pressure that can lead to a stroke

**Muscarinic receptors:** located in the most internal organs, including the cardiovascular, respiratory, gastrointestinal (GI), and genitourinary systems; when activated by acetylcholine, the affected cells may be excited or inhibited in their functions

**Mydriasis:** pupil dilation

**Nicotinic receptors:** located in motor nerves and skeletal muscles; when activated by acetylcholine, the cell membrane depolarizes and produces muscle contraction

**"Off time":** periods of the day when the medication is not working well, causing worsening of parkinsonian symptoms

**Parkinson's disease:** chronic, progressive, degenerative disorder of the central nervous system characterized by resting tremor, bradykinesia, rigidity, and postural instability

**Parkinsonism:** often defined as a parkinsonian syndrome that is idiopathic (having no known cause), although some atypical cases have a genetic origin

**Quaternary amines:** anticholinergic drugs that carry a positive charge and are lipid insoluble; they do not readily cross the cell membranes, are poorly absorbed from the GI tract, and do not cross the blood–brain barrier

**Substantia nigra:** region of the midbrain with dopamine cells

**Tertiary amines:** anticholinergic drugs that are unchanged lipid-soluble molecules, are able to cross cell membranes readily, and are well absorbed from the GI tract and conjunctiva, and they cross the blood–brain barrier

# INTRODUCTION

The first part of this chapter discusses Parkinson's disease and the medications administered to decrease the symptoms of the disease. The second part discusses anticholinergic drugs administered to decrease secretions and prevent urinary urgency.

# OVERVIEW OF PARKINSON'S DISEASE

**Parkinson's disease** (also called **parkinsonism**) is a chronic, progressive, degenerative disorder of the central nervous system (CNS) characterized by resting tremor, bradykinesia, rigidity, and postural instability. Manifestations of Parkinson's disease

also may occur with other CNS diseases, brain tumors, and head injuries. Drugs that deplete dopamine stores or block dopamine receptors, including the older antipsychotic drugs (phenothiazines and haloperidol), reserpine, and metoclopramide, can produce movement disorders such as secondary parkinsonism (which also involves **extrapyramidal reactions**; see Chap. 56). Treatment can be pharmacologic, nonpharmacologic, and/or surgical.

The Parkinson's Disease Foundation estimates that by the year 2020, approximately 930,000 people in the United States will be living with Parkinson's disease (2019). This includes about 60,000 people who are diagnosed with the disease each year, with 96% older than 50 years of age. More than 10 million people worldwide have Parkinson's disease. The disease occurs

1.5 more often in men than in women and in Caucasian and Hispanic/Latino people more often than in African Americans.

## Etiology

The cause of the nerve cell damage is unknown; age-related degeneration, genetics, and exposure to environmental toxins are possible etiologic factors. A total of nine genetic linkages and four genes have been associated with Parkinson's disease, including mutations of alpha-synuclein and parkin genes. A high incidence of mutations in the parkin-2 gene has been associated with early-onset parkinsonism.

## Pathophysiology

Idiopathic parkinsonism results from progressive destruction of or degenerative changes in dopamine-producing nerve cells in the **substantia nigra** in the **basal ganglia**, the area in the midbrain that controls smooth voluntary movement. The basal ganglia in the brain normally contain substantial amounts of the neurotransmitters dopamine and acetylcholine. The correct balance of dopamine and acetylcholine is important in regulating posture, muscle tone, and voluntary movement. People with Parkinson's disease have an imbalance in these neurotransmitters, resulting in a decrease in inhibitory brain dopamine and a relative increase in excitatory acetylcholine.

## Clinical Manifestations

The first symptom of Parkinson's disease is often a resting tremor that begins in the fingers and thumb of one hand ("pill-rolling" movements), eventually spreading over one side of the body and progressing to the contralateral limbs. Other common symptoms include inability to move (**bradykinesia**), rigid limbs (**akinesia**), shuffling gait, stooped posture, masklike facial expression, and a soft speaking voice. Less common manifestations may include depression, personality changes, loss of appetite, sleep disturbances, speech impairment, or sexual difficulty. Approximately 15% to 20% of people with Parkinson's disease

develop dementia. The severity of disease manifestations usually worsen over time. However, disease progression is often quite gradual, and patients may retain near-normal functional abilities for several years.

## Drug Therapy

Drugs used in Parkinson's disease include **dopamine receptor agonists**, which help correct the neurotransmitter imbalance by increasing levels of dopamine, and **catechol-*O*-methyltransferase (COMT) inhibitors**, which inhibit the metabolism of levodopa in the periphery. See Table 48.1. (The older belladonna alkaloids and the newer centrally acting anticholinergic agents inhibit the actions of acetylcholine in the brain. As previously stated, these medications are discussed later in this chapter.)

## DOPAMINE RECEPTOR AGONISTS

Levodopa (L-dopa), the original prototype dopamine receptor antagonist, was developed in the 1960s. It is routinely administered with the drug carbidopa; therefore, the combination medication is discussed as the prototype.  **Levodopa–carbidopa**

## TABLE 48.1

### Drugs Administered for the Treatment of Parkinson's Disease

| Drug Class | Prototype | Other Drugs in the Class |
|---|---|---|
| Dopamine receptor agonist | Levodopa–carbidopa | Amantadine (Gocovri, Osmolex ER)<br>Apomorphine hydrochloride (Apokyn)<br>Bromocriptine mesylate (Parlodel, Cycloset)<br>Pramipexole dihydrochloride (Mirapex, Mirapex ER)<br>Rasagiline (Azilect)<br>Ropinirole (Requip XL, Requip)<br>Rotigotine transdermal (Neupro)<br>Safinamide (Xadago)<br>Selegiline hydrochloride (Emsam, Zelapar) |
| Catechol-*O*-methyltransferase (COMT) inhibitors | Tolcapone (Tasmar) | Entacapone (Comtan) |
| COMT inhibitor and decarboxylase inhibitor/dopamine precursor | Levodopa, carbidopa, and entacapone (Stalevo) | |

(Sinemet, Duopa, Rytary) is well established as the most effective drug for the symptomatic treatment of idiopathic Parkinson's disease. (Carbidopa is used only in conjunction with levodopa.) The combination is particularly effective for the management of akinetic symptoms.

---

### Clinical Application 48.1

- A nurse is providing patient teaching to Mr. Stokes and his family. The family inquires about the progression of Parkinson's disease. What does the nurse tell the patient and the family with regard to disease progression?

---

## Pharmacokinetics

In peripheral tissues (e.g., gastrointestinal [GI] tract, liver), levodopa is metabolized extensively by the enzyme aromatic amino acid decarboxylase (AADC) and to a lesser extent by COMT. Because most levodopa is metabolized in peripheral tissues, large doses are required to obtain therapeutic levels of dopamine in the brain. These large amounts increase adverse drug effects. To reduce levodopa dosage and decrease adverse effects, carbidopa, an AADC inhibitor, is given to decrease the peripheral metabolism of levodopa. The combination of levodopa and carbidopa greatly increases the amount of available levodopa, so that levodopa dosage can be reduced by approximately 70%. When carbidopa inhibits the decarboxylase pathway of levodopa metabolism, the COMT pathway becomes more important (see COMT Inhibitors for a discussion of entacapone and tolcapone).

Levodopa is well absorbed from the small intestine after oral administration, reaches peak serum levels within 30 to 90 minutes, and has a short serum half-life (1–3 hours). Absorption is decreased by delayed gastric emptying, hyperacidity of gastric secretions, and competition with amino acids (from digestion of protein foods) for sites of absorption in the small intestine. Pyridoxine (vitamin $B_6$) promotes the breakdown of levodopa, reducing its effectiveness. Levodopa is metabolized to 30 or more metabolites, some of which are pharmacologically active and probably contribute to drug toxicity; the metabolites are excreted primarily in the urine, usually within 24 hours.

## Action

Dopaminergic drugs increase the amount of dopamine in the brain by various mechanisms (Fig. 48.1). If levodopa is administered alone, large doses must be taken to produce therapeutic effects. Carbidopa combined with levodopa prevents the decarboxylation of the levodopa, which makes levodopa more available for transportation to the brain. Levodopa is the metabolic precursor of dopamine, and after levodopa crosses the blood–brain barrier, it converts to dopamine in the brain. This is thought to be the mechanism whereby the drug relieves symptoms of Parkinson's disease. Carbidopa does not cross the blood–brain barrier and does not affect levodopa metabolism.

## Use

Levodopa–carbidopa is a treatment of idiopathic Parkinson's disease, postencephalitic and arteriosclerotic parkinsonism, and parkinsonism related to carbon dioxide and manganese intoxication. Prescribers may also order levodopa to reduce the symptoms of restless legs syndrome (RLS). People with RLS, also known as Ekbom's syndrome, experience paresthesias of the muscles, particularly in the calf and thighs, creating the urge to move. Movement relieves the paresthesia, which returns when the person is at rest or trying to sleep. The disorder may result in insomnia, mental distress, and, in some cases, suicide.

Levodopa and carbidopa are usually given together in a fixed-dose formulation called Sinemet. Table 48.2 gives the doses of this combination and other dopamine receptor agonists used to treat Parkinson's disease.

### Use in Children

Safety and effectiveness for use in children have not been established for most antiparkinson drugs. Parkinsonism is a degenerative disorder of adults, and antiparkinson drugs are most likely to be used in children for other purposes such as the stimulation of growth hormone in children with Down's syndrome.

### Use in Older Adults

It may be necessary to reduce dosages of levodopa–carbidopa because of an age-related decrease in peripheral AADC, the enzyme that carbidopa inhibits. The risk of hallucinations is increased in older patients who take dopamine agonist drugs.

### Use in Patients With Renal Impairment

Caution is necessary with the use of levodopa–carbidopa in patients with renal failure. Dosage adjustments are required.

### Use in Patients With Hepatic Impairment

With levodopa, cautious use in patients with hepatic impairment is warranted, and dosage reduction may be necessary. Reduced dosages are indicated with severe hepatic impairment. It is important to monitor liver transaminase enzymes frequently to assess for liver impairment. At the earliest sign of hepatotoxicity, drug withdrawal is essential, and there should be no reinstatement.

### Use in Patients With Critical Illness

Caution is necessary with the use of levodopa in patients with severe neurologic, cardiac, or hepatic injuries. Dosage adjustment to the lowest level required for therapeutic effects is essential.

### Use in Patients Receiving Home Care

The home care nurse can help patients and caregivers understand that the purpose of drug therapy is to control symptoms and that noticeable improvement may not occur for several weeks. Also, the nurse can encourage patients to consult physical therapists, speech therapists, and dietitians to help maintain their ability to perform activities of daily living. In addition, teaching about preventing or managing adverse drug effects may be necessary. Caregivers may need to be informed that most activities (e.g., eating, dressing) take longer and require considerable effort by patients with parkinsonism.

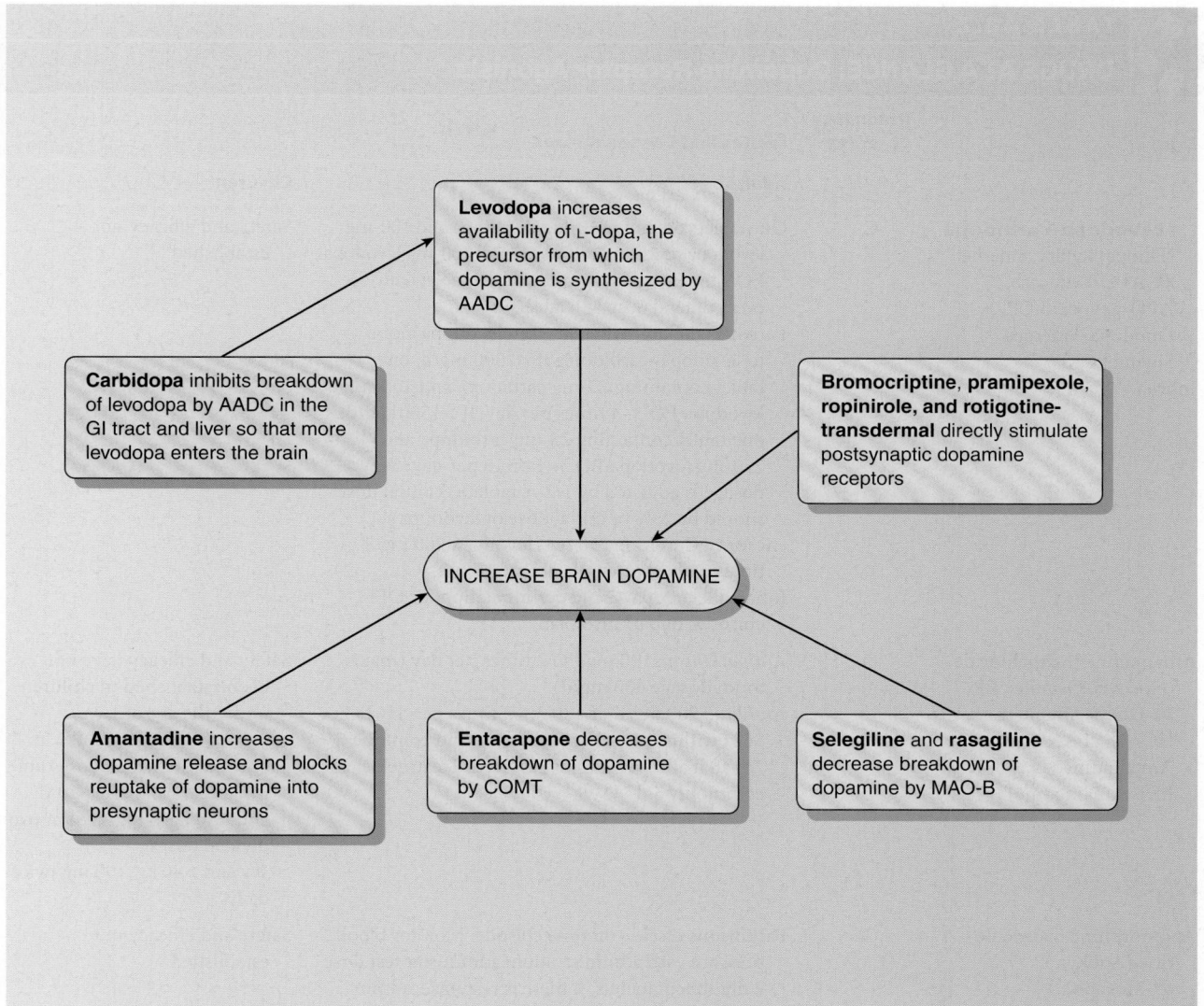

**Figure 48.1.** Mechanisms by which dopaminergic drugs increase dopamine in the brain. AADC, amino acid decarboxylase; COMT, catechol-*O*-methyltransferase; MAO-B, monoamine oxidase B.

## Adverse Effects

Because of the adverse effects and recurrence of parkinsonism symptoms after a few years of levodopa therapy, levodopa is usually reserved for patients with significant symptoms and functional disabilities. The most common CNS adverse effects are headache and anxiety. Older patients may experience problems such as hallucinations, dementia, and drowsiness. The most severe adverse effect is depression with suicidal tendencies.

Cardiovascular adverse effects include ectopic beats, tachycardia, anginal pain, palpitations, hypotension, vasoconstriction, dyspnea, bradycardia, and a widened QRS. The medication can cause orthostatic hypotension. This effect is common during the first few weeks but usually subsides. Concurrent administration of nonselective monoamine oxidase (MAO) inhibitors (used in the treatment of depression) and levodopa can result in extreme elevations in blood pressure or **hypertensive crisis**. (MAO exists in two types, MAO-A and MAO-B, both of which are found in the CNS and peripheral tissues.)

In addition, some patients report anorexia, bruxism, and nausea and vomiting. Other less common adverse effects are piloerection, azotemia, and gangrene with prolonged use. Dermatologic effects such as hypersensitivity, anaphylaxis, and urticaria occur less frequently.

## Contraindications

Contraindications to the use of levodopa–carbidopa include a known hypersensitivity to the drug. The drug can dilate pupils and raise intraocular pressure; thus, narrow-angle glaucoma is also a contraindication. Levodopa may activate malignant melanoma; people with suspicious skin lesions or a history of melanoma should not take it. To avoid the severe hypertension that may occur with concurrent use of some MAO inhibitors and levodopa, it is essential that MAO inhibitors be discontinued 14 days prior to beginning levodopa therapy. In addition, use of levodopa warrants caution in patients with severe cardiovascular, pulmonary, renal, hepatic, or endocrine disorders; depression; and peptic ulcer disease.

| | | | |
|---|---|---|---|
| **TABLE 48.2** | | | |
| **DRUGS AT A GLANCE: Dopamine Receptor Agonists** | | | |

| Drug | Pregnancy Category | Routes and Dosage Ranges | |
|---|---|---|---|
| | | **Adults** | **Children** |
| Ⓟ **Levodopa–carbidopa** (Duopa, Rytary, Sinemet; ✹ APO-Levocarb, APO-Levocarb CR, Duodopa, Sinemet, Sinemet CR) Inbrija | C | One tablet containing 10-mg carbidopa and 100-mg levodopa or 25-mg carbidopa and 100-mg levodopa PO 3 times per day; increased by 1 tablet daily or every other day up to 6 tablets/d. Patients who are switched from levodopa alone to levodopa–carbidopa: if <1500 mg/d; one tablet containing 25-mg carbidopa and 100-mg levodopa PO 3–4 times per day; if >1500 mg/d; one tablet containing 25-mg carbidopa and 250-mg levodopa PO 3–4 times per day; the dosage is adjusted by 1/2–1 tablet/d (initial dose should be 25% of initial dose of levodopa). CR form: Carbidopa 50 mg–levodopa 200 mg 2 times daily at intervals not <6 h. Inhaled levodopa 42 mg per inhalation for OFF episodes of parkinsonism | Safety and efficacy not established |
| Amantadine hydrochloride (Gocovri, Osmolex ER; ✹ DOM-Amantadine HCl, MYLAN-Amantadine, PDP-Amantadine) | C | *Antiparkinson*: 100 mg PO 2 times per day (maximum dosage 400 mg/d) *Antiviral*: 200 mg/d or 100 mg 2 times per day PO. Start within 24–48 h of exposure and continue 24–48 h after symptoms resolved. Treatment commonly 5 d | Safety and efficacy have not been established in children under the age of 1 y 1–9 y: 4.4–8.8 mg/kg/d PO in one or two divided doses not to exceed 150 mg/d >10 y and <40 kg: 5 mg/kg/d in two divided doses >10 y and >40 kg, 100 mg twice daily |
| Apomorphine hydrochloride (Apokyn; ✹ Movapo) | C | Parkinson's disease off time episode: Monitor blood pressure with administration: administer test dose 2 mg subcutaneous; if there is response, administer 2 mg and may increase dose by 1 mg every few days with max dose of 6 mg; if no response, administer the second test dose of 4 mg; if well tolerated, administer 3 mg; may increase by 1 mg every few days with max dose of 6 mg; if no response, give the third test dose 3 mg; if well tolerated, administer 2 mg for off time episodes; may increase to 3 mg after a few days | Safety and efficacy not established |
| Bromocriptine mesylate (Parlodel, Cycloset) | C | 1.25 mg PO twice daily; increase by 2.5 mg daily in 2- to 4-wk intervals as needed (max dosage: 100 mg/d) | Safety and efficacy not established |
| Bromocriptine (✹ DOM-Bromocriptine) | B | 0.25 mg PO daily initially twice weekly; may increase up to 0.25 mg twice weekly (max dosage 1 mg twice weekly) | Safety and efficacy not established |
| Pramipexole dihydrochloride (Mirapex, Mirapex ER; ✹ ACT-Pramipexole, APO-Pramipexole, Mirapex) | C | 0.125 mg PO 3 times per day gradually increase every 5–7 d to a max dose of 0.5–1.5 mg 3 times per day Extended release: 0.375 mg PO daily, may increase to 0.75 mg per dose after 5–7 d up to a max dose of 4.5 mg/d RLS: 0.125 mg taken 2–3 h before bed, dose can be increased every 4–7 d Renal impairment: CrCl 30–50 mL/min: 0.125 mg 2 times per day (max dose, 0.75 mg 3 times per day); CrCl 15–29 mL/min, 0.125 mg/d (max dosage 1.5 mg/d) | Safety and efficacy not established |

| | TABLE 48.2 | | | |
| --- | --- | --- | --- | --- |
| | **DRUGS AT A GLANCE: Dopamine Receptor Agonists** (Continued) | | | |

| Drug | Pregnancy Category | Routes and Dosage Ranges | | |
| --- | --- | --- | --- | --- |
| | | **Adults** | | **Children** |
| Rasagiline (Azilect; ✳ APO-Rasagiline, Azilect, TEVA-Rasagiline) | C | 1 mg PO daily as monotherapy; (max dose: 1 mg/d); PO; with levodopa: 0.5 mg/d with max dose of 1 mg/d based on tolerance<br>Hepatic impairment: 0.5 mg PO daily | | Safety and efficacy not established |
| Ropinirole hydrochloride (Requip, Requip XL; ✳ ACT-Ropinirole, JAMP-Ropinirole, PMS-Ropinirole) | C | 0.25 mg PO 3 times per day; titrate up by 0.25 mg/dose 3 times per day every week to a target dose of 1 mg 3 times per day; may be increased by 1.5 mg/d every week (max dosage: 9 mg/d) and then 3 mg/d weekly to a max dosage of 24 mg/d<br>Extended release: 2 mg/d for 1–2 wk and then increase by 2 mg/d at 1-wk intervals; max dosage 24 mg/d<br>RLS: 0.25 mg/d 1–3 h before bedtime for 2 d, may increase to 0.5 mg for the 1st week and then increase to 1 mg/d to a max dose of 3 mg during week 6 and to a max dosage of 4 mg starting at 7 wk | | Safety and efficacy not established |
| Rotigotine (Neupro; ✳ Neupro) | C | 2 mg/24-h transdermal patch; may increase by 2 mg weekly based on clinical response | | Safety and efficacy not established |
| Safinamide (Xadago) | C | 50 mg PO once daily; after 2 wk may increase to 100 mg once daily | | Safety and efficacy not established |
| Selegiline hydrochloride (Eldepryl, Emsam, Zelapar; ✳ APO Selegiline, DOM Selegiline, MYLAN Selegiline, PMS Selegiline, TEVA Selegiline) | C | 5 mg PO 2 times per day with breakfast and lunch; dosages >10 mg/d are associated with increased risk of toxicity due to MAO inhibition<br>Geriatric dosage: start with 5 mg in the morning ODT: 1.25 mg/d with carbidopa/levodopa therapy for 6 wk; may increase to 2.5 mg/d based on tolerance (max 2.5 mg/d); transdermal, start with 6 mg/d; may titrate by 3 mg/d every 2 wk (max 12 mg/d) | | Depression: adolescents >17 y, transdermal; refer to adult dosing |

## Nursing Implications

### Preventing Interactions

The administration of levodopa–carbidopa with an MAO inhibitor can precipitate a hypertensive crisis. Postural hypotension occurs with the administration of tricyclic antidepressants and levodopa–carbidopa. Methyldopa combined with levodopa increases CNS effects. Dysrhythmic effects are increased when combined with halogenated general anesthetics. Several drugs interact with levodopa–carbidopa, increasing or decreasing its effects (Box 48.1). A high-protein meal increases the effects of levodopa–carbidopa, and kava decreases the effects of the drug.

### Administering the Medication

The nurse ensures that: *[handwritten: don't give food w/ ↑ protein content]*

- Levodopa–carbidopa is administered with or just after food or following a meal to reduce nausea and vomiting.
- Sinemet CR is not crushed.
- Levodopa is not given with iron preparations or multivitamin–mineral preparations that contain iron.

**BOX 48.1    Drug Interactions: Levodopa–Carbidopa**

**Drugs That Increase the Effects of Levodopa–Carbidopa**
- Monoamine oxidase inhibitors
  *Increase the risk of hypertensive crisis*

**Drugs That Decrease the Effect of Levodopa–Carbidopa**
- Anticholinergics
  *Increase anticholinergic effects by delaying gastric emptying*
- Pyridoxine (vitamin B$_6$)
  *Stimulates decarboxylase, the enzyme that converts levodopa to dopamine, causing metabolism in the peripheral tissues and decreasing medication distribution to the central nervous system*
- Phenytoin, papaverine, tricyclic antidepressants, and benzodiazepines
  *Decrease drug efficacy*

- Levodopa–carbidopa is not administered with a high-protein diet. Adequate hydration is also necessary.

In addition, the nurse should ensure a temperature-controlled environment; this prevents hyperpyrexia.

> ⓘ **QSEN Alert: Patient-Centered Care**
>
> When administering levodopa, carbidopa, and other medications for Parkinson's disease, it is important that medications be given to the patient on time. Timing of medication administration is critical for optimal therapeutic effect.

### Assessing for Therapeutic Effects

With levodopa and other dopaminergic agents, the nurse observes for improvement in mobility, balance, posture, gait, speech, handwriting, and self-care ability. Elimination of drooling and seborrhea may occur. Mood elevation may result. After 2 to 5 years, the medication may lose its overall effectiveness, and the dosage may need to be increased. The nurse needs to be aware of symptoms such as ataxic gait, tremors of the hands and fingers, drooling, and masklike facial expressions.

### Assessing for Adverse Effects

The nurse assesses for anorexia, nausea, and vomiting. These symptoms usually disappear after a few months of levodopa–carbidopa therapy. As previously stated, giving the drug with food minimizes these effects. The nurse also assesses the patient's blood pressure in the sitting and standing positions to identify signs of orthostatic hypotension. This effect, too, commonly dissipates a few weeks after beginning therapy. Levodopa and its metabolites stimulate beta-adrenergic receptors in the heart. Patients with preexisting coronary artery disease may take propranolol (Inderal) to counteract cardiac dysrhythmia effects. It is necessary to assess the patient for dyskinesia. The involuntary movements of the tongue, mouth, and face are common adverse effects. Decreasing the dose of the medication decreases dyskinesia.

### Patient Teaching

Box 48.2 identifies patient teaching guidelines for levodopa–carbidopa.

## Other Drugs in the Class

Amantadine hydrochloride is an antiparkinson and antiviral agent (see Chap. 23). It increases the dopamine release in the nigrostriatal pathway of patients with Parkinson's disease. It is absorbed in the GI tract with an onset of action of 36 to 48 hours, a peak of action of 1.5 to 8 hours, and a half-life of 10 to 25 hours. It crosses the placenta and enters the breast milk. It is excreted unchanged in the urine. The most common adverse effects of amantadine are dizziness, light-headedness, and insomnia. The nurse instructs the patient to report swelling of the fingers or ankles, difficulty walking, urinary retention, tremors, slurred speech, or thoughts of suicide to the health care provider. It is important not to discontinue this drug abruptly.

Apomorphine hydrochloride (Apokyn) is an antiparkinson agent administered for "**off time**," or "off" episodes, of

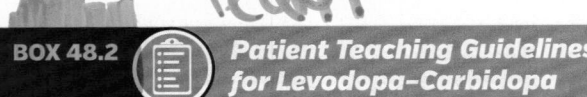

**BOX 48.2** 📋 *Patient Teaching Guidelines for Levodopa–Carbidopa*

- Take the medication as prescribed.
- Do not crush the sustained-release preparation.
- Do not take multivitamin preparations containing pyridoxine.
- Understand that there are adverse effects of medication such as drowsiness, dizziness, and orthostatic hypotension.
- Change positions slowly to prevent drop in blood pressure.
- Avoid alcohol.
- Take the medication with food to prevent nausea and vomiting.
- Do not take the medication with a high-protein meal.
- Report fainting, light-headedness, irregular heart rate, uncontrolled facial movements, urinary retention, nausea, and vomiting to the prescriber.
- Notify the prescriber of any increase in symptoms such as static gait, altered mobility, and "pill rolling."

Parkinson's disease—to assist in diminishing the symptoms of hypomobility. "Off time" is the period when the medication is not adequately controlling the patient's symptoms. Patients who suffer from "off time" episodes have advanced Parkinson's disease. Administration is subcutaneous. Doses are incremental, generally ranging from 20 to 40 mg. The most common dosage is 30 mg, or 0.3 mL, and the maximum dosage is 60 mg. The patient's blood pressure must be monitored for hypertensive crisis during the administration. When apomorphine is administered to patients with a known cardiac history, periodic electrocardiogram results should be monitored as well as serum electrolytes.

Bromocriptine mesylate (Parlodel, Cycloset) is an ergot derivative that directly stimulates dopamine receptors in the brain. It is used in the treatment of idiopathic Parkinson's disease, with levodopa–carbidopa, to prolong effectiveness and to allow reduced dosage of levodopa. Administration to patients with a history of myocardial infarction with residual dysrhythmia requires caution.

Inbrija is an orally inhaled levodopa inhalation powder and a dopamine precursor. In December 2018, the U.S. Food and Drug Administration (FDA) approved Inbrija for the intermittent treatment of OFF episodes in patients with Parkinson's disease, already treated with carbidopa/levodopa. OFF episodes in Parkinsonism are noted when levodopa's effect wears off before the next dose. Inbrija must be used concurrently with carbidopa/levodopa. OFF episodes occur in Parkinson's disease because the GI system may become delayed in the absorption of levodopa, and levels will be altered. The advantage of Inbrija is the systemic pulmonary route, which enables its effect to control parkinsonism to be more consistent than that of levodopa. Clinical trials revealed a 10-minute onset of action with an 84-mg dose of Inbrija and improvement in motor function within 30 minutes. The drug comes in a capsule form, to be administered only through the Inbrija inhaler, which comes with the medication. Each capsule dose is 42 mg; the inhaler holds one capsule at a time. Once the capsule has been placed in the haler, replace the mouthpiece, breath out, close lips around the inhaler, and take a deep, comfortable breath and you will hear the capsule spin inside the inhaler. Remove the inhaler, and take a deep breath and hold it for 5 seconds. Remove and discard the capsule. Repeat with a second capsule. Capsules should never be swallowed. The approved daily dose is 84 mg up to five times daily as needed for OFF period symptoms in Parkinson's disease. The maximum daily dose is 420 mg. Adverse reactions include cough, low blood pressure, chest discomfort, headache, hallucinations, nausea/vomiting, decreased red blood cell count, and sputum discoloration. Concerns related to adverse effects include hallucinations, thinking/behavioral changes, CNS depression, dyskinesias, and neuroleptic malignant syndrome. Oral administration of levodopa crosses the placenta and is present in the breast milk. The manufacturer of Inbrija advises caution to patients when considering breastfeeding and the risk of infant exposure.

Pramipexole (Mirapex, Mirapex ER) and ropinirole (Requip, Requip XL) stimulate dopamine receptors in the brain. The U.S. FDA has approved their use in both early and late stages of Parkinson's disease. In early stages, one of these drugs can be used alone to improve motor performance, improve ability to participate in usual activities of daily living, and delay levodopa therapy. In advanced stages, one of these drugs can be used with levodopa and perhaps other antiparkinson drugs to provide more consistent relief of symptoms between doses of levodopa and allow reduced dosage of levodopa. These drugs, which are not ergot derivatives, may not cause some adverse effects associated with bromocriptine (e.g., pulmonary and peritoneal fibrosis, constriction of coronary arteries).

Pramipexole is rapidly absorbed with oral administration. Peak serum levels are reached in 1 to 3 hours after a dose and steady-state concentrations in about 2 days. The drug is less than 20% bound to plasma proteins and has an elimination half-life of 8 to 12 hours. Most of the drug is excreted unchanged in the urine; only 10% is metabolized. As a result, renal failure may cause higher-than-usual plasma levels and possible toxicity. However, hepatic disease is unlikely to alter drug effects.

Rasagiline (Azilect) is an irreversible MAO inhibitor. It is indicated for initial treatment for idiopathic parkinsonism and as an adjunct therapy with levodopa to reduce "off time" when movements are poorly controlled. Because it has not been determined to be selective for MAO-B in humans, care must be taken to avoid tyramine-containing foods as well as sympathomimetic medications to prevent hypertensive crisis. In addition, rasagiline has the potential to increase serotonin neurotransmission. When given with other drugs that enhance stimulation of serotonergic receptors (e.g., antidepressants, St. John's wort, dextromethorphan, and meperidine), serotonin syndrome, a potential fatal CNS toxicity reaction characterized by hyperpyrexia and death, can occur. Rasagiline should be discontinued at least 14 days before beginning treatment with most antidepressants or other MAO inhibitors. Fluoxetine should be discontinued at least 5 weeks before initiating rasagiline, due to its long half-life. Rasagiline is well absorbed orally, metabolized in the liver, and excreted primarily by the kidney.

It is contraindicated with foods containing tyramine or sympathomimetic amine–containing medications (e.g., nonprescription cold preparations and anesthetics) because of the risk of hypertensive crisis and with antidepressants (e.g., tricyclic antidepressants, selective serotonin reuptake inhibitors, serotonin–norepinephrine reuptake inhibitors, mirtazapine), meperidine, and dextromethorphan because of the potential for inducing serotonin syndrome.

Ropinirole (Requip, Requip XL) is also well absorbed with oral administration. It reaches peak serum levels in 1 to 2 hours and steady-state concentrations within 2 days. It is 40% bound to plasma proteins and has an elimination half-life of 6 hours. It is metabolized by the cytochrome P450 enzymes in the liver to inactive metabolites, which are excreted through the kidneys. Less than 10% of ropinirole is excreted unchanged in the urine. Thus, hepatic failure may decrease metabolism, allow drug accumulation, and increase adverse effects. Renal failure does not appear to alter drug effects.

Rotigotine (Neupro) is an antiparkinson agent that is a dopamine agonist. It is a transdermal patch in which the mechanism of action is unknown. When starting the medication, the patient should be aware that decreases in blood pressure can place the patient at risk for falls. Instruct to cautiously change positions due to orthostatic hypotension.

Safinamide (Xadago) is a monoamine type B inhibitor that blocks the catabolism of dopamine, to increase the dopamine level and dopaminergic activity in the brain. It is administered as an adjunctive therapy with levodopa to increase motor function. It is important to monitor blood pressure with the administration of safinamide.

Selegiline (Emsam, Zelapar) inhibits the metabolism of dopamine by MAO, which exists in two types (as previously stated). These types are differentiated by their relative specificities for individual catecholamines. MAO-A acts more specifically on tyramine, norepinephrine, epinephrine, and serotonin. This enzyme is the main subtype in GI mucosa and in the liver and is responsible for metabolizing dietary tyramine. If MAO-A is inhibited in the intestine, tyramine in various foods is absorbed systemically rather than deactivated. As a result, there is excessive stimulation of the sympathetic nervous system, and severe hypertension and stroke can occur. This is sometimes called the "cheese reaction" because aged cheeses are high in tyramine. This life-threatening reaction can also occur with some medications (e.g., sympathomimetics) that are normally metabolized by MAO. MAO-B metabolizes dopamine; in the brain, most MAO activity is due to type B. At oral dosages of 10 mg/day or less, selegiline inhibits MAO-B *selectively* and is unlikely to cause severe hypertension and stroke. However, at dosages greater than 10 mg/day, selectivity is lost and metabolism of both MAO-A and MAO-B is inhibited. Dosages greater than 10 mg/day should be avoided in patients with Parkinson's disease. Selegiline inhibition of MAO-B is irreversible, and drug effects persist until more MAO is synthesized in the brain, which may take several months.

In early Parkinson's disease, selegiline may be effective as monotherapy (level A). In advanced disease, prescribers order the drug to enhance the effects of levodopa. Its addition aids symptom control and allows the dosage of levodopa–carbidopa to be reduced. Once proposed to have neuroprotective properties, authorities now believe that there is insufficient evidence to recommend the use of selegiline to confer neuroprotection in patients with Parkinson's disease (level U).

## NCLEX Success

1. The daughter of a 75-year-old woman states to the parish nurse that she has noticed her mother rolling her fingers together on her right hand. The nurse observes the patient and determines she is "pill rolling," which is a characteristic of Parkinson's disease. Which of the following factors contributes to the development of central nervous system symptom of "pill rolling?"

   A. decrease firing of the sinoatrial node
   B. conversion of angiotensin I to angiotensin II
   C. increase in excitatory acetylcholine
   D. influx of potassium through the cell membrane

2. A 65-year-old woman has been taking levodopa for several weeks for symptoms of Parkinson's disease. Which of the following symptoms indicates that she is not receiving an adequate dose for the treatment of her symptoms?

   A. edema of the feet and ankles
   B. widened QRS complex
   C. static gait
   D. increased intraocular pressure

3. The 56-year-old man is taking levodopa–carbidopa for Parkinson's disease. During the therapy, he becomes light-headed and dizzy. Which of the following is a potentially serious adverse effect of the drug treatment?

   A. orthostatic hypotension
   B. diminished fluid volume
   C. hematuria
   D. jaundice

4. A 52-year-old man is taking selegiline for the treatment of Parkinson's disease. He consumes port-wine cheese and crackers at a party. Which of the following symptoms does he develop?

   A. ataxic gait
   B. melena
   C. cardiac dysrhythmia
   D. hypertension

5. A 48-year-old man with severe akinesia develops severe symptoms of parkinsonism following the administration of his antiparkinson medications. This condition occurs only one to two times per month. Which of the following medications is the man's prescriber most likely to order?

   A. bromocriptine mesylate
   B. apomorphine hydrochloride
   C. cabergoline
   D. pramipexole dihydrochloride

### Clinical Application 48.2

- Mr. Stokes has been having "off time" symptom development. His neurologist orders rasagiline (Azilect). He develops an upper respiratory viral infection with a cough. He begins to take dextromethorphan hydrobromide (Robitussin) every 4 hours. What is Mr. Stokes at risk for developing?
- What symptom does the nurse assess Mr. Stokes for when combining rasagiline and dextromethorphan hydrobromide?

# CATECHOL-*O*-METHYLTRANSFERASE INHIBITORS

Ⓟ **Tolcapone** (Tasmar) is the prototype COMT inhibitor. COMT plays a role in brain metabolism of dopamine and metabolizes approximately 10% of peripheral levodopa. By inhibiting COMT, tolcapone increases levels of dopamine in the brain and relieves symptoms more effectively and consistently.

## Pharmacokinetics

Tolcapone is absorbed rapidly and is highly protein bound. It is metabolized in the liver and possesses a 2- to 3-hour half-life. It crosses the placenta and enters the breast milk. It is excreted in the feces and urine.

## Action

The main mechanism of action of tolcapone seems to be inhibiting the metabolism of levodopa in the bloodstream, thus increasing the plasma concentration and duration of action of the drug. It may also inhibit COMT in the brain and prolong the activity of dopamine at the synapse.

## Use

Tolcapone is useful for the treatment of signs and symptoms of idiopathic Parkinson's disease. Administration is only in conjunction with levodopa–carbidopa, and a reduction in levodopa dosage is required. If a patient does not show a clinical benefit within 3 weeks of starting treatment, discontinuation of tolcapone is necessary.

Table 48.3 presents the dosage information for tolcapone and other drugs in its class.

### Use in Older Adults

When administering tolcapone to geriatric patients, it is important to reduce the dosage and adjust it slowly to prevent adverse effects.

### Use in Patients With Renal Impairment

Caution is warranted in the administration of tolcapone to patients with renal impairment because it is excreted in the urine.

### Use in Patients With Hepatic Impairment

If liver values are greater than two times the upper limit of normal, discontinuation of tolcapone is necessary. Patients with

**TABLE 48.3**

**DRUGS AT A GLANCE: Catechol-*O*-Methyltransferase Inhibitors**

| Drug | Pregnancy Category | Routes and Dosage Ranges | |
|---|---|---|---|
| | | **Adults** | **Children** |
| Ⓟ **Tolcapone** (Tasmar) | C | 100 mg PO 3 times per day with carbidopa/levodopa (max dose: 200 mg 3 times per day); doses of levodopa >600 mg may need reduced<br><br>Because of the risk of potentially fatal acute fulminant liver failure, tolcapone should ordinarily be used in patients with Parkinson disease on L-dopa/carbidopa who are experiencing symptom fluctuations and are not responding satisfactorily to or are not appropriate candidates for other adjunctive therapies | Safety and efficacy not established |
| Entacapone (Comtan; ❁ Comtan, Mylan-Entacapone) | C | 200 mg PO administered with each dose of levodopa/carbidopa up to 8 times per day (max dose: 1600 mg daily) | Safety and efficacy not established |

moderate to severe hepatic impairment should not take tolcapone at doses exceeding 100 mg three times per day. The FDA has issued a BLACK BOX WARNING ◆ stating that patients who take tolcapone risk potentially fatal acute fulminant liver failure. It is important to monitor liver function tests before therapy begins and every 2 weeks thereafter.

## Adverse Effects

Tolcapone produces adverse effects in several major body systems, including the CNS, cardiovascular system, dermatologic system, GI system, and respiratory system. The most severe adverse effect is fulminant liver failure, which may be fatal. CNS adverse effects include disorientation, confusion, hallucinations, and psychosis. Dry mouth, dizziness, and orthostatic hypotension may also occur.

## Contraindications

Contraindications to tolcapone include a hypersensitivity to the drug. Other contraindications are liver disease, nontraumatic rhabdomyolysis, hyperpyrexia, and confusion. Caution is warranted with hypertension, hypotension, and renal impairment.

## Nursing Implications

### Preventing Interactions

It is essential that tolcapone and other COMT medications not be administered with MAO inhibitors due to the risk of hypertensive crisis.

### Administering the Medication

It is necessary to administer tolcapone in conjunction with levodopa–carbidopa and to monitor the patient's response to the medication. The addition of the drug may require a decrease in the levodopa dosage. Abrupt withdrawal of tolcapone can lead to serious complications. Tapering over 2 weeks is necessary to prevent adverse effects.

### Assessing for Therapeutic Effects

The decrease or absence of symptoms of Parkinson's disease such as improved gait and mobility, diminished tremors, and rigidity is indicative of tolcapone's therapeutic effectiveness.

### Assessing for Adverse Effects

The nurse assesses for disorientation and confusion, lightheadedness, and orthostatic hypotension. It is necessary to take blood pressure lying down, sitting, and standing up. Frequent monitoring of liver enzymes is essential.

### Patient Teaching

Box 48.3 presents patient teaching guidelines for tolcapone.

## Other Drugs in the Class

Entacapone (Comtan) is well tolerated and safer than tolcapone, and thus, prescribers more commonly order entacapone. This COMT inhibitor is well absorbed after oral administration and

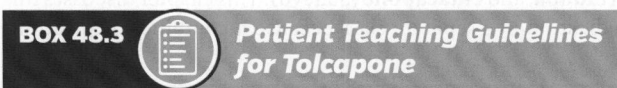

**BOX 48.3  📋  *Patient Teaching Guidelines for Tolcapone***

- Take the medication exactly as prescribed.
- Do not stop the medication abruptly; taper it over 2 weeks.
- Take the medication in conjunction with levodopa–carbidopa.
- Use barrier contraceptives while using this medication.
- Do not breast-feed while taking the medication.
- Use caution when operating machinery due to central nervous system (CNS) depression.
- Use hard candy to decrease dry mouth.
- Have liver function tests as scheduled.
- Avoid concurrent use of alcohol or other CNS depressants.

reaches a peak plasma level in 1 hour. It is highly protein bound (98%), has a half-life of about 2.5 hours, and is metabolized in the liver to an inactive metabolite. The dosage must be reduced by 50% in the presence of impaired liver function. The parent drug and metabolite are 90% excreted through the biliary tract and feces, and 10% of excretion occurs in the urine. Adverse effects include confusion, dizziness, drowsiness, hallucinations, nausea, and vomiting, which can be reduced by lowering the dose of either levodopa or entacapone. Although clinical trials report few instances of liver enzyme elevation or hemoglobin decreases, it is recommended that liver enzymes and red blood cell counts be measured periodically.

## NCLEX   Success

6. An elderly woman is taking tolcapone. She has noticed that her skin is yellow. The nurse assesses which of the following?

 A. intake of carrots
 B. temperature related to infection
 C. sclera
 D. amount of urine output

7. A 35-year-old woman has begun to take tolcapone in addition to levodopa–carbidopa for Parkinson's disease. Which of the following is the priority nursing intervention?

 A. Arrange to assess the patient for hypertension early in the morning.
 B. Evaluate the patient's ability care for herself.
 C. Have the patient take levodopa–carbidopa 2 hours after tolcapone.
 D. Instruct the patient to report tea-colored urine to the prescriber.

## CATECHOL-*O*-METHYLTRANSFERASE INHIBITOR AND DECARBOXYLASE INHIBITOR/DOPAMINE PRECURSOR

One antiparkinson drug is a combination of Ⓟ **levodopa**, **carbidopa**, and **entacapone** (Stalevo). This chapter discusses this medication in a separate class because it combines medications

from two separate classes. Administration of Stalevo allows for greater convenience and improved Parkinson symptom management. Use of the drug combination provides the patient with the convenience of one medication.

## Pharmacokinetics

The combination drug Stalevo has the same pharmacokinetics as those of levodopa–carbidopa and entacapone.

## Action

Levodopa is the metabolic precursor of dopamine. Depleted in Parkinson's disease, levodopa is circulated in the plasma and crosses the blood–brain barrier, where it is converted to dopamine by the striatal enzymes. Carbidopa inhibits the peripheral plasma breakdown of levodopa by inhibiting decarboxylation, thus increasing levodopa. Entacapone is a reversible and selective inhibitor of COMT. It alters the pharmacokinetics of levodopa, allowing for more sustained levodopa serum levels and increased concentrations for absorption across the blood–brain barrier.

## Use

Stalevo is used for the treatment of idiopathic Parkinson's disease. Table 48.4 presents the dosage information for Stalevo.

### Use in Patients With Renal Impairment

It is necessary to administer Stalevo with caution in patients with severe renal impairment. Dosage reduction to prevent further renal insufficiency may be warranted.

### Use in Patients With Hepatic Impairment

Cautious administration of Stalevo is also necessary in patients with hepatic impairment because the medication is metabolized in the liver.

## Adverse Effects

Stalevo may affect the GI, dermatologic, respiratory, and cardiovascular systems. GI adverse effects include diarrhea as well as nausea, vomiting, bruxism, dry mouth, and excess salivation.

### TABLE 48.4

### DRUGS AT A GLANCE: Catechol-*O*-Methyltransferase Inhibitor and Decarboxylase Inhibitor/Dopamine Precursor

| Drug | Pregnancy Category | Routes and Dosage Range | |
|---|---|---|---|
| | | **Adults** | **Children** |
| Ⓟ **Levodopa–carbidopa–entacapone** (Stalevo; ✳ Stalevo) | C | Dosing forms:<br>Levodopa 50 mg–carbidopa 12.5 mg–entacapone 200 mg PO daily<br>Levodopa 75 mg–carbidopa 18.75 mg–entacapone 200 mg<br>Levodopa 100 mg–carbidopa 25 mg–entacapone 200 mg<br>Levodopa 125 mg–carbidopa 31.25 mg–entacapone 200 mg<br>Levodopa 150 mg–carbidopa 37.5 mg–entacapone 200 mg<br>Levodopa 200 mg–carbidopa 50 mg–entacapone 200 mg | Safety and efficacy not established |

The development of diarrhea is indicative of drug-induced colitis, and it is necessary to discontinue Stalevo if diarrhea occurs. Somnolence has been reported in which patients fall asleep without warning. This adverse effect is linked to entacapone. Also, the risk of melanoma may increase. If dyskinesia occurs, it may be necessary to reduce the dose. As with other antiparkinson medications, hypotension is a risk, along with heart attack, stroke, and cardiovascular death. Also, there is an increased risk of cardiovascular events in patients who received Stalevo versus those who received Sinemet. However, studies show that the risk of cardiovascular events is not statistically significant, but research is continuing. In addition, postmarketing studies report that impulsivity and compulsive behaviors may occur.

*Monitor pt w/ heart defects/disease*

## Contraindications

Contraindications to the use of Stalevo include a known sensitivity to the levodopa, carbidopa, or entacapone. The concurrent use of MAO inhibitors, or use within 14 days, is also a contraindication. Levodopa may trigger melanoma; therefore, patients with a history of melanoma should not receive Stalevo. Also, it is important to note that ergot-derived dopamine agonists administered with Stalevo have been associated with fibrotic complications such as pleural effusion, pleural thickening, and pulmonary infiltrates.

## Nursing Implications

### Preventing Interactions

The administration of catecholamines such as epinephrine, dopamine, and methyldopa enhances the action of entacapone, one of the components of Stalevo.

### Administering the Medication

Patients whose medication regimen is being changed to Stalevo should be administered levodopa and the adjunctive entacapone. The levodopa dose should be adjusted prior to the conversion to Stalevo therapy. The dose should be individualized based on the therapeutic response. The presence of dyskinesia necessitates a dosage adjustment. The dose may be adjusted by changing the strength or adjusting the dosing intervals. Fractionated doses are not recommended, and only one tablet should be administered at each dosing interval. The maximum daily dose is eight 50-, 75-, 100-, 125-, and 150-mg tablets and only six 200-mg tablets. (Patients who take more than 600 mg/day of levodopa should not switch directly to Stalevo.) Patients should swallow the tablets whole—not crushed, broken, or chewed. Stalevo can be administered without regard to meals. To prevent fluctuation in levodopa absorption, it is necessary to distribute protein intake throughout the day. People should take iron, iron supplements, and multivitamins that contain minerals separately from Stalevo.

### Assessing for Therapeutic Effects

The decrease or absence of Parkinson's symptoms such as muscle rigidity, excessive salivation, "pill rolling," and tremors is indicative of Stalevo's therapeutic effectiveness.

### Assessing for Adverse Effects

The nurse assesses the patient's cardiovascular status, including heart rate and blood pressure, to determine alterations in cardiovascular symptoms. It is also necessary to assess for chest pain, confusion, and weakness of extremities related to cerebrovascular accident or myocardial infarction. In addition, the nurse assesses the patient's skin for unusual skin lesions and checks the patient's fecal elimination for drug-induced colitis. It is important to teach the family to report any statements that indicate suicidal ideations. The nurse assesses for abnormal compulsive urges.

### Patient Teaching

Patient education for Stalevo is the same as the patient education for the drug's individual components: levodopa, carbidopa, and entacapone (see Box 48.2). With entacapone, the nurse instructs the patient to report hallucinations and diarrhea. It is also necessary to tell the patient that his or her urine may become brownish orange. This is a normal reaction to the medication and is not harmful. In addition, the nurse tells the patient to protect against falls due to orthostatic hypotension; patients can stand up slowly.

---

### NCLEX Success

8. A 76-year-old woman is taking levodopa–carbidopa–entacapone. Which of the following is the priority nursing intervention?

   A. administering with a high-protein meal
   B. administering with meals only
   C. assessing for diarrhea
   D. assessing for constipation

9. An elderly man begins taking levodopa–carbidopa–entacapone. Which of the following symptoms warrants a change in the dosage? [Select all that apply.]

   A. dilated pupils
   B. increased tremors
   C. static gait
   D. edema
   E. nausea

---

### Clinical Application 48.3

● Mr. Stokes' prescriber switches him from levodopa–carbidopa to levodopa–carbidopa–entacapone. He asks his nurse what is the difference between the medication he once took and what he is now taking. What patient education does the nurse provide?

---

## OVERVIEW OF ANTICHOLINERGIC DRUGS

**Anticholinergic drugs** inhibit the actions of acetylcholine in the brain and affect the parasympathetic nervous system. Most anticholinergic drugs interact with muscarinic cholinergic receptors

## TABLE 48.5

### Common Tertiary Amine and Quaternary Amine Anticholinergic Drugs

| Tertiary Amines | Quaternary Amines |
|---|---|
| Atropine | Glycopyrrolate (Robinul, Cuvposa) |
| Benztropine mesylate (Cogentin) | Ipratropium bromide (Atrovent HFA) |
| Darifenacin hydrobromide (Enablex) | Methscopolamine bromide (Pamine) |
| Dicyclomine hydrochloride (Bentyl) | Tiotropium bromide (Spiriva) |
| Flavoxate hydrochloride | Trospium chloride |
| Oxybutynin chloride (Ditropan XL, Gelnique, Gelnique Pump) | |
| Scopolamine hydrobromide (Transderm Scop) | |
| Solifenacin succinate (Vesicare) | |
| Tolterodine tartrate (Detrol, Detrol LA) | |
| Trihexyphenidyl hydrochloride | |

Most anticholinergic medications are either **tertiary amines** or **quaternary amines** (Table 48.5). Tertiary amines are uncharged lipid-soluble molecules. Atropine and scopolamine are tertiary amines and therefore are able to cross cell membranes readily. They are well absorbed from the GI tract and conjunctiva, and they cross the blood–brain barrier. Tertiary amines are excreted in the urine.

Quaternary amines carry a positive charge and are lipid insoluble. Some belladonna derivatives and synthetic anticholinergics are quaternary amines. Consequently, they do not readily cross cell membranes. They are poorly absorbed from the GI tract and do not cross the blood–brain barrier. Quaternary amines are excreted largely in the feces.

## Clinical Use

The widespread effects of anticholinergic drugs limit their clinical usefulness. Consequently, several synthetic drugs have been developed in an effort to increase the selectivity of action on particular body tissues, especially to retain the antispasmodic and antisecretory effects of atropine while eliminating its adverse effects. This effort has been less than successful—all the synthetic drugs produce atropine-like adverse effects when doses are sufficient.

Some synthetic drugs are used for antispasmodic effects in GI disorders and overactive urinary bladder. Another group of synthetic drugs includes centrally active anticholinergics used in the treatment of Parkinson's disease; these drugs balance the relative cholinergic dominance that causes the movement disorders associated with parkinsonism. Specific body systems and conditions in which anticholinergic medications are administered are listed in Table 48.6.

## Drug Therapy

Anticholinergic drugs act by occupying receptor sites on target organs innervated by the parasympathetic nervous system, thereby leaving fewer receptor sites free to respond to

in the brain, secretory glands, heart, and smooth muscle and are sometimes called **antimuscarinic drugs**. When given at high doses, a few anticholinergic drugs are also able to block **nicotinic receptors** in autonomic ganglia and skeletal muscles. Glycopyrrolate (Robinul) is an example of such a medication. This drug class includes belladonna alkaloids and their derivatives, such as atropine, and many synthetic substitutes.

## TABLE 48.6

### Body System and Indication of Anticholinergic Use

| Body System | Indication for Anticholinergic Use |
|---|---|
| Cardiac | Bradycardia, heart block with hypotension and shock: increases heart rate and prevent vagal stimulation |
| Gastrointestinal | Peptic ulcer disease, gastritis, pylorospasm, and diverticulitis: relieves pain and relaxes gastrointestinal smooth muscle<br>Irritable bowel, colitis: reduces frequent bowel movements and abdominal discomfort |
| Genitourinary | Urinary incontinence and frequency: reduces urinary muscle spasm<br>Cystitis, urethritis, and prostatitis: decreases pain and frequency<br>Enuresis, paraplegia, and neurogenic bladder: increases bladder capacity |
| Otolaryngology | Head and neck surgery and bronchoscopy: reduces respiratory tract secretions |
| Ophthalmology | Mydriatic and cycloplegic effects: dilate pupils |
| Respiratory | Asthma, chronic bronchitis: produces bronchodilation |
| Metabolic | Mushroom poisoning and organophosphate pesticide poisoning: reduces cholinergic stimulation; salivation, urination, defecation, bronchial secretions, laryngospasm, and bronchospasm |

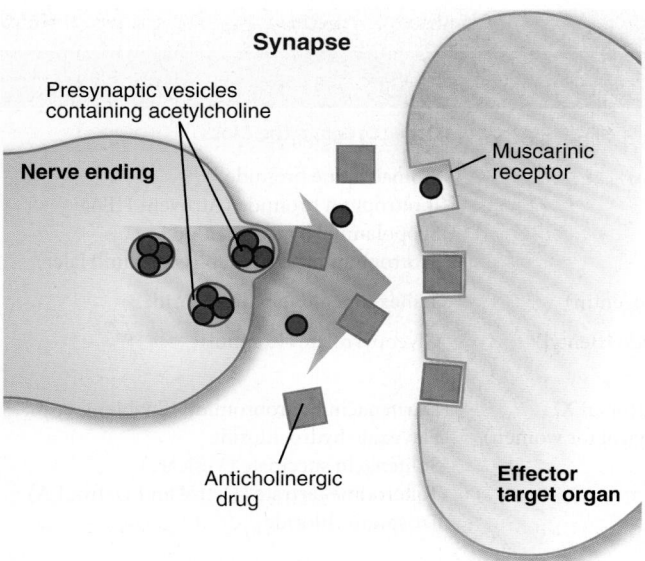

**Figure 48.2.** Mechanism of action of anticholinergic drugs. Anticholinergic (antimuscarinic) drugs prevent acetylcholine from interacting with muscarinic receptors on target effector organs, thus blocking or decreasing a parasympathetic response in these organs.

acetylcholine (Fig. 48.2). Parasympathetic response is absent or decreased, depending on the number of receptors blocked by anticholinergic drugs and the underlying degree of parasympathetic activity. Because cholinergic **muscarinic receptors** are widely distributed in the body, anticholinergic drugs produce effects in a variety of locations, including the CNS, heart, smooth muscle, glands, and the eye.

Specific effects on body tissues and organs include the following:

- CNS stimulation followed by depression, which may result in coma and death. This is most likely to occur with large doses of anticholinergic drugs that cross the blood–brain barrier (atropine, scopolamine, and antiparkinson agents).
- Decreased cardiovascular response to parasympathetic (vagal) stimulation that slows heart rate. Atropine is the anticholinergic drug most often used for its cardiovascular effects. According to the advanced cardiac life support (ACLS) protocol, atropine is the drug of choice to treat symptomatic sinus bradycardia. Low doses (less than 0.5 mg) may produce a slight and temporary decrease in heart rate; however, moderate to large doses (0.5–1 mg) increase heart rate by blocking parasympathetic vagal stimulation. Although the increase in heart rate may be therapeutic in bradycardia, it can be an adverse effect in patients with other types of heart disease because atropine increases the myocardial oxygen demand. Atropine usually has little or no effect on blood pressure. Large doses cause facial flushing because of dilation of blood vessels in the neck.
- Bronchodilation and decreased respiratory tract secretions. Anticholinergics block the action of acetylcholine in bronchial smooth muscle when given by inhalation. This action reduces intracellular guanosine monophosphate (GMP), a

bronchoconstrictive substance. When anticholinergic drugs are given systemically, respiratory secretions decrease and may become viscous, resulting in mucous plugging of small respiratory passages. Administering the medications by inhalation decreases this effect while preserving the beneficial bronchodilation effect.

- Antispasmodic effects in the GI tract due to decreased muscle tone and motility. The drugs have little inhibitory effect on gastric acid secretion with usual doses and insignificant effects on pancreatic and intestinal secretions.
- **Mydriasis** and **cycloplegia** in the eye. Normally, anticholinergics do not change intraocular pressure, but with narrow-angle glaucoma, they may increase intraocular pressure and precipitate an episode of acute glaucoma. When the pupil is fully dilated, photophobia may be uncomfortable, and reflexes to light and accommodation may disappear.
- Miscellaneous effects. These include decreased secretions from salivary and sweat glands; relaxation of ureters, urinary bladder, and the detrusor muscle; and relaxation of smooth muscle in the gallbladder and bile ducts.

Table 48.7 lists the various anticholinergic medications.

## BELLADONNA ALKALOID AND DERIVATIVES

Ⓟ **Atropine sulfate,** the prototype of the anticholinergic drugs, is a naturally occurring belladonna alkaloid that can be extracted from the belladonna plant or prepared synthetically. It is usually prepared as atropine sulfate, a salt that is very soluble in water. Atropine sulfate is also classified as a muscarinic antagonist.

## Pharmacokinetics

Atropine is well absorbed after all forms of administration. The peak effect occurs in 0.7 to 4 minutes with intravenous (IV) preparations, 30 minutes with intramuscular (IM) preparations, 1 to 2 hours with subcutaneous preparations, and 1.5 to 4 hours with inhalation preparation. The pharmacologic effects last for about 4 hours, except for ocular effects, which last for up to 2 weeks in normal eyes. The drug is absorbed systemically when applied locally to mucous membranes. Atropine crosses the blood–brain barrier and enters the CNS, where large doses produce stimulant effects and toxic doses produce depressant effects. It is metabolized in the liver and rapidly excreted in the urine. Atropine crosses the placenta and enters the breast milk.

## Action

Atropine competitively blocks the effects of acetylcholine at muscarinic cholinergic receptors that mediate the effects of parasympathetic postganglionic impulses. It also prevents the action of acetylcholine in the CNS. Atropine depresses the salivary and bronchial secretions, dilates the bronchi, and increases cardiac output. Large doses can decrease motility of the GI and

## TABLE 48.7

### Anticholinergic Medications

| Drug Class | Prototype | Other Drugs in the Class |
|---|---|---|
| Belladonna alkaloids and derivatives | Atropine sulfate (Atropen) | Homatropine bromide<br>Ipratropium bromide (Atrovent HFA)<br>Scopolamine hydrobromide<br>Tiotropium bromide (Spiriva HandiHaler) |
| Centrally acting anticholinergic agents | Benztropine mesylate (Cogentin) | Trihexyphenidyl hydrochloride |
| Gastrointestinal antisecretory/antispasmodic | Dicyclomine hydrochloride (Bentyl) | Glycopyrrolate (Robinul) |
| Urinary antispasmodic | Oxybutynin chloride (Ditropan XL, Gelnique, Oxytrol, Oxytrol for women) | Darifenacin hydrobromide (Enablex)<br>Flavoxate hydrochloride<br>Solifenacin succinate (Vesicare)<br>Tolterodine tartrate (Detrol and Detrol LA)<br>Trospium chloride |

GU tracts. In addition, it relaxes the pupil of the eye and prevents the accommodation for near vision.

## Use

In the past, atropine was used to control the symptoms of Parkinson's disease—to relieve tremors and decrease rigidity. The development of the centrally acting anticholinergic agents has replaced the use of atropine for Parkinson's disease. Impaired renal or hepatic function is a contraindication to the use of atropine.

The most common use of atropine is the restoration of cardiac rate and arterial pressure during anesthesia when vagal stimulation produced by intra-abdominal traction causes a decrease in pulse rate, lessening the degree of atrioventricular block when increased vagal tone is a factor. Atropine also relieves bradycardia and syncope due to hyperactive carotid sinus reflex. It also serves as an antidote for cardiac collapse with an overdose of parasympathomimetic drugs also known as cholinergic agents and cholinesterase inhibitors such as physostigmine.

Also, practitioners administer atropine in the preanesthesia stage to reduce respiratory tract secretions.

In addition, atropine is an antidote for mushroom poisoning (*Amanita muscaria*). Symptoms of muscarinic poisoning include salivation, lacrimation, visual disturbances, bronchospasm, diarrhea, bradycardia, and hypotension. Atropine prevents the poison from interacting with muscarinic receptors, thus reversing the toxic effects. Muscarinic poisoning can also occur from cholinergic agonist drugs, cholinesterase inhibitor drugs, and insecticides that contain organophosphates.

Table 48.8 presents the dosage information for atropine sulfate and the other belladonna alkaloids.

### Use in Children

Systemic anticholinergics, including atropine, have essentially the same indications in children of all ages as in adults. Anticholinergic drugs cause the same adverse effects in children as in adults. However, the effects may be more severe in children, who are especially sensitive to these drugs. Facial flushing is common, and skin rashes may occur. In addition, the administration of atropine sulfate to children can cause hyperpyrexia or atropine fever.

### Use in Older Adults

It is necessary to administer atropine cautiously in the geriatric population. In older adults, CNS reactions are more likely to occur.

### Use in Patients With Critical Illness

When atropine is administered for cardiovascular symptoms, it is necessary to monitor the patient's cardiac status with an electrocardiogram.

## Adverse Effects

Atropine sulfate may adversely affect several body systems. Cardiovascular adverse effects include bradycardia (low doses) and tachycardia (high doses). CNS adverse effects include blurred vision, mydriasis, cycloplegia, photophobia, and increased intraocular pressure. In the geriatric population, nervousness, weakness, confusion, and excitement are common. The most severe GI adverse effect is paralytic ileus. Genitourinary effects are urinary hesitancy and retention. The patient may also complain of decreased sweating, which leads to heat prostration.

Overdose of atropine or other anticholinergic drugs produces the usual pharmacologic effect such as decreased secretions, increased heart rate, relaxation of the bronchial smooth muscle, and decreased GI and genitourinary tone in severe and exaggerated forms. The anticholinergic overdose syndrome is characterized by hyperthermia; hot, dry, flushed skin; dry mouth; mydriasis; delirium; tachycardia; paralytic ileus; and urinary retention. Myoclonic movements and choreoathetosis may be evident. Seizures, coma, and respiratory arrest may also occur. Treatment involves the use of activated charcoal to absorb the ingested drug. Hemodialysis, hemoperfusion, peritoneal dialysis, and repeated doses of charcoal are not effective.

Physostigmine salicylate (Antilirium) (see Chap. 47), an acetylcholinesterase inhibitor, is a specific antidote for overdose of anticholinergics. It is usually given intravenously at a slow rate of 1 mg/min because rapid administration may cause bradycardia,

**TABLE 48.8**

## DRUGS AT A GLANCE: Belladonna Alkaloids and Derivatives

| Drug | Pregnancy Category | Routes and Dosage Ranges | |
|---|---|---|---|
| | | **Adults** | **Children** |
| Ⓟ **Atropine sulfate** (Atropen) **Ophthalmic atropine** (Isopto Atropine; 🍁 Dioptic's Atropine Solution, Isopto Atropine) | C | IM, SC, or IV 0.4–1 mg preoperatively; may repeat every 4–6 h (max dose 3 mg) Amblyopia and mydriasis: instill a drop in the conjunctiva 40 min maximal dilation time; may repeat up to 2 times daily | IM, IV: neonatal; 0.02 mg/kg/dose; IM, SC, IV: infant, children <12 y; 0.02 mg/kg/dose; give 30–60 min prior to the procedure, may repeat every 4–6 h (max dose 1 mg/procedure); children >12 y; 0.02 mg/kg/dose; give 30–60 min prior to procedure, may repeat every 4–6 h (max dose 2 mg/procedure) Mydriasis: infants >3 mo and children <3 y, instill one drop 1% solution 40 min prior to dilation time. Max dose of one drop per eye/d. Children >3 y and adolescents: instill 1 drop 1% solution 40 min prior to dilation time |
| Homatropine bromide (Homatropaire; 🍁 Isopto Homatropine) | C | For refraction: instill 1–2 drops of 2% or 5% solution into the affected eye before the procedure. May repeat in 5–10 min as needed For uveitis: instill one or two drops of 2% or 5% solution into the affected eye every 3–4 h | Refraction/uveitis: infants >3 mo, children, and adolescents, instill 1–2 drops of 5% solution into the affected eye up to every 3–4 h |
| Hyoscyamine sulfate (Anaspaz, Ed-Spaz, Hyosyne, Levsin; 🍁 Levsin) | C | PO, 0.125–0.25 every 4 h PRN daily before meals and at bedtime (max dose 1.5 mg/d) PO (timed-release formula): 0.375–0.75 mg every 12 h (max dose 1.5 mg/d); IM, IV, SC: 0.25–0.5 mg up to 4 times daily every 4 h | Children <2 y: oral drops 0.125 mg/mL based on age and wt repeat dose every 4 h PRN. 3.4–<5 kg, 4 drops with maximum 24 drops/daily; 5–<7 kg, 5 drops with max 30 drops/daily; 7–<10 kg, 6 drops with max 36 drops/daily; >10 kg: 8 drops with max 48 drops/daily. Children 2–12 y: tablets—0.0625–0.125 mg every 4 h PRN with max 0.75 mg/daily. Oral drops: 0.125 mg/mL; 0.03125–0.125 mg every 4 h PRN with max 0.75 mg/daily |
| Ipratropium bromide (Atrovent HFA; 🍁 Apo-Ipravent Solution, Apo-Ipravent Sterules, Atrovent HFA) | B | COPD, oral inhalation; nebulizer, 500 mcg every 6–8 h; MDI, 2 inhalations 4 times/daily with max dose 12 inhalations/daily Acute asthma exacerbation (off-label): for oral inhalation, give with short-acting beta-adrenergic agonist. Nebulizer: 500 mcg every 20 min for 3 doses and then PRN. MDI: 8 inhalations every 20 min PRN up to 3 h. Rhinorrhea: two sprays/nostril of 0.06% spray 4 times daily | COPD: <12 y—see adult dosing Acute asthma (off-label) <5 y; nebulizer 250 mcg every 20 min PRN for 1 h; ≤12 y; nebulizer 250–500 mcg every 20 min every 3 h and then PRN: MDI, <5 y; 2 inhalations every 20 min if needed for 1 h; ≤12 y; 4–8 inhalations every 20 min PRN up to 3 h Rhinorrhea: children 5–11 y, 0.06%—two sprays in each nostril 3 times/daily. Children ≥12 y and adults: 0.06%—two sprays in each nostril 4 times/daily. |
| Scopolamine (Transderm Scop; 🍁 Buscopan) | C | PO 0.4–0.8 mg daily every 8–12 h PRN Transdermal: apply disk 4 h before antiemetic effect is needed. Replace every 3 d. For refraction: instill one or two drops into the eye 1 h before refracting. For iridocyclitis: instill one or two drops into eye(s) up to 4 times daily | Apply one transdermal disk behind the ear at least 4 h prior to exposure every 3 d as needed For refraction: instill one drop of 0.25% to the eye twice daily for 2 d before the procedure For iridocyclitis: instill one drop of 0.25% to the eye up to 3 times daily |

*(Continued on page 960)*

| Drug | Pregnancy Category | Routes and Dosage Ranges | |
|---|---|---|---|
| | | **Adults** | **Children** |
| Tiotropium bromide (Spiriva HandiHaler, Spiriva Respimat; ✽ Spiriva, Spiriva Respimat) | C | Asthma: oral inhalation with Spiriva Respimat (1.25 mcg), two inhalations 2.5 mcg once daily with max two inhalations/24 h<br>COPD: oral inhalation with HandiHaler, inhale each capsule twice to ensure drug delivery; Spiriva Respimat (2.5 mcg) two inhalations (5 mcg) once daily with max 2 inhalations/24 h | Children >6 y and adolescent: oral inhalation Spiriva Respimat—see adult dosing |

hypersalivation (with subsequent respiratory distress), and seizures. The IM/IV adult dose is 0.5 to 2 mg, IM or IV, and may be repeated every 10 to 30 minutes until a response is achieved. Additional doses may be required for life-threatening anticholinergic effects. For infants, children, and adolescents, give IM or IV at an initial dose of 0.02 mg/kg, with a maximum dose of 2 mg. The drug should be administered IV no faster than 0.5 mg/min to prevent bradycardia, respiratory distress, and seizures. The pediatric dose is warranted only for life-threatening cases. For infants, children, and adolescents, give IM or IV at an initial dose of 0.02 mg/kg, with a maximum dose of 2 mg. Administer IV no faster than 0.5 mg/min to prevent bradycardia, respiratory distress, and seizures. Repeated doses may be given every 5 to 10 minutes if life-threatening dysrhythmias, convulsions, or coma occurs with anticholinergic overdose. However, the benefit of repeat dosing must be balanced against the risk of physostigmine overdose. Excessive administration of physostigmine can precipitate a cholinergic crisis, leading to seizures and dysrhythmias. Atropine is the antidote for physostigmine overdose.

Diazepam or a similar drug may be given for excessive CNS stimulation (e.g., delirium, excitement) that accompanies anticholinergic toxicity. Ice bags, cooling blankets, and tepid sponge baths may help reduce fever. Artificial ventilation and cardiopulmonary resuscitative measures are used if excessive depression of the CNS causes coma and respiratory failure. Infants, children, and the elderly are especially susceptible to the toxic effects of anticholinergic drugs.

## Contraindications

Contraindications to the use of atropine include a known hypersensitivity to anticholinergic agents. Other contraindications include glaucoma, stenosing peptic ulcer, pyloroduodenal obstruction, bronchial asthma, and bladder neck obstruction, as well as hepatic or renal disease.

## Nursing Implications

### Preventing Interactions

Drugs that increase the anticholinergic effects of atropine include amantadine, antihistamines, tricyclic antidepressants,

quinidine, disopyramide, and procainamide. Some herbs also increase the effectiveness of atropine (Box 48.4).

### Administering the Medication

Prior to administering atropine, the nurse assesses for hypersensitivity to anticholinergic agents, glaucoma, stenosing peptic ulcer, paralytic ileus, bronchial asthma, bladder neck obstruction, and cardiac dysrhythmias. The patient should be well hydrated and the environment should be cool to protect from hyperpyrexia. If the patient has a history of urinary retention, the patient should void before administration of the drug.

### Assessing for Therapeutic Effects

The nurse assesses the heart rate if atropine is administered for bradycardia. In preoperative patients, the nurse assesses for diminished secretions, particularly when the drug is administered for head and neck surgery. Patients with Parkinson's disease or Parkinson-like syndromes require assessment for decreased spasticity and tremors.

### Assessing for Adverse Effects

The nurse assesses for the following conditions, which may indicate a severe anticholinergic reaction:

- Changes in rate, quality, and rhythm of the heart that indicates ventricular tachycardia.
- Urinary retention.
- Bowel sounds for signs of paralytic ileus.
- Photophobia, mydriasis, blurred vision, and increased intraocular pressure.

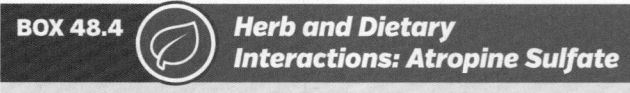

**BOX 48.4** *Herb and Dietary Interactions: Atropine Sulfate*

**Herbs and Foods That Increase the Effects of Atropine Sulfate**

- Aloe
- Cascara
- Senna

- Dry mouth.
- Increased temperature. Elderly people and children are prone to hyperpyrexia due to suppression of perspiration and heat loss.

### Patient Teaching

Box 48.5 identifies patient teaching guidelines for atropine sulfate.

## Other Drugs in the Class

Homatropine hydrobromide is a semisynthetic derivative of atropine used as eye drops to produce mydriasis and cycloplegia. Compared with atropine, homatropine may be preferable, because its ocular effects do not last as long.

Ipratropium (Atrovent HFA) is an anticholinergic drug chemically related to atropine. When given as a nasal spray, it is useful in treating rhinorrhea due to allergy or the common cold. When given in inhaled or aerosol form to patients with chronic obstructive pulmonary disease (COPD), it is beneficial as a bronchodilator. Using the respiratory route instead of the systemic route to administer anticholinergic drugs results in less thickening of respiratory secretions and therefore a reduced incidence of mucus-plugged airways.

Scopolamine has similar uses, adverse effects, and peripheral effects when compared with atropine but is different with regard to its central effects. When scopolamine is given parenterally, it depresses the CNS and causes amnesia, drowsiness, euphoria, relaxation, and sleep. Effects of the drug appear more quickly and disappear more readily than those of atropine. Scopolamine also is used in motion sickness. It is available as oral tablets and as a transdermal adhesive disk that is placed behind the ear. The disk (Transderm-V) protects against motion sickness for 72 hours.

Tiotropium bromide (Spiriva HandiHaler, Spiriva Respimat) is administered for COPD; Spiriva HandiHaler is a dry powder in capsule form intended for oral inhalation with the HandiHaler inhalation device. Spiriva Respimat is a spray in which the Spiriva Respimat cartridge is inserted in the Spiriva Respimat inhaler. This long-acting, antimuscarinic, anticholinergic, quaternary ammonium compound inhibits $M_3$ receptors in smooth muscle, resulting in bronchodilation. Tiotropium is indicated for daily maintenance treatment of bronchospasm associated with COPD. It is not indicated for acute episodes of bronchospasm (i.e., rescue therapy). Tiotropium is eliminated via the renal system, and patients with moderate to severe renal dysfunction should be carefully monitored for drug toxicity. No dosage adjustments are required for older patients or patients with hepatic impairment or mild renal impairment.

### NCLEX Success

10. A 62-year-old man is admitted to the cardiac intensive care unit. He is in sinus bradycardia with a rate of 48 beats/min. What is the drug of choice for sinus bradycardia?
    A. atropine sulfate
    B. epinephrine
    C. isoproterenol
    D. dopamine

11. A hospice patient has loud gurgling respirations that are audible without a stethoscope. Which of the following medications is the drug of choice to decrease the secretions?
    A. trihexyphenidyl
    B. tolterodine
    C. tiotropium bromide
    D. scopolamine

12. After a man takes atropine sulfate, he becomes nonresponsive and his respiratory rate drops. Based on these symptoms, what medication is administered?
    A. dicyclomine
    B. dopamine
    C. physostigmine salicylate
    D. diazepam

## CENTRALLY ACTING ANTICHOLINERGICS

Older anticholinergic drugs such as atropine are rarely used to treat Parkinson's disease because of their undesirable peripheral effects (e.g., dry mouth, blurred vision, photophobia, constipation, urinary retention, tachycardia). Newer, centrally acting synthetic anticholinergic drugs are more selective for muscarinic receptors in the CNS and are designed to produce fewer adverse effects. The prototype centrally acting anticholinergic agent is **P benztropine mesylate** (Cogentin).

## Pharmacokinetics

Benztropine is administered orally and parenterally. The oral form has an onset of action of 60 minutes and a 6- to 10-hour duration of action, with a peak effect of 7 hours.

**BOX 48.5    Patient Teaching Guidelines for Atropine Sulfate**

- Avoid excessive high temperatures.
- Drink water frequently.
- Rinse the mouth frequently.
- Maintain good dental hygiene.
- Use hard candy to decrease dry mouth.
- Void before taking the medication.
- Visit the ophthalmologist regularly.
- Notify your prescriber if fluid intake is greater or less than urine output.
- Notify your prescriber if you develop a fever.
- Notify your prescriber if weakness becomes severe.
- Avoid the use of machinery if visual acuity or alertness is impaired.

The parenteral form has an onset of action within a few minutes and a similar duration of action. The drug is absorbed from the GI tract and metabolized in the liver. It crosses the blood–brain barrier and the placenta. It is unknown how the drug is excreted.

## Action

The anticholinergic activity of benztropine takes place in the CNS. Experts believe that the drug helps normalize the imbalance of cholinergic and dopaminergic neurotransmission in the basal ganglia of the brain to reduce rigidity, akinesia, and tremor. It suppresses the secondary symptoms of parkinsonism such as excessive salivary secretions and drooling.

## Use

Benztropine mesylate is used for adjunctive therapy of all forms of parkinsonism: arteriosclerotic, idiopathic, and postencephalitic. It is also administered to control extrapyramidal disorders such as tardive dyskinesia due to neuroleptic drugs (phenothiazines). In addition, it is commonly used as a supplement with trihexyphenidyl, carbidopa, or levodopa. Table 48.9 lists the dosages of the centrally acting anticholinergic agents.

### Use in Older Adults

Use of benztropine in older adults requires caution. Prescribers and nurses must adhere strictly to dosing regulations. Patients older than 60 years of age can develop increased sensitivity to the CNS effects of all anticholinergic medications.

## Adverse Effects

CNS adverse effects of benztropine include disorientation, confusion, hallucinations, memory loss, psychoses, agitation, euphoria, light-headedness, depression, giddiness, and heaviness of the limbs. With the administration of high doses, an inability to move certain muscle groups may occur. Peripheral anticholinergic effects include tachycardia, palpitation, hypotension, orthostatic hypotension, blurred vision, dry mouth, urinary retention, decreased sweating, and elevated temperature.

## Contraindications No M.G. patients

There are several contraindications to the use of benztropine mesylate. Glaucoma is a problem because the drug can increase intraocular pressure. GI obstruction, prostatic hypertrophy, and urinary bladder neck obstruction are other complications because of the drug's effect on smooth muscle and sphincter tone. Also, myasthenia gravis is a contraindication, because blockade of acetylcholine receptor sites at neuromuscular synapses exacerbates muscle weakness.

Caution is necessary in patients with cardiovascular disorders (e.g., tachycardia, dysrhythmias, and hypertension) because parasympathetic blockade may allow a harmful increase in sympathetic dominance. Also, caution is warranted in elderly patients with pre-existing cognitive impairments because acetylcholine is an important neurotransmitter in memory function.

## Nursing Implications

### Preventing Interactions

Benztropine has the same interactions as atropine. Phenothiazines and tricyclic antidepressants combined with benztropine mesylate can cause confusion, hallucinations, and paralytic ileus.

### Administering the Medication

If the patient is experiencing GI upset, it is necessary to administer benztropine with food. The drug may be taken before meals in the presence of a dry mouth and after meals if drooling or nausea occurs. The use of ice chips or lozenges to counteract

---

**TABLE 48.9**

**DRUGS AT A GLANCE: Centrally Acting Anticholinergics**

| Drug | Pregnancy Category | Routes and Dosages | |
|---|---|---|---|
| | | **Adults** | **Children** |
| ℗**Benztropine mesylate** (Cogentin; ❋ Benztropine Omega, PMS-Benztropine) | C | 0.5–1 mg PO, IM, IV at bedtime; may increase up to 6 mg given at bedtime or in 2–4 divided doses.<br>For acute dystonia: PO, IM, IV 1–2 mg (orally) 1–2 times/daily up to 7–28 d to prevent recurrence; IM/IV is preferred over oral route for severe acute dystonic reactions | Safety and efficacy have not been established |
| Trihexyphenidyl (❋ PMS-Trihexyphenidyl) | C | 1 mg/daily PO; increase by 2-mg increments at 3- to 5-d intervals until a total of 6–10 mg is given daily in divided doses 3–4 times daily at mealtimes and bedtimes<br>PO 1 mg initially. Increase as needed to control symptoms | Safety and efficacy have not been established |

symptoms of dry mouth may help. The patient should void prior to the administration of the medication. Dosage reduction during the summer months may be necessary.

### Assessing for Therapeutic Effects

The nurse assesses for decreased rigidity and tremor. Also, he or she assesses for a decrease in oral secretions and an absence of drooling.

### Assessing for Adverse Effects

The nurse monitors the patient's intake and output. If difficulty with urination results, a dosage reduction may be necessary. The nurse assesses for signs and symptoms of paralytic ileus such as intermittent constipation, abdominal pain, diminished bowel sounds on auscultation, and distention. It is also necessary to assess the heart rate for tachycardia. In addition, the nurse assesses the inability to move certain muscle groups. Checking the patient's ambulation for signs of muscle weakness and unsteady gait helps.

### Patient Teaching

Box 48.6 identifies patient teaching guidelines for benztropine.

## Other Drugs in the Class

Trihexyphenidyl is used in the treatment of parkinsonism and extrapyramidal reactions caused by some antipsychotic drugs. This drug relieves smooth muscle spasm by a direct action on the muscle and by inhibiting the parasympathetic nervous system. It supposedly has fewer adverse effects than atropine, but approximately half of the recipients report mouth dryness, blurring of vision, and other adverse effects common to anticholinergic drugs. Trihexyphenidyl requires the same precautions as other anticholinergic drugs and is contraindicated in glaucoma.

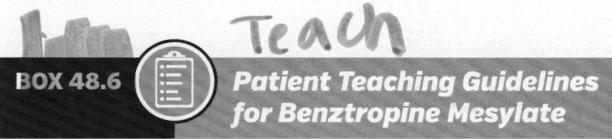

*Teach*

**BOX 48.6** — *Patient Teaching Guidelines for Benztropine Mesylate*

- Take the medication as prescribed.
- Avoid excessive high temperatures.
- Avoid alcohol, sedatives, and over-the-counter medications, including cough and cold remedies.
- Drink water frequently.
- Rinse the mouth frequently.
- Maintain good dental/oral hygiene.
- Use hard candy to decrease dry mouth.
- Void before taking the medication.
- Visit the ophthalmologist regularly.
- Notify your prescriber if fluid intake is greater or less than urine output.
- Notify your prescriber of if you develop a fever.
- Notify your prescriber if weakness becomes severe.
- Avoid the use of machinery if visual acuity or alertness is impaired.

## NCLEX Success

13. A 46-year-old woman is taking benztropine mesylate. The nurse teaches her which of the following?
    - A. Avoid overheating and stay well hydrated.
    - B. Double the dose with excess secretions.
    - C. Report diarrhea to the prescriber.
    - D. Administer benztropine with phenothiazines.

14. A patient is taking benztropine mesylate and reports gastrointestinal upset following administration of the medication. The nurse teaches the patient to do what?
    - A. Take the medication prior to eating.
    - B. Take the medication before bed.
    - C. Take the medication with food.  *Food*
    - D. Take the medication with Maalox.

## GASTROINTESTINAL ANTICHOLINERGICS (ANTISECRETORY/ANTISPASMODIC)

Dicyclomine hydrochloride (Bentyl) and glycopyrrolate (Robinul) are older medications previously administered for the treatment of peptic ulcer disease. The use of these medications has declined with the advent of the proton pump inhibitors. However, they are still prescribed for irritable bowel syndrome. Ⓟ **Dicyclomine hydrochloride** (Bentyl) is the prototype GI anticholinergic medication.

## Pharmacokinetics

Dicyclomine is available for oral and parenteral administration. Its onset of action is 1 to 2 hours, and its duration of action is 4 hours. It is metabolized in the liver and excreted by the kidneys. The drug crosses the placenta and enters the breast milk.

## Action

Dicyclomine is a GI smooth muscle relaxant. It competitively blocks the effects of acetylcholine at muscarinic cholinergic receptors that mediate the effects of the parasympathetic postganglionic impulses.

## Use

Prescribers order dicyclomine for the treatment of irritable bowel syndrome. Table 48.10 gives the dosage information for this drug and related agents.

### Use in Older Adults

The onset of adverse effects is increased in elderly people. Use of dicyclomine in older patients requires caution.

## Adverse Effects

Adverse effects of dicyclomine are blurred vision, dry mouth, altered taste perception, nausea, vomiting, dysphagia, urinary hesitancy, urinary retention, and irritation at the injection site.

## Contraindications

Dicyclomine possesses the same contraindications as the belladonna derivatives and the centrally acting anticholinergics. Contraindications to the belladonna derivatives include hypersensitivity, glaucoma, some ulcers, bronchial asthma, urinary bladder neck obstruction, and hepatic or renal disease. Contraindications to the use of centrally acting anticholinergics also include glaucoma, GI obstruction, and urinary bladder neck obstruction, as well as prostatic hypertrophy and myasthenia gravis.

## Nursing Implications

### Preventing Interactions

Dicyclomine has interactions similar to those of the previous anticholinergics. The combination of antipsychotic agents with dicyclomine results in decreased effectiveness of the antipsychotic medications. Tricyclic antidepressants and amantadine combined with dicyclomine produces increased anticholinergic effects. If dicyclomine is administered with digoxin or atenolol, there is a greater reduction in the heart rate or blood pressure then if the medications are administered alone.

### Administering the Medication

As with the other anticholinergic medications, it is necessary to have the patient void before taking dicyclomine. With the IM preparation, it is important that the patient is switched to the oral form as soon as possible because of the increased anticholinergic effects of the parenteral formulation.

### Assessing for Therapeutic Effects

If dicyclomine is working, the patient reports a decrease in abdominal pain.

### Assessing for Adverse Effects

The nurse assesses for altered taste perception, dry mouth, nausea, and vomiting, as well as for urinary retention. Administering the parenteral preparation requires assessment for injection site irritation.

### Patient Teaching

Patient teaching for dicyclomine is the same as for atropine and benztropine (see Boxes 48.5 and 48.6).

## URINARY ANTISPASMODICS

Anticholinergic drugs are the drugs of choice for their antispasmodic effects on smooth muscle to relieve the symptoms of urinary incontinence and frequency that accompany an overactive bladder. In infections, such as cystitis, urethritis, and prostatitis, the drugs decrease the frequency and pain of urination.

| TABLE 48.10 | | | |
|---|---|---|---|
| **DRUGS AT A GLANCE: Gastrointestinal Anticholinergics (Antisecretory/ Antispasmodic)** | | | |
| **Drug** | **Pregnancy Category** | **Routes and Dosage Ranges** | |
| | | **Adults** | **Children** |
| Ⓟ **Dicyclomine hydrochloride** (Bentyl; ✳ Bentylol, JAMP Dicyclomine, Protylol, RIVA-Dicyclomine) | B | 20 mg PO 4 times daily/7 d; increase to 40 mg 4 times/daily after 1 wk; if no efficacy in 2 wk or if adverse effects require a dose of <80 mg/d, discontinue therapy. Safety is not established for doses >80 mg/daily that exceed 2 wk. IM 10–20 mg 4 times/daily for 1–2 d and then to oral therapy as soon as possible | Safety and efficacy have not been established |
| Glycopyrrolate (Robinul, Cuvposa, Glycate; ✳ Cuvposa, Glycopyrrolate Injection) | B | Preoperatively to reduce secretions: 4 mcg/ kg IM 30–60 min prior to anesthesia Reversal of bradycardia/vagal reflexes intraoperatively: IV, 0.1 mg single dose, may repeat PRN at 2- to 3-min intervals Reversal muscarinic effects of cholinergic agents: 0.2 mg IV for each 1 mg of neostigmine or 5-mg pyridostigmine administered | Preoperatively to reduce secretions: <2 y, 4–9 mcg/kg IM 30–60 min prior to anesthesia Reversal of bradycardia/vagal reflexes intraoperatively (all ages): 4 mcg/ kg/dose IV (max dose, 0.1 mg); may repeat PRN at 2- to 3-min intervals Reversal muscarinic effects of cholinergic agents (all ages): See adult dosing |

The drugs are also given to increase bladder capacity in enuresis, paraplegia, and neurogenic bladder. ℗ **Oxybutynin** (Ditropan XL, Gelnique, Oxytrol), the prototype, is a urinary antispasmodic that is available in oral and transdermal forms.

## Pharmacokinetics

The oral preparation of oxybutynin has an onset of action 30 to 60 minutes, a peak of 3 to 6 hours, and a duration of 6 to 10 hours. The transdermal preparation has an onset of action of 24 to 48 hours, a variable peak, and a duration of action of 96 hours. The medication is metabolized in the liver and is excreted in the urine. It crosses the placenta and may enter the breast milk.

## Action

Oxybutynin acts directly to relax the smooth muscle and inhibits the effects of acetylcholine at muscarinic receptors. A less potent anticholinergic than atropine, oxybutynin is more potent as an antispasmodic and devoid of antinicotinic activity at the skeletal neuromuscular junctions or autonomic ganglia.

## Use

Oxybutynin is administered for the relief of bladder instability associated with voiding in patients with uninhibited neurogenic and reflex neurogenic bladder. The extended-release tablets decrease the symptoms of overactive bladder, incontinence, urgency, and frequency. Table 48.11 gives the dosage information for oxybutynin and other urinary antispasmodics.

### Use in Children

The FDA has approved the use of the extended-release formulation of oxybutynin for the treatment of symptoms of detrusor muscle overactivity associated with neurologic conditions such as spina bifida in children 6 years and older.

### Use in Older Adults

In older adults, the dosage of oxybutynin should not exceed 2.5 mg PO two to three times per day.

### Use in Patients With Renal Impairment

The use of oxybutynin in the presence of renal impairment requires caution because of its elimination in the urine.

### TABLE 48.11

## DRUGS AT A GLANCE: Urinary Antispasmodics

| Drug | Pregnancy Category | Routes and Dosages | |
|---|---|---|---|
| | | **Adults** | **Children** |
| ℗ **Oxybutynin** (Ditropan XL, Gelnique, Oxytrol, Oxytrol for women; ✤ APO-Oxybutynin, Ditropan XL, DOM-Oxybutynin, Gelnique, MYLAN-Oxybutynin) | B | PO: 5 mg 2 or 3 times daily; max dose 5 mg 4 times daily. Extended release: 5 mg increments at intervals weekly; max 30 mg/daily. Gel 10%: use contents of one sachet (100 mg/g) once/d TDS: apply one 3.9 mg/d twice weekly every 3–4 d Geriatrics: IR, start with 2.5 mg 2–3 times daily/increase with caution | PO: infants, ≤5 y 0.1–0.2 mg/kg 2–3 times per day (max 5 mg/dose) Children >5 y and adolescents: 5 mg PO twice daily (max dosage 5 mg 3 times per day) Extended release: >6 y and adolescents, 5 mg daily; dosage may be adjusted in 5 mg increments at weekly intervals up to a max dose of 20 mg/daily |
| Darifenacin hydrobromide (Enablex; ✤ Enablex) | C | 7.5 mg PO once daily. May increase to 15 mg once daily if needed to control symptoms | Safety and efficacy have not been established. |
| Flavoxate hydrochloride (✤ Apo-Flavoxate, Urispas) | B | 100–200 mg PO 3 or 4 times daily. Reduce when symptoms improve | Children >12 y: see adult dosing |
| Solifenacin succinate (Vesicare; ✤ ACT-Solifenacin, APO-Solifenacin, JAMP-Solifenacin, Vesicare) | C | 5 mg once PO daily. May increase to 10 mg once daily if needed to control symptoms | Safety and efficacy have not been established |
| Tolterodine tartrate (Detrol, Detrol LA; ✤ Detrol, Detrol LA, APO-Tolterodine, MINT-Tolterodine, MYLAN-Tolterodine) | C | IR: 2 mg PO twice daily. May decrease to 1 mg when symptoms improve. Reduce doses to 1 mg PO twice daily in the presence of hepatic impairment ER: 4 mg/daily; dose may be lowered to 2 mg/daily based on response | Safety and efficacy have not been established |
| Trospium chloride (✤ Sanctura XR, Trosec) | C | IR: 20 mg PO twice daily at least 1 h before meals or on an empty stomach ER: 60 mg/daily in morning | Safety and efficacy have not been established |

### Use in Patients With Hepatic Impairment

The use of oxybutynin in the presence of hepatic impairment requires caution because it is metabolized by the liver.

### Adverse Effects

The adverse effects of oxybutynin are consistent with the previous anticholinergic agents discussed in this chapter. The most commonly reported CNS adverse effects include drowsiness, dizziness, and blurred vision. Other adverse effects are dry mouth, nausea, urinary hesitancy, and decreased sweating.

## Contraindications

Contraindications to oxybutynin are hypersensitivity to the medication, pyloric or duodenal ulcer, obstructive intestinal lesions, intestinal atony, megacolon, colitis, obstructive uropathies, glaucoma, myasthenia gravis, cardiovascular instability, and urinary retention.

## Nursing Implications

### Preventing Interactions

Use of oxybutynin in combination with phenothiazines results in increased anticholinergic effects. The phenothiazines inhibit the cytochrome 450 enzyme CYP3A4 in the liver. This enzyme is required in the metabolism of oxybutynin. The inhibition of the enzyme results in a greater amount of oxybutynin that has not undergone first-pass metabolism contributing to oxybutynin toxicity. This same effect occurs if haloperidol is administered with oxybutynin. Also, use of oxybutynin together with haloperidol reduces the effect of the haloperidol and results in the development of tardive dyskinesia. Administration of oxybutynin with amantadine or nitrofurantoin leads to increased toxicity of oxybutynin.

### Administering the Medication

It is important that the extended-release medication is not cut, crushed, or chewed.

### Assessing for Therapeutic Effects

The nurse assesses for patient reports of decreased urinary incontinence, urgency, and frequency.

### Assessing for Adverse Effects

The nurse assesses for CNS depression. He or she also assesses for urinary hesitancy and retention as well as for impotence. In addition, it is necessary to assess for allergic reactions to the medication such as urticarial reactions.

### Patient Teaching

Box 48.7 identifies the patient teaching guidelines for oxybutynin.

## Other Drugs in the Class

Darifenacin (Enablex) is a competitive, antimuscarinic, anticholinergic agent with selective affinity for $M_3$ receptors involved in the contraction of the urinary bladder. Darifenacin is indicated for the treatment of overactive bladder, reducing symptoms of urge incontinence, urgency, and frequency. After oral administration, darifenacin is 98% protein bound and extensively metabolized in the liver by enzymes CYP3A4 and CYP2D6. A small group of people (~7% Caucasian and 2% African American) are poor metabolizers of the drug and may require

**BOX 48.7**   *Patient Teaching Guidelines for Oxybutynin Chloride*

- Take the medication as prescribed; do not cut, crush, or chew extended-release tablets.
- Apply the transdermal patch to dry intact skin over the abdomen, hip, or buttock every 3 to 4 days (twice weekly). Do not put on waistline. Remove the old system before applying a new one. Select a new site when applying a new system.
- Have periodic bladder examinations to evaluate the therapeutic response.
- Drink water frequently.
- Rinse the mouth frequently.
- Maintain good dental/oral hygiene.
- Use hard candy to decrease dry mouth.
- Avoid excessive high temperatures.
- Notify your prescriber if fluid intake is greater or less than urine output.
- Notify your prescriber if you develop a fever.

reduced dosages to avoid adverse effects. Dosage should also be reduced in people with moderate hepatic dysfunction and avoided in those with severe hepatic impairment.

Flavoxate was developed specifically to counteract spasm in smooth muscle tissue of the urinary tract. It has anticholinergic, local anesthetic, and analgesic effects. Thus, the drug relieves dysuria, urgency, frequency, and pain with genitourinary infections, such as cystitis and prostatitis.

Solifenacin (Vesicare) is a competitive, antimuscarinic, anticholinergic agent indicated for the treatment of overactive bladder with symptoms of urgency, urge incontinence, and frequency. Solifenacin is well absorbed after oral administration, 98% bound to plasma proteins, and extensively metabolized in the liver by CYP3A4 enzymes. Dosages should be reduced in people with moderate renal or hepatic impairment, and solifenacin is not recommended for those with severe hepatic impairment. Solifenacin may prolong QT intervals, especially at higher dosages, potentially resulting in dysrhythmias.

Tolterodine (Detrol, Detrol LA) is a competitive antimuscarinic, anticholinergic agent that inhibits bladder contraction, decreases detrusor muscle pressure, and delays the urge to void. It is used to treat urinary frequency, urgency, and urge incontinence. Tolterodine is more selective for muscarinic receptors in the urinary bladder than in other areas of the body, such as the salivary glands, and therefore, anticholinergic adverse effects are less marked. Reduced doses (1 mg) are recommended for patients with hepatic dysfunction. Tolterodine is also available in an extended-release form.

Trospium chloride is an antimuscarinic, anticholinergic drug for treatment of urgency, urge incontinence, and urinary frequency associated with overactive bladder. Trospium reduces the tone of smooth muscle in the bladder, exerting an antispasmodic effect. Because of its quaternary structure, less than 10% of an orally administered dose is absorbed, and food further delays absorption. Therefore, it is recommended that the medication be taken at least 1 hour before meals or on an empty stomach. Absorbed trospium is eliminated by a combination of glomerular filtration and active tubular secretion. Trospium has the potential for interaction with other drugs that are eliminated by active tubular secretion (e.g., digoxin, procainamide, pancuronium, morphine, vancomycin, metformin, tenofovir), resulting in increased serum concentration of either trospium or the coadministered drug because of competition for the urinary tubular pump. Reduced dosages of trospium are recommended for patients with renal insufficiency and those older than 75 years of age who may be less able to tolerate the adverse effects of anticholinergic drugs.

## THE NURSING PROCESS

A concept map outlines the nursing process related to drug therapy considerations in this chapter. Additional nursing implications related to the disease process should also be considered in care decisions.

**Assessment**
- Assess for signs and symptoms of Parkinson's disease and drug-induced extrapyramidal reactions, such as the following, depending on the severity and stage of progression:
- Slow movements (bradykinesia) and difficulty in changing positions, assuming an upright position, eating, dressing, and other self-care activities
- Stooped posture
- Accelerating gait with short steps
- Tremor at rest (e.g., "pill-rolling" movements of fingers)
- Rigidity of arms, legs, and neck
- Mask-like, immobile facial expression
- Speech problems (e.g., low volume, monotonous tone, rapid, difficult to understand)
- Excessive salivation and drooling
- Dysphagia
- Excessive sweating
- Constipation from decreased intestinal motility
- Mental depression from self-consciousness and embarrassment over physical appearance and activity limitations. The intellect is usually intact until the late stages of the disease process.

**Outcomes of Therapy**
The patient will
- Experience relief of excessive salivation, muscle rigidity, spasticity, and tremors.
- Experience improved motor function, mobility, and self-care abilities.
- Increase knowledge of the disease process and drug therapy.
- Take medications as instructed.
- Avoid falls and other injuries from the disease process or drug therapy.

**Nursing Interventions**
- Use measures to assist the patient and family in coping with symptoms and maintaining function. These include the following:
- Arrange for physical therapy for heel-to-toe gait training, widening stance to increase balance and base of support, and other exercises.
- Encourage ambulation and frequent changes of position, assisted if necessary.
- Help with active and passive range-of-motion exercises.
- Encourage self-care as much as possible.
- It may help to cut meat; open cartons; give frequent, small meals; and allow privacy during mealtime.
- If the patient has difficulty chewing or swallowing, chopped or soft foods may be necessary.
- Hook-and-loop-type fasteners or zippers are easier to handle than buttons.
- Slip-on shoes are easier to manage than laced ones.
- Spend time with the patient and encourage socialization with other people. Victims of Parkinson's disease tend to become withdrawn, isolated, and depressed.
- Schedule rest periods. Tremor and rigidity are aggravated by fatigue and emotional stress.
- Provide facial tissues if drooling is a problem.
- Provide appropriate patient teaching related to drug therapy (see Boxes 48.2 and 48.3).

**Evaluation**
- Interview and observe for relief of symptoms.
- Interview and observe for increased mobility and participation in activities of daily living.
- Interview and observe regarding correct usage of medications.

## KEY CONCEPTS

- Parkinsonism is a progressive neurodegenerative disorder characterized by a deficit of dopamine and a relative excess of acetylcholine.
- Classic symptoms of Parkinson's disease include resting tremor, bradykinesia, rigidity, and postural instability.
- Dopaminergic drugs increase dopamine concentrations in the brain, exerting dopaminergic activity, directly or indirectly.
- Dopamine activity can be increased by increasing dopamine release and reducing neuronal reuptake (amantadine), directly stimulating dopamine receptors (apomorphine, bromocriptine, pramipexole, ropinirole, rotigotine transdermal), replacement of dopamine or its precursor (levodopa), or inhibition of metabolism of dopamine by MAO or COMT enzymes (rasagiline, selegiline, entacapone, tolcapone).
- Carbidopa prevents levodopa breakdown in the periphery, resulting in higher brain concentrations with lower levodopa dosages.
- The FDA has issued a **BLACK BOX WARNING** ◆ stating that patients who take tolcapone risk potentially fatal acute fulminant liver failure.
- Anticholinergic drugs (e.g., benztropine, trihexyphenidyl, and diphenhydramine) decrease the effect of acetylcholine in the brain.
- Combinations of antiparkinson drugs are often given to reduce dosages and achieve better control of symptoms.
- Care must be taken to avoid serious food or drug interactions that may diminish treatment effectiveness (levodopa) or be potentially fatal (selegiline and rasagiline).
- Anticholinergic drugs block the action of acetylcholine on the parasympathetic nervous system.
- Most anticholinergic drugs interact with muscarinic cholinergic receptors in the brain, secretory glands, heart, and smooth muscle and are sometimes called antimuscarinic drugs.
- Cholinergic (muscarinic) receptors are widespread throughout the body, producing effects in a variety of locations including the CNS, heart, smooth muscle, glands, and the eye.

- Synthetic anticholinergics were developed to exert more selective effects on particular body tissues.
- Anticholinergic drugs (e.g., dicyclomine or glycopyrrolate) are indicated for antispasmodic effects in GI disorders. Historically, they have also been used to treat peptic ulcer disease; however, they are weak inhibitors of gastric acid secretion and have been largely replaced other more effective medications (e.g., proton pump inhibitors).
- Urinary antispasmodic anticholinergic drugs are the drugs of choice for treatment of symptoms of overactive bladder.
- Ophthalmic anticholinergic preparations are indicated for mydriatic and cycloplegic effects to aid in eye examination and surgery.
- Ipratropium and tiotropium are anticholinergic medications given by inhalation for bronchodilation effects in the treatment of asthma and chronic bronchitis.
- Atropine is the drug of choice to treat bradycardia.
- Anticholinergic medications are indicated in the relief of CNS symptoms of Parkinson's disease or extrapyramidal symptoms associated with some antipsychotic drugs.
- Anticholinergic drugs are given preoperatively to prevent anesthesia-associated complications such as bradycardia, excessive respiratory secretions, and hypotension.
- Anticholinergic drugs are contraindicated for patients with benign prostatic hypertrophy, myasthenia gravis, hyperthyroidism, narrow-angle glaucoma, tachydysrhythmias, myocardial infarction, heart failure, or conditions associated with esophageal reflux.
- Anticholinergic overdose is characterized by hyperthermia; hot, dry, flushed skin; dry mouth; mydriasis; delirium; tachycardia; paralytic ileus; urinary retention; myoclonic movements; seizures; coma; and respiratory arrest. Physostigmine is the specific antidote for anticholinergic overdose.
- Atropine is the antidote for muscarinic agonist poisoning.

## CLINICAL REASONING CASE STUDY

**Meet the Patient**

Henrietta Charbonier, an 85-year-old woman, lives in a senior independent living facility. The nurse practitioner there is checking the woman's blood pressure—a weekly occurrence. During the visit, the nurse notices a fine hand tremor with "pill rolling." Mrs. Charbonier also has developed static gait and has recently fallen. The nurse notifies Mrs. Charbonier's primary care provider, who, after seeing Mrs. Charbonier, confirms that she has Parkinson's disease. She is prescribed levodopa 100 mg–carbidopa 10 mg three times daily. To assist with her gait, she is prescribed trihexyphenidyl 0.5 mg once daily.

- What is the action of levodopa–carbidopa?
- What are the adverse effects of this drug?
- What patient teaching should Mrs. Charbonier be provided regarding this drug?
- What is the action of trihexyphenidyl?
- What are the adverse effects of trihexyphenidyl?

**Assessing Drug Information**

- Dopaminergic drugs increase the amount of dopamine in the brain by various mechanisms. If levodopa is administered alone, large doses must be taken to produce therapeutic effects. Carbidopa combined with levodopa prevents the decarboxylation of the levodopa, which makes levodopa more available for transportation to the brain. Levodopa is the metabolic precursor of dopamine, and after levodopa crosses the blood–brain barrier, it converts to dopamine in the brain. This is thought to be the mechanism whereby the drug relieves symptoms of Parkinson's disease. Carbidopa does not cross the blood–brain barrier and does not affect levodopa metabolism.
- The most common CNS adverse effects are headache and anxiety. Older patients may experience problems such as hallucinations, dementia, and drowsiness. The most severe adverse effect is depression with suicidal tendencies. Cardiovascular adverse effects include ectopic beats, tachycardia, anginal pain, palpitations, hypotension, vasoconstriction, dyspnea, bradycardia, and a widened QRS. The medication can cause orthostatic hypotension. This effect is common during the first few weeks but usually subsides. Less common adverse effects are piloerection, azotemia, and gangrene with prolonged use. Dermatologic effects such as hypersensitivity, anaphylaxis, and urticaria occur less frequently.
- Trihexyphenidyl relieves smooth muscle spasm by a direct action on the muscle and by inhibiting the parasympathetic nervous system. Mrs. Charbonier takes it to relax the smooth muscle in her legs. She has been experiencing static gait due to the muscle tightness.
- Trihexyphenidyl has fewer adverse effects than atropine, but approximately half of the recipients report mouth dryness, blurring of vision, and other adverse effects common to anticholinergic drugs.

**Nursing Actions**

- Assess for diminished tremors and improvement in gait. Also, patients with Parkinson's disease are prone to depression. It is important to assess the patient's sensorium.
- Assess for adverse effects of medication, particularly the development of cholinergic crisis.
- Instruct Mrs. Charbonier to take her levodopa–carbidopa on time three times per day to maintain an optimal effect.
- Instruct her about safety when changing positions due to orthostatic hypotension.
- Instruct her about the adverse effects of trihexyphenidyl. If dry mouth occurs, hard candy may provide relief.

Visit thePoint® at **http://thePoint.lww.com/Frandsen12e** for answers to NCLEX Success questions (in Appendix A), answers to Clinical Application Case Studies (in Appendix B), and more!

## REFERENCES AND RESOURCES

Anonymous. (2019). *Nursing 2019 drug handbook*. Philadelphia, PA: Lippincott Williams & Wilkins.

Hinkle, J. H., & Cheever, K. H. (2018). *Brunner & Suddarth's textbook of medical-surgical nursing* (14th ed.). Philadelphia, PA: Lippincott Williams & Wilkins.

Karch, A. M. (2019). *2019 Lippincott's pocket drug guide for nurses*. Philadelphia, PA: Lippincott Williams & Wilkins.

Kitten, A. K., Hallowell, S. A., Saklad, S. R., & Evoy, K. E. (2018). Pimavanserin: A novel drug approved to treat Parkinson's disease psychosis. *Innovations in Clinical Neuroscience, 15*(1–2), 16–22.

Norris, T. (2019). *Porth's pathophysiology: Concepts of altered health states* (10th ed.). Philadelphia, PA: Lippincott Williams & Wilkins.

Parkinson Disease Foundation. (2019). *Statistics on Parkinson's.* Retrieved June 14, 2019 from http://www.pdf.org/en/parkinson_statistics

Spindler, M. A., & Tarsy, D. (2019). Initial pharmacological treatment of Parkinson disease. In *UpToDate*. Waltham, MA.

UpToDate. (2019). *Drug information*. Lexi-Comp, Inc.

# Drug Therapy With Opioids

## LEARNING OBJECTIVES

*After studying this chapter, you should be able to:*

1. Categorize the types of pain.
2. Recognize the pathophysiology associated with pain.
3. Identify the prototype and describe the action, use, adverse effects, contraindications, and nursing implications for the opioid agonists.
4. Discuss administration of preemptive analgesia in the treatment of pain related to surgery.
5. Identify the prototype and describe the action, use, adverse effects, contraindications, and nursing implications for the opioid antagonists.
6. Implement the nursing process in the care of the patient receiving opioid medications for pain.

## CLINICAL APPLICATION CASE STUDY

Darlene Hoffman, a 50-year-old woman, is receiving treatment for ovarian cancer. After surgery, she arrives on the unit from the postanesthesia care unit [PACU] complaining of lower back pain of 2 out of 10 on a 10-point pain scale. She received a total of 10 mg of morphine sulfate in the PACU. Her vital signs are temperature 98.2°F, pulse 82 beats/min, respirations 22 breaths/min, and blood pressure 124/72 mm Hg, with an $O_2$ saturation of 94% on 2 L/min nasal cannula.

## KEY TERMS

**Breakthrough pain:** episodic bursts of intense pain that "breaks through" the pain control of the medication regime

**Ceiling effect:** a phenomenon of certain drugs that limits the ability to produce a further effect above a particular dosage level

**Endogenous analgesia system:** nerve signals that relieve pain by suppressing the transmission of pain signals from peripheral nerves; can be activated by nerve signals entering the brain or by morphine-like drugs

**Endorphins:** morphine-like neuropeptides that interact with neuroreceptors to inhibit the transmission of pain signals while also producing a sense of euphoria

**Enkephalins:** morphine-like neuropeptides that interrupt the transmission of pain signals at the spinal cord level by modulating pain perception, mood, behavior, and neuroendocrine regulation

**Nociceptors:** nerve endings that selectively respond to painful stimuli and send pain signals to the brain and spinal cord

**Opioid-naive:** patients who do not meet opioid-tolerant criteria and have not had at least 60 mg of morphine or an equianalgesic dose of another opioid for a week or longer

**Opioid-tolerant:** patient has been taking at least 60 mg of morphine or an equianalgesic dose of another opioid for a week or longer

**Patient-controlled analgesia:** any method used by patients to administer their own pain medication, typically used to indicate administration through a controlled intravenous pump

## INTRODUCTION

Pain is an unpleasant, sensory, emotional sensation associated with actual or potential tissue injury. The perception of pain is part of the clinical presentation in many acute and chronic disorders and is one of the most difficult sensations for patients to cope with across the course of a disease. It impels a person to remove the cause of the damage or seek relief from the pain. This chapter aids in the understanding of drug actions by discussing pain and pain-relieving opioid drugs.

## OVERVIEW OF IMPACT OF THE OPIOID EPIDEMIC

The United States is in the midst of an opioid epidemic. Much of the early use and abuse of the drugs resulted from the mistaken belief that opioids were not addictive. The number of deaths from accidental overdose of opioids—both prescription and nonprescription—has eclipsed that of every other drug *combined* and is now the leading cause of accidental death in the United States. In 2017, the U.S. Department of Health and Human Services declared a public health emergency and introduced a 5-point strategy to combat this crisis, focusing on better addiction, prevention, treatment, and recovery services; better data on the epidemic; better evidence-based methods of pain management;

better targeting of opioid-reversing drugs; and better research on pain and addiction. The President's Commission on Combating Drug Addiction and the Opioid Crisis, also established in 2017, serves as an advisory board to make recommendations regarding policies and practices for combating addiction, specifically the opioid crisis. Additional information can be found at https://www.hhs.gov/opioids/about-the-epidemic/index.html.

## OVERVIEW OF PAIN

Pain is the most common symptom prompting people to seek health care. When not managed effectively, pain may greatly impair quality of life and ability to perform activities of daily living. The Joint Commission includes assessment and management of pain for all patients (the fifth vital sign) in the standards by which it evaluates health care organizations. Opioid analgesics are drugs that provide pain relief by affecting people's perception and tolerance of moderate to severe pain.

### Etiology

The causes of pain include nerve damage, actual tissue injury, cancer, or surgery. Pain may be classified according to its origin in body structures (e.g., somatic, visceral, neuropathic), duration (e.g., acute, chronic), or cause (e.g., cancer). Box 49.1 describes these types of pain.

---

| BOX 49.1 | *Types of Pain* |
|---|---|

**Acute pain** may result from injury, trauma, spasm, disease processes, and treatment or diagnostic procedures that damage body tissues. Patients often describe it as sharp or cutting. The intensity of the pain is usually proportional to the amount of tissue damage, and the pain serves as a warning system by demanding the sufferer's attention and compelling behavior to withdraw from or avoid the pain-producing stimulus.

Acute pain is called fast pain because it is felt quickly after a pain stimulus is applied. It is aroused by mechanical and thermal stimuli and conducted to the spinal cord by A-delta fibers in the peripheral nerves. Glutamate is the neurotransmitter secreted in the spinal cord at the A-delta nerve fiber endings.

Acute pain is often accompanied by anxiety and objective signs of discomfort (e.g., facial expressions of distress; moaning or crying; positioning to protect the affected part; tenderness, edema, and skin color or temperature changes

in the affected part; and either restlessness and excessive movement or limited movement, if movement increases pain). It usually responds to treatment with analgesic drugs and resolves as tissue repair mechanisms heal the damaged area.

**Chronic (noncancer) pain** (i.e., lasting 3 months or longer) demands attention less urgently, may not be characterized by visible signs, and is often accompanied by emotional stress, increased irritability, depression, social withdrawal, financial distress, loss of libido, disturbed sleep patterns, diminished appetite, weight loss, and decreased ability to perform usual activities of daily living. It may occur with or without evidence of tissue damage and may include acute pain that persists beyond the typical recovery time for the precipitating tissue injury, pain related to a chronic disease, pain without an identifiable cause, and pain associated with cancer. It may arise from essentially any part of the body. It may be continuous or episodic or a combination of both.

**BOX 49.1**      *Types of Pain* (Continued)

Chronic (noncancer) pain may also be called slow pain. It can be elicited by mechanical, thermal, and chemical stimuli and is described as burning, aching, or throbbing. Slow, chronic pain is transmitted by C nerve fibers to the spinal cord and brain. Substance P is the neurotransmitter at C nerve fiber endings; it is released slowly and accumulates over seconds or minutes.

**Cancer pain** has characteristics of both acute and chronic pain, and it may be constant or intermittent. Chronic cancer pain is often caused by tumor spread into pain-sensitive tissues and the resulting tissue destruction. It usually progresses as the disease advances and can be severe and debilitating. Acute pain is often associated with diagnostic procedures or treatment measures (e.g., surgery, chemotherapy). It may also occur with disease progression, with activity, or with the development of drug tolerance.

**Somatic pain** results from stimulation of nociceptors in the skin, bone, muscle, and soft tissue. It is usually well localized and described as sharp, burning, gnawing, throbbing, or cramping. It may be intermittent or constant and acute or chronic. Sprains and other traumatic injuries are examples of acute somatic pain; the bone and joint pain of arthritis is an example of chronic somatic pain, although acute exacerbations may also occur. Somatic pain of low to moderate intensity may stimulate the sympathetic nervous system and produce increased blood pressure, pulse, and respiration; dilated pupils; and increased skeletal muscle tension, such as rigid posture or clenched fists.

**Visceral pain,** which is diffuse and not well localized, results when nociceptors are stimulated in abdominal or thoracic organs and their surrounding tissues. It includes pain associated with cholecystitis, pancreatitis, uterine disorders, and liver disease and is often described as deep, dull, aching, or cramping. It may be referred to a different part of the body (e.g., pain from the liver can be referred to the right shoulder area; ischemic pain from the heart can be referred to the left arm or neck area). Severe visceral pain stimulates the parasympathetic nervous system and produces decreased blood pressure and pulse, nausea and vomiting, weakness, syncope, and possibly loss of consciousness.

**Neuropathic pain** is caused by lesions or physiologic changes that injure peripheral pain receptors, nerves, or the central nervous system. It is characterized by excessive excitability in the damaged area or surrounding normal tissues, so that nerve cells discharge more easily. As a result, pain may arise spontaneously or from a normally nonpainful stimulus such as a light touch. It is a relatively common cause of chronic pain and is usually described as severe, shooting, burning, or stabbing. It occurs with peripheral neuropathies associated with diabetes mellitus (diabetic neuropathy), herpes zoster infections (postherpetic neuralgia), traumatic nerve injuries, and some types of cancer or cancer treatments. It is difficult to treat because standard analgesics (e.g., nonsteroidal anti-inflammatory drugs and opioids) are less effective in neuropathic pain than in other types of pain. Antidepressants and anticonvulsants are often used along with analgesics.

## Pathophysiology

Pain occurs when tissue damage activates the free nerve endings (pain receptors) of peripheral nerves. **Nociceptors,** nerve endings that selectively respond to painful stimuli, are abundant in arterial walls, joint surfaces, muscle fascia, periosteum, skin, and soft tissues; they are scarce in most internal organs. Causes of tissue damage may be physical (e.g., heat, cold, pressure, stretch, spasm, and ischemia) or chemical (e.g., pain-producing substances are released into the extracellular fluid surrounding the nerve fibers that carry the pain signal). These pain-producing substances activate pain receptors, increase the sensitivity of pain receptors, or stimulate the release of inflammatory substances.

For a person to feel pain, the signal from the nociceptors in peripheral tissues must be transmitted to the spinal cord and then to the hypothalamus and cerebral cortex in the brain. The signal is carried to the spinal cord by two types of nerve cells, A-delta fibers and C fibers. A-delta fibers, which are myelinated and found mainly in skin and muscle, transmit fast, sharp, well-localized pain signals. These fibers release glutamate and aspartate (excitatory amino acid neurotransmitters) at synapses in the spinal cord. C fibers, which are unmyelinated and found in muscle, abdominal viscera, and periosteum, conduct the pain signal slowly and produce a poorly localized, dull, or burning type of pain. Tissue damage resulting from an acute injury often produces an initial sharp pain transmitted by A-delta fibers followed by a dull ache or burning sensation transmitted by C fibers. C fibers release somatostatin and substance P at synapses in the spinal cord. Glutamate, aspartate, substance P, and perhaps other chemical mediators enhance transmission of the pain signal.

The dorsal horn of the spinal cord is the control center or relay station for information from the A-delta and C nerve fibers, for local modulation of the pain impulse, and for descending influences from higher centers in the central nervous system (CNS) (e.g., attention, emotion, memory). Here, nociceptive nerve fibers synapse with nonnociceptive nerve fibers (neurons that carry information other than pain signals). The brain also contains descending pathways that inhibit nociceptive input. Some brain nuclei are serotonergic and project to the dorsal horn of the spinal cord, where they suppress nociceptive transmission. Another inhibitory pathway is noradrenergic and originates in the pons. Thus, increasing the concentration of norepinephrine and serotonin in the synapse inhibits transmission of nerve impulses that carry pain signals to the brain and spinal cord.

In the brain, the thalamus is a relay station for incoming sensory stimuli, including pain. Perception of pain is a primitive awareness in the thalamus, and sensation is not well localized. From the thalamus, pain messages are relayed to the cerebral cortex, where they are perceived more specifically and analyzed to determine actions needed.

The CNS has its own system, the **endogenous analgesia system,** for relieving pain by suppressing the transmission of pain signals from peripheral nerves. Nerve signals entering the brain or morphine-like drugs can activate the system. Important elements include receptors and endogenous peptides with actions similar to those of morphine. Receptors are highly concentrated in some regions of the CNS, including the ascending and descending pain pathways and portions of the brain essential to the endogenous analgesia system. The opioid (morphine-like) neuropeptides (i.e., endorphins, enkephalins, and dynorphins) interact with receptors to inhibit perception and transmission of pain signals. **Endorphins** interact with receptors to inhibit the transmission of pain signals, and these peptides also produce a sense of euphoria. Excitement, stress, or aerobic exercise can trigger their release. **Enkephalins** interrupt the transmission of pain signals at the spinal cord level by inhibiting the release of substance P from C nerve fibers. Enkephalins primarily modulate pain perception, mood, behavior, and neuroendocrine regulation. Dynorphins also modulate the pain response to produce analgesia but has also been studied for their role in appetite control and as a negative feedback inhibitor of oxytocin secretion. The endogenous analgesia system may also inhibit pain signals at other points in the pain pathway.

## Clinical Manifestations

Pain is a subjective experience, and patients' self-reporting of pain is considered the gold standard of pain assessment measurements because it offers the most valid measurement of pain. However, numerous factors, including mood, sleep disturbances, fatigue, and medications, may influence self-reporting. Cultural, gender, age, and other psychosocial factors can play a role in manifestations of pain.

A variety of pain measurement tools exists, including visual analog scales, verbal or numerical rating scales, or picture scales. The pain measurement tool chosen should be appropriate to the individual patient, considering developmental, cognitive, emotional, language, and cultural factors. A mnemonic device (SOCRATES) can be used to assess the clinical manifestations of pain. Its meaning appears below:

- *Site*
- *Onset*
- *Character*
- *Radiation*
- *Associations with other symptoms*
- *Time course (pattern)*
- *Exacerbating/relieving factors*
- *Severity*

Nurses can use observational tools for patients who cannot communicate their pain for various reasons (e.g., unconsciousness, cognitive impairment). These tools involve facial expressions, limb movements, vocalization, restlessness, and guarding as indicators of pain. In patients with pain, vital signs may demonstrate tachycardia, tachypnea, and hypertension.

## Drug Therapy

Opioid analgesics relieve moderate to severe pain by inhibiting adenylate cyclase, which coordinates the transmission of pain signals from peripheral tissues to the brain, reducing the perception of pain sensation in the brain, producing sedation, and decreasing the emotional upsets often associated with pain. The drugs also inhibit the production of pain and inflammation by prostaglandins and leukotrienes in peripheral tissues. With repeated opioid use, adenylate cyclase adapts, reducing the ability of the opioids to inhibit pain signals. Thus, patients no longer respond to an opioid as they originally did and so require a higher dose of the drug to achieve the same level of response reached initially. This response is the cause of opioid tolerance.

Most of the opioids are Schedule II drugs under federal narcotics laws and may lead to drug abuse and dependence (see Chap. 1). Because opioid abuse has risen to epic proportions, the U.S. Food and Drug Administration (FDA) has approved abuse-deterrent formulations that reduce the ability to crush the tablets for three opioids—oxycodone (Xtampza ER), morphine (Mitigo), and hydrocodone (Hysingla)—to attempt to reduce the risk of abuse. Table 49.1 outlines the subgroups of opioid analgesics: the opioid agonists, agonists/antagonists, and antagonists. The larger group of agonists includes morphine and morphine-like drugs. These agents have activity at mu and kappa receptors and thus produce prototypical effects. As their name indicates, the agonists/antagonists have both agonist and antagonist activity. Antagonists are antidote drugs that reverse the effects of agonists. In addition, numerous combinations of opioid and nonopioid analgesics (see Chap. 16) are available and commonly used in most health care settings.

Health care providers are now able to take advantage of several approaches to perioperative pain management. Preemptive analgesia refers to the administration of an analgesic treatment preoperatively. Clinical trials have demonstrated no consistent postoperative benefits. Preventive analgesia, a

---

**TABLE 49.1**

### Drugs (Opioids) Administered for the Treatment of Pain

| Drug Class | Prototype | Other Drugs in the Class |
|---|---|---|
| Agonists | Morphine sulfate (Duramorph, Infumorph, Kadian, MS Contin, Mitigo) | Codeine<br>Fentanyl (Actiq, Duragesic, Subsys, Lazanda)<br>Hydrocodone (Hysingla)<br>Hydromorphone (Dilaudid)<br>Meperidine (Demerol)<br>Methadone (Dolophine)<br>Oxycodone (OxyContin, Xtampza ER)<br>Oxymorphone Tramadol (Ultram, ConZip) |
| Agonists/antagonists | Butorphanol | Nalbuphine (Nubain)<br>Pentazocine |
| Antagonists | Naloxone (Evzio, Narcan) | Naltrexone (Vivitrol) |

broader approach, works to minimize sensitization produced by noxious stimuli that occur throughout the perioperative period. Multimodal analgesia builds on that approach by simultaneously administering medications from different drug classes to suppress pain by blocking multiple pain pathways (Fig. 49.1). Many of these methods are considered opioid sparing, which

allows a clinically significant reduction in the dose of opioids given. This reduces opioid adverse effects without sacrificing pain control. In addition, properly managed pain reduces health care costs and improves postoperative outcomes.

> **⚠ QSEN Alert: Safety**
>
> Respiratory depression is a possible adverse effect for patients taking opioids, but the concern can be minimized by (1) avoiding concomitant use of other drugs such as alcohol and benzodiazepines that depress the CNS and (2) careful monitoring of the response to the drug and the dosage. It is important to use additional caution when administering narcotics to patients with underlying respiratory disorders, such as chronic pulmonary disease or sleep apnea.

> **⚠ QSEN Alert: Teamwork and Collaboration**
>
> The use of long-term opioid therapy for chronic pain has escalated. However, concerns about addiction, tolerance, and diversion often lead to suboptimal pain management that results in decreased quality of life. A position statement by the American Academy of Pain Medicine (2013) identifies considerations that minimize the potential for abuse of opioids while ensuring effective pain control.
>
> In all cases, providers must balance the possibility of addiction against the benefits of the therapy. However, addiction is a serious problem that should be considered in all patients receiving opioids. Lack of understanding of addiction and mislabeling of patients as addicts may result in unnecessary withholding of opioid medications. The management of pain in patients with a history of addiction or a coexisting psychiatric disorder requires special consideration by a pain management specialist.
>
> It was previously thought that the ability to use opioids effectively on a long-term basis for pain management was limited because of the risk of tolerance. However, experience has shown that tolerance is not a major drawback to long-term opioid use. In cancer patients, what initially appears to be tolerance is usually progression of the disease. In noncancer patients, the failure to respond to increasing doses of opioids may result from several factors, including tolerance, disease progression, and opioid-induced sensitivity to noxious stimuli.
>
> Drug diversion, or obtaining or using prescription medications illegally, is a major concern. The ability of the health care team, including the patient, to provide ongoing communication during each transition in care can reduce the risk of diversion. Activities that may help rule out diversion include urine and/or blood drug screening, pill counts, and regular patient follow-up to review treatment efficacy. State prescription monitoring program databases, where available, are useful in monitoring compliance and enhance communication. In addition, legislation and regulatory policies should not deter the use of opioids where medically indicated for moderate to severe pain and the treatment plan is reasonably designed to mitigate the risk of addiction and abuse.

**FIGURE 49.1.** Summary of the sites of action of the major drug classes used for pain management. Analgesics target various steps in pain perception, from the initiation of a pain stimulus to the central perception of that pain. Nonsteroidal anti-inflammatory drugs (NSAIDs) modulate the initial membrane depolarization (signal transduction) in response to a peripheral stimulus. Sodium channel blockers decrease action potential conduction in nociceptive fibers. Opioids, antidepressants, NSAIDs, antiepileptic drugs (anticonvulsants), and $\alpha_2$-adrenergic agonists all modulate transmission of pain sensation in the spinal cord by decreasing the signal relayed from peripheral to central pain pathways. Opioids also modulate the central perception of painful stimuli. Multimodal analgesia combines drugs with multiple sites of action to enhance effective pain management. (Reprinted with permission from Golan, D. E. [2017]. *Principles of pharmacology: The pathophysiologic basis of drug therapy* [4th ed.]. Philadelphia, PA: Wolters Kluwer.)

## OPIOID AGONISTS

ⓟ **Morphine sulfate** (Duramorph, Infumorph, Kadian, MS Contin, Mitigo), the prototype, is an opium alkaloid used mainly to relieve moderate to severe pain. A Schedule II–controlled drug, administration is most often oral or parenteral. Patient response depends on route of administration and dosage.

## Pharmacokinetics

Morphine is well absorbed after oral (PO), intramuscular (IM), subcutaneous, and intravenous (IV) administration. PO formulations undergo significant first-pass metabolism in the liver, which means that PO doses must be larger than injected doses to have equivalent therapeutic effects. After PO administration of fast-acting (e.g., immediate release) formulations, peak activity occurs in about 60 minutes. After IV injection, maximal analgesia and respiratory depression usually occur within 10 to 20 minutes. After IM injection, these effects occur in about 30 minutes. After subcutaneous injection, morphine effects may be delayed up to 60 to 90 minutes. Morphine is extensively metabolized in the liver, and metabolites are excreted in urine. Morphine is about 30% bound to plasma proteins, and its half-life is 2 to 4 hours. The duration of action is 5 to 7 hours.

## Action

Morphine relieves pain by binding to receptors in the brain, spinal cord, and peripheral tissues. When bound to the drug, receptors function like gates that close and thereby block or decrease transmission of pain impulses from one nerve cell to the next. The receptors also activate the endogenous analgesia system. The major types of receptors are mu, kappa, and delta. Most of the effects of morphine (analgesia; CNS depression, with respiratory depression and sedation; euphoria; decreased gastrointestinal [GI] motility; and physical dependence) are attributed to activation of the mu receptors. Analgesia, sedation, and decreased GI motility occur with activation of kappa receptors. The endogenous analgesia system involves the delta receptors, which may not bind with opioid drugs.

## Use

The main indication for morphine is to prevent or relieve acute or chronic pain. Specific conditions for morphine include acute myocardial infarction, biliary colic, renal colic, burns and other traumatic injuries, postoperative states, and cancer. Health care providers usually give morphine for chronic pain, such as that associated with terminal cancer, only when other measures and milder drugs are ineffective. Other clinical uses of morphine include the following:

- Before and during surgery to promote sedation, decrease anxiety, facilitate induction of anesthesia, and decrease the amount of anesthesia required
- During labor and delivery (obstetric analgesia; note that morphine crosses the placenta)
- Treatment of GI disorders, such as abdominal cramping and diarrhea
- Treatment of acute pulmonary edema
- Treatment of severe, unproductive cough (codeine may be used)
- Unlabeled use: relief of dyspnea associated with acute left ventricular failure and pulmonary edema

Table 49.2 gives dosages of morphine sulfate and other opioid agonists.

## TABLE 49.2

### DRUGS AT A GLANCE: Opioid Agonists

| Drug | Pregnancy Category | Routes and Dosage Ranges | |
|---|---|---|---|
| | | **Adults** | **Children** |
| ℗ **Morphine** (Duramorph, Infumorph, Kadian, MS Contin, Mitigo; ✽ M.O.S.-S.R, MS Contin SRT, Statex, Teva-Morphine SR) | C | PO immediate release, 5–30 mg every 4 h PRN PO controlled release, 30 mg or more every 8–12 h IM, subcutaneously 5–20 mg/70 kg every 4 h PRN IV injection, 2–10 mg/70 kg, diluted in 5 mL water for injection and injected slowly, over 5 min IV continuous infusion, 0.1–1 mg/mL in 5% dextrose in water solution, by controlled infusion pump Epidurally, 2–5 mg/24 h; intrathecally, 0.2–1 mg/24 h Rectal, 10–20 mg every 4 h PCA dosing based on institutional protocols; standard parameters: 2-mg bolus, 1-mg dose, lockout interval 10 min, 4-h maximum limit 30 mg, basal rate not recommended for starting PCA Older adult, PCA dosing per institutional protocols typically 25% of adult dose and requires more intense monitoring and dose individualization | IM, subcutaneous 0.05–0.2 mg/kg (up to 15 mg) every 4 h |

(*Continued on page 976*)

**TABLE 49.2**

# DRUGS AT A GLANCE: Opioid Agonists [Continued]

| Drug | Pregnancy Category | Routes and Dosage Ranges | |
|---|---|---|---|
| | | **Adults** | **Children** |
| Codeine (✹ Codeine Contin, PMS-Codeine, Ratio-Codeine) | C | Pain: PO, subcutaneous, IM 15–60 mg every 4–6 h PRN; usual dose 30 mg; max, 360 mg/24 h<br>Cough: PO 10–20 mg every 4 h PRN; max, 120 mg/24 h | 1 y or older, pain: PO, subcutaneous, IM 0.5 mg/kg every 4–6 h PRN<br>2–6 y, cough: PO 2.5–5 mg every 4–6 h; max, 30 mg/24 h<br>6–12 y, cough: PO 5–10 mg every 4–6 h; max, 60 mg/24 h |
| Fentanyl (Actiq, Duragesic, Subsys, Lazanda; ✹ Abstral, Fentora, Matrix Patch, PMS-Fentanyl MTX)* | C | Preanesthetic sedation: IM 0.05–0.1 mg 30–60 min before surgery<br>Analgesic adjunct to general anesthesia: IV total dose of 0.002–0.05 mg/kg, depending on surgical procedure<br>Adjunct to regional anesthesia: IM or slow IV (over 1–2 min) 0.05–0.1 mg PRN<br>Postoperative analgesia: IM 0.05–0.1 mg, repeat in 1–2 h if needed<br>General anesthesia: IV 0.05–0.1 mg/kg with oxygen and a muscle relaxant (max dose 0.15 mg/kg with open heart surgery, other major surgeries, and complicated neurologic or orthopedic procedures)<br>Chronic pain (Duragesic transdermal system): 2.5–10 mg every 72 h | Children weighing at least 10 kg: conscious sedation or preanesthetic sedation, 5–15 mcg/kg of body weight (100–400 mcg), depending on weight, type of procedure, and other factors; max dose, 400 mcg, regardless of age and weight. 2–12 y: general anesthesia induction and maintenance, IV 2–3 mcg/kg |
| Hydrocodone (Hysingla ER, Zohydro ER)<br>Hydrocodone (with acetaminophen: Paracetamol, Lortab, Vicodin HP) (with ibuprofen: Ibudone, Reprexain, Vicoprofen, Xylon; ✹ Vicoprofen) | C<br>With acetaminophen: C<br>With ibuprofen: C | Hysingla ER: 20 mg once daily and then increase 10–20 mg every 3–5 d PRN<br>Zohydro ER: 10 mg every 12 h and then increase 10 mg every 12 h every 3–7 d PRN<br>With acetaminophen: 1–2 tablets every 4–6 h as needed for pain, not to exceed 4 g of acetaminophen daily<br>With ibuprofen: 1 tablet (hydrocodone 2.5–0 mg/ibuprofen 200 mg) every 4–6 h as needed for pain, not to exceed five tablets daily; consider reducing dosing in elderly | 2–13 y or <50 kg: hydrocodone 0.1–0.2 mg/kg/dose, not to exceed 6 doses a day or the max recommended dose of acetaminophen. ≥16 y: refer to adult dosing for hydrocodone with ibuprofen. Extended-release products containing hydrocodone should not be given to children younger than 6 y of age and should be used with caution in children 6–12 y of age |
| Hydromorphone (Dilaudid; ✹ Hydromorph Contin, Jurnista) | C | PO 2–4 mg every 4–6 h PRN<br>IM, subcutaneous, IV 1–2 mg every 4–6 h PRN (may be increased to 4 mg for severe pain)<br>Rectal suppository 3 mg every 6–8 h | Dosage not established |
| Meperidine (Demerol; ✹ Demerol) | C | PO, IM, IV, subcutaneous, PO 50–150 mg every 3–4 h<br>Obstetric analgesia: IM, subcutaneous 50–100 mg when pain becomes regular; may repeat at 1- to 3-h intervals | PO, IM, subcutaneous 1.1–1.8 mg/kg/dose, up to adult dose, every 3–4 h as needed |
| Methadone (Dolophine; ✹ Metadol, Metadol-D) | C | PO (opioid naive) initial 2.5 mg every 8–12 h<br>IV, IM, subcutaneous, initial 2.5–10 mg every 8- to 12-h titrate slowly to effect | Neonatal abstinence syndrome PO, IV 0.05–0.2 mg/kg/d divided every 8 h |
| Oxycodone (OxyContin, Xtampza ER; ✹ Oxy IR, OxyNEO, PMS-Oxycodone CR, Supeudol) | B/C (based on manufacturer) | PO, immediate release, 5 mg every 6 h PRN; 10–30 mg every 4 h PRN for other formulations<br>PO, controlled release, 10 mg every 12 h, increased if necessary | Not recommended for children younger than 12 y of age |

| | | **TABLE 49.2** | |
| | | **DRUGS AT A GLANCE: Opioid Agonists** (Continued) | |

| Drug | Pregnancy Category | Routes and Dosage Ranges | |
| | | **Adults** | **Children** |
| Oxymorphone | C | PO (opioid naive), 5–10 mg every 4–6 h; conversion from stable parenteral dose 10 times the total parenteral requirement in divided doses every 4–6 h<br>PO, extended release (opioid naive), 5 mg every 12 h, increased by 5–10 mg every 12 h every 3–7 d until pain relieved; conversion from stable parenteral dose 10 times the total parenteral requirement in two divided doses<br>IM, subcutaneous 1–1.5 mg every 4–6 h PRN<br>IV 0.5 mg every 4–6 h PRN<br>Labor analgesia: IM 0.5–1 mg | Dosage not established |
| Tramadol (Ultram, ConZip;  Durela, Tridural, Ultram, Zytram XL) | C | PO 50–100 mg every 4–6 h PRN (max, 400 mg/d)<br>Renal impairment (CrCl < 30 mL/min): PO 50–100 mg every 12 h (max dose, 200 mg/d)<br>Hepatic impairment (cirrhosis): PO 50 mg every 12 h<br>Older adults (65–75 y): same as adults, unless they also have renal or hepatic impairment<br>Older adults (>75 y): <300 mg daily, in divided doses | Dosage not established |

*Actiq, Fentora are special preparations for specific uses. (Check manufacturers' instructions for dosage and administration instructions.)

## Use in Children

In general, experts do not completely understand the physiology, pathology, assessment, and management of pain in children. Many authorities indicate that in children, pain is often ignored or undertreated, including children having surgical and other painful procedures for which adults routinely receive an anesthetic, a strong analgesic, or both. This is especially true in preterm and full-term neonates. In the past, one reason for inadequate prevention and management of pain in newborns was a common belief that they did not experience pain because of immature nervous systems. However, research indicates that neonates have abundant C fibers and that A-delta fibers are developing during the first few months of life. These nerve fibers carry pain signals from peripheral tissues to the spinal cord. In addition, brain pain centers and the endogenous analgesia system are developed and functional.

Older infants and children may experience pain even when analgesics are readily available. For example, children may be unable to communicate their discomfort, or they may fear injections. It is important to question parents about their child's response to pain. Health care providers or parents may fear adverse effects of morphine, including excessive sedation, respiratory depression, and addiction.

To make the situation more complex, formulations of morphine and other opioids for children are not generally available.

Rectal suppositories, which are used more often in children than in adults, are useful when PO or parenteral routes are not indicated.

> **QSEN Alert: Safety**
>
> When children's doses are calculated based on adult doses, fractions and decimals often result, which greatly increases the risk of a dosage error. It is advisable to have two people do the calculations independently and compare results.

With all forms of opioids, it is important to note that the effects of the drugs in children may differ from those expected in adults because of physiologic and pharmacokinetic differences. Even with suppositories, the dose of medication received by the child is unknown because drug absorption is erratic and because adult suppositories are sometimes cut in half or otherwise altered. The nurse assesses children regularly and is alert for unusual signs and symptoms.

## Use in Older Adults

It is necessary to use morphine cautiously in older adults, especially if they are debilitated; have hepatic, renal, or respiratory impairment; or are receiving other drugs that depress the CNS. Older adults are especially sensitive to respiratory depression, excessive sedation, confusion, and other adverse effects.

However, they should receive adequate analgesia, along with vigilant monitoring. Specific recommendations for use in older adults include the following:

- Start with low doses and increase doses gradually, if necessary.
- Give morphine less frequently than in younger adults because the duration of action may be longer.
- Monitor carefully for sedation or confusion. In addition, monitor voiding and urine output because acute urinary retention is more likely to occur in older adults.

### Use in Patients With Renal Impairment

Patients with renal impairment should take minimal doses of morphine for the shortest effective time because usual doses may produce profound sedation and a prolonged duration of action. Morphine produces an active metabolite that may accumulate in patients with renal impairment.

### Use in Patients With Hepatic Impairment

Morphine is extensively metabolized by the liver; therefore, morphine may accumulate and cause increased adverse effects in the presence of hepatic impairment. Drug accumulation and increased adverse effects may occur if dosage is not reduced, especially with chronic use.

### Use in Patients With Critical Illness

Morphine is commonly used to manage pain associated with disease processes and invasive diagnostic and therapeutic procedures. In intensive care units, morphine and other opioid agonists are also used concurrently with sedatives and neuromuscular blocking agents, which increase the risks of adverse drug reactions and interactions. In patients with critical illness, morphine is usually given by IV bolus injection or continuous infusion. Guidelines include the following:

- Assume that all critically ill patients are in pain or at high risk for development of pain.
- When pain is thought to be present, identify and treat the underlying cause when possible.
- Prevent pain when possible. Some specific interventions include being very gentle when performing nursing care to

avoid tissue trauma and positioning patients to prevent ischemia, edema, and misalignment. In addition, give analgesics before painful procedures, when indicated.

- Consider **patient-controlled analgesia** (PCA), which is any method that allows a person in pain to administer his or her own pain relief. Commonly, an IV device regulated by programmable settings delivers morphine at a preset bolus dosage when the patient presses a button. It is possible to program a lockout period into the pump so that the frequency of administration is controlled, as well as the basal amount of drug to be delivered. When starting a continuous IV infusion of pain medication, a health care professional gives a loading dose to attain therapeutic blood levels quickly. The nurse assesses pain scores after initiation, after any change in pump setting, and periodically using a standardized pain rating scale to assess pain relief response to the PCA medication based on hospital protocol. Box 49.2 outlines specific assessment considerations prior to and throughout the administration of opioids using PCA.
- Manage pain to provide relief and prevent its recurrence. In general, morphine should be given continuously or on a regular schedule of intermittent doses, with supplemental or bolus doses when needed for breakthrough pain, episodic bursts of intense pain that "break through" the pain control provided by the pain medication.

### Use in Patients Receiving Home Care

The use of morphine is often restricted to a short period, and patients self-administer their medication. The need for strong pain medication recedes as healing occurs. The home care nurse may teach patients and caregivers safe usage of morphine (e.g., that the drugs decrease mental alertness and physical agility, so potentially hazardous activities should be avoided). It is important to consider nonpharmacologic methods of managing pain and ways to prevent adverse effects of opioids, although these do not serve as a substitute for adequate pharmacologic pain relief. Physical dependence is uncommon with short-term use of morphine for acute pain.

With some types of chronic pain, such as those occurring with low back pain or osteoarthritis, morphine is not indicated

---

**BOX 49.2**    *Assessment for Appropriateness of Patient-Controlled Analgesia*

- Preprocedure cognitive assessment (patient must be cognitively competent to actively participate in pain management)
  - Assess mental status, level of consciousness, and developmental status.
  - Assess patient's (and family's) ability to comprehend teaching regarding his or her role in managing pain, specific information on pump operation, safety measures, and when to alert a nurse.
- Is the patient opioid-tolerant or opioid naive?
  - **Opioid-tolerant**: patient has been taking at least 60 mg of morphine or an equianalgesic dose of another opioid for a week or longer.
  - Opioid naive: patients who do not meet opioid-tolerant criteria and have not had narcotics in the amounts given above for a week or more.

- Pain assessment: use a consistent standard pain assessment tool, such as the 0 to 10 pain scale or the 0 to 10 Faces Pain Scale for children.
- Sedation assessment
  - Assess sedation using a consistent tool (e.g., Pasero, Ramsay, or Richmond Agitation and Sedation Scale [RASS] sedation scales).
  - This is a critical component; sedation precedes respiratory depression because less opioid is required to produce it.
- Respiratory assessment
  - Assess rate, quality, and sounds of respirations.
  - Assess oxygen saturation using pulse oximetry.

for long-term use. Treatment involves nonopioid medications, physical therapy, and other measures. The home care nurse may need to explain the reasons for not using opioids on a long-term basis and help patients and caregivers learn alternative methods of relieving discomfort. The nurse should also assess for the effectiveness of the opioid in relieving pain as well as any signs that might indicate addiction, diversion, or tolerance.

With cancer pain, the goal of treatment is to prevent or relieve pain and keep patients comfortable. Thus, the home care nurse must assist patients and caregivers in understanding the appropriate use of morphine in cancer care, including administration on a regular schedule, storing the drugs to avoid use by people other than the patient, and avoiding theft and diversion to street use. The nurse also must be proficient in using and teaching various routes of drug administration and in arranging regimens with potentially very large doses and various combinations of drugs. In addition, the nurse must make an active effort to prevent or manage adverse effects, such as a bowel program to prevent constipation.

Additional guidelines include the following:

- Morphine should be given on a regular schedule, around the clock. Patients should be awakened, if necessary, to prevent pain recurrence.
- PO, rectal, and transdermal routes of administration are generally preferred over injections.
- When long-acting forms of morphine are given on a regular schedule, fast-acting forms also need to be available for **breakthrough pain** (acute pain that occurs spontaneously or with activity). If supplemental or "rescue" doses are needed frequently, the baseline dose of long-acting medication may need to be increased.
- In addition to morphine, other drugs may be used to increase patient comfort (see Other Drugs in the Class). In addition, multimodal anesthesia, including the use of select antidepressants and anticonvulsants to decrease neuropathic pain, may enhance the efficacy of pain management.

## Adverse Effects

Morphine has widespread pharmacologic effects, especially in the CNS and the GI system. These effects occur with usual doses and may be therapeutic or adverse, depending on the reason for use. CNS effects include analgesia; CNS depression, ranging from drowsiness to sleep to unconsciousness; decreased mental and physical activity; respiratory depression; nausea and vomiting; and pupil constriction. Sedation and respiratory depression are major adverse effects and potentially life threatening. In the GI tract, morphine slows motility, and it may cause constipation and smooth muscle spasms in the bowel and biliary tract.

## Contraindications

Contraindications and cautions are respiratory depression, acute or chronic lung disease, liver or kidney disease, prostatic hypertrophy, pregnancy, increased intracranial pressure and head injury, seizure disorders, or hypersensitivity reactions to

morphine. Lactation is a consideration (it may be safer to wait 4 to 6 hours after opioid administration to nurse an infant). Additional contraindications may include Addison's disease, severe alcoholism, and toxic psychosis.

## Nursing Implications

### Preventing Interactions

Drugs that increase the effects of morphine are found in Box 49.3. Naloxone is known to reverse the effects of morphine. Herbs such as kava, valerian, and St. John's wort may increase the sedative effect of morphine. The FDA has issued a **BLACK BOX WARNING ◆** for the combined use of morphine and other opioid analgesics with the benzodiazepines and other drugs that depress the CNS. The risk of serious adverse reactions, including slowed or difficult breathing and death, has been reported.

### Administering the Medication

Although the dose of morphine can be titrated upward for adequate analgesia, unacceptable adverse effects (e.g., excessive sedation, respiratory depression, nausea, and vomiting) may limit the dose. With PO administration, patients may take the drug without regard to food. However, if GI upset occurs, food is acceptable. It is essential that PO forms are not broken or crushed. The nurse dilutes and administers IV doses slowly to minimize likelihood of adverse effects.

It is necessary to monitor respiration closely in neonates. The antagonist naloxone should be readily available (see "Opioid Antagonists"). Other guidelines for morphine administration include:

- Assess for pain on a regular schedule around the clock (e.g., every 1 to 2 hours). It is important to use a consistent method for assessing severity, such as a visual analog or numeric scale. If the patient is able to communicate, the nurse asks about the location, severity, and so forth. If the patient is unable to communicate needs for pain relief, as

**BOX 49.3** **Drug Interactions: Morphine Sulfate**

**Drugs That Increase the Effects of Morphine Sulfate**
- Alcohol, antidepressants, antipsychotics, barbiturates, benzodiazepines, and sedatives
  *Increase the risk of drowsiness, confusion, memory loss, or respiratory distress*
- Antihistamines
  *Increase sedation and the risk of constipation and urinary retention*
- Monoamine oxidase (MAO) inhibitors
  *Increase the risk of hypotension, respiratory depression, or coma; patients should not take morphine and an MAO inhibitor within 14 days of each other.*
- Other narcotics or opiates
  *Increase the risk of hypotension, respiratory depression, or coma*

is often the case during critical illnesses, the nurse must evaluate posture, body language, risk factors, and other possible indicators of pain.

- In patients with trauma and other critical illnesses, administer morphine by IV infusion over a prolonged period. Health care providers may also give the drug by transdermal patch or by epidural infusion, depending on the patient's condition. For information about the use of PCA, see Box 49.2.
- As previously stated, the nurse administers morphine by the recommended routes (e.g., PO, IV, epidural) rather than IM injections, because IM injections are painful and frightening for children. For any child receiving parenteral medications, it is essential to assess vital signs and level of consciousness regularly.

### Assessing for Therapeutic Effects

The nurse assesses for decreased pain (patient reports) and general feeling of well-being. The nurse ensures that the patient is free from adverse effects. Tolerance (the initial dose of a substance loses its effectiveness over time) occurs with morphine and other opioids (see Chap. 2).

### Assessing for Adverse Effects

The nurse should assess for increases in respiratory distress, cardiac rhythm disturbances, and increasing somnolence. The FDA has issued **BLACK BOX WARNING ◆** for all opioid analgesics because of the potentially fatal adverse effects of respiratory depression, coma, and death, as well as the risks of drug abuse and dependence. Assessing for pruritus and urticaria, which may indicate an allergic reaction, is also important. Sweating may be a sign of tolerance and dependence in some patients taking morphine. Box 49.4 presents measures to recognize and manage toxicity. Additionally, Box 49.5 measures to recognize and manage withdrawal from opioids.

### Patient Teaching

Box 49.6 presents patient teaching guidelines for morphine sulfate and other opioids.

---

### Clinical Application 49.1

- Mrs. Hoffman complains of pain in her lower back with an intensity of 7 out of 10. Her vital signs remain stable. To manage her pain, her prescriber has ordered morphine 4 to 8 mg intravenously, every 2 to 4 hours as needed, to be given over 5 minutes, as well as oxycodone 5 mg with acetaminophen 500 mg orally (after 24 hours), every 4 to 6 hours, as needed, not to exceed six doses in 24 hours. When assessing pain in Mrs. Hoffman, what are the major considerations?
- Mrs. Hoffman tells the nurse that she does not want to take morphine because she is afraid that she will become addicted. What is the best response regarding addiction to narcotics?
- What major adverse effects of analgesics should the nurse observe for in Mrs. Hoffman once the morphine is administered?

---

### NCLEX Success

1. When caring for a patient who is receiving morphine, it is most important that the nurse regularly assess for which of the following?

   A. respiratory depression
   B. hyperactive bowel sounds
   C. frequent urination
   D. insomnia

2. A man has an order for morphine sulfate 2 mg intravenously every 2 hours following a cholecystectomy. The patient has a history of IV drug abuse. He reports that his pain is 7 out of 10 (with 10 being the worst) and requests the morphine every hour. What is the nurse's appropriate response?

   A. to instruct him about possible adverse effects
   B. to tell him that you can administer the drug only every 2 hours
   C. to use distraction techniques to help him forget his pain
   D. to notify the surgeon of his request

---

### Unfolding Patient Stories: Yoa Li • Part 2

Recall Yoa Li, a 26-year-old Asian male with appendicitis from Chapter 32. He arrived on the medical–surgical unit following an appendectomy. What are the desired outcomes for postoperative pain management? What assessments should the nurse perform when administering morphine intravenously and evaluating Yoa's response? What ethnic factors can influence the ability to provide good pain control?

Care for Yoa and other patients in a realistic virtual environment: *vSim for Nursing* (thepoint.lww.com/vSim-Pharm). Practice documenting these patients' care in DocuCare (thepoint.lww.com/DocuCareEHR).

---

## Other Drugs in the Class

Several other opioid agonists aside from morphine are available (see Table 49.2). Factors such as patient variability, the type of pain (i.e., acute vs. chronic), length of administration

---

### BOX 49.4 — Recognition and Management of Toxicity With Opioid Use

- Acute toxicity or overdose can occur from therapeutic use or from abuse by drug-dependent people.
- Overdose may produce severe respiratory depression and coma.
- The main goal of treatment is to restore and maintain adequate respiratory function.
- Managed by inserting an endotracheal tube and starting mechanical ventilation or by giving an antagonist, such as naloxone.
- Emergency supplies should be readily available in any setting where opioids are used.

| BOX 49.5 | *Prevention and Management of Withdrawal With Opioid Use* |
| --- | --- |

- Abstinence from opioids after chronic use produces a withdrawal syndrome characterized by anxiety; restlessness; insomnia; perspiration; pupil dilation; piloerection (goose bumps); anorexia, nausea, and vomiting; diarrhea; elevation of body temperature, respiratory rate, and systolic blood pressure; muscle cramps; and dehydration.
- Signs and symptoms in neonates include tremor, restlessness, increased muscle tone, screaming, fever, sweating, tachycardia, vomiting, diarrhea, respiratory distress, and possibly seizures.
- Although all opioids produce similar withdrawal syndromes, the onset, severity, and duration vary.
  - With morphine, symptoms begin within a few hours of the last dose, reach peak intensity in 36 to 72 hours, and subside over 8 to 10 days.
  - With methadone, symptoms begin in 1 to 2 days, peak in about 3 days, and subside over several weeks.
  - Heroin, meperidine, methadone, morphine, oxycodone, and oxymorphone are associated with more severe withdrawal symptoms than other opioids.
- If an antagonist such as naloxone (Narcan) is given, withdrawal symptoms occur rapidly and are more intense but of shorter duration.
- Recognition and treatment of early, mild symptoms of withdrawal can prevent progression to severe symptoms.
  - One technique is to give the opioid from which the person is withdrawing, which immediately reverses the signs and symptoms of withdrawal. Then, dosage is gradually reduced over several days.
  - Another technique is to substitute a long-acting opioid (e.g., methadone) for a short acting. Methadone is usually given in an adequate dose to control symptoms, once or twice daily, and then is gradually tapered over 5 to 10 days.
  - In neonates undergoing withdrawal, methadone or paregoric may be used.

of the previous drug, and drug tolerance may be influential. To calculate the dose of a specific opioid agonist, a prescriber may consult an equianalgesic chart, a conversion table that lists equivalent doses of these pain-relieving drugs. Table 49.3 outlines the equianalgesic dosing of common opioids.

 **QSEN Alert: Evidence-Based Practice**

Scheiber et al. (2019) explored trends and patterns of geographic variation in opioid prescribing practices in the United States by state from 2006 to 2017 and found considerable variation occurring with prescribing patterns among states. The researchers found that during this time, the number of opioids prescribed decreased but long-term prescriptions increased. One of the six measures described is the milligrams of a prescribed opioid weighted to national and state populations for each study year. This measure, expressed as MME, is based on the opioid's analgesic potency relative to morphine. The authors used an administrative database to provide these weighted estimates of the number of retail opioid prescriptions dispensed in the United States. The study reported that each year between 2006 and 2017, an estimated 233.7 million opioid prescriptions (211.0 billion MME) met the study's inclusion criteria and were filled in retail pharmacies in the United States. In 2017, pharmacies filled enough opioid prescriptions to theoretically provide every individual living in the United States with 5 mg of hydrocodone bitartrate every 4 hours around the clock for 3 weeks. States with the greatest MME per person in 2017 were Tennessee, Oklahoma, Delaware, and Alabama. Trend information in state prescribing patterns may be useful when designing state-specific intervention programs. In addition, analysis of interventions used in states with the lowest MME per person may help promote a decline in trends and patterns.

Codeine is an opium alkaloid used for analgesic and antitussive effects. This Schedule II drug has weaker analgesic and antitussive effects and milder adverse effects than morphine. Compared with other opioid analgesics, codeine is more

effective when given orally and is less likely to lead to abuse and dependence. The injected drug is more effective than the oral drug in relieving pain, but onset (15 to 30 minutes), peak (30 to 60 minutes), and duration of action (4 to 6 hours) are about the same. Half-life is about 3 hours. Larger doses are required for analgesic than for antitussive effects. Codeine is often given with acetaminophen for additive analgesic effects.

The cytochrome P450 2D6 (CYP2D6) family of enzymes metabolizes the opioid to morphine, which is responsible for codeine's analgesic effects.

 **QSEN Alert: Safety**

The CYP2D6 enzyme is inherited as an autosomal recessive trait. As many as 10% of Caucasians, 7% of African Americans, and 5% of Asians have inadequate amounts or activity of the CYP2D6 enzymes and are classified as poor metabolizers (see Chap. 2). These individuals may therefore receive less pain relief with the usual therapeutic doses of codeine and other opioids metabolized by CYP2D6. In addition, 21% of Asians, 5% of Caucasians, and 5% of African Americans are classified as ultrarapid metabolizers of the CYP2D6 enzymes and quickly metabolize codeine to its morphine, its active metabolite. This increases the risk of adverse effects, including respiratory depression and CNS depression.

The FDA has issued a **BLACK BOX WARNING ◆** regarding the cautious use of codeine in children, particularly for pain management following surgery, after reports of the death of children taking codeine who are ultrarapid metabolizers of the drug.

Prescribers sometimes order codeine for moderate pain, often with a nonopioid analgesic. The multimodal combination of opioid and nonopioid drugs produces additive analgesic effects and may allow smaller doses of opioids.

Fentanyl (Duragesic, Sublimaze, others) is a potent opioid agonist and Schedule II–controlled substance that is widely used for preanesthetic medication, postoperative analgesia, and

| BOX 49.6 | *Patient Teaching Guidelines for Opioid Analgesics* |

### General Considerations

- For acute episodes of pain that occur at irregular intervals, most opioids may be taken as needed; for acute pain that occurs daily and for chronic pain, the drugs should be taken on a regular schedule, around the clock.

- When a choice of pain-relieving medication is available, use the least amount of the mildest drug that is likely to be effective in a particular situation.

- Take only as prescribed. If desired effects are not achieved, report to your health care provider. Do not increase the dose and do not take medication more often than prescribed. Although these principles apply to all medications, they are especially important with opioid analgesics because of potentially serious adverse effects and because analgesics may mask pain for which medical attention is needed.

- Do not drink alcohol or take other drugs that cause drowsiness (e.g., some antihistamines, sedative-type drugs for nervousness or anxiety, sleeping pills) while taking opioids for pain. Combining drugs with similar effects may lead to excessive sedation and difficulty in breathing.

- Do not smoke, cook, drive a car, or operate machinery when drowsy or dizzy or when vision is blurred from medication.

- Sit or lie down at least 30 to 60 minutes after receiving an opioid by injection. Injected drugs may cause dizziness, drowsiness, and falls when walking around. If it is necessary to stand up, ask someone for assistance.

- If hospitalized, ask a health care provider about methods of pain management. For example, if anticipating surgery, ask how postoperative pain will be managed, how you need to report pain and request pain medication, and so on. It is better to take adequate medication and be able to cough, deep breathe, and walk around than to avoid or minimize pain medication and be unable to perform activities that promote recovery and healing. Do not object to having bed rails up or asking for assistance when receiving a strong narcotic analgesic. These

are safety measures to prevent falls or other injuries because these drugs may cause drowsiness, weakness, unsteady gait, and blurred vision.

- Avoid constipation, a common adverse effect of opioid analgesics. It may be prevented or managed by eating high-fiber foods, such as whole-grain cereals, fruits, and vegetables; drinking 2 to 3 quarts of fluid daily; and being as active as tolerated. If you take these medicines for more than a few days, or if you are the caregiver for someone who takes them, ask a health care provider about a bowel program to prevent constipation. A possible regimen is a daily stool softener (e.g., docusate) and a daily or every other day laxative (e.g., bisacodyl), preferably started at the same time as the narcotic. Docusate and bisacodyl are available over the counter.

### Self-administration

- Take oral opioid analgesics with 6 to 8 ounces of water, with or after food to reduce nausea.

- Do not crush or chew long-acting tablets (e.g., MS Contin, OxyContin). The tablets are formulated to release the active drug slowly, over several hours. Crushing or chewing causes immediate release of the drug, with a high risk of overdose and adverse effects, and shortens the duration of pain-relieving effects.

- You may experience these side effects: nausea, loss of appetite (take the drug with food and lie quietly), constipation (notify your health care provider if this is severe; a laxative may help), dizziness, sedation, drowsiness, and impaired visual acuity (avoid driving or performing other tasks requiring alertness, visual acuity).

- Omit one or more doses if severe adverse effects occur, and report to a health care provider. Also, report a skin rash.

- Take these drugs exactly as prescribed. Avoid alcohol, antihistamines, sedatives, tranquilizers, and over-the-counter drugs.

- Do not take any leftover medication for other disorders, and do not let anyone else take your prescription.

## TABLE 49.3

### Equianalgesic Dosing of Common Opioids

| Drug | Intravenous (IV) to Oral | Dose Equianalgesic to 1 mg IV Morphine | Comments |
|---|---|---|---|
| Morphine | 1:3 | — | Route: IV, subcutaneous, IM, PO, rectal, intrathecal |
| Oxycodone | — | — | No IV form available in the United States. Oxycodone: morphine 1:1 to 1:1.5 |
| Fentanyl patch (Duragesic) | — | 25 mcg | Also available as PO, IV, IM injection; sublingual tablets and spray; lozenges; nasal tablets; and spray buccal preparations |
| Hydromorphone | 1:4 | 0.2 mg | Sustained-release preparation available |
| Methadone | 1:2 | Ratio increases as daily morphine dose increases | Use only by experienced prescriber is suggested |

chronic pain that requires an opioid analgesic. Because of the high risk of respiratory depression, the drug is contraindicated in the use of acute pain, including management of headaches or migraines, or for postoperative pain outside the hospital setting. It should not be administered in **opioid-naive** patients (those who have not had at least 60 mg of morphine or an equianalgesic dose of another opioid for a week or longer); the FDA has issued a **BLACK BOX WARNING ◆** for fentanyl, reporting that fatal respiratory depression has occurred following use in opioid-intolerant patients and with improper dosing. In addition, the substitution of buccal fentanyl for any other fentanyl product may result in fatal overdose because the pharmacokinetic profiles are significantly different. There are numerous routes of administration, including IV and IM injection, transdermal application, sublingual tablets and spray, lozenges, and nasal spray. These formulations are not interchangeable on a microgram-per-microgram basis, and current dosages must be exchanged appropriately using a conversion table. The United States and Canadian guidelines differ, so it is necessary to consult the appropriate conversion table.

Duragesic is available as a transdermal formulation of fentanyl. Duragesic is for treatment of chronic and severe malignant pain. After deposition of active drug in the skin, systemic absorption slowly occurs. Duragesic has a slow onset of action (12 to 24 hours), but it lasts about 72 hours. When a Duragesic patch is removed, the drug continues to be absorbed from the skin deposits for 24 hours or longer.

With a transdermal formulation, a fast-acting formulation should be available for acute pain. An oral lozenge on a stick (Actiq) and a buccal tablet (Fentora) are approved to treat acute (breakthrough) pain in people who have been receiving opioids and have become opioid tolerant. Because of a risk of respiratory depression, recommended dosages must not be exceeded with any formulation.

Hydrocodone (Hysingla), a Schedule III drug, is similar to codeine in its analgesic and antitussive effects. It is available only in oral combination products for cough and with acetaminophen or ibuprofen for pain. Its half-life is about 4 hours, and its duration of action is 4 to 6 hours. Hydrocodone is metabolized to hydromorphone by the CYP2D6 enzymes.

Hydromorphone (Dilaudid) is a Schedule II, semisynthetic derivative of morphine that has the same actions, uses, contraindications, and adverse effects as morphine. It is more potent on a milligram-to-milligram basis and more effective orally than morphine. Effects occur in 15 to 30 minutes, peak in 30 to 90 minutes, and last 4 to 5 hours. Hydromorphone is metabolized in the liver to inactive metabolites that are excreted through the kidneys.

Meperidine (Demerol) is a synthetic drug similar to morphine in action and adverse effects. After injection, analgesia occurs in 10 to 20 minutes, peaks in 1 hour, and lasts 2 to 4 hours. After an oral dose, about half is metabolized in the liver and never reaches the systemic circulation. Prescribers order meperidine infrequently for therapeutic purposes, mainly because it produces a neurotoxic metabolite (normeperidine). Normeperidine accumulates with chronic use, large doses, or renal failure and produces CNS stimulation characterized by agitation, hallucinations, and seizures. The half-life of normeperidine is 15 to 30 hours, depending on renal function, and the effects of normeperidine are not reversible with opioid antagonist drugs. Meperidine is not recommended for cancer pain management or for use in older adults.

Methadone (Dolophine) is a synthetic drug similar to morphine but with a longer duration of action. It is usually given orally, and onset and peak of action occur in 30 to 60 minutes. Effects last 4 to 6 hours initially and longer with repeated use. Half-life is 15 to 30 hours, and this also lengthens with repeated use. Prescribers order methadone for severe pain and in the detoxification and maintenance treatment of opiate addicts. In 2006, the FDA issued an alert about serious adverse effects (e.g., death, overdose, and serious cardiac dysrhythmias) reported in patients taking methadone. The FDA recommended that methadone dosage for pain should be carefully selected and titrated and that patients should be taught not to exceed prescribed dosage or frequency of administration.

Oxycodone (OxyContin, Xtampza ER) is a derivative of codeine used to relieve moderate pain; its pharmacologic actions are similar to those of other opioid analgesics. It is a Schedule II drug of abuse. With oral administration, action starts in 15 to 30 minutes, peaks in 60 minutes, and lasts 4 to 6 hours. Its half-life is unknown. It is metabolized by the CYP2D6 enzymes and excreted through the kidneys.

An agonist narcotic, oxycodone is used, alone or in combination with acetaminophen, for the treatment of moderate to severe pain. The drug is available in tablets, capsules, and solutions. Immediate-release products are intended for patients who are narcotic naive. Extended-release products are intended only for patients who are opioid tolerant. When giving extended-release products every 12 hours, the goal is to relieve pain around the clock. Thus, these effects are most useful for patients with terminal cancer or other chronic pain conditions.

Unfortunately, OxyContin is a popular drug of abuse and is associated with many deaths and much criminal activity. Most deaths have resulted from inappropriate use through diversion either (1) by chewing, crushing, and snorting through the nose or (2) crushing and injecting the drug. Chewing or crushing destroys the long-acting feature and constitutes an overdose. As a result, the FDA has issued a **BLACK BOX WARNING ◆** for the extended-release tablets and capsules because of serious, life-threatening, or fatal respiratory depression. Crushing, chewing, or dissolving can cause rapid release and a potentially fatal dose. In addition, the FDA has approved an abuse-deterrent formulation that is designed to prevent the tablets from being chewed or crushed.

Oxymorphone, a Schedule II drug, is a derivative of morphine with actions, uses, and adverse effects similar to those of morphine. Used for acute and chronic pain and for analgesia during labor, administration can be administered IV, IM, and PO. Oral tablets are available in immediate-release and extended-release formulations. The FDA has issued **BLACK BOX WARNING ◆** cautioning that accidental ingestion of even one dose of extended-release oxymorphone, particularly in children, can result in a fatal overdose. Also, when taken with a high-fat meal, peak concentration is increased up to 50%; both formulations should be taken 1 hour before or 2 hours after eating.

Tramadol (Ultram, ConZip) is an oral, synthetic, Schedule IV opioid that acts at the central opioid receptors for moderate to severe pain. It is effective and well tolerated in older adults and in people with acute or chronic pain, back pain, fibromyalgia, osteoarthritis, and neuropathic pain. Because it has a low potential for producing tolerance and abuse, it may be used long term for the management of chronic pain. It is not chemically related to opioids and is not a controlled drug. Its mechanism of action includes binding to mu opioid receptors and inhibiting reuptake of norepinephrine and serotonin in the brain, actions that interfere with transmission of pain signals. Analgesia occurs within 1 hour of administration and peaks in 2 to 3 hours with immediate-release tablets. Tramadol is associated with less risk of respiratory depression and constipation than morphine but carries a risk of serotonin syndrome, especially when combined with other serotonergic agents, such as the selective serotonin reuptake inhibitors, serotonin norepinephrine reuptake inhibitors, tricyclic antidepressants, and monoamine oxidase (MAO) inhibitors.

Tramadol is available in oral immediate-release tablets alone and in combination with acetaminophen as well as an extended-release tablet that can be given once daily. The drug is well absorbed after oral administration, even if taken with food. It is minimally bound to plasma proteins, and its half-life is 6 to 7 hours. The CYP3A4 and CYP2D6 enzymes metabolize the drug, and it forms an active metabolite. About 30% of a dose is excreted unchanged in the urine, and 60% is excreted as metabolites. Dosage reduction in people with renal or hepatic impairment is necessary.

# OPIOID AGONISTS/ANTAGONISTS

Opioid agonists/antagonists act on the same pain receptors in the CNS as morphine and other opiates, resulting in interference with pain transmission and/or pain sensation. These agents have agonist activity at some receptors and antagonist activity at others. Because of their agonist activity, they are potent analgesics with a lower abuse potential than pure agonists. However, they are considered second-line drugs for treatment of moderate to severe pain. Because of their antagonist activity, they should not be given to people who have been receiving analgesics, and they may produce withdrawal symptoms in people with dependence. Pentazocine was the original prototype, but its use is marginal. Ⓟ **Butorphanol** will serve as the prototype in this discussion. Butorphanol is a synthetic, Schedule IV

agonist similar to morphine in analgesic effects and ability to cause respiratory depression. Prescribers order it for moderate to severe pain. Administration may be parenteral; after IM or IV use, analgesia peaks in 30 to 60 minutes. Alternatively, administration may be topical to nasal mucosa by a metered spray; after nasal application, analgesia peaks within 1 to 2 hours.

## Pharmacokinetics

Butorphanol is rapidly and well absorbed following IV, IM, and nasal administration. Onset of action occurs within a few minutes with IV administration and within 15 minutes with the other routes. Time to peak concentration is 20 to 40 minutes (IM) and 30 to 60 minutes (nasal), and the duration of action is usually 3 to 4 hours with IV and IM routes and 4 to 5 hours with nasal administration. Butorphanol is metabolized in the liver and excreted primarily in the urine, with a small amount excreted in feces. The drug crosses the placenta, and it also enters breast milk.

## Action

Butorphanol is an agonist of kappa opiate receptors and a partial agonist of mu opiate receptors in the CNS, causing inhibition of ascending pain pathways. The drug alters the perception of pain and produces analgesia. Like morphine, it has a sedative effect.

## Use

Butorphanol is used to treat moderate to severe pain that has not been adequately managed with alternative treatments. The drug is also used as a preoperative medication and as a supplement to multimodal anesthesia. Injection is approved for the management of pain during labor with a fetus greater than 37 weeks of gestation and in no signs of respiratory distress. Table 49.4 presents dosage information for butorphanol and the other opioid agonists/antagonists.

## TABLE 49.4

### DRUGS AT A GLANCE: Opioid Agonists/Antagonists

| Drug | Pregnancy Category | Routes and Dosage Ranges | |
|------|-------------------|--------------------------|---|
| | | **Adults** | **Children** |
| Ⓟ **Butorphanol** (🍁 Butorphanol) | C | IM, IV 1–4 mg every 3–4 h PRN<br>Nasal spray 1 mg (one spray in one nostril) every 3–4 h PRN<br>Older adults: IM 1–2 mg every 6–8 h PRN<br>Renal or hepatic impairment: IM 1–2 mg every 6–8 h | Not recommended for children younger than 18 y of age |
| Nalbuphine (🍁 Nubain) | C | IM, IV, subcutaneous 10 mg/70 kg every 3–6 h PRN; max dose in non–opioid-dependent patients: 20 mg as a single dose, max daily dose 160 mg<br>Surgical anesthesia supplement: induction IV 0.3–3 mg/kg to 5 mg/kg over 10–15 min, maintenance doses of 0.25–0.5 mg/kg as required | ≥1 y IM, IV, subcutaneous 0.1–0.2 mg/kg every 3–4 h as needed; 20 mg max as a single dose, max daily dose 160 mg |
| Pentazocine (🍁 Talwin) | C | IV, 30 mg (do not exceed) every 3–4 h (max dose 360 mg)<br>IM, subcutaneous, 30–60 mg every 3–4 h (max dose 360 mg)<br>Labor analgesia: IM, 30 mg once<br>IV, 20 mg every 2–3 h PRN (max dose 60 mg) | 5–8 y: IM 15 mg<br>9–14 y: IM 30 mg<br>1–16 y: preoperative/preanesthetic, IM 0.5 mg/kg |

### Use in Children

The safety of butorphanol has not been established in children younger than 18 years of age.

### Use in Older Adults

Cautious use of butorphanol is warranted in older adults, particularly with the intranasal route, because increased frequency of adverse effects has been reported. It is necessary to begin with low doses, which should be given at least 6 hours apart.

### Use in Patients With Hepatic Impairment

Extensive liver disease, with decreased metabolism, may predispose the patient to accentuated adverse effects. Although laboratory tests have not indicated that butorphanol causes or increases hepatic impairment, caution is important when administering butorphanol to patients with such impairment, and doses should be at least 6 hours apart.

### Use in Patients With Renal Impairment

Similarly, caution is necessary in patients with renal impairment. It is important to use the lowest dose possible and doses should be at least 6 hours apart.

## Adverse Effects

The adverse effects of butorphanol include headache, dizziness, drowsiness, vertigo, constipation, nausea and/or vomiting, dizziness, and euphoria. Reported effects with the nasal spray include nasal congestion, cough, dyspnea, and rhinitis. With both injection and intranasal routes, the type and incidence of adverse effects are similar to those of morphine, but butorphanol may be more likely to cause hallucinations. When used for pain relief during labor, butorphanol may temporarily affect the heart rate of the fetus and may cause apnea or respiratory distress in the newborn. Also, some drugs of the opioid class, including butorphanol, produce dose-related symptoms, including delusions and/or delirium, which mimic psychosis.

Unlike morphine, the respiratory depressant action of butorphanol is subject to a **ceiling effect**; there is no further effect (in this case respiratory depression) above a particular dosage level. The **BLACK BOX WARNING ◆** issued for morphine also applies to butorphanol because of its potentially fatal adverse effects of respiratory depression, coma, and death, as well as risks of drug abuse and dependence.

## Contraindications

Caution is necessary when administering butorphanol to patients with acute asthma who are unmonitored or if resuscitative equipment is not available or with patients with significant respiratory depression. The FDA has issued a **BLACK BOX WARNING ◆** regarding the risk of neonatal withdrawal syndrome in newborns that may occur with prolonged maternal use of butorphanol and other opioids during pregnancy.

## Nursing Implications

### Preventing Interactions

The FDA has issued a **BLACK BOX WARNING ◆** regarding concomitant use of intranasal butorphanol with CYP3A4 inhibitors because of the risk of increased or prolonged adverse effects, including potentially fatal respiratory depression. In addition, discontinuing a CYP3A4 inducer while taking butorphanol may result in an increased butorphanol plasma level. The nurse should be aware that alcohol and other CNS depressants add to the sedative effect of butorphanol. Concomitant use with the phenothiazines or benzodiazepines increases the risk of respiratory depression, hypotension, profound sedation, or coma.

### Administering the Medication

Administration of butorphanol is by IM and IV injection or intranasal spray. Before giving IV butorphanol and other drugs together in a syringe or at a tubing Y-site, a pharmacist needs to confirm that combination is compatible.

### Assessing for Therapeutic Effects

The nurse assesses for pain relief. However, tolerance can be a problem, and it may be necessary to adjust the dosage of butorphanol.

### Assessing for Adverse Effects

The nurse assesses for respiratory depression, CNS depression, and possible signs of withdrawal in opioid-tolerant patients. The signs of withdrawal from butorphanol include tremors and anxiety. In patients taking the nasal spray, the nurse assesses for nasal congestion cough, dyspnea, and rhinitis. When used for pain relief during labor, the nurse monitors the drug effect on the heart rate of the fetus and for the presence of apnea or respiratory distress in the newborn.

### Patient Teaching

The nurse ensures that patients are instructed to notify the prescriber if the pain does not disappear, becomes worse, or changes in location or type. Patients should not stop taking butorphanol abruptly, and they should take care when changing positions quickly or operating equipment that requires mental alertness. Box 49.6 outlines additional patient teaching guidelines.

## Other Drugs in the Class

Nalbuphine (Nubain) is a synthetic analgesic used for moderate to severe pain. It is not a controlled drug. Administration is IV, IM, or subcutaneous. After IV injection, action starts in 2 to 3 minutes, peaks in 15 to 20 minutes, and lasts for 3 to 6 hours. After IM or subcutaneous injection, action begins in less than 15 minutes, peaks in 30 to 60 minutes, and lasts for 3 to 6 hours. The half-life is 5 hours. The most common adverse effect is sedation; at recommended doses, other effects are minimal.

---

### Clinical Application 49.2

- Twenty-four hours after surgery, Mrs. Hoffman is started on oxycodone 5 mg with acetaminophen 500 mg orally, with her pain level at 3 out of 10. She is able to ambulate independently and is eating and voiding without difficulty. In planning for discharge, what instruction does the nurse provide to Mrs. Hoffman regarding the adverse effects of oxycodone with acetaminophen?

3. The patient receives butorphanol for pain. Which of the following statements by the patient indicates an adverse effect of the medication?
   A. "I feel cold all over."
   B. "My ears are ringing."
   C. "I feel like I am going to throw up."
   D. "My heart feels like it is skipping a beat."

4. A man is receiving patient-controlled analgesia (PCA), and his family questions why his pain medication is being given in this manner. The nurse is most correct in explaining that the main advantage of PCA is that it
   A. requires less nursing time
   B. causes fewer adverse effects
   C. relieves pain more effectively
   D. can be used long term

## OPIOID ANTAGONISTS

An antagonist (antidote) reverses analgesia and the CNS and respiratory depression caused by agonists. However, an opioid antagonist does not relieve the depressant effects of other drugs, such as sedative–hypnotic, antianxiety, and antipsychotic agents. The chief clinical use of an antagonist is to relieve opioid-induced CNS and respiratory depression. The prototype of this class is ℗ **naloxone** (Evzio, Narcan). It is essential that this drug be readily available in all health care settings in which opioids are given. In addition, inhaled naloxone is now available either (1) with a prescription in all states or (2) without a prescription to patients and their caregivers using narcotics for pain in many states. Some states have approved peace officers (first responders) to carry naloxone

when on duty. For the most current information on availability of naloxone, access http://www.narcan.com/.

## Pharmacokinetics

Therapeutic effects occur within minutes after injection (IV [about 2 minutes], IM [2 to 5 minutes], or subcutaneous [2 to 5 minutes]) or intranasal administration (8 to 13 minutes); they last 1 to 2 hours. Naloxone has a shorter duration of action than opioids, and repeated injections are usually necessary. To combat the effects of a long-acting drug such as methadone, patients may need injections for 2 to 3 days.

## Action

Naloxone (antidote) reverses analgesia and the CNS and respiratory depression caused by agonists. It competes with opioids for receptor sites in the brain and thereby prevents binding with receptors or displaces opioids already occupying receptor sites. When opioids cannot bind to receptor sites, they are "neutralized" and cannot exert their effects on body cells.

## Use

Naloxone has long been the drug of choice to treat respiratory depression caused by an overdose of opioids. Given intravenously, naloxone begins to reverse CNS and respiratory depression induced by opioids in minutes. However, the American Heart Association's recommendations for initial treatment of life-threatening opioid-related respiratory depression do not include the inhaled route. Table 49.5 gives dosage information for naloxone.

### Use in Children

Cautious use of naloxone is necessary in neonates and children. As usual, the dose is smaller and given according to kilogram weight. The child's renal and hepatic function also affects the

---

**TABLE 49.5**

**DRUGS AT A GLANCE: Opioid Antagonists**

| Drug | Pregnancy Category | Routes and Dosage Ranges | |
|---|---|---|---|
| | | **Adults** | **Children** |
| ℗ **Naloxone** (Evzio, Narcan; ✦ Naloxone hydrochloride injection) | C | Overdose: IV 0.4–2 mg, repeat every 2–3 min if needed. Give IM or subcutaneously (Evzio contents of 1 autoinjector [0.4 mg]) if unable to give IV; also may give 2½ times initial IV dose via endotracheal tube<br>Narcan nasal spray: 4 mg (contents of 1 nasal spray) as single dose; may repeat every 2–3 min in alternating nostrils until medical assistance available<br>Postoperative reversal: IV 0.1–0.2 mg every 2–3 min until desired level of reversal is attained | Birth to 5 y or weight <20 kg: 0.1 mg/kg; may repeat every 2–3 min if needed<br>≥5 y or weight ≥20 kg: 2 mg/dose; may repeat every 2–3 min if needed |
| Naltrexone (Vivitrol; ✦ ReVia) | C | PO initial 25 mg, if no signs of withdrawal, 50 mg every 24 h; alternate dosing can be used with supervised administration.<br>IM, 380 mg once every 4 wk | Not approved by use in children |

response to the medication. The recommended route is IV only, to control absorption.

### Use in Patients With Renal Impairment

Use of naloxone in renal impairment requires caution. If it is advised, it is necessary to give small dose. Impaired renal function leads to slower drug excretion and increased risk of accumulation.

### Use in Patients With Hepatic Impairment

Similarly, use of naloxone in hepatic impairment requires caution. It is necessary to monitor the patient's liver function closely to prevent toxicity.

### Use in Patients With Critical Illness

Critically ill patients who have increased intracranial pressure, seizure disorders, head trauma, or respiratory depression should not receive naloxone. However, people with coma of unknown origin may receive the drug to determine if the cause of the mental status change could result from opioids.

## Adverse Effects

Adverse effects of naloxone include tremors, drowsiness, sweating, decreased respirations, hypertension, and nausea and vomiting. Naloxone itself has minimal toxicity.

## Contraindications

Contraindications to naloxone include known hypersensitivity to the drug, presence of narcotic abuse, and pregnancy. The drug may precipitate withdrawal, producing tachycardia, hypertension, and violent behavior.

## Nursing Implications

### Assessing for Therapeutic Effects

The nurse assesses for reversal of opioid effects, including improved respiratory function and decreased sedation.

### Assessing for Adverse Effects

The nurse assesses for decreased reparations and elevated blood pressure. With the use of naloxone, the nurse is prepared to repeat the dose. The return of pain is a factor to be considered.

## Other Drugs in the Class

Naltrexone (Vivitrol) is an opiate antagonist that acts in the brain to prevent opiate effects (e.g., pain relief, feelings of well-being), making it effective in decreasing the desire to take opiates and in treating alcohol dependence. Professionals commonly use naltrexone as part of a complete treatment program for substance abuse (e.g., compliance monitoring, counseling, support, behavioral contract, lifestyle modification); health care providers administer the medication. The drug decreases the desire to drink alcohol, and the dose is based on the patient's medical condition and response to treatment.

Contraindications to naltrexone include concurrent use of opiates, including methadone. Such use can cause sudden withdrawal symptoms (see Box 49.5). After discontinuing opiates, at least 7 days should pass before a person starts taking naltrexone. To confirm absence of opioids, health care providers should verify self-reporting of opioid abstinence in addicted patients using urine analysis. If results for opioids are positive or there are signs of opiate withdrawal, a naloxone challenge test (administering small doses of naltrexone and observing for signs of withdrawal) is typically necessary. It is important to assess liver function in patients taking naltrexone, because liver problems may occur.

### NCLEX Success

5. A man is difficult to arouse after IV administration of morphine sulfate. He has a respiratory rate of 7 breaths/min. Which of the following (with appropriate prescriber orders) are priority nursing actions? (Select all that apply.)
   A. Administer oxygen.
   B. Administer naloxone.
   C. Insert a urinary catheter.
   D. Increase the IV fluid rate.
   E. Place the patient in semi-Fowler's position.

6. For an overdose of morphine sulfate, which drug should the nurse have on hand to counteract an overdose?
   A. phenytoin
   B. tramadol
   C. naloxone
   D. atropine sulfate

## THE NURSING PROCESS

A concept map outlines the nursing process related to drug therapy considerations in this chapter. Additional nursing implications related to the disease process should also be considered in care decisions.

**Assessment**

- Assess the patient with regard to pain, initially to determine appropriate interventions to be implemented. Assess the patient after interventions are implemented. Increase data collection by interviewing family members about the patient's pain. Specific assessment data include:
  - Location. Determine the location of the pain and whether it radiates. Intensity or severity. Have the patient rate their pain utilizing an accepted scale. Assess pain in relation to time, activities, and other signs and symptoms.
  - Assess for pain on a regular schedule around the clock (e.g., every 1–2 hours). If the patient is unable to communicate needs for pain relief, as is often the case during critical illnesses, evaluate posture, body language, risk factors, and other possible indicators of pain.
- Administer analgesics before painful procedures, when indicated. Provide nursing care that does not promote tissue or muscle damage.
- For uncontrolled or unexpected pain, reassess and consider alternative causes for the pain.

**Outcomes of Therapy**

The patient will
- Understand the use of nonpharmacological and pharmacological therapies for pain relief.
- Maintain safety with the administration of pharmacological agents to relieve pain.
- Avoid or be relieved of pain.
- Use opioid analgesics appropriately.
- Avoid preventable adverse effects.
- Be monitored for excessive sedation and respiratory depression.
- Be able to communicate and perform other activities of daily living when feasible.

The patient and caregivers will
- Verbalize expected adverse effects of pain management medications.
- Verbalize effective management of adverse effects of pain management medications.

**Nursing Interventions**

- Use measures to prevent, relieve, or decrease pain when possible. General measures include those that promote optimal body functioning and those that prevent trauma, inflammation, infection, and other sources of painful stimuli. Specific interventions include the following:
  - Use sterile technique when caring for wounds, urinary catheters, or IV lines.
  - Use exercises, ambulation, and position changes to promote circulation and musculoskeletal function.
  - Rub or massage the painful area to stimulate other nerve fibers that block the nerve fibers carrying pain signals from entering the spinal cord.
  - Handle any injured tissue gently, to avoid further trauma.
  - Prevent bowel or bladder distention.
  - Apply heat or cold, as indicated.
  - Use relaxation or distraction techniques.
- When caring for children in pain:
  - Recognize that expressions of pain may differ according to age and developmental level. Infants may cry and have muscular rigidity and thrashing behavior. Preschoolers may behave aggressively or complain verbally of discomfort. Young school-aged children may express pain verbally or behaviorally, often with regression to behaviors used at younger ages.
  - Adolescents may be reluctant to admit they are uncomfortable or need help. With chronic pain, children of all ages tend to withdraw and regress to an earlier stage of development.
- Adults and children are better able to cope with pain when they are informed about what is happening to them and are assisted in developing coping strategies.

**Evaluation**

- Ask patients about their levels of comfort or relief from pain.
- Observe behaviors that indicate the presence or absence of pain, including ability to complete activities of daily living.
- Observe for presence or absence of sedation and respiratory depression.
- Observe signs of drug-seeking behavior (possibly indicating dependence).

## KEY CONCEPTS

- Pain is a subjective experience, and a patient's self-reporting of pain is considered the gold standard for assessment because it is the most valid measure of pain.
- It is important to assess all patients for pain. If present, effective pain management, often with a combination of strategies that may include nonpharmacologic treatments, nonanalgesics, analgesics, and adjuvant drugs, is essential.
- Acute pain may be manifested verbally or by behavior that indicates discomfort. Chronic pain may not be manifested by visible signs and is often accompanied by anxiety and depression.
- Failure to properly manage pain is a significant contributor to elevated health care costs and poor postoperative outcome.
- Analgesics react with receptors in the CNS and peripheral tissues to inhibit transmission of pain signals, to reduce the perception of pain, and to reduce the emotional upsets often associated with pain.
- Most opioid analgesics are Schedule II–controlled drugs and may cause serious adverse effects (e.g., respiratory depression, sedation) and physical dependence. As a result, they all have **BLACK BOX WARNING ◆** regarding safe and appropriate use.
- In addition, the FDA has issued a **BLACK BOX WARNING ◆** for the combined use of opioid analgesics and benzodiazepines and other drugs that depress the CNS because of respiratory depression and death. The FDA has issued a **BLACK BOX WARNING ◆** concerning codeine. It should be used cautiously in children, particularly for pain management following surgery, after reports of the death of children taking codeine who are ultrarapid metabolizers of the drug.
- The FDA has issued **BLACK BOX WARNING ◆** cautioning that accidental ingestion of even one dose of extended-release oxymorphone, particularly in children, can result in a fatal overdose.
- Agonist drugs stimulate receptors; agonists/antagonists have agonist activity at some receptors and antagonist activity at others; and antagonists reverse or block the effects of agonists.
- Selection, dosage, and route of administration should be individualized according to the patient's condition.
- For most acute and chronic pain, analgesics are more effective if given on a regular schedule, on an around-the-clock basis. When acute pain has subsided or occurs at irregular intervals and when breakthrough pain occurs in patients receiving long-term analgesic therapy for chronic pain, administration of analgesics may occur as needed.
- For patients who require large doses of opioids to relieve pain, it is often necessary to use additional medications and interventions to manage adverse effects (e.g., nausea, constipation).
- Assess pain using a visual analogue scale, verbal or numerical rating scale, or picture scale. Mnemonic devices, such as SOCRATES (Site, Onset, Character, Radiation, Associations, Time course, Exacerbating/Relieving factors, and Severity), may be helpful.
- It is essential that pain-relieving interventions are documented in patient records.
- The FDA's **BLACK BOX WARNING ◆** issued for morphine also applies to the opioid agonist/antagonist butorphanol because of its potentially fatal adverse effects of respiratory depression, coma, and death, as well as risks of drug abuse and dependence.
- The FDA has issued a **BLACK BOX WARNING ◆** regarding the risk of neonatal withdrawal syndrome in the newborn, which may occur with prolonged maternal use of butorphanol and other opioids during pregnancy.
- The FDA has issued a **BLACK BOX WARNING ◆** with concomitant use of intranasal butorphanol with all CYP3A4 inhibitors as the risk of increased or prolonged adverse effects including potentially fatal respiratory depression.

## CLINICAL REASONING CASE STUDY

### Meet the Patient

Mr. Mohamed, an 80-year-old man, is hospitalized and receiving extended-release morphine sulfate (MS Contin) 30 mg every 8 hours for management of the pain associated with newly diagnosed colon cancer. He is receiving an intravenous $D_5NS$ infusion of 100 mL/h. The nurse assessing him one evening has difficulty arousing him. His vital signs are temperature 98.4°F, pulse 104 beats/min, respirations 7 breaths/min, and blood pressure 92/52 mm Hg, with $O_2$ saturation 89% on room air.

- As the nurse caring for Mr. Mohamed, what are the priority interventions at this time?
- After receiving naloxone, Mr. Mohamed arouses and is oriented to person, place, and time. He begins complaining of his usual left upper quadrant abdominal pain. His vital signs are temperature 98.4°F, pulse 90 beats/min, respirations 16 breaths/min, blood pressure 114/62 mm Hg, with an $O_2$ saturation of 96% on 2 L/min nasal cannula. His nurse practitioner is at the bedside and has called the pain management team to reassess his pain control. What additional assessment should be made over the next few hours?

### Assessing Drug Information

- Oxycodone
  - This derivative of codeine and Schedule II drug of abuse is used to relieve moderate pain.
  - Pharmacologic actions are similar to those of other opioid analgesics.
  - With oral administration, action starts in 15 to 30 minutes, peaks in 60 minutes, and lasts 4 to 6 hours. Its half-life is unknown.
  - It is metabolized by the CYP2D6 enzymes and excreted through the kidneys.
  - Adverse effects include central nervous system (CNS) depression (drowsiness, dizziness, headache), respiratory depression, pruritus, nausea, and constipation.

- Naloxone
  - This opioid antagonist competes with opioids for receptor sites in the brain. It prevents binding with receptors or displaces opioids already occupying receptor sites, neutralizing the effects of opioids.
  - It is the drug of choice to treat respiratory and CNS depression caused by an overdose of opioids and should be administered per protocol.
  - Given intravenously, it begins to reverse CNS and respiratory depression induced by opioids in minutes. Two nurses should determine the correct dose of intravenous naloxone.
  - Because it has a shorter duration of action than opioids, repeated injections are usually necessary.
  - Pain-relieving effects of morphine are eliminated once treatment with naloxone begins. It is important to enforce institutional protocols and document the event.

### Nursing Actions

- Initial assessment
  - Focus on counteracting the life-threatening depression of Mr. Mohamed's respiratory and central nervous systems. Administer and assess the effectiveness of naloxone in increasing respiratory rate and returning to baseline mental status.
  - Have available emergency resuscitation equipment, including an endotracheal tube and mechanical ventilation.
  - Notify the patient's health care provider and administer supplemental $O_2$ by nasal cannula to keep the patient's $O_2$ saturations greater than 90% per standing protocol orders.
- Ongoing assessment
  - Continue to assess Mr. Mohamed's breathing; level of consciousness; vital signs, including oxygen saturation levels; and kidney function.
  - Continue to assess for concurrent use of drugs that could have contributed to respiratory and CNS depression. Oxycodone is metabolized by the CYP2D6 enzymes, so the potential for drug interactions is significant.
  - Observe for signs of withdrawal, such as body aches, diarrhea, increased heart rate, fever, sweating, nausea or vomiting, irritability, trembling, weakness, and increased blood pressure.
  - Assess for the effectiveness of pain management once opioids are reintroduced by pain management team.
  - Instruct the patient and caregiver about the action, adverse effects, and patient teaching guidelines for opioid use.

*Visit* **thePoint** *at* **http://thePoint.lww.com/Frandsen12e** *for answers to NCLEX Success questions (in Appendix A), answers to Clinical Application Case Studies (in Appendix B), and more!*

## REFERENCES AND RESOURCES

American Academy of Pain. (2016). Use of opioids for the treatment of chronic pain. Retrieved from http://www.painmed.org/files/use-of-opioids-for-the-treatment-of-chronic-pain.pdf

Centers for Disease Control and Prevention. (2016). Guideline for prescribing opioids for chronic pain—United States, 2016. *Morbidity and Mortality Weekly Report Recommendations and Reports, 65*(1), 1–49.

Smith, L. A., Burns, E., & Cuthbert, A. (2018). Parenteral opioids for maternal pain management in labour. *Cochrane Database of Systematic Reviews, 6,* CD007396. doi: 10.1002/14651858.CD007396.pub3.

Guille, C., Barth, K. S., Mateus, J., McCauley, J. L., & Brady, K. T. (2017). Treatment of Prescription opioid use disorder in pregnant women. *The American Journal of Psychiatry, 174*(2), 208–214.

Hinkle, J. H., & Cheever, K. H. (2017). *Brunner & Suddarth's textbook of medical-surgical nursing* (14th ed.). Philadelphia, PA: Lippincott Williams & Wilkins.

Karch, A. M. (2020). *2020 Lippincott's pocket drug guide for nurses.* Philadelphia, PA: Lippincott Williams & Wilkins.

Knight, C. L., Deyo, R. A., Staiger, T. O., & Wipf, J. E. (2020). *Treatment of acute low back pain.* UpToDate. Lexi-Comp, Inc.

Lippincott. (2019). *Nursing 2020 Drug handbook* (37th ed.). Philadelphia, PA: Lippincott Williams & Wilkins.

Norris, T. L. (2019). *Porth's pathophysiology: Concepts of altered health states* (10th ed.). Philadelphia, PA: Wolters Kluwer.

Portenoy, R. K., Mehta, Z., & Ahmed, E. (2016). *Cancer pain management with opioids: Optimizing analgesia.* UpToDate. Lexi-Comp, Inc.

Riley, J., Branford, R., Droney, J., Gretton, S., Sato, H., Kennett, A., et al. (2015). Morphine or oxycodone for cancer-related pain? A randomized, open-label, controlled trial. *Journal of Pain and Symptom Management, 49*(2), 161–172.

Rosenquist, R. (2020). *Use of opioids in the management of chronic noncancer pain.* UpToDate. Lexi-Comp, Inc.

Rosero, E. B., & Joshi, G. P. (2014). Preemptive, preventive, multimodal analgesia: What do they really mean? *Plastic and Reconstructive Surgery, 134*(42S), 85S–93S.

Severtson, S. G., Bartelson, B. B., Davis, J. M., Muñoz, A., Schneider, M. F., Chilcoat, H., et al. (2013). Reduced abuse, therapeutic errors, and diversion following reformulation of extended-release oxycodone in 2010. *The Journal of Pain, 14*(10), 1122–1130.

Schieber, L. Z., Guy, P. G., Seth, P., Young, R., Mattson, C. L., Mikosz, C. A., & Schieber, R. A. (2019). Trends and patterns of geographic variation in opioid prescribing practices by state, United States, 2006-2017. *JAMA Network Open, 2*(3):e190665. doi:10.1001/jamanetworkopen.2019.0665.

UpToDate. (2020). *Drug information.* Lexi-Comp, Inc.

U.S. Department of Health and Human Services. (n.d.) *HHS.GOV/ Opioids.* Retrieved from https://www.hhs.gov/opioids/about-the-epidemic/index.html

Varndell, W., Elliott, D., & Fry, M. (2015). The validity, reliability, responsiveness and applicability of observation sedation-scoring instruments for use with adult patients in the emergency department: A systematic literature review. *Australian Emergency Nursing Journal, 18*(1), 1–23.

# Drug Therapy
# With Local Anesthetics

## CLINICAL APPLICATION CASE STUDY

Lexi Scruggs, a 7-year-old girl, was swinging from the monkey bars on the school playground. She lost her grip and fell, cutting her left knee on a piece of glass. At the emergency department, she requires 10 sutures to close the jagged cut. She receives lidocaine (Xylocaine) prior to cleaning and suturing the wound.

## KEY TERMS

**Bier block anesthesia:** regional limb anesthesia provided by local anesthesia and an extremity tourniquet

**Epidural anesthesia:** injection of local anesthetic into the epidural space

**Field block anesthesia:** subcutaneous injection of local anesthetic around the margin of the surgical or procedural site

**Local anesthetic systemic toxicity (LAST):** systemic absorption of a local anesthetic agent that results in excitation of the central nervous system

**Nerve block anesthesia:** blocking a group of nerves, called a plexus or ganglion, to a specific area of the body

**Spinal anesthesia:** injection of anesthetic into the cerebrospinal fluid, usually in the lumbar spine

**Topical anesthesia:** application of a local anesthetic on the skin or mucous membranes

# INTRODUCTION

This chapter serves two primary purposes: it (1) introduces the fundamentals of local anesthesia and (2) discusses the implementation of safe perioperative nursing care during the administration of local anesthesia.

The local anesthetic agents are classified as amides and esters. The molecular structure of the amides possesses an amide linkage, and the esters' structure contains an ester linkage. The amide group is the most commonly used clinically.

# OVERVIEW OF LOCAL ANESTHESIA

Local anesthetics, given to produce loss of sensation and motor activity, are injected into localized areas of the body. These agents decrease the permeability of the nerve cell membrane to ions, especially sodium. They stop the nerve from depolarizing, preventing the sodium ions from entering the nerve, which means that the nerve impulses can no longer be initiated or conducted by the anesthetized nerves. Thus, local anesthetics prevent the cells from responding to pain impulses and sensory stimulation. This loss of sensation occurs in the following sequence: temperature, touch, proprioception, and skeletal muscle tone. These effects diminish as the drug molecules diffuse out of the neurons into the bloodstream. The drugs are then transported to the liver for metabolism to inactive metabolites and eventual excretion in the urine.

## Methods of Administration

There are several different methods to administer local anesthesia.

- **Topical anesthesia** involves the application of ointment, lotion, cream, lotion, or drop of local anesthetic to the skin or mucous membranes in the eyes, nose, throat, mouth, urethra, anus, or rectum. These preparations are used to relieve pain and itching of dermatoses, sunburn, minor skin wounds, hemorrhoids, sore throat, and other conditions.
- **Field block anesthesia** is where nerves are blocked en masse by an anesthetic agent, not individually, to form a barrier proximal to the surgical site. This method is often used for tooth extraction.
- **Nerve block anesthesia** involves blocking a group of nerves, called a plexus or ganglion, through the injection of an anesthetic into a specific area of the body.
- Neuraxial blocks are epidural, spinal, and caudal.
- Peripheral nerve blocks involve blocking a single nerve or group of nerves such as a plexus or ganglion.

## Age-Related Considerations

Local anesthetics are used in children and older adults in much the same way as they are used in adults. Nursing care should include support and reassurance, assessing for skin breakdown related to immobility and safety precautions.

Infants are at particular risk for systemic absorption and toxicity from topically applied local anesthetics. Tight diapers and occlusive dressings can increase systemic absorption.

Older adults are more at risk for adverse effects, including neurologic, cardiovascular, and dermatologic effects. They are also more prone to developing toxicity because of possible hepatic and renal impairment and polypharmacy. Longer monitoring and regular reorientation and reassurance are important.

## Local Anesthetic Systemic Toxicity

Although the use of local anesthetics are usually safe, they have the potential to cause toxic systemic or local reactions when administered improperly and, in some cases, may cause unintended effects even when administered appropriately. **Local anesthetic systemic toxicity (LAST) is the most severe and life-threatening effect associated** with the use of any local anesthetic. The incidence of LAST is a rare but well-recognized complication that may occur with a large overdose, particularly involving inadvertent intravascular injection. The consequences may be severe, potentially resulting in death. LAST occurs when the local anesthetic is absorbed systemically, resulting in extreme central nervous system (CNS) excitation followed by cardiovascular excitation and cardiovascular collapse. Manifestations usually occur 1 to 5 minutes after the injection but may be delayed for as long as 1 hour. Initial symptoms may include analgesia, circumoral numbness, metallic taste, tinnitus or auditory changes, and agitation. These may progress to seizure activity and then lead to symptoms of CNS depression, including coma, respiratory arrest, ventricular dysrhythmias, and cardiovascular collapse.

Treatment of LAST consists of stopping the injection of the anesthetic immediately and attending to airway management, seizure suppression, and management of dysrhythmias, hypotension, and subsequent cardiac arrest. The use of lipid emulsion therapy with 20% lipid emulsion (lipid rescue therapy) is an effective antidote and should be started early in resuscitation process.

 **QSEN Alert: Safety**

Although propofol is prepared in a lipid emulsion, it should not be substituted for a 20% lipid solution for the management of LAST because the vasodilation and cardiac depression associated with a large dose of propofol may counteract resuscitation efforts.

Table 50.1 lists the common drugs administered for local anesthesia. The use of topical anesthetics is especially important in children, who are administered local anesthesia before suturing, insertion of an intravenous (IV) line, or vaccination administration. Box 50.1 summarizes the use of topical anesthesia in children.

 **QSEN Alert: Evidence-Based Practice**

Local anesthetic agents are commonly administered during labor and delivery. The most common local anesthetics used are epidural, spinal, and pudendal nerve blocks. Subcutaneous infiltration is administered before perineal tear repair. Serious adverse effects from local anesthetic agents is called local anesthetic systemic toxicity or LAST. LAST awareness has been reported worldwide. Bowsher, Deepak, and Edwards [2018] stated that the knowledge in assessing patients for adverse effects has been overlooked. Nurses need to be aware of safe maximum doses, signs and symptoms of toxicity, the immediate management of symptoms, and both the type and location of the antidote. Anesthesia providers need to inform the nurse of the maximum dose adminis-

**TABLE 50.1**

## Drugs Administered for Local Anesthesia

| Drug Class | Prototype | Other Drugs in the Class |
|---|---|---|
| Amides | Lidocaine (ReadySharp Lidocaine, Xylocaine) | Bupivacaine (Exparel, Marcaine, Sensorcaine)<br>Liposomal Bupivacaine (Exparel)<br>Dibucaine (Nupercaine)<br>Mepivacaine (Carbocaine, Polocaine)<br>Ropivacaine (Naropin) |
| Esters | Chloroprocaine (Clorotekal Nesacaine, Nesacaine-MPF) | Benzocaine (Anacaine, Anbesol, Benz-O-Sthetic, Blistex, Cepacol, Dentapaine, Topex Topical Anesthetic)<br>Tetracaine hydrochloride |

tered. Clinical features of LAST include perineal paresthesias, metallic taste in the mouth, tinnitus, dizziness, headache, muscle twitching, palpitations, seizures, confusion, cardiac arrhythmias, hypotension, shock, bradycardia, tachycardia, respiratory depression, respiratory arrest, and cardiac arrest. Anesthesia providers in this study were asked to name three clinical features. Overall, only 9% could name three symptoms. In conclusion, nurses caring for these patients in the postpartum phase should be able to assess and identify patients who are at risk for LAST and report to the patient's health care provider.

## NCLEX Success

1. A 50-year-old patient is 1-day postoperative following abdominal surgery for resection of colon cancer. Which of the following pain control devices is most effective in treating his pain?

   A. lidocaine using IV regional anesthesia
   B. bupivacaine by the epidural route
   C. benzocaine by the transdermal route
   D. fentanyl citrate by patient-controlled analgesia

2. Local anesthetics reduce the excitability neuronal cell membranes by decreasing permeability to which ion?

   A. sodium
   B. potassium
   C. chloride
   D. magnesium

## AMIDES

**Lidocaine** (ReadySharp Lidocaine, Xylocaine) is the prototype amide local anesthetic agent. The drug has a rapid effect, and when combined with epinephrine, this effect is prolonged. An additional discussion of lidocaine as a treatment for ventricular dysrhythmias is found in Chapter 27.

## Pharmacokinetics and Action

The pharmacokinetics of lidocaine depends on the route of administration. The onset of action may be almost immediate, with a peak of 2 to 5 minutes and a duration of 30 to 120 minutes. The anesthetic has an elimination half-life of 96 minutes, and therefore, a single dose should not be repeated during this period. The drug is metabolized in the liver into two active metabolites, and most is excreted in the urine.

Lidocaine diminishes pain by blocking nerve conduction. It decreases the neuronal membrane's permeability to sodium ions. This action then inhibits the depolarization and blocks nerve conduction.

## Use

Clinicians use lidocaine in its various forms to obtain local anesthesia. Specific uses include:

- Topical preparation: used to relieve pain associated with postherpetic neuralgia
- Injectable solution: used for infiltration of the skin or subcutaneous administration prior to the insertion of an IV or cen-

**BOX 50.1** *Topical Anesthesia Used in Children*

Common drugs used for topical anesthesia include:
- Eutectic mixture of local anesthetics (EMLA): This cream-based mixture of lidocaine and prilocaine is applied to intact skin. The cream penetrates intact skin to provide local anesthesia and decrease pain of vaccinations and venipuncture. The cream is applied at the injection site with an occlusive dressing at least 60 minutes before the vaccination or venipuncture. EMLA should never be applied to abraded skin or mucous membranes.
- Lidocaine, epinephrine, and tetracaine (LET): This combination of lidocaine (4%), epinephrine (0.1%), and tetracaine (0.5%) is an aqueous solution or gel that blocks the sen-

sory and motor nerves. It inhibits axonal sodium channels, thus blocking conduction of action potential. Epinephrine causes local vasoconstriction, whereas lidocaine and tetracaine produce numbness and weakness. It is used for laceration repair.
- Needle-free lidocaine delivery: Lidocaine is administered by compressed gas. It reduces pain at the site of venipunctures or intravenous line insertion.
- Liposomal lidocaine (LMX 4 or LMX 5): This solution contains lidocaine encapsulated in liposomes. It is applied to intact skin with the use of an occlusive dressing.

**TABLE 50.2**

**DRUGS AT A GLANCE: Amides**

| Drug | Pregnancy Category | Routes and Dosage Ranges | |
|---|---|---|---|
| | | **Adults** | **Children** |
| Ⓟ **Lidocaine** (ReadySharp Lidocaine, Xylocaine; ✹ Cathejell, Jelido, Lidodan, Xylocaine) | B | Maximum single dose, 300 mg, with epinephrine 500 mg; do not repeat within 2 h<br>Infiltration, 0.5% or 1%<br>Peripheral nerve block, 1% or 2%, 3–40 mL<br>Epidural, 1%, 1.5%, or 2%, 20–30 mL in 3–5 mL increments, allowing time to detect toxic manifestations<br>Saddle block, 1% with dextrose<br>Topical, 2.5%–5% jelly, ointment, cream, solution | Anesthesia, local injectable, 5 mg/kg/dose not to exceed adult maximum dose of 300 mg/dose; do not repeat within 2 h; administer lowest concentrations to allow for larger volumes |
| Bupivacaine (Exparel, Marcaine, Sensorcaine, Bupivacaine Spinal; ✹ Marcaine, Sensorcaine) | C | Maximum single dose, 175 mg, with epinephrine 200 mg<br>Local anesthesia, 0.25%<br>Spinal, 0.75% in 8.25% dextrose, 1–2 mL<br>Epidural, 0.25% or 0.5%, 20–30 mL in 3–5 mL increments, allowing time to detect toxic manifestations<br>Caudal, 0.25% or 0.5%, 15–30 mL<br>Peripheral nerve block, 0.25% or 0.5%, 3–40 mL | ≥12 y, same as adults<br>Caudal, 0.25%, 0.5–1.25 mL/kg, not to exceed 2.5 mg/kg |
| Mepivacaine (Carbocaine, Polocaine, Scandonest Plain; ✹ Carbocaine, Polocaine) | C | Maximum single dose, 300 mg, with epinephrine 500 mg<br>Infiltration, 0.5% or 1%, up to 40 mL of 1% solution<br>Therapeutic block pain management, 1–5 mL of 1% solution (max dose 50 mg)<br>Caudal and epidural block, 15–30 mL of 1% solution (max 300 mg) or 10–25 mL solution (max 375 mg) or 10–20 mL of 2% solution (max 400 mg) | Local or regional anesthesia: max single or total dose for one procedure 5–6 mg/kg (to adult max); only concentration <2% should be used in children <3 y or <14 kg |
| Ropivacaine (Naropin; ✹ Naropin) | B | Maximum single dose, 200 mg, with epinephrine 250 mg<br>Infiltration, 0.2% or 0.5%<br>Epidural, 0.5%, 0.75%, or 1%, 15–30 mL<br>Peripheral nerve block, 0.5% or 0.75%, 10–40 mL | Caudal, 0.2%, 0.5–1.25 mL/kg, not to exceed 2 mg/kg<br>Epidural, 0.2%, 0.7 mL/kg (wait 45 min for repeat dosing, reduce dose by 1/3–1/2) |

tral venous catheter, spinal, epidural, or a minor emergency procedure such as suturing or a minor surgical procedure.

- 1% to 2% solution: administered intravenously preceding administration of a painful IV medication such as propofol (Diprivan) in the surgical arena. Lidocaine 1% to 2% is also used in conjunction with other local anesthetics to achieve **epidural anesthesia**, appropriate for surgical procedures, treatment of postoperative pain, or management of labor pain. In addition, it can be administered as surface anesthesia for a diagnostic procedure of the upper respiratory tract, such as a medical thoracoscopy.
- 0.5% to 2% solution: administered for IV regional anesthesia. **Bier block anesthesia** is regional limb anesthesia produced by a local anesthetic such as lidocaine and a pneumatic extremity tourniquet. The tourniquet prevents lidocaine and blood flow from the extremity to enter the general circulation.
- 4% solution: administered through a nebulizer and inhaled into the lungs to produce anesthesia for a diagnostic procedure, such as a bronchoscopy.
- 2% and 4% viscous solution: administered for topical oropharyngeal anesthesia (gargle, or swish, and spit

for oral anesthesia, swallow for pharyngeal anesthesia), awake fiberoptic intubation and bronchoscopy, and upper endoscopy.

Table 50.2 gives route and dosage information for lidocaine and other amide local anesthetics.

## Adverse Effects

Adverse effects of lidocaine are often dose related and vary with the route of administration. They include allergic reactions (e.g., skin rash; itching; hives; swelling of the face, lips, or tongue), swelling, burning and pain at application site, headache, shivering, and nausea and vomiting.

## Contraindications

A known hypersensitivity or allergic reaction to an amide local anesthetic rules out the use of lidocaine in any form. Any patient may experience hypersensitivity reactions to any local anesthetic. If lidocaine is combined with sulfites, the patient may develop a laryngospasm. Other contraindications include severe trauma, sepsis, blood dyscrasias, and cardiac abnormalities, including heart block.

## Nursing Implications

### Preventing Interactions

Some medications interact with lidocaine, increasing or decreasing its effects (Box 50.2). St. John's wort decreases the serum concentration of the anesthetic.

### Administering the Medication

The nurse ensures that the appropriate preparation of lidocaine is administered properly. For topical anesthesia, it is necessary to:

- Apply the gel formulation to the skin of the affected area, approximately 1/8 inch thick. The area becomes numb in 20 to 60 minutes.
- Swish the oral solution in the mouth and then spit it out. When pharyngeal anesthesia is needed, the patient gargles and then swallows the medication.
- Apply Lidoderm to the most painful area of the skin. Patients should not expose this preparation to an external heat source such as a heating pad.
- Apply the lido patch (lidocaine and menthol) to the most painful area of the skin after removing the protective film. First, remove the old patch and cleanse the skin.
- Use a nebulizer following dilution in normal saline or sterile water.

>  **QSEN Alert: Safety**
>
> Although lidocaine is administered intravenously for specific conditions (e.g., to mitigate venous irritation with propofol administration and for ventricular dysrhythmias), only a qualified provider should administer the injectable form of lidocaine as a peripheral nerve block. When administering lidocaine for a peripheral nerve block, the practitioner will aspirate prior to starting injection and then every 5 mL thereafter (for larger injection volumes) to prevent accidental intravenous injection.

### Assessing for Therapeutic Effects

The therapeutic effect of lidocaine is dependent on the route of administration, concentration of the medication, vascularization of the site, and the patient's physical condition. The nurse assesses the patient's sense of touch at 2 to 5 minutes after the application of lidocaine to determine if the patient is experiencing numbness at the site. It is also important to ask the patient if he or she senses any pain, pressure, or discomfort. The nurse should ask the patient questions throughout the procedure to determine if feeling is returning to the site.

### Assessing for Adverse Effects

The nurse assesses the skin for redness, hives, or rash, indicating a hypersensitivity reaction. It is necessary to assess the respiratory status and lung sounds for signs of bronchospasm related to hypersensitivity. (Respiratory adverse effects are more common when lidocaine is administered by nebulizer.) The nurse observes for CNS symptoms (i.e., altered taste, anxiety, agitation, paresthesia), which typically occur before seizure activity. Also, she or he assesses the cardiovascular status for tachycardia and hypertension, leading to cardiovascular collapse. Ongoing patient monitoring should occur after administration of the drug for at least 12 hours because cardiovascular depression due to local anesthetics can persist or recur.

>  **QSEN Alert: Safety**
>
> Facilities that commonly administer local anesthetics in doses sufficient to produce LAST are more prepared to correct this medical emergency if they have an established and regularly reviewed plan for management of LAST as well as a readily available local anesthetic toxicity kit and instructions for its use. This kit includes 20% Intralipid (20% IV fat emulsion). Any site where regional anesthesia is administered should have this available.

### Patient Teaching

Box 50.3 identifies patient teaching guidelines for lidocaine.

## Other Drugs in the Class

Bupivacaine (Exparel, Marcaine, Sensorcaine) is used for local, regional, and **spinal anesthesia** for diagnostic and therapeutic procedures. The drug is more potent and has a longer duration of action than lidocaine, procaine, or mepivacaine. Consequently, if systemically absorbed, the drug has a higher risk of toxicity than most other local anesthetics, and patients often have seizures as the first manifestation of toxicity. It is important to administer a test dose before the full dosage and ensure that resuscitative equipment is available. Bupivacaine is contraindicated for local infiltration in pregnant women.

---

**BOX 50.2** **Drug Interactions: Lidocaine**

**Drugs That Increase the Effects of Lidocaine**
- Antidysrhythmic drugs (amiodarone, dronedarone, beta-adrenergic blockers mexiletine), barbiturates, conivaptan, and darunavir
  *Increase serum concentration*
- Procainamide
  *Increases the neurologic and cardiac effects*

---

**BOX 50.3**  **Patient Teaching Guidelines for Lidocaine**

- Report pain.
- Report tachycardia and anxiety.
- Do not drink fluids or eat after gargling with viscous lidocaine for at least 60 minutes due to risk of aspiration.
- Prior to applying lido patch, remove the old patch, cleanse the skin, and apply the new patch to the most painful site.

The U.S. Food and Drug Administration (FDA) has issued a **BLACK BOX WARNING ◆** alerting providers to the risk in obstetrical patients of cardiac arrest with difficult resuscitation or death with the use of 0.75% concentration of bupivacaine for epidural anesthesia. Caution should be used with the drug in the elderly, debilitated, and acutely ill patients. The 0.75% concentration is used for spinal anesthesia, typically for surgical procedures where a high degree of muscle relaxation and prolonged effects are necessary, including when prolonged postprocedure pain control is preferred.

Mepivacaine (Carbocaine, Polocaine) is used to produce local or regional analgesia. It is also used for local infiltration, peripheral neural, and central neural with epidural and caudal anesthesia. Adverse effects include hypersensitivity and LAST.

## NCLEX Success

3. Which of the following medications prolongs the effect of local anesthetics?

    A. propofol
    B. epinephrine
    C. calcium
    D. labetalol

4. A patient has been administered lidocaine via an epidural. Which of the following symptoms indicate the patient is having an adverse reaction to the anesthesia? (Select all that apply.)

    A. blood pressure of 130/86 mm Hg
    B. metallic taste in mouth
    C. pulse rate of 76 beats/min
    D. crackles in the right lower lobe of the lung
    E. circumoral numbness
    F. anxiety

### Clinical Application 50.1

- How does lidocaine produce numbness in Lexi's knee?
- What assessments does the nurse make to determine whether Lexi is anesthetized so that the wound can be cleaned?

## ESTERS

**Chloroprocaine hydrochloride** (Nesacaine, Nesacaine-MPF) serves as the prototype ester local anesthetic. The decreasing use of the esters has significantly decreased the frequency of anaphylaxis with local anesthetics as most allergic reactions are due to para-aminobenzoic acid, the common metabolic product of esters.

## Pharmacokinetics

Chloroprocaine is absorbed rapidly at the injection site. The onset of action is 6 to 12 minutes, with a duration of 1 hour. The serum half-life varies with the age of the patient. In adults, the half-life elimination is 20 to 25 seconds; in neonate, half-life

 neonate

elimination is about 43 seconds. The drug is rapidly metabolized in the liver into two active metabolites, and most is excreted in the urine unchanged. As a result or rapid metabolism, the drug can be used in large doses producing rapid onset of action with short duration of action.

## Action

The action of chloroprocaine is similar to that of lidocaine. Chloroprocaine reversibly decreases the influx of sodium into the nerve cell and depresses depolarization to prevent conduction of the nerve impulse.

## Use

Chloroprocaine is used to produce local anesthesia by nerve block, infiltration, caudal, or epidural blocks. The utility of chloroprocaine is generally limited to epidural anesthesia where a very rapid onset is desired (emergent cesarean section). Chloroprocaine's short duration of action limits its use otherwise.

### ! QSEN Alert: Safety

Chloroprocaine is available with and without preservatives. Chloroprocaine with preservatives should not be used for lumbar or caudal epidural anesthesia.

Table 50.3 gives route and dosage information for chloroprocaine and other ester local anesthetics.

## Adverse Effects and Contraindications

The most severe adverse effects of chloroprocaine, as with lidocaine, include LAST and hypersensitivity reactions.

Contraindications include known hypersensitivity to chloroprocaine or similar drugs that contain para-aminobenzoic acid. The drug should not be used for subarachnoid administration.

## Nursing Implications

### Preventing Interactions

Sulfonamides and antihypertensive drugs may cause hypotension. In addition, St. John's wort decreases the serum concentration of chloroprocaine.

### Assessing for Therapeutic and Adverse Effects

Assessing for the therapeutic and adverse effects of chloroprocaine is the same as for lidocaine. The therapeutic effect of chloroprocaine is dependent on the route of administration, concentration of the medication, vascularization of the site, and the patient's physical condition. It is necessary to assess the sense of touch and to ask the patient if he or she senses any pain, pressure, or discomfort.

In addition, the nurse assesses the skin for redness, hives, or rash, indicating a hypersensitivity reaction. It is necessary to assess the respiratory status and lung sounds for signs of bronchospasm related to hypersensitivity. The nurse assesses the CNS for excitability and the cardiovascular status for tachycardia and hypertension, leading to cardiovascular collapse.

**TABLE 50.3**

## DRUGS AT A GLANCE: Esters

| Drug | Pregnancy Category | Routes and Dosage Ranges | |
|---|---|---|---|
| | | **Adults** | **Children** |
| ℗ **Chloroprocaine** (Clorotekal, Nesacaine) | C | Max single dose, 800 mg, with epinephrine 1000 mg Infiltration, 1% or 2% Epidural or caudal, 2% or 3%, 15–25 mL Peripheral nerve block, 1% or 2%, 0.5–10 mL | Max dose (without epinephrine), 11 mg/kg Infiltration, 0.5% or 1% Peripheral nerve block, 1%–1.5% |
| Benzocaine (Anacaine, Anbesol, Benz-O-Sthetic, Blistex, Cepacol, Dentapaine, Topex Topical Anesthetic) | C | Topical anesthesia, 1–2 drops of 0.5% solution or 1.25–2.5 cm of ointment in the lower conjunctival fornix or 0.5% solution or ointment to the nose or throat; spray 5%, 1 spray up to four times daily | Check product insert for pediatric dosage |
| Tetracaine (🍁 Ametop) | C | Topical anesthesia, 1–2 drops of 0.5% solution or 1/25–2.5 cm of ointment in lower conjunctival fornix or 0.5% solution or ointment to nose or throat Spinal anesthesia, 2.5–15 mg; dosage varies with anesthetic procedure | Check product insert for pediatric dosage |

Do not use solutions if crystals, cloudiness, or discoloration is present.

### Patient Teaching

Box 50.4 identifies patient teaching guidelines for chloroprocaine.

## Other Drugs in the Class

Benzocaine (Anacaine, Anbesol, Benz-O-Sthetic, Blistex, Cepacol, Dentapaine, Topex Topical Anesthetic) is a topical ester local anesthetic applied for skin irritation related to minor burns, sunburns, and insect bites. There are many other trade names for benzocaine. The names listed are noted to be the most common. Application of the 5% to 20% topical solution relieves hemorrhoid pain. The use of oral solutions relieves mouth and gum irritation, such as teething pain in infants greater than or equal to 4 months of age.

Tetracaine is a topical, ophthalmic, and spinal anesthetic that is metabolized in the liver and excreted in the urine. The topical preparation can be applied to the skin prior to IV catheter placement or venipuncture. While the topical form should not be applied to the eyes, ears, mucous membranes, or broken skin, ophthalmic drops are instilled in the eye for ocular procedures. When administering the drops, care is necessary so the eye is not touched with the applicator. Spinal anesthesia is accomplished by the injection of tetracaine in the subarachnoid space. The patient is at risk for cardiac arrest if the medication is administered too rapidly. As with any neuraxial or regional nerve block, it is important to have resuscitation equipment available.

### BOX 50.4 📋 Patient Teaching Guidelines for Procaine

- Following dental procedures, do not eat or drink until numbness disappears and swallowing reflex is intact.
- When numbness dissipates following spinal anesthesia, do not ambulate without assistance until instructed to do so.
- Report anxiety, rash, hives, or redness.

### NCLEX Success

5. A child returns to school after a dental procedure requiring anesthesia. He visits the school nurse's office to take his pain medication. The most important assessment the nurse should make prior to the administration of the pain medication is to assess the
   A. prescription for an expiration date
   B. child's blood pressure and pulse
   C. child's mouth for bleeding
   D. child's mouth for numbness

6. The rationale for withholding food or fluids following the application of a local anesthetic to the mouth or throat is to
   A. prevent aspiration
   B. prevent infection
   C. minimize a hypersensitivity reaction
   D. enhance pain control

### Clinical Application 50.2

- What does the nurse teach Lexi's mother about the anesthetic?

## THE NURSING PROCESS

A concept map outlines the nursing process related to drug therapy considerations in this chapter. Additional nursing implications related to the disease process should also be considered in care decisions.

**Assessment**
- Assess the patient's status in relation to the application and response of the local anesthetic.
- Assess his or her understanding of the administration of the topical, spinal, and epidural anesthesia.
- Interview him or her regarding any past experience with anesthesia, particularly the development of LAST.
- Identify what medications, both prescription and over-the-counter or complementary and alternative therapies, he or she is taking.
- Assess his or her skin integrity.
- If the patient is to receive local anesthesia for treatment of an injury, assess his or her psychosocial response to the injury and administration of local anesthesia.
- If the patient is to receive local anesthesia for a procedure, assess his or her vital signs preprocedure, immediately following the administration of the local anesthetic, throughout the procedure, and postprocedure.

**Outcomes of Therapy**
The patient will
- Experience a reduced level of anxiety in the preprocedure and postprocedure phases.
- Understand the benefits and risks of local anesthesia.
- Have no adverse effects from local anesthesia.
- Understand the expected outcome or limitations of local anesthesia, including the following:
  - Postprocedure pain
  - Limited mobility
  - Recovery

**Nursing Interventions**
- Instruct the patient to report symptoms of redness, hives, or rash.
- Instruct the patient to report anxiety.
- Provide accurate information to the patient regarding surgery, emergency care, the diagnostic procedure, or during the obstetrical delivery.
- Assess the patient's psychosocial status.
- Monitor vital signs before, during, and after the local anesthetic has been administered.
- Instruct the patient about postanesthesia care.

**Evaluation**
- Be familiar with your institution's practice guidelines and benchmark goals to help direct therapy and evaluate recovery from anesthesia.
- Observe that patient planning/goals are met.
- Assess the effectiveness of perioperative nursing interventions and medication therapy.

## KEY CONCEPTS

- Local anesthetics are given to produce loss of sensation and motor activity. These drugs prevent the cells from responding to pain impulses and sensory stimulation.
- The loss of sensation from local anesthetics occurs in the following sequence: temperature, touch, proprioception, and skeletal muscle tone.
- Local anesthetic agents may be administered topically or through field or nerve blocks.

- LAST is the most severe and life-threatening effect with the administration of any local anesthetic.
- Lidocaine is the prototype amide local anesthetic.
- Chloroprocaine is the prototype ester local anesthetic.
- The FDA has issued a **BLACK BOX WARNING ◆** for bupivacaine, alerting providers to the risk in obstetrical patients of cardiac arrest with difficult resuscitation or death following the use of 0.75% concentration of bupivacaine for epidural anesthesia.

## CLINICAL REASONING CASE STUDY

**Meet the Patient**

Cassandra Powell, a staff nurse in the outpatient surgery center, is the preceptor of Jordan Maynor, a nursing student. Ms. Maynor is observing a bilateral inguinal herniorrhaphy under local anesthesia. The surgeon is planning to infiltrate the skin with 2% lidocaine with epinephrine prior to the skin incision followed by bupivacaine, 0.5%. Ms. Maynor asks the nurse why the surgeon is using two local anesthetics. She also asks her what nursing observations should be made to assess for therapeutic and adverse effects of the drug therapy. What is the best response by the nurse to these questions?

**Assessing Drug Information**

1. Lidocaine with epinephrine
   • Action
      • Lidocaine diminishes pain by blocking nerve conduction. It decreases the neuronal membrane's permeability to sodium ions. This action then inhibits the depolarization and blocks nerve conduction.
      • Lidocaine is the prototype amide local anesthetic agent. More than one local anesthetic can be combined to decrease onset time while providing longer lasting analgesia. Lidocaine has a rapid effect, and, when combined with epinephrine, this effect is prolonged.
      • Epinephrine works to stimulate alpha-, beta$_1$-, and beta$_2$-adrenergic receptors, resulting in relaxation of smooth muscle of the bronchial tree, cardiac stimulation, and dilation of skeletal muscle vasculature; small doses can cause vasodilation via beta$_2$-vascular receptors.
      • Tachycardia and hypertension occurring after the local anesthetic is injected indicate inadvertent injection into the vascular system; these symptoms result from epinephrine's effects.

**Assessing Drug Information**

• Uses
      • Clinicians use lidocaine in its various forms to obtain local anesthesia.
      • Epinephrine is a vasoconstrictor that has multiple uses; its use as an adjunct added to peripheral nerve blocks decreases the absorption of the local anesthetic from tissues.
   • Adverse Effects
      • Adverse effects with lidocaine are often dose-related and vary with the route of administration. In general, allergic reactions (e.g., skin rash, itching, hives, swelling of the face, lips, or tongue), swelling, burning and pain at application site, headache, shivering, and nausea and vomiting have been reported.
      • Adverse effects from epinephrine include tachycardia and a potential for ischemia to nerves and other tissues.

2. Bupivacaine
   • Action
      • Blocks both the initiation and conduction of nerve impulses by decreasing the neuronal membrane's permeability to sodium ions, which results in inhibition of depolarization with resultant blockade of conduction
      • The drug is more potent and has a longer duration of action than lidocaine, procaine, or mepivacaine.
   • Uses
      • The drug is used for local, regional, and spinal anesthesia for diagnostic and therapeutic procedures.
   • Adverse Effects
      • If systemically absorbed, the drug has a higher risk of toxicity than most other local anesthetics and patients often have seizures as the first manifestation of toxicity.
      • Greatest adverse effect is the development of local anesthetic systemic toxicity (LAST), which can occur with inadvertent injection into the vascular system.

**Nursing Actions**

• During the perioperative period, assess vital signs, state of consciousness, signs of CNS toxicity, or allergic reaction.
• Should LAST occur, stop the injection immediately and pay attention to airway management; seizure suppression; and management of dysrhythmias, hypotension, and subsequent cardiac arrest.
   • The use of lipid rescue therapy has proven successful with potent lipophilic anesthetics such as bupivacaine.
   • Immediate management includes cardiopulmonary resuscitation (CPR), advanced cardiac life support (ACLS), and treatment for ventricular fibrillation (e.g., epinephrine or vasopressin, defibrillation). Unfortunately, bupivacaine-associated cardiovascular toxicity is often very difficult to reverse.

*Visit* thePoint® *at* **http://thePoint.lww.com/Frandsen12e** *for answers to NCLEX Success questions (in Appendix A), answers to Clinical Application Case Studies (in Appendix B), and more!*

## REFERENCES AND RESOURCES

Baldor, R., & Mathes, B. M. (2017). Digital nerve block. In J. Grayzel (Ed.). *UpToDate*. Wolters Kluwer.

Balocco, A. L., Van Zumder, P. G. E., Gan, S. S., Gan, T. J., & Hadzic, A. (2018). Extended release bupivacaine formulations for postoperative analgesia: An update. *Anesthesiology, 31*(5), 636–642.

Bowsher, G. M., Deepak, S., & Edwards, A. (2018). Multidisciplinary knowledge of local anaesthetic system toxicity in maternity care: A pilot study. *British Journal of Midwifery, 26*(2), 103–108.

Butterworth, J. F. & Lahaye, L. (2018). Clinical use of local anesthetics in anesthesia. In M. Crowley (Ed.). *UpToDate*. Wolters Kluwer.

Chung, A. S., & Spangehl, M. J. (2018). Peripheral nerve blocks vs periarticular injections in total knee arthroplasty. *The Journal of Arthroplasty, 33*, 3383–3388.

Flood, P., Rathmell, J. P., & Shafer, S. (2015). *Stoelting's pharmacology & physiology in anesthetic practice* (5th ed.). Philadelphia, PA: Wolters Kluwer.

Hsu, D. C. (2018a). Subcutaneous infiltration of local anesthetics. In J. F. Wiley (Ed.). *UpToDate*. Wolters Kluwer.

Hsu, D. C. (2018b). Clinical use of topical anesthetics in children. In J. F. Wiley (Ed.). *UpToDate*. Wolters Kluwer.

Karch, A. M. (2018). *2019 Lippincott's pocket drug guide for nurses*. Philadelphia, PA: Wolters Kluwer.

Kumar, K., Kirksey, M. A., Duong, S., & Wu, C. L. (2017). A review of opioid-sparing modalities in perioperative pain management: Methods to decrease opioid use postoperatively. *Anesthesia & Analgesia, 125*(5), 1749–1760.

Miller, R. D., Cohen, N. H., Eridsson, L. I., Fleisher, L. A., Wiener-Kronish, J. P., & Young, W. L. (2015). *Miller's anesthesia* (8th ed.). Philadelphia, PA: Elsevier Saunders.

Neal, J. M., Woodward, C. M., & Harrison, R. K. (2018). The American Society of Regional Anesthesia and Pain Medicine checklist for managing local anesthetic systemic toxicity: 2017 version. *Regional Anesthesia and Pain Medicine, 43*, 150–153.

Norris, T. L. (2019). *Porth's Pathophysiology: Concepts of altered health status* (10th ed.). Philadelphia, PA: Lippincott Williams & Wilkins.

Patacsil, J. A., McAuliffe, M. S., Feyh, L. S., & Sigmon, L. L. (2016). Local anesthetic adjuvants providing the longest duration of analgesia for single-injection peripheral nerve blocks in orthopedic surgery: A literature review. *AANA Journal, 84*(2), 95–103.

Schatz, M. (2018). Allergic reactions to local anesthetics. In A. M. Fedweg (Ed.). *UpToDate*. Wolters Kluwer.

Suresh, S., Ecoffey, C., & Bosenberg, A. (2018). The European society of regional anaesthesia and pain therapy/American society of regional anesthesia and pain medicine recommendations on local anesthetics and adjuvants dosage in pediatric regional anesthesia. *Regional Anesthesia and Pain Medicine, 43*(2), 211–216.

Tayeb, B. O., Eidelman, A., Eidelman, C. L., McNicol, E. D., & Carr, D. B. (2017). Topical anaesthetics for pain control during repair of dermal laceration. *Cochrane Database of Systematic Reviews, 2*, CD005364. doi:10.1002/14651858.CD005364.pub3

Urman, R. D., & Ehrenfeld, J. M. (2016). *Pocket anesthesia* (3rd ed.). Philadelphia, PA: Wolters Kluwer Health.

Wick, E. D., Grant, J. C., & Wu, C. L. (2017). Postoperative multimodal analgesia pain management with nonopioid analgesics and techniques: A review. *JAMA Surgery, 152*(7), 691–697.

UpToDate. (2019). *Drug information*. Lexi-Comp, Inc.

# Drug Therapy
# With General Anesthetics

## LEARNING OBJECTIVES

*After studying this chapter, you should be able to:*

1. Define general anesthesia.
2. Describe the three phases of general anesthesia.
3. Identify the fundamental principles of balanced anesthesia.
4. Describe how inhalation anesthetics are delivered and describe how this process is different from intravenous anesthetics.
5. Identify the prototype and describe the action, use, adverse effects, contraindications, and nursing implications for the inhalation and intravenous general anesthetic agents.
6. Identify the prototype and describe the action, use, adverse effects, contraindications, and nursing implications for the neuromuscular blocking agents.
7. Identify the prototype and describe the action, use, adverse effects, contraindications, and nursing implications for the adjuvant medications administered to patients receiving general anesthesia.
8. Implement the nursing process in the care of patients receiving general anesthesia.

## CLINICAL APPLICATION CASE STUDY

Harriet Wilberson is a mildly obese 60-year-old woman with chronic cholecystitis and a history of allergic asthma. Despite dietary modification, she continues to have right abdomen pain, nausea, and bloating sensation. Ms. Wilberson believes that her numerous food allergies are the cause of these symptoms. She is scheduled for a laparoscopic cholecystectomy in an ambulatory surgical facility. Because Ms. Wilberson has an anaphylactic penicillin allergy, the surgeon has ordered preoperative intravenous gentamicin and clindamycin. The anesthesia practitioner has completed a preanesthetic evaluation and plans to administer a general endotracheal anesthetic. You are the nurse assigned to her care.

## KEY TERMS

**Amnesia:** memory loss (of limited duration in anesthesia)

**Analgesia:** reduction or absence of pain

**Balanced anesthesia:** four elements of general anesthesia (amnesia, analgesia, hypnosis, and muscle relaxation) achieved by a combination of medications to produce a state of physiologic and pharmacologic equilibrium

**Emergence:** return to consciousness from general anesthesia

**Fasciculation:** transitory muscle contractions that occur after the administration of a depolarizing muscle relaxant

**General anesthesia:** medication-induced reversible unconsciousness with loss of protective reflexes

**Hypnosis:** unconsciousness

**Induction:** rendering the patient unconscious by using inhalation anesthetics, intravenous anesthetics, or both

**Maintenance anesthesia:** administering a continuous level of inhalation and/or intravenous anesthetic to sustain general anesthesia until the procedure is complete

**Malignant hyperthermia:** potentially fatal hypermetabolic response after exposure to volatile inhalation anesthetics or the drug succinylcholine

**Minimum alveolar concentration:** quantitative measure of the potency of inhalation anesthetics

**Monitored anesthesia care:** sedation administered by an anesthesia practitioner

**Rapid sequence induction:** intubation procedure that uses cricoid pressure and omits face mask ventilation to reduce the risk of aspiration

**Recurarization:** residual weakness after assumed recovery from the effects of nondepolarizing muscle relaxants (also referred to as residual neuromuscular blockade)

**Total intravenous anesthesia:** a method of general anesthesia that replaces the inhalation agent with an intravenous anesthetic for the induction and maintenance of anesthesia

## INTRODUCTION

This chapter introduces the fundamentals of general anesthesia and the implementation of nursing care during the administration of general anesthesia. The administration of general anesthesia is a complex task that requires the expertise of a certified registered nurse anesthetist (CRNA), anesthesiologist (physician), or both. The CRNA and anesthesiologist may practice independently or as a team. They are physically present and actively providing care during the entire anesthetic process.

The goal of this chapter is to learn the basic aspects of anesthesia and anesthetic medications. With knowledge of anesthesia drug classes and their actions, the nurse is able to recognize adverse consequences and intervene to avoid detrimental outcomes. In some circumstances, complications arising from anesthesia can be immediately life threatening. For this reason, the operating room and postanesthesia care unit (PACU) must be a controlled environment to promote patient safety. The nurse must have an organized differential approach to clinical problems. It is necessary to provide lifesaving interventions and then seek the cause of the difficulty. Airway, breathing, circulation, and supplemental oxygen is an important approach to all clinical problems. Fortunately, present-day anesthetic medications are generally safe with rapid onset and recovery. Because this chapter is not about medication therapy for a disease process, the content focuses on understanding the medications, adverse effects (or after effects), and nursing care.

## OVERVIEW OF GENERAL ANESTHESIA

**General anesthesia** is defined as a medication-induced reversible unconsciousness with loss of protective reflexes. There is the misconception that general anesthesia is a deep sleep. It is much deeper and more like a drug-induced coma. Arousal, even to painful stimuli, cannot occur. Therefore, it is possible to perform surgery or other unpleasant therapeutic or diagnostic procedures such as endoscopy or interventional radiology that would be unreasonable or impossible to accomplish in a conscious person.

## Clinical Manifestations

The concept of using several drugs to achieve a state of physiologic and pharmacologic equilibrium under general anesthesia is called **balanced anesthesia**. Balanced anesthesia refers to the following four elements of general anesthesia designed to work collectively to produce a superior outcome:

1. **Amnesia** or memory loss (of limited duration in anesthesia)
2. **Analgesia** or a reduction or absence of pain
3. **Hypnosis** or unconsciousness
4. Muscle relaxation or immobility

Suppression of the sympathetic nervous system in response to noxious stimuli is also desired. Depending on the procedure, the anesthesia practitioner combines one or more of these elements by selecting appropriate medications. Generally, a major surgical procedure that requires tracheal intubation requires all of these elements to some degree.

## Drug Therapy

Selection of anesthesia and adjuvant medications depends on a variety of conditions. This includes the requirements of the procedure, the patient's age and health status, medical conditions, weight, drug allergies, the results of laboratory or diagnostic tests, and the patient's and/or surgeon's preferences (if relevant). Using this information, the anesthesia practitioner develops a plan of care that maintains the patients' health and physiologic homeostasis. The U.S. Food and Drug Administration (FDA) warns that lengthy or repeated use of general anesthetic and sedation drugs during surgeries or procedures in pediatric patients younger than 3 years or in pregnant women during their third trimester may affect the children's neurologic development.

The administration of a general anesthetic can be divided into three phases. The first phase is **induction**, which is rendering the patient unconscious by using inhalation anesthetics, intravenous anesthetics, or both. Adult patients usually receive a rapid-acting intravenous anesthetic medication. Pediatric patients more often breathe an inhalation anesthetic through a face mask. Called a mask induction, this allows an anesthesia practitioner or a nurse to perform the venipuncture for intravenous solutions after the patient is under general anesthesia. Before induction, the patient, whether adult or child, may receive a benzodiazepine that provides rapid anxiolytic and amnestic effects. The induction phase also includes securing and maintaining a patent airway.

The next phase is maintenance or **maintenance anesthesia**, which is administering a continuous level of inhalation and/or intravenous anesthetics until the procedure is complete. Adjunctive medications may be used at this time, such as antiemetics (see Chap. 38), opioids (see Chap. 49), nonopioid analgesics, local anesthetics, and neuromuscular blocking agents.

The concluding phase is **emergence**. As the procedure ends, the general anesthetic medications are stopped, and the patient is permitted to wake up. As the patient emerges from the anesthetic, the anesthesia practitioner may use medications to reverse the effects of neuromuscular blocking agents. The patient is then transported to the PACU or perhaps the intensive care unit (ICU) for close observation, monitoring of vital signs and neurologic status, and additional nursing or medical care.

Five drug classes are used to achieve balanced anesthesia: benzodiazepines, analgesics, inhalation anesthetics, intravenous anesthetics, and neuromuscular blocking agents. Benzodiazepines or inhalation anesthetics are used to achieve amnesia. Opioid or nonopioid medications are used to achieve analgesia. Inhalation or intravenous anesthetics are used to achieve hypnosis. Neuromuscular blocking agents and, to some extent, inhalation anesthetics are used to achieve muscle relaxation. Within each class, every medication has unique properties that determine onset, duration, elimination, and other characteristics. The anesthesia practitioner can select from several medications in each class to achieve balanced anesthesia. Knowledge of the synergistic, additive, or antagonistic effects of anesthetic medications helps decide the appropriate dose and combination.

Table 51.1 lists the general anesthetics and neuromuscular blocking agents discussed in this chapter.

## INHALATION ANESTHETICS

Inhalation anesthetics are volatile organic liquids administered by inhalation for induction and maintenance of general anesthesia. Volatile means having the ability to evaporate readily and release a gas. Today's volatile inhalation anesthetics are halogenated ethers, which contain fluorine. The stability of the fluorine carbon bond helps reduce solubility, decreasing metabolism and organ toxicity. **Isoflurane** (Forane), an extremely physically stable methyl ethyl ether, is the prototype inhalation anesthetic. Although not the first inhalation anesthetic introduced for clinical use, it deserves recognition for its wide acceptance. Its improved potency, low tissue solubility and metabolism, and chemical stability earned isoflurane the gold standard. Currently, it is the most potent inhalation anesthetic available. Isoflurane has a mild pungent or ethereal odor and can irritate

### TABLE 51.1

## General Anesthetics and Neuromuscular Blocking Agents

| Drug Class | Prototype | Other Drugs in the Class |
|---|---|---|
| Inhalation anesthetics | Isoflurane (Forane) | Desflurane (Suprane) Nitrous oxide Sevoflurane (Ultane) |
| Intravenous anesthetics | Propofol (Diprivan) | Etomidate (Amidate) Ketamine (Ketalar) Methohexital (Brevital Sodium) |
| Neuromuscular blocking agents | Vecuronium | Atracurium Cisatracurium (Nimbex) Pancuronium Rocuronium Succinylcholine (Anectine, Quelicin) |
| Adjuvant drugs | | Dexmedetomidine (Precedex) Fentanyl (Sublimaze, Abstral, Actiq, Duragesic, Fentora, Ionsys, Lazanda) Midazolam (Nayzilam) |

the airways when concentration increases. Therefore, it does not lend itself to inhalation mask inductions. However, it makes an excellent maintenance anesthetic after using an intravenous induction medication.

## Pharmacokinetics

Inhalation of isoflurane results in its delivery as a gas to the lungs. From there, it diffuses rapidly into the arterial vascular system, travels throughout the vascular system, and crosses the blood–brain barrier. As the inhaled concentration of the anesthetic increases or decreases, the depth of anesthesia also changes. Several factors determine the speed of onset, but the desired level of anesthesia can be obtained in just a few minutes. The characteristics of intermediate solubility and high potency of isoflurane allow for easy regulation of the depth of anesthesia, and it is possible to sustain its effect on the brain without significant absorption into blood or body tissues. This means that induction and emergence are rapid.

Metabolism of isoflurane principally occurs in the liver, although some metabolism takes place in the kidney. Approximately 0.2% of the anesthetic undergoes complete metabolism. Therefore, absorption (uptake) and elimination are primarily through the alveoli and involve ventilation of the lungs. At the conclusion of the anesthesia, the patient receives 100% oxygen. This creates a reverse gradient, and the lungs eliminate the anesthetic. Awakening usually takes place within 10 minutes, and the patient is coherent within 15 to 30 minutes.

## Action

Isoflurane produces amnesia, skeletal muscle relaxation, and hypnosis. It therefore blocks the perception of pain. Its ability to provide analgesia is unclear. The exact mechanism of action of inhalation anesthetics has not been established. However, the drug may amplify the effect of inhibitory neurotransmitter targets such as the gamma-aminobutyric acid (GABA) and glycine receptors. Activation of brain GABA receptors results in a loss of consciousness and amnesia, and the spinal cord glycine receptors cause immobility or absence of response to noxious stimuli. The action of inhalation anesthetics also involves the antagonism of excitatory *N*-methyl-D-aspartate (NMDA) receptors and possibly other unidentified molecular sites.

Isoflurane produces a dose-dependent change in several organ systems. As the isoflurane concentration increases, blood pressure decreases and heart rate may increase.

The respiratory rate increases, but the tidal volume diminishes resulting in an overall decrease in minute ventilation. Isoflurane produces moderate bronchodilation. Once the patient emerges from general anesthesia, the depressant effects normally resolve within 30 minutes. Therefore, residual effects may be observed in the PACU. In addition, as concentration increases, there is progressive skeletal muscle relaxation likely due to the effect on spinal cord glycine receptors. This enhances the action of neuromuscular blocking agents.

## Use

Isoflurane is indicated for the induction and maintenance of general anesthesia in people of all ages, in those who are healthy, and in those who are critically ill. It can be used alone to maintain general anesthesia or more commonly in combination with other agents to produce balanced anesthesia. Table 51.2 summarizes the use of the inhalation anesthetic agents.

### Use in Patients With Renal Impairment

Isoflurane reduces renal blood flow and urine output. Adequate hydration during the perioperative period maintains normal renal function, so the drug is considered safe in patients with renal impairment or insufficiency.

### Use in Patients With Hepatic Impairment

Isoflurane is associated with very mild and brief postoperative hepatic dysfunction, but the incidence of hepatotoxicity with its use is rare. Therefore, isoflurane can be administered to patients with hepatic disease.

## Adverse Effects

Inhalation anesthetics such as isoflurane are associated with cardiovascular and respiratory depression. They can also cause airway irritation and progress to coughing, laryngospasm, or bronchospasm in susceptible patients such as smokers or asthmatics. In addition, inhalation anesthetics are known to cause postoperative nausea and vomiting (PONV), especially after 2 or more hours of exposure.

There is also a very rare possibility of immune-mediated hepatotoxicity that can result in death. In the obstetrical patient, all volatile inhalation anesthetics, including isoflurane, decrease the tone of uterine smooth muscle, increasing the risk of bleeding during surgery such as cesarean section. Additionally, an alteration in the thermoregulatory system with or without hypothermia may cause shivering after emergence.

**Malignant hyperthermia**, a genetic disorder, is a potentially fatal hypermetabolic response after exposure to volatile inhalation anesthetics or to the neuromuscular blocking agent succinylcholine. Several myopathies such as muscular dystrophy have a predisposition to malignant hyperthermia. The symptoms and their timing vary and include hypercapnia, tachycardia, elevated temperature, body rigidity, mixed metabolic and respiratory acidosis, mottling and sweating, masseter spasm (rigid jaw), hyperkalemia, elevated creatine kinase (CK), myoglobinuria, and renal failure. Prompt treatment with intravenous dantrolene sodium (Dantrium) (see Chap. 53), oxygenation and hyperventilation, hydration, and body cooling improves outcomes. Additional medications are necessary to treat the acidosis, hyperkalemia, and dysrhythmias and to prevent renal failure.

## Contraindications

Factors that rule out the use of volatile anesthetics include a family history of malignant hyperthermia, a history of hepatic dysfunction after halogenated inhalation anesthetics, or any risk

| TABLE 51.2 | | | |
|---|---|---|---|
| **DRUGS AT A GLANCE: Inhalation Anesthetics** | | | |
| **Drug** | **Pregnancy Category** | **Routes and Dosage Ranges** | |
| | | **Adults** | **Children** |
| ℗ **Isoflurane** (Forane) | C | MAC in 100% $O_2$, 30–55 y old: 1.15% (range 0.7%–2.5%) | MAC values are generally lower in newborns but higher in infants and then progressively decrease with age |
| Desflurane (Suprane) | B | MAC in 100% $O_2$, 30–55 y old: 6% (range 3%–7%) | MAC in 100% $O_2$, 9 mo old, 10%; 3 y old, 8.9% (range 5.2%–10%); dosage must be individualized based on response |
| Nitrous oxide | D or X | MAC in 100% $O_2$, 30–55 y old: 104% (range up to 70%) | Refer to adult dosing; dosage must be individualized based on response |
| Sevoflurane (Ultane) | B | MAC in 100% $O_2$, 30–55 y old: 1.85% (range 1%–3%) | MAC in 100% $O_2$, 1–6 mo, 3%; 6 mo to ≤1 y, 2.8%; 1 to ≤3 y, 2.8%; 3–12 y, 2.5% (0.5%–3%) |

MAC, minimum alveolar concentration.

of a sensitivity reaction. In patients who have a history of severe PONV, the anesthetist may substitute the inhalation anesthetic with a technique called **total intravenous anesthesia** (TIVA). TIVA replaces the inhalation agent with a less emetic and non-malignant hyperthermia triggering intravenous anesthetic for the induction and maintenance of anesthesia.

---

 **QSEN Alert: Safety**

With the exception of cesarean section, surgery while pregnant would be performed only under urgent or emergent circumstances. The benefits of surgery must outweigh the risks. Therefore, a preoperative pregnancy test is routinely ordered before elective procedures in women of childbearing age. Should a pregnant patient require surgery, the anesthesia practitioner designs effective strategies and tailors the anesthetic to avoid the possibility of patient harm, fetal teratogenicity, and premature labor.

---

The more advanced the pregnancy, the smaller the chance that the medications and inhalation anesthetics affect the unborn child. Authorities generally agree that anesthesia and surgery after the first trimester can be conducted in a safe manner and that the risk of fetal teratogenicity is minimal to nonexistent. Both the nurse and anesthesia practitioner serve as an advocate and minimize the possibility of harm to the patient and unborn child.

## Nursing Implications

Anesthesia practitioners use inhalation anesthetics widely in their daily practice. The choice of inhalation anesthetic is based on several factors such as the pharmacokinetic profile, preexisting medical conditions, and history of previous reactions.

### Preventing Interactions

Isoflurane combined with dopamine, ephedrine, epinephrine, isoproterenol, or norepinephrine may be capable of producing cardiac dysrhythmias. Alcohol and some herbs may increase the effect of isoflurane (Box 51.1).

The administration of inhalation anesthetics requires the use of an anesthesia machine. These devices vary in features and sophistication. It only takes a very small amount of anesthetic (1%–3%) to produce general anesthesia. The mixture of agents is delivered to the patient's lungs through a plastic breathing circuit that connects to a mask, endotracheal tube, or supraglottic airway device such as the laryngeal mask airway.

---

**BOX 51.1**  *Herb and Dietary Interactions: Isoflurane and Propofol*

**Herbs and Foods That May Increase the Effect of Isoflurane and Propofol**
- Alcohol
- Kava
- St. John's wort
- Valerian root

---

The term **minimum alveolar concentration** (MAC) is a quantitative measure of the potency of an anesthetic. It is the concentration of anesthetic necessary to suppress a response to pain in 50% of patients who receive a noxious stimulus such as a surgical incision. MAC values vary with the age of the patient. Furthermore, MAC values are additive. With the addition of other medications such as benzodiazepines, opioids, intravenous anesthetics, or nitrous oxide, MAC values decrease. For example, the MAC of isoflurane is 1.15% in adults when it is administered alone. However, when in combination with 70% nitrous oxide, the MAC of isoflurane decreases to 0.5%.

### Assessing for Therapeutic Effects

Assessing the patient for the therapeutic effects of inhalation anesthetics is the responsibility of the anesthesia practitioner.

### Assessing for Adverse Effects

Because inhalation anesthetics may lead to low blood pressure and respiratory depression, it is prudent to provide oxygen and frequently assess the blood pressure and quality of breathing or ventilation early in the postoperative period. Monitoring oxygen saturation as measured by pulse oximetry helps guide therapy. The nurse may treat postoperative shivering with warm blankets or forced-air warming devices. Nausea and vomiting may occur after surgery using isoflurane. Treatment involves antiemetics (see Chap. 38). If there are symptoms suspicious of malignant hyperthermia, it is imperative that the nurse notify the anesthesia practitioner immediately.

---

 **QSEN Alert: Evidence-Based Practice**

Approximately 30% to 40% of acute care facility surgeries result in perioperative kidney injury. According to McKinlay, Tyson, and Forni (2018), comorbid conditions such as diabetes, liver disease, hypertension, and chronic kidney disease combined with the type and urgency of the procedure may increase the risk for kidney injury. The choice of anesthetic agent also contributes to renal injury. The authors recommend avoiding nephrotoxic drugs to prevent kidney injury and controlling blood pressure to prevent the development of hypotension. The nurse must also monitor blood pressure and renal function in the postoperative phase.

---

### Patient Teaching

Box 51.2 identifies patient teaching guidelines for the inhalation anesthetics, including isoflurane.

## Other Drugs in the Class

Several other inhaled anesthetic agents are available. These inhalation anesthetics further reduce body tissue solubility and allow rapid induction and emergence from anesthesia making them valuable adjuncts in ambulatory surgery.

Desflurane (Suprane) is a completely fluorinated methyl ethyl ether. Of the currently available inhalation anesthetics, it is the least soluble and least potent. These characteristics favor rapid induction, emergence, and return of protective airway reflexes and negligible metabolism. Patients benefit from faster recovery and return of normal cognition. However, desflurane

## BOX 51.2 — *Patient Teaching Guidelines for General Anesthetics*

- Ask your health care practitioner for information about the administration and effects of the general anesthetic agent(s) you may receive. Feel free to ask questions. Learn about the postoperative/postprocedural recovery phase.
- If you will be receiving an intravenous anesthetic such as propofol, be aware that there may be pain, burning, or stinging when the medication is injected into the intravenous catheter and flows into the vein. (Preinduction opioids and simultaneous administration of intravenous lidocaine also help relieve the discomfort.)
- Refrain from smoking prior to surgery.
- Discontinue complementary and alternative medicine products, including herbal supplements, for 2 weeks prior to surgery.
- Do not ingest alcohol for 24 hours prior to their scheduled surgery or procedure.
- Ask your health care practitioner about diagnostic testing to screen for malignant hyperthermia or atypical plasma cholinesterase if you have a family history.

is very pungent, making mask inhalation induction impractical. Moreover, desflurane produces airway irritation and increases the incidence of coughing, breath holding, or laryngospasm. Unlike other inhalation anesthetics, desflurane may cause mild bronchoconstriction.

Sevoflurane (Ultane) is a completely fluorinated methyl isopropyl ether that has about half the potency of isoflurane. Its solubility is extremely low. Therefore, induction, emergence, and recovery are fast. In addition, sevoflurane is nonpungent and results in the least amount of airway irritation. It provides a pleasant inhalation mask induction in both adults and children without the need of an initial intravenous anesthetic. Furthermore, it produces bronchodilation similar or perhaps greater than isoflurane. These properties make sevoflurane a popular choice for patients with reactive airway disease or chronic obstructive pulmonary disease. In young children, sevoflurane is associated with emergence or postoperative agitation but does not seem to have long-term implications.

In addition to the volatile anesthetics, the inorganic inhalation agent nitrous oxide can be used in combination with other anesthetic medications. Also known as laughing gas, it is not a volatile agent like isoflurane because it is a gas at room temperature. Unfortunately, the potency of nitrous oxide is low, and it cannot produce general anesthesia by itself. However, its additive effect will permit a lower concentration or dose of the volatile or intravenous anesthetics. Nitrous oxide produces amnesia, analgesia, and euphoria. Because it has a greater solubility in blood than nitrogen, it diffuses into closed body cavities and expands. This can place undue pressure in the bowels, middle ear, and other spaces created by surgery or disease. As a result, it is contraindicated in many types of surgeries and preexisting medical conditions.

## NCLEX Success

1. The nurse is circulating in the operating room when the anesthesia practitioner declares a malignant hyperthermia emergency. Which of the following symptoms are indicative of malignant hyperthermia? Select all that apply.
   - A. muscle rigidity
   - B. bradycardia
   - C. rash
   - D. hypercapnia
   - E. increased serum creatinine *[handwritten: creatine kinase]*
   - F. hyperkalemia

2. A 32-year-old woman is admitted to the hospital for an appendectomy. She has a history of reactive airway disease. Which of the following inhalation anesthetic agents, if any, is contraindicated?
   - A. isoflurane
   - B. sevoflurane
   - C. desflurane
   - D. nitrous oxide

### Clinical Application 51.1

- The anesthesia practitioner has decided to use sevoflurane, an inhalation anesthetic, for Ms. Wilberson's cholecystectomy. Why is this anesthetic an appropriate choice?

## INTRAVENOUS GENERAL ANESTHETICS

Intravenous general anesthetics render a patient unconscious in a fast and safe manner. Introduced in 1934, the fast-acting barbiturates revolutionized the often slow and difficult procedure of inducing the surgical patient using only an inhalation anesthetic. **Propofol** (Diprivan) is the prototype intravenous anesthetic with wide acceptance and extensive use for surgical, therapeutic, and diagnostic procedures. Unlike barbiturates, awakening from propofol is associated with negligible aftereffects such as lingering sedation, confusion, and nausea. Fortunately, no intravenous anesthetic triggers malignant hyperthermia.

### Pharmacokinetics

Following intravenous administration, propofol provides smooth hypnosis in less than 1 minute. Chiefly metabolized in the liver to water-soluble inactive metabolites, the drug is excreted by the kidneys. Elimination of the anesthetic is not altered by chronic hepatic or renal impairment. Propofol, which is very lipid soluble, easily crosses the blood–brain barrier. The cessation of the effect of propofol is dependent on its redistribution away from the central nervous system (CNS). Therefore, because of both extensive redistribution and high metabolic clearance, recovery from anesthesia is rapid, usually within 10 minutes. However, very long administration times, with large dosages, can result in delayed emergence from anesthesia.

## Action

Propofol produces amnesia, euphoria, and hypnosis. It therefore blocks the perception of pain. It does not provide analgesia. Propofol causes depression of the CNS by amplifying the inhibitory neurotransmitter GABA. The action of propofol may also involve modulation of excitatory NMDA receptors, glycine receptors, and the endocannabinoid system. Furthermore, propofol has anticonvulsant properties.

Propofol produces a dose-dependent change in several organ systems. This effect is exacerbated in hypovolemia and significant cardiac disease or in elderly patients or those who are critically ill. There are reductions in blood pressure and cardiac output. The tidal volume and respiratory rate decrease and may necessitate assisted ventilation. Unlike inhalation anesthetics, propofol does not alter the actions of neuromuscular blocking agents.

## Use

Propofol is indicated for the induction and maintenance of general anesthesia. It can be used alone to maintain general anesthesia (TIVA) or more commonly combined with other medications to produce a balanced anesthesia. Because of propofol's antiemetic properties, it is frequently used for the induction and maintenance of general anesthesia with patients at high risk for PONV.

Propofol can produce bronchodilation, which is therapeutic for patients with asthma and chronic obstructive pulmonary disease. Moreover, propofol suppresses laryngeal reflexes, making it a suitable choice when inserting a supraglottic airway device.

Propofol can be titrated and used in lesser amounts to provide light, moderate, or deep sedation, in addition to its use as a general anesthetic. When an anesthesia practitioner administers propofol or similar medications for sedation, it is called **monitored anesthesia care**. During conscious or moderate sedation, the patient can be aroused with stimulation and maintains protective airway reflexes. However, anesthesia practitioners may provide deep sedation in particularly uncomfortable procedures or minor surgery. Deeply sedated patients are not easily aroused and may partially or entirely lose protective airway reflexes. The level of deep sedation can rapidly change into general anesthesia, necessitating a clinician educated in airway management and the recognition and treatment of anesthetic-related complications.

Table 51.3 summarizes the use of the intravenous anesthetics.

### Use in Children

Propofol is used for general anesthesia and short-term sedation in infants and children.

### Use in Patients With Critical Illness

Propofol is used to sedate patients on mechanical ventilation. Propofol infusion syndrome is a rare but sometimes fatal adverse effect of long-term infusion with high doses usually observed in critically ill ICU patients. The syndrome affects both children and adults and is characterized by metabolic acidosis, rhabdomyolysis, dysrhythmias, and multiorgan failure. Along with other indicators, monitoring for elevations in lactic acidosis, CK levels, and triglyceride levels helps avoid this syndrome.

### TABLE 51.3

### DRUGS AT A GLANCE: Intravenous Anesthetics

| Drug | Pregnancy Category | Routes and Dosage Ranges | |
|---|---|---|---|
| | | **Adults** | **Children** |
| (P) **Propofol** (Diprivan; ❋ Diprivan, PMS-Propofol, ACT Propofol, Diprivan) | B | Induction: Healthy: 2–2.5 mg/kg IV or 40 mg every 10 s until hypnosis Elderly or debilitated: 1–1.5 mg/kg IV or 20 mg every 10 s until hypnosis Maintenance: 50–200 mcg/kg/min IV Sedation: 10 mg IV PRN titrated to effect or 25–75 mcg/kg/min IV | Induction: Healthy: 2.5–3.5 mg/kg Debilitated: lower dose Maintenance: 125–300 mcg/kg/min IV |
| Etomidate (Amidate) | C | Induction: 0.2–0.6 mg/kg IV, average dose 0.3 mg/kg IV | Induction: 0.2–0.4 mg/kg IV (>10 y of age) |
| Ketamine (Ketalar; ❋ Ketalar) | C | Induction: 1–2 mg/kg IV Maintenance infusion: 10–30 mcg/kg/min Sedation and analgesia: 0.2–0.5 mg/kg IV PRN | Induction: 0.5–3 mg/kg IV; 5–10 mg/kg IM Maintenance infusion: 0.5–1 mg/kg IV every 15–30 min PRN |
| Methohexital (Brevital Sodium) | B | Induction: 1–2 mg/kg IV Sedation: 5–30 mg IV PRN titrated to effect | Induction: 1–2.5 mg/kg IV |

## Adverse Effects

The rapid intravenous administration of propofol can be unpleasant because of the emulsion formula. On injection, pain, burning, or stinging at the intravenous site may occur. Occasionally, hiccups and myoclonic movements are observed during induction with propofol.

## Contraindications

The anesthesia practitioner should exercise caution in patients with disorders of lipid metabolism and pancreatitis. Patients who are allergic to soybean or soy products, or eggs or egg products, should not receive propofol. Generic formulations of propofol are preservative free, whereas the trade preparation Diprivan contains disodium edetate (EDTA or metabisulfite). Metabisulfite can cause bronchoconstriction and wheezing in susceptible patients. Therefore, the anesthetic practitioner must exercise discretion in the choice of propofol formulation in patients with a history of reactive airway disease or an allergy to sulfites.

## Nursing Implications

Similar to inhalation anesthetics, propofol is widely used in daily practice. The choice of propofol is based on several factors such as the pharmacokinetic profile, preexisting medical conditions, and allergies.

### Preventing Interactions

The same foods and herbs that interact with isoflurane may also increase the effect of propofol (see Box 51.1).

### Administering the Medication

An anesthesia practitioner administers anesthesia or sedation with propofol. It may be administered in the ICU, where the nurse managing the patient must be skilled in the care of critically ill patients and educated in advanced life support, including airway management. Propofol is an intravenous drug that is either injected manually or attached to an electronic syringe pump to provide a precise dose for continuous infusion. Electronic pumps are especially useful for maintenance anesthesia or sedation.

The administration of propofol should be individualized according to concomitant anesthetic medications and comorbidities. It should be titrated to the desired effect while maintaining cardiovascular stability. Age-appropriate doses are necessary. The handling of propofol requires aseptic technique because the emulsion-based formulation favors the growth of pathogens.

### Assessing for Adverse Effects

When caring for a patient who received propofol, the hypnosis or sedation dissipates quickly. Adverse effects are few.

### Patient Teaching

Box 51.2 identifies patient teaching guidelines for intravenous anesthetics, including propofol.

## Other Drugs in the Class

Other intravenous anesthetics with differing profiles are available for use. Etomidate (Amidate) is a short-acting anesthetic that appears to promote cardiovascular stability, even in critically ill patients. As an imidazole-containing compound, it is structurally dissimilar to the other intravenous anesthetics. Like propofol, etomidate amplifies the inhibitory neurotransmitter GABA and results in quick patient recovery because of its redistribution to other tissues. However, etomidate suppresses steroid synthesis, leading to short-term adrenocortical suppression. Symptoms may include weakness and hypotension. There is some evidence that the use of etomidate in critically ill patients results in increased mortality. The risks versus benefits of using etomidate in this patient population should be carefully considered. In addition, when compared with other intravenous anesthetics, etomidate causes more PONV. Cyclopropyl-methoxycarbonyl metomidate, or ABP-700, an analogue of etomidate that does not exhibit adrenal suppression, is undergoing clinical trials.

Ketamine is a dissociative anesthetic, which means that it produces a trancelike state or detached feeling. It causes hypnosis, amnesia, and potent analgesia. A noncompetitive NMDA receptor antagonist that blocks glutamate, it is opioid-sparing and does not rely on opioid receptors. Because of these unique properties, ketamine can be used as a sedative or total anesthetic. Ketamine has sympathomimetic effects and is commonly used in the care of critically ill patients because it maintains blood pressure and heart rate as long as catecholamine reserves are present. The anesthetic has a versatile profile, and its administration may be intravenous, intramuscular, oral, or nasal. When carefully titrated, ketamine preserves airway reflexes and adequate ventilation. It is also an excellent bronchodilator. Because ketamine increases salivation, prior administration of glycopyrrolate is recommended.

The FDA has issued a **BLACK BOX WARNING ◆** for ketamine. A phencyclidine derivative, it can produce emergence delirium, hallucinations, and unpleasant dreams. Symptoms of this effect may include confusion, agitation, and nystagmus. Psychological effects can last up to 24 hours. Reducing adverse effects involves using the lowest necessary doses and premedicating with benzodiazepines. With the exception of required nursing care and vital signs, the nurse minimizes stimulation and permits the patient to recover in a calm, quiet environment with gentle reorientation. Monitoring to ensure a complete recovery from anesthesia is essential. The anesthesia practitioner may have to treat severe reactions. A responsible adult should accompany the patient home. Esketamine (Spravato), the pure S-enantiomer of ketamine, is currently available as a nasal spray for the treatment of depression. Esketamine demonstrates better analgesic and anesthetic effects with less psychomimetic properties compared to ketamine; thus, there is increasing interest in using this preparation for analgesia, sedation, and anesthesia.

Methohexital sodium (Brevital) is an ultrashort-acting barbiturate with a fast recovery period. Although it was predominantly used to induce anesthesia before the introduction of propofol, it may be used to induce rapid anesthesia, which is then maintained with an inhaled anesthetic. The anesthetic depresses the cardiovascular and respiratory system. Patients with porphyria should not receive barbiturates. Barbiturates are highly alkaline and cause venous irritation. Venous infiltration results in local tissue damage. Incompatibility with other medications results in precipitation, so it is necessary to flush the intravenous line before and after injecting barbiturates. Methohexital does not raise the seizure threshold. Therefore, it is the drug of choice when providing short-term anesthesia prior to electroconvulsive therapy.

The FDA has issued a **BLACK BOX WARNING ◆** for methohexital. Appropriately educated clinicians should be available to continuously monitor the patient and provide age-specific resuscitative measures if necessary. The use of deep sedation requires that clinician be dedicated to patient monitoring and care and not be participating in the surgery or procedure.

### Clinical Application 51.2

- Ms. Wilberson stated in the nursing interview that she has a history of food allergies. Before administration of the anesthetic, the nurse and anesthesia practitioner need to assess for which food allergies?

### NCLEX Success

3. A patient is admitted to the diagnostic procedure center for a routine colonoscopy. Propofol is the drug of choice for sedation. Which of the following would contraindicate the use of propofol?

   A. a history of postoperative nausea and vomiting
   B. a diagnosis of hypertension
   C. an allergy to eggs
   D. the need for rapid emergence

4. What is the rationale for the administration of ketamine?

   A. It provides sedation and analgesia.
   B. It can be administered without risk.
   C. It slowly crosses the blood–brain barrier.
   D. It reduces blood pressure.

5. A seriously ill pediatric patient has been admitted to the ICU. The patient is intubated, and propofol is used for long-term sedation so the patient does not "fight" the ventilator. Which of the following laboratory values should be monitored? Select all that apply.

   A. complete blood count
   B. triglycerides
   C. alkaline phosphatase
   D. lactate
   E. creatine kinase
   F. luteinizing hormone

6. A 30-year-old woman suffering from postpartum depression is scheduled to receive electroconvulsive therapy. Which of the following anesthetic agents will most likely be administered?

   A. methotrexate sodium
   B. methohexital sodium
   C. methocarbamol
   D. methimazole

## NEUROMUSCULAR BLOCKING AGENTS

Modern neuromuscular blocking agents, or muscle relaxants, are divided into two classes, the nondepolarizing and depolarizing muscle relaxants. **Vecuronium**, a nondepolarizing aminosteroid compound, is the prototype. There are several nondepolarizing muscle relaxants. Succinylcholine is the only depolarizing agent

used in the United States. Each agent has unique characteristics (see Other Drugs in the Class), and the anesthesia practitioner makes the appropriate choice based on the health history of the patient as well as the length and type of procedure.

## Pharmacokinetics

Maximum neuromuscular blockade with vecuronium occurs within 3 to 5 minutes, and the duration of action is 25 to 40 minutes. The onset and duration are dose dependent. For example, larger doses result in faster onset and longer duration. The cessation of effect is dependent on the redistribution of the medication away from the neuromuscular junction. Vecuronium has an extensive hepatic uptake and metabolism, which accounts for a rapid decline in plasma concentration. Because of its lipid solubility, about 40% of the vecuronium is excreted in the bile. Hepatic metabolites and unchanged vecuronium are excreted in the urine. Because of the distribution to peripheral compartments, large and repeated dosing can result in accumulation of vecuronium and active metabolites.

## Action

Vecuronium acts by temporarily suspending nerve impulses at the neuromuscular junction. It can be titrated to produce weakness through complete paralysis. The inhibition of nerve transmission occurs at the postsynaptic nicotinic acetylcholine (ACh) receptors. Because vecuronium is structurally similar to ACh, it binds to the receptors on the muscle and prevents normal function of ACh, producing skeletal muscle paralysis. As vecuronium redistributes and metabolizes, ACh effectively takes over, and normal functioning of skeletal muscle resumes. Vecuronium has no abnormal effects on the cardiovascular system.

## Use

The use of vecuronium and other neuromuscular blocking agents is often necessary because inhalation or intravenous anesthetics alone may not produce the skeletal muscle relaxation a surgeon needs when performing an operation. Muscles may need to be relaxed, so that proper exposure occurs. Also, absolutely no movement is essential for delicate repairs. In addition, neuromuscular blocking agents facilitate easy tracheal intubation and mechanical ventilation by relaxing the vocal cords, jaw, and associated respiratory muscles.

Table 51.4 summarizes the use of the neuromuscular blocking agents.

### Use in Children

Children have a larger volume of distribution than adults. In addition, they have a high clearance rate. Therefore, children younger than 10 years of age may require higher initial doses and more frequent supplementation to maintain sedation. However, infants between the age of 7 weeks and 1 year are more sensitive to vecuronium and take longer to recover.

### Use in Older Adults

Cautious use of vecuronium is necessary in elderly patients. An age-related reduction in organ clearance prolongs the effect of the anesthetic.

## Clinical Application 51.3

● During laparoscopic procedures such as Ms. Wilberson's cholecystectomy, the surgeon has long metal instruments inside the body, perhaps next to major blood vessels. The anesthesia practitioner administers vecuronium during the procedure, in addition to the sevoflurane. What is the purpose of using vecuronium?

### Use in Patients With Renal Impairment

Some vecuronium is excreted unchanged in the urine. Therefore, when larger doses of vecuronium are administered and the patient has significant renal dysfunction, the clearance is inhibited. This can result in drug accumulation and prolonged muscle paralysis.

### Use in Patients With Hepatic Impairment

Because of the extensive hepatic metabolism and biliary excretion of vecuronium, patients with significant hepatic impairment such as cirrhosis or cholestasis can experience slow elimination and prolonged muscle paralysis.

### Use in Patients With Critical Illness

Vecuronium or other nondepolarizing neuromuscular blocking agents are administered in critical care situations to enhance the therapeutic effects of mechanical ventilation.

## Adverse Effects

Nondepolarizing neuromuscular blocking agents can result in allergic reactions during anesthesia such as anaphylaxis or mild dermatologic conditions such as urticaria or erythema.

## Contraindications

In the case of a patient who reports a known hypersensitivity or allergy to vecuronium or nondepolarizing neuromuscular blocking agents, the anesthesia practitioner modifies the anesthetic plan.

## Nursing Implications Airway!

The maintenance of the patient's airway and respiratory function following the administration of neuromuscular blocking agents such as vecuronium is the most important nursing implication. The anesthetist ensures respiratory function during the period of anesthesia.

### Preventing Interactions

Numerous medications interact with vecuronium (Box 51.3).

### Administering the Medication

Neuromuscular blocking agents are intravenous drugs that may be injected manually. Or, like propofol, they may be attached to an electronic syringe pump to provide a controlled continuous infusion.

## TABLE 51.4

### DRUGS AT A GLANCE: Neuromuscular Blocking Agents

| Drug | Pregnancy Category | Routes and Dosage Ranges | |
|---|---|---|---|
| | | **Adults** | **Children** |
| ⓅVecuronium | C | Intubation: 0.08–0.12 mg/kg IV<br>Rapid sequence induction: 0.2–0.4 mg/kg IV<br>Maintenance: 0.015–0.05 mg/kg IV PRN | Intubation: 0.07–0.1 mg/kg IV<br>Rapid sequence induction: 0.2 mg/kg IV<br>Maintenance: 0.02–0.03 mg/kg IV PRN |
| Atracurium | C | Intubation: 0.4–0.6 mg/kg IV<br>Rapid sequence induction: 0.75–1.5 mg/kg IV<br>Maintenance: 0.15–0.25 mg/kg IV PRN | Intubation: 0.3–0.5 mg/kg IV<br>Maintenance: 0.1–0.2 mg/kg IV PRN |
| Cisatracurium (Nimbex; ✹ Cisatracurium Omega) | B | Intubation: 0.15–0.2 mg/kg IV<br>Rapid sequence induction: 0.4 mg/kg IV<br>Maintenance: 0.03–0.05 mg/kg IV PRN | Intubation: 0.1–0.2 mg/kg IV<br>Maintenance: 0.02–0.04 mg/kg IV PRN |
| Pancuronium | C | Intubation: 0.08–0.10 mg/kg IV<br>Rapid sequence induction: 0.15–0.2 mg/kg IV<br>Maintenance: 0.015–0.06 mg/kg IV PRN | Intubation: 0.1–0.15 mg/kg IV<br>Maintenance: 0.02–0.1 mg/kg IV PRN |
| Rocuronium | C | Intubation: 0.45–0.8 mg/kg IV<br>Rapid sequence induction: 1–1.2 mg/kg IV<br>Maintenance: 0.1–0.3 mg/kg IV PRN | Intubation: 0.6–1 mg/kg IV<br>Rapid sequence induction: 1.2 mg/kg IV<br>Maintenance: 0.075–0.3 mg/kg IV PRN |
| Succinylcholine (Anectine, Quelicin; ✹ Quelicin Chloride) | C | Intubation: 1–1.5 mg/kg IV, 2.5–4 mg/kg deep IM (150 mg max) | Intubation:<br>Neonate 2 mg/kg IV<br>Infant 2–3 mg/kg IV<br>Child 1–1.5 mg/kg IV<br>Child 4 mg/kg IM |

## BOX 51.3 — Drug Interactions: Vecuronium

**Drugs That Increase the Effects of Vecuronium**

- Abobotulinumtoxin A, aminoglycosides, calcium channel blockers, cyclosporine, inhalation anesthetics, lincosamide antibiotics, lithium, local anesthetics, magnesium salts, polymyxins, quinidine, spironolactone, and vancomycin

    *Act in a complex way*

**Drugs That Decrease the Effects of Vecuronium**

- Acetylcholinesterase inhibitors; calcium; chronic use of carbamazepine, fosphenytoin, or phenytoin

    *Act in a complex way*

**Drugs That May Increase or Decrease the Effects of Vecuronium Depending on Dose and Comorbidities**

- Corticosteroids, loop diuretics

    *Act in a complex way*

After administration of vecuronium is complete, it may be necessary to reverse its effects so that the patient can regain baseline skeletal muscle function. The anesthetist uses an anticholinesterase, such as neostigmine, edrophonium, or pyridostigmine, which inhibits acetylcholinesterase, the enzyme responsible for degrading ACh. This allows an increase in synaptic ACh, which displaces the neuromuscular blocking agent, thus resulting in a regaining muscle movement. Anticholinesterases must always be given with an anticholinergic, such as glycopyrrolate or atropine, to prevent adverse effects at other cholinergic receptor sites in the body, particularly the heart (bradycardia, asystole) and lungs (bronchoconstriction). Sugammadex (Bridion) is a newer reversal agent without cholinergic effects.

### Assessing for Therapeutic Effects

Most often, anesthesia practitioners use a device called a peripheral nerve stimulator to monitor the level of paralysis. Using this as a guide, the anesthesia practitioner is better able to select the correct dosing regimen. When administered in the ICU, the nurse may be responsible for monitoring the level of paralysis. Because nondepolarizing neuromuscular blocking agents have no anesthetic or analgesic properties, medication-induced hypnosis and amnesia must be provided to ensure patient comfort.

### Assessing for Adverse Effects

The actions of nondepolarizing neuromuscular blocking agents such as vecuronium may persist after emergence from anesthesia and manifest in the PACU. This may occur after improper reversal or no reversal. This persistent or return of weakness after assumed recovery from the effects of nonpolarizing neuromuscular blocking agents is known as **recurarization.** Patients at risk include those with liver and kidney disease, acid–base or electrolyte imbalance, hypothermia, critical illness, myopathic disorders, and neuromuscular diseases such as myasthenia gravis or myasthenic (Eaton-Lambert) syndrome. In addition, elderly patients or those taking medications that may intensify or prolong the actions of neuromuscular blocking agents are at risk. Recurarization can elevate the risk of upper airway obstruction, aspiration, and hypoventilation with respiratory

acidosis and hypoxia. Therefore, it is essential to assess airway, breathing, and circulation. The nurse assesses the quality of respirations by observing the rate and depth. Subtle signs such as difficulty swallowing or double vision may be present, and patients may have a weak and ineffective cough. Difficulties with vocalization and taking a deep breath are possible. The nurse assesses the patient's ability to sustain a head lift for 5 seconds and assesses the strength of the patient's hand grip. If the patient shows any signs or symptoms of respiratory distress, the nurse immediately begins supplemental high-flow oxygen by mask and notifies the anesthesia practitioner. Reversal medications and supported ventilation are necessary.

### Patient Teaching

Box 51.2 identifies patient teaching guidelines for vecuronium.

### Clinical Application 51.4

- On admission to the PACU, Ms. Wilberson complains of difficulty breathing in a weak voice. She has trouble lifting her head. What would be the initial nursing actions?
- What aspect of Ms. Wilberson's care and anesthetic provide clues as to the cause of her symptoms?

## Other Drugs in the Class

### Nondepolarizing Neuromuscular Blocking Agents

Other aminosteroids in addition to vecuronium include the long-acting (greater than 60 minutes) pancuronium and the intermediate-acting (less than 60 minutes) rocuronium. Pancuronium is useful when prolonged paralysis is indicated. In addition, it has the ability to stimulate the vagus nerve and accelerate the heart rate. However, patients with hepatic and renal insufficiency or significant disease may experience prolonged paralysis. Rocuronium has a rapid onset in high doses and is the drug of choice when succinylcholine is contraindicated.

The isoquinoline derivative intermediate-acting nondepolarizing neuromuscular blocking agents are cisatracurium and atracurium. Cisatracurium, an isomer of atracurium, is three times as potent. Both drugs are useful when anesthetizing patients with compromised renal or hepatic function, because elimination is not dependent on enzymatic, liver, or kidney pathways. Cisatracurium has a longer duration than atracurium. At higher doses, atracurium releases histamine, whereas cisatracurium does not. Histamine can produce hypotension, bronchospasm, tachycardia, and skin flushing.

### Depolarizing Neuromuscular Blocking Agent

Succinylcholine (Anectine, Quelicin) is a rapid onset and short-duration muscle relaxant administered by intravenous or intramuscular injection. The structure of succinylcholine is two acetylcholine molecules connected by a methyl group. Succinylcholine attaches to postsynaptic nicotinic ACh receptors and activates them. The depolarization caused by succinylcholine results in momentary contractions of the muscles called **fasciculation;** the patient's entire body may twitch and move for about 5 to 10 seconds. After the fasciculation, the succinylcholine remains attached to the receptor, and there is muscle paralysis for approximately 5 to 10 minutes. Succinylcholine is metabolized by plasma cholinesterase. There are no reversal medications for succinylcholine.

The primary use for succinylcholine is paralysis for tracheal intubation, especially when it is necessary to quickly protect the airway. When tracheal intubation is combined with cricoid pressure to occlude the esophagus, it is referred to as **rapid sequence induction**. This type of induction is indicated in emergency procedures that reduces the risk of aspiration when an empty stomach cannot be guaranteed. Succinylcholine is also used to relax the vocal cords and terminate a laryngospasm.

The adverse effects of succinylcholine include bradycardia, hyperkalemia, and postoperative myalgia. Because there is a risk of abrupt hyperkalemia and cardiac arrest, it is important to avoid using succinylcholine in patients with preexisting hyperkalemia, major burns or extensive tissue damage, denervation conditions such as paraplegia, prolonged illness with immobility, stroke, or motor neuron disease. In patients at risk, serum electrolytes with potassium levels help guide therapy. Malignant hyperthermia is also possible with succinylcholine, so it is contraindicated with confirmed or suspicious history of this condition. In addition, it is avoided in disease processes associated with malignant hyperthermia. Finally, two scenarios cause prolonged paralysis after administration of succinylcholine. The first is decreased plasma cholinesterase, which can result from severe illness that may include liver disease and interactions with other medications. The prolonged effect is usually small. The other scenario is the genetic condition called atypical plasma cholinesterase. Paralysis can last from approximately 30 minutes to many hours. Patients remain intubated and are observed in the ICU until the paralysis spontaneously resolves. During this time, they receive a drug to induce hypnosis.

The FDA has issued a **BLACK BOX WARNING ◆** for succinylcholine because of the risk of sudden cardiac arrest from rapid onset rhabdomyolysis and hyperkalemia. (This condition most likely occurs in boys younger than 8 years of age with Duchenne muscular dystrophy.) Because of the possibility of undiagnosed myopathy in children, the use of succinylcholine in this population is reserved for emergency airway control and intubation to prevent aspiration.

## NCLEX Success

7. An anesthesia practitioner administers succinylcholine. What is the expected effect of this drug? Select all that apply.

   A. decrease in anxiety
   B. fasciculations
   C. muscle relaxation
   D. apnea
   E. analgesia

8. A surgical patient with which of the following conditions may experience recurarization following the administration of vecuronium?

   A. hypertension
   B. hyperthyroidism
   C. cirrhosis
   D. Parkinson's disease

9. A man is admitted to the postanesthesia care unit following surgery, where he received vecuronium. He is unable to raise his head and develops shortness of breath. What are the priority nursing interventions? Select all that apply.

   A. Draw an arterial blood gas.
   B. Notify the anesthesia practitioner.
   C. Administer furosemide.
   D. Apply high-flow oxygen.
   E. Intubate the patient.

## ADJUVANT MEDICATIONS USED IN GENERAL ANESTHESIA

The adjuvant medications are administered during the preoperative, intraoperative, and postoperative phase in support of balanced anesthesia. Table 51.5 summarizes the chief adjuvant medications administered to support balanced anesthesia.

### TABLE 51.5

### DRUGS AT A GLANCE: Adjuvant Drugs Used in General Anesthesia

| Drug | Pregnancy Category | Routes and Dosage Ranges | |
|------|----------|-------------------------|---|
| | | **Adults** | **Children** |
| ⓟ **Midazolam** (Nayzilam) | D | 0.015–0.07 mg/kg IV PRN titrated to effect; usually given in 0.5–1-mg increments | 0.25–1 mg/kg PO (15 mg max)<br>0.08–0.2 mg/kg IM<br>0.02–0.1 mg/kg IV in divided doses |
| ⓟ **Fentanyl** (Sublimaze, Abstral, Fentora, Ionsys; ❧ Abstral, Duragesic, Fentora) | C | Balanced anesthesia: 2–8 mcg/kg with 50%–75% of total dose at induction<br>Higher doses may be used for complex surgeries<br>Sedation/analgesia: 25–50 mcg IV PRN titrated to effect | Balanced anesthesia: 1–3 mcg/kg standard range<br>4–10 mcg/kg higher range for complex surgeries |
| ⓟ **Dexmedetomidine** (Precedex; ❧ Precedex) | C | Loading dose: 1 mcg/kg over 10 min<br>Maintenance: 0.2–0.7 mcg/kg/h | Loading dose: 0.5–2 mcg/kg over 10 min<br>Maintenance: 0.5–1 mcg/kg/h |

## Benzodiazepines

Benzodiazepines are a valuable adjunct to all types of anesthesia. This includes sedation, regional techniques such peripheral nerve blocks, spinal anesthetics, epidural anesthetics, and general anesthesia. Benzodiazepines produce amnesia, anxiolysis, and sedation and have anticonvulsant properties (see Chap. 54). At high doses, benzodiazepines can induce hypnosis. Ⓟ **Midazolam** (Nayzilam), the prototype drug in this class, is a short-acting intravenous medication. Midazolam is the most common medication administered prior to surgery or procedures. Furthermore, when given for procedures that only require sedation, midazolam can be continuously administered to maintain sedation. Because midazolam also can be administered in flavored syrup orally, as an intranasal spray, or intramuscularly, it is a valuable adjunct in pediatric anesthesia.

The FDA has issued a **BLACK BOX WARNING ◆** for midazolam because of profound respiratory depression that may result in hypoxia, brain damage, or death. Rapid intravenous administration to neonates has resulted in hypotension and seizures. It is essential to titrate midazolam carefully according to age and medical conditions. Following administration of midazolam, continuous monitoring for respiratory depression is required, and if necessary, age-specific resuscitative measures should be implemented. Flumazenil is a benzodiazepine antagonist that reverses the effects of midazolam.

## Opioid Analgesics

When pain is anticipated, opioid analgesics are a component of the anesthetic technique. Opioids (see Chap. 49) bind to several classes of opioid receptors in the nervous system and tissues. The prototype intravenous opioid analgesic is Ⓟ **fentanyl** (Sublimaze, Abstral, Fentora, Ionsys). A synthetic opioid that is about 100 times more potent than morphine sulfate, fentanyl can be used to supplement sedation, regional techniques, and general anesthesia. Common adverse effects of all opioids are respiratory depression, nausea and vomiting, altered mentation, urinary retention, and itching. Naloxone (Narcan) (see Chap. 49) is an antagonist that reverses the effects of opioids.

## Alpha-2 Adrenergic Agonist

Ⓟ **Dexmedetomidine** (Precedex) is an alpha-2 receptor agonist that acts on the brain and spinal cord, resulting in sedation, analgesia, and anxiolysis without respiratory depression. Dexmedetomidine is used to provide sedation for surgical, therapeutic, and diagnostic procedures and also as an adjunct to general anesthesia. Hypotension and bradycardia can occur, particularly when dexmedetomidine is used with medications that have similar effects (propofol). It is administered as a continuous infusion using an electronic pump for precise dosing. The length of the infusion will influence the time to complete recovery.

## THE NURSING PROCESS

A concept map outlines the nursing process related to drug therapy considerations in this chapter. Additional nursing implications related to the disease process should also be considered in care decisions.

**Assessment**

A systematic preoperative interview is conducted prior to the surgery or diagnostic procedure to determine the physical and psychological preparation of the patient. This helps predict the possible implications or interactions with anesthesia. Although the anesthesia provider is responsible for the assessment and treatment of the patient, the care of the patient is a team process.

• **Assess the patient's status in relation to the anesthesia administration and his or her surgical experience preoperatively.**
  • Assess the patient's understanding of the perioperative process.
  • Assess the patient's health and surgical history, including allergies to medications, eggs or soy products, latex, or anesthesia-related products.
  • Interview the patient about the surgical experience and administration of anesthetics, including a family or patient history of malignant hyperthermia or atypical plasma cholinesterase.
  • Assess medications, both prescription and over-the-counter or complementary and alternative therapies, taken in the past 2 weeks, and the day of surgery.
• **Implement preoperative assessments.**
  • Assess blood count, chemistry panel, coagulation profile, fasting blood sugar, HbA1c, ECG, chest radiation, and pregnancy test.
  • Assess baseline vital signs, level of consciousness, and orientation.
• **Assess the patient's response to general anesthesia.**
  • Assess vital signs continuously.
  • Assess physiologic response to anesthesia.
• **Implement postanesthesia/postoperative assessment.**
  • Assess airway, vital signs, level of consciousness, pain.
  • Assess for postoperative nausea and vomiting.

## THE NURSING PROCESS (Continued)

**Outcomes of Therapy**

The patient will
- Understand the expected outcome or limitations of the anesthesia, including the following:
  - Level of pain
  - Postoperative nausea and vomiting
  - Expectations during the surgery or procedure and recovery period
- Adhere to preoperative instructions (a coherent patient may be necessary for selected surgical or diagnostic procedures):
  - Cessation of alcohol, complementary and alternative therapies, and smoking
  - Essential medications day of surgery
- Experience partial or complete amnesia while in the surgical suite.
- Experience control of pain to acceptable level.
- Experience control of PONV so as not to cause excessive pain, dehydration, or disrupt the surgical repair.
- Have no adverse effects from the anesthesia.

**Nursing Interventions**

- Provide accurate information to the patient about the surgical or diagnostic procedure, the planned anesthetic, and the expected outcomes.
- Instruct the patient to report symptoms such as pain, nausea, difficult breathing, weakness, lightheadedness, itching, and chest pain.
- Assess the patient's preoperative psychological status.
- Be available to assist the anesthesia provider during tracheal intubation and extubation.
- Monitor vital signs, fluid intake or output, or perform other responsibilities in coordination with the anesthesia provider.
- Do not move or reposition an intubated patient without prior coordination with the anesthesia provider.
- Know the location of emergency equipment such as a difficult airway cart, malignant hyperthermia cart, or code cart.
- Refrain from inappropriate discussion during surgery. Even during general anesthesia or sedation, a patient may have recall of conversation or events.
- Be cognizant that anesthetics have the potential for rapid and profound changes in physiologic stability and that the nurse may be required to assist the anesthesia provider at any time.
- Assist the anesthesia provider with the transport from the operating room to the PACU or ICU.
  - Continue to evaluate airway patency, breathing, and circulation during transport and on arrival to the PACU or ICU. Supplemental oxygen may be necessary, especially for pediatric and elderly patients.
  - Information includes the anesthetic technique and medications used, time of last narcotic, intake and output, pertinent events during the surgery or procedure, length of anesthetic, stability during procedure, and whether neuromuscular blocking agents were reversed and at what time.
  - Develop a customized plan of patient care with the anesthesia provider.
- When the patient is transferred from the PACU to the division or outpatient suite, maintain and assess:
  - Pulse oximetry oxygen saturation
  - Airway, circulation, Level of consciousness and motor function
  - Temperature, pain, PONV, emotional comfort and intake and output

**Evaluation**

- Be familiar with your institution's practice guidelines and benchmark goals to help direct therapy and evaluate recovery from anesthesia.
- Observe that patient planning/goals are met.
- Assess the effectiveness of perioperative nursing interventions and medication therapy.

## KEY CONCEPTS

- General anesthesia is defined as a medication-induced reversible unconsciousness with loss of protective reflexes, much like a drug-induced coma.
- The administration of anesthesia and monitored anesthesia care requires a CRNA or anesthesiologist educated in advanced airway control and the recognition and treatment of anesthetic-related complications.

- The nurse solves clinical problems in an organized differential approach and temporizes life-threatening situations by maintaining airway, breathing, and circulation and providing supplemental oxygen.
- Three phases of general anesthesia are induction or rendering the patient unconscious, maintenance or administering a continuous level of anesthetic, and emergence or stopping

general anesthetic medications and allowing the patient to wake up.

- Balanced anesthesia combines several medications to produce amnesia, analgesia, hypnosis, and muscle relaxation, which achieves a state of physiologic and pharmacologic equilibrium while under general anesthesia.
- Volatile inhalation anesthetics are liquid halogenated hydrocarbons whose inhaled vapors produce hypnosis, amnesia, and skeletal muscle relaxation.
- Nitrous oxide is an inorganic inhalation agent in the form of a gas that produces amnesia, analgesia, and euphoria but cannot produce general anesthesia.
- Malignant hyperthermia is a genetic disorder that may trigger a potentially fatal hypermetabolic response after exposure to volatile inhalation anesthetics or succinylcholine.
- Intravenous anesthetics are used to induce hypnosis or sedation in a fast-acting manner.
- The mishandling of the propofol syringe, vial, or ampoule can result in inadvertent bacterial contamination and elevate the risk of systemic sepsis.
- The FDA has issued a **BLACK BOX WARNING** ◆ for the intravenous anesthetic ketamine. It can produce emergence delirium, hallucinations, and unpleasant dreams. Therefore, special attention is necessary during the administration of the drug in addition to providing a safe and quiet environment during recovery.
- The FDA has also issued a **BLACK BOX WARNING** ◆ for methohexital, another intravenous anesthetic. Appropriately educated clinicians should be available to continuously moni-

tor the patient and provide age-specific resuscitative measures if necessary.

- Neuromuscular blocking agents are divided into two classes according to their mechanism of action: depolarizing and nondepolarizing.
- Neuromuscular blocking agents are used to facilitate endotracheal intubation and mechanical ventilation, relax skeletal muscle to facilitate surgical exposure or repair, and maintain a motionless surgical field.
- Recurarization is defined as a postoperative weakness caused by residual nondepolarizing muscle relaxants, which requires prompt recognition and treatment.
- Succinylcholine is a rapid onset and short-duration depolarizing neuromuscular blocker that is usually given intravenously for tracheal intubation, especially when it is necessary to quickly protect the airway in rapid sequence induction.
- The FDA has released a **BLACK BOX WARNING** ◆ for succinylcholine because of the risk of sudden cardiac arrest from rapid onset rhabdomyolysis and hyperkalemia.
- The benzodiazepine midazolam produces amnesia, anxiolysis, and sedation, and it is frequently administered prior to surgery or a procedure. The FDA has issued a **BLACK BOX WARNING** ◆ for midazolam because of profound respiratory depression that may result in hypoxia, brain damage, or death. Rapid intravenous administration to neonates has resulted in hypotension and seizures.
- Opioids are used to reduce pain during and after surgery or procedures and are selected according to their pharmacokinetic and pharmacodynamic properties.

## CLINICAL REASONING CASE STUDY

### Meet the Patient

A 45-year-old woman is having a spinal cord nerve stimulator surgically implanted under monitored anesthesia care. She has a history of complex regional pain syndrome in the lower extremities and takes several opioid analgesics at home to treat the chronic pain. In addition to propofol for hypnosis, the anesthesia provider plans to administer ketamine for analgesia and amnesia.

- Why is ketamine indicated in this procedure?
- What adverse effects may be expected during the procedure?
- What intraoperative nursing interventions can help alleviate the adverse effects?
- What other class of medication would be beneficial?

### Assessing Drug Information

- Actions
  - Ketamine is a noncompetitive NMDA receptor antagonist that blocks glutamate.
  - Ketamine is a dissociative anesthetic, which means that it produces a trancelike state or detached feeling. It causes hypnosis, amnesia, and potent analgesia.
  - When carefully titrated, ketamine preserves airway reflexes and adequate ventilation. It is also an excellent bronchodilator.
- Use: Ketamine is indicated for this procedure because the patient may have developed tolerance to opioids with chronic pain. Intraoperative opioids may be less effective. The opioid-sparing ketamine does not rely on opioid receptors and will provide analgesia and amnesia.
- Adverse effects
  - Reducing adverse effects involves using the lowest necessary doses and premedicating with benzodiazepines.
  - During the procedure, ketamine can produce delirium and hallucinations. Therefore, the patient may act and sound inappropriate.
  - Permit the patient to recover in a calm, quiet environment with gentle reorientation. Monitoring to ensure a complete recovery from anesthesia is essential.
  - Psychological effects can last up to 24 hours.
  - Because ketamine increases salivation, prior administration of glycopyrrolate may be considered.
  - A responsible adult should drive the patient home and stay with them until adverse effects have resolved.

### Nursing Actions

- During the perioperative period, assess vital signs, state of consciousness, and signs of allergic reaction.
- Provision of a safe, calm, operating room environment is essential. Elimination of any unnecessary noise and gentle reorientation are necessary to minimize adverse effects.
- The benzodiazepine midazolam may help prevent adverse effects.

Visit the Point® at **http://thePoint.lww.com/Frandsen12e** *for answers to NCLEX Success questions (in Appendix A), answers to Clinical Application Case Studies (in Appendix B), and more!*

## REFERENCES AND RESOURCES

Andrade, C. (2017). Ketamine for depression, 3: does chirality matter? *Journal of Clinical Psychiatry, 78*(6), e674–e677. doi:10.4088/JCP.17f11681

Bittner, E. A. (2019). Clinical use of neuromuscular blocking medications in critically ill patients. In P. E. Parson, G. Finlay, & M. Crowley (Eds.). *UpToDate.* Wolters Kluwer.

Bruder, E. A., Ball, I. M., Ridi, S., Pickett, W., & Hohl, C. (2015). Single induction dose of etomidate versus other induction agents for endotracheal intubation in critically ill patients. *The Cochrane Database of Systematic Reviews, 8*(1), CD010225. doi:10.1002/14651858.CD010225

Falk, S. A., & Fleisher, L. E. (2019). Overview of anesthesia and anesthetic choices. In S. B. Jones, N. A. Nussmeier, & W. Chen (Eds.). *UpToDate.* Wolters Kluwer.

Feinleib, J., Kwan, L. H., & Yamani, A. (2019). Postoperative nausea and vomiting. In H. F. Holt, A. Davidson, & M. Crowley (Eds.). *UpToDate.* Wolters Kluwer.

Fernández-Guisasola, J., Gómez-Arnau, J. I., Cabrera, Y., & del Valle, S. G. (2010). Association between nitrous oxide and the incidence of postoperative nausea and vomiting in adults: A systematic review and meta-analysis. *Anaesthesia, 65*(4), 379–387.

Flood, P., Rathmell, J. P., & Shafer, S. (2014). *Stoelting's pharmacology and physiology in anesthesia practice* (5th ed.). Philadelphia, PA: Lippincott Williams & Wilkins.

Gan, T. J., Diemunsch, P., Habib, A. S., Kovac, A., Kranke, P., Meyer, T. A., et al.; Society for Ambulatory Anesthesia. (2014). Consensus guidelines for the management of postoperative nausea and vomiting. *Anesthesia and Analgesia, 118*(1), 85–113.

Karch, A. M. (2018). *2019 Lippincott's pocket drug guide for nurses.* Philadelphia, PA: Wolters Kluwer.

King, A. (2018). General anesthesia: Maintenance. In G. P. Joshi & N. A. Nussmeier (Eds.). *UpToDate.* Wolters Kluwer.

Mckinlay, J., Tyson, E., & Forni, L. G. (2018). Renal complications of anaesthesia. *Anesthesia, 73*(1), 85–94. doi:10.1111/anae.14144

Nettina, S. M. (Ed.). (2019). *Lippincott manual of nursing practice* (11th ed.). Philadelphia, PA: Wolters Kluwer.

Rosero, E. B. (2018). Monitored anesthesia care in adults. In G. P. Joshi & M. Crowley (Eds.). *UpToDate.* Wolters Kluwer.

UpToDate. (2019). *Drug Information.* Lexi-Comp, Inc.

Valk, B. I., Absalom, A. R., Meyer, P., Meier, S., den Daas, I., van Amsterdam, K., et al. (2018). Safety and clinical effect of i.v. infusion of cyclopropyl-methoxycarbonyl etomidate (ABP-700), a soft analogue of etomidate, in healthy subjects. *British Journal of Anaesthesia, 120*(6), 1401–1411. doi:10.1016/j.bja.2018.01.038

# Drug Therapy for Migraine and Other Headaches

## CLINICAL APPLICATION CASE STUDY

Tanya Van Art, who is 18 years of age, has experienced headaches since she was 13. In the past year, the headaches have been increasing in severity. While at work this past week, she developed a severe headache with nausea and vomiting and was admitted to the emergency department. On admission, her blood pressure was 180/90 mm Hg and her pain was 10 on a 10-point scale. She denied having any aura preceding the onset of the headache or any vision changes at onset or now. In the emergency department, she received ketorolac 15 mg and, in addition, prochlorperazine 10 mg plus diphenhydramine 25 mg intravenously over 5 minutes.

The diagnosis was acute migraine headache.

## KEY TERMS

**Abortive therapy:** medications administered to manage the symptoms of migraine headache

**Aura:** subjective sensation that immediately precedes a migraine headache, consisting of a breeze, odor, or light

**Cluster headache:** recurrent, severe, unilateral orbitotemporal headache

**Menstrual migraine headache:** migraine headache associated with a drop in circulating estrogen that occurs 2 to 3 days prior to the onset of menses; also called estrogen-associated headaches

**Migraine headache:** unilateral pain in the head that may or may not be accompanied by an aura; may be associated with vertigo, nausea, vomiting, and photophobia

**Orbitotemporal:** area centered around the orbit of the eye and the temple

**Preventive therapy:** administration of medications to prevent the onset of migraine headaches

**Tension-type headache:** headache associated with nervous tension or anxiety, often related to chronic contraction of scalp muscles

**Vascular constriction:** narrowing of the blood vessels

## INTRODUCTION

Headaches are among the most common disorders, yet focus on their importance as a public health concern was limited until 20 years ago. Although headache disorders can be debilitating for a relatively large minority of the population, most individuals experience a headache from time to time, the disorder is not fatal, and it does not result in permanent disability. These factors have delayed the focus on headache disorders.

This chapter discusses the various types of headaches, including cluster, migraine, and tension-type, all of which produce pain. However, the pain experienced by patients and the physiology involved varies with each type of headache. To aid understanding of drug therapy for cluster, migraine, and tension-type headaches, this chapter presents the pathophysiology and clinical manifestations of the different types of headaches. This chapter also considers the pharmacologic treatment for each of these headaches.

## OVERVIEW OF HEADACHES

**Cluster headache** belongs to a group of headache conditions, called the trigeminal autonomic cephalalgias, all of which involve unilateral, often severe headache symptoms. Cluster headache is the most common syndrome and presents with recurrent and severe **orbitotemporal** headache. Evidence suggests that the syndrome demonstrates a familial pattern and is four times more prevalent in women than men.

**Migraine headache** is a severe and disabling neurologic disorder resulting from an inherited tendency for the brain to lose control of its inputs. Annually, this condition affects approximately 20% of women and 8% of men. It occurs most commonly in persons between 25 and 55 years of age, although children may have migraine headaches. Migraine is associated with a huge socioeconomic impact when symptoms are episodic and chronic in nature. The headache involves unilateral pain in the head that may or may not be accompanied by an **aura**. An aura is a subjective sensation that immediately precedes the migraine headache consisting a breeze, odor, or light.

Migraine predominately affects women more often than men. In part, the increased incidence in women may be the result of circulating estrogen. Menstruation may be the most common and potent trigger of a migraine attack. **Menstrual migraine headaches**, also called estrogen-associated headaches, are most commonly brought on with a drop in circulating estrogen 2 to 3 days prior to the onset of menses. Nearly one in four U.S. households includes a person who experiences migraine.

**Tension-type headache**, previously described as tension or stress headache, muscle contraction headache, and psychogenic headache, is the most common headache in the general population. Many individuals do not seek help for the condition, because the headache is intermittent, mild, and often indistinctive. This type of headache is the least studied of all the primary headache disorders despite having a high socioeconomic impact. A tension-type headache was once thought to be the result of chronic contraction of the scalp muscles, but that concept is no longer considered valid.

## Pathophysiology

### Cluster Headache

The pathophysiology of a cluster headache is not completely understood. One theory, the major one, states that a primary cluster headache is characterized by hypothalamic activation with secondary activations of the trigeminal autonomic reflex. Another theory states that neurogenic inflammation of the walls of the cavernous sinus obliterates venous outflow, injuring the transverse sympathetic fibers of the intracranial internal carotid artery and its branches.

### Migraine Headaches

Authorities have proposed two theories related to the pathophysiology of a migraine headache. First, at the onset of a migraine, the trigeminal nerve is stimulated, resulting in the release of neuropeptides. This leads to painful neurogenic inflammation in the meningeal vasculature characterized by plasma protein extravasation, vasodilation, and mast cell degranulation. Second, neurogenic vasodilation of the meningeal blood vessels occurs, producing inflammation. The activations of trigeminal sensory fibers cause neurogenic dural vasodilation mediated by the calcitonin gene–related peptide. The calcitonin gene–related peptide is elevated during a migraine.

Estrogen may also play a role. It exerts its predominant effects on the central nervous system (CNS) through facilitation of the serotonergic and glutamatergic systems. When estrogen concentrations decline, serotonin concentrations also fall because of reduced production combined with an increased rate of elimination. A decline in serotonergic concentrations is accompanied by a release of calcitonin gene–related peptide and substance P from trigeminal nerves. This may produce vasodilation of cranial vessels and sensitization of meningeal afferents of the trigeminal nerve. Estrogen may also affect other chemical mediators, such as nitric oxide, magnesium, and prostaglandins, which are known to modulate the balance between excitatory and inhibitory neurotransmission.

### Tension-Type Headache

The pathophysiology of tension-type headache is multifactorial, although the exact mechanism is unclear. In episodic tension-type headaches, environmental factors appear to influence development. With chronic headaches, genetic factors seem to play an important role. Current theory of chronic tension-type headache asserts that a person experiences a sensitization of the dorsal horn neurons related to increased nociceptive inputs from pericranial myofascial tissues. Experts believe that this heightened sensitivity of pain pathways in the CNS plays a critical role in the pathogenesis and the conversion of episodic tension-type headache to the chronic form. With a decreased pain threshold, the person misinterprets normally innocuous incoming signals as pain. Decreased pain, thermal, and electrical thresholds reported in patients with chronic tension-type headache probably represent a central misinterpretation of incoming signals.

## Clinical Manifestations

### Cluster Headache

A cluster headache typically occurs up to eight times per day with pain commonly lasting 15 to 180 minutes. In the episodic form, the attacks typically occur daily for a period of 6 to 12 weeks followed by a period of remission that can last for up to a year or longer. In the chronic form, remission is not part of the cluster attack.

Cluster symptoms are indicative of both parasympathetic hyperactivity and sympathetic impairment. A person with cluster headache presents with severe orbital, supraorbital, or temporal pain accompanied by ipsilateral autonomic symptoms such as ptosis, miosis, lacrimation, conjunctival injection, rhinorrhea, and nasal congestion. Sweating and cutaneous blood flow also increase on the side of the pain, particularly in areas of sympathetic deficit. The symptoms typically resolve with the headache, but mitosis and ptosis, signs of sympathetic paralysis, can persist but intensify during attacks. In addition, patterns of circadian rhythmicity are a hallmark of the syndrome.

### Migraine Headache

A migraine headache with an aura has four phases: prodrome, aura, headache, and recovery. The prodrome phase occurs hours or days before the onset of a migraine headache. Symptoms include depression, irritability, feeling cold, cravings, loss of appetite, alterations in activity, polyuria, diarrhea, and constipation. The aura phase, which occurs only in some patients, involves an aura lasting 1 hour with focal neurologic symptoms, visual disturbances, or vision in only half of the visual field. The headache phase is characterized by vasodilation and a decline in serotonin levels. A throbbing headache becomes more intense, lasting for several hours. The headache can become incapacitating, with photophobia, nausea, and vomiting. The recovery phase involves slow subsiding of the pain. There may be muscle contractions in the neck and scalp, with localized tenderness, tiredness, and alterations in mood. The patient may sleep for hours after the recovery phase.

Symptoms in women with a menstrual headache may vary from this pattern. These headaches are not commonly associated with an aura, although women may experience an aura during periods of nonmenstrual attacks. In addition, menstrual migraines tend to be more severe, last longer, and be less responsive to abortive treatment.

Chronic migraine is diagnosed by the presence of a migraine headache without an aura for 8 days or more per month for 3 months. The headache is unilateral, pulsating with moderate to severe intensity, and aggravated by activity.

### Tension-Type Headache

A wide variation exists in the experiences of people who suffer from a tension-type headache. Characteristic signs and symptoms include bilateral, nonthrobbing head pain of mild to moderate intensity. Patients may describe pressure, head fullness, or a bandlike sensation around the head, or they may report a feeling like a heavyweight is on their head or shoulders without other associated features. Tension-type headaches are classified into three subtypes based on the frequency of headache episodes:

- Infrequent: headache less than 1 day per month
- Frequent: headache 1 to 14 days per month
- Chronic: headache 15 or more days per month

Management of the condition varies based on the subtype. Infrequent or low-frequency episodic subtype patterns are managed with acute symptomatic treatment; prophylactic treatments are added for high-frequency and chronic headaches. In addition, impact on the quality of life increases with the headache frequency of the subtype.

## Drug Therapy

### Cluster Headache

Treatment of a cluster headache involves subcutaneous sumatriptan and high-flow (100%) oxygen. Because the adverse effects of oxygen use are less than those of sumatriptan, high-flow oxygen may be administered for 15 minutes to determine effectiveness. Although oxygen may be effective in some patients, resuming the use of high-flow oxygen within a short period of time following relief of the headache should be avoided, because evidence shows that the frequency of cluster headaches may increase in some patients with overuse of high-flow oxygen. Ergot derivatives, lidocaine, and octreotide are also effective in the treatment of acute cluster headaches. Cluster headaches often are not treated as effectively as migraines. New guidelines have suggested that sumatriptan, administered subcutaneously, and zolmitriptan nasal spray, augmented by high-flow oxygen, may be effective. Steroid injections as well as calcium channel blockers may offer an option. Nonpharmacologic options include occipital and vagal nerve stimulation.

## Migraine Headaches

Drug therapy to manage a migraine is guided mainly by several factors: (1) the severity of the attacks; (2) the presence of associated symptoms, such as nausea and vomiting; (3) the type of treatment setting (outpatient or inpatient); and (4) patient-specific factors, such as the patient's medication preference and the presence of vascular risk factors. There are two specific courses of treatment for migraine headaches: abortive and preventive therapy. **Abortive therapy** is the administration of medications to treat the symptoms of migraine headache. **Preventive therapy** is the administration of medications to prevent the development of a migraine headache. Medications used in the treatment of migraine headaches are listed in Table 52.1.

The abortive agents administered for the treatment of migraine headaches include nonsteroidal anti-inflammatory agents, acetaminophen–aspirin with caffeine medication, the ergot alkaloids, and the triptans (serotonin receptor [5-HT$_{1B}$ and 5-HT$_{1D}$] agonists). Although it can produce nervousness and dizziness, caffeine was found to be an effective analgesic adjuvant in the acute treatment of migraine headache. The pharmacologic and nonpharmacologic treatment of long-term migraine is to reduce the frequency, severity, and disability. The initial pharmacotherapy for acute treatment of migraine is the administration of triptans subcutaneously. In addition, intravenous metoclopramide and prochlorperazine are also used in eligible adults who present to an emergency department with acute migraine. Metoclopramide has been shown to be highly effective in relieving migraine-associated symptoms. In children, ketorolac, administered intramuscularly or intravenously, is highly effective.

Initial abortive therapy for women who experience acute menstrual migraines is the same as that for migraine occurring at any other time. People who suffer from migraines take preventive medications, which are discussed later in this chapter.

> **⚠ QSEN Alert: Evidence-Based Practice**
>
> Cook and Newberry (2018) evaluated the effectiveness of migraine management in the emergency department. These researchers used a randomized, double-blind research design comparing prochlorperazine 10 mg plus diphenhydramine 25 mg with hydromorphone 1 mg plus a normal saline placebo. All doses were given intravenously and administered over 5 minutes. If the migraine attack was not controlled with the initial dose of medication, a subsequent dose of the same medication was offered to the patient 1 hour after the initial infusion began. Patients enrolled in the trial could only receive a maximum of two doses of a particular medication. Study participants were randomly assigned to either the control or experimental group based on a random number sequence generated online by the research pharmacist. The sample analysis consisted of 127 patients, with 63 patients receiving prochlorperazine and diphenhydramine and 64 patients receiving hydromorphone and normal saline placebo.

The primary study outcome was sustained headache relief, which was defined by two variables: a reduction in acute migraine pain to either mild or none within 2 hours and whether the headache relapsed and/or was not rated as worse than mild at 48 hours. Prochlorperazine was found to be superior when compared with hydromorphone on treatment outcomes. Only 8% of patients in the prochlorperazine group requested an additional dose of medication, whereas 31% of patients in the hydromorphone group requested an additional dose. Those who received prochlorperazine were noted to have decreased length of ED stays compared with participants receiving hydromorphone. Although prochlorperazine was superior in the treatment of acute migraine, there were no differences in headache days postdischarge, frequency of return ED visits, or functional disability.

## TABLE 52.1

### Drugs Administered for the Treatment of Migraine Headache

| Drug Class | Prototype | Other Drugs in the Class |
|---|---|---|
| Nonsteroidal anti-inflammatory drugs | Naproxen (Naprosyn) Naproxen sodium (Aleve, Anaprox DS, Naprelan) | Ketorolac tromethamine (ReadySharp Ketorolac) |
| Analgesic | Aspirin–acetaminophen–caffeine (Excedrin) | |
| Ergot alkaloids | Ergotamine tartrate (Ergomar) | Dihydroergotamine (D.H.E. 45, Migranal) |
| Triptans | Sumatriptan (Imitrex, Onzetra Xsail, others) | Almotriptan Eletriptan (Relpax) Frovatriptan (Frova) Naratriptan (Amerge) Rizatriptan (Maxalt, Maxalt-MLT) Zolmitriptan (Zomig) |
| Estrogen | Estradiol | |
| Antiemetic | Chlorpromazine hydrochloride | Metoclopramide (Reglan) Prochlorperazine (Compro) |

**Clinical Application 52.1**

- What does the nurse teach Ms. Van Art about the pathophysiology of acute migraine?
- What does the nurse discuss about auras and migraine-associated vision changes?

### Tension-Type Headaches

Acute therapy for tension-type headaches entails the use of non-pharmacologic methods such as rest, relaxation techniques, or stress reduction strategies as well as medication. Pharmacologic treatment of tension-type headaches includes acetaminophen, aspirin, and nonsteroidal anti-inflammatory agents (see Chap. 16). Studies have shown that tricyclic drugs can reverse the central sensitization and chronicity of these headaches. In addition, a meta-analysis of eight placebo-controlled clinical trials found that botulinum toxin type A led to a small decrease in number of headaches per month, although the result was not statistically significant.

### NCLEX Success

1. A patient admitted to the emergency department complains of a severe headache with nausea and vomiting received a diagnosis of an acute migraine headache. Which medication assists in decreasing the nausea and vomiting related to the acute migraine episode?
   A. intravenous ketorolac
   B. subcutaneous sumatriptan
   C. inhaled albuterol
   D. oral diclofenac

2. Which of the following medications are administered for preventive therapy in the treatment of migraine?
   A. beta-adrenergic blockers
   B. nonsteroidal anti-inflammatory agents
   C. ergot alkaloids
   D. analgesics

## NONSTEROIDAL ANTI-INFLAMMATORY AGENTS

Ibuprofen is the traditional prototype of the nonsteroidal anti-inflammatory agents (see Chap. 16). However, naproxen sodium is more commonly prescribed for the treatment of migraine headaches because it is more rapidly absorbed and produces more rapid analgesia. Thus, naproxen (Naprosyn) or **naproxen sodium** (Aleve) serves as the prototype described in detail in this chapter.

## Pharmacokinetics

There are two types of naproxen: naproxen and naproxen sodium. Naproxen has an onset of action of 1 hour, a peak of action of 2 to 4 hours, and duration of action of 7 hours or less. Naproxen sodium has an onset of action of 1 hour, a peak of action of 1 to 2 hours, and the same duration of action as naproxen. Metabolism of both agents occurs in the liver, and they have a half-life of 12 to 15 hours. Excretion is in the urine. Naproxen and naproxen sodium cross the placental barrier and enter the breast milk.

## Action

Naproxen is a nonselective inhibitor of cyclooxygenase resulting in the inhibition of prostaglandin synthesis of COX-1 and COX-2. Naproxen sodium improves the solubility of naproxen through faster absorption and rapid onset of action.

## Use

Prescribers order naproxen sodium to reduce the pain resulting from an acute migraine headache. Table 52.2 presents dosage information for naproxen and related drugs.

### Use in Older Adults

Older people should not take more than 200 mg of naproxen sodium every 12 hours.

### Use in Patients With Renal Impairment

Caution is necessary with the administration of naproxen sodium in patients with renal disease because the renal system excretes the drug. It should be avoided in patients with advanced renal disease.

### Use in Patients With Hepatic Impairment

Caution is warranted with the administration of naproxen sodium in patients with hepatic impairment because the site of metabolism is the liver.

## Adverse Effects

The most severe adverse effects of naproxen sodium include bronchospasm and anaphylaxis. Gastrointestinal (GI) adverse effects include GI bleeding, nausea, dyspepsia, and GI pain. The U.S. Food and Drug Administration (FDA) has issued a **BLACK BOX WARNING** ◆ stating that naproxen sodium may put patients at increased risk for cardiovascular events and GI bleeding.

## Contraindications

Contraindications to naproxen or naproxen sodium include a known allergy to aspirin or other nonsteroidal anti-inflammatory drugs as well as pregnancy and lactation. It is important to administer the medication cautiously to patients with asthma, cardiovascular dysfunction, hypertension, GI bleeding, and peptic ulcer.

## Nursing Implications

### Preventing Interactions

The administration of naproxen sodium with lithium results in increased lithium levels and the risk of lithium toxicity.

**TABLE 52.2**

## DRUGS AT A GLANCE: Nonsteroidal Anti-inflammatory Drugs*

| Drug | Pregnancy Category | Routes and Dosages | |
|---|---|---|---|
| | | **Adults** | **Children** |
| **Naproxen** (Naprosyn) | C | 375–500 mg PO two times per day | 10 mg/kg PO in two divided doses |
| **Naproxen sodium** (Aleve, Anaprox DS, Naprelan; 🍁 Aleve, Maxidol, Naproxen, others) | C | Prevention, 250–500 mg PO two times per day Treatment, 750 mg PO initially, an additional 250–500 mg may be given if needed 25 8 (max 1200 mg/24 h) | Safety has not been established for migraine treatment. |
| Ketorolac tromethamine (ReadySharp Ketorolac 🍁, Toradol, Toradol IM) | C (second and third trimester) D (third trimester) | 30 mg IV every 6 h to a maximum of 120 mg/d | 2–16 y: 0.5 mg/kg IV up to a maximum of 15 mg |

*Drugs used in headache treatment.

### Assessing for Therapeutic Effects

Following the administration of naproxen or naproxen sodium, the patient should exhibit diminished pain. The nurse assesses the patient's pain level using a pain scale.

### Assessing for Adverse Effects

The nurse assesses the patient for GI upset, dyspepsia, or bleeding. He or she also assesses pulmonary function and lung sounds for bronchospasm or anaphylactic reaction.

### Patient Teaching

Box 52.1 identifies patient teaching guidelines for naproxen sodium.

## Other Drugs in the Class

Migraine sufferers often seek treatment in the emergency department when the more commonly used abortive therapies are ineffective. In the emergency setting, ketorolac tromethamine is the most frequently administered intravenous drug.

### Clinical Application 52.2

- What is the rationale for administering ketorolac and prochlorperazine to Ms. Van Art?

**BOX 52.1**  *Patient Teaching Guidelines for Naproxen Sodium*

- Take the medication with meals to prevent gastrointestinal upset.
- Take medication as prescribed.
- Do not cut, crush, or chew tablets.
- Do not operate machinery if dizziness or drowsiness occurs.
- Report sore throat, fever, rash, itching, edema, visual changes, and black, tarry stools to your health care provider.

## ACETAMINOPHEN, ASPIRIN, AND CAFFEINE

The combination of 🅿 **acetaminophen**, **aspirin**, and **caffeine** may be effective for the treatment of headaches. In the United States, brand names include Anacin Advanced Headache Formula, Excedrin Extra Strength, Excedrin Migraine, and Goody's Extra Strength.

## Pharmacokinetics

To understand the pharmacokinetics of acetaminophen, aspirin, and caffeine, it is important to review each medication individually. Acetaminophen reaches a peak of action in 0.5 to 2 hours and possesses a 1- to 3-hour half-life. It crosses the placental barrier and enters the breast milk. The drug is metabolized in the liver and excreted in the urine. Aspirin has an onset of action of 5 to 30 minutes, reaches a peak of action in 15 to 120 minutes, and has a duration of action of 3 to 6 hours. The half-life of aspirin is 15 minutes to 12 hours. The drug is absorbed in the stomach and metabolized in the liver. Caffeine has an onset of action of 15 minutes and reaches a peak of action in 15 to 45 minutes. It readily crosses the placental barrier and enters breast milk. Like acetaminophen and aspirin, caffeine is metabolized in the liver. It is eliminated by the kidneys.

## Action

Acetaminophen may act as an analgesic, and its mechanism of action is unknown. Aspirin has the ability to inhibit the synthesis of prostaglandins, which are a mediator of inflammation. Caffeine increases calcium permeability in the sarcoplasmic reticulum to promote the accumulation of cyclic adenosine monophosphate (cAMP) and block the adenosine receptors, stimulating the CNS, cardiac activity, gastric acid secretion, and diuresis. It causes constriction of the blood vessels, which is known as **vascular constriction**. Migraine headaches result from the vasodilation of blood vessels. In addition, caffeine increases the effectiveness of acetaminophen and aspirin by approximately 40%.

| TABLE 52.3 | | | |
|---|---|---|---|
| **DRUGS AT A GLANCE: Acetaminophen–Aspirin–Caffeine Combinations** | | | |
| **Drug** | **Pregnancy Category** | **Routes and Dosages** | |
| | | **Adults** | **Children** |
| Ⓟ **Acetaminophen–aspirin–caffeine** (Anacin Advanced Headache Formula, Excedrin Extra Strength, Excedrin Migraine, Vanquish Extra Strength Pain Reliever | C (acetaminophen), D (third trimester; aspirin) C (caffeine) | 2 tablets PO once per 24 h (each tablet: aspirin 250 mg, acetaminophen 250 mg, caffeine 65 mg) (maximum of two tablets per 24 h) | >12 y: same as adults |

## Use

Acetaminophen–aspirin–caffeine products are administered to reduce pain related to migraine or tension-type headache. Table 52.3 presents oral dosage of information for these combination products.

### Use in Children

Children older than 12 years of age may receive the adult dose of the combination agent.

### Use in Patients With Hepatic Impairment

People with hepatic impairment should not receive this combination agent on an ongoing basis. They may not metabolize acetaminophen in this combined medication effectively, leading to hepatotoxicity.

## Adverse Effects

Each component of the combination medication has adverse effects, which will be addressed individually. Acetaminophen may result in headache, chest pain, dyspnea, myocardial damage with doses of 5 to 8 g/day, and hepatic impairment. Aspirin may lead to GI effects such as dyspepsia, heartburn, and epigastric discomfort as well as hematologic effects such as occult blood loss and hemostatic defects. Aspirin toxicity involves respiratory alkalosis, tachypnea, hemorrhage, excitement, confusion, seizures, tetany, cardiovascular collapse, and metabolic acidosis. Caffeine may result in excitement, insomnia, restlessness, tremors, headaches, and lightheadedness, as well as cardiovascular effects such as tachycardia, hypertension, extrasystole, and palpitations.

## Contraindications

Contraindications to acetaminophen include a known allergy to the drug. Caution is necessary in impaired hepatic function, chronic alcoholism, pregnancy, and lactation. Contraindications to aspirin include a known hypersensitivity to the drug or other anti-inflammatory agents. Vigilance is warranted with renal impairment. Contraindications to caffeine include duodenal ulcers, diabetes, and lactation. Caution is essential in pregnancy, renal and hepatic impairment, and cardiovascular disease.

## Nursing Implications

People most commonly take the acetaminophen–aspirin–caffeine in the home setting. It is important to be familiar with all aspects of each medication to maintain medication safety.

## Preventing Interactions

Several drug–drug interactions may occur with acetaminophen–aspirin–caffeine combinations. Box 52.2 names the specific medications that increase or decrease the effects of each of the medications in the combined drug. Other drug–drug interactions include the following:

- Oral anticoagulants combined with acetaminophen increase hypothrombinemic effects.
- Aspirin combined with sulfonylureas and insulin results in greater glucose-lowering effects.
- Valproic acid combined with aspirin puts patients at risk for seizure activity secondary to protein receptor site displacement.
- Spironolactone or furosemide combined with aspirin leads to decreased diuretic effects.
- Theophylline or clozapine combined with caffeine increases the serum levels of theophylline or clozapine.

**BOX 52.2** **Drug Interactions: Acetaminophen, Aspirin, and Caffeine**

**Drugs That Increase the Effects of Acetaminophen**
- Alcohol, barbiturates, carbamazepine, hydantoins, rifampin, sulfinpyrazone
  *Increase the risk of hepatotoxicity*

**Drugs That Increase the Effects of Aspirin**
- Alcohol, anticoagulants, nonsteroidal anti-inflammatory agents
  *Increase the bleeding risk*
- Carbonic anhydrase inhibitors
  *Increase the risk of salicylate toxicity*

**Drugs That Increase the Effects of Caffeine**
- Cimetidine, hormonal contraceptive, disulfiram, ciprofloxacin, mexiletine
  *Increase the central nervous system effects*

**Drugs That Decrease the Effects of Aspirin**
- Acetazolamide, methazolamide, antacids, alkalinizers
  *Decrease the salicylate levels*

**Drugs That Decrease the Effects of Caffeine**
- Nicotine
  *Produces vasoconstriction*

The concomitant administration of caffeine and guarana, ma huang, and ephedra is not recommended.

### Assessing for Therapeutic Effects

Following the administration of the acetaminophen–aspirin–caffeine combination, the patient should exhibit diminished pain. The nurse assesses for pain using a pain scale.

### Assessing for Adverse Effects

The nurse assesses for hepatotoxicity, allergic reaction, fluid and electrolyte imbalance, hypoglycemia, agitation, and cardiovascular effects.

## Patient Teaching

Box 52.3 identifies patient teaching guidelines for acetaminophen–aspirin–caffeine combinations.

### NCLEX Success

3. Which of the following effects occurs when the naproxen is administered in combination with lithium?
    A. increased risk of lithium toxicity
    B. increase in creatinine clearance
    C. hepatotoxicity
    D. potential gastrointestinal effects

4. An adolescent female is suffering from migraine headaches and her health care provider orders a combination of acetaminophen, aspirin, and caffeine. Prior to the administration of the medication, it is necessary to assess for which of the following?
    A. anxiety and depression
    B. history of smoking
    C. family history of migraines
    D. antacid use

## ERGOT ALKALOIDS

The ergotamine preparations are administered for abortive therapy for migraine headaches, although they have been largely replaced by the triptans (see later discussion). Clinical studies have shown that oral ergotamine plus caffeine is less effective than triptans for acute migraine. The prototype medication is **ergotamine tartrate** (Ergomar), an alpha-adrenergic antagonist.

### Pharmacokinetics

Ergotamine has a variable rate of absorption and onset of action. The peak of action is 0.5 to 3 hours. The half-life of ergotamine is 2 hours, but the effects of the medication can continue for 24 hours. The medication is metabolized by the cytochrome P450 enzyme CYP3A4 in the liver and excreted in the bile. Ergotamine is excreted in the breast milk and may cause vomiting, diarrhea, and changes in heart rate and blood pressure in the nursing infant. It has caused fetal growth retardation in animal studies.

### Action

Ergotamine produces stimulation of the cranial and peripheral vascular smooth muscles while depressing the effects of the central vasomotor centers. It is a partial agonist and antagonist that act against tryptaminergic, dopaminergic, and alpha-adrenergic receptors to constrict the cranial and peripheral blood vessels.

### Use

Prescribers order ergotamine individually or in combination with caffeine to prevent or stop migraine, cluster, or vascular headaches. Children as well as people with renal or hepatic impairment should not take ergotamine. Table 52.4 gives dosage information for the ergot alkaloids.

### Use in Older Adults

It is necessary to administer ergotamine cautiously in older adults because of the drug's vasoconstrictive properties and cardiovascular adverse effects.

### Adverse Effects

The cardiovascular adverse effects of ergotamine include absence of pulse, bradycardia, cardiac valvular fibrosis, cyanosis, edema, heart rhythm changes, gangrene, hypertension, ischemia, precordial distress, chest pain, tachycardia, and vasospasm. Musculoskeletal adverse effects include muscle pain, numbness, paresthesia, and weakness. Other side effects may include vertigo, nausea, vomiting, itching, pulmonary fibrosis, and genitourinary retroperitoneal fibrosis.

### Contraindications

Contraindications of ergotamine include a known hypersensitivity reaction to the drug or its components. Additional contraindications are the existence of peripheral vascular disease, hepatic and renal disease, coronary artery disease, hypertension, and sepsis. The FDA has issued a **BLACK BOX WARNING** ◆

| TABLE 52.4 | | | | |
|---|---|---|---|---|
| **DRUGS AT A GLANCE: Ergot Alkaloids** | | | | |
| **Drug** | **Pregnancy Category** | **Routes and Dosages** | | |
| | | **Adults** | | **Children** |
| Ⓟ **Ergotamine tartrate** (Ergomar) | X | 1–2 mg sublingual followed by 1–2 mg every 30 min until headache abates or until max dosage of 6 mg/24 h or 10 mg/wk | | Safety and efficacy have not been established. |
| Dihydroergotamine mesylate (D.H.E. 45, Migranal; 🍁 Migranal) | X | 1 mg may be repeated at 1-h intervals to a total of 3 mg IM or 2 mg IV or SC (max dosage: 6 mg/wk) 1 spray (0.5 mg) in each nostril, may repeat with additional spray in 15 min if no relief (max of 4 sprays/ attack); wait 6–8 h before treating another attack (max of sprays 8 sprays/24 h, 24 sprays/wk) | | Safety and efficacy have not been established. |

stating that ergotamine is contraindicated with potent inhibitors of CYP3A4 medications. These drugs include the protease inhibitors, azole antifungals, and some macrolide antibiotics. Concomitant use of these medications results in the risk of vasospasm, producing serious or life-threatening cerebral and limb ischemia. Pregnancy and lactation are also contraindications to the use of ergotamine.

## Nursing Implications

### Preventing Interactions

Ergot derivatives may increase the hypertensive effects of alpha 1 agonists. Ergotamine is metabolized by the cytochrome P450 enzyme CYP3A4 in the liver; therefore, it is important to avoid all CPY3A4 inhibitors. In addition, many medications and foods interact with ergotamine, increasing its effects (Boxes 52.4 and 52.5).

---

| BOX 52.4 |  | **Drug Interactions: Ergotamine** |
|---|---|---|

**Drugs That Increase the Effect of Ergotamine**

- Alpha- and beta-adrenergic blockers, sympathomimetics
  *Have additive vasoconstrictive effects*
- Erythromycin, troleandomycin
  *Increase the risk of peripheral vasospasm*
- Rizatriptan, sumatriptan, zolmitriptan
  *Increase the risk of coronary ischemia*
- Azole antifungals, nefazodone, fluoxetine, fluvoxamine, amprenavir, delavirdine, efavirenz, indinavir, nelfinavir, ritonavir, saquinavir
  *Inhibit ergotamine metabolism and increase toxicity*
- Sibutramine, dexfenfluramine, nefazodone, fluvoxamine
  *Increase the risk of muscle rigidity also known as serotonin rigidity*
- Clarithromycin, boceprevir, cobicistat, crizotinib, posaconazole
  *Increase the serum concentration of ergotamine*

---

### Administering the Medication

Administration of ergotamine is sublingual, and the tablet should be dissolved under the tongue. It is important that tablets not be crushed, chewed, or swallowed whole. Patients should not drink, eat, or smoke while the medication is being dissolved.

### Assessing for Therapeutic Effects

The nurse assesses for a decrease in headache pain.

### Assessing for Adverse Effects

Following administration of ergotamine, the nurse assesses for cardiovascular adverse effects. Measurement of pulse and blood pressure is essential. The nurse also assesses for vertigo, muscle pain, numbness, paresthesia, and weakness, as well as for signs and symptoms of a hypersensitivity reaction to ergotamine. It is important to assess the patient's fluid and electrolyte status if the patient is suffering from nausea and vomiting. In addition, the nurse assesses the patient's urinary elimination due to the adverse effect of retroperitoneal fibrosis in which the patient develops an obstruction of the ureters.

### Patient Teaching

Box 52.6 identifies patient teaching guidelines for ergotamine.

## Other Drugs in the Class

Dihydroergotamine mesylate reduces the rate of serotonin-induced platelet aggregation and has a weaker vasoconstrictive action than ergotamine. It has a greater adrenergic blocking activity to relieve migraine headaches.

---

| BOX 52.5 |  | **Herb and Dietary Interactions: Ergotamine** |
|---|---|---|

**Foods That Increase the Effect of Ergotamine**

- Cola
- Coffee
- Tea
- Grapefruit juice

## NCLEX Success

5. For the patient with migraine headaches who receives a prescription for an ergot alkaloid as abortive therapy, which of the following is a priority nursing intervention for patient education?
   A. Notify the prescriber if an aura precedes the migraine headache.
   B. Administer the medication with food.
   C. Seek emergency help if cardiac changes occur.
   D. Administer the medication with caffeinated beverages.

6. In assessing the 32-year-old woman who has been taking ergotamine tartrate as abortive therapy for migraine headache for many years, the nurse should assess for which of the following adverse effects?
   A. hypotension
   B. muscle weakness
   C. hypoventilation
   D. valvular fibrosis

## TRIPTANS

Triptans are serotonin 5-HT$_{1B}$ and 5-HT$_{1D}$ agonists that affect the pathophysiologic mechanism of migraine or cluster headaches, thus relieving the associated symptoms. The mechanism of action of the triptans, although similar to that of the ergot alkaloids, has a more selective serotonin agonist receptor profile, and it does not interact with adrenergic and dopaminergic receptors. In addition, the advantage of the administration of triptans over the ergot alkaloids is that these medications can be easily taken by patients during their daily lives. The prototype triptan is  **sumatriptan** (Imitrex, Onzetra Xsail, others).

## Pharmacokinetics

The oral preparation of sumatriptan has an onset of action of 60 to 90 minutes and a peak of action of 2 to 4 hours. The onset of action of intranasal sumatriptan is rapid, with a peak of action of

90 minutes. The onset of action of subcutaneous sumatriptan varies, with a peak of action of 5 to 20 minutes. Sumatriptan is widely distributed and is 10% to 20% protein bound. Its therapeutic half-life is 115 minutes. Metabolism occurs in the liver. Excretion is in the urine, with excretion of the oral preparation in the feces. Sumatriptan crosses the placenta and enters the breast milk.

## Action

Sumatriptan binds to the serotonin receptors 5-HT$_{1D}$, producing vascular constriction of the cranial blood vessels and relieving the pain of a migraine headache. It also relieves the nausea, vomiting, photophobia, and phonophobia that accompany the migraine headache. Figure 52.1 shows the site of action of triptans, including sumatriptan, in the relief of a migraine.

## Use

Health care providers use sumatriptan to treat acute migraine headache pain with or without an aura. They also use it to treat cluster headaches. Older adults should not take sumatriptan and other triptans. Table 52.5 gives dosage information for the triptans.

### Use in Patients With Renal Impairment

Caution is necessary when administering sumatriptan to patients with impaired renal function because elimination takes place in the renal system.

### Use in Patients With Hepatic Impairment

Caution is also warranted when administering sumatriptan to patients with impaired hepatic function because metabolism takes place in the liver.

## Adverse Effects

CNS adverse effects of all sumatriptan preparations are dizziness, vertigo, headache, anxiety, malaise, myalgia, and fatigue. Cardiovascular adverse effects include alterations in blood pressure and chest pain as well as the most severe cardiovascular adverse effect, shock. The nasal administration of sumatriptan produces nausea, nasal and throat irritation, and a bad taste in the mouth. The injectable form of the drug may cause injection site discomfort.

## Contraindications

Contraindications include a history of hypersensitivity reactions to the drug. Other contraindications are existing cerebrovascular or peripheral vascular syndromes.

## Nursing Implications

### Preventing Interactions

 **QSEN Alert: Safety**

It is important to ask the patient about recent administration ergot alkaloids. The ergot alkaloids should not be given within 24 hours of the administration of triptans. The combination of ergot-containing drugs and the triptans results in cardiac ischemia.

---

**BOX 52.6** — *Patient Teaching Guidelines for Ergotamine*

- Take ergotamine or ergot alkaloids at the onset of the migraine headache.
- Notify the prescriber if the migraine attacks occur more frequently or are not relieved.
- Rest in a dark room for 2 to 3 hours after taking the medication.
- Provide information on adverse effects and notify the prescriber if muscle pain, weakness of extremities, changes in heart rate, nausea, or vomiting develops.
- Never crush, swallow, or chew tablets.
- Do not increase dose unless indicated by the prescriber.

**Figure 52.1.** Site of action of migraine drugs. The site of action of triptans in aborting migraine attack include the following: [1] a direct contraction of dilated cranial extracerebral blood vessels; [2] suppression of neuropeptide [mainly calcitonin gene–related peptide or CGRP] release from peripheral nerve endings around blood vessels; [3] inhibition of impulse transmission centrally in the trigeminal nucleus caudalis; and [4] presynaptic blockade of synaptic transmission between axon terminals of the peripheral trigeminovascular neurons and cell bodies of their central counterparts. [Adapted with permission from Olesen, J., Tfelt-Hansen, P., Welch, K. M. A., Goadsby, P. J., & Ramadan, N. M. [2006]. *The Headaches* [3rd ed.]. [Fig. 51.4]. Philadelphia, PA: Lippincott Williams and Wilkins.]

Also, administration of monoamine oxidase (MAO) inhibitors leads to increased serum levels of sumatriptan and sumatriptan toxicity. Two weeks after an MAO inhibitor has been discontinued, it is permissible to give sumatriptan in combination with the MAO inhibitor. In addition, administration of the herb St. John's wort with triptans results in triptan toxicity.

## Administering the Medication

It is important to administer sumatriptan at the onset of migraine symptoms. Although it is appropriate to administer a second dose of the oral preparation when symptoms return, this should not occur earlier than 2 hours after the first tablet is taken. Dosages should not exceed 100 mg in a single dose or 200 mg/day. It is necessary to administer the oral preparation

## TABLE 52.5

## DRUGS AT A GLANCE: Triptans

| Drug | Pregnancy Category | Routes and Dosages | |
|---|---|---|---|
| | | **Adults** | **Children** |
| ℗ **Sumatriptan** (Imitrex, Onzetra Xsail, others; ❧ Imitrex, Sumatriptan DF) | C | 25, 50, or 100 mg PO; additional doses may be repeated in 2 h or more (max dosage 200 mg/d) 6 mg SC may be repeated in ≥1 h (max dosage 12 mg/24 h) 22 mg intranasally, half into each nostril or 10 mg divided doses of 5 mg, one in each nostril; may be repeated once after 2 h (max dosage 44 mg/24 h) 1 patch (6.5 mg/4 h) transdermal; may be repeated in ≥2 h (max 2 patches/24 h) | Safety and efficacy have not been established. |
| Almotriptan (❧ Axert, Mylan-Almotriptan, Sandoz Almotriptan) | C | 6.25–12.5 mg PO repeat after 2 h if necessary (max, 2 doses/24 h) | ≥12 y: same as adult dosing |
| Eletriptan (Relpax; ❧ Relpax) | C | 20–40 mg PO as a single dose, repeat after 2 h if necessary (max dose, 80 mg/d) | Safety and efficacy have not been established. |
| Frovatriptan (Frova; ❧ Frova) | C | 2.5 mg PO; repeat after 2 h if necessary (max dose, 7.5 mg) | Safety and efficacy have not been established. |
| Naratriptan (Amerge; ❧ Amerge) | C | 1–2.5 mg PO as a single dose; repeat in 4 h if necessary (max dose, 5 mg/d) | Safety and efficacy have not been established. |

| TABLE 52.5 | | | |
|---|---|---|---|
| **DRUGS AT A GLANCE: Triptans** (Continued) | | | |
| **Drug** | **Pregnancy Category** | **Routes and Dosages** | |
| | | **Adults** | **Children** |
| Rizatriptan (Maxalt, Maxalt-MLT; ✳ Maxalt, Maxalt RPD) | C | 5–10 mg PO as a single dose; repeat after 2 h if necessary (max dose, 30 mg/d) | ≥6 y: <40 kg 5 mg PO as a single dose; ≥40 kg 10 mg as a single dose; safety and efficacy of multiple doses in a 24-h period have not been established. |
| Zolmitriptan (Zomig, Zomig ZMT; ✳ Zomig, Zomig Nasal Spray, Zomig Rapimelt) | C | 1.25–2.5 mg PO as a single dose; may repeat after 2 h if necessary (max dose, 10 mg/d) 2.5 mg intranasal by unit-dose spray device (max dose, 5 mg/d) Orally disintegrating tablets (Zomig ZMT) 2.5–5 mg as a single dose; may repeat after 2 h if necessary (max dose, 10 mg/d) | ≥12 y: nasal inhalation, same as adult dosing |
| Sumatriptan and naproxen (Treximet) | C | 1 tablet (sumatriptan 85 mg and naproxen 500 mg) PO; if migraine is not relieved in 2 h, a second dose may be administered (max dose, 2 tablets/24 h) | ≥12 y: 1 tablet (sumatriptan 10 mg and naproxen 60 mg) PO (max dose, 85 mg naproxen/naproxen 500 mg [single adult dose]) |

with fluids and the intranasal preparation as a single dose of one spray in each nostril. With the subcutaneous preparation, administration just below the skin as soon as symptoms develop is best. If relief does not occur or if symptoms reappear, a second injection may follow 1 hour or longer after the first one. A person may have two injections in 24 hours. With the administration of all sumatriptan preparations, it is necessary to monitor the blood pressure for hypertension.

### Assessing Therapeutic Effects

The nurse assesses for diminished pain and ultimate relief of migraine headaches.

### Assessing for Adverse Effects

The nurse assesses for increased blood pressure, as well as chest pain, shock, dizziness, and vertigo. With subcutaneous administration, the nurse also assesses for irritation at the injection site.

### Patient Teaching

Box 52.7 identifies patient teaching guidelines for sumatriptan.

## Other Drugs in the Class

Almotriptan (Axert) is similar in action to other triptans; however, it can be administered with MAO inhibitors. After oral administration, it has a variable onset of action and a peak of action of 1 to 3 hours. Prior to administering almotriptan, it is necessary to determine whether the patient has received any ergot alkaloids in the past 24 hours.

Eletriptan (Relpax) has a rapid onset of action, with a 1.5- to 2-hour peak of action. It is administered orally in 20- or 40-mg doses. It is important to ensure the patient has not taken an ergot-containing compound within 24 hours and to control the environment for light and sound. The drug is usually well tolerated and causes no major harm; however, any elevation in blood pressure or chest pain requires discontinuation of the medication.

Frovatriptan (Frova) has a variable onset of action and reaches the peak of action in 2 to 4 hours. It interacts unfavorably with selective serotonin reuptake inhibitors such as fluoxetine, fluvoxamine, paroxetine, and sertraline, producing weakness, hyperreflexia, and diminished CNS effects such as alertness. Frovatriptan may lead to serotonin syndrome, and a potentially life-threatening reaction may occur when two drugs that affect serotonin levels in the body are taken concurrently. Other symptoms of serotonin syndrome include restlessness, hallucinations, fever, loss of consciousness, tachycardia, and a rapid change in blood pressure.

Naratriptan (Amerge) has a slow onset of action. Contraindications include a creatinine clearance less than 15 mL/min or severe hepatic impairment. Women of childbearing age should use barrier contraceptives due to the risk of serious birth defects.

**BOX 52.7** | **Patient Teaching Guidelines for Sumatriptan**

- Provide instruction about the administration of subcutaneous sumatriptan or use of the autoinjector.
- Do not administer more than two injections in 24 hours.
- Inject just below the skin as soon as symptoms are noted.
- Properly dispose of the autoinjector, syringes, and needles.
- Administer nasal spray as a single dose; repeat if necessary in 2 hours.
- Do not administer the medication if you are pregnant.
- Do not operate machinery after the administration of sumatriptan.
- Report symptoms of hypersensitivity such as heat, flushing, tiredness, and feeling sick to your health care provider.

Rizatriptan (Maxalt) is an oral preparation that can be swallowed or administered in a "melt-away" (orally disintegrating) formulation. It is effective in the treatment of acute migraine. The most common adverse effects are dizziness, fatigue, nausea, and somnolence. Patients with risk factors for coronary artery disease should receive the initial dose in a health care setting where their response can be evaluated.

Zolmitriptan (Zomig) is a triptan that may be administered orally or intranasally. The onset of action of the oral drug is variable, whereas that of the intranasal preparation is 15 minutes. Two large studies have found that zolmitriptan is effective for acute migraine therapy, with an optimal starting dose of 2.5 mg. The most commonly reported adverse effects were dizziness, nausea, somnolence, paresthesia, fatigue, and tightness of the throat or chest.

Sumatriptan–naproxen sodium (Treximet) is a combination drug that is administered orally. Patients should not divide, chew, or crush the tablets. This combination is effective in treating acute migraine and decreasing photophobia. The FDA has issued two **BLACK BOX WARNING** ◆: (1) cardiovascular risk from sumatriptan, with an increased risk of adverse thrombotic events, including myocardial infarction and stroke, and (2) GI risk due to naproxen sodium, with an increased risk of GI irritation, inflammation, ulceration, bleeding, and perforation.

## NCLEX Success

7. A 50-year-old woman has a subarachnoid bleed. She has received treatment for migraine headaches in the past. Which of the following patient teaching guidelines is a priority on her discharge from the rehabilitation facility?

   A. Take estrogen to prevent a menstrual migraine.
   B. Take gabapentin for neuropathic pain.
   C. Do not take sumatriptan for migraine headache.
   D. Take zolmitriptan because it has a more rapid onset of action.

8. A patient has taken sumatriptan–naproxen sodium for an acute migraine. She has also taken over-the-counter ibuprofen for menstrual cramps. Which of the following adverse effects is she at risk for developing?

   A. bronchospasm
   B. urinary retention
   C. edema
   D. gastrointestinal bleeding

Ms. Van Art is discharged from the emergency department following an acute migraine headache. Her prescriber orders sumatriptan (Imitrex) to be administered subcutaneously at the onset of an acute migraine headache.

- What education will Ms. Van Art receive prior to discharge?
- What information will Ms. Van Art need if subcutaneous medication administration is new to her?
- What medications are contraindicated with the administration of sumatriptan?

## ESTROGEN

Estrogen in the form of **estradiol** is a treatment for menstrual migraines, which are most likely 2 days prior to menses through the 3rd day of bleeding. Perimenstrual estrogen supplementation is based on evidence that the natural decline in estrogen in the late luteal phase of the menstrual cycle, prior to menstruation, is associated with the increased risk of migraine.

### Pharmacokinetics

Metabolism of estradiol occurs in the liver. Excretion takes place in the urine. The drug crosses the placenta and enters the breast milk.

### Action

Estradiol binds to intracellular receptors to form a complex that stimulates synthesis of proteins responsible for estrogenic effects. Prophylactic administration minimizes the premenstrual decline in estrogen that precipitates the development of the migraine headache.

### Use

Transcutaneous administration of estradiol increases the estrogen levels in the late luteal phase of the menstrual cycle that contribute to the development of menstrual migraine headaches. Table 52.6 and Chapter 7 give dosage information for estradiol.

### Adverse Effects

The major adverse effect associated with the administration of estrogen preparations is thromboembolic disorders. Menstrual irregularity can occur because of the suppression of endogenous estrogen during treatment.

**TABLE 52.6**

**DRUGS AT A GLANCE: Estradiol**

| Drug | Pregnancy Category | Routes and Dosages | |
|------|--------------------|--------------------|---|
| | | **Adults** | **Children** |
| ℗ **Estradiol** | X | 100-mcg patch or 1.5-mg gel | Safety and efficacy have not been established for treating migraines. |

**BOX 52.8    Drug Interactions: Estradiol**

**Drugs That Increase the Effects of Estradiol**
- Cyclosporine, theophylline, tricyclic antidepressants
  *Increase serum levels*

**Drugs That Decrease the Effects of Estradiol**
- Phenytoin and rifampin
  *Decrease serum levels*
- Nicotine
  *Reduces or cancels efficacy*

## Contraindications

Contraindications include incomplete bone growth, which occurs in adolescents. Other contraindications are the presence of neoplasms, breast cancer, thromboembolic disorders, fibroids, endometriosis, thyroid disease, and pregnancy.

## Nursing Implications

### Preventing Interactions

Some drugs interact with estradiol, increasing or decreasing its effects (Box 52.8). In addition, the combination of estradiol and bromocriptine interferes with the effects of bromocriptine.

### Administering the Medication

Prior to applying the transcutaneous preparation, it is necessary to clean and dry the skin area. It is important to apply the preparation to the trunk.

### Assessing for Therapeutic Effects

The nurse assesses for the development of migraine headache in the later luteal phase of the menstrual cycle. If a headache does not develop, the dose is adequate.

### Assessing for Adverse Effects

The nurse assesses for the development of leg pain or chest pain indicative of the development of thromboembolism. He or she also assesses for breakthrough bleeding.

### Patient Teaching

Box 52.9 identifies patient teaching guidelines for estradiol.

## PREVENTIVE THERAPY FOR MIGRAINE HEADACHES

Many medications are administered for the prevention of migraine headaches. These medications are primarily

**BOX 52.9    Patient Teaching Guidelines for Estradiol**

- Take estradiol transdermal as ordered by the prescriber.
- Notify your health care provider of intermittent breakthrough bleeding, spotting, or unexplained pain, especially calf or chest pain.

administered for the treatment of other conditions and are thoroughly covered in other chapters. Their use in the prevention of migraines medications is discussed briefly. For complete information about these drugs, one may review the information in the chapters indicated.

## Carboxylic Acid Derivative

Valproic acid (see Chap. 53) is a carboxylic acid derivative that is most commonly administered to control seizures. However, it has proved effective in the prevention of migraine headaches. Valproic acid is available in two forms. The dosage for valproic acid tablets is 250 mg orally two times per day, with a maximum dosage of 1000 mg. The dosage of the extended-release preparation is 500 mg orally once per day. Limited data suggest that valproic acid is safe for children as young as 7 years of age, and extended-release valproic acid is well tolerated by adolescents with migraine headaches. The risk of hepatotoxicity with valproic acid in children younger than 2 years has been reported.

## Gamma-Aminobutyric Acid

Gabapentin (Neurontin; see Chap. 53) is a gamma-aminobutyric acid medication commonly administered to control neuropathic pain and as an adjunctive agent for control of seizures. Studies have shown that gabapentin is effective in reducing the frequency of migraines. At the end of 12 weeks, 46% of patients who received 2400 mg/day had a 50% reduction in the 4-week rate of migraine. The most commonly reported adverse effects were dizziness and somnolence.

## Sulfamate-Substituted Monosaccharide

Topiramate (Topamax) is a sulfamate-substituted monosaccharide agent used most commonly as an antiepileptic agent (see Chap. 53). In clinical trials, the mean monthly migraine frequency decreased significantly with either 100 or 200 mg/day compared with placebo. However, with 50 mg/day, there was no statistically significant reduction in migraine frequency. The most commonly reported adverse effects include paresthesia, fatigue, anorexia, diarrhea, weight loss, altered memory, difficulty concentrating, and nausea. Limited data from comparative trials suggest that topiramate is as effective as the beta-adrenergic blocking agent propranolol; however, topiramate is much more expensive than propranolol.

## Beta-Adrenergic Blocking Agents

The most common beta-adrenergic blocking agent administered prophylactically for migraine headaches is propranolol (Inderal) (see Chap. 27). The recommended dosage is two divided doses, starting at 40 mg daily. The maintenance dosage may be increased to 160 to 240 mg/day. Studies have shown that propranolol is effective in reducing migraine frequency.

In addition, two other beta-adrenergic blockers, metoprolol (50 mg daily in two divided doses, ranging to 200 mg daily) and timolol (5 mg once daily, ranging from 10 to 30 mg daily in two divided doses), are effective for migraine prophylaxis. It takes several weeks for these drugs to become effective, and it is necessary to titrate the dose for at least 3 months to ascertain effectiveness.

A concern related to the use of beta-adrenergic blockers is the increased risk of stroke and other cardiovascular events, which limits their use in patients older than 60 and in those who smoke.

## Calcium Channel Blockers

Verapamil is the calcium channel blocker of choice for migraine prophylaxis. It takes several weeks for benefits of the medication to be noted. It seems to be the most effective calcium channel blocker for migraine prevention. It is necessary to take 120 mg in three divided doses.

Studies have also noted that tolerance may develop with calcium channel blockers. Tolerance to the medication can be overcome by increasing the dosage or switching to a different calcium channel blocker. Calcium channel blocking agents such as nifedipine (Procardia) (see Chap. 28) have been used for prevention of migraine headache. However, data supporting the efficacy of calcium channel blockers are weak and conflicting.

## Angiotensin-Converting Enzyme Inhibitors

As Chapter 26 points out, enalapril maleate is the prototype angiotensin-converting enzyme (ACE) inhibitor, but clinical trials have shown that lisinopril seems to be more effective in the prevention of migraine headaches. A study has shown that a dose of 10 mg/day for 1 week and then 20 mg/day reduced the number of hours and days with headache and headache severity compared to a placebo. However, the small sample size and design of this clinical trial and another performed by the same investigators limits any definitive conclusions regarding the use of ACE inhibitors in migraine prevention. These drugs are not widely used in migraine management. An adverse effect with ACE inhibitors is the development of a cough, which is the result of an interference with bradykinin, substance P, or tachykinin metabolism.

## Angiotensin II Receptor Blockers

Angiotensin II receptor blockers (see Chap. 26) can be effective in the prevention of migraine headache but are not commonly used. Studies on the effectiveness of candesartan have revealed that it produces favorable results in the prevention of migraine headaches. It is necessary to inform women of childbearing age that barrier contraceptives are required with this medication. The FDA has issued a **BLACK BOX WARNING ◆** stating that fetal injury and death have been reported with candesartan.

Olmesartan is effective and well tolerated as a migraine prophylactic agent for patients with comorbid hypertension and prehypertension. Researchers have studied patients with hypertension and prehypertension to determine the effectiveness of this medication.

## Tricyclic Antidepressants

Imipramine (Tofranil) and other tricyclic antidepressants (see Chap. 54) are effective in the prevention of migraine and tension headaches. Amitriptyline 10 to 50 mg at bedtime is also effective for migraine prophylaxis. Tricyclic antidepressants have a sedative effect, and to minimize this, it helps to administer the drugs at bedtime. Other side effects of tricyclic antidepressants include dry mouth, constipation, tachycardia, palpitations, orthostatic hypotension, weight gain, and urinary retention.

## Herbal and Vitamin Supplements

People with migraines may use herbal supplements to treat these headaches. Several herbs, including feverfew and butterbur, and vitamins, such as magnesium and riboflavin, have shown modest efficacy for migraine prevention. In general, it is necessary to encourage patients to try standard methods of preventing and treating migraine before taking products with uncertain benefits and risks.

Feverfew, an herbal medicine, is most widely studied for migraine prevention, but evidence of its benefit is conflicting. The main active ingredient of feverfew is thought to be parthenolide, which functions by inhibiting platelet aggregation, prostaglandin synthesis, and the release of inflammatory mediators such as histamine. Its exact mechanism in migraine prophylaxis is unknown. Study results have not established that feverfew is more effective than placebo for the prevention of migraine. Contraindications include pregnancy and lactation. The safety of the herb is unknown.

Butterbur is an extract of a perennial shrub. Two small clinical trials have shown limited efficacy in migraine prophylaxis. Concerns that the pyrrolizidine alkaloids in feverfew are hepatotoxic and potentially carcinogenic have raised concerns about their long-term safety. The most common adverse effect in the trials was burping.

Magnesium may be successful in treating and preventing migraine headaches in pregnant women. Adverse effects include diarrhea and GI discomfort.

Riboflavin, vitamin $B_2$, has demonstrated statistically significant benefit in the reduction in the frequency of headaches, the number of headache days per month, and mean headache severity. Its use is well tolerated. Riboflavin is inexpensive and produces minimal side effects. However, the benefits of the vitamin are not realized for up to 3 months of therapy. Without additional studies, it is uncertain who would most likely benefit from the administration of riboflavin and what dose produces optimal benefits.

**NCLEX  Success**

9. Which of the following factors prevents the use of estradiol for the treatment of menstrual migraines for a 14-year-old?
   A. breakthrough bleeding
   B. leg pain
   C. incomplete long bone growth
   D. anxiety

10. A 16-year-old girl develops migraine headaches. Which of the following medications is safe and effective for the treatment of migraine headaches?
   A. antiepileptic agents
   B. triptans
   C. ergot alkaloids
   D. opioids

11. Reduced dosages of zolpidem are expected in older adults and patients with renal impairment because these conditions result in an increase in which pharmacokinetic states? [Select all that apply.]
   A. first-pass effect
   B. bioavailability
   C. half-life
   D. peak plasma concentration
   E. receptor site activation

## ADJUVANT MEDICATIONS FOR MIGRAINE HEADACHES

Adjuvant medications administered for severe migraine headaches include antiemetics and opioids. Antiemetic agents are adjuvant medications administered to control the symptoms of nausea and vomiting related to migraine, tension, and cluster headaches. Table 52.7 gives dosage information for the antiemetics. Opioid use is controversial because these agents can contribute to the development of chronic daily headache and interference with preventive therapy. Opioids are not discussed in this section but are reviewed in Chapter 49.

Antiemetic agents may be useful for treatment of symptoms related to migraine headache. Chlorpromazine hydrochloride (see Chap. 56) is a phenothiazine that has been shown to be effective in treating both the headache itself and the associated nausea and vomiting. Investigators have also shown that antiemetic drugs decrease the photophobia and phonophobia that may accompany the migraine headache. The mechanism of action involved in the decrease of nausea and vomiting is related to the suppression of the chemoreceptor zone. Besides chlorpromazine, related antiemetics include metoclopramide and prochlorperazine. Parenteral preparations of these drugs appear more effective than oral preparations. When administering the antiemetic agents, it is necessary to assess the patient for relief of headache, nausea, and vomiting. Chlorpromazine also depresses the CNS, so it is important to assess the patient's level of consciousness.

Metoclopramide is a GI stimulant that is effective in reducing headache, nausea, and vomiting. It is less effective than chlorpromazine in reducing symptoms. Metoclopramide is a potent central dopamine receptor antagonist that increases esophageal sphincter tone and elevates the chemoreceptor zone threshold. Although the drug can be administered by numerous routes, the American Headache Society guidelines prefer the intravenous route for migraine relief (see Table 52.7).

Prochlorperazine has the same antiemetic action as chlorpromazine and metoclopramide. When taking prochlorperazine orally, it is important to swallow it whole and not chew or crush the tablets. When administering the medication parenterally, it is necessary to give it intramuscularly (deep) and never subcutaneously. When administering metoclopramide and prochlorperazine, it is necessary to assess the patient for signs and symptoms of dystonia, which is indicative of a hypersensitivity reaction. If the patient develops dystonia, it is necessary to administer diphenhydramine to counteract this reaction. With all of these medications, the patient should be assessed for urinary retention due to the anticholinergic effects.

### TABLE 52.7

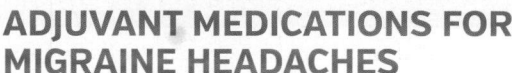

### DRUGS AT A GLANCE: Antiemetics Used for the Treatment of Headaches

| Drug | Pregnancy Category | Routes and Dosages | |
|---|---|---|---|
| | | **Adults** | **Children** |
| **Chlorpromazine hydrochloride** (Chlorpromazine Hydrochloride Injection) | C | 10–25 mg PO every 4–6 h; 50–100-mg suppository rectally every 6–8 h; 25–50 mg IM/IV every 4–6 h | >6 mo: 0.55 mg/kg PO every 4–6 h PRN up to 500 mg/d >6 mo: 0.55 mg/kg IM/IV every 6–8 h |
| Metoclopramide (Reglan; Metoclopramide Hydrochloride Injection, Metoclopramide Omega, Metonia) | B | 10–20 mg PO as a single dose; 10 mg IM/SC as a single dose; 10–20 mg IV as a single dose | 2 mg/kg IM/IV |
| Prochlorperazine (Compro) | C | 5–10 mg PO 3–4 2/d sustained release; 10–15 mg every 12 h; 5–10 mg IM every 3–4 h (max dose, 40 mg); 2.5–10 mg IV every 3–4 h (max dose, 40 mg); 25 mg per rectum two times per day | 2.5 mg PO or per rectum 1–3 times per day or 5 mg two times per day (max dose, 15 mg/d; 0.13 mg/kg IM every 3–4 h) |

A concept map outlines the nursing process related to drug therapy considerations in this chapter. Additional nursing implications related to the disease process should also be considered in care decisions.

**Assessment**
- Assess the severity, patterns (including frequency), and occurrences of cluster, tension, or migraine headaches. Include any additional symptoms such as photophobia, aura, alterations in vision (e.g., flashing lights, unilateral vision loss), and nausea or vomiting.

**Outcomes of Therapy**

The patient will
- Take medications as prescribed to routinely prevent headache.
- Take medications to abort and/or treat acute migraine with the onset of symptoms or aura.
- Avoid trigger factors that contribute to headache symptoms.
- Experience fewer and less severe attacks of migraine, tension, or cluster headaches.

**Nursing Interventions**
- Implement measures to minimize and prevent the symptoms of headache.
- Instruct the patient on medications to treat acute migraine headache pain.
- Instruct the patient on the trigger points related to migraine and strategies to decrease trigger points.
- Instruct the patient on medications to prevent migraine headaches.
- Administer medications to treat acute migraine headaches.
- Administer medications to prevent migraine headaches.
- Administer antiemetic agents to reduce nausea and vomiting during acute episodes.

**Evaluation**
- Interview and observe patient for relief of symptoms.
- Interview and observe patient's ability to provide self-care.
- Interview and observe patient regarding safe, effective use of the medications for acute and preventive treatment.
- Interview and assess patient for medication compliance.

 **KEY CONCEPTS**

- Cluster headaches are characterized by recurrent, severe, unilateral orbitotemporal headaches that are associated with a histamine reaction.
- Tension headaches are associated with nervous tension or anxiety and involve the chronic contraction of the scalp muscles.
- Migraine headache are unilateral pain in the head that may or may not be accompanied by an aura, which is a subjective sensation that immediately precedes the migraine headache.
- Menstrual migraines are associated with a drop in circulating estrogen 2 to 3 days prior to the onset of menses.
- The safest way to manage migraines, particularly in pregnant women, involve changes in lifestyle (i.e., adequate sleep, healthy meals, exercise), which may lead to a reduction in the

frequency and severity of migraine symptoms. In addition, relaxation training, yoga, and biofeedback may prove helpful. The FDA has issued a **BLACK BOX WARNING ◆** indicating serious risk of cardiovascular thrombotic events and risk of serious GI bleeding, ulceration, and perforation with naproxen use.
- Naproxen sodium is administered for the reduction pain related to an acute migraine headache.
- The combination of acetaminophen, aspirin, and caffeine has been used for the treatment of headaches.
- Ergotamine produces stimulation of the cranial and peripheral vascular smooth muscles while depressing the effects of the central vasomotor centers. It is a partial agonist and antagonist against tryptaminergic, dopaminergic, and alpha-adrenergic receptors.

- A **BLACK BOX WARNING** ◆ stresses that ergotamine is contraindicated with potent inhibitors of CYP3A4 medications. These medications include the protease inhibitors, azole antifungals, and some macrolide antibiotics. Concomitant use of these medications results in ergot toxicity.
- Triptans are serotonin 1B/1D agonists that act on the pathophysiologic mechanism of the headache. The advantage of the administration of triptans over the ergot alkaloids is that these medications are easily administered by the patient throughout their daily lives.
- For the sumatriptan/naproxen sodium combination (Treximet), the FDA has issued two **BLACK BOX WARNING** ◆: (1) cardiovascular risk from sumatriptan, which has an increased risk of adverse thrombotic events, and (2) GI effects due to naproxen sodium, which has an increased risk of GI irritation, inflammation, ulceration, bleeding, and perforation.

- Estrogen supplementation in the form of estradiol in the late luteal phase decreases symptoms of menstrual migraines.
- Abortive agents administered for the symptomatic treatment of migraine headaches include nonsteroidal anti-inflammatory agents, acetaminophen–aspirin with caffeine medication, the ergot alkaloids, and the triptans.
- Preventive agents administered to prevent the development of migraine headaches include antiepileptic agents, beta-adrenergic blockers, calcium channel blockers, and the angiotensin II receptor blockers. Antidepressants have been identified as beneficial in long-term treatment of migraine headache.
- The FDA has issued a **BLACK BOX WARNING** ◆ stating that fetal injury and death have been reported with candesartan, an angiotensin II receptor blocker.
- The adjuvant medications administered for severe migraine headaches include antiemetics and opioids.

## CLINICAL REASONING CASE STUDY

**Meet the Patient**

Jasmine Doral, a 20-year-old woman, is diagnosed with acute migraines. She receives a prescription for sumatriptan 6 mg to be administered with the onset of migraine symptoms. She experiences an aura prior to the onset of pain.

- What is the action of sumatriptan?
- What are the adverse effects of sumatriptan?
- When should sumatriptan be administered?
- What patient teaching does the nurse implement?

**Assessing Drug Information**

- Sumatriptan binds to the serotonin receptors 5-HT1D, producing vascular constriction on the cranial blood vessels to relieve the pain associated with a migraine headache. It also relieves the nausea, vomiting, photophobia, and phonophobia that accompany the pain.
- Sumatriptan is used for the acute treatment of migraine with or without aura in adults. It is also used to treat cluster headaches in adults.
- Adverse effects include:
  - Local effects
    - Nasal formulation: nausea and irritation of the nose and throat, and a bad taste in the mouth
    - Injectable formulation: possible injection site discomfort
  - Central nervous system effects: dizziness, vertigo, headache, anxiety, malaise, myalgia, and fatigue
  - Cardiovascular effects: alterations in blood pressure and chest pain. The most severe cardiovascular adverse effect is shock.

**Nursing Actions**

- Ensure that Ms. Doral knows how to administer all forms of the medication, particularly the subcutaneous preparation and autoinjector. Here are guidelines for administration:
  - Administer the drug at the onset of migraine symptoms.
  - Administer a second dose of the oral preparation when the symptoms recur but no sooner than 2 hours after the first tablet.
  - Do not exceed 100 mg in a single dose or 200 mg in a day.
  - Take the oral preparation with fluids.
  - Administer the intranasal preparation by putting one spray in each nostril.
  - Inject the subcutaneous preparation just below the skin. If relief does not occur or symptoms recur, a second injection 1 hour or longer following the first injection is necessary. A health care provider such as a nurse may give a total of two injections in 24 hours.
  - Monitor the patient's blood pressure for hypertension. This is necessary with the administration of all sumatriptan preparations.
- Educate the patient about key teaching points. These include:
  - Do not administer more than two injections in 24 hours.
  - Inject just below the skin as soon as symptoms are noted.
  - Properly dispose of autoinjector, syringes, and needles.
  - Administer nasal spray as a single dose; repeat if necessary in 2 hours.
  - Ensure that pregnant patients do not take the medication. If Ms. Doral believes she is pregnant, she must notify her prescriber as soon as possible.
  - Do not operate machinery after the administration of sumatriptan.
  - Report feelings of hypersensitivity, such as heat, flushing, tiredness, and a feeling of sickness, to your health care provider.

*Visit* thePoint® **at http://thePoint.lww.com/Frandsen12e** *for answers to NCLEX Success questions (in Appendix A), answers to Clinical Application Case Studies (in Appendix B), and more!*

## REFERENCES AND RESOURCES

Burch, R., Rizzoli, P., & Loder, E. (2018). The prevalence and impact of migraine and severe headache in the United States: Figures and trends from government health studies. *Headache, 58*(4), 496–505.

Cady, R. K., & Farmer, K. (2016). Managing migraine by patient profile: Role of frovatriptan. *Patient Preference and Adherence, 10,* 501–510.

Cook, C., & Newberry, B. (2018). Emergency department use of intravenous prochlorperazine for acute migraine. *Advanced Emergency Nursing Journal, 40*(3), 148–154.

Diamond, M. L., & Hutchinson, S. (2018). Approach to the identification and differentiation of migraine. *Journal of Family Practice, 67* (8 Suppl), S9–S12.

Fisher, M., Fran, F., Willie, G., Klein, S., Lackner, P., & Broessner, G. (2016). Triptans for acute migraine headache: Current experience with triptan use and prescription habits in a tertiary care headache outpatient clinic: An observational study. *Headache: The Journal of Head and Face Pain, 48*(6), 952–960.

Friedmann, B. W., Cabral, L., Adewunmi, V., Solorzano, C., Esses, D., Bijur, P. E., et al. (2016). Diphenhydramine as adjuvant therapy for acute migraine: An emergency department-based randomized clinical trial. *Annals of Emergency Medicine, 67*(1), 32–39.

Goadsby, P. J., Holland, P. R., Martins-Oliveira, M., Hofmann, J., Schankin, C., & Ackerman, S. (2018). Pathophysiology of migraine: A disorder of sensory processing. *Physiological Reviews, 97*(2), 553–622. doi:10.1152/physrev.00034.2015

Guilbot, A., Bangratz, M., Abdella, S. A., & Lucas, C. (2017). A combination of coenzyme Q10, feverfew and magnesium for migraine prophylaxis: A prospective observational study. *BMC Complementary and Alternative Medicine, 17*(433), 1–7.

He, A. Song, D., Zhang, L., & Li, C. (2017). Unveiling the relative efficacy, safety and tolerability of prophylactic medications for migraine: Pairwise and network-meta analysis. *The Journal of Headache and Pain, 18*(26), 1–17.

Hesami, O., Shams, M. R., Ayazkhoo, L., Assarzadegan, F., Lima, B. S., et al. (2018). Comparison of pregabalin and sodium valproate in migraine prophylaxis: A randomized double-blinded study. *Iranian Journal of Pharmaceutical Research: IJPR, 17*(2), 781–789.

Kacperski, J., & Bazarsky, A. (2017). New developments in the prophylactic drug treatment of pediatric migraine: What is new in 2017 and where does it leave us? *Current Pain and Headache Reports, 21*(38), 1–5.

Karch, A. (2020). *Focus on nursing pharmacology* (8th ed.). Philadelphia, PA: Wolters Kluwer.

Leone, M., Giustiniani, A., & Cecchini, A. P. (2017). Cluster headache: Present and future therapy. *Neurological Sciences, 38*(Suppl I), 545–550.

Lipton, R. B., Diener, H. C., Robbins, M. S., Garas, S. Y., & Patel, K. (2017). Caffeine in the management of patients with headache. *The Journal of Headache and Pain, 18*(107), 1–11.

Mannix, S., Skalicky, A., Buse, D. C., Desai, P., Sapra, S., et al. (2016). Measuring the impact of migraine for evaluating outcomes of preventive treatments for migraine headaches. *Health and Quality of Life Outcomes, 14*(143), 1–11.

Mayans, L., & Walling, A. (2018). Acute migraine headache: Treatment strategies. *American Academy of Family Physicians, 97*(4), 243–251.

Norris, T. L. C. M. (2019). *Pathophysiology: Concepts of altered health states* (10th ed.). Philadelphia, PA: Wolters Kluwer.

Orr, S. L., Friedman, B. W., Christie, S., Minen, M. T., Bamford, C., Kelley, N. E., et al. (2016). Management of adults with acute migraine in the emergency department: The American Headache Society evidence assessment of parenteral pharmacotherapies. *Headache, 56*(6), 911–940.

Papadopoulus, G. (2017). A case of migraine headache successfully treated with low-dose magnesium phosphate in a pregnant woman. *Australian Journal of Herbal Medicine, 29*(4), 136–140.

Rizzoli, P. B. (2018). What the pharmacological management of migraine can tell us about the future of migraine patient care. *Neurological Sciences, 39*(Suppl 1), 539–545.

Robbins, M. S., Starling, A. J., Pringsheim, T. M., Becker, W. J., & Schwedt, T. J. (2016). Treatment of cluster headache: The American Headache Society evidence-based guidelines. *Headache, 56*(7), 1093–1106.

Sahd-Brown, K. E. (2018). Acute migraine headache in children. *Nursing, 48*(4), 25–29.

Sheridan, D. C., & Meckler, G. D. (2016). Inpatient pediatric migraine treatment: Does choice of abortive therapy affect length of stay? *Journal of Pediatrics, 179*, 211–215.

Thompson, D. F., & Saluja, H. S. (2017). Prophylaxis of migraine headaches with riboflavin: A systematic review. *Journal of Clinical Pharmacy and Therapeutics, 42*(4), 394–403. doi:10.1111/jcpt.12548

UpToDate. (2019). *Drug information*. Lexi-Comp, Inc.

Wieckiewicz, M., Grychowska, N., Zietak, M., Wiecklewicz, G., & Smardz, J. (2018). Evidence to use botulinum toxin injections in tension-type headache management: A systematic review. *Toxins (Basel), 9*(370), 1–8.

# Drug Therapy for Seizure Disorders and Skeletal Muscle Disorders

## LEARNING OBJECTIVES

*After studying this chapter, you should be able to:*

1. Identify types of seizures as well as the potential causes and pathophysiology of seizures.
2. Identify factors that influence the choice of antiepileptic medications in treating seizure disorders.
3. Identify the prototypes and describe the actions, uses, adverse effects, contraindications, and nursing implications for antiepileptic drugs in all classes.
4. Describe strategies for prevention and treatment of status epilepticus.
5. Implement the nursing process in the care of patients undergoing drug therapy for seizure disorders.
6. Discuss the common symptoms and disorders for which skeletal muscle relaxants are used.
7. Identify the prototypes and describe the actions, uses, adverse effects, contraindications, and nursing implications for the skeletal muscle relaxants.
8. Implement the nursing process in the care of patients undergoing drug therapy for muscle spasms and spasticity.

## CLINICAL APPLICATION CASE STUDY

Two days ago, Andrew Cummings, a 7-year-old boy, was at home playing and experienced a tonic–clonic seizure, which was witnessed by his mother. On questioning the mother, a pediatric neurologist at the hospital where the boy was admitted determined that the seizure was unprovoked and had a generalized onset. The mother stated that it lasted approximately 3 minutes. The neurologist diagnoses a seizure disorder. Andrew is now taking carbamazepine (Tegretol) 50 mg orally four times per day and valproate (Depakene Syrup) 20 mg/kg/d.

## KEY TERMS

**Antiepileptic drugs:** drugs used to control seizures or convulsions; also referred to as antiseizure medications or anticonvulsants

**Clonic:** spasms that alternate between contraction and relaxation

**Clonic phase:** rapid rhythmic and symmetric jerking movements of the body

**Convulsion:** tonic–clonic type of seizure characterized by spasmodic contractions of involuntary muscles

**Epilepsy:** disease where the patient has repetitive seizures

**Gingival hyperplasia:** overgrowth of the gums related to long-term administration of phenytoin

- **Malignant hyperthermia:** rare but life-threatening complication of anesthesia characterized by hypercarbia, metabolic acidosis, skeletal muscle rigidity, fever, and cyanosis

- **Monotherapy:** use of a single drug in drug therapy; advantages include fewer drug–drug interactions, lower cost, and usually greater patient adherence

- **Muscle spasm:** sudden, involuntary, painful muscle contraction that occurs with musculoskeletal trauma or inflammation

- **Seizure:** brief episode of abnormal electrical activity in nerve cells of the brain that may or may not be accompanied by visible changes in appearance or behavior

- **Spasticity:** caused by nerve damage in the brain and spinal cord, it is a permanent condition that may be painful and disabling; involves increased muscle tone or contraction and stiff, awkward movements

- **Status epilepticus:** repeated seizures or a seizure that lasts at least 30 minutes; may be convulsive, nonconvulsive, or partial

- **Tonic:** muscle spasms with sustained contraction

- **Tonic–clonic:** most common type of seizure; often referred to as a major motor seizure

- **Tonic phase:** sustained contraction of skeletal muscles; abnormal postures, such as opisthotonos; and absence of respirations, during which the person becomes cyanotic

## INTRODUCTION

The first part of this chapter introduces the condition known as epilepsy, which is characterized by recurrent seizures, and discusses the pharmacologic care of the patient who is experiencing a seizure. Although the terms seizure and convulsion may be used interchangeably, they have different meanings. A seizure involves a brief episode of abnormal electrical activity in nerve cells of the brain that may or may not be accompanied by visible changes in appearance or behavior. It refers to all types of epileptic occurrences. A convulsion is a tonic–clonic type of seizure characterized by spasmodic contractions of involuntary muscles.

The second part of this chapter describes the role skeletal muscle relaxants play in decreasing seizures and reducing muscle spasms and spasticity associated with neurologic and musculoskeletal injuries. A muscle spasm is a sudden, involuntary, painful muscle contraction that occurs with musculoskeletal trauma (e.g., overuse or injury of skeletal muscle, twisting a joint, or tearing a ligament as with a sprain) or inflammation (e.g., bursitis, arthritis). Muscle spasm also occurs with acute and chronic low back pain. Spasms may be clonic (alternating contraction and relaxation) to tonic (sustained contraction). Muscle spasms commonly occur, sometimes causing significant disability with inflammation, edema, and poor coordination and mobility.

Spasticity involves increased muscle tone or contraction and stiff, awkward movements. It occurs in neurologic disorders such as multiple sclerosis, spinal cord injury, traumatic brain injury, cerebral palsy, and poststroke syndrome. Because spasticity is caused by nerve damage in the brain and spinal cord, it is a permanent condition that may be painful and disabling.

In patients with spinal cord injury, spasticity requires treatment when it impairs safety, mobility, and the ability to perform activities of daily living (e.g., self-care in hygiene, eating, dressing, and work or recreational activities). Stimuli that precipitate spasms vary from one individual to another and may include muscle stretching, bladder infections or stones, constipation and bowel distention, or infections. It is necessary to assess each person for personal precipitating factors, so that these factors can be avoided if possible. Treatment measures include passive range-of-motion and muscle-stretching exercises and antispasmodic medications (e.g., baclofen, dantrolene).

## OVERVIEW OF EPILEPSY

Sudden, abnormal, hypersynchronous firing of neurons is characteristic of epilepsy. Signs and symptoms of seizure activity lead to the diagnosis. On the electroencephalogram (EEG), abnormal brain wave patterns are present.

### Etiology

Seizures may occur as single events in response to hypoglycemia, fever, electrolyte imbalances, overdoses of numerous medications (e.g., amphetamine, cocaine, isoniazid, lidocaine, lithium, methylphenidate, antispasmodics, theophylline), and withdrawal from alcohol or sedative–hypnotic drugs. Alternatively, seizures may be idiopathic (having no discernible cause) or attributable to a secondary cause. Authorities also classify seizures as unprovoked (idiopathic) or provoked (secondary). Secondary causes in infancy include developmental defects, metabolic disease, or birth injury. Fever is a common secondary cause in late infancy and early childhood. Inherited forms of epilepsy usually begin in childhood or adolescence. When epilepsy begins in adulthood, it is often caused by an acquired neurologic disorder (e.g., head injury, stroke, brain tumor) or alcohol and other drug effects. Toxemia is a secondary cause of seizures in pregnancy.

Some of the identified specific causes of seizures include alterations in cell membrane permeability or the distribution of ions across the neuronal cell membranes. Genetic mutations have also been linked to epilepsy. In addition, a decrease in the inhibition of thalamic or cortical neuronal activity is a cause. Finally, imbalances in the neurotransmitters gamma-amino-butyric acid (GABA) or acetylcholine excess result in seizure disorders.

## Pathophysiology

Experts broadly classify seizures as partial or generalized. Partial seizures begin in a specific area of the brain and often indicate a localized brain lesion such as birth injury, trauma, stroke, or tumor. They produce symptoms ranging from simple motor and sensory manifestations to more complex abnormal movements and bizarre behavior. Movements are usually automatic, repetitive, and inappropriate to the situation, such as chewing, swallowing, or aversive movements (automatisms). In simple partial seizures, consciousness is not impaired; in complex partial seizures, the level of consciousness is decreased.

## Clinical Manifestations

Generalized seizures are bilateral and symmetric and have no discernible point of origin in the brain. The most common type is the **tonic–clonic** or major motor seizure. The **tonic phase** involves sustained contraction of skeletal muscles; abnormal postures, such as opisthotonos; and absence of respiration, during which the person becomes cyanotic. The **clonic phase** is characterized by rapid rhythmic and symmetric jerking movements of the body. Tonic–clonic seizures are sometimes preceded by an aura—a brief warning, such as a flash of light or a specific sound or smell. In children, febrile seizures (i.e., tonic–clonic seizures that occur with fever in the absence of other identifiable causes) are the most common form of epilepsy.

The absence seizure, which is characterized by abrupt alterations in consciousness that last only a few seconds, is a kind of generalized seizure. Other types of generalized seizures include the myoclonic type (contraction of a muscle or group of muscles) and the akinetic type (absence of movement). Some people are subject to mixed seizures.

**Status epilepticus** is a life-threatening emergency characterized by generalized tonic–clonic convulsions lasting for several minutes or occurring at close intervals. During this time, the patient does not regain consciousness. Hypotension, hypoxia, and cardiac dysrhythmias may also occur. There is a high risk of permanent brain damage and death unless prompt, appropriate treatment is instituted. In a person taking medications for a diagnosed seizure disorder, the most common cause of status epilepticus is abruptly stopping **antiepileptic drugs** (AEDs). In other patients, regardless of whether they have a diagnosed seizure disorder, causes of status epilepticus include brain trauma or tumors, systemic or central nervous system (CNS) infections, alcohol withdrawal, and overdoses of drugs (e.g., cocaine, theophylline).

## Drug Therapy

Treatment of the underlying cause or use of an AED may relieve seizures. AEDs can usually control seizure activity but do not cure the underlying disorder. Numerous difficulties, for both clinicians and patients, have been associated with

AED therapy, including trials of different drugs; consideration of **monotherapy** (using a single drug) versus combination therapy (using two or more drugs); the need to titrate dosage over time; lack of seizure control while drugs are being selected and dosages adjusted; social stigma and adverse drug effects, often leading to poor patient adherence; and undesirable drug interactions among AEDs and between AEDs and other medications.

The AEDs used in the prevention and treatment of seizures have evolved over the years. In recent years, the U.S. Food and Drug Administration (FDA) has approved newer medications in the treatment of seizure disorders. The FDA most often classifies these medications as newer or miscellaneous drugs. The medication tables identify the newer drugs primarily as derivatives. Table 53.1 summarizes the drug classes. For specific drugs, other tables identify the AEDs administered, the dosage, pregnancy category, the type of seizure they are used to treat, and the therapeutic serum drug levels. The therapeutic serum drug level is very important because of the risk of drug toxicity.

> ## ! QSEN Alert: Safety
>
> When administering AEDs requiring dosage calculation, two nurses should calculate the dosage, checking for accuracy.

> ## *Clinical Application 53.1*
>
> - According to Andrew's chart, he should receive carbamazepine [Tegretol] 50 mg four times per day. The elixir is 100 mg/5 mL. The boy weighs 56 lbs. How much carbamazepine does the nurse administer?
> - The physician has ordered valproate [Depakene] 20 mg/kg/d for Andrew. The elixir is 250 mg/5 mL. How much valproate does the nurse administer?

> ## NCLEX Success
>
> 1. A male infant is admitted to the emergency department. His parents report that he had a seizure. The infant's aural temperature is 104.3°F. What is the most likely cause of the seizure?
>
>    A. head injury
>    B. developmental delay
>    C. sepsis
>    D. fever
>
> 2. A woman is admitted to the labor and delivery unit with a blood pressure of 200/90 mm Hg. The admitting diagnosis is preeclampsia. The intravenous magnesium sulfate ordered for this patient prevents?
>
>    A. seizures
>    B. myocardial damage
>    C. tetany
>    D. hypothermia

### TABLE 53.1

## Drugs Administered for Seizures (Antiepileptic Drugs)

| Drug Class | Prototype | Other Drugs in the Class |
|---|---|---|
| **Drugs Used to Treat Seizure Disorders** | | |
| Barbiturates | Phenobarbital | Pentobarbital (Nembutal) <br> Primidone (Mysoline) |
| Benzodiazepines | Diazepam (Valium, Diastat, Acudial, Pediatric Diazepam Intensol) | Clobazam (Onfi, Sympazan) <br> Clonazepam (Klonopin) <br> Clorazepate (Tranxene) <br> Lorazepam (Ativan, LORazepam Intensol) |
| GABA structural analogs | Gabapentin (Neurontin) | Pregabalin (Lyrica, Lyrica CR) <br> Tiagabine hydrochloride (Gabitril) <br> Vigabatrin (Sabril) |
| Hydantoins | Phenytoin (Dilantin) | Ethotoin (Peganone) <br> Fosphenytoin (Cerebyx) |
| Iminostilbenes | Carbamazepine (Tegretol, TEGretol-SR) | Eslicarbazepine (Aptiom) <br> Oxcarbazepine (Oxtellar XR, Trileptal) |
| **Other Antiepileptic Drugs (AEDs)** | | |
| Carbonic anhydrase inhibitor | Acetazolamide (Diamox) | |
| Succinimide | Ethosuximide (Zarontin) | |
| Sulfonamide | Zonisamide (Zonegran) | |
| Histone deacetylase inhibitor | Valproate (Depakote, Depakote ER, Depakote Sprinkles) | |
| Functionalized amino acids | Lacosamide (Vimpat) | |
| Mineral electrolytes | Magnesium sulfate | |
| Phenyltriazine derivatives | Lamotrigine (LaMICtal) | |
| Pyrrolidine derivatives | Levetiracetam (Keppra) | |
| AMPA glutamate receptor antagonist | Perampanel (Fycompa) | |
| Sulfamate-substituted monosaccharides | Topiramate (Topamax) | |
| Triazole derivatives | Rufinamide (Banzel) | |

3. A patient is having a seizure that lasts longer than 30 minutes. What type of generalized seizure is the patient experiencing?
   A. tonic–clonic
   B. absence seizure
   C. atonic seizure
   D. status epilepticus

4. A patient is admitted to the emergency department with repeated tonic–clonic seizures. Tonic–clonic seizures may be attributed to which of following drugs?
   A. ciprofloxacin hydrochloride
   B. cimetidine
   C. cocaine
   D. morphine sulfate

## DRUGS USED TO TREAT SEIZURE DISORDERS

### BARBITURATES

**Phenobarbital** is the prototype AED of the barbiturate class. Since its development in 1912, it has been used as an antiepileptic or sedative.

## Pharmacokinetics

Phenobarbital, like all barbiturates, is absorbed rapidly through the gastrointestinal (GI) tract, usually within 1 hour. The oral drug has an onset of action of greater than 60 minutes and a duration of 10 to 12 hours. The intravenous (IV) form begins to act in 5 minutes and lasts approximately 6 hours. Phenobarbital has a half-life of 53 to 118 hours. In children, the half-life is 60 to 180 hours. The drug takes approximately 2 to 3 weeks to reach therapeutic serum levels and 3 weeks to reach a steady-state concentration. It is also lipid bound, which means that it crosses the placenta and is present in breast milk. Phenobarbital is metabolized in the liver and excreted by the renal system.

## Action

Phenobarbital depresses the CNS by inhibiting the conduction of impulses in the ascending reticular activating system, thus depressing the cerebral cortex and cerebellar function. Figure 53.1 indicates the site of action of barbiturates, along with other AEDs.

## Use

Prescribers order oral phenobarbital as a sedative and antiepileptic agent in the treatment of generalized tonic–clonic and

Barbiturates inhibit impulses in RAS to depress brainstem and cortex function

Cortex

Limbic system

RAS

Zaleplon, zolpidem affect serotonin levels in RAS

Rameiteon affects melatonin levels

Cerebellum

Mechanisms not understood:
levetiracetam

**Carboxylic acid derivatives**
↑ GABA effects, and decreases electrical activity

**Sulfonamide**
acetazolamide inhibits neuronal excitability

GABA

**Benzodiazepines, clorazepate**
↑ GABA effects, to inhibit neuron firing

**Hydantoins** delay Na⁺ influx to stabilize neuronal membrane

**Iminostilbenes**
increase GABA activity and block Na⁺ and Ca⁺ channels to stop APs

Cell firing inhibited, leading to stabilization

**Figure 53.1.** Sites of action of antiepileptic drugs. AP, action potential; GABA, gamma-aminobutyric acid; RAS, reticular activating system. [Adapted with permission from Karch, A. M. (2020). *Focus on nursing pharmacology* [8th ed., Fig. 23.2]. Philadelphia: Wolters Kluwer.]

partial seizures. Clinicians use the parenteral form to control acute seizures. Table 53.2 gives route and dosage information for phenobarbital and other barbiturates.

Older adults may experience greater sedation, due to decreased absorption and altered renal excretion of phenobarbital, placing them at risk for injury. These patients may also be at risk for adverse drug reactions related to altered metabolism and excretion.

### Use in Patients With Renal or Hepatic Impairment

Patients who have decreased creatinine clearance (CrCl) may not be able to excrete phenobarbital adequately. Patients with hepatic impairment require a lower dose to prevent adverse effects associated with the drug.

### Use in Patients With Critical Illness

When administering phenobarbital parenterally, it is best to do so in a critical care unit. This allows for constant monitoring of drug effects and early resuscitation in the event of respiratory arrest.

## Adverse Effects

As with all AEDs, CNS depression, possibly cognitive impairment with sedation, is the most common adverse effect. Other reported conditions include somnolence, agitation, confusion, vertigo, and nightmares. The most severe adverse effect is Stevens-Johnson syndrome, a hypersensitivity reaction. Respiratory problems may occur, particularly with parenteral phenobarbital. Sudden withdrawal of the medication places the patient at risk for status epilepticus. The FDA has issued a **BLACK BOX WARNING ◆** for phenobarbital. Patients who take phenobarbital are at risk for suicidal ideation. It is important to monitor the patient for statements that indicate depression and suicide.

## Contraindications

Contraindications to phenobarbital include a known hypersensitivity to barbiturates. Other contraindications include liver failure, nephritis, porphyria, respiratory depression, pregnancy, or addiction to barbiturates. Caution is necessary in acute or chronic pain, lactation, fever, hyperthyroidism, diabetes, decreased liver renal function, and pulmonary and cardiac disease.

## Nursing Implications

### Preventing Interactions

Several drugs interact with phenobarbital, increasing its effects (Box 53.1). Opioid analgesics combined with phenobarbital result in enhanced CNS depression. When administered with phenobarbital, corticosteroids, doxycycline, estrogens, hormonal contraceptives, oral anticoagulants, and tricyclic antidepressants have an increased metabolism and a decreased effect. Oil of primrose increases the effects of phenobarbital. Combined with vitamin D, phenobarbital increases the hepatic metabolism of the vitamin. In addition, it reduces calcium absorption. Because of this, it may be necessary to take supplemental vitamin D and calcium.

### Administering the Medication

Oral administration of phenobarbital may occur without regard to food. Parenteral administration may involve combining the medication with dextrose, lactated Ringer's, or normal saline. However, if a precipitate forms, administration should not take place. Also, the drug is incompatible with acidic solutions, amphotericin B, chlorpromazine, diphenhydramine, insulin, and vancomycin. The nurse always injects IV phenobarbital into large veins at an infusion rate no faster than 60 mg/minute. Inadvertent intra-arterial injection can cause spasm of the artery and gangrene. When administering the intramuscular (IM) drug, the nurse uses a large needle and injects into deep muscle.

### Assessing for Therapeutic Effects

The ultimate goal of therapy with phenobarbital is to decrease seizure effects. The patient's EEG reveals decreased brain waves consistent with seizure activity.

| | | | TABLE 53.2 | | |
|---|---|---|---|---|---|

## DRUGS AT A GLANCE: Barbiturates

| Drug | Pregnancy Category | Type of Seizure Treated | Routes and Dosage Ranges | | Therapeutic Serum Drug Level |
|---|---|---|---|---|---|
| | | | **Adults** | **Children** | |
| (P) **Phenobarbital** | D | Generalized tonic–clonic and partial seizures | Status epilepticus: IV 20 mg/kg infused 50–100 mg/min; may repeat once after 10 min with an additional 5–10 mg/kg<br>60–200 mg or 50–100 mg PO daily in 2–3 divided doses | Status epilepticus: IV 20 mg/kg infused 50–100 mg/min; may repeat once after 10 min with an additional 5–10 mg/kg<br>3–6 mg/kg PO per day | 10–40 mcg/mL |
| Pentobarbital (Nembutal) | D | Acute seizure episodes associated with anesthesia, eclampsia, meningitis, tetanus, and status epilepticus | Initial dose, 5–15 mg/kg administered at a rate of ≤50 mg/kg; may give an additional 5–10 mg/kg; follow with a continuous infusion<br>Continuous infusion: 0.5–5 mg/kg | 2–6 mg/kg; maximum 100 mg | Has not been determined |
| Primidone (Mysoline) | D | Tonic–clonic, psychomotor, and focal seizures | 100–125 mg PO at bedtime; gradually increase dosage until satisfactory dosage is attained | >8 y, adult dosage<br><8 y, day 1–3, 50 mg PO at bedtime; day 4–6, 50 mg PO 2 times/d; day 7–9, 100–125 mg PO 2 times/d; maintenance dose, 125–250 mg PO 3 times/d | 5–12 mcg/mL |

## Assessing for Adverse Effects

The nurse assesses for increases in CNS activity consistent with paradoxical excitation, as noted most often in the elderly. It is essential to assess respiratory problems such as hypoventilation, apnea, respiratory depression, laryngospasm, bronchospasm, and circulatory collapse, particularly in patients receiving parenteral phenobarbital. In addition, it is necessary to:

- Assess for bradycardia, hypotension, and syncope
- Assess the serum drug level for signs of toxicity or inadequate seizure treatment

**BOX 53.1** **Drug Interactions: Phenobarbital**

### Drugs That Increase the Effects of Phenobarbital

- Alcohol, chloramphenicol, diazepam, and monoamine oxidase inhibitors
  *May increase central nervous system and respiratory depression*
- Gabapentin and valproate
  *Increase serum level*
- Mephobarbital and primidone
  *May increase serum level*

- Assess for changes in the integumentary system indicative of the onset of Stevens-Johnson syndrome
- Assess complete blood count (CBC) and differential
- Assess blood urea nitrogen (BUN) and creatinine

### Patient Teaching

Box 53.2 identifies patient teaching guidelines for phenobarbital.

## Other Drugs in the Class

Pentobarbital (Nembutal) is a short-acting barbiturate that produces antiseizure activity by depressing the sensory cortex, decreasing motor activity, and altering cerebellar function. It should be administered cautiously in patients who have an alteration in their respiratory function. It is listed in the Beers Criteria as a drug to be avoided in patients 65 and over because of the risk of dependence and its increased risk of overdosage in low doses.

Primidone (Mysoline) is similar to phenobarbital in its action. It raises the seizure threshold and decreases neuron excitability. It is well absorbed in the GI tract and is 20% protein bound. It is metabolized in the liver to phenobarbital by oxidation and then to phenylethylmalonamide. Its half-life is 5 to 16 hours, and it is excreted in the urine. Phenobarbital and primidone concentrations should be monitored. Primidone has

## BOX 53.2 — *Patient Teaching Guidelines for Phenobarbital*

*Teach*

*CNS*

- Understand that this drug is administered long term for the treatment of seizure activity.
- Take the medication as prescribed, and do not stop the medication abruptly.
- Have regular tests to determine serum levels of the drug.
- Change positions slowly. This drug may cause drowsiness or syncope.
- Do not drive or operate machinery with central nervous system depression.
- If you are of childbearing age, use two forms of contraception.
- Notify your prescriber about the development of rashes or skin eruptions.
- Wear a medical alert bracelet or necklace stating that you have a seizure disorder and naming the medications you take.

*teratogenic*

significant hematologic adverse effects, including agranulocytosis, granulocytopenia, and megaloblastic anemia. It is important to obtain a baseline CBC before initiating therapy and at 6-month intervals.

## BENZODIAZEPINES

Drugs belonging to this class have a broad range of uses; they may act as antidepressants, antiepileptics, or skeletal muscle relaxants. The benzodiazepines potentiate the effects of GABA by increasing the attraction to the receptor sites. The prototype of this class is Ⓟ **Diazepam** (Valium, Diastat). See Figure 53.1 for the increased effects of GABA by benzodiazepines.

## Pharmacokinetics

This varies with the preparation of diazepam. For the IV drug, the onset of action is 1 to 5 minutes, with a peak of 30 minutes and a duration of 15 to 60 minutes. For the oral drug, the onset of action is 30 to 60 minutes, with a peak of 1 to 2 hours and a duration of 3 hours. For the IM drug, the onset of action is generally within 15 to 30 minutes, with a peak of 30 to 45 minutes and a duration of 3 hours. For the rectal drug, the onset is rapid, with a peak of 1.5 hours and a duration of 3 hours. Its half-life, which is longer in newborns and the elderly, is 20 to 80 hours.

Diazepam crosses the placenta and enters the breast milk. It is metabolized by the liver and excreted by the kidneys.

## Action

The exact mechanism of action of diazepam is unknown. However, authorities believe that the drug acts primarily on the limbic system and reticular formation to produce skeletal muscle relaxation. It potentiates the effect of GABA by increasing the attraction of the medication to the receptor sites.

## Use

IV diazepam is an adjunctive skeletal muscle relaxant administered for the treatment of severe recurrent convulsive seizures and status epilepticus. Oral diazepam is an adjunctive agent used for seizure disorders. Clinicians also order benzodiazepines such as diazepam for treatment of Lennox-Gastaut syndrome, a mixed seizure disorder that presents at approximately 2 years of age. Table 53.3 gives route and dosage information for diazepam and other benzodiazepines.

### Use in Children

IV diazepam is recommended for use in children age 1 month or older. Newborns require a lower dose. Oral diazepam is recommended for children older than 6 months of age. Rectal administration is not recommended in children younger than 2 years of age.

### Use in Older Adults

It is necessary to reduce the dosage of diazepam administered to older adults because the drug has an extended half-life in this population.

### Use in Patients With Renal or Hepatic Impairment

Diazepam is excreted by the kidneys after being metabolized in the liver. Thus, patients with renal or hepatic impairment should take reduced dosages of diazepam.

### Use in Patients With Critical Illness

Patients with critical illness or those in debilitated states should take reduce dosages of diazepam. During IV administration, patients should receive oxygen.

## Adverse Effects

CNS adverse effects of diazepam include depression, disorientation, restlessness, and confusion. In the first 2 weeks of treatment, paradoxical excitatory reactions may occur. The most serious cardiovascular adverse effect is cardiovascular collapse with bradycardia and hypotension. Also, potentially life-threatening tachycardia may occur. In addition, in August of 2016, the FDA issued a **BLACK BOX WARNING ◆**. The combination of a benzodiazepine such as diazepam and an opioid medication depresses the CNS, resulting in serious adverse effects, including respiratory depression or death. Other reported problems include constipation, diarrhea, incontinence, urinary retention, and changes in libido.

## Contraindications

Patients with known hypersensitivity to benzodiazepines should not receive diazepam. Contraindications also include acute narrow-angle glaucoma, shock, coma, acute alcohol intoxication, and pregnancy.

## Nursing Implications

### Preventing Interactions

Many medications and herbs interact with diazepam, decreasing or increasing its effects (Boxes 53.3 and 53.4).

**TABLE 53.3**

## DRUGS AT A GLANCE: Benzodiazepines

| Drug | Pregnancy Category | Type of Seizure Treated | Routes and Dosage Ranges | | Therapeutic Serum Drug Level |
|---|---|---|---|---|---|
| | | | **Adults** | **Children** | |
| Ⓟ **Diazepam** (Valium, Diastat Acudial, Diazepam, Diastat Pediatric, Diazepam Intensol; ❀ BIO-Diazepam, Diastat Pediatric, Valium) | D | Status epilepticus | Seizure control: 2–10 mg PO 3–4 times/d Status epilepticus: 5–10 mg IV slowly administered; may repeat every 5–10 min; maximum dose of 30 mg | Status epilepticus: older than 1 mo and younger than 5 y, 0.2–0.5 mg slowly IV every 2–5 min up to a maximum dose of 5 mg 5 y and older, 1 mg IV every 2–5 min up to a maximum dose of 10 mg | Has not been determined |
| Clobazam (Onfi, Sympazan; ❀ Apo-Clobazam, Clobazam-10, Dom-Clobazam, Frisium, Novo-Clobazam, PMS-Clobazam) | C | Lennox-Gastaut, epilepsy (adjunctive) | Lennox-Gastaut: PO ≤30 kg; initial 5 mg once daily; then increase to 5 mg twice daily for ≥1 wk; then increase to 10 mg twice daily thereafter >30 kg: initial 5 mg twice daily for ≥1 wk, then increase to 5 mg twice daily for ≥1 wk, and then increase to 10 mg twice daily; after ≥1 wk, may increase to 20 mg twice daily Epilepsy: PO; initial 5–15 mg/d; dosage may be gradually adjusted based on tolerance and seizure control to a maximum dose of 80 mg/d | Lennox-Gastaut: ≥2 y through adolescence: refer to adult dosing Epilepsy: <2 y; Initial 0.5–1 mg/kg/d 2–16 y: initial 5 mg daily; may be increased (no more frequently than every 5 d) to a maximum of 40 mg daily; daily doses of up to 30 mg may be taken as a single dose at bedtime; higher doses should be divided | 30–300 ng/mL |
| Clonazepam (Klonopin; ❀ Apo-Clonazepam, Clonapen, Clonazepam-R, Dom-Clonazepam, TEVA-ClonazePAM) | D | Myoclonic or akinetic seizures, alone or with other antiepileptic drugs (AEDs); possibly effective in generalized tonic, clonic, and psychomotor seizures | 1.5 mg PO daily increased by 0.5 mg/d every 3–7 d if necessary; maximum dose, 20 mg/d | 0.01–0.03 mg/kg/d PO, increased by 0.25–0.5 mg/d every 3–7 d if necessary; maximum dose, 0.2 mg/kg/d | 20–80 ng/mL |
| Clorazepate (Tranxene-T) | D | Partial seizures, with other AEDs | 7.5 mg PO three times daily maximum initial dose; increased by 7.5 mg every wk, if necessary; maximum dose 90 mg/d | >12 y, same as adults 9–12 y, 7.5 mg PO two times daily maximum initial dose; increased by 7.5 mg every wk, if necessary; maximum dose 60 mg/d | Has not been determined |
| Lorazepam (Ativan, LORazepam, Intensol; ❀ APO-LORazepam, Ativan, TEVA-LORazepam) | D | Status epilepticus | 18 y and older, 4 mg IV slowly at 2 mg/min; may give another 4 mg after 10–15 min if needed | Not recommended in children younger than 12 y | Has not been determined |

AED, antiepileptic drug.

## BOX 53.3 — Drug Interactions: Diazepam

**Drugs That Increases the Effect of Diazepam**
- Alcohol and omeprazole
  *Increase central nervous system depression*
- Cimetidine, disulfiram, and hormonal contraceptives
  *Increase pharmacologic effects*

**Drugs That Decrease the Effects Diazepam**
- Theophylline and ranitidine
  *Decrease pharmacologic effects*

### ⚠ QSEN Alert: Safety

A review by the FDA has shown that the combination of (1) an opioid medication and (2) a benzodiazepine or any drug that suppresses the CNS results in serious adverse effects.

### Administering the Medication

When preparing diazepam, the nurse does not mix the drug in plastic bags or tubing or combine it with other solutions. During administration, it is important to monitor pulse, blood pressure, and respiration. During parenteral administration, it is necessary to administer oxygen as well as to put the patient on bed rest for 3 hours. The nurse injects the IV form of the drug slowly into a large vein at 1 mL/minute—over at least 3 minutes in children—never intra-arterially or into small veins. Intra-arterial administration results in arterial spasm.

### Assessing for Therapeutic Effects

When administering diazepam for a seizure disorder, the goal of therapy is to control seizure activity. When administering drug for status epilepticus, the goal is to eliminate the seizure activity.

### Assessing for Adverse Effects

The nurse assesses for changes in cardiovascular status that could indicate hypotension, bradycardia, or tachycardia. He or she closely monitors the CNS response. In addition, the nurse assesses for alterations in elimination patterns.

### Patient Teaching

Box 53.5 identifies patient teaching guidelines for diazepam.

### Clinical Application 53.2

- During a hospitalization, Andrew has an episode of status epilepticus. His neurologist orders diazepam (Valium) 1 mg IV every 2 to 5 minutes, with a maximum dosage of 10 mg. How does the nurse administer the medication?
- What assessments and interventions are necessary to implement before, during, and after the administration of diazepam?

## Other Drugs in the Class

Clobazam (Onfi) is an adjunctive benzodiazepine used in treating Lennox-Gastaut syndrome and epilepsy. (Lennox-Gastaut

## BOX 53.4 — Herb and Dietary Interactions: Diazepam

**Herbs and Foods That Increase the Effect of Diazepam**
- Kava
- Valerian
- Grapefruit juice

syndrome is a severe seizure disorder that presents prior to the age of 8.) The drug potentiates the action of GABA at the postsynaptic GABA neuron. The inhibitory effect of GABA is enhanced, providing greater permeability to chloride ions. With the shift in chloride ions, hyperpolarization occurs resulting in stabilization and decreased excitability. Clobazam can be administered with or without food. Tablets can be crushed and administered with applesauce. The suspension should be shaken well and administered with an oral dosing syringe.

Clonazepam (Klonopin) is a benzodiazepine that has an unknown mechanism of action. Somnolence is an adverse effect of this medication, which can be reduced by administering the medication at bedtime. The drug is supplied in an orally disintegrating tablet. The patient should be instructed to open the pouch and peel back the foil. The patient's hands should be very dry when removing the tablet. Periodically throughout the course of treatment, the patient's CBC, liver, and renal function should be monitored, as well as suicidal ideation.

Clorazepate (Tranxene-T) is a benzodiazepine that binds to the receptors on the postsynaptic GABA neuron at several sites in the CNS. It increases the effect of GABA, resulting in increased neuronal membrane permeability. This increase in permeability allows the chloride ions to shift, leading to hyperpolarization and less excitability in the brain.

Lorazepam (Ativan) has an action similar to that of clorazepate. The administration of lorazepam requires routine monitoring of the CBC, liver enzymes, serum creatinine, BUN, and serum lactate.

## BOX 53.5 — Patient Teaching Guidelines for Diazepam

- Take the medication as prescribed and do not skip doses or stop therapy.
- Do not use alcohol or smoke. Alcohol is more potent when combined with diazepam. Smoking may constrict blood vessels, resulting in reduced elimination of the drug.
- Obtain instructions about the administration of rectal diazepam.
- Use two types of contraceptives if you are a woman of childbearing age and are sexually active.
- Ask your prescriber about safety and central nervous system (CNS) depression. Protect yourself from falls. Do not drive or operate machinery if you have CNS depression.
- Wear a medical alert bracelet or necklace stating that you have a seizure disorder and naming the medications you take.

5. Which of the following medications is administered for status epilepticus?
   A. phenytoin
   B. diazepam
   C. levetiracetam
   D. clobazam

6. A patient is taking phenobarbital for a seizure disorder. Which of the following statements indicates that the patient should be seen by a health care provider immediately?
   A. "I have a rash that started on my trunk, and now it is on my arms and legs."
   B. "I rest if I feel tired."
   C. "I take my medication routinely and do not skip doses."
   D. "I have my blood levels checked if my breathing decreases."

7. A patient stops taking clonazepam. What adverse effect will occur?
   A. status epilepticus
   B. bone marrow depression
   C. cerebral edema
   D. lethargy

## GAMMA-AMINOBUTYRIC ACID STRUCTURAL ANALOGS

In 1993, the FDA approved ℗ **Gabapentin** (Neurontin) for treatment of partial seizures. In May of 2002, the FDA approved it for treatment of postherpetic neuralgia pain.

## Pharmacokinetics and Action

Gabapentin reaches its peak in 1 hour. It binds to sites in the brain that have a high affinity for gabapentin. The drug crosses the placenta and may enter the breast milk. Metabolism occurs in the liver and elimination takes place in the urine. Structurally, gabapentin is related to GABA. Its antiepileptic action is related to its ability to inhibit postsynaptic responses and block posttetanic potentiation.

## Use

Prescribers order gabapentin as an adjunctive treatment for partial seizures and postherpetic neuralgia. There are many off-label uses, some of which include alcohol withdrawal, fibromyalgia, and neuropathic pain. Table 53.4 gives route and dosage information for gabapentin and other GABA structural analogs.

### Use in Patients With Renal Impairment

Patients with impaired renal function require the following dosage adjustment depending on their CrCl.

- CrCl ≥ 60 mL/minute: 30 to 1200 mg three times per day
- CrCl > 30 to 59 mL/minute: 200 to 700 mg twice daily
- CrCl > 15 to 29 mL/minute: 200 to 700 mg once daily
- CrCl 15 mL/minute: 100 to 300 mg once daily
- CrCl < 15 mL/minute: reduced daily dose in proportion to CrCl based on dose for CrCl of 15 mL/minute (reduce dose by half [range: 50–150 mg/day])

### Use in Patients With Hepatic Impairment

Patients with impaired liver function require monitoring for elevated liver enzymes but do not require a dosage adjustment.

## Adverse Effects

The most common adverse effects of gabapentin are associated with CNS depression and include dizziness, somnolence, insomnia, and ataxia. Other reported adverse effects are pruritus, dry mouth, dyspepsia, nausea, vomiting, and suicidal ideation.

## Contraindications

Contraindications to gabapentin include a known hypersensitivity to the medication.

## Nursing Implications

### Preventing Interactions

Antacids do not affect the serum level, but they decrease absorption of gabapentin when administered at the same time. The herb *Ginkgo biloba* decreases the effect of the drug.

### Administering the Medication

The nurse ensures that gabapentin is taken orally. People may take the drug with food to prevent GI upset. Extended-release tablets should be swallowed whole and not crushed or chewed.

### Assessing for Therapeutic and Adverse Effects

The nurses assesses for the absence of partial seizures, the most important therapeutic effect.

It is also necessary to assess changes in mood and personality in patients receiving gabapentin, as with all antiepileptic medications, because suicidal ideation is the result of CNS depression. The nurse assesses for CNS depression that could affect patient safety.

### Patient Teaching

Box 53.6 identifies patient teaching guidelines for gabapentin.

## Other Drugs in the Class

Pregabalin (Lyrica) is administered for partial-onset seizures, postherpetic neuralgia, neuropathic pain, and neuropathic pain associated with diabetes. The drug increases the neuronal GABA and decreases calcium currents in the neuronal calcium channels to stabilize and decrease excitability. This action exerts anticonvulsant activity. It is necessary to instruct the patient to monitor his or her weight because of the increased risk of peripheral edema.

Tiagabine (Gabitril) is an adjunctive therapy for partial seizures. It is an inhibitor of GABA uptake in the presynaptic neurons. This action allows for an increase of GABA in the postsynaptic neurons. Patients should understand that the herb ginkgo will decrease tiagabine effectiveness, placing the patient at risk for seizures.

### TABLE 53.4

### DRUGS AT A GLANCE: Gamma-Aminobutyric Acid Structural Analogs

| Drug | Pregnancy Category | Type of Seizure Treated | Routes and Dosage Ranges | | Therapeutic Serum Drug Level |
|------|--------------------|-----------------------|--------------------------|--|------------------------------|
| | | | **Adults** | **Children** | |
| ℗ **Gabapentin** (Neurontin, Gralise, Gralise Starter [Gralise and Gralise Starter are used for the treatment of partial seizures]; ✷ AG-Gabapentin, Auro-Gabapentin, Apo-Gabapentin, GD, Gabapentin, GLN-Gabapentin, Dom-Gabapentin, TARO-Gabapentin, Teva-Gabapentin) | C | Partial seizures | Epilepsy: 300 mg PO 3 times/d initially Maintenance: 900–1800 mg/d PO in divided doses 3 times/d; maximum interval between doses should not exceed 12 h; up to 2400–3600 mg/d has been used Postherpetic neuralgia: 300 mg/d PO initially; 300 mg PO 2 times/d on day 2, 300 mg PO 3 times/d on day 3 Renal impairment: creatinine clearance (CrCl) > 60 mL/min, 400 mg three times daily (1200 mg/d); CrCl 30–60 mL/min, 300 mg two times daily (600 mg/d); CrCl 15–30 mL/min, 300 mg once daily; CrCl < 15 mL/min, 300 mg every other day. Patients on hemodialysis: 200–300 mg after each 4 h of hemodialysis | 3–12 y, initially 10–15 mg/kg/d PO in three divided doses; 3–4 y, up to 50 mg/kg/d in three divided doses; 5 y and older, adjust upward over about 3 d to 25–35 mg/kg daily in three divided doses Maximum dose: 50 mg/kg/d | Clinical trial data indicate that monitoring serum levels is not necessary for safe use |
| Pregabalin (Lyrica, Lyrica CR; ✷ AG-Pregabalin, APO-Pregabalin, Auro-Pregabalin, Dom-Pregabalin, JAMP Pregabalin, SANDOZ-Pregabalin) | C | Partial-onset seizures with other AEDs | Epilepsy: 150–600 mg/d PO 2–3 times/d Fibromyalgia: 75–150 mg PO 2 times/d; maximum dose, 450 mg/d Postherpetic pain: 75–150 mg PO 2 times/d; maximum dose, 600 mg/d | Safety and efficacy not established | Has not been determined |
| Tiagabine (Gabitril) | C | Partial seizures, with other AEDs | 4 mg PO daily for 1 wk; increased by 4–8 mg/wk until desired effect; maximum dose 56 mg/d in 2–4 divided doses | <12 y, not recommended 12–18 y, 4 mg PO daily for 1 wk; increased to 8 mg/d in 2 divided doses for 1 wk; then increased by 4–8 mg/wk up to a maximum of 32 mg/d in 2–4 divided doses | Has not been determined |

*(Continued on page 1048)*

## TABLE 53.4

## DRUGS AT A GLANCE: Gamma-Aminobutyric Acid Structural Analogs (Continued)

| Drug | Pregnancy Category | Type of Seizure Treated | Routes and Dosage Ranges | | Therapeutic Serum Drug Level |
|---|---|---|---|---|---|
| | | | **Adults** | **Children** | |
| Vigabatrin (Sabril, Vigadrone; ❋ Sabril) | C | Infantile spasms Refractory complex partial seizures | 500 mg PO twice daily; increase daily dose by 500 mg increments at weekly intervals based on response and tolerability Recommended dose: 1.5 g/d | Infantile spasms: 1 mo–2 y; PO 50 mg/kg divided twice daily; may titrate up to 25–50 mg/kg/d increments every 3 d to a maximum of 150 mg/kg/d divided twice daily Refractory complex partial seizures: children 10–<17 y and to 25–60 kg; PO 250 mg twice daily; increase dose by 500 mg increments at weekly intervals based on response. Recommended dose: 1000 mg twice daily | Has not been determined |

AED, antiepileptic drug.

Vigabatrin (Sabril) received FDA approval for treatment of infantile spasms and as adjunctive therapy in adults who experience refractory focal seizures. The FDA issued a **BLACK BOX WARNING ◆** for vigabatrin because it can cause permanent bilateral concentric visual field constriction. This damage can include tunnel vision, damage to the central retina, and decrease visual acuity. The loss of vision can occur within weeks of beginning therapy. This adverse effect has limited the availability of the drug in the United States. The drug is part of the Share (Support, Help, and Resources for Epilepsy) Program. Participating physicians and pharmacies can provide vigabatrin to patients who are deemed to need this medication. Visual field testing should be completed before beginning the medication and every 6 months.

## HYDANTOINS

The prototype antiepileptic of the hydantoin class is **Ⓟ Phenytoin** (Dilantin). The oldest and most widely used AED, it is often the initial drug of choice, especially in adults. In addition to using it to treat seizure disorders, prescribers sometimes order it for cardiac dysrhythmias.

## Pharmacokinetics

Phenytoin is highly bound (90%) to plasma proteins, and only the free drug (the fraction not bound to plasma albumin) is therapeutically active. The oral preparation, absorbed by the GI tract, has a slow onset of action, with a peak of 2 to 12 hours and a duration of 6 to 12 hours. The IV preparation has an onset of action of 1 to 2 hours with a rapid peak and a duration of 12 to 24 hours. The drug is metabolized by the liver and excreted in the urine.

## Action

Phenytoin stabilizes the neuronal membrane by delaying the influx of sodium ions into the neurons and preventing the excitability caused by excessive stimulation. See Figure 53.1 for the site of action of hydantoins.

## Use

Clinicians use phenytoin to control tonic–clonic seizures, psychomotor seizures, and nonepileptic seizures. They also use it to prevent seizure activity in patients during and following

---

### BOX 53.6 Patient Teaching Guidelines for Gabapentin

- Take the medication as prescribed and do not stop taking it abruptly.
- Take the medication with food to decrease gastrointestinal discomfort.
- Do not cut, crush, or chew extended-release capsules. If swallowing is difficult, sprinkle the contents of the capsule over soft food.
- Notify your prescriber if seizure activity occurs.
- You may experience nausea, vomiting, insomnia, fatigue, and confusion.
- Do not drive or operate machinery with central nervous system depression.
- Report severe nausea and vomiting, changes in stool or urine color, diarrhea, or changes in neurologic function to the prescriber.

## TABLE 53.5

### DRUGS AT A GLANCE: Hydantoins

| Drug | Pregnancy Category | Type of Seizure Treated | Routes and Dosage Ranges | | Therapeutic Serum Drug Level |
|------|--------------------|-----------------------|--------------------------|--|------------------------------|
| | | | **Adults** | **Children** | |
| ℗ **Phenytoin** (Dilantin, Dilantin Infatabs, Phenytek, Phenytoin Infatabs; ✹ APO-Phenytoin Sodium, Dilantin, Dilantin Infatabs, Tremytoine) | D | Generalized tonic–clonic and some partial seizures Prevention and treatment of seizures occurring during or after neurosurgery | Status epilepticus: loading dose IV 20 mg/kg maximum rate of 50 mg/min 100 mg PO three times daily initially; 300 mg (long acting) once daily as maintenance | Status epilepticus: loading dose IV 20 mg/g at a maximum rate of 1 mg/kg/min 5–10 mg/kg 10 min after the loading dose Children and adolescents Immediate release: PO 5 mg/kg/d in 2–3 divided doses, individualize dose with dosage adjustments at no <7–10 d intervals; maintenance dose, 4–8 mg/kg/d Extended release: 5 mg/kg/d in 2–3 equally divided doses | 5–20 mcg/mL (40–80 μmol/L) |
| Ethotoin (Peganone) | D | Tonic–clonic, psychomotor seizures, used with other AEDs | 1 g/d PO; increase gradually over several days; usual maintenance dose 2–3 g/d in 4–6 divided doses; <2 g/d is ineffective in most adults | 750 mg/d PO initially in 4–6 divided doses; maintenance doses range from 500–1000 mg/d PO | 15–50 mcg/mL |
| Fosphenytoin (Cerebyx; ✹ Cerebyx) | D | Status epilepticus | Status epilepticus: IV loading dose 20 mg PE/kg administered at 100–150 PE/min | Not recommended | |

PE, phenytoin equivalent.

neurosurgery and brain injury. Table 53.5 gives route and dosage information for phenytoin and the other hydantoins.

Phenytoin is available in several forms: a capsule (Dilantin), chewable tablet, oral suspension, and injectable solution. Patients should not switch between generic and trade name formulations because of differences in absorption and bioavailability. If a patient becomes stable on a generic drug and then switches to Dilantin, there is a risk of higher serum phenytoin levels and toxicity. If a patient becomes stable on Dilantin and then switches to a generic drug, there is a risk of lower serum phenytoin levels, loss of therapeutic effectiveness, and seizures. (There may also be differences in bioavailability among generic formulations manufactured by different companies.)

### Use in Children

When used for status epilepticus, the IV phenytoin dose is determined according to the weight of the child. The recommended dosage is 15 to 20 mg/kg.

### Use in Older Adults

It is necessary to administer phenytoin cautiously to older adults. Elderly patients may have altered albumin levels, decreasing the

affinity of phenytoin for albumin and causing displacement of the drug.

### Use in Patients With Renal Impairment

Renal impairment or failure also causes displacement of the drug, placing the patient at risk for toxicity.

### Use in Patients With Hepatic Impairment

Hepatic impairment results in altered albumin levels, decreasing the affinity of phenytoin for albumin and causing displacement of the drug.

### Use in Patients With Critical Illness

The IV administration of phenytoin can result in cardiovascular collapse. It is important to assess blood pressure, pulse, and respirations. Monitoring the patient's cardiovascular status is necessary with the use of telemetry.

## Adverse Effects

The most common adverse effects of phenytoin affect the CNS (e.g., ataxia, drowsiness, lethargy) and GI tract (e.g., nausea, vomiting). **Gingival hyperplasia**, an overgrowth of gum tissue, is also common, especially in children. Long-term use may lead to an increased risk of osteoporosis because of its effect on vitamin D metabolism. Serious reactions are uncommon but may include allergic reactions, hepatitis, nephritis, bone marrow depression, and mental confusion.

## Contraindications

Contraindications to phenytoin include a known hypersensitivity to the hydantoins. Other conditions that require caution are seizures related to hypoglycemia, sinus bradycardia, heart block, and Stokes-Adams syndrome. In patients exhibiting seizures related to hypoglycemia, the primary treatment involves interventions to increase blood glucose (not the use of AEDs). Given the sedative effects associated with phenytoin, the patient is at risk for decreased heart rate; thus, frequent assessment of cardiac output is required if phenytoin is administered to these patients. Caution is also required when administering phenytoin to pregnant women. The risk of birth defects is a significant adverse effect.

## Nursing Implications

### Preventing Interactions

Several medications interact with phenytoin, increasing or decreasing its effects (Box 53.7). The effectiveness of corticosteroids, oral contraceptives, and nisoldipine is reduced when combined with phenytoin. Absorption of folic acid, calcium, and vitamin D is decreased with the administration of phenytoin. The herb *Ginkgo biloba* decreases the effect of the drug.

### Administering the Medication

The injectable solution is highly irritating to tissues. Therefore, when giving the drug intravenously, it is necessary to use special techniques.

### Assessing for Therapeutic and Adverse Effects

The nurse assess for the absence of tonic–clonic and psychomotor seizures.

The nurse assesses for the presence of a rash or skin eruption indicative of a hypersensitivity reaction; the presence of a skin eruption could be indicative of Stevens-Johnson syndrome.

---

**BOX 53.7**  **Drug Interactions: Phenytoin\***

**Drugs That Increase the Effects of Phenytoin**
- Alcohol, amiodarone, chloramphenicol, omeprazole, and ticlopidine
  *Increase phenytoin levels*

**Drugs That Decrease the Effects of Phenytoin**
- Enteral feedings
  *Decrease phenytoin absorption*

\*Complex interactions and effects may occur when phenytoin and valproate are taken together. Phenytoin toxicity may result with apparently normal serum phenytoin levels.

---

**BOX 53.8** **Patient Teaching Guidelines for Phenytoin**

- Take the drug as prescribed and do not stop taking it abruptly.
- Take the medication with food to prevent gastric upset.
- Have serum drug levels checked as ordered by your prescriber.
- Maintain good oral hygiene (regular brushing and flossing) to prevent gum disease.
- Have regular dental checkups.
- Use contraception if you are of childbearing age and are sexually active.
- Wear a medical alert bracelet or necklace stating that you have a seizure disorder and naming the medications you take.

---

In addition, the nurse assesses for cardiovascular collapse with IV administration.

### Patient Teaching

Box 53.8 identifies patient teaching guidelines for phenytoin.

## Other Drugs in the Class

Ethotoin (Peganone) stabilizes the seizure threshold. This action prevents the spread of the seizure activity. It is rapidly absorbed and metabolized in the liver to form metabolites. The half-life is 3 to 9 hours with excretion in the feces and minimally in the saliva. Blood dyscrasias have been reported, so the patient should have a CBC and urinalysis before therapy is initiated and then monthly for several months.

Fosphenytoin (Cerebyx) is administered intravenously, and the rate should not exceed 150 mg because of the risk of severe hypotension and cardiac dysrhythmias. During administration, the patient's cardiac function should be monitored. The patient's CBC, aspartate aminotransferase, alanine aminotransferase, and serum phenytoin level should be measured.

## IMINOSTILBENES

The AEDs classified as the iminostilbenes include the prototype **Carbamazepine** (Tegretol).

## Pharmacokinetics

Carbamazepine is administered orally and absorbed by the GI tract. The onset of action is slow in both the oral and oral extended-release preparations. The regular oral preparation peaks in 4 to 5 hours, whereas the oral suspension peaks in 1.5 hours. The extended-release preparation peaks in 3 to 12 hours. The half-life of the drug is 12 to 17 hours. Carbamazepine induces the liver enzymes to increase metabolism and shorten the half-life over time. The variability of the half-life is related to autoinduction, which is usually complete in 3 to 5 weeks. The drug is metabolized by the liver and excreted in the feces and urine. It crosses the placenta and enters breast milk.

## Action

The mechanism of action of carbamazepine is not understood, but its antiepileptic activity may be related to inhibition of polysynaptic responses that block posttetanic potentiation. Like the tricyclic antidepressants, the drug affects sodium channels within the cortical neurons. It has the ability to decrease action potential of the cell by inhibiting the influx of sodium into the cell. See Figure 53.1 for the site of action of the iminostilbenes.

## Use

Clinicians use carbamazepine to prevent partial seizures with complex symptoms, as in patients with psychomotor and temporal lobe epilepsy. Prescribers order the drug for generalized tonic–clonic and mixed seizures, either partial or generalized. Patients who have uncontrolled seizures or CNS depression on other AEDs use it commonly. Table 53.6 presents route and dosage information for carbamazepine and other iminostilbenes.

### Use in Older Adults

Carbamazepine may result in increased sedation and confusion. It is necessary to assess patient safety when using this medication in older adults.

### Use in Patients With Renal or Hepatic Impairment

Caution is necessary with carbamazepine in patients with renal or hepatic impairment. The drug may cause hepatic cellular necrosis.

## Adverse Effects

Carbamazepine may have serious adverse effects. The FDA has issued a BLACK BOX WARNING ◆ for carbamazepine concerning aplastic anemia and agranulocytosis. Other

## TABLE 53.6

## DRUGS AT A GLANCE: Iminostilbenes

| Drug | Pregnancy Category | Type of Seizure Treated | Routes and Dosage Ranges Adults | Children | Therapeutic Serum Drug Level |
|---|---|---|---|---|---|
| Ⓟ **Carbamazepine** (Carbatrol, Epitol, Equetro, TEGretol, TEGretol-SR; ✹ APO-CarBAMazepine, DOM-CarBAMazepine, DOM-CarBAMazepine CR) | D | Partial, generalized tonic–clonic, and mixed seizures | Epilepsy: 200 mg PO twice daily, increased gradually to 600–1200 mg daily if needed, in 3 or 4 divided doses<br>Trigeminal neuralgia: 200 mg PO daily, increased gradually<br>Bipolar disorder: 400 mg PO in divided doses, increased gradually to 1600 mg if necessary | Epilepsy: 6–12 y, 100 mg PO twice daily (tablet) or 50 mg four times daily (suspension), increase to 1000 mg daily if necessary in 3–4 divided doses; >12 y, 200 mg PO twice daily, increase to 1000 mg daily for children 12–15 y and 1200 mg for children older than 15 y | 4–12 mcg/mL |
| Eslicarbazepine (Aptiom; ✹ Aptiom) | C | Partial-onset seizures | Monotherapy: PO Initial: 400 mg once daily; may initiate treatment at 800 mg once daily; if seizure reduction outweighs risk, dosage can be increased in increments of 400–600 mg Maintenance dose: 800–1600 mg daily | Dosage not established | No established range |
| Oxcarbazepine (Oxtellar XR, Trileptal; ✹ APO-OXcarbazepine Jamp-Oxcarbazepine, Trileptal) | C | Partial seizures, as monotherapy or with other AEDs in adults, with other AEDs in children 4–16 y old | 600 mg PO twice daily (1200 mg/d); maximum dose, 2400 mg/d<br>Severe renal impairment creatinine clearance (CrCl < 30 mL/min): 300 mg PO twice daily (600 mg/d) and increased slowly until response achieved | With other AEDs, 8–10 mg/kg/d PO, not to exceed 600 mg twice daily; titrate to reach target dose over 2 wk | Monitor serum sodium levels prior to beginning therapy and periodically during drug therapy |

AED, antiepileptic drug.

*BBW* (handwritten)

adverse effects include heart block, Stevens-Johnson syndrome, respiratory depression, hepatitis, massive hepatic cellular necrosis with total loss of intact liver tissue, and suicidal ideation.

*Carbamazepine* (handwritten)

## Contraindications

Contraindications include a hypersensitivity reaction to carbamazepine or tricyclic antidepressants as well as administration of monoamine oxidase inhibitors. Caution is warranted in patients with a history of increased intraocular pressure; adverse hematologic reaction to other medications; cardiac, hepatic, or renal damage; and latent psychosis.

## Nursing Implications

### Preventing Interactions

Some medications interact with carbamazepine, increasing or decreasing its effects (Box 53.9). Warfarin combined with carbamazepine produces greater anticoagulant effects. The herb *Ginkgo biloba* decreases the effect of the drug.

### Administering the Medication

It is essential that carbamazepine not be administered within 14 days of use of a monoamine oxidase inhibitor. The nurse should tell patients never to crush or chew extended-release tablets. When the nurse administers carbamazepine suspension, he or she never mixes the preparation with other liquid medications because a precipitate may develop. The nurse ensures that the medication is taken with food to prevent GI upset.

### Assessing for Therapeutic Effects

The nurse assesses the patient for absence of partial, tonic–clonic, and mixed seizures.

### Assessing for Adverse Effects

There is a risk of aplastic anemia with the administration of carbamazepine, and hematologic assessments are most important.

The nurse also assesses the integumentary system for Stevens-Johnson syndrome. It is also important that he or she assess hepatic function to check for hepatic adverse effects, including hepatic failure.

In addition, to prevent toxicity, the nurse assesses serum levels as ordered.

### Patient Teaching

Box 53.10 identifies patient teaching guidelines for carbamazepine.

## Other Drugs in the Class

Eslicarbazepine (Aptiom) is administered as monotherapy with partial-onset seizures and as an adjunctive therapy. The action is not precisely known, but it is thought to inhibit voltage-gated sodium channels. It is important to monitor the serum sodium and chloride levels. The symptoms of hyponatremia can result. Also, the patient and family should monitor for suicidal ideations.

Oxcarbazepine (Trileptal) has two mechanisms of action that block the voltage-sensitive sodium channels to stabilize the excitability in the brain and control the seizure spread. The serum sodium level should be monitored. Patients with hyponatremia have an increased risk of seizure activity and seizure frequency.

---

### Clinical Application 53.3

- If Andrew receives a carbamazepine suspension at 9:00 AM, when will the peak serum level be reached?
- At 10 years of age, Andrew develops petechiae on his face and bruising on his arms and legs. His mother calls the pediatric nurse practitioner. What does this nurse suspect is the cause of the bruising?

---

### BOX 53.9 Drug Interactions: Carbamazepine

**Drugs That Increase the Effects of Carbamazepine**
- Erythromycin, troleandomycin, cimetidine, danazol, isoniazid, propoxyphene, and verapamil
  *Increase serum levels and manifestations of toxicity*
- Lithium
  *Increases central nervous system (CNS) toxicity*
- Isoniazid
  *Increases the risk of hepatotoxicity*

**Drugs That Decrease the Effects of Carbamazepine**
- Barbiturates
  *Decrease serum levels*
- Phenytoin and primidone
  *Increase drug metabolism without changing seizure control*

---

### BOX 53.10 Patient Teaching Guidelines for Carbamazepine

- Take the medication with food.
- Do not chew or crush extended-release tablets.
- Do not stop taking the medication abruptly.
- Avoid alcohol, sleep agents, or over-the-counter medications.
- Have hematologic testing as ordered by your prescriber.
- Use contraceptives if you are of childbearing age and are sexually active.
- Wear medical alert bracelet or necklace stating that you have a seizure disorder and naming the medications you take.
- Report symptoms of bruising or bleeding immediately to your prescriber.

# OTHER ANTIEPILEPTIC DRUGS

## CARBONIC ANHYDRASE INHIBITOR

The carbonic anhydrase inhibitor Ⓟ **Acetazolamide** (Diamox) controls fluid secretion in the CNS. A diuretic, it is useful in the treatment of seizures as an adjuvant medication.

## Pharmacokinetics and Action

Acetazolamide is absorbed by the GI tract. For regular tablets, the onset of action is 1 hour, the peak is 2 to 4 hours, and the duration of action is 6 to 12 hours. For sustained-release tablets, the onset of action is 2 hours, the peak is 3 to 6 hours, and the duration of action is 6 to 12 hours. The half-life of the drug is 5 to 6 hours. Acetazolamide is concentrated in the red blood cells, plasma, and kidneys. The drug is excreted by the kidneys and eliminated in the urine. It crosses the placenta.

The antiepileptic action of acetazolamide is unclear, but it is thought to inhibit CNS carbonic anhydrase to decrease neuronal excitability.

## Use

Clinicians use acetazolamide to control absence and tonic–clonic seizures. Table 53.7 presents route and dosage information for acetazolamide.

### Use in Older Adults

It is necessary to use acetazolamide cautiously in older adults because of an increased risk of diuresis.

### Use in Patients With Renal Impairment

In patients with a glomerular filtration rate greater than 50 mL/minute, administration of acetazolamide should occur every 6 hours. If the glomerular filtration rate is 10 to 50 mL/minute, administration should occur every 12 hours. With a glomerular filtration rate of less than 10 mL/minute, the drug is not effective, and the patient should not receive it.

### Use in Patients With Hepatic Impairment

Patients with hepatic impairment should not take acetazolamide.

## Adverse Effects

The adverse effects of acetazolamide include excessive diuresis, Stevens-Johnson syndrome, CNS depression, aplastic anemia, leukopenia, thrombocytopenia, hypokalemia, asymptomatic hyperuricemia, and hyperchloremic acidosis.

## Contraindications

Contraindications to acetazolamide include hypersensitivity to the drug, hyponatremia, hypokalemia, renal or hepatic insufficiency, and chronic noncongestive angle-closure glaucoma. Administration with thiazide diuretics or antibacterial sulfonamides should not occur.

## Nursing Implications

### Preventing Interactions

Several medications interact with acetazolamide. There is decreased renal excretion of quinidine, amphetamine,

| ![pills] **TABLE 53.7** | | | | | |
|---|---|---|---|---|---|
| **DRUGS AT A GLANCE: Other Antiepileptic Drugs** | | | | | |
| **Drug** | **Pregnancy Category** | **Type of Seizure Treated** | **Routes and Dosage Ranges** | | **Therapeutic Serum Drug Level** |
| | | | **Adults** | **Children** | |
| Ⓟ **Acetazolamide** | C | Absence and tonic–clonic seizures | 8–30 mg/kg/d PO in divided doses given in combination with other antiepileptics; starting dose 250 mg | 8–30 mg/kg/d PO in divided doses given in combination with other AEDs; starting dose 250 mg | Has not been determined |
| Ⓟ **Ethosuximide** (Zarontin; 🍁 Zarontin) | C | Absence seizures, myoclonic, and akinetic epilepsy | 500 mg/d PO initially, increased by 250 mg weekly until seizures are controlled or toxicity occurs; maximum dose, 1500 mg/d | 250 mg/d PO initially, increased at weekly intervals until seizures are controlled or toxicity occurs; maximum dose, ≈750–1000 mg/d | 40–100 mcg/mL |
| Ⓟ **Zonisamide** (Zonegran) | D | Partial seizures, with other AEDs | 100–200 mg PO daily as a single dose or as 2–3 divided doses; increase by 100 mg/d every 1–2 wk if necessary; maximum dose, 600 mg daily | <16 y, 1–2 mg/kg PO given once daily or in divided doses twice daily; increase by 0.5–1 mg/kg/d only every 1–2 wk; target range is 4–8 mg/kg/d | 10–20 mcg/mL |

(*Continued on page 1054*)

**TABLE 53.7**

## DRUGS AT A GLANCE: Other Antiepileptic Drugs (Continued)

| Drug | Pregnancy Category | Type of Seizure Treated | Routes and Dosage Ranges | | Therapeutic Serum Drug Level |
|---|---|---|---|---|---|
| | | | **Adults** | **Children** | |
| Ⓟ **Valproate** (Depakote, Depakote ER, Depakote Sprinkles; ✹ APO-Divalproex, APO-Valproic, Depakene, DOM-Divalproex, DOM-Valproic acid) | D | Absence, mixed, and complex partial seizures | PO: 10–15 mg/kg/d, increase weekly by 5–10 mg/kg/d, until seizures controlled, adverse effects occur, or maximum dose (60 mg/kg/d) is reached; give amounts >250 mg/d in divided doses; usual daily dose, 1000–1600 mg, in divided doses IV: usual dose, diluted in 5% dextrose or 0.9% sodium chloride injection | 15–30 mg/kg/d PO | 50–100 mcg/ mL (350–700 µmol/L) |
| Ⓟ **Lacosamide** (Vimpat; ✹ APO-Lacosamide, Auro-Lacosamide, MINT-Lacosamide, Pharma-Lacosamide, SANDOZ Lacosamide) | C | Adjunctive therapy for partial seizures | 17 y and older, initially 50 mg PO twice daily; increase at weekly intervals to a maxi-mum daily dosage of 100–200 mg twice daily; IV administra-tion when PO route is not feasible Hepatic impairment: 300 mg maximum dosage | 1–2 mg/kg/d PO in divided doses (maximum initial dose 50 mg/dose) | Not available |
| Ⓟ **Magnesium sulfate** | A | Preeclampsia and eclampsia paroxysms | Eclampsia, severe pre-eclampsia: total initial 10–14 g; may infuse 4–5 g in 250 mL of 5% dextrose while giving IM doses up to 10 g or may give initial dose of 4 g IV over 3–4 min; then inject 405 g IM into alternate buttocks every 4 h as needed depending on patellar reflex and respiratory function OR, after initial IV dose, 1–2 g/h by constant IV infu-sion; continue until paroxysms stop; do not exceed 30–40 g in 24 h | | 6 mg/100 mL |

**TABLE 53.7**

## DRUGS AT A GLANCE: Other Antiepileptic Drugs (Continued)

| Drug | Pregnancy Category | Type of Seizure Treated | Routes and Dosage Ranges | | Therapeutic Serum Drug Level |
|------|--------------------|-----------------------|--------------------------|--|------------------------------|
| | | | **Adults** | **Children** | |
| Ⓟ **Lamotrigine** (LaMICtal, LaMICtal ODT, LaMICtal XR, Subvenite; ✿ APO-LamoTRIgine, Auro-LamoTRIgine, LaMICtal, Mylan-Lamotrigine, PMS-LamoTRIgine, RATIO-Lamotrigine, Teva-Lamotrigine) | C | Partial seizures, with other AEDs Lennox-Gastaut syndrome, with other AEDs | With AEDs, other than valproic acid: 50 mg PO once daily for 2 wk, then 50 mg twice daily (100 mg/d) for 2 wk, then increase by 100 mg/d at weekly intervals to a maintenance dose; usual maintenance dose, 300–500 mg/d in 2 divided doses<br>With AEDs, including valproic acid: 25 mg PO every other day for 2 wk, then 25 mg once daily for 2 wk, then increase by 25–50 mg/d every 1–2 wk to a maintenance dose; usual maintenance dose, 100–150 mg/d in 2 divided doses | 2–12 y, with enzyme-inducing AEDs, initially, PO 0.15 mg/kg/d in 1 or 2 doses for 2 wk; if calculated dose is 2.5–5 mg, give 5 mg on alternate days for 2 wk, and then 0.3 mg/kg/d in 1 or 2 doses, rounded to nearest 5 mg, for 2 wk; maintenance dose, PO 5–15 mg/kg/d in 2 divided doses<br>>12 y, with enzyme-inducing AEDs, initially, PO 25 mg every other day for 2 wk, then 25 mg daily for 2 wk; maintenance dose, PO 100–400 mg daily in 1 or 2 divided doses; with valproic acid, PO 50 mg daily for 2 wk, then 100 mg daily in 2 divided doses for 2 wk; maintenance dose, PO 300–500 mg daily in 1 or 2 doses | Has not been determined |
| Ⓟ **Levetiracetam** (Keppra, Keppra XR, Roweepra, Roweepra XR, Spritam; ✿ Apo-Levetiracetam, Auro-Levetiracetam, Dom-Levetiracetam, JAMP-Levetiracetam, Keppra, PMS-Levetiracetam, PRO-Levetiracetam, RAN-Levetiracetam) | C | Myoclonic, tonic–clonic, partial seizures | Partial-onset and tonic–clonic seizures: 500 mg PO twice daily initially, increased by 500 mg/d every 2 wk, if necessary; maximum dose, 1500 mg twice daily<br>Extended release: 1000 mg once daily; increase every 2 wk by 1000 mg/d to a maximum dose of 3000 mg once daily<br>IV 500 mg twice daily; increase every 2 wk by 500 mg/dose to a maximum of 1500 mg twice daily | Myoclonic: PO immediate-release tablet or oral solution; ≥12 y, refer to adult dosing<br>Partial seizures or refractory seizures (adjunctive treatment); 1 mo–<6 mo, 7 mg/kg/dose twice daily; increase every 2 wk to a recommended dose of 21 mg/kg/dose twice daily | Has not been determined |

*(Continued on page 1056)*

## DRUGS AT A GLANCE: Other Antiepileptic Drugs (Continued)

| Drug | Pregnancy Category | Type of Seizure Treated | Routes and Dosage Ranges | | Therapeutic Serum Drug Level |
|------|---------------------|--------------------------|---------------------------|---|-------------------------------|
| | | | **Adults** | **Children** | |
| | | | Renal impairment: creatinine clearance (CrCl > 80 mL/min), 500–1500 mg; CrCl 50–80 mL/min, 500–1000 mg; CrCl 30–50 mL/min, 250–750 mg; CrCl < 30 mL/min, 250–500 mg. End-stage renal disease, on hemodialysis: 500–1000 mg, with a supplemental dose of half the total daily dose (250–500 mg) | 6 mo–<4 y: initial 10 mg/kg/dose twice daily; increase every 2 wk by 10 mg/kg/dose to a recommended dose of 25 mg/kg/dose twice daily. 4–5 y, 10 mg/kg PO twice daily; can increase the daily dose every 2 wk by increments of 10 mg/kg to recommended dose of 30 mg/kg twice daily (60 mg/kg/d) | |
| **Perampanel** (Fycompa; ✽ Fycompa) | C | Partial seizures | Patients not taking enzyme-inducing AED regimens: 2 mg PO once daily at bedtime; may increase dose by 2 mg at weekly intervals based on response and tolerability. Recommended dose: 8–12 mg once daily. Patients taking enzyme-inducing AED regimens: 4 mg PO once daily at bedtime; may increase dose by 2 mg at weekly intervals based on response and tolerability. Recommended dose: 8–12 mg once daily at bedtime | Partial-onset seizures: adjunct. ≥12 y 2 mg PO at bedtime; may increase daily dose by 2 mg increments at no more frequent than weekly intervals; recommended dose, 8–12 mg once daily at bedtime; 12 mg has shown greater efficacy for reduction of seizure rate than 8 mg; 12 mg is associated with higher adverse effects | |
| **Topiramate** (Topamax, Qudexy XR, Topamax Sprinkles, Trokendi XR; ✽ AG Topiramate, Apo-Topiramate, Auro-Topiramate, Dom-Topiramate) | C | Initial monotherapy for partial seizures or generalized tonic–clonic seizures; partial seizures, generalized tonic–clonic, and Lennox-Gastaut syndrome with other AEDs | 25–50 mg PO daily, increased by 25–50 mg/wk until response; usual dose, 400 mg daily in 2 divided doses | 2–16 y, week 1, 25 mg PO every PM, increase by 1–3 mg/kg/d at 1- or 2-wk intervals until response; usual dose 5–9 mg/kg/d, in 2 divided doses. Monotherapy: 10 y and older, 25 mg PO twice daily, titrating to maintenance dose of 200 mg PO twice daily over 6 wk | Has not been determined |

**TABLE 53.7**

**DRUGS AT A GLANCE: Other Antiepileptic Drugs** (Continued)

| Drug | Pregnancy Category | Type of Seizure Treated | Routes and Dosage Ranges | | Therapeutic Serum Drug Level |
|---|---|---|---|---|---|
| | | | **Adults** | **Children** | |
| | | | | Week 1: 25 mg twice daily Week 2: 50 mg twice daily Week 3: 75 mg twice daily Week 4: 100 mg twice daily Week 5: 150 mg twice daily Week 6: 200 mg twice daily Check package insert for dosages of extended-release brands | |
| ℗ **Rufinamide** (Banzel; ✻ Banzel) | D | Adjunctive treatment of seizures caused by Lennox-Gastaut syndrome | 400–800 mg PO in 2 divided doses; maximum dosage 3200 mg/d | <17 y: initial 10 mg/kg/d in 2 equally divided doses; increase dose by 10 mg/kg every other day to a maximum dose of 45 mg/kg/d, not to exceed 3200 mg daily in 2 equally divided doses | Not available |

procainamide, and tricyclic antidepressants with acetazolamide. Salicylates and lithium administered with acetazolamide result in diminished renal excretion of these drugs. There is also a risk of salicylate toxicity related to metabolic acidosis with acetazolamide.

### Administering the Medication

To prevent GI upset, the nurse ensures that the drug is taken with food. Crushing or chewing of regular tablets is permissible, but patients must swallow sustained-release tablets whole. It is necessary to store the oral preparation in a container with a tight-fitting lid at 59°F to 86°F.

### Assessing for Therapeutic and Adverse Effects

The patient should be without symptoms of absence or tonic–clonic seizures.

The nurse assesses the integumentary system for any sign of skin rash or eruption and fluid and electrolyte levels for metabolic acidosis. The patient should have annual eye examinations to determine if there has been an increase in intraocular pressure.

### Patient Teaching

Box 53.11 identifies patient teaching guidelines for acetazolamide.

## SUCCINIMIDES

℗ **Ethosuximide** (Zarontin) is a succinimide antiepileptic agent. The frequency of absence seizures is reduced through the depression of the motor cortex.

## Pharmacokinetics and Action

Ethosuximide is rapidly and completely absorbed orally. The drug increases the seizure threshold to suppress the paroxysmal spike and wave pattern noted in absence seizures. The half-life for children is 30 hours and 50 to 60 hours for adults. The medication reaches a peak level in 1 to 7 hours. It is metabolized by the liver into three active metabolites and excreted slowly in the urine. Ethosuximide increases the seizure threshold to suppress the paroxysmal spike and wave pattern noted in absence seizures.

## Use

Ethosuximide is used for absence seizures or in combination with other antiepileptic agents in patients with mixed type seizures. No dosage adjustments are required in patients with diminished renal or hepatic function. Table 53.7 gives route and dosage information for ethosuximide.

**BOX 53.11** 📋 *Patient Teaching Guidelines for Acetazolamide*

- Take the medication with food to prevent gastric upset.
- Have annual eye examinations to assess intraocular pressure.
- Report any changes in weight, unusual bruising or bleeding, pain, or rash to your prescriber.

## Adverse Effects and Contraindications

The most serious adverse effects of ethosuximide are its hematologic effects. Eosinophilia, leukopenia, thrombocytopenia, agranulocytosis, pancytopenia, and aplastic anemia have been reported. In the event of eosinophilia, multiorgan hypersensitivity, a potentially serious and often fatal drug reaction, can occur. Other adverse effects include anorexia, epigastric distress, abdominal pain, weight loss, diarrhea, constipation, and gingival hyperplasia. CNS effects are impaired physical and mental abilities, CNS depression, anxiety, and hyperactivity. Stevens-Johnson syndrome can result within 28 days of the onset of therapy. At the first sign of rash, the prescriber should be notified and the medication discontinued.

Ethosuximide is contraindicated in patients who experience a hypersensitivity reaction.

## Nursing Implications

### Preventing Interactions

Carbamazepine and isoniazid will decrease the serum levels of ethosuximide, placing the patient at risk for seizures. *Ginkgo biloba* will decrease the seizure threshold. Cannabis will increase CNS depression.

### Administering the Medication

Administer ethosuximide with food to decrease GI distress. The medication should be stored at 15°C to 30°C or 59°F to 86°F.

### Assessing for Therapeutic and Adverse Effects

Good control with ethosuximide is indicated by the lack of seizure activity. Assess the patient's weight on a weekly basis because of anorexia and normal weight loss. Check the drug level, which should be in the therapeutic range. Assess the patient for changes in sensorium or increased seizure activity with dosage changes. Assess CBC monthly to determine signs and symptoms of eosinophilia.

### Patient Teaching

Box 53.12 identifies patient teaching guidelines for ethosuximide.

## SULFONAMIDE

 **Zonisamide** (Zonegran) is a sulfonamide antiepileptic medication. Prescribers administer it as adjunctive therapy for partial seizures.

---

**BOX 53.12** *Patient Teaching Guidelines for Ethosuximide*

- Report a skin rash or any hypersensitivity to the prescriber.
- Have monthly complete blood count or as ordered.
- Do not drive or operate machinery with central nervous system depression.
- Report any changes in behavior.

---

 **QSEN Alert: Evidence-Based Practice**

Senadim, Baslo, Guveli, Sari, & Atakli (2018) investigated the use of zonisamide in patients with partial and generalized seizures. They sought to understand the safety and efficacy of zonisamide. The study was composed of 39 patients. Twenty of the subjects responded to treatment, with a seizure frequency of 25%. Five percent of the patients saw a decrease in seizure frequency by half. The researchers concluded that zonisamide was safe and effective for the treatment of refractory seizures.

## Pharmacokinetics and Action

Zonisamide is rapidly and completely absorbed. It is highly concentrated in erythrocytes and 40% protein bound. The hepatic cytochrome P450 isoenzyme CYP3A4 is responsible for the metabolism of zonisamide. Zonisamide does not affect GABA. Its action stabilizes the neuronal membranes. It accelerates the dopamine and serotonin neurotransmitters.

## Use

Zonisamide is used for a variety of seizures but primarily adjunctive therapy for absence seizures or partial seizures. Infantile spasms are treated with zonisamide. The titration of the medication is faster with infantile spasms. Table 53.7 gives route and dosage information for zonisamide.

## Use in Children

Oligohydrosis is an adverse effect that is commonly seen in children. It will often result in heat stroke and hyperthermia. The child should maintain hydration and protection from increased temperatures.

---

**QSEN Alert: Safety**

When administering zonisamide, instruct the patient and family on the signs of heat stroke and to maintain adequate hydration. In addition, patients living in warm climates should pay particular attention to increases in body temperature.

---

## Adverse Effects and Contraindications

CNS depression with dizziness and drowsiness has been reported. The most severe adverse effect is the development of toxic epidermal necrolysis and Stevens-Johnson syndrome. Oligohydrosis and heat stroke have been reported in adolescents receiving zonisamide therapy. Metabolic acidosis, abdominal pain, weight loss, constipation, agranulocytosis, and aplastic anemia have also been reported. The FDA has established a warning that zonisamide is contraindicated with all other sulfonamide drug classes. Zonisamide is contraindicated with a known hypersensitivity to sulfonamides.

## Nursing Implications

### Preventing Interactions

The half-life of zonisamide is decreased when combined with carbamazepine, phenobarbital, phenytoin, and valproate.

## Administering the Medication

The medication should be stored at room temperature and protected from light and moisture. The capsules should be swallowed whole with a full glass of water or other fluid. Administer without regard to food; however, the presence of food will delay maximum concentration. The dosage information is in Table 53.7.

## Assessing for Therapeutic and Adverse Effects

Assess the patient's response to the medication and decrease in seizure activity. Assess for metabolic acidosis with the onset of lethargy, confusion, headache, and weakness. If acidosis is suspected, assess arterial blood gases. Assess the patient's intake and output.

## Patient Teaching

The patient should be instructed to maintain adequate hydration and protection in warm climates. The patient should avoid the consumption of alcoholic beverages. The medication should be tapered when discontinuing and not abruptly stopped.

## HISTONE DEACETYLASE INHIBITOR

Ⓟ **Valproate** (Depakote, Depakote ER) a histone deacetylase inhibitor has been in use for approximately 40 years. A researcher identified its antiseizure ability while studying laboratory rats. The drug is synthesized from valeric acid, which is found in the herb valerian.

## Pharmacokinetics

The onset of action for oral and parenteral valproate varies, and it reaches its peak in serum in 15 minutes to 4 hours. Parenteral valproate reaches a peak of action in 1 hour. The drug is metabolized by the liver and excreted by the kidneys. It crosses the placenta and enters breast milk. See Figure 53.1 for the site of action of the carboxylic acid derivatives.

## Action

The action of valproate is not understood, but it is thought to produce antiepileptic activity by increasing GABA effects, thus decreasing electrical activity.

## Use

Clinicians use valproate alone or in combination with other AEDs for the treatment of simple and complex absence seizures, and prescribers also order the drug for the treatment of seizures related to Lennox-Gastaut syndrome. Table 53.7 presents route and dosage information for valproate.

## Use in Children

Children aged 10 years and older may receive extended-release forms (Depakote ER) for the treatment of epilepsy. Use in children younger than age 10 requires extreme caution. Fatal hepatotoxicity has occurred, and children younger than 2 years of age are at greatest risk for hepatic failure within the first 6 months of drug administration. The nurse must monitor the patient's liver function closely. In addition, caution is warranted in children younger than 18 months of age and those younger than 2 years of age with congenital abnormalities and severe mental disability.

## Use in Older Adults

When administering valproate to the elderly, it is necessary to adjust the dosage slowly.

## Use in Patients With Renal or Hepatic Impairment

Caution is necessary in renal or hepatic impairment.

## Adverse Effects

The most life-threatening adverse effects associated with valproate are pancreatitis and hepatic failure. Other significant adverse effects include altered bleeding time, thrombocytopenia, bruising, and hemorrhage. The most common GI adverse effects are nausea, vomiting, indigestion, diarrhea, and abdominal cramps. CNS adverse effects include sedation, tremor, emotional upset, weakness, and suicidal ideation, as well as brain atrophy.

The FDA has issued several **BLACK BOX WARNING ◆** for valproate. The first instructs patients to discontinue valproate at any sign of pancreatitis. The development of this condition is life threatening. The second points out that valproate is a teratogenic medication. Women of childbearing age should not take the drug without using two forms of birth control. The third instructs the patient to check for signs of bleeding or bruising. Altered bleeding times may occur. The nurse should tell the patient to have platelet counts, bleeding time determination, and clotting times according to the prescriber's orders.

## Contraindications

Contraindications to valproate include significant hepatic impairment as well as a hypersensitivity reaction to the drug.

## Nursing Implications

### Preventing Interactions

Certain medications interact with valproate, decreasing or increasing its effects (Box 53.13). Serum levels of phenobarbital, primidone, ethosuximide, diazepam, lamotrigine, and zidovudine may increase when these drugs are combined with valproate. The herb *Ginkgo biloba* decreases the effect of the drug.

### Administering the Medication

The nurse dilutes the vial in 5% dextrose, 0.9% sodium chloride, or lactated Ringer's solution for IV administration. The reconstituted medication is stable for 24 hours and does not need to be refrigerated. Infusion should occur over 1 hour, no faster than 20 mg/minute. IV administration is permissible only for 14 days, and a switch to an oral preparation is necessary. When administering Depakote to children, the nurse may open the tablets and sprinkle the contents on applesauce or pudding. It is important to note that Depakote ER should be swallowed whole and never crushed or chewed.

## BOX 53.13 — *Drug Interactions: Valproate*

**Drugs That Increase the Effects of Valproate**
- Alcohol and central nervous system depressants
  *Increase sedation*
- Chlorpromazine, cimetidine, erythromycin, felbamate, and salicylates
  *Increase serum levels and toxicity*

**Drugs That Decrease the Effects of Valproate**
- Carbamazepine, charcoal, and rifampin
  *Decrease drug levels*
- Fosphenytoin, Phenytoin
  *Valproate will decrease the protein binding of fosphenytoin and phenytoin. This leads to increase in fosphenytoin and phenytoin concentrations.*

## Assessing for Therapeutic Effects

The absence of simple and complex absent seizures is indicative that the therapeutic effects of the valproate have been attained.

## Assessing for Adverse Effects

The nurse assesses the patient for signs and symptoms of pancreatitis, which include severe abdominal pain and back pain (Hinkle & Cheever, 2018). He or she should also assess for bleeding and bruising. In addition, the nurse needs to assess the patient's liver function tests routinely. Finally, it is necessary to assess the patient's motor and cognitive function because of brain atrophy.

## Patient Teaching

Box 53.14 identifies patient teaching guidelines for valproate.

## BOX 53.14 — *Patient Teaching Guidelines for Valproate*

- Take medication at regular intervals, do not skip a dose, and do not stop abruptly. *[handwritten: thats for all these meds]*
- Do not chew or crush extended-release tablets.
- Avoid alcohol and over-the-counter sleep aids.
- Keep follow-up appointments with your prescriber.
- Keep follow-up appointments for serum blood levels, platelet counts, bleeding and clotting times, liver function, and renal function.
- Use two types of birth control if you are a woman of childbearing age and are sexually active. Notify your prescriber if you become pregnant.
- Do not operate machinery with central nervous system (CNS) depression. You may have sedation, tremors, emotional upset, weakness, or suicidal ideation.
- Know the signs and symptoms of pancreatitis, such as upper abdominal pain and nausea and vomiting, which often begins or worsens after eating.
- If you have diabetes, be aware that this medication interferes with ketones.
- Report any unusual bleeding or bruising.
- Wear a medical alert bracelet or necklace stating that you have a seizure disorder and naming the medications you take.

# FUNCTIONALIZED AMINO ACIDS

Ⓟ **Lacosamide** (Vimpat) is an AED that is available in oral and IV preparations.

## Pharmacokinetics

Lacosamide is rapidly absorbed. The oral preparation reaches its peak in 1 to 4 hours, and the IV preparation reaches its peak at the end of the infusion. The half-life of the medication is 13 hours. The drug is metabolized by the CYP3A4, CYP2C9, and CYP2C19 enzymes in the liver and excreted in the urine. It crosses the placenta and may enter the breast milk.

## Action

The mechanism of action of lacosamide is not fully understood. The drug inhibits the voltage-sensitive sodium channels, producing stabilization of the neuronal membrane and inhibition of the repetitive firing of the neuron.

## Use

Indications for oral lacosamide include the treatment of partial-onset seizures. Clinicians use the IV drug on a short-term basis when oral administration is prohibited. Table 53.7 gives route and dosage information for lacosamide.

### Use in Older Adults

A reduction in dosage in the elderly is not necessary unless renal impairment is apparent. It is important to determine the dosage based on the patient's hepatic and renal function.

### Use in Patients With Renal Impairment

Renal function regulates dosage, because the drug is eliminated in the urine. Patients with a CrCl of 30 mL/minute or less should receive 300 mg/day as the maximum dosage. In those with end-stage renal disease, the maximum dosage should be 300 mg daily or less.

### Use in Patients With Hepatic Impairment

It is necessary to titrate the dosage in patients with mild to moderate hepatic impairment. The maximum dosage is 300 mg/day. Experts do not recommend use of the drug in patients with severe hepatic impairment, because the drug possesses hepatotoxic adverse effects.

### Use in Patients With Critical Illness

Critically ill patients should receive lacosamide intravenously when oral preparation is prohibited. Caution is necessary in the presence of cardiac conduction abnormalities, myocardial ischemia, and heart failure.

## Adverse Effects and Contraindications

The adverse effects of lacosamide include a prolonged PR interval, dizziness, ataxia, diplopia, somnolence, suicidal ideation, headache, nausea, and vomiting.

Contraindications include a known hypersensitivity to the drug.

## Nursing Implications

### Preventing Interactions

It is important that lacosamide not be combined with any medication that prolongs the PR interval. Patients should not take this drug in combination with alcohol.

### Administering the Medication

The nurse may give IV lacosamide in 0.9% sodium chloride, 5% dextrose, or lactated Ringer's solution. The period of infusion is 30 to 60 minutes. Administration of lacosamide should not occur in the same IV line with other medications. The preparation is stable at room temperature for 24 hours.

### Assessing for Therapeutic and Adverse Effects

The nurse assesses the patient for CNS depression and diminished partial-onset seizure activity.

The greatest risks associated with lacosamide are suicidal ideation and cardiac conduction abnormalities. The nurse assesses the patient for sudden personality changes, signs of aggression, and severe nausea and vomiting. During parenteral administration, the nurse assesses for signs of a prolonged PR interval.

### Patient Teaching

Box 53.15 identifies patient teaching guidelines for lacosamide.

## MINERAL ELECTROLYTES: MAGNESIUM SULFATE

It is important to understand the use and administration of the mineral electrolyte ⓟ **Magnesium sulfate** because of the fetal neuroprotection it can give to pregnant women. This medication provides the opportunity to improve neurodevelopmental outcomes in infants by delaying preterm birth and decreasing maternal seizure risk. Table 53.7 contains some dosage information about this agent. Chapter 6 discusses the use of magnesium sulfate more fully.

## PHENYLTRIAZINE DERIVATIVES

ⓟ **Lamotrigine** (LaMICtal) is used for adjunctive therapy in the treatment of partial seizures.

---

**BOX 53.15** 📋 *Patient Teaching Guidelines for Lacosamide*

- Take the medication as prescribed.
- Do not discontinue the drug abruptly. If you need to stop taking it, taper the dosage.
- Report any mood changes to the prescriber.
- Keep follow-up appointments to monitor drug response and assessment of adverse effects.
- Do not drink alcohol because of the increased risk of central nervous system depression.
- If you are a woman of childbearing age and are sexually active, use contraceptives.

---

## Pharmacokinetics

Lamotrigine is administered orally. It is absorbed by the GI tract with a rapid onset of action. Lamotrigine is metabolized by the liver and excreted in the urine. It crosses the placenta and enters the breast milk. The medication is 55% protein bound and has a 25- to 30-hour half-life.

## Action

The action of lamotrigine is not well understood. It is thought to reduce the release of glutamate, an excitatory neurotransmitter, in the brain. The neurotransmitter is sensitive to sodium channels, thus decreasing seizure activity.

## Use

Clinicians use lamotrigine for partial seizures as well as for generalized tonic–clonic, absence, or myoclonic seizures. Other uses include bipolar disorder. Table 53.7 gives route and dosage information for lamotrigine.

### Use in Children

Children should receive lamotrigine in combination with valproate and other AEDs.

### Use in Patients With Renal or Hepatic Impairment

It may be necessary to reduce the dosage in patients with renal or hepatic impairment.

## Adverse Effects

Adverse effects of lamotrigine include dizziness, drowsiness, headache, ataxia, blurred or double vision, nausea and vomiting, and weakness. The FDA has issued a **BLACK BOX WARNING ◆** related to the potential development of serious dermatologic reactions. Because a serious skin rash may occur, especially in children, lamotrigine should be administered cautiously to children younger than 16 years of age and should be discontinued at the first sign of skin rash in an adult. Skin rash is more likely to occur with concomitant valproate therapy, high lamotrigine starting dose, and rapid titration rate. It may resolve if lamotrigine is discontinued, but it progresses in some patients to more severe forms, such as Stevens-Johnson syndrome or toxic epidermal necrosis.

## Contraindications

Contraindications to lamotrigine include any hypersensitivity to the drug. Patients who have signs and symptoms of suicide, as well as those who are pregnant or lactating, should not take it.

## Nursing Implications

### Preventing Interactions

Several medications and herbs interact with lamotrigine, increasing or decreasing its effects (Boxes 53.16 and 53.17).

**BOX 53.16** **Drug Interactions: Lamotrigine**

**Drugs That Increase the Effects of Lamotrigine**
- Valproate
  *Significantly increases plasma concentration*

**Drugs That Decrease the Effects of Lamotrigine**
- Carbamazepine, fosphenytoin, oral contraceptives, phenobarbital, primidone, and phenytoin
  *Decrease serum concentration*

## Administering the Medication

The nurse should ensure that chewable tablets are chewed or crushed, not swallowed. If the drug is discontinued, it is essential to taper the medication over a 2-week period.

## Assessing for Therapeutic and Adverse Effects

The nurse should assess for the lack of generalized, myoclonic, and absence seizures.

The nurse assesses the integumentary system daily for the onset of skin eruptions. He or she also questions the patient about ophthalmologic changes.

## Patient Teaching

Box 53.18 identifies patient teaching guidelines for lamotrigine.

---

### NCLEX Success

8. A 12-year-old boy comes to the school nurse's office after falling during gym class. The nurse assesses the child and notes that he has bruising and petechiae over most of his legs, arms, and torso. The child has a history of absence seizures that are treated with valproate. Based on the child's history, what would the nurse suspect?

   A. abuse
   B. leukemia
   C. adverse effect
   D. anemia

9. Which of the following places the patient at risk for toxicity following the administration of phenytoin?

   A. The patient skips a dose of phenytoin.
   B. The patient takes a different brand of phenytoin.
   C. The patient switches to a different antiepileptic agent.
   D. The patient receives phenytoin in an enteral feeding.

10. Which of the following is most important to teach a patient who is being administered lamotrigine?

    A. to report the development of edema
    B. to report anxiety
    C. to report the development of a skin rash
    D. to report anorexia

---

**BOX 53.17** **Herb and Dietary Interactions: Lamotrigine**

**Herbs and Foods That Decrease the Effect of Lamotrigine**
- *Ginkgo biloba*
- Oil of primrose

## PYRROLIDINE DERIVATIVES

*stroke pt.*

**Levetiracetam** (Keppra) is an AED that is effective in the treatment of a wide variety of seizure disorders. The use of levetiracetam has increased in treating seizure disorders in adults and children. It is approved for use in patients with myoclonic, tonic–clonic, and partial seizures. In the United States, an unlabeled use of levetiracetam is status epilepticus. A Swiss study showed that the drug was not as effective in treating status epilepticus as other approved agents.

## Pharmacokinetics

Levetiracetam is administered orally or intravenously and is rapidly absorbed, reaching its peak in 1 hour. It is 10% protein bound with minimal hepatic metabolism. It is excreted in the urine and has a 7.1-hour half-life. The half-life in older adults is 9.6 hours.

## Action

Levetiracetam is chemically unrelated to other AEDs, and its mechanism of action is unknown. It inhibits abnormal neuronal firing but does not affect normal neuronal excitability or function.

## Use

Clinicians use levetiracetam as adjunctive therapy for partial-onset and generalized tonic–clonic seizures. Table 53.7 presents route and dosage information for levetiracetam.

### Use in Patients With Renal Impairment

It is essential to reduce the dose in patients with impaired renal function, because the kidneys eliminate the majority of a dose (66%). A study conducted by Lima-Rogel et al. (2018) found that a neonate's CrCl and weight affects the pharmacokinetic properties of levetiracetam.

**BOX 53.18** **Patient Teaching Guidelines for Lamotrigine**

- Call your prescriber if a skin rash develops.
- Use protection from sunlight.
- Do not operate machinery if you have central nervous system depression.
- Use contraceptives if you are of childbearing age and are sexually active.
- Schedule eye examinations annually.
- Do not stop the medication abruptly.

## Adverse Effects and Contraindications

Common adverse effects of levetiracetam include drowsiness, dizziness, and fatigue. Others include decreases in red and white blood cell counts, double vision, amnesia, anxiety, ataxia, emotional lability, hostility, nervousness, paresthesia, pharyngitis, and rhinitis. Postmarketing research noted that there is a risk of hepatic failure, acute renal failure, and multiorgan failure. There is also a risk for the development of Stevens-Johnson syndrome.

Contraindications include a known hypersensitivity to the medication, pregnancy, lactation, and suicidal ideation.

## Nursing Implications

### Preventing Interactions

CNS depressants combined with levetiracetam may increase symptoms of sedation.

### Administering the Medication

It is essential that the IV preparation of levetiracetam be administered only on a short-term basis. The nurse tells patients not to crush extended-release forms of the drug. To prevent GI upset, the nurse administers the oral preparation with food. Although food may delay absorption, it does not affect the degree of absorption. The nurse monitors patients for psychosis and depression.

### Assessing for Therapeutic and Adverse Effects

The nurse assesses the patient for symptoms of partial-onset and generalized tonic–clonic seizures, which should be absent.

The nurse assesses the patient for ocular changes, CNS depression, and hematologic changes.

### Patient Teaching

Box 53.19 identifies patient teaching guidelines for levetiracetam.

## AMPA GLUTAMATE RECEPTOR ANTAGONIST

Ⓟ **Perampanel** (Fycompa) is an α-amino-3-hydroxy-5-methyl-4-isoxazolepropionic acid (AMPA) glutamate receptor antagonist, which is considered a miscellaneous antiepileptic agent.

---

**BOX 53.19**  📋  *Patient Teaching Guidelines for Levetiracetam*

- Take the medication as prescribed and do not crush or chew extended-release tablets.
- Do not stop taking the medication abruptly.
- Use contraceptives if you are of childbearing age and are sexually active.
- Schedule eye examinations annually.
- Do not operate machinery if you have central nervous system depression.

---

See Adverse Effects and Contraindications for more information about the serious psychiatric effects of this drug.

## Pharmacokinetics and Action

Perampanel is rapidly absorbed, but the presence of food will slow the absorption. It is 95% to 96% protein bound by albumin and alpha$_1$ acid glycoprotein. Metabolism occurs in the liver by primary oxidation with the isoenzymes CYP3A4, CYP3A5, CYP1A2, and CYP2B6 and subsequent glucuronidation.

This medication exerts an unknown antiseizure activity.

## Use

Prescribers use perampanel for adjuvant treatment of partial-onset seizures with or without generalized seizures in individuals 12 years and older. Table 53.7 gives route and dosage information for perampanel.

## Adverse Effects and Contraindications

The most serious adverse effect of perampanel is hostile behavior. The FDA issued a **BLACK BOX WARNING** ◆ that serious or life-threatening psychiatric and behavioral adverse reactions such as aggression, hostility, anger, and homicidal ideations can occur.

Other adverse effects in multiorgan hypersensitivity referred to as DRESS syndrome. DRESS is a drug reaction with eosinophilia and systemic symptoms that is life threatening. The reaction includes atypical lymphocytosis, lymphadenopathy, a skin eruption, and multiorgan failure. The metabolic adverse effect is hyponatremia and weight gain. Other less severe adverse effects are as follows: skin rash, abdominal pain, constipation, nausea, vomiting, urinary tract infection, bruising, blurred vision, diplopia, upper respiratory infection, lacerations, head trauma, and limb injury. According to the manufacturer's labeling, there are no contraindications to perampanel.

## Nursing Implications

### Preventing Interactions and Administering the Medication

According to the manufacturer, potential interactions may exist requiring a dosage or frequency adjustment. It is important to monitor the outcomes of therapy. Medications that alter CNS effects have a potential to cause enhanced adverse effects, particularly CNS depression. St. John's wort combined with perampanel also produces and increases CNS depression.

The oral formulation should be administered at bedtime.

### Assessing for Therapeutic and Adverse Effects

The nurse assesses the patient's response to the medication, including seizure activity, duration, and frequency. Also, the nurse assesses for aggressive, hostile, and homicidal behavior. In addition, it is necessary to assess serum sodium level and for changes in weight.

### Patient Teaching

Box 53.20 identifies patient teaching guidelines for perampanel.

## SULFAMATE-SUBSTITUTED MONOSACCHARIDES

**Topiramate** (Topamax) is a sulfamate-substituted monosaccharide that was identified during a research project to develop a new antidiabetic agent. The drug has many unlabeled uses, including migraine prophylaxis, alcohol dependence, and weight loss.

## Pharmacokinetics

Topiramate is absorbed in the GI tract and produces peak plasma levels about 2 hours after oral administration. The average half-life is about 21 hours, and steady-state concentrations are reached in about 4 days with normal renal function. The drug is 20% bound to plasma proteins. Topiramate is not extensively metabolized and is primarily eliminated via the kidneys.

## Action

The mechanism of action of topiramate is not understood, but the antiepileptic action may be related to the blockage of sodium channels in neurons with sustained depolarization. This action increases GABA activity at the receptors, potentiating the inhibition of the neurotransmitters blocking excitatory neurotransmitters at the neuron receptor sites.

## Use

Clinicians use topiramate as monotherapy in partial-onset or primary generalized tonic–clonic seizures as well as in adjunctive therapy for partial-onset or primary generalized seizures. Lennox-Gastaut syndrome is also an indication. In addition, prescribers order the medication as a preventive for migraine headaches. Table 53.7 gives route and dosage information for topiramate.

## Use in Patients With Renal Impairment

Patients with a CrCl less than 70 mL/minute should receive one-half of the usual dose.

### Use in Patients With Hepatic Impairment

Patients with elevated liver enzymes should receive reduced doses of topiramate, with the dosage increased slowly over time. It is necessary to monitor patients closely for increased hepatic effects.

## Adverse Effects and Contraindications

Adverse effects of topiramate include CNS effects such as ataxia, somnolence, dizziness, and nystagmus as well as GI adverse effects such as nausea and dyspepsia. The metabolic adverse effects of topiramate are a decreased serum bicarbonate and weight loss. Renal stones may develop. Other adverse effects are increased intraocular pressure and fatigue. A rare adverse effect is oligohydrosis, which is decreased sweating and hyperthermia. These adverse effects are more common in children and exposure to high environmental temperatures.

Contraindications include hypersensitivity to the drug and metabolic acidosis. Anticholinergic medications will increase the patient's risk of developing oligohydrosis and hyperthermia.

## Nursing Implications

### Preventing Interactions

Several medications interact with topiramate, increasing or decreasing its effects (Box 53.21). The drug decreases the effectiveness of oral contraceptives. The herb *Ginkgo biloba* decreases the effect of topiramate.

### Administering the Medication

Topiramate has a very bitter taste. To prevent patients from tasting the bitterness, the nurse instructs them never to chew the medication. In addition, the nurse notes that it is necessary to store topiramate in a tightly closed container at 59°F to 86°F.

### Assessing for Therapeutic and Adverse Effects

Patients are without symptoms of partial or generalized seizures. Those with Lennox-Gastaut syndrome have no seizure activity.

The nurse assesses the patient for pain or discomfort related to kidney stones. The patient should have an annual eye examination to determine the onset of increased intraocular pressure. Monitor the patient's temperature and diminished sweating when exposed to high environmental temperatures.

### Patient Teaching

Box 53.22 identifies patient teaching guidelines for topiramate.

## TRIAZOLE DERIVATIVES

**Rufinamide** (Banzel) is structurally unrelated to other AEDs. Rufinamide is effective in reducing the generalized tonic–clonic seizures related to Lennox-Gastaut syndrome.

**BOX 53.22** | *Patient Teaching Guidelines for Topiramate*

- Take the medication as prescribed.
- Do not stop taking the medication abruptly.
- Use two types of contraceptives if you are of childbearing age and are sexually active.
- Do not operate machinery with central nervous system (CNS) depression.
- Drink six to eight 8-oz glasses of water per day to decrease risk of renal stone development.

## Pharmacokinetics and Action

Rufinamide is absorbed slowly by the GI tract. Peak plasma concentrations occur between 4 and 6 hours. The drug is metabolized extensively without active metabolites. It is excreted by the kidneys.

Rufinamide decreases seizure activity by prolonging the inactive sodium channels in the cortical neurons.

## Use

Clinicians use rufinamide in the treatment of seizures in patients with Lennox-Gastaut syndrome. Table 53.7 gives route and dosage information for rufinamide.

### Use in Patients With Hepatic Impairment

It is necessary to administer rufinamide cautiously to patients with moderate hepatic impairment. Patients with severe hepatic impairment should not take the drug.

## Adverse Effects and Contraindications

The most common adverse effects of rufinamide include fatigue, headache, somnolence, vomiting, and flulike symptoms. Dermatologic effects, including Stevens-Johnson syndrome, require immediate discontinuation of rufinamide. Decreased white blood cell counts may occur.

Contraindications include short QT syndrome, severe hepatic impairment, pregnancy, and lactation.

## Nursing Implications

### Preventing Interactions

Several drugs interact with rufinamide, increasing or decreasing its effects (Box 53.23).

### Administering the Medication

To increase drug absorption, the nurse ensures that rufinamide is taken with food. It is acceptable to crush or split the medication for ease of administration.

### Assessing for Therapeutic and Adverse Effects

The patient is without seizure activity related to Lennox-Gastaut syndrome.

It is important to assess the patient's CNS response to the medication. The nurse also assesses the patient for GI upset and

**BOX 53.23** | *Drug Interactions: Rufinamide*

**Drugs That Increase the Effect of Rufinamide**
- Valproate
  *Increases plasma concentration*

**Drugs That Decrease the Effect of Rufinamide**
- Primidone
  *Decreases the serum concentration of rufinamide*
- Carbamazepine, ethinyl estradiol, and norethindrone
  *Decrease the effect of both drugs*
- Phenobarbital and phenytoin
  *May increase levels of these drugs as well as decrease rufinamide level*

flulike symptoms, as well as for hypersensitivity reactions such as Stevens-Johnson syndrome.

### Patient Teaching

Box 53.24 identifies patient teaching guidelines for rufinamide.

# OVERVIEW OF SPINAL CORD INJURY

Spinal cord injuries are classified by the spinal level at which the injury occurs. Tetraplegia, or quadriplegia, is the impairment of motor and sensory function in the arms, trunk, legs, and pelvic organs. Paraplegia is the impairment of motor and sensory function in the thoracic, lumbar, and sacral segments of the spinal cord. Upper motor neuron injuries result in spastic paralysis with hyperreflexia, preventing purposeful movement. Lower motor neuron injuries result in the flaccidity of muscles and muscle atrophy.

## Etiology

Spinal cord injury is a result of damage to the cord by trauma. The damage to the cord is related to indirect injury from vertebral fractures or contusions. The direct cause of spinal cord injury is from a penetrating wound. The indirect cause of spinal cord injury is the result of a vertebral fracture, fracture dislocations, or spinal subluxation.

## Pathophysiology

Primary spinal cord injury produces hemorrhage in the gray matter of the cord with edema of the white matter and ultimate necrosis of the neural tissue. The injury is from compression,

**BOX 53.24** | *Patient Teaching Guidelines for Rufinamide*

- Take the medication with food.
- Take the medication as prescribed.
- Do not stop taking the medication abruptly.
- Use two types of contraceptives if you are of childbearing age and are sexually active.

stretch, and shearing associated with spinal fracture or dislocation. An injury to the cord producing penetration of the cord is from laceration or a tear of the cord. The secondary spinal cord injury follows the primary injury with further tissue destruction and progressive damage of neurologic tissue.

## Clinical Manifestations

The clinical manifestations of a spinal cord injury are the result of the type and level of the injury. The level of the spinal cord injury produces greater loss of function and sensation. Clinical manifestations of complete spinal cord injury are irreversible with loss of autonomic, neural, and motor function. Incomplete spinal cord injuries vary in the severity of neurologic loss according the severity of the damage. Changes in the autonomic nervous system affect temperature regulation, bowel and bladder function, and hypotension.

## Drug Therapy

All skeletal muscle relaxants except dantrolene are centrally acting drugs. Pharmacologic action is usually attributed to general depression of the CNS but may involve blockage of nerve impulses that cause increased muscle tone and contraction. It is unclear whether relief of pain results from muscle relaxation or sedative effects. In addition, although parenteral administration of some drugs (e.g., diazepam, methocarbamol) relieves pain associated with acute musculoskeletal trauma or inflammation, it is uncertain whether oral administration of usual doses exerts a beneficial effect in acute or chronic disorders.

Baclofen and diazepam increase the effects of GABA, an inhibitory neurotransmitter. Tizanidine inhibits motor neurons in the brain. Dantrolene is the only skeletal muscle relaxant that acts peripherally on the muscle itself; it inhibits the release of calcium in skeletal muscle cells, thereby decreasing the strength of muscle contraction.

Table 53.8 summarizes the drug classes of skeletal muscle reactants, naming the prototype drug.

### TABLE 53.8

### Drugs Administered for the Treatment of Spasticity and to Relax Skeletal Muscles

| Drug Class | Prototype | Other Drugs in the Class |
|---|---|---|
| Carbamate derivatives | Carisoprodol (Soma) | |
| GABA derivatives | Baclofen (Gablofen, Lioresal) | |
| Direct-acting skeletal muscle relaxant | Dantrolene sodium (Dantrium, Revonto, Ryanodex) | |
| Tricyclic antidepressant derivatives | Cyclobenzaprine hydrochloride (Amrix) | Chlorzoxazone (Lorzone) Orphenadrine Citrate |
| Imidazole derivatives | Tizanidine hydrochloride (Zanaflex) | |

**Clinical Application 53.4**

• Andrew is now a 20-year-old college student. While living in the dorm, he has not been consistently taking his antiepileptic medications. On his trip home for the holidays, he suffers a seizure and has an automobile accident that leaves him paralyzed. The site of the spinal cord injury is T12. This injury results in muscle spasticity. Why is muscle spasticity so severe with spinal cord injuries?

## DRUGS USED TO TREAT MUSCLE SPASMS AND SPASTICITY

### CARBAMATE DERIVATIVES

**Carisoprodol** (Soma) is a centrally acting skeletal muscle relaxant. It is chemically related to meprobamate, which inhibits multineuronal spinal reflexes.

## Pharmacokinetics

The onset of action of carisoprodol is 30 minutes, with a peak in 1 to 2 hours and a duration of 4 to 6 hours. The half-life is 8 hours. The drug is metabolized in the liver by the enzyme CYP2C19 and excreted in the urine. It crosses the placenta and is present in breast milk.

## Action

The action of carisoprodol is not known, but animal studies have shown that the drug inhibits interneuronal activity in the descending reticular formation and spinal cord. It does not act directly to relax the skeletal muscles.

## Use

Clinicians use carisoprodol in the relief of discomfort associated with acute painful musculoskeletal conditions in which relief was not attained by rest, physical therapy, or alternative measures. Table 53.9 gives route and dosage information for carisoprodol.

## Adverse Effects

CNS adverse effects of carisoprodol include dizziness, drowsiness, vertigo, ataxia, tremor, agitation, and irritability. Initially, after the first, second, third, or fourth dose, patients may exhibit an allergic or idiosyncratic reaction with rash, erythema multiforme, pruritus, eosinophilia, hypotension, bronchospasm, vision and speech alterations, and the most severe adverse effect, anaphylactoid shock.

## Contraindications

Contraindications to carisoprodol include an allergic response to the drug or acute intermittent porphyria. Other contraindications are pregnancy and lactation.

**TABLE 53.9**

## DRUGS AT A GLANCE: Drugs Used to Relax Skeletal Muscles

| Drug | Pregnancy Category | Routes and Dosage Ranges | |
|---|---|---|---|
| | | **Adult** | **Children** |
| **P Carisoprodol** (Soma) | C | 12 y and older, 250–350 mg PO three times daily for maximum of 2–3 wk, with last dose at bedtime<br>Geriatric patients and patients with renal or hepatic impairment: reduce dose and monitor closely | Not recommended for children younger than 12 y |
| **P Baclofen** (Gablofen, Lioresal, Ozobax; ✽ AP-Baclofen, Dom-Baclofen, Lioresal, Lioresal Intrathecal, Mylan-Baclofen, Baclofen 10 or 20) | C | Start at a low dosage and increase gradually until optimum effect is achieved (40–80 mg/d); 5 mg PO for 3 d; 10 mg three times daily for 3 d; 15 mg three times daily for 3 d; 20 mg three times daily for 3 d; may increase to a maximum of 80 mg/d (20 mg four times daily)<br>Intrathecal, refer to manufacturer's instructions; testing is usually done with 50 mcg/mL injected into intrathecal space over 1 min; patient is observed for 4–8 h, and then a dose of 75 mcg/1.5 mL is given and patient is observed for another 4–8 h; a final screening bolus of 100 mcg/2 mL is given 24 h later if response is still not adequate. Patients who do not respond to this dose are not candidates for the implant.<br>Maintenance dose: 22–1400 mcg/d (smallest dose to achieve muscle tone without adverse effects) | Safety in children younger than 12 y of age has not been established; orphan drug use to decrease spasticity in children with cerebral palsy is being studied |
| **P Dantrolene sodium** (Dantrium, Revonto, Ryanodex; ✽ Dantrium) | C | Chronic spasticity: establish therapeutic goal before initiating therapy; titrate and individualize dosage, increasing until maximum performance is compatible to relieve dysfunction; initially 25 mg daily; increase to 25 mg three times daily for 7 d; then to 50 mg three times daily, and, if necessary, to 100 mg three times daily; most patients respond to 400 mg/d or less; maintain each dosage level for 4–7 d to evaluate response; discontinue after 45 d if benefits are not evident<br>Preoperative prophylaxis of malignant hyperthermia: 4–8 mg/kg/d PO in 3–4 divided doses for 1–2 d prior to surgery; give the last dose 3–4 h before scheduled surgery with minimum amount of water; adjust dose to prevent incapacitation due to drowsiness and excessive GI irritation<br>Postcrisis follow-up: 4–8 mg/kg/d PO in 4 divided doses for 1–3 d to prevent recurrence<br>Parenteral administration for malignant hyperthermia: discontinue all anesthetics as soon as problem is recognized; give dantrolene by continuous rapid IV push beginning at minimum dose of 1 mg/kg and continuing until symptoms subside or maximum cumulative dose of 10 mg/kg has been given; if physiologic and metabolic abnormalities reappear, repeat regimen; give continuously until symptoms subside<br>Preoperative prophylaxis of malignant hyperthermia: 2.5 mg/kg IV 1 h before surgery infused over 1 h | Safety for children <5 y has not been established<br>Chronic spasticity: initially 0.5 mg/kg once daily for 7 d, followed by 0.5 mg/kg three times daily for 7 d; then 1 mg/kg three times daily for 7 d; then 2 mg/kg three times daily if necessary; do not exceed 100 mg four times daily |

*(Continued on page 1068)*

**TABLE 53.9**

## DRUGS AT A GLANCE: Drugs Used to Relax Skeletal Muscles (Continued)

| Drug | Pregnancy Category | Routes and Dosage Ranges | |
|---|---|---|---|
| | | **Adult** | **Children** |
| P **Cyclobenzaprine hydrochloride** (Amrix, Fexmid; 🍁 Apo-Cyclobenzaprine, Auro-Cyclobenzaprine, Dom-Cyclobenzaprine, JAMP-Cyclobenzaprine, Mylan-Cyclobenzaprine) | B | 5 mg PO three times daily up to 10 mg PO three times daily, not to exceed 60 mg/d; do not use longer than 2–3 wk; extended-release capsules: 15 mg daily; some patients may require 30 mg/d | Safety and efficacy not established in children younger than 15 y |
| Chlorzoxazone (Lorzone) | Animal reproductive studies have not been conducted | 250–500 mg PO three times per day | 20 mg/kg/d PO in 3–4 divided doses |
| Orphenadrine citrate | Animal reproductive studies have not been conducted | 100 mg PO two times per day 60 mg IV or IM every 12 h | Safety and efficacy not established in children |
| P **Tizanidine hydrochloride** (Zanaflex; 🍁 Gen-Tizanidine, Pal-Tizanidine) | C | 4 mg PO daily, increased in 2–4 mg increments as needed over 2–4 wk; usual maintenance dose, 8 mg PO every 6–8 h; maximum dose, 36 mg/d in divided doses; reduce dose in patients with renal impairment | Safety and efficacy not established |

## Nursing Implications

### Preventing Interactions

CNS system depressants and alcohol combined with carisoprodol increase CNS depression.

### Administering the Medication

The nurse administers carisoprodol with food to prevent GI upset, giving the last dose of medication at bedtime. It is necessary to store the mediation in a container with a tight-fitting lid.

### Assessing for Therapeutic Effects

The nurse assesses the musculoskeletal area for relief of pain and spasms associated with the musculoskeletal injury.

### Assessing for Adverse Effects

The nurse assesses the integumentary system for signs and symptoms of an idiosyncratic reaction after the fourth to fifth doses of carisoprodol. It is also important to observe for visual changes, speech difficulties, bronchospasm, hypotension, and anaphylaxis. Carisoprodol is habit forming and should not be stopped abruptly. Abrupt withdrawal results in headache, nausea, insomnia, and abdominal cramping.

### Patient Teaching

Box 53.25 identifies patient teaching guidelines for carisoprodol.

## GAMMA-AMINOBUTYRIC ACID DERIVATIVES

The GABA derivative P **Baclofen** (Gablofen, Lioresal) is an agonist-specific inhibitor to GABA_B receptors located in the spinal cord. It restricts the influx of calcium to reduce the presynaptic neurotransmitter release in the excitatory spinal pathways.

## Pharmacokinetics

Oral baclofen begins to act in 1 hour, peaks in 2 hours, and lasts 4 to 8 hours. It is metabolized in the liver and excreted in urine; its half-life is 3 to 4 hours. Intrathecal baclofen has an onset of action of 30 to 60 minutes, peaks in 4 hours, and, like oral baclofen, has a duration of action of 4 to 8 hours. The drug crosses the placenta and enters the breast milk.

## Action

The exact mechanism of action of baclofen is unknown. It appears to reduce impulse transmissions from the spinal cord to the skeletal muscle, thus decreasing muscle spasms.

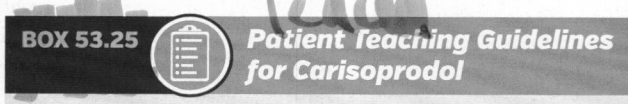

**BOX 53.25** *Patient Teaching Guidelines for Carisoprodol*

- Do not operate machinery with central nervous system [CNS] depression.
- Do not combine with other CNS depressants or alcohol.
- Take the medication with food.
- Do not combine with over-the-counter cold remedies without approval from the prescriber.
- Do not stop the medication abruptly.
- Know the idiosyncratic effects of the drug and how to maintain safety when CNS effects are evident.
- Report signs and symptoms of idiosyncratic adverse effects.

## Use

Clinicians use baclofen to alleviate signs and symptoms of spasticity in patients with multiple sclerosis. It is particularly effective against flexor spasms, concomitant pain, and muscular rigidity. Other indications include the treatment of spinal cord injuries and other diseases of the spinal cord. Table 53.9 gives route and dosage information for baclofen.

### Use in Older Adults

Older adults who take baclofen require close monitoring. Dosage reduction to prevent excessive CNS depression may be necessary.

### Use in Patients With Renal Impairment

Dosage reduction is necessary in patients with renal impairment.

## Adverse Effects and Contraindications

The most common adverse effects of baclofen are transient drowsiness, dizziness, weakness, fatigue, confusion, headache, insomnia, hypotension, and urinary frequency. Elevated blood sugar may occur, requiring the administration of an oral hypoglycemic agent.

Contraindications include known hypersensitivity to the drug and skeletal muscle spasms resulting from rheumatic disorders.

## Nursing Implications

### Preventing Interactions

When baclofen is combined with alcohol or other CNS depressants, patients experience increased CNS depression.

### Administering the Medication

Administration of baclofen is oral or intrathecal. The nurse starts with a low dose that he or she increases slowly, using the smallest dose possible to achieve muscle tone without adverse effects. If the benefits of the medication are not evident during a trial period, then the medication is withdrawn gradually.

Intrathecal administration involves an implantable pump. It is best to consult the manufacturer's literature concerning the pump instructions and initiation of long-term infusions.

### Assessing for Therapeutic Effects

The nurse assesses the affected musculoskeletal region for decrease in symptoms of spasticity.

### Assessing for Adverse Effects

It is important to assess the degree of CNS depression. The nurse assesses the patient's blood pressure for hypotension, particularly with position changes. Genitourinary assessments include the patient's level of urinary frequency and dysuria. Other adverse effects noted are weight gain, increased aspartate aminotransferase, blood sugar, and alkaline phosphatase.

### Patient Teaching

Box 53.26 identifies patient teaching guidelines for baclofen.

**BOX 53.26** | *Patient Teaching Guidelines for Baclofen*

- Do not stop taking the drug abruptly; abrupt discontinuation may cause hallucinations or other serious side effects.
- Avoid alcohol and other central nervous system depressants.
- Do not take if you are pregnant or breast-feeding.
- Do not operate machinery.
- Report painful or frequent urination, constipation, headache, insomnia, or confusion.

### Clinical Application 53.5

- Andrew is receiving baclofen (Lioresal) to treat the spasticity. He and his parents are to receive instruction about the administration of intrathecal baclofen. What aspects of the medication administration does the nurse teach?
- His parents ask the nurse why he is taking baclofen (Lioresal) and not diazepam (Valium), which he has taken in the past. What is the best response to this question?

## NCLEX Success

11. A nurse administers a peripherally acting muscle relaxant to a patient with a spinal cord injury. Which of the following drugs does the nurse administer?
    A. dantrolene
    B. baclofen
    C. methocarbamol
    D. diazepam

12. A patient is taking carisoprodol for back spasms related to an occupational injury. Which of the following is most important to teach the patient?
    A. to take the medication at 8:00 AM, 2:00 PM, and 8:00 PM
    B. to know the signs and symptoms of an idiosyncratic reaction
    C. to take the medication between meals
    D. to stop the medication with the first sign of abdominal cramping

13. A nurse administers baclofen to a young man for a back injury. Which of the following interventions is most important related to the administration of baclofen?
    A. Assess heart rate.
    B. Assess for edema.
    C. Assess blood sugar.
    D. Assess for increased spasticity.

# DIRECT-ACTING SKELETAL MUSCLE RELAXANTS

**Ⓟ Dantrolene sodium** (Dantrium, Revonto, Ryanodex) is a drug administered for spasticity related to multiple sclerosis, cerebral palsy, spinal cord injury, and stroke.

## Pharmacokinetics

Oral dantrolene is absorbed by the GI tract, reaching a peak in 4 to 6 hours. The duration of action is 8 to 10 hours, and the half-life is 9 hours. IV dantrolene has a rapid onset of action with a peak in 5 hours, a duration of action of 6 to 8 hours, and a half-life of 4 to 8 hours. The drug is metabolized by the liver and excreted in the urine. Dantrolene crosses the placenta and enters the breast milk.

## Action

Dantrolene interferes with the release of calcium from the sarcoplasmic reticulum to relax skeletal muscle. It does not interfere with neuromuscular transmission or affect the surface membrane of the skeletal muscle.

## Use

*primary use*

Dantrolene controls spasticity caused by upper motor neuron disorders, such as spinal cord injury, cerebrovascular accident, cerebral palsy, and multiple sclerosis. Clinicians may use it to prevent and manage **malignant hyperthermia**, a rare but life-threatening complication of anesthesia characterized by hypercarbia, metabolic acidosis, skeletal muscle rigidity, fever, and cyanosis. Table 53.9 gives route and dosage information for dantrolene.

### Use in Older Adults

Aging increases the risk of liver damage as a result of the administration of dantrolene. Administration of dantrolene necessitates the close monitoring of liver enzyme levels.

### Use in Patients With Hepatic Impairment

It is important not to administer dantrolene to patients with active liver disease. The development of hepatocellular damage can be fatal. As in the elderly, close monitoring of liver enzymes is necessary.

## Adverse Effects

Common adverse effects of dantrolene include drowsiness, dizziness, diarrhea, and fatigue. The most serious adverse effect is potentially fatal hepatitis, with jaundice and other symptoms that usually occur within 1 month of starting drug therapy. Liver function tests should be monitored periodically in all patients receiving dantrolene. These adverse effects do not occur with short-term use of IV drug for malignant hyperthermia. The FDA has issued a **BLACK BOX WARNING ◆** stating that the patient should have liver function tests and that dantrolene be discontinued at the first indication of hepatic impairment.

## Contraindications

Contraindications to dantrolene include active liver disease. Other contraindications include spasticity used to maintain an upright position and balance with locomotion as well as spasticity from rheumatic conditions.

## Nursing Implications

### Preventing Interactions

The patient is at risk for hyperkalemia and myocardial depression if dantrolene is combined with verapamil.

### Administering the Medication

When administering dantrolene intravenously, the nurse monitors the injection sites and ensures that extravasation does not occur. Dantrolene is an alkaline agent that is irritating to the tissues.

When administering dantrolene orally, the nurse consults with other health care professionals to determine interventions that enhance mobility. Withdrawal of the oral medication should occur over 2 to 4 days. If diarrhea occurs, discontinuance of dantrolene is necessary.

If malignant hyperthermia develops, it is essential to discontinue all triggering drugs. In addition, the nurse assesses for metabolic acidosis and electrolyte imbalances. It may be necessary to use a cooling blanket.

### Assessing for Therapeutic Effects

The nurse assesses the patient's response to dantrolene. The patient should have a decrease in muscle spasticity that does not affect the ability to perform activities of daily living. The IV administration for the treatment of malignant hyperthermia results in a reverse of symptoms, including decreased temperature and fluid and electrolyte balance without signs and symptoms of metabolic acidosis.

### Assessing for Adverse Effects

It is necessary to check the patient's liver enzymes with the administration of oral dantrolene. The nurse assesses the patient for diarrhea, dizziness, and fatigue. Headache, anorexia, and nervousness are potentially serious adverse effects in people older than 35 years of age who have taken the drug for 60 days or longer. Women in this age group who take estrogens have the highest risk of developing these adverse effects. Hepatotoxicity can be prevented or minimized by administering the lowest effective dose, monitoring liver enzymes during therapy, and discontinuing the drug if no beneficial effects occur in 45 days.

### Patient Teaching

Box 53.27 identifies the patient teaching guidelines for dantrolene.

| BOX 53.27 |  | *Patient Teaching Guidelines for Dantrolene* |
|---|---|---|

- Do not alter positions when experiencing dizziness.
- Report gastrointestinal upset and eat small frequent meals.
- Avoid alcohol and other central nervous system depressants.
- Report severe diarrhea, headache, and anorexia.

# TRICYCLIC ANTIDEPRESSANT DERIVATIVES

Ⓟ **Cyclobenzaprine hydrochloride** (Flexeril) is a centrally acting skeletal muscle relaxant administered on a short-term basis for the relief of muscle spasm.

## Pharmacokinetics

Cyclobenzaprine is administered orally and is well absorbed by the GI tract. The onset of action is 1 hour, with a peak in 3 to 8 hours, and the duration of action is 12 to 24 hours. The half-life is 1 to 3 days. The drug is highly protein bound. It is metabolized in the liver to inactive metabolites and is excreted in the urine, with some eliminated in the feces. Cyclobenzaprine crosses the placenta and is excreted in the breast milk.

## Action

The mechanism of action of cyclobenzaprine is not known, but it appears to produce relaxation by acting at the brainstem and spinal cord to depress motor activity.

## Use

Clinicians use cyclobenzaprine as an adjunctive to other measures such as physical therapy to relieve muscle spasm. Table 53.9 gives route and dosage information for cyclobenzaprine.

### Use in Older Adults

Conventional 5-mg tablets are used in older adults, with the dosage adjusted slowly upward. Use of extended-release capsules is not recommended.

### Use in Patients With Hepatic Impairment

The same recommendations for older adults apply to patients with hepatic impairment.

## Adverse Effects and Contraindications

Common adverse effects of cyclobenzaprine are drowsiness, dizziness, and anticholinergic effects (e.g., dry mouth, constipation, urinary retention, tachycardia). *like sympathic*

Contraindications include known hypersensitivity to the drug. Other contraindications include acute myocardial infarction, dysrhythmia, heart block, conduction disturbances, heart failure, and hyperthyroidism. Caution is necessary with urinary retention, increased intraocular pressure, and mild hepatic impairment.

## Nursing Implications

### Preventing Interactions

Increased CNS depression occurs when cyclobenzaprine is combined with alcohol or other CNS depressants.

### Administering the Medication

Because of the risk of inconsistent doses, the nurse does not split the generic 10-mg tablets when administering cyclobenzaprine. He or she administers extended-release capsules whole.

### Assessing for Therapeutic and Adverse Effects

The nurse assesses the patient's response to the medication, which should indicate relief of the skeletal muscle spasm, decreased pain, and increased activity.

---

**BOX 53.28** 📋 *Patient Teaching Guidelines for Cyclobenzaprine*

- Avoid alcohol and other central nervous system (CNS) depressants.
- Do not operate machinery with CNS depression.
- Report effectiveness of therapy to prescriber.

---

The nurse assesses for increased CNS depression, which will place the patient at risk for falls and injury. It is necessary to assess the patient's cardiovascular status, including pulse and blood pressure. The medication places the patient at risk for hypotension. Anticholinergic effects occur. The nurse assesses the patient for urinary retention.

### Patient Teaching

Box 53.28 identifies patient teaching guidelines for cyclobenzaprine.

## Other Drugs in the Class

Chlorzoxazone is a centrally acting skeletal muscle relaxant used to treat muscle spasms and pain associated with musculoskeletal conditions. It should be administered cautiously in patients with drug allergies, CNS depression, and altered liver and renal function. Chlorzoxazone should be administered with food to prevent gastric upset. Do not combine with alcohol or CNS depressants. Assess the patient for injury due to CNS depression. Monitor the patient's liver function tests. Instruct the patient the medication may discolor urine orange or purple/red.

Orphenadrine citrate is also a centrally acting skeletal muscle relaxant that has tertiary amine anticholinergic effects. It is contraindicated in narrow angle glaucoma, duodenal obstruction, prostatic hypertrophy, and bladder neck obstruction. Use cautiously in older adults due to urinary hesitancy or retention.

---

## NCLEX Success

14. An 18-year-old man is having an open reduction external fixation of a hip following a football injury. During surgery, he develops a fever of 105°F. Which of the following medications is administered?

    A. cyclobenzaprine hydrochloride
    B. dexamethasone sodium phosphate
    C. phenytoin
    D. dantrolene sodium

15. Which of the following interventions assists the patient in decreasing the anticholinergic effects of cyclobenzaprine?

    A. Have the patient void before the administration of cyclobenzaprine.
    B. Give the patient lemon juice mixed with warm water to prevent constipation.
    C. Give the patient hard candy to suck on.
    D. Assess the patient's pulse and blood pressure.

# IMIDAZOLINE DERIVATIVES

**P** **Tizanidine hydrochloride** (Zanaflex) is a centrally acting alpha$_2$-adrenergic agonist administered for acute and intermittent management of increased muscle tone with spasticity.

## Pharmacokinetics

Tizanidine is absorbed rapidly in the GI tract. The medication has an onset of action in 30 to 60 minutes, peak in 1 to 2 hours, and duration of action in 3 to 6 hours. It is metabolized by the liver with a 2.7- to 4.2-hour half-life, and the drug is excreted in the urine. Tizanidine crosses the placenta and enters the breast milk.

## Action

Tizanidine is a centrally acting alpha$_2$-adrenergic agonist that produces antispasmodic effect as a result of indirect depression of postsynaptic reflexes by blocking the excitatory actions of spinal interneurons.

## Use

Clinicians use tizanidine as indicated for use in patients who have acute and intermittent management of increased muscle tone associated with spasticity. Table 53.9 gives route and dosage information for tizanidine.

## Adverse Effects and Contraindications

Common adverse effects of tizanidine include drowsiness, dizziness, constipation, dry mouth, and hypotension. Hypotension may be significant and occur at usual doses. The drug may also cause psychotic symptoms, including hallucinations.

Contraindications include hypersensitivity to the medication. Other contraindications include use of fluvoxamine and ciprofloxacin.

# Nursing Implications

## Preventing Interactions

The administration of alcohol, baclofen, or CNS depressants with tizanidine can increase the patient's susceptibility to symptoms of depression. Hormonal contraceptives may increase the plasma concentration of tizanidine. Administration with other alpha$_2$ agonists may have hypotensive effects. Kava and valerian may decrease the effect of the drug.

## Administering the Medication

Patients may take tizanidine with or without food. However, consistent administration of the drug assists in absorption of the drug and its effect.

## Assessing for Therapeutic and Adverse Effects

The nurse assesses the patient for a reduction of skeletal muscle spasms and decreased muscle tone.

The nurse assesses patients for somnolence, sedation, dizziness, and hallucinations. He or she also assesses the cardiovascular patient's status for bradycardia and hypotension. In addition, it is necessary to assess the patient's liver and renal function.

## Patient Teaching

Box 53.29 identifies patient teaching guidelines for tizanidine.

---

**BOX 53.29**  **Patient Teaching Guidelines for Tizanidine**

- Do not alter positions when experiencing dizziness.
- Do not operate machinery.
- Report unusual sensory effects such as hallucinations or delusions.

---

## THE NURSING PROCESS

A concept map outlines the nursing process related to drug therapy considerations in this chapter. Additional nursing implications related to the disease process should also be considered in care decisions.

**Assessment**

- Assess the patient status in relation to seizure activity and other factors.
  - Interview the patient about the seizure disorder and AEDs.
    - How long has the patient had the seizure disorder, and when was the last seizure?
    - What is the frequency of the seizures, and will something precipitate its development?
    - How does the seizure affect the patient (loss of consciousness, body part or parts affected, drowsiness after the seizure)?
    - What AEDs are prescribed, and what effect do they produce?
    - Does the patient take the AEDs as prescribed? What other medications have been prescribed?
    - What is the patient's attitude toward the seizure disorder?
  - Assess serum levels of AEDs.
  - Identify risk factors for seizure disorders (previous seizure activity, brain surgery, head injury, hypoxia, hypoglycemia, drug overdosage, withdrawal of AEDs or CNS depressants).
  - Observe and document seizure activity accurately; location (localized or general); and specific characteristics of abnormal movements or behavior, duration, and concomitant events (loss of consciousness, incontinence, and postseizure behavior).
  - Assess for risk of status epilepticus (recent changes in AED therapy, chronic alcohol ingestion, use of drugs known to cause seizures, and infection).

## THE NURSING PROCESS (Continued)

**Outcomes of Therapy**

The patient will
- Take the medication as prescribed, and do not discontinue abruptly.
- Experience control of seizures, and avoid serious adverse effects.
- Verbalize knowledge of the disease process and treatment regimen.
- Keep follow-up appointments with the primary care provider.

**Nursing Interventions**

- Assist the patient in identifying the conditions under which seizures are likely to occur. Precipitating factors may include ingestion of alcoholic beverages or stimulant drugs; fever; severe physical or emotional stress; and sensory stimuli, such as flashing lights and loud noises. Identifying lifestyle changes (e.g., reducing stress, reducing alcohol and caffeine intake, increasing exercise, improving sleep, and diet) and treating existing disorders can reduce the frequency of seizures.
- Discuss the seizure disorder, the plan of treatment, and the importance of adhering to prescribed drug therapy with the patient and family members.
- Involve the patient in decision making when possible.
- Inform the patient and family that seizure control is not gained immediately when drug therapy is started.
- Protect the patient experiencing a generalized tonic–clonic seizure by
  - Placing a small pillow or piece of clothing under the head to prevent injury from the ground or floor. Never restrain the patient's movements; fractures may result.
  - Loosening tight clothing, especially around the neck and chest, to promote respirations.
  - Turning the patient to one side so that accumulating secretions can drain from the mouth and throat when paroxysms stop. Most of these seizures subside within 3 to 4 minutes, and the patient starts responding and regaining normal skin color. If the patient has one seizure after another (status epilepticus), has trouble breathing or continued cyanosis, or has sustained an injury, further care is needed, and a physician should be notified immediately.
- If an aura or smell is noted prior to the onset of seizure, be sure the patient notifies a nurse.

**Evaluation**

- Interview and observe for decrease in or absence of seizure activity.
- Interview and observe for avoidance of adverse drug effects, especially those that impair safety.
- When available, check laboratory reports of serum drug levels for the therapeutic ranges or evidence of underdosing or overdosing.

## KEY CONCEPTS

- Seizures are idiopathic or secondary (caused by tumors, metabolic disorders, overdoses of numerous drugs, or withdrawal of alcohol or sedative–hypnotic drugs).
- When seizures occur in a chronic, recurrent pattern, they characterize a disorder known as epilepsy, which usually requires long-term drug therapy.
- Types of seizures include generalized (generalized tonic–clonic seizures) and partial (simple or complex, depending on whether consciousness is altered).
- Status epilepticus is a life-threatening emergency that may result in hypotension, hypoxia, cardiac dysrhythmias, permanent brain damage, and death unless prompt, appropriate treatment is instituted.
- The FDA has issued a **BLACK BOX WARNING** ◆ for phenobarbital. Patients who take phenobarbital are at risk for suicidal ideation. It is important to monitor the patient for statements that indicate depression and suicide.

- The FDA issued a **BLACK BOX WARNING** ◆ for diazepam. The combination of benzodiazepines and opioid medications depresses the CNS, resulting in serious adverse effects, including respiratory depression or death.
- The FDA has issued a **BLACK BOX WARNING** ◆ for diazepam. The combination of any benzodiazepine and an opioid medication depresses the CNS, resulting in serious adverse effects, including respiratory depression or death.
- The **BLACK BOX WARNING** ◆ for vigabatrin warns that it can cause permanent bilateral concentric visual field constriction.
- Side effect profiles vary with individual AEDs; potential teratogenic adverse effects, drug interactions, hypersensitivity reactions, and blood dyscrasias have been reported.
- The FDA has issued several **BLACK BOX WARNING** ◆ for valproate. The first instructs patients to discontinue valproate at any sign of pancreatitis; the development of this condition

is life threatening. The second points out that valproate is a teratogenic medication. The third instructs the patient to check for signs of bleeding or bruising. Altered bleeding times may occur.

- The FDA has issued a **BLACK BOX WARNING** ◆ for carbamazepine concerning aplastic anemia and agranulocytosis.
- Newer AEDs have better adverse effect profiles with enhanced seizure control and are classified as derivatives.
- The FDA has issued a **BLACK BOX WARNING** ◆ related to the potential development of serious dermatologic reactions with lamotrigine. Because a serious skin rash may occur, especially in children, lamotrigine should be administered cautiously to children younger than 16 years of age and should be discontinued at the first sign of skin rash in an adult.
- Monotherapy should guide initial management of seizure disorders.
- When an AED is being discontinued, its dosage should always be tapered gradually, usually over 1 to 3 months.

Abruptly stopping an AED may exacerbate seizures or cause status epilepticus.

- Monitoring of serum drug levels is useful for most AEDs and must be interpreted in relation to clinical responses.
- Muscle spasms usually result from trauma to the affected skeletal muscle.
- Spasticity results from damage to nerves in the brain and spinal cord.
- Both muscle spasms and spasticity can cause pain and disability.
- Physical therapy and other nonpharmacologic treatments are useful in treating muscle spasm and spasticity.
- Most muscle relaxant drugs are CNS depressants; only dantrolene acts on the muscle.
- The FDA has issued a **BLACK BOX WARNING** ◆ stating that the patient should have liver function tests and that dantrolene be discontinued at the first indication of hepatic impairment.

## CLINICAL REASONING CASE STUDY

**Meet the Patient**

Gene Hamerlink is a 57-year-old man who is status post-craniotomy for brain cancer. He has received a diagnosis of glioblastoma and has a seizure disorder as a result of the brain tumor. He takes lamotrigine (Lamictal) 250 mg PO twice daily and levetiracetam (Keppra XR) 3000 mg once daily. When giving his history, he states that he smells a scent similar to ammonia prior to experiencing a seizure.

- What is the action of lamotrigine?
- What is the action of levetiracetam?
- What are the adverse effects of lamotrigine?
- What are the adverse effects of levetiracetam?
- What patient teaching should the nurse provide to Mr. Hamerlink regarding his medications?
- What should the nurse teach him about the adverse effects of each medication?

**Assessing Drug Information**

- Lamotrigine is thought to reduce the release of glutamate, which is an excitatory transmitter in the brain. The neurotransmitter is sensitive to sodium channels, thus decreasing seizure activity.
- Levetiracetam is chemically unrelated to other AEDs, and its mechanism of action is unknown. It inhibits abnormal neuronal firing but does not affect normal neuronal excitability or function.
- The most significant adverse effect of lamotrigine is the potential development of serious dermatologic reactions, and a severe rash may occur leading to Stevens-Johnson syndrome or toxic epidermal necrosis. Other adverse effects of lamotrigine include dizziness, drowsiness, headache, ataxia, blurred or double vision, nausea and vomiting, and weakness.
- Common adverse effects of levetiracetam include drowsiness, dizziness, and fatigue. Other effects include decreases in red and white blood cell counts, double vision, amnesia, anxiety, ataxia, emotional lability, hostility, nervousness, paresthesia, pharyngitis, and rhinitis. Postmarketing research has shown that a risk of hepatic failure, acute renal failure, and multiorgan failure is possible. There is also a risk for the development of Stevens-Johnson syndrome.

**Nursing Actions**

- Educate Mr. Hamerlink about all adverse effects of lamotrigine and levetiracetam. Be sure both he and his family are aware of the adverse effect of Stevens-Johnson syndrome.
- Make sure he understands that at the first sign of a rash or any type of skin eruption, he should notify his prescriber.
- Tell him to have frequent eye examinations and to notify the prescriber about any ocular changes.
- Educate him about the administration of his extended-release medication. Make sure he understands that it should not be chewed or crushed.
- Stress that he should not stop his medication abruptly.
- Teach him to not operate machinery because of central nervous system depression.

*Visit* the Point® *at* **http://thePoint.lww.com/Frandsen12e** *for answers to NCLEX Success questions (in Appendix A), answers to Clinical Application Case Studies (in Appendix B), and more!*

## REFERENCES AND RESOURCES

Abrams, G. M., & Wakasa, M. (2020). Chronic complications of spinal cord injury and disease. In *UpToDate*. Lexi-Comp, Inc.

Hinkle, J. H., & Cheever, K. H. (2018). *Brunner & Suddarth's textbook of medical-surgical nursing* (14th ed.). Philadelphia: Wolters Kluwer.

Kuhn, M. A., & Winston, D. (2008). *Herbal therapy supplements a scientific and traditional approach* (2nd ed.). Philadelphia: Lippincott Williams & Wilkins.

Lima-Rogel, V., Lopez-Lopez, E. J., Medllin-Garibay, S. E., Gomez-Ruiz, L. M., Romero-Mendex, C., Milan-Segovia, R. C., et al. (2018). Population pharmacokinetics of levetiracetam in neonates with seizures. *Journal of Clinical Pharmacy and Therapeutics, 43*, 422–429. doi:10.1111/jcpt.12658

Norris, T. L. (2019). *Porth's pathophysiology concepts of altered health states* (10th ed.). Philadelphia: Wolters Kluwer.

*Nursing 2020 drug handbook*. (2020). Philadelphia: Lippincott William & Wilkins.

Schachter, S. (2020). Antiseizure drugs: Mechanism of action, pharmacology, and adverse effects. In *UpToDate*. Lexi-Comp, Inc.

Senadim, S., Baslo, S. A., Guveli, B. T., Sari, H., & Atakli, D. (2018) Safety and efficacy of zonisamide in refractory epilepsy patients: clinical experience from a tertiary center. *Epilepsi: Journal of the Turkish Epilepsi Society, 24*(1), 27–32.

UpToDate. (2020). *Drug information*. Lexi-Comp, Inc.

# Drug Therapy for Anxiety and Insomnia

## LEARNING OBJECTIVES

*After studying this chapter, you should be able to:*

1. Discuss the pathophysiology and clinical manifestations of anxiety.
2. Discuss the pathophysiology and clinical manifestations of sleep and insomnia.
3. Identify the prototype and describe the action, use, adverse effects, contraindications, and nursing implications for the benzodiazepines.
4. Discuss the various nonbenzodiazepines used to reduce anxiety and produce hypnosis in terms of their action, use, contraindications, adverse effects, and nursing implications.
5. Implement the nursing process in the care of the patient being treated for anxiety and insomnia.

## CLINICAL APPLICATION CASE STUDY

Lorraine Terrence, an 83-year-old widow who has lived alone since her husband died 6 months ago, is in the early stages of Alzheimer's disease. She has a history of cardio-vascular disease and hypertension and has been admitted to the local hospital for observation after complaints of chest pain. At present, she is very anxious and agitated. The admitting nurse received a telephone call from Mrs. Terrence's daughter, who lives out of town. The daughter states that her mother has experienced anxiety and depression for many years and her symptoms have worsened since her father died. The daughter does not know what medications her mother currently takes, and she is concerned that her mother lives alone and wants her to move to a nursing home. The provider orders the following medications: alprazolam for anxiety, citalopram for depression, and zolpidem for sleep.

## KEY TERMS

**Anterograde amnesia:** short-term memory loss

**Anxiety:** common disorder that may be referred to as nervousness, tension, worry, or other terms that denote an unpleasant feeling

**Anxiety disorder:** severe anxiety that is prolonged and impairs the ability to function in usual activities of daily living

**Anxiolytics:** antianxiety drugs

**Hypnotics:** drugs that produce sleep

**Insomnia:** prolongs difficulty in going to sleep or staying asleep long enough to feel rested

**Sedatives:** drugs that promote relaxation and ease agitation

# INTRODUCTION

This chapter introduces the pharmacologic care of the patient who is experiencing anxiety and/or insomnia. Antianxiety and sedative–hypnotic drugs are central nervous system (CNS) depressants that have similar effects. **Anxiolytics** are antianxiety drugs, **sedatives** promote relaxation and ease agitation, and **hypnotics** produce sleep. The difference between the effects depends largely on dosage. Large doses of antianxiety and sedative drugs produce sleep, and small doses of hypnotics have anxiolytic or sedative effects. Also, therapeutic doses of hypnotics taken at bedtime may have residual sedative effects ("morning hangover") the following day. Because these drugs produce varying degrees of CNS depression, some are also used as anticonvulsants and anesthetics.

# OVERVIEW OF ANXIETY

To promote understanding of the uses and effects of both benzodiazepines and nonbenzodiazepines, anxiety and insomnia are described in the following sections. The clinical manifestations of these disorders are similar and overlapping; that is, daytime anxiety may be manifested as nighttime difficulty in sleeping because the person cannot "turn off" worries, and difficulty in sleeping may be manifested as anxiety, fatigue, and decreased ability to function during usual waking hours. Many individuals with an anxiety disorder often go unidentified and untreated.

## Etiology

**Anxiety** is a common disorder that may be referred to as nervousness, tension, worry, or other terms that denote an unpleasant feeling. It occurs when a person perceives a situation as threatening to physical, emotional, social, or economic well-being. Anxiety may occur in association with everyday events related to home, work, school, social activities, and chronic illness, or it may occur episodically, in association with acute illness, death, divorce, losing a job, starting a new job, or taking a test. Situational anxiety is a normal response to a stressful situation. It may be beneficial when it motivates the person toward constructive, problem-solving, coping activities. Symptoms may be quite severe, but they usually last only 2 to 3 weeks.

Although there is no clear boundary between normal and abnormal anxiety, when anxiety is severe or prolonged and impairs the ability to function in usual activities of daily living, it is called an **anxiety disorder**. The American Psychiatric Association (2013) delineates anxiety disorders as medical diagnoses in the *Diagnostic and Statistical Manual of Mental Disorders, 5th edition (DSM-5)*, the universal authority for psychiatric diagnoses. There are several types of anxiety disorders, as described in Box 54.1. Although the *DSM-5* has reclassified posttraumatic stress disorder (PTSD) as a trauma and stress-related disorder and not an anxiety disorder, the condition is included in this chapter because of mutual clinical manifestations, drug therapy, and nursing considerations. Generalized anxiety disorder (GAD) is emphasized in this chapter.

**Concept Mastery Alert**

Anxiety disorders have distinctive characteristics, but all involve an excessive and irrational fear and dread. Some patients, but not all, experience physiologic symptoms, lack insight into their worrying, or have difficulty identifying the source and trigger for their anxiety.

## Pathophysiology

The pathophysiology of anxiety disorders is unknown, but there is evidence of a biologic basis and possible imbalances among several neurotransmission systems. A simplistic view involves an excess of excitatory neurotransmitters (e.g., norepinephrine) or a deficiency of inhibitory neurotransmitters (e.g., gamma-aminobutyric acid [GABA]).

The noradrenergic system is associated with the hyperarousal state experienced by patients with anxiety (i.e., feelings of panic, restlessness, tremulousness, palpitations, hyperventilation), which is attributed to excessive norepinephrine. Norepinephrine is released from the locus coeruleus (LC) in response to an actual or a perceived threat. The LC is a brainstem nucleus that contains many noradrenergic neurons and has extensive projections to the limbic system, cerebral cortex, and cerebellum. Certain observations lend support to the role of the noradrenergic system in anxiety. Drugs that stimulate activity in the LC (e.g., caffeine) may cause symptoms of anxiety, and drugs used to treat anxiety (e.g., benzodiazepines) decrease neuronal firing and norepinephrine release in the LC.

Neuroendocrine factors also play a role in anxiety disorders. Perceived threat or stress activates the hypothalamic–pituitary–adrenal axis and corticotropin-releasing factor (CRF), one of its components. CRF activates the LC, which then releases norepinephrine and generates anxiety. Overall, authorities consider CRF important in integrating the endocrine, autonomic, and behavioral responses to stress.

GABA is the major inhibitory neurotransmitter in the brain and spinal cord. Gamma-aminobutyric acid$_A$ (GABA$_A$) receptors are attached to chloride channels in nerve cell membranes. When GABA interacts with GABA$_A$ receptors, chloride channels open, chloride ions move into the neuron, and the nerve cell is less able to be excited (i.e., generate an electrical impulse).

The serotonin system, although not as well understood, also may play a role in anxiety. Both serotonin reuptake inhibitors and serotonin receptor agonists are now used to treat anxiety disorders. Research has suggested two possible roles for the serotonin receptor HT$_{1A}$. During embryonic development, stimulation of HT$_{1A}$ receptors by serotonin may contribute to the development of normal brain circuitry necessary for normal anxiety responses. However, during adulthood, some serotonin reuptake inhibitors act through HT$_{1A}$ receptors to reduce anxiety responses.

Additional causes of anxiety disorders include medical conditions (anxiety disorder due to a general medical condition according to the *DSM-5*), psychiatric disorders, and substance abuse. Almost all major psychiatric illnesses may be associated with symptoms of anxiety (e.g., dementia, major depression, mania, schizophrenia). Anxiety related to substance abuse is categorized in the *DSM-5* as substance-induced anxiety disorder (see Chap. 58).

**BOX 54.1** *Generalized Anxiety Disorder*

## Generalized Anxiety Disorder

Major diagnostic criteria for generalized anxiety disorder (GAD) include excessive and exaggerated anxiety and worry about everyday life circumstances and multiple symptoms for 6 months or more after elimination of disease processes or drugs as possible causes. The frequency, duration, or intensity of the worry is unrealistic or out of proportion to the actual situation. Symptoms are related to motor tension (e.g., muscle tension, restlessness, trembling, fatigue), overactivity of the autonomic nervous system (e.g., dyspnea, palpitations, tachycardia, sweating, dry mouth, dizziness, nausea, diarrhea), and increased vigilance (feeling fearful, nervous, or keyed up, difficulty concentrating, irritability, insomnia, being easily startled).

Symptoms of anxiety occur with many disease processes, including medical disorders (e.g., hyperthyroidism, cardiovascular disease, cancer) and psychiatric disorders (e.g., mood disorders, schizophrenia, substance use disorders). They also frequently occur with drugs that affect the CNS. With CNS stimulants (e.g., nasal decongestants, antiasthma drugs, nicotine, caffeine), symptoms occur with drug administration; with CNS depressants (e.g., alcohol, benzodiazepines), symptoms are more likely to occur when the drug is stopped, especially if stopped abruptly.

When the symptoms are secondary to medical illness, they may decrease as the illness improves. However, most people with GAD experience little relief when one stressful situation or problem is resolved. Instead, they quickly move on to another worry. Additional characteristics of GAD include its chronicity, although the severity of symptoms fluctuates over time; its frequent association with somatic symptoms (e.g., headache, gastrointestinal complaints, including irritable bowel syndrome); and its frequent coexistence with depression, other anxiety disorders, and substance abuse or dependence.

## Obsessive–Compulsive Disorders and Related Conditions

An obsession involves an uncontrollable desire to dwell on recurring, unwanted thoughts, ideas, or sensations; a compulsion involves repeated performance of some act to relieve the fear and anxiety associated with an obsession. Obsessive–compulsive disorder (OCD) is characterized by obsessions or compulsions that are severe enough to be time consuming (e.g., take more than an hour per day), cause major distress, or impair the person's ability to function in usual activities or relationships. The compulsive behavior provides some relief from anxiety but is not pleasurable. Many people recognize that the obsessions or compulsions are not true; others may think that their obsessions could be true (known as poor insight). Even if people know their obsessions are not true, people have a hard time keeping their focus off the obsessions or stopping the compulsive actions. When patients resist or are prevented from performing the compulsive behavior, they experience increasing anxiety and often abuse alcohol or antianxiety, sedative-type drugs in the attempt to relieve anxiety.

## Panic Disorder

Panic disorder involves acute, sudden, and recurrent attacks of anxiety, with feelings of intense fear, terror, or impending doom. It may be accompanied by such symptoms as palpitations, sweating, trembling, shortness of breath or a feeling of smothering, chest pain, nausea, or dizziness. Symptoms usu-

ally build to a peak over about 10 minutes and may require medication to be relieved. Afterward, the person usually lives in fear of another attack and may avoid places where an attack has occurred. For some people, the fear takes over their lives, and they cannot leave their homes.

A significant number (50%–65%) of patients with panic disorder are thought to also have major depression. In addition, some patients with panic disorder also develop agoraphobia, a fear of having a panic attack in a place or situation where one cannot escape or get help. Combined panic disorder and agoraphobia often involves a chronic, relapsing pattern of significant functional impairment and may require lifetime treatment.

## Posttraumatic Stress Disorder

Posttraumatic stress disorder (PTSD) is a trauma- and stress-related disorder that associates the condition with highly stressful events that may involve actual or threatened death or serious injury (e.g., natural disasters, military combat, violent acts such as rape or murder, explosions or bombings, serious automobile accidents). The person responds to such an event with thoughts and feelings of intense fear, helplessness, or horror and develops symptoms such as hyperarousal, irritability, outbursts of anger, difficulty sleeping, difficulty concentrating, and an exaggerated startle response. These thoughts, feelings, and symptoms persist as the traumatic event is relived through recurring thoughts, images, nightmares, or flashbacks in which the actual event seems to be occurring. The intense psychic discomfort leads people to avoid situations that remind them of the event, become detached from other people, have less interest in activities they formerly enjoyed, and develop other disorders (e.g., anxiety disorders, major depression, alcohol, or other substance abuse).

The response to stress is highly individualized and the same event or type of event might precipitate PTSD in one person and have little effect in another. Thus, most people experience major stresses and traumatic events during their lifetimes, but many do not develop PTSD. This point needs emphasis because many people seem to assume that PTSD is the normal response to a tragic event and that intensive counseling is needed. For example, counselors converge on schools in response to events that are perceived to be tragic or stressful. Some authorities take the opposing view, however, that talking about and reliving a traumatic event may increase anxiety in some people and thereby increase the likelihood that PTSD will occur. It is also important to note that many PTSD sufferers who need medical attention do not seek treatment.

## Social Anxiety Disorder

Social anxiety disorder (SAD) involves excessive concern about scrutiny by others, which may start in childhood and be lifelong. Affected people are afraid that they will say or do something that will embarrass or humiliate them or that will cause them to be judged, negatively evaluated, or rejected. As a result, they try to avoid certain situations (e.g., public speaking) or experience considerable distress if they cannot avoid them. Many with SAD experience physical symptoms including tachycardia, nausea, and sweating. They are often uncomfortable around other people or experience anxiety in many social situations. SAD may be inherited; there is a threefold increase in the occurrence of SAD in related family members.

# Clinical Manifestations

Clinical manifestations of anxiety include motor tension, such as muscle tension, restlessness, trembling, and fatigue; they also include overactivity of the autonomic nervous system, such as dyspnea, palpitations, tachycardia, sweating, dry mouth, dizziness, nausea, and diarrhea. Other clinical manifestations include increased vigilance, such as feeling fearful, nervous, or keyed up; difficulty concentrating; irritability; and insomnia. Box 54.1 summarizes the clinical manifestations of specific anxiety disorders.

# Drug Therapy

Benzodiazepines are widely used to treat anxiety disorders (Table 54.1). These drugs are useful in the short-term treatment of symptoms of acute anxiety in response to stressful situations. However, they may not be appropriate in all cases (see the discussion of benzodiazepines for more details). Antidepressants (i.e., selective serotonin reuptake inhibitors, tricyclic antidepressants, and newer miscellaneous drugs) are preferred as first-line drugs for long-term treatment of most chronic anxiety disorders, with benzodiazepines considered second-line drugs. Chapter 55 discusses antidepressant medications in more detail.

The barbiturates, a historically important group of CNS depressants, are obsolete for most uses, including treatment of anxiety and insomnia. A few may find use as intravenous (IV) general anesthetics (see Chap. 51), as treatment for seizure disorders (phenobarbital; see Chap. 53), and as drugs of abuse (see Chap. 58).

## TABLE 54.1

### Drugs Administered to Reduce Anxiety and Produce Hypnosis

| Drug Class | Prototype | Other Drugs in the Class |
|---|---|---|
| Benzodiazepines | Diazepam (Valium) | Alprazolam (Xanax, Xanax XR) Clonazepam (Klonopin) Chlordiazepoxide (Librium, Librax) Clorazepate (Gen-xene, Tranxene) Flurazepam Lorazepam (Ativan) Midazolam Oxazepam Temazepam (Restoril) Triazolam (Halcion) |
| Sedative–hypnotics | | Eszopiclone (Lunesta) Ramelteon (Rozerem) Suvorexant (Belsomra) Tasimelteon (Hetlioz) Zaleplon (Sonata) Zolpidem (Ambien, Zolpimist) |

**! QSEN Alert: Evidence-Based Practice**

In the pediatric population, current guidelines do not recommend benzodiazepines for acute management of anxiety disorders. In practice settings, prior to an invasive procedure, benzodiazepines are commonly used to relieve preprocedure stress in the pediatric population. A meta-analysis by Kuangm, Johnson, Mulqueen, and Bloch (2017) examined the effectiveness of benzodiazepines as short-term anxiolytics in children. The authors examined twenty-one randomized controlled trials, involving 1416 participants, assessing the efficacy of benzodiazepines as short-term anxiolytics in pediatric patients. A fixed effects model was used to examine the improvement in anxiety levels compared to control conditions. The effects of the specific agents, dosages, timing, and setting of benzodiazepine treatment were reviewed. A significant benefit was seen for benzodiazepines compared to the control group. Positive outcomes were seen when benzodiazepines were used in dental or nonoperating room procedures, and the researcher conclusions were that benzodiazepines are effective and well-tolerated when used as short-term anxiolytics in procedural settings for pediatric patients. The authors also suggested further research is needed to determine whether benzodiazepines are effective in pediatric anxiety disorders. Nurses working with pediatric patients can advocate for their patients in the use of preprocedure benzodiazepines in a variety of procedures and settings

# OVERVIEW OF SLEEP AND INSOMNIA

Sleep is a recurrent period of decreased mental and physical activity during which a person is relatively unresponsive to sensory and environmental stimuli. Normal sleep allows rest, renewal of energy for performing activities of daily living, and alertness on awakening.

## Etiology

**Insomnia**, prolonged difficulty in going to sleep or staying asleep long enough to feel rested, is the most common sleep disorder. Occasional sleeplessness is a normal response to many stimuli and is not usually harmful. Insomnia is said to be chronic when it lasts longer than 1 month. As in anxiety, several neurotransmission systems are apparently involved in regulating sleep–wake cycles and producing insomnia. Chronic insomnia affects 57% of older adults in the United States and impairs quality of life and health. Older adults with poor sleep quality have almost twice the mortality rate from stroke, cancer, and heart disease than those that sleep well.

Insomnia has many causes. Medical disorders, such as chronic pain syndromes and fibromyalgia, and neurologic disorders, such as movement disorders or headaches, may lead to sleep disturbances. Psychiatric conditions and substance abuse may also play a role. Other causes of insomnia include environmental factors (e.g., light, temperature, noise, uncomfortable mattress) or stress-related factors (e.g., stressful life events, deadlines, new job, personal losses). Certain medications, including stimulants such as caffeine, some antidepressants, beta-adrenergic blockers, and over-the-counter (OTC) and herbal medications, can cause sleep difficulties. Evidence supports the genetic susceptibility to factors such as light and stress on sleep hygiene.

Also, research has demonstrated that patients with insomnia show evidence of increased brain arousal, higher day and night body temperatures, and increased levels of adrenocorticotropic hormone. In addition, patients with insomnia have higher rates of depression and anxiety.

## Pathophysiology

When a person retires for sleep, there is an initial period of drowsiness or sleep latency, which lasts about 30 minutes. After the person is asleep, cycles occur approximately every 90 minutes during the sleep period. During each cycle, the sleeper progresses from drowsiness (stage I) to deep sleep (stages III and IV). These stages are characterized by depressed body functions, non-rapid eye movement (non-REM), and nondreaming, and they are thought to be physically restorative. Activities that occur during these stages include increased tissue repair, synthesis of skeletal muscle protein, and secretion of growth hormone. At the same time, there is decreased body temperature, metabolic rate, glucose consumption, and production of catabolic hormones. A period of 5 to 20 minutes of REM, dreaming, and increased physiologic activity follows stage IV.

Experts believe that REM sleep is mentally and emotionally restorative; REM deprivation can lead to serious psychological problems, including psychosis. It is estimated that people spend about 75% of sleeping hours in non-REM sleep and about 25% in REM sleep. However, older adults often have a different pattern, with less deep sleep, more light sleep, more frequent awakenings, and generally more disruptions.

## Clinical Manifestations

Clinical manifestations of insomnia include fatigue, lack of energy, and irritability. Patients with insomnia report diminished work performance and decreased concentration. Generally, patients with insomnia do not complain of daytime sleepiness. They tend to be overconcerned about their inability to fall asleep; the more they try to sleep, the more agitated they become, and the less they are able to fall asleep.

## Drug Therapy

The main drugs used to treat insomnia are the benzodiazepines and the nonbenzodiazepine hypnotics (see Table 54.1). However, it is important to note that drug companies market only a few benzodiazepines for the treatment of insomnia, although all are effective sedative–hypnotics. People also use OTC medications as

sleep aids; these medications include antihistamines alone or in combination with pain relievers. A new hypnotic agent, suvorexant (Belasomra), is a dual orexin receptor antagonist approved to treat sleep onset and sleep maintenance insomnia. Along with OTC medications, many herbal supplements are consumed to decrease stress and anxiety and induce sleep. Box 54.2 summarizes herbal supplements that are commonly taken and may interact with other prescription medications administered for anxiety and sleep induction. In addition, contamination with undesirable substances may make such herbal remedies less trustworthy.

### Clinical Application 54.1

- Mrs. Terrence's two sons come to visit her in the hospital. They complain to the nurse that their mother seems oversedated. In denial about her mental status, the sons request that their mother's medication be discontinued, but the nurses are concerned that if she is agitated, she may pull out her IV lines and Foley catheter as well as possibly strike out at staff. How does the nurse handle this situation while respecting the family's concerns, based on his or her knowledge and skills of patient-centered care according to the Quality and Safety Education for Nurses [QSEN] project?

## BENZODIAZEPINES

Benzodiazepines are widely used for anxiety and insomnia and are also used for several other indications. These drugs have a wide margin of safety between therapeutic and toxic doses, and they are rarely fatal, even in overdose, unless combined with other CNS depressant drugs, such as alcohol. Practitioners have used benzodiazepines to manage the anxiety and hyperarousal caused by PTSD, but research does not support their efficacy. With the high prevalence of substance abuse in patients with PTSD, judicious monitoring and consideration of alternate drug therapy would enhance safety in patients with a history of substance use. In addition, limited data

**BOX 54.2** *Herbal Supplements Commonly Used to Reduce Anxiety and Insomnia*

**Kava**

This supplement is derived from the root of a shrub found in many South Pacific islands. The major active ingredients of kava extract are kavalactones, which have psychoactive properties. The extract is claimed to be useful in numerous disorders and has been used or studied most often for treatment of anxiety, stress, and restlessness. Although the mechanism of action is not known, it is believed that the herb modulates gamma-aminobutyric acid (GABA) activity and inhibits noradrenaline and dopamine reuptake. Effects include analgesia, sedation, diminished reflexes, impaired gait, and pupil dilation. Multiple research studies have demonstrated that the herb has reduced anxiety in patients with increased symptom levels. However, additional high-quality studies are needed because most of the clinical trials had methodologic flaws, with small sample sizes, and there were conflicts of interest. Limited clinical trials have shown that kava is not effective in the treatment of insomnia.

Adverse effects of kava include impaired thinking, judgment, motor reflexes, and vision. Serious adverse effects may

occur with long-term, heavy use, including decreased plasma proteins, decreased platelet and lymphocyte counts, dyspnea, and pulmonary hypertension. The extract should not be taken concurrently with other CNS depressant drugs [e.g., benzodiazepines, ethanol], antiplatelet drugs, or levodopa [increases Parkinson symptoms]. Kava may increase the sedative effects of anesthetics and should be discontinued at least 24 hours prior to surgery. In addition, it should not be taken by women who are pregnant or lactating or by children under 12 years of age. Finally, it should be used cautiously by patients with renal disease, thrombocytopenia, or neutropenia. Recently, the U.S. Food and Drug Administration issued a warning that products containing kava have been implicated in many cases of severe liver toxicity [e.g., hepatitis, cirrhosis, liver failure].

**Melatonin**

This hormone is produced by the pineal gland, an endocrine gland in the brain. Endogenous melatonin is derived from the amino acid tryptophan, which is converted to serotonin,

| BOX 54.2 | *Herbal Supplements Commonly Used to Reduce Anxiety and Insomnia* (Continued) |

which is then enzymatically converted to melatonin in the pineal gland. Exogenous preparations are produced synthetically and may contain other ingredients. Melatonin products are widely available. Recommended doses on product labels usually range from 0.3 to 5 mg.

Melatonin influences sleep–wake cycles; it is released during sleep, and serum levels are very low during waking hours. Prolonged intake of exogenous melatonin can reset the sleep–wake cycle. As a result, it is widely promoted for prevention and treatment of jet lag (considered a circadian rhythm disorder) and treatment of insomnia. It is thought to act similarly to the benzodiazepines in inducing sleep. In several studies of patients with sleep disturbances, those taking melatonin experienced modest improvement compared with those taking a placebo. Other studies suggest that melatonin supplements improve sleep in older adults with melatonin deficiency and decrease weight loss in people with cancer. Large, controlled studies are needed to determine the effects of long-term use and the most effective regimen when used for jet lag.

Melatonin supplements are contraindicated in patients with hepatic insufficiency because of reduced clearance. They are also contraindicated in people with a history of cerebrovascular disease, depression, or neurologic disorders. They should be used cautiously by people with renal impairment and those taking benzodiazepines or other CNS depressant drugs. Adverse effects include altered sleep patterns, confusion, headache, hypothermia, pruritus, sedation, and tachycardia.

**Valerian**

This herb is a perennial flowering plant, and the root has been used for centuries as a treatment for anxiety and insomnia. It is believed that valerian increases the amount of GABA in the brain, probably by inhibiting the transaminase enzyme that normally metabolizes GABA. Increasing GABA, an inhibitory neurotransmitter, results in calming, sedative effects. However, there is a lack of evidence to support the use of valerian for treating insomnia or anxiety. In a meta-analysis of 11 clinical trials, there was no significant difference found in sleep benefit between valerian and placebo. In addition, valerian was associated with a greater number of adverse events per person compared with placebo. A small clinical trial did not find that valerian reduced anxiety compared to a placebo.

Adverse effects with acute overdose or chronic use of valerian include blurred vision, cardiac disturbance, excitability, headache, hypersensitivity reactions, insomnia, and nausea. There is a risk of hepatotoxicity from overdosage and from using combination herbal products containing valerian. Valerian should not be taken by people with hepatic impairment (risk of increased liver damage) or by pregnant or breast-feeding women (effects are unknown). The herb should not be taken concurrently with any other sedatives, hypnotics, alcohol, or CNS depressants because of the potential for additive CNS depression.

---

suggest that benzodiazepines may impair the therapeutic effects of certain behavioral therapies, such as exposure therapy.

Benzodiazepines are Schedule IV drugs under the Controlled Substances Act. Drugs of abuse, they may cause physiologic dependence; therefore, withdrawal symptoms occur if these drugs are stopped abruptly. To avoid withdrawal symptoms, it is necessary to taper benzodiazepines gradually before discontinuing them completely. The Food and Drug Administration (FDA) has issued a **BLACK BOX WARNING ◆** for the combined use of benzodiazepines and opioid analgesics. The risk of serious adverse reactions, including slowed or difficult breathing and deaths, has been reported.

Although benzodiazepines are effective anxiolytics, long-term use is associated with concerns over tolerance, dependency, withdrawal, lack of efficacy for treating the depression that often accompanies anxiety disorders, and the need for multiple daily dosing with some agents. These drugs differ mainly in their plasma half-lives, production of active metabolites, and clinical uses. **Diazepam** (Valium) is the prototype benzodiazepine.

## Pharmacokinetics

Diazepam has a long half-life (20–100 hours) if the contribution from metabolites is included. The drug requires 5 to 7 days to reach steady-state serum levels. It is well absorbed, highly lipid soluble, widely distributed in body tissues, and highly bound to plasma proteins (85%–98%). The high lipid solubility allows the drug to easily enter the CNS and perform its actions. After IV injection, diazepam may act within 1 to 5 minutes. However, the duration of action of a single IV dose is short (30–100 minutes). Thus, the pharmacodynamic effects (e.g., sedation) do not cor-

relate with plasma drug levels because the drugs move in and out of the CNS rapidly. This redistribution allows a patient to awaken even though the drug may remain in the blood and other peripheral tissues for days or weeks before it is completely eliminated.

Diazepam is mainly metabolized in the liver by the cytochrome P450 enzymes (CYP3A4 subgroup) and glucuronide conjugation. Metabolites are excreted through the kidneys.

## Action

Diazepam enhances the inhibitory effect of GABA to relieve anxiety, tension, and nervousness and to produce sleep. The decreased neuronal excitability also accounts for its usefulness as a muscle relaxant, hypnotic, and anticonvulsant.

## Use

Health care providers mainly use diazepam for antianxiety, hypnotic, and anticonvulsant purposes. They also give the drug for preoperative sedation, prevention of agitation and delirium tremens in acute alcohol withdrawal, and treatment of anxiety symptoms associated with depression, acute psychosis, or mania. Thus, patients often take it concurrently with antidepressants, antipsychotics, and mood stabilizers. However, use of diazepam contraindicates the use of some antidepressants. Experts do not advise using the drug for long periods, because it may cause excessive sedation and respiratory depression.

Investigators have extensively studied diazepam, and it has more approved uses than other drugs in its class. Table 54.2 gives route and dosage information for diazepam and the other benzodiazepines. Larger-than-usual doses may be necessary for

**TABLE 54.2**

# DRUGS AT A GLANCE: Benzodiazepines

| Drug | Pregnancy Category | Routes and Dosage Ranges | |
|---|---|---|---|
| | | **Adults** | **Children** |
| Diazepam (Valium) | D | 2–10 mg PO 2–4 times daily; 5–10 mg IM or IV. Give IV slowly, no faster than 5 mg (1 mL)/min repeated in 3–4 h if necessary<br>Older or debilitated adults: 2–5 mg PO once or twice daily. Increased gradually if needed and tolerated | 0.12–0.8 mg/kg/d in divided doses every 6–8 h |
| Alprazolam (Xanax, Xanax XR; ❊ Jamp-Alprazolam, Xanax) | D | Anxiety: 0.25–0.5 mg PO three times daily; maximum 4 mg daily in divided doses. Older or debilitated adults: 0.25 mg PO 2–3 times daily. Increased gradually if necessary<br>Panic disorder: 0.5 mg PO three times daily initially. Gradually increase to 4–10 mg daily.<br>Xanax XR, 0.5–1 mg PO daily; gradually increase PRN to maximum dose of 3–6 mg daily | <18 y: dosage not established<br>≥18 y: same as adult dosage |
| Chlordiazepoxide (Librium, Librax; ❊ Chlordiazepoxide) | D | Anxiety: 5–10 mg PO daily in 3–4 divided doses<br>Older or debilitated adults: 5 mg PO 2–4 times daily | <6 y: not recommended<br>≥6 y: 5 mg PO 2–4 times daily. Dose may be increased to 10 mg 2–3 times daily |
| Clonazepam (Klonopin; ❊ Accel-Clonazepam, Teva-Clonazepam) | D | Panic disorder: 0.25 mg PO two times daily, increasing to 1 mg daily after 3 d; max 4 mg/d | >10 y: same as adult dosage |
| Clorazepate (Gen-xene, Tranxene) | D | 30 mg PO in divided doses or 15 mg PO at bedtime; dose adjusted based on response; range 15–60 mg daily; max 90 mg/d | 9–12 y: 7.5 mg PO two times daily, increased by no more than 7.5 mg/wk; maximum 60 mg daily<br><9 y: not recommended |
| Flurazepam (❊ PMS-Flurazepam) | D | 15–30 mg PO at bedtime | Not for use in children <15 y of age |
| Lorazepam (Ativan; ❊ Apo-Lorazepam, Ativan) | D | 2–6 mg/d PO in 2–3 divided doses; 0.05 mg/kg IM to a maximum of 4 mg; 2 mg IV, diluted with 2 mL of sterile water, sodium chloride, or 5% dextrose injection. Do not exceed 2 mg/min; older or debilitated adults, 1–2 mg/d PO in divided doses | <12 y: PO, IV 0.05 mg/kg/dose, maximum 2 mg dose every 4–6 h<br>≥12 y: PO 0.25–2 mg/dose 2 to 3 times daily, maximum 2 mg/dose |
| Midazolam (❊ PMS-Midazolam) | D | Preoperative sedation: 0.05–0.08 mg/kg IM ~1 h before surgery<br>Prediagnostic test sedation: 0.1–0.15 mg/kg IV or up to 0.2 mg/kg IV initially; maintenance dose, ~25% of initial dose; reduce dose by 25%–30% if an opioid analgesic is also given<br>Induction of anesthesia: 0.3–0.35 mg/kg IV initially, then reduce dose as above for maintenance; reduce initial dose to 0.15–0.3 mg/kg if a narcotic is also given | Preoperative or preprocedure sedation and induction of anesthesia: syrup 0.25–1 mg/kg PO; maximum of 20 mg as a single dose |
| Oxazepam (❊ Oxazepam) | D | 10–30 mg PO 3–4 times daily; older or debilitated adults, 10 mg PO three times daily, gradually increased to 15 mg three times daily if necessary | |
| Temazepam (Restoril) | X | 15–30 mg PO | Not for use in children <18 y of age |
| Triazolam (Halcion) | X | 0.125–0.25 mg PO | Not for use in children <18 y of age |

patients who are severely anxious or agitated. Also, large doses are usually required to relax skeletal muscle, control muscle spasm, control seizures, and provide sedation before surgery, cardioversion, endoscopy, and angiography. When using benzodiazepines with opioid analgesics, it is important to reduce the analgesic dose initially and increase it gradually to avoid excessive CNS depression.

### Use in Children

Prescribers often order diazepam for children with anxiety and sleepwalking or night terrors. Use of the drug requires caution. Children may be more sensitive to the effects of this drug, namely, mood and/or mental changes. They may have unanticipated or variable responses, including paradoxical CNS stimulation and excitement rather than CNS depression and calming. Children should take diazepam and other benzodiazepines only when clearly indicated, in the lowest effective dose, and for the shortest effective time. Diazepam should not be used in children younger than 1 month of age.

### Use in Older Adults

In older adults, most benzodiazepines are metabolized more slowly, and half-lives are longer than in younger adults. Caution is necessary. The elderly may be sensitive to its effects, especially drowsiness, poor coordination, and mental and/or mood changes caused by the drug. Adverse effects may contribute to falls and other injuries unless patients are carefully monitored and safeguarded. It is important to make the initial dose of any antianxiety or sedative–hypnotic drug small and to increase doses gradually. Diazepam and other benzodiazepines may produce paradoxical excitement and aggression in adults older than 50 years of age who have a history of psychosis. Current studies suggest a relationship between benzodiazepine use and cognitive declines.

### Use in Patients With Renal or Hepatic Impairment

In impaired renal excretion, active metabolites may accumulate, causing excessive sedation and respiratory depression. Hepatic impairment also rules out use of diazepam.

### Use in Patients With Critical Illness

Antianxiety and sedative–hypnotic drugs are often useful in critically ill patients to relieve stress, anxiety, and agitation. Their calming effects decrease cardiac workload (e.g., heart rate, blood pressure, force of myocardial contraction, myocardial oxygen consumption) and respiratory effort. Additional benefits include improving tolerance of treatment measures (e.g., mechanical ventilation); keeping confused patients from harming themselves by pulling out IV catheters, feeding or drainage tubes, wound drains, and other treatment devices; and allowing more rest or sleep. In addition to sedation, the drugs often induce amnesia, which may be a desirable effect in the critically ill.

Caution is necessary with the use of diazepam in patients with critical illness. Patients should provide a comprehensive list of all medications to their health care provider, including antiretrovirals, certain antibiotics, and blood pressure medications. Use of many drugs is a contraindication to taking diazepam.

### Use in Patients Receiving Home Care

Most patients take diazepam at home, and the home care nurse shares the responsibility for teaching patients how to use the drug effectively and how to recognize medication responses that should be reported to the health care provider. Accurate dosing is vitally important because underuse may cause the recurrence of the symptoms and overuse may cause toxicity, which may be life threatening. The nurse tells the patient and any caregivers that if symptoms of withdrawal or overdose develop, it is necessary to seek medical attention immediately. The nurse also monitors the patient's response to the drug and any changes in the patient's condition.

## Adverse Effects

Both therapeutic effects and adverse effects of diazepam are more likely to occur after 2 or 3 days of therapy than initially. Such effects accumulate with chronic usage and persist for several days after the drug is discontinued. Many of the adverse effects associated with diazepam are related to its CNS depressant effects. They include drowsiness, problems with memory, confusion, disinhibition, depressed mood with or without suicidal ideation, slurred speech, dizziness, shallow breathing, restlessness, irritability, loss of bladder control, and diminished sexual interest. Other effects may include new or worsening seizures, nausea, constipation, drooling or dry mouth, mild skin rash, and itching. Diazepam and other benzodiazepines exert effects on the GABA receptors and can lead to overdose. Signs of overdose include blurred or double vision, labored breathing, weakness, stupor, and coma. Flumazenil is a benzodiazepine antagonist that interacts with the GABA receptors to reverse overdose (see Chap. 58).

## Contraindications

Contraindications to diazepam include severe respiratory disorders, such as chronic obstructive pulmonary disease or sleep apnea, severe liver or kidney disease, hypersensitivity reactions, and a history of alcohol or other drug abuse. People with narrow-angle glaucoma or who are pregnant or breast-feeding should not take diazepam. The concurrent use of diazepam and any other CNS depressants warrants caution.

### NCLEX Success

1. Which teaching fact is the priority for the woman receiving treatment for acute short-term anxiety with a benzodiazepine?
   A. Monitor serum glucose levels.
   B. Avoid alcohol when taking these medications.
   C. Take medications with food.
   D. Expect a delay in therapeutic effects of several weeks.

2. Which baseline laboratory tests should a patient receive prior to starting the benzodiazepine?
   A. blood glucose level
   B. liver enzymes
   C. lipid profile
   D. thyroid panel

# Nursing Implications

## Preventing Interactions

Smaller-than-usual doses of diazepam and other benzodiazepines may be necessary in patients receiving cimetidine or other drugs that decrease the hepatic metabolism of benzodiazepines.

## Administering the Medication

There are various preparations of diazepam, for both oral and parenteral use. The nurse adheres to the following guidelines:

- Ensure that the patient has swallowed sustained-release tablets whole. It is important not to chew these tablets.
- Ensure that the patient consumes the entire dose of medication.
- Do not abruptly withdraw the medication. This places the patient at risk for alterations in mood.
- Administer the intramuscular preparation in a large muscle. Inject it slowly and rotate injection sites.
- Administer the IV form undiluted IV push at a rate of 5 mg/minute. In children, inject it at a rate of 0.25 mg/kg over 3 minutes.

## Assessing for Therapeutic Effects

The nurse observes for a relaxed, but easily aroused, appearance. The nurse interviews the patient to assess response to the medication. For example, the patient should verbalize that he or she feels less worried and more relaxed. Nonverbal behavior is important; response to the medication includes decreased heart rate and blood pressure and a relaxed posture. It is necessary to assess the level of drowsiness and sleep pattern.

## Assessing for Adverse Effects

The nurse monitors the patient's blood pressure. It is necessary to make sure that the patient does not experience paradoxical responses, which include anger, aggression, and hallucinations, to the diazepam.

The nurse assesses for symptoms of diazepam dependence, overdose, and withdrawal. The presence of withdrawal symptoms when the drug is stopped indicates physical dependence, which is associated with longer use and higher doses. Common signs and symptoms of withdrawal include increased anxiety, psychomotor agitation, insomnia, irritability, headache, tremor, and palpitations. Less common but more serious signs include confusion, abnormal perception of movement, depersonalization, psychosis, and seizures. Symptoms usually occur 4 to 5 days after stopping a long-acting drug such as diazepam. Relief requires administration of a benzodiazepine.

## Patient Teaching

Box 54.3 identifies guidelines for teaching patients who are taking diazepam and other benzodiazepines for anxiety and insomnia.

# Other Drugs in the Class

Alprazolam (Xanax, Xanax XR) is administered orally to reduce anxiety and panic disorders. Elderly patients are more sensitive to the effects of the drug and may experience ataxia and oversedation. The immediate-release preparations can be given sublingually if the patient cannot swallow. Alprazolam is preferred over diazepam due to its immediate onset of action. Calcium channel blockers decrease the metabolism of alprazolam and other benzodiazepines, leading to increased adverse drug effects.

Chlordiazepoxide (Librium, Librax) is most commonly administered for the control of withdrawal symptoms related to acute alcoholism. As with many drugs, it is important that this drug not be administered with grapefruit juice. The combination decreases drug metabolism and increases drug toxicity. Also, the herbs St. John's wort, kava, and valerian, if given in combination with chlordiazepoxide, increase CNS depression.

Clorazepate (Gen-xene, Tranxene) has a longer onset of action than diazepam. This drug is commonly administered for anxiety, alcohol withdrawal, and epilepsy.

> ## ! QSEN Alert: Safety
>
> It is important not to confuse clorazepate with clonazepam; both drugs are used to control seizure activity but dosages differ significantly. For instance, in adults the maximum daily dosage of clorazepate is 90 mg; with clonazepam, the maximum daily dosage is 4 mg.

Flurazepam is administered on a short-term basis for patients who suffer from insomnia characterized by difficulty in falling asleep, frequent nocturnal awakenings, or early morning awakenings. Patients should take it only at bedtime. Adverse effects include dizziness, drowsiness, light-headedness, staggering, and loss of coordination and falling, particularly in elderly or debilitated persons. It is necessary to observe the patient for dizziness and orthostatic hypotension.

Lorazepam (Ativan) is probably the benzodiazepine of first choice. The drug provides rapid tranquilization of patients experiencing agitation. Administered intravenously, it reduces nausea and vomiting as well as anxiety and induces procedural amnesia. Administered orally, it helps combat anxiety disorders and the anxiety associated with depressive symptoms or anxiety- or stress-associated insomnia. Lorazepam has a slow onset of action (5–20 minutes) because of delayed brain penetration but an intermediate to prolonged duration. In addition, there is little accumulation, and its elimination is not significantly affected by hepatic or renal disease. As with all benzodiazepines, there is a risk of dependence. Rapid discontinuation of the drug can produce withdrawal symptoms.

Midazolam (see Chap. 51) is a short-acting IV medication and the most common medication administered prior to surgery or procedures. Furthermore, when given for procedures that only require sedation, midazolam can be continuously administered to maintain sedation. Because midazolam can be administered in flavored syrup orally, it is a valuable adjunct in pediatric anesthesia.

The FDA has issued a **BLACK BOX WARNING ◆** for midazolam because of profound respiratory depression that may result in hypoxia, brain damage, or death. Rapid IV administration to neonates has resulted in hypotension and seizures. It is essential to titrate midazolam carefully according to age and medical conditions. Following administration of midazolam, continuous monitoring for respiratory depression is required; and if necessary, age-specific resuscitative measures should be implemented. The benzodiazepine antagonist flumazenil reverses the effects of midazolam.

Oxazepam is administered for the reduction of anxiety including anxiety associated with depression. The drug is also

**BOX 54.3** *Patient Teaching Guidelines for Benzodiazepines*

- "Nerve pills" and "sleeping pills" can relieve symptoms temporarily, but they do not cure or solve the underlying problems. With rare exceptions, these drugs are recommended only for short-term use. For long-term relief, counseling or psychotherapy may be more beneficial because it can help you learn other ways to decrease your nervousness.

- Try to identify and avoid factors that cause nervousness, such as caffeine-containing beverages and stimulant drugs. This may prevent or decrease the severity of nervousness. If the drugs are used, these factors can cancel or decrease the drugs' effects. Stimulant drugs include asthma and cold remedies and appetite suppressants.

- Most pills to control anxiety belong to the same chemical group and have similar effects, including the ability to decrease nervousness, cause drowsiness, and cause dependence. Thus, there is no logical reason to take a combination of the drugs for anxiety or to take one drug for daytime sedation and another for sleep. Xanax, Ativan, and Restoril are commonly used examples of this group, but there are several others as well.

- Inform all health care providers when taking a sedative-type medication, preferably by the generic and trade names. This helps avoid multiple prescriptions of drugs with similar effects and reduces the risk of serious adverse effects from overdose.

- Do not perform tasks that require alertness if drowsy from medication. The drugs often impair mental and physical functioning, especially during the first several days of use, and thereby make routine activities potentially hazardous. Avoid smoking, ambulating without help, driving a car, operating machinery, bathing, and other potentially hazardous tasks. These activities may lead to falls or other injuries if undertaken while alertness is impaired.

- Avoid alcohol and other depressant drugs (e.g., OTC antihistamines and sleeping pills, narcotic analgesics, sedating herbs such as kava and valerian, and the dietary supplement melatonin) while taking any antianxiety or sedative–hypnotic drugs (except buspirone). An antihistamine that causes drowsiness is the active ingredient in OTC sleep aids (e.g., Compoz, Nytol, Sominex, Unisom) and in many pain reliever products with "PM" as part of their names (e.g., Tylenol PM). Because these drugs depress brain functioning when taken alone, combining them produces additive depression and may lead to excessive drowsiness, difficulty breathing, traumatic injuries, and other potentially serious adverse drug effects.

- Store drugs safely, out of reach of children and adults who are confused or less than alert. Accidental or intentional ingestion may lead to serious adverse effects. Also, do not keep the drug container at the bedside, because a person sedated by a previous dose may take additional doses.

- Do not share these drugs with anyone else. These mind-altering, brain-depressant drugs should be taken only by those people for whom they are prescribed.

- Do not stop taking a diazepam-related drug abruptly. Withdrawal symptoms can occur. When being discontinued, dosage should be gradually reduced, as directed by and with the supervision of a health care provider.

- Follow instructions carefully about how much, how often, and how long to take the drugs. These drugs produce more beneficial effects and fewer adverse reactions when used in the smallest effective doses and for the shortest duration feasible in particular circumstances. Omit one or more doses if excessive drowsiness occurs to avoid difficulty breathing, falls, and other adverse drug effects.

- Take oral benzodiazepines with a glass of water. Take them with food if stomach upset occurs.

- Take Xanax XR once daily, preferably in the morning. Take the tablet intact; do not crush, chew, or break it.

---

used for the management of alcohol withdrawal. It does not have analgesic, antidepressant, or antipsychotic properties. Oxazepam is slowly but completely absorbed, with 96% to 98% of the drug protein bound; the time to peak drug effect is about 3 hours. The drug is a class IV controlled substance. Respiratory depression may occur with use, so respiratory and cardiovascular status should be assessed.

Temazepam (Restoril) appears to act at the subcortical levels of the CNS. The drug's main site of action is the limbic system and mesencephalic reticular formation. It potentiates the effects of GABA. Temazepam is eliminated by conjugation and excreted through the kidneys. Thus, it is the drug of choice for elderly patients, those patients who have liver disease, or those who take medications that interfere with hepatic drug–metabolizing enzymes. The adverse effects of temazepam are similar to those of other benzodiazepines. The most severe adverse effect is cardiovascular collapse.

Triazolam (Halcion) has a very rapid onset of action, and it is necessary to administer the drug while patients are in bed. Cirrhosis of the liver or hepatic insufficiency is a contraindication. If patients are receiving protracted therapy, diagnostic testing with routine complete blood counts, urinalysis, and blood chemistry is required because of possible decreases in the hematocrit level and development of blood dyscrasias. Patients should not combine triazolam with ketoconazole or itraconazole.

### Clinical Application 54.2

Mrs. Terrence receives alprazolam 0.25 mg PO at 2:00 PM. Later, when the nurse brings in her supper tray, the patient seems relaxed. The supper tray contains roast beef, salad, chocolate pie, and hot tea. Visitors arrive at 5:00 PM and remark to the nurse that Mrs. Terrence is agitated and wringing her hands. She says that she is afraid to verbalize her anxiety to the nursing staff. The nurse prepares to give Mrs. Terrence another dose of medication.

- What does the nurse prepare and why?
- What foods on the supper tray contribute to the patient's anxiety?
- What patient teaching is necessary?

3. Oxazepam can be used in the treatment for patients who have which conditions? (Select all that apply.)

   A. severe agitation
   B. schizophrenia with hallucinations
   C. anxiety with depression
   D. opioid dependence
   E. alcoholism

4. The nurse is conducting patient teaching for a patient who will be taking alprazolam for treatment of anxiety. Which medication increases the amount of alprazolam in the body?

   A. diltiazem
   B. timolol
   C. albuterol inhaler
   D. bosentan

5. Benzodiazepines are thought to work through which action?

   A. exciting the central nervous system
   B. stimulating the reticular activating system
   C. increasing inhibitory feelings
   D. enhancing the effects of gamma-aminobutyric acid

6. Which medication can be administered to the elderly, accumulates to a small extent in the brain, and is not affected by diminished hepatic function?

   A. diazepam
   B. lorazepam
   C. clonazepam
   D. chlordiazepoxide

7. When a patient is prescribed chlordiazepoxide for acute alcohol withdrawal, which herbal supplement may increase the risk of increased central nervous system depression?

   A. garlic
   B. ginger
   C. St. John's wort
   D. *Ginkgo biloba*

# NONBENZODIAZEPINE SEDATIVE–HYPNOTIC AGENTS

The nonbenzodiazepine sedative–hypnotics produce sleep. People may receive them prior to diagnostic or surgical procedures or take them nightly. Table 54.1 lists the most commonly administered nonbenzodiazepines that produce sleep. This classification lacks a specific prototype, so each drug in the class will be discussed individually.

In general, people should use sedative–hypnotics only when insomnia causes significant distress and resists management by nonpharmacologic means. The drugs are not indicated for occasional sleeplessness. The goal of treatment is to relieve anxiety or sleeplessness without permitting sensory perception, responsiveness to the environment, or alertness to drop below safe levels. The drugs of choice for most patients are the benzodiazepines and the nonbenzodiazepine hypnotics, eszopiclone, ramelteon, zaleplon, and zolpidem. However, for patients with insomnia associated with major depression, antidepressants are preferred (see Chap. 55).

The use of sedative–hypnotics every night should not occur unless absolutely necessary. Intermittent administration helps maintain drug effectiveness and decreases the risks of drug abuse and dependence. It also decreases disturbances of normal sleep patterns. For chronic insomnia, only eszopiclone is recommended for long-term treatment (≤12 months). To restore the sleep-producing effect, administration of the hypnotic drug must be interrupted for 1 to 2 weeks. Table 54.3 gives route and dosage information for the sedative–hypnotics. Box 54.4 identifies guidelines for teaching patients who are taking sedative–hypnotics for anxiety and insomnia.

## Eszopiclone

Eszopiclone (Lunesta) is the first oral nonbenzodiazepine hypnotic to receive FDA approval for long-term use (≤12 months). During testing, researchers did not observe tolerance to the hypnotic benefits of the drug over a 6-month period. It increases total sleep time and reduces the amount of time needed to fall asleep. Studies show that eszopiclone does not reduce nighttime awakenings. The drug is a Schedule IV controlled substance.

Supposedly, the hypnotic effect of eszopiclone is due to interaction with the $GABA_A$ receptor at a location close to or coupled with the benzodiazepine receptors. The drug is rapidly absorbed after oral administration, reaching peak plasma levels 1 hour after administration. It has a half-life of 6 hours. It is metabolized in the liver and eliminated primarily by the renal system.

People should take eszopiclone immediately prior to going to bed due to its rapid onset of action.

> **!  QSEN Alert: Safety**
>
> It is important to instruct patients not to engage in any activities following the administration of the medication.

Also, people should not take the medication following a high-fat meal, because the onset of action may be delayed by approximately 1 hour, or prior to bathing. In addition, geriatric people should not use the drug according to the Beers criteria.

Adverse reactions to eszopiclone include behavioral changes such as reduced inhibition, aggression or bizarre behavior, worsening depression and suicidal ideation, hallucinations, and **anterograde amnesia** (short-term memory loss). A commonly reported reaction to the drug is an unpleasant taste. Contraindications include hypersensitivity reaction. Caution is necessary during pregnancy and lactation, in depression, and with impaired hepatic or respiratory function. Elderly patients, those with hepatic impairment or debilitating conditions, and those taking drugs that inhibit CYP3A4 enzymes (e.g., antidepressants, antifungals, erythromycin, grapefruit, protease inhibitors, others) require lower dosages to reduce adverse effects. People who take eszopiclone should not take alcohol or other CNS depressants to avoid additive effects.

**TABLE 54.3**

## DRUGS AT A GLANCE: Sedative–Hypnotics

| Drug | Pregnancy Category | Routes and Dosage Ranges | | Children |
|---|---|---|---|---|
| | | **Adults** | | **Children** |
| Eszopiclone (Lunesta) | C | 2 mg PO at bedtime; may be increased to 3 mg if needed; for initial dose, debilitated patients, and those with hepatic impairment, 1 mg PO at bedtime; may be increased to 2 mg if needed | | Not recommended |
| Ramelteon (Rozerem) | C | 8 mg PO at bedtime | | Not recommended |
| Suvorexant (Belsomra; ✳ Belsomra) | C | 10–20 mg PO within 30 min of bedtime | | Safety and efficacy not established |
| Tasimelteon (Hetlioz) | C | 20 mg PO before bedtime at the same time each night | | Dosage not established |
| Zaleplon (Sonata) | C | 10 mg PO at bedtime; 5 mg for adults who are elderly and of low weight or have mild to moderate hepatic impairment | | Dosage not established |
| Zolpidem (Ambien, Zolpimist; ✳ APO-Zolpidem, Sublinox) | C | Immediate-release tablet, spray 5 mg (females) or 5–10 mg (males) PO at bedtime<br>Extended-release tablet, 6.25 mg (females) or 6.25–12.5 mg (males) PO at bedtime | | ≥18 y, same as adult dosage |

## Ramelteon

Ramelteon (Rozerem), a melatonin agonist, is used for the long-term treatment of insomnia characterized by difficulty with sleep onset. Unlike other nonbenzodiazepine hypnotics, which bind to GABA$_A$ receptors, ramelteon binds to melatonin receptors in the CNS. Stimulation of melatonin receptors by ramelteon, like endogenous melatonin, is thought to play a role in the maintenance of the circadian rhythm, which helps regulate the normal sleep–wake cycle. Ramelteon does not appear to cause rebound insomnia posttreatment. Because it does not produce physical dependence, ramelteon is not classified as a controlled substance.

**BOX 54.4**  *Patient Teaching Guidelines for Nonbenzodiazepine Sedative–Hypnotics*

- Sleeping pills, like antianxiety drugs, can relieve symptoms temporarily, but they do not cure or solve the underlying problems. With rare exceptions, these drugs are recommended only for short-term use. For long-term relief, counseling or psychotherapy may be more beneficial because it can help you learn other ways to decrease your difficulty in sleeping.
- Avoid alcohol and other depressant drugs (e.g., OTC antihistamines and sleeping pills, narcotic analgesics, sedating herbs such as kava and valerian, and the dietary supplement melatonin) while taking sedative–hypnotic drugs. An antihistamine that causes drowsiness is the active ingredient in OTC sleep aids (e.g., Compoz, Nytol, Sominex, Unisom) and in many pain reliever products with "PM" as part of their names (e.g., Tylenol PM). Because these drugs depress brain functioning when taken alone, combining them produces additive depression and may lead to excessive drowsiness, difficulty breathing, traumatic injuries, and other potentially serious adverse drug effects.
- Do not perform tasks that require alertness if drowsy from medication. The drugs often impair mental and physical functioning, especially during the first several days of use, and thereby make routine activities potentially hazardous. Avoid smoking, ambulating without help, driving a car, operating machinery, bathing, and other potentially hazardous tasks. These activities may lead to falls or other injuries if undertaken while alertness is impaired.
- Store drugs safely, out of reach of children and adults who are confused or less than alert. Accidental or intentional ingestion may lead to serious adverse effects. Also, do not keep the drug container at the bedside, because a person sedated by a previous dose may take additional doses.
- Take nonbenzodiazepine hypnotics on an empty stomach, at bedtime, because fatty heavy meals delay onset of action.
- Do not take herbal supplements with nonbenzodiazepine sedative–hypnotics.
- Do not take most "sleeping pills" every night. Many sleeping pills lose their effectiveness in 2 to 4 weeks if taken nightly and cause sleep disturbances when stopped. If longer drug therapy for insomnia is needed, eszopiclone and ramelteon are approved for long-term use.
- Use nondrug measures to promote relaxation, rest, and sleep when possible. Physical exercise, reading, craft work, stress management, and relaxation techniques are safer than any drug.
- Take sleeping pills just before going to bed so that you are lying down when the expected drowsiness occurs.
- Do not take zolpidem concurrently with alcohol or other CNS depressant drugs because of increased risk of excessive sedation and respiratory depression.
- Prime zolpidem oral spray prior to initial use. Compress the container five times, hold the container upright, and aim it directly into the mouth.
- Report adverse effects such as hypersensitivity reactions, complex sleep-related behaviors, or thoughts of suicide to the prescriber.

Ramelteon is rapidly absorbed orally, reaching peak plasma levels in about 45 minutes. Ramelteon is moderately protein bound (82%) and undergoes rapid hepatic first-pass metabolism by cytochrome P450 enzyme systems, including CYP3A4. Ramelteon is excreted primarily in the urine and does not accumulate in the body due to the short half-life of the drug (1–2.6 hours). Patients should avoid taking ramelteon with a high-fat meal because food may delay the onset of action.

Common adverse effects of ramelteon include headache, fatigue, dizziness, nausea, diarrhea, arthralgia/myalgia, and taste changes. The drug may affect endocrine hormones, resulting in decreased testosterone levels, increased prolactin levels, and decreased cortisol levels. Contraindications include severe hepatic impairment if combined with fluvoxamine. Caution is warranted in depression or impaired respiratory function. People should not take ramelteon with alcohol because of resulting excessive sedation and respiratory depression.

Tasimelteon (Hetlioz), a drug in the same class as ramelteon, has been approved for the treatment of non–24-hour sleep–wake disorder in adults, a circadian sleep–wake rhythm disorder that occurs primarily affecting blind individuals.

## Zaleplon

Zaleplon (Sonata) is an oral, nonbenzodiazepine hypnotic approved for the short-term treatment (7–10 days) of insomnia. Overall, this drug is effective in helping people get to sleep and has several advantages as a hypnotic, including the rapid onset, absence of active metabolites, absence of clinically significant CYP450 drug interactions, rapid clearance from the body, and absence of major memory impairments. However, it may not increase total sleep time or decrease the number of awakenings during sleeping hours.

Zaleplon is well absorbed, but bioavailability is only about 30% because of extensive presystemic or first-pass hepatic metabolism. Onset of action is rapid, with a peak in 1 hour. A high-fat, heavy meal slows absorption and may reduce the drug's effectiveness in inducing sleep. It is 60% bound to plasma proteins, and its half-life is 1 hour. The drug is metabolized mainly in the liver to inactive metabolites. The metabolites and a small amount of unchanged drug are excreted in the urine.

Zaleplon apparently enhances the inhibitory effects of GABA, as do the benzodiazepines. A few studies indicate that it has abuse potential similar to that of the benzodiazepines; zaleplon is a Schedule IV controlled substance.

No dosage adjustment with zaleplon is necessary in mild to moderate renal impairment. However, to reduce the risk of adverse effects, it is necessary to decrease the dosage in mild to moderate hepatic impairment and avoid using the drug in severe hepatic impairment. It is also important to decrease the dosage in older adults.

Adverse effects associated with zaleplon include depression, drowsiness, nausea, dizziness, headache, hypersensitivity, impaired coordination, and short-term memory impairment. Contraindications include hypersensitivity reactions and lactation. Caution is warranted during pregnancy and in impaired hepatic or respiratory function.

Use of zaleplon with alcohol or other CNS depressant drugs should not occur because of the increased risk of excessive sedation and respiratory depression. There is also a risk of increased serum zaleplon levels if people take the hypnotic concurrently with cimetidine. It is very important that patients taking zaleplon

be taught about this interaction because cimetidine is available without prescription, and the patient may not inform the health care provider who prescribes zaleplon about taking cimetidine.

## Zolpidem

Zolpidem (Ambien, Zolpimist) is a nonbenzodiazepine hypnotic that differs structurally from the benzodiazepines but produces similar effects. This drug is a Schedule IV drug approved for short-term treatment (7–10 days) of insomnia. It is well absorbed with oral administration and has a rapid onset of action, usually within 20 to 30 minutes. The half-life of zolpidem is 2.5 hours, and its hypnotic effects last 6 to 8 hours. A newer controlled-release form (Ambien CR) contains a rapid-releasing layer, which promotes falling asleep, and a slow-releasing layer, which promotes sleep all night. The drug is metabolized to inactive metabolites in the liver; these are then eliminated by renal excretion.

Dosage reductions with zolpidem are not necessary in renal impairment, but this condition requires close monitoring. Increased bioavailability, peak plasma concentration, and half-life occur in older adults and in patients with impaired hepatic function. Thus, dosage reduction is essential for these groups. People should not take zolpidem concurrently with alcohol or other CNS depressant drugs because of the increased risk of excessive sedation and respiratory depression.

Adverse effects of zolpidem include daytime drowsiness, dizziness, nausea, diarrhea, and anterograde amnesia. Hallucinations have been reported in some patients. Older adults may experience headache, somnolence, and dizziness. Caution is necessary with signs and symptoms of major depression because of increased risk of intentional overdose. Rebound insomnia may occur for a night or two after stopping the drug, and withdrawal symptoms may occur if it is stopped abruptly after approximately a week of regular use.

## NCLEX Success

8. Zolpidem is the most appropriate choice for patients with which condition?
   A. difficulty in initiating and maintaining sleep
   B. morning awakening
   C. agitation and violent outbursts
   D. obstructive sleep apnea and respiratory problems

9. When a 5-year-old child is scheduled for a sleep electroencephalogram (EEG), which medication is a drug of choice prior to the diagnostic test?
   A. diazepam
   B. lorazepam
   C. zolpidem
   D. diphenhydramine

10. When a patient receives a prescription for zolpidem, which teaching point is most important?
   A. Take the medication with a high-fat meal.
   B. Only take the medication if acetaminophen PM does not produce sleep.
   C. Go to bed immediately after taking the medication.
   D. Take the medication if nondrug relaxation has not produced sleep.

## THE NURSING PROCESS

A concept map outlines the nursing process related to drug therapy considerations in this chapter. Additional nursing implications related to the disease process should also be considered in care decisions.

**Assessment**

- Assess the patient's subjective and objective data regarding anxiety and insomnia.
- Assess the patient's sleep patterns.
- Assess physiological aspects of anxiety (e.g., increased heart rate and respiratory rate).
- Obtain a careful drug history, including the use of alcohol and sedative–hypnotic drugs, and assess the likelihood of drug abuse and dependence.
- Assess for use of CNS stimulants (e.g., appetite suppressants, bronchodilators, nasal decongestants, caffeine, cocaine) and herbs (e.g., St John's Wort, ephedra).
- Identify coping mechanisms used in managing previous situations of stress, anxiety, and insomnia.

**Outcomes of Therapy**

The patient will
- Feel more calm, relaxed, and comfortable with anxiety; experience improved quantity and quality of sleep with insomnia.
- Be monitored for excessive sedation and impaired mobility to prevent falls or other injuries (in health care settings).
- Verbalize and demonstrate nondrug activities to reduce or manage anxiety or insomnia.
- Demonstrate safe, accurate drug usage.
- Notify a health care provider if he or she wants to stop taking a benzodiazepine; agree to not stop taking a benzodiazepine abruptly.
- Avoid preventable adverse effects, including abuse and dependence.

**Nursing Interventions**

- Use nondrug measures to relieve anxiety or to enhance the effectiveness of antianxiety drugs.
- Assist patients to identify and avoid or decrease situations that cause anxiety and insomnia, when possible. In addition, help them to understand that medications do not solve underlying problems.
- Implement therapeutic communication skills.
- Instruct on the overall treatment plan, including medical treatments, diagnostic tests, medication and treatment measures, and any aspects of care.
- When a benzodiazepine is used with diagnostic tests or minor surgery, provide instructions for postprocedure care to the patient or to family members, preferably in written form.
- Implement measures to decrease the need for or increase the effectiveness of sedative-hypnotic drugs, such as the following:
- Modify the environment to promote rest and sleep (e.g., reduce noise and light).
- Plan care to allow uninterrupted periods of rest and sleep, when possible.
- Relieve symptoms that interfere with rest and sleep. Drugs such as analgesics for pain or antitussives for cough are usually safer and more effective than sedative–hypnotic drugs. Nondrug measures, such as positioning, exercise, and back rubs, may be helpful in relieving muscle tension and other discomforts. Allowing the patient to verbalize concerns, providing information so that he or she knows what to expect, or consulting other personnel (e.g., social worker, chaplain) may be useful in decreasing anxiety.
- Help the patient modify lifestyle habits to promote rest and sleep (e.g., limiting intake of caffeine-containing beverages, limiting intake of fluids during evening hours if nocturia interferes with sleep, avoiding daytime naps, having a regular schedule of rest and sleep periods, increasing physical activity, not trying to sleep unless tired or drowsy).
- Boxes 54.3 and 54.4 present patient guidelines for antianxiety and sedative-hypnotics.

**Evaluation**

- Decreased symptoms of anxiety or insomnia and increased rest and sleep are reported or observed.
- Excessive sedation and motor impairment are not observed.
- The patient reports no serious adverse effects.
- Monitoring of prescriptions (e.g., "pill counts") does not indicate excessive use.

- Anxiety is a common disorder that occurs when a person perceives a situation as threatening to physical, emotional, social, or economic well-being.
- When anxiety is severe or prolonged and impairs the ability to function in usual activities of daily living, it is called an anxiety disorder. The American Psychiatric Association delineates anxiety disorders as medical diagnoses in the *DSM-5*.
- Examples of anxiety disorders include GAD, OCD, panic disorder, separation anxiety disorder, and SAD (see Box 54.1).
- Patients with PTSD often have anxiety and insomnia and typically are treated with the drugs included in this chapter.
- Insomnia is a prolonged difficulty in going to sleep or staying asleep long enough to feel rested.
- Benzodiazepines are used as sedatives–hypnotics, antianxiety agents, muscle relaxants, and anticonvulsants.
- The FDA has issued a **BLACK BOX WARNING ◆** for the combined use of benzodiazepines and opioid analgesics. The risk of serious adverse reactions, including slowed or difficult breathing and deaths, has been reported.
- Benzodiazepines and some nonbenzodiazepine hypnotics are Schedule IV drugs under the Controlled Substance Act and can cause physical dependence and withdrawal syndromes.

- The choice of benzodiazepine for a particular purpose and patient depends on the pharmacokinetics of the drug. Benzodiazepines differ in terms of plasma half-life, production of active metabolites, and metabolism.
- Benzodiazepines and most nonbenzodiazepine hypnotics are indicated for short-term use only; tolerance develops after approximately 2 weeks.
- The FDA has issued a **BLACK BOX WARNING ◆** for midazolam because of profound respiratory depression that may result in hypoxia, brain damage, or death. Rapid intravenous administration to neonates has resulted in hypotension and seizures.
- Contraindications to most antianxiety and sedative–hypnotics include severe respiratory disorders, severe liver or kidney disease, hypersensitivity reaction, and a history of drug or alcohol abuse.
- The concurrent use of antianxiety or sedative–hypnotics with other CNS depressants should be avoided to prevent respiratory depression and excessive sedation.
- Generally, older adults should take the lowest effective doses of antianxiety and sedative–hypnotic drugs.

**CLINICAL REASONING CASE STUDY**

**Meet the Patient**

Dwight Rossi, a 43-year-old man, has been seen in the clinic with complaints of difficulty falling asleep and waking up repeatedly at night. He lost his job two months ago. He is starting a new job in 2 weeks and asks for something to help him sleep so he is able to be effective in his new job. The nurse practitioner prescribes flurazepam 15 mg orally at bedtime and wants to see him in the clinic in 1 week.

- What patient teaching does the nurse provide Mr. Rossi regarding the administration of flurazepam?
- What assessments should the nurse make when he returns to the clinic?

**Assessing Drug Information**

- Flurazepam enhances the inhibitory effect of gamma-aminobutyric acid to relieve anxiety, tension, and nervousness and to produce sleep.
- Flurazepam is administered on a short-term basis for patients who suffer from insomnia characterized by difficulty in falling asleep, frequent nocturnal awakenings, or early morning awakenings.
- Adverse effects include dizziness, drowsiness, light-headedness, staggering, loss of coordination, and falling.

**Nursing Actions**

- The nurse instructs Mr. Rossi regarding administration of flurazepam.
  - Take the drug right before going to bed.
  - Do not drink alcohol or take other medications that cause drowsiness.
  - Do not engage in any hazardous occupations requiring complete mental alertness, such as operating machinery or driving a car, until you know how the drug will affect you.
  - Side effects of the drug include dizziness, drowsiness, light-headedness, and loss of coordination, so change positions slowly and make sure your balance is good before you try walking.
- The nurse also encourages Mr. Rossi to modify his lifestyle habits to promote rest and sleep (e.g., limiting intake of caffeine-containing beverages, limiting intake of fluids during evening hours if nocturia interferes with sleep, avoiding daytime naps, setting a regular schedule of rest and sleep periods, increasing physical activity).
- On return to the clinic, the nurse observes Mr. Rossi for his reported level of daytime drowsiness and sleep pattern. The nurse interviews him to assess his perception of his response to the medication. The nurse should assess for known adverse effects, including dizziness, orthostatic hypotension, respiratory rate, balance, and behavior profile.

Visit thePoint® at **http://thePoint.lww.com/Frandsen12e** *for answers to NCLEX Success questions (in Appendix A), answers to Clinical Application Case Studies (in Appendix B), and more!*

## REFERENCES AND RESOURCES

Abad, V. C., & Guillenminault, C. (2018). Insomnia in elderly patients: Recommendations for pharmacological management. *Drugs & Aging, 35*, 791–817.

American Psychiatric Association. (2013). *The diagnostic and statistical manual of mental disorders (DSM-5)*. Washington, DC: Author.

Atkin, N., Vickerstaff, V., & Candy, B. (2017). "Worried to death": The assessment and management of anxiety in patients with advanced life-limiting disease, a national survey of palliative medicine physicians. *BMC Palliative Care, 16*(69), 1–10.

Bernardy, N. C., & Friedman, M. J. (2017). Pharmacological management of posttraumatic stress disorder. *Current Opinion in Psychology, 14*, 116–121.

Bradly, H. G. (2018). Post-traumatic stress disorder in veterans. Treatments and risk factors for nonadherence. *JAAPA, 31*(11), 21–24.

Buck, M. J. L., Kritjenberg, P., Kox, M. (2016). Preoperative use of anxiolytic-sedative agents; are we on the right track? *Journal of Clinical Anesthesia, 33*, 135–140.

Chapdelaine, A., Carrier, I. J. D., Fournier, L., Duhoux, A., & Roberge, I. P. (2018). Treatment adequacy for social anxiety disorder in primary care patients. *PLoS One, 13*(11), e0206357. doi:10.1371/journal.pone.0206357

Crocco, E. A., Jaramillo, S., Cruz-Ortiz, C., & Camfield, K. (2017). Pharmacological management of anxiety disorders in the elderly. *Curr Treat Options Psychiatry, 4*, 33–46.

Duncan, C., & Sheppard, K. (2019). Implications and recommendations for addressing insomnia disorders. *The Nurse Practitioner, 44*(1), 19–25.

El-Sohl, A. A., Riaz, U., & Roberts, J. (2018). Sleep disorders in post-traumatic stress disorder. *Chest Journal, 154*(2), 427–439.

Friedman, M. J., & Bernardy, N. C. (2017). Considering future pharmacotherapy for PTSD. *Neurosci Lett, 649*, 181–185.

Kahmen, D. (2018). Emerging pharmacological treatment for post-traumatic stress disorder. *Joining Forces, 26*(2), 10–11.

Kuangm, H., Johnson, J. A., Mulqueen, J. M., & Bloch, M. H. (2017). The efficacy of benzodiazepines as acute anxiolytics in children: A meta-analysis. *Depression and Anxiety, 17*(34), 888–889.

Maguire, A., Moriarty, J., O'Reily, D., McCann, M. (2017). Education as a predictor of antidepressant and anxiolytic medication use after bereavement: a population-based record linkage study. *Quality of Life Research, 26*, 1251–1262.

Miller, M. W. (2018). Leveraging genetics to enhance the efficacy of PTSD pharmacotherapeutics. *Neuroscience Letters*, 133562. doi:10.1016/j.neulet.2018.04.039

Picton, J., Marino, A. B., & Neely, K. L. (2018). Benzodiazepine use and cognitive decline. *American Journal of Health-System Pharmacy, 75*(1), 36.e12.

Quang, A., Doctor, J. A., Zoellner, L. A., & Feeny, N. C. (2018). Effects of treatment of choice, and preference on health-related quality-of-life outcomes in patients with posttraumatic stress disorder (PTSD). *Quality of Life Research, 27*, 1555–1562.

Sorscher, A. J. (2017). Insomnia, getting to the cause, facilitating relief. *The Journal of Family Practice, 66*(4), 216–225.

Strawn, J. R., Dobson, D. T., & Giles, L. L. (2017). Primary pediatric care psychopharmacology: Focus on medications for ADHD, depression and anxiety. *Current Problems in Pediatric and Adolescent Health Care, 47*(1), 3–14.

Strohle, A., Gensichen, J., & Domschke, K. (2018). The diagnosis and treatment of anxiety disorders. *Deutsches Ärzteblatt International, 115*, 611–620.

# Drug Therapy for Depression and Mood Stabilization

## LEARNING OBJECTIVES

*After studying this chapter, you should be able to:*

1. Discuss the etiology and pathophysiology of depression and bipolar disorder.
2. Describe the major features of various mood disorders.
3. Compare and contrast the different categories of antidepressants: tricyclic antidepressants, selective serotonin reuptake inhibitors, mixed serotonin–norepinephrine reuptake inhibitors, monoamine oxidase inhibitors, and other atypical antidepressants.
4. Discuss the drugs used to treat depression in terms of prototype, action, indications for use, adverse effects, and nursing implications.
5. Discuss the drugs used to treat bipolar disorder in terms of prototype, action, indications for use, adverse effects, and nursing implications.
6. Implement the nursing process in the care of patients undergoing drug therapy for mood disorders.

## CLINICAL APPLICATION CASE STUDY

While in the hospital, Carl Mehring, a 70-year-old man, receives a diagnosis of chronic depression secondary to chronic heart failure, hypertension, diabetes mellitus, and renal insufficiency. As his health has declined, so has his interest in his family, friends, and hobbies. His physician prescribes sertraline 50 mg orally at bedtime.

## KEY TERMS

**Antidepressant discontinuation syndrome:** condition that occurs with sudden termination of most antidepressant drugs. Typical symptoms may occur more rapidly and may be more intense with drugs that have a short half-life and/or are used for long periods

**Bipolar disorder:** mood disorder characterized by episodes of depression alternating with episodes of mania

**Cyclothymia:** mild type of bipolar disorder involving periods of hypomania and depression that do not meet the criteria for mania and major depression

**Depression:** most common mental illness, which is characterized by depressed mood, feelings of sadness, or emotional upset; occurs in people of all ages

**Dysthymia:** chronically depressed mood and at least two other symptoms of depression for 2 years

**Enuresis:** bed wetting or involuntary urination resulting from a physical or psychological disorder

**Hypomania:** persistent irritable mood but absence of psychotic symptoms characteristic of true mania

**Mania:** emotional disorder characterized by euphoria or irritability; usually occurs in bipolar disorder

**Postpartum depression:** major depressive episode occurring after the birth of a child

**Seasonal affective disorder:** depressive episode occurring in a certain season, usually the winter

**Serotonin syndrome:** serious and sometimes fatal reaction due to combined therapy with a selective serotonin reuptake inhibitor or serotonin–norepinephrine reuptake inhibitor and a monoamine oxidase inhibitor or another drug that potentiates serotonin neurotransmission

# INTRODUCTION

Mood disorders include depression, dysthymia, bipolar disorder, and cyclothymia (Box 55.1). Major depressive disorder is relatively common in adults, and it also occurs in children and adolescents. This chapter focuses on depression and antidepressant drugs as well as bipolar disorder and mood-stabilizing drugs.

# OVERVIEW OF DEPRESSION

**Depression** is a mood disorder in which feelings of sadness, loss, anger, or frustration interfere with everyday life for several weeks or longer. The condition affects people of all ages. It is difficult to determine the overall incidence of depression in the United States, because only 50% of the people who meet the criteria for depression (see Box 55.1) seek help. Generally, major depression affects women

---

**BOX 55.1** · *Types and Symptoms of Mood Disorders*

## Depression

Depression, often described as the most common mental illness, is characterized by depressed mood, feelings of sadness, or emotional upset, and it occurs in all age groups. Mild depression occurs in everyone as a normal response to life stresses and losses and usually does not require treatment; severe or major depression is a psychiatric illness and requires treatment. Major depression also is categorized as unipolar, in which people of usually normal moods experience recurrent episodes of depression.

## Major Depression, Seasonal Affective Disorder, and Postpartum Depression

Major depression is noted to be present for 2 weeks with the patient having a distinct change in the previous level of functioning. The symptoms of depression include

- Feelings of hopelessness or sadness
- Lack of interest in daily activities
- Loss of sleep or excessive sleep
- Weight loss or weight gain
- Fear and anxiousness
- Lack of self-worth
- Agitation
- Unexplained physiologic symptoms
- Suicidal ideations

   **Seasonal affective disorder** is episodes of major depression, mania, or hypomania that occurs during a particular season. Most commonly, this occurs in winter and resolves in spring and summer. However, it can also occur in spring and summer. Treatment generally involves the use of psychotherapy and/or antidepressants; however, there is limited information available to guide the selection of the most efficacious antidepressants for treatment of postnatal depression.

- Fall and winter onset: The patient experiences increased sleep and appetite with carbohydrate craving and increase weight.
- Spring and summer onset: The patient experiences insomnia, decreased sleep, decreased appetite and weight loss.

Postpartum unipolar major depression is a condition in which a postpartum woman develops depressive symptoms. These symptoms can be mild and termed the baby blues or present as major depression. Risk factors for **postpartum depression** include previous depression, antenatal depression, and high levels of postnatal stress. Additional factors that can contribute to postpartum depression are stressful life events, such as martial conflict, single parenting, multiparity, intimate partner violence, lack of financial and social support, or unwanted pregnancy. Treatment for postpartum depression is psychotherapy and antidepressants.

## Dysthymia

Dysthymia involves a chronically depressed mood and at least two other symptoms (e.g., anorexia, overeating, insomnia, hypersomnia, low energy, low self-esteem, poor concentration, feelings of hopelessness) for 2 years. Although the symptoms may cause significant social- and work-related impairments, they are not severe enough to meet the criteria for major depression.

## Bipolar Disorder

Bipolar disorder involves episodes of depression alternating with episodes of mania. Mania is characterized by excessive central nervous system (CNS) stimulation with physical and mental hyperactivity (e.g., agitation, constant talking, constant movement, grandiose ideas, impulsiveness, inflated self-esteem, little need for sleep, poor concentration, racing thoughts, short attention span) for at least 1 week. Symptoms are similar to those of acute psychosis or schizophrenia. Hypomania involves the same symptoms, but they are less severe, indicate less CNS stimulation and hyperactivity, and last 3 or 4 days.

## Cyclothymia

Cyclothymia is a mild type of bipolar disorder that involves periods of hypomania and depression that do not meet the criteria for mania and major depression. Symptoms must be present for at least 2 years. It does not usually require drug therapy.

twice as often as men. According to the National Institutes of Health (2020), depression is not a normal part of aging. However, it is a common problem among older adults. Life changes are great contributors to depression in the older adult—for example, acute and chronic health problems, or the death of a spouse, significant others, relatives, or close friends. Depression has no particular racial affinity.

## Etiology and Pathophysiology

Extensive study has demonstrated that depression results from interactions among several complex factors. Causes involve the immune system, monoamine neurotransmitter dysfunction, and neuroendocrine factors, as well as genetic and environmental factors.

### Immune Factors

Immune cells (e.g., T lymphocytes, B lymphocytes) produce cytokines (e.g., interleukins, interferons, tumor necrosis factor), which affect neurotransmission. Possible mechanisms of cytokine-induced depression include increased corticotropin-releasing factor (CRF) and activation of the hypothalamic–pituitary–adrenal (HPA) axis, alteration of monoamine neurotransmitters in several areas of the brain, or cytokines functioning as neurotransmitters and exerting direct effects on brain function.

### Monoamine Neurotransmitter Dysfunction

Depression is thought to result from a deficiency of norepinephrine and/or serotonin. This hypothesis has stemmed from studies demonstrating that antidepressant drugs increase the amounts of norepinephrine and/or serotonin in the central nervous system (CNS) synapse by inhibiting their reuptake into the presynaptic neuron. Serotonin helps regulate mood, sleep, appetite, energy level, and cognitive and psychomotor functions, which are disturbed in depression.

Emphasis shifted toward receptors because the neurotransmitter view did not explain why the amounts of neurotransmitter increased within hours after single doses of a drug, but relief of depression occurred only after weeks of drug therapy. Researchers identified desensitization in norepinephrine and serotonin receptors (down-regulation) with chronic antidepressant drug therapy. Apparently, long-term administration of antidepressant drugs produces complex changes in the sensitivities of both presynaptic and postsynaptic receptor sites.

Overall, there is increasing awareness that balance, integration, and interactions among norepinephrine, serotonin, and possibly other neurotransmission systems (e.g., dopamine, acetylcholine) are probably more important etiologic factors than single neurotransmitter or receptor alterations.

### Neuroendocrine Factors

In addition to monoamine neurotransmission systems, researchers have identified nonmonoamine systems that influence neurotransmission and are significantly altered in depression. A major nonmonoamine is CRF, whose secretion is increased in people with depression. CRF-secreting neurons are widespread in the CNS, and CRF apparently functions as a neurotransmitter and mediator of the endocrine, autonomic, immune, and behavioral responses to stress as well as a releasing factor for corticotropin. The subsequent increase in cortisol by the adrenal cortex (part of the normal physiologic response to stress) is thought to decrease the numbers or sensitivity of cortisol receptors

(down-regulation) and lead to depression. This alteration of cortisol receptors takes about 2 weeks, the approximate time interval required for the drugs to improve symptoms of depression. Extrahypothalamic CRF is also increased in depression. Secretion of both hypothalamic and extrahypothalamic CRF apparently returns to normal with recovery from depression.

### Other Factors

Genetic factors are important because the link between genetics and depression suggests that a close relative of a depressed person is more likely to inherit the disease than the general population. Twin studies support this conclusion.

Environmental factors include stressful life events, such as physical or sexual abuse in childhood, which apparently alter brain structure and function and contribute to the development of depression in some people. Experts have identified changes in CRF, the HPA axis, and the noradrenergic neurotransmission system, which are thought to cause a hypersensitive or exaggerated response to later stressful events, including mild stress or daily life events.

## Clinical Manifestations

Box 55.1 outlines the clinical manifestations of depression. Behavioral changes, especially anxiety, agitation, panic attacks, insomnia, irritability, hostility, impulsivity, akathisia, hypomania, and mania, may indicate worsening depression or suicidality.

## Drug Therapy

Antidepressant therapy may be indicated if depressive symptoms persist at least 2 weeks, impair social relationships or work performance, and occur independently of life events. Antidepressants are used to regulate mood specifically affecting serotonin, norepinephrine, and dopamine. Antidepressant effects are attributed to changes in receptors rather than changes in neurotransmitters. Although some of the drugs act more selectively on one neurotransmission system than another initially, this selectivity seems to be lost with chronic administration. Drugs used in the pharmacologic management of depressive disorders are derived from several chemical groups. Older antidepressants include the tricyclic antidepressants (TCAs) and the monoamine oxidase (MAO) inhibitors. Newer drugs include the selective serotonin reuptake inhibitors (SSRIs), the serotonin–norepinephrine reuptake inhibitors (SNRIs), and several adjuvant atypical antidepressant drugs that differ from TCAs and MAO inhibitors. As the name implies, reuptake inhibitors block the reuptake of certain neurotransmitters (serotonin with the SSRIs and serotonin and norepinephrine with the SNRIs). Table 55.1 lists the drugs used to treat depression. The mood-stabilizing section lists some atypical antipsychotics.

General characteristics of antidepressants include the following:

- All are effective in relieving depression, but they differ in their adverse effects.
- People must take them for 2 to 4 weeks before depressive symptoms improve.
- Administration is oral. Absorbed from the small bowel, they enter the portal circulation and circulate through the liver, where they undergo extensive first-pass metabolism before reaching the systemic circulation.

## TABLE 55.1

## Drugs Administered for the Treatment of Depression

| Drug Class | Prototype | Other Drugs in the Class |
|---|---|---|
| **Antidepressants** | | |
| Tricyclic antidepressants | Imipramine | Amitriptyline<br>Amoxapine<br>Clomipramine (Anafranil)<br>Desipramine (Norpramin)<br>Doxepin (Silenor)<br>Nortriptyline (Pamelor)<br>Protriptyline hydrochloride<br>Trimipramine |
| Selective serotonin reuptake inhibitors (SSRIs) | Fluoxetine (PROzac, Sarafem) | Citalopram (Celexa)<br>Escitalopram (Lexapro)<br>Fluvoxamine (Luvox)<br>Paroxetine (Paxil, Paxil CR, Brisdelle, Pexeva)<br>Sertraline (Zoloft)<br>Vilazodone (Viibryd, Viibryd Starter Pack) |
| Serotonin–norepinephrine reuptake inhibitors (SNRIs) | Venlafaxine (Effexor XR) | Desvenlafaxine (Pristiq)<br>Duloxetine (Cymbalta, Drizalma Sprinkle)<br>Levomilnacipran (Fetzima, Fetzima Titration)<br>Milnacipran (Savella, Savella Titration Pack)<br>Nefazodone |
| Monoamine oxidase (MAO) inhibitors | Phenelzine (Nardil) | Isocarboxazid (Marplan)<br>Selegiline hydrochloride (Emsam, Zelapar)<br>Tranylcypromine (Parnate) |
| Atypical antidepressants | | Bupropion (Aplenzin, Wellbutrin SR, Wellbutrin XL)<br>Mirtazapine (Remeron)<br>Trazodone |
| Mood-stabilizing agents | Lithium carbonate (Lithobid) | Aripiprazole (Abilify, Abilify Maintena, Abilify MyCite)<br>Olanzapine (ZyPREXA, ZyPREXA Relprew, ZyPREXA Zydis)<br>Quetiapine (Seroquel)<br>Olanzapine–fluoxetine (Symbyax)<br>Risperidone (Perseris, RisperDAL, RisperDAL Consta)<br>Ziprasidone (Geodon) |

- Metabolism is by the cytochrome P450 (CYP) enzymes in the liver. Thus, antidepressants may interact with each other and with a wide variety of drugs that are normally metabolized by the same subgroups of enzymes. Additionally, there is a documented ethnic variation (ethnopharmacology) in response to antidepressants (Box 55.2).

Because the available drugs have similar efficacy in treating depression, the choice of an antidepressant depends on the patient's age; medical condition; previous history of drug response, if any; and the specific drug's adverse effects. Also, prescribers often use the side effect profile to help determine the best choice for a specific patient. In addition, cost is a factor to consider. Although the newer drugs are much more expensive than the TCAs, they may be more cost-effective overall because TCAs are more likely to cause serious adverse effects, they require monitoring of plasma drug levels and electrocardiograms (ECGs), and patients are more likely to stop taking them.

It is important to note that sudden termination of most antidepressants results in **antidepressant discontinuation syndrome**. In general, symptoms, which include flulike symptoms,

insomnia, nausea, imbalance, sensory disturbances, and hyperarousal, develop more rapidly and may be more intense with drugs that have a short half-life and/or that are given for long periods. As with other psychotropic drugs, to avoid this syndrome, it is essential to taper the dosage of the antidepressant and discontinue it gradually, over 6 to 8 weeks, unless severe drug toxicity, anaphylactic reaction, or another life-threatening condition is present. The occurrence of withdrawal symptoms may indicate skipped doses or abrupt discontinuation of the drug.

## OVERVIEW OF BIPOLAR DISORDER

**Bipolar disorder** is a condition in which people alternate between periods of depression and overexcitement. There are two subtypes of this disorder, which are defined by the presentation of the mood disorder. Bipolar disorder type I is characterized by episodes of major depression plus **mania** (euphoria or irritability) and occurs equally in men and women. Bipolar disorder type II is characterized by episodes of major depression plus episodes of **hypomania** (persistent irritable mood but absence of euphoria) and occurs more frequently in women. Bipolar spectrum disorder broadens the definition of bipolar disorder to include conditions such as **cyclothymia** (a mild type of bipolar disorder) and **dysthymia** (chronically depressed mood). Bipolar disorders may affect an estimated 4.4% of people in the United States.

## Etiology and Pathophysiology

Like depression, mania, and hypomania, the hallmarks of bipolar disorder have historically been associated with abnormal functioning of neurotransmitters or receptors, such as a relative excess of excitatory neurotransmitters (e.g., norepinephrine) or a relative deficiency of inhibitory neurotransmitters (e.g., gamma-aminobutyric acid [GABA]). Another more recent proposed etiology for bipolar disorder is alteration in neuronal growth and survival in areas of the brain (e.g., subgenual precortex, hippocampus) involved with mood and memory. Secondary causes of manic and hypomanic behavior include drugs that stimulate the CNS, CNS diseases and infections, and electrolyte or endocrine disorders. Patients with acute bipolar major depression or mania may require maintenance therapy with medications and psychotherapy. Patients may also require neuromodulation therapies, which include electroconvulsive therapy, magnetic seizure therapy, repetitive transcranial magnetic stimulation, or cranial electrical stimulation.

## Clinical Manifestations

Bipolar disorder manifests with unpredictable mood swings. In the manic phase, clinical manifestations include excessive happiness and energy, excitement, racing thoughts, restlessness, decreased need for sleep, high sex drive, and a tendency to make grandiose statements and unattainable plans. During a depressive episode, manifestations include sadness, lack of energy, increased need for sleep, uncontrollable crying, changes in appetite, and thoughts of suicide. Box 55.1 outlines additional symptoms.

## Drug Therapy

Research has shown that mood-stabilizing drugs such as lithium stimulate neuronal growth and reduce brain atrophy in people with long-standing mood disorders. Table 55.1 lists some mood-stabilizing drugs.

## TRICYCLIC ANTIDEPRESSANTS

TCAs are the oldest antidepressants, although they are now second-line drugs for the treatment of depression. ⓟ **Imipramine** is the prototype. A patient's previous response or susceptibility to adverse effects may be the basis for initial selection of TCAs. For example, if a patient (or a close family member) once responded well to a particular drug, that drug is probably the drug of choice for repeated episodes of depression. The response of family members to individual drugs may be significant because there is a strong genetic component to depression and drug response. If therapeutic effects do not occur within 4 weeks, it is probably necessary to discontinue or change the TCA, because some patients tolerate or respond better to one TCA than to another. For patients with suicidal tendencies, beginning an SSRI or another newer drug is preferred over a TCA due to the safety profile.

## Pharmacokinetics

Imipramine is well absorbed after oral administration, and the drug is widely distributed in body tissues. Peak levels occur in 2 to 6 hours, and the duration of action is unknown. Its half-life is 8 to 21 hours. Imipramine is metabolized in the liver by CYP2D6 enzymes to the active metabolite, desipramine, and inactive metabolites. It goes through significant first-pass metabolism. Imipramine is excreted primarily in the urine as metabolites.

## Action

Imipramine blocks the reuptake of norepinephrine and serotonin at the presynaptic nerve endings, increasing the action of both neurotransmitters. The drug's use in enuresis may be due to the fact that imipramine also blocks acetylcholine receptors.

## Use

Imipramine may be useful in the treatment of depression. Prescribers may order it for children and adolescents in the management of **enuresis** (bed wetting or involuntary urination resulting from a physical or psychological disorder) after physical causes (e.g., urethral irritation, excessive intake of fluids) have been ruled out. Table 55.2 contains route and dosage information for imipramine and the other TCAs.

**TABLE 55.2**

## DRUGS AT A GLANCE: Tricyclic Antidepressants

| Drug | Pregnancy Category | Routes and Dosage Ranges | |
|---|---|---|---|
| | | **Adults** | **Children** |
| Ⓟ Imipramine | D | 75 mg PO daily initially in divided doses or a single bedtime dose, gradually increased to 150 mg daily if necessary; maintenance dose, 05–150 mg PO daily; max dosage of 200 mg daily<br>Older adults: PO 25–50 mg daily at bedtime, increased to max dosage of 100 mg daily if necessary | ≥8 y: 1.5 mg/kg/d in 2–3 divided doses; max daily dosage 5 mg/kg/d<br>Adolescents: 25–50 mg PO daily in divided doses, increased to max dosage of 100 mg daily if necessary<br>Children >6 y (enuresis): 25–50 mg PO 1 h before bedtime |
| Amitriptyline (✹ AG-Amitriptyline, Amitriptyline-10, Amitriptyline-25, APO-Amitriptyline, JAMP-Amitriptyline) | C | 25–50 mg PO initially once daily at bedtime or in divided doses, gradually increased to 100–300 mg daily if necessary<br>Older adults: 10 mg PO three times daily and 20 mg at bedtime | Adolescents: 10 mg PO three times daily and 20 mg at bedtime |
| Amoxapine | C | 50 mg PO three times daily; may be increased to 100 mg 2–3 times daily by the end of the first week based on response and tolerability; may be titrated to 600 mg daily in divided doses | Not approved for use in children |
| Clomipramine (Anafranil; ✹ Anafranil) | C | Obsessive–compulsive disorder: 25 mg PO daily, increased to 100 mg daily by end of 2 wk, in divided doses, with meals; give maintenance dose in a single dose at bedtime; max dose 250 mg daily | ≥10 y: 25 mg PO initially daily, increased to 3 mg/kg/d or 200 mg/d, whichever is less, over 2 wk. Give maintenance dose in a single dose at bedtime. Max dose 3 mg/kg or 200 mg, whichever is less |
| Desipramine (Norpramin; ✹ Dom-Desipramine, Nu-Desipramine) | C | 25–50 mg PO daily in divided doses or as a single daily dose; usual maintenance dose 100–200 once daily or in divided doses; max dose 300 mg/d<br>Older adults: 25–100 mg PO daily in divided doses or as a single daily dose; max dose 150 mg/d | Not approved in pediatric patients (children)<br>Adolescents: 25–100 mg PO daily in divided doses or as a single daily dose; max dose 150 mg/d |
| Doxepin (Silenor; ✹ NOVO-Doxepin, Silenor, SINEquan) | C | 25–50 mg PO initially daily in divided doses or a single dose at bedtime; max dose 300 mg/d | 7–11 y: 1–3 mg/kg/d in single or divided doses<br>≥12 y: 25–75 mg/d PO initially at bedtime or in 2–3 divided doses; max single dose 150 mg or 300 mg daily |
| Nortriptyline (Pamelor; ✹ APO-Nortriptyline, Aventyl) | D | 25 mg PO three or four times daily or in a single dose (75–100 mg) at bedtime; max dose 150 mg/d<br>Older adults: 30–50 mg/d PO in divided doses or a single dose once daily | 6–12 y: 1–3 mg/kg/d in 4 divided doses; max dose 150 mg/d<br>Adolescents: 30–50 mg/d PO in 3–4 divided doses or a single dose once daily; max dose 150 mg/d |
| Protriptyline hydrochloride | Adverse events have not been reported in animal reproduction studies | 10–20 mg PO divided in 3–4 doses; gradually increase based on response | Adolescents: 5 mg PO three times per day; gradually titrate based on response; maximum dose 60 mg/d |
| Trimipramine (✹ APO-Trimipramine) | C | 25–50 mg PO daily at bedtime or in divided doses; initial doses 100 mg PO daily for hospitalized patients | Not recommended for children |

### Use in Children

TCAs are more toxic in overdose than other antidepressants, and suicide is a leading cause of death in adolescents. The U.S. Food and Drug Administration (FDA) has issued a BLACK BOX WARNING ◆ alerting health care providers to the increased risk of suicidal ideation in children, adolescents, and young adults 18 to 24 years of age who are taking antidepressants, including imipramine.

However, in clinical trials, imipramine and other TCAs have not been shown to be superior to placebo for the treatment of depression in children and adolescents. TCAs are not recommended as first-line agents, although they may be beneficial in patients with attention deficit hyperactivity disorder or enuresis.

### Use in Older Adults

Imipramine may cause or aggravate conditions common in older adults (e.g., cardiac conduction abnormalities, urinary retention, narrow-angle glaucoma). In addition, impaired compensatory mechanisms make older adults more likely to experience anticholinergic effects, confusion, orthostatic hypotension, and sedation. It is important to monitor vital signs, serum drug levels, and ECGs regularly.

### Use in Patients With Hepatic Impairment

Hepatic impairment leads to higher plasma levels of imipramine. Thus, caution is necessary in patients with severe liver impairment.

**QSEN Alert: Evidence-Based Practice**

In a study conducted by Stanford, Jones, and Hudson (2018), a longitudinal community sample was obtained to examine the complexity in adolescent self-harm risk factors. The researchers compared new self-harm rates over a 6-month period across different psychological profiles. Adolescent self-harm poses concerns for a young adult's general mental health. In this study, three components of individual psychological variables were identified: poor coping, impulsivity, and high anxiety. To assist adolescents in coping strategies, mental health providers and school officials should build supportive environments. Multifaceted mental health programs should be developed for adolescents. One important factor to include is the effect bullying has on the adolescent's mental health.

### Use in Patients With Critical Illness

Adverse effects common with imipramine use (e.g., confusion, dysrhythmias, tachycardia, orthostatic hypotension, urinary retention) are a concern and may further compromise patients who are critically ill. Antidepressants, including imipramine, warrant very cautious use perioperatively because of the risk of serious adverse effects and interactions with anesthetics and other commonly used drugs. It is necessary to discontinue imipramine several days before elective surgery and resume it several days after surgery.

### Use in Patients Receiving Home Care

The nurse who sees a patient taking imipramine in the home setting should assess him or her for improvement of symptoms, appropriate administration of the drug, and management of adverse effects, particularly safety factors. A nurse visiting the home for other reasons should observe for signs of depression; health concerns may precipitate symptoms.

## Adverse Effects

Adverse effects of imipramine include sedation, orthostatic hypotension, cardiac dysrhythmias, anticholinergic symptoms (e.g., blurred vision, dry mouth, constipation, urinary retention), and weight gain. Symptoms of TCA overdose occur 1 to 4 hours after drug ingestion. They consist primarily of CNS depression and cardiovascular effects (e.g., nystagmus, tremor, restlessness, seizures, hypotension, dysrhythmias, myocardial depression). Death usually results from cardiac, respiratory, and circulatory failure.

TCAs are associated with clearly defined withdrawal syndromes, and these drugs also have strong anticholinergic effects. When they are abruptly discontinued, cholinergic rebound may occur. Symptoms include hypersalivation, diarrhea, urinary urgency, abdominal cramping, and sweating.

## Contraindications

Contraindications to imipramine include known sensitivity to the drug and immediately postacute myocardial infarction.

## Nursing Implications

### Preventing Interactions

Several drugs interact with imipramine. The drug may inhibit the metabolism of other drugs, including antidepressants, phenothiazines, carbamazepine, flecainide, and propafenone. The use of imipramine and MAO inhibitors concurrently may have serious effects, including severe seizures and death. Alcohol may increase the sedative effects of imipramine. The herb St. John's wort may reduce the blood levels of imipramine and other TCAs. Grapefruit juice can inhibit the metabolism of imipramine and other TCAs.

### Administering the Medication

People should take imipramine at bedtime to aid sleep and decrease daytime sedation. Overall, with TCAs, it is best to begin with small doses, which are increased to the desired dose over 1 to 2 weeks. Administration once or twice daily is possible because the drug has a long elimination half-life. Measurement of plasma levels is helpful in adjusting drug dosages. Imipramine, like other TCAs, should not be administered with grapefruit juice.

### Assessing for Therapeutic Effects

The nurse is aware of patient statements about feeling better or less depressed. He or she observes for increased appetite, physical activity, and interest in surroundings; improved sleep patterns; improved appearance; decreased anxiety; and decreased somatic complaints. Mood elevation may take 2 to 3 weeks or longer. Note that it may even take 4 to 8 weeks of treatment before a patient may experience a response, partial response, or no response to imipramine.

### Assessing for Adverse Effects

The nurse observes for CNS effects, gastrointestinal (GI) effects, cardiovascular effects, and other effects. Because imipramine may have adverse effects on the heart, especially in overdose, experts recommend baseline and follow-up ECGs for all patients. In addition, it is important to assess for suicidal thoughts or plans, especially at the beginning of therapy or when dosages are increased or decreased.

### Patient Teaching

Box 55.3 presents patient teaching guidelines for the antidepressants, including the TCAs.

## Other Drugs in the Class

Commonly used TCAs include amitriptyline, clomipramine (Anafranil), desipramine (Norpramin), doxepin (Silenor), and nortriptyline (Pamelor). Amitriptyline, desipramine, and nortriptyline are the TCAs most commonly prescribed to treat

---

 **BOX 55.3**    *Patient Teaching Guidelines for Antidepressants*

**General Considerations**

- Take antidepressants as directed to maximize therapeutic benefits and minimize adverse effects. Do not alter doses when symptoms subside. Antidepressants are usually given for several months, perhaps years.
- Therapeutic effects (relief of symptoms) may not occur for 2 to 4 weeks after drug therapy is started. As a result, it is very important not to think the drug is ineffective and stop taking it prematurely. Continue to take the drug even if you feel better to prevent the return of depression.
- Do not take other prescription or over-the-counter drugs, including cold remedies, without consulting a health care provider. Potentially serious drug interactions may occur.
- Do not take the herbal supplement St. John's wort while taking a prescription antidepressant. Serious interactions may occur.
- Inform any physician, surgeon, dentist, or nurse practitioner about the antidepressants being taken. Potentially serious adverse effects or drug interactions may occur if certain other drugs are prescribed.
- Avoid activities that require alertness and physical coordination (e.g., driving a car, operating other machinery) until reasonably sure the medication does not make you drowsy or impair your ability to perform the activities safely.
- Avoid alcohol and other CNS depressants (e.g., any drugs that cause drowsiness). Excessive drowsiness, dizziness, difficulty breathing, and low blood pressure may occur, with potentially serious consequences.
- Learn the name and type of the prescribed antidepressant to help avoid undesirable interactions with other drugs or a physician prescribing other drugs with similar effects. There are several different types of antidepressants, with different characteristics and precautions for safe and effective usage.
- Do not stop taking any antidepressant without discussing it with a health care provider. If a problem occurs, the type of drug, the dose, or other aspects may be changed to solve the problem and allow continued use of the medication.
- Counseling, support groups, relaxation techniques, and other nonpharmacologic treatments are recommended along with drug therapy.
- Notify your physician if you become pregnant or intend to become pregnant during therapy with antidepressants.

**Self or Caregiver Administration**

- With a tricyclic antidepressant (e.g., amitriptyline), take at bedtime to aid sleep and decrease adverse effects.

Also, report urinary retention, fainting, irregular heartbeat, seizures, restlessness, and mental confusion. These are potentially serious adverse drug effects.

- With a selective serotonin reuptake inhibitor, take the drug in the morning because it may interfere with sleep if taken at bedtime.
  - In addition, notify a health care provider if a skin rash or other allergic reaction occurs. Allergic reactions are uncommon but may require that the drug be discontinued.
  - Recognize the importance of follow-up and seeking professional help for the signs of dizziness or insomnia or other symptoms that negatively affect your life.
- Realize that escitalopram (Lexapro) is a derivative of citalopram (Celexa). The two medications should not be taken concomitantly.
- With venlafaxine (Effexor), take as directed or ask for instructions. This drug is often taken twice daily. Notify a health care provider if a skin rash or other allergic reaction occurs. An allergic reaction may require that the drug be discontinued.
- With venlafaxine, use effective birth control methods while taking this drug. Pregnancy is a contraindication.
- With duloxetine and desvenlafaxine, swallow the medication whole; do not crush, chew, or sprinkle capsule contents on food.
- With phenelzine and other monoamine oxidase inhibitors, foods that contain tyramine or tyrosine may have to be avoided altogether to prevent the risk of hypertensive crisis. This includes aged cheeses, coffee, chocolate, wine, bananas, avocados, fava beans, and most fermented and pickled foods.
- Bupropion is a unique drug prescribed for depression (brand name, Wellbutrin) and for smoking cessation (brand name, Zyban). It is extremely important not to increase the dose or take the two brand names at the same time (as might happen with different physicians or filling prescriptions at different pharmacies). Overdoses may cause seizures as well as other adverse effects. When used for smoking cessation, Zyban is recommended for up to 12 weeks if progress is being made. If significant progress is not made by approximately 7 weeks, it is considered unlikely that longer drug use will be helpful.
- There are short-, intermediate-, and long-acting forms of bupropion that are taken three times, two times, or one time per day, respectively. Be sure to take your medication as prescribed by your physician.
- Make sure that you and the people you live with are familiar with the signs and symptoms of worsening depression and know how to seek help for signs of overdose.

depression in children older than 12 years of age although they are not first-line agents. The FDA has approved clomipramine for treatment of obsessive–compulsive disorder in children. In general, amitriptyline, clomipramine, desipramine, doxepin, and nortriptyline are similar to imipramine in terms of adverse effects. Amitriptyline and doxepin are more likely to cause weight gain. Desipramine is more likely to cause drowsiness. These TCAs are effective; however, antidepressants that produce fewer adverse effects are increasingly replacing them.

Amoxapine is used to relieve symptoms of depression in patients with reactive or neurotic disorders. It is also effective in treating endogenous and psychotic disorders. According to the Beers criteria, amoxapine should be avoided in patients older than 65 years because this drug has strong anticholinergic properties that produce sedation and orthostatic hypotension.

Trimipramine is used for depression in adults. This drug also has strong anticholinergic properties. It can be used in the geriatric population; the dose is 50 mg daily, which can be increased to 100 mg daily. The lowest effective dose should be administered at bedtime. It is necessary to monitor blood pressure and pulse rate with initial therapy.

## NCLEX Success

1. Which of the following adverse effects of the imipramine is considered the most serious?
   A. dry mouth
   B. constipation
   C. urinary retention
   D. orthostatic hypotension

2. A man has been taking imipramine for 1 week for depression. He tells the nurse that he is going to stop taking this medication because it is not working. The best response is which of the following?
   A. "Contact your prescriber about taking a different antidepressant medication."
   B. "It may take up to 4 weeks before this medication makes you feel better."
   C. "You should slowly taper rather than suddenly discontinue this medication."
   D. "You should take an extra dose today to build up your blood level and get faster results."

## SELECTIVE SEROTONIN REUPTAKE INHIBITORS

SSRIs, of which **fluoxetine** (PROzac, Sarafem) is the prototype, produce fewer serious adverse effects than the TCAs. (SSRIs are called "selective" because they seem to primarily affect serotonin and not other neurotransmitters.) The drugs of first choice in the treatment of depression, SSRIs are effective and usually produce fewer and milder adverse effects than other antidepressants. There are no guidelines for choosing one SSRI over another.

## Pharmacokinetics

Fluoxetine is well absorbed with oral administration, with a peak of action of 6 to 8 hours. The half-life of elimination for the parent drug is 2 to 3 days; this may lead to accumulation with chronic administration. (An active metabolite has a half-life of 7 to 9 days.) Thus, steady-state blood levels are achieved slowly, over several weeks, and drug effects decrease slowly (over 2 to 3 months) when fluoxetine is discontinued. The drug is present in breast milk. Metabolism takes place in the liver, and excretion predominately occurs in the kidneys.

## Action

Fluoxetine blocks the reabsorption of the neurotransmitter serotonin in the brain. This helps elevate the patient's mood. Fluoxetine has no effect on the norepinephrine or dopamine.

## Use

Uses for fluoxetine include the treatment of depression and its associated anxiety, obsessive–compulsive disorder, bulimia nervosa, and premenstrual dysphoric disorder. Table 55.3 gives the route and dosage information for fluoxetine and other SSRIs.

### Use in Children

The FDA has issued a **BLACK BOX WARNING ◆** alerting health care providers to the increased risk of suicidal ideation in children, adolescents, and young adults 18 to 24 years of age when taking antidepressant medications, including fluoxetine.

### Use in Older Adults

Fluoxetine and other SSRIs are the drugs of choice in older adults because they produce fewer sedative, anticholinergic, cardiotoxic, and psychomotor adverse effects than the TCAs and related antidepressants. Elimination may be slower, and smaller or less frequent doses may be prudent in older adults. Weight loss is often associated with SSRIs and may be undesirable in older adults. Use of maintenance antidepressant therapy is beneficial to prevent recurrence of depression in older adults.

### Use in Patients With Hepatic Impairment

Hepatic impairment leads to reduced first-pass metabolism of fluoxetine and most antidepressant drugs, resulting in higher plasma levels. Thus, caution is warranted in severe liver impairment.

### Use in Patients With Critical Illness

Patients who are critically ill may need a drug to combat the depression that often develops with major illness. The decision to start fluoxetine should involve a thorough assessment of the patient's condition, other drugs being given, and potential adverse drug effects.

Antidepressants, including imipramine, warrant caution perioperatively because of the risk of serious adverse effects and adverse interactions with anesthetics and other commonly used drugs.

## Adverse Effects

Adverse effects of fluoxetine include a high incidence of GI symptoms (e.g., nausea, diarrhea, and weight loss) and sexual dysfunction (e.g., delayed ejaculation in men, impaired orgasmic ability in women). Most SSRIs also cause some degree of CNS stimulation (e.g., anxiety, nervousness, insomnia), which is most prominent with fluoxetine. These drugs are also associated

**TABLE 55.3**

## DRUGS AT A GLANCE: Selective Serotonin Reuptake Inhibitors (SSRIs)

| Drug | Pregnancy Category | Routes and Dosage Ranges | |
|---|---|---|---|
| | | **Adults** | **Children** |
| **Fluoxetine** (PROzac, Sarafem; ❈ AG-Fluoxetine, APO-Fluoxetine) | C | 20 mg PO once daily in the morning, increased after several weeks if necessary. Give doses larger than 20 mg once in the morning or in two divided doses, morning and noon. Max daily dose 60 mg <br> Prozac weekly (delayed-release capsules) 90 mg PO once each week, starting 7 d after the last 20-mg dose | 8–17 y for depression: 10–20 mg/d PO; may increase to 20 mg/d after 1 wk if necessary |
| Citalopram (Celexa; ❈ ACCEL-Citalopram, ACT-Citalopram, AG-Citalopram, AURO-Citalopram) | C | 20 mg PO initially once daily, morning or evening, increased to max dose of 40 mg daily in 1 wk, if necessary <br> Elderly/hepatic impairment: 20 mg PO daily | Not approved for use in children and adolescents |
| Escitalopram (Lexapro; ❈ ACH-Escitalopram, Cipralex) | C | 10 mg PO once daily; may increase to max dose of 20 mg after minimum of 1 wk of therapy | ≥12 y: 10 mg PO once daily; may increase to max dose of 20 mg if symptoms do not lessen within 3 wk of therapy |
| Paroxetine (Paxil, Paxil CR, Brisdelle, Pexeva; ❈ ACT-PARoxetine, AG-Paroxetine, APO-PARoxetine, Auro-PARoxetine, DOM-PARoxetine, Paxil, Paxil CR, Sandoz PARoxetine) | D | 20 mg PO once daily in the morning, increased at 1 wk or longer intervals, if necessary; usual range 20–50 mg/d; max dose 50 mg/d <br> Controlled-release (CR) tablets: 25 mg PO once daily in the morning, increase up to 62.5 mg/d max if necessary <br> Elderly or debilitated adults: 10 mg PO once daily, increase if necessary; maximum dose 40 mg <br> Severe renal or hepatic impairment: same as for older adults | Not approved for use in children and adolescents |
| Sertraline (Zoloft; ❈ AG-Sertraline, APO-Sertraline, Auro-Sertraline MINT-Sertraline, Mylan-Sertraline, Zoloft) | C | Depression, OCD: 50 mg PO once daily morning or evening, increase at 1-wk or longer intervals to a max daily dose of 200 mg <br> Panic disorder, PTSD: 25 mg PO once daily, increase after 1 wk to 50 mg once daily; max dosage 200 mg daily | OCD: ≥6 y, 25 mg PO once daily, increase dose in increments of 25–50 mg to a max daily dose of 200 mg <br> Adolescents: 50 mg PO once daily, increase dose in increments of 25–50 mg to a max daily dose of 200 mg |
| Vilazodone (Viibryd, Viibryd Starter Pack; ❈ Viibryd, Viibryd Starter Pack) | Nonteratogenic effects in the newborn following SSRI exposure | Major depressive disorder: 10 mg PO once daily for 7 days, then increase to 20 mg once daily, maximum dose: 40 mg once daily | Not approved in children |

OCD, obsessive–convulsive disorder; PTSD, posttraumatic stress disorder.

with increased risk of GI bleeding. For patients with diabetes mellitus, SSRIs may have a hypoglycemic effect.

**Serotonin syndrome**, a serious and sometimes fatal reaction characterized by hypertensive crisis, hyperpyrexia, extreme agitation progressing to delirium and coma, muscle rigidity, and seizures, may occur due to combined therapy with an SSRI and an MAO inhibitor or another drug that potentiates serotonin neurotransmission. It is important not to take an SSRI or SNRI

and an MAO inhibitor concurrently or within 2 weeks of each other. In most cases, if a patient taking an SSRI is transferred to an MAO inhibitor, it is necessary to discontinue the SSRI at least 14 days before starting the MAO inhibitor. However, the patient should discontinue fluoxetine at least 5 weeks before starting an MAO inhibitor due to the prolonged half-life.

As previously discussed, antidepressant discontinuation syndrome can occur with sudden termination of the SSRIs.

Withdrawal symptoms include dizziness, GI upset, lethargy or anxiety/hyperarousal, dysphoria, sleep problems, and headache, which can last from several days to several weeks. More serious symptoms may include aggression, hypomania, mood disturbances, and suicidal tendencies. Fluoxetine, with its long half-life, has not been associated with withdrawal symptoms.

## Contraindications

Contraindications to fluoxetine include known sensitivity to the drug as well as the use of MAO inhibitors or thioridazine.

 **QSEN Alert: Safety**

People of any age who have attempted suicide should not receive fluoxetine.

## Nursing Implications

### Preventing Interactions

Because fluoxetine and other SSRIs are highly bound to plasma proteins, they compete with endogenous compounds and other medications for binding sites, resulting in drug interactions. Several drugs increase the effects of fluoxetine (Box 55.4). Also, CYP2D6 enzymes metabolize fluoxetine; therefore, the drug may cause accumulation of other drugs using this enzyme system (e.g., amitriptyline, imipramine, desipramine, thioridazine).

 **QSEN Alert: Safety**

In addition, fluoxetine can prevent the conversion of codeine to its active form, resulting in lack of pain relief when the drugs are used concurrently.

### Administering the Medication

People typically take SSRIs, including fluoxetine, once daily in the morning to prevent interference with sleep. They may take the drug with food to avoid GI upset. The nurse advises the patient to use sugar-free gum or hard candies to counteract dry mouth.

 **BOX 55.4** **Drug Interactions: Fluoxetine**

**Drugs That Increase the Effects of Fluoxetine**
- Alcohol
  *Increases the sedative effect*
- Amiodarone, cimetidine, ciprofloxacin, cytochrome P450 2D6 inhibitors [e.g., opioid analgesics, beta-adrenergic blockers, promethazine], and macrolide antibiotics
  *Increase the risk of toxicity*
- Haloperidol
  *Increases the risk of neurologic toxicity*
- 5-Hydroxytryptophan
  *Increases the risk of serotonin syndrome*

### Assessing for Therapeutic Effects

The nurse assesses for statements of improved depression. He or she assesses improvement in appetite, physical activity, and interest in surroundings; improved sleep patterns; improved appearance; decreased anxiety; and reduced somatic complaints. The patient response to fluoxetine can significantly vary from patient to patient. The full response of the medication may not be seen for 8 to 12 weeks. Therapeutic serum levels of fluoxetine range from 100 to 800 ng/mL.

### Assessing for Adverse Effects

The nurse assesses for dizziness, headache, nervousness, insomnia, nausea, diarrhea, dry mouth, sedation, skin rash, and sexual dysfunction.

 **QSEN Alert: Safety**

It is essential to assess for suicidal thoughts or plans, especially at the beginning of therapy or when dosages are increased or decreased.

### Patient Teaching

Box 55.3 contains patient teaching guidelines for the antidepressants, including the SSRIs.

## Other Drugs in the Class

Other SSRIs include citalopram (Celexa), escitalopram (Lexapro), paroxetine (Paxil), sertraline (Zoloft), and vilazodone (Viibryd, Viibryd Starter Pack).

Sertraline and citalopram also have active metabolites, but paroxetine, like fluoxetine, is more likely to accumulate. Escitalopram, paroxetine, and sertraline reach steady-state concentrations in 1 to 2 weeks. People may take the drugs in the morning or evening (but at the same time each day). An evening dose may interfere with sleep. The SSRIs are strong inhibitors of the CYP enzyme system, which metabolizes many drugs. As a result, serum drug levels and risks of adverse effects are greatly increased. Most significantly, fluoxetine, paroxetine, and sertraline slow metabolism of bupropion, codeine, desipramine, dextromethorphan, flecainide, metoprolol, nortriptyline, phenothiazines, propranolol, risperidone, and timolol. Vilazodone can produce discontinuation syndrome; its abrupt discontinuation or interruption will produce symptoms including nausea, vomiting, diarrhea, headache, lightheadedness, sweating, chills, tremors, paresthesias, somnolence, and sleep disturbances. Discontinuation of antidepressant treatment should last for >3 weeks.

 **QSEN Alert: Safety**

With citalopram and escitalopram, poor metabolizers of CYP2C19 or concurrent use of moderate-to-strong CYP2C19 inhibitors [e.g., cimetidine, chloramphenicol, omeprazole] should receive half the maximum dose [20 mg] daily.

Paroxetine, which has a half-life of approximately 24 hours and does not produce active metabolites, may be associated with antidepressant discontinuation syndrome even when discontinued gradually, over 7 to 10 days. Symptoms may include a flulike syndrome with nausea, vomiting, fatigue, muscle aches, dizziness, headache, and insomnia.

- Mr. Mehring visits the physician again 2 weeks later. His wife complains that she sees no improvement in her husband's mood and that he is taking too many drugs. How should the nurse respond?

# SEROTONIN–NOREPINEPHRINE REUPTAKE INHIBITORS

Like the SSRIs, the SNRIs, of which Ⓟ **venlafaxine** (Effexor XR) is the prototype, inhibit the neuronal uptake of serotonin. In addition, they also inhibit the uptake of norepinephrine, increasing the activity of these neurotransmitters in the brain. The SNRIs are similar to SSRIs in terms of therapeutic effects.

## Pharmacokinetics and Action

Venlafaxine is well absorbed, extensively metabolized in the liver, and excreted in urine. It crosses the placenta and may enter breast milk.

The drug increases the levels of serotonin and norepinephrine in the brain by preventing the reuptake of these neurotransmitters known to play an important part in mood. The drug also weakly inhibits dopamine reuptake.

## Use

SNRIs are a standard first-line treatment for depression and anxiety disorders. Uses for venlafaxine include the treatment of depression, as well as generalized anxiety disorder, social phobia, and panic disorder. Table 55.4 gives route and dosage information of venlafaxine and the other SNRIs.

## TABLE 55.4

### DRUGS AT A GLANCE: Serotonin–Norepinephrine Reuptake Inhibitors

| Drug | Pregnancy Category | Routes and Dosage Ranges | |
|---|---|---|---|
| | | **Adults** | **Children** |
| Ⓟ **Venlafaxine** (Effexor XR; ✴ ACT-Venlafaxine, APO-Venlafaxine XR, Auro-Venlafaxine, DOM-Venlafaxine XR, MYLAN-Venlafaxine XR) | C | Immediate-release tablets: 37.5–75 mg/d PO initially in 2–3 divided doses with food; increase by ≤75 mg/d (4 d or longer between increments); usual dosage 75–225 mg/d; max dose 375 mg/d<br>Extended-release (XR) capsules: initially, 37.5 or 75 mg/d PO in a single dose, morning or evening; increase by ≤75 mg/d (4 d or longer between increments) usual dosage 75–225 mg/d; max dose 225 mg/d<br>Hepatic or renal impairment: reduce dose by 50% and increase very slowly | Not approved for use in children and adolescents |
| Desvenlafaxine (Pristiq; ✴ APO-Desvenlafaxine, Pristiq) | C | 50 mg PO once daily; increases >100 mg daily not recommended | Not approved for use in children and adolescents |
| Duloxetine (Cymbalta, Drizalma Sprinkle; ✴ AG-Duloxetine, APO-Duloxetine, Auro-Duloxetine, Cymbalta, JAMP-Duloxetine) | C | 40–60 mg PO daily. Dose may be divided. Increase to 60 mg once daily; max daily dose 120 mg daily<br>Renal impairment: decrease doses | 7–17 y: 30 mg once daily; increase to 60 mg once daily; max daily dose 120 mg daily |
| Levomilnacipran (Fetzima Titration; ✴ Fetzima) | C | 20 mg PO once daily for 2 days; increase to 40 mg once daily; may then be increased in increments of 40 mg at intervals of 2 or more days<br>Maintenance: 40–120 mg once daily<br>Maximum dose: 120 mg daily | Not approved for use in children and adolescents |
| Milnacipran (Savella, Savella Titration Pack) | C | 50 mg PO twice daily<br>Titration schedule: 12.5 mg once on day 1; 12.5 mg twice daily on days 2–3; 25 mg twice daily on days 4–7; then, 50 mg twice daily thereafter. Dose may be increased to 100 mg twice daily, based on individual response | Not approved for use in children and adolescents |
| Nefazodone | C | Depression: 100 mg PO twice daily, alternatively, depression treatment guidelines suggest starting doses of 50–100 mg/d; gradually increase dose in increments of 100–200 mg/d (in two divided doses) and intervals ≥1 week to a usual dose of 150–600 mg in two divided doses | Not approved for use in children |

### Use in Children

The FDA has issued a **BLACK BOX WARNING ◆** alerting health care providers to the increased risk of suicidal ideation in children, adolescents, and young adults 18 to 24 years of age when taking antidepressant medications, including venlafaxine. Children who take the drug are quite likely to experience weight loss.

### Use in Older Adults

Venlafaxine and other SNRIs are suitable for use in older people, although the weight loss often associated with these drugs may be undesirable. Authorities recommend using smaller initial doses and dosing increments. In addition, there is an increased risk of the syndrome of inappropriate antidiuretic hormone or hyponatremia in older adults. It is necessary to monitor sodium levels frequently.

### Use in Patients With Renal Impairment

Venlafaxine is excreted by the kidneys; thus, dosage adjustment is necessary in patients with renal impairment.

### Use in Patients With Hepatic Impairment

Caution is warranted in patients with hepatic impairment. Prescribers should consider lower doses, longer intervals between doses, and slower dose increases than usual.

### Use in Patients With Critical Illness

Patients who are critically ill may need a drug such as venlafaxine to combat the depression that often develops with major illness. It is necessary to make a thorough assessment of the patient's condition, other drugs being given, potential adverse drug effects, and other factors before starting the drug.

## Adverse Effects

Adverse effects of venlafaxine, which may be greater than with the SSRIs, include the following:

- CNS effects: anxiety, dizziness, dreams, insomnia, nervousness, somnolence, and tremors
- GI effects: anorexia, weight loss, nausea, vomiting, constipation, and diarrhea
- Cardiovascular effects: hypertension, tachycardia, and vasodilation
- Genitourinary effects: abnormal ejaculation, impotence, and urinary frequency. (The negative effect of venlafaxine on sexual function is less than that reported with the SSRIs.)
- Dermatologic effects: sweating, rash, and pruritus

## Contraindications

Contraindications to venlafaxine include known sensitivity to the drug, use of an MAO inhibitor, and pregnancy.

## Nursing Implications

### Preventing Interactions

Venlafaxine and other SNRIs interact with MAO inhibitors, leading to increased serum levels and the risk of serotonin syndrome. It is necessary to discontinue the MAO inhibitor at least 14 days before starting venlafaxine.

### Administering the Medication

People should take venlafaxine with food to decrease its GI effects (e.g., nausea and vomiting). They should take the extended-release formulation in the morning and evening, at approximately the same time. For patients who have difficulty swallowing extended-release capsules, they can be opened and sprinkled on applesauce. The nurse instructs patient to swallow the applesauce and medication without chewing and to follow this by drinking a glass of water. This will ensure all pellets are swallowed.

### Assessing for Therapeutic Effects

The nurse assesses for improvement in mood, including improvement in anxiety level, reduced agitation or irritability episodes, decreased number of panic attacks, and ability to sleep through the night.

### Assessing for Adverse Effects

The nurse observes for dizziness, headache, nervousness, insomnia, nausea, diarrhea, dizziness, dry mouth, sedation, and skin rash. Also, it is necessary to assess for altered sexual function and provide options and resources for the patient and the significant other. In addition, the nurse evaluates for the occurrence of weight loss. Finally, it is important to monitor for signs of suicidal ideation and hostility.

### Patient Teaching

Box 55.3 presents patient teaching guidelines for the antidepressants, including the SNRIs.

## Other Drugs in the Class

Desvenlafaxine (Pristiq) also inhibits the neuronal uptake of serotonin. A synthetic form of the major active metabolite of venlafaxine, desvenlafaxine is used to treat major depressive disorder in adults. The drug, which is metabolized by CYP3A4 and not CYP2D6 enzymes, is associated with fewer drug interactions than other SNRIs. It is generally well tolerated and is formulated as an extended-release product taken once a day. Adverse effects include constipation or diarrhea, decreased sexual desire, drowsiness, dry mouth, headache, and trouble sleeping.

Duloxetine (Cymbalta, Drizalma Sprinkle), like duloxetine, inhibits the neuronal uptake of serotonin. The drug is commonly used in the treatment of neuropathic pain and relieves painful physical symptoms (e.g., overall pain, backache, shoulder pain) associated with depression, thereby reducing remission rates, and reduces depression-associated anxiety. It may result in hepatic toxicity, leading to increased liver transaminases and bilirubin. Use of alcohol with duloxetine increases the risk of liver damage, and thus, it is not recommended for patients with significant alcohol use. Overall, the adverse effects of duloxetine and venlafaxine are similar. Significant drug interactions with SSRIs, MAO inhibitors, TCAs, lithium, St. John's wort, phenylpiperidine opioids, dextromethorphan, and tryptophan may potentiate the risk of serotonin syndrome with duloxetine.

Levomilnacipran (Fetzima, Fetzima Titration) is administered with or without food at the same time every day. Its primary use is the treatment of major depressive disorder. If a patient is taking nonsteroidal anti-inflammatory drugs or any anticoagulants with levomilnacipran, the nurse instructs the patient that the risk of bleeding is incrsseased. Also, levomil-nacipran has the potential to increase blood pressure and pulse rate. It is necessary to monitor pulse and blood pressure closely. If hypertension and tachycardia occur, a dosage reduced is warranted.

Milnacipran (Savella, Savella Titration Pack) is a potent inhibitor of norepinephrine and serotonin reuptake. As with other drugs in this class, it is important to monitor blood pressure and pulse rate. In addition, it is necessary to check periodically for increases in intraocular pressure in any patient who has a history of intraocular pressure elevation or glaucoma.

Nefazodone is administered for depression. It can cause life-threatening hepatic failure, resulting in death or transplant, in 1 out of 250,000 to 300,000 patients treated with nefazodone. The patient must be instructed on the risk of liver dysfunction. Nefazodone may be administered with or without food. However, administration with food may decrease absorption and the effectiveness of the medication. In patients who have a history of orthostatic hypotension, the administration of nefazodone may result in transient hypotensive episodes. Instruct patient to use caution when changing positions.

## MONOAMINE OXIDASE INHIBITORS

MAO inhibitors are third-line agents for the treatment of depression and are rarely used in clinical practice today, mainly because they may interact with some foods and drugs to produce severe hypertension and possible heart attack or stroke. Prescribers are most likely to order MAO inhibitors when a patient does not respond to other antidepressant drugs or when electroconvulsive therapy is refused or contraindicated. The prototype MAO inhibitor is **phenelzine** (Nardil).

## Pharmacokinetics and Action

Phenelzine is well absorbed and widely distributed. The drug reaches peak levels in 2 to 4 hours, but mood elevation may take 2 to 8 weeks. It is metabolized in the liver and excreted by the kidneys. The drug improves mood by binding irreversibly to MAO, increasing the concentrations of epinephrine, norepinephrine, serotonin, and dopamine in the CNS.

## Use

Phenelzine is used to treat depression when other antidepressants have been unsuccessful in symptom management. Table 55.5 gives route and dosage information for this drug and other MAO inhibitors.

### Use in Older Adults

Phenelzine and other MAO inhibitors may be more likely to cause hypertensive crises in older adults because their cardiovascular, renal, and hepatic functions are often diminished.

### Use in Patients With Renal or Hepatic Impairment

Caution is necessary with phenelzine and other MAO inhibitors in people with renal or hepatic impairment.

### Use in Patients With Critical Illness

Phenelzine interacts with numerous drugs and could potentially complicate the condition of patients with critical illness. If it is necessary to continue phenelzine, its use must be cautious and slow and careful monitoring of patients' responses is warranted; patients with critical illness are often frail and unstable, with multiple organ dysfunctions.

**TABLE 55.5**

**DRUGS AT A GLANCE: Monoamine Oxidase Inhibitors**

| Drug | Pregnancy Category | Routes and Dosage Ranges | |
|---|---|---|---|
| | | **Adults** | **Children** |
| **Phenelzine** (Nardil; Nardil) | C | 15 mg PO three times daily; not to exceed 90 mg/d | Not approved for use in children and adolescents |
| Selegiline (Emsam, Zelapar; APO-Selegiline, TEVA-Selegiline) | C | Depression: 6 mg/24 hours transdermal, target dose 6 mg/24 hours once daily; may titrate based on clinical response in increments of 3 mg/d every 2 weeks up to a maximum of 12 mg/24 hours. Parkinson disease: 5 mg PO twice daily at breakfast and lunch with concomitant carbidopa/levodopa therapy; maximum 10 mg/d | Depression: Adolescents >17 years: Same as adult dosing |
| Isocarboxazid (Marplan) | C | 10 mg PO 2–4 times daily; increase to 40 mg by the end of the first week to a max daily dose of 60 mg/d | Not approved for use in children and adolescents |
| Tranylcypromine (Parnate; Parnate) | C | 10 mg PO initially; increase in 10-mg intervals every 1–3 wk; usual dosage range 30–60 mg PO daily in divided doses, not to exceed 60 mg/d | Younger than 16 y: not recommended. 16 y of age or older: same as adults |

## Adverse Effects

The most serious adverse effect associated with phenelzine is hypertensive crisis, which can be precipitated by intake of foods containing tyramine. Other reported effects include dysrhythmias, drowsiness, dizziness, sexual dysfunction, and orthostatic hypotension.

## Contraindications

Contraindications to phenelzine include known sensitivity to the drug. Patients should not have elective surgery requiring general anesthesia or spinal anesthesia or use local anesthesia containing sympathomimetic vasoconstrictors. Patients who take other MAO inhibitors or weight-reduction and over-the-counter cold or hay fever preparations containing vasoconstrictors should not take phenelzine.

## Nursing Implications

### Preventing Interactions

Phenelzine interacts with many drugs and some herbs and foods, increasing its effects (Boxes 55.5 and 55.6). It is important that SSRIs and phenelzine are not taken concurrently or close together because serious and fatal reactions may occur. Other critical interactions occur with foods that contain tyramine, a monoamine precursor of norepinephrine. Normally, tyramine is deactivated in the GI tract and liver, so that large amounts do not reach the systemic circulation. When deactivation is blocked by MAO inhibitors, tyramine is absorbed systemically and transported to adrenergic nerve terminals, where it causes a sudden release of large amounts of norepinephrine.

---

**BOX 55.5** **Drug Interactions: Phenelzine**

**Drugs That Increase the Effects of Phenelzine**
- Alcohol (red wine, beer)
  *Increases central nervous system depression*
- Altretamine
  *Increases the risk of orthostatic hypotension*
- Antidepressants (tricyclic antidepressants, selective serotonin reuptake inhibitors, serotonin–norepinephrine reuptake inhibitors), buspirone, carbamazepine, dextromethorphan, 5-hydroxytryptophan
  *Increase the risk of serotonin syndrome*
- Levodopa
  *Increases the risk of hypertensive reactions*
- Monoamine oxidase inhibitors
  *Increase the risk of serotonin syndrome and hypertensive crisis*
- Narcotic analgesics
  *Increase the risk of hypotension, respiratory depression, or coma*
- Selegiline, sibutramine, tramadol
  *Increase the risk of hypertensive crisis*

---

**BOX 55.6** **Herb and Dietary Interactions: Phenelzine**

**Herbs and Foods That Increase the Effects of Phenelzine**
- Caffeine
- Kava kava
- Phenylalanine
- St. John's wort
- Tryptophan (e.g., game meats, soy products, seaweed, seafood, sesame seeds, aged cheeses and meats, brewer's yeast, sauerkraut, fava beans)
- Tyrosine (e.g., meat, seafood, wheat products, oatmeal)
- Valerian

### Administering the Medication

Phenelzine is taken orally three times a day, which may require a reminder system for accurate administration. The drug may be crushed and mixed with fluids or food for patients with difficulty swallowing.

### Assessing for Therapeutic and Adverse Effects

The nurse assesses for improvement in symptoms of depression, including improvement in anxiety level, reduced agitation or irritability episodes, decreased number of panic attacks, and ability to sleep through the night. It is important to monitor the patient for severe headache, nausea, vomiting, neck stiffness, photophobia, and sweating.

In addition, it is necessary to observe for blurred vision, constipation, dizziness, dry mouth, hypotension, urinary retention, and hypoglycemia. If the patient eats any foods containing tyramine, hypertensive crisis may occur. The treatment for hypertensive crisis is phentolamine.

### Patient Teaching

Box 55.3 contains patient teaching guidelines for the antidepressants, including the MAO inhibitors.

## Other Drugs in the Class

Isocarboxazid, selegiline, and tranylcypromine have the same adverse effects as phenelzine, and they interact with drugs and foods in the same way.

Selegiline, a MAO inhibitor, is an antiparkinsonian drug (Chapter 48). For depression, the transdermal preparation can be prescribed. The initial dose is 6 mg/24 h once daily, with a maximum dose of 2.5 mg/d. It is a potent, irreversible monoamine oxidase inhibitor with a great affinity for MAO-B in the brain. Selegiline increases dopaminergic activity by interfering with dopamine reuptake at the synapse. The metabolites of amphetamine and methamphetamine are also affected and interfere with neuronal uptake and enhance the release of the neurotransmitters, norepinephrine, dopamine, and serotonin.

## NCLEX Success

3. A patient is beginning a new drug regimen of escitalopram for depression. Before administering this medication, it is necessary to assess for which of the following?

   A. prior recent use of monoamine oxidase (MAO) inhibitors
   B. prior diet high in tyramine-containing foods
   C. history of cigarette use
   D. history of seizure disorders

4. Monoamine oxidase (MAO) inhibitors are indicated in which of the following?

   A. in patients who have previously developed serotonin syndrome
   B. in patients who are first beginning treatment of depression
   C. in patients who are having trouble sleeping
   D. in patients who have not responded successfully to selective serotonin reuptake inhibitors and tricyclic antidepressants

5. Fluoxetine achieves its effects by

   A. blocking the uptake of monoamines
   B. inhibiting monoamine oxidase A (MAO-A) enzyme in nerve terminals
   C. selectively inhibiting serotonin reuptake
   D. directly stimulating serotonin receptors

# ATYPICAL ANTIDEPRESSANTS

Other drugs used to treat depression include bupropion, mirtazapine, and trazodone. Table 55.6 gives route and dosage information for these drugs. People also use the herbal preparation St. John's wort as an antidepressant (Box 55.7).

## Bupropion

Bupropion (Aplenzin, Wellbutrin SR, Wellbutrin XL, Zyban) inhibits the reuptake of dopamine, norepinephrine, and serotonin. After an oral dose, peak plasma levels are reached in about 2 hours. The drug is metabolized in the liver and excreted primarily in the urine. Several metabolites are pharmacologically active. Bupropion is useful in the treatment of depression, seasonal affective disorder (SAD) (see Box 55.1), and smoking cessation. Prescribers often add it to a drug regimen when an SSRI does not provide a complete response. Acute episodes of depression usually require several months of drug therapy. It is necessary to reduce the dosage in patients with impaired hepatic or renal function.

Bupropion may have significant adverse effects. Seizures are likely to occur with doses above 450 mg/d and in patients known to have a seizure disorder. The drug has few adverse effects on cardiac function and does not cause orthostatic hypotension or sexual dysfunction. However, in addition to seizures, the drug has CNS stimulant effects (agitation, anxiety, excitement, increased motor activity, insomnia, restlessness) that may require a sedative during the first few days of administration. These effects may increase the risk of abuse. Other common adverse effects include dry mouth,

## TABLE 55.6

### DRUGS AT A GLANCE: Atypical Antidepressants

| Drug | Pregnancy Category | Routes and Dosage Ranges | |
|---|---|---|---|
| | | **Adults** | **Children** |
| Bupropion (Aplenzin, Wellbutrin SR, Wellbutrin XL; ❋ ACT-BuPROPion XL MYLAN-BuPROPion XL, PMS-BuPROPion SR, SANDOZ-BuPROPion, Wellbutrin SR, Wellbutrin XL, Zyban) | C | Immediate-release tablets: 100 mg PO twice daily; increase to 100 mg three times daily (at least 6 h apart) if necessary; max single dose 450 mg daily<br>Sustained-release (SR) tablets: 150 mg PO once daily in the morning; increase to 150 mg twice daily (at least 8 h apart); max daily dose 200 mg twice daily<br>Wellbutrin XL: 150 mg PO once daily in the morning; may increase to target dose of 300 mg on or after 4th day of therapy; max single dose 450 mg | Not recommended for use in children |
| Mirtazapine (Remeron, Remeron Sol, Tab; ❋ Remeron, Teva-Mirtazapine, ZYM-Mirtazapine) | C | 15 mg/d PO initially, not to exceed 45 mg/d; usual dosage range 15–45 mg daily | Not recommended for use in children |
| Trazodone (❋ APO-TraZODone, APO-TraZODone D, DOM-TraZODone, TraZODone-50, TraZODone-100, TraZODone-150) | C | 150 mg PO initially daily in divided doses; increase to a max dose of 600 mg daily if necessary | 6–12 y: 1.5–2 mg/kg/d PO initially; increase to a max dose of 6 mg/kg/d if necessary<br>Adolescents: 25–50 mg PO initially; increase to 100–150 mg daily in divided doses |

St Johns Wart

| BOX 55.7 | *Use of St. John's Wort as an Antidepressant* |

St. John's wort (*Hypericum perforatum*) is a herb that is widely used for depression. However, evidence for the efficacy with St. John's wort is modest at best. Most authorities agree that there is insufficient evidence to support the use of St. John's wort for mild to moderate depression and that more studies are needed to confirm the safety and effectiveness of this herb.

Drug interactions may be extensive. People should not combine St. John's wort with alcohol, antidepressants, nasal decongestants, or other over-the-counter cold and flu medications, bronchodilators, opioid analgesics, or amino acid supplements containing phenylalanine and tyrosine. All of these interactions may result in hypertension, possibly severe.

For patients who report use of St. John's wort, it is necessary to teach them to purchase products from reputable sources; to avoid taking antidepressant drugs, alcohol, and cold and flu medications while taking the herb; to avoid using the herb during pregnancy because effects are unknown; and to use sunscreen lotions and clothing to protect themselves from sun exposure.

headache, nausea and vomiting, and constipation. The FDA has issued a **BLACK BOX WARNING ◆** for bupropion, because serious neuropsychiatric reactions have been reported with the administration of the drug for smoking cessation. These reactions are more common with the discontinuation of the medication.

## Mirtazapine

Mirtazapine (Remeron), another atypical antidepressant, blocks presynaptic alpha₂-adrenergic receptors (which increase the release of norepinephrine), serotonin receptors, and histamine H₁ receptors. Consequently, the drug decreases anxiety, agitation, insomnia, and migraine headaches as well as depression. (Note that the drug is now classified as a tetracycline antidepressant.)

Mirtazapine is well absorbed after oral administration, and it is metabolized in the liver, mainly to inactive metabolites. Common adverse effects include drowsiness (with accompanying cognitive and motor impairment), increased appetite, weight gain, dizziness, dry mouth, and constipation. The drug does not cause sexual dysfunction. Mirtazapine should not be taken concurrently with other CNS depressants (e.g., alcohol, benzodiazepine, antianxiety, or hypnotic agents) because of additive sedation. In addition, it should not be taken concurrently with an MAO inhibitor.

It is necessary to monitor patients for agranulocytosis or severe neutropenia. Patients should report sore throat, stomatitis, or any signs of an infection to the prescriber.

## Trazodone

Trazodone is used more often for sedation and sleep than for depression because high doses (greater than 300 mg/d) are required for antidepressant effects, and these amounts cause excessive sedation in many patients. The drug is often given concurrently with a stimulating antidepressant, such as bupropion, fluoxetine, sertraline, or venlafaxine.

Trazodone should be administered with food for maximum absorption. The drug is metabolized in the liver and excreted primarily by the kidneys. Adverse effects include sedation, dizziness, edema, cardiac dysrhythmias, and priapism (prolonged and painful penile erection).

## MOOD-STABILIZING AGENTS: DRUGS USED TO TREAT BIPOLAR DISORDER

 **Lithium carbonate** (Lithobid), the prototype, is a naturally occurring metallic salt that is used in patients with bipolar disorder, mainly to treat and prevent manic episodes. When used therapeutically, lithium is effective in controlling mania in 65% to 80% of patients. When used prophylactically, the drug decreases the frequency and intensity of manic cycles.

### Pharmacokinetics

Lithium is well absorbed after oral administration, with peak serum levels in 1 to 3 hours after a dose and steady-state concentrations in 5 to 7 days. The drug is not metabolized; it is entirely excreted by the kidneys.

### Action

The exact mechanism of action of lithium is unknown. However, the drug is known to affect the synthesis, release, and reuptake of several neurotransmitters in the brain, including acetylcholine, dopamine, GABA, and norepinephrine. It also stabilizes postsynaptic receptor sensitivity to neurotransmitters, probably by competing with calcium, magnesium, potassium, and sodium ions for binding sites. Lithium may also stimulate neuronal growth, exerting a neuroprotective effect on areas of the brain involved with mood.

### Use

Lithium is the drug of choice for use in the treatment of manic episodes of bipolar disorder and as a maintenance treatment to decrease the number and intensity of manic episodes. Long-term therapy is the usual practice because of the high recurrence rate of bipolar disorder if the drug is discontinued. The prescriber may add an antiepileptic agent to the regimen.

| ！ | QSEN Alert: Safety |

Gradually tapering the dose over 2 to 4 weeks delays the recurrence of symptoms.

It is important to note that doses should be relatively low initially and may increase gradually according to regular measurements of serum drug levels. Dosage is based on serum drug levels, control of symptoms, and occurrence of adverse effects. Measurements of serum levels are required for two reasons: (1) therapeutic doses are only slightly lower than toxic doses and (2) patients vary widely in rates of lithium absorption and excretion. Thus, a dose that is therapeutic in one patient may be toxic in another.

Table 55.7 gives route and dosage information for lithium and other mood-stabilizing drugs.

## TABLE 55.7

## DRUGS AT A GLANCE: Mood-Stabilizing Agents

| Drug | Pregnancy Category | Routes and Dosage Ranges | |
|---|---|---|---|
| | | **Adults** | **Children** |
|  **Lithium carbonate** (Lithobid, ✿ APO-Lithium Carbonate, DOM-Lithium Carbonate Carbolith, Lithane, PMS-Lithium Carbonate) | D | Immediate-release: 300 mg PO three times daily or less; usual dosage 900–1800 mg PO daily in 3–4 divided doses<br>Extended-release: 450 mg two times daily or less; usual dosage 900–1800 mg PO daily in 2 divided doses. Maintain a serum lithium level of 0.6–1.2 mEq/L | ≥6 y: <30 kg initially 300 mg PO twice daily; ≥30 kg 300 mg PO three or four times daily<br>>12 y: same as adults<br>Maintenance dose: 15–60 mg/kg/d PO three times daily<br>Maximum daily dose 40 mg/kg/d<br>Maintain a serum lithium level <1.4 mEq/L |
| Aripiprazole (Abilify, Abilify Maintena, Abilify MyCite; ✿ Abilify, APO-ARIPiprazole, Abilify Maintena, AURO-ARIPiprazole) | C | 30 mg PO daily | Mania: ≥10–17 y, 2 mg PO daily for 7 days and then 5 mg daily for 2 days to 10 mg daily, not to exceed 30 mg daily; close monitoring in children with depression |
| Olanzapine (ZyPREXA, ZyPREXA Relprew, ZyPREXA Zydis; ✿ ACT-OLANZapine, JAMP-OLANZapine ODT, Teva-OLANZapine, Zyprexa, XyPEXA Zyds) | C | 10–15 mg/d PO initially; may increase by 5 mg daily at no <24 intervals to max dose of 20 mg/d<br>Elderly or debilitated adults: 5 mg/d PO | 13–17 y: 2.5–5 mg/d PO initially; may increase by 2.5–5 mg daily to max dose of 20 mg/d |
| Quetiapine (Seroquel, SEROquel XR; ✿ Dom-Quetiapine, Seroquel, Seroquel QR) | C | Acute mania: 50 mg PO twice daily on day 1; 100 mg PO twice daily on day 2; 150 mg PO twice daily on day 3; 200 mg PO twice daily on day 4. If needed, may continue to increase max dose 800 mg/d.<br>Depressive episodes: 50 mg PO at bedtime; may increase by 50 mg/d to max dose 600 mg at bedtime | 13–17 y: 25 mg PO twice daily on day 1; 50 mg PO twice daily on day 2; 100 mg PO twice daily on day 3; 150 mg PO twice daily on day 4; 200 mg PO twice daily on day 5. If needed, may continue to increase in increments of no >100 mg/d to max dose 400–600 mg/d |
| Olanzapine–fluoxetine (Symbyax) | C | Depressive episodes: 6 mg/25 mg PO in evening; usual dose 6–12 mg/25–50 mg; may increase to max 18 mg/75 mg daily | 10–17 y: 3 mg/25 mg PO in evening; usual dose 6–12 mg/25–50 mg daily |
| Risperidone (Perseris, RisperDAL, RisperDAL Consta; ✿ AG-Risperidone, RAN-Risperidone, RisperDAL, RisperDAL Consta) | C | Acute mania: 2–3 mg/d PO initially; may increase 1 mg/d to max dose of 6 mg/d<br>Elderly or debilitated adults: 0.5 mg/d PO initially, may increase by 0.5–3 mg/d, and then may increase by 1 mg/wk to max dose of 6 mg/d<br>Maintenance (RisperDAL Consta): 25 mg IM every 2 wk; max dose 50 mg every 2 wk | 10–17 y: 0.5 mg/d PO initially; titrate 0.5–1 daily to a target dose of 2.5 mg/d; dosage range 0.5–6 mg/d |
| Ziprasidone (Geodon; ✿ AURO-Ziprasidone, Zeldox) | C | Acute mania: 40 mg PO initially twice daily; usual dose 40–80 mg twice daily; max dose 80 mg twice daily | Not recommended for use in children with bipolar disorder |

## Use in Patients With Renal Impairment

Adequate renal function is a prerequisite for lithium therapy. The proximal renal tubules reabsorb approximately 80% of a lithium dose, and the amount of reabsorption depends on the concentration of sodium in the tubules. A sodium deficit causes more lithium to be reabsorbed and increases the risk of lithium toxicity. A sodium excess causes more lithium to be excreted (i.e., lithium diuresis) and may lower serum lithium levels to nontherapeutic ranges.

## ! QSEN Alert: Safety

Therefore, if a patient with renal impairment or unstable renal function receives lithium, it is essential that the dose be markedly reduced and that plasma serum levels be closely monitored.

## Use in Patients With Hepatic Impairment

Caution is necessary when lithium is used in patients with hepatic impairment.

### Use in Patients With Critical Illness

Lithium warrants caution in patients with critical illness. Lower doses are necessary in patients with conditions that impair lithium excretion (e.g., diuretic drug therapy, dehydration, low-salt diet, renal impairment, decreased cardiac output). It is necessary to discontinue lithium 1 to 2 days before surgery and resume it when full oral intake of food and fluids is allowed.

**QSEN Alert: Safety**

Lithium may prolong the effects of anesthetics and neuromuscular blocking drugs.

## Adverse Effects and Contraindications

Common adverse effects of lithium include metallic taste, hand tremors, nausea, polyuria, polydipsia, diarrhea, muscular weakness, fatigue, edema, and weight gain.

Contraindications include known sensitivity to the drug as well as pregnancy. (Lithium is a pregnancy category D medication.) Cardiac malformations are a common anomaly when lithium is administered in the first trimester.

### Preventing Interactions

Several drugs interact with lithium, increasing or decreasing its effects (Box 55.8). No herbal interactions exist.

### Administering the Medication

Before beginning lithium therapy, it is important to obtain baseline studies of renal, cardiac, and thyroid status because adverse drug effects involve these organ systems. Baseline electrolyte studies are also necessary.

When lithium therapy begins, it is necessary to measure the serum drug concentration two or three times weekly in the morning, 12 hours (trough) after the last dose of the drug. For most patients, the therapeutic range of serum drug levels is 0.5 to 1.2 mEq/L (SI units, 0.5 to 1.2 mmol/L). Serum lithium levels should not exceed 1.5 mEq/L because of the risk of serious drug toxicity. Doses of lithium should decrease after mania is controlled. During long-term maintenance therapy, it is necessary to measure serum lithium levels at least every 3 months.

---

**BOX 55.8    Drug Interactions: Lithium**

**Drugs That Increase the Effects of Lithium**

- Alcohol and diuretics
  *Increase the risk of dehydration, increasing the risk of lithium toxicity*
- Angiotensin-converting enzyme inhibitors, angiotensin II receptor blockers, indomethacin, and some other nonsteroidal anti-inflammatory drugs
  *Increase the serum level and the risk of toxicity*
- Selective serotonin reuptake inhibitors
  *Increase the risk of adverse effects such as confusion, drowsiness, and issues with coordination*

**Drugs That Decrease the Effects of Lithium**

- Theophylline
  *Increases renal excretion*

---

People should take lithium with food to decrease the risk of nausea and vomiting.

### Assessing for Therapeutic and Adverse Effects

The nurse observes for decreases in manic behavior and stability in mood swings. Therapeutic effects do not occur until approximately 7 to 10 days after therapeutic serum drug levels are attained (1 to 1.5 mEq/L with acute mania; 0.6 to 1.2 mEq/L for maintenance therapy). In mania, a person usually takes a benzodiazepine or an antipsychotic drug to reduce agitation and control behavior until the lithium takes effect.

The nurse also observes for the presence of a metallic taste, hand tremors, nausea, polyuria, polydipsia, diarrhea, muscular weakness, fatigue, edema, and weight gain.

### Patient Teaching

Box 55.9 contains patient teaching guidelines for lithium.

## Other Drugs in the Class

Atypical antipsychotics (see Chap. 56) are used to decrease dopamine activity in the treatment of the mania phase of bipolar disorder, including reducing acute mania, psychomotor agitation, and psychosis. Currently, aripiprazole, olanzapine (monotherapy or combination with fluoxetine), quetiapine, risperidone, and ziprasidone are approved by the FDA for this indication. Additionally, there is a potential risk for extrapyramidal signs and withdrawal symptoms in newborns whose mothers took these drugs during the third trimester of pregnancy.

Aripiprazole (Abilify, Abilify Maintena, Abilify MyCite) is used to treat acute manic and mixed bipolar disorder adults and in children and adolescents aged 8 to 17 years. The drug is well absorbed with oral administration; is highly protein bound, metabolized in the liver; and is excreted in the urine and feces. Adverse effects include headache, somnolence, sedation, fatigue, dizziness, nausea, and vomiting. In May 2016, the FDA issued a **BLACK BOX WARNING ◆** regarding aripiprazole; use placed the patient at risk for the development of compulsive or uncontrollable urges to gamble, shop, binge eat, or have sex. The nurse must educate the patient and family about this risk.

Olanzapine (ZyPREXA, ZyPREXA Relprew, ZyPREXA Zydis) is prescribed as monotherapy for the treatment of acute, mixed, or manic episodes associated with bipolar disorder and in combination with fluoxetine (Symbyax) for the treatment of depressive episodes associated with bipolar disorder. The drug is predominantly excreted in the urine and feces. Reported adverse effects, which are dose dependent, include somnolence, extrapyramidal symptoms, dizziness, weight gain, constipation, and xerostomia. In May 2016, the FDA issued **BLACK BOX WARNING ◆** concerning olanzapine because it can cause a drug reaction with eosinophilia and systemic symptoms. DRESS (drug reaction with eosinophilia and systemic symptoms) consists of a rash or exfoliative dermatitis. In addition, the patient may develop pancreatitis, nephritis, or pneumonitis.

Quetiapine (Seroquel) is an atypical antipsychotic used for the treatment of bipolar disorder and schizophrenia. This drug is not recommended for dementia-related psychosis. It has antagonist effects on serotonin and dopamine. Excretion is in the urine and feces. Quetiapine may cause drowsiness, dizziness, decreased vision, fatigue, and weight gain. It should be administered without food or with 300 calories or less. Administration with food increases the peak serum concentration.

**BOX 55.9** · *Patient Teaching Guidelines for Lithium*

**General Considerations**

- Take lithium as directed to maximize therapeutic benefits and minimize adverse effects. Do not alter doses when symptoms subside. Lithium therapy may be lifelong.
- Keep scheduled office or clinic visits for blood tests. Regular measurements of blood lithium levels are necessary for safe and effective lithium therapy. Report for measurements of lithium blood levels as instructed and do not take the morning dose of lithium until the blood sample has been obtained. Accurate measurement of serum drug levels requires that blood be drawn approximately 12 hours after the previous dose of lithium.
- Do not take diuretic medications without consulting a health care provider. Diuretics cause loss of sodium and water, which increases lithium toxicity.
- Maintain a normal diet, including consistent salt and adequate fluid intake. Loss of salt in sweat increases the risk of adverse effects from lithium. Minimize activities that cause excessive perspiration, such as sweating during heavy exercise, sauna use, or outdoor activities during hot summer days. Loss of salt in sweat increases the risk of adverse effects from lithium.

- Lithium can harm an unborn baby. If you are a woman of childbearing age, use an effective form of birth control during treatment, and notify your prescriber immediately if you become pregnant.
- If signs of overdose occur (e.g., vomiting, diarrhea, unsteady walking, tremor, drowsiness, muscle weakness), stop taking lithium and contact the prescriber or other health care provider immediately.

**Self or Caregiver Administration**

- Take with food or milk or soon after a meal to decrease stomach upset.
- Do not alter dietary salt intake. Decreased salt intake (e.g., low-salt diet) increases risk of adverse effects from lithium. Increased intake may decrease therapeutic effects.
- Drink 8 to 12 glasses of fluids daily; avoid excessive intake of caffeine-containing beverages. Excessive intake of such beverages may decrease levels of lithium and reduce the effectiveness of the drug. Also, caffeine has a diuretic effect, and dehydration increases lithium toxicity.

Risperidone (Perseris, RisperDAL, RisperDAL Consta) is an atypical antipsychotic used alone or in combination with lithium or valproate for the treatment of acute mania or mixed episodes. The drug is approved by the FDA for use in adolescents aged 10 to 17 years with type I bipolar disorder. It is administered orally and intramuscularly and is well absorbed after oral administration. Risperidone is metabolized in the liver and predominately excreted in the urine. The drug enters breast milk. Adverse effects include significant weight gain, insomnia, sexual dysfunction, and photosensitivity. Neuroleptic malignant syndrome and tardive dyskinesia reportedly occur. Orthostatic hypotension may be present during the first few weeks of therapy. A **BLACK BOX WARNING ◆** for risperidone reports that increasing mortality occurs in elderly patients with dementia-related psychosis.

Ziprasidone (Geodon) is another atypical antipsychotic used for the treatment of bipolar disorder in adults. The exact mechanism of action is unknown. The drug is well absorbed, is highly protein bound, and is excreted in feces and urine. Adverse effects include dizziness, drowsiness, and lightheadedness.

## OTHER MEDICATIONS USED TO TREAT BIPOLAR DISORDER

Anticonvulsants (see Chap. 53) are also used as mood-stabilizing agents in bipolar disorder because they modify nerve cell function. Carbamazepine (Carbatrol, Epitol, TEGretol, TEGretol-SR), lamotrigine (LaMICtal, LaMICtal ODT, LaMICtal Starter, LaMICtal, and others), and valproate (Depakote, Depakote ER, Depakote Sprinkles) are currently approved by the FDA for treating bipolar disorder. The drugs are typically used for patients who do not respond to lithium. Other anticonvulsants (e.g., gabapentin, topiramate, oxcarbazepine) are being studied and used off-label for their effects in bipolar disorder, but they do not have FDA approval for this use.

## NCLEX Success

6. A nurse is teaching the importance of proper diet to a patient taking the MAO inhibitor tranylcypromine for depression. Which of the following food selections by the patient indicates that further teaching is needed?

   A. a tossed salad and a bowl of vegetable soup
   B. a salami and Swiss cheese sandwich and a banana
   C. a hamburger and French fries
   D. a cold plate with cottage cheese, chicken salad, and grapes

7. A patient taking lithium is having problems with coordination and unstable gait. The patient's lithium level is 2.3 mEq/L. The nurse should do which of the following?

   A. Continue to administer the lithium three times per day.
   B. Skip a dose of lithium and then resume the regular medication schedule.
   C. Administer an extra dose of lithium.
   D. Withhold the lithium, offer fluids, and notify the prescriber of the lithium level.

8. A nurse practitioner plans to order lithium for a patient with bipolar disorder. Lithium is contraindicated in a patient with an impairment of which of the following systems?

   A. respiratory system
   B. cardiac system
   C. endocrine system
   D. renal system

9. A woman who is stable on lithium therapy for her bipolar disorder is shortly going to be receiving a drug for her hypertension. Which drug would be of greatest concern if added to the treatment regimen?

A. a vasodilator
B. an angiotensin-converting enzyme inhibitor
C. a diuretic
D. a calcium channel blocker

### *Clinical Application 55.2*

- Mr. Mehring reports that he is having difficulty sleeping. What measures should the nurse initiate?

### ! QSEN Alert: Safety

Institute suicide precautions for at-risk patients. These usually involve close observation, often on a one-to-one basis, and removal of potential weapons from the environment. For patients hospitalized on medical–surgical units, transfer to a psychiatric unit may be necessary.

## THE NURSING PROCESS

A concept map outlines the nursing process related to drug therapy considerations in this chapter. Additional nursing implications related to the disease process should also be considered in care decisions.

**Assessment**

- Identify patients at risk for current or potential depression. Areas to assess include health status, family and social relationship, and work status. Severe or prolonged illness, impaired interpersonal relationships, inability to work, and job dissatisfaction may precipitate depression. Depression also occurs without an identifiable cause.
- Observe for signs and symptoms of depression. Clinical manifestations are nonspecific and vary in severity. For example, fatigue and insomnia may be caused by a variety of disorders and range from mild to severe. When symptoms are present, try to determine their frequency, duration, and severity.
- When a patient appears depressed or has a history of depression, assess for suicidal thoughts and behaviors. Statements indicating a detailed plan, accompanied by the intent, ability, and method for carrying out the plan, place the patient at high risk for suicide.
- Identify the patient's usual coping mechanisms for stressful situations. Coping mechanisms vary widely, and behavior that may be helpful to one patient may not be helpful to another. For example, one person may prefer being alone or having decreased contact with family and friends, whereas another may find increased contact desirable.

**Outcomes of Therapy**

The patient will
- Experience improvement of mood and depressive state.
- Receive or self-administer the drugs correctly.
- Identify signs and symptoms of suicidal ideation (or caretakers will). If present, caretakers will implement safety measures.
- Show improvement in activities of daily living, nutrition, exercise habits, and social interaction by the end of the hospital stay.
- Maintain self-care activities after discharge.
- Identify preventable adverse drug effects. If present, patients and/or caregivers can take action.

**Nursing Interventions**

The nurse will use general measures to prevent or decrease the severity of depression such as supportive. psychotherapy and reduction of environmental stress. Specific measures include the following:
- Support the patient's usual mechanisms for handling stressful situations, when feasible. Helpful actions may involve relieving pain or insomnia, scheduling rest periods, and increasing or decreasing socialization.
- Call the patient by name, encourage self-care activities, allow him or her to participate in setting goals and making decisions, and praise efforts to accomplish tasks. These actions promote a positive self-image.
- When signs and symptoms of depression are observed, initiate treatment before depression becomes severe.
- Provide patient teaching regarding drug therapy (see Boxes 55.3 and 55.9).

**Evaluation**

- Observe for behaviors indicating lessened depression.
- Interview regarding feelings and mood.
- Observe and interview regarding adverse drug effects.
- Observe and interview regarding suicidal thoughts and behaviors.

Remember Jermaine Jones, a 34-year-old African American male diagnosed with depression in Chapter 35. He is prescribed sertraline (Zoloft) 50 mg PO daily. What patient education would the nurse provide on sertraline? When comparing sertraline with other antidepressant drugs, how would the nurse differentiate drug classifications, actions, adverse effects, and ethnic variations in drug response?

Care for Jermaine and other patients in a realistic virtual environment: *vSim for Nursing* (thepoint.lww.com/vSimPharm). Practice documenting these patients' care in DocuCare (thepoint.lww.com/DocuCareEHR).

## KEY CONCEPTS

- Major depression is associated with impaired ability to function in usual activities and relationships. Other types of depression include SAD and postnatal depression.
- Bipolar disorder is a mood disorder characterized by episodes of depression alternating with episodes of mania. There are two subtypes of this disorder, type I (characterized by episodes of major depression plus mania) and type II (characterized by episodes of major depression plus episodes of hypomania).
- SSRIs are considered to be first-line medications in the treatment of depression because they have a more favorable side effect profile (e.g., GI symptoms, sexual dysfunction, CNS stimulation, and increased risk of GI bleeding).
- SNRIs are similar to SSRIs in terms of therapeutic effects but exhibit more anticholinergic, CNS sedation, and cardiac conduction abnormalities.
- TCAs, second-line medications in the treatment of depression, produce a high incidence of adverse effects (e.g., sedation, orthostatic hypotension, cardiac dysrhythmias, anticholinergic effects, and weight gain).
- MAO inhibitors are used in the treatment of depression only if other antidepressants are not effective; there is a high incidence of food and drug interactions that potentially lead to hypertensive crisis.
- Serotonin syndrome, a serious and sometimes fatal reaction characterized by hypertensive crisis, hyperpyrexia, extreme agitation progressing to delirium and coma, muscle rigidity, and seizures, may occur due to combined therapy with an SSRI or SNRI and an MAO inhibitor or other drug that potentiates serotonin neurotransmission. An SSRI or SNRI and an MAO inhibitor should not be given concurrently or within 2 weeks of each other. Fluoxetine, because of a long half-life, must be discontinued at least 5 weeks before starting an MAO inhibitor.
- Antidepressants must be taken for 2 to 4 weeks before depressive symptoms improve.
- Some antidepressant drugs are highly toxic and potentially lethal when taken in large doses.
- A **BLACK BOX WARNING ◆** alerts health care providers to the increased risk of suicidal ideation in children, adolescents, and young adults 18 to 24 years of age when taking antidepressant medications.
- Antidepressant discontinuation syndrome has been reported with sudden termination of most antidepressant drugs.
- Most authorities agree that there is insufficient evidence to support the use of St. John's wort for treatment of depression.
- The FDA has issued a **BLACK BOX WARNING ◆** for bupropion, because serious neuropsychiatric reactions have been reported with the administration of the drug for smoking cessation.
- Lithium is the drug of choice to treat bipolar disorder. Lithium has a narrow therapeutic index, and serum drug levels determine dosage, control of symptoms, and occurrence of adverse effects. The therapeutic range for the serum lithium level is 0.5 to 1.2 mEq/L.
- Lithium is retained in the absence of sodium; thus, patients on a low-sodium diet are at greater risk of lithium toxicity.
- Other drugs useful in the treatment of bipolar disorder include atypical antipsychotics and some anticonvulsants.
- The FDA has issued a **BLACK BOX WARNING ◆** for aripiprazole; use places the patient at risk for the development of compulsive or uncontrollable urges to gamble, shop, binge eat, or have sex.
- The FDA has issued a **BLACK BOX WARNING ◆** concerning olanzapine because it can cause a drug reaction with eosinophilia and systemic symptoms.
- A **BLACK BOX WARNING ◆** for risperidone reports occurrence of increasing mortality in elderly patients with dementia-related psychosis.

## CLINICAL REASONING CASE STUDY

**Meet the Patient**

Mrs. Alexandra Greene is a 49-year-old woman who suffers from depression. She is being seen by the nurse practitioner, who works with a primary care provider. She states she is dragging, sleeps a lot, has no appetite, and says, "I can't seem to do anything right." She has been taking St. John's wort, but it has not helped her to feel better. Recently her mother passed away, and her twin daughters have entered college. The nurse practitioner has prescribed fluoxetine (Prozac) 20 mg once daily.

• What is the dosing schedule of fluoxetine, and when will Mrs. Greene's dosage be increased?
• How long will it take for her to respond to the initial dose?
• What is the action of fluoxetine?
• What are the adverse effects of fluoxetine?
• What patient teaching will you provide?

**Assessing Drug Information**

• Fluoxetine blocks the reabsorption of the neurotransmitter serotonin in the brain. This helps elevate the patient's mood. Fluoxetine has no effect on norepinephrine or dopamine.
• The dosing schedule for fluoxetine is as follows: 20 mg PO once daily in the morning, which is increased after several weeks if necessary. Give doses larger than 20 mg once in the morning or in two divided doses, morning and noon, to a maximum daily dose of 60 mg. For fluoxetine in the form of Prozac Weekly (delayed-release capsules), give 90 mg PO once each week, starting 7 days after the last 20-mg dose.
• The patient response to fluoxetine can significantly vary from patient to patient. The full response of the medication may not be seen for 8 to 12 weeks. Therapeutic serum levels of fluoxetine range from 100 to 800 ng/mL.
• Adverse effects of fluoxetine include nausea, diarrhea, weight loss, and sexual dysfunction (e.g., delayed ejaculation in men, impaired orgasmic ability in women). Most SSRIs also cause some degree of CNS stimulation (e.g., anxiety, nervousness, insomnia), which is most prominent with fluoxetine. SSRIs are also associated with increased risk of GI bleeding. For patients with diabetes mellitus, these drugs may have a hypoglycemic effect. Suicidal ideation may occur; it is more common in children and adolescents.
• Serotonin syndrome (a serious and sometimes fatal reaction characterized by hypertensive crisis, hyperpyrexia, extreme agitation progressing to delirium and coma, muscle rigidity, and seizures) may also occur. This results from combined therapy with an SSRI and an MAO inhibitor or another drug that potentiates serotonin neurotransmission.

**Nursing Actions**

• Instruct Mrs. Greene to discontinue St. John's wort. The combination of this herbal preparation with fluoxetine can lead to serotonin syndrome.
• Make sure she understands that it may take 8 to 12 weeks for her to experience an improvement in her mood.
• Assess her ability to complete her activities of daily living and reduction of depressive behaviors.
• Assess her for suicidal ideations and adverse drug reactions.

---

*Visit* thePoint® *at* **http://thePoint.lww.com/Frandsen12e** *for answers to NCLEX Success questions (in Appendix A), answers to Clinical Application Case Studies (in Appendix B), and more!*

## REFERENCES AND RESOURCES

American Psychiatric Association. (2016). *Series: DSM-5 Selections.* Arlington, VA: American Psychiatric Association Publishing. eBook. Database: eBook Clinical Collection (EBSCOhost).

Avery, D. *Seasonal affective disorder: Treatment.* UpToDate. Lexi-Comp, Inc.

Boyd, M. A. (2018). *Psychiatric nursing: Contemporary practice* (6th ed.). Philadelphia, PA: Wolters Kluwer.

Hirsch, M., & Birnbaum, R. J. (2020). *Selective serotonin reuptake inhibitors: Pharmacology, administration, and side effects.* UpToDate. Lexi-Comp, Inc.

Hirsch, M., & Birnbaum, R. J. (2020). *Tricyclic and tetracyclic drugs: Pharmacology, administration, and side effects.* UpToDate. Lexi-Comp, Inc.

Holtzheimer, P. E. (2020). *Bipolar disorder in adults: Overview of neuro-modulation procedures.* UpToDate. Lexi-Comp, Inc.

National Institutes of Health. (2020). Your guide to understanding genetic conditions: Bipolar disorder. *Genetics Home Reference.* Retrieved from: https://ghr.nlm.nih.gov/condition/bipolar-disorder#statistics

National Institutes of Health. (2020). Depression and older adults. National Institute on Aging. Retrieved from: https://www.nia.nih.gov/health/depression-and-older-adults

Nelson, C. (2020). *Serotonin-norepinephrine reuptake inhibitors (SNRIs): Pharmacology, administration, and side effects.* UpToDate. Lexi-Comp, Inc.

*Nursing 2020 drug handbook.* (2020) (40th ed.). Philadelphia, PA: Wolters Kluwer.

Stanford, S., Jones, M. P., & Hudson, J. L. (2018). Appreciating complexity in adolescent self-harm risk factors: psychological profiling in a longitudinal community sample. *Journal of Youth Adolescence, 47,* 916–931. doi: 10.1007/s10964-017-0721-5

UpToDate. (2020). *Drug information.* Lexi-Comp, Inc.

Viguera, A. (2020). *Postpartum unipolar major depression: Epidemiology, clinical features, assessment, and diagnosis.* UpToDate. Lexi-Comp, Inc.

# Drug Therapy for Psychotic Disorders

## LEARNING OBJECTIVES

*After studying this chapter, you should be able to:*

1. Discuss common manifestations of psychotic disorders, including schizophrenia.
2. Identify the prototype and describe the action, use, adverse effects, contraindications, and nursing implications for the first-generation antipsychotics.
3. Recognize the significance of the level of potency of first-generation antipsychotics.
4. Identify the prototype and describe the action, use, adverse effects, contraindications, and nursing implications for the second-generation antipsychotics.
5. Implement the nursing process in the care of the patient being treated with antipsychotics.

## CLINICAL APPLICATION CASE STUDY

Caroline Jones, a 20-year-old college student, is brought to the university's mental health clinic by a friend. The friend says that Caroline has been talking to the television set and has complained that the voices from the television are telling her that she is ugly. In addition, she has become more withdrawn and reclusive. Caroline has not taken care of her personal hygiene for some time, and she looks disheveled. She receives a diagnosis of psychosis. The treatment plan involves supportive psychotherapy and haloperidol 10 mg twice daily.

## KEY TERMS

**Akathisia:** motor restlessness and inability to be still, usually occurs in the first few months of treatment with antipsychotic agents

**Alogia:** poverty or lack of speech

**Anhedonia:** inability to experience pleasure

**Asociality:** social withdrawal

**Avolition:** lack of motivation

**Catatonia:** grossly disorganized or abnormal motor behavior

**Delusions:** false beliefs that persist in the absence of reason or evidence

**Disorganized thinking:** speech so disorganized that it substantially impairs communication

**Drug-induced parkinsonism:** loss of muscle movement, muscular rigidity and tremors, shuffling gait, masked facies, and drooling

**Dystonias:** uncoordinated, twisting, and repetitive movements

**Extrapyramidal effects:** movement disorders such as tardive dyskinesia, akathisia, dystonia, and drug-induced parkinsonism that may occur with usage of antipsychotic drugs

**Hallucinations:** sensory perceptions of people or objects that are not present in the external environment

**Neuroleptic malignant syndrome:** a rare but potentially fatal adverse effect; characterized by rigidity, severe hyperthermia, respiratory failure, and acute renal failure

**Paranoia:** belief that other people control their thoughts, feelings, and behaviors or seek to harm them

**Psychosis:** severe mental disorder characterized by disorganized thought processes, hallucinations, and delusions

**Tardive dyskinesia:** irreversible late extrapyramidal effect of some antipsychotic drugs that include lip smacking, tongue protrusion, facial grimaces, and choreic movements of trunk and limbs

# INTRODUCTION

This chapter introduces the pharmacologic care of the patient who is experiencing psychosis. **Psychosis** is a severe mental disorder characterized by disorganized thought processes. Emotional responses may be blunted or inappropriate. Behavior may be bizarre and range from hypoactivity to hyperactivity with agitation, aggressiveness, hostility, and combativeness; it also may involve social withdrawal in which a person pays less than normal attention to the environment and other people, deterioration from previous levels of occupational and social functioning (poor self-care and interpersonal skills), hallucinations, and paranoid delusions. This chapter focuses primarily on schizophrenia as a chronic psychosis.

Several features are characteristic of psychosis. **Hallucinations** are sensory perceptions of people or objects that are not present in the external environment. More specifically, people see, hear, or feel stimuli that are not visible to external observers, and they cannot distinguish between these false perceptions and reality. Hallucinations occur in delirium, dementias, schizophrenia, and other psychotic states. In schizophrenia or bipolar affective disorder, they are usually auditory; in delirium, they are usually visual or tactile; and in dementia, they are usually visual. **Delusions** are false beliefs that persist in the absence of reason or evidence. Deluded people are often fearful and exhibit **paranoia**, the belief that other people control their thoughts, feelings, and behaviors or seek to harm them. Delusions indicate severe mental illness. Although they are commonly associated with schizophrenia, delusions also occur with delirium, dementias, and other psychotic disorders.

# OVERVIEW OF PSYCHOSIS

Psychosis may be acute or chronic. Acute episodes, also called confusion or delirium, have a sudden onset over hours to days and may be precipitated by physical disorders (e.g., brain damage related to cerebrovascular disease or head injury, metabolic disorders, infections); drug intoxication with adrenergics, antidepressants, some anticonvulsants, amphetamines, cocaine, and others; and drug withdrawal after chronic use (e.g., alcohol, benzodiazepine antianxiety or sedative–hypnotic agents). In addition, acute psychotic episodes may be superimposed on chronic dementias and psychoses, such as schizophrenia.

## Etiology

Although schizophrenia is often referred to as a single disease, it includes a variety of related disorders. The lifetime prevalence of schizophrenia in the United States is approximately 1%. Males and females are equally affected; however, the disorder manifests itself earlier in males (early 20s for males as compared with late 20s to early 30s for females).

The etiology of schizophrenia is unknown. The neurodevelopmental model proposes that schizophrenia results when abnormal brain synapses are formed in response to an intrauterine insult during the second trimester of pregnancy, when neuronal migration is normally taking place. Intrauterine events such as upper respiratory infection, obstetric complications, and neonatal hypoxia have been associated with schizophrenia. The emergence of psychosis in response to the formation of these abnormal circuits in adolescence or early adulthood corresponds to the time period of neuronal maturation. Some studies of patients with schizophrenia have shown early neurologic abnormalities in infancy and early childhood, such as abnormal movements or motor developmental delays in infancy and psychological abnormalities as early as 4 years of age. This early onset of abnormalities coupled with emergence of schizophrenia in young adulthood suggests a neurodegenerative etiology for schizophrenia as well.

Genetics may play a role in the development of schizophrenia. Family studies identify increased risk if a first-degree relative has the illness (10%), if a second-degree relative has the illness (3%), if both parents have the illness (40%), and if a monozygotic twin has the illness (48%). Adoption studies of twins suggest that heredity rather than environment is a key factor in the development of schizophrenia.

Many genetic studies are underway to identify the gene or genes responsible for schizophrenia. Possible genes linked to schizophrenia include mutations in *WKL1* on chromosome 22, which may play a role in catatonic schizophrenia; mutations in *DISC1*, which cause delays in migration of brain neurons in mouse models; and mutation in the gene responsible for the glutamate receptor, which regulates the amount of glutamine in synapses.

## Pathophysiology

There is evidence of abnormal neurotransmission systems in the brains of people with schizophrenia, especially in the dopaminergic, serotonergic, and glutamatergic systems. There is also evidence of extensive interactions among neurotransmission systems. In addition, illnesses or drugs that alter neurotransmission in one system are likely to alter neurotransmission in other systems. The dopaminergic, serotonergic, and glutamatergic systems have been the focus of the most studies.

Researchers have studied the dopaminergic system more extensively studied than other systems, because, historically, scientists have attributed schizophrenia to increased dopamine activity in the brain. Stimulation of dopamine can initiate psychotic symptoms or exacerbate an existing psychotic disorder. Two findings further support the importance of dopamine: (1) antipsychotic drugs exert their therapeutic effects by decreasing dopamine activity (i.e., blocking dopamine receptors) and (2) drugs that increase dopamine levels in the brain (e.g., bromocriptine, cocaine, levodopa) can cause signs and symptoms of psychosis.

In addition to the increased amount of dopamine, dopamine receptor subtypes and their location also play a role. In general, authorities believe that overactivity of dopamine$_2$ (D$_2$) receptors in the basal ganglia, hypothalamus, limbic system, brainstem, and medulla accounts for the positive symptoms of schizophrenia (e.g., hallucinations, delusions, confused thought and speech, trouble concentrating, movement disorders). These experts also believe that underactivity of dopamine$_1$ (D$_1$) receptors in the prefrontal cortex accounts for associated negative symptoms including inability to experience pleasure (**anhedonia**), lack of motivation (**avolition**), diminished emotional expression, poor grooming and hygiene, poor social skills, poverty or lack of speech (**alogia**), and social withdrawal (**asociality**).

The serotonergic system, which is widespread in the brain, is mainly inhibitory in nature. In schizophrenia, serotonin apparently decreases dopamine activity in the part of the brain associated with negative symptoms, causing or aggravating these symptoms.

The glutamatergic neurotransmission system involves glutamate, the major excitatory neurotransmitter in the central nervous system (CNS). Glutamate receptors are widespread and possibly located on every neuron in the brain. They are also diverse, and their functions may vary according to subtypes and their locations in particular parts of the brain. When glutamate binds to its receptors, the resulting neuronal depolarization activates signaling molecules (e.g., calcium, nitric oxide) within and between brain cells. Thus, glutamatergic transmission may affect every CNS neuron and is considered essential for all mental, sensory, motor, and affective functions. Dysfunction of glutamatergic neurotransmission has been implicated in the development of psychosis.

In addition, the glutamatergic system interacts with the dopaminergic and gamma-aminobutyric acid (GABA) systems and possibly other neurotransmission systems. In people with schizophrenia, evidence indicates the presence of abnormalities in the number, density, composition, and function of glutamate receptors. During brain development, glutamate receptors are genetically encoded and can interact with environmental factors (e.g., stress, alcohol, and other drugs). Thus, glutamatergic dysfunction may account for the roles of genetic and environmental risk factors in the development of schizophrenia as well as the cognitive impairments and negative symptoms associated with the disorder.

## Clinical Manifestations

Symptoms of psychosis may begin gradually or suddenly, usually during adolescence or early adulthood. The American Psychiatric Association's *Diagnostic and Statistical Manual of Mental Disorders,* 5th edition (DSM-5), stipulates that characteristic psychotic symptoms must have been present during a 1-month period, with presence of some overt psychotic symptoms for at least 6 months, before schizophrenia can be diagnosed. There are five domains that comprise the clinical features of psychotic disorders: delusions, hallucinations, disorganized speech that impairs communication (**disorganized thinking**), grossly disorganized or abnormal motor behavior (**catatonia**), and negative symptoms. Two negative symptoms most often seen with schizophrenia include diminished emotional expression and avolition. Criteria changes for substance use disorders in the *DSM-5* provide for the ability to assign a diagnosis (unspecified schizophrenia spectrum and other psychotic disorder) to individuals who are experiencing symptoms of schizophrenia or other psychotic symptoms but do not meet the full diagnostic criteria for schizophrenia or another more specific psychotic disorder. Antipsychotic drugs are generally more effective in treating positive symptoms than negative symptoms, although the newer, atypical medications have been effective at treating the negative symptoms.

## Drug Therapy

Overall, the goal of drug treatment is to relieve symptoms with minimal or tolerable adverse effects. In patients with acute psychosis, the goal during the first week of treatment is to decrease symptoms (e.g., aggression, agitation, combativeness, hostility) and normalize patterns of sleeping and eating. The next goals may be increased ability for self-care and increased socialization. Therapeutic effects usually occur gradually, over 1 to 2 months. Long-term goals include increasing the patient's ability to cope with the environment, promoting optimal functioning in self-care and activities of daily living, and preventing acute episodes and hospitalizations. With drug therapy, patients often can participate in psychotherapy, group therapy, or other treatment modalities; return to community settings; and return to their preillness level of functioning.

Schizophrenia in children is often characterized by more severe symptoms and a more chronic course than in adults. Drug therapy in children has been largely empiric. However, research establishing an evidence base for treatment decisions in children and adolescents is growing. Dosage regulation is difficult because children may require lower plasma levels for therapeutic effects, but they also metabolize antipsychotic drugs more rapidly than do adults.

The American Academy of Child and Adolescent Psychiatry has updated established practice guidelines that advocate for high-quality assessment of the child or adolescent receiving antipsychotic medications. The purpose of the practice guidelines is to promote the appropriate use of antipsychotic medications and to enhance safety in the pediatric population. Box 56.1 lists major recommendations.

Table 56.1 summarizes the drugs used in the treatment of psychosis, which are also known as neuroleptics because of the increased risk of extrapyramidal neurologic effects with their

| BOX 56.1 | *Guidelines for the Use of Antipsychotic Medications in Children and Adolescents* |
|---|---|

Before starting therapy:

- Assess the general mental health of the family.
- Conduct a thorough psychiatric and physical examination.
- Explore strategies for pharmacologic and psychosocial treatment based on the best evidence.
- Choose a drug based on potency, adverse effect profile, and the patient's response.
- Educate the patient and family about the treatment and monitoring plan.
- Explain all risks and benefits of the treatment plan to the parents.
- Respond to any questions the parents or patient may have.
- Document the consent of the parents to the treatment plan.
- Assess the response to treatment and discuss with the patient and family the ongoing treatment plan.

use. As a class, antipsychotics are also effective in the treatment of acute agitation, bipolar mania, and other psychiatric conditions. These drugs may be broadly categorized as (1) "typical," "conventional," or first-generation agents and (2) "atypical" or second-generation agents. Typical antipsychotic drugs fall into five different major chemical categories, including two that are discussed in this chapter—the phenothiazines, such as chlorpromazine, and older nonphenothiazines, such as haloperidol. In addition, the typical, first-generation drugs can be classified by potency. The level of potency refers to the size of the dose needed to produce a given response; all first-generation antipsychotics have the same ability to relieve symptoms of psychosis.

- Low potency: chlorpromazine, thioridazine
- Medium potency: loxapine, perphenazine
- High potency: fluphenazine, haloperidol, pimozide, thiothixene, trifluoperazine

 **QSEN Alert: Safety**

Although the atypical antipsychotic agents have replaced the typical agents in the treatment of psychiatric disorders, they remain widely used in the treatment of nausea. See Chapter 38 for additional information.

Second-generation drugs, including clozapine and other related drugs, generally have lower risk of extrapyramidal adverse effects and tardive dyskinesia compared with the typical first-generation antipsychotics. Both generations of these drugs bind to $D_2$ dopamine receptors and block the action of dopamine (Fig. 56.1). However, binding to the receptors does not account for antipsychotic effects because binding occurs within a few hours after a drug dose, and antipsychotic effects may not occur until the drugs have been given for a few weeks.

Prescribers caring for patients with psychosis have a greater choice of drugs than ever before. Some general factors to consider include the patient's age and physical condition, the severity and duration of illness, the frequency and severity of adverse effects produced by each drug, the patient's use of and response to antipsychotic drugs in the past, the supervision available, and the prescriber's experience with a particular drug.

 **QSEN Alert: Safety**

All antipsychotics are identified in the Beers criteria as potentially inappropriate medications in patients 65 years and older with dementia. Antipsychotics should be avoided because they increase risk of mortality and cerebrovascular accidents as well as lead to a greater rate of cognitive decline.

People with schizophrenia usually need to take antipsychotics for years because there is a high rate of relapse (acute psychotic episodes) when drug therapy is discontinued,

## TABLE 56.1

### Drugs Administered for the Treatment of Psychosis

| Drug Class | Prototype | Other Drugs in the Class |
|---|---|---|
| First-generation (typical) antipsychotics | Chlorpromazine Haloperidol (Haldol) | Fluphenazine Loxapine Perphenazine Pimozide Thioridazine Trifluoperazine Thiothixene |
| Second-generation (atypical) antipsychotics | Clozapine (Clozaril, Versacloz) | Aripiprazole (Abilify, Abilify Maintena) Asenapine (Saphris, Secuado) Iloperidone (Fanapt) Lurasidone (Latuda) Olanzapine (Zyprexa, Zyprexa Relprevv) Paliperidone (Invega, Invega Sustenna, Invega Trinza) Quetiapine (Seroquel, Seroquel XR) Risperidone (Risperdal, Perseris, Risperdal Consta) Ziprasidone (Geodon) |

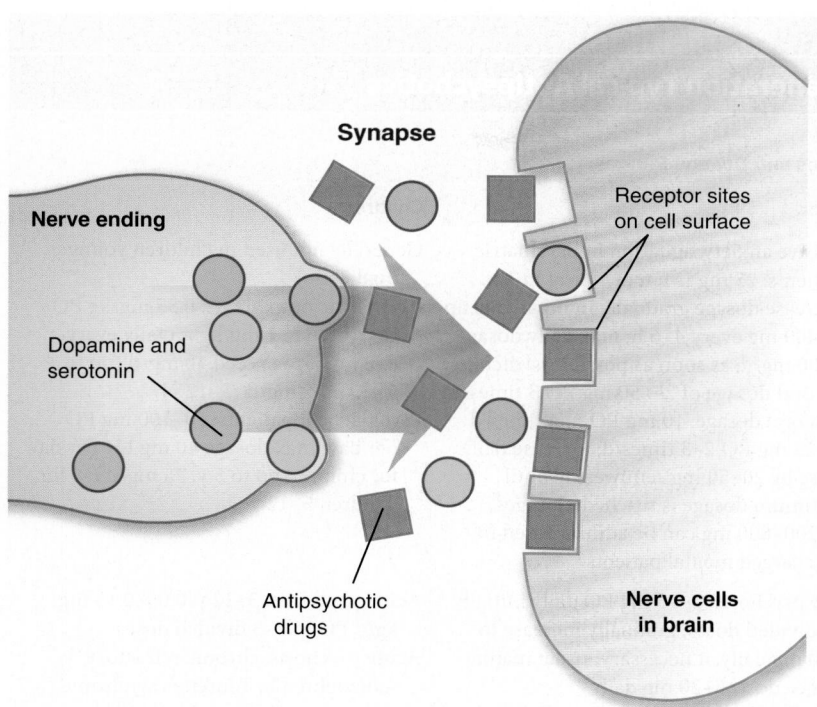

**Figure 56.1.** Antipsychotic drugs prevent dopamine and serotonin from occupying receptor sites on neuronal cell membranes and exerting their effects on cellular functions. This action leads to changes in receptors and cell functions that account for therapeutic effects (i.e., relief of psychotic symptoms). Other neurotransmitters and receptors may also be involved.

most often by patients who become unwilling or unable to continue taking their medication. With wider use of maintenance therapy and the newer, better-tolerated antipsychotic drugs, patients may experience fewer psychotic episodes and hospitalizations.

Most antipsychotics are available in oral formulations. Patients who are unable or unwilling to take daily doses of an antipsychotic may receive periodic injections of long-acting forms of aripiprazole, fluphenazine, haloperidol, olanzapine, risperidone, or paliperidone. These long-acting injectable (LAI) antipsychotics may be an important therapeutic option for patients with schizophrenia; it allows a prescriber to tailor pharmacotherapy to each patient's needs. The LAI form may serve to replace oral medications for patients who may have difficulty with medication adherence. These first- and second-generation antipsychotic LAIs are administered via "depot" injections. Depot refers to the way the drug is deposited and stored in the muscle before being absorbed. The injected drug takes time to move out of the muscle into the bloodstream, extending its action. However, extrapyramidal symptoms may be more problematic with depot injections of antipsychotics. Although some LAIs are expensive because they have been recently approved for use, they potentially reduce the financial burden of schizophrenia and improve quality of life.

## Clinical Application 56.1

- Describe the positive and negative symptoms that Caroline is experiencing.
- What neurotransmitter system is involved in Caroline's psychosis?
- How do antipsychotic drugs decrease Caroline's psychotic symptoms?

## NCLEX Success

1. A man is diagnosed with schizophrenia. He exhibits anhedonia, which is defined as which of the following?

   A. seizure activity
   B. inability to experience pleasure
   C. wormlike movements
   D. depression

2. A man is hospitalized because of a relapse of his psychotic disorder. He states, "I quit taking my medicines because I always forget to take them at least one time a day." Which of the following regimens for his antipsychotic medications will increase medication adherence?

   A. monthly injection by a home care nurse
   B. low-dose daily therapy
   C. daily visits to the clinic to receive his medications
   D. once-a-week drug therapy

## FIRST-GENERATION ANTIPSYCHOTICS

Health care providers have used the first-generation antipsychotics, including phenothiazines and nonphenothiazines, to treat psychosis since the 1950s. Although these drugs are historically significant, their usage and clinical importance have waned in recent years. Two drugs are identified as prototypes in this chapter. **Chlorpromazine hydrochloride** is the prototype drug of the phenothiazine groups, and **Haloperidol** (Haldol) is the prototype nonphenothiazine first-generation antipsychotic. Table 56.2 gives route and dosage information for the first-generation typical antipsychotics.

**TABLE 56.2**

## DRUGS AT A GLANCE: First-Generation Typical Antipsychotics

| Drug | Pregnancy Category | Routes and Dosage Ranges | |
|---|---|---|---|
| | | **Adults** | **Children** |
| ℞ **Chlorpromazine** (❋ Chlorpromazine Hydrochloride Injection, Teva-Chlorpromazine) | C | Excessive anxiety, agitation in psychiatric patients: 25 mg IM; may repeat in 1 h; increase dosage gradually in inpatients up to 400 mg every 4–6 h; max daily dosage 2000 mg/d; as soon as possible, switch to an oral dosage of 25–50 mg PO 3 times/d<br>Initial oral dosage: 10 mg PO 3–4 times/d or 25 mg PO 2–3 times/d; increase daily dose by 20–50 mg semiweekly until optimum dosage is reached; dosages of 200–800 mg can be administered in discharged mental patients | Generally not used in children younger than 6 mo<br>Psychiatric outpatients: 0.55 mg/kg PO every 4–6 h, 1 mg/kg rectally every 6–8 h not to exceed 40 mg/d (up to 5 y), or 75 mg/d (5–12 y)<br>Psychiatric inpatients: 50–100 mg PO per day; max dosage 40 mg IM per day for children up to 5 y; 75 mg/d IM for children 5–12 y |
| ℞ **Haloperidol** (Haldol, Haldol decanoate; ❋ Novo-Peridol, PMS-Haloperidol, PMS-Haloperidol LA) | C | Acute psychosis: 1–15 mg PO daily initially in divided doses; gradually increase to 100 mg daily, if necessary; usual maintenance dose, 5–20 mg daily<br>Chronic schizophrenia: 6–15 mg PO daily; max 100 mg daily; dosage is reduced for maintenance, usually 15–20 mg daily.<br>Haloperidol decanoate IM, initial dose up to 100 mg, depending on previous dose of oral drug, then titrated according to response; usually given every 4 wk | Acute psychosis: 3–12 y, 0.05–0.15 mg/kg/d PO in 2–3 divided doses<br>Acute psychosis, chronic refractory schizophrenia, Tourette's syndrome, mental retardation with hyperkinesia: 13 y and older, same as adults<br>Chronic refractory schizophrenia: dosage not established<br>Tourette's syndrome: 1.5–6 mg PO daily initially in divided doses; usual maintenance dose, 1.5 mg daily<br>Mental retardation with hyperkinesia: 1.5 mg PO initially, in divided doses, gradually increase to a max of 15 mg daily, if necessary; when symptoms are controlled, dosage is gradually reduced to the minimum effective level; IM dosage not established |
| Fluphenazine (❋ Apo-Fluphenazine, Fluphenazine Omega) | C | 2.5–10 mg PO initially, gradually reduced to maintenance dose of 1–5 mg (doses above 3 mg are rarely necessary)<br>Acute psychosis: 1.25 mg initially, increased gradually to 2.5–10 mg daily in 3–4 divided doses | 5–12 y, 0.75–10 mg PO daily; no IM dosage established |
| Loxapine (❋ Loxapac, PHL-Loxapine, Xylac) | | Schizophrenia, 10 mg PO twice daily; usual dosage 60–100 mg daily in divided doses 2–4 times daily; max dosage not to exceed 250 mg daily<br>Acute agitation with schizophrenia or bipolar disorder, 10 mg once daily; max dosage 10 mg in 24-h period | Safety and efficacy not established |
| Perphenazine (❋ Apo-Perphenazine) | C | Outpatients: 4–8 mg PO 3 times/d; reduce dose as soon as possible to minimum effective dosage; max dosage 64 mg/d<br>Inpatients: 8–16 mg PO 2–4 times/d; max dosage 64 mg/d | 4 mg PO 2–4 times/d; max dosage 16 mg/d |
| Pimozide (❋ Apo-Pimozide, Orap) | | 1–2 mg PO daily initially; max dosage 10 mg daily or 0.2 mg/kg/d (whichever is less) | 2–12 y, 0.05 mg/kg PO initially at bedtime; usual dosage 2–4 mg daily; max dosage 0.2 mg/kg/d not to exceed 10 mg daily |

| **TABLE 56.2** | | | |
| --- | --- | --- | --- |
| **DRUGS AT A GLANCE: First-Generation Typical Antipsychotics** (Continued) | | | |
| **Drug** | **Pregnancy Category** | **Routes and Dosage Ranges** | |
| | | **Adults** | **Children** |
| Thioridazine | C | 50–100 mg PO initially three times daily; usual dosage 300–5800 mg in 2–4 divided doses; max dosage 800 mg daily | ≥6 y: 0.5 mg/kg/d PO; max daily dose 3 mg/kg/d |
| Thiothixene (✹ Navane) | C | 6–10 mg PO daily in divided doses; usual dosage 20–30 mg daily; max 60 mg daily Elderly or debilitated adults, PO one third to one half the usual adult dosage | <12 y, dosage not established ≥12 y, same as adults |
| Trifluoperazine | | 2–5 mg PO initially daily in divided doses; usual dosage 15–20 mg daily; max dosage 50 mg daily | 6–12 y: 1 mg initially 1–2 times daily; max dosage 15 mg daily Adolescents: same as adults |

## Pharmacokinetics

Chlorpromazine is well absorbed and distributed to most body tissues, and it reaches high concentrations in the brain. After oral administration, the onset of action is 30 to 60 minutes, with a peak of 2 to 4 hours and a duration of 4 to 6 hours. After intramuscular (IM) administration, the onset of action is 10 to 15 minutes, with a peak at 15 to 20 minutes and a duration of 4 to 6 hours. The half-life is 2 to 30 hours. The drug is metabolized in the liver and excreted in urine.

## Action

The mechanism of action of chlorpromazine is not fully understood. When the drug produces antipsychotic effects, it blocks the postsynaptic dopamine receptors in the brain.

## Use

The major clinical indication for chlorpromazine and other phenothiazine antipsychotics is schizophrenia. Other uses include treatment of psychotic symptoms associated with brain impairment induced by head injury, tumor, stroke, alcohol withdrawal, overdoses of CNS stimulants, and other disorders.

It is necessary to individualize the dosage and route of administration of chlorpromazine according to the patient's condition and response; in some cases, prescribers may exceed the recommended maximum dosage approved by the U.S. Food and Drug Administration (FDA).

### Use in Children

Chlorpromazine is administered for the treatment of psychosis. The drug is not routinely administered to children under the age of 6 months. It is also used preoperatively for the control of restlessness and apprehension. In addition, it is administered rectally or intramuscularly for the control of nausea and vomiting.

### Use in Older Adults

Chlorpromazine should be administered cautiously to older adults. The dosage of chlorpromazine should be started at one fourth to one third of the level for younger adults. Older adults

are more likely to have problems for which chlorpromazine and other antipsychotic agents are contraindicated (e.g., severe cardiovascular disease, liver damage, Parkinson's disease) or must be used very cautiously (diabetes mellitus, glaucoma, prostatic hypertrophy, peptic ulcer disease, chronic respiratory disorders).

### Use in Patients With Renal Impairment

Excretion of chlorpromazine takes place in the kidneys, and therefore, caution is necessary when using the drug in patients with impaired renal function. It is necessary to monitor renal function periodically during long-term therapy and lower the dosage or discontinue the drug altogether if test results (e.g., blood urea nitrogen) become abnormal.

### Use in Patients With Hepatic Impairment

Chlorpromazine undergoes extensive hepatic metabolism, which means that caution is warranted in patients with hepatic impairment. In the presence of liver disease (e.g., cirrhosis, hepatitis), metabolism may be slowed and drug elimination half-lives prolonged, with resultant accumulation and increased risk of adverse effects.

### Use in Patients With Critical Illness

Antipsychotic medications have been used for decades to treat symptoms associated with delirium in critically ill patients. Undesirable adverse effects caused by chlorpromazine include anticholinergic symptoms, hypotension, tachycardia, cardiac dysrhythmias, and extrapyramidal symptoms, which limit its use (see Adverse Effects). In addition, chlorpromazine has been shown to lower the seizure threshold. Because of these serious problems, chlorpromazine is generally not recommended for critically ill patients. There are other antipsychotic medications that have a lower adverse effect profile that may be more effective.

### Use in Patients Receiving Home Care

People with chronic mental illness, such as schizophrenia, are among the most challenging in the caseload of the home care nurse. Major recurring problems include failure to take antipsychotic medications as prescribed and the concurrent use of alcohol and other drugs of abuse. Either problem is likely to lead to acute psychotic episodes and hospitalizations. The nurse must assist and support caregivers' efforts to administer medications and manage adverse effects, other aspects of daily care, and follow-up psychiatric care. In addition, the nurse may need to coordinate the efforts of several health and social service agencies or providers.

## Adverse Effects

Chlorpromazine has several adverse effects, including

- CNS effects: excessive sedation, with drowsiness, lethargy, fatigue, slurred speech, impaired mobility, and impaired mental processes. **Extrapyramidal effects** may also occur. Symptoms include movement disorders such as tardive dyskinesia, akathisia, dystonia, and drug-induced parkinsonism.

  - **Tardive dyskinesia** occurs as the result of long-term chlorpromazine use. Patients may experience lip smacking, tongue protrusion, and facial grimaces and may have choreic movements of trunk and limbs. This condition is usually irreversible, and there is no effective treatment.
  - **Akathisia** (motor restlessness and inability to be still), the most common extrapyramidal reaction, may occur about 5 to 60 days from the start of drug therapy.
  - **Dystonias** are uncoordinated bizarre movements of the neck, face, eyes, tongue, trunk, or extremities. These adverse effects may occur suddenly 1 to 5 days after drug therapy is started and may be misinterpreted as seizures or other disorders.
  - **Drug-induced parkinsonism** is loss of muscle movement (akinesia), muscular rigidity and tremors, shuffling gait, masked facies, and drooling.
  - **Neuroleptic malignant syndrome** is a rare but potentially fatal reaction, which may occur hours to months after initial drug use. Symptoms of fever, muscle rigidity, respiratory failure, and confusion develop rapidly.

- Cardiovascular effects: prolonged QT and PR interval, T-wave blunting, and depression of the ST interval.
- Hematologic effects: agranulocytosis and pancytopenia.
- Other effects: antiadrenergic effects, such as hypotension, dizziness, fatigue, and faintness, as well as respiratory depression, endocrine effects, photosensitivity, and difficulty with temperature regulation.

## Contraindications

Because of wide-ranging adverse effects, chlorpromazine may cause or aggravate a number of conditions. Contraindications include liver damage, coronary artery disease, cerebrovascular disease, parkinsonism, bone marrow depression, severe hypotension or hypertension, coma, and severely depressed states. Caution is warranted in seizure disorders, diabetes mellitus, glaucoma, prostatic hypertrophy, peptic ulcer disease, and chronic respiratory disorders, as well as in pregnancy, especially during the first trimester.

## Nursing Implications

### Preventing Interactions

Many medications interact with chlorpromazine, increasing or decreasing its effects (Box 56.2). The combination of the herbal supplement with kava results in increased dystonia.

## Administering the Medication

For acute psychotic episodes, therapy with chlorpromazine may require IM administration and hospitalization. Control of symptoms usually occurs within 48 to 72 hours, after which the person takes the oral drug. It is necessary to obtain a baseline electrocardiogram (ECG) prior to administering the drug, because of associated risk of alterations in the cardiac rhythm. The nurse needs to check doses carefully, especially when starting or stopping an antipsychotic drug or substituting one for another. The dosages are often changed during the course of treatment. When the drug is started, it is usually necessary to titrate initial doses upward over days or weeks and then reduce them for maintenance. Discontinuation of the drug requires a gradual reduction in dosage.

For IM administration, the nurse adheres to the following guidelines:

- Determine the dose, which is approximately half of an oral dose. IM doses avoid first-pass metabolism and produce serum drug levels approximately double those of oral doses.
- Change the needle after filling the syringe with the injectable medication.
- Give the injection in the ventrogluteal muscle with a 1½-inch needle.
- Have the patient lie down for 30 to 60 minutes after the injection to prevent orthostatic hypotension.
- Watch for idiopathic edema and muscle necrosis, which may occur with IM administration.

For oral administration, the nurse adheres to the following guidelines:

- Give doses 1 to 2 hours before bedtime; peak sedation occurs in about 2 hours.
- Mix liquid concentrations with at least 60 mL of fruit juice. Avoid contact with skin because the liquid forms can cause contact dermatitis.

**BOX 56.2** **Drug Interactions: Chlorpromazine**

**Drugs That Increase the Effects of Chlorpromazine**
- Barbiturates, lithium
  *May decrease phenothiazine effect*
- Central nervous system [CNS] depressants, narcotics
  *Produce additive CNS depression and hypotension*
- Anticholinergic drugs
  *Increase anticholinergic effects such as decreased secretions and urinary retention*
- Beta-adrenergic blockers, centrally acting hypertensives
  *Produce tachycardia, may decrease antihypertensive effect*
- Epinephrine, norepinephrine
  *Produce hypotension*

**Drugs That Decrease the Effects of Chlorpromazine**
- Antacids
  *Decrease absorption*
- Anticholinergic drugs
  *Decrease antipsychotic effects*

- Administer the oral preparation with food to reduce gastric upset.
- Use divided doses.

### Assessing for Therapeutic Effects

With acute psychotic episodes, the nurse observes for decreased agitation, combativeness, and psychomotor activity. The sedative effects of chlorpromazine, considered to be therapeutic, occur within 48 to 72 hours. With acute or chronic psychosis, the nurse observes for decreased psychotic behaviors, such as decreased hallucinations and delusions.

### Assessing for Adverse Effects

The nurse assesses the fluid and electrolyte status for a possible fluid volume deficit. It is also necessary to measure the patient's weight daily and assess for signs of dehydration. In addition, the nurse assesses for increased anticholinergic effects, such as diminished fluid status and urinary retention.

The nurse assesses for aspiration related to depressed cough reflex. It is important to monitor renal and hepatic function along with the complete blood count. A depression in white blood cell count requires discontinuation of the medication.

The nurse monitors for increased CNS depression that could result in falls or altered safety. He or she assesses for extrapyramidal effects such as dystonia, tardive dyskinesia, and akathisia.

### Patient Teaching

Box 56.3 identifies patient teaching guidelines for chlorpromazine.

## Other Drugs in the Class

Although all of these agents are equally effective, symptomatic relief varies from one drug to another.

---

**BOX 56.3**  *Patient Teaching Guidelines for Chlorpromazine*

- Take the medication as prescribed.
- Do not combine the medication with over-the-counter medications or alcohol.
- Be sure to drink enough fluids, especially during hot weather.
- If you go outdoors, wear protective clothing and use sunscreen.
- Use caution when changing positions. It may be necessary to lie down for approximately an hour after taking your medication, because faintness and dizziness may occur.
- Do not overexercise and reduce body fluids.
- Do not drive a car or operate dangerous machinery. Dizziness or decreased mental alertness may occur.
- Report dark urine, pale stools, and yellowing of the eyes or skin to a health care provider.
- If you are a woman of childbearing age and intend to become pregnant, discuss chlorpromazine use with a health care provider.

---

Fluphenazine is a high-potency antipsychotic used in the management of schizophrenia. The most common adverse effect seen is extrapyramidal symptoms. Other effects include menstrual irregularities, gynecomastia, and galactorrhea. Relative to other antipsychotics, fluphenazine has a low potential of anticholinergic effects (constipation, xerostomia, blurred vision, urinary retention). The drug can be administered orally or intramuscularly. Two injectable preparations are available; the decanoate injection is a depot preparation and intended for use in the management of patients who require prolonged therapy.

Pimozide is a high-potency agent approved only for the treatment of Tourette's syndrome. The drug suppresses severe motor and phonic tics that have not responded to standard treatment. Adverse effects include sedation, akathisia, drowsiness, akinesia, and visual disturbances. More rarely, neuroleptic malignant syndrome and prolongation of the QT interval can occur. Pimozide can also prolong the QT interval on the ECG, which increases the risk of fatal dysrhythmias. Concurrent administration with citalopram (Celexa), escitalopram (Lexapro), or sertraline (Zoloft) should be avoided because the combination can increase the risk of dysrhythmias. An ECG should be performed baseline and periodically thereafter, especially during dosage adjustment to observe for prolongation of the QT interval.

Because the drug is highly metabolized by CYP1A2, CYP2D6, and CYP3A4 of the cytochrome P-450 system, major drug interactions are possible.

> **! QSEN Alert: Safety**
>
> In adults and children, if drug therapy with pimozide exceeds a dose of 4 mg/day, CYP2D6 genomic testing is recommended; CYP2D6 poor metabolizers should receive incremental dose changes over greater time (14 days) and should not receive doses in excess of 4 mg/day.

Trifluoperazine is a high-potency antipsychotic that is used to treat schizophrenia and other psychotic disorders. The drug leads to early extrapyramidal symptoms most commonly, and it has a moderate potential for anticholinergic effects.

Perphenazine and loxapine are medium-potency agents used to treat schizophrenia. Perphenazine is also used to manage other psychotic disorders. The adverse effect profile of both drugs is similar to fluphenazine.

Thioridazine is a low-potency antipsychotic that is now reserved for use in patients with schizophrenia who have not responded to safer agents. The drug prolongs the QT interval, which increases the risk of fatal dysrhythmias. The most common adverse effects relate to its anticholinergic effects. Weight gain and inhibition of ejaculation may also occur.

## NCLEX Success

3. The nurse should administer chlorpromazine in which of the following ways?

   A. intramuscularly into the deltoid muscle
   B. subcutaneously into the abdomen
   C. intramuscularly in the ventrogluteal muscle
   D. subcutaneously in the small of the back

4. In monitoring the status of a patient on a course of a phenothiazine antipsychotic, the nurse needs to be most aware that an adverse effect of phenothiazine antipsychotics is the development of which of the following?

   A. glaucoma
   B. akathisia
   C. hypertension
   D. diabetes

5. A man is taking chlorpromazine. He develops a high fever, respiratory depression, and diminished level of consciousness. What condition has the patient developed?

   A. neuroleptic malignant syndrome
   B. dystonia
   C. anhedonia
   D. akathisia

6. A 68-year-old man is seen by a home care nurse. He has been taking chlorpromazine since 1969 for schizophrenia. Which of the following adverse effects are most commonly seen after use of chlorpromazine for long periods?

   A. lethargy
   B. amnesia
   C. tardive dyskinesia
   D. dystonia

# FIRST-GENERATION NONPHENOTHIAZINES

Nonphenothiazines include the first-generation antipsychotics, which are similar to phenothiazines in many ways. They were introduced approximately 50 years ago and are effective in treating acute psychosis, chronic psychotic disorders, and other psychiatric conditions. They are effective in treating both psychotic disorders and nonpsychotic depression.

The first-generation antipsychotic medication **Haloperidol** (Haldol) is the prototype "typical" nonphenothiazine. This butyrophenone is a frequently used, long-acting antipsychotic.

## Pharmacokinetics

Haloperidol is well absorbed after oral or IM administration. For the oral drug, the onset of action is 2 hours, with a peak of 2 to 6 hours and a duration of 8 to 12 hours. For the IM drug, the onset of action is 20 to 30 minutes, with a peak of 30 to 45 minutes and a duration of 4 to 8 hours. The half-life of the drug is 21 to 24 hours. It is metabolized in the liver and is excreted in urine and bile.

## Action

The mechanism of action of haloperidol is not fully understood, but experts believe that the drug produces antipsychotic effects by blocking the postsynaptic dopamine receptors in the brain.

## Use

Prescribers order haloperidol to control the symptoms of schizophrenia and psychotic disorders.

### Use in Children

The FDA has issued a **BLACK BOX WARNING ◆** regarding extrapyramidal and withdrawal symptoms in newborns who have been exposed to haloperidol. Withdrawal symptoms occur in newborns born to women who take haloperidol during the third trimester of pregnancy.

### Use in Older Adults

It is important to note that the FDA has not approved haloperidol for treatment of dementia-related psychosis. A **BLACK BOX WARNING ◆** alerts health care practitioners that older patients who suffer from dementia and dementia-related psychosis and receive haloperidol have an increased risk of death compared with those patients who receive a placebo. (The deaths were related to cardiovascular or infectious diseases.)

### Use in Patients With Renal Impairment

Excretion of haloperidol takes place in the kidneys, and therefore, caution is necessary when using the drug in patients with impaired renal function. It is necessary to monitor renal function periodically during long-term therapy and lower the dosage or discontinue the drug altogether if test results (e.g., blood urea nitrogen) become abnormal.

### Use in Patients With Hepatic Impairment

Haloperidol undergoes extensive hepatic metabolism. In the presence of liver disease (e.g., cirrhosis, hepatitis), metabolism may be slower, with resultant accumulation and increased risk of adverse effects. Thus, caution is necessary.

### Use in Patients With Critical Illness

Haloperidol has relatively weak sedative effects and does not cause respiratory depression. However, it can cause hypotension in patients who are volume depleted or receiving antihypertensive drugs. It can also cause cardiac dysrhythmias, including life-threatening torsade de pointes, in patients who are receiving large doses (greater than 50 mg/day) or who have abnormal serum electrolyte levels (e.g., calcium, potassium, magnesium). Patients should be on a cardiac monitor, and it is necessary to check the ECG for a prolonged QT interval.

### Use in Patients Receiving Home Care

Major recurring challenges face patients with psychosis and their caregivers in the home. Supporting efforts to stabilize positive and negative symptoms and cognitive function, take medications as prescribed, manage adverse effects, and follow-up psychiatric care may require the coordinated efforts of several health and social service agencies or providers.

## Adverse Effects

Haloperidol has several adverse effects, including

- Cardiovascular effects: abnormal T waves, prolonged ventricular depolarization, QT prolongation, torsade de pointes, tachycardia, and sudden death

- CNS effects: akathisia, hyperthermia, dystonia, extrapyramidal symptoms, neuroleptic malignant syndrome, parkinsonism, seizures, and vertigo
- Dermatologic effects: photosensitivity, hyperpigmentation, contact dermatitis, and alopecia
- Genitourinary effects: anticholinergic adverse effects such as urinary retention, sexual dysfunction, amenorrhea, breast engorgement and galactorrhea (women), and priapism and gynecomastia (men)
- Metabolic effects: hyperglycemia, hypoglycemia, and hyponatremia
- Respiratory effects: bronchospasm or laryngospasm

## Contraindications

Contraindications to haloperidol include Parkinson's disease, seizure disorders, and severe mental depression.

## Nursing Implications

### Preventing Interactions

Many medication and herbs interact with haloperidol (Boxes 56.4 and 56.5), increasing or decreasing its effects.

### Administering the Medication

Oral administration of haloperidol tablets requires taking the tablets with a full glass of water or milk. People should take them with food to decrease gastric upset. IM administration of haloperidol decanoate requires that the nurse gives the drug intramuscularly deep in the ventrogluteal muscle. (The amount injected should not exceed 3 mL.) During administration of the IM preparation, the patient should be in the recumbent position and remain recumbent for 1 hour following the administration. It is necessary to keep the preparation in a light-protected container.

**BOX 56.4** **Drug Interactions: Haloperidol**

**Drugs That Increase the Effects of Haloperidol**

- Alcohol, central nervous system depressants, anticholinergic drugs, antidepressants, antihistamines
  *Increase sedation and anticholinergic effects*
- Nonsteroidal anti-inflammatory drugs
  *Increase drowsiness and confusion*
- Propranolol and angiotensin-converting enzyme inhibitors, lithium
  *Enhance neurotoxic effect of antipsychotics and increase extrapyramidal symptoms*
- Antifungals, buspirone, macrolides
  *May increase haloperidol level*

**Drugs That Decrease the Effects of Haloperidol**

- Antacids
  *Inhibit absorption*
- Carbamazepine, rifampin
  *May decrease haloperidol level*

**BOX 56.5** **Herb and Dietary Interactions: Haloperidol**

**Herbs and Foods That Increase the Effects of Haloperidol**

- American and Asian ginseng
- Kava
- Gotu kola
- Scotch broom
- St. John's wort
- Valerian
- Yohimbine

When discontinuing haloperidol, it is essential to taper the dosage to prevent extrapyramidal symptoms. If the medication is abruptly discontinued, the patient is at risk for this condition.

### Assessing for Therapeutic Effects

When haloperidol is given for acute psychotic episodes, the nurse observes for sedation, decreased agitation, combativeness, and psychomotor activity. When the drug is given for acute or chronic psychosis, he or she observes for decreased psychotic behaviors, such as decreased hallucinations and delusions.

### Assessing for Adverse Effects

The nurse assesses the ECG for tachycardia and other abnormalities. Also, he or she assesses the patient's temperature for the onset of neuroleptic malignant syndrome. In addition, the nurse assesses for laryngospasm. Finally, it is necessary to monitor for the development of parkinsonism and extrapyramidal signs and symptoms, most notably tardive dyskinesia.

### Patient Teaching

Box 56.6 identifies patient teaching guidelines for haloperidol.

**BOX 56.6** **Patient Teaching Guidelines for Haloperidol**

- Take the medication as prescribed.
- Report sore throat or fever to the prescriber.
- Notify the prescriber of any adverse effects such as tardive dyskinesia, dystonia, or akathisia.
- Do not drive a car or operate dangerous machinery. Dizziness or decreased mental alertness may occur.
- If you go outdoors, wear protective closing and use sun screen.
- Maintain adequate hydration.
- Use lozenges to counteract anticholinergic effects.
- Realize that dark-colored urine (pink or red-brown) is normal.
- If you are a woman of childbearing age and intend to become pregnant, discuss haloperidol use with a health care provider.

## Other Drugs in the Class

Thiothixene is a high-potency antipsychotic used in the management of schizophrenia. The most common adverse effect seen is extrapyramidal symptoms. Other effects include menstrual irregularities, gynecomastia, and galactorrhea. Use with other anticholinergic agents or drugs that are CNS depressants can enhance adverse effects.

### Clinical Application 56.2

- After 6 weeks of therapy, Caroline has far fewer symptoms. She has withdrawn from her university classes to focus on her treatment and recovery. However, her friends observe that she has a gradual loss of muscle movement and a shuffling gait. What adverse reaction is likely to be occurring?
- Caroline has decided that she no longer wants to take the medication because of the adverse effects, despite experiencing a decrease in psychotic thinking. How would the nurse handle this situation?

### NCLEX Success

7. An elderly woman with dementia is receiving haloperidol. What adverse effect is this woman at increased risk for developing?

   A. anorexia
   B. increased temperature
   C. infection
   D. tardive dyskinesia

8. A patient is receiving haloperidol decanoate 100 mg intramuscularly. What assessment should the nurse make before and after the administration of the medication?

   A. pulse rate
   B. respiratory rate
   C. blood pressure
   D. mental status

9. A patient is taking thiothixene. Which of the following outcomes is desirable with this medication?

   A. decreased heart rate and diminished agitation
   B. blood pressure within normal limits and diminished psychosis
   C. heart rate of 60 beats/min with increased pulse pressure
   D. a widened QT complex and normal ST segment

## SECOND-GENERATION "ATYPICAL" ANTIPSYCHOTICS

The "atypical" antipsychotics are the drugs of choice, especially for patients who are newly diagnosed with schizophrenia. These second-generation antipsychotics differ from first-generation agents in that they have a broader range of action due to their effects on the serotonergic, noradrenergic, and dopaminergic systems. They may be more effective in relieving some symptoms, they usually produce milder adverse effects, and patients seem to take them more consistently. Better adherence to the drug regimen helps prevent acute episodes of psychosis and repeated hospitalizations, thereby reducing the overall cost of health care, according to studies. A major drawback is the high cost of these drugs, which may preclude their use in some patients. **Clozapine** (Clozaril, Versacloz) is the prototype "atypical" antipsychotic.

## Pharmacokinetics

Clozapine is an oral drug. Its onset of action is unknown, with a peak of 1 to 6 hours and a duration of weeks. The half-life is 12 hours. Clozapine crosses the placenta and enters the breast milk. The drug is metabolized in the liver, and it is excreted in the urine and in the feces.

## Action

The mechanism of action of clozapine is not clearly understood. Apparently, the drug blocks the dopamine receptors in the brain, depressing the reticular activating system. It also blocks the serotonin and glutamate receptors. In addition, clozapine has anticholinergic, antihistamine, and alpha-adrenergic blocking activity.

## Use

Clinicians consider clozapine and other "atypical" antipsychotics to be first-line therapy for schizophrenia. Prescribers use the drug to manage patients with severe schizophrenia who have not responded to standard antipsychotic medications. Other uses in psychosis include reducing the risk of recurrent suicidal behavior in patients with schizophrenia or with schizoaffective disorder. Clozapine is available only through a distribution system that ensures monitoring of white blood cell count and absolute neutrophil count. Table 56.3 presents route and dosage information for atypical antipsychotics, including clozapine.

### Use in Children

Despite the wide range of benefits associated with clozapine treatment, use of this drug has been reserved for treatment-resistant children and adolescents because of its greater propensity to cause serious hematologic adverse events (agranulocytosis) compared with other first- and second-generation antipsychotic medications. The safety and effectiveness of clozapine in children have not been established.

### Use in Older Adults

The FDA has issued a **BLACK BOX WARNING** ◆ related to the administration of clozapine and other second-generation antipsychotics to elderly patients with dementia. The risk of death is increased in these patients. The FDA has not approved the drug for use in dementia-related psychosis.

## Use in Patients With Renal Impairment

Although renal complications of clozapine use are very rare, it is essential that psychiatrists using clozapine are aware of the

**TABLE 56.3**

## DRUGS AT A GLANCE: Atypical Antipsychotics

| Drug | Pregnancy Category | Routes and Dosage Ranges | |
|---|---|---|---|
| | | **Adults** | **Children** |
| **Clozapine** (Clozaril, Versacloz; ❋ Clozaril, AA-Clozapine, GEN-Clozapine) | B | 12.5 mg PO once or twice daily; increase by 25–50 mg daily every 3–7 d up to a max dose of 900 mg daily. | ≥6 y, 6.25–12.5 mg once daily<br>Adolescents, 12.5 mg PO initially once or twice daily; increase to a target dose of 125–475 mg/d in divided doses |
| Aripiprazole (Abilify, Abilify Maintena; ❋ Abilify, Abilify Maintena, TEVA-ARIPiprazole) | C | Acute agitation: 9.75 mg PO initially as a single dose; range 5.25–15 mg PO daily initially; repeat doses may be given at ≥2-h intervals to maximum of 30 mg daily<br>Schizophrenia: 10–15 mg once daily; may be increased to a max dosage of 30 mg once daily; extended release 400 mg IM once monthly<br>Older adults: 12.5–25 mg PO daily, increase in 2.5-mg increments to desired response | ≥8 y, 10–15 mg PO once daily initially; efficacy has not been established above 10–15 mg daily |
| Asenapine (Saphris, Secuado; ❋ Saphris) | C | Schizophrenia: 5 mg SL 2 times/d<br>Secuado (patch): 3.8 mg/24 h once daily; may increase to 5.7 mg/24 h or 7.6 mg/24 h after 1 wk<br>Bipolar disorder: 10 mg SL 2 times/d; may be decreased to 5 mg/d as needed | ≥10 y, 2.5 mg SL 2 time/daily, maximum 20 mg/d |
| Iloperidone (Fanapt) | C | 12–24 mg PO daily; titrate based on orthostatic hypotension tolerance; initially 1 mg PO 2 times/d then 2, 4, 6, 8, 10, and 12 mg PO 2 times/d on days 2, 3, 4, 5, 6, and 7, respectively | Safety and efficacy not established |
| Lurasidone (Latuda; ❋ Latuda) | C | 40 mg PO initially once daily; max recommended dose is 160 mg/d; take with food (≥350 calories)<br>Elderly: do not give to older patients with dementia-related psychosis | 13–17 y, 40 mg PO initially once daily; max recommended dose is 80 mg/d<br>>17 y, same as adult |
| Olanzapine (Zyprexa; ❋ Teva-Olanzapine ODT, APO-Olanzapine, Zyprexa) | C | 5–10 mg PO initially once daily at bedtime; increase over several weeks to 20 mg daily, if necessary | 4–<6 y, 1.25 mg PO once daily titrated to target of 10 mg/d<br>6–12 y, 2.5 mg PO once daily titrated to target of 10 mg/d<br>Adolescents, initial: 2.5–5 mg PO once daily titrated to target of 10 mg/d once daily |
| Paliperidone (Invega, Invega Sustenna, Invega Trinza; ❋ Invega, Invega Sustenna, Invega Trinza) | C | 6 mg PO daily in the morning; may be increased over several weeks to max of 12 mg daily<br>Maintenance dose of 39–234 mg (as palmitate) or 25–150 mg (as base) every month IM monthly (Invega Sustenna) or every 3 mo (Invega Trinza) | ≤18 y, 6 mg PO once daily or 78–234 mg IM monthly |
| Quetiapine (Seroquel, Seroquel XR; ❋ Dom-Quetiapine, Seroquel, Seroquel XR, BIO-Quetiapine) | C | 25 mg PO 2 times/d initially; increase by 25–50 mg two or three times daily on 2nd and 3rd days, as tolerated, to 300–400 mg, in two or three divided doses on the 4th day; additional increments or decrements can be made at 2-d intervals; max dose 800 mg/d<br>Elderly or debilitated adults: use lower initial doses and increase more gradually, to a lower target dose than for other adults<br>Hepatic impairment: same as for elderly or debilitated adults | ≥10 y, titrate 25 mg PO 2 times/d until clinical response 25 mg PO 2 times/d initially; increase by 25–50 mg two or three times daily on 2nd and 3rd days, as tolerated, to usual dose range 200–300 mg, in two or three divided doses on the 4th day; additional increments or decrements can be made at 2-d intervals; max dose 600 mg/d |

*(Continued on page 1128)*

**TABLE 56.3**

## DRUGS AT A GLANCE: Atypical Antipsychotics (Continued)

| Drug | Pregnancy Category | Routes and Dosage Ranges | |
|---|---|---|---|
| | | **Adults** | **Children** |
| Risperidone (Risperdal, Perseris; ❋ APO-Risperidone, DOMRisperidone, MINT-Risperidone) | C | 1 mg twice daily PO, initially; increase to 2 mg/d twice daily on the 2nd day; increase to 3 mg twice daily on the 3rd day, if necessary; usual maintenance dose, 4–8 mg/d; after initial titration, dosage increases or decreases should be made at a rate of 1 mg/wk<br><br>Elderly or debilitated adults: initially 0.5 mg twice daily; increase in 0.5-mg increments to 1.5 mg twice daily<br><br>Renal or hepatic impairment: same as for elderly or debilitated adults | Schizophrenia 13–17 y, initially 0.5 mg/d PO; increase 0.5–1 mg/d for a target dose of 3 mg/d; doses range is 0.5–3 mg daily<br>Bipolar mania: 10–17 y, initially 0.5 mg/d PO; increase 0.5–1 mg/d for a target dose of 1–2.5 mg/d; dosage range is 1–6 mg/d<br>Autism spectrum disorder, <20 kg, 0.25 mg PO initially, and increased to maintenance dose of 0.5 mg daily<br>≥20 kg, 0.5 mg PO initially, and increased to maintenance dose of 1.0 mg daily |
| Risperidone (Risperdal Consta; ❋ Risperdal Consta) | C | 25 mg IM every 2 wk; max dose not to exceed 50 mg/2 wk; oral risperidone should be continued for first 3 wk of therapy to ensure adequate blood levels are maintained | <18 y, dosage not established |
| Ziprasidone (Geodon; ❋ Zeldox, Auro-Ziprasidone) | C | 20 mg PO twice daily with food, initially; gradually increased up to 80 mg twice daily, if necessary<br>Acute agitation in schizophrenia: 10–20 mg IM every 4 h up to a max of 40 mg/d, not to exceed 3 d | Schizophrenia (acute agitation): 5–11 y, 10 mg IM<br>12 y 10–20 mg<br>Autism: ≥8 y, 20–160 mg/d divided twice daily |

potential for this adverse reaction in order to instigate prompt treatment if necessary. Dose reduction may be necessary in patients with impaired renal functioning, and the drug should not be used in patients with severe kidney disorders. There have been a few cases of clozapine-induced acute renal faculty that have been reported. This may indicate that this hypersensitivity reaction is very rare but may also indicate that it has not been recognized or reported.

## Use in Patients With Hepatic Impairment

Clozapine is extensively metabolized by the liver, partially via the cytochrome P-450 system. For patients with significant hepatic impairment, dose reduction may be warranted. In rare instances, use has been linked to clinically apparent acute liver injury. Several cases of acute liver failure caused by the drug have been reported, although there have been no instances of chronic liver disease or vanishing bile duct syndrome. Clozapine should not be given to patients with active liver disease associated with nausea, loss of appetite or jaundice, or worsening liver disease or liver failure.

## Use in Patients With Critical Illness

Because of the many possible adverse effects of clozapine (see Adverse Effects), the drug should be used with caution or not used at all in persons with critical illness.

## Use in Patients Receiving Home Care

People with chronic mental illness, such as schizophrenia, are among the most challenging for the home care nurse. Major recurring problems include failure to take antipsychotic medications as prescribed and the concurrent use of alcohol and other drugs of abuse. Either problem is likely to lead to acute psychotic episodes and hospitalizations. The nurse must assist and support caregivers' efforts to administer medications and manage adverse effects, other aspects of daily care, and follow-up psychiatric care. In addition, the nurse may need to coordinate the efforts of several health and social service agencies or providers.

## Adverse Effects

Clozapine has several adverse effects, including

- Cardiovascular effects: orthostatic hypotension, tachycardia, ECG changes, and increased risk of myocarditis (greatest during the 1st month of treatment). The patient is also at risk for myocardial infarction, pericarditis, cardiomyopathy, mitral insufficiency, heart failure, and pericardial effusion.
- Gastrointestinal effects: The patient is at risk for severe constipation.
- CNS effects: increased risk of seizures in patients with a known seizure disorder. An FDA-issued **BLACK BOX WARNING ◆** alerts users of clozapine that the drug increases the risk of seizure activity as the dose increases.

- Hematologic effects: agranulocytosis. Clozapine can decrease the number of neutrophils, a type of white blood cell, that function in the body to fight off infections. When neutrophils are significantly decreased, severe neutropenia may result and the body may become prone to infections. Also, the FDA has issued a **BLACK BOX WARNING** ◆ regarding the potential risk of fatal agranulocytosis in patients who take clozapine.
- Metabolic effects: hyperglycemia and weight gain. The FDA has issued a **BLACK BOX WARNING** ◆ regarding the risk of hyperglycemia in patients who take clozapine. (In some extreme cases, there have been reports of ketoacidosis, hyperosmolar coma, and death.)

## Contraindications

Contraindications to clozapine include a known allergy to the drug, a history of clozapine-induced agranulocytosis or severe granulocytopenia, CNS depression, and a history of seizure disorders. Caution is warranted in cardiovascular disease, narrow-angle glaucoma, diabetes mellitus, and/or pulmonary disease. Conditions that rule out drug use include pregnancy, especially the first trimester, immunosuppression, and coma.

**BOX 56.7    Drug Interactions: Clozapine**

**Drugs That Increase the Effects of Clozapine**
- Alcohol
  *Increases central nervous system depression*
- Cimetidine, caffeine, other cytochrome P-450 inhibitors [SSRIs], ritonavir
  *Increase the risk of toxicity*
- Anticholinergics
  *May potentiate the anticholinergic effects of clozapine*

**Drugs That Decrease the Effects of Clozapine**
- Phenytoin, ethotoin, other cytochrome P-450 inducers
  *Decrease the serum concentration*

### Clinical Application 56.3

- Caroline's family has read some literature about the newer atypical antipsychotic medications and the success they have had in treating patients with positive and negative symptoms of schizophrenia. Consequently, her physician has prescribed clozapine 12.5 mg twice daily. What safety patient teaching should the nurse conduct?

## Nursing Implications

### Preventing Interactions

Many medications and herbs interact with clozapine, increasing or decreasing its effects (Boxes 56.7 and 56.8).

### Administering the Medication

Prior to beginning the administration of clozapine, it is necessary to obtain a baseline white blood cell count and neutrophil count. Also, it is important to monitor the blood glucose level regularly for hyperglycemia, especially if signs and symptoms of diabetes mellitus or risk factors are present.

If clozapine is to be discontinued, gradual tapering over a 2-week period is essential. If the drug is discontinued abruptly, the nurse monitors for symptoms of acute psychosis.

### Assessing for Therapeutic Effects

When clozapine is given for acute psychotic episodes, the nurse observes for sedation, decreased agitation, combativeness, and psychomotor activity. When the drug is given for acute or chronic psychosis, the nurse observes for decreased psychotic behaviors, such as decreased hallucinations and delusions.

### Assessing for Adverse Effects

The nurse implements a thorough assessment of the cardiovascular and cardiopulmonary status to check for orthostatic hypotension, heart failure, and cardiovascular adverse events. It is essential to monitor the complete blood count due to the risk of fatal agranulocytosis. Also, it is necessary to monitor the intraocular pressure for increased pressure and potential development of glaucoma. In January 2020, the FDA strengthened an existing safety warning that constipation caused by clozapine can progress to serious bowel complications, such as intestinal ischemia and necrotizing colitis, which could require hospitalization or lead to death.

### Patient Teaching

Box 56.9 identifies patient teaching guidelines for clozapine.

## Other Drugs in the Class

Aripiprazole (Abilify, Abilify Maintena) is the first of a new class of drugs called the dopamine system stabilizers. In its oral form, the drug is used to treat schizophrenia, bipolar disorder, major depressive disorder, irritability associated with autistic disorder, and Tourette's syndrome; the injectable immediate-release formulation is used to treat agitation associated with schizophrenia or bipolar mania, and the extended-release injection (Abilify Maintena) is used to treat schizophrenia. The injectable products are not interchangeable. Aripiprazole may not be as effective as

**BOX 56.8    Herb and Dietary Interactions: Clozapine**

**Herbs and Foods That Increase the Effects of Clozapine**
- American and Asian ginseng
- Guarana
- Gotu kola
- Kava
- St. John's wort
- Valerian
- Yerba mate
- Yohimbine

**BOX 56.9** *Patient Teaching Guidelines for Clozapine*

- Obtain weekly blood tests to determine the safe and effective dosage.
- Keep appointments for white blood cell count monitoring.
- Keep counseling appointments.
- Be aware that only 1 week of medication will be dispensed at a time.
- Do not drive a car or operate dangerous machinery. Dizziness or decreased mental alertness may occur.
- Do not stop the medication abruptly.
- You may experience drowsiness, dizziness, and decreased alertness.
- You may experience constipation and a stool softener may need to routinely be administered if constipation occurs.
- If you are a woman of childbearing age and intend to become pregnant or are pregnant, discuss clozapine use with a health care provider.
- Notify the prescriber of increased heart rate.
- Report lethargy, weakness, or flulike symptoms to the prescriber.

other agents. Adverse effects include headache, extrapyramidal reaction, drowsiness, akathisia, sedation, agitation, weight gain, nausea, vomiting, constipations, and tremors. The drug does not prolong the QT interval. The FDA has announced a safety alert, confirming that compulsive or uncontrollable urges to gamble, binge eat, shop, and have sex have been reported with the use of aripiprazole.

**! QSEN Alert: Safety**

Numerous drug interactions are possible with aripiprazole because the drug and its metabolite are metabolized hepatically by CYP2D6 and CYP3A4 enzymes of the cytochrome P-450 system, respectively. Drugs that inhibit CYP2D6 (e.g., quinidine, paroxetine, fluoxetine) and CYP3A4 (e.g., erythromycin, fluconazole, ketoconazole, itraconazole) can raise the drug's serum level, increasing the risk of adverse effects. Drugs that induce CPY3A4 (e.g., barbiturates, carbamazepine, phenytoin, rifampin) can speed up the metabolism of aripiprazole and can lower the serum level, reducing the efficacy of the drug at that dosage.

Asenapine (Saphris) is used to manage acute and chronic schizophrenia and manic or mixed episodes of bipolar disorder. The risk of dyslipidemia, diabetes, or weight gain is low. Adverse effects include drowsiness, insomnia, and increased creatine phosphokinase. Few drug interactions are noted. Sublingual tablets should be allowed to completely dissolved and should not be split, crushed, chewed, or swallowed. Patients should not eat or drink for at least 10 minutes after taking asenapine; this decreases the bioavailability of the drug.

Iloperidone (Fanapt) is used to treat schizophrenia in adults. The drug is better tolerated than some, but common adverse

effects include prolonged QT interval, hypotension, and weight gain. Other dose-related adverse effects include tachycardia, dry mouth, fatigue, drowsiness, and increased serum prolactin level. The drug is metabolized by the liver by the CYP2D6 and CYP3A4 enzymes, so numerous drug interactions are possible.

**! QSEN Alert: Safety**

The dose of iloperidone should by decreased by 50% in patients while concurrently taking strong CYP2D6 inhibitors (e.g., paroxetine, fluoxetine, quinidine) or strong CYP3A4 inhibitors (e.g., ketoconazole, clarithromycin) because the drugs can increase levels of iloperidone and increase adverse effects, including prolongation of the QT interval. In addition, a decrease in iloperidone dose by 50% is necessary in patients who are poor metabolizers of CYP2D6.

Olanzapine (Zyprexa) is also used to manage schizophrenia and manic or mixed episodes of bipolar disorder. The drug can cause leukopenia and neutropenia, which increases the risk of infection. Other adverse effects include drowsiness, extrapyramidal symptoms, akathisia, Parkinson-like syndrome, dizziness, headache, increased serum prolactin, increased appetite, xerostomia, increased serum aspartate aminotransferase (AST), decreased serum bilirubin, and increased serum alanine aminotransferase (ALT). The drug is highly metabolized by CYP1A2 and CYP2D6 of the cytochrome P-450 system. About 40% of the drug is removed via first-pass metabolism. Drug interactions are likely with drugs that induce CYP1A2 (e.g., nafcillin, omeprazole, modafinil) or inhibit this enzyme (e.g., ciprofloxacin, verapamil, cimetidine). In addition, vegetables such as chargrilled meat, cabbages, broccoli, and cauliflower are known to increase levels of CYP1A2. Conversely, St. John's wort, echinacea, peppermint, German chamomile, and dandelion teas, as well as tobacco, are inhibitors of CPY1A2. Drugs that induce (e.g., haloperidol, dexamethasone, glutethimide) or inhibit (e.g., quinidine, paroxetine, fluoxetine) CYP2D6 are known to interact with olanzapine.

Lurasidone (Latuda) is used to treat schizophrenia and bipolar depression. The FDA has issued a **BLACK BOX WARNING ◆** stating that older patients who suffer from dementia and dementia-related psychosis treated with lurasidone have an increased risk of death. The drug is not approved for the treatment of dementia-related psychosis. Administering the drug with food greatly increases absorption. Reported adverse effects include somnolence, Parkinson's syndrome, and akathisia. The drug does not cause prolonged QT interval, orthostatic hypotension, or cholinergic effects. Because lurasidone is metabolized by CYP3A4, drug interactions will occur with concurrent use of drugs that are strong inhibitors of CYP3A4 (ketoconazole), and strong inducers (rifampin) are contraindicated.

Risperidone (Risperdal, Perseris) is prescribed for the treatment of schizophrenia and acute bipolar mania. The drug is also used to manage children with autism spectrum disorders to reduce irritability-associated symptoms, including self-injury, aggression, tantrums, and mood swings. In schizophrenia, relief of positive and negative symptoms and improved cognitive function may occur in as little as 1 week. Generally, adverse effects are mild and include weight gain, diabetes, and dyslipidemia. A dose-related increase in extrapyramidal symptoms may occur with increased oral doses and the long-term formulation (Risperdal Consta), a depot preparation.

Paliperidone (Invega) is used in the treatment of schizophrenia and other psychoses. As major active metabolite of risperidone, it has the same therapeutic and adverse effects. The drug is available in three forms, a short-acting oral form (Invega), a LAI form (Invega Sustenna; to be taken monthly), and a LAI form (Invega Trinza; to be taken every 3 months). Common adverse effects include akathisia, headache, Parkinson-like syndrome, dystonia, and tremor.

Quetiapine (Seroquel, Seroquel XR) is prescribed to treat schizophrenia, depressive disorder, and manic episodes with bipolar disorder. Extended-release Seroquel XR is for use only in adults and should not be given to patients younger than 18 years old. Adverse effects include tachycardia, increased systolic and/or increased systolic and diastolic blood pressure, drowsiness, headache, agitation, dizziness, weight gain, increased serum total cholesterol, low-density cholesterol, triglycerides, and decreased high-density cholesterol, as well as xerostomia, constipation, and increased appetite. As with many atypical antipsychotic agents, the potential for clinically relevant drug interactions exists because the drug is metabolized by CYP2D6 and CYP3A4.

### ! QSEN Alert: Evidence-Based Practice

Kishimoto, Hagi, Nitta, Kane, and Currell (2019) completed a systematic review and meta-analysis of 59 randomized trials and 45,787 participants comparing drug effectiveness and safety in two or more second-generation antipsychotics (SGAs) in the long-term treatment of schizophrenia. No one SGA proved superior over another in terms of overall effectiveness and tolerability. However, clozapine, olanzapine and risperidone demonstrated less all-cause discontinuation while quetiapine more frequently required termination as compared to other SGAs. Since there were limited trials that directly compared an SGA to an existing standard of care, the results must be interpreted cautiously. The use of a specific SGA needs to be tailored to optimize the individual patient's treatment outcomes.

Ziprasidone (Geodon) is indicated for schizophrenia, bipolar mania, and autism spectrum disorder in children. The drug produces fewer extrapyramidal symptoms than other second-generation agents and reportedly leads to improvement in positive and negative symptoms and cognitive function. Because ziprasidone prolongs the QT interval, the drug should not be administered with other drugs (e.g., tricyclic antidepressants that have the potential to prolong QT interval). Like olanzapine, ziprasidone can cause leukopenia and neutropenia that increases the risk of infection. Numerous drug interactions are possible with ziprasidone as the drug and its metabolite are metabolized hepatically by CYP2D6 and CYP3A4, respectively. Drugs that inhibit CYP2D6 (e.g., quinidine, paroxetine, fluoxetine) and CYP3A4 (e.g., erythromycin, fluconazole, ketoconazole, itraconazole) can raise the drug's serum level, increasing the risk of adverse effects. Drugs that induce CPY3A4 (e.g., barbiturates, carbamazepine, phenytoin, rifampin) can speed up the metabolism of aripiprazole and can lower the serum level, reducing the efficacy of the drug at that dosage.

### Clinical Application 56.4

Caroline has not adhered to her daily antipsychotic regimen. She states that she feels her symptoms are under control, and because she feels "normal" again, she no longer needs to take the medication. She has dropped out of the university and has moved home with her parents. She spends her free time in her room and she is isolating herself again.
- What does the nurse discuss with the patient and her family?
- What medication alternatives does the nurse suggest at this point, considering her history of nonadherence?

### NCLEX Success

10. A woman reports to the prescriber that she has developed a fever, sore throat, and malaise after starting clozapine therapy. Which of the following interventions is most important?
    A. Treat the patient with a broad-spectrum antibiotic.
    B. Discontinue the clozapine and obtain a complete blood count with differential.
    C. Inform the patient that this is normal when taking clozapine.
    D. Assess the patient for diminished mental alertness.

11. Which statement made by a man indicates that he requires further patient teaching regarding adherence to his medication regimen?
    A. "If I experience muscle spasms in my neck, I must report that to the health care provider."
    B. "If I experience sudden fever and difficulty breathing, I must report that to the health care provider."
    C. "If I experience sedation, I must cut down on my medication."
    D. "If I experience dizziness, I must report that to the health care provider."

### Clinical Application 56.5

- Caroline has been taking clozapine for 6 months, and she has all the necessary blood tests for white blood cell count monitoring. Her psychotic symptoms have decreased. Adverse effects have been minimal. Caroline is eager to return to the university next semester and asks how long she needs to take this medication. What response is appropriate?

## THE NURSING PROCESS

A concept map outlines the nursing process related to drug therapy considerations in this chapter. Additional nursing implications related to the disease process should also be considered in care decisions.

**Assessment**

- Assess the patient's mental health status, history of psychotic behavior, need for antipsychotic drugs, and response and compliance to drug therapy. Some assessment directives include the following:
  - Interview the patient and family members. Attempts to interview an acutely psychotic person will yield little useful information.
  - Assess the patient's level of orientation and presence of positive and negative symptoms and cognitive status, if possible.
  - Determine from family members what predisposing factors precipitated the event (e.g., increased environmental stress, ingestion of alcohol or drugs).
  - Ask the family if the patient seems to be a hazard to self or others.
  - Have the family provide some description of preillness personality traits, level of social interaction, and ability to function in usual activities of daily living.

**Outcomes of Therapy**

The patient will
- Become less agitated within a few hours of the start of drug therapy, and less psychotic within 1 to 3 weeks.
- Be kept safe while sedated from drug therapy.
- Be cared for by staff in areas of nutrition, hygiene, exercise, and social interactions when unable to provide self-care.
- Improve in ability to participate in self-care activities.
- Avoid preventable adverse drug effects, especially those that impair safety.
- Be helped to take medications as prescribed and return for follow-up appointments with health care providers.

**Nursing Interventions**

- Use nondrug measures when appropriate to increase the effectiveness of drug therapy and to decrease adverse reactions.
- Answer questions or provide information about drug therapy and other aspects of the treatment plan.
- Devise a schedule of administration times that is as convenient as possible for the patient.
- Assist the patient or caregiver in preventing or managing adverse drug effects (see Boxes 56.3, 56.6, and 56.9).
- Supervise ambulation to prevent falls or other injuries if the patient is drowsy or elderly or has postural hypotension.
- Instruct the patient to lie down for approximately 1 hour after a large oral dose or an injection of antipsychotic medication.
- Apply elastic stockings, and instruct the patient to change positions gradually, elevate legs when sitting, avoid standing for prolonged periods, and avoid hot baths (hot baths cause vasodilation and increase the incidence of hypotension).
- Instruct the patient on oral hygiene. The effects of the medications can lead to dry mouth and oral infections.
- Instruct the patient about strategies to decrease dry mouth such as chewing sugarless gum, frequently brushing teeth, and rinsing the mouth with water.
- Instruct the patient about measures to increase fluid intake, dietary fiber, and exercise, which can help prevent constipation.
- Instruct the patient regarding the importance of keeping medical appointments and taking medications as prescribed.

**Evaluation**

- Interview the patient to determine the presence and extent of hallucinations and delusions.
- Observe the patient for decreased signs and symptoms.
- Document abilities and limitations in self-care.
- Note whether any injuries have occurred during drug therapy.
- Interview the caregiver about the patient's behavior, medication response, and compliance with drug therapy and follow-up care.

## KEY CONCEPTS

- Antipsychotic drugs are indicated to treat psychosis, including disorders such as schizophrenia and the manic phase of bipolar disorder.
- First-generation antipsychotics, or "typical antipsychotics," include the phenothiazines and older nonphenothiazines such as haloperidol and thiothixene.
- The mechanism of action of first-generation antipsychotic drugs is blockade of $D_2$ receptors.
- All first-generation antipsychotics are considered equal in terms of their ability to relieve symptoms of psychosis; however, they differ in potency and adverse effects.
- The FDA has issued a **BLACK BOX WARNING** ◆ for haloperidol regarding extrapyramidal and withdrawal symptoms in newborns exposed to the drug during the third trimester of the pregnancy.
- The FDA has issued a **BLACK BOX WARNING** ◆ stating that older patients who suffer from dementia and dementia-related psychosis treated with haloperidol have an increased risk of death.
- Second-generation antipsychotics, or "atypical antipsychotics," include newer nonphenothiazine drugs. They are also considered first-choice therapy for schizophrenia because they have a more favorable adverse effect profile, producing fewer extrapyramidal movement disorders.
- The mechanism of action of second-generation antipsychotics is blockade of dopamine and serotonin receptors.
- The FDA has issued a **BLACK BOX WARNING** ◆ related to the administration of clozapine to elderly patients with dementia. These patients are at risk for death.
- The FDA has issued a **BLACK BOX WARNING** ◆ regarding the risk of fatal agranulocytosis with clozapine.
- The FDA has issued a **BLACK BOX WARNING** ◆ for clozapine regarding the risk of hyperglycemia.
- The FDA has issued a **BLACK BOX WARNING** ◆ stating that use of clozapine increases the risk of seizure activity as the dose increases.
- Positive symptoms of schizophrenia respond to drug therapy more readily than negative symptoms. The second-generation "atypical" nonphenothiazine drugs may be slightly more effective in treating negative symptoms of schizophrenia.
- Therapeutic effects to antipsychotics may take several weeks to achieve maximum therapeutic effect.
- Adverse effects occurring more frequently in low-potency drugs as compared with high-potency drugs include anticholinergic effects, antiadrenergic effects (orthostatic hypotension), and CNS depression (sedation).
- Adverse effects more common to high-potency drugs as compared with low-potency drugs include early extrapyramidal effects (acute dystonia, akathisia, parkinsonism).
- Early extrapyramidal effects are treated by reducing dosage, changing to a second-generation antipsychotic, or use of anticholinergic medications. Akathisia may also be treated with benzodiazepines and beta-adrenergic blockers to reduce the urge to move.
- Tardive dyskinesia, a late extrapyramidal effect, may occur with all phenothiazine and typical nonphenothiazine drugs and is generally considered to be irreversible. Prevention through early detection is key.
- Neuroleptic malignant syndrome is a potentially fatal adverse effect characterized by rigidity, severe hyperthermia, agitation, confusion, delirium, dyspnea, tachycardia, respiratory failure, and acute renal failure.
- The FDA has issued a **BLACK BOX WARNING** ◆ for lurasidone stating that older patients who suffer from dementia and dementia-related psychosis treated with this drug have an increased risk of death.

## CLINICAL REASONING CASE STUDY

**Meet the Patient**

Dmytro Shevchenko, a 54-year-old man, received a diagnosis of schizophrenia when he was 23 and was expelled from college. He has a long history of nonadherence to antipsychotic medications; he has taken haloperidol, risperidone, clozapine, and quetiapine. He had to stop taking the clozapine as the result of a lowered white blood cell count. Because of his limited insight into his illness, he does not believe he needs to take medication because he does not perceive he is ill. Recently, his psychotic symptoms have returned and he needs to be hospitalized.

- Patient teaching regarding medication adherence has not worked. What are some treatment options for this patient?
- The provider has considered prescribing a long-acting injectable form (LAI) of paliperidone. Discuss the nursing assessments and interventions that the nurse should implement to ensure adherence to the LAI treatment regimen.
- What additional patient teaching should the nurse take to minimize adverse effects from Mr. Shevchenko's LAI medication?

**Assessing Drug Information**

- Paliperidone is a second-generation atypical antipsychotic medication used in the treatment of schizophrenia and other psychoses.
- Paliperidone may antagonize both central dopamine ($D_2$) and serotonin type 2 receptors, as well as $alpha_1$, $alpha_2$, and $H_1$ receptors. It is a major active metabolite of risperidone and demonstrates the same therapeutic and adverse effects.
- The drug comes in three forms: a short-acting oral form (Invega), a long-acting injectable form (Invega Sustenna; to be taken every month), and a long-acting injectable (LAI) form (Invega Trinza; to be taken every 3 months).
- Common adverse effects include akathisia, headache, Parkinson-like syndrome, dystonia, and tremor.

**Nursing Actions**

- Recognize that prior to beginning paliperidone LAI, the nurse should obtain baseline data to help monitor the Mr. Shevchenko's response to drug therapy, including baseline laboratory tests of liver, kidney, and blood and metabolic functions, as well as ECG. Such tests may assist in early detection and treatment of adverse drug effects. Baseline blood pressure readings also may be helpful.
- Continue assessing his response to drug therapy and his ability to function in activities of daily living, whether he is an inpatient or an outpatient.
- Answer questions or provide information about drug therapy and other aspects of the treatment plan. Use nondrug measures when appropriate to increase the effectiveness of drug therapy and to decrease adverse reactions.
- Devise a schedule of administration times that is as convenient as possible for him.
  - Because he is taking the LAI form of the medication, it is necessary to schedule initial injection in the deltoid muscle and repeat in one week. Do not give the injection subcutaneously.
  - After the second dose, give the monthly maintenance doses in deltoid or gluteal muscle. Then make adjustments monthly or every three months, as necessary.
- Regularly monitor the skin for possible injection site reaction.
- Assist the patient or caregiver in preventing or managing adverse drug effects (see Boxes 56.3, 56.6, and 56.9). (Most adverse effects are less likely to occur or be severe with the newer atypical drugs than with phenothiazines and other older drugs.)
- Supervise ambulation to prevent falls or other injuries if the patient is drowsy or has postural hypotension.
- Provide additional teaching related to drug therapy and medications to avoid, including herbal supplements and alcohol.

---

*Visit* thePoint® *at* **http://thePoint.lww.com/Frandsen12e** *for answers to NCLEX Success questions (in Appendix A), answers to Clinical Application Case Studies (in Appendix B), and more!*

## REFERENCES AND RESOURCES

American Psychiatric Association. (2013). *Diagnostic and statistical manual of mental disorders* (5th ed.). Washington, DC: American Psychiatric Association.

Arango, C., Ng-Mak, D., Finn, E., Byrne, A., & Loebel, A. (2019). Lurasidone compared to other atypical antipsychotic monotherapies for adolescent schizophrenia: A systematic literature review and network meta-analysis. *European Child & Adolescent Psychiatry*. doi:10.1007/s00787-019-01425-2

Bonner, A. F., Field, T. S., Lemay, C. A., Mazor, K. M., Anderson, D. A., Compher, C. J., et al. (2015). Rationales that providers and family members cited for the use of antipsychotic medications in nursing home residents with dementia. *Journal of the American Geriatrics Society, 63*, 302–308.

Brooker, D. J., Latham, I., Evans, S. C., Jacobson, N., Perry, W., Bray, J., et al. (2016). FITS into practice: Translating research into practice in reducing the use of anti-psychotic medication for people with dementia living in care homes. *Aging & Mental Health, 20*(7), 709–718. doi:10.0180/13607863.2105.1063102

Fischer, B. A., & Buchanan, R. W. (2020). Schizophrenia in adults: Clinical manifestations, course, assessment, and diagnosis. In *UpToDate*. Lexi-Comp, Inc.

Green, C. A., Yarborough, B. H., Leo, M. C., Stumbo, S. P., Perrin, N. A., Nichols, G. A., et al. (2015). Weight maintenance following the STRIDE lifestyle intervention for individuals taking antipsychotic medications. *Obesity, 23*(7), 1995–2001. doi:10.1002/oby.21205

Jibson, M. (2020a). First generation antipsychotic medications: Pharmacology, administration, and comparative side effects. In *UpToDate*. Lexi-Comp, Inc.

Jibson, M. (2020b). Second generation antipsychotic medications: Pharmacology, administration, and side effects. In *UpToDate*. Lexi-Comp, Inc.

Karch, A. M., & Tucker, R. (2019). *2020 Lippincott's pocket drug guide for nurses*. Philadelphia, PA: Wolters Kluwer.

Kishimoto, T., Hagi, K., Nitta, M., Kane, J. M., & Currell, C. U. (2019). Long-term effectiveness of oral second-generation antipsychotics in patients with schizophrenia and related disorders: A systematic review and meta-analysis of direct head-to-head comparisons. *World Psychiatry, 18*(2), 208–224. doi:10.1002/wps.20632

Lippincott Williams & Wilkins. (2019). *Nursing 2020 drug handbook* (40th ed.). Philadelphia, PA: Wolters Kluwer.

Lorberg, B., Davico, C., Martsenkovskyi, D., & Vitiello, B. (2019). Principles in using psychotropic medication in children and adolescents. In J. M. Rey, & A. Martin (Eds.), *IACAPAP e-textbook of child and adolescent mental health*. Geneva: International Association for Child and Adolescent Psychiatry and Allied Professions.

Malla, A., Chue, P., Jordan, G., Stip, E., Koczerginski, D., Milliken, H., et al. (2016). An exploratory, open-label, randomized trial comparing risperidone long-acting injectable with oral antipsychotic medication in the treatment of early psychosis. *Clinical Schizophrenia & Related Psychoses, 9*(4), 198–208.

Stone, J. M., Roux, S., Taylor, D., & Morrison, P. D. (2018). First-generation *versus* second-generation long-acting injectable antipsychotic drugs and time to relapse. *Therapeutic Advances in Psychopharmacology, 8*(12), 333–336. doi:10.1177/2045125318795130

UpToDate. (2020). *Drug Information*. Lexi Comp, Inc.

Walkup, J.; the Work Group on Quality Issues. (2009). Practice parameter on the use of psychotropic medication in children and adolescents. *Journal of the American Academy of Child and Adolescent Psychiatry, 48*(9), 961–973.

Wu, H. E., & Okusaga, O. O. (2015). Antipsychotic medication-induced dysphoria: Its meaning, association with typical vs. atypical medications and impact on adherence. *Psychiatric Quarterly, 86*, 199–205. doi:10.1007/s11136-014-9319-1

Zaim, N., Findling, R. L., & Sun, A. (2020). Antipsychotics for treatment of adolescent onset schizophrenia: A review. *Current Treatment Options in Psychiatry, 7*, 23–38. doi:10.1007/s40501-020-00198-9

# Drug Therapy for Attention Deficit Hyperactivity Disorder and Narcolepsy

## LEARNING OBJECTIVES

*After studying this chapter, you should be able to:*

1. Understand the etiology, pathophysiology, and clinical manifestations of attention deficit hyperactivity disorder.
2. Understand the etiology, pathophysiology, and clinical manifestations of narcolepsy.
3. Describe the general characteristics of the central nervous system stimulants.
4. Identify the prototypes and discuss the action, use, adverse effects, contraindications, and nursing implications for the stimulants used in the treatment of attention deficit hyperactivity disorder and narcolepsy.
5. Implement the nursing process in the care of patients who take central nervous stimulants for attention deficit hyperactivity disorder and narcolepsy.

## CLINICAL APPLICATION CASE STUDY

Brian Connor received a diagnosis of attention deficit hyperactivity disorder at 7 years of age. He is now 9 years old and is taking methylphenidate (Ritalin) 15 mg daily, which he takes each morning before school. With drug therapy and individual counseling, his attention span and school performance have improved. However, Brian's most recent physical examination shows that his height and weight are less than normal for his age and that he has lost weight since his examination last year. The school nurse talks with Brian's teachers, who report that he seems more restless in class after lunch. He has had more difficulty getting along with his classmates due to his impulsive behaviors.

## KEY TERMS

**Attention deficit hyperactivity disorder:** relatively common disorder of childhood onset characterized by inattention, impulsiveness, and overactivity

**Cataplexy:** episodic loss of sudden loss of muscle tone ranging from slight weakness to complete body collapse in response to strong emotion

**Drug holiday:** temporary drug-free period to allow some return of normal functions, to maintain sensitivity to a drug, and to reduce the likelihood of adverse effects.

**Hypnagogic hallucinations:** vivid, often frightening, dreamlike experiences that occur while dozing, falling asleep, or awakening

**Narcolepsy:** sleep disorder in which a person goes to sleep at any place or at any time

# INTRODUCTION

This chapter introduces the pharmacologic care of attention deficit hyperactivity disorder (ADHD) and narcolepsy. Clinicians use drugs that stimulate the central nervous system (CNS) to treat these disorders.

# OVERVIEW OF ATTENTION DEFICIT HYPERACTIVITY DISORDER

To adequately understand the pharmacologic treatment of **attention deficit hyperactivity disorder**, or ADHD, it is important to understand the causes, pathophysiology, and clinical manifestations of ADHD. This condition is characterized by persistent hyperactivity, short attention span, difficulty completing assigned tasks or schoolwork, restlessness, and impulsiveness.

## Etiology and Pathophysiology

ADHD is the most common psychiatric or neurobehavioral disorder in children. Although the cause is not fully understood, evidence suggests that subtle dysfunction in the frontal lobe and functionally related subcortical structures plays an essential role in the core symptoms of ADHD. Research has suggested that ADHD is a highly heritable, neurobiologic disorder partially attributed to dopamine and norepinephrine transport dysfunction in the brain.

ADHD is usually diagnosed between 3 and 7 years of age and may affect as many as 8% of school-aged children. Children with ADHD find it difficult to get along with others (e.g., family members, peer groups, teachers) and to function in situations requiring controlled behavior (e.g., classrooms). Approximately three to five percent of children and adolescents are affected by ADHD, and the prevalence is higher in boys. Approximately 10% to 20% of children with ADHD also have a diagnosed learning disability, causing further academic and emotional difficulties.

ADHD continues into adolescence and adulthood in approximately 50% of cases and may affect about 4% of adults in the United States. In adolescents and adults, hyperactivity is not prominent, but impulsiveness, inattention, and difficulties in structured settings such as school or work may continue. Some studies indicate that children with ADHD are more likely to have mood disorders and substance abuse disorders as adolescents and adults. A major criterion for diagnosing later ADHD is a previous diagnosis of ADHD by 7 years of age. Some authorities believe this age limit is too restrictive. The diagnosis of ADHD in adults has greatly increased in recent years, with a concomitant increase in the use of prescribed CNS stimulants for its treatment.

## Clinical Manifestations

Clinical manifestations of ADHD usually occur in various or multiple environments in a child's life, including school, home, church, or recreational activities. The level of problems typically varies, but symptoms generally worsen in situations that require sustained attention, such as listening to teacher, performing repetitive tasks, or reading lengthy materials.

Hyperactivity in children presents as fidgeting or squirming in their seats, excessive running or climbing when it is dangerous or inappropriate, disruptive playing during quiet activities, and demonstrating a driven verbal or motor quality. Impulsivity manifests as impatience, blurting out answers, and frequently interrupting others. Inattention manifests as messy work, careless mistakes, and appearance of daydreaming. Based on the behaviors associated with ADHD, affected people also may have low self-esteem and strained peer relations. Early diagnosis and treatment are essential. Evidence suggests that behavior management combined with pharmacotherapy yields the best outcomes.

## Drug Therapy

Drug therapy is indicated when symptoms are moderate to severe; are present for several months; and interfere in social, academic, or behavioral functioning. Counseling and psychotherapy (e.g., parental counseling, family therapy) are recommended along with drug therapy for effective treatment and realistic expectations of outcomes. Young children may not require treatment until starting school. Then, the goal of drug therapy is to control symptoms, facilitate learning, and promote social development. Table 57.1 summarizes the drugs used in the treatment of ADHD, and Figure 57.1 identifies the mechanisms of action of these drugs. Treatment is based on individual signs and symptoms.

## TABLE 57.1

### Drugs Administered for the Treatment of Attention Deficit Hyperactivity Disorder and Narcolepsy

| Drug Class | Prototype | Other Drugs in the Class |
|---|---|---|
| Amphetamines | Dextroamphetamine (Dexedrine) | Dextroamphetamine and amphetamine (Adderall XR, Adderall) Lisdexamfetamine (Vyvanse) Methamphetamine (Desoxyn) |
| Amphetamine-related CNS stimulants | Methylphenidate (Ritalin, Ritalin LA, Concerta, Daytrana, Metadate CD, Metadate ER, Methylin, QuilliChew ER, Aptensio XR) | Dexmethylphenidate (Focalin, Focalin XR) Armodafinil (Nuvigil) Modafinil (Provigil) |
| Selective norepinephrine reuptake inhibitors | Atomoxetine (Strattera) | |
| Sympatholytics | Guanfacine (Intuniv, Tenex) | |
| CNS depressant | Sodium oxybate (Xyrem) | |

CNS, central nervous system.

Ventral tegmental area
Substantia nigra
Locus ceruleus

——— Noradrenergic neurons    ⋯⋯⋯ Dopaminergic neurons
——— Postsynaptic neuron receptors that receive noradrenergic innervation

**Figure 57.1.** Mechanisms of action for commonly used drugs to treat ADHD. Amphetamine, amphetamine-related CNS stimulants, and selective norepinephrine reuptake inhibitors act on noradrenergic neurons originating in the locus ceruleus and projecting throughout the cerebral cortex, hypothalamus, cerebellum, and spinal cord (*yellow*). Amphetamine also acts on dopaminergic neurons originating in the ventral tegmental area and projecting to the cerebral cortex, hypothalamus, and nucleus accumbens (*black solid lines*). Other dopaminergic neurons originating in the substantia nigra and projecting to the striatum (*black dashed lines*) help initiate intended movement. Sympatholytics, such as guanfacine, preferentially bind postsynaptic alpha$_{2A}$-adrenoreceptors in the prefrontal cortex (*pink solid lines*), which is theorized to improve delay-related firing of prefrontal cortex neurons, improving symptoms associated with ADHD. [Adapted with permission from Golan, D. E., Tashjian, A. H., Armstrong, E. J. (2008). *Principles of Pharmacology: The Pathophysiologic Basis of Drug Therapy* (2nd ed., Fig. 17.9). Baltimore: Wolters Kluwer Health.]

## OVERVIEW OF NARCOLEPSY

To adequately understand the pharmacologic treatment of the chronic sleep disorder narcolepsy, it is important to understand the causes, pathophysiology, and clinical manifestations of narcolepsy. This condition is characterized by excessive sleepiness and sleep attacks at inappropriate times, such as at work. Narcolepsy affects men and women equally and usually begins during the teenage or young adult years. Nearly half of affected patients report that the sleepiness substantially interferes with their daily lives, including school, work, marriage, and social life.

### Etiology and Pathophysiology

**Narcolepsy** is one of the most common chronic sleep disorders. It affects about 1 in 2000 people in the United States. However, the disorder may be underdiagnosed, particularly in people with mild symptoms. It disrupts the normal sleep–wake cycle, causing daytime sleepiness. It is most likely the result of a combination of genetic and environmental factors; although some of these have been identified, others remain unknown. Most people diagnosed with narcolepsy also have cataplexy (episodic, sudden loss of muscle tone in response to strong emotion, such as laughing, surprise, or anger). However, some people do not, which has led

researchers to identify two major forms of the condition: type 1, or narcolepsy with cataplexy, and type 2, narcolepsy without cataplexy. Type 1 is associated with the significant loss of neurons and orexin neuropeptides, and type 2 has an unknown etiology.

### Loss of Orexin Signaling

Some people with narcolepsy have a loss of the neuropeptides orexin-A and orexin-B (also called hypocretin-1 and hypocretin-2), which are made by neurons in the hypothalamus. These neuropeptides have excitatory effects when released during wakefulness and increase other brain activity involved in promoting wakefulness. Loss of orexins may allow rapid-eye movement sleep-related phenomena to intrude into wakefulness. It is unclear what triggers the death of orexin-producing neurons, although evidence increasingly points to an abnormality of the immune system.

### Genetic Abnormalities

Variations in several genes are associated with the development of narcolepsy. The most well studied of these genes is *HLA-DQB1*, part of a family of genes called the human leukocyte antigen (HLA) complex. This gene provides instructions for making part of a protein that plays an important role in how the immune system reacts to a range of foreign proteins. A specific variation *HLA-DQB1*06:02* has been linked with narcolepsy, particularly in people who also have cataplexy and a loss of orexins. Other genetic and environmental factors likely influence a person's risk of developing narcolepsy, including bacterial or viral infections such as colds, strep throat, and influenza.

A small percentage of people who have narcolepsy have family members who also have the disorder. Although the condition does not clearly appear to be inherited, first-degree relatives (parents, siblings, and children) of people with narcolepsy type 1 have a 40 times greater risk of developing the disorder compared to the general population.

## Clinical Manifestations

People with narcolepsy often experience disturbed nocturnal sleep and an abnormal daytime sleep pattern; it is important not to confuse this pattern with insomnia. Excessive daytime drowsiness (even after an adequate night's sleep) and fatigue are characteristic. People are likely to become drowsy or fall asleep or just be very tired. The hazards of drowsiness during normal waking hours and suddenly going to sleep in unsafe environments restrict activities of daily living.

**Cataplexy** is another common feature of narcolepsy. This episodic condition features the loss of muscle function, ranging from slight weakness to complete body collapse. These episodes may be triggered by emotional reactions such as laughter, anger, or fear, lasting from a few seconds to minutes. Cataplexy can cause an affected person to fall, which may lead to injury. Episodes of cataplexy vary in frequency from several times a day to a few times a year. Other signs and symptoms of narcolepsy include hypnagogic hallucinations and sleep paralysis. **Hypnagogic hallucinations** are vivid, often frightening, dreamlike experiences that occur while dozing, falling asleep, or awakening. Sleep paralysis is the temporary inability to move or talk on waking.

## Drug Therapy

Treatment of narcolepsy is based on individual symptoms and therapeutic response. In addition to drug therapy, prevention of sleep deprivation, regular sleeping and waking times, avoiding shift work, and short naps may be helpful in reducing daytime sleepiness. Also, avoiding large meals, alcohol, and caffeine-containing beverages before bedtime may enhance sleep quality. However, even adequate amounts of nighttime sleep do not produce full alertness. Table 57.1 summarizes the medications used in the treatment of narcolepsy.

### Clinical Application 57.1

Brian has been disrupting class, most notably after lunch. The teachers have contacted his parents regarding this situation. His parents have made an appointment with his health care provider, who changed his medication to methylphenidate [Metadate ER 20 mg]. This new medication comes in capsule form, and Brian and his parents are afraid that he cannot swallow the large capsule.

- Is this an appropriate medication change?
- Brian's mother asks if she can empty the contents of the capsule in applesauce. What patient teaching should the nurse implement?
- What strategies might the nurse suggest to Brian and his parents to help him with taking this new medication?

### NCLEX Success

1. A child with attention deficit hyperactivity disorder would most likely exhibit which of the following symptoms?
   A. anxiety
   B. positive peer relationships
   C. hostility
   D. restlessness

2. Which behavior would a nurse expect in the child who takes methylphenidate every morning?
   A. sitting and playing with toys for 90 minutes
   B. getting along well with peers
   C. expressing anger in an appropriate manner
   D. not throwing toys across the room

## STIMULANTS

CNS stimulants act by facilitating initiation and transmission of nerve impulses that excite other cells. The drugs are somewhat selective in their actions at lower doses but tend to involve the entire CNS at higher doses. Stimulant drugs and stimulant-like drugs (e.g., methylphenidate) are generally the first-line treatment for ADHD in school-aged children and adolescents. These drugs are generally available in short-, intermediate-, and long-acting formulations. In ADHD, the drugs improve academic performance, behavior, and interpersonal relationships. In narcolepsy, stimulants significantly improve the performance of daily activities. The major groups of stimulants are amphetamines, amphetamine-related drugs, and xanthines.

The main goal of therapy with CNS stimulants is to relieve symptoms of the disorders for which they are given. A secondary goal is to have patients use the drugs appropriately. Misuse and abuse of stimulants often occur when people who want to combat fatigue and delay sleep, such as long-distance drivers, students, and athletes, take the drugs. College students reportedly use stimulants as study aids; this is not justified. These drugs are dangerous for drivers and those involved in similar activities, and they have no legitimate use in athletics.

When a prescriber orders a CNS stimulant, the dose starts low and then increases as necessary, usually at weekly intervals, until the drug becomes effective or the dose reaches a maximum. It is also necessary to limit the number of doses that can be obtained with one prescription. This action reduces the likelihood of drug dependence or diversion (use by people for whom the drug is not prescribed). For additional information on substance abuse and diversion, see Chapter 58.

Overdoses may occur with acute or chronic ingestion of large amounts of a single stimulant, combinations of stimulants, or concurrent ingestion of a stimulant and another drug that slows the metabolism of the stimulant. Signs of toxicity may include severe agitation, cardiac dysrhythmias, combativeness, confusion, delirium, hallucinations, high body temperature, hyperactivity, hypertension, insomnia, irritability, nervousness, panic states, restlessness, tremors, seizures, coma, circulatory collapse, and death.

## AMPHETAMINES

Amphetamines produce mood elevation or euphoria, increasing mental alertness and capacity for work, decreasing fatigue and drowsiness, and prolonging wakefulness. They are prescribed as single salts (dextroamphetamine) or mixed dextroamphetamine–amphetamine salts. Large doses can lead to signs of excessive CNS stimulation (e.g., agitation, confusion, hyperactivity, difficulty concentrating on tasks, hyperactivity, nervousness, restlessness) and sympathetic nervous system stimulation (e.g., increased heart rate and blood pressure, pupil dilation, slowed gastrointestinal [GI] motility, and other symptoms). Overdoses can result in psychosis, convulsions, stroke, cardiac arrest, and death. Amphetamines are schedule II drugs under the Controlled Substances Act; they have a high potential for drug abuse and dependence. Widely sold on the street, they are commonly abused. **Dextroamphetamine** (Dexedrine) is the prototype amphetamine.

### Pharmacokinetics

Dextroamphetamine has a rapid absorption and onset of action. The drug reaches its peak in 1 to 5 hours, and the duration is between 8 and 10 hours. It is metabolized by the liver and excreted in the urine. Dextroamphetamine may cross the placenta and has been found in breast milk.

### Action

Dextroamphetamine acts in the CNS to release norepinephrine from nerve terminals and increases the amounts of norepinephrine, dopamine, and possibly serotonin in the brain. Dopamine is released in higher doses. Dextroamphetamine suppresses appetite, increases alertness, elevates mood, and improves physical performance. The drug's effectiveness and efficacy in ADHD are paradoxical, and its action is not well understood.

## TABLE 57.2

## DRUGS AT A GLANCE: Amphetamines

| Drug | Pregnancy Category | Routes and Dosage Ranges | |
|---|---|---|---|
| | | **Adults** | **Children** |
| Ⓟ **Dextroamphetamine** (Dexedrine, 🍁 Dexedrine) | C | Narcolepsy: start with 10 mg/d PO in divided doses; increase in increments of 10 mg/d at weekly intervals. Reduce dose if adverse effects occur. Usual dose is 5–60 mg/d PO in divided doses. Long-acting forms can be given once daily | ADHD, 3–5 y, start with 2.5 mg/d PO; increase in increments of 2.5 mg/d at weekly intervals until optimal response is obtained ≥6 y, start with 5 mg PO twice daily; increase in increments of 5 mg/d until optimal response is obtained; dosage will rarely exceed 40 mg/d; long-acting forms may be used once a day Narcolepsy, 6–12 y, start with 5 mg/d PO; increase in increments of 5 mg at weekly intervals until optimal response is obtained; max dose 60 mg daily ≥12 y: same as adults |
| Dextroamphetamine and amphetamine (Adderall XR, Adderall; 🍁 Adderall) | C | Narcolepsy, 10 mg/d PO initially, increased if necessary ADHD, extended-release 20 mg/d | ADHD, 3–5 y, 2.5 mg/d PO; increased if necessary 6–12 y, 5 mg PO 1–2 times daily; increase if necessary; max dose 40 mg/d in 1–3 divided doses; extended-release 5–10 mg/d PO, increase at weekly intervals if necessary; max dose 30 mg/d 13–17 y, 10 mg PO once daily; increase to 20 mg if necessary |
| Lisdexamfetamine (Vyvanse; 🍁 Vyvanse) | C | ADHD, 30 mg PO once daily in morning; increased if necessary; max dose 70 mg daily | ADHD, ≥6 y, 30 mg PO once daily; increased if necessary; max dose 70 mg/d |
| Methamphetamine (Desoxyn; 🍁 Desoxyn) | C | Narcolepsy, 20–60 mg PO administered within 1 h of awakening | ≥6 y, 5 mg PO 1–2 times daily initially, increased if necessary; usual dose 20–25 mg/d, in 2 divided doses |

ADHD, attention deficit hyperactivity disorder.

## Use

The clinical indications for use of dextroamphetamine include the management of ADHD and narcolepsy. Amphetamines are useful in both acute and chronic conditions. Table 57.2 summarizes the route and dosage information for dextroamphetamine and other amphetamines.

### Use in Children

Parents need to monitor their children's use of medications for ADHD, and it is necessary to titrate the dosage carefully to avoid excessive CNS stimulation, anorexia, and insomnia. Suppression of weight and height (e.g., less than the estimated average of 2 inches per year) may occur, and the nurse ensures that growth is monitored during drug therapy. In children with psychosis or Tourette's syndrome, CNS stimulants may exacerbate symptoms. In children and adolescents with preexisting heart disease, usual doses of dextroamphetamine may cause sudden death.

In ADHD, careful documentation of baseline symptoms over approximately 1 month is necessary to establish the diagnosis and evaluate outcomes of treatment. This may involve videotapes of behavior, observations and ratings by clinicians familiar with the condition, and interviewing the child, parents, or caretakers. Some authorities believe that ADHD is overdiagnosed and that stimulant drugs are prescribed unnecessarily.

### Use in Older Adults

The use of dextroamphetamine warrants caution in older adults. As with most other drugs, slowed metabolism and excretion increase the risks of accumulation and toxicity. Older adults are likely to experience anxiety, confusion, insomnia, and nervousness from excessive CNS stimulation. In addition, older adults often have cardiovascular disorders (e.g., angina, dysrhythmias, hypertension) that may be aggravated by the cardiac-stimulating effects of the drug. In general, reduced doses are safer in older adults.

### Use in Patients With Renal or Hepatic Impairment

Dextroamphetamine is excreted in the urine after being metabolized in the liver. Thus, caution is necessary in patients with renal and/or hepatic impairment. The nurse monitors such patients for adverse effects and helps ensure that lower doses are used.

## Adverse Effects

Dextroamphetamine has several adverse effects.

• Cardiovascular effects: tachycardia, other dysrhythmias, and hypertension. A BLACK BOX WARNING ◆ makes users aware of the drug's high abuse potential; misuse may cause sudden death or serious cardiovascular events. It is essential to obtain a baseline electrocardiogram (ECG) and blood pressure reading.

- CNS effects: excessive CNS stimulation. Possible anxiety, hyperactivity, nervousness, insomnia, tremors, convulsion, and psychotic behavior may occur. These reactions are more likely with larger doses.
- GI effects: gastritis, nausea, diarrhea, and constipation
- Other effects: anorexia and weight loss

## Contraindications

Contraindications to dextroamphetamine include cardiovascular disorders (e.g., angina, dysrhythmias, hypertension), which are likely to be aggravated by the drug. Other contraindications include anxiety or agitation, glaucoma, and hyperthyroidism, as well as a history of drug abuse, pregnancy, or lactation. People with Tourette's syndrome and children with motor tics should not take the drug.

## Nursing Implications

### Preventing Interactions

Many medications interact with dextroamphetamine, increasing or decreasing its effects (Box 57.1). In addition, the use of the herb, ephedra, increases the effect of dextroamphetamine, while caffeine and acidic foods and juices decrease the drug's effect.

### Administering the Medication

People should take the first dose of dextroamphetamine on awakening or early in the day and the last dose at least 6 hours before bedtime. Children with ADHD should take the drug 30 to 45 minutes before meals to minimize the appetite-suppressing effects. It is important not to crush, chew, or bite the long-acting form; this destroys the extended-release feature and may result in an overdose. For young children who have difficulty swallowing pills, the capsules may be opened and taken with pudding or ice cream.

Dextroamphetamine often causes loss of appetite, and the health care provider may stop the medication during the months when the child is not in school. This temporary drug-free period

---

**BOX 57.1** 🗌 **Drug Interactions: Dextroamphetamine**

**Drugs That Increase the Effects of Dextroamphetamine**

- Albuterol, pseudoephedrine, tricyclic antidepressants
  *Increase stimulant effects of dextroamphetamine*
- Antacids
  *Decrease the excretion of amphetamines*
- Monoamine oxidase inhibitors
  *Enhance the hypertensive effects of amphetamines*

**Drugs That Decrease the Effects of Dextroamphetamine**

- Ammonium chloride
  *Decreases the serum concentration of dextroamphetamine*
- Antipsychotics, lithium, alcohol
  *Diminish the stimulant effect of dextroamphetamine*
- Gastrointestinal acidifying agents
  *Decrease the serum concentration of dextroamphetamine*

---

is used to allow some return of normal functions, to maintain sensitivity to a drug, and to reduce the likelihood of adverse effects. A **drug holiday**, as this is called, helps decrease weight loss and growth suppression in children who take dextroamphetamine. It may not be appropriate for every child.

### Assessing for Therapeutic Effects

For patients with ADHD, the nurse assesses for improved behavior and performance of cognitive and psychomotor tasks. For patients with narcolepsy, the nurse assesses for fewer sleep attacks, increased mental alertness, and decreased mental fatigue.

### Assessing for Adverse Effects

The nurse assesses for signs and symptoms of excessive CNS stimulation as evidenced by an inability to complete tasks due to nervousness and hyperactivity. It is necessary to check the patient's cardiovascular status for tachycardia and elevation in blood pressure. The nurse assesses the patient's diet for inability to eat and the patient for loss of weight. He or she should monitor the patient's growth regularly. It is also important to assess the GI system for constipation or diarrhea.

### Patient Teaching

Box 57.2 identifies patient teaching guidelines for drugs used in ADHD or narcolepsy.

### Other Drugs in the Class

Dextroamphetamine–amphetamine (Adderall) is a mixed salt drug that is available in immediate- and sustained-release preparations. The immediate-release form has an onset of action of 20 to 60 minutes and a duration of up to 6 hours. The extended-release form extends the duration to at least 10 hours. It is the only stimulant with U.S. Food and Drug Administration (FDA) approval for use in children younger than 3 years of age who meet the established criteria.

Lisdexamfetamine (Vyvanse) is a prodrug of dextroamphetamine that is pharmacologically activated after oral ingestion and was designed to discourage drug misuse. Lisdexamfetamine has an onset of action within 60 minutes and lasts up to 10 hours. As with dextroamphetamine, many of the adverse effects are mild, of short duration, and reversible with adjustment to the dose or dosing interval. They include anorexia, poor growth or weight loss, social withdrawal, agitation, and sleep disturbances. Growth should be monitored regularly.

---

**Clinical Application 57.2**

Brian has been taking methylphenidate (Metadate ER) every morning for 2 months, and the teachers have noticed that his concentration and his behavior have improved after lunch. However, his appetite has decreased dramatically and he has lost 4 lbs. The teachers have noticed that he does not eat his lunch and skips his afternoon snack. His parents are concerned and schedule a visit to the health care provider. The health care provider is hesitant to change Brian's medication regimen because his behavior at school has improved. What patient teaching can the school nurse provide to Brian and his parents to increase his weight?

**BOX 57.2**   *Patient Teaching Guidelines for Drugs Used in Attention Deficit Hyperactivity Disorder and Narcolepsy*

**General Considerations**

- When diagnosed with ADHD and before taking any medication for it, adult patients and parents of affected children should inform the health care provider about any other stimulant drugs being taken, involvement in strenuous activities of any kind, any heart disease, or any family history of sudden cardiac death. All drugs for ADHD stimulate the heart and blood vessels. The effects are usually a faster heartbeat and increased blood pressure, but cardiac arrest, stroke, or sudden death may occur.
- Use caution while driving or performing other tasks requiring alertness. These drugs may mask symptoms of fatigue, impair physical coordination, and cause dizziness or drowsiness.
- Notify a health care provider of nervousness, insomnia, heart palpitations, vomiting, fever, or skin rash. These are adverse drug effects and dosage may need to be reduced.
- Avoid other stimulants, including caffeine.
- Record weight at least weekly; report excessive losses.
- The drugs may cause weight loss; caloric intake (of nutritional foods) may need to be increased, especially in children.
- Insufficient intake of long-chain polyunsaturated fatty acids plays a role in the development of ADHD. Zinc, iron, and magnesium supplementation may reduce symptoms of ADHD in children.
- Take stimulant drugs only as prescribed:
  - Accurate dosing is important because underuse may cause the recurrence of symptoms and overuse may cause toxicity.

- Do not increase the dosage without consulting with your health care provider. These drugs have a high potential for abuse. The risks of serious health problems and drug dependence are lessened if they are taken correctly. The likelihood of medical problems is greatly increased when ADHD medication is used improperly or in combination with other drugs.
- Get adequate rest and sleep. Do not take stimulant drugs to delay fatigue and sleep; these are normal, necessary resting mechanisms for the body.
- Keep these medications away from children, preferably in a locked cabinet. Parents (or a school nurse) need to dispense each dose and to be sure the drug is taken only by the child for whom it was prescribed.

**Self or Parental Administration**

- Take (or give) regular tablets approximately 30 to 45 minutes before meals.
- Take (or give) the last dose of the day in the afternoon, before 6:00 PM, to avoid interference with sleep.
- Ensure that long-acting/extended-release CNS stimulants are swallowed whole, without crushing or chewing.
- Apply the Daytrana skin patch to the hip area as prescribed. Patch should be removed after 9 hours; alternate hips. See the manufacturer's instructions for opening, applying, removing, and disposing of the skin patch.
- If excessive weight loss, nervousness, or insomnia develops, ask the prescribing physician if the dose can be reduced or taken on a different schedule to relieve these adverse effects.

## NCLEX Success

3. **What is the expected outcome for a central nervous system stimulant in a child?**
   A. increased behavioral problems
   B. improved performance in schoolwork
   C. decreased ability to complete a task
   D. increased hyperactivity

4. **When the nurse is caring for a child receiving a central nervous system stimulant for attention deficit hyperactivity disorder, which assessment is most important to monitor?**
   A. liver function
   B. weight loss
   C. fever
   D. seizure activity

5. **Which finding is indicative of an adverse effect of dextroamphetamine?**
   A. increased appetite
   B. respiratory depression
   C. sedation
   D. cardiac dysrhythmias

6. **Which of the following are expected adverse effects of amphetamine sulfate? (Select all that apply.)**
   A. weight loss
   B. anorexia
   C. dry mouth
   D. bradycardia
   E. constipation

7. **When a 7-year-old child, already of short stature, is prescribed amphetamine sulfate, which intervention will promote growth?**
   A. administering growth hormone
   B. encouraging daily exercise
   C. maintaining a 2200-calorie diet
   D. drug holidays when on school breaks

## AMPHETAMINE-RELATED DRUGS

Amphetamine-related drugs, which resemble amphetamines, have essentially the same stimulant effects as the amphetamines and are also schedule II drugs. **Methylphenidate** (Ritalin, others) is the prototype. This drug, marketed under generic and trade names, is available in several dosage forms, including immediate-release and chewable tablets, extended-release capsules, and a transdermal patch. These dosage forms are not interchangeable.

The FDA has issued a **BLACK BOX WARNING ◆** regarding the risk of drug dependence with amphetamine-related drugs. Methylphenidate has become a drug of abuse, and its nonmedical use, alone or with other drugs, has been associated with increased visits for emergency departments by adolescents and young adults.

## Pharmacokinetics

Methylphenidate is well absorbed after oral administration. Depending on the formulation, the onset of action varies, with a peak in 1 to 8 hours and a duration of action of 3 to 12 hours (longer for transdermal and long-acting preparations). The drug is mostly metabolized in the liver and excreted in the urine.

## Action

Methylphenidate is a mild cortical stimulant that acts on the CNS-like amphetamines. The drug suppresses appetite, increases alertness, elevates mood, and improves physical performance. The efficacy in ADHD is paradoxical and not well understood.

## Use

The clinical indications for use of methylphenidate include the management of ADHD and narcolepsy. The drug may be useful for the treatment of both acute and chronic conditions. Table 57.3 gives route and dosage information for methylphenidate and other amphetamine-related drugs.

### Use in Children and in Older Adults

The use of methylphenidate in both children and older adults is similar to that for dextroamphetamine. This information is available in "Use."

 **QSEN Alert: Evidence-Based Practice**

Osland, Steeves, and Pringsheim (2018) reviewed eight randomized controlled trials (four of which were cross-over trials) with 510 participants (443 boys, 67 girls). Participants were children with both ADHD and chronic tic disorders. All studies took place in the United States and ranged in duration from 3 to 22 weeks. Several of the trials assessed multiple agents including methylphenidate, clonidine, desipramine, dextroamphetamine, guanfacine, atomoxetine, and deprenyl. The results suggested there was low-quality support for the use of methylphenidate, atomoxetine, and clonidine, and very low support for the use of desipramine, dextroamphetamine, guanfacine, and deprenyl in the treatment of ADHD in children with tics. However, all studies reported improvement in symptoms of ADHD. Appetite suppression or weight loss occurred with methylphenidate, dextroamphetamine, atomoxetine, and desipramine, insomnia with methylphenidate and dextroamphetamine, and sedation with clonidine. Methylphenidate, clonidine, guanfacine, desipramine, and atomoxetine appeared to reduce ADHD symptoms in children with tics, but the quality of the available evidence was low to very low. Finally, the researchers suggested that although there is evidence that desipramine may improve ADHD in children, safety concerns will likely continue to limit its use in this population.

### Use in Patients With Renal or Hepatic Impairment

Methylphenidate is excreted in the urine after being metabolized by the liver. Thus, it is necessary to use the drug with caution in patients with renal or hepatic impairment. The nurse should help ensure that lowest possible dose is used.

## Adverse Effects

Methylphenidate has several adverse effects:

- Cardiovascular effects: tachycardia, other dysrhythmias, and hypertension. It is necessary to obtain a baseline ECG and blood pressure.
- CNS effects: excessive CNS stimulation as well as anxiety, hyperactivity, nervousness, insomnia, tremors, convulsion, and possibly psychotic behavior. These reactions are more likely with larger doses of medication.
- GI effects: gastritis, nausea, diarrhea, and constipation.
- Dermatologic effects: rash, exfoliative dermatitis, and loss of scalp hair.
- Hematologic effects: leukopenia and anemia. It is important to obtain a baseline complete blood count and platelet count.
- Other effects: anorexia and weight loss.

It is important to note that in recent years, warnings have been added to all drugs used to treat ADHD and narcolepsy about the associated risks of sudden death, serious cardiovascular problems (e.g., heart attack, hypertension), and psychiatric illnesses (e.g., psychosis, aggression, mania).

## Contraindications

Contraindications to methylphenidate include cardiovascular conditions (e.g., angina, dysrhythmias, hypertension) that are likely to be aggravated by the drug. Other contraindications are anxiety or agitation, glaucoma, or hyperthyroidism. Conditions such as a history of drug abuse or pregnancy or lactation usually preclude use of the drug. Caution is necessary with seizure disorders.

## Nursing Implications

### Preventing Interactions

Methylphenidate may increase effects of phenytoin, tricyclic antidepressants, selective serotonin reuptake inhibitors, and oral anticoagulants. Also, methylphenidate may decrease effects of antihypertensive drugs.

### Administering the Medication

People should take the first dose of methylphenidate on awakening or early in the day, and they should take the last dose at least 6 hours before bedtime. Children with ADHD should take the drug 30 to 45 minutes before meals to minimize the appetite-suppressive effects. It is important not to crush, chew, or bite the long-acting form of methylphenidate; this destroys the extended-release feature and may result in an overdose. Extended-release tablets (Concerta) are coated with immediate-release methylphenidate (for initial dosing) and use an osmotic pump to gradually release methylphenidate to approximate a three-times-a-day dosing schedule. They, too, should be taken whole. Like dextroamphetamine, methylphenidate often causes loss of appetite. Thus, the health care provider may stop the medication during

**TABLE 57.3**

## DRUGS AT A GLANCE: Amphetamine-Related Central Nervous System Stimulants

| Drug | Pregnancy Category | Routes and Dosage Ranges | |
|---|---|---|---|
| | | **Adults** | **Children** |
| ℗ **Methylphenidate** (Ritalin, Ritalin LA, Concerta, Daytrana, Metadate CD, Metadate ER, Methylin, QuilliChew ER, Aptensio XR; ❋ Biphentin, Ritalin) | C | ADHD, 10–60 mg/d PO two or three times daily, preferably 30–45 min before meals. If insomnia is a problem, drug should be taken before 6:00 PM. Timed-release tablets (duration of 8 h) may be used ER forms (Concerta), 18 mg PO daily in the morning; may be increased by 18 mg/d at 1-wk intervals to a max of 54 mg/d (Aptensio XR); increments of 10 mg/d to a max of 60 mg/d (Metadate CD, Ritalin LA) Narcolepsy: immediate release 5 mg twice daily; increase in increments of 5–10 mg/d to a max of 60 mg/d Extended and sustained release may be given in place of immediate release tab when dosage amount corresponds to max of 60 mg/d | ADHD, 6–12 y, start with 5 mg PO before breakfast and lunch with gradual increase 13–17 y, start in the morning without regard to food. Titrate to a max of 72 mg/d. Do not exceed 2 mg/kg/d Transdermal patch (Daytrana) 10–30 mg/d. Apply patch 2 h before effect needed and remove after 9 h in increments of 5–10 mg/wk. Daily dosage exceeding 60 mg/d is not recommended. Discontinue use after 1 mo if no improvement Extended-release forms, use adult dosage |
| Dexmethylphenidate (Focalin, Focalin XR) | C | 5–10 mg/d PO, increased if necessary, max dose 20 mg/d | 6 y and older, 2.5–5 mg/d PO, increased if necessary, max dose 20 mg/d |
| Armodafinil (Nuvigil) | C | Narcolepsy, 150–250 mg once daily in the morning | Safety and effectiveness not established in children |
| Modafinil (Provigil, ❋ Alertec, Auro-Modafinil) | C | Narcolepsy, 200 mg once daily in the morning ADHD, 100–400 mg once daily | Safety concerns in children reported |

the months when the child is not in school. A drug holiday, as this is called, helps decrease weight loss and growth suppression. It may not be appropriate for every child. Ongoing research regarding the long-term impact of these drugs on the developing brains in children is necessary. The overall goal is to improve behavior so that school success is more achievable.

### Assessing for Therapeutic Effects

For patients with ADHD, the nurse assesses for improved behavior and performance of cognitive and psychomotor tasks. For patients with narcolepsy, the nurse assesses for fewer sleep attacks, as well as for increased mental alertness and decreased mental fatigue.

### Assessing for Adverse Effects

The nurse assesses the blood pressure and pulse for hypertension and tachycardia related to the stimulant effects. It is necessary to assess the patient's CNS response for increased anxiety and hyperactivity that impairs the ability to perform activities of daily living. The nurse checks the patient's sleep patterns and inability to sleep restfully. It is also important to assess the patient's GI status for reflux and pain leading to gastritis. In addition, the nurse checks the complete blood count and platelet count for the onset of anemia.

### Patient Teaching

Box 57.2 identifies patient teaching guidelines for medications administered for the treatment of ADHD or narcolepsy.

### Clinical Application 57.3

Brian has been maintaining his weight with his current dosage of methylphenidate and continues to drink two nutritional supplement drinks per day. It is now late spring, and his health care provider wants to try a drug holiday in the summer. Brian's parents are concerned about their son's being able to function at summer camp without any pharmacologic intervention. They voice their worries to the school nurse. What information should the school nurse provide to Brian's parents? What are the advantages and disadvantages of their decision to support a drug holiday?

## Other Drugs in the Class

Dexmethylphenidate (Focalin, Focalin XR), a schedule II controlled drug, is used in the treatment of ADHD. Adverse effects include headache, insomnia, restlessness, anxiety, decreased appetite, and weight loss. The FDA has issued a **BLACK BOX WARNING ◆** regarding caution with the use of dexmethylphenidate in patients with a history of drug dependence or alcoholism. Chronic, abusive use can lead to marked tolerance and psychological dependence with varying degrees of abnormal behavior. Contraindications and the drug interaction profile are similar to methylphenidate.

Modafinil (Provigil) and armodafinil (Nuvigil) are used to treat narcolepsy and to improve wakefulness in other sleep disorders (e.g., obstructive sleep apnea/hypopnea syndrome, shift work sleep disorder). Modafinil is also used to treat ADHD and to decrease the fatigue associated with multiple sclerosis and other disorders. Armodafinil is the R-enantiomer of modafinil, which means that both drugs have identical chemical and physical properties but may interact differently in the body. The FDA requires that a specific warning against the use of modafinil in children be included on the label as serious dermatologic adverse effects and psychiatric events have been reported. Modafinil and armodafinil's ability to promote wakefulness is similar to that of amphetamines and methylphenidate, but their mechanism of action is unknown. Like other CNS stimulants, modafinil and armodafinil have psychoactive effects that alter mood, perception, and thinking; they are schedule IV controlled drugs. Both drugs are rapidly absorbed and reach peak plasma levels in 2 to 4 hours. Modafinil and armodafinil are metabolized by the liver and are major substrates of CYP3A4, making drug interactions likely. The drugs are excreted in the urine. Adverse effects include anxiety, chest pain, dizziness, dyspnea, dysrhythmias, headache, nausea, palpitations, and nervousness. Serious dermatologic and psychiatric drug-related reactions may occur.

## NCLEX Success

8. Patient teaching for children taking methylphenidate for attention deficit hyperactivity disorder should include which of the following?

   A. Give the child the drug at bedtime.
   B. Drowsiness may be a side effect.
   C. If necessary, the child may take over-the-counter cold products without problems.
   D. Provide for periodic drug-free holidays.

9. A boy comes to the school nurse's office and states, "I did not take my Ritalin today." Which of the following is the most appropriate nursing intervention?

   A. Call the child's parent or guardian to try to find out if the boy has taken his medicine.
   B. Give the child his morning dose because it is in the office.
   C. Send him back to class and tell him it is not necessary to take the medication.
   D. Call the child's physician to obtain a one-time dose of methylphenidate.

## OTHER MEDICATIONS USED TO TREAT ATTENTION DEFICIT HYPERACTIVITY DISORDER AND NARCOLEPSY

Three other drugs are commonly administered for the treatment of ADHD or narcolepsy. These drugs include the selective norepinephrine reuptake inhibitor atomoxetine and the antihypertensive drug guanfacine. Table 57.4 gives route and dosage information for these medications.

**Atomoxetine** (Strattera), a second-line drug for the treatment of ADHD in children and adults, acts to inhibit reuptake of norepinephrine in nerve synapses. It has a low risk of abuse and dependence compared with the other drugs used for ADHD and is not a controlled substance. The drug is rapidly absorbed with oral administration, with peak plasma levels in 1 to 2 hours. Atomoxetine is metabolized in the liver and is excreted mainly in urine. People may take the drug with or without food. Dosage adjustment is necessary in patients receiving strong CYP2D6 inhibitors (e.g., paroxetine, fluoxetine, quinidine) or patients known to be CYP2D6 poor metabolizers. Common adverse effects include weight loss, abdominal pain, anorexia, cough, dry mouth, headache, insomnia, irritability, nausea, and vomiting. A **BLACK BOX WARNING ◆** advises that suicidal ideation may occur in children and adolescents with ADHD who take atomoxetine; it is necessary to balance risk with clinical need.

**Guanfacine** (Intuniv), a selective alpha$_{2A}$-adrenoreceptor agonist used in ADHD, preferentially binds postsynaptic alpha$_{2A}$-adrenoreceptors in the prefrontal cortex. The drug is thought to improve delay-related firing of prefrontal cortex neurons affecting underlying working memory and behavioral inhibition. In addition, guanfacine reduces sympathetic nerve impulses resulting in reduced sympathetic outflow and a subsequent decrease in vasomotor tone and heart rate, making it useful in the treatment of hypertension. It is available in an extended-release form that is usually reserved for children and adolescents in whom atomoxetine has not been effective or produces unacceptable adverse effects. No response may occur for up to 2 weeks. Guanfacine is metabolized by the liver and excreted in the urine. It crosses the placenta and enters the breast milk. Adverse effects include sedation, weakness, dizziness, vision disturbance, and headache, as well as cardiovascular conditions (bradycardia and hypotension) and GI problems (dry mouth, constipation, and abdominal pain). Caution is necessary in cardiovascular disease, in hepatic and renal insufficiency, and in pregnancy or during lactation. The extended-release and immediate-release forms are not interchangeable on a milligram-per-milligram basis because of differences in bioavailability.

**Sodium oxybate** (Xyrem), the sodium salt of gamma hydroxybutyrate (GABA), is prescribed to treat cataplexy and excessive daytime sleepiness in individuals with narcolepsy. The drug is a CNS depressant that can cause significant respiratory depression and decreased level of consciousness. The FDA has issued a **BLACK BOX WARNING ◆** regarding the risk of CNS depression and possible abuse and misuse. Because of the risks, the drug is available only through a restricted Risk Evaluation and Mitigation Strategy program.

## NCLEX Success

10. Which of the following groups are most commonly used for drug management of the hyperactive child?

    A. central nervous system (CNS) depressants
    B. CNS stimulants
    C. anticonvulsants
    D. major tranquilizers

11. Which of the following groups are most commonly used for drug management of the patient with narcolepsy?

    A. central nervous system (CNS) depressants
    B. CNS stimulants
    C. anticonvulsants
    D. major tranquilizers

12. Which of the following statements indicate the patient is in need of further patient teaching regarding medication for attention deficit hyperactivity disorder?

    A. I should not crush my tablets.
    B. I can skip doses when I am feeling good.
    C. I should not change my dosage without consulting my health care provider.
    D. I should consult with my health care provider before taking any new medications.

13. An 8-year-old boy has been taking dexmethylphenidate 5 mg daily for 3 months. His mother is concerned that this dosage is not adequately treating his symptoms of attention deficit hyperactivity disorder. Which of the following behaviors would support the mother's concerns?

    A. increased concentration during school
    B. weight gain of 8 lbs over the past 3 months
    C. increased activity
    D. bradycardia

14. A mother who calls the clinic to report that her son has recently started medication to treat attention deficit hyperactivity disorder (ADHD) fears her son is experiencing side effects of the medication. Which of the following side effects are typically related to medications used for ADHD?

    A. poor appetite
    B. frequency of urination
    C. weight gain
    D. sedation

15. Which characteristics would the nurse recognize as primary symptoms of narcolepsy? (Select all that apply.)

    A. excessive daytime drowsiness
    B. fatigue
    C. cataplexy
    D. hypnagogic hallucinations
    E. sleep paralysis

## TABLE 57.4

### DRUGS AT A GLANCE: Other Drugs Administered for Attention Deficit Hyperactivity Disorder

| Drug | Pregnancy category | Routes and dosage ranges | |
|---|---|---|---|
| | | **Adults** | **Children** |
| **Selective norepinephrine reuptake inhibitors** | | | |
| Ⓟ **Atomoxetine** (Strattera; 🍁 Teva-Atomoxetine, Strattera) | C | Adults and children more than 70 kg: start with 40 mg/d PO; increase after a minimum of 3 d to a target daily dose of 80 mg PO daily given as a single dose in the morning or 2 evenly divided doses during the day. Dosage may be increased to 100 mg/d after 2–4 wk if needed | 32 kg or less, start with 0.5 mg/kg/d PO and increase after a minimum of 3 d to a target daily dose of 1.2 mg/kg/d as a single daily dose in the morning; may be given in 2 evenly divided doses throughout the day. Do not exceed 1.4 mg/kg/d or 100 mg/d, whichever is less <br> ≥6 y and ≤70 kg: start with 0.5 mg/kg/d increase after minimum of 3 d to 1.2 mg/kg/d |
| **Sympatholytics** | | | |
| Ⓟ **Guanfacine** (Intuniv, Tenex; 🍁 Intuniv XR) | B | | ADHD, 6–12 4 mg/d <br> 13–17 y 7 mg/d <br> >17 y, 1 mg/kg/d PO in ER tablet; increase by 1 mg/d/wk to a max of 4 mg/d |
| **Central nervous system depressant** | | | |
| Ⓟ **Sodium oxybate** (Xyrem; 🍁 Xyrem) | C | Narcolepsy, PO 2.25 g at bedtime initially after the patient is in bed, and 2.25 g 2.5–4 h later (4.5 g per night). Titrate dose by 1.5 g per night (0.75 g at bedtime and 0.75 g 2.5–4 h later) in weekly intervals (max dose: 9 g per night) | Narcolepsy, ≥7 y <br> 20 to <30 kg: PO, up to 1 g at bedtime initially after the patient is in bed, and up to 1 g 2.5–4 h later (up to 2 g per night). Titrate dose by 1 g per night (0.5 g at bedtime and 0.5 g 2.5–4 h later) in weekly intervals; max dose, 3 g/dose; 6 g per night <br> 30 to <45 kg, PO, up to 1.5 g at bedtime initially after the patient is in bed, and up to 1.5 g 2.5–4 h later (up to 3 g per night). Titrate dose by 1 g per night (0.5 g at bedtime and 0.5 g 2.5–4 h later) in weekly intervals; maximum dose; 3.75 g/dose; 7.5 g per night <br> ≥45 kg, PO up to 2.25 g at bedtime initially after the patient is in bed, and up to 2.25 g 2.5–4 h later (up to 4.5 g per night). Titrate dose by 1.5 g per night (0.75 g at bedtime and 0.75 g 2.5–4 h later) in weekly intervals; max dose, 4.5 g/dose; 9 g per night |

## THE NURSING PROCESS

A concept map outlines the nursing process related to drug therapy considerations in this chapter. Additional nursing implications related to the disease process should also be considered in care decisions.

**Assessment**

- Assess use of stimulant and depressant drugs (prescribed, over-the-counter, or street drugs).
- Assess caffeine intake as a possible cause of anxiety, nervousness, insomnia, or tachycardia, alone or in combination with other CNS stimulants. Heavy users of caffeine may also be taking other psychoactive medications, especially CNS depressants such as antianxiety and sedative-hypnotic drugs.
- Try to identify potentially significant sources of caffeine intake.
- Assess for conditions that are aggravated by CNS stimulants.
- For a child with possible ADHD, assess behavior as specifically and thoroughly as possible.
- For any patient receiving amphetamines or methylphenidate, assess behavior for signs of tolerance and abuse.

**Outcomes of Therapy**

The patient will
- Take CNS stimulants safely and accurately.
- Improve attention span and task performance (children and adults with ADHD) and decrease hyperactivity (children with ADHD).
- Function appropriately in social interactions with other children.
- Maintain appropriate height and weight for age.
- Have fewer sleep episodes during normal waking hours (for patients with narcolepsy).

**Nursing Interventions**

- For a child receiving a CNS stimulant, assist parents in scheduling drug administration to increase beneficial effects and help prevent drug dependence and stunted growth. In addition, ask parents to control drug distribution and monitor the number of pills or capsules available and the number prescribed. The goals are to prevent overuse by the child for whom the drug is prescribed and to prevent the child from sharing his medication with other children who wish to take the drug for nonmedical purposes.
- Record weight at least weekly.
- Promote nutrition to avoid excessive weight loss.
- Provide information about the condition for which a stimulant drug is being given and the potential consequences of overusing the drug.

**Evaluation**

- Ask parents and teachers of children with ADHD to report on behavior and academic performance.
- For adolescents and adults with ADHD, ask the patient or family about the patient's ability to function in work, school, or social environments.
- Ask parents and older children about weight loss and decreased nutritional status.
- Assess for decreased inappropriate sleep episodes in patients with narcolepsy.

## KEY CONCEPTS

- ADHD is characterized by hyperactivity, impulsivity, and a short attention span.
- ADHD usually starts in childhood and may persist through adulthood.
- CNS stimulants improve behavior and attention in patients with ADHD.
- Narcolepsy is characterized by daytime drowsiness and unpredictable "sleep attacks."
- Prescribed CNS stimulants are also abused and used for nonmedical purposes.
- All of the CNS stimulants can cause life-threatening health problems with excessive intake.
-  **BLACK BOX WARNING ◆** makes users aware of dextroamphetamine's high abuse potential; misuse may cause sudden death or serious cardiovascular events.

- **BLACK BOX WARNING ◆** states that there is a risk of drug dependence with amphetamine-related drugs.
- The FDA has issued a **BLACK BOX WARNING ◆** regarding caution with the use of dexmethylphenidate in patients with a history of drug dependence or alcoholism. Chronic, abusive use can lead to marked tolerance and psychological dependence with varying degrees of abnormal behavior.
- **BLACK BOX WARNING ◆** advises that suicidal ideation may occur in children and adolescents who take atomoxetine.
- The FDA has issued a **BLACK BOX WARNING ◆** regarding the risk of CNS depression and the concern over abuse and misuse with the use of sodium oxybate.

## CLINICAL REASONING CASE STUDY

**Meet the Patient**

The nurse practitioner has prescribed immediate-release methylphenidate (Ritalin) 5 mg orally twice daily for 27-year-old Miguel Martinez, after a sleep study confirmed a diagnosis of narcolepsy. Mr. Martinez reports that he has disrupted nocturnal sleep with vivid nightmares and a tendency to fall asleep while at work. The condition is interfering with his job and marriage. The nurse is conducting some patient teaching.

- What are the major adverse effects of central nervous system (CNS) stimulants, such as methylphenidate, and how is it possible to minimize them?
- What patient teaching considerations would be appropriate for the nurse to include?

**Assessing Drug Information**

- Methylphenidate is an amphetamine-related CNS stimulant, which is a schedule II drug. The drug is used to treat narcolepsy and attention deficit hyperactivity disorder.
- The main adverse effects of CNS stimulants are cardiovascular and gastrointestinal, including tachycardia, cardiac dysrhythmias, nervousness, palpitations, decreased appetite, and weight loss. Additional specific adverse effects of methylphenidate include dermatologic effects, such as rash, exfoliative dermatitis, loss of scalp hair, and hematologic effects, such as leukopenia and anemia.

**Nursing Actions**

- To minimize these adverse effects, it is important to teach Mr. Martinez to
  - Take the drug exactly as prescribed; dosage forms are not interchangeable.
  - Take the first dose daily shortly after arising and the second dose before 6 PM.
  - Avoid taking over-the-counter medications because they may alter effects of methylphenidate.
  - Use the drug appropriately and not share the drug with others to decrease the risk of abuse.
  - Use nutritional supplements to increase caloric intake should weight loss occur.
  - Report any new adverse effects to the nurse practitioner.
- Educate Mr. Martinez about obtaining a baseline and periodic electrocardiogram and blood pressure, complete blood count and platelet count, and weight and height.

---

Visit thePoint° at **http://thePoint.lww.com/Frandsen12e** for answers to NCLEX Success questions (in Appendix A), answers to Clinical Application Case Studies (in Appendix B), and more!

## REFERENCES AND RESOURCES

Abad, V. C., & Guilleminault, C. (2018). Insomnia in elderly patients: Recommendations for pharmacological management. *Drugs and Aging, 35,* 791–817.

Altszuler, A., Morrow, A., Merrill, B., Bressler, S., Macphee, F., & Elizabeth Gnagy, E. (2017). The effects of stimulant mediation and training on sports competence among children with ADHD. *Journal of Clinical Child and Adolescent Psychology, 46,* 1–13. doi:10.1080/15 374416.2016.1270829

Alvarado, C., & Modesto-Lowe, V. (2016). Improving treatment in minority children with attention deficit/hyperactivity disorder. *Clinical Pediatrics, 56*(2), 171–176.

Centers for Disease Control and Prevention. (2015). Less than half of children with ADHD received therapy. *Mental Health Weekly, 24*(15), 3–5.

Childress, A. C. (2016). A critical appraisal of atomoxetine in the management of ADHD. *Therapeutics and Clinical Risk Management, 12,* 27–39.

Eugenia, C., Folger, J. M., & Hammerness, P. G. (2016). Treatment of attention-deficit/hyperactivity disorder in adolescents: A systematic review. *Journal of the American Medical Association, 315*(16), 1997–2008.

Lange, K. W., Hauser, J., Lange, K. M., Makuiska-Gerturda, E. Nakamura, A., et al. (2017). The role of nutritional supplements in the treatment of ADHD: What the evidence says. *Current Psychiatry Reports, 19*(8), 1–9.

McLennan, J. D. (2018). Returning to stimulants in children with treatment resistant ADHD: A case study. *Journal of the Canadian Academy of Child and Adolescent Psychiatry, 27*(1), 50–56.

Osland, S. T., Steeves, T. D. L., & Pringsheim, T. (2018). Pharmacological treatment for attention deficit hyperactivity disorder (ADHD) in children with comorbid tic disorders. *Cochrane Database of Systematic Reviews, 6,* CD007990. doi:10.1002/14651858.CD007990.pub3

Padilha, S., Virtuoso, S., Tonin, F. S., Borba, H. H. L., & Pontarolo, R. (2018). Efficacy and safety of drugs for attention deficit hyperactivity disorder in children and adolescents: a network meta-analysis. *European Child and Adolescent Psychiatry, 27,* 1335–1345.

Ryan-Krause, P. (2017). Preschoolers with ADHD and disruptive behavior disorder. *The Journal for Nurse Practitioners, 13*(4), 284–290.

Woon, L. S., Hazil, Z., & Gan, L. L. Y. (2018). Pharmacology for comorbid adult attention-deficit hyperactivity disorder and stimulant dependence: A systematic review. *IIUM Medical Journal Malaysia, 17*(2), 149–162.

Zinnow, T., Banaschewsk, T., Fallgatter, A. J., Jenkner, C., Phillipp-Wiegmann, F. P., et al. (2018). ESCAlate—adaptive treatment approach for adolescents and adults with ADHD: Study protocol for a randomized controlled trail. *Trials, 19*(1), 1–15.

UpToDate. (2019). *Drug information.* Lexi-Comp, Inc.

# 58

# Drug Therapy for Substance Use Disorders

## LEARNING OBJECTIVES

*After studying this chapter, you should be able to:*

1. Describe the etiology, pathophysiology, and clinical manifestations of substance use disorders.
2. Identify the central nervous system (CNS) depressants of abuse.
3. Identify the prototypes and describe the action, use, adverse effects, contraindications, and nursing implications for the treatment of alcohol withdrawal and for the maintenance of sobriety.
4. Identify commonly abused CNS stimulants.
5. Identify commonly abused psychoactive medications.
6. Implement the nursing process for patients who may be abusing CNS depressants, CNS stimulants, or other psychoactive substances.

## CLINICAL APPLICATION CASE STUDY

Bryan Wilson is a 24-year-old man who regularly uses marijuana, alcohol, and tobacco. He was involved in a physical altercation at a local nightclub, and the owner called the police. The police brought Mr. Wilson to the emergency department, where he received a diagnosis of acute alcohol intoxication. He is admitted for treatment of alcohol withdrawal.

## KEY TERMS

**Intoxication:** development of a reversible substance-specific syndrome caused by the recent ingestion of or exposure to a substance

**Physical dependence:** cluster of cognitive, behavioral, and physiologic symptoms, indicating a person continues to use a substance of abuse despite significant substance-related problems

**Psychological dependence:** overwhelming desire to repeat the use of a particular drug to produce pleasure or avoid discomfort

**Substance use disorder:** maladaptive pattern of substance use manifested by recurrent and significant adverse consequences related to repeated use of the substance

**Tolerance:** need for increasingly larger or more frequent doses of a substance to obtain the desired effects originally produced by a lower dose

**Withdrawal:** development of a substance-specific maladaptive behavioral change, with physiologic and cognitive concomitants due to the cessation of or reduction in heavy and prolonged substance use

# INTRODUCTION

This chapter introduces the pharmacologic care of the patient who is experiencing substance use disorders, which include the conditions of substance abuse and substance dependence in the *Diagnostic and Statistical Manual of Mental Disorders,* 5th Edition: DSM-5 (2013). It describes commonly abused substances, characteristics of substance-related disorders, and drugs used to treat substance-related disorders. A **substance use disorder** is a maladaptive pattern of substance use, leading to clinically significant impairment or distress. This abuse involves self-administration of a drug for prolonged periods or in excessive amounts. It produces physical or psychological dependence, impairs functions of body organs, reduces the ability to function in usual activities of daily living, and decreases the ability and motivation to function as a productive member of society.

Substance use is a significant health, social, economic, and legal problem. It is often associated with substantial damage to the user and society (e.g., crime, child and spouse abuse, traumatic injury, chronic health problems, death).

# OVERVIEW OF SUBSTANCE USE

Most drugs associated with substance use disorder are those that affect the central nervous system (CNS) and alter the state of consciousness. Commonly used drugs include CNS depressants (e.g., alcohol, antianxiety and sedative–hypnotic agents, opioid analgesics), CNS stimulants (e.g., cocaine, methamphetamine, methylphenidate, nicotine), and other mind-altering drugs (e.g., marijuana, "ecstasy"). The overwhelming desire to repeat the use of a particular drug to produce pleasure or avoid discomfort is known as substance dependence. Many of these commonly abused drugs have clinical usefulness and are discussed elsewhere: anxiolytics and sedative–hypnotics (see Chap. 54), opioids

(see Chap. 49), and CNS stimulants (see Chap. 57). Although they produce different effects, they are associated with feelings of pleasure, positive reinforcement, and compulsive self-administration.

**Psychological dependence** involves feelings of satisfaction and pleasure from taking a drug. These feelings, perceived as extremely desirable by the drug-dependent person, contribute to acute **intoxication** (symptoms caused by recent ingestion of a substance), development and maintenance of drug abuse patterns, and return to drug-taking behavior after periods of abstinence.

**Physical dependence** involves physiologic adaptation to chronic use of a drug so that **withdrawal** or unpleasant symptoms occur when the drug is stopped, when its action is antagonized by another drug, or when its dosage is decreased. Withdrawal or abstinence produces specific manifestations according to the type of drug and does not occur as long as adequate dosage is maintained. Attempts to avoid withdrawal symptoms reinforce psychological dependence and promote continuing drug use.

Characteristics of drug dependence include craving a drug, often with unsuccessful attempts to decrease its use; compulsive drug-seeking behavior; physical dependence; and continuing to take a drug despite adverse consequences (e.g., drug-related illnesses, mental or legal problems, job loss or decreased ability to function in an occupation, impaired family relationships). Box 58.1 describes other characteristics of substance use disorder.

**Tolerance**, which may be associated with many drugs if used repeatedly, is often an element of drug dependence. Increasing doses are required to obtain psychological effects or avoid physical withdrawal symptoms. The body "adjusts" to the drugs, and higher doses are needed to achieve feelings of pleasure ("reward") or to stave off withdrawal symptoms ("punishment"). Both reward and punishment serve to reinforce continued substance use.

---

**BOX 58.1** | *Characteristics of Substance Use Disorders*

- Substance use disorders involves all socioeconomic levels and affects all age groups. It is especially prevalent among adolescents and young adults. Patterns of use may vary by age group. For example, adolescents and young adults are more likely to use illicit drugs, and older adults are more likely to abuse alcohol and prescription drugs. Health care professionals (e.g., physicians, pharmacists, nurses) are also considered at high risk for development of substance use disorders, at least partly because of easy access.
- A person who abuses one drug is likely to abuse others.
- Multiple drugs are often used concurrently. Alcohol, for example, is often used with other drugs, probably because it is legal and readily available. In addition, alcohol, marijuana, opioids, and sedatives are often used to combat the anxiety and nervousness induced by cocaine, methamphetamine, and other CNS stimulants.
- Users of alcohol and other drugs are not reliable sources of information about the types or amounts of drugs used. Most users understate the amount and frequency of substance use; heroin addicts may overstate the amount used in attempts to obtain higher doses of methadone. In addition, those who use illegal street drugs may not know

what they have taken because of varying purity, potency, additives, contaminants, names, and substitutions of one drug for another.
- Substance users rarely seek health care unless circumstances force the issue. Thus, most substance use comes to the attention of health care professionals when the user experiences a complication such as acute intoxication, withdrawal, or serious medical problems resulting from chronic drug overuse, misuse, or abuse.
- Smoking or inhaling drug vapors is a preferred route of administration for cocaine, marijuana, and nicotine because the drugs are rapidly absorbed from the large surface area of the lungs. Then, they rapidly circulate to the heart and brain without dilution by the systemic circulation or metabolism by enzymes.
- Substance users who inject drugs intravenously are prey to serious problems because they use impure drugs of unknown potency, contaminated needles, poor hygiene, and other dangerous practices. Specific problems include overdoses, death, and numerous infections (e.g., hepatitis, human immunodeficiency virus infection, endocarditis, phlebitis, cellulitis at injection sites).

## Etiology

Researchers have identified a number of factors, especially genetics, in the predisposition to substance use. With genetics, the connection is not straightforward. This is evident with many substances, especially with alcohol. For example, studies indicate that children of alcoholics have a fourfold increased risk of becoming alcoholics as adults when compared with the general population. The tendency to develop substance use disorders runs in families, although certain personality traits are thought to contribute to addictive behavior. Personality characteristics, such as low self-esteem, depression, and the inability to delay gratification, have been found in people with substance use.

Other factors important in developing drug dependence include the specific drug; the amount, frequency, and route of administration; and environmental or circumstantial characteristics. The environment in which a person uses a substance may contribute to the reinforcement. Moreover, the pleasurable effect of the substance itself may encourage the user to repeat it.

Cultural and ethnic influences may also play a role in substance use disorders, related to patterns of consumption of substance and cultural acceptance of substance use. In addition, peer pressure is often an important factor in initial and continuing drug ingestion. Although patterns of drug use vary in particular populations and in geographic areas, continuing trends seem to include increased use of methamphetamines, "club drugs," prescription drugs, and using multiple drugs at the same time. Internet Web sites have become an important source of the drugs, and in some instances, instructions for manufacturing particular drugs are available.

 **QSEN Alert: Evidence-Based Practice**

The annual National Youth Tobacco Survey explores tobacco use patterns and associated factors in middle school and high school students. Wang et al. (2019) reported the findings from the 2019 survey that involved completed and weighted responses of approximately 27 million students. An estimated 24.3% of middle school students and 53.3% of high school students reported having ever tried a tobacco product. In addition, 12.5% of middle school students and 31.2% of high school students reported using a tobacco product (e.g., electronic cigarettes, cigarettes, cigars, smokeless tobacco, hookahs, pipe tobacco, bidis) in the past 30 days. Tobacco products have grown to include various smoked, smokeless, and electronic products. However, since 2014, electronic cigarettes were the most cited tobacco product currently used in these age groups. Over half of students currently using tobacco product reported they were seriously thinking about quitting the use of all tobacco products and over half reported they had stopped using all tobacco products for one or more days because they were trying to quit. Factors that influence initiation and establishment of tobacco-use patterns included the availability of flavors of electronic cigarettes, exposure to tobacco product marketing, curiosity and susceptibility, and misperceptions about the lack of harm from tobacco product use.

## Pathophysiology

Many drugs of abuse activate the pleasure or reward system in the brain by altering neurotransmission systems. Prolonged drug abuse damages nerve cells in the brain and alters brain functions. The damage is long lasting.

Drug dependence is a complex phenomenon. Although the cause is unknown, one theory is that drugs stimulate or inhibit neurotransmitters in the brain to produce pleasure and euphoria or to decrease unpleasant feelings such as anxiety. For example, dopaminergic neurons in the limbic system are associated with the brain's reward system and are thought to be sites of action of alcohol, amphetamines, cocaine, nicotine, and opiates. These major drugs of abuse increase dopaminergic transmission and the availability of dopamine. These actions are believed to stimulate the brain's reward system and lead to compulsive drug administration and abuse.

The noradrenergic neurotransmission system, which uses norepinephrine as its neurotransmitter, is often involved as well as the dopaminergic system. Noradrenergic neurons innervate the limbic system and cerebral cortex and are important in setting mood and affect. Drugs that alter noradrenergic transmission have profound effects on mood and affect. Amphetamines and cocaine increase noradrenergic transmission, as with dopaminergic transmission, by promoting the release of norepinephrine and/or inhibiting its reuptake. Increased norepinephrine leads to mood elevation and euphoria, which promotes continued drug abuse. Increased norepinephrine also leads to major adverse effects of amphetamines and cocaine, including myocardial infarction, severe hypertension, and stroke, as well as profound mood swings from euphoria to depression.

## Clinical Manifestations

Drug effects vary according to the type of substance being abused, the amount, route of administration, duration of use, and phase of substance use (e.g., acute intoxication, withdrawal syndromes, organ damage, medical illness). Thus, acute intoxication often produces profound behavioral changes, and chronic abuse often leads to serious organ damage and impaired ability to function in work, family, or social settings. Withdrawal symptoms are characteristic of particular types of drugs and are usually opposite to the effects originally produced. For example, withdrawal symptoms of alcohol and sedative-type drugs are mainly agitation, nervousness, and hyperactivity.

## Therapy

### General Approach

The major goals of treatment for substance use disorder are detoxification, initiation of abstinence, and prevention of relapse. Patients who are likely to benefit from treatment are those who recognize that substance use is negatively influencing their problems and causing significant problems in their ability to function. Despite advances in treatment and the many adverse consequences of substance abuse, relapses to drug-taking behavior are common among people who have been detoxified or even abstinent for varying periods of time.

Treatments for substance use are limited but increasing, and more treatment facilities are needed. For most health professionals, contact with substance users is more likely to occur in acute situations, such as with intoxication or overdose,

| BOX 58.2 | *Sources of Information About Substance Abuse* |
|---|---|

- The National Institute on Drug Abuse (NIDA) of the National Institutes of Health supports most of the world's research on the health aspects of drug abuse and addiction.
    - 6001 Executive Blvd.
    - Bethesda, MD 20892–9561
    - (301) 443–1124
    - www.drugabuse.gov
    - www.nida.nih.gov
- Substance Abuse and Mental Health Services Administration (SAMHSA)
    - PO Box 2345
    - Rockville, MD 20847–2345
    - (877) 726–4727
    - www.samhsa.org
    - SAMHSA's National Clearinghouse for Alcohol and Drug Information (NCADI): http://ncadi.samhsa.gov
- The National Institute on Alcohol Abuse and Alcoholism (NIAAA) conducts and supports research on the causes, consequences, prevention, and treatment of alcohol abuse and disseminates research findings to general, professional, and academic audiences. Publications and research information are available at www.niaaa.nih.gov.

withdrawal syndromes, or various medical–surgical illnesses associated with the substance use. In general, treatment depends on the type, extent, and duration of drug-taking behavior and the particular situation for which treatment is needed.

Psychological rehabilitation efforts should be part of any treatment program for a drug-dependent person. Several approaches may be useful, including inpatient and outpatient psychotherapy, voluntary self-help groups (e.g., Alcoholics Anonymous, Narcotics Anonymous), and other types of emotional support and counseling. Box 58.2 gives sources of information about substance use disorders.

## Use of Drugs

Drug therapy for treatment of drug dependence is limited for several reasons. First, specific antidotes are available only for benzodiazepines (flumazenil) and opioid narcotics (naltrexone). Second, there is a high risk of substituting one abused drug for another. Third, there are significant drawbacks to giving CNS stimulants to reverse effects of CNS depressants and vice versa. Fourth, there is often inadequate information about the types and amounts of drug taken. Two of the more successful drug therapy regimens are methadone administration for heroin dependence and nicotine replacement (or other drugs [e.g., bupropion or varenicline]) for nicotine dependence. With both treatments, however, a combination of drug therapy and counseling is more effective than either method alone. Treatment programs for substance use emphasize sobriety, which is complete abstinence from substance use. Combined with psychotherapy, there are pharmacologic interventions that can assist the patient with sobriety. Table 58.1 lists the specific drugs that may be used to treat substance-related disorders.

## NCLEX Success

1. The nurse who is caring for a patient who has been abusing alcohol may expect to see what symptom as the patient enters withdrawal?
   - A. sleep
   - B. muscle relaxation
   - C. euphoria
   - D. agitation

2. The nurse is taking care of an adolescent male with a history of compulsive drug use. His parents have questioned him about the reasons behind such drug use. What factor is attributed to compulsive drug use?
   - A. drug stimulation of the "reward" center in the brain
   - B. a belief that the drugs are not harmful
   - C. parental pressure to do well in school
   - D. a permissive attitude toward taking drugs by parents and society

### TABLE 58.1

### Drugs Administered for the Treatment of Substance Use Disorders

| Drug Class | Representative Drugs |
|---|---|
| Antialcoholic drug; enzyme inhibitor | Disulfiram (Antabuse) |
| Benzodiazepine | Chlordiazepoxide (Librium) Lorazepam (Ativan) |
| GABA agonist/glutamate antagonist | Acamprosate (Campral) |
| Centrally acting alpha-agonist antihypertensive | Clonidine (Catapres, Duraclon) |
| Benzodiazepine receptor antagonist | Flumazenil |
| Opioid antagonist | Naloxone (Narcan, Evzio) |
| Opioid antagonist | Naltrexone (Vivitrol) |
| Opioid agonist–antagonist analgesic | Buprenorphine (Buprenex, Belbuca, Butrans, Sublocade) Naltrexone–buprenorphine (Suboxone) |
| Opioid agonist analgesic | Methadone (Methadose) |
| Antipsychotic; dopamine blocker | Haloperidol (Haldol) |
| Nicotine receptor agonist | Varenicline (Chantix) |
| Atypical antidepressant; smoking deterrent | Bupropion (Zyban, Welbutrin SR, Contrave) |
| Smoking deterrent | Nicotine (Nicoderm CQ, Nicorette mini, Nicotrol NS) |

# CENTRAL NERVOUS SYSTEM DEPRESSANT USE: DRUG THERAPY

CNS depressants are drugs that slow down or "depress" brain activity. These drugs are capable of inducing varying degrees of CNS depression ranging from tranquilizing relief of anxiety to anesthesia, coma, and even death. Effects produced by these substances depend on the size of dose and potency of the drug administered. They include alcohol, benzodiazepines (antianxiety drugs), and opioids. Box 58.3 summarizes information about these drugs.

## BENZODIAZEPINES FOR TREATMENT OF ALCOHOL WITHDRAWAL

Benzodiazepines are the drugs of choice for treating withdrawal from alcohol and other CNS depressants. ⓟ**Chlordiazepoxide** (Librium), the prototype benzodiazepine for treatment of such substance use, provides adequate sedation and has a significant anticonvulsant effect. The drug may also make it easier for the patient to participate in rehabilitation programs and allow for the gradual reduction and discontinuation of the abused substance.

## Pharmacokinetics

The oral form of chlordiazepoxide has a rapid onset of action, with a peak of 1 hour. The intramuscular (IM) form has an onset of action within 10 to 15 minutes and peaks within 15 to 30 minutes. The IV form has an immediate onset of action and peaks within 30 minutes. For all forms, the duration is 48 to 72 hours. Metabolism occurs in the liver, and excretion is in the urine.

## Action

The exact mechanism of action of chlordiazepoxide is not understood; however, the drug acts mainly at the subcortical levels of the CNS. The main sites of action may be the limbic system and reticular formation.

---

| **BOX 58.3** | *Central Nervous System Depressants of Abuse* |

### Alcohol (Ethanol)

Alcohol is commonly abused around the world. It is legal and readily available, and its use is accepted in most societies. Excessive amounts and long-term abuse damage essentially all organ systems of the body. Alcohol is thought to exert its effects on the CNS mainly by enhancing the activity of gamma-aminobutyric acid, an inhibitory neurotransmitter, or by inhibiting the activity of glutamate, an excitatory neurotransmitter.

The clinical manifestations of acute alcohol intoxication include impaired thinking, judgment, and psychomotor coordination, which may lead to poor work performance and accidents. There is a loss of conscious control of behavior, and exhibitionism and aggressiveness often result. Chronic ingestion may cause severe organ damage and mental problems.

Psychological dependence, physical dependence, tolerance, and cross-tolerance with other CNS depressants may occur with chronic alcohol consumption. People who are alcohol dependent are unlikely to seek treatment for alcohol abuse unless an acute illness or other situation forces the issue. However, they are likely to seek treatment for other disorders, such as agitation and anxiety. Delirium tremens, the most serious form of alcohol withdrawal, is characterized by confusion, disorientation, delusions, visual hallucinations, and other signs of acute psychosis. Treatment with psychological counseling, referral to a self-help group such as Alcoholics Anonymous, and drug therapy with disulfiram or naltrexone may be useful.

### Benzodiazepines

Benzodiazepines, commonly used for their anxiolytic and sedative–hypnotic effects (see Chap. 54), are also widely abused, mainly by people who also abuse alcohol and/or other drugs. Benzodiazepines rarely cause respiratory depression or death, even in overdose, unless taken with alcohol or other drugs. However, they may cause oversedation, memory impairment, poor motor coordination, and confusion. Withdrawal reactions can be extremely uncomfortable. Unfortunately, abusers often combine drugs in their quest for a greater "high" or to relieve the unpleasant effects of CNS stimulants and other street drugs.

With mild benzodiazepine overdose, the patient usually sleeps off the effects of the drug. More severe overdoses cause respiratory depression and coma.

Flumazenil is a specific antidote that can reverse benzodiazepine-induced sedation, coma, and respiratory depression. The drug competes with benzodiazepines for benzodiazepine receptors. It has a short duration of action, and repeated intravenous (IV) injections are usually necessary. Close observation is required, because symptoms of overdose may recur when the effects of a dose of flumazenil subside and because the drug may precipitate acute withdrawal symptoms (e.g., agitation, confusion, seizures). A **BLACK BOX WARNING ◆** alerts practitioners about the risk of seizures associated with the use of flumazenil.

### Opioids

Opioids are potent analgesics extensively used in pain management (see Chap. 49). They are also commonly abused. Legal opioid analgesics are increasingly being diverted from their appropriate use and bought and sold as street drugs. The focus here is on heroin, a common drug of abuse. A Schedule I drug in the United States, it is not used therapeutically. Heroin produces the same effects as naturally occurring endorphins and other opioid drugs. The drug rapidly enters the brain, where it is converted to morphine. Morphine stimulates opioid receptors in the reward system of the brain, which causes greater amounts of dopamine to be released.

Opioids produce tolerance and high degrees of psychological and physical dependence. Most other drugs that produce dependence do so with prolonged usage of large doses, but morphine-like drugs produce dependence with repeated administration of small doses. Medical usage of these drugs produces physical dependence and tolerance but rarely leads to use or abuse for mind-altering effects. Thus, "addiction" should not be an issue when the drugs are needed for pain management in patients with cancer or other severe illnesses.

Treatment may be needed for overdose or withdrawal syndromes. Overdose may produce severe respiratory depression and coma. Insertion of an endotracheal tube and mechanical ventilation may be necessary. Drug therapy consists of an opioid antagonist, such as naloxone, to reverse opioid effects. In addition to profound respiratory depression, pulmonary edema, hypoglycemia, pneumonia, cellulitis, and other infections often accompany opioid overdose and require specific treatment measures.

## Use

Prescribers may order chlordiazepoxide for acute alcohol withdrawal as well as for the management of anxiety disorders. The drug is useful in symptomatic relief of acute agitation, tremors, and delirium tremens. Treatment with chlordiazepoxide for alcohol withdrawal should begin as soon as the clinician identifies that the patient needs it. Table 58.2 gives route and dosage information for chlordiazepoxide and other drugs used to treat substance use.

### TABLE 58.2

### DRUGS AT A GLANCE: Drugs Used to Treat Substance Use Disorders

| Drug | Pregnancy Category | Routes and Dosage Ranges | |
|------|--------------------|--------------------------|---|
| | | **Adults** | **Children** |
| **Chlordiaze-poxide** (Librium) | D | 50–100 mg PO followed by repeated doses up to 300 mg/d; subsequent doses reduced to lowest effective dose | Not recommended in children younger than 6 y<br>≥6 y, 5 mg PO two to four times daily; may be increased to 10 mg PO two to three times daily |
| **Disulfiram** (Antabuse) | C | Initially, 500 mg/d PO once daily for 1–2 wk (maximum 500 mg daily)<br>Maintenance, 125–500 mg PO daily (maximum 500 mg daily) | Safety and efficacy in patients younger than 18 y not established |
| Acamprosate (✹ Campral) | C | 666 mg PO 3 times daily | Safety and efficacy not established in children |
| Buprenorphine (Buprenex, Belbuca, Butrans, Sublocade; ✹ Butrans) | C | 12–16 mg/d SL; use as induction with switch to Suboxone for maintenance (same dosage) | Ages 2–12 y, 2–6 mcg/kg IM or slow IV injection every 4–6 h<br>≥13 y, same as adult dosage |
| Buprenorphine–naloxone (Suboxone, Bunavail, Zubsolv; ✹ Mylan-Buprenorphine/Naloxone, Suboxone) | C | Short-acting opioid dependency:<br>Suboxone film, day 1, initial buprenorphine 2–4 mg/naloxone 0.5–1.0 mg film sublingually approximately every 2 h to control acute withdrawal symptoms up to total dose of buprenorphine 8 mg/naloxone 2 mg; day 2 up to buprenorphine 16 mg/naloxone 4 mg<br>Zubsolv, day 1, initial sublingual tablet, buprenorphine 1.4 mg/naloxone 0.36 mg and to control withdrawal symptoms increase in those increments every 1.5–2 h to a total day 1 dose up to buprenorphine 5.7 mg/naloxone 1.4 mg; day 2, up to buprenorphine 4.2 mg/naloxone 2.9 mg once daily<br>Maintenance:<br>Bunavail, buccal film, buprenorphine 8.4 mg/naloxone 1.4 mg | ≥16 y, same as adult dosage |
| Bupropion (Zyban, Welbutrin SR, Contrave; ✹ Bupropion SR, Zyban) | C | Smoking cessation: 150 mg PO once daily for 3 d, then increase to 150 mg twice daily, at least 8 h apart; maximum dose, 300 mg/d; treat for 7–12 wk | Safety and efficacy in patients younger than 18 y not established |
| Clonidine (Catapres, Duraclon; ✹ Catapres, Novo-Clonidine) | C | Methadone withdrawal: 0.1 mg PO three times daily up to a maximum of 1 mg daily<br>Nicotine withdrawal: 0.1 mg PO twice daily, increased by 0.1 mg daily every 7 d<br>0.1 mg/24 patch transdermal applied once every 7 d, increased by 0.1 mg daily at 1 wk intervals | Neonatal abstinence syndrome (opioid withdrawal; limited data available):<br>GA < 35 wk, 0.5–1.0 mcg/kg/dose PO every 6 h until stable and tapered as tolerated<br>GA ≥ 35 wk, 0.5–1.0 mcg/kg/dose PO every 4–6 h until stable and tapered as tolerated |

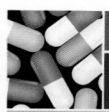

| Drug | Pregnancy Category | Routes and Dosage Ranges | |
|---|---|---|---|
| | | **Adults** | **Children** |
| Flumazenil | C | Suspected benzodiazepine overdose: 0.2 mg IV over 30 s; repeat with 0.3 mg IV every 30 s to maximum dose of 3 mg | Reversal of benzodiazepine when used in conscious sedation: ≥1 y, 0.01 mg/kg IV over 15 s to maximum 0.2 mg; repeated as needed at 1-min intervals to maximum 4 doses or 1 mg or 0.05 mg/kg, whichever lower |
| Haloperidol (Haldol; ❦ PMS-Haloperidol, Novo-Peridol) | C | 0.5–2 PO mg two to three times daily with moderate symptoms, 3–5 mg PO two to three times daily for more resistant patients; 2–5 mg IM daily every 60 min or 4–8 h as needed | 3–12 y or 15–40 kg, 0.5 mg/d (25–50 mcg/kg/d) as initial dose; may increase in 0.5-mg increments |
| Lorazepam (Ativan; ❦ Apo-Lorazepam) | D | Alcohol withdrawal hallucinations or seizures: 1–4 mg IV, every 5–15 min until calm, repeat as necessary 1–4 mg IM, every 30–50 min until calm, repeat as necessary Benzodiazepine withdrawal: 2 mg PO every 6–8 h initially, then tapered over 1–2 wk | No recommendations for treatment of withdrawal in children |
| Methadone (Methadose; ❦ Metadol, Methadose) | C | Withdrawal: 20–30 mg daily initially PO or parenteral; increase dose to suppress withdrawal signs; 40 mg/d in single or divided doses is an adequate stabilizing dose; gradually reduce dosage every day after 2–3 d of stabilization dose Maintenance: 20–120 mg PO daily | Neonatal opioid withdrawal syndrome: 0.05–0.2 mg/kg/dose PO, IV every 12–24 h or 0.5 mg/kg/d divided every 8 h |
| Naloxone (Narcan, Evzio; ❦ Naloxone hydrochloride injection) | C | Initial dose, 0.4–2 mg IV; additional doses may be repeated at 2–3-min intervals; if no response after 10 mg, question the diagnosis; IM, subcutaneous, endotracheal routes may be used if IV route is unavailable | <5 y or ≤20 kg, 0.1 mg/kg/dose IV; additional 0.1 mg/kg every 2–3 min as needed; may be given intraosseous or endotracheally ≥5 y or >20 kg, 2 mg IV, may repeat every 2–3 min; IM, subcutaneous, endotracheal routes may be used if IV route is unavailable |
| Naltrexone (Vivitrol; ❦ APO-Naltrexone, ReVia) | C | Alcohol dependence: 50 mg PO daily or 380 mg IM every 4 wk Opioid dependence: initial dose, 25 mg PO; observe for 1 h; if no signs or symptoms are seen, complete dose with 25 mg PO; usual maintenance dose is 50 mg/24 h; flexible dosing can include 100 mg PO every other day or 150 mg PO every 3 d or 380 mg IM every 4 wk | Safety and efficacy in patients <18 y not established |
| Nicotine (Nicoderm CQ, Nicorette mini, Nicotrol NS; ❦ Habitrol, Nicoderm, Nicorette, Nicotrol) | D | Transdermal, apply system (5–21) mg once every 24 h; dosage based on response and stage of withdrawal Nicotine chewing gum, 1 piece (2 or 4 mg) every 1–2 h for wk 1–6 with an urge to smoke; gradual reduction over next 6 wk Nasal lozenge, 2 mg or 4 mg dose within 30 min of awakening, then every 1–2 h for wk 1–6; gradual reduction over next 6 wk (max 5 lozenges every 6 h or 20 lozenges daily) Nasal spray, 1–2 sprays each hour, up to 10 sprays/h or 80 total sprays per day Nasal inhaler, 6–16 cartridges daily for first 6–12 wk, then gradual reduction over next 6–12 wk | Safety and efficacy in patients younger than 18 y who smoke not established |
| Varenicline (Chantix; ❦ Champix) | C | Patient should pick a date to stop smoking and begin drug therapy 1 wk before that date; d 1–3, 0.5 mg/d PO; d 4–7, 0.5 mg PO twice daily; d 8 until the end of treatment, 1 mg PO twice daily; treatment should last 12 wk | Not recommended for children younger than 18 y |

GA, gestational age.

## Use in Patients With Renal or Hepatic Impairment

Chlordiazepoxide is excreted in the urine after being metabolized in the liver. Thus, caution is warranted in patients with renal or hepatic impairment.

## Use in Patients With Critical Illness

Patients who abuse alcohol or other CNS depressants often have comorbid critical illnesses. Thus, chlordiazepoxide requires caution in patients with critical illness.

## Use in Patients Receiving Home Care

Alcohol detoxification through pharmacologic means generally takes place in a hospital setting but may occur in the home. The home care nurse shares the responsibility for teaching patients how to use chlordiazepoxide effectively and how to recognize medication responses that should be reported to the health care provider. The nurse instructs the patient and/or caregivers to recognize signs and symptoms of alcohol withdrawal and reviews the pharmacologic treatment regimen with them. Also, the nurse monitors the patient's response to the drug. If the patient is unable to take the medication for any reason or is not responding to current dosage, it is essential to notify the health care provider.

## Adverse Effects

CNS adverse effects of chlordiazepoxide include sedation, depression, lethargy, disorientation, and delirium. Patients taking high dosages may experience paradoxical excitatory reactions during the first few weeks of treatment. Other adverse effects include alterations in pulse and blood pressure, urticaria, constipation, diarrhea, dry mouth, jaundice, changes in libido, and blood dyscrasias.

The U.S. Food and Drug Administration (FDA) has issued a **BLACK BOX WARNING ◆** for the combined use of benzodiazepines and opioid analgesics. Serious adverse reactions, including slowed or difficult breathing and death, have been reported.

## Contraindications

Contraindications to chlordiazepoxide include hypersensitivity to benzodiazepines, psychosis, acute narrow-angle glaucoma, shock, coma, acute alcoholic intoxication with depression of vital signs, pregnancy, labor and delivery, and lactation.

## Nursing Implications

### Preventing Interactions

Some medications and herbs interact with chlordiazepoxide, increasing its effects (Boxes 58.4 and 58.5).

### Administering the Medication

Chlordiazepoxide is available in capsule form for oral use and powder form for parenteral use. For adults, the dosage is individualized and is often based on institution-specific protocol. It is necessary to increase the dosage carefully to avoid adverse effects. The nurse gives IM injections slowly in the upper outer quadrant of the gluteus muscle. He or she should take the patient's vital signs regularly during this period, especially when giving the IV form of the drug, as well as observe and document subjective and objective reports by the patient. It is important

**BOX 58.4** **Drug Interactions: Chlordiazepoxide**

**Drugs That Increase the Effect of Chlordiazepoxide**

- Antiepileptic drugs, central nervous system depressants, cimetidine, phenytoin
  *Increase central nervous system depression*
- Levodopa
  *Increases parkinsonian symptoms*

to taper the drug gradually based on the patient's response to treatment.

### Assessing for Therapeutic Effects

The nurse assesses the patient's vital signs; they should stabilize to within normal parameters. In addition, the nurse observes for the presence of cognitive impairment and/or thought disturbances and assesses for signs and symptoms of agitation and/or restlessness. The patient should not appear restless or confused and should not complain of thought disturbances.

### Assessing for Adverse Effects

The nurse assesses the patient for signs and symptoms of CNS depression. It is necessary to check the blood pressure for fluctuations from hypertension to hypotension. The nurse assesses the skin for redness, itching, and signs of bruising as well as the skin and sclera for jaundice. It is also necessary to interview the patient regarding the following:

- Frequency and amount of bowel movements
- Desire for sexual intercourse

**Clinical Application 58.1**

Mr. Wilson admits to the nurse in the emergency department that he consumes alcohol on a daily basis. He admits to smoking tobacco in the form of cigarettes (one pack per day) and to smoking marijuana (average, two times per week). The health care providers in the emergency department are concerned that he may experience alcohol withdrawal, and a physician subsequently prescribes a short-acting benzodiazepine.

- Is a benzodiazepine the pharmacologic treatment of choice for this condition?
- What are some symptoms for which the nurse should monitor?

**BOX 58.5** **Herb and Dietary Interactions: Chlordiazepoxide**

**Herbs and Foods That Increase the Effects of Chlordiazepoxide**

- Kava
- Valerian

### Patient Teaching

With chlordiazepoxide, it is necessary to instruct the patient and/or caregiver to

- Take the drug as prescribed and not to stop taking it without consulting the health care provider.
- Understand what adverse effects are associated with use of the drug.

In addition, it is important that females do not become pregnant while taking chlordiazepoxide.

## ENZYME INHIBITORS FOR MAINTENANCE OF ALCOHOL SOBRIETY

Drug therapy for maintenance of sobriety is limited, mainly because of poor adherence. One of the drugs approved for this purpose is Ⓟ **disulfiram** (Antabuse).

## Pharmacokinetics and Action

Disulfiram is quickly absorbed in the gastrointestinal tract. It has a slow onset of action, with a peak of up to 12 hours and a duration of 1 to 2 weeks. The medication is deposited in fat. It is metabolized slowly by the liver and excreted by the lungs and in the feces.

Disulfiram inhibits the enzyme aldehyde dehydrogenase to block the oxidation of alcohol. This allows acetaldehyde to accumulate in the blood to concentrations that are 5 to 10 times higher than normally achieved during alcohol metabolism. This accumulation of acetaldehyde produces an unpleasant reaction when disulfiram is consumed with alcohol.

## Use

Prescribers order disulfiram for people with chronic alcoholism to maintain a state of sobriety. Table 58.2 gives route and dosage information for disulfiram and other drugs used to treat substance use.

### Use in Patients With Hepatic Impairment

Hepatitis and hepatic failure may occur with disulfiram. This reaction may be severe, resulting in death in patients with hepatic impairment.

## Adverse Effects

The combination of disulfiram with alcohol may result in headaches, confusion, seizures, chest pain, flushing, palpitations, hypotension, sweating, blurred vision, nausea, vomiting, and a garlic-like aftertaste. More severe effects (with alcohol) include dysrhythmias, cardiovascular collapse, heart failure, myocardial infarction, and death.

## Contraindications

Contraindications to disulfiram include use with alcohol, metronidazole, or paraldehyde, as well as multiple drug dependence. A **BLACK BOX WARNING** ◆ states that the drug should not be given to a patient who has consumed alcohol in the past 12 hours or without his or her full knowledge. It is important that disulfiram never be administered to patients with myocardial

disease, coronary occlusion, or psychosis. Also, patients who are known to be allergic to the drug should not take it.

## Nursing Implications

### Preventing Interactions

Nitroglycerin, paraldehyde, metronidazole, and cotrimoxazole produce a reaction similar to that of alcohol; the accumulation of acetaldehyde produces an unpleasant reaction accompanied by nausea and vomiting. Isoniazid and disulfiram produce neurologic effects such as changes in behavior and coordination. Warfarin, paraldehyde, and phenytoin combined with disulfiram result in increased serum blood levels of the drugs.

### Administering the Medication

Administration of disulfiram at bedtime allows the patient to sleep, because the drug has a sedative effect.

### Assessing Therapeutic and Adverse Effects

The nurse determines whether the patient has remained sober. In the event disulfiram is consumed with alcohol, the nurse assesses for cardiovascular effects. In a patient who presents with a severe reaction, it is essential to monitor for shock and hypokalemia.

### Patient Teaching

With disulfiram, it is necessary to instruct the patient to

- Take the medication daily—at bedtime if dizziness and drowsiness occur.
- Never consume alcohol in any form, including liniments, mouthwash, over-the-counter cough and cold aids, vinegars, sauces, and colognes.
- Not take the medication if alcohol has been consumed.
- Have periodic liver function tests.
- Wear a medical alert bracelet.

## DRUGS USED TO REDUCE CRAVINGS IN ALCOHOL USE

Acamprosate (Campral) and oral naltrexone (Vivitrol) are used for relapse prevention and are considered anticraving agents. These drugs have different mechanisms of action and target different neurotransmitter systems that may provide effectiveness for different aspects of alcohol use behavior. In treatment for alcohol use disorders, acamprosate has been found to be slightly more effective in promoting abstinence and naltrexone slightly more effective in reducing heavy drinking and craving.

Alcohol use stimulates opioid receptors and releases endorphins in the brain, and naltrexone, an opioid antagonist, is thought to reduce the incentive to drink and decrease craving by blocking the rewarding effect of alcohol. Acamprosate is a GABA agonist/glutamate antagonist used in the treatment of alcohol abuse. Although the exact mechanism is unclear, the drug is thought to normalize the dysregulation of $N$-methyl-D-aspartate (NMDA)-mediated glutamatergic excitation that occurs in alcohol withdrawal and early abstinence, restoring balance to GABA and glutamate. Unlike naltrexone, acamprosate does not appear to affect alcohol consumption after the first drink and does not cause a disulfiram-like reaction following alcohol ingestion. Among the two, acamprosate has low abuse potential, is better tolerated, and is safer in overdose.

## NCLEX Success

3. A patient is admitted to the chemical dependence unit. The nurse receives an order to administer flumazenil. Clinicians use flumazenil to treat overdoses with which of the following?

   A. alcohol
   B. benzodiazepines
   C. opioids
   D. amphetamines

4. A patient is admitted to the chemical dependence unit with chronic alcohol abuse. For which of the following symptoms does the nurse assess during alcohol withdrawal?

   A. euphoria, hyperactivity, and insomnia
   B. depression, suicidal ideation, and hypersomnia
   C. diaphoresis, nausea, vomiting, and tremors
   D. unsteady gait, nystagmus, and profound disorientation

5. Which of the following medications is the health care provider most likely to prescribe for a patient who is experiencing alcohol withdrawal?

   A. haloperidol
   B. chlordiazepoxide
   C. propoxyphene
   D. phenytoin

### *Clinical Application 58.2*

Mr. Wilson is scheduled to be discharged after completing an alcohol withdrawal protocol for several days. After discharge, he is scheduled to attend outpatient chemical dependency treatment. His health care provider has prescribed disulfiram (Antabuse) for the patient to take on an outpatient basis.

- Is this an appropriate treatment choice for the patient?
- What symptoms will Mr. Wilson have if he drinks alcohol and takes disulfiram?
- What patient teaching should the nurse provide to Mr. Wilson regarding his treatment plan with disulfiram?

## OPIOID AGONISTS AND ANTAGONISTS FOR TREATMENT OF OPIOID ABUSE

Ideally, the goal of treatment for opioid abuse is abstinence from further opioid use. However, because opioid users rarely meet this goal, long-term drug therapy may be used to treat heroin dependence.

The first option uses opioid substitutes to prevent withdrawal symptoms and improve a lifestyle that revolves around obtaining, using, and recovering from a drug. The substitute is methadone, an agonist at specific opioid receptors in the CNS. This drug has long been used as a detoxification and/or as maintenance therapy for opioid addiction. It is usually given in a single, daily oral dose at an outpatient methadone clinic. The FDA has issued a **BLACK BOX WARNING ◆** concerning methadone, stating that it should be part of an approved program for opioid addiction. Deaths have been reported during the initiation of treatment. It is essential that emergency services be on standby. Another **BLACK BOX WARNING ◆** for methadone stipulates that monitoring for QT interval prolongation on an electrocardiogram is necessary. Methadone is also used in the treatment of neonatal abstinence syndrome. However, the long elimination half-life makes tapering difficult, and an alternate drug should be considered.

Proponents say that methadone blocks the euphoria produced by heroin, acts longer, and reduces preoccupation with drug use. This effect allows a more normal lifestyle for the patient and reduces morbidity and mortality associated with the use of illegal and injected drugs. Opponents say that methadone maintenance only substitutes one type of drug dependence for another. In addition, a substantial percentage of those people receiving methadone maintenance therapy abuse other drugs, including cocaine.

A second option uses naltrexone, a pure opioid antagonist that blocks opioids from occupying receptor sites, thereby preventing their physiologic effects. (As discussed previously, this drug is also used to combat alcohol abuse.) Used to maintain opioid-free states in the opioid addict, it is recommended for use in conjunction with psychological counseling to promote patient motivation and adherence. If the patient taking naltrexone has mild or moderate pain, he or she should receive a nonopioid analgesic (e.g., acetaminophen or a nonsteroidal anti-inflammatory drug). If the patient has severe pain and requires an opioid, administration of the naltrexone should occur in a setting staffed and equipped for cardiopulmonary resuscitation because respiratory depression may be deeper and more prolonged than usual. The FDA has issued a **BLACK BOX WARNING ◆** about naltrexone and the risk of hepatocellular injury. It is necessary to obtain periodic liver function tests during therapy and discontinue the drug at signs of increasing hepatic impairment.

A third option is buprenorphine (Buprenex, Belbuca, Butrans, Sublocade), an opioid agonist–antagonist analgesic that is occasionally injected therapeutically to relieve moderate to severe pain. The drug is given sublingually to treat opioid dependence. It is essential that the pill be dissolved under the tongue and not swallowed. Serious and potentially deadly adverse effects may occur if a patient combines this drug with other CNS depressant medications. Suboxone, a buprenorphine–naloxone combination, is preferred therapy over buprenorphine alone for induction treatment and for maintenance therapy for short-acting opioid dependence. Naloxone has poor transmucosal bioavailability, but if the combination product is injected, naloxone will compete with buprenorphine at the receptor and reduce any euphoric effects of the injection. However, naloxone's action of shutting off opioid receptors and signals in the body can trigger withdrawal symptoms in people who are currently taking an opioid. Naloxone administration places individuals with chronic addiction to an opioid agonist (such as heroin) at risk for developing seizures and respiratory failure, which can be fatal.

Physicians who prescribe buprenorphine for outpatient use must meet several restrictions and are required to have special training. The FDA has issued a **BLACK BOX WARNING ◆** for buprenorphine because use of buccal and transdermal routes increases the risk of addiction, abuse, and misuse and the risk of life-threatening respiratory depression. In addition, there is a risk of fatal overdose with accidental exposure by children of buprenorphine administered by buccal film or a transdermal patch. In addition, prolonged use of the buccal or transdermal routes of buprenorphine during pregnancy has been known to cause neonatal opioid withdrawal syndrome.

>  **QSEN Alert: Safety**
>
> Opioids should not be abruptly discontinued in a patient who is physically dependent. Patients taking opioid pain medications long term should be instructed not to stop taking their medicine suddenly; they should first develop a plan with their health care prescriber for how to slowly decrease the dose of the opioid while continuing to manage their pain.

## CENTRAL NERVOUS SYSTEM STIMULANT ABUSE: DRUG THERAPY

CNS stimulants are identified by the behavioral stimulation and psychomotor agitation that they produce. The amount of CNS stimulation caused by a certain drug depends on both the area in the brain or spinal cord that is affected by the drug and the cellular mechanism fundamental to the increased excitability. CNS stimulants include amphetamines and related drugs, caffeine (discussed in Chap. 57), cocaine, and nicotine. Box 58.6 discusses these substances in more detail. For the most part, few proven pharmacologic treatments are effective in the treatment of CNS stimulant use, because most of the cravings patients experience are psychological in nature.

### NCLEX Success

6. A construction worker sees the company's occupational health nurse. He inquires about smoking cessation medications. Which of the following drug products can be used to aid smoking cessation?
   A. naltrexone
   B. disulfiram
   C. bupropion
   D. dronabinol

7. The nurse who is caring for a patient admitted with an acute overdose of cocaine. What physiologic response should the nurse expect?
   A. severe lung damage
   B. anaphylaxis
   C. myocardial infarction
   D. hypotension

8. A teenager is taking a central nervous system (CNS) stimulant. Which of the following is a common effect of CNS stimulant medications?
   A. hypotension
   B. anorexia
   C. sedation
   D. hypouricemia

9. What is the most common cause of death from opioids?
   A. hypertension
   B. central nervous system stimulation
   C. respiratory depression
   D. myocardial infarction

10. A nurse working in the emergency department is caring for a patient who has been brought in with suspected opioid overdose. What is the appropriate treatment to administer?
   A. disulfiram
   B. naloxone
   C. amitriptyline
   D. chlordiazepoxide

## PSYCHOACTIVE SUBSTANCE USE: DRUG THERAPY

Other psychoactive substances include marijuana, hallucinogens, "club" and "date-rape" drugs, and inhalants. Box 58.7 contains information about these substances. Few proven pharmacologic treatments are effective in the treatment of psychoactive substance abuse and dependence.

| BOX 58.6 | *Central Nervous System Stimulants of Abuse* |

### Amphetamines

Amphetamines and related drugs [see Chap. 57] are used therapeutically for narcolepsy and attention deficit hyperactivity disorder (ADHD). However, amphetamines are more important as drugs of abuse than therapeutic agents. These drugs may be part of a pattern of polydrug use in which CNS depressants such as alcohol or sedative-type drugs ("downers") are alternated with CNS stimulants, such as amphetamines ("uppers").

Amphetamines and related drugs produce stimulation and euphoria. Small amounts produce mental alertness, wakefulness, and increased energy for a few hours. Tolerance develops rapidly. Methamphetamine is a commonly abused drug that is often manufactured in illegal "meth labs." Inhalation or IV injection produces a pleasurable sensation that lasts only a few minutes. Methylphenidate (Ritalin, others), a prescription drug used to treat ADHD, is increasingly being used for nonmedical purposes. The pattern of abuse is similar to that of other CNS stimulants, with episodes of binge use followed by severe depression and continued use despite serious adverse consequences.

Symptomatic treatment includes sedation, lowering of body temperature, and administration of an antipsychotic drug. Sedative-type drugs must be used with great caution,

*(Continued on page 1160)*

| BOX 58.6 | *Central Nervous System Stimulants of Abuse* (Continued) |
| --- | --- |

however, because depression and sleep usually follow amphetamine use, and these aftereffects can be aggravated by sedative administration.

### Cocaine

Cocaine is a popular drug of abuse. It produces strong CNS stimulation by preventing reuptake of catecholamine neurotransmitters (e.g., dopamine, norepinephrine), which increases and prolongs neurotransmitter effects. The two main drug forms are cocaine hydrochloride powder and "crack." In addition to intense euphoria, acute use of cocaine produces increased energy and alertness, sexual arousal, tachycardia, increased blood pressure, and restlessness. High doses can cause cardiac dysrhythmias, convulsions, myocardial infarction, respiratory failure, stroke, and death. Cocaine is not thought to produce physical dependence. However, it may lead to psychological dependence.

Drug therapy of cocaine dependence is largely symptomatic. Thus, agitation and hyperactivity may be treated with a benzodiazepine antianxiety agent, psychosis may be treated with haloperidol (Haldol) or another antipsychotic agent, cardiac dysrhythmias may be treated with usual antidysrhythmic drugs, myocardial infarction may be treated by standard methods, and so forth. Initial detoxification and long-term treatment are best accomplished in centers or units that specialize in substance use disorders. A **BLACK BOX WARNING** ◆ warns about the increased mortality in older adults with dementia-related psychosis who take haloperidol.

### Nicotine

Nicotine, one of many active ingredients in tobacco products, is the ingredient that promotes compulsive use, abuse, and dependence. Inhaling smoke from a cigarette produces CNS stimulation in a few seconds. Nicotine produces its effects by increasing levels of dopamine and other substances in the brain.

Nicotine dependence is characterized by compulsive use and the development of tolerance and physical dependence, including mental depression. Cigarette smokers may smoke to obtain the perceived pleasure of nicotine's effects, avoid the discomfort of nicotine withdrawal, or both. Evidence indicates a compulsion to smoke when blood levels of nicotine become low. Abstinence from smoking leads to signs and symptoms of withdrawal (e.g., anxiety, irritability, difficulty concentrating, restlessness, headache, increased appetite, weight gain, sleep disturbances).

Most tobacco users who quit do so on their own. For those who are strongly dependent and unable or unwilling to quit on their own, there are two main methods of treatment. One method is NRT with drug formulations of nicotine. The other method involves smoking cessation drugs for nicotine dependence.

Nicotine is available in a transdermal patch, chewing gum, an oral inhaler, lozenges, and a nasal spray. Nicotine products are intended to be used for limited periods of 3 to 6 months, with tapering of dosage and discontinuation. They are effective in helping smokers achieve abstinence, but many users resume smoking with long-term quit rates ranging from 19% to 36.5%.

Drugs include the antidepressant bupropion (see Chap. 55); the smoking cessation formulation is Zyban, a sustained-release tablet. Varenicline (Chantix) blocks some nicotine receptors and thereby decreases the ability of nicotine to stimulate dopamine activity in the brain (the "reward" system). It also stimulates some other nicotine receptors and thereby decreases symptoms of nicotine withdrawal (the "punishment" system). Both medications are generally well tolerated. The most common adverse effects are insomnia with bupropion and nausea with varenicline.

| BOX 58.7 | *Other Psychoactive Medications of Abuse* |
| --- | --- |

### Marijuana

Marijuana and other cannabis preparations are obtained from *Cannabis sativa*, the hemp plant, which grows in most parts of the world, including the entire United States. Marijuana and hashish are the two cannabis preparations used in the United States. Delta-9-tetrahydrocannabinol (THC) is the main psychoactive ingredient.

Use of marijuana results in a dose-dependent impairment of memory, thought, concentration, time and depth perception, and coordinated movement. THC may cause serious cardiovascular (e.g., hypertension, bradycardia, vasoconstriction; hypotension may occur with high doses) as well as respiratory effects (e.g., chronic bronchitis with cough and wheezing, respiratory infections, possibly increased risk of lung cancer).

The legal status of cannabis for medical and recreational use varies nationally. Marijuana is a Schedule I substance under federal narcotic laws. However, nearly two thirds of U.S. states allow medical marijuana to be used by registered, qualified patients who would likely benefit from it so long as they have a prescription. Marijuana does have demonstrated modest antiemetic activity. However, concern about its abuse

potential and its rather unfavorable side effect profile, especially in older adults, has limited its clinical utility.

The cannabinoid dronabinol (Marinol, Syndros) is approved in patients who have failed to respond adequately to conventional antiemetic treatments, and national clinical practice guidelines propose that this agent be considered as a rescue antiemetic for refractory nausea and vomiting. The drug may cause a withdrawal syndrome when abruptly discontinued. Withdrawal symptoms (e.g., insomnia, irritability, restlessness) are most likely to occur with high doses or prolonged use, and sleep disturbances may persist for several weeks. These adverse effects make dronabinol a Schedule III drug.

### Hallucinogens

Hallucinogenic drugs include a variety of substances that cause mood changes, anxiety, distorted sensory perceptions, hallucinations, delusions, depersonalization, pupil dilation, elevated body temperature, and elevated blood pressure.

Dextromethorphan is a cough suppressant found in many over-the-counter multisymptom cold and cough remedies. It is a CNS depressant but is usually classified as a hallucinogen because of dissociative effects similar to those of phencyclidine

**BOX 58.7**    *Other Psychoactive Medications of Abuse* (Continued)

and ketamine (see below) when it is taken in the high doses characteristic of abuse. Adverse effects include blurred vision, brain damage, confusion, dizziness, drowsiness, excessive sweating, hallucinations, impaired breathing, impaired judgment and mental functioning, loss of consciousness, loss of physical coordination, muscle twitches, nausea and vomiting, paranoia, rapid and irregular heartbeat, seizures, slurred speech, and death.

Lysergic acid diethylamide (LSD) is a synthetic, potent derivative of a naturally occurring compound. The exact mechanism of action is unknown, and effects cannot be predicted accurately. LSD alters sensory perceptions and thought processes; impairs most intellectual functions; distorts perception of time and space; and produces sympathomimetic reactions, including increased blood pressure, heart rate, and body temperature, as well as pupil dilation. Adverse reactions include self-injury and possibly suicide, violent behavior, psychotic episodes, "flashbacks," and possible chromosomal damage.

Mescaline is an alkaloid of the peyote cactus. It is the least active of the commonly used psychotomimetic agents but produces effects similar to those of LSD.

The dissociative anesthetic phencyclidine (PCP) produces excitement, delirium, hallucinations, and other profound psychological and physiologic effects; altered sensory perceptions; impaired thought processes; impaired motor skills; psychotic reactions; sedation and analgesia; nystagmus and diplopia; and pressor effects that can cause hypertensive crisis, cerebral hemorrhage, convulsions, coma, and death. Tolerance develops, but there is no apparent physical dependence or abstinence syndrome. Psychological dependence probably occurs but is usually not intense.

### "Club" and "Date-Rape" Drugs

"Ecstasy" or "Molly" (3,4-methylenedioxymethamphetamine; MDMA) is an illegal, Schedule I derivative of amphetamine. Structurally similar to methamphetamine and mescaline, it produces stimulant and hallucinogenic effects. Developed as an appetite suppressant, MDMA first became popular with adolescents and young adults as a commonly abused drug at "raves," but its use has spread to a variety of settings and age groups. Users report increased energy and perception, euphoria, and feelings of closeness to others. MDMA is extremely dangerous, and usage is gaining popularity particularly in adolescents and young adults who may erroneously believe that MDMA produces a safe "high." Adverse effects include acute psychiatric symptoms (e.g., anxiety, panic, depression, paranoid thinking), cardiac dysrhythmias, coma, dehydration, delirium, hypertension, hyperthermia, hyponatremia, rhabdomyolysis, seizures, tachycardia, and death. These effects have occurred with a single use. MDMA is not thought to cause dependence or withdrawal syndromes.

Flunitrazepam (Rohypnol) is an intermediate-acting benzodiazepine with general properties similar to those of diazepam (Valium). However, its effects are estimated to be 7 to 10 times more powerful than diazepam. It is a Schedule IV drug that produces dependence; the drug is not approved for medical use or manufactured in the United States, where it is not available legally. However, it is available legally internationally as Rohypnol. In addition to intentional use, it has reportedly been added to punch and other drinks at fraternity parties and other social events, leading to its designation as a "date-rape" drug. The drug has also been associated with

human trafficking. Federal penalties for trafficking Rohypnol are the same as those for Schedule I, II, and III substances, depending on quantity. In relatively low doses, flunitrazepam can cause muscle relaxation, general sedative and hypnotic effects, and the appearance of intoxication. It also leads to confusion, dizziness, drowsiness, hypotension, memory impairment, and visual disturbances. Combining the drug with alcohol increases its adverse effects.

Gamma-hydroxybutyrate (GHB) is classed as Schedule I controlled drug when used for illicit purposes and is available for medical use as the Schedule III drug sodium oxybate (Xyrem). A CNS depressant, this drug is structurally related to the inhibitory neurotransmitter gamma-aminobutyric acid. Illicit use of GHB has increased in recent years, mainly in the party or dance club setting, and is increasingly involved in poisonings, overdoses, date rapes, visits to hospital emergency departments, and fatalities. GHB is also sometimes used by body builders for alleged anabolic effects. The FDA has issued a **BLACK BOX WARNING** ◆ for sodium oxybate because the drug alone or in combination with other CNS depressants produces adverse reactions, including respiratory depression, seizures, unconsciousness, hypoxia, and death. With chronic use, GHB reportedly induces tolerance and produces dependence. Because of these risks, sodium oxybate is available only through a restricted distributed program.

Ketamine (Ketalar, Spravato) is a general anesthetic that is chemically related to PCP and used during induction or maintenance of general anesthesia. The drug is a Schedule III controlled substance. It has become a "recreational" drug, with effects similar to those of PCP and LSD (e.g., distorted senses and perceptions, dissociative reactions). These effects are associated with a high risk of injuries.

### Inhalants

These drugs include volatile solvents such as acetone, toluene, and gasoline, substances that produce chemical vapors that can be inhaled to induce mind-altering effects. These solvents may be constituents of some types of glues, plastic cements, aerosol sprays, butane lighters, spray paints, degreasers or cleaning fluids, paint thinners and removers, felt-tip marker fluids, and other products. Some general inhalation anesthetics, such as nitrous oxide, have also been abused to the point of dependence. Volatile solvents frequently the first drugs abused by preadolescents and adolescents because the inhalants are readily accessible and inexpensive. For example, this age group squeezes glue into a plastic bag and sniffs the fumes. Suffocation sometimes occurs when the sniffer loses consciousness while the bag covers the face.

Inhalants produce symptoms comparable with those of acute alcohol intoxication, including initial mild euphoria followed by ataxia, confusion, and disorientation. Some substances in gasoline and toluene also may produce symptoms similar to those produced by the hallucinogens, including euphoria, hallucinations, recklessness, and loss of self-control. These substances can harm the brain, liver, heart, kidneys, and lungs, and abuse of any drug during adolescence may interfere with brain development. Inhalants can also produce psychological dependence and physiologic withdrawal. Experts believe that education about prevention and treatment is responsible for a significant decrease in inhalant abuse.

**THE NURSING PROCESS**

A concept map outlines the nursing process related to drug therapy considerations in this chapter. Additional nursing implications related to the disease process should also be considered in care decisions.

**Assessment**
- Interview the patient regarding alcohol and other drug use to help determine immediate and long-term nursing care needs.
- Assess behavior that may indicate drug abuse, such as alcohol on the breath, altered speech patterns, staggering gait, and other signs of excessive CNS depression or stimulation.
- Assess for disorders that may be caused by substance abuse. These disorders may include infections, liver disease, accidental injuries, and psychiatric problems of anxiety or depression.
- Assess liver function, complete blood count (hypocalcemia, hypomagnesemia, and acidosis are common in alcoholics), and alcohol and drug levels in the blood.

**Outcomes of Therapy**
The patient will
- Maintain safety if impaired by alcohol and drug abuse.
- Remain current on information regarding drug effects and treatment resources.
- Maintain efforts toward stopping drug usage be recognized and reinforced.

**Nursing Interventions**
- Decrease environmental stimuli for the person undergoing drug withdrawal.
- Record vital signs; cardiovascular, respiratory, and neurologic functions; mental status; and behavior at regular intervals.
- Support use of resources for stopping drug abuse (psychotherapy, treatment programs).
- Request patient referrals to psychiatric/mental health physicians, nurse clinical specialists, or self-help programs when indicated.
- Use therapeutic communication skills to discuss alcohol or other drug-related health problems, health-related benefits of stopping substance use or abuse, and available services or treatment options.
- Teach nondrug techniques for coping with stress and anxiety.
- Provide positive reinforcement for efforts toward quitting substance abuse.
- Inform smokers with young children in the home that cigarette smoke can precipitate or aggravate asthma and upper respiratory disorders in children.
- Inform smokers with nonsmoking spouses or other members of the household that secondhand smoke can increase the risks of cancer and lung disease in the nonsmokers as well as in the smoker.
- For smokers who are concerned about weight gain if they quit smoking, emphasize that the health benefits of quitting far outweigh the disadvantages of gaining a few pounds and discuss ways to control weight without smoking.

**Evaluation**
- Observe for improved behavior (e.g., less impulsiveness, improved judgment and thought processes, commits no injury to self or others).
- Observe for use or avoidance of nonprescribed drugs while hospitalized.
- Interview to determine the patient's insight into personal problems stemming from drug abuse.
- Verify enrollment in a treatment program.
- Observe for appropriate use of drugs to decrease abuse of other drugs.

## KEY CONCEPTS

- Substance use disorder is a maladaptive pattern of substance use, leading to clinically significant impairment or distress.
- Commonly abused drugs include CNS depressants (e.g., alcohol, antianxiety and sedative–hypnotic agents, opioid analgesics), CNS stimulants (e.g., cocaine, methamphetamine, methylphenidate, nicotine), and other mind-altering drugs (e.g., marijuana, "ecstasy").
- CNS depressants are drugs that slow down or "depress" brain activity. These types of drugs are capable of inducing varying degrees of CNS depression, ranging from tranquilizing relief of anxiety to anesthesia, coma, and even death. They include alcohol, antianxiety and sedative–hypnotic agents, and opiates.
- Benzodiazepines are the drugs of choice for treating alcohol withdrawal and withdrawal from other CNS depressant drugs. Chlordiazepoxide is the prototype.
- The FDA has issued a **BLACK BOX WARNING ◆** for the combined use of benzodiazepines and opioid analgesics. Serious adverse reactions, including slowed or difficult breathing and death, have been reported.
- Methadone acts as an agonist at specific opioid receptors in the CNS to produce analgesia, euphoria, and sedation. This drug has long been used as a detoxification and/or as maintenance therapy for opioid addiction, usually given in a single, daily oral dose at an outpatient methadone clinic.
- **BLACK BOX WARNING ◆** states that methadone used for treatment of opioid addiction should be part of an approved program. Deaths have been reported during the initiation of treatment. The nurse ensures that emergency services are on standby. Another **BLACK BOX WARNING ◆** states that it is necessary to monitor the patient taking methadone for QT interval prolongation, especially with higher doses.
- **BLACK BOX WARNING ◆** states that it is necessary to obtain periodic liver function tests during naltrexone therapy and discontinue therapy at signs of increasing hepatic impairment.
- The FDA has issued a **BLACK BOX WARNING ◆** for buprenorphine because use of buccal and transdermal routes increases the risk of addiction, abuse, and misuse and the risk of life-threatening respiratory depression. In addition, the risk of fatal overdose with accidental exposure by children of buprenorphine administered by buccal film or a transdermal patch and the risk of neonatal withdrawal syndrome with prolonged use of buccal or transdermal buprenorphine during pregnancy pose significant concern.
- Drug therapy for maintenance of sobriety is limited, mainly because of poor adherence. The drugs approved for this purpose include disulfiram (Antabuse), naltrexone (Vivitrol), and acamprosate (Campral).
- A **BLACK BOX WARNING ◆** states that it is essential never to administer the disulfiram to a patient who has consumed alcohol in the past 12 hours.
- A **BLACK BOX WARNING ◆** alerts practitioners about the risk of seizures associated with the use of flumazenil.
- A **BLACK BOX WARNING ◆** cautions about the increased mortality in older adults with dementia-related psychosis who take haloperidol.
- A **BLACK BOX WARNING ◆** for sodium oxybate alone or in combination with other CNS depressants produces adverse reactions, including respiratory depression, seizures, unconsciousness, hypoxia, and death.
- Treatment for nicotine dependence involves nicotine products and certain drugs.

## CLINICAL REASONING CASE STUDY

**Meet the Patient**

Thomas Giordano, a 66-year-old man with arteriosclerotic cardiovascular disease, has recently undergone a four-vessel coronary artery bypass graft. Part of his cardiac rehabilitation program includes exercise training, nutrition counseling, and smoking cessation. He has smoked two packs of cigarettes a day for 30 years. He is motivated to try to stop smoking, but he has failed every time he has tried to quit because of his intense craving for tobacco. Mr. Giordano asks the nurse to explain some possible treatment options to help with smoking cessation. After determining his options, Mr. Giordano and the prescriber decide to use varenicline (Chantix), nicotine patches, and counseling.

**Assessing Drug Information**

Nicotine transdermal patch
- Action: The nicotine patch supplements the nicotine previously inhaled with smoking and binds to nicotine receptors, thereby maintaining and then reducing nicotine levels with tapering.
- Use: This patch aids smoking cessation by providing nicotine to a smoker without using tobacco, thereby managing nicotine withdrawal symptoms as the smoker breaks the behavior of cigarette smoking.
- Adverse effects: These include nausea, vomiting, abdominal pain, diarrhea, headache, and local irritation at the site of patch application.

Varenicline (Chantix)
- Action: This drug blocks nicotine receptors in the brain, thereby decreasing the ability of nicotine to stimulate dopamine activity in the brain resulting in decreased craving and withdrawal symptoms.
- Use: This drugs aids smoking cessation.
- Adverse effects: These include shortness of breath, feelings of confusion, hallucinations, behavioral changes, nausea and vomiting, sleepwalking, and seizures.

**Nursing Actions**

- Instruct Mr. Giordano about options for smoking cessation.
  - There are two main methods of treatment:
    - Nicotine replacement therapy includes transdermal patches, chewing gum, oral inhalers, lozenges, and nasal spray. Many of these products are available without a prescription. It is necessary to apply the patch once daily and use the other treatments intermittently. People should use nicotine products for a limited period (average, 3–6 months), with tapering dosage and eventual discontinuation.
    - Other pharmacological treatments, such as bupropion (Zyban), an antidepressant, and varenicline (Chantix), block some dopamine receptors, thereby decreasing the ability of nicotine to stimulate dopamine activity in the brain.
      - Patients who take Zyban must quit smoking within the first 2 weeks of treatment.
      - It is necessary to begin Chantix treatment 1 week before stopping smoking. This treatment option usually lasts 12 weeks, and dosing increases will likely occur throughout the treatment period.
  - Counseling added to either of these options increases the effectiveness of the drug therapy.

With Chantix:
- Instruct Mr. Giordano that because there is an increased risk of cardiovascular events, he needs to seek medical attention and report the following conditions:
  - Signs of a heart attack, such as chest pain that may spread to the arms, neck, jaw, back, or stomach; sweating that is not normal; or feeling sick or throwing up
  - Signs of a stroke, such as a change in strength on one side is greater than the other; eyesight, speech, or balance problems; change in thinking clearly; or very bad headache.
- Tell Mr. Giordano that he should notify his prescriber if he experiences agitation, depression, suicidal behavior, or suicidal ideation.
- Make sure that he understands that he should take the medication after eating with a full glass of water.
- Varenicline may enhance the toxic effects of alcohol. Therefore, instruct him to speak to his prescriber before drinking alcohol.
- Tell him to avoid driving and performing other tasks or actions that require alertness until he understands how this drug affects him.
- Instruct him not take this drug for longer than instructed without discussing it with his prescriber.

With nicotine patches:
- Instruct Mr. Giordano that the nicotine patch helps decrease nicotine in the body over time, without the presence of carcinogens found in cigarettes and breaks the behavior of smoking.
- Tell him that to control cravings and withdrawal symptoms, he may use a short-acting form (e.g., gum or lozenge) repeatedly throughout the day.
- Make sure that he understands that if he has insomnia or vivid dreams, he can minimize them by removing the patch at bedtime. If the patch is removed, it may take 30 minutes to 3 hours for nicotine levels to be reached after a new patch is applied. It is possible to manage morning cravings with a short-acting form of nicotine while waiting for the patch to take effect.
- Suggest that given his two-pack per day history, the higher dosage of the drug may be appropriate at the beginning. With some nicotine patches, this would be step 1 (21 mg/24 hours).

*Visit* thePoint® *at* **http://thePoint.lww.com/Frandsen12e** *for answers to NCLEX Success questions (in Appendix A), answers to Clinical Application Case Studies (in Appendix B), and more!*

## REFERENCES AND RESOURCES

American Psychiatric Association. (2013). *Diagnostic and statistical manual of mental disorders* (5th ed.). Washington, DC: Author.

Apollonio, D., Phillips, R., & Bero, L. (2016). Interventions for tobacco use cessation in people in treatment for or recovery from substance use disorders. *Cochrane Database of Systematic Reviews, 11,* CD010274. doi:10.1002/14651858.CD010274.pub2

Bukstein, O. (2020). Approach to treating substance use disorder in adolescents. In *UpToDate,* Lexi-Comp, Inc.

Castells, X., Cunill, R., Perez-Mana, C., & Capella, D. (2016). Psychostimulants drugs for cocaine dependence. *Cochrane Database of Systematic Reviews,* (9), CD007380. doi:10.1002/14651858.CD007380.pub4

Cullen, K. A., Liu, S. T., Bernat, J. K., Slavit, W. I., Tynan, M. A., King, B. A., et al. (2019). Flavored tobacco product use among middle and high school students—United States, 2014-2018. *MMWR Morbidity and Mortality Weekly Report, 68*(39), 839.

Dogosh, K. L., Cacciola, J. S., & Jarvis, M. E. (2019). Clinical assessment of substance use disorders. In *UpToDate,* Lexi-Comp, Inc.

Goerlick, D. A. (2017). Cannabis use and disorder: Clinical manifestations, course, assessment, and diagnosis. In *UpToDate,* Lexi-Comp, Inc.

Hinkle, J. H., & Cheever, K. H. (2018). *Brunner & Suddarth's textbook of medical-surgical nursing* (14th ed.). Philadelphia, PA: Wolters Kluwer.

Hsiao, R. C., & Riggs, P. D. (2016). The changing landscape of adolescent substance treatment. *Child Adolescent Psychiatric Clinics of North America, 25*(4), xv–xvi. doi:10.1016/j.chc.2016.07.002

Karch, A. M. (2019). *Focus on nursing pharmacology* (8th ed.). Philadelphia, PA: Wolters Kluwer.

Lippincott Williams & Wilkins. (2019). *Nursing 2020 drug handbook* (40th ed.). Philadelphia, PA: Wolters Kluwer.

Maisel, N. C., Blodgett, J. C., Wilbourne, P. L., Humphreys, K., & Finney, J. W. (2012). Meta-analysis of naltrexone and acamprosate for treating alcohol use disorders: When are these medications most helpful? *Addiction, 108*(2), 275–293. doi:10.1111/j.1360-0443.2012.04054.x

McCarty, D. A. (2019). Changing landscape for treatment of alcohol and drug use disorders. *American Journal of Public Health, 109*(6), 838–839. doi:10.2105/AJPH.2019.305080

Norris, T. L. (2019). *Pathophysiology: Concepts of altered health status* (10th ed.). Philadelphia, PA: Wolters Kluwer.

Reus, V. I., Fochtmann, L. J., Bukstein, O., Eyler, A. E., Hilty, D. M., Horvitz-Lennon, M., et al. (2018). The American Psychiatric Association practice guideline for the pharmacological treatment of patients with alcohol use disorder. *American Journal of Psychiatry, 175*(1), 86–90. doi:10.1176/appi.ajp.2017.1750101.

Rigotti, N. A. (2020). Pharmacotherapy for smoking cessation in adults. In *UpToDate,* Lexi-Comp, Inc.

Roberts, W., Shi, J. M., Tetrault, J. M., & McKee, S. A. (2018). Effects of varenicline alone and in combination with low-dose naltrexone on alcohol-primed smoking in heavy-drinking tobacco users: A preliminary laboratory study. *Journal of Addiction Medicine, 12*(3), 227–233. doi:10.1097/ADM.0000000000000392

Saitz, R. (2020). Approach to treating alcohol use disorder. In *UpToDate,* Lexi-Comp, Inc.

UpToDate. (2020). *Drug information.* Lexi-Comp, Inc.

Wang, T. W., Gentzke, A. S., Creamer, M. R., Cullen, K. A., Holder-Hayes, E., Sawdey, M. D., et al. (2019). Tobacco product use and associated factors among middle and high school students-United States, 2019. *MMWR Surveillance Summary, 68*(12), 1–22. doi:10.15585/mmwr.ss6812a1

# Drugs Affecting the Eye, Ear, and Skin

# Drug Therapy for Disorders of the Eye

## LEARNING OBJECTIVES

*After studying this chapter, you should be able to:*

1. Describe the basic structures and functions of the eye.
2. Describe the pathophysiology of glaucoma and other ocular disorders.
3. Identify the prototypes and describe the action, use, adverse effects, contraindications, and nursing implications for medications administered for diagnosis and treatment of ocular disorders.
4. Identify the prototypes and describe the action, use, adverse effects, contraindications, and nursing implications for medications administered for glaucoma.
5. Identify the prototypes and describe the action, use, adverse effects, contraindications, and nursing implications for medications administered for ocular infections and inflammation.
6. Implement the nursing process in the care of the patient with an ocular disorder.

## CLINICAL APPLICATION CASE STUDY

Irene Molnar is a 75-year-old woman who has open-angle glaucoma. Her physician has prescribed the following: acetazolamide [Diamox], 250 mg orally, every 6 hours; timolol [Timoptic], one drop in each eye, twice daily; and pilocarpine [Isopto Carpine], one drop of 2% solution in each eye, three times daily. You are a home care nurse visiting Mrs. Molnar.

## KEY TERMS

**Blepharitis:** chronic infection of glands and lash follicles on the margins of the eyelids

**Conjunctiva:** mucous membrane lining the eyelids

**Conjunctivitis:** inflammation of the conjunctiva

**Glaucoma:** group of diseases characterized by optic nerve damage and changes in visual fields, which is characterized by increased intraocular pressure (IOP) (greater than 22 mm Hg), although it may also occur with normal IOP (less than 21 mm Hg); one of the leading causes of blindness in the United States

**Intraocular pressure (IOP):** pressure inside the eye; normally less than 21 mm Hg (average 15–16 mm Hg)

**Keratitis:** inflammation of the cornea

**Lacrimation:** production of tears

**Miosis:** pupil constriction

**Mydriasis:** pupil dilation

**Nasolacrimal occlusion:** application of pressure to the tear duct

**Refraction:** deflection of light rays in various directions according to the density of the ocular structures through which they pass

• **Tonometry:** diagnostic test to measure the pressure inside the eye to determine if glaucoma is present

## INTRODUCTION

This chapter introduces the eye and its disorders. It addresses the drug therapy implemented to enhance visualization of the eye for eye examination and the drug therapy for ocular disorders, including glaucoma, ocular infection, and ocular inflammation.

## BASIC STRUCTURE AND FUNCTION OF THE EYE

The eye is the major sensory organ through which a person receives information about the external environment. Extensive discussion of vision and ocular anatomy is beyond the scope of this chapter, but some characteristics and functions are described to facilitate understanding of ocular drug therapy.

The eyelids and lacrimal system function to protect the eye. The eyelid is a barrier to the entry of foreign bodies, strong light, dust, and other potential irritants. The **conjunctiva** is the mucous membrane lining the eyelids. The canthi (singular, canthus) are the angles where the upper and lower eyelids meet. The lacrimal system produces a fluid that constantly moistens and cleanses the anterior surface of the eyeball. The fluid drains through two small openings in the inner canthus and flows through the nasolacrimal duct into the nasal cavity. When the conjunctiva is irritated or certain emotions are experienced (e.g., sadness), the lacrimal gland produces more fluid than the drainage system can accommodate. The excess fluid overflows the eyelids and becomes tears. Production of tears is known as **lacrimation**.

The eyeball is a spherical structure composed of the sclera, cornea, choroid, and retina, plus special refractive tissues. The sclera is a white, opaque, fibrous tissue that covers the posterior five sixths of the eyeball. The cornea is a transparent, special connective tissue that covers the anterior sixth of the eyeball. It contains no blood vessels. The choroid, composed of blood vessels and connective tissue, continues forward to form the iris. The iris is composed of pigmented cells, the opening called the pupil, and muscles that control the size of the pupil by contracting or dilating in response to stimuli. Pupil constriction is called **miosis**, and pupil dilation is called **mydriasis**. The retina is the innermost layer of the eyeball.

For vision to occur, light rays must enter the eye through the cornea; travel through the pupil, lens, and vitreous body (discussed below); and be focused on the retina. Light rays do not travel directly to the retina. Instead, they are deflected in various directions according to the density of the ocular structures through which they pass. This process, called **refraction**, is controlled by the aqueous humor, lens, and vitreous body. The optic disk is the area of the retina where ophthalmic blood vessels and the optic nerve enter the eyeball.

The structure and function of the eyeball are further influenced by the lens, aqueous humor, and vitreous body. The lens is an elastic, transparent structure; its function is to focus light rays to form images on the retina. It is located behind the iris and is held in place by ligaments attached to the ciliary body.

The aqueous humor is a clear fluid produced by capillaries in the ciliary body. Most of the fluid flows through the pupil into the anterior chamber (between the cornea and the lens and anterior to the iris). A small amount flows into a passage called Schlemm's canal, from which it enters the venous circulation.

Nearly 60% to 80% of the aqueous humor is drained through the trabecular meshwork outflow pathways, as seen in Figure 59.1. In the healthy eye, the pressure inside the eye, **intraocular pressure (IOP)**, is maintained through a balance between the amount of aqueous humor produced in the ciliary body epithelium and the amount drained from the anterior chamber. Impaired drainage of aqueous humor causes increased IOP. The vitreous body is a transparent, jellylike mass located in the posterior portion of the eyeball. It functions to refract light rays and maintain the normal shape of the eyeball.

## OVERVIEW OF DISORDERS OF THE EYE

The eye is subject to many disorders that threaten its structure, function, or both. Some disorders in which ophthalmic drugs play a prominent role are discussed in this section.

### Specific Disorders of the Eye

#### Refractive Errors

Refractive errors include myopia (nearsightedness), hyperopia (farsightedness), presbyopia, and astigmatism. These conditions impair vision by interfering with the eye's ability to focus light rays on the retina. Ophthalmic drugs are used only in the diagnosis of the conditions; treatment involves prescription of eyeglasses or contact lenses.

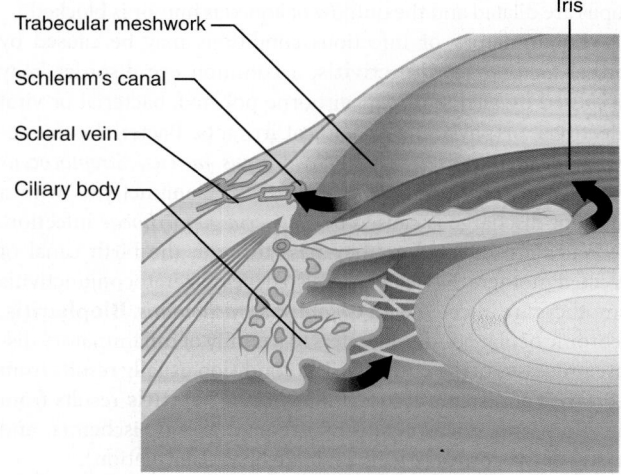

**FIGURE 59.1.** Ocular anatomy concerned with control of intraocular pressure. [Reprinted with permission from Barash, P. G., Cullen, B. F., Stoelting, R. K., et al. [2017]. *Clinical anesthesia* [8th ed.]. Philadelphia, PA: Wolters Kluwer.]

### Glaucoma

**Glaucoma** is one of the leading causes of blindness in the United States and the most common cause of blindness in African Americans. It is a group of diseases characterized by optic nerve damage and changes in visual fields. It is often characterized by increased IOP (above 22 mm Hg) but may also occur with normal IOP (below 21 mm Hg; average 15–16 mm Hg). Diagnostic tests for glaucoma include ophthalmoscopic examination of the optic disk; measurement of IOP, or **tonometry**; and testing of visual fields.

### Ocular Infections and Inflammation

Ocular infections may result from foreign bodies, contaminated hands, contaminated eye medications, or infections in contiguous structures (e.g., nose, face, sinuses). Causes of ocular inflammation include bacteria, viruses, allergic reactions, and irritating chemicals. These conditions include the following:

- Conjunctivitis, which is inflammation of the conjunctiva
- Blepharitis, which is a chronic infection of glands and lash follicles on the margins of the eyelids
- Keratitis, which is inflammation of the cornea
- Corneal ulcers
- Fungal infections

## Etiology

Refractive errors of the eye result in impaired vision. Light rays cannot focus sharply on the retina if the eyeball is lengthened or shortened. When the distance to the eyeball is shortened, the visual image is focused at the front of the retina, resulting in myopia. If the focus is beyond the retina, the result is hyperopia. The most common cause of refractive errors is astigmatism or an irregular curve of the cornea.

The cause of open-angle glaucoma is unknown, but contributing factors include advanced age, ethnic background, family history of glaucoma and elevated IOP, diabetes mellitus, hypertension, myopia, long-term use of corticosteroid drugs, and previous eye injury, inflammation, or infection. Elevated IOP is the most important risk factor and the most likely cause. The incidence of glaucoma in African Americans is about three times higher than in non–African Americans. Closed-angle glaucoma may occur when pupils are dilated and the outflow of aqueous humor is blocked.

Inflammatory or infectious conditions may be caused by several factors. **Conjunctivitis**, a common eye disorder, may be caused by allergens (e.g., airborne pollens), bacterial or viral infections, or physical or chemical irritants. Bacterial conjunctivitis is often caused by *Staphylococcus aureus*, *Streptococcus pneumoniae*, or *Haemophilus influenzae*. Conjunctivitis with a purulent discharge is caused by *Neisseria gonorrhoeae* infection. Neonates are infected as they pass through the birth canal of infected mothers. Neonates can also develop keratoconjunctivitis if mothers are infected with *Chlamydia trachomatis*. **Blepharitis**, a chronic ocular condition, refers to a family of inflammatory disease processes of the eyelid(s). The condition usually results from seborrhea and staphylococcal infections. **Keratitis** results from infection with microorganisms, trauma, allergy, ischemia, and drying of the cornea (e.g., from inadequate lacrimation).

Corneal ulcers may be bacterial, fungal, or viral. Bacterial ulcers most often occur because of infections with pneumococci and staphylococci. Pseudomonal ulcers are less common. Fungal ulcers may follow topical corticosteroid therapy or injury with plant matter, such as a tree branch. Viral ulcers are usually caused by the herpesvirus. Other fungal infections may often be attributed to frequent use of ophthalmic antibiotics and corticosteroids.

## Pathophysiology

As previously stated, refractive errors impair vision by interfering with the eye's ability to focus light rays on the retina. When the dimension of the eyeball is too short, near images are blurred. Conversely, if the eyeball dimension is too long, distant objects will be blurred.

Glaucoma is characterized by increased IOP, possibly damaging the optic nerve, which transmits images to the brain. If damage to the optic nerve from high IOP continues, glaucoma leads to loss of vision. The most common type of glaucoma is open-angle glaucoma, which is characterized by increased IOP. In this type of glaucoma, there is no obstruction at the iridocorneal angle. This form of open-angle glaucoma most commonly occurs due to an abnormality of the trabecular meshwork that controls the flow of aqueous humor into the canal of Schlemm. The tissues of the trabecular outflow pathway are avascular and rely on the aqueous humor to supply nutrients, growth factors, and antioxidants. If left untreated, elevated IOP will lead to loss of retinal ganglion cells resulting in irreversible vision loss. A secondary form of open-angle glaucoma occurs with the formation of red cell fragments after trauma or iris pigment epithelial granules clogging the trabecular mesh. Closed-angle glaucoma is usually an acute situation requiring emergency surgery. It may occur when pupils are dilated and the outflow of aqueous humor is blocked.

Inflammatory or infectious conditions may lead to conjunctivitis, blepharitis, keratitis, bacterial corneal ulcers, or fungal infections of the eye. Conjunctivitis typically is a self-limited process. However, depending on the immune status of the patient and the etiology, conjunctivitis can progress to more severe and sight-threatening infections. Blepharitis involves bacterial colonization of the eyelids, which results in direct microbial invasion of tissues, immune system–mediated damage, or damage caused by the production of bacterial toxins, waste products, and enzymes. Keratitis may not initially affect vision. However, if the condition is not treated effectively, corneal ulceration, scarring, and impaired vision may result. In nonulcerative keratitis, the layers of the epithelium are affected but remain intact. Ulcerative keratitis affects the epithelium, stroma, or both. Chronic ulcerative keratitis will result in deformities of the eyelid, paralysis of the lid muscles, or severe exophthalmos.

## Clinical Manifestations

Refractive errors are manifested by loss of near or far vision. Glaucoma is characterized by blurred vision, halos around lights, difficulty focusing, difficulty adjusting to low lighting, loss of peripheral vision, headache, and aching around the eye. Conjunctivitis involves redness, tearing, itching, edema, and burning or gritty sensations. Blepharitis is an inflammation of the anterior or posterior structures of the eyelids. Anterior blepharitis presents with burning, redness, and itching of the anterior eyelids. Posterior blepharitis is eyelid inflammation with inflammation of the meibomian glands. An infected sebaceous gland is noted as a hordeolum or stye-producing pain, redness, and swelling of the site. Keratitis is characterized by irritation, increased tear production, and photophobia. Corneal ulcers and fungal infections also produce eye pain, discharge, changes in vision, swelling, and redness.

## Clinical Application 59.1

- Mrs. Molnar has been diagnosed with open-angle glaucoma. What is the pathophysiology of this disease?
- If untreated, what is the outcome of this disease?

## NCLEX Success

1. A nursing student is reviewing a 72-year-old man's chart. In the diagnostic section of the chart, the student notices that the man's intraocular pressure is 23 mm Hg. What should the student suspect regarding this pressure?

   A. glaucoma
   B. blepharitis
   C. diminished vision
   D. macular degeneration

2. When applying mascara, a woman may have scratched her cornea. She states she does not have time to go to the ophthalmologist. What ocular disorder could this result in?

   A. corneal redness
   B. corneal ulceration
   C. blepharitis
   D. conjunctivitis

## Drug Therapy

Drug therapy of ophthalmic conditions is unique because of the location, structure, and function of the eye. Many systemic drugs are unable to cross the blood–eye barrier and achieve therapeutic concentrations in ocular structures. In general, penetration is greater if the drug achieves a high concentration in the blood, is fat soluble, and is poorly bound to serum proteins and if inflammation is present.

Because of the difficulties associated with systemic therapy, various methods of administering drugs locally have been developed. The most common and preferred method is topical application of ophthalmic solutions or suspensions (eyedrops) to the conjunctiva. Drugs are distributed through the tear film covering the eye and may be used for superficial disorders (e.g., conjunctivitis) or for relatively deep ocular disorders (e.g., glaucoma). Topical ophthalmic ointments may also be used. In addition, ophthalmologists may inject medications (e.g., antibiotics, corticosteroids, local anesthetics) into or around various eye structures. A major use of topical ophthalmic drugs in children is to dilate the pupil and paralyze accommodation for ophthalmoscopic examination. As a general rule, practitioners prefer the short-acting mydriatics and cycloplegics (e.g., cyclopentolate, tropicamide) because they cause fewer systemic adverse effects than atropine and scopolamine. In addition, children usually receive lower drug concentrations (given empirically) because of their smaller size and the potential risk of systemic adverse effects.

## DRUG THERAPY FOR THE DIAGNOSIS AND TREATMENT OF OCULAR DISORDERS

Drugs used to diagnose or treat ophthalmic disorders represent numerous therapeutic classifications, most of which are discussed in other chapters. This chapter describes the major classes of drugs used in ophthalmology. Later, the chapter discusses drugs used in the treatment of glaucoma. Table 59.1 summarizes the medications used to diagnose and treat some ocular disorders. Ocular medications are administered topically with limited systemic effects.

## ANTICHOLINERGIC DRUGS

Anticholinergic drugs dilate the pupil to provide greater observation of the inner aspect of the eye. The prototype of this class is **atropine sulfate** (Isopto Atropine: ophthalmic).

## Pharmacokinetics and Action

The onset of action of atropine (ophthalmic) is 5 to 10 minutes, with a peak of action in 30 to 40 minutes and a duration of action of 7 to 14 days. Metabolism occurs in the liver, and excretion takes place in the urine.

Atropine (ophthalmic) blocks the effects of acetylcholine in the central nervous system (CNS). It produces mydriatic effects by relaxing the pupil of the eye and prevents accommodation of near vision.

## Use

Diagnostic use of atropine (ophthalmic) involves production of mydriasis and cycloplegia–pupillary dilation in acute and inflammatory conditions of the iris and uveal tract. Other uses include measurement of refractive errors and treatment of uveitis. Table 59.2 presents route and dosage information for atropine and related drugs in adults and children.

| TABLE 59.1 | | |
| --- | --- | --- |
| **Drugs Administered for Diagnosis and Treatment of Ocular Disorders** | | |
| **Drug Class** | **Prototype** | **Other Drugs in the Class** |
| Anticholinergic drugs | Atropine sulfate (Isopto Atropine) | Cyclopentolate (Cyclogyl) Homatropine (Homatropaire) Scopolamine Tropicamide (Mydriacyl) |
| Adrenergic agonists | Phenylephrine hydrochloride (Altafrin) | |
| Local anesthetic drugs | Lidocaine (Akten) | Proparacaine (Alcaine) Tetracaine (Altacaine, Tetcaine, TetraVisc) |

**TABLE 59.2**

## DRUGS AT A GLANCE: Drugs for the Diagnosis and Treatment of Ocular Disorders

| Drug | Pregnancy Category | Routes and Dosage Ranges | |
|---|---|---|---|
| | | **Adults** | **Children** |
| **Anticholinergic Drugs** | | | |
| ℗ **Atropine sulfate** (ophthalmic) (Isopto Atropine; ❋ Isopto Atropine, Minims Atropine Sulfate, Odan-Atropine) | C | Prior to evaluation: 1–2 drops of 1.0% solution 1 h before procedure | ≥3 mo: 1 drop of 1.0% solution 40 min before procedure<br>≥3 y: 1–2 drops of 1.0% solution 40 min before procedure |
| Cyclopentolate (Cyclogyl; ❋ Cyclogyl, Minims Cyclopentolate HC, Odan-Cyclopentolate) | C | 1–2 drops of 0.5%, 1%, or 2% solution; may repeat in 5–10 min; instill 2% in heavily pigmented iris | Infants: 1 drop of 0.5% solution as a single-dose cyclopentolate and phenylephrine combination formulation is the preferred agent for use in infants<br>Children and adolescents: 1–2 drops of 0.5%, 1%, or 2% solution; may repeat with 0.5% or 1% solution in 5–10 min |
| Homatropine | C | 1–2 drops of 2% or 5% solution; may repeat in 5–10 min if necessary before refraction<br>Uveitis: 1–2 drops of 2% or 5% solution every 3–4 h | ≥3 mo: same as for adults |
| Scopolamine | C | Procedure: 1–2 drops of 0.25% 1 h before refraction<br>Iridocyclitis: 1–2 drops up to 4 times daily | Procedure: 1 drop of 0.25% to eye twice daily for 2 d before |
| Tropicamide (Mydriacyl; ❋ Mydriacyl, Odan-Tropicamide) | C | Cycloplegia: 1–2 drops of 1% solution 20–30 min before refraction<br>Mydriasis: 1–2 drops of 0.5% solution 15–20 min before | Cycloplegia, mydriasis, same as adult dosage |
| **Adrenergic Agonists** | | | |
| ℗ **Phenylephrine** (Altafrin; ❋ Minims Phenylephrine HCl) | C | Mydriasis, 1 drop of 2.5% or 10% solution every 3–5 min as needed (max 3 drops per eye) | Mydriasis: Infants 1 drop of 2.5% solution every 3–5 min as needed (max 3 drops per eye)<br>Children and adolescents: same as adult dosage |
| **Local Anesthetic Drugs** | | | |
| ℗ **Lidocaine** (Akten) | B | Anesthesia, 2 drops to ocular surface in the area of procedure; may repeat to maintain effect | Refer to adult dosage |
| Proparacaine (Alcaine) | C | Ophthalmic surgery: 1 drop of 0.5% solution in the eye every 5–10 min for 5–7 doses<br>Tonometry, gonioscopy, suture removal: 1 drop of 0.5% solution in eye prior to procedure | Same as adult dosage |
| Tetracaine (Altacaine, Tetcaine, TetraVisc) | C | Short-term anesthesia: 1–2 drops in the affected eye before examination<br>Minor surgical procedure: 1–2 drops every 5–10 min for up to 3 doses<br>Prolonged surgical procedure: 1–2 drops every 5–10 min for up to 5 doses | Safety and efficacy not established |

## Adverse Effects and Contraindications

Atropine (ophthalmic) may cause local transient stinging. The systemic effects of this medication depend on the amount of medication absorbed and rarely lead to an inhibition of vagal stimulation affecting the heart or diminished bronchial or gastric secretions.

Contraindications to atropine (ophthalmic) include the presence of glaucoma or the tendency to this condition.

## Nursing Implications

### Administering the Medication

For uveitis, it is necessary to instill one to two drops of atropine (ophthalmic) in the eye 1 hour prior to examination or three times per day to decrease inflammation of the iris and uveal tract. The nurse uses **nasolacrimal occlusion** to prevent the systemic absorption of the ophthalmic medication. In this process, he or she applies finger pressure over the lacrimal sac for 1 to 2 minutes after instillation to decrease the risk of absorption and systemic effects. Box 59.1 presents general nursing guidelines for the topical administration of eye medications.

### Assessing for Therapeutic and Adverse Effects

One hour following administration, the ophthalmologist uses an ophthalmic scope to assess the ability to visualize the inner aspect of the eye. In the treatment of uveitis, the nurse assesses for diminished blurred vision and diminished photophobia.

It is necessary to assess for pain and stinging. In addition, the nurse assesses for blurred vision and sensitivity to light. These effects should diminish and are reversible over time.

### Patient Teaching

The nurse instructs patients about the effects of the medication such as photophobia and stinging on administration. It is essential to tell patients not to drive if their vision is impaired. The nurse should tell them to wear sunglasses. Box 59.2 presents additional patient teaching guidelines for ophthalmic medications, including atropine.

### Other Drugs in the Class

Cyclopentolate (Cyclogyl) is useful when given prior to ophthalmic examinations that involve diagnostic testing. It increases the papillary size so the fundus of the eye can be thoroughly examined. Five minutes before the examination, the ophthalmologist or nurse administers the drug (2% solution) to patients who have a heavily pigmented iris. To avoid excessive systemic absorption, it is necessary to use nasolacrimal occlusion during and for 1 to 2 minutes following administration. Patients who have uveitis should receive cyclopentolate in combination with atropine (ophthalmic). Caution is important in the elderly due to increased IOP. Psychotic reactions and behavioral disturbances have occurred in children. It is important to withhold infant feeding for 4 hours after ophthalmic examination due to feeding intolerance.

3. A nurse is administering cyclopentolate to a patient with uveitis. What is the most important nursing intervention when administering the medication?

   A. Touch the inner canthus of the eye with the medication applicator.
   B. Evaluate the redness and inflammation prior to administering the medication.
   C. Ask the patient to blink to enhance absorption of the medication.
   D. Apply pressure to the lacrimal sac for 2 minutes after medication administration.

4. An elderly patient is receiving cyclopentolate for visualization of the eye. What is the patient at risk for developing?

   A. cataracts
   B. retinal detachment
   C. increased intraocular pressure
   D. cerebral edema

---

**BOX 59.1**  *General Nursing Guidelines for the Administration of Topical Ophthalmic Medications*

- Topical application is the most common route of administration for ophthalmic drugs, and correct administration is essential for optimal therapeutic effects.
- Systemic absorption of eyedrops can be decreased by closing the eye and applying pressure over the tear duct (nasolacrimal occlusion) for 3 to 5 minutes after instillation.
- When multiple eyedrops are required, there should be an interval of 5 to 10 minutes between drops because of limited eye capacity and rapid drainage into tear ducts.
- Absorption of eye medications is increased in eye disorders associated with hyperemia and inflammation.
- Many ophthalmic drugs are available as eyedrops (solutions or suspensions) and ointments. Ointments are administered less frequently than drops and often produce higher concentrations of drug in target tissues. However, they also cause blurred vision, which limits their daytime use, at least for ambulatory patients. For some patients,

  drops may be used during waking hours and ointments at bedtime.
- Topical ophthalmic medications should not be used after the expiration date; cloudy, discolored solutions should be discarded.
- Topical eye medications contain a number of inactive ingredients, such as preservatives, buffers, tonicity drugs, antioxidants, and so on. Some contain sulfites, to which some people may have an allergic reaction.
- Some eyedrops contain benzalkonium hydrochloride, a preservative, which is absorbed by soft contact lenses. The medications should not be applied while wearing soft contacts and should be instilled 15 minutes or longer before inserting soft contacts.
- To increase safety and accuracy of ophthalmic drug therapy, the labels and caps of eye medications are color coded.

## BOX 59.2 · *Patient Teaching Guidelines for Topical Eye Medications*

**General Considerations**

- Prevent eye disorders, when possible. For example, try to avoid long periods of reading and computer work; minimize exposure to dust, smog, cigarette smoke, and other eye irritants; and wash hands often and avoid touching the eyes to decrease risk of infection. Use protective eyewear when indicated.

- Do not use nonprescription eyedrops (e.g., Murine, Visine) on a regular basis for longer than 48 to 72 hours. Report persistent eye irritation and redness to a health care provider.

- Have regular eye examinations and testing for glaucoma after 40 years of age.

- Eyedrop preparations often contain sulfites, which can cause allergic reactions in some people.

- If you have glaucoma, do not take any drugs without your ophthalmologist's knowledge and consent. Many drugs given for purposes other than eye disorders may cause or aggravate glaucoma. Also, wear a medical alert bracelet or carry identification that states you have glaucoma. This helps avoid administration of drugs that aggravate glaucoma or to maintain treatment of glaucoma, in emergencies.

- If you have an eye infection, wash your hands before and after contact with the infected eye to avoid spreading the infection to the unaffected eye or to other people. Also, avoid touching the unaffected eye.

- If you wear contact lenses, wash your hands before inserting them and follow instructions for care (e.g., cleaning, inserting, or removing, and duration of wear). Improper or infrequent cleaning may lead to infection. Overwearing is a common cause of corneal abrasions and should be avoided to prevent the development of ulcers.

- If you wear soft contact lenses, do not use any eye medication without consulting a specialist in eye care. Some eyedrops contain benzalkonium hydrochloride, a preservative, which is absorbed by soft contacts. The medication should not be applied while wearing soft contacts and should be instilled 15 minutes or longer before inserting soft contacts.

- Never use eye medications used by someone else and never allow your eye medications to be used by anyone else. These preparations should be used by one person only, and they are dispensed in small amounts for this purpose. Single-person use minimizes cross-contamination and risks of infection.

- Many eyedrops and ointments cause temporary blurring of vision. Do not use such medications just before driving or operating potentially hazardous machinery.

- Avoid straining at stool (use laxatives or stool softeners if necessary), heavy lifting, bending over, coughing, and vomiting when possible. These activities increase IOP, which may cause eye damage in glaucoma and after eye surgery.

**Self-Administration**

- If using more than one eye medication, be sure to administer the correct one at the correct time. Benefits depend on accurate administration.

- Check expiration dates; do not use any eye medication after the expiration date and do not use any liquid medication that has changed colors or contains particles.

- Shake the container if instructed on the label to do so. Suspensions should be shaken well to ensure the drug is evenly dispersed in the liquid and not settled in the bottom of the container.

- Wash hands thoroughly.

- Tilt the head back or lie down and look up.

- Pull the lower lid down to expose the conjunctiva (mucous membrane).

- Place the dropper directly over the eye. Avoid contact of the dropper with the eye, finger, or any other surface. Such contact contaminates the solution and may cause eye infections and serious damage to the eye, with possible loss of vision.

- Look up just before applying a drop; look down for several seconds after applying the drop.

- Release the eyelid, close the eyes, and press the inside corner of the eye with a finger for 3 to 5 minutes. Closing the eyes and blocking the tear duct helps the medication be more effective by slowing its drainage out of the eye.

- Do not blink for 30 seconds after the administration of eye medications and during the eye examination.

- Do not rub the eye; do not rinse the dropper.

- If more than one eyedrop is ordered, wait 10 minutes before instilling the second medication.

- Use the same basic procedure to insert eye ointments.

## ADRENERGIC AGONIST

Ⓟ **Phenylephrine** (Altafrin), the prototype ophthalmic adrenergic agonist, is used for its mydriatic effects. Unlike anticholinergic drugs, it does not produce cycloplegic effects.

### Pharmacokinetics and Action

The mydriatic effects of phenylephrine (ophthalmic) occur 15 to 30 minutes after administration. Peak plasma effects occur in less than 20 minutes, and the duration of action is 1 to 3 hours. Systemic absorption is minimal.

Phenylephrine (ophthalmic) causes contraction of the dilator muscles of the pupil. It produces mydriasis, vasoconstriction, and increased outflow of aqueous humor.

## Use

Uses of phenylephrine (ophthalmic) include mydriasis prior to ophthalmic procedures and therapy of wide-angle glaucoma. It can also provide relief of redness with eye irritation. Table 59.2 presents route and dosage information for phenylephrine.

## Adverse Effects and Contraindications

With phenylephrine (ophthalmic), systemic adverse effects are rare, but dysrhythmia, hypertension, myocardial infarction, syncope, and subarachnoid bleeding may occur. Ocular effects are reversible and include burning, irritation, visual changes, floaters, and rebound miosis.

Contraindications include hypersensitivity reactions, hypertension, ventricular tachycardia, and narrow-angle glaucoma.

## Nursing Implications

### Preventing Interactions

Phenylephrine combined with atomoxetine enhances the effects of hypertension and tachycardia. Taking phenylephrine with monoamine oxidase (MAO) inhibitors and sympathomimetic drugs also contributes to the effects of hypertension.

### Administering the Medication

Box 59.1 lists general nursing guidelines for the administration of ophthalmic medications. Patients should take phenylephrine for no longer than 72 hours. To administer the ophthalmic solution, the nurse has the patient lie down with the head tilted back. Then he or she takes the following steps:

- Holds the dropper above the eye and drops the medication inside the lower lid, without touching the dropper to the eye
- Has the patient keep the eye open and avoid blinking for 30 seconds
- Applies pressure to the inside corner of the eye for 1 minute

### Assessing for Therapeutic and Adverse Effects

The nurse assesses whether the inner aspect of the eye can be visualized 15 minutes after administration.

The nurse measures the blood pressure and the heart rate and checks for hypertension for dysrhythmia. He or she also asks the patient about visual floaters. In addition, it is necessary to assess for burning and irritation of the eye.

### Patient Teaching

Box 59.2 presents patient teaching guidelines for topical ophthalmics, including phenylephrine.

### NCLEX Success

5. A patient is receiving phenylephrine eyedrops for wide-angle glaucoma. What assessment should be made following administration?
   A. peripheral edema
   B. lung sounds
   C. visual changes
   D. blood pressure

6. The nurse instructs a patient on the procedure to occlude the tear ducts for 5 minutes after administering eyedrops. What is the purpose of this patient teaching?
   A. It prevents eye infections.
   B. It prevents systemic absorption of the medication.
   C. It makes self-administration easier.
   D. It allows for the administration of a smaller dose.

## LOCAL ANESTHETIC DRUGS

Ⓟ **Lidocaine** (Akten) is the prototype local anesthetic drug for ophthalmic use.

## Pharmacokinetics and Action

The onset of action of lidocaine is 20 seconds to 5 minutes, with a median onset of 40 seconds. The duration of action is 5 to 30 minutes, with a median of 15 minutes.

Lidocaine blocks the initiation and conduction of nerve impulses. It decreases the neuronal membrane's permeability to sodium ions, resulting in an inhibition of depolarization and blocking of conduction.

## Use

Lidocaine produces local anesthesia of the ocular surface during ophthalmic procedures such as surgery, tonometry, and gonioscopy. Table 59.2 presents route and dosage information for lidocaine and other ophthalmic local anesthetics.

## Adverse Effects

Local adverse effects of lidocaine include burning. Specific ocular effects include conjunctival hyperemia, corneal epithelial changes, diplopia, and changes in vision.

## Nursing Implications

### Administering the Medication

It is important not to administer solution if it is crystallized. The nurse is certain not to touch the eye with the tip of the applicator.

### Assessing for Therapeutic and Adverse Effects

The physician performing the procedure assesses for adequate anesthesia. The nurse may assess for opacity of the lens and loss of vision with prolonged use.

## DRUG THERAPY FOR THE TREATMENT OF GLAUCOMA

At present, the goal of drug therapy for chronic open-angle glaucoma is to slow disease progression by reducing IOP. For monotherapy, the prostaglandin analogs and beta-adrenergic blockers are first-line drugs. The prostaglandin analogs may be preferred because they are generally more effective at lowering IOP, show a better tolerated adverse effect profile than nonselective drugs, and offer a once-daily dosing regimen. Older drug classes, including the beta-adrenergic blockers, alpha agonists, and carbonic anhydrase inhibitors, lower IOP by decreasing the production of aqueous humor. These drugs are commonly used either alone or in combination for the treatment of chronic open-angle glaucoma and are outlined in Table 59.3.

## PROSTAGLANDIN ANALOGS

The prostaglandin analogs are the most widely prescribed glaucoma drugs, and lower IOP by increasing the aqueous drainage by a mechanism of action different from other drugs, namely, by increasing the uveoscleral outflow; aqueous inflow is not affected. Of the prostaglandin analogs, Ⓟ **bimatoprost** (Latisse, Lumigan) is the prototype. Bimatoprost is classified as a prostamide, whereas latanoprost, travoprost, and tafluprost are prostanoids.

### TABLE 59.3

## Drugs Administered for the Treatment of Open-Angle Glaucoma

| Drug Class | Prototype | Other Drugs in the Class |
|---|---|---|
| Prostaglandin analogs | Bimatoprost (Latisse, Lumigan) | Latanoprost (Xalatan)<br>Tafluprost (Zioptan)<br>Travoprost (Travatan Z) |
| Beta-adrenergic blocking drugs | Timolol maleate (Betamol, Istalol, Timoptic, Timoptic Ocudose, Timoptic-XE) | Betaxolol (Betoptic S)<br>Carteolol<br>Levobunolol<br>Metipranolol |
| Alpha$_2$-adrenergic agonists | Brimonidine (Alphagan P, Lumify) | Apraclonidine hydrochloride (Iopidine) |
| Cholinergic drugs | Pilocarpine (Isopto Carpine)<br>Pilocarpine Ocular System (Ocusert Pilo-20 or Pilo-40) | |
| Carbonic anhydrase inhibitors | Acetazolamide | Brinzolamide (Azopt)<br>Dorzolamide (Trusopt) |
| Alpha$_2$-adrenergic agonists and carbonic anhydrase inhibitors | | Brinzolamide and Brimonidine (Simbrinza) |
| Osmotic drugs | Mannitol (Osmitrol, Resectisol) | |

## Pharmacokinetics

The onset of action of bimatoprost is approximately 4 hours, with maximum reduction of IOP in 8 to 12 hours. It is 88% protein bound and undergoes oxidation, *N*-deethylation, and glucuronidation after reaching systemic circulation to form metabolites. Excretion is primarily in the urine, with 25% excreted in the feces.

## Action

Bimatoprost produces ocular hypotensive effects to decrease IOP and to increase outflow of aqueous humor. (Latisse formulation can also increase the percent and duration of hairs in the growth phase to increase eyelash growth.)

## Use

In patients with open-angle glaucoma and ocular hypertension, health care providers use bimatoprost to reduce IOP. Treatment of hypotrichosis of the eyelashes is another use. Table 59.4 contains route and dosage information for bimatoprost and other prostaglandin analogs.

## Adverse Effects and Contraindications

Ocular adverse effects of bimatoprost include iris and eyelid hyperpigmentation and eyelash changes. Use of the Latisse formulation may result in erythema of the eyelid, allergic conjunctivitis, blepharitis, burning, cataract formation, conjunctival edema, pain, photophobia, tearing, and visual disturbances. Contraindications include hypersensitivity.

## Nursing Implications

### Administering the Medication

When applying Latisse to the eyelid, patients who are wearing contacts should remove them; in addition, it is necessary to remove makeup and wash the face thoroughly with soap and water. Patients should apply the medication with a sterile applicator and use a new applicator for each eye. It is important that contacts not be reinserted for 15 minutes.

### Assessing for Therapeutic and Adverse Effects

It is important to assess IOP. In patients taking the medication for hypertrichosis of the eyelashes, the nurse assesses for increased growth of eyelashes.

The nurse assesses for ocular changes, including pruritus, blepharitis, and visual disturbances.

### Patient Teaching

The nurse instructs the patient about the importance of keeping regularly scheduled medical appointments to check IOP. Box 59.2 contains additional patient teaching information.

## Other Drugs in the Class

Other prostaglandin analogs include latanoprost (Xalatan), travoprost (Travatan Z), and tafluprost (Zioptan). Like bimatoprost, they act to lower IOP. Tafluprost is the only topical prostaglandin analog that does not contain the widely used preservative, benzalkonium chloride.

### ! QSEN Alert: Evidence-Based Practice

El Hajj Moussa, Farhat, Nehme, Sahyoun, Schakal, Jalkh, Abi Karam, and Azar (2018) compared the efficacy of bimatoprost, latanoprost, travoprost, and tafluprost. The study examined 32 patients with primary open-angle glaucoma. All patients received a complete ophthalmologic examination initially and at 1, 3, and 6 months. The researchers found that all four drugs equally and significantly reduced intraocular pressure. There was a greater reduction in intraocular pressure with bimatoprost.

**TABLE 59.4**

## DRUGS AT A GLANCE: Antiglaucoma Drugs

| Drug | Pregnancy Category | Routes and Dosage Ranges | |
|---|---|---|---|
| | | **Adults** | **Children** |
| **Prostaglandin Analogs** | | | |
| ⓟ **Bimatoprost** (Latisse, Lumigan; 🍁 Latisse, Lumigan, Vistitan) | C | Glaucoma: 1 drop at bedtime<br>Hypotrichosis of eyelashes: 1 drop on applicator applied evenly along the skin of the upper eyelid at the base of the eyelashes at bedtime | ≥16 y: IOP reduction (Lumigan), refer to adult dosage. Not recommended under age of 16 due to hyperpigmentation<br>≥5 y, hypotrichosis of eyelashes (Latisse). Same as adult dosage |
| Latanoprost (Xalatan; 🍁 APO Latanoprost, GD Latanoprost, JAMP Latanoprost, MED-Latanoprost, Xalatan) | C | Elevated IOP: 1 drop at bedtime | Safety and efficacy not established |
| Tafluprost (Zioptan) | C | Elevated IOP: 1 drop at bedtime | Safety and efficacy not established |
| Travoprost (Travatan Z; 🍁 APO-Travoprost, Sandoz-Travoprost, Travatan Z) | C* | Elevated IOP: 1 drop at bedtime | ≥16 y: elevated IOP: refer to adult dosage. |
| **Beta-Adrenergic Blocking Drugs** | | | |
| ⓟ **Timolol maleate** (Betamol, Istalol, Timoptic, Timoptic Ocudose, Timoptic-XE; 🍁 APO-Timop, SANDOZ-Timolol, Timoptic, Timoptic-XE) | C | Solution, 1 drop of 0.25% solution twice daily; mat increase to 1 drop of 0.5% solution twice daily if response inadequate<br>Gel, 1 drop of 0.25% or 0.5% solution once daily | Same as for adults |
| Betaxolol (Betoptic S; 🍁 Betoptic S) | C | Solution and suspension, 1 or 2 drops twice daily | Suspension, 1 drop twice daily |
| Carteolol | C | 1 drop twice daily | Safety and efficacy not established |
| Levobunolol (🍁 APO-Levobunolol, Betagen) | C | 1 or 2 drops of 0.25% solution twice daily; 1 or 2 drops of 0.5% solution once daily (doses >1 drop of 0.5% solution twice daily are generally not more effective) | Safety and efficacy not established |
| Metipranolol | C | Glaucoma, 1 drop twice daily | Safety and efficacy not established |
| **Alpha₂-Adrenergic Agonists** | | | |
| ⓟ **Brimonidine** (Alphagan P, Lumify; 🍁 Alphagan P, Brimonidine P) | B | 1 drop 3 times daily, every 8 h | ≥2 y: same as for adults |
| Apraclonidine hydrochloride (Iopidine; 🍁 Iopidine) | C | Open-angle glaucoma: 1 drop 0.5% solution every 12 h<br>Intraoperative and postoperative increased IOP: 1–2 drops of 1% solution 1 h before surgery and immediately after surgery | Safety and efficacy not established |
| **Cholinergic Drugs** | | | |
| ⓟ **Pilocarpine** (Isopto Carpine; 🍁 Isopto Carpine, Odan-Pilocarpine) | C | Elevated IOP: 1 drop of 1% or 2% solution up to 4 times daily<br>Glaucoma: 1 drop of 1% or 2% solution up to 3 times over a 30-min period<br>Miosis: 1 drop (or 2 drops 5 min apart) | <2 y: 1 drop of 1% solution up to 3 times daily<br>≥2 y: same as for adults |

*(Continued on page 1178)*

**TABLE 59.4**

**DRUGS AT A GLANCE: Antiglaucoma Drugs** (Continued)

| Drug | Pregnancy Category | Routes and Dosage Ranges | |
|---|---|---|---|
| | | **Adults** | **Children** |
| Pilocarpine Ocular System (Ocusert Pilo-20 or Pilo-40) | C | Miosis: one system in conjunctival sac per week | Same as for adults |
| **Carbonic Anhydrase Inhibitors** | | | |
| Ⓟ **Acetazolamide** | C | Glaucoma: 250 mg PO 1–4 times daily; preoperatively: 5–10 mg/kg/d IV, IM in divided doses, every 6 h | <12 y, glaucoma: 10–30 mg/kg/d PO divided every 6–8 h (max 1000 mg/d); preoperatively: 5–10 mg/kg IV every 6 h |
| Brinzolamide (Azopt; ❋ Azopt) | C | IOP reduction: 1 drop 3 times daily | Safety and efficacy not established |
| Dorzolamide (Trusopt; ❋ APO-Dorzolamide, JAMP-Dorzolamide, RIVA-Dorzolamide, Trusopt, SANDOZ-Dorzolamide) | C | IOP reduction: 1 drop 3 times daily | Same as adults |
| **Alpha₂-Adrenergic Agonists and Carbonic Anhydrase Inhibitors** | | | |
| Brinzolamide and brimonidine (Simbrinza; ❋ Simbrinza) | C | IOP: 1 drop each eye 2–3 times per day | 1 drop each eye 2–3 times per day |
| **Osmotic Drugs** | | | |
| Ⓟ **Mannitol** (Osmitrol, Resectisol; ❋ Osmitrol, Resectisol) | B | IOP reduction: 1.5–2 g/kg as a 20% solution over 45 min twice daily for IOP > 35 mm Hg | Infants, children, adolescents: 1–2 mg IV over 20–30 min |

*Contact with contents of vial should be avoided by women who are pregnant or are trying to become pregnant. In case of accidental exposure to skin, wash the exposed area thoroughly with soap and water.

IOP, intraocular pressure.

## BETA-ADRENERGIC BLOCKING DRUGS

The purpose of the administration of beta-adrenergic blocking drugs is to decrease the IOP. Although the prototype medication in this class is propranolol (see Chap. 26), it is not formulated in an ophthalmic preparation. The drug Ⓟ **timolol maleate** (Betamol, Istalol) was the first drug developed in this class for the treatment of open-angle glaucoma.

## Pharmacokinetics and Action

The onset of action of timolol is 30 minutes, with a peak action in 1 to 2 hours. The duration of action for intraocular effects is 24 hours.

Timolol blocks the beta₁- and beta₂-adrenergic receptors to reduce the IOP by reducing aqueous humor production and increasing outflow.

## Use

Uses for timolol include chronic open-angle glaucoma, aphakic glaucoma, secondary glaucoma, and ocular hypertension.

Table 59.4 presents route and dosage information for timolol and other beta-adrenergic blocking drugs.

## Adverse Effects and Contraindications

The most common adverse effects associated with timolol are burning and stinging. Most adverse effects of systemic beta-adrenergic blockers may also occur with ophthalmic preparations, and patients with respiratory or cardiac disease may not be able to take them.

Contraindications include asthma and chronic obstructive pulmonary disease, as well as heart failure, bradycardia, atrioventricular block, left ventricular dysfunction, and cardiogenic shock. Known hypersensitivity to timolol is also a contraindication.

## Nursing Implications

### Preventing Interactions

Many medications and herbs interact with timolol maleate, increasing its effects (Boxes 59.3 and 59.4).

## BOX 59.3    *Drug Interactions: Timolol*

**Drugs That Increase the Effect of Timolol**
- Amifostine, amiodarone, antihypertensives, beta-adrenergic blockers, calcium channel blockers, cardiac glycosides, monoamine oxidase inhibitors, reserpine
  *Increase hypotensive and bradycardic effects*

## Administering the Medication

Administration of the ophthalmic form of timolol necessitates the following:

- Have patients who wear contact lenses remove the lenses prior to administration.
- When administering more than one ophthalmic medication, wait 10 minutes between each medication.
- Use good hand hygiene before administering ophthalmic drugs.
- Always invert the bottle of timolol and shake it before use.
- Have the patient tilt the head back. Use the index finger of one hand to pull the lower lid down to form a pocket for the eyedrop. Place the dispenser tip close to the eye and gently squeeze the bottle to administer one drop.
- Have patients who wear contact lenses wait 15 minutes before inserting them. The product can contain benzalkonium chloride, which can be absorbed into the soft contact lens.

## Assessing for Therapeutic and Adverse Effects

The nurse helps ensure that the patient keeps regularly scheduled appointments with the ophthalmologist to assess the IOP. In addition, the nurse asks the patient about stinging and burning of the eyes.

## Patient Teaching

Box 59.2 contains additional patient teaching information for topical ophthalmic medications, including timolol.

### Clinical Application 59.2

- Mrs. Molnar has received prescriptions for timolol and pilocarpine eyedrops. What patient teaching regarding these medications should the nurse provide?
- What is the action of timolol?

## BOX 59.4    *Herb and Dietary Interactions: Timolol*

**Herbs and Foods That Increase the Effects of Timolol**
- Garlic
- Ginger
- Ginseng
- Goldenseal
- Nettle

## ALPHA₂-ADRENERGIC AGONISTS

Alpha₂-adrenergic agonists are administered when a patient's IOP is not lowered adequately with a beta-adrenergic blocker or when a beta-adrenergic blocker is contraindicated. Ⓟ **Brimonidine** (Alphagan P, Lumify) is the prototype. Practitioners, who consider this group of medications to be as effective as timolol, use it in conjunction with other antiglaucoma drugs such as beta-adrenergic blockers or carbonic anhydrase inhibitors when multiple drugs are required.

## Pharmacokinetics and Action

Brimonidine has a rapid onset of action, with a half-life of 2 hours. Extensive metabolism occurs in the liver. The drug reduces aqueous humor production and increases uveoscleral outflow.

## Use

Brimonidine is used to lower IOP in patients with open-angle glaucoma or ocular hypertension. Table 59.4 presents route and dosage information for brimonidine and the other alpha₂-adrenergic agonists.

### Use in Children

Administration to children can result in a higher risk of adverse effects. Children are at greatest risk for CNS depression from brimonidine, with somnolence and diminished alertness.

## Adverse Effects

Several adverse effects may occur with brimonidine use. Cardiovascular effects include hypertension, bradycardia, hypotension, and tachycardia. CNS effects include headache, dizziness, somnolence, diminished attention and alertness, and insomnia. Respiratory effects are bronchitis, cough, dyspnea, sinusitis, nasal dryness, and apnea. Local reactions such as stinging and burning of the eye may occur. Other ocular effects are blepharitis, conjunctival edema, conjunctival hemorrhage, dryness, irritation, and eye pain. In addition, allergic conjunctivitis, hyperemia, and pruritus affect approximately 10% to 20% of patients.

## Contraindications

Contraindications to brimonidine include known hypersensitivity to the drug or use within 14 days of an MAO inhibitor. Caution is warranted in patients with advanced cardiovascular disease.

## Nursing Implications

### Preventing Interactions

Many medications and herbs interact with brimonidine, increasing or decreasing its effects (Boxes 59.5 and 59.6).

## BOX 59.5    *Drug Interactions: Brimonidine*

**Drugs That Increase the Effects of Brimonidine**
- Hypotensive drugs, monoamine oxidase inhibitors
  *Increase hypotensive effects*
- Hydroxyzine, selective serotonin reuptake inhibitors, central nervous system (CNS) depressants
  *Increase CNS depression*

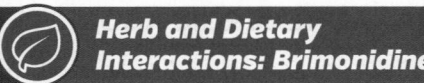

## BOX 59.6 — *Herb and Dietary Interactions: Brimonidine*

**Herbs and Foods That Increase the Effects of Brimonidine**
- Bayberry
- Blue cohosh
- Cayenne
- Ephedra
- Ginger
- Ginseng
- Licorice

**Herbs and Foods That Decrease the Effects of Brimonidine**
- Black cohosh
- California poppy
- Coleus
- Goldenseal
- Hawthorne
- Mistletoe

### Administering the Medication

Box 59.1 lists general guidelines for the administration of topical ophthalmic medications.

### Assessing for Therapeutic and Adverse Effects

It is necessary to assess the IOP.

The nurse monitors the blood pressure and assesses for hypertension and hypotension, and he or she checks the heart rate and monitors for bradycardia or tachycardia. The nurse also assesses the CNS for depressive effects such as dizziness, somnolence, and diminished alertness. In addition, the nurse assesses the respiratory status for cough and dyspnea and checks for nasal dryness, sinus infection, and sinusitis. It is necessary to assess for hypersensitivity reactions as well.

### Patient Teaching

The nurse ensures that the patient keeps regularly scheduled appointments with the ophthalmologist to assess the IOP. Box 59.2 contains additional patient teaching information for the topical ophthalmic medications, including brimonidine.

## CHOLINERGIC DRUGS

Ophthalmic cholinergic drugs increase the outflow of aqueous humor to reduce IOP. The prototype of this class is **P pilocarpine** (Isopto Carpine), which is administered for glaucoma and as a miotic drug.

## Pharmacokinetics and Action

Following administration of pilocarpine, miosis begins in 10 to 30 minutes, with reduction in IOP in 1 hour. The miotic duration of action is 4 to 8 hours. Metabolism occurs in the liver.

Pilocarpine stimulates the cholinergic receptors in the eye, causing miosis, loss of accommodation, and lowering of the IOP.

## Use

Pilocarpine is used for chronic simple glaucoma as well as for chronic and acute angle-closure glaucoma. Table 59.4 gives route and dosage information for pilocarpine.

## Adverse Effects

Several adverse effects may occur with pilocarpine. Ocular conditions include burning, ciliary spasm, conjunctival vascular congestion, lacrimation, lens opacity, retinal detachment, myopia, and diminished visual acuity. CNS problems may include headache. Cardiopulmonary manifestations are hypertension, tachycardia, bronchial spasm, and pulmonary edema. Gastrointestinal (GI) effects include nausea, vomiting, diarrhea, and increased salivation.

## Contraindications

Contraindications include known hypersensitivity to the drug or acute inflammation of the anterior chamber of the eye.

## Nursing Implications

### Preventing Interactions

Acetylcholinesterase inhibitors may enhance the adverse effects of pilocarpine.

### Administering the Medication

If the solution and gel have been prescribed together, it is necessary to administer the solution first and then give the gel 5 minutes later. Following the administration of the solution, the nurse or patient should provide pressure on the lacrimal sac for 1 to 2 minutes. Box 59.1 lists general guidelines for the administration of topical ophthalmic medications.

### Assessing for Therapeutic and Adverse Effects

It is necessary to check the IOP.

### Assessing for Adverse Effects

The nurse assesses for ocular burning, lens opacity, diminished visual acuity, and headache over the affected eye. He or she monitors the patient's blood pressure and heart rate and assesses for signs of hypertension and tachycardia. The nurse also assesses for bronchial spasm and pulmonary edema as well as for nausea, vomiting, diarrhea, and increased salivation.

### Patient Teaching

The nurse helps ensure that the patient keeps regularly scheduled appointments with the ophthalmologist to assess the IOP. Box 59.2 provides patient teaching information for pilocarpine.

## NCLEX Success

7. A patient with Parkinson's disease is taking selegiline hydrochloride. He receives a diagnosis of increased IOP. His ophthalmologist prescribes brimonidine drops. What recommendation does the nurse make to the prescriber?

   A. Stop the selegiline hydrochloride for 2 weeks before starting the brimonidine.
   B. Suggest that because administration of brimonidine increases blood pressure, another alpha₂-adrenergic agonist should be prescribed.
   C. Ask the prescriber whether levobunolol would be more stable and cause fewer adverse effects.
   D. Increase the selegiline hydrochloride to prevent the increase in Parkinson's-related symptoms.

8. A patient with glaucoma is receiving pilocarpine. What patient teaching does the nurse provide to decrease the possible cardiac adverse effects?
   A. Administer the medication at bedtime.
   B. Apply pressure to the lid after application.
   C. Apply pressure to the lacrimal sac after application.
   D. Administer the medication every 3 hours.

# CARBONIC ANHYDRASE INHIBITORS

Ⓟ **Acetazolamide**, the prototype ocular carbonic anhydrase inhibitor, is an oral drug. Prescribers use it for the management of glaucoma.

## Pharmacokinetics and Action

Oral acetazolamide has an onset of action in 1 hour. Absorption occurs in the GI tract. Intravenous (IV) administration has an onset of action of 15 minutes. Distribution takes place throughout the body, concentrating in the red blood cells, plasma, and kidneys. Elimination is in the urine.

Acetazolamide inhibits carbonic anhydrase in the eye to reduce the rate of aqueous humor formation and lower the IOP.

## Use

Uses for acetazolamide include open-angle glaucoma and secondary glaucoma. Practitioners also use it preoperatively for the treatment of acute closed-angle glaucoma. Table 59.4 presents route and dosage information for acetazolamide and other carbonic anhydrase inhibitors.

## Adverse Effects

The major adverse effects associated with acetazolamide are Stevens-Johnson syndrome, flaccid paralysis, agranulocytosis, hemolytic anemia, aplastic anemia, leukopenia, pancytopenia, and metabolic acidosis.

## Contraindications

Contraindications to acetazolamide include known hypersensitivity to carbonic anhydrase inhibitors, renal and hepatic disease, and Addison's disease, as well as electrolyte imbalance. Caution is necessary in older adults. Specialists do not recommend the drug for the treatment of chronic noncongestive angle-closure glaucoma.

## Nursing Implications

### Preventing Interactions

Many medications and herbs interact with acetazolamide, increasing its effects (Boxes 59.7 and 59.8).

### Administering the Medication

To reduce GI upset, it is necessary to administer acetazolamide with food or meals. Patients should not crush or chew sustained-release preparations.

**BOX 59.7    Drug Interactions: Acetazolamide**

**Drugs That Increase the Effect of Acetazolamide**
- Alcohol, central nervous system (CNS) depressants, droperidol, hydroxyzine, selective serotonin reuptake inhibitors
  *Enhance CNS depression*
- Alfuzosin, amifostine, antihypertensives, diazoxide, pentoxifylline, phosphodiesterase five inhibitors (sildenafil), prostacyclin analogs (treprostinil)
  *Enhance antihypertensive effects*
- Salicylates
  *Act by unknown mechanism*

### Assessing Therapeutic and Adverse Effects

It is necessary to assess the IOP.

The nurse assesses the patient's skin for signs of redness, blisters, or swelling that may indicate Stevens-Johnson syndrome. In addition, he or she checks the complete blood count for signs of anemia and the electrolytes for signs of acidosis.

### Patient Teaching

The nurse helps ensure that the patient keeps regularly scheduled appointments with the ophthalmologist to assess the IOP. Box 59.9 presents patient teaching guidelines for acetazolamide.

## Other Drugs in the Class

Brinzolamide (Azopt) reduces IOP in patients with ocular hypertension or open-angle glaucoma. The drug is contraindicated in patients with a known hypersensitivity to brinzolamide, sulfonamides, or any component of the formulation. It reaches peak effect in 2 hours and has an 8- to 12-hour duration of action. It can be absorbed in the systemic circulation and accumulates in the red blood cells. It is excreted unchanged in the urine.

Dorzolamide hydrochloride (Trusopt) is a carbonic anhydrase inhibitor administered for increased IOP or open-angle glaucoma. One drop is inserted into each eye three times per day. It decreases the aqueous humor secretion by slowing

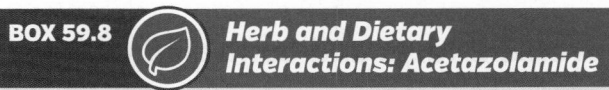

**BOX 59.8    Herb and Dietary Interactions: Acetazolamide**

**Herbs and Foods That Increase the Effects of Acetazolamide**
- Garlic
- Ginger
- Ginseng
- Goldenseal
- Nettle

bicarbonate ions to reduce sodium and fluid transport, thus reducing IOP. Adverse reactions are bitter taste, ocular burning and stinging, photophobia, and superficial punctuate keratitis.

# ALPHA₂-ADRENERGIC AGONISTS AND CARBONIC ANHYDRASE INHIBITORS

Brinzolamide and brimonidine (Simbrinza) is an anti-glaucoma medication that combines an alpha₂ agonist and carbonic anhydrase inhibitor ophthalmic agent. The combination of two agents enhances the ability to reduce IOP better than with one agent alone.

## Pharmacokinetics, Action, and Use

The action of brinzolamide inhibits carbonic anhydrase, leading to a decrease in aqueous humor secretion. Brimonidine is the alpha₂-adrenergic receptor agonist that reduces aqueous humor formation and increases uveoscleral outflow. The absorption of brinzolamide is topical and enters the systemic circulation. It is 60% protein bound and metabolized to *N*-desethyl brinzolamide. It is excreted primarily unchanged in the urine. Brimonidine accumulates in the red blood cells to bind with carbonic anhydrase. It is metabolized in the liver and excreted in the urine. The half-life of brinzolamide is 111 days; brimonidine's half-life is 2 to 3 hours. This combination ophthalmic medication is used to reduce IOP. Tables 59.3 and 59.4 provide the dosage and administration of brinzolamide and brimonidine.

### Use in Children

There are no dosage adjustments for children. In children age 2 to 6 years, brinzolamide and brimonidine may cause somnolence and decrease alertness. It is contraindicated in infants and toddlers under the age of 2 years.

## Adverse Effects and Contraindications

The adverse reactions of brinzolamide and brimonidine are minimal, with gastrointestinal effects of dysgeusia and xerostomia. Hypersensitivity reactions of the eye have been noted, along with blurred vision and eye irritation. Brinzolamide may be absorbed systemically, placing the patient at risk for acid-based balance disturbances. If a patient has developed a hypersensitivity reaction to either medication or the combination medication, then the use of the medication is contraindicated. It is also contraindicated in neonates, infants, and children <2 years of age.

## Nursing Implications
### Assessing for Therapeutic and Adverse Effects

The nurse should assess the patient for hypersensitivity reactions. The patient should be assessed by the ophthalmologist or optometrist for lowered IOP.

# OSMOTIC DRUGS

Osmotic diuretics are used to reduce IOP when the pressure cannot be lowered by other means. The drugs in this class are especially useful for treating acute episodes of angle-closure, absolute, or secondary glaucoma and for lowering IOP prior to intraocular surgery. Chapter 34 provides additional information on the prototype osmotic diuretic Ⓟ **mannitol** (Osmitrol, Resectisol), which is discussed in this section as it relates to reducing IOP.

## Pharmacokinetics and Action

After IV administration of mannitol, absorption is immediate, and the drug begins to work in 15 to 30 minutes. When used preoperatively to reduce IOP, administration 60 to 90 minutes prior to surgery allows the drug to reach its peak of action to achieve maximum IOP reduction. The drug's half-life is approximately 1 to 1.6 hours. Excretion is primarily as unchanged drug in the urine. Mannitol reduces the IOP by creating an osmotic gradient in between the plasma and ocular fields.

## Use

Mannitol temporarily reduces IOP in acute attacks of glaucoma. Prescribers also order it for reduction of IOP prior to surgery. Table 59.4 contains route and dosage information for mannitol.

## Use in Older Adults

It is important to start mannitol at the low end of the dosing range in older adults because of age-related decreases in hepatic, renal, and cardiac function and concomitant disease and polypharmacy.

## Adverse Effects and Contraindications

Adverse effects of mannitol relate to decreased fluid volume. The most serious of these conditions is hyperosmolar nonketotic coma. Other adverse effects include confusion, headache, syncope, cardiac dysrhythmias, nausea, vomiting, and severe dehydration.

Contraindications include severe dehydration, abdominal pain, appendicitis, pulmonary edema, and severe cardiac decompensation.

## Nursing Implications
### Assessing for Therapeutic and Adverse Effects

It is important to check for therapeutic effects, indicated by a reduction in IOP. In addition, the nurse checks fluid and electrolytes and assesses for signs and symptoms of dehydration. He or she monitors blood pressure, pulse, and respirations. The nurse assesses for hyperglycemia, adventitious breath sounds, and pupillary reflexes. It is also necessary to assess for hypersensitivity to mannitol.

**QSEN Alert: Safety**

If extravasation occurs at the injection site, stop the infusion of mannitol and leave the IV cannula in place. Aspirate the IV line gently, and initiate the antidote, hyaluronidase, as per institutional protocol.

## Patient Teaching

The nurse instructs the patient about the importance of keeping regularly scheduled medical appointments to check IOP. In addition, the nurse reminds the patient to report severe headache, chest pain, confusion, rapid respirations, and violent diarrhea to his or her prescriber. Box 59.2 contains additional patient teaching information for the ophthalmologic medications.

## NCLEX Success

9. A patient's ophthalmologist has prescribed mannitol intravenously for the treatment of glaucoma. Which of the following aspects of patient teaching will provide the patient with information about the action of the medication?

A. It competitively blocks the effects of acetylcholine.
B. It selectively binds to serotonin receptors to block the release of serotonin.
C. It stimulates the alpha$_2$-adrenergic receptors to reduce intraocular pressure (IOP).
D. It reduces the IOP by creating an osmotic gradient in between the plasma and ocular fields.

10. A 14-year-old girl visits the school nurse's office. The girl wants longer eyelashes after watching a commercial for Latisse. What information should the school nurse provide the girl regarding this form of bimatoprost?

A. "This medication is only given to patients with glaucoma."
B. "This medication is not recommended for anyone under the age of 16."
C. "You do not need this medication—your eyelashes are long enough."
D. "You should talk to your guidance counselor about ways to build your self-esteem."

# DRUG THERAPY FOR OCULAR INFECTIONS AND INFLAMMATION

Previous chapters have presented information about the medications administered to treat viral, fungal, and bacterial infections and the inflammation that often accompanies an infection. This section of the chapter addresses the anti-infective medications administered for the treatment of ocular infections and the anti-inflammatory drugs used to decrease inflammation. The nonsteroidal anti-inflammatory drugs (NSAIDs) and corticosteroids are administered to decrease the inflammatory response. Table 59.5 lists the drugs administered to treat ocular infections and to reduce ocular inflammation.

## TABLE 59.5

### Drugs Administered for the Treatment of Ocular Infections and Inflammation

| Drug Class | Prototype | Other Drugs in the Class |
|---|---|---|
| Antibacterial drugs | Ciprofloxacin ophthalmic (Ciloxan) | Erythromycin 5% ointment<br>Gatifloxacin (Zymaxid)<br>Gentamicin 3 mg/mL solution or 3 mg/g ointment (Gentak)<br>Levofloxacin 5 mg/mL solution<br>Moxifloxacin (Moxeza, Vigamox)<br>Ofloxacin (Ocuflox)<br>Sulfacetamide (Bleph-10)<br>Tobramycin (0.3% solution and 3 mg/g ointment) (Tobrex) |
| Antiviral drugs | Trifluridine 1% solution | Ganciclovir (Zirgan) |
| Antifungal drugs | Natamycin 5% suspension (Natacyn) | |
| Antiallergic drugs | Cromolyn | Lodoxamide (Alomide) |
| H$_1$ receptor antagonists: second generation | Emedastine difumarate | Azelastine<br>Epinastine (Elestat)<br>Ketotifen (Alaway Children Allergy, Claritin Eye, Zaditor)<br>Olopatadine (Pataday, Pazeo) |
| Corticosteroids | Dexamethasone (Dextenza, Dexycu, Maxidex, Ozurdex) | Fluorometholone (Flarex, FML, Liquifilm)<br>Loteprednol (Alrex)<br>Prednisolone (Pred Forte, Pred Mild)<br>Rimexolone |
| Anti-inflammatory drugs | Diclofenac | Flurbiprofen (Ocufen)<br>Ketorolac (Acular, Acuvail) |
| Immunosuppressants | Cyclosporine emulsion (Restasis) | |

## ANTIBACTERIAL DRUGS

Various antibacterial drugs have ophthalmic uses. The most common prescribed drug is the prototype fluoroquinolone (P) **ciprofloxacin** (Ciloxan).

## Pharmacokinetics and Action

The amount of ciprofloxacin absorbed by the body is so small that its pharmacokinetic properties are inconsequential.

Ciprofloxacin ophthalmic inhibits DNA gyrase and the relaxation of supercoiled DNA, which promotes breakage of double-stranded DNA in the target bacteria.

## Use

Uses of ciprofloxacin include the treatment of corneal ulcer and bacterial conjunctivitis. It is essential that contact lenses not be worn during drug therapy. Table 59.6 presents route and dosage information about ciprofloxacin and other antibacterial ophthalmic drugs.

**TABLE 59.6**

**DRUGS AT A GLANCE: Antimicrobial Drugs**

| Drug | Pregnancy Category | Routes and Dosage Ranges Adults | Children |
|---|---|---|---|
| **Antibacterial Drugs** | | | |
| (P) **Ciprofloxacin** Ophthalmic (Ciloxan; Ciloxan) | C | Corneal ulcer: day 1, 2 drops every 15 min for 6 h, then every 30 min for rest of day; day 2, 2 drops every hour; day 3–14, 2 drops every 4 h. Conjunctivitis: 1 or 2 drops every 2 h while awake for 2 d, then 1 or 2 drops every 4 h while awake for 5 d | Safety and efficacy not established in infants <1 y; ≥1 y: same as for adults |
| Erythromycin 5% ointment (EURO-Erythromycin, PDP-Erythromycin) | B | Ocular infection: instill 1 cm ribbon up to 6 times daily | Ocular infection: same as adult dosage. Prevention of neonatal gonococcal or chlamydial conjunctivitis: 1 cm in each lower conjunctival sac |
| Gatifloxacin (Zymaxid; Zymar) | C | Conjunctivitis: 1 drop every 2 h while awake, up to 8 times daily for 2 d, then 1 drop up to 4 times daily while awake for 5 d | ≥1 y: same as for adults |
| Gentamicin 3 mg/mL solution or 3 mg/g ointment (Gentak; Odan-Gentamicin) | D | Infection: Solution, 1–2 drops every 4 h up to 2 drops every hour for severe infections. Ointment, apply 0.5 inch, 2 or 3 times daily to every 3–4 h | Same as for adults |
| Levofloxacin 5 mg/mL solution | C | Conjunctivitis: 1 or 2 drops every 2 h up to 8 doses/d for 1 or 2 d, then every 4 h up to 4 doses/d for 5 d | Conjunctivitis: ≥1 y, same as adult dosage. Corneal ulcer: ≥6 y, 1.5% solution, 1 or 2 drops every 30 min to 2 h while awake and 4 and 6 h after retiring, then on day 4 through completion 1 or 2 drops every 4 h while awake |
| Moxifloxacin (Moxeza, Vigamox; PMS-Moxifloxacin, Vigamox) | C | Conjunctivitis: Vigamox, 1 drop 3 times daily for 7 d. Moxeza, 1 drop 2 times daily for 7 d | Conjunctivitis: ≥1 y: Vigamox, same as for adults; ≥4 mo: Moxeza, same as for adults |
| Ofloxacin (Ocuflox; APO-Ofloxacin, Ocuflox) | C | Conjunctivitis: 1 or 2 drops every 2–4 h while awake for 2 d and then 4 times daily for 3–5 d. Corneal ulcer: 1 or 2 drops every 30 min while awake, every 4–6 h during sleep for 1–2 d, then every hour while awake for 4–6 d, and then every 4 h while awake until healed | Conjunctivitis, corneal ulcer: ≥1 y, same as for adults |
| Sulfacetamide (Bleph-10; Odan-Sulfacetamide) | C | Conjunctivitis, corneal ulcers, or other superficial infections caused by susceptible organisms: 1 or 2 drops every 2–3 h or 0.5-inch ointment 3 or 4 times daily and at bedtime for 7–10 d | ≥2 mo: same as for adults |

**TABLE 59.6**

**DRUGS AT A GLANCE: Antimicrobial Drugs** (Continued)

| Drug | Pregnancy Category | Routes and Dosage Ranges | |
|---|---|---|---|
| | | **Adults** | **Children** |
| Tobramycin (0.3% solution and 3 mg/g ointment) (Tobrex; ❋ Tobrex, SANDOZ-Tobramycin) | D | Infection:<br>Solution, 1 or 2 drops every 4 h, up to 2 drops every hour<br>Ointment, 0.5 inch ribbon 2–3 times daily, up to every 3–4 h until improvement | Infection: ≥2 mo, same as for adults |
| **Antiviral Drugs** | | | |
| ⓟ **Trifluridine** (❋ APO-Trifluridine, Viroptic) | C | Keratoconjunctivitis or corneal ulcers caused by herpes simplex virus: 1 drop every 2 h while awake (maximum, 9 drops/d) until corneal ulcer heals and then 1 drop every 4 h (minimum, 5 drops/d), for 7 d | ≥6 y: same as for adults |
| Ganciclovir (Zirgan) | C | Herpetic keratitis: 1 drop every 3 h while awake (maximum, 5 drops/d) until corneal ulcer heals and then 1 drop 3 times daily for 7 d | ≥2 y: same as adults |
| **Antifungal Drugs** | | | |
| Natamycin 5% suspension (Natacyn) | C | 1 drop every 1–2 h for 3–4 d and then every 3–4 h for 14–21 d | Safety and efficacy not established |

## Adverse Effects

Ciprofloxacin ophthalmic has adverse effects that include hypersensitivity reactions and superinfection. When ciprofloxacin ophthalmic is administered concurrently with any of the quinolones, hypersensitivity reactions, tendon inflammation, and tendon rupture may occur. There have been reports of superinfections with prolonged use, with possible fungal or bacterial infections.

## Contraindications

Patients with a known hypersensitivity to ciprofloxacin or any quinolone should not receive the drug.

## Nursing Implications

### Preventing Interactions

The only interaction identified with ciprofloxacin ophthalmic is anaphylaxis when administered with quinolones.

### Administering the Medication

Ciprofloxacin ophthalmic is for topical use only. It is important not to contaminate the tip of the applicator.

### Assessing for Therapeutic Effects

The nurse assesses for decreased conjunctival redness and eye drainage.

### Patient Teaching

Box 59.2 contains patient teaching information for topical ophthalmic medications.

## Other Drugs in the Class

An ophthalmic form of erythromycin can produce edema, urticaria, dermatitis, and angioneurotic edema. Long-term topical use may lead to superinfection, and patients with viral, fungal, or mycobacterial infections of the eye should not use this drug.

## ANTIVIRAL DRUGS

The prototype ⓟ **trifluridine** is the most commonly administered antiviral ophthalmic drug. A locally active drug, it is available as an ophthalmic ointment.

## Pharmacokinetics and Action

Systemic absorption of trifluridine is negligible. The drug does not affect liver or kidney function.

Trifluridine interferes with viral replication. It incorporates viral DNA in place of thymidine to inhibit thymidylate synthetase, causing formation of defective viral proteins.

## Use

Uses of trifluridine include treatment of primary keratoconjunctivitis and recurrent epithelial keratitis caused by herpes simplex virus types 1 and 2. Table 59.6 presents route and dosage information for trifluridine.

## Adverse Effects and Contraindications

The most common adverse effects associated with trifluridine are burning and stinging. Rare adverse effects include epithelial keratopathy, increased IOP, palpebral edema, and stromal edema.

Contraindications include known hypersensitivity to trifluridine or its components.

# Nursing Implications

## Administering the Medication

Trifluridine is a hazardous drug, and it is important to wear gloves when administering the medication. If trifluridine is being used with other ophthalmic medications, it is necessary to wait several minutes between applications. Storage of the medication in the refrigerator at 2°C to 8°C or 36°F to 48°F is required. Disposal in accordance with biohazard procedures should occur.

## Assessing for Therapeutic and Adverse Effects

It is necessary to assess for decreased erythema of the conjunctiva. Complete healing of the corneal ulcer should occur in 1 to 2 weeks.

The nurse assesses for transient burning, stinging, and irritation of the eye. He or she also assesses for photophobia, increased IOP, epithelial keratopathy, keratitis, palpebral edema, and stromal edema.

## Patient Teaching

The nurse provides instruction to the patient on medication administration, including safe handling of the drug. He or she also teaches the patient about the importance of keeping regularly scheduled medical appointments for eye examinations. In addition, the nurse tells the patient that herpetic eye infections often recur and, if not treated, lead to damage of the cornea. Box 59.2 contains additional patient teaching information.

# Other Drugs in the Class

Ganciclovir (Zymaxid) is an antiviral ophthalmic agent used to treat herpetic keratitis. Gloves and a protective gown should be worn for administering the drug topically. Current guidelines for the use of antiretroviral agents in HIV-1–infected adults and adolescents (Department of Health and Human Services) includes recommendations on the HIV-related uses of ganciclovir for progressive outer retinal necrosis and acute retinal necrosis both of which are infections and necrotizing inflammation associated with a high rate of blindness.

---

11. A male college student receives a diagnosis of bacterial conjunctivitis. His physician orders ciprofloxacin to be instilled every 4 hours for 5 days. On day 3, the student visits to the campus health center. He states, "My tongue is swollen." He is having trouble speaking clearly. What is the possible cause of the swollen tongue?
    A. He is allergic to a food.
    B. He has a bacterial infection of the mouth.
    C. He is having a hypersensitivity reaction.
    D. He has a fungal or bacterial superinfection.

12. Which of the following is the most important aspect of patient teaching with the administration of trifluridine?
    A. Tell the patient to instill the medication by pulling the upper lid toward the forehead.
    B. Tell the patient that he or she will be cured of herpetic eye infections.
    C. Tell the patient to use safe handling of the drug and wear gloves when administering.
    D. Tell the patient not to take acetazolamide due to a drug interaction.

# ANTIFUNGAL DRUGS

ⓟ **Natamycin** (Natacyn) is the prototype ophthalmic antifungal drug.

# Pharmacokinetics and Action

Approximately 2% of natamycin administered topically is absorbed systemically. It is distributed by adhering to the cornea and is retained in the conjunctival fornices. It does not affect intraocular fluid concentrations.

Natamycin increases cellular permeability to susceptible fungi.

# Use

Uses of natamycin include the treatment of blepharitis, conjunctivitis, and keratitis. It is effective against common fungi such as *Aspergillus, Candida, Cephalosporium, Fusarium,* and *Penicillium.* Table 59.6 presents route and dosage information for natamycin.

# Adverse Effects

Reported adverse effects of natamycin may be numerous. These conditions may include hypersensitivity and allergic reactions, chest pain, opacity of the cornea, eye pain, edema, dyspnea, hyperemia, irritation, foreign body sensation of the eye, paresthesia, tearing, and alteration in visual acuity.

# Contraindications

Patients who have exhibited a hypersensitivity reaction to natamycin should not take the drug.

# Nursing Implications

## Administering the Medication

It is important that contact lenses are not worn when signs and symptoms of the fungal infection are visible. In any case, the natamycin solution contains benzalkonium chloride, which can be absorbed by the lens; thus, it is necessary to remove the lenses prior to administration of the medication. Reinsertion of the lenses should not occur for 15 minutes. The nurse shakes the medication well and then administers it without touching the applicator tip to the eye.

### Assessing for Therapeutic and Adverse Effects

The nurse assesses for decreased eye pain, redness, and tearing. Also, the patient should also have increased visual acuity with a decrease in blurring and cloudiness.

It is also necessary to assess for signs and symptoms of a hypersensitivity reaction such as hyperemia, dyspnea, edema, or chest pain. The nurse also assesses for paresthesia and visual changes.

### Patient Teaching

The nurse tells the patient to discontinue wearing contacts during the acute phase of the fungal infection. Also, the nurse emphasizes that even when the patient is wearing contacts, he or she should not reinsert them for 15 minutes after instillation of the medication. In addition, it is important to maintain good hand hygiene and prevent contamination of the applicator tip. Box 59.2 contains additional patient teaching information.

## ANTIALLERGIC DRUGS

Ⓟ **Cromolyn sodium** (Opticrom) is the prototype antiallergic ophthalmic drug.

## Pharmacokinetics and Action

The onset of action varies. The half-life of the drug is 80 to 90 minutes. Cromolyn is excreted unchanged in the urine and feces with small amounts in exhaled gases.

Cromolyn reduces the release of leukotrienes, thus decreasing or stopping the body's reaction to an allergen.

## Use

Uses of cromolyn include the treatment of vernal keratitis, vernal conjunctivitis, and vernal keratoconjunctivitis. Table 59.7 presents route and dosage information for cromolyn and other ophthalmic antiallergy medications.

---

### TABLE 59.7

### DRUGS AT A GLANCE: Anti-inflammatory Drugs

| Drug | Pregnancy Category | Routes and Dosages Ranges | |
|---|---|---|---|
| | | **Adults** | **Children** |
| **Antiallergic Drugs** | | | |
| Ⓟ **Cromolyn sodium** | B | 1–2 drops in each eye 4–6 times per day | ≥4 y, same as for adults |
| Lodoxamide (Alomide; 🍁 Alomide) | B | 1–2 drops 4 times a day for up to 3 mo | ≥2 y, same as for adults |
| **H₁ Receptor Antagonists: Second Generation** | | | |
| Ⓟ **Emedastine difumarate** (Emadine) | C | 1 drop 4 times per day | ≥3 y, same as for adults |
| Azelastine | C | 1 drop twice daily | ≥3 y, same as for adults |
| Epinastine (Elestat) | C | 1 drop 2 times per day even when symptoms subside | ≥3 y, same as for adults |
| Ketotifen (Alaway, Claritin Eye, Zaditor; Zaditor) | C | 1 drop 2 times a day at least 8 h apart | ≥3 y, same as for adults |
| Olopatadine (Pataday, Patanol, Pazeo; ACT-Olopatadine, Pataday, Patanol) | C | Patanol, 1 drop 2 times per day at least 6 h between doses<br>Pataday and Pazeo, 1 drop once daily | Patanol, ≥3 y, same as adult dosage<br>Pataday, ≥2 y, same as adult dosage |
| **Corticosteroids** | | | |
| Ⓟ **Dexamethasone** (Dextenza, Dexycu, Maxidex, Ozurdex; 🍁 Maxidex, Odan Dexamethasone, Ozurdex) | C | Ophthalmic solution, 1–2 drops into conjunctival sac every hour during the day and every other hour during the night; gradually reduce dose to 1 drop every 3–4 times per day<br>Ophthalmic suspension, 1–2 drops into conjunctival sac 4–6 times per day; may use hourly in severe disease; taper dose during discontinuation<br>Macular edema or noninfective uveitis: Ophthalmic injection, ocular implant with Ozurdex, intravitreal 0.7-mg implant injected in affected eye | Ophthalmic solution, 1–2 drops into conjunctival sac every hour during the day and every other hour during the night; gradually reduce dose to every 3–4 h, then 3–4 times per day<br>Ophthalmic suspension, 1–2 drops into conjunctival sac up to 4–6 times per day; may use hourly in severe disease in older children; taper dose during discontinuation; following strabismus surgery: 2–4 times per day |

*(Continued on page 1188)*

**TABLE 59.7**

## DRUGS AT A GLANCE: Anti-inflammatory Drugs (Continued)

| Drug | Pregnancy Category | Routes and Dosages Ranges | |
|---|---|---|---|
| | | **Adults** | **Children** |
| Fluorometholone (Flarex, FML, Liquifilm; ❋ Flarex, SANDOZ-Fluorometholone) | C | Ointment, 1/2-inch ribbon to conjunctival sac 1–3 times daily; may increase to every 4 h during the initial 24–48 h<br>Suspension, 1 drop into the conjunctival sac 2–4 times per day | ≥2 y of age, same as for adults |
| Loteprednol (Lotemax, Alrex; ❋ Alrex Lotemax) | C | Seasonal allergic conjunctivitis: 0.2% suspension 1 drop 4 times per day<br>Inflammatory conditions: 0.5% suspension 1–2 drops into the conjunctival sac 4 times per day; during the first week the dose may be increased by 1 drop every hour; do not discontinue therapy prematurely; if signs and symptoms do not improve in 2 d, the patient should be reevaluated<br>Postoperative inflammation: 0.5% suspension 1–2 drops into the conjunctival sac 4 times per day beginning 24 h after surgery and continue for 2 wk | Safety and efficacy not established |
| Prednisolone (Pred Forte, Pred Mild; ❋ PMS-Prednisolone, Pred Forte, Sandoz Prednisolone) | C | 1–2 drops into conjunctival sac 2–4 times daily; dosing frequency first 48 h may be increased if necessary | 1–2 drops into conjunctival sac 3–6 times daily |
| **Anti-inflammatory Drugs** | | | |
| Ⓟ **Diclofenac** | C | Cataract surgery: 1 drop 4 times per day beginning 24 h after surgery and continuing for 2 wk<br>Corneal refractive surgery: 1–2 drops within the hour prior to surgery and continuing 4 times daily for up to 3 d | Safety and efficacy of ophthalmic preparation not established |
| Flurbiprofen | C | 1 drop every 30 min starting 2 h prior to surgery (total of 4 drops to each affected eye) | Same as for adults |
| Ketorolac (Acular, Acuvail, Acular LS; ❋ Acular, Acuvail, Acular LS) | C | Seasonal allergic conjunctivitis: 1 drop 4 times per day<br>Postoperative inflammation: 1 drop 4 times per day starting 24 h after cataract surgery and through 14 d after surgery<br>Postoperative pain: 1 drop times per day as needed up to 4 d after corneal refractive surgery<br>Postoperative pain and photophobia: 1 drop 2 times per day as needed beginning 24 h before and for up to 2 wk after incisional refractive surgery | Seasonal allergic conjunctivitis: ≥2 y, same as adult dosage<br>Postoperative ocular pain: ≥3 y, same as for adults<br>Postoperative pain: ≥3 y, same as for adults |
| **Immunosuppressants** | | | |
| Ⓟ **Cyclosporine emulsion** (Cequa, Restasis; Restasis Multidose; ❋ Restasis, Restasis MultiDose, TEVA-CycloSPORINE, Verkazia) | C | 1 drop every 12 h | ≥16 y, same as for adults |

## Adverse Effects and Contraindications

Cromolyn is associated with several adverse effects, including hypersensitivity reactions. Eye effects include edema, dryness, irritation, itching, puffiness, rash, and tearing. Styes may also develop.

Contraindications include a known hypersensitivity to the drug or its formulations.

## Nursing Implications

### Assessing for Therapeutic Effects

The nurse assesses for a reduction in allergic conjunctivitis, keratitis, or keratoconjunctivitis. Response to treatment with cromolyn may occur in a few days. However, treatment for up to 6 weeks is routinely necessary.

### Assessing for Adverse Effects

The nurse assesses for hypersensitivity response to the medication as well as ocular effects that include edema, dryness, irritation, itching, swelling, rash, or tearing. It is necessary to ask the patient about feelings of a foreign body, which could indicate a stye. Withdrawal may result in the exacerbation of symptoms.

### Patient Teaching

Box 59.2 contains additional patient teaching information.

## H₁-RECEPTOR ANTAGONISTS: SECOND GENERATION

Allergic rhinitis produces ocular pruritus. The second-generation antihistamines block the H₁ receptors to relieve ocular pruritus. The prototype of this class of ophthalmic medications is Ⓟ **emedastine difumarate**.

## Pharmacokinetics, Action, and Use

Emedastine difumarate is a selective histamine H₁ receptor antagonist for topical ophthalmic use. It is minimally absorbed systemically. Emedastine difumarate is used for adult and pediatric patients to relieve seasonal allergic conjunctivitis.

## Adverse Effects and Contraindications

Emedastine difumarate produces a headache in 11% of the patients. A smaller proportion of patients have reported hyperemia, abnormal dreams, dermatitis, pruritus, weakness, blurred vision, corneal infiltrates, corneal staining, keratitis, transient burning, rhinitis, or sinusitis. Emedastine difumarate is contraindicated in patients who have signs and symptoms of hypersensitivity with the ophthalmic solution.

## Nursing Implications

### Administering the Medication

Check the solution for clarity before administering it. Prior to and following the administration of the medication, wash hands for a minimum of 20 seconds. Shake the emedastine difumarate prior to administration. Instill one drop in the conjunctival sac.

Never touch the eye with the eye dropper tip. The patient should close the eye for 1 to 2 minutes after instillation. Wait 10 minutes to insert contact lenses.

### Assessing for Therapeutic and Adverse Effects

Assess the patient for decreased ocular redness, watering, and inflammation. Adverse effects of emedastine difumarate include a hypersensitivity reaction with increased redness, edema, and pruritus.

### Patient Teaching

The patient should be taught to wash hands for 20 seconds prior to and following the administration of emedastine difumarate. Instill the medication in the conjunctival sac without touching the medication tip to the eye. The patient should close the eye for 1 to 2 minutes after the medication administration. Emedastine difumarate contains benzalkonium, which can damage soft contact lenses. Contact lenses should not be inserted for a minimum of 10 minutes after instillation. Instruct the patient on the signs and symptoms of hypersensitivity.

## Other Drugs in the Class

Azelastine hydrochloride treats ocular pruritus. Epinastine (Elestat), Ketotifen (Alaway Children's Allergy, Claritin Eye, Zaditor), and Olopatadine (Pataday, Pazeo) treat allergic conjunctivitis.

## CORTICOSTEROIDS

The prototype corticosteroid ophthalmic drug is Ⓟ **dexamethasone** (Dextenza, Dexycu, Maxidex, Ozurdex).

## Pharmacokinetics

The onset of action of dexamethasone ophthalmic drops is unknown. The half-life and duration of action are unknown. The onset of action of the implant is 20% to 30% within the first 2 months following intravitreal injection. The duration of action is 1 to 3 months.

## Action

Dexamethasone decreases inflammation by suppressing the migration of neutrophils and decreasing the production of the mediators of inflammation. It reverses the increase in capillary permeability and suppresses the normal immune response.

## Use

Uses of dexamethasone include a decrease of symptoms of allergic conjunctivitis, iritis, and cyclitis. It is a treatment of corneal injury from chemical, radiation, and thermal burns or penetrating foreign bodies. Dexamethasone in the form of an intravitreal implant (Ozurdex) is used for the treatment of macular edema following retinal vein occlusion or central retinal vein occlusion, as well as for noninfective uveitis. Table 59.7 presents dosage information for the corticosteroid ophthalmic drugs.

## Adverse Effects

Ocular adverse effects associated with dexamethasone include blurred vision, increased IOP, photophobia, vitreous detachment, conjunctival edema, corneal edema, eye pain, dryness, irritation, and eye discharge.

## Contraindications

Contraindications to dexamethasone include corneal or conjunctival viral disease caused by herpes simplex, vaccinia, or varicella. Also, other contraindications are mycobacterial and fungal infection of the eye as well as advanced glaucoma and hypersensitivity to corticosteroids. In addition, patients who are taking corticorelin, a synthetic hormone that is administered to diagnose Cushing's disease, should not receive ophthalmic forms of dexamethasone.

## Nursing Implications

### Preventing Interactions

The dexamethasone decreases the therapeutic effects of corticorelin. If patients who are taking the chelating drug deferasirox combine it with corticosteroids, there is an increased risk of GI ulceration, irritation, and bleeding.

### Administering the Medication

> **❗ QSEN Alert: Safety**
>
> It is important to double check medications before administration. The nurse should not confuse medications with similar names. For example, it is easy to confuse dexamethasone [Maxidex] with triamterene/hydrochlorothiazide [Maxzide].

The solution and suspension contain benzalkonium chloride. Thus, a nurse may administer dexamethasone solutions and suspensions, but an ophthalmologist gives the implant (Ozurdex) under aseptic conditions. Prior to injection of Ozurdex, a broad-spectrum bactericidal drug is administered. If administered to both eyes, a different applicator is used for each application. Box 59.1 lists general guidelines for the administration of topical ophthalmic medications.

### Assessing for Therapeutic Effects

The nurse assesses for decreased pain, irritation, redness, and eye drainage. An ophthalmologist evaluates patients who have received Ozurdex for decreased macular edema and inflammation of the uveal tract.

### Assessing for Adverse Effects

The nurse assesses for eye pain, blurred vision, photophobia, increased IOP, photophobia, vitreous detachment, conjunctival edema, eye dryness, or eye discharge.

### Patient Teaching

For patients who use the ophthalmic implant (Ozurdex), it is important to instruct them about the sterile procedure for administration and the rationale for the implant. Box 59.2 contains additional patient teaching information.

## ANTI-INFLAMMATORY DRUGS

The prototype ophthalmic NSAID is  **diclofenac**, an analgesic, non-narcotic drug.

## Pharmacokinetics and Action

Very little systemic absorption of diclofenac occurs. Mainly, it has local effects.

This cyclooxygenase 1 and 2 inhibitor decreases the formation of prostaglandin, thus resulting in an anti-inflammatory action.

## Use

Diclofenac reduces inflammation following cataract extraction. It is administered to relieve pain and photophobia associated with corneal refractive surgery. Table 59.7 provides route and dosage information about diclofenac and other NSAIDs.

## Adverse Effects

Diclofenac may produce facial edema, dizziness, fever, headache, pain, and insomnia. Associated ocular adverse effects are burning, stinging, increased IOP, keratitis, and lacrimation. Less frequently occurring ocular conditions include disturbances in vision, inflammation, corneal deposits and edema, corneal lesions or opacity, discharge, swelling, iritis, itching, and allergy. In addition, rhinitis, muscle pain and weakness, abdominal pain, nausea, vomiting, and viral infection may follow use.

## Contraindications

Contraindications to diclofenac include hypersensitivity to any NSAID.

## Nursing Implications

### Preventing Interactions

Any ophthalmic NSAID combined with latanoprost diminishes the therapeutic effect of latanoprost.

### Administering the Medication

As with other ophthalmic medications, it is necessary to prevent contamination of the applicator tip. In addition, it is important to wait at least 5 minutes before administering any other eyedrops.

### Assessing for Therapeutic and Adverse Effects

The nurse assesses for decreased inflammation and pain related to surgery.

In addition, the nurse assesses for tearing, inflammation, and pain or discomfort of the eye, as well as for facial edema and rhinitis. It is necessary to assess for increased IOP. Also, the nurse assesses for GI conditions and viral infections.

### Patient Teaching

Box 59.2 contains patient teaching information.

# IMMUNOSUPPRESSANTS

The prototype ophthalmic immunosuppressant drug is Ⓟ **cyclosporine emulsion** (Restasis).

## Pharmacokinetics and Action

No systemic concentrations of cyclosporine are detected in blood samples.

The drug increases tear production.

## Use

Cyclosporine emulsion increases tear production in keratoconjunctivitis sicca, which is an ocular inflammation. Table 59.7 presents route and dosage information for the cyclosporine emulsion.

## Adverse Effects and Contraindications

The adverse effects of cyclosporine emulsion are burning, hyperemia, ocular pain, and pruritus.

Contraindications include active eye infections or hypersensitivity to the medication.

## Nursing Implications

### Administering the Medication

It is important to invert the medication bottle to mix the emulsion adequately prior to administration. In addition, patients should remove contact lenses before administration and not reinsert them for 15 minutes. The instillation of other ocular medications should occur at 15-minute intervals.

### Assessing for Therapeutic and Adverse Effects

The nurse interviews the patient to determine if the dryness of the eye has resolved.

In addition, the nurse assesses for discomfort of the eye, pruritus, and hyperemia.

### Patient Teaching

It is important to instruct the patient about medication administration, including inversion of the bottle to mix the medication, removal of contacts, and waiting 15 minutes between the administration of other ocular medications. Box 59.2 contains additional patient teaching information.

## THE NURSING PROCESS

A concept map outlines the nursing process related to drug therapy considerations in this chapter. Additional nursing implications related to the disease process should also be considered in care decisions.

**Assessment**
- Assess visual acuity and the ability to complete activities of daily living and work-related activities.
- Identify risk factors for eye disorders. These include trauma, allergies, infection in one eye (a risk factor for infection in the other eye), use of contact lenses, infections of facial structures or skin, and occupational exposure to chemical irritants or foreign bodies.
- Assess subjective and objective data related to eye pain, inflammation of the eye, purulent or mucous discharge from the eye, pruritus, or photosensitivity.

**Outcomes of Therapy**
The patient will
- Administer ophthalmic medications as prescribed.
- Follow safety precautions to protect eyes from trauma and disease.
- Experience improvement in signs and symptoms (e.g., decreased drainage with infections, decreased intraocular pressure with glaucoma).
- Avoid injury from impaired vision (e.g., falls).
- Avoid systemic effects of ophthalmic drugs.
- Have regular eye examinations.

**Nursing Interventions**
- Instruct the patient to have regular eye examinations; including annual monitoring of intraocular pressure at the age of 40 years.
- Instruct patients who have glaucoma not to take any medications without a physician's knowledge. Many drugs given for purposes other than eye disorders may cause or aggravate glaucoma. Also, suggest that patients wear a medical alert bracelet stating that they have glaucoma.
- Assist patients at risk of eye damage from IOP (e.g., those with glaucoma; those who have had intraocular surgery, such as cataract removal) to avoid straining at stool (use laxatives or stool softeners if needed), heavy lifting, bending over, coughing, and vomiting when possible.
- Promote handwashing and keeping hands away from eyes to prevent eye infections.
- Cleanse contact lenses or assist patients in lens care, when needed.
- Apply warm, wet compresses; they are often useful in ophthalmic inflammation or infections.

**Evaluation**
- Observe and interview for compliance with instructions regarding drug therapy and follow-up care.
- Observe and interview for relief of symptoms.
- Observe for systemic adverse effects of ophthalmic drugs (e.g., tachycardia and dysrhythmias with adrenergic drugs; bradycardia or bronchoconstriction with beta-adrenergic blockers).

## KEY CONCEPTS

- Drug therapy for eye disorders is unique because of the location, structure, and function of the eye.
- Eye medications represent several different drug classes.
- Most eye medications are administered as drops.

- Therapeutic effects of eye drops depend on accurate administration.
- Eye medications should be kept sterile to avoid infection.
- Local eye medications may cause systemic effects.
- Systemic drugs may affect eye function.

## CLINICAL REASONING CASE STUDY

| | |
|---|---|
| **Meet the Patient** | Rosaria Gomez, a 55-year-old woman, is being treated for open-angle glaucoma. She has received a prescription for timolol (Timoptic), 1 drop of a 0.25% solution into both eyes daily. She wears contact lenses on occasion.<br><br>• What should the nurse understand regarding the etiology of open-angle glaucoma?<br>• What patient education related to her drug therapy and glaucoma should the nurse provide Mrs. Gomez? |
| **Assessing Drug Information** | • Timolol blocks the beta$_1$- and beta$_2$-adrenergic receptors to reduce the intraocular pressure (IOP) by reducing aqueous humor production and increasing outflow.<br>• Timolol is used to treat chronic open-angle glaucoma, aphakic glaucoma, secondary glaucoma, and ocular hypertension.<br>• The most common adverse effects associated with timolol are burning and stinging. Most adverse effects of systemic beta-adrenergic blockers may also occur with ophthalmic preparations, and patients with respiratory or cardiac disease may not be able to take them. |
| **Nursing Actions** | • Recognize that the most common type of glaucoma is open-angle glaucoma, which is characterized by an increase in IOP. In this type of glaucoma, there is no obstruction at the iridocorneal angle; it most commonly results from an abnormality of the trabecular meshwork that controls the flow of aqueous humor into the canal of Schlemm. A secondary form of open-angle glaucoma occurs when the formation of red cell fragments after trauma or epithelial granules of iris pigment clog the trabecular mesh.<br>• Reinforce compliance with the treatment plan because there is a potential loss of peripheral vision with a lack of treatment.<br>• Ensure that Mrs. Gomez administers timolol correctly and can demonstrate the appropriate instillation of eye drops. Key teaching points include the following:<br>  • Remove contact lenses prior to administration.<br>  • Use good hand hygiene before administering ophthalmic drugs.<br>  • Always invert the bottle of timolol and shake it before use.<br>  • Tilt head back and use the index finger of one hand to pull the lower lid down to form a pocket for the eye drop. Place the dispenser tip close to the eye and gently squeeze the bottle to administer one drop.<br>  • Wait 15 minutes after drug administration before reinserting contact lenses. The product can contain benzalkonium chloride, which can be absorbed into the soft contact lens.<br>• Instruct Mrs. Gomez to report decreased visual acuity, diplopia, or visual disturbances or signs of hypersensitivity, bronchoconstriction, or difficulty swallowing to her health care provider.<br>• Encourage Mrs. Gomez to keep regularly scheduled appointments with her ophthalmologist to assess her IOP. |

*Visit* thePoint® *at* **http://thePoint.lww.com/Frandsen12e** *for answers to NCLEX Success questions (in Appendix A), answers to Clinical Application Case Studies (in Appendix B), and more!*

## REFERENCES AND RESOURCES

DHHS Panel on Antiretroviral Guidelines for Adults and Adolescents. Guidelines for the use of antiretroviral agents in HIV-1-infected adults and adolescents. Department of Health and Human Services. Retrieved from http://aidsinfo.nih.gov/contentfiles/lvguidelines/AdultandAdolescentGL.pdf

DHHS Panel on Opportunistic Infections in HIV-Exposed and HIV-Infected Children. Guidelines for the prevention and treatment of opportunistic infections in HIV-exposed and HIV-infected children. Department of Health and Human Services. Retrieved November 2013, from http://aidsinfo.nih.gov/contentfiles/lvguidelines/oi_guidelines_pediatrics.pdf

Hinkle, J. H., & Cheever, K. H. (2018). *Brunner & Suddarth's textbook of medical-surgical nursing* (14th ed.). Philadelphia, PA: Wolters Kluwer.

Jacobs, D. S. (2020). Open-angle glaucoma: Treatment. *UpToDate.* Lexi-Comp, Inc.

El Hajj Moussa, W. G., Farhat, R. G., Nehme, J. C., Sahyoun, M. A., Schakal, A. R., Jalkh, A. E., et al. (2018). Comparison of efficacy and ocular surface disease index score between bimatoprost, latanoprost, travoprost, and tafluprost in glaucoma patients. *Journal of Ophthalmology,* 1–7. Article ID 1319628. Retrieved from https://doi.10.1155/2018/1319628

Norris, T. L. (2019). *Porth's pathophysiology concepts of altered health states* (10th ed.). Philadelphia, PA: Wolters Kluwer.

Lippincott Williams & Wilkins. (2020). *Nursing 2020 drug handbook* (40th ed.). Philadelphia, PA: Wolters Kluwer.

Reynolds, J. D. & Reynolds, A. L. (2020). Overview of glaucoma in infants and children. *UpToDate.* Lexi-Comp, Inc.

UpToDate. (2020). *Drug information.* Lexi-Comp, Inc.

# Drug Therapy for Disorders of the Ear

## LEARNING OBJECTIVES

*After studying this chapter, you should be able to:*

1. Recognize the etiology, pathophysiology, and clinical manifestations of both acute otitis externa and necrotizing otitis externa.
2. Identify the prototype and describe the action, use, adverse effects, contraindications, and nursing implications for topical medications used to treat otitis externa.
3. Identify the prototype and describe the action, use, adverse effects, contraindications, and nursing implications for systemic medications used to treat necrotizing otitis externa.
4. Identify the prototype and describe the action, use, adverse effects, contraindications, and nursing implications for systemic medications used to treat otitis media.
5. Identify the adjuvant drugs used to treat otitis externa and otitis media.
6. Implement the nursing process in the care of the patient with otitis externa or otitis media.

## CLINICAL APPLICATION CASE STUDY

Derrick Washington is a member of the high school swim team. He has been swimming two times per day for the past 3 months. The swim team has been very successful this season; it has qualified for the state finals. One morning well before the state meet, Derrick awakens with a severe earache. His mother makes an appointment with a pediatric nurse practitioner, who diagnoses acute otitis externa (swimmer's ear). The nurse prescribes neomycin–polymyxin B–hydrocortisone suspension.

## KEY TERMS

**Necrotizing otitis externa:** invasive soft tissue infection of the external auditory canal and skull; also called malignant external otitis

**Otalgia:** ear pain

**Otic:** relating to the ear

**Otitis externa:** inflammation of the external ear that occurs as a mild allergic dermatitis or as a severe cellulitis

**Otitis media:** inflammation of the middle ear

**Otorrhea:** any discharge from the ear (clear to purulent) following perforation of the tympanic membrane

# INTRODUCTION

This chapter discusses some ear-related disorders and their pharmacologic treatment. Infections, whether bacterial or fungal, or allergic reactions result in ear pain–related inflammation. **Otitis externa** is a disorder of the external ear that produces inflammation. This condition, most commonly known as swimmer's ear, is more likely to occur in the summer months. People whose ears are frequently exposed to moisture are more prone to the development of this disorder. Malignant necrotizing otitis externa (also called malignant otitis externa) most commonly affects elderly patients with diabetes mellitus and patients with the human immunodeficiency virus. The disease is rare in children. **Otitis media** is an acute infection or inflammation of the middle ear. Acute otitis media is the most common ailment for which anti-infective agents are prescribed in children.

The pharmacologic therapy of choice for disorders of the ear is **otic** preparations. These medications, which are discussed elsewhere in this book, have special uses in the treatment of ear conditions.

# OVERVIEW OF DISORDERS OF THE EAR

## Etiology

### Otitis Externa

Causes of otitis externa include moisture in the ear canal (as seen with a history of ear irrigations), allergic reactions such as psoriasis, or trauma of the ear canal related to itching or scratching. *Pseudomonas aeruginosa, Proteus,* and *Staphylococcus aureus* are bacteria that may play a causal role. *Aspergillus* is the fungus that thrives in the most ear canal. Malignant necrotizing otitis externa in patients infected with the human immunodeficiency virus implicates a compromised immune system as a predisposing factor in the disease.

### Otitis Media

Otitis media, one of the most common infections in early infancy and childhood, is more prevalent in children than adults. By 3 years of age, most children have had at least one episode of acute otitis media. Although this condition usually resolves without treatment, health care providers often prescribe antibiotics. The causative pathogens include *Haemophilus influenzae, Streptococcus pneumoniae,* and *Moraxella catarrhalis.* The organisms enter the middle ear as a result of an alteration in the eustachian tube. Upper respiratory congestion, inflammation, or an allergic reaction may allow this to happen. Bacteria may enter the middle ear from the contaminated secretions of the nasopharynx or perforation of the tympanic membrane of the middle ear.

## Pathophysiology

### Otitis Externa

Otitis externa involves the presence of moisture in the external ear canal, leading to the development of inflammation of the pinna and canal. The canal becomes itchy, red, and tender, and increased swelling makes it narrower. Ear pain occurs with movement because of the inflammation. There may be watery or purulent drainage, and intermittent hearing loss may result.

**Necrotizing otitis externa** is an invasive soft tissue infection of the external auditory canal and skull. The epidermis becomes thickened and inflamed, and the underlying dermis exhibits chronic inflammation. Involvement of the osseous portion of the external auditory canal can lead to temporal bone osteomyelitis. The infection is progressive causing rapid debilitation. If the infection spreads to the base of the skull, it can be fatal.

### Otitis Media

In otitis media, infection causes an obstruction of the eustachian tube, resulting in fluid retention and suppuration of retained secretions. This infection is more common in children because the eustachian tube is straighter, allowing the pathogen to enter the ear more easily.

## Clinical Manifestations

### Otitis Externa

In acute otitis externa, the patient complains of **otalgia** (ear pain) and **otorrhea** (drainage from the external auditory canal). The discharge may be yellow or green, with a foul odor most likely due to *P. aeruginosa.*

The patient may also report a feeling of "fullness" in the ear, decreased hearing, and pruritus.

In necrotizing otitis externa, the presenting symptoms are otalgia and otorrhea with purulent drainage. The pain is primarily experienced at night and may extend to the temporomandibular joint when chewing. The advancement of the infection results in osteomyelitis of the skull and temporomandibular joint that can be associated with cranial nerve palsies.

### Otitis Media

In acute otitis media, marked fluid and inflammation in the mucosa lining the middle ear space are present (Fig. 60.1). These cause pain and general symptoms of illness such as fever, irritability, and problems feeding and sleeping. Otalgia and diminished

**Figure 60.1.** Acute otitis media. [Reprinted with permission from Weber, J., & Kelly, J. H. (2014). *Health assessment in nursing* [6th ed., image in Abnormal Findings 17-2 table]. Philadelphia, PA: Wolters Kluwer Health | Lippincott Williams & Wilkins.]

**TABLE 60.1**

**Drugs Administered for the Treatment of Disorders of the Ear**

| Drug Class | Prototype | Other Drugs in the Class |
|---|---|---|
| Acute otitis externa | | |
| Anti-infective, antiseptic, glucocorticoid, and acidifying agents | Neomycin–polymyxin B–hydrocortisone | Coly-Mycin S Otic<br>Cipro HC Otic<br>Ofloxacin |
| Necrotizing otitis externa | | |
| Fluoroquinolones | Ciprofloxacin (Cipro) | |
| Acute otitis media | | |
| Penicillin | Amoxicillin | |

hearing occur. An upper respiratory tract infection or seasonal allergic rhinitis commonly precedes acute otitis media. Changes in equilibrium may occur. If the tympanic membrane ruptures, patients report a reduction or relief of ear pain.

## Drug Therapy

Table 60.1 lists the various drugs used to treat ear disorders.

### Otitis Externa

For acute otitis externa, use of topical agents, as opposed to systemic agents, is more common. Systemic medications are indicated only if a deep tissue infection develops outside the external canal or if immunocompromised status is an issue. Topical drugs are more effective because they deliver higher concentrations of medication to the infected, inflamed tissue. The use of these agents also reduces adverse effects.

When the infection extends to the pinna, prescribers order oral anti-infective agents. For necrotizing otitis externa, the primary treatment is systemic antipseudomonal antimicrobial agents. Ciprofloxacin is the drug of choice for adults, whereas cephalexin (Keflex) is the preferred drug for children (see Chaps. 18 and 19). The otic solutions most commonly prescribed for acute otitis externa are combination solutions. These medications contain an anti-infective agent, antiseptic, glucocorticoid, and acidifying agent.

### Otitis Media

Oral amoxicillin is the drug of choice for the treatment of acute otitis media (see Table 60.3). Patients who are allergic to penicillins may take cephalosporins.

 **QSEN Alert: Evidence-Based Practice**

A Cochrane Review [2020] explored whether topical antibiotics are effective in treating chronic necrotizing otitis externa and whether one type of topical antibiotic treatment is more effective than any other. It is unclear whether topical antibiotics contribute to the resolution of ear discharge in patients with chronic otitis media. There is some evidence that indicates that using topical antibiotics may be effective when compared to a placebo or when added to treatment with a systemic antibiotic, but certainty of evidence is very low. In addition, the type of topical antibiotic that would be the most effective is unclear.

## ANTI-INFECTIVE, ANTISEPTIC, GLUCOCORTICOID, AND ACIDIFYING AGENTS

Health care providers use the combination drug Ⓟ **neomycin–polymyxin B–hydrocortisone** for the treatment of acute external otitis media. Neomycin and polymyxin B are antibiotics, which combat bacterial infections. Hydrocortisone is a steroid, which reduces the actions of chemicals in the body that cause inflammation, redness, and swelling.

### Pharmacokinetics

The metabolism and transport effects of polymyxin and neomycin are unknown. Hydrocortisone is metabolized in the liver, and excretion occurs in the urine.

### Action

Each component of neomycin–polymyxin B–hydrocortisone suspension has its own mechanism of action. Neomycin, an aminoglycoside, inhibits bacterial protein synthesis by irreversibly binding to the 30S ribosome of the susceptible bacteria. Polymyxin B, a miscellaneous anti-infective agent, binds to the lipid phosphates in the bacterial cell membrane, which changes the membrane permeability to prevent leakage of cytoplasm from the bacterial cell wall, contributing to cell death. Hydrocortisone, a steroid, decreases inflammation by stabilizing the leukocyte lysosome membrane, inhibiting phagocytosis and release of allergic substances.

### Use

Health care providers use neomycin–polymyxin B–hydrocortisone suspension for the treatment of acute otitis externa caused by *P. aeruginosa, Proteus,* and *S. aureus.* Table 60.2 presents route and dosage information for neomycin–polymyxin B–hydrocortisone suspension.

### Use in Children

Authorities recommend neomycin–polymyxin B–hydrocortisone suspension in children only for bacterial infections of the external auditory canal due to the adverse effect of ototoxicity. The hydrocortisone may cause suppression of the hypothalamic–pituitary–adrenal axis in younger children.

| TABLE 60.2 |||||
| :--- | :--- | :--- | :--- | :--- |
| **DRUGS AT A GLANCE: Anti-infective, Antiseptic, Glucocorticoid, and Acidifying Drugs** |||||
| **Drug** | **Pregnancy Category** | **Routes and Dosage Ranges** || |
| | | **Adults** | **Children** |
| **Neomycin–polymyxin B–hydrocortisone** (✳ Odan-Spor-HC) | C | Instill 4 drops three to four times daily for no more than 10 d | 6 mo and older, 3 drops into affected ear three to four times daily for no more than 10 d |
| Neomycin–colistin–hydrocorti-sone–thonzonium (Coly-Mycin S Otic) | C | 5 drops in affected ear three to four times daily for no more than 10 d | 4 drops in affected ear three to four times daily for no more than 10 d |
| Ciprofloxacin–hydrocortisone (Cipro HC Otic; ✳ Cipro HC) | C | 3 drops in affected ear twice daily for 7 d | ≥1 y, 3 drops in affected ear twice daily for 7 d |
| Ofloxacin | C | Otitis media, chronic suppurative: 10 drops into affected ear twice daily for 14 d<br>Otitis externa: 10 drops into affected ear twice daily for 7 d | 1–12 y, 5 drops into affected ear twice daily for 10 d<br>≥13 y, same as adult |

## Adverse Effects and Contraindications

Adverse effects of neomycin–polymyxin B–hydrocortisone suspension include burning, stinging, and ototoxicity.

Contraindications include a known hypersensitivity to the drug's components. Prescribers should not order it for viral, fungal, or mycobacterial infections.

## Nursing Implications

### Preventing Interactions

Neomycin–polymyxin B–hydrocortisone suspension is associated with no significant drug or herbal interactions.

### Administering the Medication

Administration of neomycin–polymyxin B–hydrocortisone suspension is directly in the external ear canal. Prior to administering the otic suspension, it is necessary to shake the medication well. In addition, if cerumen is present, cleaning of the ear canal with a cotton swab is important.

> **! QSEN Alert: Safety**
>
> It is necessary to assess the tympanic membrane with an otoscope before inserting neomycin–polymyxin B–hydrocortisone suspension. If the tympanic membrane is torn, then the medication is absorbed directly by the inner ear, leading to hearing loss.

The proper administration of eardrops requires tilting the head toward the opposite shoulder, pulling the superior aspect of the auricle upward, and instilling the eardrops into the ear canal. The patient should then lie on the side opposite the side of administration for 20 minutes. To maximize medication absorption, the patient should have a cotton ball placed in the ear canal.

### Assessing for Therapeutic and Adverse Effects

The nurse assesses for decreased ear pain and itching as well as for decreased drainage from the ear canal.

It is also necessary to assess for signs of hearing loss due to ototoxicity. He or she also assesses for burning and stinging.

### Patient Teaching

Box 60.1 lists patient teaching guidelines for Cortisporin.

> **BOX 60.1** **Patient Teaching Guidelines for Neomycin–Polymyxin B–Hydrocortisone Suspension**
>
> • Use the eardrops properly. Put them directly in the ear canal. Prior to administering the otic suspension, it is necessary to shake the medication well. If any earwax is present, use a cotton swab to remove it.
>   • Tilt your head toward the opposite shoulder, pull the top of your outer ear upward, and put the eardrops into the ear canal.
>   • Then lie on the side opposite the side of administration for 20 minutes. To maximize medication absorption, place a cotton ball in your ear for that time.
> • Refrain from inserting anything in the ear canal.
> • Do not let water enter the ear canal during the treatment period. If you swim, use ear plugs, shake the ear dry after swimming, and use a blow dryer on the low setting 12 inches away to dry the ear canal.
> • Stop using the medication after 10 days.
> • Have a follow-up assessment in 1 to 2 weeks.

## Other Drugs in the Class

The otic drug Coly-Mycin, a combination of neomycin, colistin, hydrocortisone, and thonzonium, is an antibiotic and corticosteroid administered for ear inflammation and infection. Contraindications include a known hypersensitivity to aminoglycosides as well as the presence of herpes simplex, vaccinia, or varicella. The neomycin may cause cutaneous sensitization, with itching, redness, edema, and diminished healing.

The combination drug Cipro HC contains ciprofloxacin and hydrocortisone. Its twice-daily administration makes it more convenient for parents with young children.

Ofloxacin (otic form), which health care providers use for treatment of otitis externa and otitis media, is suitable for administration to a patient with a perforated tympanic membrane. This medication does not contain neomycin; therefore, there is no risk of ototoxicity.

### Clinical Application 60.1

- What does the nurse tell Derrick and his mother about the pathophysiology of otitis externa?
- What is the reason for the development of otitis externa in this case?
- With what signs and symptoms of otitis externa does the nurse expect Derrick to present?

### NCLEX Success

1. Which of the following patients are at risk for the development of otitis externa?
   A. a patient who wears ear plugs while swimming
   B. a patient who has hearing loss
   C. a patient who wears a hearing aid
   D. a patient with labyrinthitis

2. What is the duration of therapy for neomycin–polymyxin B–hydrocortisone?
   A. 5 days
   B. 8 days
   C. 10 days
   D. 14 days

3. Which of the following medications is administered for otitis externa and otitis media?
   A. ofloxacin
   B. Burow's solution
   C. benzyl alcohol
   D. acetic acid and hydrocortisone

4. Which of the following nursing actions should be implemented when instilling eardrops?
   A. Tilt the head toward the opposite shoulder.
   B. Lay on the affected ear after instillation.
   C. Apply the medication on a cotton ball and insert in the outer auricle.
   D. Apply ear plugs after instilling eardrops.

5. Which nursing action should be implemented prior to instilling eardrops?
   A. Evaluate the patient's pain level.
   B. Assess the amount of hearing loss.
   C. Instruct the patient to lie on the affected ear.
   D. Assess if cerumen is visible.

### Clinical Application 60.2

- What patient teaching does the nurse need to provide to Derrick and his mother?
- The state swim meet is in 2 weeks. Will Derrick be able to participate?
- What does the school nurse need to teach the swim coach to prevent further outbreaks of otitis externa?

## FLUOROQUINOLONE: CIPROFLOXACIN

The fluoroquinolone **ciprofloxacin** (Cipro) is the drug of choice for necrotizing otitis externa. Initially, administration is intravenous, until symptoms decrease; then it is oral. A suspension is available, as indicated.

### Pharmacokinetics

The intravenous preparation has an onset of action in 10 minutes, with a peak of action in 30 minutes and duration of 4 to 5 hours. Onset of action for the oral preparation varies, with a peak of action in 60 to 90 minutes, and the same duration of action. The intravenous and oral preparations are absorbed rapidly and distributed to the kidneys, gallbladder, liver, lungs, gynecologic or prostate tissue, and cerebrospinal fluid. It is 20% to 40% protein bound, and partial metabolism takes place in the liver. The serum half-life is 3 to 5 hours with normal renal function. The excretion of the drug occurs in the urine and feces.

### Action

Ciprofloxacin inhibits DNA gyrase in susceptible organisms and inhibits the supercoiled DNA, promoting breakage of the double-stranded DNA.

### Use

Health care providers use ciprofloxacin for the treatment of *P. aeruginosa* in patients with necrotizing otitis externa. The cure rate with fluoroquinolones is approximately 90%. (If the causative agent is *Aspergillus*, amphotericin B is the drug of choice [see Chap. 24].) Table 60.3 gives route and dosage information for ciprofloxacin and other oral anti-infective drugs.

#### Use in Patients With Renal Impairment

Dosage adjustment is necessary for patients with renal impairment (see Chap. 19).

### Adverse Effects

Patients generally tolerate ciprofloxacin well. The most frequent adverse effects are gastrointestinal (GI) and include nausea,

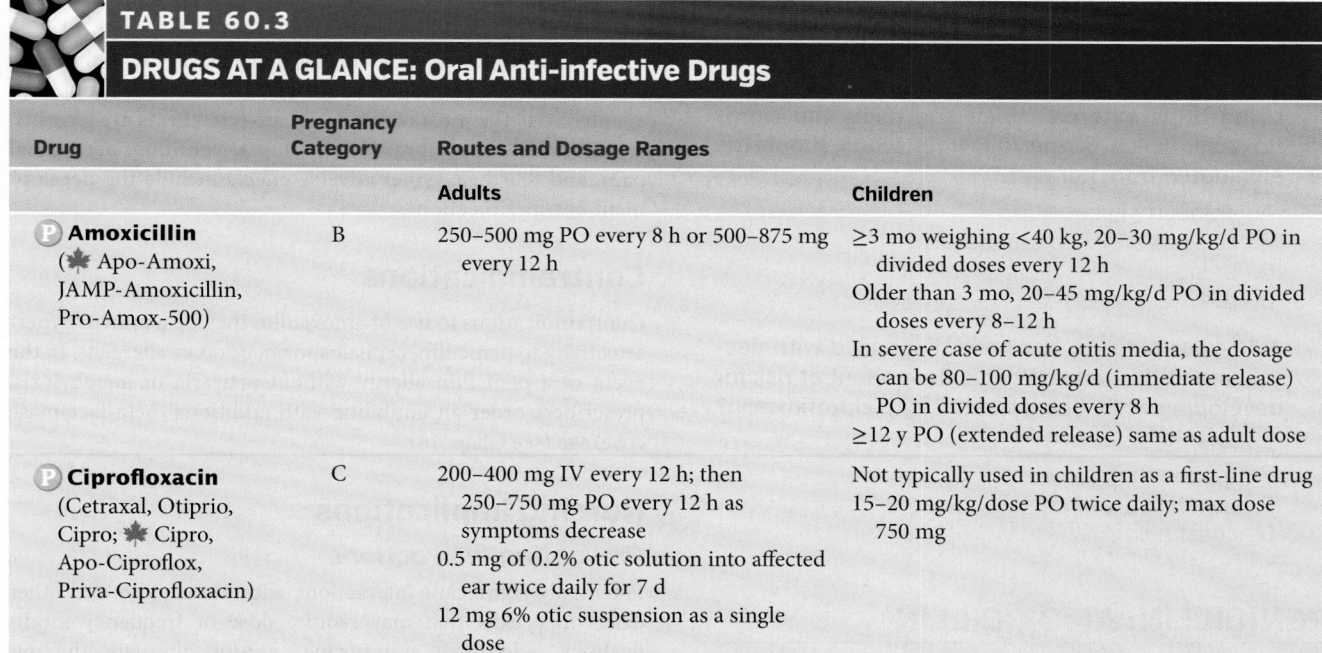

### TABLE 60.3
### DRUGS AT A GLANCE: Oral Anti-infective Drugs

| Drug | Pregnancy Category | Routes and Dosage Ranges | |
|------|--------------------|-------------------------|---|
| | | **Adults** | **Children** |
| Ⓟ **Amoxicillin** (✸ Apo-Amoxi, JAMP-Amoxicillin, Pro-Amox-500) | B | 250–500 mg PO every 8 h or 500–875 mg every 12 h | ≥3 mo weighing <40 kg, 20–30 mg/kg/d PO in divided doses every 12 h Older than 3 mo, 20–45 mg/kg/d PO in divided doses every 8–12 h In severe case of acute otitis media, the dosage can be 80–100 mg/kg/d (immediate release) PO in divided doses every 8 h ≥12 y PO (extended release) same as adult dose |
| Ⓟ **Ciprofloxacin** (Cetraxal, Otiprio, Cipro; ✸ Cipro, Apo-Ciproflox, Priva-Ciprofloxacin) | C | 200–400 mg IV every 12 h; then 250–750 mg PO every 12 h as symptoms decrease 0.5 mg of 0.2% otic solution into affected ear twice daily for 7 d 12 mg 6% otic suspension as a single dose | Not typically used in children as a first-line drug 15–20 mg/kg/dose PO twice daily; max dose 750 mg |

vomiting, and abdominal discomfort. Dizziness and mild headache may occur. There are reports of allergic and skin reactions. Photosensitivity can occur while taking ciprofloxacin with exposure to direct or indirect sunlight. Artificial light or sun lamps may also precipitate photosensitivity reactions. The U.S. Food and Drug Administration (FDA) has expanded the current **BLACK BOX WARNING ◆** for fluoroquinolones, including ciprofloxacin, not only alerting health professionals to the increased disabling risk of tendinitis and tendon rupture but also the significant risk of peripheral neuropathy, central nervous system and cardiac effects, and dermatologic and hypersensitivity reactions. The risk is greater for people older than 60 years of age; those with heart, kidney, and lung transplants; and those taking corticosteroid medications. Adverse effects can occur up to weeks after beginning fluoroquinolones and may potentially be permanent. Discontinuation of the drug is necessary with the development of adverse effects. Another **BLACK BOX WARNING ◆** exists for fluoroquinolones, including ciprofloxacin, because the drugs in this class may exacerbate muscle weakness in persons with myasthenia gravis; their use should be avoided in these patients. QT interval prolongation may occur, and the degree of severity varies by agent.

## Contraindications

Patients with a known sensitivity to ciprofloxacin should not receive the drug or any other fluoroquinolone. Administration of ciprofloxacin with tizanidine is contraindicated.

## Nursing Implications

### Preventing Interactions

Many medications, herbs, and foods interact with ciprofloxacin, increasing or decreasing its effects (see Boxes 19.2 and 19.3).

### Administering the Medication

Parenteral administration of ciprofloxacin should occur over 60 minutes through a verified patent intravenous line. If signs

and symptoms of hypersensitivity develop, it is important to discontinue the medication. Patients may take the oral preparation with food to reduce GI upset. However, they should not take it within 2 hours of eating dairy products, calcium-fortified juices, antacids, zinc, or iron. Enteral feedings should be discontinued for 1 to 2 hours prior to and after ciprofloxacin administration because drug absorption is decreased by more than 30% with enteral feedings.

### Assessing for Therapeutic and Adverse Effects

The nurse assesses for diminished pain with chewing, otalgia, and otorrhea. He or she also assesses the patient's renal function during the course of treatment. It is also important to observe for any signs or symptoms of hypersensitivity to the medication.

### Patient Teaching

Patient teaching guidelines for ciprofloxacin are listed in the Box 60.2.

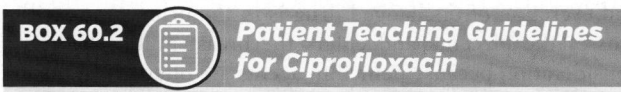

**BOX 60.2**    **Patient Teaching Guidelines for Ciprofloxacin**

- Avoid exposure to sunlight and apply sunscreen during the course of drug treatment.
- Do not operate machinery or drive if experiencing dizziness or light-headedness occurs.
- Stay well hydrated during the course of treatment.
- Do not drink calcium-fortified juices or dairy products while taking the drug.
- Do not take antacids, zinc, or iron supplements during the course of drug treatment.
- Report tendon pain to the primary care provider.
- Report nausea, vomiting, or diarrhea.

# PENICILLIN: AMOXICILLIN

**(P) Amoxicillin**, a penicillin, is the preferred antibacterial agent for the treatment of acute otitis media unless a child has received the drug within 30 days, also has purulent conjunctivitis, or is allergic to the drug. A consensus group convened by the Centers for Disease Control and Prevention recommended increasing the dose used for empiric treatment because of concerns about increasingly resistant strains of *S. pneumoniae,* which are theoretically susceptible to a higher dose. Combination of amoxicillin with clavulanic acid reestablishes amoxicillin's activity against beta-lactamase–producing bacteria, including *H. influenzae* and penicillinase-producing anaerobes.

Many people with acute otitis media do not benefit from antibiotics because the cause of their illness is not bacterial in origin, or their immune system clears the infection without the use of a drug. Unfortunately, no clinical criteria currently distinguish people with acute otitis media who require antibiotic therapy from those who do not.

## Pharmacokinetics

Amoxicillin has a variable onset of action; it reaches a peak in 1 hour. The duration of action is 6 to 8 hours. The therapeutic half-life is 1 to 1.4 hours. Metabolism occurs in the liver, and excretion of unchanged drug is in the urine. Amoxicillin crosses the placenta and enters the breast milk, which is a consideration because penicillin agents are often given during pregnancy.

## Action

Amoxicillin has bactericidal properties. It inhibits cell wall synthesis of sensitive organisms, resulting in cell death.

## Use

Amoxicillin is administered for the treatment of acute otitis media. It is active against *S. pneumoniae, H. influenzae,* and *Streptococcus pyogenes.*

## Adverse Effects

The most common adverse effect is hypersensitivity to the medication, with the development of a rash or severe reactions with anaphylaxis. The most common GI adverse effects are glossitis, stomatitis, gastritis, sore throat, nausea, vomiting, abdominal pain, and diarrhea. Other adverse effects include the development of superinfections.

## Contraindications

Contraindications to use of amoxicillin include a known hypersensitivity to penicillin, cephalosporin, or other allergens. In the event of a penicillin allergy without urticaria or anaphylaxis, prescribers order an antibiotic with additional beta-lactamase coverage (see Chap. 18).

## Nursing Implications

### Preventing Interactions

Potentially significant interactions with amoxicillin and other drugs may exist that may require dose or frequency modifications, additional monitoring, and/or alternate therapy. Amoxicillin may diminish or enhance the therapeutic effects of other drugs. Amoxicillin may diminish the therapeutic of several vaccines (i.e., cholera, bacillus Calmette-Guérin, and typhoid), mycophenolate, lactobacillus, and estriol. The drug may enhance the anticoagulant effects of vitamin K antagonists (e.g., warfarin) and methotrexate. Box 60.3 lists drugs that increase or decrease the effect of amoxicillin. No significant herbal interactions have been identified.

### Administering the Medication

Amoxicillin is administered orally. It is necessary to take amoxicillin in divided doses around the clock within 1 hour of a meal. The patient should take the full course of antibiotics and not discontinue them, even if the otitis media seems to be improving.

### Assessing for Therapeutic Effects

The nurse assesses for otalgia and otorrhea. Both pain and drainage may decrease with antibiotic therapy. It is also necessary to assess the patient's hearing. As the fullness of the tympanic membrane decreases, the patient reports improvement in hearing. The nurse inspects the tympanic membrane for bulging (see Fig. 60.1). As the infection resolves, the tympanic membrane becomes shiny gray with a visible cone of light from the otoscope (Fig. 60.2).

**BOX 60.3** **Drug Interactions: Amoxicillin**

**Drugs That Decrease the Effects of Amoxicillin**
- Chloramphenicol and tetracycline
  *Cause inhibition of the activity of amoxicillin*

**Drug That Increases the Effects of Amoxicillin**
- Probenecid
  *Prolongs the serum concentration and activity of amoxicillin*

**Figure 60.2.** Normal tympanic membrane, after resolution of otitis media. [Adapted with permission from Moore, K. L., Dalley, A. F., & Agur, A. M. R. (2018). *Essential clinical anatomy* (8th ed., Fig. B8.42). Philadelphia, PA: Wolters Kluwer Health.]

---

### ⚠ QSEN Alert: Evidence-Based Practice

Approximately 95% of children in the United States with acute otitis media receive antibiotic therapy. In an update of a previous review, Venekamp, Sanders, Glasziou, Del Mar, and Rovers (2015) assessed the effects of antibiotics compared to a placebo on relief of symptoms of acute otitis media and complications of the disease in children. The authors judged that evidence from combined results from thirteen randomized control trials meeting eligibility criteria was of high quality for most of the outcomes in the review. Findings indicated that antibiotics were not particularly useful for most children with acute otitis media, did not decrease the number of children with pain at 24 hours (when 60% of children were better anyway), and reduced the number of children with pain after 24 hours only slightly. In addition, adverse events (e.g., vomiting, diarrhea, rash) occurred more often in children taking antibiotics. In a subset of included trials, a meta-analysis of individual patient data found antibiotics to be most beneficial in children younger than 2 years with bilateral acute otitis media or with both acute otitis media and otorrhea.

## Assessing for Adverse Effects

The nurse assesses the patient for signs and symptoms of hypersensitivity, with symptoms of wheezing, rash, or difficulty breathing. It is also important to assess for GI adverse effects such as nausea, vomiting, stomatitis, mouth irritation, sore throat, abdominal pain, and diarrhea. In addition, the nurse assesses for signs of superinfection.

## Patient Teaching

Box 60.4 lists patient teaching guidelines for amoxicillin.

---

## NCLEX Success

8. A child receives a diagnosis of acute otitis media. His physician orders amoxicillin. The onset of which of the following adverse effects warrants the discontinuation of the medication?
   A. diarrhea
   B. abdominal pain
   C. diminished appetite
   D. wheezing

9. Which of the following assessment findings reveals that the amoxicillin is decreasing the symptoms of acute otitis media?
   A. retracted tympanic membrane
   B. otalgia
   C. otorrhea
   D. visible cone of light

10. A 76-year-old woman is receiving amoxicillin for acute otitis media. She also has gout. Which of the following antigout medications increases the effect of amoxicillin?
    A. allopurinol
    B. probenecid
    C. aspirin
    D. acetaminophen

---

### Unfolding Patient Stories: Toua Xiong • Part 2

Think back to Toua Xiong, a 64-year-old male with emphysema from Chapter 33. He presents to the clinic with left ear pain and fever following an upper respiratory infection. The provider prescribes amoxicillin for acute otitis media. What patient education would the nurse provide on amoxicillin and the treatment options for fever and pain relief? How would the nurse differentiate a hypersensitivity reaction to amoxicillin from worsening respiratory symptoms associated with an acute exacerbation of emphysema?

Care for Toua and other patients in a realistic virtual environment: *vSim for Nursing* (thepoint.lww.com/vSim-Pharm). Practice documenting these patients' care in DocuCare (thepoint.lww.com/DocuCareEHR).

---

### BOX 60.4 📋 *Patient Teaching Guidelines for Amoxicillin*

**Self or Caregiver Administration**

• Ensure that the child takes the entire course of the drug.
• Administer the drug around the clock.
• Take the medication within an hour of completing a meal.
• Report persistent ear pain or diminished hearing.

# ADJUVANT MEDICATIONS TO TREAT PAIN AND FEVER RELATED TO INFECTIONS OF THE EAR

Infections of the ear produce pain and may result in fever. The adjuvant medications most commonly administered for relief of pain and fever include agents such as aspirin, acetaminophen (Tylenol), or ibuprofen (Motrin) (see Chap. 16).

## Salicylates

**P Aspirin** is the prototype of the salicylates. Children should not take this drug. Aspirin has the ability to inhibit prostaglandin synthesis (a cause of the inflammatory effect). Its role in fever reduction, or antipyretic action, is not understood. Experts believe that aspirin acts on the thermoregulatory center of the hypothalamus, blocking the effects of the endogenous pyrogens and inhibiting the synthesis of prostaglandins. Administration is oral or rectal. To prevent gastric irritation, it is necessary to take the oral preparation with food.

## Nonnarcotic Analgesic Antipyretic

Acetaminophen is equivalent to aspirin in analgesic and antipyretic effects, and it possesses weak anti-inflammatory properties. This drug is safe for children. It acts directly on the hypothalamus to increase vasodilation and sweating. Although the primary mechanism of action of acetaminophen is not fully understood, it is believed to inhibit cyclooxygenase (COX), with a predominant effect on COX-2. Acetaminophen is oral or rectal. Alternating acetaminophen and ibuprofen every 4 hours over a 3-day period to control fever in young children (ages 6–36 months) has been shown to be more effective than monotherapy with either agent. A discussion of the prototype considerations is found in Chapter 16.

## Propionic Acid Derivatives

Ibuprofen (Motrin, Advil) is a nonsteroidal anti-inflammatory agent that inhibits prostaglandin synthesis in both the central and peripheral nervous systems. There are two forms of cyclooxygenase, COX-1 and COX-2. Ibuprofen blocks prostaglandin synthesis and modulates T-cell production, inhibiting the chemotaxis of the inflammatory cells and increasing their destruction. The drug blocks COX-1 and COX-2 and is more selective with COX-1. It is administered to reduce pain, inflammation, and fever. Ibuprofen is administered orally or intravenously. For treatment of otalgia and fever, the drug is administered orally. Chapter 16 describes ibuprofen as a prototype.

## THE NURSING PROCESS

A concept map outlines the nursing process related to drug therapy considerations in this chapter. Additional nursing implications related to the disease process should also be considered in care decisions.

**Assessment**
- Assess for diminished hearing and signs of ear infection.
- Inspect the external ear and palpate the auricle and surrounding tissue.
- Inspect for alterations in skin integrity of the outer ear.
- Inspect the tympanic membrane with an otoscope.
- Assess for fluid in the eardrum and absence of the cone of light.
- Interview the patient related to fullness of the ear, diminished hearing, or pain.
- Assess temperature.

**Outcomes of Therapy**
The patient will
- Take the entire course of anti-infective agents safely and accurately.
- Take anti-inflammatory/antipyretic agents as ordered to reduce pain and fever.
- Not insert any items in the ear.
- Use earplugs when swimming.
- Dry the ear carefully following bathing or swimming.

**Nursing Interventions**
- Instruct the patient on the administration of ear drops.
- Instruct on the medication regimen and about administration of anti-infective agents around the clock.
- Assess the tympanic membrane for signs of infection.
- Assess the lesion of the external ear for signs of healing.
- Instruct parents to never let a baby sleep drinking a bottle (this promotes the development of otitis media).
- Administer pain and fever reducers as needed.
- Assess for ear drainage.

**Evaluation**
- Interview the patient for relief of symptoms with the completion of the course of anti-infective agents.
- Interview the patient regarding compliance with the medication regimen.
- Assess the external and middle ear for signs of infection or inflammation.

## KEY CONCEPTS

- Otitis externa is a disorder of the external ear that produces inflammation.
- Malignant necrotizing otitis externa occurs in elderly patients with diabetes or in patients who are immunocompromised. The causative agent is *P. aeruginosa*.
- Anti-infective, antiseptic, glucocorticoid, and acidifying agents such as neomycin–polymyxin B–hydrocortisone suspension are administered to treat otitis externa.
- Antipseudomonal antimicrobial agents are the primary therapy for malignant necrotizing otitis externa.
- Otitis media is inflammation of the middle ear and is most common in children but can also occur in adults.
- Oral amoxicillin is the drug of choice for the treatment of acute otitis media.
- Infections of the ear produce pain and may result in fever. The adjuvant medications most commonly administered for

relief of pain and fever include agents such as aspirin, acetaminophen (Tylenol), and ibuprofen (Motrin).
- The FDA has expanded the current **BLACK BOX WARNING ◆** for fluoroquinolones, including ciprofloxacin, alerting health professionals to not only the increased disabling risk of tendinitis and tendon rupture but also the significant risk of peripheral neuropathy, central nervous system and cardiac effects, and dermatologic and hypersensitivity reactions.
- Another **BLACK BOX WARNING ◆** exists for fluoroquinolones, including ciprofloxacin, because the drugs may exacerbate muscle weakness in persons with myasthenia gravis; their use should be avoided in these patients. QT interval prolongation may occur, and the degree of severity varies by agent.

## CLINICAL REASONING CASE STUDY

### Meet the Patient

Cara Hwang calls the pediatric division at the local children's hospital seeking information. She says her 3-month-old daughter, Liliana, has been up all night crying and pulling on her right ear. She thinks the baby may have a fever, but she does not have a thermometer.

- What information does the nurse convey to the mother?
- What does the nurse suspect is wrong with the baby?
- What patient teaching should the emergency department nurse provide to the mother regarding the administration of amoxicillin (Moxatag), as well as acetaminophen (Tylenol) and ibuprofen (Motrin, Advil) if ordered for Liliana?

### Assessing Drug Information

Amoxicillin
- This drug has bactericidal properties. It inhibits cell wall synthesis of sensitive organisms, resulting in cell death.
- Amoxicillin is used to treat infections due to beta-lactamase-negative *Streptococcus* (alpha- and beta-hemolytic isolates only), *S. pneumoniae, Staphylococcus,* or *H. influenzae.*
- Adverse effects include rash (and other signs of hypersensitivity), glossitis, stomatitis, gastritis, sore throat, nausea, vomiting, abdominal pain, and diarrhea.

Acetaminophen
- Actions of acetaminophen are as follows:
  - Although the primary mechanism of action of this drug is not fully understood, it is believed to inhibit cyclooxygenase (COX), with a predominant effect on COX-2. It acts directly on the hypothalamus to increase vasodilation and sweating.
  - This drug has antipyretic and analgesic actions but very weak anti-inflammatory activity.
- This drug may relieve mild to moderate otalgia and fever.
- Adverse effects include skin rash and metabolic and electrolyte imbalances.

Ibuprofen
- Actions of ibuprofen are as follows:
  - This drug reversibly inhibits COX-1 and COX-2 enzymes, which results in decreased formation of prostaglandin precursors.
  - It has antipyretic, analgesic, and anti-inflammatory properties.
- This drug may relieve mild to moderate otalgia and fever.
- Adverse effects include dizziness, skin rash, epigastric pain, heartburn, and tinnitus.

### Nursing Actions

- The nurse should inform the mother to take the infant to the emergency department to be assessed for acute otitis media. Given the infant's age and lack of information about the presence of a fever, it is important that the infant be checked. Infants younger than 1 year of age are at risk for febrile seizures.
- If Liliana is diagnosed with acute otitis media and is placed on amoxicillin, acetaminophen, and ibuprofen, the nurse teaches the mother to
  - Use strategies to enhance the administration of the amoxicillin suspension, such as administration with an oral syringe.
  - Administer the medication around the clock after feeding.
  - Keep the appointment for an ear recheck. Provide the date and time, if necessary.
  - Notify the prescriber if the amoxicillin is not effective. It may be necessary to switch to amoxicillin-clavulanate.
  - For a temperature of more than 101°F, alternate acetaminophen with ibuprofen every 2 hours. Explain that alternating acetaminophen and ibuprofen every 4 hours over a 3-day period to control fever in young children (ages 6–36 months) has been shown to be more effective than monotherapy with either agent.

---

*Visit* thePoint® *at* **http://thePoint.lww.com/Frandsen12e** *for answers to NCLEX Success questions (in Appendix A), answers to Clinical Application Case Studies (in Appendix B), and more!*

## REFERENCES AND RESOURCES

Brennan-Jones, C. G., Head, K., Chong, L. Y., Burton, M. J., Schilder, A. G. M., & Bhutta, M. F. (2020). Topical antibiotics for chronic suppurative otitis media. *The Cochrane Database of Systematic Reviews,* (1), CD013051. doi:10.1002/14651858.CD013051.pub2

Gandis, J. R., & Yu, V. L. (2020). Malignant (necrotizing) external otitis. In *UpToDate,* Lexicomp, Inc.

Goguen, L. A. (2020). External otitis: Treatment. In *UpToDate,* Lexicomp, Inc.

Hinkle, J. H., & Cheever, K. H. (2018). *Brunner & Suddarth's textbook of medical-surgical nursing* (14th ed.). Philadelphia, PA: Wolters Kluwer.

Karch, A. M., & Tucker, R. (2019). *2020 Lippincott's pocket drug guide for nurses* (8th ed.). Philadelphia, PA: Lippincott Williams & Wilkins.

Limb, C. J., Lustig, L. R., & Durand, M. L. (2020). Acute otitis media in adults. In *UpToDate,* Lexicomp, Inc.

Norris, T. L. (2019). *Porth's pathophysiology: Concepts of altered health states* (10th ed.). Philadelphia, PA: Wolters Kluwer.

Sjoukes, A., Venekamp, R. P., van de Pol, A. C., Hay, A. D., Little, P., Schilder, A. G., et al. (2016). Paracetamol (acetaminophen) or nonsteroidal anti-inflammatory drugs, alone or combined, for pain relief in acute otitis media in children. *The Cochrane Database of Systematic Reviews,* (12), CD011534. doi:10.1002/14651858.CD011534.pub2

UpToDate. (2020). *Drug information.* Lexi-Comp, Inc.

Venekamp, R. P., Sanders, S. L., Glasziou, P. P., Del Mar, G. B., & Rovers, M. M. (2015). Antibiotics for acute otitis media in children. *The Cochrane Database of Systematic Reviews,* (23), CD000219. doi:10.1002/14651858

# Drug Therapy for Disorders of the Skin

## LEARNING OBJECTIVES

*After studying this chapter, you should be able to:*

1. Identify the disorders of the skin.
2. Recognize age-related considerations in children and adolescents with acne vulgaris.
3. Identify drug therapy for the treatment of acne vulgaris and drug therapy for other skin disorders.
4. Identify the prototype and describe the action, use, adverse effects, contraindications, and nursing implications for the retinoids.
5. Implement the nursing process in the care of the patient with disorders of the skin.

## CLINICAL APPLICATION CASE STUDY

Gerard Aylward is a 16-year-old high school sophomore who has a history of asthma. As a child, he received allergy shots on a weekly basis. He now has a severe case of acne vulgaris. He has been taking tetracycline hydrochloride 500 mg orally every 12 hours. His acne remains severe, and his dermatologist has decided to discontinue the tetracycline and start isotretinoin 35 mg orally two times per day for 15 weeks.

## KEY TERMS

**Acne vulgaris:** common disorder characterized by excessive production of sebum and obstruction of hair follicles, which normally carry sebum to the skin surface

**Dermatitis:** general term denoting an inflammatory response of the skin to injuries, irritants, allergens, or trauma; also referred to as eczema

**Erythema:** redness of the skin

**Pruritus:** itching

**Psoriasis:** scaling, dry, erythematous skin eruptions on the elbows, knees, scalp, and trunk

**Rosacea:** chronic disease characterized by erythema, telangiectases (fine, red, superficial blood vessels), and acne-like lesions of facial skin

**Tinea pedis:** common type of ringworm infection; also called athlete's foot

**Toxic epidermal necrolysis:** Wide spread sloughing of the skin with severe mucositis

**Urticaria:** inflammatory response characterized by a skin lesion called a wheal, a raised edematous area with a pale center and red border, which itches intensely; also known as hives

# INTRODUCTION

This chapter discusses the disorders of the skin. In addition, it introduces acne vulgaris and the drugs administered for their treatment.

# DISORDERS OF THE SKIN

Dermatologic disorders may be primary (i.e., originate in the skin or mucous membranes) or secondary (i.e., result from a systemic condition, such as measles or adverse drug reactions).

## Inflammatory Disorders

### Dermatitis

**Dermatitis**, also called eczema, is a general term denoting an inflammatory response of the skin to injuries from irritants, allergens, or trauma. Whatever the cause, dermatitis is usually characterized by **erythema** (redness), **pruritus** (itching), and skin lesions. It may be acute or chronic.

Atopic dermatitis is a common disorder characterized by dry skin, pruritus, and lesions that vary according to the extent of inflammation, stages of healing, and scratching. Scratching damages the skin and increases the risk of secondary infection. Acute lesions are reddened skin areas containing papules and vesicles; chronic lesions are often thick, fibrotic, and nodular. The cause is uncertain but may involve allergic, hereditary, or psychological elements. Exposure to possible causes or exacerbating factors such as allergens, irritating chemicals, foods, and emotional stress are factors to consider.

Contact dermatitis results from direct contact with irritants (e.g., soaps, detergents) or allergens (e.g., clothing materials or dyes, jewelry [nickel], cosmetics) that stimulate inflammation. Irritants cause tissue damage and dermatitis in anyone with sufficient contact or exposure. Allergens cause dermatitis only in sensitized or hypersensitive people. The most common sensitizer in North America is the plant oleoresin urushiol found in poison ivy, poison oak, and poison sumac. The fruit of ginkgoes and the skin of mangoes also contain urushiol and can cause an allergic contact dermatitis. The location of the dermatitis may indicate the cause (e.g., facial dermatitis may indicate an allergy to cosmetics). Hypersensitivity to drugs, including topical hydrocortisone, benzocaine, and topical bacitracin and neomycin, can also cause an allergic contact dermatitis.

Seborrheic dermatitis is a chronic, relapsing disease involving the sebaceous glands. The cause of the condition is unknown but tends to worsen with stress and during the cold, dry winter months. The disease is characterized by excessive production of sebum by the scalp, face, external ear, or trunk. A simple form involving the scalp is dandruff, which is characterized by flaking and itching of the skin. More severe forms are characterized by greasy, yellow scales or crusts with variable amounts of erythema and itching. Repeated or long-term treatment is often necessary. Available treatment options include topical corticosteroids (see Chap. 17), topical antifungal drugs (see Chap. 24), and several topical agents with nonspecific, antimicrobial, anti-inflammatory, or keratolytic actions.

Drug-induced skin reactions can occur with virtually any drug and can resemble the signs and symptoms of virtually any skin disorder. Topical drugs usually cause a localized, contact dermatitis type of reaction, and systemic drugs cause generalized skin lesions. Skin manifestations of serious drug reactions include erythema, facial edema, pain, blisters, necrosis, and urticaria. Systemic manifestations may include fever, enlarged lymph nodes, joint pain or inflammation, shortness of breath, hypotension, and leukocytosis. Drug-related reactions usually occur within the 1st or 2nd week of drug administration and subside when the drug is discontinued.

### Urticaria

**Urticaria** (hives) is an inflammatory response characterized by a skin lesion called a wheal, a raised edematous area with a pale center and red border, which itches intensely. Histamine, the most common mediator of urticaria, causes vasodilation, increased vascular permeability, and pruritus. Mast cells and basophils release histamine as a result of both allergic (e.g., insect bites, foods, drugs) and nonallergic (e.g., radiocontrast media, opiates, heat, cold, pressure, ultraviolet [UV] light) stimuli. An important difference between allergic and nonallergic reactions is that many allergic reactions require prior exposure to the stimulus, whereas nonallergic reactions can occur with the first exposure.

### Psoriasis

**Psoriasis** is a chronic, inflammatory disorder attributed to activated T lymphocytes, which produce cytokines that stimulate abnormal growth of affected skin cells and blood vessels. The abnormal growth results in excessively rapid turnover of epidermal cells. Instead of 30 days from formation to elimination of normal epidermal cells, epidermal cells involved in psoriasis are abnormal in structure and have a life span of about 4 days. Skin lesions of psoriasis are erythematous, dry, and scaling. The lesions may occur anywhere on the body but commonly involve the skin covering bony prominences, such as the elbows and knees. Skin lesions may be tender, but they do not usually cause severe pain or itching. However, the lesions are unsightly and usually cause embarrassment and mental distress.

This skin disease is characterized by remissions and exacerbations. Exacerbating factors include infections, winter weather, some drugs (e.g., beta-adrenergic blockers, lithium), and possibly stress, obesity, and alcoholism.

### Rosacea

**Rosacea** is a chronic disease characterized by erythema, telangiectases (fine, red, superficial blood vessels), and acne-like lesions of facial skin. Hyperplasia of the nose (rhinophyma) eventually develops. The disorder usually occurs in middle-aged and older people, and it is more common in men. The etiology is thought to be excessive production of certain inflammatory proteins. Spicy foods, heat, alcohol, and embarrassment can worsen the condition.

## Toxic Epidermal Necrolysis and Stevens-Johnson Syndrome

**Toxic epidermal necrolysis** is the widespread sloughing of the skin and development of severe mucositis that is associated with a risk of sepsis. The patient has acute or chronic symptoms of systemic illness with generalized blisters. Stevens-Johnson syndrome is a generalized blistering with skin sloughing. The most common cause of Stevens-Johnson syndrome is related to an adverse effect of a medication. The patient experiences a prodromal period with fever and flulike symptoms. Following the prodromal period, the patient develops diffuse macular erythema that progress to vesicles, bullae, and skin sloughing.

The onset of toxic epidermal necrolysis is 4 days to 8 weeks of continuous use of a drug. Common drugs that result in Stevens-Johnson syndrome are allopurinol, lamotrigine, sulfasalazine, nevirapine, and oxicam. Amoxicillin and ampicillin have also been linked to Stevens-Johnson syndrome.

## Dermatologic Infections

### Bacterial Infections

Bacterial infections of the skin are common; they are most often caused by streptococci or staphylococci.

- Cellulitis is characterized by erythema, tenderness, and edema, which may spread to subcutaneous tissue. Generalized malaise, chills, and fever may occur.
- Folliculitis is an infection of the hair follicles that most often occurs on the scalp or bearded areas of the face.
- Furuncles and carbuncles are infections usually caused by staphylococci. Furuncles (boils) may result from folliculitis and tend to recur. They usually occur in the neck, face, axillae, buttocks, thighs, and perineum. Carbuncles involve many hair follicles and include multiple pustules. Carbuncles may cause fever, malaise, leukocytosis, and bacteremia. Healing of carbuncles often produces scar tissue.
- Impetigo is a superficial skin infection caused by streptococci or staphylococci.

### Fungal Infections

Fungal infections of the skin and mucous membranes are most often caused by *Candida albicans*.

- Oral candidiasis (thrush) involves mucous membranes of the mouth. It often occurs as a superinfection after the use of broad-spectrum systemic antibiotics.
- Candidiasis of the vagina and vulva occurs with systemic antibiotic therapy and in women with diabetes mellitus.
- Intertrigo involves skin folds or areas where two skin surfaces are in contact (e.g., groin, pendulous breasts).
- Tinea infections (ringworm) are caused by fungi (dermatophytes). These infections may involve the scalp (tinea capitis), the body (tinea corporis), the foot (tinea pedis), and other areas of the body. **Tinea pedis**, commonly called athlete's foot, is a type of ringworm infection.

### Viral Infections

Viral infections of the skin include verrucae (warts) and herpes infections. There are two types of herpes simplex infections: type 1 usually involves the face or neck (e.g., fever blisters or cold sores on the lips) and type 2 involves the genitalia. Other herpes infections include varicella (chickenpox) and herpes zoster (shingles).

## Trauma

Trauma refers to a physical injury that disrupts the skin. When the skin is broken, it may not be able to function properly. The major problem associated with skin wounds is infection. Common wounds include lacerations (cuts or tears), abrasions (shearing or scraping of the skin), puncture wounds, surgical incisions, and burns.

## Ulcerations

Cutaneous ulcerations are usually caused by trauma and impaired circulation. They may become inflamed or infected.

- Pressure ulcers (also called decubitus ulcers) may occur anywhere on the body when external pressure decreases blood flow. Older adults often have thin, dry skin and are at risk of pressure ulcers. Pressure ulcers are most likely to develop in patients who are immobilized, incontinent, malnourished, and debilitated. Common sites include the sacrum, trochanters, ankles, and heels. In addition, abraded skin is susceptible to infection and ulcer formation.
- Venous stasis ulcers, which usually occur on the legs, result from impaired venous circulation. Other signs of venous insufficiency include edema, varicose veins, stasis dermatitis, and brown skin pigmentation. Bacterial infection may occur in the ulcer.

## Anorectal Disorders

Hemorrhoids and anal fissures are common anorectal disorders characterized by pruritus, bleeding, and pain. Inflammation and infection may occur.

## Acne

Acne is a common disorder characterized by excessive production of sebum and obstruction of hair follicles, which normally carry sebum to the skin surface. As a result, hair follicles expand and form comedones (blackheads and whiteheads). Acne lesions vary from small comedones to **acne vulgaris**, the most severe form, in which follicles become infected and irritating secretions leak into surrounding tissues to form inflammatory pustules, cysts, and abscesses. Most patients have a variety of lesion types at one time. At least four pathologic events take place within acne-infected hair follicles: (1) androgen-mediated stimulation of sebaceous gland activity; (2) abnormal keratinization leading to follicular plugging (comedone formation); (3) proliferation of the bacterium *Propionibacterium acnes* within the follicle; and (4) inflammation.

Acne occurs most often on the face, upper back, and chest because there are large numbers of sebaceous glands in these areas. One etiologic factor is increased secretion of male hormones (androgens), which occurs at puberty in both sexes. This leads to increased production of sebum and proliferation of *P. acnes*, which depend on sebum for survival. *P. acnes* bacteria contain lipase enzymes that break down free fatty acids and produce inflammation in acne lesions. Other causative factors may include medications (e.g., phenytoin, corticosteroids) and stress (i.e., the stress mechanism may involve stimulation of androgen secretion).

 **QSEN Alert: Safety**

The development of acne is not related to a lack of facial hygiene. The use of harsh astringents, abrasives, or vigorous scrubbing can worsen acne and the likelihood of inflammation and scarring.

Scientists have explored the role of diet in acne development for decades. Several research trials have noted that a low dietary glycemic load provides superior reduction in the number of inflammatory acne lesions in teenagers. Previous studies found no evidence that the ingestion of certain foods or dietary constituents (e.g., chocolate, zinc, antioxidants) play a role in acne development. However, based on a variety of emerging data, there is renewed interest in reinvestigating the effects of diet on acne development and management.

## NCLEX Success

1. Androgens play a role in the development of acne vulgaris by increasing production of which of the following?
   A. testosterone
   B. estrogen
   C. sebum
   D. facial oil

2. A woman is taking dexamethasone for increased pain and inflammation in her right heel. She states that she has developed acne. The best response to this patient's statement is to teach the patient that dexamethasone
   A. should decrease acne, not cause it
   B. may cause acne
   C. has no effect on acne or contact dermatitis
   D. should be combined with tetracycline to prevent acne

3. A 30-year-old man has been asthmatic since age 2 years. Which of the following dermatologic disorders is this man prone to developing?
   A. rosacea
   B. atopic dermatitis
   C. external otitis media
   D. impetigo

4. Which of the following foods contributes to the development of rosacea?
   A. milk
   B. high-protein foods
   C. alcohol
   D. ice creams

# DRUG THERAPY

Many different drugs are used to prevent or treat dermatologic disorders. General treatment goals for many skin disorders are to relieve symptoms (e.g., dryness, pruritus, inflammation, infection), eradicate or improve lesions, promote healing and repair, restore skin integrity, and prevent recurrence. Specific goals often depend on the condition being treated. With acne, for example, treatment aims to minimize as many pathogenic factors as possible by reducing sebum production, preventing the formation of microcomedones, suppressing *P. acnes*, and reducing inflammation that may lead to scarring.

Topical drugs are used primarily for local effects of skin and mucous membranes, and systemic absorption is undesirable. Major factors that increase systemic absorption of topical medications include damaged or inflamed skin, high concentrations of drug, and application of drug to the face or mucous membranes, to large areas of the body, or for prolonged periods. With topical medications, cautious use is recommended with infants and young children due to the fact they have more permeable skin and are more likely to absorb the topical drugs. Box 61.1 presents general patient teaching information for topical medications for skin disorders.

 **QSEN Alert: Safety**

Mupirocin is administered for surgical prophylaxis in methicillin-resistant *Staphylococcus aureus* (MRSA) carriers. Intranasal mupirocin is administered twice daily for 5 days prior to surgery.

 *Concept Mastery Alert*

Avoid applying a dressing over a topical corticosteroid. Covering the ointment, especially with an impervious dressing, increases the likelihood that localized adverse reactions will occur.

## General Guidelines

Most of the drugs used to treat dermatologic disorders fit into one or more of the following categories:

- Antimicrobials are used to treat infections caused by bacteria, fungi, and viruses (see Section 4). When used in dermatologic

**BOX 61.1**    *Patient Teaching Guidelines for Topical Medications for Skin Disorders*

**General Considerations**

- Promote healthy skin by a balanced diet, personal hygiene measures, avoiding excessive exposure to sunlight, avoiding skin injuries, and lubricating dry skin. Healthy skin is less susceptible to inflammation, infections, and other disorders. It also heals more rapidly when disorders or injuries occur.

- Prevent actinic keratosis and skin cancer by minimizing sun exposure, wearing sun-protective clothing, and using sunscreen. Such measures should begin in early childhood.

- Common symptoms of skin disorders are inflammation, infection, and itching, and the goal of most drug therapy is to relieve these symptoms and promote healing. Systemic medications (e.g., oral antihistamines, antibiotics, and corticosteroids) may be used for severe disorders, at least initially, but most medications are applied directly to the skin. There is a wide array of topical products, both prescription and over the counter.

- It is important to use the correct topical medication and the correct amount for the condition being treated. Topical corticosteroids, for example, come in many vehicles (e.g., creams, lotions, ointments) that cannot be used interchangeably. In addition, they should not be covered with occlusive dressings unless instructed to do so.

- For patients who have wounds secondary to burns, drugs are to be applied using sterile gloves or sterile applicators with cotton tips.

- Adverse effects of topical medications may involve the skin (e.g., irritation, infection) where the drug is applied or the entire body, when the drug is absorbed into the bloodstream. Systemic absorption is increased when the drug is highly potent; applied to inflamed skin, over a large surface area, or frequently; or covered with an occlusive dressing (e.g., plastic wrap). Systemic absorption is of most concern with corticosteroid preparations.

- Some ways to prevent or decrease skin disorders include the following:
  - Identifying and avoiding, when possible, substances that cause skin irritation and inflammation (e.g., harsh cleaning products, latex gloves, cosmetics, pet dander).
  - Bathing in warm water with a mild cleanser (e.g., Cetaphil), patting skin dry, and applying lotions or oils (e.g., Eucerin, mineral oil) to lubricate skin and decrease dryness.
  - Avoiding scratching, squeezing, or rubbing skin lesions. These behaviors cause additional skin damage and increase risks of infection. Fingernails should be cut short; cotton gloves can be worn at night.
  - Maintaining a cool environment; preventing sweating.
  - Applying cold compresses to inflamed, itchy skin.
  - Using baking soda or colloidal oatmeal (Aveeno) in bath water to relieve itching.

- If you are taking an oral antihistamine to relieve itching, take it on a regular schedule, around the clock, for greater effectiveness.

- Unavoidable skin lesions or scars can often be hidden or rendered less noticeable with makeup or clothing.

- Women can wear cosmetics over most topical medications. If unclear, ask a health care provider whether makeup is permissible. With acne, use noncomedogenic makeup, moisturizers, and sunscreens.

**Self-Administration**

- Use topical medications only as prescribed or according to the manufacturer's instructions (for over-the-counter products). Use the correct preparation for the intended area of application (i.e., skin, ear, vagina).

- For topical application to skin lesions, cleanse the skin and remove previously applied medication to promote drug contact with the affected area of the skin.

- Wash the skin and pat it dry.

- Apply a small amount of the drug preparation and rub it in well. A thin layer of medication is effective and decreases the incidence and severity of adverse effects. With acne and rosacea, preventing skin lesions is easier than eliminating lesions that are already present. As a result, topical medications should be applied to the general area of involvement rather than individual lesions.

- Wash hands before and after application. Wash before to avoid infection; wash afterward to avoid transferring the drug to the face or eyes and causing adverse reactions.

- With azelaic acid (Azelex) for acne, use for the full prescribed period, do not use occlusive dressings or wrappings, and keep away from mouth, eyes, and other mucous membranes (if it gets into eyes, wash eyes with a large amount of water).

- With benzoyl peroxide for acne:
  - With cleansing solutions, wash affected areas once or twice daily. Wet skin areas to be treated before applying the cleanser. Rinse thoroughly and pat dry. Reduce use if excessive drying or peeling occurs.
  - With other dosage forms, apply once daily initially and gradually increase to two or three times daily if needed. Cleanse skin, let dry completely, and apply a small amount over the affected area. Reduce dosage if excessive drying, redness, or discomfort occurs. If excessive stinging or burning occurs after any single application, remove with mild soap and water and resume use the next day. Keep away from eyes, mouth, and inside of nose. Rinse with water if contact occurs with these areas. Avoid other sources of skin irritation (e.g., sunlight, sunlamps, other topical acne medications).

infections, antimicrobials may be administered locally (topically) or systemically (orally or parenterally). Topical antibacterials are used to treat superficial skin disorders such as acne and skin infections. Systemic antibacterials (e.g., cephalosporins) are used for soft tissue infections such as cellulitis and postoperative wound infections. Tetracyclines are used for

acne and rosacea; fluoroquinolones (e.g., ciprofloxacin) may be used to treat soft tissue infections caused by gram-negative organisms.

- Antiseptics kill or inhibit the growth of bacteria, viruses, or fungi. They are used primarily to prevent infection. Skin surfaces should be clean before application of antiseptics.

- Corticosteroids (see Chap. 17) are used to treat the inflammation present in many dermatologic conditions. They are most often applied topically but also may be given orally or parenterally. The choice of a corticosteroid depends on the acuity, severity, location, and extent of the condition being treated.
- Emollients and moisturizers (e.g., lanolin) are lubricants used to relieve dry skin and pruritus.
- Enzymes may be used to débride burn wounds, decubitus ulcers, and venous stasis ulcers. They promote healing by removing necrotic tissue.
- Immunosuppressants (see Chap. 13) may be used to treat inflammatory skin disorders. Two topical agents, tacrolimus (Protopic) ointment and pimecrolimus (Elidel) cream, are used for moderate to severe atopic dermatitis. However, the U.S. Food and Drug Administration (FDA) has issued BLACK BOX WARNING ◆ for these drugs because both medications may cause a possible increased risk of skin cancer and lymphoma. Precautions include using them only when other drugs are ineffective and avoiding long-term use. Several systemic drugs, including alefacept (Amevive), etanercept (Enbrel), and infliximab (Remicade), are used for the treatment of severe psoriasis. The FDA has issued BLACK BOX WARNING ◆ for these drugs concerning the increased risks of infection, and their long-term effects are unknown.

- Keratolytics are used to treat keratin-containing skin conditions. Alpha hydroxy acids (e.g., glycolic acid) are used to treat wrinkles and sun-damaged skin. These acids are a component of many "antiaging" cosmetics and other products. Salicylic acid is used to remove warts, corns, and calluses.
- Sunscreens are used to protect the skin from the damaging effects of UV radiation, thereby decreasing skin cancer and signs of aging, including wrinkles. Dermatologists recommend sunscreen preparations that block both UVA and UVB and have a "sun protection factor," or SPF, of 30 or higher.

Tables 61.1 and 61.2 list antimicrobial drugs as well as other drugs used in the therapy of skin disorders, including acne vulgaris.

## TABLE 61.1

## DRUGS AT A GLANCE: Antimicrobial Drugs for Skin Disorders

| Drug | Pregnancy Category | Indications | Route and Dosage Ranges |
|---|---|---|---|
| **Antibacterial Drugs** | | | |
| Azelaic acid (Azelex, Finacea; ❋ Finacea) | B | Acne (20% cream) Rosacea (15% gel) | To lesions, twice daily |
| Bacitracin | C | Bacterial skin infections | To affected area, one to three times daily |
| Benzoyl peroxide (Acne-Clear, Benziq, others; ❋ Benzac W Wash 10 Nettoyant) | C | Acne | To affected areas, once or twice daily |
| Clindamycin (Cleocin, Cleocin T, Clindamycin ETZ, Clindacin Pac, Clindacin-P, Clindagel, Clindesse, Evoclin; ❋ Dalacin T, Dalacin Vaginal, TARO-Clindamycin) | C | Acne | To affected areas, twice daily |
| Erythromycin (Ery, Erygel) | C | Acne | To affected areas, twice daily |
| Gentamicin | D if significantly absorbed systemically with topical application | Skin infections caused by susceptible organisms | To infected areas, three to four times daily |
| Metronidazole (MetroCream, MetroLotion, Noritate, Nuvessa Rosadan, Vandazole; ❋ Flagyl, Metrogel, Nidagel, Noritate) | B | Rosacea | To affected area, once or twice daily |
| Mupirocin (Centany, Centany AT) | B | Impetigo caused by *Staphylococcus aureus*, beta-hemolytic streptococci, or *Streptococcus pyogenes* Eradication of nasal colonization with methicillin-resistant *S. aureus* | Impetigo: ointment, to affected areas, three times daily Other skin lesions: cream, three times daily for 10 d Eradication of nasal colonization: ointment from single-use tube, one half in each nostril, morning and evening for 5 d |

**TABLE 61.1**

## DRUGS AT A GLANCE: Antimicrobial Drugs for Skin Disorders (Continued)

| Drug | Pregnancy Category | Indications | Route and Dosage Ranges |
|---|---|---|---|
| Retapamulin (Altabax) | B | Impetigo | To affected area, twice daily for 5 d |
| Silver sulfadiazine (Silvadene; ❋ Flamazine) | B | Prevent or treat infection in burn wounds caused by *Pseudomonas* and many other organisms | To affected area, once or twice daily, using sterile technique |
| **Combination Products** | | | |
| Bacitracin and polymyxin B (Polysporin) | C | Bacterial skin infections | To lesions, one to three times daily |
| Erythromycin/benzoyl peroxide (Benzamycin; ❋ Benzamycin) | C | Acne | To affected areas, twice daily |
| Neomycin, polymyxin B, and bacitracin (Neosporin Original, Triple Antibiotic) | C | Bacterial skin infections | To lesions, two or three times daily |
| **Antifungal Drugs** | | | |
| Butenafine (Mentax, Lotrimin Ultra) | C | Tinea pedis | To affected area, once daily for 2–4 wk |
| Ciclopirox (Ciclodan, Loprox, Penlac; ❋ Apo-Ciclopirox, Penlac) | B | Tinea infections Cutaneous candidiasis | To affected area, twice daily for 2–4 wk |
| Clotrimazole (Lotrimin AF, Shopko Athletes Foot; ❋ Canesten Topical, Clotrimaderm) | B | Tinea infections Cutaneous candidiasis | To affected areas, twice daily for 2–4 wk |
| Econazole (Ecoza) | C | Tinea infections Cutaneous candidiasis | To affected areas, once daily for tinea infections, twice daily for candidiasis |
| Ketoconazole (Nizoral, Ketodan; ❋ Ketoderm) | C | Tinea infections Cutaneous candidiasis Seborrheic dermatitis | Tinea infections and candidiasis: to affected areas, once daily for 2–4 wk Seborrheic dermatitis: twice daily for 4 wk |
| Miconazole (Micatin, Podactin, others; ❋ Dermazole, Micatin, Micozole) | B | Tinea infections Cutaneous candidiasis | To affected area, once daily for 2–4 wk |
| Naftifine (Naftin) | B | Tinea infections | To affected areas, once daily with cream, twice daily with gel |
| Nystatin (Nyamyc, Nystop) | A: vaginal C: topical | Candidiasis of skin and mucous membranes | To affected areas, two or three times daily until healed |
| Oxiconazole (Oxistat) | B | Tinea infections | To affected areas, once or twice daily for 2–4 wk |
| Terbinafine (Lamisil; ❋ Lamisil) | A | Tinea infections | To affected areas, twice daily for 1–4 wk |
| Tolnaftate (Tinactin, Fungoid-D) | A | Tinea infections | To affected areas, twice daily for 2–4 wk |
| **Antiviral Drugs** | | | |
| Acyclovir (Zovirax; ❋ APO-Acyclovir, TEVA-Acyclovir, Zovirax) | B | Herpes genitalis Herpes labialis in immunosuppressed patients | To lesions, every 3 h six times daily for 7 d |
| Penciclovir (Denavir) | B | Herpes labialis | To lesions, every 2 h while awake for 4 d |

**TABLE 61.2**

**DRUGS AT A GLANCE: Other Drugs Used for Skin Disorders**

| Drug | Pregnancy Category | Indications | Route and Dosage Ranges |
|---|---|---|---|
| **Enzymes** | | | |
| Trypsin (TBC) | B | Débridement of infected wounds (e.g., decubitus and varicose ulcers) | Topically by spray twice daily |
| **Immunomodulators** | | | |
| Pimecrolimus (Elidel; ❋ Elidel) | C | Atopic dermatitis | Topically to affected skin, twice daily |
| Tacrolimus (Protopic; ❋ Protopic) | C | Atopic dermatitis | Topically to affected skin, twice daily |
| **Retinoids** | | | |
| Ⓟ **Isotretinoin** (Absorica, Claravis, Amnesteem, Myorisan; ❋ Accutane, Clarus, Epuris) | X | Severe cystic acne Disorders characterized by excessive keratinization (e.g., pityriasis, ichthyosis) Mycosis fungoides | 1–2 mg/kg/d PO, in 2 divided doses, for 15–20 wk |
| Acitretin (Soriatane; ❋ Soriatane) | X | Severe psoriasis | 25–50 mg/d PO |
| Adapalene (Differin; ❋ Differin, Differin XP) | C | Acne vulgaris | Topically to skin lesions once daily at bedtime |
| Tazarotene (Avage, Fabior, Tazorac; ❋ Tazorac) | X | Acne Psoriasis | Topically to skin, after cleansing, once daily at bedtime |
| **Other Drugs** | | | |
| Becaplermin (Regranex) | C | Diabetic skin ulcers | Topically to ulcer; amount calculated according to size of the ulcer |
| Calcipotriene (Calcitrene, Dovonex, Sorilux; ❋ Dovonex) | C | Psoriasis | Topically to skin lesions twice daily |
| Capsaicin (Aleveer, Captracin, Zostrix-HP; ❋ Zostrix, Zostrix H.P.) | B | Relief of pain associated with rheumatoid arthritis, osteoarthritis, and neuralgias | Topically to affected area, up to three or four times daily |
| Coal tar (Beta Care Betatar Gel, DSH Tar. Pentrax Gold, Psoriasin) | A | Psoriasis Dermatitis | Topically to skin, in various concentrations and preparations |
| Colloidal oatmeal (Aveeno) | A | Pruritus | Topically as a bath solution (1 cup in bathtub of water) |
| Fluorouracil (Carac, Efudex, Fluoroplex, Tolak; ❋ Efudex, Tolak) | X | Actinic keratoses Superficial basal cell carcinomas | Topically to skin lesions twice daily for 2–6 wk |
| Salicylic acid (Bensal HP, Gordofilm, Clear Away One Step Wart Remover; ❋ Keralyt Keralyt 5, Medplast) | C | Removal of warts, corns, calluses Superficial fungal infections Seborrheic dermatitis Acne Psoriasis | Topically to skin lesions |
| Selenium sulfide (Anti-Dandruff, Dandrex) | C | Dandruff Tinea versicolor | Topically to scalp as shampoo once or twice weekly |

## Herbal Preparations

Many supplements are promoted for use in skin conditions. Most of these formulations have not been tested adequately to ensure effectiveness. At the same time, however, topical use rarely causes serious adverse effects or drug interactions. Two topical agents for which there is some support of safety and effectiveness are aloe and oat preparations (Box 61.2).

- Aloe is often used as a topical remedy for minor burns and wounds (e.g., sunburn, cuts, abrasions) to decrease pain, itching, and inflammation and to promote healing. Its active ingredients are unknown. Wound healing is attributed to moisturizing effects and increased blood flow to the area. Reduced inflammation and pain may result from inhibition of arachidonic acid metabolism and formation of inflammatory prostaglandins. Reduced itching may result from inhibition of histamine production.
- Commercial products are available for topical use, but fresh gel from the plant may be preferred. When used for this purpose, a clear, thin, gellike liquid can be squeezed directly from a plant leaf onto the burned or injured area several times daily if needed.
- Oats, a cereal, a good source of dietary fiber, and a well-documented cholesterol-lowering product, is used topically to treat minor skin irritation and pruritus associated with common skin disorders. They contain gluten, which forms a sticky mass that has emollient effects and holds moisture in the skin when it is mixed with a liquid. Oats are contained in bath products, cleansing bars, and lotions (e.g., Aveeno products) that can be used topically once or twice daily. They should not be used near the eyes or on inflamed skin. After use, it is important to wash bath products off with water.

## NCLEX Success

5. A patient has been diagnosed with atopic dermatitis. She receives a prescription for pimecrolimus cream. What is she at increased risk for developing?

A. skin cancer
B. infection
C. papilledema
D. joint pain

6. A 22-year-old man has developed a soft tissue cellulitis on his right heel. He has been swimming in the ocean and been in the hotel hot tub. It is cultured as a gram-negative organism. Which anti-infective agent will he receive?

A. fluconazole
B. acetazolamide
C. ampicillin
D. ciprofloxacin

## Acne Vulgaris

Several prescription and nonprescription antiacne products are available for acne vulgaris.

Antimicrobial drugs include both topical and systemic agents. Topical drugs are indicated for mild to moderate acne, often in combination with a topical retinoid to maximize reduction in severity and number of lesions. The goal is to eliminate the *P. acnes* colonizing the skin, thus reducing the inflammatory response. The most commonly used topical antimicrobials include benzoyl peroxide, clindamycin, and erythromycin. Azelaic acid (Azelex) has antibacterial activity against

*P. acnes* and is reportedly as effective as benzoyl peroxide, topical erythromycin, or tretinoin (a retinoid) in the treatment of acne vulgaris. Benzoyl peroxide is an effective topical agent that is available in numerous preparations (e.g., gel, lotion, cream, wash) and concentrations (e.g., 2.5%–10%). Low-concentration forms and lotion and cream preparations are the least irritating. Clindamycin and erythromycin are also available in topical dosage forms. These drugs reduce *P. acnes* with comparable efficacy. Combination products of topical clindamycin or erythromycin and benzoyl peroxide are more effective than antibiotics alone, and the benzoyl peroxide also decreases the development of antibiotic resistance. Best results require 8 to 12 weeks of therapy, and maintenance therapy is usually required.

Adverse effects of topical antibiotics include erythema, peeling, dryness, and burning as well as development of resistant strains of *P. acnes*. Recommendations for reducing drug resistance include using topical retinoids or benzoyl peroxide or both when using topical antibiotics. It is important to avoid long-term use of topical or oral antibiotics when feasible. Benzoyl peroxide can also cause an irritant dermatitis and bleach hair, clothes, and bed linens.

Oral antibiotics are first-line treatment for patients with moderate to severe inflammatory acne because they produce more rapid clinical improvement than topical preparations. These drugs have both antimicrobial and anti-inflammatory effects. Tetracycline also has direct anti-inflammatory properties. It reduces *P. acnes* organisms and thereby inhibits production of *P. acnes*–induced inflammatory cytokines. Commonly used oral antibiotics include tetracycline, doxycycline, minocycline, trimethoprim–sulfamethoxazole, clindamycin, azithromycin, and erythromycin. Tetracycline, clindamycin, azithromycin, and erythromycin suppress leukocyte chemotaxis and bacterial lipase activity. Minocycline and doxycycline inhibit cytokines and proteinase enzymes that contribute to inflammation and tissue breakdown. Trimethoprim–sulfamethoxazole interferes with bacterial folic acid synthesis and inhibits dihydrofolic acid reduction to tetrahydrofolate, resulting in sequential inhibition of enzymes of the folic acid pathway. Resistance is commonly reported with erythromycin. Resistance to minocycline is rare but may be emerging in the United States. All oral antibiotics require at least 6 to 8 weeks of use. Although there are no established guidelines for duration of use, some clinicians encourage using the drugs for shorter periods and avoiding long-term use as maintenance therapy, to decrease the development of resistant *P. acnes* and the occurrence of adverse effects such as vaginal candidiasis and gastrointestinal (GI) distress.

Retinoids, in both systemic and topical forms, may be used for moderate to severe acne. All topical retinoids (isotretinoin, acitretin, adapalene, tazarotene) reduce acne lesions, usually within 12 weeks. Isotretinoin is often used with other products.

> **! QSEN Alert: Evidence-Based Practice**
>
> Wiznia, Stevenson, and Nagler (2017) conducted a review of literature regarding the use of laser treatments in conjunction with medical treatment for acne vulgaris. Various types of lasers are used for the treatment of acne. The review concluded that laser therapies in conjunction with medical therapy offer the greatest benefit for treatment of acne vulgaris. Many of the lasers used provided favorable treatment of acne for months even years after the treatment.

## NCLEX Success

7. A 15-year-old girl receives a prescription for tetracycline twice daily for an outbreak of acne. How does tetracycline decrease the girl's acne?

    A. It suppresses the cell membrane.
    B. It suppresses leukocyte cytokines.
    C. It blocks the development of sebum.
    D. It produces isotonic changes in the cell.

8. The mother of a boy being treated for acne vulgaris asks a nurse why her son is being treated with doxycycline and a topical benzoyl peroxide agent. Which of the following is the best response the nurse can make to the patient's mother?

    A. "Benzoyl peroxide cannot be administered without doxycycline."
    B. "Doxycycline should be administered only until the acne vulgaris improves."
    C. "If your son's acne does not improve in 2 weeks, then one of the two agents will be stopped."
    D. "Doxycycline orally and benzoyl peroxide topically will provide better treatment of the acne vulgaris."

### Clinical Application 61.1

- Gerard first took tetracycline for his acne vulgaris. How does tetracycline work against this disorder?
- What are some topical applications that he could use to assist in clearing his acne vulgaris?

## RETINOIDS

Retinoids are vitamin A derivatives that are active in proliferation and differentiation of skin cells. These drugs are commonly used to treat acne, psoriasis, aging and wrinkling of skin from sunlight exposure, and skin cancers. The prototype drug in this class is Ⓟ **Isotretinoin** (Absorica, Amnesteem, Claravis, Myorisan).

## Pharmacokinetics

Isotretinoin dissolves slowly in the GI tract, and the drug is then absorbed rapidly. It crosses the placenta. Isotretinoin is metabolized in the liver and excreted in equal amounts in the feces and urine.

## Action

The antiacne effects of isotretinoin include suppression of sebum production, inhibition of comedone formation, and inhibition of inflammation. The drug normalizes keratinization, reversibly decreases the size of sebaceous glands, and makes sebum less viscous and less likely to plug follicles. The decrease in sebum results in the inhibition of the sebum-dependent bacterium *P. acnes*, which is a key promoter of inflammation in acne vulgaris. Researchers have often found that isotretinoin also decreases cell proliferation and induces differentiation in neuroblastoma.

## Use

Uses of isotretinoin include treatment of severe recalcitrant nodular acne that is unresponsive to other treatments in adolescents and adults.

## Adverse Effects

Isotretinoin has severe adverse effects. Therefore, in the United States, the FDA has imposed restrictions on who may prescribe and distribute the drug. These adverse effects, which may limit its use, include:

- Reproductive effects: severe life-threatening congenital malformations and spontaneous abortions.
- Psychiatric effects (serious): depression, psychosis, aggressive or violent behavior, and changes in mood; rarely, suicidal thoughts and actions have been reported. It is important to observe closely all patients for symptoms of depression or suicidal thoughts; it may be necessary to discontinue therapy and make appropriate referrals to mental health professionals.
- Dermatologic effects (most common): dryness and swelling of the lips (cheilitis), dry skin and mucous membranes, nasal dryness, epistaxis, dry mouth, conjunctivitis, peeling skin, skin fragility, rash, and pruritus.
- GI effects (potential): nausea, vomiting, and, rarely, inflammatory bowel disease and pancreatitis.
- Musculoskeletal effects (common): arthralgia, myalgia (particularly with vigorous exercise), weakness, increased creatine phosphokinase (CPK), and back pain in some children and also bone abnormalities, decreased bone mineral density, and premature epiphyseal closure.
- Metabolic effects: hyperlipidemia (elevated triglycerides in 45% of patients, elevated total cholesterol, and low-density lipoprotein in 30% of patients: usually transient elevations).
- Other effects: decreased night vision, corneal opacities, hepatotoxicity, and bone marrow suppression.

## Contraindications

Contraindications to isotretinoin include hypersensitivity to the drug, parabens (used as a preservative), vitamin A, or other retinoids, as well as pregnancy. As reported earlier, the FDA has issued a **BLACK BOX WARNING** ◆ stating that isotretinoin, in pregnancy category X, causes both spontaneous abortions and severe life-threatening congenital malformations. In addition, women of childbearing potential should not take isotretinoin unless they have had two negative pregnancy test results before beginning therapy, will begin drug therapy on the 2nd or 3rd day of the next menstrual period, and will comply with stringent contraceptive measures for 1 month before therapy, during therapy, and for 1 month after therapy. Box 61.3 describes the measures put in place by the iPLEDGE program developed by the FDA. The FDA has established a computer-based risk evaluation and mitigation strategy (REMS) to prevent fetal exposure to isotretinoin.

### ! QSEN Alert: Safety

All patients receiving isotretinoin, as well as all prescribers, dispensing pharmacies, and wholesale distributors of the medication, are required to register with the iPLEDGE program and strictly follow its requirements.

## BOX 61.3    *iPLEDGE Program*

- The iPLEDGE program is a risk management program designed to prevent fetal exposure to isotretinoin. Registration, activation, and additional information are provided at https://www.ipledgeprogram.com/iPledgeUI/home.u or by calling 866-495-0654. The program requires that
  - All patients (female and male) who are able to become pregnant or father a child must use two forms of birth control for at least 1 month prior to starting therapy, during therapy, and for 1 month after therapy. Patients are allowed to avoid the contraceptive requirements if they agree to abstain completely from sex; this commitment must be made in writing.
  - All female patients who are able to become pregnant must have two negative blood or urine pregnancy tests before receiving the initial prescription. It is essential that the second pregnancy test be conducted in a certified

laboratory. During each month of therapy and 1 month after completing therapy, patients must see their health care provider for evaluation, counseling, and education. They must also have a negative pregnancy test in a certified laboratory monthly and 1 month after completing therapy.
- Every month, prescribers must document in the iPLEDGE system the results of the pregnancy test and the two forms of birth control in use. The prescriber must also document the counseling and education. All patients, even if not able to become pregnant, must be counseled about the iPLEDGE program and the risk of birth defects.
- Health care providers can prescribe only a maximum 30-day supply at each monthly visit.
- Physicians must certify their expertise in the diagnosis and treatment of acne.

---

Cautious use is also advisable with a history of mental illness or a family history of psychiatric disorders. Other conditions that warrant caution are asthma, liver disease, diabetes, heart disease, osteoporosis, history of childhood osteoporosis, genetic predisposition for age-related osteoporosis, weak bones, anorexia nervosa, osteomalacia, and other disorders of bone metabolism.

## Nursing Implications

### Preventing Interactions

Many medications interact with isotretinoin, increasing its effects (Box 61.4). Isotretinoin may decrease the therapeutic effect of estrogen and progestin contraceptives. Microdosed progesterone-only preparations, in particular, may be ineffective.

### Administering the Medication

Before starting isotretinoin, it is necessary to perform a complete blood cell count (CBC), a fasting lipid profile, and liver function tests to obtain a baseline. People should take the drug with or shortly after a meal to improve absorption. It is necessary to swallow capsules whole with a full glass of liquid. The contents of the capsule may irritate the esophagus if removed from the

capsule. Females of childbearing age should have a pregnancy test. Women should avoid coming in contact with the contents of the capsules because the drug is teratogenic.

### Assessing for Therapeutic Effects

The nurse assesses for a decrease in total cyst count. The ideal value is a 70% decrease.

### Assessing for Adverse Effects

With oral retinoids, the nurse observes for hypervitaminosis. Nausea and vomiting; headache; blurred vision, eye irritation, and conjunctivitis; skin disorders; musculoskeletal pain (any evidence of osteoporosis, osteopenia, or fractures); and depression and suicidal ideation are common signs of hypervitaminosis. Although adverse effects commonly occur with usual doses, they are more severe with higher doses. Most adverse effects can be managed without stopping the drug.

Also, the nurse monitors laboratory tests. It is important to conduct repeat tests (CBC, lipid profile, liver function tests) at 4 and 8 weeks. If the repeat tests are normal and the dose is stable, monitoring is no longer necessary.

### Patient Teaching

Box 61.5 identifies patient teaching guidelines for isotretinoin.

## BOX 61.4  *Drug Interactions: Isotretinoin*

**Drugs That Increase the Effects of Isotretinoin**
- Alcohol
  *Increases triglycerides*
- Corticosteroids
  *Increase the risk of osteoporosis*
- Phenytoin
  *Increases the risk of osteomalacia*
- Tetracycline
  *Increases the risk of cerebri pseudotumor*
- Vitamin A
  *Produces toxic effects associated with isotretinoin*

### Clinical Application 61.2

- How does isotretinoin work to reduce acne vulgaris?
- Isotretinoin may cause severe psychiatric adverse effects, such as depression, psychosis, or violent behavior. What are some strategies the nurse can teach Gerard's parents about looking for psychosocial abnormalities?

## Other Drugs in the Class

Adapalene and tazarotene are effective topical retinoids used to treat both noninflammatory and inflammatory acne. Adapalene

**BOX 61.5**  *Patient Teaching Guidelines for Isotretinoin*

- Understand that acne is not caused by dirt, that washing does not improve acne, and that vigorous scrubbing may worsen acne lesions. There is also no evidence that acne is caused by eating chocolate or other foods.
- If you are a woman of childbearing age, it is essential that you adhere to all requirements of the iPLEDGE program.
  - Use two forms of birth control.
  - Adhere to mandatory pregnancy testing requirements.
- Take the drug with or shortly after meals.
- Report bone, muscle, or joint pain or visual disturbances immediately, as well as persistent headaches or GI pain.
- Report depression or suicidal thoughts immediately.
- Do not take oral vitamin A supplements.
- Avoid using abrasives, medicated soaps and cleansers, acne preparations containing peeling drugs, and topical products containing alcohol (e.g., cosmetics, aftershave). These products will exacerbate skin dryness and irritation.
- Avoid prolonged sun exposure. Use sun block.
- Do not donate blood during therapy and up to 1 month after therapy.

is the only topical retinoid available without a prescription. A combination gel product (Epiduo, Epiduo Forte) containing adapalene and benzoyl peroxide is available by prescription. Traditionally, administration of most topical retinoids takes place at bedtime because of initial reports of drug instability in the presence of light; newer formulations are less affected by exposure to light.

## NCLEX Success

9. A 13-year-old girl has developed a mild case of acne vulgaris. Which of the following medications will be prescribed?
   A. doxycycline
   B. benzoyl peroxide
   C. isotretinoin
   D. fluconazole

10. A 17-year-old boy is seen in the school nurse's office. He has been taking tretinoin for 6 months. He is complaining of nausea and visual changes. What should the nurse suspect the symptoms may be related to?
    A. an adverse effect of the medication
    B. the development of a pseudotumor cerebri
    C. the development of the flu
    D. an occurrence of migraine headaches

## THE NURSING PROCESS

A concept map outlines the nursing process related to drug therapy considerations in this chapter. Additional nursing implications related to the disease process should also be considered in care decisions.

**Assessment**

- When a skin rash is present, inspect the area and interview the patient to determine the following: location, appearance, distribution, accompanying symptoms, and history of development.
- Some etiologic factors include the following:
  - Drug therapy. Many commonly used drugs may cause skin lesions, including anti-infective agents, narcotic analgesics, and thiazide diuretics. Skin rashes due to drug therapy are usually generalized and appear abruptly.
  - Irritants or allergens that may cause contact dermatitis.
  - Communicable diseases (e.g., measles, chickenpox), which cause characteristic skin rashes and systemic signs and symptoms.
- When assessing the skin, consider the age of the patient. Infants are likely to have "diaper" dermatitis, miliaria (heat rash), and tinea capitis (ringworm infection of the scalp). School-aged children have a relatively high incidence of measles, chickenpox, and tinea infections. Adolescents often have acne. Older adults are more likely to have dry skin, actinic keratoses (lesions on sun-exposed skin formerly thought to be premalignant but now considered early-stage squamous cell cancer), and skin cancer.
- Assess for skin neoplasms. Basal cell carcinoma may initially appear as a pale nodule, most often on the head and neck. Squamous cell carcinomas may appear as actinic keratoses or ulcerated areas. Malignant melanoma is the most serious skin cancer. It involves melanocytes, the pigment-producing cells of the skin. Malignant melanoma may occur in pigmented nevi (moles) or previously normal skin. In nevi, malignant melanoma may be manifested by enlargement and ulceration. In previously normal skin, lesions appear as irregularly shaped.

**Outcomes of Therapy**

The patient will
- Apply topical drugs correctly.
- Experience relief of symptoms.
- Use techniques to prevent or minimize skin damage and disorders.
- Avoid scarring and disfigurement when possible.
- Be encouraged to express concerns about acute and chronic body-image changes.

**Nursing Interventions**

- Use measures to prevent or minimize skin disorders, including good personal hygiene.
- Maintain adequate nutrition, rest, and exercise.
- Practice safety measures to avoid injury to the skin. Injury with a disruption of skin integrity increases the likelihood of skin infections.
- Avoid known irritants or allergens, such as:
  - Use measures to relieve dry skin and pruritus. Alternate complete and partial baths.
  - Liberal use of lubricating creams and lotions. Creams and lotions may be applied several times daily.
- Prevent pressure ulcers by avoiding trauma to the skin and prolonged pressure on any part of the body. Implement frequent position changes and correct lifting techniques. Daily inspection of the skin is needed for early detection and treatment of beginning pressure ulcers.
- Avoid excessive exposure to sunlight and other sources of UV light.
- Apply sunscreen daily.
- When skin rashes are present, cool, wet compresses or baths are often effective in relieving pruritus. A cool environment also tends to decrease pruritus. Keep the patient's fingernails cut short.
- For relief of severe itching, a systemic antihistamine may be needed.

**Evaluation**

- Observe and interview regarding use of dermatologic drugs.
- Observe for improvement in skin lesions and symptoms.
- Interview regarding use of measures to promote healthy skin and prevent skin disorders.

## KEY CONCEPTS

- Many dermatologic medications are applied topically to skin and mucous membranes. The drugs may improve barrier function, soften and remove scaly lesions, alter inflammation in the skin, alter blood flow, exert antimicrobial effects, or affect proliferating cells.

- Immunosuppressants such as tacrolimus and pimecrolimus are used for moderate to severe atopic dermatitis. The drugs have **BLACK BOX WARNING** ◆ regarding a possible increased risk of skin cancer and lymphoma. Several systemic biologic drugs, alefacept, etanercept, and infliximab, are used for the treatment of severe psoriasis. **BLACK BOX WARNING** ◆ for these drugs alert clinicians about increased risks of developing infections and their unknown long-term effects.

- Acne is a common disorder characterized by excessive production of sebum and obstruction of hair follicles, which normally carry sebum to the skin surface. As a result, hair follicles expand and form comedones (blackheads and whiteheads).

- Acne lesions vary from small comedones to acne vulgaris, the most severe form, in which follicles become infected and irritating secretions leak into surrounding tissues to form inflammatory pustules, cysts, and abscesses.

- With acne, treatment goals include minimizing as many pathogenic factors as possible by reducing sebum production, preventing the formation of microcomedones, suppressing *P. acnes*, and reducing inflammation to prevent scarring.

- Retinoids are vitamin A derivatives that are active in proliferation and differentiation of skin cells. These drugs are commonly used to treat acne, psoriasis, aging and wrinkling of skin from sunlight exposure, and skin cancers.

- Isotretinoin should not be prescribed to women who are or are likely to become pregnant while using the drug. A **BLACK BOX WARNING** ◆ cautions that isotretinoin causes both spontaneous abortions and severe life-threatening congenital malformations.

## CLINICAL REASONING CASE STUDY

**Meet the Patient**

Kyra Sidana, a 17-year-old female, has a severe case of acne vulgaris. She has received a prescription for isotretinoin, and the nurse is providing patient teaching to Kyra and her parents. The nurse is giving them information about iPLEDGE.

- What hygienic practices decrease acne vulgaris?
- When taking isotretinoin, what is important about its administration?
- How should the nurse best describe iPLEDGE ?

**Assessing Drug Information**

- Action
  - Isotretinoin suppresses sebum production, inhibits comedone formation, and inhibits inflammation. The drug normalizes keratinization, reversibly decreases the size of sebaceous glands, and makes sebum less viscous and less likely to plug follicles.
  - The decrease in sebum results in the inhibition of the sebum-dependent bacterium *P. acnes*, which is a key promoter of inflammation in acne vulgaris.
- Use: Isotretinoin is used in adolescents and adults to treat severe recalcitrant nodular acne unresponsive to other treatments.
- Adverse effects
  - Adolescents and women who are pregnant or who may become pregnant should not take isotretinoin. If pregnancy occurs while any amount of the drug is taken, even for a short period, there is an extremely high risk of severe birth defects.
  - Additional adverse effects are significant and include
    - Psychiatric effects (serious): depression, psychosis, aggressive or violent behavior, and changes in mood; rarely, suicidal thoughts and actions have been reported. It is important to observe closely all patients for symptoms of depression or suicidal thoughts; it may be necessary to discontinue therapy and make appropriate referrals to mental health professionals.
    - Dermatologic effects (most common): dryness and swelling of the lips (cheilitis), dry skin and mucous membranes, nasal dryness, epistaxis, dry mouth, conjunctivitis, peeling skin, skin fragility, rash, and pruritus
    - GI effects (potential): nausea, vomiting, and, rarely, inflammatory bowel disease and pancreatitis
    - Musculoskeletal effects (common): arthralgia, myalgia (particularly with vigorous exercise), weakness, increased creatine phosphokinase, and back pain in some children; also bone abnormalities, decreased bone mineral density, and premature epiphyseal closure
    - Metabolic effects: hyperlipidemia (elevated triglycerides in 45% of patients, elevated total cholesterol, and low-density lipoprotein in 30% of patients: usually transient elevations)

**Nursing Actions**

- Instruct Kyra and her parents that the iPLEDGE program affects all female patients of childbearing age taking isotretinoin, as well as their partners. The iPLEDGE program states all these patients must use two forms of birth control for at least 1 month before starting isotretinoin. Carrie must have two negative blood or urine tests for pregnancy before starting the medication. Additional information is found in Box 61.3.
- Instruct Kyra to wash her face gently every day with a mild soap. It is not necessary to scrub the face; this might spread the infection.
- Instruct Kyra to take the isotretinoin with food to improve absorption. It is important to swallow the capsule whole to prevent esophageal irritation. Additional patient teaching information is found in Box 61.5.

Visit thePoint® *at* **http://thePoint.lww.com/Frandsen12e** *for answers to NCLEX Success questions (in Appendix A), answers to Clinical Application Case Studies (in Appendix B), and more!*

## REFERENCES AND RESOURCES

Goldner, R., & Fransway, A. F. (2020). Irritant contact dermatitis in adults. In *UpToDate*. Lexi-Comp, Inc.

Graber, E. (2020). Treatment of acne vulgaris. In *UpToDate*. Lexi-Comp, Inc.

Hinkle, J. H., & Cheever, K. H. (2018). *Brunner & Suddarth's textbook of medical-surgical nursing* (14th ed.). Philadelphia, PA: Lippincott Williams & Wilkins.

Hugh, W. A. (2019). Stevens-Johnson syndrome and toxic epidermal necrolysis: pathogenesis, clinical manifestations, and diagnosis. In *UpToDate*. Waltham, MA.

Hull, C., & Zone, J. J. (2019). Approach to the patient with cutaneous blisters. In *UpToDate*. Waltham, MA.

iPLEDGE: Committed to Pregnancy Prevention. U.S. Food and Drug Administration–approved program for use of isotretinoin. Retrieved from http://www.ipledgeprogram.com

Lippincott Williams & Wilkins. (2019). *Nursing drug handbook* (39th ed.). Philadelphia, PA: Wolters Kluwer Publishers.

Norris, T. L. (2019). *Porth's pathophysiology: Concepts of altered health states* (10th ed.). Philadelphia, PA: Wolters Kluwer.

Sasseville, D. (2020). Seborrheic dermatitis in adolescents and adults. In *UpToDate*. Lexi-Comp, Inc.

UpToDate. (2020). *Drug Information*. Lexi-Comp, Inc.

Weston, W. L., & Howe, W. (2020). Overview of dermatitis. In *UpToDate*. Lexi-Comp, Inc.

Wiznia, L. E., Stevenson, M. L., & Nagler, A. R. (2017). Laser treatments of active acne. *Lasers in Medical Science, 32*, 1647–1658.

# Index